Abbreviations Commonly Used for Drug Orders

$\overline{\text{aa}}$	of each
a.c.	before meals
ad lib.	freely, as desired
admov.	apply
agit.	shake, stir
b.i.d.	two times daily
b.i.n.	twice a night
bol.	bolus
c.	with
caps.	capsules
d. or da.	day
dil.	diluted
dim.	one-half
div.	divide
dos.	dose
dr.	dram
elix. or el.	elixir
emp.	plaster
emul.	emulsion
ext.	extract
g or gm	gram
garg.	a gargle
gr.	grain
gt.	a drop; plural gtt.
h.	hour
hor. som. or h.s.	bedtime
id.	the same
I.M.	intramuscular
inf.	let it infuse
I.V.	intravenous
lin.	liniment
liq.	a solution
M.	mix
m	minim
man. prim.	first thing in the morning
med.	medicine
m. et n.	morning and night
ml	milliliter
mm	millimeter
non rep. or n r.	not to be repeated
nunc	now
O.D.	right eye
omn. bih.	every second hour
omn. hor. or o.h.	every hour
omn. noct. or o.n.	every night
O.S.	left eye
os	mouth
O.U.	both eyes
oz.	ounce
p.	after
p.c.	after meals
P.O.	by mouth
P.R.	by rectum
p.r.n.	as required
q.	every
q.d.	every day
q.h.	every hour
q.i.d.	four times a day
q.o.d. or A.D.T.	every other day
q.s.	as much as required
s	without
S.C. or S.Q.	subcutaneously
Sig.	indicate on label
sing.	of each
s.o.s.	if necessary
sp.	spirits
ss.	one half
stat.	immediately
sum.	take
suppos.	a suppository
tab.	tablet
T.	take one
t.i.d.	three times daily
tr. or tinct.	tincture
ung.	ointment
ut dict.	as directed

Conversion Factors

Weight

1 milligram	=	1000 micrograms
1 milligram	=	1,000,000 nanograms
1 milligram	=	0.015432 grain
1 milligram	=	32.15 apothecaries' ounces
1 gram	=	15.432 grains
1 gram	=	0.25720 dram
1 grain	=	64.7989 milligrams
1 grain	=	0.0648 gram
1 dram	=	3.8879 gram
1 apothecaries' ounce	=	31.1035 grams
1 pound	=	435.5924 gm

Volume

1 milliliter	=	16.23 minims
1 milliliter	=	0.2705 fluid dram
1 milliliter	=	0.0338 fluid ounce
1 liter	=	33.8148 fluid ounces
1 liter	=	2.1134 pints
1 liter	=	1.0567 quarts
1 liter	=	0.2642 gallon
1 fluid dram	=	60 minims
1 fluid dram	=	3.697 milliliters
1 teaspoon	=	4–5 milliliters
1 tablespoon	=	3 teaspoons
1 fluid ounce	=	2 tablespoons
1 fluid ounce	=	8 drams
1 fluid ounce	=	29.573 milliliters
1 cup	=	8 fluid ounces
1 pint	=	2 cups
1 pint	=	473.166 milliliters
1 quart	=	2 pints
1 quart	=	946.332 milliliters
1 gallon	=	4 quarts
1 gallon	=	3.785 liters

Temperature

Celsius degrees × 9/5 + 32 = Fahrenheit degrees

(Fahrenheit degrees − 32) × 5/9 = Celsius degrees

Nursing Pharmacology

Nursing Pharmacology

AN INTEGRATED APPROACH TO DRUG THERAPY AND NURSING PRACTICE

Alvin K. Swonger, PhD
College of Pharmacy
University of Rhode Island

Myrtle P. Matejski, BSN, MSN Ed, AM, PhD
College of Nursing
University of Delaware

Scott, Foresman/Little, Brown College Division
Scott, Foresman and Company
Glenview, Illinois Boston London

Library of Congress Cataloging-in-Publication Data

Swonger, Alvin K.
Nursing pharmacology.

Includes bibliographies and index.
1. Chemotherapy. 2. Nursing. I. Matejski, Myrtle P.
II. Title. [DNLM: 1. Drug Therapy—nurses' instruction.
2. Pharmacology—nurses' instruction. QV 4 S979n]
RM262.S94 1987 615.5'8 87-17073
ISBN 0-673-39752-1

1 2 3 4 5 6 7 8 9 10 —VHJ— 93 92 91 90 89 88 87

Printed in the United States of America

The table "Classification of Canadian Drugs" on the inside back cover is reproduced (with minor changes) by permission from Julia B. Clark, Sherry F. Queener, and Virginia Burke Karb, *Pharmacological Basis of Nursing Practice,* 2nd ed., St. Louis, 1986, The C.V. Mosby Co.

Nursing Pharmacology is dedicated to:

Elsie C. Swonger
Krishna M. Swonger
Joline L. Swonger
Matthias W. Swonger
Alina R. Swonger
and
Stanley F. Matejski

Preface

The professional nurse needs to be knowledgeable about pharmacology as much as any of the other medical sciences, because most clients for whom nurses provide care receive at least one drug as part of their medical regimen. Nurses not only need to understand how drugs fit into the overall therapeutic plan but also the special responsibilities that are part of the drug regimen. One of the nurse's vital contributions is in early identification of drug side effects and in teaching clients and their families to recognize such reactions to medication. Nurses can often facilitate beneficial effects or reduce adverse effects of medication. Frequently, nurses have the most thorough knowledge about all the drugs a client is receiving or self-administering and thus are uniquely able to recognize potential danger in drug interactions. Often nurses actually administer a prescribed drug and are especially responsible for educating clients in all aspects of the drug regimen, with the ultimate objective of promoting safe and efficacious drug therapy.

Nursing Pharmacology: An Integrated Approach to Drug Therapy and Nursing Practice provides an introduction to pharmacology tailored to the nursing student's needs. The complexity and great bulk of drug information currently available rules out an approach based on memorization. Instead, we advocate an integrated approach, interweaving pharmacology with other medical sciences and with nursing practice. To facilitate the integrative approach, we organize units around body systems. For each system, the student progresses from physiology and other basic medical sciences to pathophysiology, to pharmacotherapeutics, and finally to nursing process. A concise review of how the body system functions is followed by a review of the principal pathological conditions that are the clinical indications for the drugs to be discussed. Next, in each chapter we cover pharmacology itself — the mechanisms and effects, pharmacokinetics, clinical indications, adverse effects and contraindications, interactions, and the preparation and administration requirements for each drug likely to be encountered in clinical practice. All this information forms the foundation for understanding the nurse's role in caring for clients receiving drug therapy. Our basic strategy is to link pharmacology at two ends to the rest of the nursing student's education: on the one end to basic biomedical sciences and on the other to nursing practice.

The first two units of the book differ from the rest, presenting a foundation to prepare the student for studying pharmacology. In Chapter 1 we set up a historical perspective linking the study of pharmacology to the college student's general education. Chapter 2 is designed to ease the student's passage into the language of drug terminology. Chapter 3 presents the principles of pharmacology, forming a rational basis for understanding drug actions. In Chapter 4, we consider the technical and in Chapter 5 the legal and ethical aspects of drug administration. In Chapters 6 and 7 we delve into special applications of pharmacological and drug-administration principles to clients at either end of the age spectrum — pediatric and geriatric individuals. Chapter

8 serves the student as a bridge between the science of pharmacology and the nursing profession, introducing concepts that are recalled and reinforced in the drug chapters that make up the rest of the book.

The drug chapters have many useful features. Each begins with a chapter outline to help the student understand the overall logic of the subject. Drug discussions are presented in a standardized format, except for the few variations that require special consideration. This standard presentation will help the student organize information for study. The many useful tables facilitate comparisons between drugs within a group or summarize drugs known to produce important actions. Extensive illustrations help students visualize physiological processes, clinical disorders, and drug mechanisms.

Information specific to the nursing role appears in the chapters in three standard places. First, nursing implications related to a drug are incorporated into the drug discussions so that the student sees the relationship between the drug's effects and the nursing actions that result. This information is italicized for easy reference. Second, a list of "Important Nursing Implications" for each drug or drug group summarizes key information. Finally, two boxes, "Nursing Observations" and "Nursing Diagnoses and Interventions," show how the steps in the nursing process apply to the study of pharmacology. Rather than merely paying lip service to the concept of nursing process, these boxes are focused on the points of contact between nursing process and pharmacology to provide the student with information that is relevant to the real issues of practice. The "Nursing Observation" boxes are focused on preadministration assessment and evaluation of drug response. The "Nursing Diagnoses and Interventions" boxes are focused on nursing diagnoses and related interventions that enhance drug benefits and minimize adverse effects and interactions.

At the end of each chapter, case studies illustrate how pharmacological knowledge is applied to clinical settings. The lists of recommended readings provided with each chapter are especially designed to be useful to students, with many references to the nursing journals most often used by practicing nurses.

All major topics in pharmacology are covered in this book. Compared with other texts, you will find added emphasis on nonprescription drugs. Instead of the usual single chapter on over-the-counter drugs, we discuss fully all significant nonprescription drugs, incorporating the coverage in comprehensive chapters pertaining to headaches, the gastrointestinal system, the respiratory system, the skin, the eye, and the ears and sinuses. We also provide more comprehensive discussions of drug effects on human sexual and reproductive function, pediatric and geriatric pharmacology, and interactions of drugs with nutrition than any other pharmacology text with which we are familiar.

In selecting topics we have kept in mind that nursing students are not only future nursing professionals but also members of society at large. They are keenly interested in topics in pharmacology that today are particularly relevant socially: drug abuse, drug testing, treatment of AIDS, treatment for Alzheimer's disease, athletes' use of performance-enhancing drugs, pollutants, food additives, health foods and herbal remedies, teratogenic effects of drugs, appearance of drugs in breast milk, new treatments for cancer, and so on. Our policy is to give full coverage to such topics. Linking the study of pharmacology to what is happening in the news and in students' lives has priceless motivational value. For the same reason, we reserve a little space for interesting historical matters, entertaining anecdotes, and social perspectives that could not be justified solely by the future nurse's professional requirements.

Every effort has been made to ensure an up-to-date text. All drugs newly approved by the FDA right up until *Nursing Pharmacology* went to press are incorporated. Many of the most important drugs currently undergoing clinical trials are also mentioned. We will also supplement the text book with a semiannual *Update*, with information on new drugs as well as new uses for old drugs. Because *Nursing Pharmacology* is up to date, comprehensive, and filled with useful nursing implications, it is the one pharmacology textbook you will want your students to keep for reference after they have used it as a text in their pharmacology coursework.

Faculty who adopt *Nursing Pharmacology* are invited to make use of the ancillaries developed by the publisher. An Instructor's Manual provides learning objectives, ideas for lectures and discussion, applications to clinical experience, and a test bank that includes multiple-choice, true-false, matching, and essay questions. The test bank is also available in software format for use on Apple, IBM, or IBM-compatible computers. And the Study Guide helps students master an amount of information that can seem formidable by providing terms to know, short-answer and multiple-choice questions, and nursing applications for self-testing.

Acknowledgments

Nursing Pharmacology owes its existence to the hard work of many fine people at Little, Brown and Company. Ann West, a bright spirit, provided impetus to the project from its inception to its completion. Sue Warne, all that one could ever ask for in a development editor, devoted countless hours to reviewing every chapter, each at several stages of preparation. The consistent soundness and insightfulness of her ideas for changing content, wording, or organization were truly remarkable. We are grateful both for her forcefulness and her ability to compromise. Victoria Keirnan supervised the book's production with both efficiency and consideration. Carolyn Woznick was very helpful in the tedious business of collecting permissions for use of previously published artwork. Cynthia Wheeler provided much help in the production of the ancillaries. Collectively, the folks in the Little, Brown College Division exhibited an uncommon wealth of professional competence and congeniality that made the project a real pleasure for the authors. We want also to acknowledge with gratitude the help of Rosalyn Tolbert in preparing the Instructor's Manual, Debi Osnowitz for writing the Study Guide, and Shirley Corvo for help with the editing of the manuscript. We are also grateful to Dean Edith Anderson of the College of Nursing at the University of Delaware for providing Dr. Matejski with the time and support needed for this project and to Stanley Matejski for his constant encouragement and support.

Elsie Swonger sacrificed many, many wee hours of the morning to painstakingly prepare most of the illustrations appearing in the book. Her care for detail and clarity was always evident and she readily accepted each request for adjustments.

In the personal domain, we want to thank our families for their support during the book's long preparation. This book is their love transformed.

Reviewers for *Nursing Pharmacology*

We want to thank the reviewers who spent long hours reading manuscript and provided many valuable suggestions.

Steven F. Bauwens, PharmD
University of Wisconsin, Madison

Larry E. Boh, MSc, RPh
University of Wisconsin, Madison

Chester A. Bond, PharmD
University of Wisconsin, Madison

Robert M. Breslow, BS, RPh
University of Wisconsin Hospital and Clinic, Madison

Barbara Buchen, MA, RN
Seton Hall University, South Orange, NJ

Helen A. Bush, RN, PhD
Texas Women's University, Denton, TX

Mary Lou Cheatham, RN, MSN
Ball State University, Muncie, IN

Vivian Hayes Churness, RN, DNSc
University of Southern California, Los Angeles, CA

Ruth A. Crabbe, RN, MS, CNRN, CRRN
University of Southern California, Los Angeles, CA

Elizabeth Davis, RNC, MEd
University of Texas at El Paso

Susan C. deWit, RN, MSN
El Centro Community College, Dallas, TX

Linda F. Garner, RN, MS
Baylor University, Dallas, TX

Elizabeth Glassman, RN, BSN, MA
Mt. St. Mary College, Newburgh, NY

Kathryn L. Grant, PharmD
University of Wisconsin, Madison

Marion F. Hale, RN, MN, BSN
Georgia State University, Atlanta

Mary Beth Hayward, RN, MSN
Medical College of Ohio, Toledo, OH

Lorrie N. Hegstad, RN, PhD
University of Texas at Arlington

Sr. Grace Henke, RN, EdD
St. Vincent Hospital, New York, NY

Tenza Housel, BSN, MSN
Mississippi University of Women, Columbus

Curtis, A. Johnson, PharmD
University of Wisconsin, Madison

Susan Jones, BSN, MSN
Western Kentucky University, Bowling Green

Barbara MacDermott, MS, RN
Syracuse University, Syracuse, NY

Sharon H. Moses, RPh
University of Wisconsin, Madison

Susan Murray, RN, MPh
New England Medical Center, Boston, MA

Kay O'Neal, RN, MSN
El Centro Community College, Dallas, TX

Michael Pitterle, MS, RPh
University of Wisconsin, Madison

Pamela Ploetz, BS
University of Wisconsin Hospital and Clinic, Madison

Debrynda A. Price, RN, EdD
Delta State University, Cleveland, MS

Beth Purdue, RNC, MSN
El Centro Community College, Dallas, TX

Kathy Roan, RN, MSN
McNeese State University, Lake Charles, LA

Pamela Rossé, RN, MS
University of Colorado Health Science Center, Denver

Angela M. Rossington, MN
Alfred University, Alfred, NY

Betsy Shenkman, RN, MSN
University of Florida, Gainesville

Judith Shockley, RN, MSN
University of Texas at San Antonio

Rosalyn B. Tolbert, RN, PhD
University of Texas at Arlington

Andrea S. Vivian, PharmD
Eastern Michigan University, Ypsilanti

Sheila Watkins, RN, MSN
Gonzaga University, Spokane, WA

Contents

UNIT III
Drugs and the Central Nervous System

PART A
Introduction to Central Nervous System Pharmacology 125

PART B
Arousal, Sleep, and Drugs 163

PART C
Anesthesia and Anesthetics 227

PART D
Drug Treatment of Psychiatric Disorders 253

PART E
Drug Treatment of Neurologic Disorders 317

UNIT IV
Drugs and the Peripheral Nervous System

UNIT V
Drugs and the Endocrine System

UNIT VI
Drugs and the Cardiovascular System

UNIT VII
Drugs, Metabolism, and Nutrition

UNIT VIII
Drugs and Inflammation

UNIT IX
Drugs and the Immune System

UNIT X
Drugs and the Systems That Interface with the External Environment

UNIT XI
Drugs and the Special Sensory Organs

UNIT XII
Cancer Chemotherapy

UNIT XIII
Toxicology

To the Reader

The authors and publisher have made every effort to ensure the accuracy and appropriateness of the drug dosages presented in this textbook. The medications described do not necessarily have specific approval by the Food and Drug Administration for use in the diseases and dosages for which they are recommended. The package insert for each drug should be consulted for use and dosage as approved by the FDA. Because standards for usage change, it is advisable to keep abreast of revised recommendations, particularly those concerning new drugs. We urge you to check the dosage information on the manufacturer's package insert before you administer any drug.

INTRODUCTION

How to Use This Book

Part of the challenge in learning about drugs is the multitude of drugs encountered in clinical practice and the enormous number of facts about each drug that may be relevant at one time or another. Furthermore, every year new drugs are introduced. How is the nursing student, and even the established professional nurse, to cope with this abundance of detail? Obviously, memorizing such a large body of facts is out of the question. The key to dealing effectively with drug information is to understand the broad concepts forming the foundations of pharmacology that enable the nurse to understand the range of possibilities in a clinical situation. The particulars about specific drugs employed by a client can be and will need to be reviewed from time to time. But only the nurse who has mastered the basic concepts and who is acquainted with the range of possible implications can use these particulars effectively to guide nursing activities.

Nursing Pharmacology: An Integrated Approach to Drug Therapy and Nursing Practice is designed to facilitate such an approach to pharmacology. Throughout the text, you will find the actions of drugs explained in terms of the normal processes in the body and pathological changes. Nursing actions are introduced in the context of the drug effects that justify them. Understanding the reasons behind nursing actions will help you to remember them.

Nursing students encountering pharmacology for the first time will find it helpful to remember that drugs can be grouped into pharmacological classes. You can reduce the mass of memorization required by first learning the properties of a drug class. Once you thoroughly command these class characteristics, you can study the individual drugs from the point of view of characteristics that distinguish each from the class as a whole. Studying drug classes also helps you learn about new drugs as they are introduced.

Organization of *Nursing Pharmacology*

In the first two units of this book we present the foundation that will prepare you for studying pharmacology. Chapter 1 sets a historical perspective that will link your study of pharmacology to your general education. Chapter 2 introduces you to drug terminology. Chapter 3 discusses the principles of pharmacology. Thoroughly understanding this chapter will profoundly help in your study of pharmacology because these principles find frequent application in the study of specific drugs. Chapter 4 acquaints you with one of the nurse's areas of special responsibility: drug administration. In Chapter 5 we discuss the legal and ethical issues facing the nurse administering drugs. Chapters 6 and 7 extend the concepts introduced in Chapters 3 and 4 to children and older adults. Finally, Chapter 8 links pharmacology and nursing practice by introducing the concepts that will serve as the basis for the nursing implication sections throughout subsequent chapters.

Each of the remaining units of the book is built around a major organ system of the body so that you will be able to integrate newly acquired knowledge of each drug's beneficial and adverse effects into your understanding of how each system of the body works or fails to work in disease. The larger units dealing with the central nervous system, the peripheral nervous system, the endocrine system, the cardiovascular system, and the immune system begin with an introductory chapter reviewing the physiology of the system. This chapter is followed by several drug chapters organized around particular drug classes. In the smaller units, each chapter is concentrated on a bodily system and includes both the physiology and the drugs that act on that system.

Organization of Drug Chapters

As your study progresses, you will recognize a common four-step pattern in the approach to each topic. First, we briefly review how the body system works. Then we describe how the system goes wrong in pathological states. We then discuss how the drug interacts with the system to produce its effects. And finally, we consider the nursing actions required by this interaction between drug and body system. The first two of these four steps — the review of normal functions and pathology — are designed to reinforce, refresh, and update knowledge that you acquire in your basic science courses. You will probably find that some of these reviews cover ground which is largely familiar; in others, though, you will delve into topics not covered in your earlier coursework. The time you spend studying each review will need to be adjusted accordingly.

Most of the information in the remaining sections in each chapter will be new to you. The pharmacology sections in each chapter take up first the pharmacology of the drug class collectively, then the pharmacology of specific drugs. The drug discussions follow a standard format to help organize your study. *Mechanisms and effects* describe the interaction between the drug and the body. Next, you will take up the *pharmacokinetic* characteristics, such as the time required for absorption, how long the drug can be expected to remain in the body, and how the drug is inactivated. You will then study the *clinical indications* for the drug or drug class, the diagnostic categories for which the drug is proven effective. Next, we consider *adverse effects and contraindications,* often covering many specific nursing implications. Then you will review the drug's *interactions* with other drugs and, if applicable, with the diet or laboratory tests. We conclude each drug discussion by summarizing *preparations and administration,* listing specific drug products and recommended doses.

Specific responsibilities of the nurse in drug therapy are discussed throughout the text, in three ways. First, nursing implications for specific drugs are incorporated into the drug discussions to help you see the relationship between the drug's effects and the resulting actions required of the nurse. This information is *italicized* for easy reference. Second, we list "Important Nursing Implications" for each drug or drug group, a convenient summary ending each section. Finally, two boxed displays, "Nursing Observations" and "Nursing Diagnoses and Interventions," show you how to apply the steps in the nursing process in studying pharmacology.

At the end of each chapter, you will encounter case studies, each providing an opportunity to apply the knowledge you have gained from the chapter to a practice situation. Each case lists information about a client, followed by questions asking you to apply principles outlined in the chapter to that case. You will gain more from the case studies by working out the answers before consulting those offered at the back of the book.

The recommended readings following each chapter are especially designed for students. Here you will find many suggestions for materials readily assimilated by nursing students or practicing nurses rather than professional pharmacologists.

Knowledge of pharmacology is a daily requirement for today's professional nurse. That need is likely to be even greater in the years ahead. More and more patients are briefly hospitalized and discharged for extended recovery in their homes. Nurses working in the community have become the major contact for such people with the health-care team. Nurses provide primary care, of course, but they must also act as the eyes and ears of the health-care team. Only the nurse with a solid foundation of drug knowledge will know what to watch for in the way of side effects, interactions, and errors in compliance. It is our hope that this text will provide the foundation you need to prepare you for this indispensable role.

UNIT I

Introduction to Pharmacology

CHAPTER 1

Historical Perspectives

Pharmacology — The study of the effects of chemicals (commonly referred to as drugs) on humans and animals — is a relatively young science, dating from the middle of the nineteenth century. Pharmacology is an offshoot of pharmacy; it draws upon physiology and biochemistry and provides, in turn, a foundation for clinical medicine. Drug utilization may well be the most important component of modern therapeutics. Though drugs are used to some extent for diagnosis, their chief value lies in prevention, treatment, and symptomatic relief of disease.

Claude Bernard (1813–1878), who experimented on the action of curare, is generally credited with being the father of pharmacology. The history of pharmacology prior to 1850 is embedded in the profession of pharmacy. Pharmacy, in turn, was an offshoot of medicine, existing as an independent discipline only after the beginning of the sixteenth century. Thus the early roots of pharmacology are interwoven with the history of medicine itself.

The Early History of Medicine

We know little about pathology or the practice of medicine in prehistoric times. What is known relates principally to pathological conditions involving the bones and teeth, since these alone have survived to modern times. There are indications in fossilized bones of such diseases as arthritis, dental caries, and osteomyelitis. Some bones of neolithic man (from about 12,000 years ago) show signs of tuberculosis, rickets, and poliomyelitis as well as clearer indications of arthritis, fractures, and tumors.

Study of the medical activities of modern primitive tribes also gives us some insight into ancient practices. As in modern Western civilization, medical care in such tribes begins with the attendance of family members and the application of home remedies. If the condition persists, the tribal medical specialist is summoned. Since primitive people view disease and sickness as supernatural processes caused by spirits or related to moral transgressions, it is not surprising that the medicine man is essentially a magician skilled in techniques for dealing with supernatural agencies. He uses sacred objects, incantations, dances, ceremonies, magic preparations, blood-letting, sucking out of small bones or pebbles from the victim's body, or other such procedures. Sometimes a taboo is imposed, meaning that the patient is prohibited from some activity, or the patient may be ostracized or called upon to confess transgressions.

There is evidence from artifacts and art works that the activity of certain botanical extracts was recognized by some of the ancient tribes (Table 1–1). Toxins such as curare, strophanthin (ouabain), picrotoxin, reserpine, and veratrine were known. Medicinals included dermatological preparations from leaves of the North American sassafras tree and chaulmoogra oil from several East Indian trees, cinchona bark for malaria, opium as an analgesic and euphoriant, parts of the tropical creeping plant ipecac as an antiameboid agent, various antipyretics such as willow bark, dogwood, and goldenseal, emetine as an emetic, and cocaine as a stimulant.

Considerably more is known about medicine in the ancient civilizations beginning with Egypt. Not only have written records been preserved, but the study of Egyptian mummies has provided the earliest information we have concerning diseases of soft tissues. Egyptian art also conveys valuable information concerning the practice of medicine of that time. The courts of the pharaohs had physicians and dentists as early as 2700 BC, of whom most were priests as well, trained in the temples. Thus, medicine retained its orientation toward the supernatural and religion. Papyri and scrolls that have survived contain not only formulas and prescriptions, but also many invocations and magical elements. Some of the formulas mentioned include the use of figs, senna, aloe, and castor oil as cathartics, squill (a Mediterranean bulbous herb) as a cardiac glycoside, wormwood and peppermint as antipyretics and analgesics, and opium as an analgesic. Diseases involving parasites were common in the Nile valley, so a special emphasis on cathartics is not surprising.

In Babylonia, the series of empires that flourished in Mesopotamia, physicians existed as early as 3000 BC. Among the drugs known to these people were opium and hyoscyamine (from which atropine and scopolamine are derived). India had an early system of secularized medicine with medical sciences established at the universities as early as 550 BC. Smallpox vaccination was apparently employed in India during this period. The ancient Peruvian civilizations made widespread use of cocaine. The use of ephedrine for breathing difficulties, mercuric and arsenic salts as antiseptics, camphor as a rubefacient, and cod liver oil as an emollient began in ancient China, along with the use of marihuana and opium as sedatives.

The Greek Influence

The Greeks were largely responsible for freeing Western medicine from superstition and religious rites and for transforming it into a rational science. Hippocrates (460–379 BC) is generally regarded as the father of medicine. His medical writings emphasize the role of diet, climate, and other natural influences and outline the doctor's role as aiding the body's inherent recuperative processes. Medical ethics became a central issue. Perhaps most important, Hippocrates denied that disease was supernatural in origin and focused instead on the importance of observations, inductive reasoning, and natural law. For the first time we find physicians stressing the value of careful observation as a tool of diagnosis and the need for a rationale as the basis for therapy.

Hippocrates' physiology, pathology, and therapeutics were based largely upon the doctrines of his Greek predecessors, who believed that four body "humors" — blood, yellow bile, black bile, and phlegm — determined the bodily state of health or disease. A proper and evenly balanced mixture of the humors was thought to result in a healthy body and mind, while an imbalance resulted in disease.

The influence of Greek physicians on medicine persisted even as civilization began to shift geographically toward the Roman Empire and Arab cities such as Alexandria. Many of the court physicians of Rome and Alexandria were Greeks trained in hippocratic medicine. During this period, the Greeks produced the first treatises describing medicines. Theophrastus wrote *The History of Plants* in approximately 300 BC. Dioscorides in AD 57 wrote the first *Materia Medica,* classifying some 600 agents by substance rather than disease for the first time. This volume was the standard source of pharmaceutical information until the sixteenth century.

Table 1-1
Histories of Use for Principal Drug Classes

Class Name	Antiquity	1000 BC	0 AD	500	1000	1200	1400	1500	1550	1600	1650	1700	1750	1800	1840	1860	1880	1900	1910	1920	1930	1940	1950	1955	1960	1965	1970	1975	1980	1985
Antimicrobial Drugs																														
Amantadine																										*	*	*	*	*
Aminoglycosides																							*	*	*	*	*	*	*	*
Cephalosporins																									*	*	*	*	*	*
Chloramphenicol																							*	*	*	*	*	*	*	*
Chloroquine																							*	*	*	*	*	*	*	*
Cinchona											*	*	*	*	*	*	*	*	*	*	*	*	*	*	*	*	*	*	*	*
Griseofulvin																									*	*	*	*	*	*
Isoniazid																								*	*	*	*	*	*	*
Penicillin																						*	*	*	*	*	*	*	*	*
Quinine															*	*	*	*	*	*	*	*	*	*	*	*	*	*	*	*
Smallpox vaccine														*	*	*	*	*	*	*	*	*	*	*	*	*	*	*	*	*
Sulfonamides																						*	*	*	*	*	*	*	*	*
Tetracyclines																							*	*	*	*	*	*	*	*
Cardiovascular																														
Alpha-blockers																								*	*	*	*	*	*	*
Belladonna alkaloids	*	*	*	*	*	*	*	*	*	*	*	*	*	*	*	*	*	*	*	*	*	*	*	*	*	*	*	*	*	*
Beta-blockers																											*	*	*	*
Calcium-channel blockers																														*
Cardiac glycosides		*	*	*	*	*	*	*	*	*	*	*	*	*	*	*	*	*	*	*	*	*	*	*	*	*	*	*	*	*
Heparin																						*	*	*	*	*	*	*	*	*
High-ceiling diuretics																										*	*	*	*	*
Hydralazine																								*	*	*	*	*	*	*
Mercurial diuretics																							*	*	*	*	*	*	*	*
Methyldopa																										*	*	*	*	*
Nitrites																	*	*	*	*	*	*	*	*	*	*	*	*	*	*
Norepinephrine																							*	*	*	*	*	*	*	*
Oral anticoagulants																							*	*	*	*	*	*	*	*
Potassium-sparing diuretics																									*	*	*	*	*	*
Quinidine											*	*	*	*	*	*	*	*	*	*	*	*	*	*	*	*	*	*	*	*
Thiazides																								*	*	*	*	*	*	*
Central Nervous System																														
Acetaminophen																							*	*	*	*	*	*	*	*
Alcohol	*	*	*	*	*	*	*	*	*	*	*	*	*	*	*	*	*	*	*	*	*	*	*	*	*	*	*	*	*	*
Amphetamines																						*	*	*	*	*	*	*	*	*
Antipyretics	*	*	*	*	*	*	*	*	*	*	*	*	*	*	*	*	*	*	*	*	*	*	*	*	*	*	*	*	*	*
Antidepressants																									*	*	*	*	*	*
Antipsychotics																								*	*	*	*	*	*	*
Barbiturates																		*	*	*	*	*	*	*	*	*	*	*	*	*
Benzodiazepines																									*	*	*	*	*	*
Cocaine	*	*	*	*	*	*	*	*	*	*	*	*	*	*	*	*	*	*	*	*	*	*	*	*	*	*	*	*	*	*
Coffee											*	*	*	*	*	*	*	*	*	*	*	*	*	*	*	*	*	*	*	*
Ether																*	*	*	*	*	*	*	*	*	*	*	*	*	*	*
Levodopa																										*	*	*	*	*
Lithium																								*	*	*	*	*	*	*
Local anesthetics																			*	*	*	*	*	*	*	*	*	*	*	*
LSD																						*	*	*	*	*	*	*	*	*
Marihuana	*	*	*	*	*	*	*	*	*	*	*	*	*	*	*	*	*	*	*	*	*	*	*	*	*	*	*	*	*	*
Meprobamate																							*	*	*	*	*	*	*	*
Narcotic analgesics		*	*	*	*	*	*	*	*	*	*	*	*	*	*	*	*	*	*	*	*	*	*	*	*	*	*	*	*	*
Nitrous oxide															*	*	*	*	*	*	*	*	*	*	*	*	*	*	*	*
Phenytoin																						*	*	*	*	*	*	*	*	*
Salicylates																		*	*	*	*	*	*	*	*	*	*	*	*	*
Strychnine															*	*	*	*	*	*	*	*	*	*	*	*	*	*	*	*

Class Name	Antiquity	1000 BC	0 AD	500	1000	1200	1400	1500	1550	1600	1650	1700	1750	1800	1840	1860	1880	1900	1910	1920	1930	1940	1950	1955	1960	1965	1970	1975	1980	1985
Tea										*	*	*	*	*	*	*	*	*	*	*	*	*	*	*	*	*	*	*	*	*
Tobacco								*	*	*	*	*	*	*	*	*	*	*	*	*	*	*	*	*	*	*	*	*	*	*
Dermatologics																														
Antiseptics	*	*	*	*	*	*	*	*	*	*	*	*	*	*	*	*	*	*	*	*	*	*	*	*	*	*	*	*	*	*
Emollients	*	*	*	*	*	*	*	*	*	*	*	*	*	*	*	*	*	*	*	*	*	*	*	*	*	*	*	*	*	*
Rubefacients	*	*	*	*	*	*	*	*	*	*	*	*	*	*	*	*	*	*	*	*	*	*	*	*	*	*	*	*	*	*
Endocrine Drugs																														
Androgens																						*	*	*	*	*	*	*	*	*
Antithyroid drugs																						*	*	*	*	*	*	*	*	*
Estrogens																						*	*	*	*	*	*	*	*	*
Glucocorticoids																							*	*	*	*	*	*	*	*
Insulin																				*	*	*	*	*	*	*	*	*	*	*
Iodine					*	*	*	*	*	*	*	*	*	*	*	*	*	*	*	*	*	*	*	*	*	*	*	*	*	*
Oral hypoglycemics																								*	*	*	*	*	*	*
Progestins																								*	*	*	*	*	*	*
Thyroid hormones																						*	*	*	*	*	*	*	*	*
Gastrointestinal Drugs																														
Antacids																						*	*	*	*	*	*	*	*	*
Cathartics	*	*	*	*	*	*	*	*	*	*	*	*	*	*	*	*	*	*	*	*	*	*	*	*	*	*	*	*	*	*
Cholinomimetic																							*	*	*	*	*	*	*	*
H_2-blockers																												*	*	*
Nutrients																														
Vitamin A																			*	*	*	*	*	*	*	*	*	*	*	*
B-complex vitamins																			*	*	*	*	*	*	*	*	*	*	*	*
Vitamin C/citrus													*	*	*	*	*	*	*	*	*	*	*	*	*	*	*	*	*	*
Vitamin D																				*	*	*	*	*	*	*	*	*	*	*
Respiratory System																														
Ephedrine	*	*	*	*	*	*	*	*	*	*	*	*	*	*	*	*	*	*	*	*	*	*	*	*	*	*	*	*	*	*
Isoproterenol																							*	*	*	*	*	*	*	*
Nasal decongestants																						*	*	*	*	*	*	*	*	*
Other																														
Colchicine																*	*	*	*	*	*	*	*	*	*	*	*	*	*	*
Curare	*	*	*	*	*	*	*	*	*	*	*	*	*	*	*	*	*	*	*	*	*	*	*	*	*	*	*	*	*	*
H_1-blockers																					*	*	*	*	*	*	*	*	*	*
Physostigmine																	*	*	*	*	*	*	*	*	*	*	*	*	*	*

The last great Greek influence was a physician named Galen (c. AD 130–201), born in Asia Minor, the son of an architect. Galen studied medicine in Alexandria and practiced in Rome. He devised a system of medicine based on speculative theories of human physiology, polypharmacy, alchemy, and a system of teleological reasoning. His remedies often entailed as many as 25 drugs for a single condition. He developed many new preparations, including cold cream (rosewater ointment). In addition, he was an experimentalist, conducting studies using lesioning techniques and dissection. Galen's system of medicine became the dogma of the Dark Ages (400–1100), when opposition to galenism was considered heretical. Medicine once again assumed its close association with superstition and religion, and very little progress occurred during this period. Monasteries became the chief repositories of medical lore, and monks cultivated the botanical gardens that became the sources of drugs such as absinthe (from wormwood), hellebore, belladonna, and various alkaloids from *Mandragora*.

Medieval and Renaissance Medicine

During the Dark Ages, the few small steps that occurred in medicine can be credited mainly to Arab peoples. The first study of smallpox was conducted by an Arab physician, Al Rhazi (860–932). Ibn Sina, also known as Aricenna (980–1037), wrote a medical textbook, the *Canon,* that was used for a century in Europe as well as in Arab countries. The Arabs established the first apothecaries and the first pharmaceutical formulary. Among the preparations that were used in the Arab world were senna, camphor, cannabis, and alcohol. The use of syrups also was an Arab contribution.

It is not surprising, then, that the rise of Western Europe out of the shroud of the Dark Ages was triggered in part by the crusades to the Middle East (1096–1272) and that the earliest European centers of learning were located close to the Arab world. During this period, mercury for syphilis and skin diseases and iodine for goiter were introduced. In the thirteenth century, pharmacies were opened throughout Europe. Dissection was carried out with increasing frequency, expanding the knowledge of anatomy and physiology. In the fourteenth century, awareness of the contagious nature of certain diseases developed. The bubonic plague (black death) killed about 25% of the population of Western Europe in the mid-1300s. The notion of quarantine was developed, prostitution came under legal sanction, and leprosy was dealt with by isolation of patients in leper houses.

With the beginning of the Renaissance, a number of physicians began to rebel against the traditionalist influences of Arab medicine and of galenism. Alchemy flourished, leading to new skills and knowledge in chemistry. Printing was invented in 1438, greatly facilitating the dissemination of knowledge. In the 1500s, pharmacy began to develop as an independent discipline. Cordus compiled and had printed the first pharmacopoeia, or official formulary, which he based on Greek, Roman, and Arab materials. In the late 1600s, woman healers, the forerunners of modern nurses, became increasingly prevalent and some compiled recipes for laxatives, suppositories, enemata, and broths.

Fracastorius (1484–1553), an Italian physician, presented a theory of contagious disease. The Flemish anatomist and physicist, Vesalius (1515–1564), working with an artist-illustrator named Kalkar, originated the modern science of anatomy. The foremost Renaissance leader, however, was Paracelsus (1493–1541), who dealt the death blow to the theory of the four humors. Paracelsus traveled widely throughout Europe, gathering knowledge of local medical practices. He was quite radical in his approach to teaching, lecturing in everyday language, German, rather than in Latin, the language of scholars of that day. Legend has it that he publicly burned a book by Galen when he began teaching in Basel, Switzerland. He was an accomplished alchemist and introduced sulfur, lead, arsenic, copper, and calomel (mercurous chloride) into clinical use. He also observed the effects of ether during experiments with chickens. His most important contribution was the concept of diseases as distinct entities rather than as excesses or deficiencies of one of the four traditional humors. Some of his original, if primitive, ideas contribute to psychiatry, to germ theory, and to our understanding of metabolism.

The sixteenth century brought with it the age of navigation and worldwide trade in drug-containing agricultural products. Columbus himself was provided with a gift of tobacco on his birthday in 1492 by North American natives. Tobacco importation into Europe began in 1550 with the shipping of tobacco leaves from Brazil to Portugal and by the end of the sixteenth century, tobacco was in use throughout Europe. Cocoa importation had begun even earlier, with the return of Cortez to Spain in 1528, but its use spread slowly. Coffee and tea likewise reached Europe during this period. Tea first arrived in Europe from China in 1610, and it was widely used by the end of the century. Coffee houses appeared in England in 1650 and in France in 1671.

Medicines in the Seventeenth through Nineteenth Centuries

William Harvey's (1578–1657) discovery of the circulation of blood paved the way for the introduction of intravenous injections (1656) and transfusions (1667), although technical difficulties prevented adoption of these measures until the nineteenth century. Robert Boyle (1627–1691) demonstrated the dependence of life on a constituent of air (later found to be oxygen) rather than on air in general. Also during the seventeenth century, tincture of benzoin (a topical skin preparation), laudanum (the alcohol tincture of opium), cocaine, cinchona (used in malaria), and ipecac (originally introduced as a remedy for dysentery) found their way into European medicine.

The eighteenth century brought with it the first

inoculations. On May 14, 1776, Edward Jenner carried out the first public inoculations with a vaccine derived from cowpox as a protection against smallpox. Digitalis, derived from the foxglove plant, was introduced into medicine by William Withering in 1785. Oxygen was identified by Carl Scheele in 1772, and hydrogen by Henry Cavendish in 1766. Antoine Lavoisier not only was the first to understand the significance of oxygen in respiration but also did much to clarify the nature of respiration itself. James Lind (1716–1794) demonstrated the importance of citrus fruit in the treatment of scurvy, thereby initiating an awareness of the essential nutrients that we call vitamins. In the eighteenth century, administration of drugs in English hospitals was already a duty of nursing "sisters."

Beginning in the nineteenth century, knowledge of chemistry began to play a major role in the advancement of drug knowledge. Morphine was extracted from opium in 1806 by Frederick W. A. Serturner and identified as its major active ingredient. This was soon followed by isolation of the active constituents of other botanical preparations, including strychnine (1818), quinine (1820), veratrine, emetine, atropine (1831), and codeine (1832). Much of this work was done by pharmacists. François Magendie, Claude Bernard's teacher, investigated strychnine, emetine, morphine, iodine, and bromides. Oswald Schmiedeberg carried out studies of digitalis and histamine, while curare, ether, opium, and nicotine were studied by Bernard. These three men were perhaps the first true pharmacologists. The Calabar bean was imported into England in 1840, and its active ingredient, physostigmine, was isolated in 1864.

Another major advance in the use of drugs was the development of anesthesia in America. Crawford Long, a Georgian physician, used ether as an anesthetic in 1842 but did not publish his experiences. Horace Wells, a Connecticut dentist, initiated use of nitrous oxide in 1844, and William Morton conducted a dramatic public demonstration of the usefulness of anesthesia for surgery at the Massachusetts General Hospital in 1846.

Twenty-two years later, in 1868, A. Crum-Brown and T. R. Frazer discovered one of the earliest principles of pharmacology — the relationship between the structure of a chemical compound and its activity. T. Lauder Brunton conducted studies of cardiac drugs that led to the introduction of amyl nitrite to relieve the pain of heart disease in 1867. Cocaine was used as the first local anesthetic in 1884 by Karl Köller, an associate of Sigmund Freud.

Another impressive breakthrough in medicine occurred with the nineteenth-century discovery that microorganisms are the causative agents in infectious disease. Certain fungi had been identified as causing contagious diseases as early as 1835. Then, in 1850, Rayer discovered the bacterial agent of anthrax and demonstrated its transference from one animal to another. Louis Pasteur, through many years of research, developed vaccines effective against anthrax, chicken cholera, and rabies. Many other vaccines were to follow in the nineteenth and early twentieth centuries. Joseph Lister developed the technique of aspetic surgery and demonstrated the potency of phenol as an antiseptic in 1867.

Another nineteenth-century landmark was the work of Sir William Perkin with coal-tar products, from which were developed salicylic acid, benzoic acid, acetanilid, and antipyrine. Just before the turn of the century, aspirin, derived from salicylic acid, was introduced into medicine by Dreser.

Medicines in the Twentieth Century

Early in the twentieth century, in 1905, J. N. Langley introduced what was to become one of the cornerstones of the then infant field of pharmacology — the receptor theory. This important notion is discussed in detail in Chapter 3. In 1933 A. J. Clark's formulation of the dose-response principle advanced the foundations of pharmacology as an empirical science. In 1948 R. P. Ahlquist introduced the classification of adrenergic receptors based on his studies of potencies of various agonists. This paved the way for the classification of other kinds of receptors and the development of drugs of greater specificity of action.

New Anesthetics and Hypnotics

Barbital became the first barbiturate in medical use in 1903, with phenobarbital added in 1912. Phenobarbital has retained great clinical importance, though many other barbiturates have also come into use. Pentobarbital was added in 1941 to the list of important barbiturates available to medicine. Nonbarbiturate sedative-hypnotics were developed during the 1950s, with glutethimide, methyprylon, ethchlorvynol, and meprobamate all being marketed in 1955.

Procaine became the standard local anesthetic after its introduction in 1905 until the introduction of lidocaine in 1949. Cyclopropane was discovered in 1929 and soon found its way into the catalogue of general anesthetics. Halothane, introduced in 1958, remains one of the best of the general anesthetics.

Vitamins and Hormones

The early decades of the twentieth century brought important discoveries about vitamins. Vitamin A was discovered in 1913 and vitamin B in 1916. Vitamin D became known in 1922. The deficiency diseases related to vitamin B (pellagra) and D (rickets) were soon identified.

A major breakthrough in endocrine pharmacology came in 1922 with the discovery of insulin as a treatment for diabetes mellitus. Oral hypoglycemic therapy became an alternative to insulin in the late 1950s. Second-generation oral hypoglycemic agents were added during the 1980s.

In the 1930s, the adrenal corticosteroids were isolated and identified. Cortisone was used in clinical practice in 1948, followed by other steroids. Several other important advances in hormone medication marked the early 1940s; androgens (methyltestosterone, 1941), estrogens (estradiol, 1940), and thyroglobulin (1940) became available. Thiouracil, the first antithyroid medication, came into use in 1946. The purified thyroid hormones, levothyroxine (1953) and liothyronine (1956) were made available during the 1950s. Norethindrone (1957) and other progestins paved the way for introduction of "the pill."

Anti-infective Agents

Few drugs existed at the turn of the century for combating infections — only cinchona and quinine for malaria and the smallpox vaccine. In 1907 the use of arsenicals in the treatment of syphilis was added to the list of drug treatments for specific microbes. Then, in the 1930s, Gerhart Domagk observed that sulfanilamide (discovered in 1908) protected mice infected with streptococcal septicemia. This and other sulfa drugs became the first agents found to possess general antibacterial properties. They were introduced clinically in 1935. Penicillin had been discovered in 1929 by Alexander Fleming, but appreciation and development of its potential awaited the efforts of Howard Florey, which began in 1938 and culminated in 1941 with the first clinical administration. Numerous antibiotics followed shortly thereafter, including streptomycin (1945), chlortetracycline (1948), and chloramphenicol (1949).

Chloroquine in 1943 replaced quinine as the antimalarial of choice. Griseofulvin became the first effective systemic antifungal agent when introduced in 1959. In 1966, amantadine became the first antiviral drug, albeit one of limited spectrum. During the 1980s second- and third-generation penicillins and cephalosporins, topical antiviral agents, and additional systemic and topical antifungal agents were added to the arsenal of anti-infective agents.

Psychotropic Drugs

The stimulant, amphetamine, found its first application in narcolepsy in 1935. In 1938 two additional classes of psychotropic drugs were originated, with the preparation of the antiepileptic, diphenylhydantoin (now phenytoin), by H. H. Merritt and T. J. Putnam and the synthesis of the psychedelic, lysergic acid diethylamide (LSD), by Albert Hofmann. In 1946 trimethadione was introduced for petit mal epilepsy. Although both meprobamate and lithium were described during the 1940s, they were not introduced into clinical use until later. Meperidine and methadone were added to the list of useful narcotic analgesics in 1944 and 1947, respectively. Propoxyphen, introduced in 1957, provided a weak narcotic analgesic. Acetaminophen became an alternative to aspirin as an analgesic in 1950 and ibuprofen, naproxen, and other nonsteroidal anti-inflammatory drugs became alternatives for anti-inflammatory applications during the 1970s.

Trihexyphenidyl was marketed for parkinsonism in 1949 and benztropine in 1954. Levodopa therapy of parkinsonism, begun in 1965, was considered a "miracle" treatment; it was approved for the U.S. market by the Food and Drug Administration in 1970.

The 1950s provided the first truly effective drug treatments for psychiatric disorders. The first neuroleptics were introduced in 1953 (reserpine) and 1954 (chlorpromazine). Other phenothiazines followed close on the heels of chlorpromazine, including members of the piperazine subgroup (prochlorperazine, 1956; trifluoperazine, 1958) and the piperadine subgroup (thioridazine, 1959). Haloperidol (1967) offered a nonphenothiazine neuroleptic and greater selectivity for dopamine receptors. Imipramine and isocarboxazid came into use as antidepressants in the United States in 1959, followed closely by amitriptyline (1961).

The 1960s began with the discovery of a remarkable class of drugs, the benzodiazepines. Chlordiazepoxide was marketed in 1960 and diazepam in 1963, and within a decade these two drugs had climbed to the top of the most prescribed-drugs list. The first benzodiazepine hypnotic agent — flurazepam — was marketed during the early 1970s. The 1960s also ushered in a new era of drug abuse as a greatly expanded phenomenon. LSD and then marihuana became focal points of social controversy, setting the stage for increased societal awareness in the next decade of the larger drug abuse problems involving alcohol and tobacco.

During the first half of the 1980s, developments in psychopharmacology included second-generation antidepressants and new benzodiazepines.

Peripheral Nervous System Drugs

Phenylpropanolamine was introduced as a nasal decongestant in 1941. Isoproterenol became available as a bronchodilator in 1948 and bethanechol as a cholinomimetic in 1949. Two drugs joined curare during the 1950s as effective skeletal muscle relaxants: gallamine (1951) and succinylcholine (1952). In the 1980s, selective beta-agonists and beta-antagonists became available.

Cardiovascular Drugs

The mercurials became the first truly effective diuretics when introduced in 1943. Both heparin (1942) and dicumarol (1944) became available as the first anticoagulants. Several important cardiovascular drugs — procainamide (1950), levarterenol (1951), and the antihypertensive agents hydralazine (1952) and phenoxybenzamine (1953) — came into use during the early 1950s. Chlorthiazide heralded the era of thiazide diuretics in 1957, and spironolactone became available two years later as a means of reducing the potassium ion depletion caused by thiazides. New and better antihypertensive agents, including guanethidine (1960), methyldopa (1963), and clonidine (1974), replaced older drugs during the sixties and seventies. The high-ceiling diuretics, furosemide (1966) and ethacrynic acid (1967), extended the maximum efficacy of diuretic therapy. The first of the beta-blockers, propranolol, became available in the 1970s. Calcium channel blockers and other new antidysrhythmic drugs were added in the 1980s.

Gastrointenstinal, Respiratory, and Dermatological Agents

The first antihistamine, diphenhydramine, was discovered in 1933 and introduced before the end of the decade. Aluminum salts were introduced as antacids in 1942. In 1954 dextromethorphan replaced codeine as the safest, most effective antitussive. Cimetidine was introduced as the first clinically useful H_2-blocker for ulcers during the 1970s. Isotretinoin was introduced for acne during the 1980s.

Federal Drug Legislation

In the twentieth century, both state and federal agencies have undertaken regulation of drug manufacturing and sales. Federal laws pertain whenever a drug enters interstate commerce, which applies to nearly all drug products. Federal regulation of drugs began with the Pure Food and Drug Act of 1906 (Table 1–2), the law that is the basis for federal jurisdiction over drug standards and labeling. Other laws have addressed specific problems that have arisen. Thus, the Sherley Amendment of 1912 established requirements regarding claims of efficacy; the Harrison Narcotic Act established the basis for regulating drugs of abuse; the Food, Drug, and Cosmetic Act established standards of testing for safety; the Durham-Humphrey Amendment established the roles of the physician and pharmacist in prescribing and dispensing drugs respectively; the Kefauver-Harris Amendment of 1962 provided standardization of drug names and requirements for proof of efficacy for existing drugs; the Controlled Substances Act classified drugs of abuse (see Chapter 10); and the Orphan Drug Act provided incentives for development and marketing of drugs with therapeutic value but little economic promise.

Changing Roles for Nurses with Emergence of Pharmacotherapeutics

The first nursing textbook (authored by Anna Caroline Maxwell and Amy Elizabeth Pope) was published in 1910 and the first guideline for nursing curricula, *Standard Curriculum for Schools of Nursing*, in 1919. These sources reveal the expectations that existed at the beginning of the century with respect to the nurse's role in drug therapy. The guidelines for nursing curricula provided for two courses dealing with medicines to be taken by nursing students. Nurses were expected to weigh and measure accurately, make up solutions, recognize pharmaceutical symbols, understand the basis for each drug's action, administer drugs competently, observe for therapeutic and adverse effects, anticipate interactions between drugs and food, and be able to recognize and treat overdosages. A decade later, a nursing text by Bertha Harmer published in 1928 added additional expectations that nurses know normal dosage ranges, factors that modify drug response, and potential idiosyncratic reactions.

In the 1930s, increased emphasis was placed on the nurse's role in educating clients about medications. For example, nurses were expected to teach clients how to measure and administer drugs properly and how to handle and store drugs to prevent

Table 1–2
U.S. Federal Drug Legislation

Year	Title of legislation	Major provisions
1906	Pure Food and Drug Act	Established United States Pharmacopoeia (USP) and NF (National Formulary) as official standards; established requirement for accurate labeling of drug products
1912	Sherley Amendment	Prohibited fraudulent claims of efficacy
1914	Harrison Narcotic Act	Regulated and restricted importation, manufacture, sales, and use of opium, cocaine, marihuana, and other drugs that the act defined as *narcotics*
1938	Food, Drug, and Cosmetic Act (Wheeler-Lea Act)	Required proof of safety before marketing of a new drug; added Homeopathic Pharmacopoeia of the United States as a third official drug standard
1945	Amendment to Pure Food and Drug Act	Required governmental certification of biological products, such as insulin and antibiotics
1952	Durham-Humphrey Amendment	Designated certain drugs as *legend* (prescription) drugs, requiring that they be prescribed by a physician and dispensed by a pharmacist
1962	Kefauver-Harris Amendment	Required proof of efficacy for drugs to remain on market; gave federal government the authority to standardize drug names
1970	Comprehensive Drug Abuse Prevention and Control Act (or Controlled Substances Act)	Classified drugs into five schedules according to abuse liability and medical value; established the Drug Enforcement Administration (DEA) as the sole drug enforcement agency; established education and treatment programs
1978	Drug Regulation Reform Act	Shortened the time period required for developing new drugs, speeding release of new drugs to the public
1983	Orphan Drug Act	Provided incentives (tax relief and protection from competition for 7 years) for marketing of orphan drugs (therapeutically valuable drugs with little economic potential)

contamination or deterioration. In the late 1930s, the practice was begun of keeping "physician sheets" at nursing stations as a permanent record of therapy and as a guard against medication errors. Increased emphasis was also now being placed on safeguarding supplies of habit-forming drugs.

By the 1950s, administration of medicines had become a major part of the responsibilities of the professional nurse. Legal and ethical issues relating to drug administration were now addressed more directly. The technical proficiencies of nurses in providing injections and initiating infusions advanced during this period. The concept of the five "rights" (see Chapter 4) was standardized during the 1960s and the centralized unit dose system was put into effect. In the 1970s, nurses responded to increased societal interest in preventative health with intensified activities in education of clients for self-care and promoting wellness.

During the 1970s and early 1980s, the role of nurses with respect to drugs has continued to expand. Nurses in many settings consult more directly than ever before with physicians regarding needed changes in medications or doses. In some states, nurse practitioners have been granted authority to write prescriptions, although frequently with constraints such as limiting their selections to an established list of drugs or requiring supervision by a physician. Nursing has also expanded in the direction of participating in drug research, either as primary investigators or co-investigators.

Recommended Readings

Ackerknecht EH: *A Short History of Medicine.* New York, Ronald Press, 1955.

Dolan JA: *Nursing in Society: A Historical Perspective,* ed 14. Philadelphia, WB Saunders, 1978.

Elliott J: *Outline of Greek and Roman Medicine.* Boston, Milford House, 1971.

Leake CD: *An Historic Account of Pharmacology to the 20th Century.* Springfield, Ill, Charles C Thomas, 1975.

Ray O: *Drugs, Society and Human Behavior,* ed 3. St Louis, CV Mosby Co, 1978.

Rogers F: *A Syllabus of Medical History.* Boston, Little Brown & Co, 1972.

Rosenberg CE: The practice of medicine in New York a century ago, in Leavitt JW and Numbers RL (eds): *Sickness and Health in America.* Madison, Wisc, The University of Wisconsin Press, 1978, pp 55–74.

Shryock RH: *Medicine and Society in America. 1660–1860.* New York, NY University Press, 1960.

Shryock RH: Nursing emerges as a profession: the American experience, in *Sickness and Health in America,* Madison, Wisc, The University of Wisconsin Press, 1978, pp 203–215.

Sonnedecker G: *History of Pharmacy,* ed 3. Philadelphia, JB Lippincott, 1963.

Stewart IM, Austin AL: *A History of Nursing from Ancient to Modern Times: A World View,* ed 5. New York, GP Putnam's Sons, 1962.

CHAPTER 2

Drug Names, Sources, Classifications, and Standards

Drug Names

Many drugs have more than one name. This has the unfortunate effect of complicating matters for the nursing student who is encountering a large number of drug names for the first time. Faced with the task of learning the pharmacology of 200–500 drug substances, the student often does not look gleefully on the fact that most of these substances have two or more names. Nevertheless, the various names of a substance have different meanings and each name is appropriate to its purpose.

The **chemical name** of a substance is a precise but often unwieldy description of the chemical structure of the compound. For example, a chemical often used in medical practice has the chemical name 7-chloro-2-methyl-amino-5-phenyl-3H-1,4-benzodiazepine 4-oxide. A medicinal chemist could diagram the structure of this compound simply by examining its chemical name:

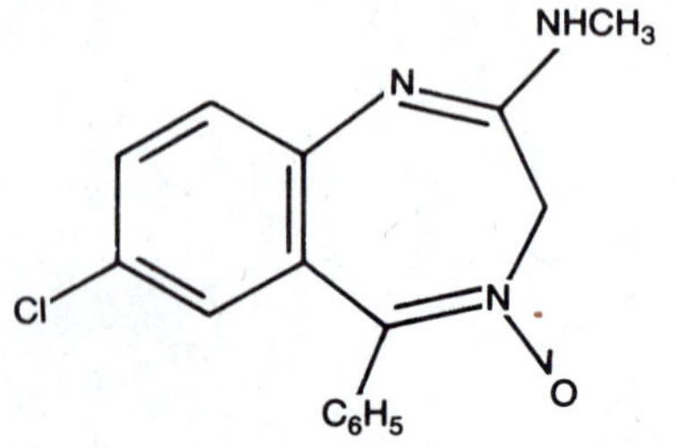

But chemical names are obviously too cumbersome for everyday use. Thus, each drug substance is given a simpler **generic name** that is used worldwide. The generic name for the example drug mentioned above is chlordiazepoxide. The generic name is selected by the original manufacturer and is usually designed to suggest relationships with preexisting drugs of similar chemical structure. Since the generic name refers to the particular chemical regardless of how it is made or by whom, the generic name is said to be a **nonproprietary name** (not owned by any particular proprietor). There is no legal restriction in the form of a trademark on use of the generic name. Any pharmaceutical company that subsequently begins production of the drug would use the same generic name.

If a company wishes to emphasize that a drug product originates from its laboratories, it can give the product an additional name — a **trade name**, or brand name. The trade name is a proprietary name, owned by the company that creates it and registered as a trademark. Unlike the chemical or generic name, it begins with a capital letter. The trade name selected for chlordiazepoxide by its original manufacturer was Librium. No other company can employ the same trade name. Trade names are usually selected to be short, catchy, and easy to pronounce, and sometimes to evoke images of benefit. In this textbook, chemical names will not be listed, but generic names *and* trade names will be used for each drug.

Sometimes a company will choose to market a drug under its generic name without designation of a trade name. Such drugs are known as **generics.** But if a drug is marketed by more than one company, it is likely to be available under more than one trade name. Recently, chlordiazepoxide has been marketed as a generic by several companies (Squibb, Abbott, to name two) and under various new trade names, including A-poxide, SK-Lygen, Sereen, Murcil, Zetran, Tenax, and Chlordiazachel. Sereen is an example of a trade name designed to evoke images of the drug's benefits.

There is considerable controversy concerning the extent to which a drug substance sold under one trade name is equivalent to the same drug substance sold under another trade name or as a generic. The products are chemically equivalent by definition but may or may not be biologically or therapeutically equivalent. Two drug products that contain the same active ingredients are said to be chemically equivalent but may produce different biological and therapeutic effects because of differences in formulation. For example, differences in compaction pressure in preparing tablets, presence of a buffering substance, or use of special coatings all may alter the absorption of the active ingredient(s), bioavailability, and ultimately therapeutic action. These issues are discussed more completely in Chapter 3.

Manufacturers, especially those marketing expensive formulations, may overstate the extent to which chemically equivalent products are therapeutically inequivalent. On the other hand, naive consumer advocates, concerned primarily with costs of medications, may overlook significant differences in biological activity when two or more chemically equivalent formulations are compared. The fact is that there are examples to support both sides of the argument. For some drugs, formulation characteristics play a significant role in determining bioavailability and, ultimately, the therapeutic benefit, for reasons that will be discussed in Chapter 3. For many other drugs, preparations from various manufacturers are not only chemically equivalent, but also biologically and therapeutically equivalent. The rational position is to determine for each drug whether it fits the first or second case. Among the drugs most likely to exhibit significant differences in bioavailability due to formulation factors are antibiotics (chloramphenicol, griseofulvin, nitrofurantoin, tetracyclines, sulfadiazine), digoxin, diuretics (hydrochlorthiazide, triamterene), phenylbutazone, phenytoin, prednisone, thyroid extract, and tolbutamide. *Nurses should advise clients not to switch brands if the drug is one for which bioavailability varies from one manufacturer's product to another's.*

Drug Sources

Drug sources can be classified as natural, semisynthetic, or synthetic. Natural sources of drugs include plants, animals, and minerals. Synthetic drugs are made in the laboratory, whereas semisynthetic drugs are derived by chemical modification of natural substances.

A new method of production of drugs based on recombinant DNA technology (genetic engineering) blurs the classic distinctions between natural and synthetic origins of drugs. In coming years, an increasing number of drugs will probably be produced by this method, utilizing the synthetic machinery of microorganisms to produce desired substances. Some of the insulin used clinically is currently made by this process (see Chapter 33).

Drugs Derived from Natural Sources

One branch of the pharmaceutical sciences, **pharmacognosy,** deals with the sources, procurement, and chemistry of natural products. It is the study of drugs that originate in the plant or animal kingdoms, encompassing matters of the history, occurrence, distribution, procurement, cultivation, preparation, identification, evaluation, preservation, and use of such substances. Although the importance and variety of synthetic drugs are expanding at a rapid rate in modern pharmaceutical development, traditional drugs from plant and animal sources continue to dominate therapeutic practice in many areas. One need only think of the cardiac glycosides, steroids, thyroid extracts, vitamins, and of course, the antibiotics, to recognize the continuing importance of natural drug sources. Natural drugs include carbohydrates, lipids, oils, resins, proteins, steroids, glycosides, tannins, alkaloids, vitamins, and antibiotics.

Carbohydrates (sugars and their derivatives), the preliminary products of photosynthesis, are abundant in plants. Sucrose, dextrose, fructose, and lactose are sugars of great importance in nutrition. Dextrose solutions are frequently employed in intravenous fluid therapy. Citric acid, lactic acid, and ferrous fumerate are drugs with a sugar base. The first two are used as acidifiers and the last as a source of iron. Another class of carbohydrates important to pharmacology are the **alcohols.** The importance of ethanol (ethyl alcohol or common alcohol), as the single most widely used drug worldwide, is obvious. Another alcohol, mannitol, is a useful osmotic diuretic and is also used for evaluating glomerular filtration rate. Sorbitol is an alcohol that has a sweet taste but is not absorbed. It is currently in use as a sweetener, but if ingested in large amounts it can act as an osmotic laxative. Some carbohydrates are polysaccharides, polymers made up of numerous sugar units. Important **polysaccharides** include starch (as a nutrient), inulin (as a diagnostic aid in measuring glomerular filtration), and dextran (as a plasma expander). Some plant polysaccharides form translucent, amorphous, hydrocolloidal masses, called **gums.** Gums such as karaya gum, agar, carrageenan, plantago (psyllium), and guar gum are sometimes employed as bulk laxatives (see Chapter 51). Other gums, such as gum tragacanth, gum arabic (acacia), and xanthan gum find use in pharmaceutical formulations as binders in tablets, as ingredients in dental adhesives, and as emulsifying agents.

Lipids, substances that dissolve readily in organic solvents such as ether or alcohol, are abundantly available from both animal and plant sources. Lipids in solid form are called fats, while those in liquid form are called oils. Castor oil, olive oil, and sesame oil are useful as laxatives. Almond oil is used as an emollient base for cosmetics, corn oil as a solvent for injections, peanut oil and sesame oil as solvents for intramuscular depot injections, cacao butter (theobroma oil) as a base for suppositories, and lanolin as an emollient base. Safflower oil, rich in unsaturated fatty acids (linoleic and oleic acids), is used in margarines: its substitution for butter reduces cholesterol intake. The **fatty acid** undecylenic acid is an effective antifungal agent for controlling tinea pedis. **Waxes** (esters of high-molecular weight alcohols and high-molecular weight fatty acids) obtained from whales (spermaceti), bees (beeswax), or plants (jojoba oil, for example) find use mainly as emulsifying agents and stiffening agents in pharmaceutical preparations. **Prostaglandins** are lipid derivatives that occur in humans as well as various plants and animals.

Volatile oils may be employed as aromatics and as flavoring agents. In this category are peppermint, spearmint, menthol, cinnamon, lemon oil, camphor, anise oil, nutmeg, eucalyptus, and wintergreen oil. Wintergreen oil is, in addition, the source of methlysalicylate, a drug used topically as an antiseptic and for rubs. Phenol volatile oils are useful as antiseptics as well as aromatic agents. Agents in this category are thymol and carvacrol (derived from thyme oil), eugenol (found in clove oil) and creosol and guaiacol (which occur in pine tar and creosote).

Resins are complex substances of plant origin that are amorphous in structure and insoluble in water. Podophyllum (mandrake) is a resin that has been used as a laxative. The resin from the *Cannabis sativa* plant is known as hashish and is a familiar illicit drug, smoked for its euphoriant effect. The resin ginger is a popular flavoring agent. Peruvian balsam is an astringent used in certain hemorrhoidal preparations. Another resin, benzoin, is an antiseptic and expectorant.

Steroids, a group of substances sharing a common four ring structure, come from both plant and animal sources. The steroids produced by the adrenal cortex in humans include glucocorticoids, mineralocorticoids, androgens, estrogens, and progestins. The latter three groups are also produced by the gonads of men and women and by the placenta. Steroidal drugs include the cardiac glycosides, vitamin D and its precursors, and spironolactone. All of these substances are cholesterol derivatives. Other endocrine substances that may be obtained from plant or animal sources include **proteins** such as insulin, pepsin, pancreatin, and trypsin, and **peptides** such as oxytocin, vasopressin, and adrenocorticotropic hormone (ACTH).

Glycosides are compounds that consist of sugar units, usually glucose, and a nonsugar component called an aglycone. Common aglycone constituents include sterols, saponins, tannins, carotenoids, and anthroquinones. Cardiac glycosides are steroidal glycosides. Many of the anthraquinone glycosides are laxatives, including cascara sagrada, aloe, rhubarb, senna, and danthron. Licorice (glycyrrhiza) is a saponin glycoside used as a flavoring agent. It has anti-inflammatory, demulcent, and expectorant properties but can cause sodium and water retention accompanied by potassium depletion. It has been used to treat peptic ulcer and Addison's disease. Wild cherry is a flavoring agent and a cyanophore glycoside. Mustard, the familiar condiment, is an isothiocyanate glycoside. Vanilla is an aldehyde glycoside and vanillin the corresponding aglycone. Lactone glycosides include coumarin and dicumarol (bishydroxycoumarin) — both anticoagulants — and cantharides, the urinary tract irritants falsely reputed to possess aphrodisiac properties.

Tannins are a class of complex substances widely distributed in nature. Their presence in many herbal teas as well as ordinary tea has been linked to occurrence of esophageal cancer. Tannins are used in the tanning process by which animal hides are converted to leather. Tannic acid is a tannin that has been used as an antiseptic and astringent for bedsores.

Alkaloids are among the most important of the drugs of natural origin. Alkaloids are a diverse group of bitter-tasting, alkaline organic chemicals, of limited distribution in plants and animals. Most are specific to a given plant species. Alkaloidal drugs are generally given names that end in "ine." Most alkaloids are poorly soluble in water but form salts that are more soluble. The nicotinic agonist drugs, arecoline, lobeline, and nicotine are **alkaloids of pyridine and piperidine bases. Tropane alkaloids** are also known as belladonna alkaloids due to their occurrence in *Atropa belladonna.* These substances are the important antimuscarinic agents, atropine and scopolamine. Henbane and stramonium are other botanical sources of tropane alkaloids. Cocaine, obtained from the coca plant, is also a tropane alkaloid.

Quinoline alkaloids derive from chichona, the bark of a Peruvian tree. Cinchona alkaloids include quinidine and quinine, important antidysrhythmic and antimalarial drugs. A number of **isoquinoline alkaloids** are used in medicine. Emetine is the principal alkaloid of ipecac, a common emetic agent. Tubocurarine chloride is an isoquinoline alkaloid long used by South American natives as an arrow poison and now used as a neuromuscular blocking agent. **Opium alkaloids** include morphine and codeine. Heroin and hydromorphone are synthesized from these. **Ergot alkaloids,** such as ergotamine and lysergic acid, **Rauwolfia alkaloids,** such as reserpine, the **catharanthus alkaloids,** vincristine and vinblastine, and physostigmine, the cholinesterase inhibitor of the ordeal bean, are all **indole alkaloids.** Pilocarpine, a cholinomimetic, is an **imidazole alkaloid.** Veratrum, a vasodilator with sedative properties, is a **steroidal alkaloid** derived from the dried roots of veratrum viride. The family of drugs known as the xanthines, including caffeine, theophylline, and theobromine, are **alkaloids of purine.** Other important drug classes of natural origins include the **vitamins** (Chapter 44) and the **antibiotics** (Chapter 47).

Synthetic Drugs

In recent years, an increasing percentage of drugs employed in the clinic have originated in the laboratory as synthetic substances. **Medicinal chemistry** is the branch of the pharmaceutical sciences most directly concerned with the synthesis of new drug substances. Medicinal chemistry concerns itself with the modification of structures having known physiological or pharmacological effects as well as the study of the relationship between structure and activity of drugs. If a systematic relationship is found to exist between structural changes within a series of molecules and their biological activity, this relationship can be used to design new molecules with predictable characteristics. The physical-chemical properties of a drug that may be relevant in determining its biological activity can include its solubility, ionization, surface activity, partition coefficient (relative solubility in aqueous and organic media), and oxidation-reduction potentials; its occurrence as isomers or stereoisomers; its ability to form various kinds of bonds with other molecules; and the interatomic distances between functional groups.

For some types of drugs, including most hypnotics, general anesthetics, and some bactericidal agents, biological activity correlates mainly with physical properties such as solubility and partition coefficients and has little to do with the specific chemical structure. These drugs are therefore said to be **structurally nonspecific.** Most drugs, however, are **structurally specific,** meaning that certain chemical features of the drug are principally responsible for its ability to interact with specific cellular receptor sites and thereby to produce biological effects.

Drug Classifications

Drugs can be classified in a variety of ways. The pharmacognocist, botanist, or biologist might use a **taxonomic** classification for natural drugs based on evolutionary relationships among the plants and animals from which the drugs are obtained. The medicinal chemist is likely to find a **chemical** classification most useful, grouping together drugs of like structure regardless of differences in source or pharmacological activity. The pharmacologist often chooses a **pharmacological** classification that groups drugs by physiological activities and mechanisms of action. The clinician is most interested in a **therapeutic** classification that groups drugs with similar therapeutic indications. For the purposes of this book, all of these classification methods are used where appropriate. Pharmacological and therapeutic groupings provide the fundamental organization of the book. Some chapters center around a grouping of drugs based on clinical indications. The chapters on general and local anesthetics, antihypertensive agents, and drugs used for headaches, for example, are organized around clinical indications. Other chapters, such as those relating to the autonomic nervous system, are organized around pharmacological mechanisms. Chemical and taxonomic classifications are used only for subdividing a large family of clinically or pharmacologically similar agents. Thus, the sedative-hypnotics include barbiturate and piperidinedione drugs grouped by chemical structure; antimuscarinic drugs include the belladonna alkaloids, a group determined by a common botanical source. It is generally more useful for the nurse to attend to classifications based on therapeutic applications and pharmacological effects than on chemical or taxonomic features.

The study of drugs by classes is an invaluable tool for learning in the field of pharmacology. For one thing it provides a basis for organizing into a coherent pattern drug information that would otherwise appear as an endless sea of detail. Just as important, the study of drug classes assures nursing students that their knowledge of drugs will not become quickly obsolete. Of the new drugs introduced each year, very few represent new drug categories without precedent among drugs already available. In most cases, given the class identity of a new drug, the nurse who has mastered pharmacology as a student will already know most of the pertinent information relating to the new drug. The drug may differ in its absorption rate or duration of action, in its adverse effects, or in its interactions. But more often than not, the drug will have much in common with others in its class. The wise student will approach the study of each class of drugs in two stages; first learning the common characteristics of the class, and only then taking note of the special characteristics of individual drugs that set them apart from the class.

Drug Standards

The *United States Pharmacopeia* (USP) and the *National Formulary* (NF) were established as the official standards for drug formulations by the Pure Food Drug Act of 1906. Since 1975 the two have been published as a single volume. The designation of USP following a drug name indicates that the drug meets the standards established by the *United States Pharmacopeia* with respect to efficacy, safety, strength, quality, purity, dosage form, packaging, and labeling. Other countries have their own official standards (examples are the British Pharmacopoeia in Britain and the Canadian Formulary in Canada). The World Health Organization has published the *Pharmacopoea Internationalis* since 1951.

Prior to 1938, drugs were not rigorously tested for either safety or efficacy; some of these drugs continue to be available today without having met modern standards. The Food, Drug, and Cosmetic Act of 1938 required that safety be demonstrated before a new drug could be marketed and the Kefauver-Harris Amendment of 1962 added a requirement for demonstration of efficacy. Thus, drugs introduced since 1962 have met rigorous standards of safety and efficacy before reaching the market. The Food and Drug Administration assigned to the National Research Council of the National Academy of Sciences the task of reviewing the efficacy of all drugs introduced between 1938 and 1962. Drugs from this period are rated according to four categories of effectiveness:

Effective: Substantial evidence of effectiveness exists.

Probably effective: Additional evidence is required to establish efficacy.

Possibly effective: Effectiveness may be established eventually, but little evidence exists currently.

Ineffective: No substantial evidence of effectiveness is available.

Drugs with ratings of ineffective have been withdrawn; drugs rated as probably or possibly effective must be withdrawn after a designated time limit unless efficacy is substantiated. When applicable, the categories established by the National Research Council are used in discussing clinical indications for drugs that appear in this book.

One important loophole in the current legislation is that it allows physicians to prescribe approved drugs for uses that have not been approved by the FDA. Thus, phenytoin (Dilantin), which is approved for use in grand mal epilepsy, is often prescribed for alleviating cardiotoxicity of digitalis. There is currently no financial incentive for manufacturers to underwrite clinical trials to establish the efficacy of approved drugs for unapproved applications.

Recommended Readings

British Pharmacopoeia, ed 10. London, Pharmaceutical Press, 1980.

La Bare C: Filling in the blanks on prescription writing. *Amer J Nurs* 1986;10(1):31–33.

Miller LC: Doctors, drugs, and names. *JAMA* 1961;177:27–33.

Tyler VE et al: *Pharmacognosy,* ed 8. Philadelphia, Lea & Febiger, 1981.

United States Pharmacopeia, ed 21, *and the National Formulary,* ed 26. Rockland, Md, The United States Pharmacopeial Convention Inc, 1985.

CHAPTER 3

Principles of Drug Action

Traditionally, one of the major responsibilities of the nurse has been the administration of drugs to clients. In most clinical settings, the primary legal, moral, and ethical responsibility for drug administration rests with nurses. In addition, the nature of nursing responsibilities is gradually evolving in many practice settings, placing increasing demands on the nurse for assessment, management, and evaluation skills. Knowledge about drug administration is expanding rapidly, posing a challenge for the conscientious nurse who hopes to be more than just adequately prepared for the responsibility of administering drugs. This chapter presents the basic principles on which the science of pharmacology is built.

Rational therapeutics begins with the establishment of a therapeutic objective (the goal of treatment). Drug administration may help achieve that objective if the drug is able to produce a therapeutic effect and if that effect is not offset by adverse drug reactions to an unacceptable extent. The principles of pharmacology presented in this chapter provide a framework for understanding how drugs produce therapeutic and adverse effects, and for evaluating and adjusting therapeutic regimens. Drug activity occurs in three phases. The **pharmaceutical phase** includes the formulation of the drug into the dosage form best suited to deliver the drug to its site of action, the administration of the drug to the client, and then the disintegration and dissolution of the drug. The **pharmacokinetic phase** includes the absorption of the drug, the distribution of the drug through the circulatory system to its site of action, and the inactivation of the drug by metabolism or excretion. The

pharmacodynamic phase is the actual effect of the drug on the body. This chapter discusses these phases of drug action and concludes with a section on adverse drug reactions.

Pharmaceutics

Because there are often many different drug preparations available for treatment of a given disease, the question naturally arises as to what extent such drug formulations are interchangeable. Two drugs may be more or less equivalent or they may differ in action in one or more of the three phases of drug action. If two formulations contain the same active ingredient, they are said to be **chemically equivalent.** Chemical equivalence does not, however, ensure that the two products will have identical pharmacological activity, because generally a drug must be absorbed into the blood stream and distributed to its site of action before it can produce its effect. A drug is said to be **bioavailable** to the extent that it is absorbed into the central body fluid compartment, and bioavailability is an important factor in the effectiveness of a drug product. Plasma levels of a drug are commonly accepted as an approximate measure of bioavailability. If two drugs are not only chemically equivalent but also have similar bioavailability, they are said to be **bioequivalent.** Two drug products that are not bioequivalent nor even chemically equivalent may nevertheless be **therapeutically equivalent** if they produce similar therapeutic benefits in a particular class of clients.

The bioavailability of a drug is influenced by its pharmaceutical composition. **Pharmaceutics** is the science of formulating drug products and the study of the influence of formulation characteristics on the ability of an administered drug product to be dissolved in a body fluid. Administration serves as the connecting link between formulation and dissolution. Administration is treated separately in Chapter 4 because of its special importance to nurses. If the drug product being administered is a tablet, an additional step between administration and dissolution is disintegration. **Disintegration** is the breakup of a tablet into small fragments; this sets the stage for **dissolution** of the drug, which is the dispersal of the substance as solute particles in the body fluid with which the drug is in contact. The step leading up to bioavailability that occurs most slowly for a given drug product will determine the overall rate at which the drug becomes bioavailable, and is thus said to be the **rate-limiting** step.

In the case of orally administered drugs, there are several ways in which formulation affects where and how quickly the active drug substance is dissolved. Drugs given in liquid form are immediately available for absorption, unlike drugs given as capsules or tablets (see Figure 3–1). Capsules dissolve rapidly and the contents become available for dissolution and then absorption nearly as quickly as liquid drugs. Tablets are absorbed least rapidly because they must pass through the additional step of disintegration before they can be dissolved and then absorbed.

Some capsules and tablets are **enteric coated,** covered with a substance that resists disintegration in gastric acid, so that the capsule or tablet does not disintegrate until it reaches the alkaline environment of the small intestines. Occasionally, the enteric coated preparation may disintegrate in the stomach in spite of its enteric coating, resulting in relatively poor absorption. In practice, enteric coated preparations are less reliable than uncoated dosage forms, especially with respect to time of onset. If gastric emptying time is prolonged, the enteric coated capsule or tablet may remain inactive in the stomach for hours. Also, absorption of the drug may sometimes be further delayed, even when the dosage form reaches the intestines if the coating does not dissolve promptly. In fact, individuals will sometimes pass the dosage form intact in the stools. *For these reasons, enteric coated preparations should not be employed when an immediate effect is required. The nurse may need to advise clients not to eat fatty meals just prior to taking enteric coated drugs.*

Sustained-release or spansule capsules contain many small particles of drug coated with substances that require varying amounts of time to be dissolved. In theory, spansules allow the drug to be absorbed gradually (typically over 8–12 hours) and provide a steadier blood level and therapeutic effect (Figure 3–2). However, most drug preparations typically reach the end of the small intestine within 3–4 hours after oral adminstration. Since most drug absorption occurs in the small intestine, a substantial fraction of the drug contained in a sustained-release preparation may be excreted in the feces without ever being absorbed. Sustained-release preparations are more convenient for the client and therefore often improve compliance (adherence with the drug regimen). Sustained-release preparations are most useful for drugs that are metabolized or excreted rapidly, and which would otherwise have to be administered frequently. Such preparations are not employed when a drug can be harmful in amounts not much higher than the therapeutic dose because a spansule capsule contains more total drug than a single dose tablet or capsule, and irregular absorption of the active drug from a spansule could result

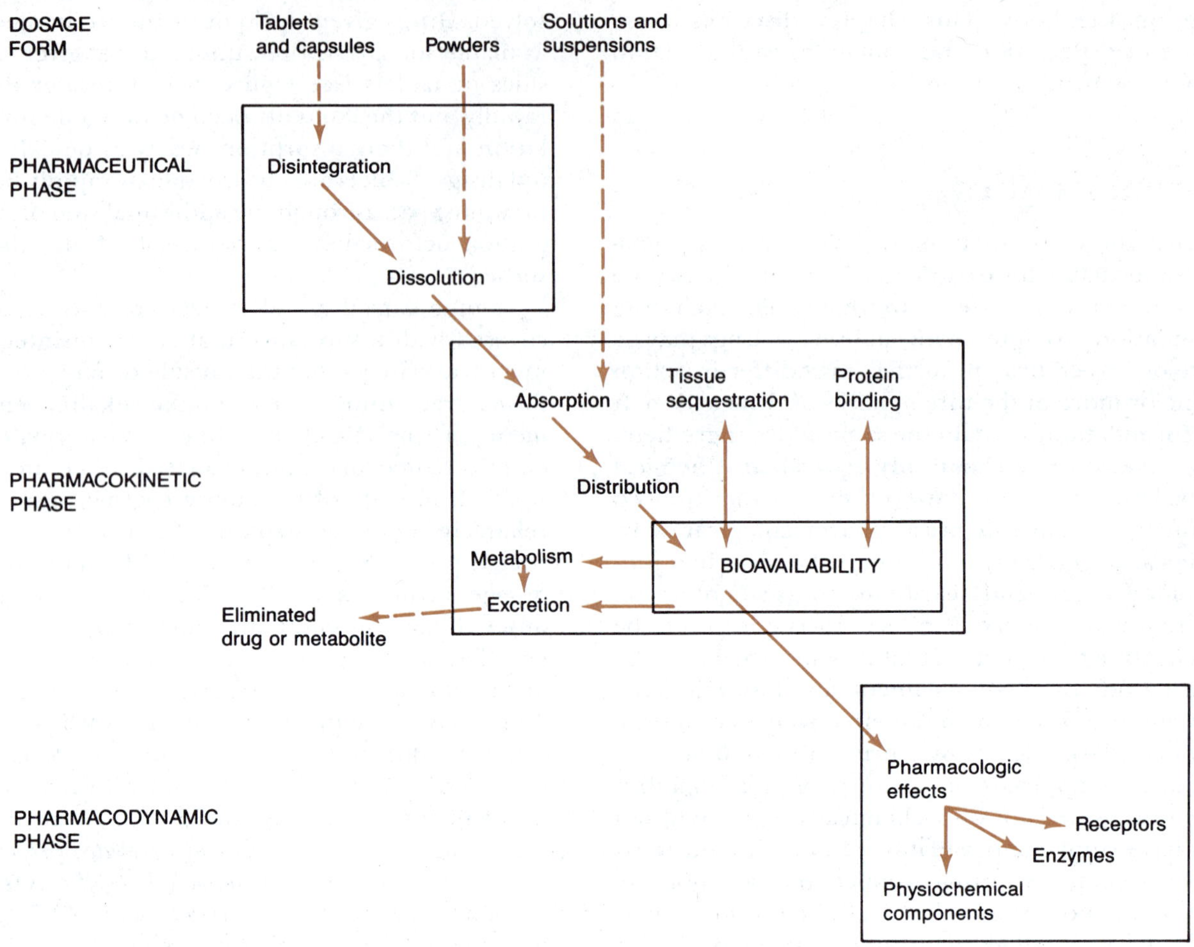

Figure 3–1
The three phases of drug activity.

in toxic consequences. Sustained action can also be achieved when drugs are injected by using repository dosage forms — oil suspensions or esters of drugs that release the drug slowly into the surrounding tissue. Examples of such preparations are protamine zinc insulin and fluphenazine esters (enanthate or decanoate).

Tablets are perhaps the most complex of the common dosage forms. A typical tablet contains, in addition to the active drug, a diluent (or filler), a binder, a disintegrator, and a lubricant. In addition, some tablets contain preservatives, pH stabilizers, coatings, flavoring, or coloring. The characteristics of the binder, the lubricant, the disintegrator, and the coatings are especially likely to influence rate of disintegration. For example, lubricants may form complexes with the active drug, reducing its availability for absorption. If a tablet is poorly formulated, bioavailability may be severely compromised. Excessive compaction during manufacture may slow disintegration. Not all tablets store well over extended periods — some deteriorate, especially in humid conditions, while others may harden enough to impair disintegration. *Clients need to be encouraged to confer with the pharmacist as to the most appropriate methods and temperature for drug storage.* Because of the complexity of tablets in comparison with capsules, bioavailability of drugs administered in tablet form is often lower and more variable; however, some well-formulated tablets actually result in more complete absorption than capsules of the same drug. Tablets, like capsules, may be enteric coated to protect the drug from the acid environment of the stomach or to protect the stomach from an irritant effect of the drug.

Dissolution rate is usually rate-limiting (that is, the slowest step) for drugs given as powders or when disintegration of a tablet or capsule results in solid

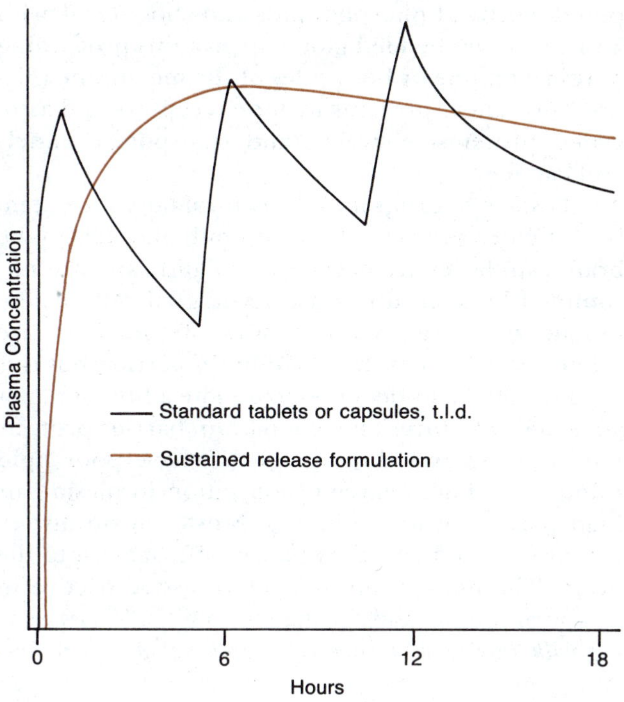

Figure 3–2
Comparison of blood levels occurring for a hypothetical drug during administration of a once-daily spansule capsule versus regular tablets or capsules administered three times a day.

particles. Particle size is an important determinant in solubility. If particle size is reduced, the surface area of the drug is increased, and absorption is hastened. The case of spironolactone illustrates the importance of particle size for poorly soluble drugs. When spironolactone was introduced, the typical dose was 500 mg, of which less than 5% was absorbed. When preparations utilizing micronization (conversion of the drug into very tiny particles) were introduced, the typical therapeutic dose was reduced twentyfold to 25 mg because of improved dissolution.

Generally, salts of weak acids or bases are more rapidly dissolved than the acid or base itself. Thus, the sodium salts of barbiturates or salicylates, the potassium salt of penicillin, and the sulfate salt of morphine dissolve and are absorbed more rapidly than the nonsalt forms. Some drugs exist in amorphous (unstructured) and one or more crystalline or hydrated forms. Often one such form is dissolved most rapidly. *Knowledge of solubility and absorption rates is critical to accurate teaching, especially when clients are to administer the medications to themselves.* These factors influence the expected onset of action, time of peak effect, duration of action, and time of administration of the drug in relation to mealtime.

Ideally, then, a dosage form is designed to optimize bioavailability of the active constituent for absorption. Dosage forms are justifiably referred to as "drug delivery systems."

On a more mundane level, bioavailability may be significantly influenced by the adequacy of drug storage procedures. Drugs given parenterally (by other than oral or rectal administration) are often provided as solutions in ampuls, vials, or other containers. Many drugs in solution are sensitive to degradation by light. Sometimes such degradation is made obvious by discoloration of the solution or formation of a precipitate. Some of the parenteral drugs that are light sensitive are listed in Table 3–1. *Nurses responsible for drug storage should ensure that light-sensitive drugs are stored away from light and dispensed in amber or opaque containers. Nurses need to teach clients how to handle light-sensitive drugs and how to know when a drug has deteriorated. Perhaps most important, once the drug is no longer to be used by the client, the remaining supply should be discarded.*

Pharmacokinetics

The pharmacokinetic phase of drug action begins after dissolution. **Pharmacokinetics** is the study of how the body *absorbs* the drug into the bloodstream, *distributes* it to its site of action, and finally *inactivates* the drug.

Individuals differ widely in their responses to drugs, and that variability is most often related to pharmacokinetic differences. Therefore, the refine-

Table 3–1
Parenteral Drugs That Are Light Sensitive

Aminophylline	Isoproterenol
Amphotericin B	Levarterenol
Chlorpheniramine	Methadone
Chlorpromazine	Morphine sulfate
Cisplatin	Multivitamins
Diazepam	Naloxone
Diazoxide	Neostigmine
Digoxin	Nitroglycerin
Diphenhydramine	Nitroprusside sodium
Dopamine HCl	Phenylephrine HCl
Droperidol	Prochlorperazine
Epinephrine	Propranolol
Fluorouracil	Streptomycin sulfate
Folic acid	Testosterone cypionate
Furosemide	Vinblastine
Haloperidol	Vincristine
Hydrocortisone	

ment of therapeutic protocols to meet the needs of the individual client requires mastery of current pharmacokinetic concepts. This section will first consider some important general mechanisms of pharmacokinetics and will then consider separately the three processes that contribute to drug kinetics — absorption, distribution, and inactivation (Figure 3–3).

Pharmacokinetic Mechanisms

Penetration Barriers

Except for those drugs given intravenously, drugs must pass across one or more penetration barriers to move from the site of application to the systemic circulation. The penetration barriers consist of semipermeable biological membranes, some simple in structure (most capillary walls and cell membranes of individual cells), some rather complex (the multicellular intestinal epithelium or the multiple layers of cells of the skin). Biological barriers are remarkably similar in composition and arrangement. Membranes consist of a two-molecule mosaic composed mostly of phospholipids and cholesterol, with a variety of embedded globular proteins protruding outward on one or both sides of the membrane (Figure 3–4). These proteins include receptors and associated proteins, enzymes, and transport channels and carriers.

Passage of drugs into the central nervous system is a bit more restricted because epithelial cells in the brain capillaries are packed very tightly and are surrounded by a sheath of astrocytic glial cells. These unique structural characteristics of the brain are often referred to as the **blood-brain barrier,** but this term should be understood to denote a function, not an actual structure. The blood-brain barrier protects the brain by excluding drugs that have poor lipid solubility, a high degree of ionization in plasma, or high plasma protein binding. Most neurotransmitters are ionized and thus poorly diffusable into the brain. The blood-brain barrier is less restrictive in newborn infants and during meningitis. *Nurses working with infants who have meningeal inflammation from*

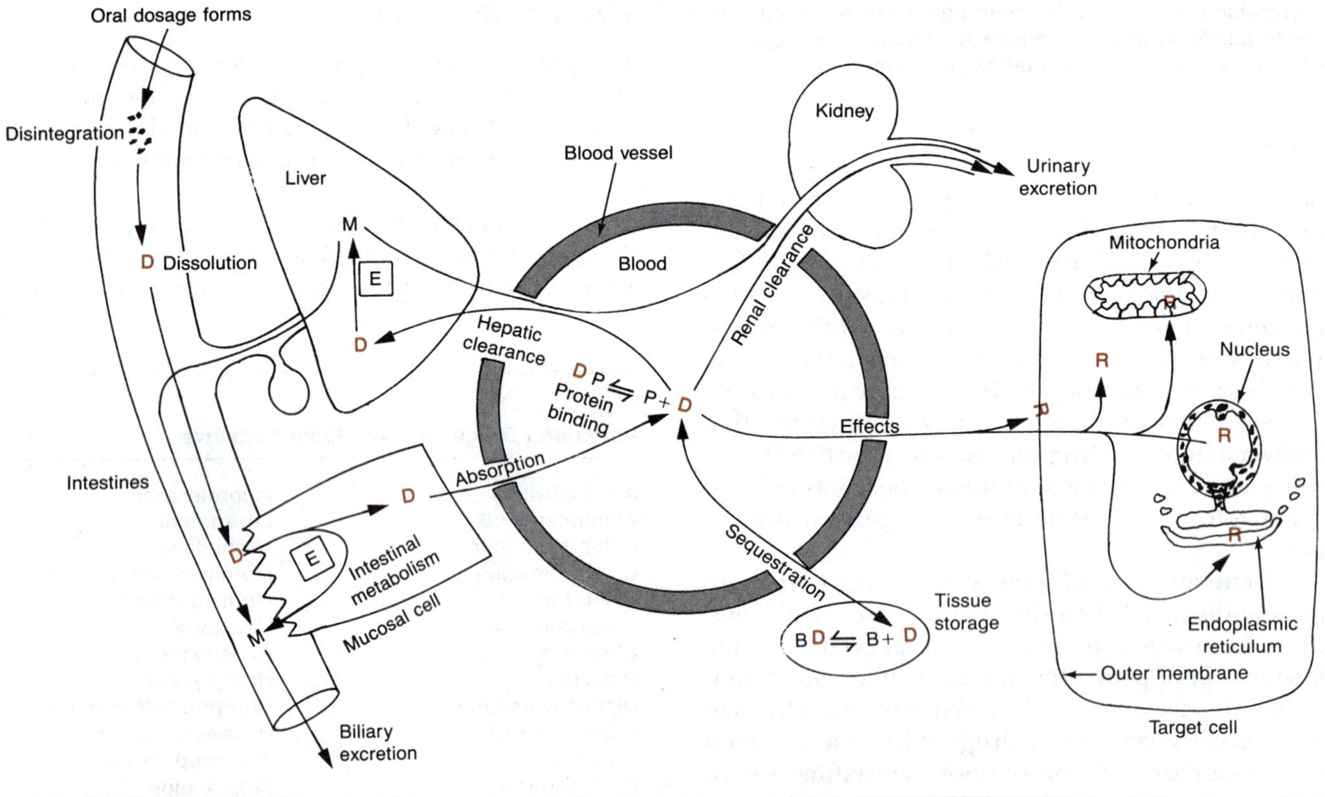

Figure 3–3
Schematic illustration of pharmacokinetic mechanisms discussed in the rest of the chapter: binding sites (B) in storage tissues, drug (D), enzyme (E), metabolite (M), plasma proteins (P), receptor (R).

Figure 3–4
Structure of a cell membrane showing double thickness of lipid molecules with their hydrophilic heads pointing outward and their hydrophobic tails pointing inward. Associated with the membrane are protein molecules, seen as larger bodies penetrating the membrane or embedded in one side or the other. From D. C. Tosteson, Lithium and mania. *Sci. Am. 244:*166, 1981.

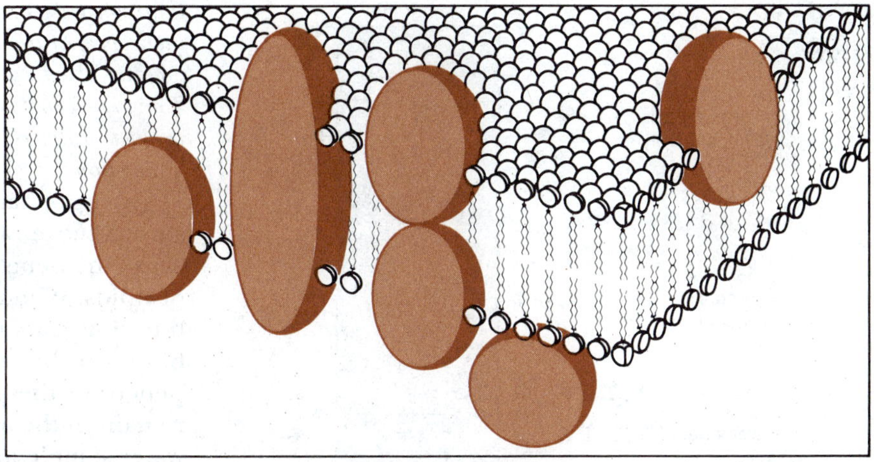

any cause need to keep in mind the increased potential for central nervous system drug toxicity in this situation.

Passage of drugs across the placenta to the fetus during pregnancy occurs commonly, especially when the drug has high lipid solubility. Low ionization and low protein binding likewise increase transfer. Narcotics, barbiturates, local and general anesthetics, steroids, oral hypoglycemic drugs, and sulfonamides are among the drugs noted to appear in fetal blood after maternal administration. Administration of drugs during pregnancy can lead to birth defects (also known as teratogenic effects) (see Chapter 34). *Nurses need to know which drugs have the potential for crossing the placental barrier and for producing teratogenic effects. Nurses need to question female clients as to whether there is any possibility that they are pregnant, whether they have intentions of becoming pregnant, and whether they are employing adequate precautions to avoid inadvertent pregnancy. This nursing responsibility is discussed more fully in Chapter 34.*

Types of Passage

The passage of substances across biological barriers can occur by a limited number of mechanisms (Figure 3–5): (1) passive diffusion, (2) facilitated or active transport by carrier mechanisms, or (3) endocytosis.

Passive diffusion is the passage of a substance along its chemical gradient, or if it is a charged substance, its electrochemical gradient, without expenditure of cellular energy. A gradient is an uneven distribution of a particular chemical substance (a chemical gradient) or electrical charges (an electrical gradient). Substances move from an area of higher concentration to one of lower concentration; if the substance is ionized (carries an electrical charge), it also tends to move from an area of higher concentration of like charges (positive or negative) to an area of higher concentration of opposite charges. Passive diffusion is not saturable (its capacity cannot be exceeded by even very high concentrations of a substance), it is not subject to inhibition by competing substances, and it is not significantly affected by temperature.

Small, water-soluble substances, including most simple ions, amino acids, and some sugars, cross biological membranes mainly through aqueous channels created by certain proteins, called *permeases,* that transverse the entire width of the membrane. Passive diffusion of ions through such ion channels can sometimes be manipulated by drugs. For example, quinidine decreases flow of sodium through channels while calcium channel blockers decrease calcium flow. Molecules larger than these aqueous pores can penetrate the barrier only to the extent that they can cross the lipid portion of the membrane. Five factors determine the rate of passive diffusion through the lipid portion: the concentration gradient, the surface area for absorption, the lipid solubility of the substance, its size, and its degree of ionization.

Diffusion is usually more rapid if a higher dose is administered because this will produce a greater **concentration gradient.** The concentration gradient of an orally administered drug is determined largely by the dose administered because the concentration of the drug on the systemic side of the intestinal mucosa remains negligible as the drug rapidly distributes throughout the central compartment. Thus ab-

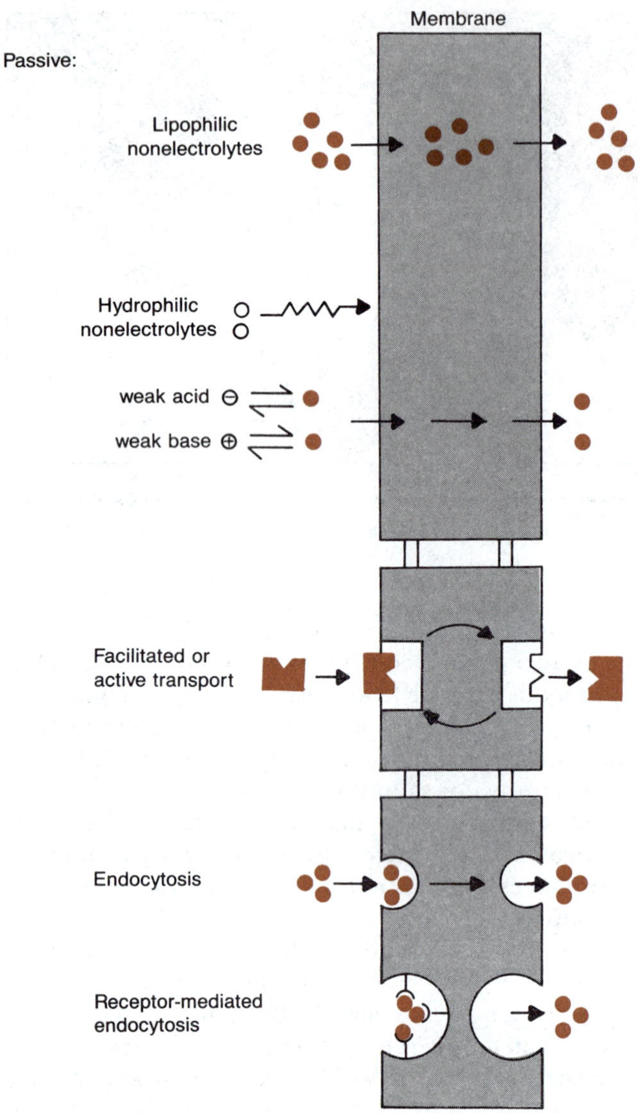

Figure 3–5
Kinds of membrane passage.

sorption across the gastrointestinal epithelium is essentially unidirectional.

The **surface area** for absorption is usually determined by the route of administration. The intestines and the lungs provide two of the largest surface areas for absorption. The surface area of the skin is, of course, still larger but is considerably more resistant to penetration unless compromised by cuts, burns, or abrasions. The extent of perfusion (the amount of blood flow through the tissue) at the site of drug application is a major determinant of how fast a drug will be absorbed by a given area. *If a patient is in shock, intramuscular injection may be ineffective because of poor perfusion of the muscle tissue. Pressor drugs (agents that constrict blood vessels) are often added to local anesthetic preparations to retard systemic absorption, thus prolonging the local effect and minimizing systemic toxicity. Tourniquets or cooling can be utilized to retard absorption of venoms or drugs; massage or heat can be employed to hasten absorption.*

Drugs that have high **lipid solubility** are absorbed more rapidly than those soluble in water because the penetration barriers are largely composed of lipids. When the desired locus of action is within the alimentary tract itself, drugs with poor lipid solubility can be especially useful because they cannot penetrate the gastrointestinal membrane and thus remain in the alimentary tract. Neomycin is a highly water-soluble antibacterial drug that can be used in this way for treatment of intestinal bacterial infections. **Size** of a molecule is another important factor in absorption. Small molecules penetrate membranes more rapidly.

Most drugs are weak organic acids or bases, existing in both **ionized and nonionized forms.** Ionization is the reversible conversion of an acid or base from its nonionized to its ionized form. Only the nonionized form of a weak acid or base can participate in passive absorption. The ionized form of a drug has very low lipid solubility and does not participate significantly in diffusion. The extent to which a substance is ionized is determined in part by the pH of the solution in which it is dissolved. In the stomach, where pH is typically an acidic 1.4, weak organic acids, such as barbiturates, phenytoin (Dilantin), or theophylline, are largely nonionized and well absorbed. Weak bases, such as morphine and diazepam, are ionized and poorly absorbed in the stomach, but better absorbed in the intestinal environment where pH is higher (from 4 to 8). *Neutralization of stomach acidity with bicarbonate can increase absorption of weak bases.*

Certain substances pass through penetration barriers at rates that exceed what can be reasonably attributed to passive diffusion. Glucose, for example, is not lipid soluble and is too large to pass through the small aqueous channels. Nevertheless, it is rapidly accumulated by most kinds of cells. It is believed that a membrane carrier molecule attaches to a molecule of glucose, forming a complex. The complex diffuses across the membrane, and the glucose is detached in the cell interior. This kind of transport process, called **facilitated diffusion,** operates only on particular substances (that is, it is *selective*), and there is an upper limit to how fast it can transport glucose (that is, it is *saturable*), but it does not use cellular energy. Facilitated diffusion always occurs in the direction of the concentration gradient.

Active transport, like facilitated diffusion, involves a carrier that attaches to the molecule, carries it across the membrane, and then releases it. This type of transport is also selective and saturable, but unlike facilitated diffusion, it requires cellular energy and often transports substances against the electrochemical gradient. The sodium pump, which maintains polarity of cells, is an active transport process. Active transport is fundamental to life itself, since it is the process that enables a living organism (in the words of Lewis Thomas) "to hold out against equilibrium, maintain imbalance, [and] bank against entropy." Active transport permits the organism to accumulate selectively those substances that are crucial for its survival. Active transport is generally limited to substances of small to moderate size.

Larger molecules and particles can be brought across lipid membranes by a process called **endocytosis.** Endocytosis is the engulfment by a cell of a droplet of the surrounding fluid, complete with all its contents. The two kinds of endocytosis that contribute to drug transfer are pinocytosis and receptor-mediated endocytosis. **Pinocytosis** is a nonselective process by which membranes trap a small quantity of adjacent fluid. The membrane invaginates to form a pocket and then closes to engulf a bead of fluid complete with whatever solutes it might contain. **Receptor-mediated endocytosis** is similar in appearance to pinocytosis but is highly specific. The receptors, consisting of membrane proteins, cluster in pits in the membrane and bind a specific substance (called the ligand) from the surrounding fluid. Binding of the ligand triggers invagination of the membrane, and incorporation of the receptor-ligand complex. Once inside the cell, the ligand is released from the receptor and the receptor is recycled for additional activity.

First-Order versus Zero-Order Kinetics

Both absorption and elimination of drugs can exhibit two distinctive types of kinetics, called first-order and zero-order kinetics. The kinetics of absorption or elimination are said to be **first-order** if the rate of transfer of drug into or out of the systemic circulation is proportional to the amount of drug remaining — that is, the more drug there is, the faster it will be absorbed or eliminated. In first-order kinetics, rate of absorption will be equal to the amount remaining to be absorbed times the absorption rate constant for that drug. The **half-life** — the time required for one-half of the drug remaining to be absorbed or eliminated — will be the same regardless of the concentration of the drug. Thus the time required to reduce the drug concentration from the full amount to one-half will be the same as the time required to further reduce the remaining drug from one-half to one-quarter, one-quarter to one-eighth, and so forth. It is generally reasonable to assume that absorption, metabolism, and renal excretion of most drugs obey first-order kinetics, unless there is evidence to the contrary.

Occasionally absorption or elimination of certain drugs is observed to follow **zero-order** kinetics; that is, the rate of drug transfer or elimination is constant and independent of the concentration of drug remaining to be acted upon. Zero-order kinetics occur when the concentration of drug is very high relative to the capacity of the system for absorption, metabolism, or extraction of the drug; the mechanism is saturated. Thus, zero-order kinetics are likely to apply when the rate of absorption, renal extraction, or metabolism is unusually low for a substance, or when the substance is typically employed at a high concentration. When the drug concentration drops to a relatively low level, kinetics typically revert to first-order mechanics. Alcohol metabolism is a classic example of a metabolic process that exhibits zero-order kinetics.

Some drugs exhibit changes in kinetics over time or at different doses. **Dose-dependent kinetics** occur whenever a drug is used at doses that saturate one or another mechanism contributing to its pharmacokinetics, causing a shift from first-order to zero-order kinetics. **Time-dependent kinetics** occur when a drug alters its own kinetics over time. Induction of liver enzymes is the major established example. *Drugs that do not exhibit dose-dependent or time-dependent kinetics should be used in preference to drugs that do, other things being equal.*

Absorption

Absorption is the process by which a drug passes from the site of application into the central compartment of circulating fluids — the bloodstream and lymphatic system. All drugs, except those applied topically, must be absorbed before they can produce their characteristic actions on the body.

Measurement of serum concentrations of a drug over time provides a good indication of the extent of absorption (Figure 3–6). The area under such a curve is a measure of bioavailability, the end result of absorption. Peak serum concentration is not as reliable an indicator of bioavailability as the area under the curve but is often used as a simpler approximation. Drugs that are bioequivalent have serum concentration time curves that are nearly identical.

Measurement of Plasma Concentrations

Monitoring plasma concentrations provides a convenient method for isolating drug response var-

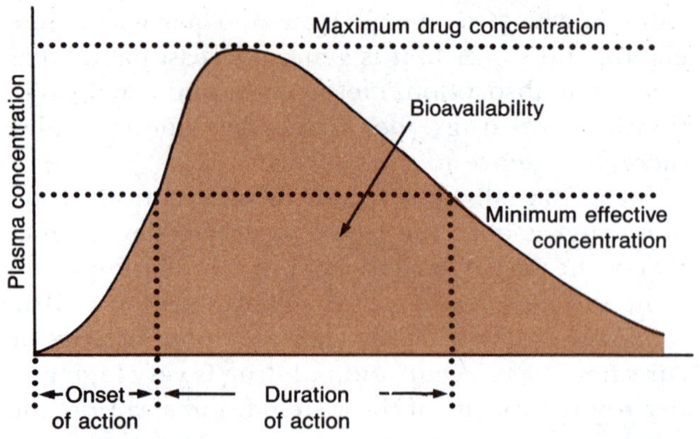

Figure 3–6
The time-concentration curve after administration of a hypothetical drug in relation to onset and duration of action.

iability that is related to absorption or preceding steps (disintegration and dissolution) from variability due to idiosyncrasies of distribution, elimination, or pharmacodynamic mechanisms. Monitoring plasma concentrations is of great value for some drugs but virtually useless for others; Table 3–2 lists criteria helpful in determining when measurement of plasma concentrations is likely to be useful. Monitoring is useful when the relationship between plasma levels and clinical response is a consistent one but the relationship between the dose administered and plasma concentrations is inconsistent. Under these circumstances, variability is related either to idiosyncrasies of absorption or pharmaceutical factors (disintegration or dissolution), and the variability can be substantially reduced by adjusting doses until the desired serum concentration is achieved.

For most drugs, excessively low plasma concentrations are ineffective while excessively high concentrations are toxic and sometimes ineffective as well. The range of plasma concentrations that produce the greatest therapeutic benefit is called the **therapeutic window** (Figure 3–7).

Measurement of plasma levels is most useful for drugs that have a narrow **therapeutic index** (the ratio between the typically lethal dose and the typically therapeutic dose), a relatively sustained plasma level, and an established therapeutic window (Table 3–3) of effective plasma concentrations. Also, when drugs are being used prophylactically, there may be no good alternative guide to therapeutic effectiveness. This is the case when antiepileptic medication is instituted for control of low-frequency seizures. Plasma monitoring is especially indicated when the nurse or physician suspects over- or undercompliance, when factors complicating pharmacokinetics are known or suspected to be present (Table 3–4), or when therapeutic complications are anticipated. Unusual plasma concentrations can be due to anomalies of dosage, dosage form, route or time of administration, compliance problems, concurrent disease states (especially hepatic, renal, gastrointestinal, or cardiovascular), weight, sex, or age, unusual protein bind-

Table 3–2
Indications for Monitoring Plasma Levels of Drugs

Plasma levels of a drug should be monitored when:

- The relationship between the dose administered and plasma levels is poor.
- The relationship between plasma levels and clinical response is good.
- The drug is being used prophylactically, so that changes in target symptoms are not easy to measure.
- The therapeutic range is narrow; the difference between the therapeutic and toxic blood levels is small.
- Overuse or lack of compliance is suspected.
- Factors modifying normal pharmacokinetics are suspected or known to be present (for example, tolerance, renal or kidney disease, drug interactions).

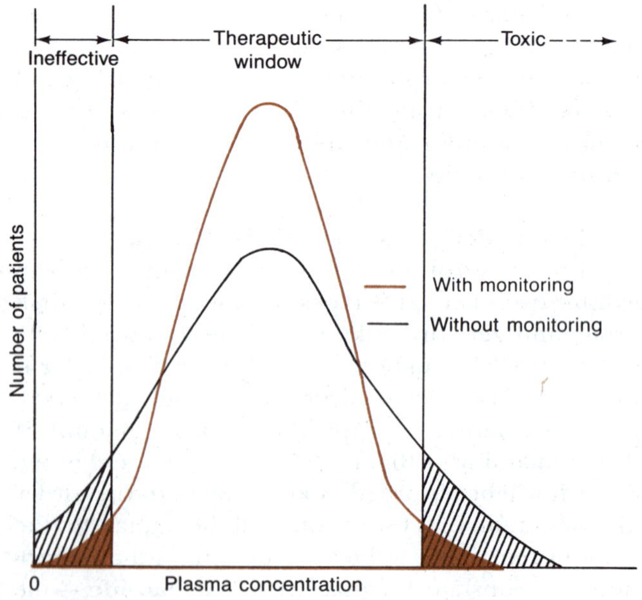

Figure 3–7
Percentage of clients with serum concentrations within therapeutic range, with and without previous monitoring (at least twice) of serum levels.

Table 3-3
Drugs with Established Effective Plasma Concentrations

Drug	Target plasma concentrations	Drug	Target plasma concentrations
Antiasthmatic		**Antihypertensives with beta-blockers**	
Theophylline	5-15 mg/L	Aprenolol	≈.03 mg/L
		Atenolol	≈1.3 mg/L
Antidysrhythmics		Clonidine	≈.001 mg/L
Lidocaine	1.4-6.0 mg/L	Hydralazine	≈1 mg/L
Procainamide	4-8 mg/L	Pindolol	≈.06 mg/L
Quinidine	3-7 mg/L	Propranolol	0.02-0.2 mg/L
Antibiotics		**Cardiac glycosides**	
Amikacin	12-25 mg/L	Digitoxin	0.01-0.03 mg/L
Ampicillin	1.5-3 mg/L	Digoxin	0.0006-0.002 mg/L
Cephalexin	9-18 mg/L	**Nonsteroidal anti-inflammatory drugs**	
Chloramphenicol	10-13 mg/L		
Erythromycin	0.3-1.9 mg/L	Acetaminophen	10-20 mg/L
Gentamicin	4-10 mg/L	Indomethacin	0.5-3.0 mg/L
Kanamycin	12-25 mg/L	Salicylates	100-300 mg/L
Penicillin G	0.01-10 mg/L		
Penicillin V	≈3 mg/L	**Oral hypoglycemics**	
Streptomycin	25-30 mg/L	Tolbutamide	80-240 mg/L
Tetracycline	≈3 mg/L		
Tobramycin	5-8 mg/L	**Psychotropics**	
		Amitriptyline	0.16-0.24 mg/L
Anticoagulants		Chlordiazepoxide	> 0.7 mg/L
Heparin	1,000-3,000 units/L	Chlorpromazine	0.03-0.35 mg/L
Warfarin	1.8-2.6 mg/L	Desipramine	> 0.225 mg/L
		Diazepam	> 0.6 mg/L
Antiepileptics		Doxepin	0.03-0.15 mg/L
Carbamazepine	4-10 mg/L	Imipramine	> .22 mg/L
Clonazepam	0.005-0.07 mg/L	Lithium	0.7-1.4 mEq/L
Ethosuximide	40-90 mg/L	Meprobamate	5-20 mg/L
Phenobarbital	15-50 mg/L	Nortriptyline	0.05-0.14 mg/L
Phenytoin	> 10 mg/L	Protriptyline	0.07-0.25 mg/L
Primidone	8-12 mg/L		
Valproic acid	55-100 mg/L		

ing, drug or diet interactions, variable absorption, clearance, or volume of distribution, dose-dependent kinetics, or delayed equilibration (Table 3-5).

Absorption after Oral Administration

Oral administration of drugs is the most commonly employed route, accounting for more than 80% of all prescription and nonprescription drug adminstrations. The mucosal membrane along the entire length of the alimentary tract is a potential absorptive surface, and the relatively thin epithelial wall and high degree of vascularity favors rapid absorption. Absorption from the mouth and esophagus is usually minimal because of the limited time the substance spends there.

Absorption in the stomach is variable, depending mainly on the acid environment, the presence or absence of foods, the amount and composition of gastric secretions, gastric motility, and gastric emptying time (Figure 3-8). The low pH of the stomach fluids promotes absorption of weak acids but inhibits absorption of weak bases because of the relationship between pH and ionization. Food constituents may form complexes with or trap certain drugs and severely curtail absorption. Food may also buffer the stomach pH or alter gastric emptying time. *Nurses need to know which drugs are to be taken with meals and which on an empty stomach, and must provide specific instructions to clients as to when drugs are to be taken in relation to food ingestion.* Some drugs are, in effect, subject to digestion. Insulin and other drugs

Table 3–4
Complicating Pharmacokinetics That May Necessitate Monitoring of Plasma Concentrations

Pharmacokinetic characteristic	Example drugs
Variable absorption after oral administration	Digoxin, phenytoin, procainamide, propranolol, quinidine
Variable volume of distribution	Digitoxin, digoxin, lidocaine, phenytoin, procainamide, propranolol, quinidine, salicylates
Variable rate of clearance	Digoxin, lidocaine, phenytoin, procainamine, propranolol, salicylates, theophylline
Variable protein binding	Benzodiazepines, oral anticoagulants, phenytoin, propranolol, salicylates, sulfonylureas
Dose-dependent kinetics	Alcohol, aspirin, griseofulvin, penicillin, phenylbutazone, phenytoin, propranolol, sulfonamides
Delayed equilibration	Digitoxin, digoxin, lithium

that are proteins are broken down by digestive enzymes and thus are ineffective if given orally. Penicillin is unstable in acid and can therefore be destroyed by gastric acid. Gastric motility is variable and promotes disintegration of tablets to a variable extent.

The stomach serves as a reservoir for ingested foods and substances, periodically opening its pyloric valve to empty a portion of its contents into the initial segment of the intestines. The rate of **gastric emptying** obeys first-order kinetics, with a usual half-life of 20–60 minutes. A normal meal typically transits the stomach in about 4 hours, but many factors alter the rate of gastric emptying. Gastric emptying is slowed by vigorous exercise, emotional stress, pain, hot meals, hypothyroidism, and certain drugs, including sympathomimetics, anticholinergics, and narcotics. Acids and electrolytes also slow gastric emptying. Gastric and duodenal ulcers are often associated with pyloric obstruction and delayed gastric emptying. *Any factor that slows gastric emptying time will decrease and prolong the absorption of most drugs.* The time that a pill remains in the stomach can range from 15 minutes to 7 hours.

Gastric emptying time can be hastened by mild exercise, hunger or fasting, ingestion of dilute liquids, cold meals, lying on the right side, and certain drugs, notably metaclorpramide. *Many drugs are given on an empty stomach with sufficient water to ensure rapid passage into the intestines. The nurse should know how to schedule administration of medications with respect to mealtime (see Chapter 44). When it is necessary to give a drug orally under conditions where gastric emptying time can be predicted to be prolonged, a useful nursing measure is to instruct the client to lie on the right side.*

All in all, the stomach is an unreliable environment for absorption. Furthermore, absorption in the stomach is slow compared to absorption that takes place in the intestines, most obviously for basic drugs, but even for weak acids because of the greater surface area for absorption in the intestines. The

Table 3–5
Some Typical Causes of Abnormal Steady-State Plasma Concentrations

Values higher than normal could be due to	Values lower than normal could be due to
Overcompliance (occurs frequently with drugs having abuse potential)	Undercompliance (a frequent problem with many drugs)
Increased absorption (can occur if the drug is normally poorly absorbed or if a factor interfering with absorption is eliminated)	Poor absorption (can occur as a result of malabsorption syndromes, an effect of diet or other drugs, time of administration in relation to meals, and other factors)
Decreased renal clearance (only if renal clearance is the major route of elimination; could be due to a change in pH, renal disease, or competition with another drug for a secretory mechanism)	Increased renal clearance (only if renal clearance is the major route; could be due to a change in pH of the urine, diuresis; not a usual explanation)
Decreased hepatic clearance (occurs in hepatic disease, drug inhibition of liver enzymes, increased protein binding, or decreased hepatic blood flow; significant only if hepatic clearance is the major route)	Increased hepatic clearance (occurs with induction of liver enzymes; significant only when hepatic clearance of the drug is the major route)
Increased plasma protein binding (not a likely possibility)	Decreased plasma protein binding (Competitive displacement is a common drug-drug interaction; also occurs in hypoalbuminemia, hepatic or renal disease.)

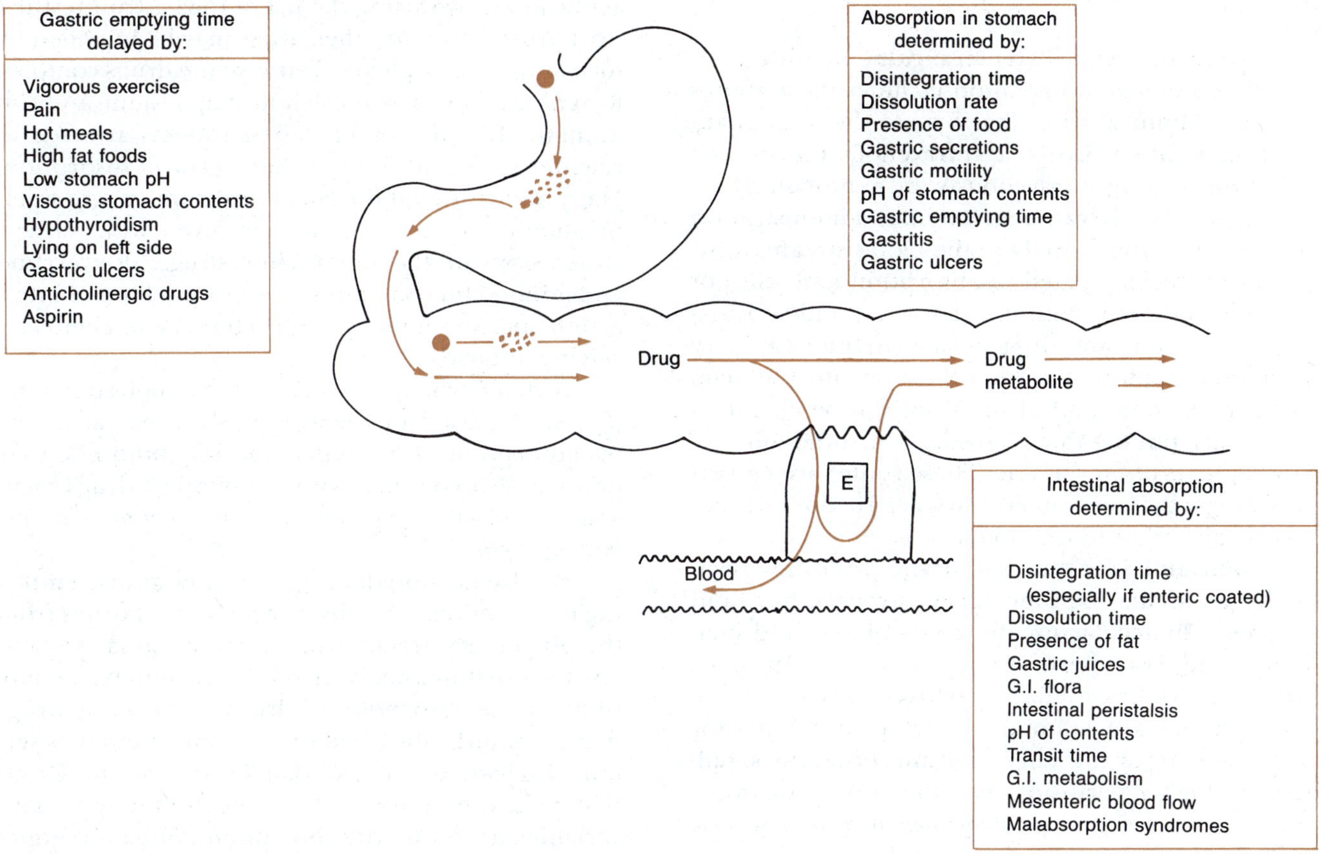

Figure 3–8
Factors altering absorption after oral administration of a drug.

sooner a drug completes passage through the stomach into the intestines, the more rapidly it will be absorbed.

In the intestines, drug absorption depends on intestinal motility, composition of intestinal fluids, perfusion, gastrointestinal flora, gastrointestinal metabolism, and disease. Increased intestinal peristalsis promotes tablet disintegration and thus enhances absorption if disintegration is rate limiting. On the other hand, increased motility may hasten passage through the intestines, reducing the time of contact between the drug and mucosal surface. This factor will be most significant for poorly soluble substances. The pH of the intestines is about 4–5 in the duodenum but becomes increasingly alkaline further along the tract. Basic drugs are better absorbed as they progress. Intestinal absorption of drugs normally follows first-order kinetics, but if the intestinal interstitium is poorly perfused (as in shock) accumulation of drug on the inside of the penetration barrier will diminish the concentration gradient and impair absorption.

Some drugs are metabolized by the commensal flora of the intestine. The wall of the intestines contains metabolic enzymes that can substantially destroy certain drugs before they ever reach the central blood supply. Drugs that are subject to significant biotransformation within the intestinal lumen include aspirin, aldosterone, chlorpromazine (Thorazine), cortisone, dexamethasone (Decadron), levodopa (Aldomet), estrogens, hydrocortisone, isoproterenol (Isuprel), meperidine (Demerol), methadone, methyldopa (Aldomet), organic nitrates, pentazocine (Talwin), progesterone, propoxyphene (Darvon), salicylamide, sulfonamides, testosterone, and terbutaline (Brethine). Intestinal diseases including achlorhydria and malabsorption syndromes can significantly impair drug absorption in the intestines. Drug-induced malabsorption syndromes provide a mechanism for a pharmacokinetic type of drug-drug and drug-food interaction (see Chapter 44).

Absorption after Parenteral Administration

Parenteral administration includes those routes of drug administration that bypass the alimentary tract, most often involving intravenous infusion or injection of drug intravenously, intramuscularly, or subcutaneously. Because intravenous administration delivers the drug directly to the blood stream, it bypasses problems related to absorption and will not be discussed here. With intramuscular and subcutaneous injection, the drug must penetrate capillary membranes before it reaches the circulatory system. With these routes, all of the drug will be absorbed eventually, but the rate of absorption, although usually rapid, is often variable. These routes are chosen for drugs that are subject to destruction or are poorly absorbed in the stomach or intestines.

Ionization is of little importance for drugs given by intramuscular or subcutaneous routes, but lipid solubility, molecular size (for drugs of low lipid solubility), and tissue perfusion are important. In shock or congestive heart failure, perfusion, and therefore absorption, may be diminished. Of the usual sites for subcutaneous or intramuscular injections, the shoulder has higher perfusion than the buttock or thigh. *Rubbing or warming the site of injection increases blood flow and absorption.*

If sustained action is desired, absorption of drugs can be retarded by use of parenteral depot forms such as the crystalline form of insulin, which dissolves slowly. Similarly, a suspension of the poorly soluble benzathine salt of penicillin can be given intramuscularly for an extended effect. Oil suspensions of drugs delay absorption by limiting contact of the drug with the surrounding aqueous environment.

Other parenteral routes include topical administration to the skin, sublingual or rectal administration, administration to other mucosal surfaces, and inhalation. The main factors determining absorption by these routes are (1) the composition, surface area, and vascularity of the penetration barrier at the site of entry, (2) the contact time, and (3) the physiochemical properties of the drug: size, lipid solubility, and ionization.

Drug-Drug and Drug-Diet Interactions Affecting Absorption

Interactions that involve a drug or nutrient altering the absorption of a drug may either slow the rate of absorption or reduce the total amount of drug absorbed. Such interactions occur due to alterations in pH of the gastrointestinal tract, formation of complexes, and changes in gastric emptying time.

Antacids may delay or reduce the absorption of acidic drugs by raising the pH of the gastrointestinal tract. Absorption of other drugs may be impeded by formation of complexes. Tetracycline drugs complex with metal ions such as calcium, magnesium, and aluminum. Milk and other dairy products are rich in calcium and will inhibit tetracycline absorption. Many antacids contain salts of calcium, magnesium, or aluminum and must not be given with tetracyclines. Two of the tetracycline drugs, doxycycline and minocycline, are not subject to this kind of interaction, and should be given preference in clients receiving antacids.

Anion-exchange resins such as cholestyramine (Questran), used in therapy of diarrhea caused by malabsorption of bile salts, not only bind bile salts but will also complex with many other drugs. *Most drugs should not be given within 4 hours after use of an ion-exchange resin.*

As already noted, drugs that slow gastric emptying time diminish the absorption of most drugs from the alimentary tract. Drugs such as cathartics and laxatives that markedly increase gastrointestinal motility reduce absorption of drugs, particularly drugs that are poorly absorbed or are administered as sustained release or enteric coated formulations. Drugs that reduce motility, such as anticholinergics, have variable effects on drug absorption. Anticholinergics tend to decrease absorption of formulations for which disintegration is rate limiting but increase absorption of drugs when exposure time to the absorptive surface is rate limiting.

Distribution

Even as a drug is being absorbed into the blood supply, the process of distribution is underway. Theoretically, the presence of the drug in the blood supply makes the drug available to all parts of the body, but distribution in the various fluid and tissue compartments is unlikely to be uniform because of (1) differences in permeability of various penetration barriers, (2) regional variations in pH and perfusion, (3) differences in solubility of the drug in blood and various tissues, and (4) sequestering of drug by protein binding or carrier-mediated transport into specific tissues. The distribution of a drug is important because it determines which tissues will be potential sites of action for the drug and the volume of fluid into which the drug will be diluted.

Apparent Volume of Distribution

Apparent volume of distribution is a measure of the extent to which a drug can penetrate into the various fluid and tissue compartments. A drug with a small volume of distribution is most likely contained within the plasma; the total plasma volume is about 3 liters (3 L). The total volume of extracellular fluid is about 12 L, and drugs that have apparent volumes of distribution close to 12 L are contained mainly within the extracellular fluid. Drugs with apparent volumes of distribution larger than 12 L penetrate cells in at least some tissues. When the volume of distribution of a drug is great, the range of potential target sites for action is increased, but the fraction of a drug available at any one site is decreased.

Volume of distribution, and hence drug concentration, is influenced by body mass, and drug dosage must therefore be adjusted in relation to body mass. Men and women have different proportions of fat and water; so predictably drug distribution will also differ by sex. This is even more evident during pregnancy, when the placenta and fetus provide additional potential tissue depots for certain drugs.

Protein Binding

In the plasma, many drugs bind to proteins (mainly albumin proteins). For such drugs, a fraction of the total plasma concentration is bound to proteins and the remainder is unbound or free. Binding is reversible, and an equilibrium exists between the unbound and bound plasma fractions (Figure 3–3). Protein binding slows absorption of a drug out of the plasma into tissues by reducing the effective concentration of the drug. Only the unbound fraction is immediately available for further distribution into tissues by passive diffusion. Carrier-mediated transport processes can operate on protein-bound drug as well as the unbound fraction. As free drug is removed from the circulation by absorption into tissues or elimination, some of the bound drug is released to restore equilibrium.

Protein-binding of drugs is saturable, so that at high doses further addition of drug adds only to the free fraction. When plasma concentrations of a drug are monitored, most assay procedures measure the total bound and unbound concentration. Protein binding increasingly influences distribution, elimination, and intensity of pharmacological activity as the percentage binding approaches 100%. Generally when a drug is bound in excess of 90%, factors that modify binding will significantly impact on activity and kinetics. Table 3–6 lists some drugs that are highly bound.

One factor that influences protein binding of drugs is competitive displacement (Figure 3–9). This is a common type of drug-drug interaction that occurs whenever two drugs capable of protein binding are given concurrently. The number of protein binding sites in the plasma are limited, so two drugs that are both bound displace each other. This will increase the unbound fraction of each drug, their pharmacological activity, and their rate of elimination. The effect is most significant for drugs that are highly bound and that have low therapeutic indexes — notably warfarin (Coumarin) and digitoxin.

Some drugs, including some of the vitamin precursors, are effectively transported through the blood only if the corresponding binding protein is available. The distribution of such drugs is dependent on an adequate level of proteins in the plasma. In hypoalbuminemia, plasma proteins are low and

Table 3–6
Some Drugs That Are Highly Bound to Plasma Proteins

Drug	Approximate percentage bound
Diazepam	99
Phenylbutazone	99
Warfarin	99
Amitriptyline	97
Chlordiazepoxide	97
Clofibrate	96
Desipramine	96
Furosemide	96
Chlorpromazine	95
Chlorthiazide	95
Dicloxacillin	95
Nortriptyline	95
Clindamycin	94
Diazoxide	94
Dicloxacillin	94
Lorazepam	93
Propranolol	93
Tolbutamide	93
Valproic acid	93
Imipramine	92
Protriptyline	92
Digitoxin	90
Indomethacin	90
Oxazepam	90
Sulfisoxazole	90
Phenytoin	89
Rifampin	89
Hydralazine	87
Nafcillin	87
Alprenolol	85
Methadone	85
Carbamazepine	80
Methaqualone	80
Erythromycin	72
Quinidine	71
Phenobarbital	70
Trimethoprim	70
Theophylline	60
Meperidine	58
Lidocaine	50
Aspirin	49

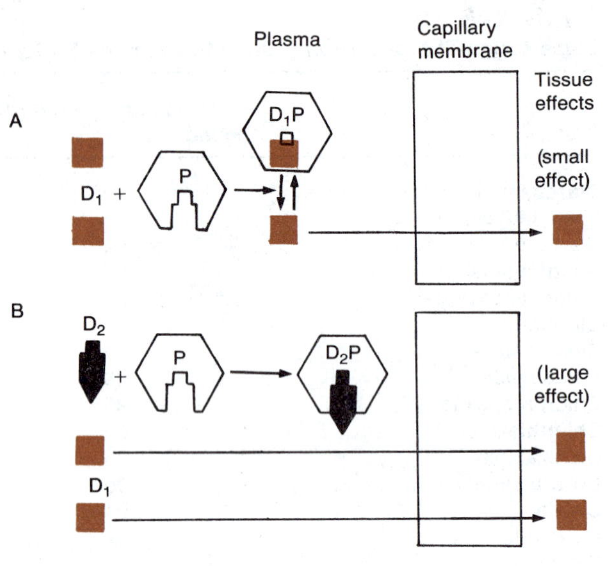

Figure 3–9
Protein (P) binding and the effect of displacement of one drug (D_1) by another (D_2). A. When D_1 is present alone, a portion of the drug is bound to plasma proteins; only the unbound portion can be absorbed into tissues to produce pharmacological effects. B. When D_2 is added, it occupies some of the binding sites, increasing the unbound portion of D_1 and consequently its absorption and pharmacological activity.

hence drug binding is reduced. *If protein binding is crucial for distribution, albumin replacement should be instituted in hypoalbuminemia.*

Sequestering and Secondary Redistribution

Some drugs are preferentially accumulated, or sequestered, in particular tissues. For example, ultra-short-acting barbiturates, marihuana, and chlorinated insecticides accumulate in fat tissue, tetracyclines accumulate in bone, and chloroquine accumulates in the eye and liver. Muscle tissue is another common depot for drugs. As plasma levels begin to drop during the elimination phase, drug stored in peripheral tissues is gradually returned to the plasma. This type of secondary redistribution contributes little to prolonging the action of the drug, since rate of release from tissue stores into the plasma is slow. These deposits of drug may, however, play a role when a drug is administered repeatedly. When an equal second dose is given as the effect of a first dose is wearing off, the response to the second dose may be greater than that to the first because the total amount of drug in the body includes the second dose and the residual deposit of drug from the first dose. Subsequent equal doses will continue to produce larger and longer effects until the level of accumulated drug is such that the amount metabolized between doses is equal to the amount of drug added by each dose (Figure 3–10). This kind of effect is observed with repeated use of methadone, marihuana, cardiac glycosides, lithium, and certain other drugs. If it is crucial that the early doses produce an effect comparable to subsequent doses, larger loading doses can be employed initially to hasten the saturation of tissue depots. This can also be done to reduce the number of doses required to reach the equilibrium where elimination between doses equals the incremental increase of bioavailable drug from each subsequent dose. Loading doses are often employed with digitalis preparations and lithium.

Inactivation

Drugs are inactivated by metabolism and excretion. Removal of drug from the plasma by either process is called **clearance; renal clearance** is that accomplished by the kidneys, while **metabolic clearance** is accomplished by metabolism, mainly in the liver. The most useful pharmacokinetic measure for describing total clearance from all sources is the half-life, the time required to reduce the remaining drug concentration in the plasma by 50%. Half-life is the most reasonable guide for establishing the dosage interval (and reciprocally, the frequency of administration) for therapies requiring repeat dosing and continuously effective plasma concentrations of the drug.

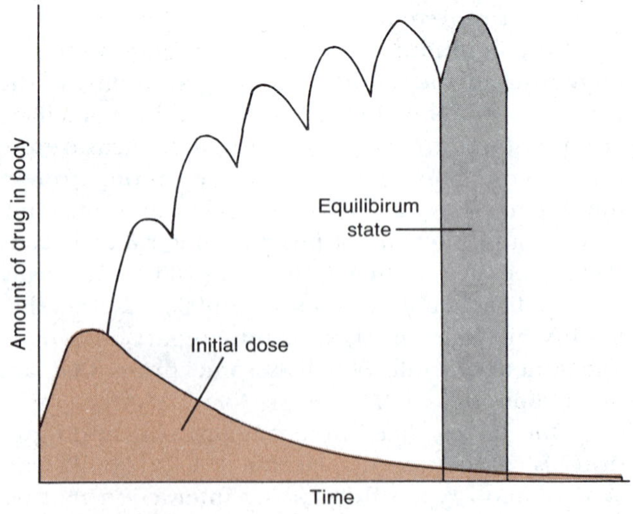

Figure 3–10
Drug accumulation with chronic administration.

Metabolism

Metabolism is the breakdown of a substance through chemical reactions that are controlled by enzymes. Metabolism of many drugs occurs largely in the liver, although some drugs are metabolized in other tissues, including the nervous system, the lungs, the intestines, the placenta, the kidneys, and plasma.

Liver metabolism can affect the activity of drugs in several ways (Table 3–7). More often than not, hepatic metabolism decreases the activity of drugs. Most drugs are at least somewhat lipid soluble (a necessity for absorption), but liver metabolism tends to yield products that are more water soluble and therefore more likely to be excreted by the kidneys. Less commonly, substances enter the body as inactive **prodrugs** and are converted in the liver into active metabolites.

Drugs (and foods) absorbed from the gastrointestinal tract enter the enterohepatic portal circulation, vessels that lead directly to the liver. Thus newly absorbed substances initially pass to the liver before entering the systemic circulation. This phenomenon is called the **hepatic first-pass effect.** Some drugs, such as morphine and lidocaine, are almost completely cleared from the plasma as a result of this first pass and therefore have little oral effectiveness. Drugs that are largely cleared by first-pass extraction (Table 3–8) have short durations of action. Extraction of such drugs is sensitive to changes in liver blood flow. Drugs that are not significantly cleared by first-pass extraction have longer durations of action unless other elimination processes clear them significantly. For these drugs, hepatic blood flow is not a factor, but changes in protein binding of the drug in plasma are important, because the concentration of poorly extracted drugs in the liver tissue (where the drug is available to the metabolic enzymes) is not materially different from the concentration of unbound drug in the plasma. Therefore, a decrease in protein binding will increase rate of metabolism for such drugs.

Most drugs at low or moderate doses are metabolized according to first-order kinetics, but drugs that have poor affinity for the metabolic enzymes or that are present in high concentration may be metabolized according to zero-order kinetics. The biotransformation of drugs in the liver can involve synthetic or nonsynthetic reactions. **Synthetic reactions,** or **conjugations,** involve the coupling of an endogenous substrate with the drug. Synthetic reactions include glucuronidation, amino acid conjugation, acetylation, sulfate conjugation, and methylation. Glucuronidation is conducted by the microsomal enzyme system; the other synthetic reactions by nonmicrosomal enzymes. The products of synthetic reactions are highly water soluble and readily ex-

Table 3–7
Examples of the Effects of Metabolism of Drugs

Prodrugs metabolized to active drugs	
Prodrug	***Metabolite***
Acetylsalicylic acid	Salicylic acid
Chloral hydrate	Trichloroethanol
Chlorguanide	A triazine derivative
Parathion	Paraoxon
Phenacetin	Acetaminophen
Prednisone	Prednisolone
Most vitamins	See Chapter 44
Active drugs metabolized to active metabolites	
Drug	***Metabolite***
Acetohexamide	Hydroxyhexamide
Amitriptyline	Nortriptyline
Chlordiazepoxide	Desmethylchlordiazepoxide
Codeine	Morphine
Diazepam	Desmethyldiazepam
Digitoxin	Digoxin
Flurazepam	Desmethylflurazepam
Glutethimide	4-Hydroxyglutethimide
Imipramine	Desipramine
Lidocaine	Desethyllidocaine
Meperidine	Normeperidine
Mephobarbital	Phenobarbital
Phenylbutazone	Oxyphenbutazone
Primidone	Phenobarbital
Procainamide	N-Acetylprocainamide
Propranolol	4-Hydroxypropranolol
Trimethadione	Dimethadione
Drugs metabolized to more toxic metabolites	
Drug	***Metabolite***
Ethanol	Acetaldehyde
Mesantoin	Nirvanol
Methanol	Formaldehyde

Table 3–8
Some Drugs That Exhibit Extensive First-Pass Extraction

Alprenolol	Morphine
Aspirin	Nitroglycerin
Chlorpromazine	Pentazocine
Desipramine	Propoxyphene
Dopamine	Propranolol
Isoproterenol	Reserpine
Lidocaine	Salicylamide
Meperidine	Serotonin
Methylphenidate	Tryptophan

creted by the kidneys. **Nonsynthetic reactions** include oxidation, reduction, and hydrolysis. Most oxidative and reductive reactions are conducted by the microsomal enzymes, but hydrolysis is catalyzed by nonmicrosomal enzymes.

The activity of liver enzymes can be inhibited or stimulated (induced). Some drugs are given expressly for their ability to inhibit specific liver enzymes. Disulfiram (Antabuse) inhibits aldehyde dehydrogenase and is used in alcohol treatment programs to increase alcohol toxicity. Allopurinol (Zyloprim), useful in gout, inhibits xanthine oxidase, the enzyme responsible for production of uric acid. Some drugs compete for the same enzymes. For example, alcohol will inhibit the metabolism of meprobamate (Miltown) and vice versa when the two are present in the body. Some other inhibitors of liver enzymes include anabolic steroids, estrogens, monoamine oxidase (MAO) inhibitors, nitrofurans, phenothiazines, and sulfonylureas.

Liver diseases including obstructive jaundice and especially hepatic cirrhosis are associated with decreased activity of metabolic enzymes. Hepatic function is not fully developed in young infants and degenerates in aged clients. *Nurses need to recognize that clients in these categories are likely to experience intensified responses to drugs that are normally cleared mainly by liver metabolism. Nurses should question such drug orders if the prescribed doses are not substantially less than those normally employed.*

Induction (or stimulation) of liver enzymes occurs with chronic use of many drugs, typically after a period of a few days. Important inducers include alcohol, barbiturates, and most other hypnotics (but not benzodiazepines), phenytoin and several other antiepileptic drugs, analgesics, antihistamines, anticoagulants, steroids, xanthines, insecticides including dichlorodiphenyltrichloroethane (DDT), many preservatives, dyes, and polycyclic hydrocarbons in cigarette smoke. Induction of liver enzymes affects the drug itself, causing drug-disposition tolerance (see Chapter 10). Induction also provokes drug interactions, some of real clinical significance. For example, inducers will elevate the rate of metabolism of warfarin (Coumadin), resulting in a diminished anticoagulant response. The dose of the anticoagulant will need to be increased to compensate for the faster rate of metabolism. If later the drug responsible for enzyme induction is withdrawn, serious toxicity may occur unless the dose of warfarin is reduced appropriately. Other drugs significantly affected by induction are digitoxin and steroids. Drugs with small therapeutic indices are most critically affected by induction.

Excretion

The kidney is the second major avenue for drug elimination. The kidneys rapidly excrete most of the products of liver metabolism that have been reabsorbed into the blood, but they also excrete many drugs unchanged.

Briefly, the kidney removes substances from the blood by two mechanisms: filtration and active secretion. In filtration, small molecules pass by passive diffusion from the blood vessels in the kidney into the tubule that collects the materials that ultimately form the urine. In active secretion, molecules are transferred from the blood to the tubule by a mechanism requiring energy. Substances removed by either filtration or active secretion may later be reabsorbed back into the blood stream.

Molecules smaller than about 40,000 molecular weight, which includes most drugs, are passively filtered. Drugs bound to plasma proteins cannot be filtered because the plasma proteins are too large for filtration, but unbound drug is filtered in proportion to the glomerular filtration rate (GFR). Once filtered, a polar drug or metabolite is not reabsorbed unless a specific transport mechanism exists for its reabsorption. If not reabsorbed, the filtered portion of a drug is excreted in the urine. Drugs that are filtered but not reabsorbed or secreted have a renal clearance rate equal to the GFR. About one-fifth of the plasma entering the kidney is filtered with each pass under normal circumstances, so that a drug that is fully unbound from plasma proteins, and which is filtered but not reabsorbed or secreted, should have a renal extraction ratio of about 0.2. Drugs with extraction ratios below this value (Table 3–9) are either significantly bound to plasma protein or reabsorbed. In the former case, factors altering the extent of protein binding will significantly impact on rate of excretion. Substances with large renal extraction ratios (>0.7) are actively secreted and their rate of excretion depends mainly on renal blood flow.

Active secretion is the energy-dependent removal of a drug from the renal circulation into the tubule. It is a saturable and selective process that exists for removal of certain natural metabolites but which operates on certain drugs as well. Penicillins, salicylic acid, procainamide, and many of the synthetic metabolites of drugs are examples of substances subject to rapid active secretion. Each substance can be secreted up to a maximal rate that is determined by the intrinsic capacity of the transport system and its affinity for the particular substance. If the rate of presentation of the drug is below the maximum capacity for its secretion, extraction is governed by first-order kinetics; at higher concentra-

Table 3-9
Elimination of Representative Drugs

Drug	Major route(s) of elimination	Renal extraction ratio	Mean half-life and/or range (hours)
Acetaminophen	Hepatic	Intermediate	2.0 (0.9–3.3)
Alprenolol	Hepatic	High	3.1
Amitriptyline	Hepatic	Intermediate	41–45
Amobarbital	Hepatic	Low	14–42
Amoxicillin	Renal/hepatic	Intermediate	1.0
Ampicillin	Renal	Low	1.3
Aspirin	Hepatic	Intermediate	0.25 (but 2.4–19 for active metabolite)
Carbamazepine	Hepatic	Low	20–37
Cephalexin	Renal	Low	0.9
Chloramphenicol	Hepatic	Low	2.7
Chlordiazepoxide	Hepatic	Low	9.9 (6–34)
Chlorthiazide	Renal	Intermediate	1.5
Chlorpromazine	Hepatic	Intermediate	30 (11–58)
Chlorpropamide	Renal	Low	36
Cimetidine	Renal	Intermediate	2.1
Clofibrate	Hepatic	Low	13
Clonazepam	Hepatic	Low	39 (22–53)
Clonidine	Renal/hepatic	Low	8.5
Desipramine	Hepatic	High	18
Diazepam	Hepatic	Low	27–87
Digitoxin	Hepatic/renal	Low	6.9
Digoxin	Renal	Low	42
Doxepin	Hepatic	Intemediate	17
Erythromycin	Hepatic	Intermediate	1.1–3.5
Ethanol	Hepatic	Low	0.24 (0.15–0.35)
Ethosuximide	Renal	Low	33 (30–56)
Furosemide	Renal	Low	0.85
Gentamicin	Renal	Low	2–3
Glucuronides (many)	Renal	High	—
Glycine conjugates	Renal	High	—
Heparin	Hepatic	Low	1–2.5
Hydralazine	Hepatic	Intermediate	2.2–2.6
Imipramine	Hepatic	High	3.5–13
Indomethacin	Hepatic	Low	2.4–11.2
Isoniazid	Hepatic	Low-intermediate	1.1–3.0
Isoproterenol	Hepatic	High	?
Isosorbide	Hepatic	High	0.5
Kanamycin	Renal	Low	2.1
Lidocaine	Hepatic	Intermediate	1.8
Lithium	Renal	Low	22 (7–24)
Lorazepam	Hepatic	Low	14 (10–20)

(continued)

Table 3–9
Elimination of Representative Drugs (*continued*)

Drug	Major route(s) of elimination	Renal extraction ratio	Mean half-life and/or range (hours)
Meperidine	Hepatic	High	3.2
Meprobamate	Hepatic	?	6–16
Methicillin	Renal	Intermediate	0.85
Methotrexate	Renal	Low	8.4
Methyldopa	Renal/hepatic	Low	1.8
Morphine	Hepatic	High	3.0 (1.3–3.4)
Nadolol	Renal	Low	16
Nafcillin	Hepatic	Intermediate	0.9–22
Neostigmine	Renal	Intermediate	1.3
Nitroglycerin	Hepatic	High	—
Nitroglycerin active metabolite	Hepatic	Low	1.8
Nortriptyline	Hepatic	Intermediate	31 (18–35)
Penicillins	Renal	High	—
Pentazocine	Hepatic	High	2.5–6.0
Phenobarbital	Hepatic	Low	86
Phenylbutazone	Hepatic	Low	50–100
Phenytoin	Hepatic	Intermediate	7–42
Prazosin	Hepatic	Low	2.9
Prednisolone	Hepatic	Low	2.1–4.0
Prednisone	Hepatic	Low	3.6
Primidone	Hepatic/renal	Low	8.0
Procainamide	Renal/hepatic	Intermediate	3.0
Propoxyphene	Hepatic	High	1.6–4.1
Propranolol	Hepatic	High at low doses Intermediate at high doses	3.9
Protriptyline	Hepatic	Low	78
Quaternary ammonia compounds	Renal	Intermediate	—
Quinidine	Hepatic	Intermediate	6.2
Rifampin	Hepatic	Intermediate	2.1
Sulfamethoxazole	Hepatic/renal	Low	8.6
Sulfates (many)	Renal	High	—
Sulfisoxazole	Renal/hepatic	Low	5.9
Tetracycline	Hepatic/renal	Low	9.9
Δ^9-Tetrahydrocannabinol	Hepatic	Low	5.6
Theophylline	Hepatic	Low	9.0
Tolbutamide	Hepatic	Low	5.9
Triamterene	Hepatic	Intermediate	2.8
Trimethoprim	Renal/hepatic	Low	11.0
Tubocurarine	Hepatic/renal	Low	2.0
Valproic acid	Hepatic	Low	16
Warfarin	Hepatic	Low	37

tions, extraction becomes zero-order. One secretory mechanism operates on organic anions, including the liver conjugates and penicillin (Table 3–10). The various substrates for this mechanism must compete for secretion. Probenecid is sometimes administered simultaneously with penicillin to decrease secretion of penicillin in this manner in order to prolong the antibiotic's effect. A second mechanism operates on organic cations. Cimetidine reduces renal clearance of procainamide by competing with it for the organic cation carrier system.

Table 3–10
Drugs Transported by the Organic Anion and Organic Cation Proximal Tubule Carrier Systems

Organic anion carrier systems	Organic cation carrier systems
Antimicrobials	**Antimicrobials**
Dapsone	Quinacrine
Penicillin	**Antiulcer drug**
Rifampin	Cimetidine
Sulfonamides	**Autocoids**
Antineoplastics	Histamine
6-Mercaptopurine	**Autonomic drugs**
Methotrexate	Hexamethonium
Thiotepa	Mecamylamine
Diagnostic agents	Pempidine
5-Hydroxyindole acetic acid	Tetramethylammonium
Iodopyracet (Diodrast)	Tolazoline
Para-aminohippurate	**Cardiac drugs**
Phenolsulfonphthalein	Procainamide
Diuretics	**Local anesthetics**
Acetazolamide	Procaine
High-ceiling diuretics	**Nutrient**
Thiazides and related diuretics	Choline
Liver metabolites	
Glucuronides	
Uric acid	
Nonsteroidal anti-inflammatory drugs	
Indomethacin	
Naproxen	
Phenylbutazone	
Salicylates	
Oral hypoglycemics	
Chlorpropamide	
Tolbutamide	
Uricosurics	
Probenecid	
Sulfinpyrazone	

Renal **reabsorption** is another factor in rate of elimination. After a weak organic acid or base has been filtered, it may be reabsorbed to the extent that it is nonionized. Tubular pH therefore exerts a major influence on excretion of such substances. Urinary pH varies from 4.5 to 8.0. Acidification of the urine promotes elimination of weak bases while alkalinization of the urine promotes elimination of weak acids. If a drug is substantially cleared by renal extraction, modification of urinary pH is a useful tactic for hastening elimination of a drug after an overdose. *Aspirin or phenobarbital excretion can be hastened by alkalinization of the urine by administering bicarbonate. Acidification of the urine can be used to speed excretion of methamphetamine.* Dialysis can be used to support inadequate kidney function temporarily when drug overdose has precipitated acute renal failure. Dialysis is effective in removing the same kinds of drugs from the plasma that are normally extracted by the kidneys.

Renal clearance of drugs depends on the adequacy of renal function; excretion of most drugs diminishes in proportion to overall impairment of function in renal diseases. Renal function in young infants is not fully developed and renal function after age 20 deteriorates at a rate of about 1% per year on the average. When renal function is poor, preference should be given to drugs cleared by liver metabolism rather than by kidney extraction (Table 3–9).

Although the kidney is the main organ responsible for excretion of most drugs, volatile drugs (such as many of the general anesthetics) may be excreted primarily through the lungs. Excretion in the bile, saliva, sweat, and breast milk contribute to excretion of certain drugs as well. Drugs and their metabolites are likely to undergo **biliary excretion** if they are polar or of high molecular weight (>300). Some substances excreted in the bile are reabsorbed, resulting in enterohepatic cycling. Biliary excretion depends on active transport by liver cells from plasma to bile. The adequacy of these transport systems can be assessed by administration of a substance such as bromsulfophthalein that is known to be actively transported into the bile. Excretion of drugs in breast milk may have important adverse consequences for the developing infant (Chapter 34).

Summary of Pharmacokinetic Considerations

We have discussed in this section the three pharmacokinetic stages that influence drug action: absorption, distribution, and elimination. At each of these stages, the drug's ability to produce the desired result can be influenced by disease, drug-drug interactions, and just plain individual variability. The ability to control pharmacotherapeutic interventions depends on an appreciation of the fundamental pharmacokinetic processes. A summary of the kinds of drug-drug interactions in relation to the three pharmacokinetic processes is provided in Table 3–11.

Table 3–11
Pharmacokinetic Drug Interactions

Drug A may exhibit	if drug B
altered absorption	forms a complex with drug A within the alimentary tract.
	sequesters drug A, promoting its excretion in the feces.
	changes intestinal pH.
	competes with drug A for an active transport or facilitated diffusion mechanism.
	changes intestinal transit time (motility).
	causes a nonspecific impairment in absorptive capacity of the gut.
	alters solubility of drug A.
	alters contact of drug A with the absorptive surface.
altered distribution	competes for plasma protein binding sites with drug A.
	inhibits uptake or release of drug A from one or more tissue compartments.
	alters blood flow or fluid compartments significantly.
altered elimination	induces liver enzymes.
	inhibits degratory enzymes.
	inhibits enzymes that convert prodrug A into an active metabolite.
	competes for same enzymes.
	impairs hepatic function.
	competes for renal secretory mechanism.
	competes for renal reabsorptive mechanism.
	alters urinary pH.
	impairs renal function.
	competes for first-pass extraction.
	alters biliary excretion of drug A.
	alters pulmonary excretion of drug A.
	alters excretion of drug A in breast milk.

Pharmacodynamics

Our discussion of the pharmacokinetic phase of drug action followed the progress of the drug from the point of dissolution in a body fluid to the delivery of the drug to its site of biological activity and then to its subsequent removal. The pharmacodynamic phase begins with the availability of the drug at its site of action. **Pharmacodynamics** is the physiological and biochemical operation of a drug on the body. Drugs act by manipulating the body's own natural processes. They can inhibit a process, they can activate a process, or they can replace a missing element. Drug effects are produced either by physiochemical influences or by interactions with specific receptors.

Physiochemical Influences

A relatively small number of drugs act by altering the physiochemical character of a body fluid or structural component. Osmotic diuretics, metal chelators, antacids, and antiseptics all act by altering the chemistry of a body system. Osmotic diuretics act to increase the osmolarity of filtrate in the renal nephron, holding water in the tubule and ultimately enhancing formation of urine. Metal chelators form chemical complexes with metal ions with the result that the metal is chemically inactivated and more readily eliminated from the body. Antacids produce a chemical neutralization of acid, thereby raising pH. Antiseptics often act by promoting denaturation of the chemical constituents of microbial cell membranes.

Furthermore, it is likely that the action of general anesthetics and alcohol, as well as part of the pharmacology of barbiturates and marihuana, are based on physiochemical interactions with the lipids in cell membranes, leading to changes in membrane fluidity. Membrane fluidity has a major influence on the activity of membrane proteins and their ability to interact with one another.

Receptor Theory

More frequently, drugs interact with specific sites, called **receptors,** in or on target cells. Receptors are cellular components with which the body's own hormones (and sometimes drugs) interact to produce characteristic effects. The body of knowledge and hypotheses concerning interactions betweeen drugs and receptors is called **receptor theory.**

Most, if not all, receptors are cellular proteins or nucleic acids that regulate the physiological and metabolic activities of the cell. Some receptors, called **recognition proteins,** exist solely for the purpose of transmitting an influence to a target cell or tissue in response to the presence of a control substance — a hormone, neurotransmitter, or a drug that mimics the natural substance. This kind of receptor is likely to consist of several elements which together form a **receptor complex.** The recognition protein identifies the presence of hormone or drug activator and triggers a cascade of events that may involve activity of coupling proteins, effector proteins, and secondary messengers that convey the influence into the cell interior. In addition, the ability of receptors to bind the control substances may be regulated by associated modulatory proteins as well as local conditions of the cell membrane. This kind of receptor complex, then, is an intricate mechanism that is primed to respond to a regulatory substance.

Other proteins and nucleic acids are receptors only incidentally. They may be primarily involved in conducting the ordinary business of the cell: some are ion channels regulating passive diffusion of small, water-soluble substances; others are carrier proteins or enzymes involved in metabolism; still others are nucleic acids involved in protein synthesis. The attachment of a drug can either stimulate or (more commonly) inhibit activity of these incidental receptors as they go about their business. Enzyme inhibitors, antimetabolites, uptake blockers, channel blockers, and drugs affecting the sodium pump are examples of drugs acting on receptor sites not specifically primed to receive chemical influences.

Specific chemical substances bind to each type of receptor to enhance or inhibit the activity that is characteristic of the particular receptor. A given receptor binds only certain chemical substances, typically a group of compounds that are similar in structure or steric configuration. These chemical substances are the ones that possess the required geometrical shape and charge distribution to match up with the shape and charge distribution of the receptor site. Thus, receptors exhibit **specificity.** Sometimes receptors even exhibit **stereospecificity,** binding more readily with one of the two stereoisomers (levorotatory or dextrorotatory) of a drug than with the other. Among the compounds that bind to a given type of receptor, some bind more readily than others; they are said to have higher **affinity** for the receptor.

Drugs interact with receptors in either of two fundamentally different ways: (1) as **agonists** (also called **activators**) or (2) as **antagonists** (known as **blockers**). Agonists bind to the receptor and modify it to produce a pharmacological effect. Antagonists bind to the receptor and prevent it from producing an effect.

Theoretically, four steps are involved in agonist-receptor interaction (Figure 3–11): (1) first the agonist **binds** to the receptor by forming chemical bonds with it; (2) the formation of these bonds **activates** the receptor to produce its effect; (3) the agonist **dissociates** from the receptor, leaving it in a still modified and unexcitable state; and (4) the receptor **regenerates,** returning to its original excitable "ground" state. *Affinity* is the capacity of a drug to engage in the first step, binding, while *efficacy* is the capacity of a drug to initiate the second step, activation.

Antagonists bind to the receptor in the manner of agonists but are not able to activate it; in other words, they have affinity but lack efficacy for the receptor. The binding of the antagonist with the receptor prevents that receptor from being activated by an agonist. Thus the action of an antagonist is indirect and preventive; it interferes with agonistic activity of either a bodily substance or a drug. Whether

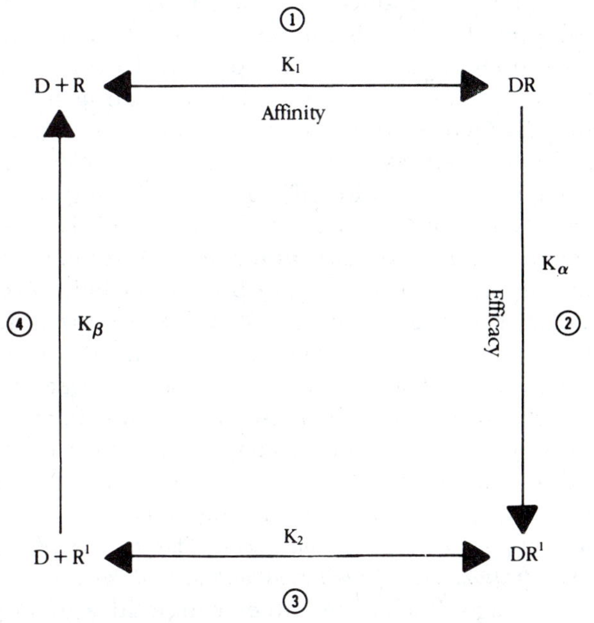

Figure 3–11
The interactions of a drug and receptor: drug (D), receptor in the ground state (R), receptor in the modified or activated state (R′). (1) Binding; (2) activation; (3) dissociation; (4) regeneration of activatable receptor.

an antagonist drug will produce a measurable pharmacological effect always depends on the preexisting level of agonist activity for the specific receptor. If agonist activity is elevated, a blocking drug will have a large impact; if ongoing agonist activity is low, the effect of the blocker will be negligible.

Dose-Response Relationship

The response of a biological system to a drug usually increases as drug concentration increases until it levels off at a point that reflects the intrinsic limits of the response system and the efficacy of the particular drug. This kind of graded **dose-response curve** is shown in Figure 3–12A. A drug that produces a greater effect at a lower dose than another is said to have greater **potency;** potency is an indication of the overall ability of an agonist to activate a receptor and is the product of its affinity and efficacy. The dose-response curve of a more potent drug will lie to the left of that of a less potent drug.

The intensity of a biological response to a drug is presumed to be related either to the number of activated receptors or the rate of their activation (step 2 in Figure 3–11). In either case, the concentration of the drug in the vicinity of the receptor as well as the number, affinity, and sensitivity of the receptors themselves will determine the magnitude of the response.

All drugs produce multiple effects, some beneficial, some harmful. Some responses are all-or-none, rather than graded. For example, every drug causes death at some dose. Each effect of a drug has its own distinctive dose-response relationship. For all-or-none responses, response is measured as the percentage of a population of subjects exhibiting the all-or-none response at each dosage level. This is called a **quantal dose-response curve** and is useful in determining the effective dose or **ED_{50}** and the lethal dose (LD_{50}) of a drug (Figure 3–13). These are the doses that produce the therapeutic effect and death, respectively, in 50% of subjects. The ratio between the two (LD_{50}/ED_{50}) is called the **therapeutic index,** a term we met earlier in the chapter. The therapeutic index is the most widely employed general indicator of the margin of safety for a drug. *A large therapeutic index is favorable; a small one means that doses or plasma concentrations must be adjusted with special care.*

Antagonists can be either competitive or noncompetitive. **Competitive** antagonists compete with agonists for the same receptor sites; the total number of sites occupied by each (the balance of competition) will be determined by the relative concentrations and the relative affinities of the two. In the presence of competitive antagonists, a greater concentration of agonist is required to produce an effect, resulting in a parallel shift in the dose-response relationship for agonist drugs (Figure 3–12B). The greater the concentration of antagonist, the further the dose-response curve shifts to the right. Most antagonists are competitive. **Noncompetitive** antago-

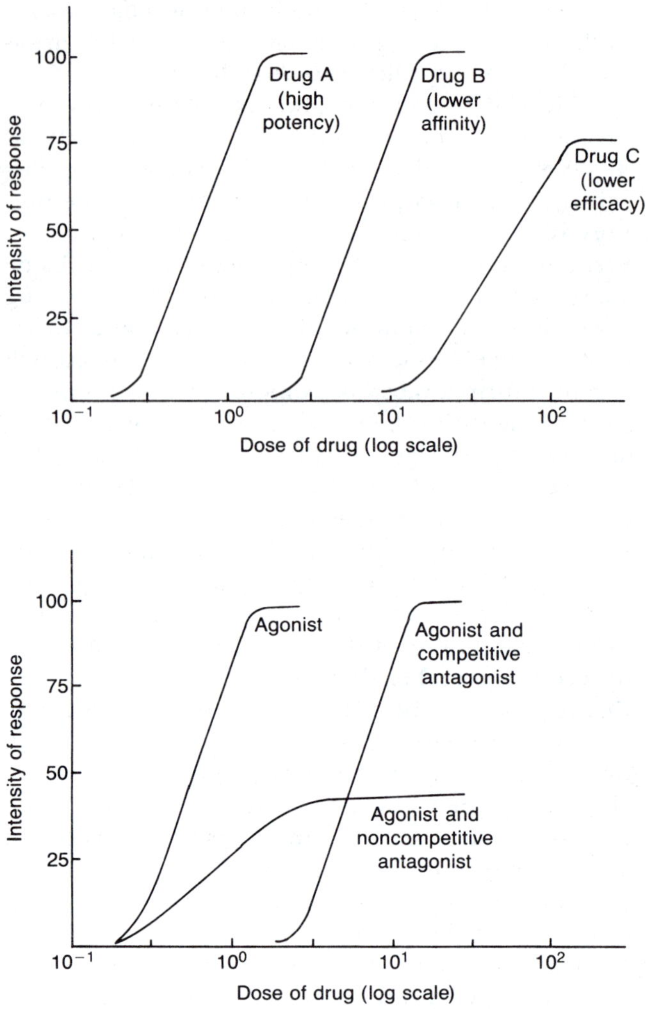

Figure 3–12
Intensity of response is a function of the dose of a drug.
Top: Comparison of dose response curves for a high potency agonist (drug A), an agonist having lower affinity for the receptor (drug B), and an agonist having lower efficacy (drug C).
Bottom: Comparison of dose response curves for a given agonist in the absence of inhibitor and in the presence of a competitive or a noncompetitive inhibitor. The competitive inhibitor causes a parallel shift in the dose-response curve, but the noncompetitive antagonist reduces the maximal intensity of response.

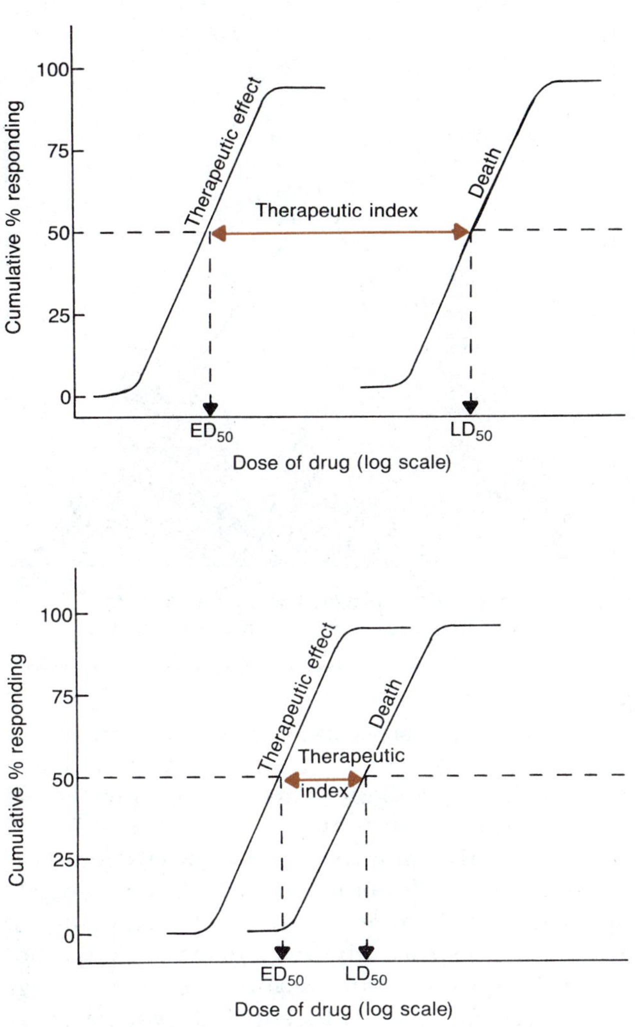

Figure 3–13
Quantal dose-response curves illustrating how such curves are used to determine an ED_{50} (effective dose in 50% of population) or an LD_{50} (lethal dose in 50% of population). The curves on the top illustrate a drug with a large therapeutic index while the curves on the bottom would indicate a drug with a small therapeutic index.

nists bind preferentially to the receptor and prevent agonists from binding, no matter what the concentration of agonist. Noncompetitive antagonists have the effect of reducing the available pool of receptors, causing a downward shift in the ceiling response (Figure 3–12).

Some substances that bind to receptors are called **partial agonists** or **partial antagonists.** These terms are really interchangeable in the same sense that a glass that is half empty is also half full. A partial agonist is a drug with good affinity but little efficacy. A partial agonist alone produces a dose-response curve with a low ceiling. For example, pentazocine (Talwin), a partial agonist at narcotic receptors, produces a low-grade analgesic effect in people not using other narcotics. But a fixed, maximally effective dose of the partial agonist will cause a downward shift in the maximal response to a pure agonist (Figure 3–14). Thus, pentazocine blocks or reverses the effects of more potent agonists, like heroin, when used by addicts. In this situation, pentazocine is acting as an antagonist.

Factors Influencing Pharmacodynamics of Drug Action

The action of drugs in living organisms is substantially more complex than is suggested by simple dose-response curves. Pharmacological effects are complicated by a number of factors: (1) the pharmaceutical and pharmacokinetic factors discussed in previous sections of this chapter, (2) circadian rhythms, (3) pathology, (4) genetic factors, (5) pharmacodynamic drug interactions, (6) compensatory and adaptive responses, and (7) psychological factors (addressed in Chapter 8).

Circadian rhythms (daily body rhythms) may influence drug effects, especially those related to cyclic functions. Daily fluctuations in arousal of the central nervous system related to the sleep-wake cycle will determine susceptibility to the effects of CNS de-

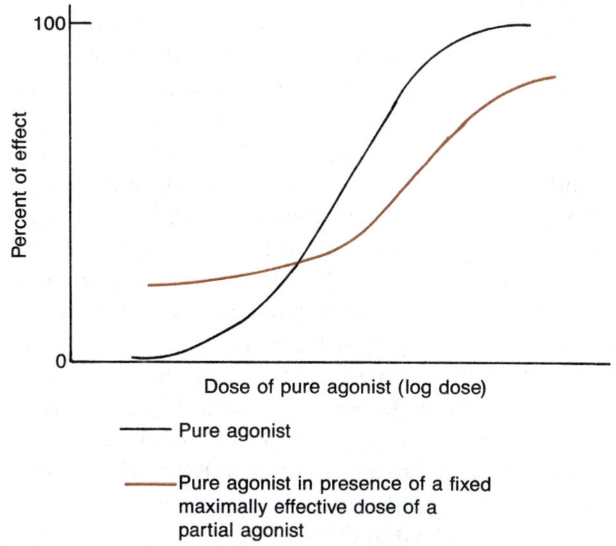

Figure 3–14
The effect of addition of a partial agonist on the dose-response curve for a pure agonist.

pressants. Steroids and drug-metabolizing enzymes of the liver likewise exhibit daily rhythms that can have an impact on drug efficacy and adverse reactions.

Some drug effects characteristically occur only in **pathological states.** Aspirin lowers temperature in fever but not when temperature is normal. Digitalis improves cardiac output in a failing heart but not in a healthy heart. Analgesics, antipsychotic drugs, antidepressants, and antimicrobial drugs, to name a few, produce their characteristic effects only when the corresponding pathological condition is present. Alpha-blockers dramatically lower blood pressure that is due to elevated catecholamines but are less effective for essential hypertension. Clients with marginal physiological dysfunctions in any organ are disproportionately susceptible to drug side effects that further impair the weakened function. So, more often than not, clinical pharmacology of drugs is tied in with pathophysiology. Since diagnostic groupings are, at best, only approximations, clients with a similar diagnosis will often respond differently to drugs. This variation in response is termed **diagnostic heterogeneity.** For example, there is evidence that the classification of major depression subsumes a "serotonin type," which is responsive to 5-hydroxytryptophan, and a "norepinephrine type," which is not.

Genetic influences are generally best characterized as random individual variability within a normal response distribution. But genetic anomalies at times result in idiosyncratic reactions. Response curves for some populations exhibit clear discontinuities — bimodal or multimodal distributions (Figure 3–15). Such curves often indicate distinct genetic subpopulations with differential sensitivity to the drug. For example, approximately 1 in every 2,500 individuals has a genetic deficiency of the enzyme pseudocholinesterase. These clients will have inordinate sensitivity to succinylcholine, which is metabolized in part by pseudocholinesterase. Roughly half of the U.S. population has a defect in isoniazid acetylase, a liver enzyme that ordinarily inactivates isoniazid, hydralazine, and sulfamethazine, among other drugs. Rarely, phenytoin metabolism may be constitutionally deficient. Some clients are genetically resistant to warfarin and others to insulin. About 5% of the U.S. population has an inherited sensitivity to corticosteroids that is expressed as increased intraocular pressure when these drugs are given. Immune system drug sensitivities are highly individualistic and almost surely at least partly determined by genetics.

Pharmacodynamic interactions take place in a number of ways. One drug can alter the effect of

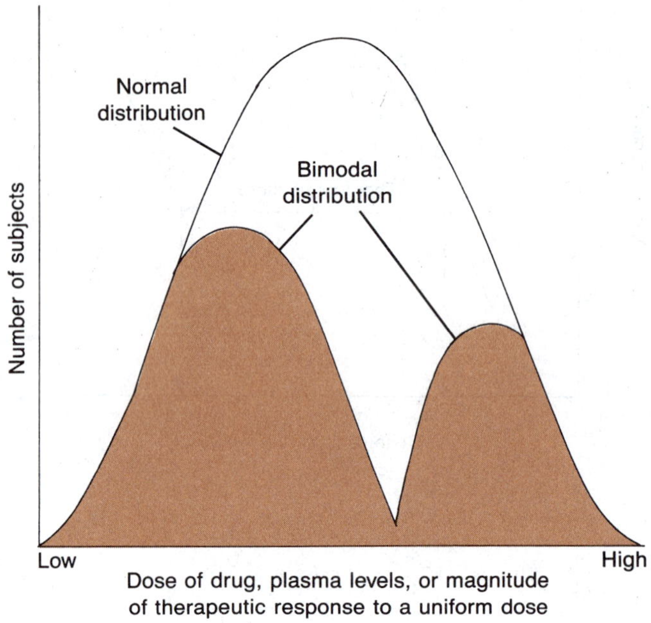

Figure 3–15
Bimodal versus normal population-response curves.

another in three basic ways: (1) by altering its bioavailability; (2) by a pharmacological interaction between agonists, antagonists, and partial agonists at the level of the receptor; or (3) by a physiological interaction. The latter two types of interaction lie within the pharmacodynamic domain. A **physiological interaction** is the relationship of two drugs that affect the same physiological parameter by means of two different receptors. If the drugs have an effect in the same direction, the interaction is **additive;** if the net effect is greater than the sum of the individual effects, the interaction is **synergistic.** All CNS depressants, from the same or different classes, have at least additive, and in some cases synergistic, depressant influence on the brain. The relationship between pentobarbital (a depressant) and strychnine (a convulsant) is one of **physiological antagonism** because they operate on different receptors to produce their opposing actions.

The total effect of a drug is substantially more (and in a way less) than just its primary effects, because the body is not passive but rather is an exquisitely modulated physiological system. Even with short-term administration, the body's **compensatory responses** tend to counteract the primary drug effect. For example, intravenous infusion of norepinephrine constricts blood vessels and stimulates the heart, which raises blood pressure, which in turn activates the parts of the autonomic nervous system that slow the heart, thereby partly offsetting the primary pressor effect of the drug. Thus, although tachycardia is the direct effect of norepinephrine on heart rate in an isolated heart preparation, bradycardia is observed in intact organisms. Neurotransmitter systems also exhibit compensatory mechanisms. Drugs may elevate neurotransmitter levels in the synapse, but this will activate presynaptic (as well as postsynaptic) receptors, which will have the effect of suppressing further transmitter release. Administration of hormones typically suppresses the body's production of those hormones. Compensatory mechanisms are important in the clinical pharmacology of digitalis, calcium channel blockers, psychotropic drugs, hormones, and antihypertensives, just to name a few.

When drugs are given chronically, **adaptive mechanism** may come into play as well. More often than not, adaptive mechanisms result in diminished drug effectiveness, or **tolerance.** The adaptation may be in pharmacokinetic factors, as with induction of liver enzymes (**drug-disposition tolerance**), or it may be at the level of the receptor, receptor complex, or response system (**pharmacodynamic tolerance**). Tolerance is especially important with respect to central nervous system drugs but has been noted also with antianginal drugs, antihypertensives, and laxatives. Pharmacodynamic tolerance to CNS drugs (discussed in Chapter 10) is based mainly on adaptive changes in neurotransmission, including up- and down-regulation of receptors, induction or repression of synthetic or degratory enzymes, and changes in transport capacity for transmitter precursors.

If, with chronic administration, the compensatory responses of the body to a drug undergo adaptive tolerance to a greater extent than the primary effects of the drug, overall response magnitude may actually increase gradually with time. This may well be the basis for the gradual development of clinical responsiveness to antipsychotics and antidepressants over 2–3 weeks of chronic administration.

A different kind of adaptation to drug action is the development of **resistance** by microorganisms to antimicrobial drugs or by cancer cells to anticancer drugs, whereby the responsiveness of the target cells to the drug gradually decreases.

Adverse Drug Reactions

The term **adverse drug reactions** covers a host of undesirable effects of drugs. For purposes of classification, adverse drug reactions can be divided into those that appear with acute (one-time) or subacute (repeated regularly up to about 3 weeks) administration and those that come into play only after chronic (long-term) administration. The former category can be further divided into toxic effects that are predictable and those that are unpredictable.

Predictable, Acute Adverse Drug Reactions

Side effects are predictable adverse drug reactions that occur within the normal range of therapeutic doses for a given drug. Unless the drug is being used in clinical trials or is quite new, it is likely that its characteristic side effects will be well documented. Some side effects occur almost inevitably with proper dosing. Some occur commonly at the upper end of the normal range of therapeutic doses. Most side effects that develop acutely are dose dependent and can be reversed by eliminating the drug, if not by reducing the dose. Some side effects are called **early side effects** because the client tends to develop tolerance to the effect with long-term use. *Identification of side effects is a major part of the nurse's role, as is educating the client to anticipate and recognize the telltale signs and symptoms.*

Overdose toxicity is the predictable consequence of excessive drug effect due to administration of doses above the normal limit. A **functional overdose** is one produced when the dose administered is within the normal range, but when unusual pharmacokinetics produce a higher than normal plasma concentration. One example is the **cumulation toxicity** that occurs when repeated dosing is used and drug elimination between doses is less than the drug made available from each additional dose. Overdose toxicity may involve an exaggeration of the characteristic side effects of the drug or additional toxic effects not observed at lower doses. Death is a possible consequence of overdose with any drug, since every drug is fatal at some dose. In practice, death from overdose is most common with barbiturates and narcotics. Overdose deaths most often result from respiratory arrest or vasomotor collapse from excess central nervous system depression, or from convulsions, hemorrhages, aplastic anemia, liver or kidney failure, massive infection, or anaphylaxis. About 6,500 drug-related fatalities occur in the United States each year. About half of these are suicides and most of the rest involve self-administered drugs.

Unpredictable, Acute Adverse Drug Reactions

Two kinds of adverse reactions are unpredictable and often not dose related: drug allergies and idiosyncratic reactions. **Drug allergies,** or **drug hyper-**

sensitivity reactions, occur unpredictably in a small percentage of clients. Drugs can function as antigens themselves or they can function as haptens, binding to endogenous proteins to create antigenic complexes. Allergic reactions are relatively frequent with antimicrobial drugs, local anesthetics, neuroleptics, and antidepressants but can occur with most drugs that are not also endogenous substances (that is, substances produced by the body). Cross-sensitivity is usually observed with drugs of related structure. Skin tests can predict allergic reactions with certain drugs, notably penicillin. Drug allergies are most commonly manifested as skin rashes or eruptions but may also take the form of jaundice, anaphylaxis, anemia, or other disorders.

Idiosyncratic reactions are reactions of unusual intensity in an individual client, outside of the normal range of responses. Idiosyncrasy is usually genetically determined. Examples include inability to metabolize certain drugs such as succinylcholine (Succinyl), isoniazid, hydralazine (Apresoline), phenytoin (Dilantin), or sulfur drugs; unusual resistance to warfarin (Coumadin) or insulin; or unusual sensitivity to glucocorticoids. Idiosyncratic intoxication is a recognized diagnostic category of reactions to alcohol, but it is not clear whether the unusual response is due to genetics, predisposing organic pathology, or psychological set.

Chronic Adverse Drug Reactions

Many adverse reactions occur only after long-term use of a medication or drug of abuse. **Tolerance and dependence** seldom develop in less than a few months of regular drug use. Tolerance and dependence are discussed more fully in Chapter 10 in relation to drug abuse.

Iatrogenic diseases are diseases caused by drugs that are part of medical treatment. The five most common types of iatrogenic diseases are blood dyscrasias (alterations in levels of blood cells), liver damage, kidney damage, teratogenic effects (fetal damage caused by maternal exposure), and skin eruptions such as porphyria, purpura, striae, acne, and abnormal pigmentation. Side effects that occur only after long-term use are called **late side effects.** An example is the tardive dyskinesias that may result from long-term use of neuroleptics. Other drug-induced diseases can occur as a result of damage to bodily tissues caused by long-term self-administration of nonprescription, social, or illicit drugs. Among drugs of abuse, significant damage to bodily tissues is most often associated with alcohol and tobacco but may occur with any of the commonly abused drugs.

Recommended Readings

Benet LZ, Massoud N, Gambertoglio JG (eds): *Pharmacokinetic Basis for Drug Treatment.* New York, Raven Press, 1984.

Gibaldi M, Perrier D: *Pharmacokinetics,* ed 2. New York, Marcel Dekker Inc, 1982.

Goldstein A, Aronow L, Kalman SM: *Principles of Drug Action: The Basis of Pharmacology,* ed 2. New York, John Wiley & Sons, 1974.

Hussar DA: Drug interactions — think about them before administering medications. *Nursing* 1986;16(8):34–39.

Levine RR: *Pharmacology: Drug Actions and Reactions,* ed 3. Boston, Little Brown & Co, 1983.

Melmon, KL, Morelli HF (eds): *Clinical Pharmacology,* ed. 2. New York, Macmillan Inc, 1978.

Stillwell S: Ensuring safe, effective drug therapy. *Nursing Life* 1986;6(6):33–39.

UNIT II

Pharmacotherapeutics in Nursing Practice

CHAPTER 4

Drug Administration

Nurses in contemporary practice must be able to perform a wide variety of activities that are related to drug administration. This chapter discusses issues that pertain to drug administration, including dosage units and calculations, storage and preparation of medications, guidelines for administering drugs, and techniques for administering drugs by various routes. Readers may want to refer also to the description of dosage forms in Chapter 2 and the discussion of ethical and legal considerations in Chapter 5.

Dosage Units

Traditionally, health care agencies stocked drugs in clinical units. There were stock supplies of the most commonly used items whether oral tablets, liquid medications, or ones for injection. The drug could be a sleeping medication in oral form (tablet or liquid) or injection form, aspirin, certain cathartics, or even antibiotics — unmixed in their powdered form. It was the responsibility of the nurse to calculate correct dosages of medicine and prepare the drug for administration at the appropriate interval of time according to the doctor's orders. The individual patient's medication was poured from the stock supply. Over time, it was realized that stock supply items were not cost effective. Medications that were infrequently used became outdated and had to be discarded. Another danger arose because stock supply bottles often so resembled one another that a nurse on a busy clinical unit could easily pick up the wrong bottle or vial. To improve the method of supplying drugs and accuracy, clinical agencies adopted the unit dose system.

In the unit dose system, few if any stock drugs are kept in clinical departments. Medications are individually prepared in the pharmacy for each client and put into packages labeled with the patient's name and sent to the clinical department. There the packages are kept in individualized compartments. Usually only a 24-hour supply of medication is sent to the clinical department for each client. There is no waste of medication. Since the calculation of dosages and amounts are performed in the pharmacy away from the bustle of clinical activity and by someone for whom this is the major job, the incidence of medication error is lessened. However, nurses still have the responsibility of making certain that the appropriate prepackaged medications are correctly administered to the right patient.

Storage of Medications

Each hospital, outpatient clinic, emergency room, or walk-in clinic has an area designated for storing drugs. It may be a wall cabinet, a medication room, or a medication cart. In addition, there are special storage areas for drugs that must be refrigerated or kept from sunlight.

Narcotics and other controlled substances are kept inside a double-locked cabinet. The keys to the cabinet must at all times be in the possession of one nurse designated to have them on each shift of duty. Every time a narcotic or other controlled substance is taken from the cabinet, the nurse administering the drug must record in the designated record book and on the patient's chart the name of the individual to whom the drug was given, the amount given, the time, the name of the physician prescribing the drug, and the name of the nurse administering it.

At times, a controlled drug may be wasted accidentally (dropped on the floor, for example), or a patient may refuse the drug once it has been prepared. When this occurs the nurse must record the information in the record book and on the patient's chart. In these instances, most institutions require a second person to witness the destruction of the medication — co-signing the record after seeing that it was crushed or flushed down the sink. In other institutions, the unused drug must be returned to the pharmacy and destroyed there.

In addition to recording the use of drugs such as opiates, barbiturates, and other scheduled substances, the numbers of pills, capsules, vials, or ampuls of such substances must be counted at each change of nursing shift by the nurse who is leaving the unit and the one assuming responsibility for these substances for the next shift. Both nurses must sign the narcotic drug record stating that they agree with the amount and type of drugs as recorded. If any drug or amount is missing and cannot be accounted for, this fact must be reported immediately to the nursing supervisor. The storage and recording of administration of narcotics, barbiturates, and other scheduled drugs are under the authority of the federal government. Periodically, the records are checked for thoroughness and credibility.

Dose Calculations

It is crucial for nurses to be able to calculate dosage requirements accurately and to prepare solutions for administration carefully. Obviously, misplacement of a decimal point or other kinds of errors in a calculation of a dose can be fatal. In this section we briefly review the methods employed for calculating doses. Calculation of dosages for pediatric and geriatric populations is considered more specifically in Chapters 6 and 7.

Systems of Measurement

The most commonly used system of weights and measures is the metric system. Nurses can expect that the metric system will gradually replace other systems in drug applications. In the meantime, nurses must recognize units from other commonly encountered systems, including the apothecaries' system and the household system.

The **metric system** is a decimal system (based on multiples of 10) that facilitates mathematical calculations. The units of the metric system are the meter for linear measurements, the gram for weight, and the liter for volume. Larger and smaller units of measure are constructed by adding prefixes to the three basic units. For example, a millimeter is one-thousandth of a meter, and a kilometer is 1,000 meters. The commonly encountered prefixes and their meanings are

micro	one-millionth	1/1,000,000
milli	one-thousandth	1/1,000
centi	one-hundredth	1/100
deci	one-tenth	1/10
deca	ten	10
hecto	one-hundred	100
kilo	one-thousand	1,000

The units of the metric system are interrelated in that a milliliter (ml) is essentially equivalent to a cubic centimeter (cc), and a gram is the weight of 1.0 milliliter of water at 4°C.

The **apothecaries' system** is a much older and less coherent system of volume and weight measurements. For volume measurement, 60 minims equals 1 fluid dram (fʒ); 8 fluid drams equals 1 fluid ounce (f℥); and 16 fluid ounces equals 1 pint. A minim roughly approximates a drop. For weight measurements, 60 grains (gr) equals 1 dram (ʒ); 8 drams equals 1 ounce (℥); and 12 (not 16!) ounces equals 1 pound (lb ap).

In the **household system** of volume measurements, one encounters the teaspoonful, the tablespoonful, and the cup. A tablespoon equals 3 teaspoonfuls; 2 tablespoonfuls equals 1 ounce; and a cup (or glassful) is 8 ounces. One teaspoonful is equivalent to 1 fluid dram of the apothecaries' system.

Table 4–1 gives some of the commonly used approximate equivalencies between the metric, apothecaries', and household systems that can be used to convert units from one system to another.

Calculating Doses in Unlike Units of Measure

It is often necessary for nurses to convert dosage requirements from one system of units to another. This happens when the dose specified by the physician is not in the same units as the product on hand. To convert a volume or weight from one system of units to another, the simplest method is to set up a proportion using the units you have and the units you want. A known equivalency (such as those listed in Table 4–1) goes on one side of the equal sign (traditionally the left) and the unknown goes on the other. For example, to convert 3 fluid ounces to a metric value, we first set up an equivalency between the units we have (ounces) and the units we want (milliliters) on the left side of the equal sign:

$$\frac{30 \text{ ml}}{1 \text{ fluid ounce}} = \frac{?}{?}$$

This is an equivalency because we know that 30 ml is equal (approximately) to 1 fluid ounce. Next, the given weight or volume value (3 fluid ounces in the current problem) is placed on the other side of the equation. The trick that must be remembered in setting up proportions is whether to place the given value on the top or bottom of the right side. The given value is always placed in the same relative position (top or bottom) as the value of the same units in the equivalency on the left side of the equation. In the current problem, fluid ounce appears on the bottom of the left side, so the given value of 3 fluid ounces is placed on the bottom on the right side. So now we have:

$$\frac{30 \text{ ml}}{1 \text{ fluid ounce}} = \frac{?}{3 \text{ fluid ounces}}$$

It is traditional to let the letter x stand for the unknown quantity, so the full equation reads:

$$\frac{30 \text{ ml}}{1 \text{ fluid ounce}} = \frac{x}{3 \text{ fluid ounces}}$$

This equation is solved by cross-multiplying (multiplying the pairs that are diagonally across from each other) to get

$$x \text{ (1 fl oz)} = \text{(30 ml) (3 fl oz)}$$

Table 4–1
Commonly Used Equivalents

Metric system	Apothecary system	Household measures
Weights		
1,000 microgram (μg) = 1 milligram (mg)	1/60 grain	
60 mg	1 grain	
1 gram (g)	15 grains	
4 g	60 grains = 1 dram	
30 g	1 ounce	
454 g	1 pound (lb)	
1,000 g = 1 kilogram (kg)	2.2 lb	
Volume		
1 milliliter (1 ml or 1 cc)	15 minims (mns)	20 drops
4–5 ml	1 dram	1 teaspoon (tsp)
15 ml		1 tablespoon (tbsp)
30 ml	1 fluid ounce (fl oz)	2 tablespoons
60 ml	2 fluid ounces	
250 ml	8 fluid ounces	1 measuring cup
500 ml	1 pint = 16 fluid ounces	
1,000 ml	1 quart (qt) = 32 fluid ounces	
4,000 ml	1 gallon = 4 quarts	

Dividing both sides of the equation and cancelling out the units gives you the final result:

$$x = \frac{(30\text{ ml})\ (3\ \cancel{\text{fl oz}})}{1\ \cancel{\text{fl oz}}}$$

$$x = \frac{90\text{ ml}}{1}$$

or

$$x = 90\text{ ml}$$

Thus 3 fluid ounces is equal to 90 ml.

Another example, involving units of weight, may help to reinforce the method. You are told to administer 30 grains of a drug and wish to convert this value to milligrams. For this conversion, the relevant equivalency from Table 4–1 is 1 gram (g) = 15 grains. Thus:

$$\frac{1\text{ g}}{15\text{ grains}} = \frac{?}{?}$$

Then, inserting the given value in the same relative position as the value of the same units in the equivalency:

$$\frac{1\text{ g}}{15\text{ grains}} = \frac{x}{30\text{ grains}}$$

$$x\ (15\text{ grains}) = (1\text{ g})\ (30\text{ grains})$$

$$x = \frac{(1\text{ g})\ (30\ \cancel{\text{grains}})}{15\ \cancel{\text{grains}})}$$

$$x = \frac{30\text{ g}}{15}$$

$$x = 2\text{ g}$$

So, 30 grains is equivalent to 2 grams.

SAMPLE PROBLEMS

1. The prescription written by Dr. A. calls for administration of 16 grains (gr) of a medication. You wish to convert this to the metric system.
2. A client has been instructed to take 20 milliliters (ml) of a syrup but would like this value converted to teaspoons. How many teaspoons should he take?

Answers to the SAMPLE PROBLEMS appear on page 71.

Calculating Oral Doses

The same basic methods are employed when the nurse needs to determine how many tablets or capsules, or what part of a scored tablet, to administer to an individual in order to provide the ordered dose. In this case, the equivalency used on the left side of the equation is the weight of drug in a single tablet or capsule. For example, the order is for 30 mg of chlorpromazine (Thorazine), which is available in 10, 25, and 50 mg tablets. How many 10 mg tablets would be required? First the equivalency is established on the left side of the equation:

$$\frac{1 \text{ tablet}}{10 \text{ mg}} = \frac{?}{?}$$

Then the given value, 30 mg, is placed in the corresponding position on the right side of the equation:

$$\frac{1 \text{ tablet}}{10 \text{ mg}} = \frac{x}{30 \text{ mg}}$$

$$x\,(10 \text{ mg}) = (1 \text{ tablet})\,(30 \text{ mg})$$

$$x = \frac{(1 \text{ tablet})\,(30\ \cancel{\text{mg}})}{(10\ \cancel{\text{mg}})}$$

$$x = \frac{30 \text{ tablets}}{10}$$

$$x = 3 \text{ tablets}$$

Thus, solving the equation, we find that three 10 mg tablets are required to provide 30 mg. If we perform the same process with respect to 25 mg or 50 mg tablets, we find that fractional tablets will be required, namely, one and one-fifth of a 25 mg tablet or three-fifths of a 50 mg tablet. Since it is not practical to break tablets except those that are scored for this purpose, the nurse should try to find an alternate dosage form that will avoid the need for fractional tablets.

The number of milliliters of a solution or concentrate required can be calculated by a similar process. If the strength of the solution is stated as a percentage, this can be translated as the number of grams per 100 ml. Thus, a 10% solution contains 10 g/100 ml. If the desired dose is 0.6 g and the solution is 20%, how many milliliters should be administered? The equivalency is

$$\frac{20 \text{ g}}{100 \text{ ml}} = \frac{?}{?}$$

Inserting the given value and solving, we find that

$$\frac{20 \text{ g}}{100 \text{ ml}} = \frac{0.6 \text{ g}}{x}$$

$$x\,(20 \text{ g}) = (100 \text{ ml})\,(0.6 \text{ g})$$

$$x = \frac{(100 \text{ ml})\,(0.6\ \cancel{\text{g}})}{(20\ \cancel{\text{g}})}$$

$$x = \frac{60 \text{ ml}}{20}$$

$$x = 3 \text{ ml}$$

SAMPLE PROBLEMS

3. A doctor has prescribed 500 mg of tetracycline qid. The capsules on hand contain 250 mg of tetracycline. How many capsules will be required at each administration?
4. A client is prescribed 120 mg of propanolol bid. You note that there are tablets of 10 mg, 20 mg, 40 mg, and 80 mg on hand. You have decided that you want to provide the prescribed dosage using the fewest number of tablets, without breaking tablets, and without using more than one tablet strength. Which tablet strength should you employ?

Sometimes it is necessary to calculate oral doses in two successive steps: one step to convert the prescribed value from one system of measurement to another, and a second step to determine the number of tablets or capsules required. For example, a prescription might call for oral administration of one-third grain of morphine sulfate. If the tablets on hand are 10 mg each, it will be necessary to first convert the prescribed value to milligrams and then to calculate the number of tablets required. In the first step, the relevant equivalency from Table 4–1 is 60 mg = 1 grain. Thus:

$$\frac{60 \text{ mg}}{1 \text{ grain}} = \frac{x}{1/3 \text{ grain}}$$

$$x\,(1 \text{ grain}) = (60 \text{ mg})\,(1/3 \text{ grain})$$

$$x = \frac{(60 \text{ mg})\,(1/3\ \cancel{\text{grain}})}{(1\ \cancel{\text{grain}})}$$

$$x = \frac{20 \text{ mg}}{1}$$

$$x = 20 \text{ mg}$$

So, ⅓ grain is equivalent to 20 milligrams. Now, in the second step of the calculation, it is necessary to determine how many 10 mg tablets will be required to furnish the dose of 20 mg. The relevant equivalency is

$$\frac{1 \text{ tablet}}{10 \text{ mg}} = \frac{?}{?}$$

Then the given value, 20 mg, is placed in the corresponding position on the right side of the equation:

$$\frac{1 \text{ tablet}}{10 \text{ mg}} = \frac{x}{20 \text{ mg}}$$

$$x\ (10 \text{ mg}) = (1 \text{ tablet})\ (20 \text{ mg})$$

$$x = \frac{(1 \text{ tablet})\ (20 \cancel{\text{mg}})}{(10 \cancel{\text{mg}})}$$

$$x = \frac{20 \text{ tablets}}{10}$$

$$x = 2 \text{ tablets}$$

SAMPLE PROBLEMS

5. Dr. A. orders that a client receive phenytoin (Dilantin) at a dose of 1.5 grains per administration. The tablets that are available are 25 mg/tablet. How many tablets will be required per administration?
6. Dr. S. orders meprobamate to be given at a dose of 0.4 grams. The tablets available are 200 mg/tablet. How many will be required per dose?
7. Dr. M. orders sulfadiazine to be given to a client at a dose of 3 grains. The tablets available are 0.1 grams each. How many tablets should be given?

Calculations for Preparing Solutions

Nurses are frequently required to prepare a predetermined volume of a solution of a particular strength. In this event, the appropriate weight of drug can be determined by use of proportions. If 20 ml of a 10% solution (10 g/100 ml) is required, the following proportion would be set up:

$$\frac{10 \text{ g}}{100 \text{ ml}} = \frac{x}{20 \text{ ml}}$$

$$x\ (100 \text{ ml}) = (10 \text{ g})\ (20 \text{ ml})$$

$$x = \frac{(10 \text{ g})\ (20 \cancel{\text{ml}})}{(100 \cancel{\text{ml}})}$$

$$x = \frac{200 \text{ g}}{100}$$

$$x = 2 \text{ g}$$

SAMPLE PROBLEM

8. Dr. F. has ordered administration of 25 ml of a 5% solution of an electrolyte. How many grams of electrolyte should be dissolved in the 25 ml of water in preparing the solution to the correct concentration?

If, on the other hand, a given weight of drug (say, 1 g) is to be made into a 20% solution, the equation would be

$$\frac{20 \text{ g}}{100 \text{ ml}} = \frac{1 \text{ g}}{x}$$

$$x\ (20 \text{ g}) = (100 \text{ ml})\ (1 \text{ g})$$

$$x = \frac{(100 \text{ ml})\ (1 \cancel{\text{g}})}{(20 \cancel{\text{g}})}$$

$$x = \frac{100 \text{ ml}}{20}$$

$$x = 5 \text{ ml}$$

SAMPLE PROBLEM

9. What volume of sterile water is required to make 5 g of a drug into a 30% solution?

Directions for reconstituting medications are usually furnished on medication labels. For example, a vial containing 3 g of ticarcillin disodium (Ticar) instructs the nurse to prepare intramuscular injection solutions as follows: "Add 6 ml of sterile water for injection, USP, or 1% lidocaine HCl solution (without epinephrine) and use promptly. Each 2.6 ml of solution will then contain 1 g of ticarcillin." If the physician's order calls for 2 g of ticarcillin, the following proportion would be solved to determine the required volume of reconstituted solution that would need to be injected:

$$\frac{1 \text{ g}}{2.6 \text{ ml}} = \frac{2 \text{ g}}{x}$$

$$x\ (1 \text{ g}) = (2.6 \text{ ml})\ (2 \text{ g})$$

$$x = \frac{(2.6 \text{ ml})\ (2 \cancel{\text{g}})}{(1 \cancel{\text{g}})}$$

$$x = \frac{5.2 \text{ ml}}{1}$$

$$x = 5.2 \text{ ml}$$

SAMPLE PROBLEMS

10. Nafcillin Powder for Oral Solution (Unipen) provides a solution having a concentration of 250 mg/5 ml when reconstituted as directed in 100 ml of sterile water. If the physician has ordered that 500 mg be given orally, what volume will be required?
11. Amikacin sulfate (Amikin) is provided in 2 ml vials containing 500 mg for reconstitution and IM or IV administration. If a doctor orders

administration of 500 mg IM, what volume will be required for each injection?

12. Dr. S. orders injection of 4 mg of thiothixene (Navane) IM for an individual exhibiting severe psychotic manifestations and belligerence. The label of the preparation on hand indicates a concentration of 5 mg/ml after reconstitution in 2 ml of sterile water for injection. What volume should be injected?

Intravenous Infusions

The preparation of solutions for intravenous administration follows the same rules as for oral solutions and solutions for intramuscular or subcutaneous injection. However, when fluids are being administered intravenously, frequently a particular rate of infusion over time is specified. The volume of a drop varies according to the make of administration equipment being employed. Let us suppose that a particular administration set delivers 15 drops per milliliter and the desired infusion rate is 5 ml/minute. How many drops would have to be administered per minute? The equivalency is

$$\frac{15 \text{ drops}}{1 \text{ ml}} = \frac{?}{?}$$

Since 5 ml per minute is the desired rate, we write

$$\frac{15 \text{ drops}}{1 \text{ ml}} = \frac{x}{5 \text{ ml/minute}}$$

$$x \text{ (1 ml)} = \text{(15 drops) (5 ml/minute)}$$

$$x = \frac{\text{(15 drops) (5 } \cancel{\text{ml}}\text{/minute)}}{\text{(1 } \cancel{\text{ml}}\text{)}}$$

$$x = \frac{\text{75 drops/minute}}{1}$$

$$x = \text{75 drops/minute}$$

SAMPLE PROBLEMS

13. Oxytetracycline HCl (Terramycin) for injection comes in vials containing 250 mg of powder. Nurses are instructed to reconstitute this powder in 10 ml of sterile water for injection, USP or 5% dextrose injection, USP, then redilute to make at least 100 ml. Assume that the nurse chooses to redilute to exactly 100 ml, how much volume will need to be infused to fulfill the physician's order for 500 mg every 12 hours?

14. Dr. F. orders that the patient receive 1,000 ml of D5W (5% dextrose in water) to be infused over 10 hours. The apparatus provides 10 drops per milliliter. What would be the appropriate flow rate?

Special Types of Units

Milliequivalents (mEq) are a unit of measure that takes into account the number of ionic charges (valence) that a molecule possesses. Usually, drugs ordered in milliequivalents will also be identified on their labels in mEq per liter. The principles of calculation are the same as for other solutions.

SAMPLE PROBLEMS

15. A physician orders that the patient receive 2 mEq of KCl per 100 ml of IV infusate. The KCl solution on hand is 20 mEq/ml. How much will need to be added to a 500 ml bag of infusion solution?

16. A patient is to be given 4 mEq of KCl per 100 ml of intravenous D5W. The KCl on hand is 40 mEq/10 ml. How much of this solution should be added to a 500 ml bag of D5W?

A unit (U) of a drug is a value that is unique for any given drug. Some examples of drugs frequently ordered in units are insulin, penicillin, and heparin. A United States Pharmacopeia (USP) unit of insulin is the amount of the drug that will promote the metabolism of 1.5 g of dextrose. A unit of penicillin is defined in terms of a reference standard of penicillin. Insulin is commonly administered using a special syringe calibrated in units. If the order is for 40 units of insulin, and the available concentration is 80 units per milliliter, the equation would read

$$\frac{100 \text{ units}}{1 \text{ ml}} = \frac{40 \text{ units}}{x}$$

$$x \text{ (100 units)} = \text{(1 ml) (40 units)}$$

$$x = \frac{\text{(1 ml) (40 } \cancel{\text{units}}\text{)}}{\text{(100 } \cancel{\text{units}}\text{)}}$$

$$x = \frac{\text{40 ml}}{100}$$

$$x = \text{0.4 ml}$$

SAMPLE PROBLEMS

17. Dr. K. orders a dose of 600,000 units of penicillin for her patient. The penicillin on hand is 500,000 units/ml. How many milliliters of this preparation will be required?

18. Dr. B. orders 2,500 units of heparin for his patient. The heparin that is available is 5,000 units/ml. How much should be given?
19. Mrs. S. is to be given 75 units of regular insulin by order of her physician. The regular insulin that is on hand is 100 units/ml. The only syringe available is measured in minims. How many minims will be required?

General Guidelines for Administering Medications

Chapter 5 will discuss the legal and ethical responsibilities of the nurse administering drugs. Here we consider some general guidelines before moving on to a discussion of the various routes of administration.

The Five Rights

The nurse is responsible for what are commonly called the **five rights** of drug administration: The nurse must verify that the **right drug** is given to the **right patient** by the **right route** at the **right time** and in the **right dose.** Thus there should be constant attention and repeated checking for accuracy to assure that the correct drug in the correct amount is being prepared for the right client. This means that the nurse preparing to give the drug should not be interrupted in the process. And because the nurse who prepares the medication is legally liable if there is an error, he or she should also be the one to administer it.

Medicines are usually prescribed by a physician, a dentist, or, in some areas, by pharmacists or by family nurse practitioners working with the guidance of a physician. However, the nurse is legally and morally responsible for providing safe care, which includes assuring that the drug prescribed is actually used by the particular client and that the dosage and route of administration are accurate. A nurse who administers a drug based on an erroneous order is legally responsible for any harm that the client experiences. This means, of course, that nurses cannot carry out an order automatically because it is written on a chart. This is especially important in those facilities where medical students practice. Medical students' orders must be countersigned to become legal. It is also important in those facilities where there are a number of interns who may not be entirely knowledgeable about the drugs they are ordering.

Upon approaching the patient, the nurse should ask the individual to state his or her name and check the patient's identification band to assure that the correct person is receiving the medication. While it would seem unlikely that a patient would give a wrong name, some people have been known to do just that, describing it as a "practical joke." Others may not be listening or think that the nurse has forgotten their name. The name provided by the individual, the name on the identification bracelet, and the one on the medicine card should be compared to be certain all contain the same information. In the absence of a name band, the patient's identity must be verified by a third person.

After determining beyond doubt that the patient is the individual for whom the medication is intended, the nurse must assure that the drug being given is the right drug. Nurses must know the abbreviations used for administration instructions (Table 4–2) and for specifying particular medications and laboratory tests (Table 4–3). Nurses must also know how to interpret and explain these terms to patients. The drug card should be compared with the medication sheet, with the card file, and the drug container. The nurse must know the action, dosage, side effects, precautions, and method of administration. If there is a question, information should be obtained before proceeding. If there is no urgency to the drug administration, the nurse should look up the information about the drug. If it is an emergency, he or she should check with the pharmacist or physician and follow through as soon as possible with researching the needed information about drug action, side effects, and expected responses.

To administer drugs safely, nurses must know the classification of the drug, the range of safe dosage, usual methods of administration, and expected therapeutic and adverse responses. This is the ultimate reason why nurses must develop a sound understanding of the pharmacology of the various drugs utilized in clinical practice. Nurses should make certain that medication ordered is appropriate for the client's condition. Nurses are expected to assume ethical, moral, and professional responsibility in carrying out orders for drugs. This means that they must question incomplete orders, illegible orders, and inappropriate orders. They should check to be sure that the drug is compatible with the client's condition and other medications the client may be taking, including over-the-counter drugs, which are often taken without any advice from physicians or pharmacists. Nurses should determine if the client has any history of allergic reactions to the medication or similar agents.

Table 4–2
Abbreviations Commonly Used for Drug Orders

aa	of each
ac	before meals
ad lib	freely, as desired
bid	two times daily
c	with
cap	capsule
d or da	day
dr	dram
elix or el	elixir
ext	extract
g or gm	gram
gr	grain
gtt	drop
h	hour
hs	hour of sleep—bedtime
IM	intramuscular
IV	intravenous
m	minum
ml	milliliter
OD	right eye
o.h.	every hour
o.n.	every night
OS	left eye
os	mouth
OU	both eyes
oz	ounce
p	after
pc	after meals
PO	by mouth
PR	by rectum
PRN	when required
q	every
qd	every day
qh	every hour
qid	four times a day
qod or ADT	every other day
qs	as much as required
s	without
SC or SQ	subcutaneously
sig	indicate on label
sos	one dose if necessary
sp	spirits
ss	one-half
stat	immediately
tab	tablet
T	take one
tid	three times daily
tr or tinct	tincture
ung	ointment

Nurses are often in a position of deciding whether or not to administer a given drug because of a patient's condition or because of the way the patient is responding to the drug. Because nurses work closely with patients and have more frequent contact with them than other members of the health care team, they are in a prime position to detect early indications of adverse reactions and make recommendations to physicians concerning drug dosage, drug choices, or even whether to omit medication. Nurses may recommend reduction in amount of drug to reduce adverse responses or to maximize the benefits. Nurses may be required to administer drugs in emergency situations. To perform these duties appropriately, nurses need knowledge about how drugs are classified, the purposes for which they are used, how they are absorbed and metabolized by the body, the correct dosage, and the margin of safety. Nurses need to understand the local and systemic effects of the drugs being administered, the potential side effects, toxic effects, and synergistic and antagonistic interactions with other medications. They need to understand factors that can modify a patient's therapeutic response to drug therapy and ways of countering adverse responses.

When necessary, the nurse should be prepared to withhold medication from a patient or recommend that the patient refrain from taking medication until he or she has contacted the physician. If a drug dosage is contaminated by whatever means, the nurse must discard the drug and request a replacement from the pharmacy, even though this may result in a delay in administering the drug, possibly upsetting drug schedules for the patient. It may also be necessary to withhold medication due to the patient's status. For example, if a patient's respirations are below 14 per minute, it may be inadvisable to administer a narcotic that will further slow respiration. A patient with a head injury should not receive drugs that will depress respiration because this will prevent the health care team from accurately assessing neurological status by monitoring respiration. In other circumstances, withholding medication designed to relieve pain may be advisable if giving it would hamper diagnosis of the cause of the pain. When medications are withheld in such circumstances, nurses must accurately explain the rationale for denying medications desired by the patient.

The Status of Verbal Orders

If the nurse is giving medications based on verbal orders, he or she should record the order on the patient's chart, including the date and time ordered, the name of the physician, the name of the drug, the name of the client, the amount to be given, the route of administration, the time, the frequency, and any special orders pertaining to the medication. The nurse must make sure the physician signs the order later. Routine orders may be given according to the physician's instructions until the order is cancelled by another order. Such orders can be used for medi-

Table 4–3
Other Abbreviations Used in Drug Therapy

ACh	acetylcholine	MBD	minimal brain dysfunction
ACTH	adrenocorticotropic hormone	μCi (μC)	microcurie
ADH	antidiuretic hormone	mCi (mC)	millicurie
ADT	alternate day therapy	mcg (μg)	microgram
ANA	antinuclear antibodies	mEq	milliequivalent
APTT	activated partial prothrombin time	mic	minimal inhibitory concentration
BSP	bromsulphalein	NAPA	N-acetylprocainamide
BBT	basal body temperature	ng	nanogram
BUN	blood urea nitrogen	NPN	nonprotein nitrogen
BT	bleeding time	NSAID	nonsteroidal antiinflammatory drug
COMT	catechol-O-methyltransferase	NSR	normal sinus rhythm
COPD	chronic obstructive pulmonary disease	17-OHCS	17-hydroxycorticosteroids
CPK	creatinine phosphokinase	OTC	over-the-counter
CSF	cerebrospinal fluid	PABA	para-aminobenzoic acid
CT	clotting time	PAWP	pulmonary artery wedge pressure
CTZ	chemoreceptor trigger zone	PBI	protein bound iodine
CVP	central venous pressure	PPI	patient pellet insert
DL	deciliter (100 ml or cc)	PPT	partial thromboplastin time
EPS	extrapyramidal symptoms	PSP	phenolsulfophthalein
ER	estrogen receptor	PSVT	paroxysmal supraventricular tachycardia
GABA	gamma-aminobutyric acid	PVC	premature ventricular contraction
GFR	glomerular filtration rate	RAI	radioactive iodine
G6PD	glucose-6-phosphate dehydrogenase	RDA	recommended daily allowance
HCG	human chorionic gonadotropin	REM	rapid eye movements
Hct	hematocrit	RTA	renal tubular acidosis
HDL	high-density lipoprotein	SBE	self breast examination
5-HIAA	5-hydroxyindoleacetic acid	SGOT	serum glutamic-oxaloacetic transaminase
HMG	human menopausal gonadotropin	SGPT	serum glutamin-pyruvic transaminase
HPA	hypothalamic-pituitary-adrenocortical	SIADM	syndrome of inappropriate antidiuretic hormone
IOP	intraocular pressure	SLE	systemic lupus erythematosus
IU	international unit	SMA	sequential multiple analysis
IVH	intravenous hyperalimentation	TCA	tricyclic antidepressant
17-KGS	17-ketogenic steroids	TPN	total parenteral nutrition
17-KS	17-ketosteroids	VMA	vanilmandelic acid
LDH	lactic dehydrogenase		
LDL	low-density lipoprotein		
LVEDP	left ventricular end-diastolic pressure		
MAOI	monoamine oxidase inhibitor		

cations to be given when the client needs the medicine (as needed, or prn).

Charting Medications

Medications should be charted only after they have been administered. The nurse should not chart the drug prior to giving it or preparing it, for there is no assurance that the patient will take the medication. Further, since a nursing assessment should precede dispensing of the medication, it is conceivable that the patient's condition does not warrant giving the drug at all or the condition may be such that the dosage of drug should be changed. The patient who has been having pain that required round-the-clock medication may now be responding sufficiently to the medical and nursing therapies so that it may be appropriate either to reduce the drug dosage, change the order to "when needed" (or prn), or to change to a less potent drug.

Each health care facility has its particular system for recording medication administration. However, regardless of the method used or the system followed, all include essentially the same information: the name of the drug, the dosage, route of administration, time of administration, and the name of the administrator. If the drug was injected, the site of injection should be included. If there are to be repeated administrations of the same drug, a diagram may well be included and sites marked as they are used so that rotation of the site can proceed in an orderly manner. If the medication is to be given as needed (prn), the basis for the decision to administer the drug is recorded.

If a patient refuses to take a medication, the nurse should attempt to learn why. The patient may object to the taste, dislike the effect of the drug, or feel there is no need for it. All refusal of drugs, regardless of the identity of the drugs, should be recorded and reported to the physician along with the patient's reasons for refusal.

Some health care units have developed self-administration systems. With this system, drugs are kept at the patient's unit and the individual takes the medication as prescribed. He or she may record this on a special chart provided for the purpose, or the nurse may make rounds to see that the drug(s) have been taken. This method is useful for encouraging people in long-term health care facilities to be responsible for self-care. It also is helpful in teaching patients about self-administration of medications. It provides patients with a feeling of participation and control over their environment. It is obvious, however, that this method is not appropriate for all patients. A patient in the hospital may be too sick to participate in self-care. Whether in a hospital or at home a person may be mentally incompetent and thus unable to participate. Therefore, before instituting the program, the nurse must conduct careful assessment to assure that the individual will be reliable both in self-administration and in self-reporting in the event of adverse drug reactions.

Since many clients will be taking their medications on their own at home, it is extremely important that they understand the significance of adhering to a schedule so that they will not forget to take their drugs as prescribed. Part of nursing management, then, demands that clients be helped to develop a schedule they can adhere to as they assume responsibility for taking their own medications. It also involves educating them as to the symptoms that indicate when they are getting into difficulty. Teaching clients about their medication and their responsibility for self-care helps to assure that their comfort, safety, and survival needs are being met, and promotes personal and social integrity. One method of meeting this obligation is to record nursing observations under headings as indicated in Table 4–4. It is just as important for clients to follow a planned pattern of assessment and evaluation of drug therapy as it is for nurses. Providing a sample chart along with explanations of terms encourages clients to become knowledgeable reporters of their condition and responses to therapy.

Topical Administration

Drugs can be administered topically to any externally accessible tissue. Drugs can be topically applied with success to the skin, cornea, respiratory tract, or mucosal membranes of the mouth, nose, throat, external ear canal, conjunctiva, vagina, uterus, urethra, or rectum. A variety of dosage forms are available for topical applications, including lotions, creams, ointments, liniments, gels, foams, aerosols, plasters, powders, tinctures, drops, solutions, inhalants, and nebulizers.

Administration to the Skin

Semisolid preparations are often selected for application to the skin. **Creams** are water-soluble preparations usually applied by rubbing the preparations into the skin. They are often used as moisturizers for dry skin. **Ointments** are applied similarly but are oily or fatty suspensions of drugs. The most commonly used ointment bases are lanolin and petrolatum. Because of the low solubility of these bases in water, they are not easily washed away by water or sweat.

Table 4–4
Sample Chart for Nursing Assessment or Self-Assessment of Clients

	Client Status		
Client Needs	Physical status	Emotional status	Social status
Affiliative needs			
Comfort needs			
Developmental needs			
Physiological needs			
Safety needs			
Survival needs			
Self-actualization needs			
Social esteem needs			

Ointments that are especially thick and viscous and that do not soften substantially from body heat are called **pastes.** Pastes are absorbed into the skin to a lesser extent than other topical dosage forms. **Gels,** aqueous suspensions of hydrated particles, are sometimes applied topically to the skin. **Lotions** are aqueous suspensions of drugs, and should be dabbed, not rubbed, onto the skin. **Liniments** are thinner than ointments, consisting of fluid mixtures of drugs with water, oil, soap, and other constituents. Liniments are applied by rubbing and are often marketed expressly for use in body rubs or massages. Liniments often contain rubefacients (or counterirritants) such as methyl salicylate, or topical anesthetics.

Plasters and **powders** are solid dosage forms applied to the skin. Plasters usually have a rubber mixture as their base. They soften in response to body heat and thus tend to adhere to the skin. Powders usually consist of fine mineral dusts, such as talc, and are applied by dusting. They are usually employed to absorb moisture from the skin, thereby altering conditions favorable to growth of microorganisms. **Patches,** another solid dosage form for application to the skin, are used to provide gradual transfer of drug from the patch to the skin, usually for drugs that will be absorbed through the skin to provide systemic effects.

Tinctures are solutions of drugs in alcohol. They are often applied to the skin by painting. **Aerosols** are used for topical application of drugs to both the skin and the respiratory tract. Aerosols consist of liquids applied under air pressure as sprays. **Foams** are aerated semisolid preparations applied under pressure in a manner similar to aerosols. **Baths** and **soaks** provide thorough and direct contact of the skin with water or other fluids for a limited time period.

Drugs applied topically to the skin, called **dermatologics,** are typically employed for their local effects, but systemic absorption may occur to a lesser or greater extent. Factors influencing absorption include formulation characteristics, application parameters, and characteristics of the skin at the site of application. For example, rubbing or massaging the skin creates friction, dilates the capillaries, increases flow of blood to the surface of the skin, and enhances absorption of topically applied agents. Nurses should also realize that local application to damaged or denuded skin can result in systemic absorption. The factors influencing absorption of drugs applied topically to the skin are addressed more fully in Chapter 53.

Dermatologics are used for a wide variety of purposes. The dermatologics include antiacne drugs, antiseptics, antibacterial agents, antifungals, anti-inflammatory drugs, antipruritics, antisporiatics, drugs for herpes simplex, burn products, sunburn products, emollients, dusting powders, local anesthetics, and scabicides. All of these agents are discussed in Chapter 53.

Before applying skin preparations, the nurse needs to assess the client for open lesions, rashes, known allergies, or changes in the skin resulting from use of other local agents. Unless specifically contraindicated, the skin at the site of application should be cleansed with soap and water and dried before applying the medication. Methods of application depend upon the consistency of the drug preparation and the reason it is being prescribed. Ointments may be applied with a tongue blade, finger, or gauze pad. The nurse should apply lotions or liniments with gauze, using firm, gentle pressure. Application of a dressing to prevent inadvertent spreading or removal of the drug may be necessary. After application, the nurse should watch for skin irritation, burning sensations, and allergic responses. If the client is to apply the medication at home, the nurse should teach appropriate methods for application and self-assessment.

Administration to Mucosal Membranes

Drug preparations commonly applied to mucosal membranes include ointments, creams, and drops. Drugs may be applied directly or indirectly to the mucosal surfaces of the urethra, vagina, conjunctiva, nose, oropharynx, rectum, or mouth. Absorption usually occurs readily from mucosal membranes. Drugs applied to mucosal membranes therefore have both local and systemic activity. The various mucosal membranes differ in sensitivity to irritation by drugs.

The mucosal membrane surfaces of the mouth are routinely in contact with a wide range of substances, including foods and dentifrices and have considerable tolerance for even highly concentrated dosage forms of drugs. Gargles and mouthwashes are sometimes used for application of substances to the oral membranes. Lozenges are sometimes placed under the tongue (**sublingually**) or between the cheek and gum (**buccally**) for absorption through mucosal surfaces.

The **nasal mucosa** are somewhat more delicate than the oral mucosa. Maximum tolerable drug concentrations are typically half what can be safely applied to the oral mucosa. Mucosal membranes of the eye and urethra are the most sensitive in the body and tolerate only dilute drug formulations.

Drugs are sometimes applied to the mucosal membranes of the vagina in the form of **vaginal suppositories.** Vaginal suppositories are usually supplied with an applicator to facilitate easy and effective insertion. Prior to administering the medication, the woman should be assisted into a supine position with her knees elevated. A draw sheet or bath blanket should be placed over her abdomen and upper torso, exposing only the vaginal area. The vulva should be spread gently; any excessive vaginal discharge should be wiped away and any accumulations on the vulva removed prior to inserting the applicator.

In instilling the suppository, the nurse should use sterile technique to avoid introducing microorganisms into the vagina. These could spread to the uterus and be lethal. If the client is going to insert vaginal suppositories herself, the nurse should teach her proper methods of instillation. In inserting the suppository the nurse or client should take care to touch only the distal tip that does not enter the vagina. If the applicator is not prelubricated, sterile petroleum jelly may be used. The first drop of jelly should be discarded before dropping lubricant onto the applicator. The applicator should then be inserted and directed downward toward the client's back, following the anatomical slant of the vagina. Following the procedure, any excess lubricant should be wiped with sterile gauze. The client should be encouraged to lie flat on her back for 15 minutes to assure that the suppository is not expelled. Ambulatory patients should be instructed to wear a sanitary pad to avoid drainage and staining of garments.

Inhalation and Insufflation

Drugs can be administered to the respiratory tract for either topical or systemic purposes. Both liquids and gases can be administered by inhalation. General anesthetics that are gaseous or volatile liquids and therapeutic gases, such as oxygen and carbon dioxide, are conveniently administered in this manner. Liquids are administered by inhalation either by use of a nebulizer or in the form of aerosols. Fine powders can also be administered to the respiratory tract, by blowing or spraying into the nose, a method of application called insufflation. The respiratory mucosa provides a large surface for absorption. In addition, the lungs are designed to permit exchange of materials between the air in the lungs and the blood. Therefore, drugs administered to the lungs by insufflation or inhalation will be substantially absorbed and will produce systemic effects. Nurses must assess clients carefully to be certain there is no adverse condition that would preclude the use of inhalants. When treatment is undertaken, the nurse will need to supply clients with specific information concerning the appropriate means of using drugs by inhalation or insufflation since these methods of application are not commonly understood by clients. Procedures for administration of beta-agonists and cromolyn (Intal, Nasalcrom) by inhalation are discussed in Chapter 52.

Ocular Instillations

The usual dosage forms for topical administration to the eyes are drops and ointments. Drops are solutions or, less commonly, suspensions, that are instilled in the eye by use of a dropper. Ophthalmic solutions and suspensions must be kept sterile. Ointments are usually placed on the inner mucosal surface of the lower eye lid or in the conjunctival sac in the inner canthus. Care must be taken to avoid trauma to the eye when installing ophthalmic medications. The tip of the dropper should not come in contact with the eye or the lid. Special care is required when the recipient of the medication is a child, because children are prone to rapid head movements. The hand holding the dropper should rest on the client's head so that the dropper will move synchronously with any head movements (Figure 4–1). Refrigerated drops should be warmed to room temperature before application to minimize reflex movements of the lids or head that might be caused by the cold.

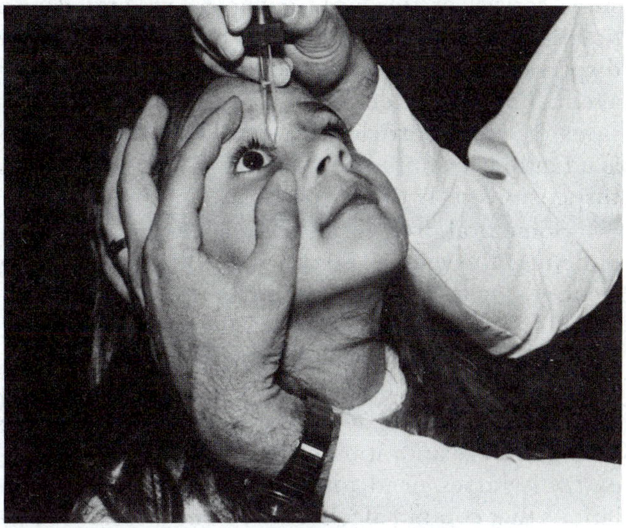

Figure 4–1
Proper technique for instillation of eye, ear, or nose drops into a child. The hand holding the dropper must rest firmly on the child's head, so that in the event of any rapid head movement, the dropper will move with it. The other hand is used to hold the head firmly and the eye (or ear or nose) in position to receive the drops.

Enteral Administration

Enteral administration is administration via the alimentary tract for systemic purposes. It includes the oral, rectal, sublingual, and buccal routes. Each of these routes is also rarely used for topical application of drugs to the mucosal membranes of the alimentary tract, but usually these routes are employed for systemic drug applications.

Oral Administration

Oral administration of drugs is the most convenient and most frequently used route. It is also generally the least expensive and safest method. However, nurses need to be aware that some clients (particularly the very young and elderly) find it difficult to swallow tablets or capsules and this needs to be determined before administration. Oral dosage forms include both solid and liquid formulations. Solid oral preparations include tablets and capsules. Capsules consist of powders or liquids in a gelatin container. They cannot be reliably divided. Tablets are complex formulations containing various fillers in addition to the active drug. The influence of tablet constituents other than the active chemical on disintegration and absorption of drugs from tablets was discussed in Chapter 3. Tablets are sometimes "scored" to aid in subdividing the tablets to achieve intermediate doses. Some tablets or capsules have enteric coating, which resists dissolution in the acid medium of the stomach. Enteric coated medications must not be crushed prior to administration and the client should be told not to chew them and not to take them with hot liquids.

Liquid dosage forms for oral administration include solutions, syrups, suspensions (including emulsions, magmas, and gels), spirits, elixirs, and extracts. **Solutions** consist of substances dissolved in water. **Syrups** are sugar solutions used as vehicles for various drugs. Syrups, especially if flavored, provide a means of disguising ill-tasting medications. **Suspensions** consist of fine drug particles suspended in a liquid vehicle. **Emulsions** consist of a lipid substance dispersed in water by the action of an emulsifying agent. **Magmas,** often called milks, are thick suspensions of white particles in water. Milk of magnesia is a familiar example of a magma. **Gels** are aqueous suspensions of hydrated particles.

Some oral drug forms include alcohol as a component of the vehicle. **Elixirs** are vehicles containing alcohol, sugar, and water. **Spirits** are alcohol solutions of volatile substances. **Tinctures** consist of drugs dissolved in alcohol or alcohol and water. **Fluid extracts** are liquid extracts, typically in alcohol, of drugs from plant or animal sources. **Extracts** are obtained by evaporation of the vehicle from a fluidextract. Nurses need to be aware that oral formulations that contain alcohol are sometimes abused by alcohol troubled individuals; some have been known to drink entire bottles of medication, thereby becoming inebriated and simultaneously overdosing on the other drug(s) contained in the formulation.

After oral administration, absorption of drugs occurs mainly from the small intestines, but the stomach and bowel participate to a lesser extent. Oral administration typically provides slower onset and more prolonged action than when drugs are given parenterally. Effects of some drugs are variable after oral administration because of the variety of factors that can influence absorption from the alimentary tract (see Chapter 3). Prior to the administration of oral preparations, the nurse must consider and advise clients about any special requirements regarding when the medication is to be given in relation to food or fluid intake or particular foods that must be avoided. In addition to the delay and the variability in drug action associated with the oral route, other disadvantages include risks of irritation to the gastric or intestinal mucosa, occurrence of gastrointestinal side effects such as nausea, vomiting, or cramps, and unpleasant odor or taste of the drug.

Sublingual and Buccal Administration

Relatively few systemic drugs are given by these routes. Nitroglycerin, however, is commonly employed by sublingual administration. Placed under the tongue, a tablet of nitroglycerin rapidly disintegrates and is absorbed quickly through the thin epithelium into the blood vessels on the underside of the tongue. One advantage of this route is that the drug enters the systemic circulation without the first-pass liver extraction that occurs when drugs are absorbed from the intestines. Another advantage is that any residual part of the dosage can be expelled when target symptoms are alleviated or if significant adverse effects appear.

When applying drugs sublingually, it is important that the nurse first examine the area under the tongue to assure that it is healthy. The client should be instructed to put the medication under the tongue but not to take any fluids. The medication should remain under the tongue until it is dissolved. When working with senile or retarded clients, it is important that the nurse check the client's mouth to assure the drug is in place and that the nurse remain with the client until the drug has dissolved.

Rectal Suppositories

Suppositories are mixtures of drugs in a base, such as cocoa butter, that is solid at room temperature but which melts at body temperature and dissolves in the body fluids. Suppositories can be molded to appropriate shapes for insertion into a body cavity, usually the rectum or vagina. Small suppositories, called **bougies,** are made for insertion into the urethra. Rectal administration is usually reserved for circumstances when oral administration cannot be employed because of gastrointestinal trauma or irritation, or for drugs that would be digested or are especially ill-tasting. The rectal route may be a suitable substitute for oral administration in comatose patients. It is usually advisable to evacuate the rectum by enema before administering drugs by the rectal route. Otherwise, the entire dose may become encapsulated in feces and excreted without absorption. Nurses are usually advised to insert the suppository to the length of the finger beyond the anal sphincter to assure the drug's position against the rectal wall. Once the suppository has been inserted, the nurse should hold the client's buttocks together for a few minutes to aid the client in retaining the drug.

It is extremely important that nurses use gentle pressure when inserting rectal medications, especially if the client has hemorrhoidal tissues, since these can be extremely painful. Also, nurses should be aware that clients feel embarrassed by having rectal medications administered. It is therefore important to provide as much privacy as possible when performing the procedure and to expose only the buttock area when inserting the drug.

The nurse needs to observe the client closely for evidence of mucosal irritation when rectal medications are used. At times, some drugs so irritate the rectal mucosa that the client feels he or she needs to defecate. If a client complains of needing to go to the bathroom more frequently, or if the nurse observes this behavior, she or he should suspect mucosal irritation.

Parenteral Administration

Parenteral administration means literally "not through the gastrointestinal tract." In modern usage, it is reserved for administration of drugs by hypodermic injection or intravenous catheter for systemic effects. Drugs given parenterally must be sterile in order not to introduce pathogenic organisms into the body fluids. The drug must be at least slowly absorbable from the site of administration and at least somewhat soluble in fluids bathing the site of administration. In comparison to oral administration, parenteral routes usually provide for a more rapid onset of action and more rapid termination of effect. Depot injections are an exception, providing slow, sustained absorption of drug from an intramuscular site of injection.

Parenteral doses of drugs are usually lower than oral doses because 100% of an injected dose is ultimately absorbed whereas absorption after oral administration is often less than complete. The ratio between effective oral and intramuscular doses is often taken as an index of oral effectiveness of a given drug. For example, codeine, with a 3 : 2 ratio of orally to intramuscularly effective doses is said to be orally effective while morphine, with a 6 : 1 ratio, is said to have poor oral effectiveness. Parenteral administration is indicated in preference to oral administration for drugs that are poorly absorbed from the alimentary tract, digestible by enzymes within the stomach or intestines, or especially irritating to the gastrointestinal mucosa. Parenteral administration is often required when a rapid effect is needed.

For several reasons, the cost of parenteral administration of drugs is greater than that of oral administration. The drugs themselves must be sterile and provided in special containers (vials, ampuls, or preloaded syringes) that maintain sterility. Parenteral administration of drugs usually requires the aid of specially trained personnel to ensure that the injection is administered safely and effectively. Exceptions occur in conditions such as insulin-dependent diabetes mellitus for which patients are frequently trained to self-administer the therapeutic agent by injection. The exact roles of the nurse and the physician in parenteral administration of drugs vary from one medical facility to another. In general, nurses administer many of the drugs given parenterally, but a few drugs, for example, *d*-tubocurarine, are given only by the physician. Regardless of who administers the drug, it is the nurse's responsibility to monitor the efficacy and report any unusual side effects.

Injections are performed with a syringe and needle. Syringes consist of a hollow barrel that holds the fluid that is to be administered and a plunger that forces the fluid through the needle. Syringes made of glass are reusable but must be sterilized before each use. Glass syringes have generally been replaced by disposable plastic syringes, which are sterilized and sealed in an envelope or plastic wrap. Selection of an appropriate needle is an important step in preparing for an injection. Needles employed for injections are classified by **gauge,** or diameter. Needle gauges that are encountered clinically range from 14 to 28. The larger the number of the gauge, the smaller the diameter of the needle. Drug formulations that are viscous or that contain suspended particles must be given through needles of larger diameter (low gauge number). Intramuscular injections require needles that are longer than those used for subcutaneous or intradermal injections.

Before a solution is withdrawn from a vial or ampul, a volume of air equal to the volume of drug to be withdrawn must be injected into the container. Otherwise, a negative pressure develops in the container and will interfere with filling of the syringe. After injecting the appropriate volume of air, the container is inverted, the tip of the needle is immersed in the fluid, and the designated volume of solution is drawn into the syringe by drawing back on the plunger.

Prior to any parenteral injection, the nurse should assess the condition of the site to be used for administration. The area should be checked for lesions, rash, inflammation, lipid dystrophy, or ecchymosis (a form of macula that appears as a large, irregularly formed hemorrhagic area on the skin). Nurses need to assess for evidence of prior tissue damage from other injections and past history of allergic reactions.

Parenteral administration of drugs requires special care. Techniques for withdrawing a drug dosage from a vial or ampul are illustrated in Figure 4–2. Nurses should practice rigorous aseptic technique. Tablets or powders used in making up parenteral solutions must not be allowed to come into contact with the hands before dissolving. Similarly, the parts of the hypodermic syringe — needle, plunger, and inside of the barrel — must remain sterile. For intravenous injections, single-dose containers are always utilized in order to avoid contamination. The surface of the skin at the site of injection or infusion should be cleansed with an antiseptic agent.

Clients are often fearful of receiving injections, or "shots." The nurse should explain the reason for parenteral administration of the drug and provide reassurance if the client shows undue anxiety.

Accurate drug dosage, always a matter of impor-

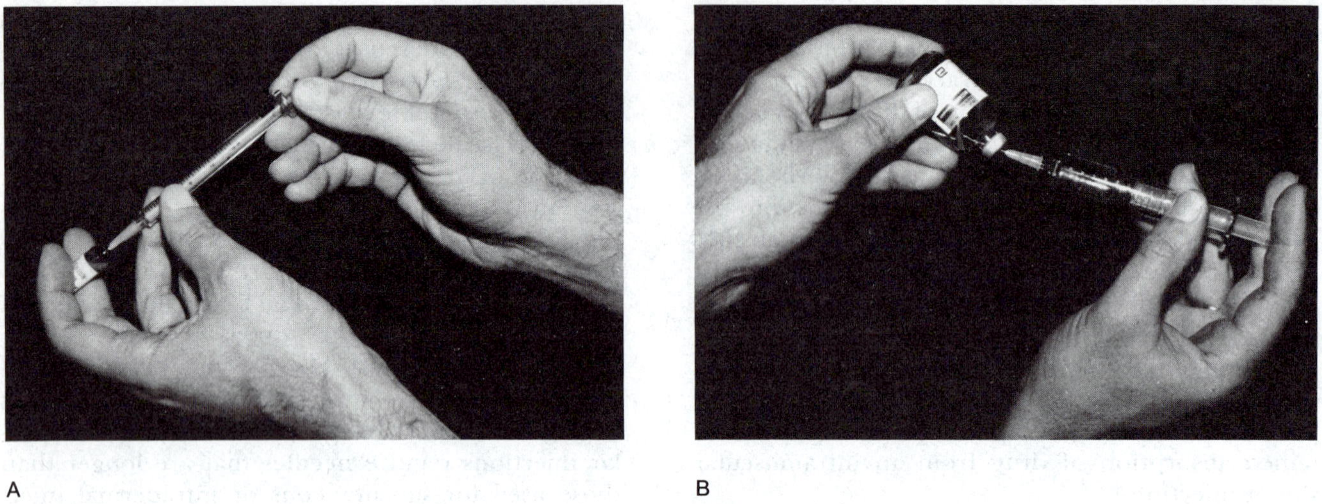

Figure 4–2
Technique for withdrawing medication from an ampul (A) or vial (B). When withdrawing medication from a stoppered vial, an equal volume of air is first injected into the vial.

tance, is especially crucial when drugs are given parenterally. Injected drugs are irretrievable since there are no techniques equivalent to gastric lavage or emesis for eliminating the unabsorbed portion of an administered dose. In the following sections, consideration is given to six common parenteral routes of administration: intradermal injection, subcutaneous injection, intramuscular injection, intraarticular injection, intravenous injection, and intravenous infusion. Seldom used parenteral routes requiring special techniques will not be discussed: intraspinal, intraventricular, and intraperitoneal injections.

Intradermal Injection

Intradermal injections are injections into the upper layers of the skin (Figure 4–3A). This is the most superficial form of parenteral administration. Absorption of drug is slow. Intradermal injections are limited to small volumes of drug. Intradermal injections are commonly employed in conducting skin patch tests to determine allergic sensitivities. Fine, short needles and small-barrelled syringes are used. The back and the medial surface of the forearm are frequently employed sites for intradermal injections. The needle is inserted immediately below the skin surface and the fluid is injected to form a small pocket, or wheal.

Subcutaneous Administration

Subcutaneous (SC or SQ) administration is simple but provides considerable variability in drug effect. Drugs introduced subcutaneously should be nonirri-

Figure 4–3
Injections: intradermal, subcutaneous, intramuscular.

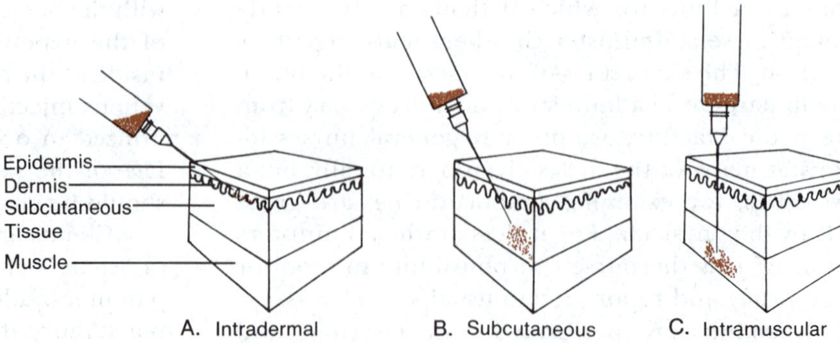

tating. Usually they are highly soluble. The drug is injected into the subcutaneous layer of fatty and connective tissue that underlies the skin (Figure 4–3B). Common sites for SC injections are the upper part of the arms, the thighs, and the abdomen. The skin at the site of injection should be cleansed with an antiseptic, and the needle (usually 25-gauge and $\frac{3}{8}$ to $\frac{5}{8}$ inches in length) is usually inserted at an angle of about 45 degrees. The hypodermic syringe should be aspirated after insertion and before injection of the drug to ensure that the tip of the needle is not in a blood vessel. Aspiration consists of drawing back the plunger slowly and slightly. If blood is drawn into the barrel, the syringe should be withdrawn, a new solution prepared, and the needle inserted into an alternative site. The site of injection is gently massaged after completing an SC injection to stimulate blood flow and drug absorption. Usually, the volume of injection should be less than 2 ml when the SC route is used. Absorption is slow and dependent on local perfusion and the lipid solubility of the drug. Subcutaneous administration is usually undesirable when peripheral circulation is compromised or when drugs are highly irritating to the tissues.

Nurses should observe the site of injection for evidence of impaired circulation, scar tissue, or hardened areas from previous subcutaneous injections that might affect the rate of absorption. If a repeated series of injections is to be used, a written plan should be established to assure that sites are rotated systematically.

The absorption and dispersion of drugs administered subcutaneously can be improved by coadministration of the drug **hyaluronidase** (Wydase). This enzyme hydrolyzes hyaluronic acid, a constituent of subcutaneous fat that obstructs diffusion of injected or invasive substances. Hyaluronidase promotes rapid spreading of coadministered drugs and hence more rapid absorption. Usually 150 units of hyaluronidase are added to an injection solution. Adverse reactions to hyaluronidase consist of occasional hypersensitivity reactions and effects attributable to overly rapid absorption of coadministered drugs (for example, hypovolemia from hypotonic injection solutions, hypertension from epinephrine). Hyaluronidase is provided as a lyophilized powder (150 units/1 ml vial or 1,500 units/10 ml vial) or as an injection solution (150 units/ml in 1 or 10 ml vials).

Sometimes it is desirable to slow absorption of a drug after SC administration if the desired locus of action is limited to the site of administration. Thus, epinephrine is often employed with local anesthetics given subcutaneously to constrict blood vessels at the site of injection and thus to slow absorption and prolong the action of the local anesthetic. Similarly, insulin may be given in a colloidal suspension or heparin in a gelatin solution to slow absorption of these drugs after SC injection.

Intramuscular Injection

The intramuscular (IM) injection route provides good versatility. Drugs that would be too irritating if given subcutaneously can often be given intramuscularly without difficulty. Drugs with only slight solubility may be suspended and administered intramuscularly. IM injection of drugs ensures that they will not be counteracted by food, digestive juices, or malabsorption. The IM route is indicated for injection of volumes of drug in excess of 2 ml, the upper limit for subcutaneous injections.

Next to intravenous administration, intramuscular injection provides the most rapid onset of action. The rate of absorption after IM injection is, however, highly dependent on tissue perfusion and will be exceedingly slow if circulatory collapse or shock has occurred. Because drugs are usually rapidly absorbed after IM injection, clients receiving drugs by this route need to be monitored with special care to assure that any adverse reactions are quickly detected and reported.

Intramuscular injections are less likely to cause pain at the site of injection than are SC or intradermal injections because pain receptors are less abundant in muscle than in skin. There is less risk of tissue necrosis with IM administration. Nevertheless, the nurse should watch for any unusual redness at the site of injection or generalized skin responses and report these to the physician immediately.

Needles employed for IM injections are selected in relation to the site of injection and the liquid being injected. The length of the needle is determined by the site of administration. Needles $\frac{5}{8}$–1 inch long are appropriate for deltoid injections. Needles 1–1.5 inch long are usually appropriate for gluteal injections, but needles as long as 3 inches may be required for obese patients. The needle diameter for intramuscular injections ranges from gauge 20 to gauge 25. Large-diameter needles (lower gauge numbers) are required for oily solutions and suspensions in oil or water. Smaller needles (higher gauge numbers) are sufficient for aqueous solutions. Injection volumes up to 2 ml are appropriate in the deltoid area; larger volumes up to about 5 ml can be given in the gluteal area.

For IM injections, the needle is inserted through the dermis into the underlying muscle at an angle of 90 degrees (Figure 4–3C). The exact site of injection must be carefully selected. Techniques for selection of appropriate sites will be demonstrated to you as part of your clinical experience.

The three most frequently used sites for IM injections are illustrated in Figure 4–4. Injection into the deltoid muscle (Figure 4–4A) should be carried out only after careful selection of the site, ensuring that bone, blood vessels, and nerves are avoided. The middle third of the lateral aspect of the deltoid muscle is used. The deltoid muscle has substantially greater perfusion than the gluteal muscle and is therefore the area of choice for most intramuscular injections. However, the volume of injection should not exceed 2 ml.

The two preferred sites in the gluteal muscle are (1) the **dorsogluteal site** — the upper, outer quadrant of the gluteus maximus muscle or the gluteus medius muscle (Figure 4–4B) — and (2) the **ventrogluteal site** — the lateral portion of the gluteus medius muscle or the gluteus minimus muscle (Figure 4–4C). The fleshy portion of the gluteus maximus muscle, though it may seem a likely site for injection, can be a risky site because the sciatic nerve runs diagonally under this area. The exact position of the sciatic nerve varies from one individual to another, so there is a risk of damaging the nerve, possibly producing permanent leg paralysis. When injections are made into the gluteus medius muscle, the nurse should instruct clients to report immediately any pain or burning sensations at sites other than where the needle is inserted. This information is important because it may indicate that the material is being injected at a point close to the sciatic nerve. Uninformed clients have been known to assume that such burning sensations, even when extending down the leg, are expected consequences of the injection.

The ventrogluteal site has the advantage of being relatively distant from major blood vessels and nerves. In addition, the injection can be made with the patient sitting or prone, on his back or on his side. A commonly employed method is to have the patient lie prone, with the head turned to one side, and a pillow under the legs below the knees. Relaxation of the gluteal muscle can be promoted by having the client point his or her toe inward.

When injecting a drug into an adult who has well-developed muscles, the nurse may elect either to spread the area, making the skin over the muscle taut, or pick up the muscle. If the client is elderly, thin, or emaciated, the nurse should draw the skin taut over the area rather than attempting to pick up the muscle since this latter approach makes penetration into the muscle difficult and painful. After insertion, the hypodermic syringe should be aspirated. If blood enters the syringe, a new solution and site should be prepared.

For drugs known to be irritating or staining to the skin, a **Z-track injection** method can be employed. In this procedure, the skin is stretched to one side before injection. After removal of the needle, the skin will rebound and the track through the skin will be out of line with the track into the muscle, preventing reflux of drug. The site of injec-

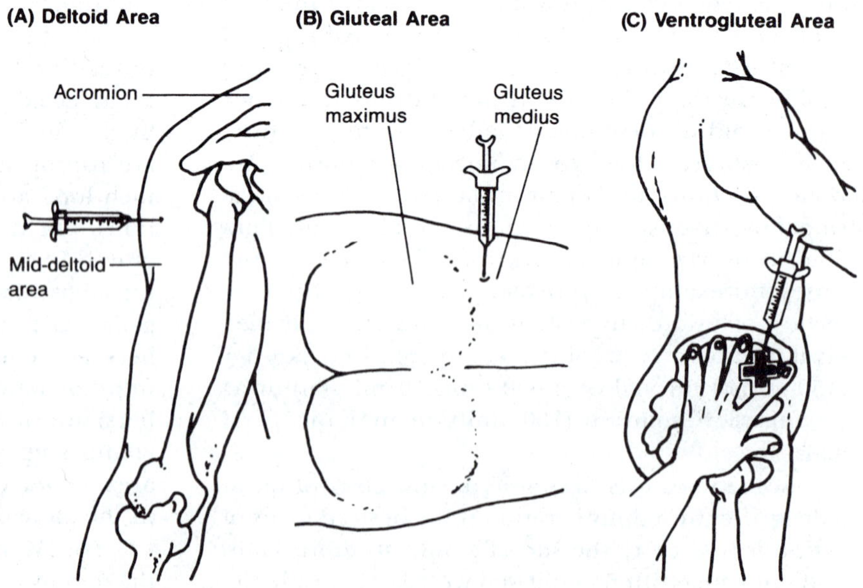

Figure 4–4
Common sites for intramuscular injection: (A) the deltoid muscle, (B) the dorsogluteal site, (C) the ventrogluteal site.

tion is not massaged in this method. The Z-track method is employed for injection of iron salts and for necrotizing or highly irritating substances.

In giving IM injections, the nurse should prepare the client by explaining what is to be done, where the nurse proposes to inject the material, and why this particular method has been chosen. Before proceeding, the nurse should give the client an opportunity to participate in the decision. The client may know of an anatomical anomaly that would necessitate using another site for injection. Or the client may already have had a number of injections at the proposed site and may feel that another injection there would be intolerable. If this is the case, the nurse might ask the client to suggest a preferable site. This kind of opportunity for choice helps to assure conservation of dignity, acknowledges client autonomy, and tends to gain client cooperation.

After a site has been selected, the nurse should inspect it for skin lesions, hardened, lumpy areas, discomfort, heat, redness, bruises, unusual texture, or discoloration. Just prior to inserting the needle, the nurse should tell the client what to expect. If the material to be injected tends to burn or sting, advise the client of this. Providing truthful information can be especially important when dealing with children. A child who knows in advance that something might hurt will be more cooperative than one who receives no information or who has been lied to previously. The tone of voice employed by the nurse is also important: a relaxed, quiet tone suggests confidence and reassures the individual.

Pain associated with injections is due to penetration of the skin and stretching of tissue to accommodate the injected fluid. Proper injection technique minimizes the pain of needle penetration (Figure 4–5). Touching the areas to be injected prior to needle insertion and keeping one hand on the skin (either as it is held taut or picked up) seem to help clients psychologically. Another technique is to ask the client to take a deep breath and hold it. This may help the client relax.

Oily suspensions or solutions and aqueous suspensions injected intramuscularly produce a drug depot from which the drug is only gradually absorbed. This method can be used to produce effects lasting up to several weeks. Examples of drugs given in this manner include fluphenazine (Prolixin), esters of steroids, and poorly soluble salts of penicillin. One hazard is that oily vehicles are sometimes not completely absorbed and may have to be removed by incision and drainage. Also, if an allergic reaction should occur, supportive treatment may have to be continued for several weeks.

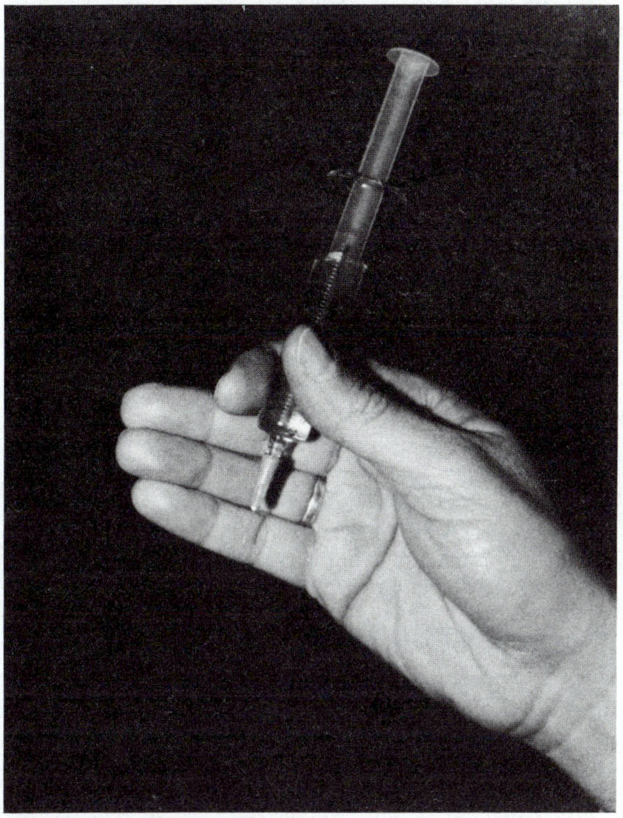

Figure 4–5
Proper technique for making an injection. With the syringe held in this manner, the side of the hand strikes the taut skin a fraction of a second before the needle so that the prick of the needle is almost imperceptible.

Intraarticular Injection

Intraarticular injections (Figure 4–6) are used mainly for administration of steroidal anti-inflammatory drugs. This method of application increases the fraction of the administered dose reaching the required site of action for relieving joint inflammation and pain. Although systemic distribution ultimately occurs, the ratio between therapeutic effects on the joint and adverse systemic effects is considerably improved. The use of this route for administration of corticosteroids is discussed in Chapter 45.

Intravenous Injection

Intravenous (IV) injections, also called IV push or bolus injection, provide rapid delivery of drug, control over the bioavailable dose, and rapid onset of

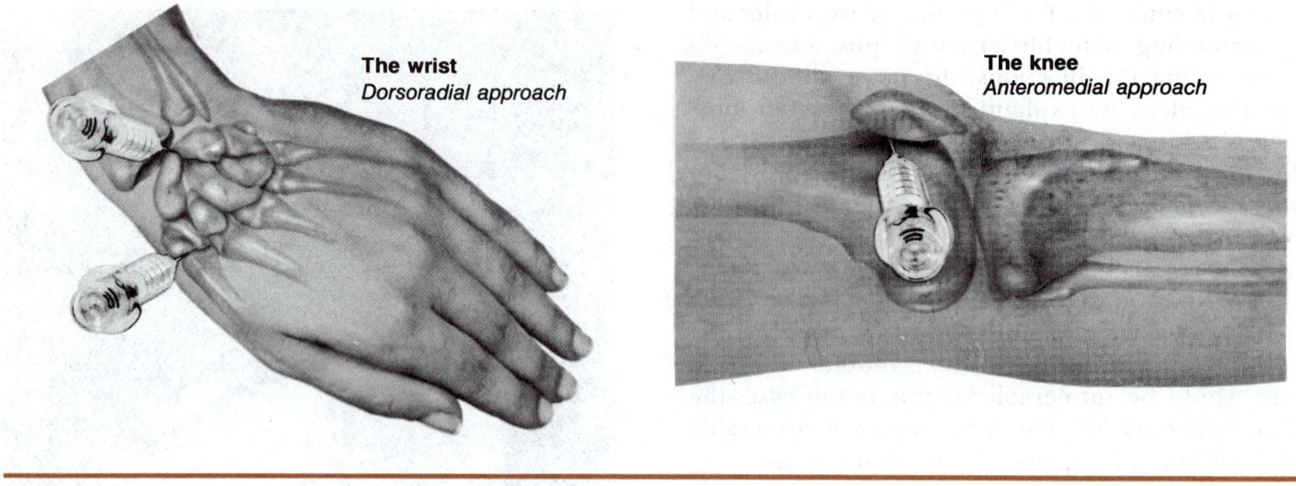

Figure 4–6
Examples of intraarticular injection. From *Complete Manual of Therapy with the Meti-Steroids.* Reproduced with the permission of Schering Corporation, Kenilworth, New Jersey 07033, Copyright © 1956 Schering Corporation. All Rights Reserved.

therapeutic benefit. The intravenous route is also the most potentially hazardous. The nurse must be alert to the patient's condition before, during, and after IV injections because of the rapidity of response to medication administered by this route. Strict asepsis must be observed. All drugs given intravenously must be highly soluble and able to survive techniques for sterilization. Vehicles for intravenous injection must be isotonic (usually saline or 5% dextrose).

Before an intravenous injection is undertaken, the nurse should have a clear idea of how rapidly the injection is to be conducted. Typically drugs are given over a 1–3 minute period, but some drugs are ineffective if given this slowly. Overly rapid delivery of large volumes can lead to embolisms, pulmonary edema, elevated blood pressure, or excessive pharmacological responses. Intravenous injections may be given directly into a vein or through a previously established cannulation. The most frequently used veins for injection are the median cephalic and median basilic veins, located on the inner surface of the elbow. A tourniquet is applied tightly around the middle of the arm in order to distend the vein. The needle is introduced pointing proximally (toward the heart). The site is aspirated — a few drops of blood are drawn back into the syringe — to ensure that proper placement in the vein has occurred. The tourniquet is removed prior to injection and the solution is pushed in at the appropriate rate, usually slowly.

Care should be taken in performing IV injections to avoid extravasation of fluid into the surrounding tissue. Many drugs given intravenously are irritating to cutaneous and subcutaneous tissue. The site of injection should be observed for indications of swelling or infiltration during injection and inflammation following injection.

Intravenous Fluid Therapy

Intravenous infusions provide a means of delivering larger volumes of fluids than could be administered conveniently by injection. Up to 1,000 ml can be given over each 8 hours of infusion. Water, electrolytes, and minerals can be given by intravenous infusion to correct abnormalties and to meet both basal and special requirements. Infusions are most commonly employed for four purposes: (1) to correct hypovolemia, disturbances of osmolarity, or acid-base imbalance, (2) to dilute toxins in the blood and other body fluids, (3) to administer electrolytes, nutrients, or drugs, and (4) to provide an emergency line for rapid drug administration. Normal saline and 5% dextrose solution are the two most commonly used fluids for IV infusions. The electrolyte and nutrient preparations commonly added are described in appropriate sections of Chapters 42 and 44. This section will address some principles of IV fluid therapy.

Mechanics of Intravenous Infusions

Infusions are used when fluids, electrolytes, nutrients, or drugs are to be given in large volume, slowly, or to achieve a steady plasma concentration. Infusions may be set up and run slowly to provide an IV line if a need for rapid drug administration or fluid adjustment is anticipated. The usual maximum flow rate is 1 liter over 8 hours, but actual flow rate depends on the therapeutic objective, patient's condition, and the nature of the fluid. For children, maximum flow rates are less and are determined by age and weight.

Flow is maintained either by gravity or an infusion pump. In the former case, the fluid is contained in a graduated bottle or bag that is elevated and connected by a plastic tube to the IV needle or catheter. Infusion pumps provide more precise and sophisticated control of fluid delivery but are expensive and require regular maintenance. Infusion pumps are routine for patients on total parenteral nutrition (see Chapter 44).

Infusion needles consist of either stainless steel scalp-vein needles or plastic cannulae (or catheters). Stainless steel needles are less likely to cause infection or phlebitis, but plastic cannulae are less likely to permit infiltration. Cannulae are generally selected if infusion is anticipated for an extended period of time.

Particulate matter and microorganisms may find their way into IV solutions in spite of well-intended precautions. These pose a real hazard for the patient, contributing to infection, phlebitis, and clotting. In-line filtering devices are used to eliminate or reduce such contaminants. Filters are available with varying pore sizes. A 5 μm filter removes gross particles, a 0.5 μm filter retains fungi, bacteria, and most particles, and a 0.22 μm filter (a so-called sterilizing filter) will remove all particulate matter and microorganisms except viruses and Pseudomonas.

The usual base solutions for IV infusions are normal saline or 5% dextrose. Both of these are approximately isotonic with plasma. Alternatives include dextran (a plasma expander) or multiple salt solutions such as Ringer's. To these base infusion fluids can be added single salt solutions, amino acids, fats, vitamins, and trace elements for total parenteral nutrition (see Chapters 42 and 44). When a drug is added to an intravenous fluid, care must be taken to ensure that the drug and solution are compatible. If a precipitate is observed to form, infusion must be immediately terminated and the solution discarded.

Pharmacokinetics

Intravenous infusions have the special advantage of providing a means of achieving a constant concentration of an electrolyte or other drug in the plasma. A steady blood level is the ideal for many therapeutic situations, but it is a goal seldom achieved by any other technique of drug administration. Even with IV infusion, plasma levels will be constant only if the rate of infusion is constant and only when the plateau concentration has been reached. The plateau occurs when the concentration of drug is such that the rate of elimination by all means is just equal to the rate of infusion. The time required to reach the plateau concentration depends solely on the elimination half-life and is always equal to 3.3 half-lives.

Complications

Complications with IV fluid therapy are common. It is frequently the nurse who must intervene quickly and wisely to avoid disastrous consequences. The usual complications are infiltration, extravasation, clotting, phlebitis, pain at the site of catheterization, infection, pyrogenic reactions, and iatrogenic imbalances of fluids, electrolytes, or nutrients.

Infiltration

Infiltration is flow of fluid into the tissue surrounding the site of infusion. It occurs when the infusion needle or cannula is dislodged or loosely inserted in the vein or when the lip of the needle has punctured the wall of the vessel and is protruding. When infiltration occurs, the infusion site appears pale and rounded from edema caused by fluid accumulation. The patient will probably report pain at the site and it will be cool or cold. Flow rate will usually be diminished. If infiltration occurs, the nurse should apply a tourniquet, discontinue the infusion, elevate the infusion site, and call the physician or IV team. Usually it is necessary to initiate infusion at a new site.

Extravasation

Extravasation is escape of fluid from the cannulated vein. If caused by distention of the vein, reduction of flow rate may eliminate the problem. Sometimes extravasation is due to osmotic and hydrostatic forces promoting an outward movement of fluid from the blood vessel. Or it could indicate a leaky cannulation that will require transferring the infusion to a new site and sterilizing the old site. When infusion is discontinued, the nurse must ensure that the venous wall seals itself, preventing leakage of blood into the space surrounding the vein. This can be accomplished by applying pressure to the site for a minute or two following removal of the cannula.

Clotting

Clotting may occur in the cannula or the blood vessel but most commonly occurs at the tip of the cannula. A thrombus may form, plugging the vessel and arresting flow. If clotting occurs, flow rate is reduced or stopped, but the cannulation site does not exhibit color change or edema. When a clot occurs, it may be possible to aspirate the clot into the needle, but it is unwise to attempt to dislodge the clot by forcing fluid into the vein. This latter technique could displace a small clot, which could then be carried by the blood to the lungs to cause a pulmonary embolism. It may be necessary to change the site of infusion.

Phlebitis and Infection

Inflammation at the site of injection is common with prolonged infusions. It may be due to contaminants, infection, or the infusion fluids themselves. The site will appear red, warm, and swollen. The patient will probably experience pain and reduced mobility. It will normally be necessary to stop the infusion and change sites. The risk of phlebitis is minimized by proper sterile technique and appropriate flow rates. The skin should be disinfected prior to needle insertion. Equipment and solutions should be checked for contamination and debris. Fluid bottles should be changed daily.

Pain at the Infusion Site

This may be due to phlebitis or infiltration but may also be caused by mechanical pressure of the needle against the venous wall. Adjustment of the angle of the tubing to relieve tension may be helpful.

Pyrogenic Reactions

Pyrogenic contaminants sometimes occur in intravenous fluids. Sudden fever, chills, headache, body aches, nausea, and vomiting are symptomatic. The infusion should be stopped immediately. The hospital pharmacist should be informed so that the batch of solutions can be checked for contamination. The IV team should be informed of the reaction.

Iatrogenic Imbalances

Overly vigorous treatment of electrolyte deficiencies, acid-base imbalance, or fluid disturbances trigger opposite conditions. Hypertonic expansion is usually iatrogenic, a result of infusion of too much normal saline. Excessive sodium bicarbonate given for metabolic acidosis may cause metabolic alkalosis. Hypercalcemia, hyperkalemia, and hypermagnesia are all often due to excess administration of the respective salts. In other cases, treatment may be inappropriate rather than overly vigorous. Hypotonic contraction develops when dextrose solutions are used instead of normal saline for isotonic contraction. Deficiencies in essential nutrients are often the result of extended parenteral nutrition without provision of one or another requirement.

Recommended Readings

Bates GF, Fitch GE, Larson MA, Mooney MP: *Basic Drug Therapy and Arithmetic Review,* ed 5. New York, Macmillan Publ Co, 1986.

Brent NJ: Medication administration: avoiding the latest legal pitfalls. *Nursing Life* 1986;6(5):53–55.

Brown M, Mulholland J: *Basic Drug Calculations,* ed 2. St. Louis, CV Mosby Co, 1984.

Channer K, Virjee J: Effect of posture and drink volume on swallowing capsules. *Br Med J* 1982;285:1702.

Chapin G, Shull H, Welk PC: Potential for error using textbook technique for intramuscular administration. *Am J Hosp Pharm* 1983;40:385.

Chaplin G et al: How safe is the air bubble technique in I.M. injections? *Nursing* 1985;85(7):59.

Coblio NA: Don't combine those drugs. *Nursing* 1981;11(8):48–51.

Cohen MR: Medication errors. *Nursing* 1985;15(5):84.

Dalgas P: Understanding drugs that affect the autonomic nervous system. *Nursing* 1985;15(10):58–63.

Gever L: Administering drugs through the skin: The new transdermal route. *Nursing* 1982;12(3):88.

Hickman RA: When you have to reconstitute meds. *RN* 1981;41(5):40–43.

Jerrett MD: Taking the ouch out of injections. *Can Nurse* 1983;79(1):24–27.

Keen MF: Comparison of intramuscular injection techniques to reduce site discomfort and lesions. *Nurs Res* 1986;35(4):207–210.

Kruszewski AZ, Lang SH, Johnson JE: Effect of positioning on discomfort from intramuscular injections in the dorsogluteal site. *Nurs Res* 1979;28:103–105.

McConnell EA: The subtle art of really good injections. *RN* 1982;45:25–34.

Peck N: Perfecting your I.V. therapy technique: Part I. *Nursing* 1986;15(5):38–43.

Petty T: Drug strategies for airflow obstruction. *Amer J Nurs* 1987;87(2):181–184.

Plumer AL: *Principles and Practice of Intravenous Therapy,* ed 4. Boston, Little, Brown, 1986.

Radany MH, Perry S, McCallum D: Is it safe to reuse disposables? *Amer J Nurs* 1987;87(1):35–38.

Rapp PR, Elgert JF, Piecoro JJ: Guidelines for the administration of commonly used intravenous drugs. *Drug Intell Clin Pharm* 1980;14:193–208.

Rosenberg JM, Sangkachand P: 'Take with meals' ... or not? Quick answers to a pesky question (parts 1 & 2). *RN* 1981;44(5):46–52, 44(6):60–65.

Shepherd, MJ, Swearington PL: Z-track injections: A step-by-step how-to for an underused IM technique. *Am J Nurs* 1984;84(6):746–747.

Sklar C: Nursing negligence in the administration of medication . . . could it happen to you? *Can Nurse* 1979;75:51–53.

Speciale JL, Kaalaas J: Infuse-a-port: new path for I.V. chemotherapy. *Nursing* 1985;15(10):40–43.

Stubbs LP: Verbal orders: A self-defense guide. *RN* 1982;82(4):104C–104F.

Todd B: Using eye drops and ointments safely. *Geriatr Nurs* 1983;4(1):53–57.

Winfrey A: Single-dose I.M. injections: How much is too much? *Nursing* 1985;15(7):38–39.

Wong DL: Significance of dead space in syringes. *Am J Nurs* 1982;82:1237.

Answers to Dosage Calculation Problems

1. Fifteen grains equals approximately 1g, so sixteen grains is 1.07 g.
2. Table 4–1 indicates that one teaspoon equals 4–5 ml, so 20 ml is 4 or 5 teaspoons.
3. Capsules required at each administration: 2.
4. The dose of 120 mg of propranolol can be provided with the fewest number of tablets (without breaking tablets or mixing tablets of different strength) by using 3 of the 40 mg tablets.
5. Table 4–1 indicates that 15 grains equals 1 g. The dose of 1.5 grains is equal to 100 mg, which can be provided by 4 tablets of 25 mg.
6. Two tablets of 200 mg will provide the dose of 0.4 g.
7. Fifteen grains is approximately equivalent to 1 g. The prescribed dose of 3 grains will require 0.2 g, or 2 of the 0.1 g tablets.
8. A 5% solution has 5 g in 100 ml. To prepare a 5% solution in 25 ml, 1.25 g of drug would be required.
9. A 30% solution has 30 g in 100 ml. Since only 5 g is to be dissolved, the volume required will be 100/6 ml, or 16.67 ml.
10. The volume required of a 250 mg/5 ml solution to deliver 500 mg is 10 ml.
11. Two milliliters.
12. The volume of a 5 mg/ml solution required to yield a dose of 4 mg is 0.8 ml.
13. The volume of a 250 mg/100 ml solution required to provide a dose of 500 mg is 200 ml.
14. At 10 drops per milliliter, it will require 10,000 drops to provide 1,000 ml. A rate of 1,000 drops per hour will provide the required volume over 10 hours. One thousand drops per hour is 167 drops per minute.
15. It will require 10 mEq of KCl in a 500 ml bag of infusion solution to provide the prescribed concentration of 2 mEq/100 ml. The 10 mEq can be provided using 0.5 ml of the 20 mEq/ml solution that is on hand.
16. It will require 20 mEq of KCl in a 500 ml bag of D5W to provide the desired concentration of 4 mEq/100 ml. The 20 mEq of KCl can be provided from a volume of 5.0 ml of the 40 mEq/10 ml solution on hand.
17. It will require 1.2 ml of the 500,000 units/ml penicillin preparation to provide the required dose of 600,000 units.
18. The required dose of 2,500 units of heparin can be provided using 0.5 ml of the 5,000 units/ml heparin that is available.
19. The 75 units of regular insulin prescribed for Mrs. S. can be provided with 0.75 ml of the 100 units/ml preparation that is on hand. 0.75 ml is equal to 11.25 minims.

CHAPTER 5

The Legal and Ethical Responsibilities of the Nurse Administering Drugs

A full discussion of the legal and ethical aspects of nursing practice is, of course, beyond the scope of a pharmacology text. But nurses administering drugs have certain responsibilities that have practical implications for how they perform their jobs. Professional ethics, as well as state and federal laws, dictate that the nurse follow certain guidelines to ensure fulfilling his or her obligations to the client. This chapter begins with a brief look at some of the legal issues involved in drug administration and then considers the nurse's ethical responsibilities.

The Legal Aspects of Drug Administration

The legal basis of nursing practice rests on the concept that a contract exists between the nurse and the client. Each time the nurse enters a client's room and performs such tasks as counseling the client, administering drugs, or performing procedures, the nurse and the client enter into a contract. A contract exists whenever there is an exchange of something of value between two or more people who are legally capable of making a binding agreement. In this case, the client receives the service the nurse performs and the nurse receives payment for work.

Contracts may be oral or written, signed or unsigned. In the case of an agreement between a nurse and a client, contracts are frequently oral. At times, courts have even declared that a contract has been agreed to by body movements or by one party remaining silent. For example, if a nurse approaches a hospital patient with a syringe, identifies the patient by reading out the name on the wrist band, and explains what she is about to do, and the client holds out an arm or otherwise moves into a position suggesting acceptance, the client has in fact agreed to receive the service. Despite the apparent casualness of such contracts, the nurse is responsible for obtaining the consent of the client. The law protects the individual from unpermitted contact with others. Therefore, if a nurse approaches a client for the purpose of injecting material via a hypodermic needle and the client refuses the injection, the nurse may not administer the medication. If the nurse administers the medication without the client's consent, the nurse's action constitutes assault and battery.

The law recognizes that medicine is not an exact science and that health care personnel cannot guarantee the recovery of health to anyone. But at the same time, the law requires that nurses perform at a level appropriate to their educational background and experience. How is this level determined? Hospitals and other health care agencies have established guidelines that can be found in policy and procedure manuals that serve as both administrative and educational tools. They define standards of practice for meeting the basic needs of clients. For example, policy manuals as well as most texts on the fundamentals of nursing stress the need to use siderails for elderly or disoriented clients, especially if an individual has been sedated. If a nurse administers a sedative to an elderly client and fails to raise the siderails, and the client falls out of bed, the question asked would be whether the nurse used the degree of skill and knowledge normally expected of a competent nurse with similar education and experience in a similar situation. If a procedure manual and nursing text can be used to demonstrate that a reasonable and prudent nurse would know that siderails are necessary when working with sedated elderly and disoriented persons, the nurse may be shown to have failed to perform at the required level of competence.

Legal liability extends to student nurses as well. Student nurses are expected to perform in a manner appropriate to their background and experience. Thus the student nurse is responsible for applying the knowledge obtained in the classroom to the care of clients in the clinical setting.

Nurses are legally, as well as morally, required to be familiar with the drugs they administer. This means that it is the nurse's legal responsibility to know the minimum and maximum dosage of drugs, the circumstances under which each is recommended, the usual route of administration, and any special precautions that should be taken, especially if the route of administration is one not commonly used. Nurses are also responsible for accurate assessment of the client's condition after the drug has been given. Responsible drug administration includes adhering to the **five rights:** the *right drug* must be given to the *right client* at the *right time,* at the *right dose,* and by the *right route.* These were discussed more fully in Chapter 4; here we will concentrate on aspects of particular legal significance.

Verifying Orders

Nurses may be sued for negligence if they misread a medication label, fail to check labels and client identification and thus administer the drug to the wrong client, or fail to adhere to the prescribed methods of administration, all of which may cause a client to suffer adverse effects. But nurses can also be sued for carrying out medication orders that are in error. For example, a nurse working in the newborn nursery of a community hospital had an order to inject vitamin K, intramuscularly, into a 5 lb infant. The nurse was told that hospital procedure dictated that all IM injections must be performed using a 2-inch needle injected into the gluteal region. The nurse questioned the standing order. After further review of the professional literature and consultation with her supervisor, the nurse selected a shorter needle and injected the material into the anterior quadriceps femoris of the infant. To do otherwise would have threatened the infant's safety, because a long needle penetrating into the gluteal musculature might have caused damage to the sciatic nerve. Had this occurred, the nurse would have been held liable for that damage.

The nurse is responsible for verifying that medication orders are not only correct but also complete. Incomplete orders are a more common problem than incorrect orders. For example, a nurse assigned to administer medication to all the clients in one unit of the hospital discovered that the medication cards for one client did not include the route of administration. The nurse first investigated the physician's order book to identify the route ordered by the physician, but no administration route was indicated. The nurse was familiar with the drug ordered and its usual route of administration but did not presume to know how the physician intended the drug to be given. To avoid any possibility of harm to the client, the nurse asked the physician to specify the route of administration. If the nurse had not acted prudently and had administered the drug by the usual route without contacting the physician, the nurse would be liable for any injury sustained by the client.

Incorrect orders, though less common, are a more difficult problem for the nurse. The nurse must be satisfied that a medication order is reasonable before administering the drug; if not satisfied, it is the nurse's responsibility to challenge the order. For example, an intern left an order for a client to receive digitalis (Digifortis), a cardiac glycoside, 100 mg PO daily. When the nurse assigned to the client's care checked the medication orders, she also found an order for digoxin (Lanoxin), another cardiac glycoside, 0.5 mg PO to be given at 10:00 A.M. and 10:00 P.M. The nurse called the intern and questioned the Lanoxin order, since the client also was taking Digifortis once a day. The intern insisted that the client be given the Lanoxin as prescribed. Acting in a reasonably prudent manner, the nurse then contacted the resident in charge of clients with cardiopulmonary dysfunction; the resident promptly cancelled the Lanoxin order. Legally, the nurse is *expected* to be familiar with the drugs she administers and to know (in this instance) that Digifortis and Lanoxin are both cardiac glycosides and that administering both drugs in the manner prescribed would cause overdose and adverse reactions.

In this case, the nurse's persistence resulted in resolution of the problem. If, however, no resolution can be reached, the nurse has a legal and ethical right to refuse to follow an order he or she recognizes is contrary to good nursing practice and the client's best interest. Legally, the nurse can base the decision on what a prudent nurse would do. As client-advocate, the nurse can base refusal to carry out an order on the ethical principle of nonmaleficence, discussed later in the chapter.

When executing oral orders, given in person or on the telephone, the nurse must be sure to record the order on the client's chart and have the physician initial the order as soon afterward as possible. It is especially important that the nurse make sure oral orders are complete and unambiguous. The nurse should read the order back to the prescriber to make sure it is accurate. It is a good idea to have the patient's chart at hand while taking such an order, so that the nurse can remind the prescriber of other medications the patient is taking.

The Responsibility to Keep Informed: Sources and Drug Information

As we have indicated, nurses are responsible for knowing about the drugs they administer. In addition, the law in some states now allows nurse practitioners to prescribe certain categories of drugs. The law recognizes that continuing education is necessary for assuring standards of client care. As technology becomes more complex and as newer drugs are developed, nurses must continue to update their knowledge about drug therapy. Courts have increasingly held nurses responsible for following instructions regarding drug administration and for recognizing obvious and dangerous signs of medication errors and common side effects that indicate a drug should be discontinued. As the number and variety of drugs increase, courts have, at times, held that nurses should be knowledgeable about all drugs administered and have held nursing responsibility to include *not* administering drugs with which they are unfamiliar (Fiesta, 1983). Juries also have been instructed to hold nurses responsible for knowing the fatal dose of all drugs. Where the potential for death or serious injury is great, the nurse's responsibility and accountability increases correspondingly.

The nurse therefore faces the formidable task of keeping up with the rapidly expanding field of pharmacology. To help meet this challenge, there are several reliable sources of drug information nurses may use to become familiar with the drugs they administer.

The United States Food and Drug Administration (FDA) recognizes the *United States Pharmacopeia* (U.S.P.) as an official source of information on the composition, efficacy, and safety of drugs. All drugs included in the *Pharmacopeia* have met standards of efficacy and safety. (Such drugs are indicated by the letters U.S.P. following their names.) The U.S.P. is revised every five years by a committee chosen from the American Medical Association, the American Pharmaceutical Association, and other groups. In 1980 the U.S.P. was merged with the *National Formulary* (N.F.), another listing of drugs of recognized efficacy and safety.

If the U.S.P. is not available, there are a number of other sources a nurse can turn to for drug information. The drug manufacturer supplies a **package insert** with each of its products, listing the composition, action, dosage, and adverse effects. Since the FDA approves these inserts, they can be relied on as accurate. Nurses should be sure to read the insert for any drug they are not familiar with, since the law holds the nurse responsible for knowing such information.

The *Physicians' Desk Reference* (PDR), published annually by the Medical Economics Company, is a listing of basic drug information. Much of the information is supplied by the manufacturer and often is identical to the package insert. The PDR contains no nursing implications of drugs discussed. It does contain a section of color photographs of tablets and capsules that can be helpful in identifying medications. *Drug Facts and Comparisons,* published annually by J.B. Lippincott, is a compendium of drug information that includes patient education information. The drugs are listed by drug class. The *American Hospital Formulary Service,* published by the American Society of Hospital Pharmacists, contains monographs on individual drugs.

Drug handbooks for nurses list drugs alphabetically, giving actions, clinical indications, pharmacokinetics, adverse reactions, routes, dosages, and nursing implications.

Several *nursing journals* contain information on the new drugs and techniques of administration. *American Journal of Nursing* (AJN) contains a monthly newsletter called *Nurses' Drug Alert. Nursing 88, RN,* and *Nursing Life* frequently contain information on new drugs.

Informed Consent

Clients are autonomous agents; they have independence, freedom of choice, self-reliance, and the ability to make decisions. The nurse is legally responsible for making sure the client has enough information to make informed decisions. Thus clients have a legal right to know about any drug therapy prescribed and have the right to refuse it.

Courts are consistently holding physicians, rather than nurses, liable for obtaining consent from clients, although nurses have a responsibility to remind physicians to obtain consent for therapy. It is a nursing responsibility, however, to clarify what physicians have said to clients; whenever possible, nurses should be present when physicians explain drug therapy to clients. Nurses can be held liable if they know that there has not been an adequate disclosure of facts.

The question of who is primarily responsible for providing information to clients varies from one clinical setting to another. Some hospitals, for example, have policies specifying that physicians are primarily responsible for providing information. The nurse should become familiar with policies of the institution for which she or he works. At the very least, however, the nurse is responsible for calling to the physician's attention any client who asks for more information or who appears confused about his or her therapy.

Where minor children are concerned, questions arise as to the legitimacy of informed consent. If a minor is judged mature or is emancipated and parents are unavailable to provide consent, courts have held such consent is informed and valid. However, the definition of *emancipated minor* varies from state to state; nurses should be familiar with the legal interpretation in the state where they are practicing. Some states require that the minor reside outside the parents' home to be considered emancipated. An employed minor married to someone of legal age is considered emancipated. Some states' laws also allow minors to consent to treatment for venereal disease, drug or alcohol dependence, or pregnancy. Nurses should consult legal authorities to assure that the consent being given is lawful.

The federal government has established strict guidelines about consent to administration of experimental drugs. Nurses should be familiar with these guidelines. Debate arises as to whether or not parents can consent to an experimental drug therapy for a minor child.

If clients are mentally incompetent, consent must be obtained from a legally authorized guardian. State statutes determine these matters, and when there is any doubt, nurses should seek legal advice about their legal rights and responsibilities.

If a client does not speak English, the nurse should attempt to contact a reliable translator. If such a person is not available, special foreign language cards and books may be of assistance in assuring the client's understanding.

If a client refuses therapy, nurses then have a responsibility to discuss with the individual the reason for the refusal and to ascertain if the client would take the same medicine in some other form (liquid as opposed to tablet; oral as opposed to injection). Although the nurse should encourage the client to take the medication, the nurse cannot force the client except in very rare instances (for example, when a client has been declared mentally incompetent or when there is strong evidence that without the medication the client is a danger to him- or herself or others). Once a medication has been refused, the nurse must record the reason for refusal and notify the physician immediately.

Recording Medications

Recording medications is an essential part of sound nursing practice. The patient's chart serves not only as a major means of communication among health team members but also as a legal record of the care the individual has received. In any legal proceeding the patient's chart would be a crucial source of evidence.

The nurse must therefore carefully record all medications and the times they are given. Medications should never be charted before they are actually given. If the drug is given as needed (PRN), the nurse must chart the factors that led to the decision to give the drug. All relevant physical data must be recorded, for example the pulse when administering atropine and respiration rate when administering morphine.

In addition the nurse must carefully record any unusual incidents that occur. If a patient refuses a medication, the nurse must record the attempt to administer the drug and the patient's reasons for refusing. Any medication errors must be carefully recorded, whether they seem important at the time or not. Errors should also be reported to the nurse in charge and, if serious, to the physician. Nurses are often required to fill out incident reports on errors. Full and careful reporting is not only best for the patient but also helps the institution keep track of the kinds of errors that occur and devise policies to help avoid them.

Nursing care plans are also evidence courts may use to determine whether a nurse has acted appropriately. In the past, institutions often discarded such plans when the patient was discharged, but increasingly today courts are requesting these plans as evidence of the appropriateness of nursing judgments and actions. Nursing assessment and actions taken are important in establishing proof that a particular standard of care was provided.

Handling of Controlled Substances

Narcotics and other drugs that have the potential for drug dependence are regulated by the Harrison Narcotics Act, which covers the manufacture, importation, sale, and use of narcotics or their derivatives. The law was amended in 1970 by the Controlled Substance Act. This act classifies drugs according to their medical uses and their potential for abuse and is discussed in Chapter 10, "Drug Abuse and Misuse" (see especially Table 10–3, which gives the categories or "schedules" of controlled substances). Nurses are expected to know which drugs are covered by this act.

It is illegal to administer a drug listed in schedule II, III, or IV of the Controlled Substance Act to anyone other than the person for whom the drug is prescribed. It is also illegal to possess controlled substances unless the individual has a valid prescription for the drug or is holding the drug temporarily for someone else; for example, a nurse administering the drug is acting legally. Nurses are required by law to account for all scheduled drugs they administer while on duty in a hospital or other agency. Scheduled drugs are listed on separate forms; the records must be accurate, and all such drugs must be fully accounted for. On most nursing units such drugs are counted, and the count is recorded as each group of nurses report off duty to those who will be replacing them. All controlled medications used during the shift (including any spilled or otherwise wasted medications) must be recorded. The schedules must be signed and dated by one nurse from each group and include the hour of the sign-off. Any violation of this accountability can result in revocation of the nursing license, fine, or imprisonment.

The Ethical Aspects of Drug Administration

The ethical dilemmas facing the health care professions grow steadily along with advances in understanding and treating disorders of the body's systems. We now face issues that were unthinkable as little as a quarter century ago. The questions of when life begins and ends and the lengths to which we will go to preserve it are widely debated in society today.

Although these broad issues are beyond the scope of this book, we will touch briefly here on the general principles of ethics that guide the nurse's behavior. Ethical decisions are often difficult to make because there are few, if any, absolutes that hold for all situations. They can be especially difficult to make in clinical situations where nurses are expected to be advocates for patients, promoting their interests in maintaining or regaining health. For example, suppose a physician orders a narcotic to be administered to a terminally ill oncology patient who is having severe pain. The client's respirations are 8, and the nurse is aware that the prescribed drug is contraindicated in this situation. The nurse calls the physician and reports the depressed respiratory rate, but the physician notes that the client is terminally ill and should receive the drug. Legally, the nurse may be held liable if she administers the medication and the client's respirations cease. What would a prudent professional nurse do in this case? What is in the client's best interest — reducing pain or prolonging life?

The American Nurses' Association has developed a code of ethics for nurses (see the box on page 77) with which all nurses should be familiar. The nurse's responsibilities to clients as defined by this code of ethics are to promote health, prevent illness, restore health, and alleviate suffering. Inherent in nursing is a respect for life, dignity, and the rights of human beings. Thus nurses are obligated to respect the wishes of clients and to treat them with dignity. The client's right to respect from the nurse is independent of nationality, race, creed, color, age, sex, politics, physical status, or social status.

Nursing ethics is based on the principles of **nonmaleficence** (that is, the duty to do no harm), **beneficence** (the duty to do good) **client autonomy, veracity,** and **justice.** For example, Mrs. L., a 29-year-old

American Nurses' Association Code of Ethics

Standard 1
The nurse provides services with respect for human dignity and the uniqueness of the client, unrestricted by considerations of social or economic status, personal attributes, or the nature of health problems.

Standard 2
The nurse safeguards the client's right to privacy by judiciously protecting information of a confidential nature.

Standard 3
The nurse acts to safeguard the client and the public when health care and safety are affected by the incompetent, unethical, or illegal practice of any person.

Standard 4
The nurse assumes responsibility and accountability for individual nursing judgments and actions.

Standard 5
The nurse maintains competence in nursing.

Standard 6
The nurse exercises informed judgment and uses individual competence and qualifications as criteria in seeking consultation, accepting responsibilities, and delegating nursing activities to others.

Standard 7
The nurse participates in activities that contribute to the ongoing development of the profession's body of knowledge.

Standard 8
The nurse participates in the profession's efforts to implement and improve standards of nursing.

Standard 9
The nurse participates in the profession's efforts to establish and maintain conditions of employment conducive to high quality nursing care.

Standard 10
The nurse participates in the profession's effort to protect the public from misinformation and misrepresentation and to maintain the integrity of nursing.

Standard 11
The nurse collaborates with members of the health professions and other citizens in promoting community and national efforts to meet the health needs of the public.

woman in her third month of pregnancy, has a serious infection that should be treated immediately. The drug the physician chooses, however, has been associated with harming fetal development, but there are no alternative drugs available. The nurse believes she should do nothing that would harm the unborn child (nonmaleficence). She also knows that unless Mrs. L. receives the drug (beneficence), she may succumb to the infection, which would of course hurt the fetus. The nurse may proceed with the therapy on the principle of beneficence in that there is no intentional harm to the fetus but that there will certainly be harm to the mother and the fetus if the mother is denied therapy.

Nurses must safeguard a client's right to privacy, which means protecting information of a confidential nature. It also means that in administering medications (or performing other nursing functions) clients should not be physically exposed unnecessarily.

The nurse's primary obligation is to the client, and this includes respecting the client's values. The nurse may not impose her own morals or opinions on a client. Except in cases where the client is declared incompetent, the locus of decision-making is always with the client. Values direct actions, thereby prescribing the desires an individual feels should be fulfilled and those that should be subverted. Thus, an individual may so value life and family that he or she is willing to suffer any pain and discomfort to live. In contrast, other individuals may value life but at some point may decide that a prescribed therapy designed to prolong life is so painful that they must subvert the value of life to a greater value — namely relief from pain and suffering. This value may dominate to the extent that the individual finally refuses all further drugs or therapy. Whether or not a nurse agrees with the client's decision, the nurse's primary ethical obligation is to support the individual's decision.

For example, Mr. D.'s physician left an order for meperidine (Demerol) 100 mg IM every 4 hours PRN to relieve his pain and discomfort after abdominal surgery. Mr D., however, considers taking pain medication unmanly and therefore refuses medication, even though it is apparent that his discomfort is great. The nurse in this situation may attempt to persuade Mr. D. to alter his decision by explaining the benefits of the drug, but the nurse must accept his final decision. Mr. D. is an autonomous agent, and unless he has been legally determined to be mentally incompetent and a danger to himself or others, the nurse may not impose her values on him nor can she administer the medication.

While the nurse may not impose her own values on the client, it is her responsibility to help the client clarify his or her own values when facing decisions about therapy. Within the limits agreed on by the health team, the nurse must make sure the client understands the therapy: the chances for successful outcome, the possible adverse effects, and so on.

Nurses must maintain a cooperative relationship with co-workers in nursing and other fields. Where there are problems with patients and physicians regarding drug therapies, the client's adherence to drug modalities, or where nursing ethical principles seem to conflict with the client's interest, nurses must establish the necessary relationship to sustain the client's health care.

Nurses have an obligation to provide health services to individuals, families, and the community and to coordinate their services with those of related groups. A hospital patient who will require daily injections of insulin when discharged and who has no one at home to perform the service should be able to rely on the nurse to procure the service. Nurses also participate in their profession's effort to protect the public from incompetent, unethical, or illegal health care practices. As an example, Mr. W., who had rheumatoid arthritis for years, asked Mrs. C., a nurse and neighbor, about the use of a new drug for arthritis. Before responding, Mrs. C. investigated the drug. She discovered it was an herb available in health food stores and that there was no scientific evidence that it could alleviate rheumatoid arthritis. Mrs. C. returned to Mr. W. and reported her findings, thus fulfilling her obligation to provide the client with information that would protect him from buying a useless remedy that would not relieve his arthritis. Should Mr. W. later decide to try the new drug he would do so as an autonomous agent making an informed choice.

The nurse has the right to refuse to participate in treatment that violates his or her ethical principles, but the nurse also has an overriding duty not to abandon a client in this case. Thus the nurse who does not want to participate must make her wishes known before the treatment begins and must transfer care of the client to someone else. While the client is in the nurse's care, the nurse's primary ethical responsibility is to give the client the best care possible, regardless of her opinion.

Case Study: The Right to Refuse Treatment

Mrs. R. was diagnosed as having acute myelogenous leukemia. The physician caring for Mrs. R. had, over the course of her therapy, treated her with the various chemotherapeutic agents at his disposal, and Mrs. R. had been able to spend much time at home. After a 2-year remission, however, Mrs. R. began to show signs of a recurrence of leukemia and was admitted to the hospital. The physician embarked on a new chemotherapy protocol in an attempt to reestablish her remission. The drugs made Mrs. R. very ill, more so than prior therapies, and her blood studies revealed no alteration in the course of her disease.

At each step of the procedure, the physician explained to Mrs. R. the purpose of the treatment and the results. The nurse assigned to Mrs. R. shared the physician's view that Mrs. R. and her family should have full knowledge of her progress and thus was able to support the medical protocols. When asked by a fellow co-worker how she could feel morally and ethically "right" watching Mrs. R. endure the suffering caused by the therapy, the nurse pointed out that Mrs. R. had voluntarily entered the hospital to receive the therapy. She was well informed about the possible results of her therapy, that is, extreme physical discomfort, remission, or possibly death from the side effects of the drug. It was clear that the intent of the therapy (to promote remission) was to benefit Mrs. R.

The nurse had reviewed the risks to Mrs. R. of no further therapy and, in her view, the balance of potential benefit justified the harm produced. However, as the nurse each day reviewed Mrs. R.'s progress, she began to note several changes in Mrs. R.'s responses. Mrs. R. was unable to retain food and fluid, and the drugs currently being used seemed to make her more ill than those used in prior protocols. As a result, Mrs. R. found it increasingly difficult to perform self-care and was so weak and ill that she found it difficult to communicate. The need for fluids was met by providing intravenous fluids, but the continual anorexia, nausea, and vomiting left Mrs. R. feeling dependent and anxious.

The nurse grouped the data into categories and began analyzing each section, comparing it with prior findings. In her nursing diagnosis, she wrote that Mrs. R. had alterations in bowel elimination, comfort, and ability to communicate, that the weakness had left Mrs. R. with impaired mobility, and that she was depressed and expressed fear about the status of her health. At this point Mrs. R. began expressing a desire to terminate the therapy.

The basic needs of Mrs. R. (food, water, sleep) were being met, as were safety needs and the need to belong and feel loved. Ethically and morally, all her needs were being considered. However, when the nurse entered Mrs. R.'s room one afternoon, she was confronted with a tearful patient who adamantly refused to allow an injection and requested that the intravenous fluids be discontinued. Clearly, Mrs. R.'s primary value of regaining health at all cost had changed. Now the focus of decision-making was Mrs. R. When the nurse sat down to discuss this decision with Mrs. R., she realized that the patient had been reviewing her status as explained by the physician and had concluded she could tolerate no further therapy.

For Mrs. R. there was more involved than personal comfort. She also was considering the effect of her continued illness and therapy upon her family. Being careful not to impose her views on the client, the nurse explored the question further with Mrs. R. and helped her to weigh the costs and risks against the benefits of further treatment. Finally, Mrs. R. stated that she had concluded that her children needed a more normal life than could be had with a parent who was "always ill" and that she would refuse all medication. While the nurse herself did not accept this view, she honored Mrs. R.'s autonomous decision to refuse further therapy.

The nurse recorded the event and reported the discussion to the physician who, in turn, met with Mrs. R. At that point Mrs. R. requested that she be discharged to "die in my own bed." The physician acceded to her wishes, and the nurse provided essential emotional support to Mrs. R. and her family. The nurse also encouraged the physician to contact the community health agency and to arrange for a nurse to follow Mrs. R.'s progress at home.

Points for Discussion

1. If you were providing care for Mrs. R. how would you determine if the principles of benefiscence and non-malefiscence were being addressed? In what ways were these and principles of veracity and autonomy being applied?
2. From this narrative what values do you think were operating for Mrs. R. as she progressed in her therapy? What values appear to be operating for other members of this health team?
3. If you were working on a team where the team members did not share your philosophy concerning drug therapy for cancer patients or your moral values how would you handle the situation? How would you handle the situation if the client or a family member questioned the ethics of chemotherapy for Mrs. R.?

Case Study: Competing Rights

Miss B. was assigned to work with Ms. C., a 17-year-old high school senior diagnosed as having lymphoma. The physical examination had also revealed that Ms. C. was 3 months pregnant. The physician explained to Ms. C. that the most effective therapy in treating her illness is the use of chemotherapeutic drugs and possibly whole body radiation therapy, both of which pose serious threats to the fetus. As a consequence, the physician suggested that Ms. C. have an abortion. Ms. C. did not agree with the physician and declared that the idea of abortion was abhorrent to her personally since her belief in the right to life precluded any such recommendation. Ms. C. also stated that the father of the baby had a right to be included in any discussions concerning her treatment since it would affect the fetus. She therefore did not wish to have chemotherapy or radiation therapy. The parents disagreed with their daughter. Although they did not want her to consider abortion, they did want her to proceed with the prescribed therapy. Accordingly, the physician ordered chemotherapy to begin and left orders for the nurse about the regimen. The nurse opposed abortion, but she recognized the necessity for the prescribed therapy.

Points for Discussion

1. If you were the nurse, which ethical rules or principles would provide the basis for your decision? Whose rights and values take precedence? The rights of parents, who are financially responsible for the daughter? The rights of the daughter, who is pregnant? Or the rights of the fetus?
2. How could you assist Ms. C. in making an ethical choice?

Case Study: Importance of Accurate Charting of Medications

Ms. P. was assigned to provide care to 10 clients on a neurologic unit. At lunchtime the head nurse asked Ms. P. to monitor all patients assigned to the unit while she went to lunch and to administer all the medications assigned to be given at 12:00 noon. Ms. P. was unfamiliar with the rest of the unit and the patients. Therefore, in preparing medications she made special note of each drug she poured; one drug was unfamiliar to her so she looked it up in the PDR. She checked all patients' wrist bands as she administered the drugs and charted them.

At 1:00 P.M. the head nurse returned and Ms. P. went to lunch. Upon her return she noted a group of physicians, the head nurse, and a client in conference at the head nurse's station. The head nurse, noting Ms. P.'s return, called her to the station and asked if she had administered all drugs assigned to be dispensed at 12:00 noon. Ms. P. assured her she had, pointing out that all orders were properly initialed by her (following that hospital's procedure) and charted. A physician then noted that one of the patients claimed she had not received her Mebaral at noon, and he demanded that Ms. P. administer the drug. Ms. P. refused, stating she had given Mebaral at noon. She clearly recalled the incident because she had found it necessary to look up the drug in the PDR and she was able to back up her assertion with the notes she had recorded at noon. Two hours later the client stated she remembered receiving the drug at noon.

1. What were Ms. P.'s legal responsibilities?
2. What steps did she take that would ensure that she could not be sued?
3. What legal grounds would support her decision?

Answers appear at the end of the book.

Recommended Readings

American Nurses' Association: *Code for Nurses With Interpretive Statements.* Kansas City, Mo., American Nurses' Association, 1976.

American Nurses' Association Committee on Ethics: *Ethical Dilemmas Confronting Nurses.* Kansas City, Mo., American Nurses' Association, 1982.

Bandman EL, Bandman B.: There is nothing automatic about rights. *Amer J Nurs* 1977;77(5):867–872.

Benjamin M, Curtis J: *Ethics in Nursing.* New York, Oxford Univ. Press, 1981.

Creighton H: *Law Every Nurse Should Know.* Philadelphia, W. B. Saunders Co., 1981.

Curtis L, Flaherty MJ: *Nursing Ethics: Theories and Pragmatics.* Bowie, Md., Robert J. Brady Co., 1982.

Davis A, Krueger JC: *Patients, Nurses, Ethics.* New York, American Journal of Nursing Company, 1980.

Davis A, Krueger JC: Dilemmas in practice: to tell or not. *Amer J Nurs* 1981;81(1):156–158.

Fiesta J: *The Law and Liability: A Guide for Nurses.* New York, John Wiley and Sons, 1983.

Flaherty MJ: Ethical decision-making in an interdisciplinary setting, in *Ethics in Nursing Practice and Education.* Kansas City, Mo., American Nurses' Association, 1980, pp 3–10.

Greenlaw J: Reporting incompetent colleagues: Will I be sued for defamation? *Nursing Law and Ethics* 1985;1(5):5.

Hemelt JD, Mackert ME: *Dynamics of Law in Nursing and Health Care,* ed. 2. Reston, Va, Reston Publ. Co., 1982.

Isler C: Six mistakes that could land you in jail. *RN* 1964;2:79.

Matejski MP: Ethical issues, nursing and the health care system. *Nursing Leadership* 1981;4:27–33.

Mills DH: Malpractice and the administration of drugs. *Medical Times* 1965;6:93.

Rabinow E: Six legal safeguards vs. drug errors. *Nursing Life* 1984;4(1):50–53.

CHAPTER 6

Pediatric Pharmacology

Children have been described as "therapeutic orphans" because most drugs have not been tested for safety and efficacy in children. In fact, more than half of all drugs released in the last 15 years carry specific disclaimers to this effect. Yet children are often susceptible to adult disorders, and the pediatrician must prescribe agents for which little or no pediatric dosage information is available. The major reason for the problem of "therapeutic orphaning" is the difficulties inherent in designing clinical studies in children that meet acceptable standards.

Thus one of the biggest problems confronting physicians who work with children is determining an appropriate dose and dosage interval when specific information is lacking from experience or studies in children. It is clear that children, and especially neonates, differ substantially from adults in pharmacokinetic matters, including drug metabolism, protein binding, volume of distribution, renal secretion, and elimination half-life of drugs. Thus, when drugs are administered to children, each drug and dosage becomes, in effect, an experiment, more so than when giving drugs to adult populations. When faced with the problem of selecting a dose and dosing interval in children, the physician can draw on four sets of guidelines: (1) rules for dosage selection, (2) knowledge of pharmacokinetic differences between neonates, children, and adults, (3) a slowly accumulating set of standard pediatric doses for commonly employed drugs, based on clinical experience, and (4) monitoring of plasma levels when indicated.

The nurse is especially important in pediatric pharmacology. The nurse's role in administration of drugs is often a challenging one when the drug is to be given to a child. The nurse also plays an especially important role in educating both the child and the parents and needs to understand the unusual effects of drugs in infants and children and the guidelines for determining pediatric doses so as to provide meaningful advice.

Rules for Selecting Pediatric Doses

There are a number of alternative rules for calculating doses for children, no one of which is entirely satisfactory. These rules calculate pediatric doses as a fraction of adult dose, based on weight, age, surface area, or body water.

The first rules for pediatric dosage were based on weight and age. Clark's weight rule is intended for use in children over 2 years of age:

$$\frac{\text{Weight in pounds}}{150} \times \text{Adult dose} = \text{Approximate dose for children over 2 years of age}$$

Two rules based on age are Young's and Fried's rules, the former for children over 2 years of age, the latter for children under 1 year of age. Young's rule is

$$\frac{\text{Age in years}}{\text{Age in years} + 12} \times \text{Adult dose} = \text{Approximate dose for children over 2 years of age}$$

Fried's rule is

$$\frac{\text{Age in months}}{150} \times \text{Adult dose} = \text{Approximate dose for children under 1 year of age}$$

Neither age nor weight proved very effective as guidelines for dosage selection in children. Currently, the rule considered to be the best first approximation is based on surface area. Clark's surface area rule is

$$\frac{\text{Surface area of the child's body}}{\text{Surface area of adult's body (c. 173 m}^2\text{)}} \times \text{Adult dose} = \text{Approximate children's dose}$$

Surface area can be rapidly estimated by use of a West nomogram if height and weight of the child are known (Figure 6–1). Since weight has more bearing on surface area than does height, a nurse can obtain a fairly reliable estimate of surface area based on weight alone, if the ratio of the child's weight to height is not extraordinary. The conversion from weight to surface area can be made directly using the boxed in portion of the West nomogram.

A number of newer rules have been offered, such as Gill and Udea's rule based on an estimate of body water volume. This formula is unwieldy and offers no advantage over Young's surface area rule.

The weakness of all of the widely used rules for calculating pediatric doses is their reliance on a definition of the average adult dose — a dose that may produce a wide range of responses in adults and bears little relationship in most cases to effects in children. Ideally, normal pediatric dosage ranges should be established, and nurses should consult these for each drug used in children. This goal has been met for many drugs, though many others await codification. A compilation of drugs with established pediatric dosage ranges is given in the appendix at the end of this chapter. Such doses are given as milligrams per kilogram of body weight or milligrams per square meter of surface area. In some instances, the best approach to dosing in children may be monitoring plasma concentrations. This is especially the case for drugs with established effective plasma concentrations, low therapeutic indexes, and considerable pharmacokinetic variability.

As difficult as dosage selection may be in children, selection of an appropriate dosing interval is both more important and more difficult because of the unique pharmacokinetics of neonates and children. At best, dosage rules give a general idea of what the pediatric dose should be. Dose, and especially dosage interval, must always be adjusted according to the effect that the immaturity of body systems has on the pharmacokinetics of the specific drug.

Pharmacokinetics in Neonates and Infants

Pharmacokinetic factors governing drug availability in neonates (newborns up to 6 weeks of age) are qualitatively the same as those that apply to adults, but substantial quantitative differences exist in all three pharmacokinetic phases: absorption, distribution, and elimination. Pharmacokinetic variability imposed by disease, diet, other drugs in use, and genetics are compounded in the neonate by the immaturity of their body systems. Many compounds are more potent and toxic in the neonate; a smaller number are less effective and require relatively higher doses than in adults. Even within a given class of drugs, some agents may be more toxic while others may be less toxic or equitoxic in neonates (Table 6–1). Thus, the health team must consider each drug individually when assessing dosage requirements in children.

Figure 6–1

West nomogram for estimating surface area from height and weight. The surface area is the point of intersection on the surface area scale of a line connecting the child's height on the left with the child's weight on the right. For children having a normal height/weight ratio, a simpler method is to find the surface area corresponding to the child's weight using the scale in the central, boxed-in area. From H. C. Shirkey, Drug therapy. From Appendix in R. E. Behrman and V. C. Vaughan (Eds.), *Nelson Textbook of Pediatrics, 12th ed.* Philadelphia: W. B. Saunders Co., 1983.

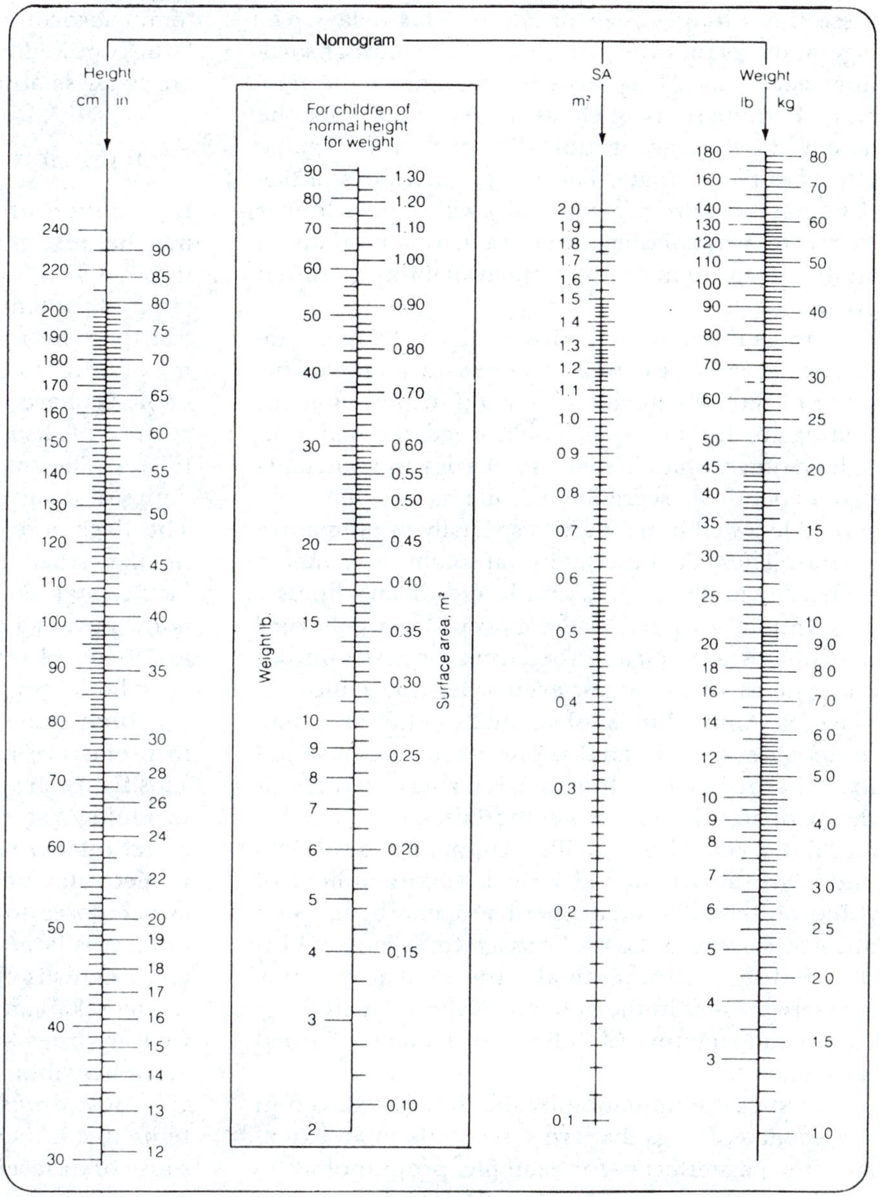

Table 6–1

Relative Toxicity of Certain Drugs in Neonates and Adults

More toxic in neonates	Less toxic or equitoxic in neonates
Aspirin	Atropine
Chlorpromazine	Codeine
Coumadins	Dextroamphetamine
Curare	Digitalis
Desipramine	Halothane
Meprobamate	Meperidine
Morphine	Phenylephrine
Phenobarbital	Succinylcholine

Absorption

Of the three pharmacokinetic arenas, absorption is the least distinctive in neonates, but some significant differences occur. At birth, pH in the stomach is approximately 6, but this declines rapidly to the typical 1–2 within the first 24 hours. Acid secretion in the stomach remains low for up to 10 days after birth in the infant born at term or for longer times in premature infants. For this reason, a drug like penicillin exhibits greater absorption in the neonate, because a smaller portion of the dose is destroyed by stomach acid in the neonate than in the adult.

Gastric emptying time in neonates is two to three times longer than in adults. This delays passage of drugs into the intestines where most absorption takes place. Peristalsis is irregular in the neonate. Formulations such as tablets that must be dissolved before absorption will have unpredictable effects in the neonate. Therefore, nurses can anticipate that most drugs given orally will require longer to reach peak plasma levels in neonates than in adults, even though total bioavailability is often greater.

Drugs that require active transport from the intestines may be less well absorbed in neonates because of the immaturity of active transport systems. Riboflavin, for example, is absorbed far better in older children than in neonates. Drugs and nutrients that depend on secretion of bile salts will be absorbed less well in neonates, especially in premature infants. These include many fat-soluble substances such as vitamins A, D, E, and K and dietary lipids.

Antibiotics, perhaps the most widely used drugs in neonates, are well absorbed from the gastrointestinal systems of neonates, even when the child has diarrhea. Ampicillin is substantially better absorbed in neonates than in adults, presumably because immaturity of hepatic drug-metabolizing activities in the neonates greatly slows the breakdown of this antibiotic. Penicillin, nafcillin (Unipen), and sulfonamides are also better absorbed. Chloramphenicol (Chloromycetin), on the other hand, may be less well absorbed because the oral dosage form must be hydrolyzed by gastrointestinal enzymes that are only sparsely present in the neonate. Nalidixic acid (NegGram) and rifampin (Rifadin) are less well absorbed in neonates.

First-pass elimination by the liver is reduced in the neonate. Drugs that are susceptible to an extensive first-pass effect — for example, propranolol (Inderal) — will produce greater effects in neonates. When propranolol is used chronically in infants, monitoring of plasma concentrations is desirable.

Neonates and infants have intensified susceptibility to nitrate-induced methemoglobinemia. One reason for this is the presence in the upper gastrointestinal tract of higher levels of bacteria that convert nitrates to nitrites. These bacteria thrive in the less acidic intestinal environment of the neonate. Nitrites are well absorbed and are responsible for the conversion of normal hemoglobin to methemoglobin. In older children and adults, ingested nitrates are largely excreted unchanged in the feces.

Passive diffusion is usually similar in neonates and adults. Exceptions exist when drugs are applied topically to penetration barriers that are incompletely formed in neonates. For example, atropine applied to the eye will undergo much greater systemic absorption in the neonate than in the adult. Drugs applied to the skin (such as hexachlorophene) are likewise absorbed more readily in the neonate.

Distribution

Distribution of an absorbed drug differs in a neonate because of differences in (1) blood flow, (2) relative mass of various tissues, (3) total body water, (4) lipid content, (5) penetration barriers that govern transport into various compartments, and (6) binding of drugs to plasma proteins. Compared to adults, neonates have lower blood pressure and a different pattern of distribution of blood flow to the various tissues. The role of such factors in the pharmacokinetics of drugs in neonates is not fully determined. The liver and brain are proportionately larger in neonates than in adults and receive a higher fraction of the total blood flow. Body fat is typically 15% of body mass in a full-term neonate but may be as little as 1% in a premature infant. Thus, distribution of fat-soluble drugs may be markedly altered.

Body water averages about 85% of body weight in premature infants, and 75% in full-term babies. This figure drops to 60% in older children and 55% in adults. Water-soluble drugs therefore have a much larger relative volume of water in which to distribute in neonates and thus must be given in relatively larger doses to achieve a given plasma concentration. This larger volume of distribution in neonates and infants is observed with antibiotics such as gentamicin, kanamycin (Kantrex), and sulfonamides, as well as drugs such as phenobarbital, theophylline, and phenylbutazone (Azolid).

Most drugs are less well bound to plasma proteins in the neonate than in the normal adult because of differences in blood composition. Neonates have a different form of albumin that has fewer binding sites and higher levels of endogenous substances, including bilirubin, free fatty acids, and steroids, that bind to the smaller number of sites. Reduced binding capacity has been reported for aspirin, phenobarbital, pentobarbital, phenytoin (Dilantin), phenylbutazone, benzylpenicillin, ampicillin, nafcillin, cephalosporins, sulfonamides, imipramine (Tofranil), desmethylimipramine, theophylline, and lidocaine (Xylocaine). Because these drugs are less protein-bound, the concentration of free drug is higher, and neonates are therefore at greater risk of toxicity from the higher concentration. Nurses need to be especially alert to subtle changes in the neonate that could signify onset of toxicity.

The blood-brain barrier is not fully developed in the neonate. Most drugs therefore penetrate into the brain more readily when given to young infants. The only exception is the relatively small number of drugs that move into the brain by active transport. Depressant effects of drugs on respiration are often greater in neonates than older children or adults even after corrections for weight or surface area are taken into account. Nurses need to be vigilant for neurological changes when depressant drugs are given to neonates.

Taken together, the differences in distribution in neonates generally result in greater tissue concentrations for many drugs, due to enhanced penetration and low protein binding, in spite of the diluting effect of the enlarged volume of distribution.

Elimination

The most significant pharmacokinetic difference between neonates and adults relates to drug elimination. These differences pertain to both metabolism by the liver and excretion by the kidneys.

Liver metabolic pathways are not fully mature in the neonate or infant. The various metabolic pathways develop at different times. For example, oxidative and reductive pathways are present at birth but proceed at a reduced rate for the first few weeks of life. Most conjugative pathways are operative early in life and develop rapidly, while N-dealkylation and glucuronidation are late-developing mechanisms. As a result of reduced liver metabolism of drugs, many drugs have a prolonged plasma half-life in neonates (Table 6–2). However, most liver pathways are probably as active after 12 months of life as they will ever be.

Excretion of drugs by the kidneys is also affected in a variety of ways by the conditions that exist in neonates. For one thing, because the large volume of distribution in neonates decreases drug concentration in the blood, the rate at which the drug reaches the kidney is decreased. Also, the volume of blood flowing through the kidney per unit time as a proportion of total body water is less in the infant. Glomerular filtration rate as a fraction of total body weight or surface area in neonates is only 30–40% of that in adults. Drugs having prolonged half-lives due mainly to reduced glomerular filtration rate include aminoglycosides, indomethacin (Indocin), salicylates, acetaminophen, digoxin, nitrofurantoin (Furadantin), thiazides, and furosemide. Renal excretion is even more affected if the drug utilizes active secretory mechanisms since these are only about 20% operational in neonates. Thus, excretion of penicillin, ampicillin, methicillin, oxacillin, and cephaloridine is greatly reduced. Renal function increases by more than 50% during the first week of life, reaching half the adult level by the seventh day postpartum. Full renal function is achieved between 9 and 12 months of age.

Table 6–2
Drugs with Prolonged Half-Lives in Neonates

Analgesics	**Cardiac glycosides**
Acetaminophen	Digoxin
Indomethacin	**Diuretics**
Phenylbutazone	Furosemide
Salicylates	Thiazides
Antidepressants	**Local anesthetics**
Nortriptyline	Lidocaine
Antiepileptics	Mepivacaine
Diazepam	**Oral hypoglycemics**
Phenobarbital	Tolbutamide
Phenytoin	**Sedative hypnotics**
Antimicrobials	Amobarbital
Ampicillin	**Xanthines**
Carbenicillin	Caffeine
Cephalosporins	Theophylline
Chloramphenicol	
Gentamicin	
Kanamycin	
Methicillin	
Nalidixic acid	
Nitrofurantoin	
Oxacillin	
Penicillin	
Streptomycin	
Sulfonamides	
Tobramycin	

The net result of these differences in hepatic and renal extraction of drugs in neonates is that drug half-life is markedly prolonged relative to that in adults, typically by from twofold to fivefold longer but by more than twentyfold for some drugs (caffeine, for example). Nurses can anticipate that effective drug levels will persist for longer periods. An increase in the duration of action of a single dose of a drug is not by itself necessarily harmful. The risk lies in the increased potential for cumulative toxicity if the interval between doses is not adjusted to take into account the greater half-life of the drug in neonates. If the doses are too close together, each dose will increase the blood level of the drug. The **gray baby syndrome** occurs in response to chloramphenicol (Chloromycetin) in precisely this way, possibly resulting in cardiovascular collapse and death. The half-life of chloramphenicol is about 26 hours in the neonate but only 4 hours in children and 2.3 hours in adults.

Pharmacokinetics in Older Children

Pharmacokinetic parameters in children who are beyond infancy are closer to those of adults than of neonates. The one significant distinction between pharmacokinetics in children and adults is that children metabolize drugs faster than adults. This may necessitate shorter dosage intervals for drugs that are eliminated mainly by hepatic metabolism. Some drugs with shorter half-lives in children than in adults include cephalothin (Keflin), doxycycline (Vibramycin), sulfonamides, phenylbutazone (Azolid), diazoxide (Hyperstat IV), diazepam (Valium), ethosuximide (Zarontin), phenytoin (Dilantin), and theophylline.

Adverse Drug Reactions in Children

Although children respond to drugs in much the same manner as adults, they may experience unique side effects not evident in adults because of the special physiological factors that are present during this period of rapid growth and maturation (Table 6–3). A child is especially likely to react uniquely to drugs that affect the endocrine system. Drugs that inhibit release of growth hormone (such as neuroleptics), or that inhibit epiphyseal closure (corticosteroids) may suppress growth. Androgens may cause virilization in females or premature pubescence in males. Children may also suffer paradoxical hyperactivity reactions to depressants such as barbiturates and narcotics, depression in response to certain nasal decongestants (naphazoline and tetrahydrozoline), rickets from the antivitamin effect of phenytoin, extreme anticholinergic reactions, the gray baby syndrome caused by chloramphenicol, kernicterus in response to displacers of bilirubin binding to plasma proteins (sulfonamides and vitamin K), and lactic acidosis in salicylate overdoses.

The child may also be exposed to drugs administered to the mother prenatally (via placental transfer) or postnatally (via breast milk). Prenatal administration of drugs to the mother can have a variety of adverse effects on the neonate, such as hemorrhage from anticoagulants or salicylates; congenital defects from a variety of teratogens (see Chapter 34); ototoxicity from aminoglycosides or chloroquine (Aralen); the gray baby syndrome from chloramphenicol; teeth and bone abnormalities from tetracyclines; neonatal depression from benzodiazepines, narcotics, neuroleptics, hypnotics, local anesthetics, or beta-blockers; electrolyte imbalances from diuretics; goiter or hypothyroidism from antithyroid drugs; feminization from estrogens; virilization from androgens; and hypoglycemia from sulfonylureas. Excretion of drugs in breast milk is addressed in Chapter 34. Some drugs, such as chloramphenicol, nalidixic acid, sulfonamides, and tetracyclines, are expressly contraindicated for use in nursing mothers because of potential risks to the infant.

Drug Administration to Children

Children present a number of special problems with respect to drug administration, regardless of route but dependent on the age of the child. When working with children the nurse must place special emphasis on maintaining an effective working relationship with both the child and the parents.

The Nurse's Relationship with the Child

Concern for psychological factors is especially important when drugs must be administered to children, because children are more psychologically vulnerable and often fearful of drug administration. Nurses should be careful to maintain an honest relationship with children. Nurses should not bribe children to take medication. It may work the first time, but on subsequent occasions the child will not succumb to the bribe or will expect a bigger one. It is equally important to urge parents not to offer bribes.

Children may require more emotional support during drug administration. They should not be threatened. Suggesting that the medication must be swallowed quickly or it will be given as a "shot" makes the child fearful of medication, and often the threat cannot be followed through if the child still does not cooperate.

An older child may be assisted in self-care by the nurse explaining (for example) that a particular drug of a particular color should be taken before meals, or after meals, or at bedtime, or suggesting that the child let someone know if the drug has not been given. If the child can understand printing, a nurse might supply a card that has drug times allocated and ask the youngster to put a checkmark when he or she takes the drug. Careful teaching when the child is in the hospital can encourage appropriate self-care and compliance once the child returns home.

Table 6–3
Adverse Drug Effects in Children

Drug	Adverse effects in neonates due to maternally administered drugs	Adverse reactions to drugs administered to neonates: Unique to children	Adverse reactions to drugs administered to neonates: Exaggerated but not unique to children
Anticholinergics			
Atropine, scolamine, methantheline		Extreme reactions of agitation, hyperthermia, tachycardia, tachypnea	Hallucinations
Anticoagulants			
Phenindione	Neonatal hemorrhage		Nephritis, acute renal failure
Antidepressants			
Tricyclics			Extrapyramidal disorders, photophobia, agranulocytosis
MAO inhibitors			Hypoglycemia
Antiepileptics			
Phenobarbital		Hyperactivity	
Phenytoin	Congenital defects, neonatal hemorrhage	Rickets due to increased metabolism of vitamin D; folic acid deficiency anemia	Nephritis, hyperglycemia, lupus syndrome
Trimethadione			Nephrotic syndrome, photophobia
Antihistamines			Hallucination, blurred vision
Antimicrobials			
Aminoglycosides	ototoxicity		Acute renal failure
Amphotericin B			Acute renal failure, tubular dysfunction
Ampicillin		Diarrhea, rash, monilial diaper rash	Acute renal failure, interstitial nephritis
Antimalarials			
Chloroquine	Retinopathy, ototoxicity		
Quinine	Thrombocytopenia		
Bacitracin			Acute renal failure
Cephalosporins			Acute renal failure
Chloramphenicol	Gray baby syndrome, cardiovascular collapse	Gray baby syndrome, cardiovascular collapse	Hematological disorders
Colistin			Acute renal failure, interstitial nephritis
Erythromycin			Acute nephritis
Gentamicin			Acute renal failure
Griseofulvin			Lupus syndrome
Hexachlorophene		Central edema	
Isoniazid			Lupus syndrome
Kanamycin			Acute renal failure
Methicillin			Acute renal failure
Nalidixic acid		Intracranial hypertension	Photophobia

(continued)

Table 6–3
Adverse Drug Effects in Children (*continued*)

		Adverse reactions to drugs administered to neonates	
Drug	**Adverse effects in neonates due to maternally administered drugs**	**Unique to children**	**Exaggerated but not unique to children**
Nitrofurantoin	Hemolytic anemia in glucose-6-phosphate dehydrogenase deficient neonates		
Novobiocin		Hyperbilirubinemia	
Penicillin			Acute renal failure, nephritis, lupus syndrome
Polymyxin			Acute renal failure, blurred vision
Streptomycin			Acute renal failure, lupus syndrome
Sulfonamides	Kernicterus, hemolytic anemia in glucose-6-phosphate dehydrogenase deficient neonates	Hyperbilirubinemia, kernicterus	Acute renal failure, nephritis, hypoglycemia, hematological disorders, lupus syndrome
Tetracyclines	Teeth abnormalities	Impaired bone growth, increased intracranial pressure, dental staining	Acute renal failure, tubular dysfunctions
Antimigraine drugs			
Methysergide			Renal damage
Antineoplastics			
Antimetabolites	Congenital abnormalities		Hematological disorders, lupus syndrome, acute renal failure
Anxiolytics	Neonatal depression		Blurred vision
Cardiovascular drugs			
Beta-blockers	Neonatal depression, bradycardia		Hypoglycemia
Diazoxide			Hypoglycemia, lens opacities
Hydralazine			Lupus syndrome
Methyldopa			Extrapyramidal reactions, lupus syndrome
Procainamide			Nephrotic syndrome, lupus syndrome
Reserpine	Nasal stuffiness, lethargy		Extrapyramidal reactions, blurred vision
Contrast media			Acute renal failure
Diuretics			
Acetazolamide			Renal damage
Furosemide	Electrolyte imbalances		Enhanced nephrotoxicity of aminoglycosides, hyperglycemia
Thiazides	Electrolyte imbalances		Enhanced nephrotoxicity of aminoglycosides, hyperglycemia

Table 6–3
Adverse Drug Effects in Children (*continued*)

Drug	Adverse effects in neonates due to maternally administered drugs	Adverse reactions to drugs administered to neonates: Unique to children	Adverse reactions to drugs administered to neonates: Exaggerated but not unique to children
Gastrointestinal drugs			
Laxatives			Renal damage
Pancreatic enzymes		Hyperuricemia	
Heavy metals			
Bismuth			Acute renal failure
Gold			Nephrotic syndrome, acute renal failure
Lead			Lead poisoning
Mercury			Nephrotic syndrome, nephritis, hypertension
Thallium			Acute renal failure
Hormones and antihormones			
Androgens	Virilization of female fetus		
Antithyroid drugs			
Iodides	Goiter		Nephritis
Radioiodine	Hypothyroidism		
Thiouracils	Goiter		Agranulocytosis, lupus syndrome
Corticosteroids	Risk of prematurity	Suppression of epiphyseal closure, increased intracranial pressure, increased systemic absorption after topical administration	Lens opacities, hypertension
Estrogens	Adenocarcinoma of cervix, feminization of male fetus		
Glucagon			Hyperglycemia
Growth hormone			Hyperglycemia
Insulin			Hypoglycemia
Oral contraceptives			Hyperglycemia, photophobia, hypertension
Oral hypoglycemics	Hypoglycemia		Nephrotic syndrome, hypoglycemia
Local anesthetics	Bradycardia, depression		
Narcotics	Neonatal depression, withdrawal syndrome	Excitation, restlessness	Hyperglycemia
Neuroleptics			
Haloperidol	Extrapyramidal reactions	Growth suppression	Lens opacities, extrapyramidal reactions
Phenothiazines	Neonatal depression, extrapyramidal reactions, retinopathy	Growth suppression	Hyperglycemia, lens opacities, agranulocytosis, extrapyramidal reactions

(continued)

Table 6–3
Adverse Drug Effects in Children (*continued*)

		Adverse reactions to drugs administered to neonates	
Drug	**Adverse effects in neonates due to maternally administered drugs**	**Unique to children**	**Exaggerated but not unique to children**
Nonsteroidal anti-inflammatory drugs			
Aspirin	Transient coagulation defects	Acute intoxication lactic acidosis	Acute renal failure, hypoglycemia
Indomethacin		Sudden death, corneal opacities	Blurred vision
Pyrazolones			Blurred vision, agranulocytosis, lupus syndrome
Sympathomimetics			
Ephedrine			Hypertension
Isoproterenol		Death	
Naphazoline and tetrahydrozoline		CNS depression and coma	Hypertension
Uricosurics			
Probenecid			Nephrotic syndrome
Vitamins			
A		Intoxication	
D		Hypercalcemia	Hypertension, renal damage
K		Kernicterus	

If the nurse is teaching an older child how to take his or her own medication, a medication chart may be helpful. When the child takes the medication, a star or some similarly appealing sticker can be placed on the chart. (This method was used by one parent to encourage improved eating habits along with the taking of medication. Thus the child put silver stars on the chart when she ate fruit, a red star when she ate her vegetables, blue stars for drinking milk, and a gold star when the child reminded mom to give her her medicine. The parent rewarded the child verbally and periodically, as a special treat, took the child to the zoo, a movie, or allowed the child to participate in some activity especially prized.)

Monitoring drug response in children can be particularly difficult since children cannot necessarily articulate what they experience. Nurses need continually to reassess drug responses in children, determining the extent to which therapeutic effects have actually occurred. When working with children, nurses must include parents' observations, children's expressions of concern or change, as well as their own observations.

The Nurse's Relationship with the Parents

Nurses administer drugs to children in a variety of settings, and nurses are often the health professional responsible for teaching parents how to administer medications to their child. Thus, it is particularly important that nurses recognize that they are working with the parent or guardian as a team. Each person must assume responsibility for components of the team effort to achieve a satisfactory response. This means that not only must nurses teach parents as much as possible about the drug and drug protocol, but that they encourage parental compliance with all phases of the child's therapy, including recording and reporting any changes whether physical or behavioral. Noting behavioral changes in children is especially critical since small, incremental changes can be evidence of serious, underlying problems.

As an active coordinator on the health care team, the nurse also must spend considerable time making sure that the efforts of the team are carried out systematically. He or she must assure that confusing information is clarified, that misinformation is corrected and made understandable. Thus, when parents are informed of their child's illness and the prescription for cure, nurses need to be certain that the parents comprehend the nature of the health care problem and, when drugs are deemed necessary by the physician, all aspects of the drug regimen.

When providing instructions to parents, nurses should arrange the information step by step according to the sequence of events to be followed. For example, if an injection is invalid, the instructions would be as follows:

1. Assemble all essential equipment. (A list of equipment should be provided by the nurse.)
2. Draw up the appropriate amount of drug into the sterile syringe.
3. Change the needle if necessary prior to injection.
4. Select the appropriate site for injection and record any rotation of sites required.
5. Clean the selected site with antiseptic.
6. Tell the child when the needle is going to be inserted and ask the child to take a deep breath and look away from the area to be injected.
7. Insert the needle and pull back on the plunger.
8. Inject the solution.
9. Withdraw the needle.
10. Massage the area (if required).
11. Give the child reassurance and comfort.

When a child requires medication, the nurse needs to teach the parent how to identify problems that may occur either as a result of the illness, the drug(s), or both. With infants and very young children, this can be a special problem since responses occur so quickly. Furthermore, because infant's bodies are immature, they tend to respond to illness and drug therapy systematically. A child who has had fever, diarrhea, and vomiting may be responding to an underlying health problem or experiencing an adverse reaction to drug therapy. Gastrointestinal responses to medication in the child can create additional problems, such as nutritional deficiencies, or fluid and electrolyte imbalance. Nurses need to stress the importance of immediately reporting minor changes so as to avoid larger problems. Because they lack adequate communication skills, children cannot accurately report how they feel. Therefore, just as nurses need to rely upon their skills in observation, so must they teach parents observation skills and what to do when relevant observations are made.

A very young child cannot monitor his or her own care. Therefore, when a child is discharged from a hospital unit, nurses need to assist parents in monitoring care and response to drug therapy. If a child is taking medication that will cause altered coloration of urine, for example, or if the medication can cause mood swings, altered behavior, skin rash, or headache, the parent or guardian should be so informed. The information should be stated in lay terms, printed, and reviewed with the responsible adult prior to the child's discharge.

When a child is very ill, it is easy for the parent to remember to give the prescribed medication. However, as the child responds to the therapy and his or her physical condition improves, it is easy for parents to forget the medication or to give it late. Nurses need to remind parents that the effects of medicine are cumulative. Thus, if an antibiotic is given only until the symptoms of infection subside, it is unlikely to have fully destroyed the causative organism. Not only is the infection likely to return, but the new population of organisms may be more resistant to drug treatment. Nurses need to make certain that parents understand that the prescription was written for the specific amount of drug to be taken and that utilizing all drugs in the regimen is essential.

In order to encourage that parents remember to give a child medication, the nurse can suggest that a chart be taped on a refrigerator door or in some other conspicuous place. There should also be a pencil at hand, and each time the drug is given, it should be recorded on the chart.

Finally, the nurse should make certain that parents know whom to contact if there are questions or problems. The nurse should also make sure that adequate provisions are made for follow-up care such as laboratory examinations or urinalysis.

Enteral Administration

Oral Administration

Oral administration is generally the most acceptable route in children, but it presents special challenges for the nurse. Nurses should usually give oral medications in liquid form to children under 5 years of age. Children under 3 months of age can be given drugs orally through a nipple, syringe, or dropper. The nurse should place the drug in the back of the mouth. It is important to support the child's head during this maneuver because infants have little head control. The nurse should administer the drug slowly to avoid choking the infant. Droppers should be of soft plastic to prevent breakage should the infant clench his jaws. Placing rubber tubing on the end of a medicine dropper also provides a safe method of administration.

Nurses should not crush tablets to provide liquid drug forms for administration to infants. Crushed tablets and capsules lose much of their effectiveness since particles formed in this way seldom mix well with water, and much of the dose ends up adhering to the vessel. Such medications cannot be given safely to infants even when mixed with formula. A pharmacist should be asked to prepare special liquid formulations when required.

From 3 months to 1 year, children may take medications from a cup, spoon, or other suitable device. When feasible, accurate pipette-type measuring devices should be used in preference to droppers or teaspoons to avoid variability in dosing. At this age, the child needs to be controlled during administration and requires reassurance and comforting before, during, and after the procedure. It is important for the nurse to sit and hold the child to comfort him or her. It is also important to make certain the child has taken all the medication. From age 1 to 2.5, the drug may be mixed with a small amount of food, but care must be taken to avoid food-drug interactions. Nurses should note incidences of vomiting since children may vomit medication immediately or as long as 8 hours after administration. Parents need to be alerted to this problem as well.

After 2.5 years of age, chewable tablets or suspensions can be used successfully. One of the child's parents may be able to accomplish drug administration better than medical personnel. A skillful nurse often devises special techniques that work with particular children. The child's nose should never be held to force swallowing of orally applied medicines since this can result in aspiration.

Children should always be told the truth about medication. Honesty and consistent behavior help the nurse gain the child's confidence. In the case of oral medications, children should be given ample warning if the medication has an unpleasant taste that cannot be masked. The child should be told to expect it to be bitter or sour, sweet or salty, or the unpleasant taste should be otherwise described.

Some children may need to be taught how to swallow pills or capsules. Prior to giving medications to a child, the nurse needs to clarify with parent and child whether or not the child has ever been given medication in pill form. The nurse can hand the child a small piece of candy (such as M & M's) or a small piece of ice and instruct the child immediately to take a sip of water. Once the child has mastered the skill, the nurse should be certain to praise the accomplishment.

Rectal Administration

The rectal route is seldom indicated, especially in children. It provides erratic absorption, since it is difficult to predict whether the child's rectal ampulla will be full or empty at any given moment. It is therefore useless to insert a suppository unless the rectum is examined and evacuated of any feces using a small saline enema.

Children often find rectal administration very stressful. Nurses should remember that the child cannot see what the nurse is doing and can easily be frightened by this type of intrusion, particularly if the child has been warned about child molestation. Therefore, it is very important to explain what is to happen and how. The child should be shown the suppository so he or she can be certain of what the nurse is saying. If there is a doll present, the nurse might demonstrate what he or she is about to do, showing where the suppository is to be inserted. Any questions the child asks should be addressed truthfully. The child can be told, for example, that the procedure will not be painful but there will be pressure.

Once questions have been answered and the nurse has reassured the child about the procedure, the nurse can proceed. The suppository should be well lubricated. Using the little finger and a finger cot, the nurse should insert the suppository until it reaches beyond the rectal sphincters. The finger should be inserted as far as the first knuckle, then withdrawn and the child's buttocks pressed firmly together until the urge to evacuate is past. The nurse should be certain to explain what is being done as it is being done. Once placement of the suppository has been accomplished, the nurse should be sure to praise the child for cooperating.

If the medication is to be administered as a retention enema, the nurse should use as little solution as possible, a maximum of 4 fluid ounces. Again there should be an explanation of what is to happen, and in this situation the child needs to be told not to expell the material even if he or she feels a need to. Once the medication has been administered, it is important to press the child's buttocks together to prevent expelling the solution and losing the medication.

Topical Administration

Topical administration also provides special challenges in children. Sublingual and buccal routes should not be utilized in younger children because they frequently swallow the medication and cannot be relied upon to keep the medication in place. Nasal inhalants also require a degree of cooperation that is seldom provided by children under 6. Topical application to the eyes, ears, or nose is difficult and risky in children because they move quickly. In addition, since most children have been taught not to insert anything in eyes, ears, or nose, it may be difficult to assure the child that what is to be done is all right. It is helpful if the parent assists in reassuring the child.

Ointments, Creams, and Lotions

When ointments, creams, or lotions are applied topically to the skin of a child, care must be taken to prevent the child from spreading the medication from fingers to mouth or eyes. The diaper provides a handy covering when medications are applied to the groin. Plastic wrap can be used as an occlusive dressing over other skin areas.

Nose Drops and Eye Drops

Having drops put into the nose is not pleasant. Therefore it is extremely important for the nurse to explain to the child that the nose drops will be uncomfortable but that the medication will make him or her feel better. It is important to tell the child how many drops or squirts will be put into each nostril and to tell him or her to sniff to assure the medication goes to the proper location. It is very important for the nurse to demonstrate how to sniff and to answer any questions the child may have.

When ready to put the drops into the nose, the nurse should have the child lie on his or her back. If the nurse is working with an infant, a mummy restraint is recommended. In this instance, a draw sheet or towel is brought over one arm and anchored underneath the child by his or her own body weight. The other side of the restraint is brought up over the top of the child's body and anchored underneath the other side by the weight of the body. The restraint is used for the duration of the procedure. If the youngster is a preschooler, it is wise to put a pillow under the shoulders so that the head can extend over the pillow and rest downward. If the youngster is school-age, he or she can be instructed to extend the head over the side of the bed so that the head is lower than the trunk.

The appropriate number of drops or a squirt is placed in one nostril. If in the left nostril, the head is turned left; if in the right nostril, the head is turned right. The nurse then instructs the child to sniff the medicine further and has the youngster remain with his or her head flat for at least a minute. This allows the medicine to come into contact with the mucous membranes of the nose. Once the procedure is successfully completed, the nurse should praise the child for cooperation.

If nose drops are frightening, having drops placed in the eyes is more so because of the discomfort and fear instilled in children in the process of warning them not to put things into the eye. For the young child, a mummy restraint is recommended. The procedures followed are the same as with adults, as described in Chapter 4.

Drops should be warmed to body temperature before application to reduce the shock of application. It is usually better to apply the full dose in a single squirt than one drop at a time because it is difficult to keep the child still for the torturous drop by drop method. In applying medications to these delicate tissues, the nurse should press gently downward over the lower bony ridge of the eye socket to open the eye. No pressure must be placed on eye tissues. The nurse should rest the hand that holds the dropper or other implement on the child's head. This technique ensures that the hand will move synchronously with the child's head in the event of a sudden movement and risk of trauma is minimized. Drops or ointment should be placed on the lower everted lid. Then the eye is allowed to close.

Ear Drops

Children who are to have ear drops usually have had a painful earache and are afraid that anything put in their ears will cause more pain. The nurse needs to tell the child that the ear drops will not hurt but they will feel funny — a kind of tickling in the ear. The nurse may demonstrate by dropping water onto the child's skin. The child's concept of what "tickles" may differ from an adult's, and the nurse needs to understand the child's interpretation so that trust and honesty persist.

Once the child understands the procedure, the nurse can have the child lie on his or her back. A mummy restraint may be required for the very young child. If the youngster is under 2 years of age, the nurse should straighten the external ear canal by pulling the ear lobe down and back. If the child is over 2 years, the pinna of the ear should be pulled gently up and back. This may be painful in the case of ear infection or mastoiditis. The drops should then be placed into each ear and the child's head held with the ear facing up for at least a full minute so that the medication fills the entire ear canal. Again, praising the child for a good performance is important.

Refrigerated fluid should not be instilled in the ear until warmed to room temperature. Cold against the tympanic membrane causes pain and also perhaps dizziness and nausea. The time spent warming the medication can be well spent reassuring the child or teaching the parent or guardian how to perform the procedure at home, if necessary.

Parenteral Routes

Parenteral routes provide the most reliable drug delivery in young children and should be used preferentially when accurate drug therapy is critical. Children should always be correctly informed about injections they are to receive. They should be told if the medication is painful and the type of pain it may cause. They should be instructed to tell the nurse immediately if they feel anything different from what the nurse has described. The explanation should be short; lengthy explanations may only increase the child's anxiety. The nurse needs to validate with the child that each is interpreting the concept of "pain," "bee sting," "mosquito sting," "burning," and so forth in the same way. Otherwise, the child may believe he or she has been lied to. Letting the youngster know you are concerned for his or her comfort, speaking in soothing tones, and handling the child gently but firmly all serve to encourage confidence in the nurse's behavior.

Subcutaneous and Intramuscular Injections

Subcutaneous and intramuscular injections are more difficult in neonates and young children because of the small mass of subcutaneous and muscle tissue. There is a risk of neuropathy in these patients if the needle penetrates a nerve. The buttocks in particular should be avoided for intramuscular injections in infants; the sciatic nerve occupies a larger portion of this space than in adults because the gluteal muscle does not become well developed until a child can walk. Therefore, frequent use of intragluteal injections sooner or later results in damage to the sciatic nerve with permanent crippling. The deltoid area or the lateral surfaces of the thighs are preferred sites for intramuscular injections in children. The usual site of intramuscular injection in infants is the lateral portion of the quadriceps muscle of the thigh. The medial section of this muscle should be avoided since it is very tender, as is the medial aspect of the thigh.

In children over 1 year of age, a ventrogluteal site may be chosen because this area has no major nerves or blood vessels. To inject into this area, the nurse puts the thumb on the child's anterior superior iliac crest. The hand is spread so that the fingers rest along the iliac crest. The space between finger and thumb is the site for injection. It may be necessary to restrain the child to perform this procedure.

When intramuscular or subcutaneous injections must be given repeatedly, rotation of sites helps to ensure complete absorption of drug and recovery of the tissue. The syringe should be held in such a manner that the side of the hand strikes the skin adjacent to the site of injection a fraction of a second before the needle penetrates to provide a distraction.

Intravenous Therapy in Children

Intravenous therapy is an effective means of administering fluids and medication to infants and children. However, there are certain precautions and rules that apply to children more than adults. For one thing, the choice of infusion site differs from infant to older child and adult.

Infants have very small veins. Therefore veins over the temporal area of the scalp are frequently chosen for IV infusion because they are fairly large. This is a particularly disturbing procedure for parents; nurses should reassure them that the use of veins in the scalp will in no way affect the brain or cause neurological damage (a frequent concern). It is important to explain that needles inserted into veins in the scalp are less likely to be dislodged than needles put into an arm, that there is less apt to be infiltration into tissues, and that, since the scalp is a particularly insensitive skin area, needles placed in the scalp create the least discomfort for the child. The nurse also needs to explain how the procedure will be performed.

Usually the area to be used is over the temporal bone. The site should be lathered with a mild soap solution, rinsed, and washed with an antiseptic to reduce the possibility of infection.

Once the site has been prepared, a rubber band is placed around the forehead and a small scalp vein needle is inserted. This is a special needle with protruding plastic "wings" on the sides allowing for easy manipulation. Once the needle is in place, the nurse must prevent the child from brushing it out. A paper medicine cup taped over the needle provides protection. In addition, nurses may restrain infants by pinning their shirt sleeves to the sides of the diapers. Sandbags placed on either side of the head also help.

Because the child has been frightened and forced to endure pain, if only briefly, it is important for the nurse to provide reassurance. Holding the infant, rocking, talking to the child, smiling, lightly touching him or her, stroking or humming softly seems to provide comfort. If the parent is present, it often helps to encourage the parent to hold the baby.

Veins on the back of the hand or flexor surface of the wrist are also sites frequently chosen for IV infusions. Generally infusion materials flow better in these sites than, say, the antecubital area (just below the elbow). In addition, children tend to keep the arms flexed. Therefore, a needle inserted in the antecubital area would be most likely to infiltrate, creating yet another problem for the child.

Among older children, there may be a choice of sites, and when the child has a preference, it should be considered. During IV therapy, a child should be encouraged to be somewhat self-sufficient in such tasks as feeding him or herself, for example. As an advocate for the child, the nurse should call this to the attention of whoever is assigned to begin the infusion. When the IV cannula is put into the hand or arm, it is important to be sure the arm is immobilized so as not to dislodge the infusion.

Utmost care must be taken to ensure that IV solutions are neither contaminated nor decomposed. Any solution that exhibits clouding or abnormal coloration should be discarded.

Intravenous fluids must not be allowed to flow too quickly into a child since a child's heart and circulatory system are small and easily overloaded. For this reason, automatic rate-flow infusions have proven ideal because they regulate the flow accurately. A pediatric infusion set allows only 50–100 mL of fluid into the drip chamber at a time. If the child's movement should suddenly increase the flow of fluid, only the amount in the drip chamber will actually enter the child's circulation. Some units may use a minidropper, a device that reduces the size of drops in the control chamber. The smaller drop size allows the same amount of fluid to be infused per hour, but the rate is easier to regulate.

Nurses need to monitor the rate of flow and check the infusion site frequently (at least once an hour) to assure that fluid is flowing appropriately. In addition, because response rates (whether favorable or unfavorable) occur rapidly in children, nurses need to check children frequently for their response to drugs used in the IV solution. The nurse should encourage parents to report immediately any changes they may notice in their child.

Congestive heart failure can result from overloading a child's circulatory system. The nurse would at first notice an increase in the child's pulse rate and blood pressure. As the situation worsens, however, the blood pressure falls and the child would show signs of edema. Therefore, vital signs must be checked at least every hour to assure that such changes have not occurred.

When a child is to have IV infusions over a long period of time, often the physician will use a cutdown (Intracath). With this procedure, the child can move about more freely without dislodging the needle. In the long run, the procedure may well prove far less painful for the child than other infusion methods. Nurses need to explain this to worried parents. A cutdown also allows the child more freedom to enter into some of the ward activities with other youngsters, thereby taking his or her mind off the physical disability and encouraging companionship and, often, solace from others in similar circumstances.

Intravenous injections should be given especially slowly in children to avoid overly high peak drug concentrations. Scalp veins should not be used since this can result in scalp necrosis and permanent baldness.

Case Study: Altered Pharmacokinetics in a Child

Q. S., a 7-year-old boy, was diagnosed as having grand mal seizures. He was initially treated with phenobarbital and seizure occurrence was eliminated. However, Q. S. experienced excessive sedation with phenobarbital, which interfered with his performance in school. The pediatrician decided to switch Q. S. to phenytoin (Dilantin) pediatric suspension, prescribing 6 mg/kg,day, PO, to be taken in the morning. After 1 month on this new regimen, Q. S. experienced a seizure, then another one a week later. Q. S. was brought to the pediatrician after school for evaluation.

The nurse discussed compliance with the parents and was assured that all doses had been given as prescribed. The nurse asked the mother, who had been administering the medication, to demonstrate the technique she employed. The mother accurately measured the prescribed dose but failed to shake the container before pouring the dose. The nurse explained to her the importance of shaking suspensions.

A blood sample was taken for determination of serum phenytoin concentration. The concentration was found to be 6 μg/ml, well below the minimum therapeutic concentration of 10 μg/ml. The physician reviewed the literature on phenytoin and then altered the regimen so that the same total daily dose was to be given in two divided doses, one upon arising in the morning, the other 12 hours later. After 2 weeks on the new regimen, blood samples were taken at midmorning and late in the afternoon. Serum concentrations of phenytoin in both samples were 12 μg/ml.

1. Was the dose originally selected for Q. S. appropriate?
2. Based on the information provided, name two factors that may have contributed to the occurrence of subtherapeutic serum concentrations of phenytoin?
3. Why did the pediatrician reduce the dosing interval? Why didn't she increase the total dose instead?

Answers appear at the back of the book.

Recommended Readings

Benitz WE, Totro DS: *The Pediatric Drug Handbook.* Chicago, Year Book Medical Publishers, 1981.

Briggs L, Beyda D: Giving pediatric code drugs: No longer a calculated risk. *Nursing* 1986;16(7):56.

Evans ML, Hansen BD: Administering injections to different-aged children. *Matern Child Nurs J* 1981;6:194–199.

Lovejoy FH, Berenberg W: Poisoning in children under age 5. *Postgrad Med* 1978;63:79–89.

Ormond EAR, Caulfield CA: A practical guide to giving oral medications to young children. *Matern Child Nurs J* 1976;1:320–325.

Rimar JM: Guidelines for the intravenous administration of medications used in pediatrics. *Matern Child Nurs J* 1982;7:184–197.

Appendix
Recommended Doses of Common Drugs in Children

Class and drug	Patient population	Indication	Route	Dose	Interval (hours)
Antienuretic					
Imipramine	> 4	Enuresis	PO	25–75 mg/day	24 (1 hour before bedtime)
Antiepileptics					
Carbamazepine	CH	Antiepileptic	PO	10 mg/kg/day	8–12
Clonazepam	CH	Initial	PO	0.01–0.03 mg/kg/day	8
	CH	Maximum	PO	0.3 mg/kg/day	8
Diazepam	NEO, IN, CH	Status epilepticus	IV	0.3 mg/kg/dose	May be repeated twice at 5-minute intervals
Ethosuximide	CH	Petit mal	PO	20 mg/kg/day	12
Phenobarbital	IN, CH	Antiepileptic	PO	1.5–6 mg/kg/day	12
Phenytoin	IN, CH	Antiepileptic	PO	3–8 mg/kg/day	12
Primidone	CH	Antiepileptic	PO	3–8 mg/kg/day	8–12
Trimethadione	CH	Petit mal	PO	20–40 mg/kg/day	8
Valproate	CH	Antiepileptic	PO	15–30 mg/kg/day	8–12
Antihistamines					
Brompheniramine	CH	Antiallergic	PO	0.5 mg/kg/day	6
Chlorpheniramine	CH	Antiallergic	PO	0.35 mg/kg/day	6
Dimenhydrinate	CH	Motion sickness	PO	5 mg/kg/day	6
Diphenhydramine	IN, CH	Antiallergic	PO, IM, IV	5 mg/kg/day	6–8
Tripelennamine	CH	Antiallergic	PO	5 mg/kg/day	6
Antimicrobials					
Amikacin	LBW and/or < 8 days	Antibacterial	IM, IVI	15 mg/kg/day	12
	NBW and > 7 days	Antibacterial	IM, IVI	15–22.5 mg/kg/day	8
Amoxicillin	CH	Antibacterial	PO	20–40 mg/kg/day	8
Ampicillin	< 8 days	Antibacterial	IM, IVI	50 mg/kg/day	12
	< 8 days	Meningitis	IVI	100 mg/kg/day	4
	> 7 days	Antibacterial	IM, IVI	75 mg/kg/day	8
	> 7 days	Meningitis	IVI	200 mg/kg/day	4
	IN	Antibacterial	PO	50–100 mg/kg/day	6
	IN	Septicemia	IVI	100–200 mg/kg/day	4
	IN	Septicemia	IM	100–200 mg/kg/day	6
	IN	Meningitis	IVI	400 mg/kg/day	4
Carbenicillin	NEO	Initial	IM, IVI	100 mg/kg	Once
	LBW or < 8 days	Maintenance	IM, IVI	225 mg/kg/day	8
	LBW > 7 days	Maintenance	IM, IVI	400 mg/kg/day	6
	NBW < 8 days	Maintenance	IM, IVI	300 mg/kg/day	6
	NBW > 7 days	Maintenance	IM, IVI	400 mg/kg/day	6
	IN, CH	Maintenance	IV	400–600 mg/kg/day	4
	IN, CH	Maintenance	IM	400–600 mg/kg/day	6

(continued)

Appendix
Recommended Doses of Common Drugs in Children (*continued*)

Class and drug	Patient population	Indication	Route	Dose	Interval (hours)
Cephalosporins					
Cefadroxil	CH	Antibacterial	PO	30 mg/kg/day	12
Cefazolin	NEO	Antibacterial	IM, IVI	40 mg/kg/day	12
	IN, CH	Antibacterial	IM, IVI	50–100 mg/kg/day	6
Cephalexin	IN, CH	Antibacterial	PO	25–50 mg/kg/day	6
Cephalothin	NEO < 7 days	Antibacterial	IM, IVI	40 mg/kg/day	12
	NEO > 7	Antibacterial	IM, IVI	60 mg/kg/day	8
	IN, CH	Antibacterial	IM, IVI	80–160 mg/kg/day	4
Cephapirin	CH	Antibacterial	IM, IVI	40–80 mg/kg/day	6
Cephradine	CH	Antibacterial	IM, IVI	50–300 mg/kg/day	6
	CH	Antibacterial	PO	50–100 mg/kg/day	6
Chloramphenicol	NEO < 15 days	Antibacterial	IV	25 mg/kg/day	4
	NEO 15–30 days, LBW	Antibacterial	IV	25 mg/kg/day	4
	NEO 15–30 days, NBW	Antibacterial	IV	50 mg/kg/day	4
	IN, CH	Antibacterial	PO	50–100 mg/kg/day	6
	IN, CH	Antibacterial	IV	100 mg/kg/day	4
Clindamycin	IN, CH	Antibacterial	PO	10–25 mg/kg/day	6–8
	IN, CH	Antibacterial	IM, IVI	25–40 mg/kg/day	6–8
Cloxacillin	IN, CH	Antibacterial	PO	50–100 mg/kg/day	6
Dicloxacillin	IN, CH	Antibacterial	PO	12.5–25 mg/kg/day	6
Erythromycin	IN, CH	Antibacterial	PO	30–50 mg/kg/day	6
	IN, CH	Antibacterial	IV	15–20 mg/kg/day	6
Gentamicin	NEO < 8 days	Antibacterial	IM, IVI	5 mg/kg/day	12
	NEO > 7 days	Antibacterial	IM, IVI	7.5 mg/kg/day	8
	CH	Antibacterial	IM, IVI	6–7.5 mg/kg/day	8
Griseofulvin	CH	Antifungal	PO	10 mg/kg/day	24
Isoniazid	IN, CH	TB	PO, IM	10–20 mg/kg/day Max.: 500 mg/day	8–12
Kanamycin	NEO, LBW, < 8 days	Antibacterial	IM, IVI	15 mg/kg/day	12
	NEO, LBW, > 7 days	Antibacterial	IM, IVI	20 mg/kg/day	12
	NEO, NBW, < 8 days	Antibacterial	IM, IVI	20 mg/kg/day	12
	NEO, NBW, > 7 days	Antibacterial	IM, IVI	30 mg/kg/day	8
	IN, CH	Antibacterial	IM, IVI	6–15 mg/kg/day	8–12
Lincomycin	CH	Antibacterial	PO	30–60 mg/kg/day	8
	CH	Antibacterial	IM, IVI	10–20 mg/kg/day	8–12
Methenamine	CH	UTI	IM, IVI	50–100 mg/kg/day	6
Methicillin	NEO, LBW, < 15 days	Antibacterial	IM, IVI	50 mg/kg/day	12
	NEO, LBW, 15–30 days	Antibacterial	IM, IV	75 mg/kg/day	8

Appendix

Recommended Doses of Common Drugs in Children (*continued*)

Class and drug	Patient population	Indication	Route	Dose	Interval (hours)
	NEO, NBW, < 15 days	Antibacterial	IM, IVI	75 mg/kg/day	8
	NEO, NBW, > 15 days	Antibacterial	IM, IVI	100 mg/kg/day	6
	IN, CH	Antibacterial	IVI	200–400 mg/kg/day	4
	IN, CH	Antibacterial	IM	200–400 mg/kg/day	6
Miconazole	CH	Antifungal	IVI	20–40 mg/kg/day	8
Nafcillin	NEO < 7 days	Antibacterial	IM, IVI	40 mg/kg/day	12
	NEO > 7 days	Antibacterial	IM, IVI	60 mg/kg/day	8
	IN, CH	Antibacterial	PO	50–100 mg/kg/day	6
	IN, CH	Antibacterial	IM	100–200 mg/kg/day	6
	IN, CH	Antibacterial	IVI	100–200 mg/kg/day	4
Nalidixic acid	IN > 3 months, CH	Antibacterial	PO	55 mg/kg/day	6
Neomycin	IN, CH	Antibacterial	PO	50–100 mg/kg/day	6–8
Nitrofurantoin	IN > 3 months, CH	UTI	PO	5–7 mg/kg/day	6
Nystatin	NEO LBW	Antifungal	PO	200,000–400,000 units/day	4–6
	NEO NBW, IN	Antifungal	PO	400,000–800,000 units/day	4–6
	CH	Antifungal	PO	800,000–2,000,000 units/day	4–6
Oxacillin	IN, CH	Antibacterial	PO	50–100 mg/kg/day	6
	IN, CH	Antibacterial	IV	100–200 mg/kg/day	4
	IN, CH	Antibacterial	IM	100–200 mg/kg/day	6
Penicillin G, benzyl-penicillin	NEO < 7 days	Antibacterial	IV, IM	50,000 units/kg/day	12
	NEO < 7 days	Meningitis	IV, IM	100,000–150,000 units/kg/day	4
	NEO > 7 days	Antibacterial	IV, IM	75,000 units/kg/day	8
	NEO > 7 days	Meningitis	IV, IM	150,000–250,000 units/kg/day	4
	IN, CH	Antibacterial	PO, IM, IV	25,000–50,000 units/kg/day	4–6
	IN, CH	Severe infection	IV	200,000–400,000 units/kg/day	2–4
Penicillin V	IN	Antibacterial	PO	25,000–100,000 units/kg/day	4–8
Rifampin	IN, CH	Antibacterial	PO	10–20 mg/kg/day	24
Streptomycin	CH	Antibacterial	IM	20–40 mg/kg/day	12
Sulfamethoxazole	IN, CH	Antibacterial	PO	50–60 mg/kg	1st dose
		Maintenance	PO	50–60 mg/kg/day	12
Sulfonamides	IN, CH	Antibacterial	PO	75 mg/kg	1st dose
(sulfadizine,		Maintenance	PO	120–150 mg/kg/day	4–6
sulfisoxazole, tri-sulfapyrimidines)	IN, CH	Antibacterial	SQ	100–110 mg/kg/day	4–6

(continued)

Appendix

Recommended Doses of Common Drugs in Children (*continued*)

Class and drug	Patient population	Indication	Route	Dose	Interval (hours)
Trimethoprim/ Sulfamethoxazole	IN > 2 months, CH	Antibacterial	PO	8 mg TMP and 40 mg SMX/kg/day	12
Tetracyclines					
Chlortetracycline	CH	Antibacterial	PO	25–50 mg/kg/day	6
Demeclocycline	CH	Antibacterial	PO	7–13 mg/kg/day	6–12
Doxycycline	CH	Antibacterial	PO	5 mg/kg/day	12
Methacycline	CH	Antibacterial	PO	7–13 mg/kg/day	6–12
Minocycline	CH	Antibacterial	PO	4 mg/kg/day	12
Oxytetracycline	CH	Antibacterial	PO	25–50 mg/kg/day	8
Tetracycline	CH	Antibacterial	PO	25–50 mg/kg/day	8
	CH	Antibacterial	IM	15–25 mg/kg/day	8–12
	CH	Antibacterial	IV	10–20 mg/kg/day	12
Anxiolytics					
Diazepam	CH	Anxiety	PO	0.2–0.3 mg/kg/day	6
Hydroxyzine	CH	Anxiety	PO	2 mg/kg/day	6–8
Autonomic drug					
Atropine	IN, CH	Various	PO, SQ	0.01 mg/kg/dose	2
Cardiovascular drugs					
Diazoxide	CH	Acute hypertension	IV	5 mg/kg/dose	2nd dose after 30 minutes
Digitoxin	NEO	Digitalization	IV, IM	0.035 mg/kg	Half initially; $\frac{1}{4}$ at 8 and 16 hours
	IN	Digitalization	IV, IM	0.05 mg/kg	Same as NEO
	IN	Digitalization	PO	0.07 mg/kg	Same as NEO
	CH	Digitalization	IM, PO	0.03 mg/kg	Same as NEO
	NEO, IN, CH	Maintenance	IV, IM, PO	0.1 × digitalizing dose	24
Digoxin	NEO	Digitalization	IV, IM	0.035 mg/kg	Half initially; $\frac{1}{4}$ at 8 and 16 hours
	IN	Digitalization	IV, IM	0.05 mg/kg	Same as NEO
	IN	Digitalization	PO	0.07 mg/kg	Same as NEO
	CH	Digitalization	IV, IM, PO	0.035 mg/kg	Same as NEO
	NEO	Maintenance	PO	0.01 mg/kg/day	12
	IN, CH	Maintenance	PO	0.017 mg/kg/day	12
Hydralazine	CH	Antihypertensive	PO	0.75–3.5 mg/kg/day	6
Lidocaine	IN, CH	Antidysrhythmic	IVI	0.02–0.5 mg/kg/minute Max.: 5 mg/kg/day	
Methyldopa	CH	Antihypertensive	PO	10 mg/kg/day	6–12
Minoxidil	CH	Antihypertensive	PO	0.5–1.0 mg/kg/day	24
Procainamide	IN, CH	Antidysrhythmic	IV	2–5 mg/kg/dose	Repeat at 20 minute intervals up to 30 mg/kg
			IM	20–30 mg/kg/day	6
			PO	40–60 mg/kg/day	4–6
Propranolol	CH	Antidysrhythmic	IV	0.02–0.03 mg/kg/dose	PRN after 20 minutes

Appendix
Recommended Doses of Common Drugs in Children (*continued*)

Class and drug	Patient population	Indication	Route	Dose	Interval (hours)
		Antidysrhythmic	PO	0.3–1.2 mg/kg/day	6
		Antihypertensive	PO	1–5 mg/kg/day	6
Reserpine	CH	Antihypertensive	PO	0.005–0.02 mg/kg/day	12
Corticosteroids					
Cortisone[a]	CH	Replacement	PO	1 mg/kg/day	8
			IM	0.5 mg/kg/day	24
		Anti-inflammatory	PO	10 mg/kg/day	6–8
			IM	3–6 mg/kg/day	12
		Status asthmaticus	IV	10–20 mg/kg/day	6
		Endotoxic shock			
		Initial	IV	50 mg/kg	Once
		Maintenance	IV	50–75 mg/kg/day	6
Diuretics					
Chlorthiazide	IN, CH	Diuretic	PO	20 mg/kg/day	12
Ethacrynic acid	CH	Diuretic	PO	1 mg/kg/dose	24
Furosemide	IN, CH	Diuretic	PO	2–6 mg/kg/dose	6–8
			IV	1–6 mg/kg/dose	2 or more
Mannitol	CH	Diuretic	IV	0.75–2.5 — g/kg/dose	-
Spironolactone	CH	Diuretic	PO	1.5–3 mg/kg/day	4–8
Triamterene	CH	Diuretic	PO	4 mg/kg/day	12
Gastrointestinal drugs					
Bisacodyl	CH	Cathartic	PO	0.3 mg/kg/dose	Once
Cascara sagrada	IN	Cathartic	PO	1–2 ml/dose	Once
	CH	Cathartic	PO	2–8 ml/dose	Once
Cimetidine	CH	Antiulcer	PO	20–40 mg/kg/day	At meals and bedtime
Magnesium sulfate	CH	Cathartic	PO	250 mg/kg/dose	Once
Minerals					
Calcium gluconate	2–12 years	Hypocalcemia	PO	500 mg/kg/day	4–8
Calcium lactate	2–12 years	Hypocalcemia	PO	500 mg/kg/day	4–8
Iron	IN, CH	Daily requirement	PO	0.5 mg/kg/day	Single or divided
		Deficiency anemia	PO	6 mg/kg/day	Divided with meals
Narcotic agonists and antagonists					
Codeine	CH	Antitussive	PO	1–1.5 mg/kg/day	4
		Analgesic	PO	4 mg/kg/day	4–6
		Analgesic	SQ	3 mg/kg/day	4–6
Meperidine	CH	Analgesic	PO, IM, SQ	6 mg/kg/day	4–6
Morphine	CH	Analgesic	SQ	0.6–1.2 mg/kg/day	4
Naloxone	NEO, IN, CH	Narcotic antagonist	IV, IM, SQ	0.01 mg/kg/dose	Can be repeated up to 3 times at 2- to 3-minute intervals
Propoxyphene	CH	Analgesic	PO	2–3 mg/kg/day	6

(continued)

Appendix

Recommended Doses of Common Drugs in Children (*continued*)

Class and drug	Patient population	Indication	Route	Dose	Interval (hours)
Neuroleptics					
Chlorpromazine	CH	Antipsychotic	PO	2 mg/kg/day	4–6
	CH	Antipsychotic	IM	1.6 mg/kg/day	6–8
Prochlorperazine	CH > 2 years	Antipsychotic	PO	0.4 mg/kg/day	6–8
	CH > 2 years	Antipsychotic	IM	0.2 mg/kg/day	8–12
Thioridazine	CH	Antipsychotic	PO	1 mg/kg/day	8
Respiratory system drugs					
Cromolyn	CH > 5 years	Asthma prophylaxis	INH	1 capsule/dose	6
Dextromethorphan	IN, CH	Antitussive	PO	1 mg/kg/day	6–8
Ephedrine	CH	Antiasthama	PO	3.0 mg/kg/day	4–6
Epinephrine	CH	Antiasthama	SQ	0.01 mg/kg/dose	Can be repeated twice at 20-minute intervals
Pseudoephrine	CH	Nasal decongestant	PO	4 mg/kg/day	6
Terbutaline	CH	Asthma	PO	0.10–0.5 mg/kg/day	8
Theophylline	CH	Maintenance for asthma	PO	10–20 mg/kg/day	6
	CH	Status asthmaticus	IV	7 mg/kg/dose	—
Sedative-hypnotics					
Amobarbital	CH	Sedative	PO	1–2 mg/kg/day	6
	CH	Hypnotic	PO	2–3 mg/kg/day	12–24
Pentobarbital	IN, CH	Sedative	PO, IM	1–2 mg/kg/day	6
	IN, CH	Hypnotic	PO, IM	2–3 mg/kg/day	12–24
Secobarbital	IN, CH	Sedative	PO, IM	1–2 mg/kg/day	6
	IN, CH	Hypnotic	PO, IM	2–3 mg/kg/day	12–24
Stimulants/antimigraine drugs					
Caffeine	CH	Migraine	PO	10 mg/kg/day	4–6
Dextroamphetamine	CH > 3 years	Attention deficit disorder Narcolepsy	PO	2.5–5.0 mg/dose	At onset of daily activities and 4–6 hours later
Ergotamine	CH, ADOL	Migraine	IM, SQ, PO, SL	0.25–0.5 mg/dose 1 mg/dose	At first sign of attack
Methylphenidate	CH > 3 years	Attention deficit disorder	PO	5 mg/dose	At onset of daily activities and 4–6 hours later
Pemoline	CH > 3 years	Attention deficit disorder	PO	1–3 mg/day	24 (single morning dose)
Uricosuric					
Probenecid	CH	Hyperuricemia or to increase action of antibiotics	PO	25–40 mg/kg/day	6

[a]Doses of other corticosteroids can be calculated based on their potencies relative to cortisone.

Key to abbreviations:
Patient Population: ADOL, adolescents; CH, children; IN, infants; LBW, low body weight infants; NBW, normal body weight infants; NEO, neonates.
Indication: TB, tuberculosis; UTI, urinary tract infection.
Route: IM, intramuscular; INH, inhalation; IV, intravenous; IVI, intravenous infusion; PO, oral; SL, sublingual; SQ, subcutaneous.
Dose: mg/kg/day, milligram per kilogram per day.

CHAPTER 7

Geriatric Pharmacology

There are currently some 27 million Americans (11% of the total population) age 65 or over, and this number will approximately double in the next 25 years. Eighty percent of these people live in the community. Like the very young, the elderly seldom have the benefit of being prescribed drugs that have been tested specifically in people of their age group. Developing rational drug regimens presents a real challenge for the medical team engaged in therapy for elderly clients.

Pharmacotherapeutics in geriatric clients is complicated by several characteristics of the elderly. For one thing, the incidence of many diseases increases with age; about 85% of elderly individuals have at least one chronic ailment and 50% have two or more. Thus, the elderly are more likely to require multiple drug regimens for multiple disorders, and the many drugs frequently interact with pathophysiological conditions to alter drug action. Nurses working with elderly clients must watch for adverse effects of drugs that can be additive with or mistaken for manifestations of disease. The elderly are especially likely to use cardiovascular agents (61% of the elderly take these), sedatives (17%), antiarthritic agents (12%), and gastrointestinal drugs (11%). This increases the likelihood of significant drug interactions. An important part of nursing management involves helping the elderly to become knowledgeable consumers of health care and to avoid harmful drug interactions.

Pharmacokinetics in the elderly is substantially different than in younger adults and more variable from client to client. The effect of altered pharmacokinetics on drug efficacy and toxicity is specific for each drug, posing a further challenge to the medical team. The pharmacodynamic aspect of drug action may also be altered in the elderly, as certain tissues become more or less responsive to the influences of particular drugs. The psychological factors in drug utilization are also distinctive in the elderly resulting in less frequent compliance with prescribed regimens. As a result of these factors, nurses might reasonably predict an increase in adverse drug reactions among the elderly, and in fact, clinical observations show a twofold to threefold increase.

Most elderly people want to care for themselves as long as possible. As a result, many delay seeking health care, worrying about cost, hospitalization, and possible ailments that might prevent them from returning to their homes. An important nursing responsibility in working with elderly clients is to assist them in adjusting activities to enable them to remain self-sufficient and independent. An important point for nurses to remember is that physiological aging does not exactly parallel chronological aging. Therefore, nurses need to individualize the treatment of elderly clients.

Altered Pharmacokinetics and Pharmacodynamics in Geriatric Patients

Drug effects are often different in geriatric clients than in younger adults (Table 7–1) due to either pharmacokinetic or pharmacodynamic factors. All three phases of drug-handling — absorption, distribution, and elimination — are altered by aging, although elimination undergoes the most clinically significant changes.

Absorption

Aging is accompanied by a general involution of the alimentary tract. The mucosal membranes of the intestines and stomach gradually lose cells, and the effective surface area for absorption is gradually reduced. In addition, the decrease in cardiac output that accompanies aging results in a 40–50% reduction in perfusion of the gastrointestinal tract, since blood flow to the alimentary canal must be sacrificed

Table 7–1
Age-Dependent Drug Kinetics

Increased effects due to		Decreased or delayed effects due to
Decreased renal extraction		**Decreased plamsa binding/ increased extraction**
Ampicillin	Penicillin	
Digoxin	Practolol	Phenytoin
Doxycycline	Streptomycin	
Kanamycin	Tetracycline	**Decreased active absorption**
Lithium		Calcium
		Galactose
Decreased hepatic metabolism		Thiamine
Amobarbital	Phenobarbital	**Decreased passive absorption**
Benzodiazepines	Phenylbutazone	
Lidocaine	Propoxyphene	Most drugs
Meperidine	Propranolol	
Meprobamate	Warfarin	**Decreased tissue responsivity**
Morphine		Amphetamine
		Isoproterenol
Decreased plasma protein binding		Norepinephrine
Digoxin	Salicylates	Quinidine
Meperidine	Sulfonamides	
Phenylbutazone	Warfarin	
Decreased red blood cell binding		
Acetazolamide	Meperidine	
Increased tissue responsivity		
Anticholinergics	Benzodiazepines	
Antihistamines	CNS depressants	
Barbiturates	Digitalis	
(paradoxical	Hypotensive agents	
excitation)	Lidocaine	

in order to maintain coronary and cerebral flow. As a result, removal of substances from the intestinal lumen is delayed, less complete, and less reliable.

Gastric emptying time is prolonged in the elderly because of diminished activity of the sphincters. In addition, elderly clients secrete less hydrochloric acid than younger people. The diminished acidity of the stomach contents alters absorption of weak acids and bases. Weak acids such as barbiturates are more ionized in the gastrointestinal tracts of the elderly and less well absorbed; weak bases are less ionized and better absorbed. Consequently, elderly clients may not respond to barbiturates as quickly as people in other age groups.

Substances that are absorbed actively from the intestines are often absorbed more slowly in the elderly. This has been noted in the case of galactose, calcium, iron, thiamine, and vitamin B_{12}. However, passive absorption is not significantly affected except as related to slowed gastric emptying and pH effects. Intestinal motility is diminished in the elderly, resulting in slower disintegration of solid dosage forms such as tablets.

The elderly are more likely than others to use laxatives and antacids. Interaction of these drugs with other orally administered agents is common and often significant. For example, preparations containing kaolin or pectin, magnesium hydroxide, or aluminum hydroxide significantly decrease absorption of digoxin (Lanoxin) from the intestines if taken concurrently. Tetracyclines, chlordiazepoxide (Librium), and vitamin A are similarly affected. Nursing assessment of elderly clients must include questions about the frequency with which antacids or laxatives are taken. Nurses should direct clients to consult a physician if they are using laxatives more than rarely. Many elderly people develop nutritional problems that result from long-term use of laxatives. Nurses should warn such clients about this problem when teaching them how to stay healthy and suggest ways in which regularity can be achieved through dietary adjustments.

The net result of these circumstances in the elderly is that most drugs are absorbed more slowly and less completely than in younger adults. Onset of drug action is generally slower, and in some cases total bioavailability is significantly impaired.

Distribution

Aging alters many of the factors that influence drug distribution, including protein binding, volume of distribution, the extent of the lipid tissue, and patterns of regional perfusion.

Drugs that are normally highly bound to plasma proteins in young adults are substantially less bound in the elderly. The ratio of free to bound drug increases. Since free drug is responsible for pharmacological activity, the relative lack of plasma protein binding sites in the elderly can increase effective drug concentrations at sites of drug action. Nurses who work with the elderly need to recognize that as a result of this mechanism, phenylbutazone (Azolid), salicylates, and sulfonamides achieve higher tissue concentrations and produce exaggerated effects in the elderly. On the other hand, if a drug is eliminated largely by renal filtration, the lack of plasma protein binding sites in the elderly may result in more rapid renal extraction since only the free portion of drug in the plasma can be filtered. This effect is seen when phenytoin (Dilantin) is given to elderly clients. It is a rare example of a drug that has a shorter half-life in the elderly than in young adults.

The lack of plasma protein binding sites and the frequency of multidrug regimens in the elderly makes older people more vulnerable to drug interactions involving competition for plasma protein binding sites. An elderly client who is taking both warfarin (Coumadin) and a sulfonamide, for example, is likely to experience an increase in the effects of warfarin. The likely result is hemorrhage. Digoxin effects can be greatly increased if the digoxin is displaced from binding sites by quinidine or heparin. Nurses should anticipate that a physician would reduce the digoxin dose by half when quinidine is employed concurrently.

Binding to red blood cells can play a significant role in distribution for some drugs. Meperidine (Demerol) binds significantly to red blood cells in young adults but much less in elderly clients. As a result, free concentrations of meperidine are elevated in the plasma of elderly individuals and pharmacological activity increases. Acetazolamide (Diamox) is another drug that is more potent in the elderly for this reason.

Older adults have 10–15% less total body water than adults at age 30. As people age they have a tendency to become dehydrated, as often as not because they may not drink enough fluid. Nurses, in their assessment, need to identify reasons for limited fluid intake or other factors contributing to dehydration. Body fat, on the other hand, increases as a fraction of total body mass. Therefore, water-soluble drugs have a reduced volume of distribution and a higher concentration. Fat-soluble drugs, on the other hand, are stored more extensively in the larger amount of fatty tissue in the elderly and therefore have prolonged activity and more potential for cumulation toxicity. This may be a factor in the exaggerated effect of many psychotropic drugs (including neuroleptics, barbiturates, benzodiazepines) in older people, because psychotropics are usually highly fat soluble.

Finally, the inevitable decrease in cardiac output with age causes a gradual redistribution of blood flow. Blood flow is shunted away from the splanchnic artery (supplying the alimentary canal) in favor of the coronary and cerebral vasculature. Nurses can expect that this change in the pattern of blood flow will not only decrease absorption of drugs from the gastrointestinal lumen but also reduce delivery of drugs to the major organs of drug elimination — the liver and kidney.

Elimination

Both major facets of elimination — metabolism by the liver and excretion by the kidneys — are significantly affected by aging. The rate of liver metabolism of most drugs depends on blood flow to the liver and, for highly bound drugs, the extent of binding to plasma proteins. The changes in blood flow and binding brought about by aging have opposite effects on metabolism. Blood flow to the liver, as previously noted, is often reduced in the elderly. Reduced blood flow causes reduced metabolism and therefore longer half-lives for such drugs as morphine, meperidine (Demerol), propoxyphene (Darvon), propranolol (Inderal), lidocaine (Xylocaine), phenylbutazone (Azolid), warfarin (Coumadin), amobarbital (Amytal), and benzodiazepines. Drugs such as propranolol that are normally subject to considerable first-pass extraction are especially likely to produce exaggerated effects in older people. The opposite is true for drugs that are highly bound. The reduction in protein binding means that more drug is freely available for metabolization. Thus drugs like phenytoin are more rapidly eliminated in the elderly.

Changes in kidney function are probably the most important factor contributing to age-dependent pharmacokinetics in the elderly. After age 30, renal function declines at a rate of nearly 1% per year or 6–10% per decade. Renal perfusion decreases (1.5% per year or 40–50% from age 25 to 65), as does glomerular filtration rate (45% from age 25 to 65). The loss of renal function accelerates after age 65. The ability to concentrate urine and the secretory mechanisms of the tubules are also diminished. The consequence of this decline in renal function is impaired efficiency in renal extraction of drugs among elderly clients. Drugs such as penicillin, streptomycin, tetracycline, and kanamycin exhibit prolonged half-lives and elevated peak plasma levels. Nurses need to be especially alert to the toxic levels of drugs that can occur among the elderly when kidney degeneration has occurred. It should be noted that impairments of renal function may occur in the absence of abnormal serum levels of creatinine or blood urea nitrogen.

Pharmacodynamic Alterations with Age

Aging influences tissue responsiveness to local concentration of drug in a number of ways. For one thing, functional capacity of many of the organs declines with aging so that the margin of unused functional capacity is less. Therefore, any adverse drug effects on the organs are felt more keenly. Drugs that produce impairments in liver, kidney, or cardiac function that might go unnoticed in the younger client can be dangerous in the elderly. Thus, nurses must be especially diligent in monitoring their clients' responses to drug therapy when such impairments are apt to occur. In addition, the vitality of control mechanisms is reduced in the elderly, their maintenance of homeostasis is less vigorous, and compensatory responses to primary drug effects are less significant. For example, drugs that raise blood pressure often do so to a greater extent in elderly clients since the vagal reflex is less efficient in generating a compensatory reduction in cardiac output.

Cardiac glycosides are noted for their small therapeutic index in all clients, but older adults are especially prone to digitalis intoxication. Elderly clients also exhibit reduced pharmacodynamic responsivity to quinidine but an increased sensitivity to lidocaine. Vascular responses to norepinephrine and cardiac response to isoproterenol are somewhat diminished.

The elderly are more sensitive to both the central and peripheral effects of anticholinergic drugs. For example, atropinic psychosis is a common reaction. Older clients are more sensitive to depressant influences of sedative-hypnotics and anxiolytics but also are more prone to exhibit paradoxical excitatory reactions characterized by restlessness, disorientation, and confusion. Nurses who discover that an older person becomes disoriented when given a sedative need to ensure that this information becomes part of the client's permanent record. The effects of stimulants such as amphetamine on locomotor activity are less in the gerontological client, but the anorexic effect is enhanced. Thus nurses should be especially vigilant to complaints of upset stomach or nausea.

Older clients frequently exhibit resistance to insulin and require higher doses of this hormone. On the other hand, the elderly are more vulnerable to diabetogenic chemicals, such as alloxan, or the hypoglycemic drugs, such as sulfonylureas. Warfarin

(Coumadin) produces its anticlotting effect in the elderly at lower doses.

Adverse Effects in Geriatric Patients

Adverse effects of drugs in the elderly are qualitatively the same as in other adults but are often quantitatively greater in severity and frequency. This is especially the case when the adverse effect relates to an organ that has reduced functional capacity as a result of aging. The elderly are more susceptible to excess depression, psychiatric disturbances, anticholinergic symptoms, or extrapyramidal disorders involving the central nervous system; heart failure, dysrhythmias, orthostatic hypotension, or hypertension in relation to the cardiovascular system; gastrointestinal disturbances, clotting defects, blood dyscrasias, ototoxicity, electrolyte or fluid imbalances, or nephrotoxicity (Table 7–2).

Antibiotics are more likely to cause adverse effects in elderly clients than in others, yet they are often selected for treating elderly clients who have, for example, a fever of unknown origin. Antibiotics are usually excreted by the kidneys; reduced renal function in older adults may result in toxic accumulation of these drugs. Nurses need to watch for signs of alterations in kidney function of clients taking antibiotics and report these to the physician.

The elderly are also more likely to experience drug interactions since they purchase more than 13 prescription drugs per year on the average, along with many nonprescription medications.

Drug Administration in the Elderly

Administration of drugs is sometimes more difficult in elderly clients because of changes in anatomy, physiology, and psychosocial environment. Some older individuals are no longer capable of administering their own medications because of blindness, arthritis, chronic organic brain syndrome, or other limitations. Problems may also occur with respect to administration of drugs by the nurse. For example, most elderly individuals have a reduced muscle mass. Finding an appropriate site for intramuscular injections may be more difficult and require more careful preliminary palpation. Some elderly clients may have difficulty swallowing. Use of liquid dosage forms may be helpful. Solid medications may need to be crushed and added to foods that are easy to swallow such as applesauce or gelatin. Massage or slight pressure on the larynx may facilitate swallowing.

Promoting Compliance among Elderly Clients

Over- and undercompliance are more common in elderly clients than in other groups of clients. In an effort to promote compliance, the nurse should take care to explain thoroughly the purpose of each medication along with the consequences of noncompliance. The fewest possible number of drugs should be prescribed and at the lowest effective doses, and unneeded medications should be discontinued as soon as they are no longer required. Every effort should be made to avoid complicated dosage schedules such as alternate days or twice a week. Once a day provides optimum compliance. Twice a day or once a week are also easy-to-remember schedules. Nurses who carefully monitor client progress can often see to it that unnecessary medications are eliminated from the regimen by discussing the possibility with the physician.

When drugs are prescribed to elderly clients, the nurse should take special care that instructions are understood. The client should be told clearly why each drug is being taken, when the drug is to be taken in relation to meals, food, or beverages, and any special precautions and storage instructions. After completing all instructions, the nurse should ask the client to repeat and explain them. The instructions should also be provided in writing to the client and responsible family members.

It is important to determine the extent to which the client in question will be able to follow instructions. Two major physical problems common to elderly people are visual impairment and hearing impairment, both of which can interfere with effective communication. Therefore nurses must assess clients for evidence of either problem.

In providing oral information, it is important to remember that many words sound the same, especially to the hearing impaired. When possible, information should be given when a responsible family member is present to verify that the client does know what has been said. When providing verbal information, the nurse needs to speak slowly, enunciating words and syllables clearly. Noting evidence of hearing deficits can also be critical when it is necessary to employ drugs that can contribute to hearing loss.

Many elderly people have visual problems as well. Nurses should make certain that instructions are printed in letters large enough for fairly easy reading. The cards or paper should not be shiny, and because older people tend to have difficulty seeing

Table 7–2
Adverse Effects in the Elderly

Common adverse effects in geriatric patients	Causative agents	
Central nervous system		
Excess depression (respiratory depression, confusion, ataxia, drowsiness, weakness, fatigue, depression)	Antihistamines	Methyldopa
	Antipsychotics	Narcotics
	Anxiolytics	Phenytoin
	Cardiac glycosides	Reserpine
	Lithium	Sedative-hypnotics
	Local anesthetics	
Psychiatric disturbances		
Psychosis	Cardiac glycosides, corticosteroids, levodopa	
Anticholinergic syndrome (impaired attention, disorientation, anxiety, confusion, hallucination, psychosis, agitation, delirium, memory impairment, combativeness, tachycardia, mydriasis, flushed face, decreased sweating, urinary retention, decreased salivation, decreased bronchial secretion, hyperpyrexia)	Antidepressants	
	Antiparkinsonian agents	
	Antipsychotic drugs	
Extrapyramidal symptoms	Antidepressants, antipsychotics, lithium	
Cardiovascular system		
Heart failure	Beta-blockers	
Dysrhythmias	Antidepressants, cardiac glycosides, phenytoin	
Hypotension (syncope, dizziness, headache, vertigo)	Antidysrhythmics	Benzodiazepines
	Antidepressants	Diuretics
	Antihistamines	Narcotics
	Antihypertensives	Phenytoin
	Antipsychotics	Vasodilators
Hypertension	Anorexics, nasal decongestants, stimulants	
Nephrotoxicity	Aminoglycosides	
Ototoxicity	Aminoglycosides	
Hemorrhage	Oral anticoagulents, heparin	
Gastrointestinal dysfunctions	Cardiac glycosides	Hyperlipemic drugs
	Colchicine	Laxatives
	Corticosteroids	Narcotics
	Diuretics	Nonsteroidal anti-inflammatory drugs
Electrolyte imbalances	Corticosteroids, diuretics	
Blood dyscrasias	Antineoplastics	Oxyphenbutazone
	Antipsychotics	Phenylbutazone

black on white background, other colors should be used. For example, large white letters on a black background or yellow letters on a green background are easier to read than are black letters on a white background.

Careful consideration of the special needs of particular geriatric clients may serve to improve compliance. Older clients with motor impairments may have difficulty opening containers that are "child-proof." They should be provided with easy-to-open containers. A system for notifying clients when a prescription should be renewed may also help in promoting compliance. Nurses need to inform elderly clients who have difficulty keeping track of their medication schedule about commercial containers in which drugs are put into separate compartments that make it easier to determine if a given dose has already been taken. For example, if a client has to take three different pills at 10:00 A.M., 2:00 P.M., and bedtime, three pills would be placed in each of three compartments to represent each time of administration. It is important that nurses make sure that at least one other person in the household or nearby can help the client identify what is to be taken, when, and in what order, and when to call the health care professional regarding symptoms indicative of drug-related problems.

Case Study: Increased Drug Sensitivity in a Geriatric Client

H. B., a 175 lb, 82-year-old man, was to be given meperidine (Demerol) for pain during recovery following a surgical procedure. The drug order called for 100 mg, IM, every 3 or 4 hours as needed. One hour after the nurse administered the first dose, H. B. became noticeably confused and weak, and his respirations were slow. A blood test revealed that the level of meperidine in his serum was 1.1 μg/ml (therapeutic range: 0.4–0.7 μg/ml). The nurse reported the reaction to the physician, who altered the drug order to read 50 mg, IM, every 4–6 hours as needed. The nurse monitored H. B. closely for the next few hours, observing that his neurological functioning and respiration gradually returned to normal over a 5-hour period.

1. How did the dose of 100 mg, IM, compare with the normal therapeutic dosage range for meperidine?
2. What was the probable reason for H. B.'s exaggerated reaction to meperidine?

Answers appear at the end of the book.

Recommended Readings

Adamson L: Drug treatment in the elderly, *Nurs Times* 1978;74:973–974.

Allen MD: Drug therapy in the elderly. *Am J Nurs* 1980;80(8):1474–1475.

Bishop T: Drugs and the elderly: A breeding ground for mishaps. *Nurs Mirror* 1978;147:49–50.

Coleman JH, Dorevitch AP: Rational use of psychoactive drugs in the geriatric patient. *Drug Intell Clin Pharm* 1981;15(12):940–944.

Dall CE et al: Promoting effective drug-taking behaviors in the elderly. *Nurs Clin North Am* 1982;17(2):283–290.

Ellor JR, Kurz DJ: Misuse and abuse of prescription and nonprescription drugs by the elderly. *Nurs Clin North Am* 1982;17:319–330.

Goldberg PB: Why do older adults need different dosages? *Geriatr Nurs* 1980;1:74.

Gotz BE, Gotz VP: Drugs and the elderly. *Am J Nurs* 1978;78:1347–1351.

Hayter J: The older adult and drug therapy. Why response to medication changes with age. *Geriatr Nurs* 1981;2(6):411–416.

Hudson MF: Drugs and the older adult take special care. *Nursing* 1984;14(8):46–51.

Kim KK, Grier MR: Pacing effects on medication instruction for the elderly. *J Gerontol Nurs* 1981;79(1):24–27.

Lenhart DG: The use of medications in the elderly population. *Nurs Clin North Am* 1976;11:135–143.

Lerner R: Sleep loss in the aged: Implications for nursing practice. *J Gerontol Nurs* 1982;8:323–326.

Oppeneer C, Vervoren A: *Gerontological Pharmacology: A Resource for Health Practitioners.* St Louis, CV Mosby Co, 1983.

Roe DA: Drug-nutrient interactions in the elderly. *Geriatrics* 1982;41(3):57–74.

Santora G: Communicating better with the elderly. *Nursing Life* 1986;6(4):25–27.

Saxton DF, Ercolano NH, Walter JF: *Programmed Instruction in Arithmetic, Dosages, and Solutions,* ed 5. St Louis, CV Mosby Co, 1982.

Shomaker DM: Use and abuse of OTC medications by the elderly. *J Gerontol Nurs* 1980;6(1):21–24.

Todd B: Drugs and the elderly: Using eye drops and ointments safely. *Geriatr Nurs* 1983; 53–57.

Vervoren TM, Oppeneer J: *Gerontology Pharmacology: A Resource for Health Practitioners.* St Louis, CV Mosby Co., 1983.

Vervoren TM, Oppeneer JE: *Workbook for Solutions and Dosage of Drugs, Including Mathematics,* ed 12. St Louis, CV Mosby Co, 1983.

CHAPTER 8

Nursing Process and Drug Therapy

The Role of the Nurse

Nursing and Holistic Care

Nursing practice is an encounter of a nurse with a client for the purpose of helping the client to achieve or maintain health, to control disease, and to adapt to disability or disorders that cannot be corrected. It involves personal, family, and community services that help to promote health: sustaining life, maintaining integrated functions, promoting normal growth and development, and preventing or controlling disease and its effects on people. Nursing is a subsystem of the larger system of health care and is thus both integral and distinctive. The integral quality of nursing is its links with the other health professions. The nurse collaborates with other members of a health-care team and contributes to the therapeutic objectives established by the team. The distinctive quality of nursing derives from the simple fact that the nurse is the one member of the health care team with the most continuous contact with the client. The nurse has several kinds of opportunities and responsibilities that are either completely unique or most fully developed for the nurse among the health professionals. It is the nurse who ultimately cares for persons in ill health, in the broadest sense.

For the nurse more than any other health professional, health care occurs in the context of holistic care: concern for the caring, nurturing, and comforting aspects of human care, recognition of the importance of basic human needs, and consideration of the factors that motivate people to achieve health.

All people have needs for safety, belonging, love, social esteem, and self-actualization, in addition to the fundamental physiological requirements such as food, water, and oxygen. Some of these needs are obvious; others are less apparent and must be identified through inferences and cues provided by clients, families, or significant others. In the context of drug therapy, the nurse's attention to the needs of clients can significantly affect both the therapeutic and adverse effects of drug therapy. Maintaining a comfortable environment and a confident attitude toward the efficacy of the therapeutic plan can increase the effectiveness of the drug regimen. At the same time, nursing measures can reduce potential threats to the safety needs of clients posed by drug side effects. For example, some drugs can cause people to become confused and disoriented. Other drugs can cause drowsiness, ataxia, impairment of reflexes, or bleeding. Some drugs tend to cause dizziness and fainting spells, and still other drugs cause distortion in sensory perceptions, increase susceptibility to sunburn, or elevate risks of cold exposure or heat exhaustion. Using side rails and other restraints, evaluating home environments for hazards to safety, teaching the client about safety, and involving the client's family in observation of the client's behavior may help to promote safety.

The Changing Roles of the Nurse

Increasingly, the nurse's role has been extended into nonclinical sites (homes and schools) and into an expanded range of health care concerns, including health education, monitoring the client's physical and emotional status and responses to medications, assessing the client's ability to cope, and determining strategies to enable clients and families to achieve health. The nursing process has always been central to achieving these goals. However, it is now especially critical to a client's well-being as hospitals and clinics throughout the country begin to utilize the new Medicare prospective payment system known as the diagnosis related groups (DRGs). Clients now enter hospitals closer to the time of scheduled therapy and remain for shorter periods of time. As a consequence, many people are now being discharged at an earlier stage in treatment and frequently require home care. These changes in the delivery of health care are designed to reduce hospital and medical costs, but clients often have little time to adapt to prescribed changes in their lives and to receive teaching and demonstrate understanding of prescribed therapies. In the newly evolving approach to health care, the nurse has an increased responsibility for teaching clients and promoting self-care.

Nurses employed by community health agencies are now confronted with increasing numbers of people at all developmental stages requiring intense assistance after hospitalization. At the same time, there is a growing population of older people and others with long-term disabilities who need home health care. In addition, the current trend toward more and more nurses establishing independent practices has increased the autonomy of the nursing profession. Increased autonomy also means increased personal responsibility for the in-depth knowledge of normal basic physiology required to assess the client's condition and the client's response to drug therapy.

Nursing Process

To facilitate understanding of the nurse's role and how it is best fulfilled, nursing can be conceptualized as a process involving a series of analyzable phases called the **nursing process.** The concept of nursing process is a relatively new one and continues to evolve. We utilize the approach that views the nursing process as five sequential and cyclical phases (Figure 8–1): (1) assessment, (2) analysis, (3) planning, (4) implementation, and (5) evaluation.

Assessment is the collection of relevant information that defines the current health situation for the particular client. Assessment encompasses the medical and drug history, physical examination, psychological, social, cultural, and environmental factors, laboratory tests, and current drug and nondrug

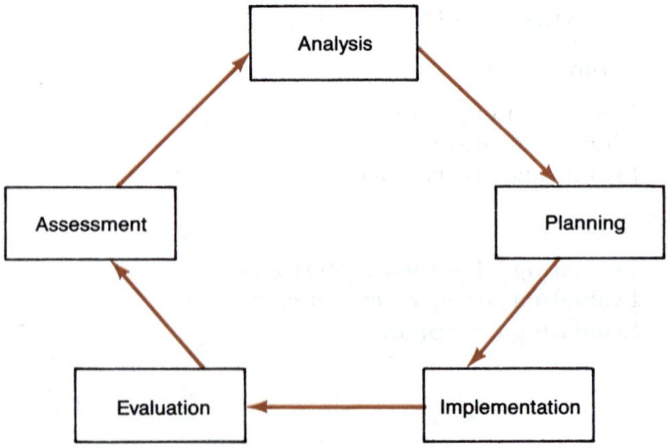

Figure 8–1
Diagram of the Nursing Process

orders and interventions. Assessment involves both review of information already available and the generation of additional information not available but deemed important.

Analysis is the critical study of the assessment data for the purposes of identifying the client's needs and establishing nursing goals. Included in this phase is the determination of appropriate nursing diagnoses and identification of requirements for referral to other health care providers.

Planning is the designing of strategies, in cooperation with the client or some person responsible for the client, that will help to achieve the established nursing goals. Nursing plans are individualized to the unique requirements and capabilities of each client. They are also dynamic, requiring frequent adjustments as the client's condition changes. Implementation is the initiation and completion of the strategies developed during the planning stage.

Evaluation is the process of determining the effects of the plan of care, both the extent to which the goals have been achieved and the occurrence of any unfavorable consequences. Because they are the health care professionals most likely to see clients on a regular basis, nurses play an especially important role in evaluation. Nurses observe and measure the extent to which the client is responding to drug treatments, any side effects the client may be experiencing, and any changes in physiological or psychological functioning.

Nursing process is cyclical; the information gathered during evaluation serves much the same role as that gathered during assessment, feeding into the next phase of analysis, nursing diagnosis, and goal-setting. The nurse may need to report some of his or her evaluation findings to the physician and other health team members. In the subsequent sections, we consider the phases of nursing process with special emphasis on their relation to drug therapy.

Assessment

Nurses assessing clients about to receive drugs must examine all aspects of the clients' condition: the clients' medical history, drug history, current prescription and nonprescription medications, and dietary habits; their physical condition; their attitudes, cultural practices, capacity for self-care, and social and financial supports; and their educational level and ability to understand language in general and medical terminology in particular. Nurses should use all available sources of information: the client, the client's family or significant others, the medical record, and consultation with other health professionals who have interacted with the client.

History

When drug therapy is anticipated, one important aspect of the medical history is to determine if there are **contraindications** for any drugs being considered for use. Contraindications are conditions that preclude or limit the use of a particular drug. Contraindications can be either absolute or relative. Presence of an absolute contraindication means that the drug should not be used for that client; presence of a relative contraindication means that the drug should be avoided if possible and used with great caution when necessary. For example, lithium carbonate, a drug often used for manic depressive (bipolar) disorder, is absolutely contraindicated for use in clients with acute myocardial infarctions, myasthenia gravis, or in their first trimester of pregnancy; it is relatively contraindicated for use in clients with organic brain syndrome, psoriasis, or acne. Contraindications are specific for each drug class and sometimes even for individual drugs. Contraindications are an important part of what nurses need to know about the pharmacology of drug classes and specific agents.

Next the nurse will need to examine the medical history for the presence of disorders that might alter the activity of drugs, causing so-called drug-disease interactions. For example, impaired liver function or altered kidney function may change the actions of drugs that are normally inactivated by these organs. Dysfunction in these tissues will slow the inactivation of drugs, allowing them to accumulate in the blood or tissues. The result is an increase in the effects of the drug. For example, digoxin (Lanoxin) a cardiotonic drug, is inactivated by liver metabolism. People who have inflammatory diseases affecting the liver, cirrhosis, or other conditions of liver insufficiency are at risk of digoxin toxicity. Digoxin is also inactivated in part by renal excretion, so clients with impaired kidney function may also suffer toxic reactions. Thus, the nurse's knowledge of a client's general health is critical for effective monitoring of the client's response to drugs. Other diseases, including intestinal obstruction, infection, inflammation, and diarrhea, can alter absorption of medications. Changes in levels of plasma proteins can alter the activity of drugs that are normally highly bound to these proteins.

Nurses are often responsible for obtaining a current drug history; that is, a record of drugs taken within the last 6 weeks. The drug history should be comprehensive, covering any evidence of drug allergies, drugs prescribed by any health care professional, use of nonprescription medications, use of the social drugs (nicotine, caffeine, and alcohol), and use of street (or illegal) drugs. Clients who cannot accurately name their medications should be asked to produce a sample for inspection. The drug history is important for determining the potential for interactions between drugs already being used by the client and those that are being considered for the current medical problem.

When allergies are reported, care must be taken to determine if the client is, in fact, allergic to the drug or if, on the other hand, the client is using the term *allergy* to indicate an untoward drug reaction that does not have an allergic mechanism. While identifying the presence of drug allergies, the nurse should review evidence of allergies to foods, pollens, dander, or other allergens, since individuals prone to such allergies have an increased likelihood of drug allergies as well.

Another component of history taking is the dietary history. This provides a basis for determining possible contributions of dietary habits to the medical problem as well as a means for anticipating drug-diet interactions. A typical form for taking a dietary history is found in Chapter 44 along with discussion of interactions between drugs and nutrients. Other matters of history that should be covered include elimination patterns and sleep patterns.

Physical Examination and Laboratory Tests

Predrug physical assessment not only contributes to assessment of the medical condition but also serves as a baseline for evaluation of the responses to drug therapy. The parameters to be assessed will be dictated by the nature of the disorder, anticipated therapeutic benefits of the drug regimen, and potential adverse reactions. Physical assessment always includes an evaluation of the client's age, weight, height, and vital signs — data essential for appropriate drug administration. Physical examination frequently involves use of four common assessment techniques: visual inspection, palpation (feeling with the hands), auscultation (listening), and percussion (listening for sounds in body parts struck by the examiner's fingers). Laboratory tests needed vary with the client's circumstances but often include x-rays, analysis of culture specimens, blood cell counts, or measurements of various substances in the blood or urine. Nurses need to know the normal value ranges for the most common tests and to have access to charts showing normal ranges for the less frequently encountered ones.

Assessing the Client's Capacity for Self-Care and Compliance

Self-care can be defined as the client's contribution to his or her own health and well-being. Self-care is often a practical and positive approach to health care, but nurses must assess the client's needs for therapeutic self-care and whether there are significant limitations for performing self-care. Based on this assessment, the nurse must determine if the client's health care is to be **wholly compensatory** (the client is unable to perform any deliberate self-care), **partly compensatory** (the client performs some activities and is gradually taught to perform others), or **supportive-educative** (where the client performs most of his or her own care). In assessing the client's capacity for self-care, the nurse should consider the client's ability in three domains: physical, intellectual, and psychological. In the physical domain, the nurse will need to identify factors such as blindness or motor disabilities that limit the client's ability to reliably self-administer drugs. In the intellectual domain, the nurse will need to assess the client's knowledge, experience, and understanding of the therapeutic regimen. In the psychological domain, the nurse must assess the client's willingness to engage in self-care. Values regarding self-determination and control can be important factors in determining the client's capacity for self-care. A dependent type of person may have no wish to participate in self-care. If such a client is required to divide pills to achieve the prescribed dosage of drug, he or she may insist that others perform the task or that the regimen be altered.

As the nurse develops a relationship with the client, there is potential for exploring more fully the client's attitudes toward health and illness. The nurse who gains this understanding is better able to enlist the client's cooperation in establishing goals and direct the client's own abilities toward recovery from illness and maintenance of health. The nurse is also in a better position to anticipate problems in compliance and to negotiate with clients to improve their compliance with drug regimens. For example, some clients fear that any drug can produce dependence. As a consequence, they will not take the amounts of medication prescribed or, in some instances, will refuse to take medicine at all. Other clients may respond adequately to treatment in the hospital but fail to follow the prescribed protocol once they are discharged. Expressions of feelings by clients that the future is hopeless and death inevitable because of the particular disease they have should also alert nurses to the likelihood that the client may not adhere to drug therapies. If the client sees drug therapy as a sign of weakness, or subscribes to a value system or religious belief that precludes all but "natural healing," he or she may be unwilling to adhere to the prescribed methods of therapy. Accurate assessment of such attitudes may suggest a need for extra time teaching the client and family in the hope of encouraging compliance.

The nurse may begin to explore attitudes toward health care by asking the following kinds of questions:

1. What is the client's experience with prior health problems? How did he or she handle them?
2. What does the client know about his or her current illness?
3. What role does the client expect to play in managing his or her own health care?
4. What significance does the client attach to personal control of health care?
5. Are there family members or friends who can contribute important information to the client's history?

Answers to these and similar questions should be part of the nursing history and assessment. Accurate assessment depends upon the development of a nurse-client relationship that encourages the client to share important information such as social and cultural values.

Analysis

Analysis is the processing of the information gathered during assessment in light of the nurse's knowledge and experience. When drug treatment is anticipated, analysis entails a consideration of the possible drug actions and interactions, how these might affect the client's health and safety needs, and how drug effects may be altered by the presence of disease. How effective has the drug been when used in similar situations? What are the expected benefits? What adverse effects are anticipated? When drugs are used in combination, what are the potential interactions? How might the drugs interact with dietary requirements? How is the action of the drug altered by the nature of the disease process or altered tissue function in the individual client? The nurse's ability to answer such questions depends upon knowledge of pharmacokinetics, adverse drug reactions, and drug interactions with other drugs, nutrients, and disease states. These issues are discussed in Chapter 3 and for specific drugs throughout the book.

Nursing Diagnosis

The analysis of the information collected during assessment leads to the formulation of one or more nursing diagnoses. The **nursing diagnosis** is a statement that defines the client's actual or potential health problems that can be addressed by nursing interventions. For the purposes of this book, we utilize a set of nursing diagnoses (Table 8–1) accepted by the American Nurses' Association and a small number of additional ones suggested by L. J. Carpenito. Nursing diagnoses serve to direct nursing activities toward achievement of specific health benefits. Nursing diagnoses are not a substitute for the medical diagnosis that is established by the physician or by the health care team. The medical diagnosis defines the primary health care problem; nursing diagnoses identify elements of the physiological or psychosocial status of the individual that can be addressed fully or in part by nursing activities.

Establishing Goals

The goals for client care flow from the medical and nursing diagnoses. Thus, the goals for nursing care are (1) to promote the goals established by the health care team and (2) to prevent or correct the health care deficits suggested by the nursing diagnoses. Generally, goals should be client-oriented, should be defined in such a way as to provide for measurement, and should include a specified time-frame. Overall therapeutic goals are typically established by the health care team, in conjunction with the client and family, to the extent that is feasible given the age and mental status of the client. Clients are best served when all members of the health care team, as well as the clients, are involved in establishing the therapeutic goals. Each member has a unique contribution to make. Each has learned something about the client's life-style, expectations, views of health and illness, and physical condition. Nursing goals related to drug therapy are specifically designed to enhance therapeutic benefits, reduce requirements for the drug, minimize side effects and adverse interactions, and educate clients and family members in all facets of the prescribed drug regimen.

Table 8–1
Nursing Diagnoses[a]

Physiological	Psychosocial
Activity intolerance	Anxiety
Airway clearance, ineffective	Comfort, alteration in — pain
Bowel elimination, alterations in—constipation	Communication, impaired verbal
Bowel elimination, alterations in—diarrhea	Coping, ineffective individual
Breathing patterns, ineffective	Coping, ineffective family
Cardiac output, decreased	Diversional activity deficit
Fluid volume deficit	Family processes, alterations in
Fluid volume excess	Fear
Gas exchange, impaired	Grieving
Infection, potential for	Health management, alterations in
Mobility, impaired physical	Home maintenance management, impaired
Nutrition, alterations in—intake less than body requirements	Injury, potential for
Nutrition, alterations in—intake more than body requirements	Knowledge deficit
Oral mucous membrane, alterations in	Noncompliance
Respiratory function, alterations in	Parenting, alterations in
Sexual dysfunction	Powerlessness
Skin integrity, impairment of	Rape trauma syndrome
Tissue perfusion, alteration in	Self-care deficit
Urinary elimination, alteration in patterns of	Self-concept, disturbance in
	Sensory-perceptual alterations
	Sleep pattern disturbance
	Social interactions, impaired
	Social isolation
	Spiritual distress
	Thought processes, alterations in
	Violence, potential for

[a]Nursing diagnoses accepted by the American Nurses' Association and a small number of additional ones suggested by Carpenito LJ: *Handbook of Nursing Diagnoses,* Lippincott: Philadelphia, 1985.

Planning

The planning phase of nursing process is the development of a plan of action that will promote the achievement of the nursing goals. A **plan of action** is developed on the basis of what the nurse can do to enable the client to achieve or maintain health. Planning may require consideration of alternative courses of action, weighing short-range and long-range results, identifying risks, and weighing potential outcomes. Attention should be given during the planning phase to issues of time, energy, and financial costs to clients. The nurse must determine which facets of care should be delegated or shared with the client, family, or other health team members.

Planning of therapies often involves assigning priorities to problems identified during the assessment. High-priority problems are often life-threatening, and can result in hospitalization of the client. Severe oxygen deprivation, anaphylactic shock, obstruction of the airway, sudden precipitous loss of fluids and electrolytes, severe drug reactions (whether from prescribed drugs or one procured illegally) are but a few examples. Each of these situations requires immediate medical attention for survival.

Once life-threatening problems have been addressed, the focus of care shifts to needs of lesser priority. Clients should participate both in identifying these needs and in planning ways to resolve the health problems. Whenever possible, the priorities of the client should be considered, enabling the individual to become a full partner in managing the health care regimen. This is important since clients must continue to manage their daily existence once they are back in the home and community. When health care providers recommend objectives that differ from those of the client, it should not be assumed that the client will accept them.

Often clients require a range of treatments. A client who is constipated, for example, may require immediate relief achieved by administering a laxative, a suppository, or an enema, as well as longer term treatment. If the constipation is a recurring problem and represents a change in bowel habits, the nurse would refer the client to a physician for a complete examination to assure that a persistent disease process is not present. Once disease processes have been ruled out, the nurse, physician, and nutritionist may enter into a collaborative relationship with the client and family to assess nutrition and health practices. Should these need correction, the health professionals could then teach appropriate nutrition and exercise habits.

The Nurse and Drug Strategy

Criteria for beginning, continuing, and discontinuing drug treatment, as well as determining the size, frequency, and number of doses, together comprise the drug strategy and should be established from the outset as the health team develops its goals for the client. Though matters of drug strategy are ultimately the responsibility of the physician, the nurse must be fully aware of the drug strategy in order to fulfill the roles of health care team member, client advocate, and health care provider.

Adverse reactions to drugs usually limit the maximum dose that can be employed for each therapeutic agent. The optimum dose of a medication strikes a balance between therapeutic effects and adverse effects. Ideally, the dose of a drug should be titrated against plasma concentrations, but practical considerations limit this method to a few drugs that meet certain criteria (see Chapter 3). More typically, the dose is evaluated against the preestablished objectives for improvement, against the appearance of side effects, or against other well-established, though perhaps unrelated, pharmacological actions, such as signs of sympathetic inhibition (hypotension or decreased heart rate) with monoamine oxidase (MAO) inhibitors. The actions and efficacy of drugs may be different in early and late stages of treatment, necessitating either upward or downward adjustments in dosage.

Some drugs are properly used only for short-term treatments. Most hypnotic agents (sleeping pills), for example, are ineffective if used nightly for more than 2 weeks, and even the agents with the longer period of usefulness (the benzodiazepines) are ineffective if used chronically for more than about 2 months. Such information must be passed along to clients, since people who have been hospitalized often ask about being sent home on the same hypnotic medication, assuming that it would prove helpful indefinitely in promoting sleep.

Termination of drug therapy is too often given less consideration than is the initiation of therapy. The therapeutic plan should include clear-cut criteria for termination of drug therapy which should be established as nearly as possible to the time when the plan of action is initially developed. Otherwise, drug use is too often continued without adequate review of the necessity for it. Nurses should realize that all drugs have the potential for causing toxic reactions. Sometimes the reaction is the result of drug accumulation in specific tissues. Some adverse effects occur only after many months of drug administration and others as a result of long-term chronic treatment. For these reasons, unnecessary continuation of drug regimens is not in the client's best interest. Continued assessment and communication with the physician is essential.

Implementation

Implementation includes those activities that are necessary to accomplish the goals established for the client. The implementation phase involves the administration of drugs to fulfill drug orders, nursing interventions to promote therapeutic objectives or to address nursing diagnoses, and the education of the client. Administration of drugs is discussed in Chapter 4; here we will discuss nursing interventions and client education.

Nursing Interventions

An important facet of nursing care is the implementation of nondrug interventions. Such measures may be designed to facilitate the effectiveness of medications or to promote therapeutic or nursing goals directly. These activities derive from nursing diagnoses or medical orders. Examples of important nursing measures that accompany drug therapy are provided in the "Nursing Diagnoses and Interventions" boxes that appear in the various drug chapters throughout this text. Here we cite just a few examples.

Nursing actions designed to facilitate the action of medication are often important in dealing with pain. For example, the nurse could attempt to relieve stress by bathing the client's face, hands, and back with warm water, tightening the bed linen, adjusting the bed to a comfortable position, and rearranging pillows. If there is disturbing noise or if the room is especially bright, the nurse might dim the lights and close the door. These actions must be done in consultation with the client, however. Attention to such physical needs will typically enhance the effectiveness of an analgesic.

In emergency rooms, nurses should attempt to reduce both physical and psychological stress for the client. Providing privacy when possible, addressing clients gently and courteously, and conveying respect for the individual's dignity and personal worth are measures that reassure clients and often encourage compliance.

Client Education

Nurses often have the primary responsibility for educating clients and their families about drug therapy. The information to be included will vary according to the client's capacity for understanding and the nature of the regimen, but generally will encompass the following:

1. The nature of the disorder and prognosis
2. The rationale for the therapeutic regimen including each prescribed medication
3. The name, action, dosage, and schedule of administration for each drug
4. Special instructions related to storage, preparations, or administration of each drug
5. Expected responses to drug therapy and potential untoward reactions
6. Comfort measures to alleviate adverse effects
7. Safety measures to prevent injury or poisonings to the client or others
8. Potential interactions of the medication with other prescription drugs, nonprescription drugs, social and illicit drugs, the diet, or laboratory tests
9. Signs and symptoms indicating adverse effects or interactions and instructions about what to do should these occur
10. Special restrictions regarding use of other drugs or discontinuation of medications included in the regimen
11. Expectations regarding the latency between initiation of drug therapy and therapeutic benefit

It is best to supplement verbal instructions with written information that includes the expectations for each medication and the directions for proper administration so that the client can have the information available at all times for ready reference. Table 8–2 provides a sample of a comprehensive set of written guidelines for self-administration that might be provided. The instructions should be written at a level the client can understand, without medical jargon.

For a variety of reasons, clients do not always actually learn what health professionals may think they have taught them. Stress associated with new health problems often interferes with the ability of clients to absorb information, regardless of how well it is presented. The sheer complexity of medical information for lay people tends to inhibit their understanding. Some clients feel intimidated by the seemingly superior level of knowledge of health care professionals. As a consequence, they may not ask questions about their therapy or the drugs they are receiving for fear of appearing stupid. Nurses should not assume that information has been understood or retained by the client. It is best to require clients to demonstrate their understanding of important points by having them repeat back the information or demonstrate to the health care professional tech-

Table 8–2
Guidelines for Self-Administration of Medications

1. Take prescription drugs only as prescribed.
2. Use a minimum of over-the-counter drugs and only after conferring with the pharmacist, physician, or nurse.
3. Make sure to tell the pharmacist all the medications being taken.
4. Never take a medication unless you understand its action, dosage, adverse drug reactions, and rules for safe storage.
5. Store medicines in their original container
6. When pouring drugs, do not allow the label to become obscured by spilled drug to guard against possible medication error.
7. Do not store unused portion of drugs. Their composition may change over time. Check for expiration dates and do not use drugs that have passed expiration.
8. Do not discard unused medications in garbage or trash. Children might find and ingest them.
9. Avoid taking medication in the presence of children.
10. Keep oral medications stored separately from drug preparations intended for external use (such as ointments) to avoid inadvertent ingestion of the topical medications.
11. Refrigerate all drugs that require refrigeration.
12. Insist that the pharmacist put the name of the drug on the label. This helps prevent errors and allows proper intervention if the drug causes poisoning or produces adverse drug response.
13. Do not take drugs in the dark. You must be able to read the label and identify the drug as the appropriate one.
14. If you have poor vision, have a reliable family member or other support person set up the medicines in a prefilled dispenser kit. Also, mark the bottle with a form of identification that you can feel with your fingertips.
15. If you have a problem remembering to take medication, make out a reminder chart that allows you to check off medications as you take them.
16. If you have a response to the drug that you were not warned about, do not take the drug until you contact your physician.

niques such as mixing a drug, administering a drug, or determining the dosage.

The nurse shares responsibility for educating the client with physicians, pharmacists, and other members of the health care team. Various institutions and health care agencies differ in their philosophies about the extent to which professional staff can inform people about their therapy or otherwise teach about the prescribed medication regimen. These positions may be found in procedure manuals, handbooks, and similar materials, explaining nursing responsibilities in that particular institution. Usually, nurses have the primary responsibility for client education, but some institutional policies defer all discussions about the rationale for the therapeutic regimen to the physician. In these circumstances, nurses are limited in the amount of information they can give to clients about their medications. However, in these circumstances nurses still have an obligation to clients to record and report their observations of the client's needs, including any need for additional information. If the physician's policy is to instruct the client personally, the nurse will need to indicate to the physician if the client appears to be confused about the medication regimen. Confusion about instructions is likely to result in the client failing to follow the drug plan.

Promoting Compliance

Psychological factors such as the client's satisfaction and attitudes toward the treatment are important in determining the extent to which they will adhere to health care advice. If clients perceive the health team members as warm, caring, and concerned, they will be encouraged to follow treatment plans and otherwise comply with recommendations for health improvement. Compliance with therapeutic regimens by clients increases when health professionals spend more time with them. Often improving compliance can be accomplished by periodic telephone calls to assure that the person is having no difficulty with his or her medication. People appreciate concern for their welfare. Treating clients with dignity also tends to encourage compliance. For example, many people prefer to be addressed as Mr., Miss, Ms., or Mrs. Using first names would violate such clients' concept of self or affront their sense of dignity and worth.

Drugs and drug taking assume different meanings to different people. Some expect drug therapy to cure ailments immediately. When client response to therapy is such that cure or amelioration of the disease can be expected to take several months (as is often the case with certain fungal infections) clients tend either to reject the therapy or to follow the regimen in a halfhearted manner. In such situations, nurses need to offer constant encouragement. Nurses and others on the health team need to identify those symptoms the client considers most important and to be alert to minor alterations in physical response that could indicate improvement in those symptoms. Unless precautionary measures are planned early and useful strategies for encouraging clients to continue taking their medication are identified, clients may prematurely discontinue drugs, such as antibiotics, once symptoms they consider important have been eliminated.

Social factors are also important to compliance. The support of family members and close friends is often the key to compliance. It has been repeatedly documented that people who are isolated socially are less likely to follow medication orders, keep clinical appointments, or eat nutritious meals than are those who are close to their families and friends. Thus, a part of the nursing process may be implementing plans to reduce the client's social isolation. This is particularly important when working with elderly people who live alone, with no family nearby to provide either psychological or social support. For these people, it might be important to include a close friend in the discussions concerning care plans. Compliance is more likely to be achieved when individuals have support, when they perceive that noncompliance can create serious problems, and where they can see benefits to be gained. For example, a client who is receiving anti-infective drug therapy needs to know the importance of following the drug protocol, and that rest, adequate nutritional and fluid intake, and practicing good hygiene will all contribute to a return to health.

People in lower educational and socioeconomic levels tend to be less apt to adhere to drug therapies than other people. This, of course, suggests that nurses need to be particularly attentive to issues of compliance to assure that the poorer, less well-educated people receive the support necessary to motivate them to adhere to a regimen and to achieve successful treatment of their health care problems. On the other hand, older people who have been treated with drugs in the past and who have chronic health problems tend to be more compliant.

In some situations, nurses may improve client compliance by making a contract with the client to develop a specific behavior. This involves the client in planning and formalizing a commitment to a health care regimen. It also individualizes care and tends to improve self-concept. The result is improved incentive to achieve important health goals.

Another method of improving client participation in health care and encouraging compliance involves self-monitoring. Clients are asked to record their own behavior and events in their lives. This allows nurses to identify areas where there may be a lack of understanding of what is required and what is being done. For example, asking a client to keep a diary for a week, recording events and medications taken, may serve to assist the individual and the nurse to identify what may interfere with compliance. It may also assist the nurse and client to tailor the taking of medications according to the client's living patterns, routines, and abilities. This would be especially important for those people who must give themselves injections, such as those with diabetes.

Three factors concerning drug orders that contribute to noncompliance are (1) the number of drugs prescribed; (2) the frequency with which the drugs must be taken; and (3) the complexity of the procedure. Fewer numbers of drugs, once-a-day regimens, and simple instructions tend to foster adherence to prescribed regimens. As client-advocates, nurses need to discuss the client's medication protocols with the physician and to indicate those factors that might interfere with a client's compliance, including any social or cultural taboos that have been identified. Certainly, drugs of marginal value ought not be included in the health care regimen.

In summary, clients tend to adhere to prescribed drug regimens in the following circumstances: (1) when they have faith and trust in the physician prescribing the drug; (2) when they know that the drug has been effective in treating others who have had the same ailment; (3) when there is personal evidence that the drug regimen controls symptoms or the disease itself; (4) when the client experiences no frightening side effects and does not know others who have had bad experiences with the drug; (5) when side effects are outweighed either by relief of disease symptoms or by fear of the disease itself; (6) when the regimen will not interfere with important daily activities of the client or significant family members and friends; and (7) when provided with encouragement and teaching by the health team.

Evaluation

The nurse is responsible for evaluating not only the therapeutic benefit of the nursing measures but also that of the medical regime in general. The therapeutic and nursing plans must entail means of systematic evaluation that include (1) the extent to which therapy has produced a level of improvement that is acceptable to the client; (2) the extent to which success has been achieved in the nursing goals and therapeutic objectives established by the team; (3) adverse consequences of the therapeutic intervention; and (4) the extent of the client's compliance with prescribed therapy. The nurse compares the data gathered at this stage with the baseline data gathered earlier in the assessment phase. Nurses are responsible for observing the client's response to therapy, for identifying clues concerning potential problems, and for recording their observations and sharing them with other members of the health team. Sometimes, the client will not report symptoms he or she considers unimportant. The nurse should look for and inquire about minor changes and symptoms that clients consider unimportant but that may be crucial indicators of improvement or deterioration in the client's condition.

Evaluating Therapeutic Response

Effective evaluation of the therapeutic benefit provided by a drug regimen requires that the nurse have a thorough understanding of the therapeutic goals and the rationale for use of each drug in the regimen. The parameters evaluated to determine the extent of benefit are as varied as the many kinds of disorders and drug therapies. Evaluation for efficacy may center on reduction of target symptoms, decreased frequency of attacks if the condition is episodic, elimination of pathogenic microorganisms, or improvements in physiological functions.

Whenever possible, evaluation should include objective measurements as well as subjective observations. For example, evaluation should include measuring the ankles or urine output during diuretic therapy, measurements of blood pressure when antihypertensive regimens are employed, measurements of hand-grip strength when treating myasthenia gravis, measurement of intraocular pressure when drugs are used for glaucoma, and microbial cultures when antibiotics are used. Frequently the tests utilized during evaluation are ones that were also employed during the assessment phase, the earlier measurements providing baseline values for purposes of comparison. While it might seem obvious that objective measurements should be used routinely to guide ongoing therapy, all too often, medical personnel rely on clinical impressions as the sole means of evaluating drug responses. Objective measurements are commonly underutilized for certain medical conditions, sometimes even though the relevant parameter is an easy one to evaluate. For example, clinical studies have repeatedly shown that many, perhaps even most, individuals under medical care for hypertension are not receiving drug regimens that lower their blood pressure to an adequate extent as evidenced by intensified monitoring of blood pressure.

When laboratory tests are used to evaluate the effects of a drug, nurses and physicians need to review the drug regimen for presence of other drugs that might interfere with the particular test. For example, thyroid function tests may be altered by oral contraceptives, iodide-containing drugs, or heavy metals. Interactions of drugs with laboratory tests are included in the interactions sections for each drug or drug class discussed in later chapters.

Evaluating Adverse Drug Reactions

Anticipating adverse reactions to drugs requires sound knowledge of the pharmacology of the drugs being used and the frequency of occurrence of the various side effects. Nurses especially need to be alert to potential adverse effects because they often have the first opportunity to recognize their occurrence. The client and the client's family may spot side effects even sooner if the nurse has made them aware of the indications of adverse reactions. The nurse should keep in mind the factors that alter liability to side effects: the age and sex of the client, aspects of the disease state that can modify drug toxicity, the psychological set of the client, and the route and rate of drug administration. When a medication will be taken over a prolonged period of time, the focus of the nurse's surveillance will gradually shift from the early side effects to those that tend to occur late in treatment, after several weeks, months, or years.

Evaluating Compliance

Nurses have a particular responsibility for evaluating clients' compliance with drug therapy. For one thing, nurses are most likely to have access to the kind of information that can reveal whether or not a particular person is following instructions given by medical personnel. For example, a nurse may learn by talking with clients and their families that the individual has ceased taking the medication because the symptoms of illness have disappeared. While such behavior is appropriate when, for example, medication is being taken for insomnia, it can be dangerously inappropriate when clients are placed on antibiotic therapy, since premature discontinuation of medication increases risks that resistance will develop or that infection recur. Discontinuation of medication is often a problem when medications are being used prophylactically (such as antiepileptics or lithium) or for symptomless conditions (medications for hypertension) because benefits are not readily visible. When noncompliance is suspected, the most conclusive means of assessing compliance is by measurement of plasma concentrations of the drug, if the drug is being used by a route of administration that provides for systemic absorption.

Nurses can also anticipate that medications that produce annoying side effects are likely to be ones that clients do not employ as instructed. For example, medications that cause nausea are often discontinued by the clients. Noncompliance also increases when medications cause side effects that are psychologically unacceptable. For example, men who must take antihypertensive agents often have a decrease in sexual response, which may cause them to stop taking the drug. Sometimes clients will, on their own, increase the dosage of medication, thinking that if a little will be good for them, twice the amount will be better. The result is overdosage. Some other common problems for which nurses should evaluate clients include taking drugs that counteract each other, improperly spacing doses, forgetting medications altogether, and borrowing drugs from friends.

Determining compliance among outpatients can be especially difficult. Nurses in these settings need to keep accurate records of when clients keep appointments and the circumstances under which they fail to keep them. For some drugs, compliance can be evaluated by measurements of drug levels in the blood or urine. Another means of determining if clients are adhering to drug regimens is to count the pills an individual has at each clinic visit. This, of course, means that the client needs to have appointments scheduled on a regular basis and that nurses need to be aware of when prescriptions have been filled. By handling the situation with tact and concern, nurses can convey an attitude of caring and concern for the client's well-being that encourages complying with prescribed treatment modalities.

In the home care situation, nurses need to take special note of client needs for further education regarding the drugs that they use. If a client is diabetic and lives alone, the nurse needs to be alert to evidence that the client may not be adhering to prescribed dietary restrictions. Presence of candy and other foods normally forbidden the diabetic client should cause the nurse to question the client about their use as well as compliance with other aspects of prescribed therapy. Is the client taking insulin as prescribed? Has the client had any evidence of too much insulin and does he or she know the symptoms of hyperinsulinism? Is the client following the methods of administration taught prior to hospital discharge?

When a nurse suspects that an individual is not following the prescribed drug protocol, an effort should be made to confirm suspicions by asking nonaccusatory questions. For example, "Many busy people find they forget to take their medicines when they are supposed to. Have you had that problem?" By acknowledging that such problems are common and suggesting a logical excuse, the nurse encourages client disclosure and gives the nurse an opportunity to reinforce teaching about the medicine the client is taking. Clients tend to admit to noncompliance when they are confident that the health care provider will not chastise them, demean them, or desert them because of their behavior.

Case Study: Assessment of a Client's Preparedness for Client Education

M. R., age 60, was admitted to the hospital complaining of excessive thirst, weight loss in spite of increased appetite, fatigue, frequent voiding, and a sore on his heel that would not heal. After a series of tests it was determined that M. R. had diabetes mellitus and would be treated by diet and insulin. The diagnosis was at first difficult for the client to accept.

The nurse noted that M. R. had only a ninth grade education and often mispronounced common words. Yet the reading material he had brought with him to the hospital suggested a level of understanding beyond his level of academic preparation. She also noted that M. R.'s questions indicated he had read some material about diabetes prior to his hospitalization and had some idea of the health problems he faced. This assessment enabled the nurse to tailor her teaching to the patient's level of understanding, taking advantage of his ability to relate new information to what he already knew.

In addition the nurse assessed M. R.'s socioeconomic status and determined that he might need some help in learning how to purchase appropriate foods required in his diet. She went over, in detail, how to purchase foods that would be within his budget, how to interpret labels on the foods, and how to adjust his diet to the necessities of his condition. She recorded information she had given M. R. on the referral sheet supplied to the community health nurse who would now follow M. R.'s progress at home. She also reviewed all information with M. R.'s wife and gave her a copy of the instructions she had given.

1. What nursing diagnoses might be appropriate in this case?
2. What factors should the nurse take into consideration in preparing directions for M. R. in order to maximize the likelihood of compliance?

Answers appear at the end of the book.

Case Study: Noncompliance

A nurse who was visiting a client (Ms. L. T., age 72) was informed by the neighbor that the client was taking "a lot of medication" and was acting "funny." The nurse noted that only two drugs had been prescribed when L. T. was discharged from the hospital, so she asked L. T. what else she was taking. L. T. pointed to a tray on the refrigerator, which contained a variety of medications. Some of the bottles had labels on them and some did not. Some bottles had screw tops while others had tops designed to prevent children from opening the bottles. In questioning L. T., the nurse learned that she was taking many prescription medications in addition to those prescribed by the physician at the hospital. She was also taking a number of over-the-counter drugs. While the client knew about her prescribed medicines, she did not know that some of the over-the-counter drugs could alter her responses to the drugs required for her particular health problem. In addition, the nurse learned that L. T. was having prescriptions filled at a number of different pharmacies so that the pharmacists were unable to keep accurate records of what she was taking and alert her to any potential dangers. Finally the nurse discovered that L. T. had found opening the child-proof drug bottles difficult so she had taken the drugs from those bottles and put them into easy-to-open bottles but had not changed the labels. As a result, she sometimes forgot which bottles contained which medications and was not always sure what she had taken. The nurse recognized that this was possibly one reason for L.T.'s "strange" behavior. The client was in danger and an accurate evaluation of her response to therapy would not be possible. Thus, the nursing assessment had disclosed critical information pertaining to health and safety needs.

The nursing history also revealed other important facts. L. T. had a baccalaureate degree in education but no knowledge of physiology or the role of her prescribed drugs in achieving recovery. L. T. stated that she had complete confidence that health professionals would "do the right thing," but had no idea of the role she needed to play to assure recovery. She had only a limited idea of the problems she imposed on herself by taking nonprescription medications without first learning if they would interfere with the actions of prescribed medications. This action was consistent with L. T.'s lack of understanding concerning the dangers to which she exposed herself by having prescriptions filled at a number of different pharmacies and written by a number of different physicians, each of whom knew nothing of what the others had planned.

To address the many problems, it was necessary for the nurse to explain to L. T. how her behavior contributed to ill health rather than to recovery. The nurse explained the prescribed therapy to the client, writing out directions for taking medications. She encouraged L. T. to discard drugs in unlabeled bottles or mislabeled bottles since L. T. could not recall what they were for or when or where they had been purchased. The nurse also communicated the problem and her planned solution to the physician and other members of the health team. Encouraged by the nurse, L. T. arranged to have all prescriptions filed at one pharmacy. She discussed with the pharmacist the drugs that she knew she was taking and the fact that she needed medications put into easy-to-open bottles. Together, the health team members worked out a system of health planning and sharing information that assured the client's compliance.

1. List the factors identified by the nurse in her assessment that were contributing to inappropriate drug use by L. T. and the nursing measures that were implemented in each case.
2. What nursing diagnoses might the nurse have made in this case?

Answers appear at the end of the book.

Recommended Readings

Edel M: Noncompliance: An appropriate nursing diagnosis? *Nursing Outlook* 1985;33(4):183–185.

Henrich AP: What's really bothering your patient? 5 Ways to find out. *Nursing Life* 1984;1:62–64.

Kieffer JS: Nursing diagnosis can make a diffference. *Nursing Life* 1984;4(3):18–21.

Malasanos L, Barkauskas V, Moss M, Stoltenberg-Allen K: *Health Assessment.* St. Louis, CV Mosby Co., 1981.

Neel CJ: Make nursing diagnoses work for you every day. *Nursing* 1986;16(5):56–57.

Orem D: *Nursing Concepts of Practice.* New York, McGraw-Hill, 1982.

Segal ET: Modern nursing practice does require nurses to make independent judgments about a patient's condition. *Nursing* 1985;15(6):43.

Tartaglia M: Nursing diagnosis: Keystone of your care plan. *Nursing* 1985;15(3):34–37.

Todd B: What does a good drug history include? *Geriatr Nurs* 1981, pp 63–64.

Walker L: Nursing diagnoses and interventions: New tools to define nursing's unique role. *Nursing Health and Care* 1986;7(6):323–326.

Yura H, Walsh MB: *The Nursing Process* ed 4. Norwalk, Conn., Appleton-Century-Crofts, 1983.

UNIT III

Drugs and the Central Nervous System

PART A
Introduction to Central Nervous System Pharmacology

CHAPTER 9

Introduction to the Central Nervous System

Overview of the Central Nervous System

Drugs may alter central nervous system functioning (such as mood, arousal state, muscle tone, relay of sensory inputs, memory, learning, or motor coordination) by interacting either with specific regions or systems of the brain or with chemicals that serve as neurotransmitters. A basic knowledge of both neuroanatomy and neurochemistry is therefore necessary for understanding the action of drugs that affect the central nervous system (CNS). This chapter reviews the essentials of neuroanatomy and neurochemistry, with the goal of providing a general description of (1) how the central nervous system receives and processes information and generates behaviors, (2) how the most important brain regions and systems contribute to the regulation of various functions, and (3) how nerve cells transmit information.

The major brain regions (Figure 9–1 and Table 9–1) from lowest to highest are the medulla oblongata, pons, cerebellum, midbrain, hypothalamus, thalamus, corpus striatum, limbic system, and cerebral cortex. Locations within the nervous system are designated as follows: the top of the brain is designated *anterior,* or *rostral;* the lower part is designated *posterior* or *caudal;* the back of the brain is *dorsal* and the front is *ventral; medial* means toward the middle and *lateral* means toward the side, left or right.

The activities of the CNS can be divided into three categories (Figure 9–2): (1) inputs, the flow of information into brain centers; (2) outputs, control of muscles, organs, and glands; and (3) processing

Figure 9–1
Major brain regions

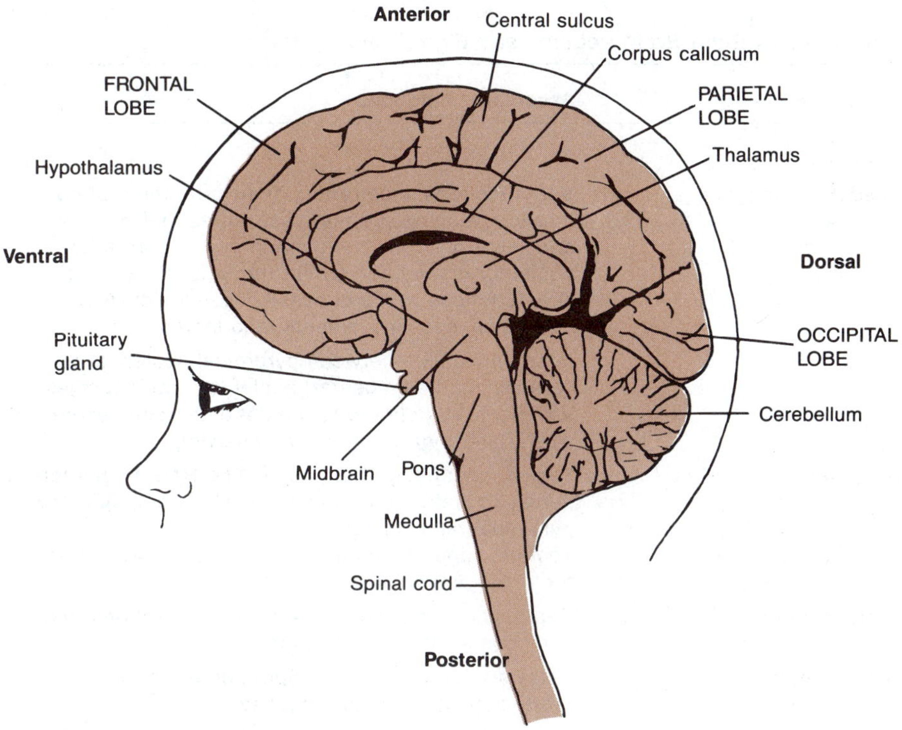

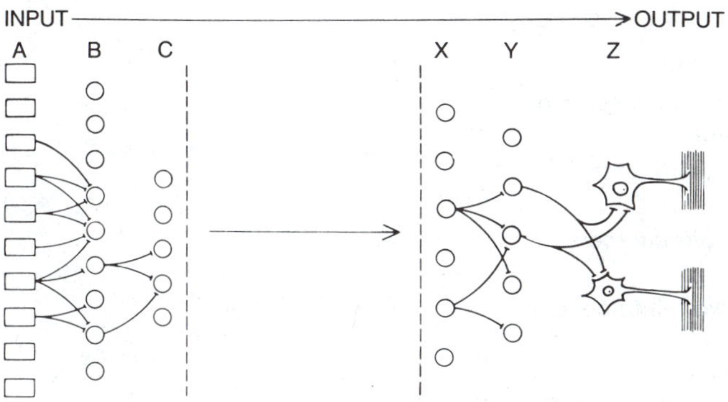

Figure 9–2
Overall organization of the brain is indicated in a rough caricature that suggests the flow of information from the input of sensory signals by receptor cells (A) to the eventual output by motor neurons (Z) terminating on muscle cells. The outputs of receptors and neurons usually branch to send diverging signals to the next stage. Most neurons receive converging inputs, both excitatory and inhibitory, from earlier stages. Something is known about the significance of the connections near the input end of the brain (B, C) and near the output end (X, Y). Far less is known about the workings of regions in between, which make up most of the brain. From D. H. Hubel. The brain. *Sci. Am.* 241:51, 1979 © *1979 by Scientific American. Inc.* All rights reserved.

which includes all intervening steps. Some inputs and outputs (carried by sensory and motor systems) relate to the interaction of the organism with the environment while others (physiochemical and autonomic inputs, autonomic and endocrine outputs) provide for maintenance of organ functions and the internal fluid environment.

Inputs

We obtain information about the physical environment through specialized sensory receptors: rods and cones in the retina of the eye, hair cells of the ear, taste buds on the tongue, dendrites of olfactory neurons, touch and pain receptors in the skin; spindle organs of muscles and tendons, and hair cells of the vestibular system in the inner ear. Impulses generated by the action of appropriate stimuli on these receptors are conducted along **afferent** nerve fibers toward the brain. Neither the generation nor the conduction of these nerve impulses is particularly susceptible to the influences of drugs, with the exception of the action of aspirin-like drugs on pain receptors.

Information about the status of the internal fluid environment and organ function reaches the

Table 9–1
Functions of Eight Brain Regions and Eight Brain Systems

Region or system	Associated functions
Regions	
Medulla oblongata	Vital functions: respiration, heart rate, force of contraction, vasomotor tone, gastrointestinal motility and secretory activity; vomiting and cough reflexes; nuclei for cranial nerves VIII through XII (relating to vital functions, visceral sensibility, swallowing and phonetion, neck movements, and lacrimation)
Pons	Interconnections between pyramidal system and cerebellum; dream center; nuclei for cranial nerves V through VII (relating to cranial pain, facial expressions, lateral gaze, taste, and chewing)
Midbrain	Tegmentum: integration, ascending RAS, nuclei for nerves III and IV (controlling eye movements), extrapyramidal relay nuclei Tectum: superior and inferior colliculi (relay nuclei for visual and auditory systems)
Cerebellum	Rapid, phasic patterns of muscle contractions that compose skilled movements
Dorsal thalamus	Relay station for sensory inputs entering the cerebral cortex; pacemaker for the cortex
Hypothalamus	Homeostatic functions: energy balance, water balance, temperature regulation, sexual functioning Neural regulation of endocrine system
Corpus striatum	Regulation of muscle tone and slow movements
Cerebral cortex	Consciousness, cognitive processes, volitional behavior, conscious sensations, verbal capabilities
Systems	
Pyramidal system	Conscious, volitional control of movement
Extrapyramidal system	Subconscious, involuntary motor control
Reticular activating system (RAS)	Cortical arousal, beta wave activity, increased motor activity, externalization of attention
Raphé system	Sleep-wave cycle, gating of sensory afferents, habituation
Reward system	Modification of behavior by positive reinforcers, pleasure
Punishment system	Suppression of behavior by negative reinforcers, anxiety
Diffuse thalamic system (DTS)	Projection of thalamic pacemaker impulses throughout the cerebral cortex; internalization of conscious focus
Limbic system	Emotional behavior (aggression, fear, pleasure), sense of smell, memory, goal-directed behavior

brain as physiochemical signals, coming from receptors that lie peripherally or in the brain itself. Peripheral receptors include the baroreceptors, which monitor blood pressure, and the carotid bodies, which monitor oxygenation of the blood. Receptors within the brain include those in the hypothalamus, which monitor hydration, core temperature, and glucose levels, and those on the surface of the medulla, which keep track of carbon dioxide. Levels of many endocrine substances are also monitored by the brain.

Outputs

Outputs from the brain involve the motor, endocrine, and autonomic systems. Motor outputs provide most behavioral responses (interactions of the organism with the environment), while endocrine and autonomic influences control the internal environment and organs.

Within the CNS, motor control is divided between two systems, the pyramidal and the extrapyramidal. The **pyramidal system** is a distinct tract arising in the motor cortex that is responsible for conscious, voluntary motor actions. Pyramidal cells in the cortex, called **upper motor neurons,** give rise to axons that descend to the spinal cord without intervening synapses, ultimately reaching the lower motor neurons of the somatic nervous system (see Chapter 27) at all levels of the spinal cord. **Lower motor neurons** are the final link for all motor outputs from the CNS and form the connections with skeletal muscles (called neuromuscular junctions) that are the site of action for neuromuscular blockers (Chapter 29). Thus, as few as two neurons are required to transmit a nerve impulse from the cerebral cortex to a skeletal muscle. Since most drugs that affect the nervous system alter transmission at synapses, the pyramidal system is relatively insensitive to drugs.

The **extrapyramidal system,** which is responsible for subconscious, involuntary motor control, is far more complex in its organization. Included in the extrapyramidal system are the cerebellum, the vestibular system, the corpus striatum, and a number of brainstem nuclei (such as the red nucleus, subthalamic nucleus, substantia nigra, and zona incerta). The extrapyramidal system is vulnerable to disruption by disease and offers numerous sites that can be influenced by drugs. Drugs that influence the extrapyramidal system or that are used to treat extrapyramidal disorders are discussed in Chapter 22.

The outputs that regulate the internal processes are conveyed by the endocrine and autonomic systems. The activity of these systems is influenced by many different drugs; thus the physiology and pharmacology of these systems are of vital importance to clinical medicine. The endocrine system is discussed in Unit VI, the autonomic nervous system in Unit V.

Processing: Special Functions of the Principal Brain Regions and Systems

The Brainstem

The brainstem includes the medulla oblongata, the pons, and the midbrain. It contains numerous ascending and descending pathways and regulates vital functions, facilitates and suppresses behavioral responses, directs the flow of inputs, integrates and relays motor outputs, activates higher brain centers, and regulates the sleep-wake cycle. Although the functional capabilities of the brainstem are quite limited in comparison with higher brain regions, the rich diversity of behaviors organized by higher centers can be accomplished ultimately only through the manipulaton of brainstem control centers. These control centers (nuclei) include (1) aminergic nuclei (with cells containing norepinephrine, dopamine, or serotonin); (2) cranial nerve nuclei (both motor and sensory); (3) extrapyramidal relay nuclei; and (4) nuclei of the reticular formation.

The portion of the brainstem immediately above the spinal cord is the **medulla oblongata.** A dorsal zone in the medulla includes several control centers which together regulate the principal vital functions. Respiration is controlled by the **respiratory center.** Blood vessel tone is regulated by the **vasomotor center.** Heart rate and contractile strength are regulated by the **cardiac center.** Gastrointestinal function is also regulated by the medulla oblongata. Another specialized area of the medulla, called the **chemoreceptor trigger zone,** is sensitive to certain noxious chemical substances and elicits vomiting when stimulated. Many drugs profoundly influence the vital centers of the medulla. Sedatives and narcotics depress the respiratory center. Other drugs, such as certain antihypertensive agents and neuroleptics, depress the vasomotor center, causing low blood pressure. Death occurs if doses of depressant drugs suppress the functioning of the medulla too much.

The **pons** lies just above the medulla and provides the massive bridges (the **cerebellar peduncles**) that connect the brainstem with the cerebellum. Thus, the pons is a major point of interconnection between the pyramidal system and the cerebellum. One pontine reticular nucleus (nucleus reticularis pontis caudalis) is responsible for stimulating dreaming.

The **midbrain** is one of the chief areas of integration within the brain. One part of the midbrain reticular formation gives rise to the ascending reticular activating system, exerting widespread influence on the activity of the cerebral cortex. Two extrapyramidal nuclei (the red nucleus and substantia nigra) reside mainly in the midbrain. The red nucleus is a center that integrates signals from the cerebellum and corpus striatum; the substantia nigra helps to regulate activity of the corpus striatum. Two pairs of midbrain nuclei (the inferior and the superior colliculi) are located on the dorsal surface of the midbrain (called the tectum). These nuclei act as relay stations for afferent impulses of the auditory and visual systems respectively.

Cranial nerve nuclei lie throughout the brainstem. The afferent (input) nuclei process cranial nerve inputs while the efferent (output) nuclei provide the final processing of regulatory signals. In the medulla are cranial nuclei that control the neck muscles, tongue movements, swallowing and vocal sounds, lacrimation, and the vital functions already described. Cranial nerve nuclei that lie in the pons include those that serve the muscles and sensory receptors of the face, jaw, and sinuses; the salivary glands; the taste receptors on the front of the tongue; and the auditory and vestibular systems. Several cranial nerve nuclei that control eye movements lie in the midbrain between the tectum and midbrain reticular formation.

The Reticular Activating System

The reticular activating system (RAS) (Figure 9–3), is divided into ascending and descending portions. The ascending part originates in the midbrain reticular formation and the descending part in the reticular formation of the medulla and pons. The descending RAS increases motor activity, while the ascending RAS serves as a general alarm system that alerts the cerebral cortex to significant events in the environment. Sensory pathways give off collateral axons to the reticular formation. When input signals representing significant stimuli pass along the sensory pathways of the brainstem, impulses reach the RAS via the collateral axons, and the RAS shifts the individual's focus of attention toward the source of the stimulation. The highly complex, multisynaptic organization of the reticular formation provides numerous target sites for the action of drugs, including stimulants and depressants. This important system is further discussed in Chapter 11.

The Raphé System

The raphé nuclei consist of eight midline nuclei scattered throughout the brainstem. Seven of the raphé nuclei contain cells that release the transmitter serotonin, the other dopamine. There are two other serotonergic cell clusters outside the raphé system, making a total of nine serotonergic nuclei (labeled B_1 through B_9; see Figure 9–4). One of these, the dorsal raphé nucleus (B_7), is the brain center that has the most direct control over the **sleep-wake cycle.** Serotonin levels in the brain exhibit diurnal (daily) fluctuations, reaching peak levels in the late evening, near bedtime, to promote sleepiness. Two other raphé nuclei are involved in regulating a process called **gating,** which is the determination of which sensory signals will be given precedence in conscious experience. Another raphé nucleus is involved in the psychophysiological phenomenon called **habituation.** The raphé system is important in understanding the action of psychedelic drugs, such as LSD (see Chapter 15).

The Reward and Punishment Systems

The reward and punishment systems are fundamental to learning controlled by positive and nega-

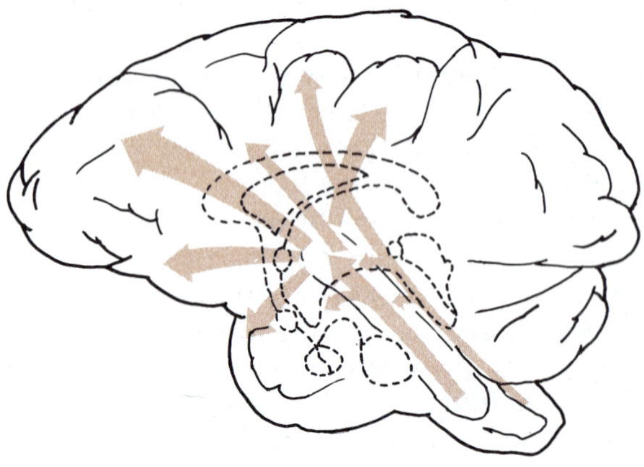

Figure 9–3
The reticular activating system. From D. B. Lindsley. The reticular system and perceptual integration. In H. H. Jasper et al. (Eds.), *The Reticular Formation of the Brain.* Boston: Little, Brown, 1958.

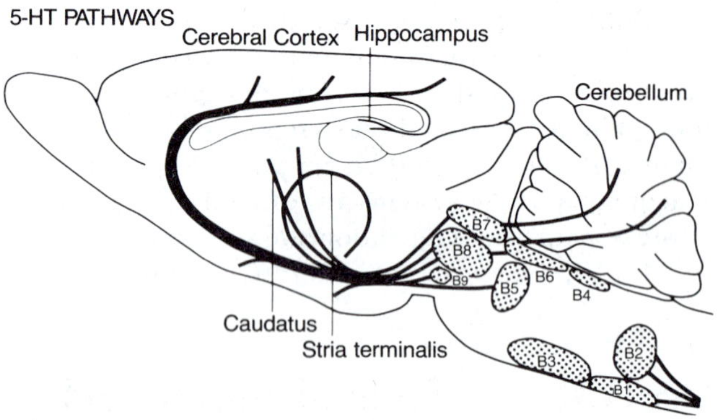

Figure 9–4
Serotonergic pathways of the raphé system. B_1–B_4 are in the medulla, B_5–B_6 in the pons, and B_7–B_9 on the boundary of the pons and midbrain. B_7 is the dorsal raphé nucleus. Modified from K. Fuxe and G. Jonsson, Further mapping of central 5-hydroxytryptamine neurons. *Adv. Biochem. Psychopharmacol. 10*:2, 1974. © 1974 by Raven Press, Publishers/New York.

tive reinforcements. The reward system, which carries out the effects of positive reinforcement, is closely associated with the two catecholamines, norepinephrine and dopamine. The reward system is important in regulating the changes in synaptic connections that occur as a result of positive experiences. Drugs that stimulate the reward system (amphetamines and similar stimulants, for example) are called primary reinforcers because of their ability to promote changes in a person's behavior.

The punishment system, associated with the periventricular gray matter of the brainstem, suppresses behaviors in response to actual or anticipated negative reinforcement (physical or emotional pain). Activity of this system is related to the psychophysiological concept of anxiety, although the precise relationship is unknown. Antianxiety drugs are especially effective in suppressing the punishment system.

The abuse potential of drugs, particularly psychological dependence, is closely associated with the effect of drugs on the reward and punishment systems — either activation of the reward system or inhibition of the punishment system. Stimulants activate the reward system, sedative-hypnotics and anxiolytics suppress the punishment system, and narcotics do both.

The Diencephalon

The diencephalon includes the dorsal thalamus, epithalamus, subthalamus, and hypothalamus. The epithalamus and subthalamus are of minor importance for interpreting drug effects on the brain. The epithalamus includes the habenulae, which are involved in olfactory circuits, and the pineal gland, which is attached to, but distinct from, the brain. The pineal gland participates in diurnal cycles, biochemical responsiveness to light, and sexual maturation. The subthalamus is a transitional zone between the midbrain and the thalamus. Some midbrain nuclei extend into the subthalamus, and some additional extrapyramidal relay nuclei are found exclusively in this region (the subthalamic nucleus and the nucleus of Forel's field). The basal nucleus (of Meynert) in the subthalamus is one of the areas first affected in Alzheimer's disease (see Chapter 24).

The Dorsal Thalamus and Diffuse Thalamic System

The dorsal thalamus (or thalamus) is a central egg-shaped collection of nuclei that act as relay stations between the lower brain and the cortex. Some of the nuclei relay sensory inputs from the visual, auditory, and somatosensory systems. Another group of nuclei belongs to the diffuse thalamic projection system (Figure 9–5), which generates the waves of electrical discharge in the cerebral cortex that provide consciousness. A third set of nuclei interconnects with other thalamic nuclei.

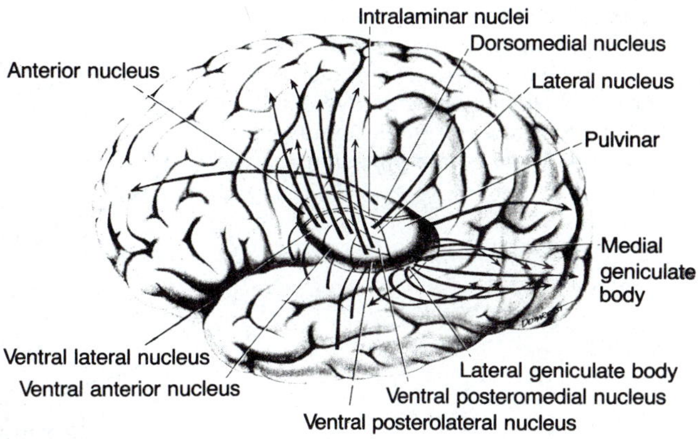

Figure 9–5
The diffuse thalamic projection system. From S. R. Noback, *The Human Nervous System.* © 1974 by McGraw-Hill Book Company, New York. Used with permission.

The diffuse thalamic system is a functional system that arises from the associative nuclei of the thalamus and spreads nerve impulses from the thalamic pacemaker to the cerebral cortex. The diffuse thalamic system is instrumental in maintaining consciousness and attention and important in the genesis of petit mal epilepsy and in the pharmacology of drugs that produce sleep or coma. The diffuse thalamic system is discussed further in Chapter 11.

The Hypothalamus

The hypothalamus (Figure 9–6), which lies at the base of the brain just above the pituitary gland, is a tightly packed cluster of nuclei. It serves as the principal discharge center for the limbic system, relaying emotional behaviors regulated by the limbic system and participating in the limbic system circuits that consolidate experience into long-term memory.

Four **homeostatic** (balance-maintaining) processes come under the domain of the hypothalamus: water balance, energy balance, temperature regulation, and sexual functioning. The hypothalamus uses the autonomic and endocrine systems for its various homeostatic functions.

The hypothalamus is the chief communication center between the nervous system and the endocrine system, providing the principal neural regulation of the pituitary gland, which is the master gland of the endocrine system. Reciprocal feedback regula-

Figure 9–6
The hypothalamus and major interconnecting fiber bundles. From S. R. Noback, *The Human Nervous System.* © 1974 by McGraw-Hill Book Company, New York. Used with permission.

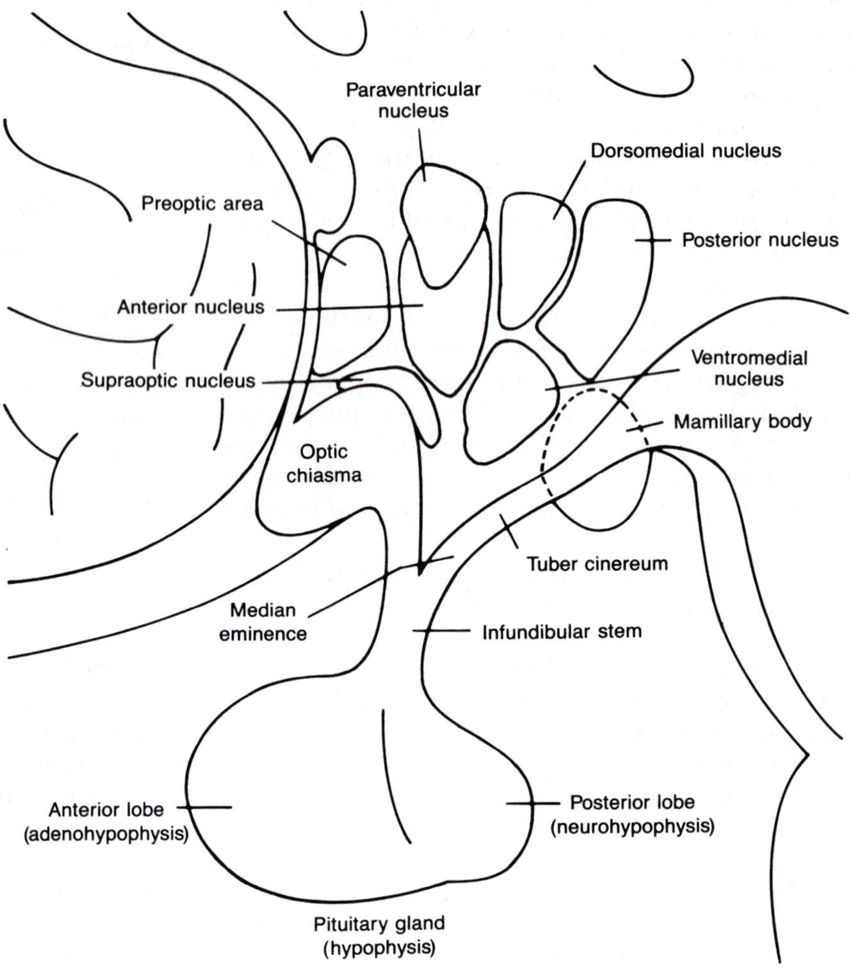

tion is exerted over the hypothalamus by the endocrine glands that it controls. Regulation of the **posterior pituitary gland** by the hypothalamus is a direct neural control. Neurons lying in the supraoptic and paraventricular nuclei of the hypothalamus synthesize antidiuretic hormone and oxytocin respectively, which then flow down the axons of these cells into the posterior pituitary gland. Stimulation of one of these nuclei causes release of its hormone from the posterior pituitary. Antidiuretic hormone increases reabsorption of water in the tubules of the kidney and helps to regulate water balance. Oxytocin controls uterine contractions and lactation.

The hypothalamus exerts endocrine control over the **anterior pituitary gland** through releasing factors. The releasing factors are secreted near the base of the hypothalamus and are transported in the blood to the anterior pituitary, stimulating the release of anterior pituitary hormones: growth hormone, thyrotropin, corticotropin, and sex hormones.

The Cerebellum and Corpus Striatum

The cerebellum and corpus striatum are the two major brain areas that contribute to the extrapyramidal system. The cerebellum is located behind the brainstem and stands apart as a distinct brain structure, although it is richly interconnected with other brain areas. The upper surface of the cerebellum receives somatosensory and proprioceptive inputs from the skeletal muscles. The rest of the cerebellum organizes the rapid, phasic patterns of muscle contractions that make up skilled movements. The cerebellum does not initiate these movements but responds instead to commands from the cerebral cortex. The cerebellum has few kinds of synapses and thus provides little opportunity for drug influences. It is seldom impaired by disease. The classic sign of cerebellar dysfunction is ataxia.

The corpus striatum controls the slow, tonic aspects of subconscious motor activity. Its nuclei are the caudate, putamen, and globus pallidus. The corpus striatum uses many different neurotransmitters and is thus susceptible to disruption by a wide variety of psychotropic drugs. The extrapyramidal side effects of neuroleptics and antidepressants are due to actions on the corpus striatum. Several important extrapyramidal diseases also relate to the corpus striatum, including parkinsonism, Huntington's disease, and Wilson's disease. Disturbances in the function of the corpus striatum lead to motor symptoms, such as tremor, hyperkinesias, muscle rigidity, or muscle weakness. The corpus striatum is discussed more completely in Chapter 22.

The Limbic System

The limbic system lines the inner wall of the cerebral cortex (Figure 9–7) and includes the amygdala, the septal region, the hippocampus, and the cingulate gyrus. This system is closely related to the olfactory system, which has led to use of the term **rhinencephalon** ("nose-brain") to describe the limbic system.

The limbic system is critical in generating emotional behaviors. For example, aggression is closely related to the amygdala and pleasure to the septal region. The limbic system is important in emotional disorders, including schizophrenia, depression, and anxiety. Drugs that are used to treat emotional disorders generally have profound effects on the limbic system.

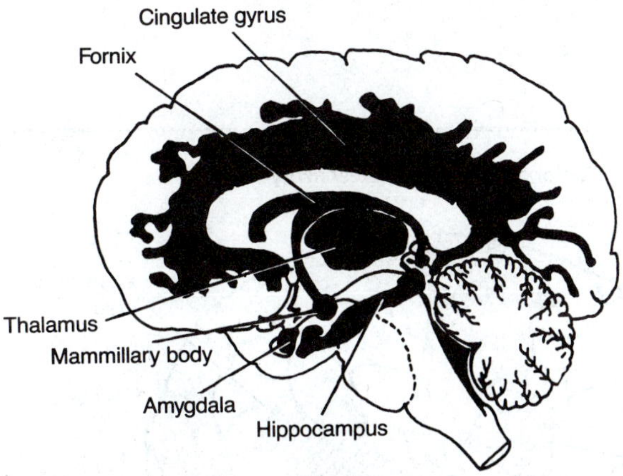

Figure 9–7
Brain regions constituting the limbic system. Modified from J. R. Smythies, *Brain Mechanisms and Behaviour.* Oxford: Blackwell Scientific Publications Ltd., 1970.

The limbic system aids in the process of selecting responses from the behavioral repertoire for use in specific circumstances. Behaviors generated by the limbic system are typically appetitive (reducing drives such as hunger, thirst, or sexual desire) or avoidance (warding off pain). The limbic system also participates in short-term memory and consolidation of memories into long-term stores. Each limbic system center contributes distinct capabilities.

The Amygdala

The amygdala, lying at the base of the temporal lobe, is functionally divisible into corticomedial and basolateral regions. The corticomedial portion modulates appetitive behaviors related to olfactory cues, especially eating and sexual responses to species-specific chemicals (called pheromones) that guide sexual attraction. The basolateral portion of the amygdala provides defensive or aggressive behaviors that include orienting responses, aggression, flight, and sympathetic activation.

The Hippocampus

The hippocampus, also located deep in the temporal lobe, is interconnected with the mammillary bodies of the hypothalamus by a large fiber bundle called the **fornix.** When activated, the hippocampus exhibits a characteristic **theta rhythm.** The hippocampus contributes to memory and selection of behavioral responses for achievement of drive reduction or avoidance. When people suffer hippocampal damage from head injury, surgery, degeneration, or drug-induced damage, their memories already established remain intact, but new events cannot be recorded.

The Septal Region

The septal region, a complex of nuclei lining the inner cortex anterior to the thalami, has been called the *pleasure center* because stimulation of this area in humans produces feelings described as "peaceful euphoria" or "well-being." Part of the septal region acts as a pacemaker for the hippocampal theta rhythm.

Adjacent to the septal complex are two nuclei that are currently receiving attention because of their possible relationship to major diseases. One of these, the nucleus accumbens septi, is considered a likely area for involvement in the etiology of schizophrenia. Many dopaminergic nerve terminals of the mesolimbic pathway end in this nucleus. The basal nucleus (of Meynert), or substantia innominata, gives rise to and receives cholinergic fibers that are among the first neurons to undergo degeneration in the progression of Alzheimer's disease (see Chapter 24).

The Cerebral Cortex

In humans, the cerebral cortices constitute about 80 percent of the mass of the brain. Many behaviors and mental processes that are especially highly developed in humans have been attributed to the cortex. The surface area of the human cortex is about 200,000 sq. in., and it varies in thickness from 1.5 cm in the visual area to about 4.5 cm in the motor area. The cortex is involved with the more complex and modifiable aspects of behavior.

The cerebral cortex is divided into two hemispheres interconnected by a small number of networks of crossing fibers called **commissures.** There are substantial differences in the functions of the two hemispheres. The left hemisphere in most individuals appears to be organized for linear thought and verbal logic, while the right hemisphere is oriented toward intuitive, holistic, aconceptual thinking. Verbal function is largely limited to the left hemisphere in most people. The roles of the two hemispheres are reversed in some left-handed individuals.

Anatomists divide each hemisphere into four lobes: the frontal, parietal, occipital, and temporal. Each lobe is further divided into gyri, which are the protrusions formed by the convolutions of the cortex. The cortical surface can also be divided into functional zones (Figure 9–8). The cortex is also organized vertically into six or seven differentiated layers of cells in most regions.

At the microscopic level, the cerebral cortex is organized into columns of cells that span the layers and make up the functional units of the cerebral cortex. As a gradual consequence of sensory experience, each cell column becomes attuned to a particular stimulus complex, gaining the ability to recognize and then represent that complex. Each impulse generated by the diffuse thalamic system activates some of the cell columns in the cortex to generate conscious experience.

The Frontal Lobe

The region at the back of the frontal lobe is the primary motor cortex. This region is the origin of the pyramidal motor system. Immediately in front of the primary motor cortex is the premotor area, which operates with the primary motor cortex to generate coordinated patterns of muscular activity. An area at the base of prefrontal cortex, called **Broca's area** (Figure 9–8), produces speech. It is found only on the left side of the brain in most individuals.

Further forward is the prefrontal, or granular, cortex, which is shallow and undifferentiated. The prefrontal cortex sends outputs to the limbic system for cortical suppression of limbic-regulated behaviors. The frontal lobes are important for initiative, willful behavior, and higher intellectual skills, such as reasoning.

The Parietal Lobe

The **postcentral gyrus** in the front of the parietal lobe receives sensory inputs of the somatosensory system, providing conscious perception of pain, temperature, touch, and body position. Each hemi-

Figure 9–8
Lateral view showing cortical subdivisions.

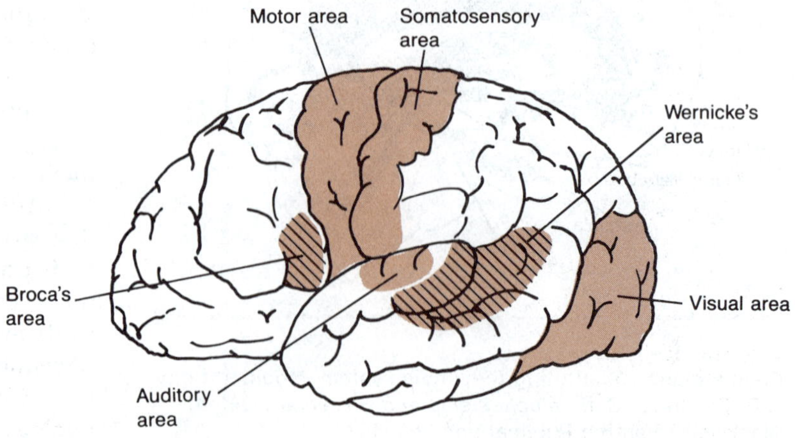

sphere receives this information from the opposite side of the body.

Immediately behind the primary somatosensory cortex is the sensory association cortex. The back of the parietal lobe is functionally linked with the occipital lobe and control of eye movements. Other parietal associative areas have a high degree of lateralization (difference in function on the left and right sides). In the dominant hemisphere (usually the left), much of the parietal associative cortex is involved with language: speech, reading comprehension, and writing skills. There is little, if any, verbal ability in the nondominant hemisphere, but the parietal lobe on that side is related to orientation in space and time. Lesions of the parietal lobe in the nondominant hemisphere result in distorted body image and an inability to find one's way around, to count backward, or to order historical events.

The Occipital Lobe

Much of the occipital lobe is concerned with the visual system. The occipital pole constitutes the primary visual cortex. The associative areas of the occipital lobe function in color vision and eye movements. Lesions may produce visual agnosia, in which objects can be seen but not named.

The Temporal Lobe

The temporal lobe receives auditory signals. Certain cells are sensitive to particular frequencies. Medial regions of the temporal lobe, including the amygdala, the hippocampus, and associated cortex, are part of the limbic system. Wernicke's area (Figure 9–8) is required for comprehension of spoken language. Other portions of the temporal lobe provide auditory-visual associations.

The Physiology of Nerve Cells

Characteristics of the Neuron

The nervous system is made up of hundreds of billions of nerve cells, called **neurons,** and associated **neuroglia,** or supporting cells. Neurons differ from other cells in size and shape. Each neuron has a large single nucleus that contains one or more nucleoli. The neuron, like other cells, contains free ribosomes and rough endoplasmic reticulum (both associated with protein synthesis) and a Golgi apparatus (involved in the packaging of secretory products). Like other cells, neurons contain mitochondria (the "powerhouse" of the cell) and microtubules (which provide organization to the cytoplasm).

The membranes of nerve cells maintain the integrity of the cell over a range of external environmental conditions and contribute to communication. Nerve cell membranes, like those of other cells, consist of a fluid mosaic — a double layer of lipid (fat) molecules in which are embedded various proteins (Figure 4–4). The fatty character of the membrane provides a cell surface that is largely impermeable to water-soluble molecules. Drugs such as anesthetics, sedative-hypnotics, alcohol, and marihuana produce their effects partly through alterations in the fluidity of membrane lipids.

Nerve cells are able to engage in their special activities because they possess specialized structures called *cytoplasmic processes.* Each nerve cell has one or more of these processes extending from its body, or **soma.** A **monopolar** cell has only one process, an axon. An **axon** specializes in rapid conduction of nerve impulses (outputs) away from the cell. Some axons are covered by an insulating layer of fatty neuroglial cells called the **myelin sheath** that increases conduction velocity. Conduction velocity also increases with axon diameter. A **bipolar** nerve cell has an axon and a single large dendritic process. **Dendrites** are specialized for receiving and integrating chemical influences (inputs) from other nerve cells or sensory receptors. **Multipolar** nerve cells (Figure 9–9) possess multiple, branching dendrites.

Highly specific interconnections, called **synapses,** occur between adjacent nerve cells and between nerve cells and the tissues they innervate — muscles, organs, and glands. Within each synapse there is a very small gap, the **synaptic cleft,** usually about 1/1,270,000 of an inch in width, that separates the two nerve cells or the nerve cell and effector tissue. Because of this space, neurons do not directly contact other neurons or effector tissues, and electrical impulses cannot be passed directly from one cell to another. Rather, the transfer of information from neurons to other neurons or to effector cells is performed by chemicals called **neurotransmitters.**

Communication at synapses is carried out in a manner that minimizes the risk of exposing the cells to challenges that could not be met adequately. The neurotransmitter molecules that carry the messages do not gain entrance into the target cell, but act instead on proteins, called *receptors,* that are embedded in the cell membrane. Stimulation of membrane receptors triggers a cascade of chemical reactions whose character is defined by the identity of the messenger, type of receptor, and subsequent effector mechanisms.

Proteins in a cell membrane vary in size, location, and function. They may be (1) **receptors,** which bind chemical messengers, (2) **modulating proteins,**

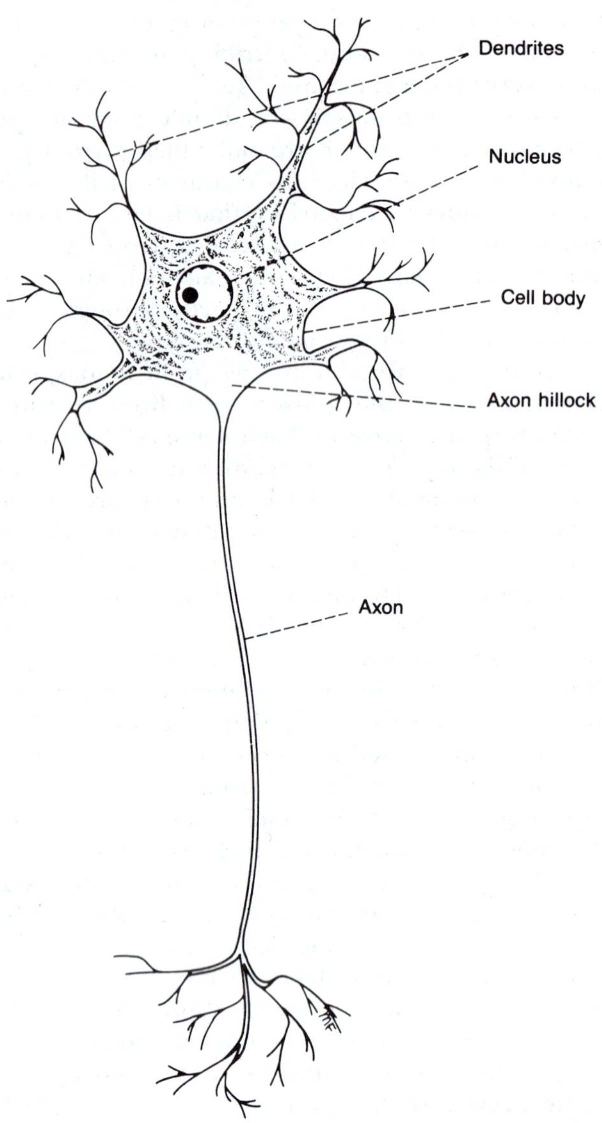

Figure 9–9
A neuron. From R. S. Snell, *Clinical Neuroanatomy.* Boston: Little, Brown, 1980.

which adjust the activities of other membrane proteins, (3) **coupling proteins,** which link together the activities of other membrane proteins, or (4) **effector proteins,** which produce changes in the target cell. This last category includes (1) **carriers,** which transport needed chemicals into the cell and escort unwanted molecules out, (2) **ion channels,** which allow limited transfer of water and small ions across the lipid barrier, and (3) **catalytic enzymes,** which regulate important metabolic activities.

Resting State

When a neuron is in its resting state, there is a small difference (about 70 mv) between the electrical charge inside and outside the cell — the inside of the cell being more negative. This polarization of electrical charge is brought about by the ability of the cell to control the distribution of ions, especially sodium. Cells are able to control the distribution of small ions because the lipid membrane limits passage of ions, and the carrier proteins, powered by cellular energy, pump the ions into or out of the cell. The pump that is most responsible for the resting potential is the **sodium-potassium exchange pump,** which carries sodium out of the cell in exchange for potassium. The sodium-potassium exchange pump produces a substantial imbalance in sodium and potassium distribution across the membrane, concentrating sodium outside the cell and potassium inside the cell. This disequilibrium can be maintained only if the cell membrane remains largely impermeable to these ions.

Nerve Cell Function: Conduction

Conduction is the movement of bioelectrical impulses along the axons of nerve cells, often over long distances, without loss of signal strength. Conduction is accomplished by an **action potential,** a propagated impulse that forms initially at the boundary between a nerve cell body and its axon, a region called the axon hillock. An action potential is triggered when the change in polarization of the cell produced by neurotransmitters is sufficiently excitatory to open sodium channels at the axon hillock. For a split second, there is a complete loss and even reversal of polarization. This depolarization excites adjacent sections of the axon, causing them to depolarize in turn, and the process repeats itself in a chain reaction down the length of the axon. The result is a propagated electrical discharge along the axon. A recording of an action potential as it passes by a particular point along the axon is diagrammed in Figure 9–10. The depolarization of the membrane (represented by the upswing of the action potential in Figure 9–10) is due to the influx of sodium. The subsequent recovery of the resting potential (the downswing of the action potential) is due to efflux of potassium in response to the initial sodium current. Potassium ions flowing outward carry positive charges and cause the interior of the cell to become more negative. As the cell returns to its resting state, the ion channels close and the membrane regains its

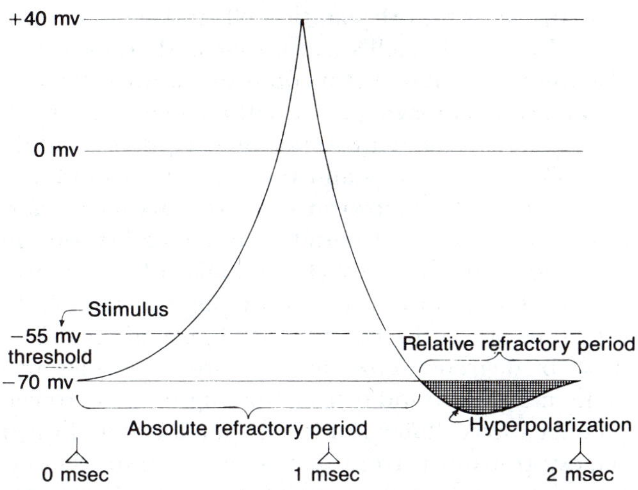

Figure 9–10
Hypothetical schema of an action potential indicating refractory periods. From A. K. Swonger and L. L. Constantine, *Drugs and Therapy*, 2d ed. Boston: Little, Brown, 1983.

normal state of impermeability. The cell resists occurrence of an additional action potential until it regains its resting potential. The action potential is all-or-nothing and electrically initiated. Action potentials are influenced by only a few kinds of drugs (most notably, local anesthetics). When a propagated action potential reaches the nerve terminal, or bouton, it dissipates, but not before initiating the other important nerve cell function: neurotransmission.

Nerve Cell Function: Neurotransmission

Mechanisms of Synaptic Transmission

Synaptic transmission is a communication between neurons or a neuron and an effector tissue (Figure 9–11). It occurs across the synapse in only one direction. The message sender is the **presynaptic** neuron, and the recipient is the **postsynaptic** neuron or effector. Message sending is a function of the nerve terminal of the presynaptic neuron. The capacity to transmit messages depends on the ability of the presynaptic neuron to maintain a resting potential and to synthesize and store neurotransmitter.

Synthesis of neurotransmitter occurs in one or more steps regulated by synthetic enzymes. The precursors, or building blocks, used to make neurotransmitters are molecules that are widely available in the body, such as an amino acid or metabolic intermediary of glucose metabolism, made available to the nerve cell by active transport from the extracellu-

Figure 9–11
Neurotransmission mechanisms: (1) Synthesis, including (1a) precursor uptake, (1b) transmitter synthesis, and (1c) vesicular uptake. (2) Storage in a (2a) vesicle (composed of protein mesh and gangliosides) and (2b) movement of full vesicle onto membrane. (3) Release, including (3a) arrival of a propagated action potential, (3b) influx of calcium through divalent ion channel, and (3c) exocytosis of transmitter. (4) Interaction with a receptor protein (RP) associated with a large ion channel, including (4a) binding, (4b) activation, resulting in an excitatory postsynaptic potential (EPSP), (4c) dissociation, and (4d) regeneration of the receptor. (5) Interaction with an adenylatecyclase (AC)-linked receptor, including (5a) binding, which may be modified by a modulatory protein (MP), (5b) activation of AC via a coupling protein (CP) to stimulate production of cyclic adenylate monophosphate (cAMP) from adenosine triphosphate (ATP), and (5c) metabolism of cAMP to AMP by phosphodiesterase (PD). (6) Feedback control of synthesis and release by action of the transmitter on a presynaptic receptor (PreR). (7) Inactivation of transmitter by (7a) reuptake, (7b) diffusion, or (7c) enzymatic degradation.

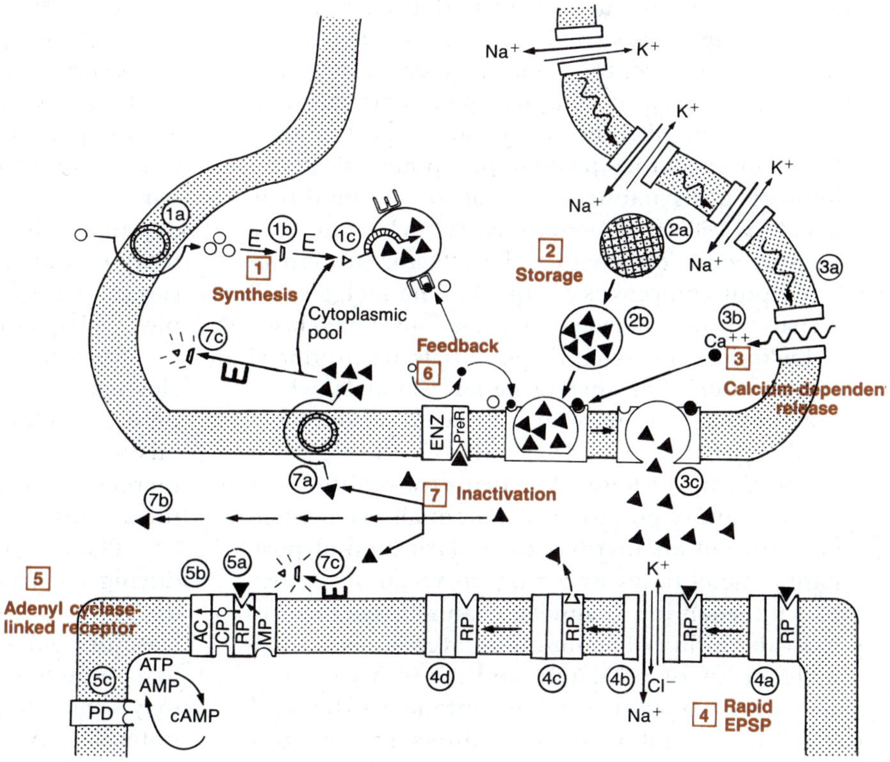

lar fluid. Whichever step in the synthesis of a neurotransmitter is the slowest is the rate-limiting step and is especially vulnerable to drug inhibition. The final step in synthesis is typically associated with storage of the neurotransmitter in vesicles. Storage protects the transmitter from destruction by cytoplasmic enzymes and sets the stage for transmitter release. After a vesicle is filled with transmitter, it moves into position on the interior face of the presynaptic cell membrane.

Transmission is triggered by the arrival of an action potential at the nerve terminal. Since an action potential results from the conduction process, the sequence of events that follows its arrival at the nerve terminal is called **conduction-transmission coupling.** Arrival of the action potential is accompanied by a sharp increase in the permeability of the cell membrane as ion channels momentarily open. The increase in membrane permeability allows calcium ions (among others) to flow into the cell, where they can bind to vesicles. Under the influence of calcium, vesicles that are filled with neurotransmitter and positioned on the presynaptic membrane fuse with the cell membrane and the neurotransmitter is released into the synapse by exocytosis.

The released neurotransmitter flows outward from the site of release and contacts the postsynaptic cell membrane and its proteins. Some of the proteins of the postsynaptic membrane are receptors for the neurotransmitter, having structures that allow them to bind the neurotransmitter. These receptors are often associated with other membrane proteins in a receptor complex. Activation of a postsynaptic receptor complex by a neurotransmitter leads to one of three effects on the postsynaptic cell: (1) an excitatory postsynaptic potential, (2) an inhibitory postsynaptic potential, or (3) modifications of the cell's metabolic activities. Which of these occurs depends on whether the effector protein in the receptor complex is a large ion channel, a small ion channel, or an enzyme (such as adenylate cyclase).

Excitatory postsynaptic potentials are produced by transmitters that open **large ion channels,** which permit influx of sodium into the cell, producing a partial depolarization (or excitation) in the region of the membrane where the neurotransmitter has acted. Inhibitory postsynaptic potentials occur when neurotransmitters increase the polarization of postsynaptic membranes by acting on receptors associated with **small ion channels,** channels too small to permit the influx of sodium but large enough to allow the efflux of potassium and the influx of chloride. An area of a nerve cell membrane may be bombarded by several neurotransmitters at the same time, some with excitatory and others with inhibitory effects. If the overall influence of the various transmitters is sufficiently excitatory, a nerve impulse will develop in the postsynaptic cell and will be conducted along the cell's axon. Released transmitters also interact with receptors on presynaptic cell membranes, called **presynaptic receptors,** exerting a feedback effect on the neurotransmission process, inhibiting further synthesis and release of transmitter.

Even as the neurotransmitter is acting on various receptors, it is also undergoing **inactivation.** Inactivation can occur by (1) reuptake of the neurotransmitter into the presynaptic nerve terminal, (2) diffusion out of the synapse, or (3) enzymatic breakdown by degratory enzymes. Degratory enzymes may be membrane-bound or free-floating in the extracellular or intracellular fluids. Reuptake occurs in two stages: transport from the synapse into the cytoplasm, and then transport from the cytoplasm into the vesicle.

Drug Effects on Synaptic Transmission

The ultimate function of transmission is to produce an effect on a postsynaptic cell. Drugs can alter transmission acutely by primary interactions (Table 9–2) or by triggering compensatory adjustments in the neurons. They can act either to increase or decrease transmission. When given chronically, drugs may also initiate adaptive changes in neurotransmission.

Acute Primary Drug Effects That Increase Transmission

Every phase of transmission can be influenced by drugs. Synthesis can be increased by administering the **precursor** required for transmitter synthesis (if the substance is one that can cross the blood-brain barrier). For example, levodopa, a precursor of dopamine, is used for parkinsonism to increase activity of dopamine receptors. Dietary supplements can increase the availability of precursors, for example tryptophan, the precursor of serotonin.

Storage of a neurotransmitter in synaptic vesicles may be inhibited by a **depletor,** such as reserpine. Depletors cause a prolonged decrease in transmission, but this may be preceded by a transient increase as neurotransmitter initially spills out into the synapse.

The amount of calcium that enters the neuron during each action potential can be increased by drugs that promote opening of calcium channels. Release of neurotransmitters is usually tightly coupled to conduction, but certain drugs, called **releasers,** may stimulate release even in the absence of action potentials. Administration of amphetamine releases norepinephrine and dopamine in this manner.

Some drugs **increase binding** of a transmitter to

Table 9–2
Potential Alterations in Synaptic Transmission by Drugs or Diet

Alterations that increase activity	Alterations that decrease activity
Administration of precursor	Inhibition of synthesis
Diet enriched with precursor	Diet deficient in precursor
Interference with storage (initial response)	Interference with storage (main response)
Decreased firing rate of presynaptic cell	Increased firing rate of presynaptic cell
Increased Ca^{++} influx per action potential	Decreased Ca^{++} influx per action potential
Release of transmitter (uncoupling of transmission from conduction)	Blockage of transmitter release
Increased affinity of postsynaptic receptor for transmitter (via modulatory protein)	Decreased affinity of postsynaptic receptor for transmitter (via modulatory protein)
Increased receptor-effector coupling (via coupling protein)	Decreased receptor-effector coupling (via coupling protein)
Inhibition of degradation of second messenger	Inhibition of effector protein
Administration of postsynaptic receptor agonist	Administration of postsynaptic receptor antagonist
Inhibition of reuptake	Stimulation of reuptake
Inhibition of transmitter degradation	Activation of degratory enzymes
Administration of presynaptic receptor antagonist	Administration of presynaptic receptor agonist

its postsynaptic receptor by influencing a modulatory protein adjacent to the transmitter receptor site. Benzodiazepines produce this effect on gamma-aminobutyric acid (GABA) binding. Receptor activity can also be increased by administering a neurotransmitter **mimic,** a drug that acts as agonist at the postsynaptic receptor. An **agonist** binds to the receptor and activates it in the same manner as the neurotransmitter itself. For example, phenylephrine is an agonist at alpha-adrenergic receptors and bethanechol at cholinergic receptors. Some agonists are many times more potent than the natural transmitter.

Postsynaptic effector activity can be increased also by interfering with the inactivation of the transmitter. Drugs such as imipramine (Tofranil) **block reuptake** of norepinephrine or serotonin, while certain other antidepressants (called MAO inhibitors) **inhibit the degradative enzyme** monoamine oxidase, which acts on several neurotransmitters.

Synaptic transmission can also be enhanced by preventing the feedback regulation exerted by the presynaptic receptor. A drug that is a selective **antagonist at presynaptic receptors** will free the presynaptic cell from feedback inhibition; yohimbine (Yohimex) has this effect on noradrenergic neurons. An **antagonist** is a drug that binds to a receptor but does not activate it, denying the neurotransmitter access to the receptor.

Acute Primary Drug Effects That Decrease Transmission

Neurotransmission can be decreased by interfering with the various steps in the process. One approach to decreasing transmission is by **inhibition of synthesis,** such as the inhibition of norepinephrine synthesis by alpha-methyl-para-tyrosine or inhibition of GABA synthesis by isoniazid (Nydrazid). Inhibition of the rate-limiting step of synthesis is most effective. If the precursor happens to be an essential dietary constituent, as in the case of tryptophan, synthesis can be inhibited by **dietary restrictions** that eliminate sources of the precursor. **Depletion** of stored transmitter also prevents transmission.

Some very potent toxins act by **preventing release** of neurotransmitter. For example, the release of acetylcholine is prevented by *Clostridium botulinum* toxins. A very common mechanism for decreasing effector activity is the use of a **postsynaptic receptor antagonist.** Neuroleptics are antagonists at dopamine receptors, preventing dopamine from reaching those sites.

The affinity of neurotransmitter for postsynaptic receptors may be decreased by modulatory proteins associated with the receptor. Nicotinic receptors exhibit **decreased affinity** for acetylcholine in the presence of peptide modulators. **Uncoupling** of receptors from their effector proteins can sometimes be achieved by drugs: narcotics uncouple dopamine receptors from adenylate cyclase, producing a *functional blockade* of dopamine receptors.

Stimulation of presynaptic receptors by a **selective presynaptic receptor agonist** will diminish synthesis and release of a neurotransmitter. The administration of the drug clonidine has this effect on norepinephrine. Release of a transmitter can also be decreased by drugs that **slow the firing rate** of the presynaptic neuron.

Compensatory and Adaptive Changes in Synaptic Mechanisms

Even when a drug is given acutely (once or a few times), its effects are sometimes substantially more than the primary effects because of **compensatory responses** on the part of the body, occurring within minutes or hours. Compensatory responses are adjustments that tend to counteract the primary effect of an administered drug. For example, when a drug is given that increases blood pressure, the initial rise in blood pressure tends to stimulate baroreceptors in blood vessels, which then signal the brain centers that control blood pressure, causing these centers to decrease cardiac output and vasomotor tone. Thus, the body opposes the primary effect of the drug with compensatory adjustments in its effort to maintain homeostasis. Similar compensatory mechanisms come into play in neurotransmission, including changes in activity of synthetic enzymes, in the firing rate of presynaptic cells, and in the affinity of postsynaptic receptors or the extent of their coupling with effector proteins.

When a drug is given for an extended period of time, its effects on neurotransmission may involve a third component in addition to the primary effects and compensatory responses: **adaptive mechanisms,** which come into play over periods of 6 days to 3 weeks. When a drug is given chronically, neurons have time to adjust to its presence by altering the synthesis of proteins. A neuron might increase or decrease its complement of synthetic enzymes, degratory enzymes, precursor transport proteins, receptors, modulatory proteins, or coupling proteins. Adaptive changes in neurotransmission may offset the primary effects of a drug, producing **tolerance,** or, conversely, might increase or decrease the compensatory responses to the drug. Adaptive changes often involve receptors or coupling proteins. A decrease in the number of either receptors or coupling proteins results in the cell being less sensitive to the action of a drug. This is called **down-regulation.** When there is an increase in receptors or coupling proteins, a cell becomes supersensitive, a process called **up-regulation.** Down-regulation is involved in the tolerance that develops to narcotics and sedative-hypnotics. Adaptive changes that occur when antidepressants or neuroleptics are administered over several weeks contribute to the fact that chronic effects of these drugs exceed the acute effects. Adaptive changes are also involved in the occurrence of tardive dyskinesias after long-term administration of neuroleptics.

The Major CNS Transmitters

Most (if not all) neurons release one, and only one, of the classical neurotransmitters. Some neurons also release one or more peptide transmitters. Each neurotransmitter has a distinctive distribution within the brain. Most drugs interact more or less specifically with one or two neurotransmitters and therefore tend to influence those parts of the brain where the particular transmitters are most abundant. Knowledge of the distribution and synaptic mechanisms of specific neurotransmitters therefore provides a basis for understanding the effects of drugs on the brain.

Acetylcholine

Acetylcholine is synthesized in the body in a one-step reaction requiring acetylcoenzyme A and choline as substrates. Acetylcoenzyme A, an intermediate in the metabolism of glucose, is readily available. Choline is obtained mainly from the diet and must be actively accumulated by cholinergic (acetylcholine-containing) nerve cells. Uptake of choline is the rate-limiting step in synthesis of acetylcholine. The synthesis is catalyzed by the enzyme **choline acetylase.** Release of acetylcholine is triggered by influx of calcium during action potentials. Its destruction is carried out by enzymes called **cholinesterases,** including *acetylcholinesterase* (which has a high degree of preference for acetylcholine over other substrates and is found in neural tissue and erythrocytes) and *pseudocholinesterase* (which metabolizes acetylcholine only slowly and is found in plasma and nonneural tissue). Cholinesterases hydrolyze acetylcholine, producing acetate and choline. Cholinesterase inhibitors are of importance in pharmacology of the autonomic nervous system (see Chapter 29).

Cholinergic receptors are of two general types: nicotinic and muscarinic. The nicotinic type is associated with large ion channels and produces excitatory postsynaptic potentials. The muscarinic type decreases activity of adenylate cyclase by increasing levels of guanidine nucleotides.

In the brain, acetylcholine is fairly widely distributed. Two important reticular nuclei of the midbrain are cholinergic, each the control center for a major system of ascending projections to diffuse targets (Figure 9–12). Brain regions particularly rich in acetylcholine include the cerebral cortex, the caudate nucleus of the corpus striatum, and the limbic system.

Cholinergic blocking drugs, such as atropine, produce a characteristic anticholinergic syndrome marked by memory impairment, slurred speech, drowsiness, ataxia, disorientation, and hallucinations, as well as numerous symptoms related to the peripheral nervous system (see Chapter 29).

Norepinephrine

Norepinephrine synthesis is a three-reaction sequence that begins with the amino acid L-tyrosine. L-Tyrosine is converted by the enzyme, tyrosine hydroxylase, to dihydroxyphenylalanine (dopa), thence by dopa-decarboxylase to dopamine. Finally, in noradrenergic neurons, dopamine is converted to norepinephrine by dopamine-β-hydroxylase. Two enzymes contribute to the breakdown of norepinephrine: monoamine oxidase (MAO) and catechol-O-methyltransferase (COMT). MAO inhibitors, such as tranylcypromine, are used in clinical medicine as antidepressants; COMT has no clinically important inhibitors. Reuptake of norepinephrine is inhibited by many of the tricyclic antidepressants and by cocaine.

Like acetylcholine, norepinephrine is released in response to the calcium influx that accompanies depolarization of nerve cell terminals. Release can also be brought about by catecholamine-releasing stimulants, such as amphetamine, leading to overstimulation, restlessness, nervousness, and agitation. Guanethidine, an antihypertensive drug, and bretylium, an antidysrhythmia agent, have the opposite effect, preventing neuronal release of norepinephrine even when the cell is depolarized. Reserpine inhibits the storage of norepinephrine within vesicles. The use of these drugs can lead to psychiatric depression.

Adrenergic receptors are classified into four types (called α-1, α-2, β-1, and β-2) based on different susceptibilities to various stimulating and blocking drugs. Drugs that mimic the effect of norepinephrine on some or all of these receptors are called **sympathomimetics** or **adrenergic agonists.** They have little effect on the brain (since they do not cross the blood-brain barrier), but they have profound effects on the sympathetic nervous system (see Chapter 28).

Noradrenergic pathways and nuclei are more limited in number and distribution than those for acetylcholine. The major noradrenergic pathways of the CNS are depicted in Figure 9–13. Norepineph-

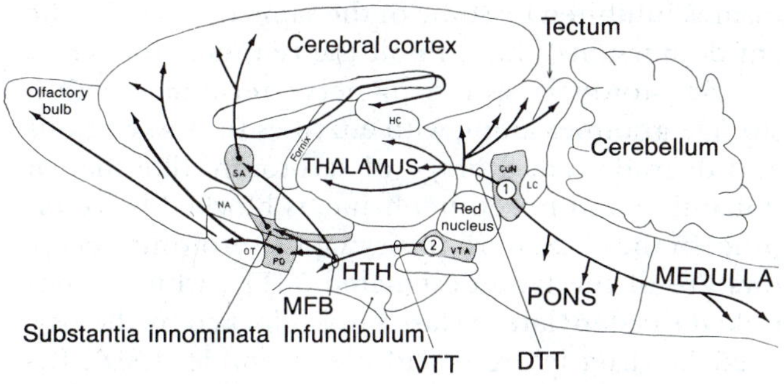

Figure 9–12
Ascending cholinergic systems. (1) Projections from the cuneiform nucleus (CuN) of the midbrain reticular formation. (2) Projections from the ventral tegmental area (VTA). DTT, dorsal tegmental tract; HC, hippocampus; HTH, hypothalamus; LC, locus ceruleus; MFB, medial forebrain bundle; NA, nucleus accumbens; OT, olfactory tubercle; PO, preoptic area; SA, septal area; VTT, ventral tegmental bundle. From A. K. Swonger and L. L. Constantine, *Drugs and Therapy,* 2d ed. Boston: Little, Brown, 1983.

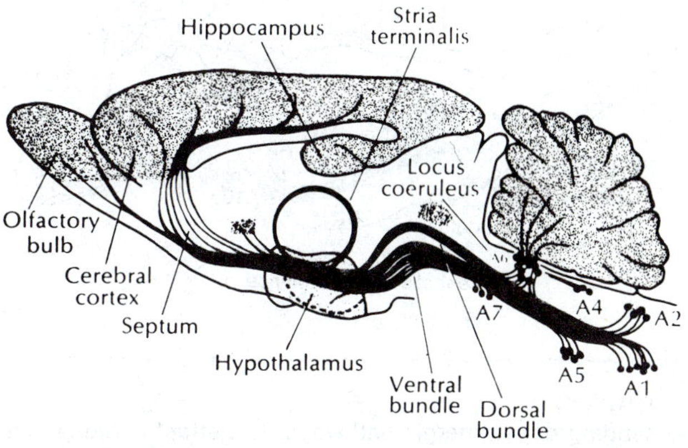

Figure 9–13
Ascending norepinephrine pathways. The stibbled regions indicate the major nerve terminal areas. A_1–A_3 are in the medulla and A_4–A_7 in the pons. A_6 is the locus ceruleus, the central control nucleus of the reward system. Modified from J. R. Cooper et al., *The Biochemical Basis of Neuropharmacology,* 3d ed. New York: Oxford University Press, 1978.

rine is important in regulating arousal, motor activity, and reward, and in the pathogenesis of affective disorders (see Chapter 20).

Dopamine

Dopamine metabolism closely parallels that of norepinephrine. In dopaminergic neurons, the pathway originating with tyrosine simply stops with the formation of DA. Dopaminergic cells lack the enzyme required for further conversion to norepinephrine. Dopamine is destroyed by the same two enzymes (MAO and COMT) that degrade norepinephrine. Like acetylcholine and norepinephrine, dopamine is released by the influence of calcium entering the cell during nerve cell depolarization.

Despite the similarities between dopamine and norepinephrine, the two transmitters have different receptors. Dopaminergic receptors are found peripherally in the renal and mesenteric vascular beds, where dopamine produces vasodilation. Dopamine-induced vasodilation is not blocked by either α- or β-adrenergic blockers but is readily blocked by specific dopamine-blocking drugs, such as haloperidol (Haldol). Dopaminergic receptors are divided into two main types, D_1 and D_2. The D_1-receptor is linked to adenylate cyclase, but the D_2-receptor is not. Chronic use of dopamine-blocking drugs (the neuroleptic agents) causes dopamine receptors to develop supersensitivity. Some of the dopaminergic pathways in the CNS (Figure 9–14) are intricately controlled by feedback regulatory mechanisms, including presynaptic receptors and multineuronal feedback loops.

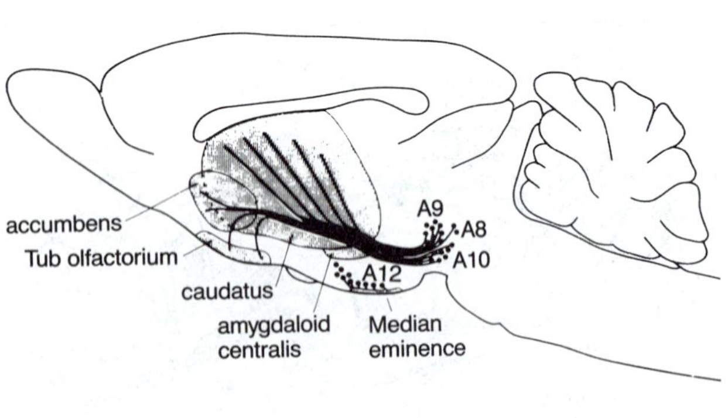

Figure 9–14
Ascending dopaminergic pathways. The stippled regions indicate the major nerve terminal areas. A_8–A_{10} are in the midbrain and A_{11}–A_{14} (only A_{12} is shown) are in the hypothalamus. A_9 is part of the substantia nigra and gives rise to the nigrostriatal dopamine pathway. Modified from K. E. Moore and P. H. Kelly, Biochemical pharmacology of mesolimbic and mesocortical dopamine neurons. In M. A. Lipton et al. (Eds.), *Psychopharmacology:* A Generation of Progress. © 1978 by Raven Press, Publishers/New York.

Clients who receive drugs that mimic dopamine or have neurologic disorders involving an excess in dopamine (such as Huntington's chorea) may be overly aggressive since dopamine regulates aggression. Stereotypy, a pattern of repetitious acts, such as gnawing, head-swinging, and biting, is another effect of overstimulation of dopamine receptors.

Serotonin

Serotonin (5-hydroxytryptamine, or 5-HT) synthesis is a two-step process beginning with the amino acid, tryptophan. Tryptophan cannot be synthesized by mammalian cells and is thus an essential dietary constituent; dietary tryptophan can influence brain levels of serotonin. Both carbohydrates and proteins contain significant amounts of tryptophan. Carbohydrates have been found to be effective in promoting sleepiness in babies and adults when ingested in the evening. However, most protein-rich foods do not elevate brain serotonin because tryptophan in protein must compete with the other amino acids for uptake into the brain, and this competition does not favor tryptophan.

Tryptophan that reaches the brain is actively transported into nerve terminals. There it is converted by the enzyme tryptophan-5-hydroxylase to 5-hydroxytryptophan, which is then converted by l-aromatic amino acid decarboxylase (the same enzyme that converts dopa to dopamine) to serotonin. Like norepinephrine and dopamine, serotonin is broken down by MAO, to produce mainly 5-hydroxyindoleacetic acid. Serotonin can also be inactivated by reuptake or diffusion. The serotonin reuptake mechanism is inhibited by some of the same drugs (tricyclic antidepressants) that inhibit the reuptake for NE.

Serotonin is stored in nerve terminals within storage granules along with enzymes for its synthesis and degradation. Storage of serotonin, like that of dopamine and norepinephrine, is blocked by reserpine. In the CNS, most postsynaptic serotonin receptors are of the type designated 5-HT_1, which is not linked to adenylate cyclase but is blocked by the psychedelic drug lysergic acid diethylamide (LSD). Receptors of the 5-HT_2 variety are linked to adenylate cyclase. A third type of serotonin receptors, called autoreceptors, are located on the cell bodies of serotonin neurons; LSD is an agonist at these receptors.

Like the catecholamines, serotonin is largely contained in a limited number of pathways (Figure 9–4), which regulate spinal reflexes, the sleep-wake cycle, the flow of sensory afferents, and habituation. A deficiency in serotonin may contribute to some instances of affective disorders (mania and depression).

Gamma-Aminobutyric Acid

The metabolic pathway leading to production of **gamma-aminobutyric acid** (**GABA**) is known as the GABA shunt because it occurs as an offshoot of the Krebs' cycle, a major metabolic pathway in the metabolism of glucose. The GABA shunt begins and ends with intermediates of the Krebs' cycle. GABA is formed from glutamic acid by the enzyme glutamic acid decarboxylase, an enzyme found only in the CNS and of primary importance in regulating GABA levels. GABA is metabolized by GABA-transaminase (GABA-T) into succinic semialdehyde. Both GABA-T and glutamic acid decarboxylase require a coenzyme, pyridoxal phosphate, for maximal activity, but drugs that decrease the availability of pyridoxal phosphate decrease the activity of glutamic acid decarboxylase more than GABA-T and hence decrease GABA levels. Glial cells play an important role in metabolism of GABA. There are several types of GABA receptors; the $GABA_A$ type is part of a receptor complex which includes modulatory proteins that are the principal receptors for barbiturates and benzodiazepines.

GABA is widely distributed throughout the brain and produces exclusively inhibitory influences on target cells. Some neuroscientists believe that up to 90% of all synapses in the brain may utilize GABA as a neurotransmitter. Most GABA neurons are intrinsic (or local circuit) neurons (contained within a given brain region); both the cerebral cortex and the cerebellum contain vast numbers of these intrinsic GABA neurons. GABA provides a background of inhibition against which the excitatory influences are registered and ensures that excitatory signals to the brain will be confined to appropriate pathways. When GABA function is compromised by inhibition of its synthesis or blockade of its receptors, the brain becomes hyperexcitable, which leads ultimately to seizure.

Neuropeptides

Neuropeptides function differently than the neurotransmitters. Our knowledge of these substances is rapidly expanding at present, and the number of peptides possibly involved in neuroregulation is rapidly increasing. It is possible that some peptides are neurotransmitters, but most of them probably serve as neuroregulators or cotransmitters. A **neuroregulator** produces slower but longer-lasting effects than a neurotransmitter, such as influences on metabolic processes. The term **contransmitter** is used to describe the ability of certain peptides to modulate the binding of a primary neurotransmitter. A peptide-releasing neuron is illustrated in Figure 9–15. The packaging of peptide neuroregulators is performed by the Golgi body and associated rough endoplasmic reticulum within the cell body, rather than in the nerve terminal, a distinctive characteristic of peptide neurons.

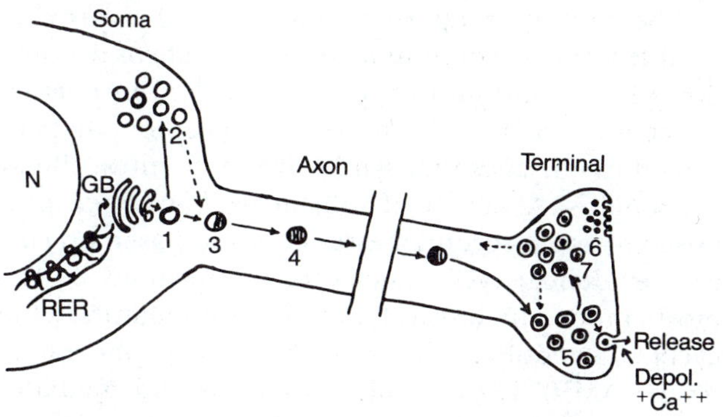

Figure 9–15
Hypothetical diagram of the intracellular processes of synthesis, storage, processing, transport, and release of peptides (or proteins) in a peptidergic neuron. GB, Golgi body; N, nucleus; RER, rough endoplasmic reticulum. (1) Newly formed granule; (2) granule pool (in soma) available for axoplasmic transport; (3 and 4) various stages of maturation of granules during transport; (5) granule pool in the axon terminal containing fully processed proteins ready for release; (6) recycled granule membranes in form of small vesicles; (7) pool of stored granules in terminal in non-releasable form. Modified from H. Gainer, Peptides and neuronal function. *Adv. Biochem. Psychopharmacol. 15*:202, 1976. © 1976 by Raven Press, Publishers/New York.

One kind of neuropeptide, the **endorphins,** is of great interest to researchers today. These peptides are the endogenous agonists for the receptors acted on by narcotic analgesics (see Chapter 25) and are important in regulating the flow of pain sensations.

Another peptide, **substance P,** released in the spinal cord by cells carrying pain signals from peripheral pain receptors, contributes to transmittal of pain sensations to higher brain centers. Other peptides under investigation as brain neuroregulators are growth-hormone inhibitory factor, vasoactive intestinal polypeptide, cholecstokinin, adrenocorticotropic hormone, thyrotropin-releasing factor, melanocyte-stimulating hormone, neurotensin, angiotensin II, antidiuretic hormone, and oxytocin.

Second Messengers

Second messengers are molecules that provide for intracellular communication. The rate of production of a second messenger is controlled in part by the action of neurotransmitters on receptors that are linked to enzymes that synthesize these intracellular messengers. A variety of substances have been proposed to act as second messengers, but based on current evidence, cyclic nucleotides appear to be the most important intracellular neuroregulators. One cyclic nucleotide, adenosine 3′,5′-cyclic phosphate (**cyclic AMP**), is especially important and mediates many hormonal effects in peripheral tissues. For example, many of the actions of epinephrine are related to cyclic AMP, including insulin release and sugar and fat utilization. Cyclic AMP is synthesized by the enzyme adenylate cyclase (Figure 9–16). This enzyme is the effector protein in many CNS receptor complexes.

Cyclic AMP is formed from adenosine triphosphate, a universal cellular constituent. Destruction of cyclic AMP is catalyzed by the enzyme phosphodiesterase. A group of drugs called xanthines, including theophylline and caffeine, are effective inhibitors of phosphodiesterase, potentiating the effects of cyclic AMP. Acetylcholine has no direct effect on cyclic AMP levels in any tissue studied, but it does elevate levels of another cyclic nucleotide, cyclic guanosine monophosphate (cyclic GMP). In some cells, cyclic GMP and cyclic AMP appear to have antagonistic roles. Several of the important psychotropic drugs produce effects on levels of cyclic AMP.

Recommended Readings

Neuroanatomy and Its Nursing Implications

Angevine JR Jr, Cotman CW: *Principles of Neuroanatomy,* New York, Oxford University Press, 1981.

Carpenter MB: *Human Neuroanatomy,* ed 8. Baltimore, Williams & Wilkins Co, 1983.

Hickey J: *The Clinical Practice of Neurological and Neurosurgical Nursing.* Philadelphia, JB Lippincott, 1981.

General Sources for Neurotransmission

Cooper JR, Bloom FE, Roth RH: *The Biochemical Basis of Neuropharmacology,* ed 4. New York, Oxford University Press, 1982.

Creese I, Sibley DR: Receptor adaptations to centrally acting drugs. *Annu Rev Pharmacol Toxicol* 1981;21:357–391.

Stewart CM: Neurochemical transmission, neurotransmitters, and clinical correlations. *J Neurosurg Nursing* 1982;14(6):303–308.

Acetylcholine

Cheney DL, Costa E: Biochemical pharmacology of cholinergic neurons, in Lipton, MA et al (eds): *Psychopharmacology: A Generation of Progress.* New York, Raven Press, 1978, pp 283–291.

Kuhar MJ: Central cholinergic pathways, in Lipton, MA et al (eds): *Psychopharmacology: A Generation of Progress.* New York, Raven Press, 1978, pp 199–203.

Lewis PR, Shute CCD: Cholinergic pathways in CNS, in Iversen LL et al (eds): *Handbook of Psychopharmacology,* 9. New York, Plenum Press, 1978, pp 315–355.

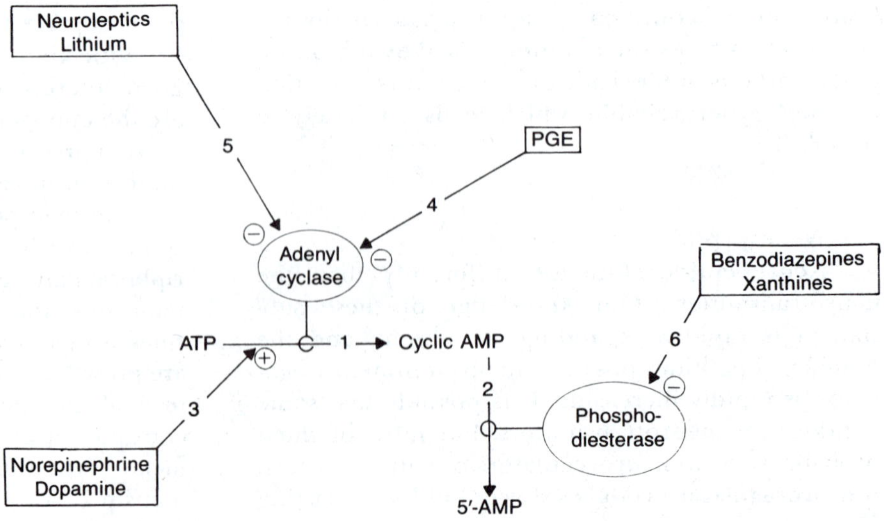

Figure 9–16
Metabolism of cyclic AMP (cAMP) indicating known and postulated drug modifications. AMP, adenosine monophosphate; ATP, adenosine triphosphate; PgE, prostaglandin E. (1) Synthesis of cAMP by adenyl cyclase; (2) degradation of cAMP by phosphodiesterase; (3) mediation of norepinephrine and dopamine effects by cAMP; (4) PgE inhibition of adenyl cyclase; (5) inhibition of adenyl cyclase as proposed mechanism for lithium and neuroleptics; (6) inhibition of phosphodiesterase by xanthines and as proposed mechanism of anxiolytics. From A. K. Swonger and L. L. Constantine, *Drugs and Therapy,* 2d ed. Boston: Little, Brown, 1983.

Dopamine

Moore RY, Bloom FE: Central catecholamine neuron systems: Anatomy and physiology of the dopamine systems. *Annu Rev Neurosci* 1978;1:129–169.

Roberts PJ, Woodruff GN, Iversen LL (eds): *Advances in Biochemical Psychopharmacology.* New York, Raven Press, 1978, vol. 19: *Dopamine.*

Gamma-Aminobutyric Acid

Defeudis FV, Mandel P (eds): *Advances in Biochemical Psychopharmacology.* New York, Raven Press, 1981, vol. 29: *Amino Acid Neurotransmitters.*

Johnston GAR: Neuropharmacology of amino acid inhibitory transmitters. *Annu Rev Pharmacol Toxicol* 1978;18:269–289.

Norepinephrine

Lindvall O, Bjorklund A: Organization of catecholamine neurons in the rat central nervous system, in Iversen LL et al (eds): *Handbook of Psychopharmacology,* 9. New York, Plenum Press, 1978, pp 139–231.

Moore RY, Bloom FE: Central catecholamine neuron systems: Anatomy and physiology of the norepinephrine and epinephrine systems. *Annu Rev Neurosci* 1979;2:113–168.

Peptides

Loh HH, Ross DH (eds): *Advances in Biochemical Psychopharmacology.* New York, Raven Press, 1979, vol. 20: *Neurochemical Mechanisms of Opiates and Endorphins.*

Martin JB, Reichlin S, Bick KL (eds): *Advances in Biochemical Psychopharmacology.* New York, Plenum, 1981, vol 28: *Neurosecretion and Brain Peptides.*

Snyder SH, Childers SR: Opiate receptors and opiate peptides. *Annu Rev Neurosci* 1979;2:35–64.

Serotonin

Aghajanian GW, Wang RY: Physiology and pharmacology of central serotonin neurons, in Lipton, MA et al (eds): *Psychopharmacology: A Generation of Progress.* New York, Raven Press, 1978, pp 171–183.

Fuller RW: Pharmacology of central serotonergic neurons. *Annu Rev Pharmacol Toxicol* 1980;20:111–127.

CHAPTER 10

Drug Abuse and Misuse

This chapter is concerned with the general principles that pertain to abuse and misuse of drugs. The pharmacology of specific drugs of abuse is reserved for subsequent chapters in this unit since many of these drugs are also employed for clinical purposes.

What Is Drug Abuse?

The term *drug abuse* is used in different ways, depending on context. Broadly speaking, the term encompasses all instances in which drugs are misapplied to the detriment of good health or well-being. For clarity, however, we will use the term *drug misuse* for this broad range of drug misapplications that includes misguided self-administration of drugs for expected health benefits and errors in medical judgment leading to erroneous drug selection, administration, dosage, or duration of use (Table 10–1). We will reserve the term *drug abuse* for those instances of misuse in which three conditions are met: (1) the drug has been self-administered, (2) the motivation for using the drug is to produce an altered mental state, and (3) the use of the drug impairs (or can be anticipated to impair) the user's physical or mental health or ability to function in a social context.

These criteria take no account of the source of the drug (prescription, over-the-counter, recreational), its legality, or its social acceptability. Alcohol, although legal, remains the source of the largest drug abuse problem in America — whether viewed in terms of economic loss, numbers of people afflicted, physiological damage, family disruption, or

Table 10–1
Characteristics of Drug Misuse and Drug Abuse

Characteristic	Drug misuse	Drug abuse
Relationship of terms	Includes drug abuse and other drug misapplications	A subcategory of drug misuse
Administration	Self or others	Self
Intended effect	Health benefit Improved performance Cosmetic benefit Altered mental state	Altered mental state
Nature of error	Benefit overvalued relative to costs or risks Erroneous drug selection, route of application, dosage, frequency of use, duration of treatment, etc.	Altered mental state overvalued relative to extent of actual or potential costs
Examples	Routine use of aspirin for minor pain Excessive use of fat-soluble vitamins Premature discontinuation of an antibiotic regimen Failure to comply with an appropriate drug regimen Excessive use of cold remedies Suppression of productive cough with cough remedies Use of androgens for body building Error in dosage calculation Extended, daily use of sleeping pills or antianxiety drugs by prescription	Habitual use of alcohol, nicotine, cocaine, psychedelics, sedatives, stimulants, narcotics, or other centrally active drugs that impair or are likely to impair physical or psychological health or the ability to function in a social context

psychological impact. Tobacco smoking is also legal, and although only minimally disruptive to social functioning until medical problems develop, it may actually outrank alcohol as a preventable cause of premature death. These two drugs, alcohol and nicotine, make it clear that drug abuse cannot be defined by legality or social acceptance.

Other terms used to describe drug abuse are addiction and habituation. These terms are used inconsistently, but generally the term **addiction** is reserved for instances of drug abuse in which physical dependence is present and psychological dependence is strong enough to create an intense craving for the drug and a compulsion to obtain it. Since addiction usually involves physical as well as psychological dependence, there are identifiable deficits in social functioning. The term **habituation,** by contrast, usually describes a psychological dependence limited to a desire to use the drug if it is available. Physical dependence is generally absent or slight, and the costs of the habitual drug use are mainly costs to the physical and psychological well-being of the user, affecting society only minimally.

Who Abuses Drugs?

Every person has a potential for drug dependency if he or she reaches a point where usual coping mechanisms fail. Social scientists, however, have begun to isolate traits that occur frequently in drug abusers, that render the individual prone to compulsive, self-destructive behavior. And while there is no uniform personality profile for all abusers, the following traits occur frequently in people who become addicted to a variety of things, ranging from work to gambling to heroin: rebelliousness, impulsiveness, desire for instant gratification, sensation-seeking, nonconformity, disregard for generally approved goals of achievement, alienation, acceptance of deviance, greater than usual stress, tendency toward depression, dependent behavior, focus on short-term goals rather than long-term goals, lack of self-esteem, and heightened anxiety. Other characteristics noted among teenage drug abusers in particular are lack of close family relationships, close friends who use drugs, parents who use drugs, nonparticipation in sports, school, or civic activities, cigarette smoking,

Drug Testing

There continues to be much public interest in drug testing (from urine samples) for air traffic controllers, police officers, firemen, bus drivers, athletes, teachers, government employees, employees of private companies, applicants for employment, and others. A 1987 survey indicated that some 30% of Fortune 500 companies screen employees for drug use and an even larger percentage test applicants for employment. The trend toward increased drug testing raises both legal and scientific questions.

The courts have generally struck a balance between the rights of the employer to maintain a safe environment and the quality of its products and services and the constitutional rights of employees to privacy and freedom from illegal searches. The courts have been more likely to uphold the right to test when testing is for cause (such as evidence of intoxication following accidents) than when testing is conducted randomly. However, even random testing has been allowed when the employee is directly responsible for the safety of others. The courts have allowed broader latitude in the testing of applicants for employment than in testing of current employees. The courts are more likely to uphold testing programs if employees have been fully informed of the program, if they are given opportunity to contest the results, and if reasonable assistance is provided to the employee to overcome drug problems that are identified. The courts have generally rejected employee suits asserting that drug testing does not accurately reflect the present level of impairment of the individual or that the tests themselves are unreliable.

The scientific questions relate to the issue of reliability, in particular, the likelihood of *false positives* — test results erroneously indicating presence of a drug — that might jeopardize a person's livelihood or reputation. Drug screening based on urinalysis is completely reliable if the following conditions are met: (1) the laboratory personnel are well trained; (2) all positives from the initial testing are retested in confirmation assays; (3) urine samples are carefully labeled and tracked to prevent samples from being mixed up; and (4) a quality assurance procedure is implemented using standard samples (having known quantities of drug added) and blank samples (controls known to have no drug). The initial screen in most laboratories is an immunoassay. The two most widely employed systems are EMIT, sold by SYVA Co., and ABUSCREEN, marketed by Roche Diagnostics. In conducting these tests, the *detection limit,* which defines a sample as positive or negative for presence of a drug, is set well above the *sensitivity limit,* which is the minimum concentration of drug that can be detected. This virtually eliminates the possibility of false positives from, for example, passive inhalation of marihuana smoke, but still permits false positives caused by presence of a *cross-reactive substance* — a drug resembling the one for which the test is intended. Therefore, it is essential for accuracy that a confirmation test be conducted when positives are found in the initial screen. The tests used for confirmation, including gas chromatography, gas chromatography/mass spectrometry, and high performance liquid chromatography, are too expensive for routine use in initial screening but provide virtually complete discrimination between various drugs and a high degree of certainty. To protect the rights of those being tested, it is essential that samples that are not confirmed as positives in the confirmation test always be reported as negatives, never as "unconfirmed positives."

The detection limit and *detection period* (the length of time after use that the drug can be detected in the urine) varies from drug to drug. In addition, the detection period can be influenced by a person's rate of metabolism, the amount of fluid imbibed prior to the test, and whether the drug has been used chronically or only once. For example, in most individuals, marihuana metabolites are detectable for about 2–5 days (10 days maximum) after a single smoking session, but for 3–4 weeks or more after a period of heavy chronic use. Typical detection limits and periods are as follows:

Drug class and drug	Detection limit	Detection period
Sedative-Hypnotics		
Alcohol	0.02%	very short
Barbiturates	200 ng/ml	
amobarbital		medium
butabarbital		medium/long
pentobarbital		medium
phenobarbital		long
secobarbital		medium
Benzodiazepines	300 ng/ml	
chlordiazepoxide		medium/long
diazepam		long
Methaqualone	750 ng/ml	long
Stimulants		
Amphetamines	1.0 μg/ml	
amphetamine		medium
methamphetamine		medium
Cocaine	300 ng/ml	short
Narcotics	300 ng/ml	
codeine		medium
hydromorphone		short/medium
morphine/heroin		medium
Psychedelics		
Cannabinoids	50–100 ng/ml	medium/long
Phencyclidine	25 ng/ml	medium

Key: Very short: 6–18 hrs; short 12–48 hrs; medium: 2–5 days; long: 6–30 days.

and lack of religious practice. Health care professionals, and physicians and nurses in particular, are among the occupational groups with the very highest incidence of drug abuse problems.

Because nurses work closely with clients on a sustained basis, they are in a prime position to identify early symptoms of drug abuse and to attempt to deter it. Drug abusers are often people who feel they have been lied to, humiliated, shamed, or dealt with inconsistently by their parents, receiving praise one minute and destructive criticism the next. Using these clues, nurses, in working with children and adolescents, need to be perceived as truthful. They need also to be consistent in their praise and approval of constructive behaviors. While nurses do not replace parents, it is important that they be identified as people upon whom one can depend for truth and support.

Pharmacological Aspects of Drug Abuse

Psychological and physical dependence are qualitatively distinct phenomena. The notion held by many lay people that psychological dependence means a weak dependence while physical dependence is a more severe one is simply wrong. Psychological dependence is far more central to the concept of drug abuse than is physical dependence. It is not too much to say that psychological dependence is at the heart of drug abuse.

Psychological Dependence

A person is psychologically dependent if he or she thinks taking a drug is necessary to maintain an acceptable feeling of well-being. The psychologically dependent individual is preoccupied with procuring and taking a drug to an extent that is detrimental to psychological health and social functioning.

The attribute of a drug that most contributes to its *abuse liability* (likelihood that it will be abused) is its ability to reinforce the drug-taking behavior rather than its ability to produce physical dependance. Reinforcement of the drug-taking behavior is a result of the ability of a drug to stimulate the brain's reward system, or to suppress the punishment system, or both. The user need not be aware of this reinforcement. Nicotine, for example, is a much more effective reinforcer than its mild subjective effects would indicate. But regardless of whether the user is aware of the reinforcement, the ability of a drug to reinforce drug-taking behavior is the principal factor contributing to initial drug-taking. Once the drug habit is established, the drug's ability to postpone withdrawal symptoms becomes a second drug-related factor that helps maintain the drug habit.

It is usually not difficult to predict how likely a new drug is to be abused. The single best test is whether laboratory animals (monkeys are the best subjects for this test) will self-administer the drug and maintain its use. Animals can be taught to self-administer all of the drugs that are abused by humans, with the sole exception of alcohol. The ability of a drug to produce physical dependence or to substitute for known addictive drugs can also be determined but does not indicate abuse liability since abuse can occur without physical dependence.

Physical Dependence

Physical dependence is best understood as a component in the triad consisting of pharmacodynamic tolerance, physical dependence, and withdrawal. Physical dependence is the craving for a drug that results from the devlopment of pharmacodynamic tolerance; it leads directly to withdrawal when the drug is discontinued. There can be no physical dependence without tolerance, although there can be tolerance without physical dependence. Nurses need to understand that drugs producing the greatest physical dependence do not necessarily produce the highest degree of tolerance. Physical dependence is not a prerequisite for either abuse or addiction.

Tolerance occurs when the effect of a given dose of a drug diminishes on repeated administration. To counter the influence of tolerance, a user wanting to maintain a constant level of effect must increase the drug dosage or advance to a stronger drug. The term *tolerance* is reserved for diminished responsiveness that occurs on a time scale of hours or days and should not be confused with tachyphylaxis, which is a diminished responsiveness lasting seconds or minutes after a large dose of a drug.

There are two mechanisms that can result in tolerance, but only one can contribute to physical dependence. **Drug disposition tolerance** is an increase in the ability of the body to dispose of a drug through increased metabolism or excretion. This type of tolerance contributes about 20% to overall tolerance with sedative-hypnotics and narcotics. Drug disposition tolerance is not a factor in physical dependence. **Pharmacodynamic tolerance,** on the other hand, is an adjustment in the neurochemistry of the brain, in response to chronic presence of a drug, that offsets that drug's effect. Because of the adjustment, the subsequent absence of the drug elicits the withdrawal syndrome. In effect, the presence of the drug becomes the norm, and its absence becomes a challenge to the system. This may be the pharmacological analogue of a statement commonly heard from heroin addicts, that they take the drug not to feel high but to feel "normal."

Two variations on the tolerance theme are reverse (or negative) tolerance and acute tolerance. In **reverse tolerance,** the central nervous system becomes increasingly sensitive (rather than less sensitive) to a drug with repeated administrations. This should not be confused with a "hypersensitivity reaction," which is an immunological response to a drug. Reverse tolerance has been reported to occur to the psychic effects of THC, the active principle in cannabis. **Acute tolerance** is said to occur when the effects (subjective or objective) of a single dose of a drug diminish faster than the decline in blood levels. Acute tolerance has been observed with cocaine and hypnotics.

Withdrawal is the withholding of a drug from a person who has developed pharmacodynamic tolerance to the drug. A **withdrawal syndrome** is the set of behavioral and physiological symptoms that accompany the withdrawal. The withdrawal of the drug causes an unmasking of the pharmacodynamic changes that have occurred during chronic administration. The withdrawal syndromes associated with amphetamines, sedative-hypnotics, and narcotics are each distinctive for that class of drugs, and nurses must be able to recognize the symptoms of both addiction and withdrawal for each class. For drugs within a given class, withdrawal syndromes are similar in quality but may vary in intensity, latency to onset, and duration. Not all drugs that produce tolerance have associated withdrawal symptoms. LSD, for example, produces a high degree of tolerance of short duration but no apparent withdrawal symptoms.

Although acute withdrawal syndromes subside within a week or two at most, some neurological indications of previous physical dependence may persist for up to six months after drug use is discontinued. These symptoms include impairments of abstract thinking, conceptualization, concentration, and memory storage and retrieval, overreaction to and incapacity to tolerate stress, poor self-image, increased

Table 10–2
Comparative Hazards of Common Drugs of Abuse

Drug	Tolerance	Physical dependence	Psychological dependence	Damage to body tissues	Acute psychosis	Death from overdose	Controlled substance
Sedative-hypnotics							
Barbiturates	++	+++	+++	0/+	+	++	Yes
Alcohol	++	+++	+++	+++	+	+	No
Benzodiazepines	+	+	+++	0	+	0	Yes
Stimulants							
Amphetamines	+++	0/+	++++	++	++++	0	Yes
Cocaine	+	0/+	+++ or +[a]	+	++	+	Yes
Caffeine	+	0	+	+	0	0	No
Nicotine	++	0/+	+++	+++	0	0	No
Narcotics	++++	++++	++++	0/+	0	++++	Yes
Psychedelics							
LSD	++++	0	0/+	0	+++	0	Yes
PCP	+	0	0/+	0/+	+++	++	Yes
Marihuana	+ and –	0	++	0/+	+	0	Yes

Key: 0, not occurring or not established; 0/+, little or none; + to ++++, from mild or occasional to intense or frequent occurrence; –, increased CNS sensitivity (negative tolerance) for certain effects.

[a]Severity of psychological dependence with cocaine is related to route of utilization: +++ if administered IV or by inhalation (smoked); + if administered orally or intranasally (snuffed).

emotionality, and overconcern about discomfort. Together, these long-term neurological deficits comprise the **post-acute withdrawal syndrome,** which contributes to occurrence of relapse after apparently successful treatments for drug abuse.

During the postacute withdrawal phase, environmental stimuli previously associated with drug taking or with drug withdrawal can intensify drug craving. For example, a former heroin addict may experience recurrence of withdrawal-like symptoms months after the last drug experience when returning to an old haunt where he or she "shot up" or when coming across an old syringe in a drawer. Such conditioning phenomena contribute to relapse after initially successful treatment of drug abuse.

Other Hazards of Drug Abuse

Apart from the risks of psychological and physical dependence, the abuse of any given drug may carry with it one or more additional hazards: damage to bodily tissues, precipitation of acute or chronic toxic psychoses, or death from overdose. The drugs of abuse differ markedly from one another in the extent to which each hazard is a factor (see Table 10–2). Damage to bodily tissues is most likely to occur with chronic abuse of alcohol, nicotine, amphetamine-like stimulants, and occasionally with cocaine, caffeine, narcotics, and marihuana. Acute toxic psychoses are commonly a consequence of amphetamine, cocaine, LSD, or PCP use and rarely occur with use of sedative-hypnotics or marihuana.

In total, all drugs cause about 6,500 overdose fatalities annually in the United States. Nondrug chemicals, including solids, liquids, and gases, add another 6,000 substance-induced deaths. CNS drugs account for the lion's share of the drug-related fatal overdoses. Barbiturates and narcotics most often cause overdose fatalities, but other drugs with significant liability in this respect include benzodiazepines, antidepressants, alcohol, nonbarbiturate sedative-hypnotics, aspirin, acetaminophen, cocaine, and amphetamines.

Drugs Commonly Misused

The drugs that are commonly abused come from four pharmacological categories: sedative-hypnotics, stimulants, narcotics, and psychedelics (Table 10–2). Except for the three major recreational drugs — alcohol, nicotine, and caffeine — all of the principal drugs of abuse are controlled sustances; that is, their distribution is restricted by law (Table 10–3). Sedative-hypnotics include barbiturates (discussed in Chapter 12), benzodiazepines (Chapters 12 and 19), and alcohol (Chapter 13). The major hazards of sedative-hypnotics include psychological dependence, physical dependence, and, in the case of alcohol, damage to bodily tissues.

The stimulants (discussed in Chapter 14) range from the rather weak drug, caffeine, to the very potent drug, amphetamine. Stimulants produce little risk of physical dependence. Caffeine promotes only

Table 10–3
Classification of Controlled Substances

Classification	Definition	Example drugs
Schedule I	Drugs with a high potential for abuse and no accepted medical uses	Heroin; LSD, marihuana, other psychedelics; methaqualone
Schedule II	Drugs with a high potential for abuse but accepted medical uses; may produce both physical and psychological dependence	Strong narcotics; most short-acting barbiturates; amphetamine, methylphenidate
Schedule III	Medically accepted drugs that may cause dependence but with lower abuse liability than drugs in schedule I or II	Preparations containing limited amounts of codeine, opium, or other narcotics; weaker barbiturates (e.g., butabarbital and hexobarbital); nonbarbiturate, nonbenzodiazepines sedative-hypnotics (e.g., methyprylon); amphetamine-like anorexics (e.g., chlorphentermine and mazindol)
Schedule IV	Medically accepted drugs that may produce mild dependence	Anxiolytics (benzodiazepines and meprobamate); chloral hydrate; phenobarbital; weak narcotics (e.g., pentazocine); weak anorexics (e.g., fenfluramine)
Schedule V	Medically accepted drugs with very limited potential for causing dependence	Drug formulations containing small quantities of codeine or other narcotics for coughs or diarrhea

weak psychological dependence, but amphetamine can cause psychological dependence as severe as occurs with any drug. Psychological dependence produced by cocaine depends on how it is used; smoking or intravenous injection can result in severe psychological dependence but intranasal or oral administraton seldom causes more than habituation.

Narcotics (Chapter 25) can result in a high-grade psychological and physical dependence. There is also a high risk of death from overdose when narcotics are abused. Psychedelics (Chapter 15) do not produce physical dependence and only marihuana in this group produces significant psychological dependence. An important risk with LSD and PCP is toxic psychosis.

A common misconception about drug misuse is that the drugs involved are obtained for the most part from the black market. An analysis of the hazards of drug misuse in relation to the four sources of drugs (prescription medications, over-the-counter medications, illicit drugs, and recreational drugs) reveals some surprising facts. For example, about two-thirds of overdose cases coming to emergency rooms involve drugs obtained by prescription. Most of the remaining one-third involve illicit drugs or alcohol. Among over-the-counter medications, only aspirin and acetaminophen are frequently involved in overdoses, and the advent of childproof packaging has reduced this problem in recent years.

Adverse drug reactions severe enough to re-

Table 10–4

Eleven Categories of Prescription Drugs Commonly Misused

Drug category	Nature of misuse	Frequency of severe adverse reactions	Frequency of emergency room treatments for overdose	Approximate yearly fatalities in the United States
Antibiotics	Use for nonresponsive organisms; determination not conducted; inappropriate dose or duration; allergic reaction not anticipated	+++	–	20–30
Anticoagulants	Unrecognized drug interactions	+	–	Few
Antihypertensives	Less than optimal drug selection; unanticipated drug interactions	++	–	Few
Antipsychotics/ antidepressants	Use for nonresponsive conditions; unnecessary use of multiple drug regimens; dosage titration not systematically conducted	+	+	500
Anxiolytics	Unnecessary use; use for nonresponsive conditions; duration of treatment too long	–	++++	700
Digitalis	Inappropriate dosage; drug interactions	+++	–	50–100
Diuretics	Unnecessary use; K^+ depletion not anticipated	++	–	Few
Hypnotics	Unnecessary use; duration of treatment too long	–	+++	1,500
Narcotics	Unnecessary use when nonnarcotic analgesics, antitussives, or antidiarrheal would suffice; overuse	–	+++	300–1800
Steroids	Unnecessary use; duration of treatment too long; use of androgens for body-building	++	–	20–30
Stimulants	Use as anorexics; too frequent use of stay-awake pills; excessive use for mild attention deficit disorder	–	++	800

Key: ++++, most frequent; +++, very frequent; ++, moderately frequent; +, occasional; –, seldom.

quire hospitalization or extension of hospitalization are almost always in response to prescription drugs. Antibiotics, digitalis, steroids, diuretics, and antihypertensives head the list of agents most frequently responsible for severe reactions. Eighteen to 30% of hospitalized patients will have a severe drug reaction while hospitalized, and such reactions are responsible for approximately 5% of hospital admissions. Seventy to 80% of severe drug reactions are caused by poor medical practice. Only 20 to 30% are unpredictable allergic or idiosyncratic reactions. Table 10–4 lists the 11 categories of prescription drugs most often misused and the nature of the misuse. Nonprescription drugs most widely misused are itemized in Table 10–5.

Chronic toxicity and increased risk of mortality, by contrast, are hazards associated most commonly with recreational drugs. All three of the widely used recreational drugs — alcohol, nicotine, and caffeine — are linked to significant hazards of tissue damage and mortality (Table 10–6), though caffeine less so than the other two agents. Other drugs with significant risks in the area of chronic toxicity include stimulants, aspirin, and steroids.

Psychological and physical dependence are hazards associated with recreational, prescription, and illicit drugs alike. The recreational drugs account for the vast majority of instances of dependence. In the United States, alcohol dependence is estimated to affect 10–20 million Americans and nicotine dependence about 34% of adults. Illicit drugs such as marihuana and cocaine are other frequent causes of psychological dependence. Narcotics, stimulants, sedative-hypnotics, and anxiolytics used in dependent behavior are far more often obtained by prescription than from illegal sources. Withdrawal syndromes may be associated with drugs of abuse such as sedative-hypnotics and narcotics, but also with a variety of prescription drugs (Table 10–7).

Toxic psychoses occur mainly with illicit drugs, notably psychedelics, amphetamines, cocaine, and depressants, but alcohol, steroids, and digitalis are potential causes. Other impairments of psychological functioning include drug-induced depression and drug-induced anxiety states. Alcohol may be involved in over 50% of cases of depression. Prescription or illicit sedative-hypnotics and anxiolytics can also contribute to depression. Caffeine is frequently implicated in anxiety disorders; other stimulants less commonly.

Clearly, misuse of drugs is a far broader problem than simply the control of illegal drug traffic.

Table 10–6
Some Relationships Between Recreational Drugs and Mortality

Likelihood of heart disease and heart failure is increased by alcohol, nicotine, and caffeine.

Nicotine and alcohol each increase the likelihood of stroke.

Alcohol contributes to atherosclerosis. Nicotine and caffeine can cause peripheral vascular disorders. All three contribute to hypertension.

Tobacco smoke contains 15 identified carcinogens. Caffeine use has been linked to cancer of the pancreas.

Alcohol can cause or aggravate chronic organic brain syndrome.

Most cases of emphysema are related to tobacco smoking.

Most cases of liver cirrhosis are related to chronic alcohol ingestion.

More than 50% of motor vehicle fatalities are alcohol-related.

Alcohol is involved in 18% of home accidents leading to death and in 13% of occupational fatalities.

Fires started by cigarettes account for more than 33% of all burn fatalities.

Alcohol use is a factor in over half of cases of clinical depression, a condition often associated with suicides.

Ninety percent of cases of physical dependence are dependence on alcohol.

Alcohol use aggravates diabetes. Caffeine, nicotine, and alcohol all can cause ulcers.

Table 10–5
Over-the-Counter Drugs That Are Widely Misused

Drug	Misuse
Aspirin and Acetaminophen	Aspirin produces about 150 fatalities per year; acetaminophen is involved in about 75 fatalities per year (apart from drug tampering). There is a general overuse of these drugs and a failure to appreciate the risk of adverse effects.
Laxatives/Cathartics	Widely overused. There are very few valid clinical indications.
Antihistamines	Excessive use, especially for colds.
Cough suppressants	Inappropriate use for "productive" cough.
Anorexics	Long-term value is dubious; addiction likely.
Sleep aids	Dubious value; overuse.

Table 10–7
Drug Withdrawal Syndromes

Drug class	Onset	Duration	Symptoms	Clinical management
Sedative-hypnotics				
Barbiturates and similar drugs	8–12 hours	5–10 days	Anxiety, irritability, insomnia, REM elevation, weakness, tremor, nausea, vomiting, hypotension, hallucinations, delirium, convulsions, cardiovascular collapse, possible death	Gradual withdrawal and symptomatic treatment; supportive and psychiatric treatment
Benzodiazepines	2–12 days	9–14 days		
Alcohol	12–72 hours	5–7 days		For alcohol, in addition to the above, substitution of chlordiazepoxide; vitamins (especially thiamine), fluid and electrolytes as needed, diazepam for convulsions
Narcotics	2–24 hours	7–10 days	Lacrimation, rhinorrhea, perspiration, mydriasis, yawning, anxiety, irritability, insomnia, REM elevation, anorexia, nausea, vomiting, diarrhea, piloerection, slight hypertension, muscle spasms	Methadone substitution and gradual withdrawal, or clonidine substitution; symptomatic treatment; supportive and psychiatric treatment
Stimulants				
Amphetamine-like drugs	12–24 hours	3–7 days	Fatigue, depression, suicidal ideation, decreased appetite, disturbed sleep, REM elevation	Supportive therapy and tricyclic antidepressants for depression if necessary
Caffeine	8–12 hours	1–2 days	Headache, drowsiness, poor concentration, irritability, lethargy	Gradual withdrawal
Cocaine	?	?	Lethargy, somnolence, depression, irritability, psychomotor retardation, nausea, and vomiting	Supportive therapy; imipramine, bromocriptine
Nicotine	3–24 hours	1–20 wk	Anxiety, irritability, restlessness, poor concentration, headache, drowsiness, nausea, anorexia	Supportive therapy; nicotine gum
Psychiatric drugs				
Antipsychotics	2–3 days	12–14 days	Withdrawal dyskinesias, nausea, vomiting, diarrhea, sweating, rhinorrhea, increased appetite, insomnia, agitation, delirium, headache, schizoid symptoms	Gradual withdrawal
Tricyclic antidepressants	1–2 days	A few days	Malaise, chills, headache, dizziness, nausea, vomiting, muscle aches, akathisias, anxiety	Resume medication and withdraw gradually.
Neurological drugs				
Antiepileptics	1–2 days	A few days	Seizures, status epilepticus	Resume medication and withdraw gradually.
Methysergide	1–2 days	A few days	Headaches	Resume drug and withdraw over 2–3 weeks.
Endocrine drugs				
Glucocorticoids	A few days	Indefinite	Depression, fatigue, hypotension, anorexia, nausea, vomiting	Resume drug and withdraw gradually over several months.
Cardiovascular drugs				
Antihypertensives	2–3 hours	1–2 days	Agitation, insomnia, headache, nausea, hypertension	Resume drug and withdraw gradually; treat hypertension.
Antianginal drugs	10 minutes to 2 weeks	Variable	Angina attacks, anxiety, trepidation, increased blood pressure	Resume drug and taper slowly.

Nursing Process and Drug Abuse

Importance of the Nursing History

Nursing histories can be especially important in cases of drug abuse because clients are often unwilling to reveal drug dependence or may not even recognize that they are dependent. In taking nursing histories, it is important to ask the client about substances that are easily obtained but not necessarily thought of as addictive, such as the use of coffee, tea, and tobacco. Nurses also should ask about household products such as glue, cleaning fluids, and solvents. Although the adult client may not use these products to produce euphoria, children or adolescents may. Nurses should ask parents about the frequency with which such substances need to be replaced.

Community health nurses are in a good position to recognize potential drug abuse problems in a family, since they see the family in the home. Once considered a problem mainly for college and high school students, drugs have become increasingly available to children in grade school. Nurses need to educate parents and teachers about symptoms of various forms of drug abuse (Table 10–8).

Among adolescents, signs of drug or alcohol abuse are often subtle if the person involved is using drugs in low dosages. School nurses are in a good position to identify such problems. Diminished academic performance and changes in activities or friendships sometimes indicate drug problems. A careful nursing history and assessment can assist in identifying the cause of the problem. It is vital for the nurse to encourage student trust; otherwise, the student will reveal little about his or her drug-taking behavior.

One way of promoting responsiveness is to meet in small groups. Nurses can use a chart such as the one in Table 10–9 to help clients determine if they have a drug problem and the extent to which drug taking has become a habit.

Drug abuse can often mask other medical problems. For example, a youngster with appendicitis may be unaware of the problem because of the strong analgesic effects of drugs he or she is taking. If the youngster comes to the clinic complaining of nausea, vomiting, diarrhea, and fever but no pain, it would be easy to make a wrong nursing or medical diagnosis. If the youngster is hospitalized and receives no further medication, the pain he or she experiences may be misinterpreted as pain due to withdrawal rather than pain due to appendicitis. Thus people who use narcotics are at risk for many medical problems quite apart from their addiction.

Nursing Observations for Drug Abuse

THERAPEUTIC GOAL	Detoxification; control of toxic psychoses; client and public safety and support of vital functions during intoxication; prevention of subsequent abuse.
PREADMINISTRATION ASSESSMENT	
Baseline Data	Observe for changes in level of consciousness, orientation, behavior, judgment, affect, pupillary diameter, respiration, blood pressure, pulse, motor coordination, speech, and skin color, temperature, or moisture. Observe for client's utilizing multiple physicians, seeking drug treatment under false pretenses, or refusing tests of compliance. Evaluate neurological status, cardiovascular and respiratory function, and renal and hepatic function. Obtain laboratory tests indicating serum concentrations of abused drug, blood cell counts, and other measurements dictated by the drug identity and health status.
EVALUATION OF DRUG RESPONSE	
For Therapeutic Benefit	Monitor for resolution of withdrawal symptoms, acute toxic psychoses, or intoxication. Monitor for decreased incidence of drug abuse and improved ability to cope successfully with life stresses.
For Compliance	Evaluate the client's compliance with all facets of the therapeutic regimen by careful observation, interviewing, and review of progress. Report compliance problems to the physician and act as client-advocate when changes in the therapeutic regimen seem indicated.

Table 10–8
Identifying Drug Users

Drug	Physical symptoms	Assessment	Dangers
Glue sniffing	Violence Drunken appearance Dreamy, blank expression	Glue smears on clothing or fingers Tubes of glue Paper bags	Lung, brain, or liver damage Death by suffocation or choking Anemia
Heroin and other narcotics	Stupor Drowsiness Loss of appetite Runny nose Constricted pupils Watery eyes	Needle or hypodermic syringe Cotton Tourniquet string Burnt bottle caps or spoon Glassine envelopes Empty cough medicine bottle Needle marks on body Blood-stained shirt sleeve	Death from overdose Addiction Liver dysfunction Systemic infection
Cocaine	Euphoria or severe depression Breakdown of mucosal lining of nose Weight loss Hallucinations Convulsions Dilated pupils	Pipe (water) Bags of cocaine	Breakdown of nasal membrane Severe weight loss Anemia Vitamin deficiency Psychological dependence
Marihuana	Sleepy Ptosis Mind wanders Lacks coordination	Strong odor of burnt leaves Cigarette papers Discolored fingers Small seeds in pocket	Psychological dependence
Hallucinogens	Speech incoherent Cold hands and feet Laughing and crying Vomiting Feels detached from surroundings Dilated pupils	Cube of sugar with discolored center Strong body odor	Suicidal tendencies Unpredictable behavior Possible neurological effects
Amphetamines	Aggressive behavior Giggling Silliness Rapid speech Confused thinking	Pills or capsules of various colors Chain smoking	Death from overdose Hallucinations Psychosis Psychological dependence

Table 10-8
Identifying Drug Users (*continued*)

Drug	Physical symptoms	Assessment	Dangers
	Lack of appetite Extreme fatigue Shakiness Insomnia Dry mouth Dilated pupils		
Sedative-hypnotics	Drowsy Stuporous Dull Slurred speech Appears drunk Vomiting	Pills or capsules of varying colors	Unconsciousness or death from overdose Addiction Convulsions from withdrawal

Source: Adapted from the *New York State Journal of Medicine, 73,* 946. Copyright 1973 by the Medical Society of the State of New York.

Infectious hepatitis is a problem common among those who use injectable drugs. Such clients appear jaundiced. A physical examination would reveal an enlarged liver (hepatomegaly) and tenderness in the right upper quadrant of the abdomen. Clients with hepatitis also often complain of nausea and anorexia. In the event that a patient is a chronic drug user and also requires surgery, it is important to have the individual undergo liver function studies. Halothane anesthesia, as well as other drugs that are metabolized or excreted by the liver, cannot be used in patients with liver dysfunction. Recently, it has also become evident that people who self-administer drugs intraveneously have a high risk of contracting the virus responsible for acquired immune deficiency syndrome (AIDS).

Adults who are drug dependent frequently suffer respiratory problems such as pneumonia, asthma, and even tuberculosis. Thus, in taking a client history, be sure to ask about the propensity to respiratory infections, the conditions under which they occur, and how they are treated. Clients who inject drugs often use fillers such as starch or talc that may cause pulmonary hypertension and right ventricular failure from thrombosis. Thrombi may also be caused by injected lint from cotton used to strain heroin.

Cutaneous symptoms of drug abuse may not always be present. Among older adolescents, there may be cutaneous scars or "tracks" along the veins used regularly for injections. Sometimes there is a tense bulla, containing clear yellow fluid, that indicates drug overdose, usually involving barbiturates. Usually the drug can be aspirated from the fluid in the lesion.

Psychiatric and neurological symptoms of drug abuse vary widely. Clients may appear anxious, apprehensive, aggressive, lethargic, jittery, or sad. Nurses need to note symptoms such as dilated pupils, which could indicate abuse of stimulants or hallucinogens. Narcotics, on the other hand, constrict the pupils, making them look like pinpoints. Some drugs that are mixed with anticholinergic agents cause an absence of sweating.

In obtaining drug histories, nurses are often in a situation requiring them to interview clients or their friends in efforts to identify further the cause of an individual's presenting symptoms. Nurses are often at the focal point of rehabilitation of clients who have been drug abusers. Thus, nurses need to be knowledgeable about the problems, sympathetic to the causes, reassuring and supportive as the user tries to recover, and they need to provide assistance to those family members most likely to be of aid in the client's rehabilitative process.

Nursing Interventions for Minimizing Iatrogenic Drug Abuse

Nurses who work in hospital settings can reduce the incidence of drug dependence by exercising restraint in the administration of narcotics and hypnotics. For example, in assessing a patient's complaint of pain, the nurse needs to determine if a

Table 10–9
Are You In Control?

		Frequency of use		
Category of substance	None	Infrequent (1-4 × yearly)	Occasional (1 × monthly)	Frequent (>1 × weekly)
I. Alcoholic beverages				
a. Beer (12 oz)				
b. Wine (4 oz)				
c. Spirits (1.5 oz)				
II. Caffeinated beverages				
a. Coffee				
b. Tea				
c. Colas				
III. OTC drugs				
a. Sleep aids				
b. Digestive aids				
c. Vitamin supplements				
d. Laxatives				
e. Painkillers				
IV. Prescription drugs				
a. Painkillers				
b. Stimulants				
c. Hypnotics				
d. Anxiolytics				
V. Illegal drugs				
a. Heroin				
b. Cocaine				
c. LSD				
d. PCP				
e. Marihuana				

Source: Modified from J. LaPace, *Health,* 4th ed. Englewood Cliffs, N.J.: Prentice-Hall, 1984, p. 349.

nonnarcotic agent would work as well as a narcotic and if nursing measures would be effective in reducing the amount of medication required. A patient who has had abdominal surgery may be especially uncomfortable for the first day or two and require narcotics for the relief of pain. However, by rubbing the patient's back and helping the patient assume a comfortable position in bed, the nurse may potentiate the effectiveness of the drug being used, and also enable the individual to have longer intervals without medication. As the patient's recovery progresses, the nurse can either gradually reduce the amount of narcotic given or substitute a nonnarcotic agent according to physicians' orders. Above all, the nurse should not give the patient a narcotic to induce sleep (an all too often unfortunate occurrence), for while narcotics may promote sleep, appropriate nursing measures are more effective in assisting clients to restore normal sleep patterns.

In both inpatient and outpatient settings, nurses should maintain current records of the prescribed and over-the-counter drugs the client is taking. The nurse should also assume responsibility for communicating with local pharmacists when there is suspicion that a client might be procuring the same drugs from different pharmacies.

Drug Abuse Education

Some deaths from overdoses and medical emergencies are caused in part by ignorance about matters such as dosage, routes of administration, fluctuating tolerance, misrepresentations of drug identity, and presence of impurities. And certainly, no matter how much the age of drug innocence recedes, there will always be an age group on the threshold between innocence and sophistication who can profit from an effective education program.

Educators in the field of drug abuse have evolved a handful of principles that may contribute to the effectiveness of communication about drugs.

1. Know your facts about illicit and social drugs, but be prepared to admit ignorance when unsure. Nothing undercuts credibility more quickly than making statements the audience knows to be incorrect.

Nursing Diagnoses and Interventions for Drug Abuse

Nursing Diagnoses	*Related Interventions*
Alteration in comfort: pain related to malaise, arthralgia, headache, and abdominal distress during withdrawal	Provide comfort measures such as back rubs and warm blankets.
Alteration in family processes: marital discord or inability to perform role functions related to drug abuse	Refer for family or marital counseling or drug abuse clinic.
Alteration in nutrition: intake less than requirements related to anorexia	Provide vitamin supplements as required.
Anxiety related to loss of control and withdrawal	Provide detoxification; encourage entry into treatment program.
Fluid volume deficit related to vomiting	Encourage intake of appropriate fluids to correct deficits.
Impaired social interaction related to intoxication	Encourage socialization with others having similar drug problems.
Impaired social interaction related to intoxication	Encourage discontinuation of drug use and entry into treatment program.
Increased risk of injury related to impaired judgment and coordination during intoxication	Provide safety measures; emphasize importance of not driving while under the influence of drugs.
Ineffective individual coping: denial, anger, and inability to manage life stresses	Encourage discussion with someone who has been successfully rehabilitated.
Potential for violence related to idiosyncratic intoxication, disinhibition of aggressive impulses, paranoia, or drug-induced belligerence or combativeness	Provide necessary measures to ensure protection of public and staff. Discuss potential behavior problems and preventive measures with the family and significant others.
Sensory-perceptual alterations: mental distortions related to intoxication; hallucinations, delusions, or delirium during toxic psychosis; delirium during withdrawal	Provide supportive care for intoxication, supportive care or antipsychotic drugs for toxic psychosis; appropriate class-specific management for withdrawal syndrome. Ensure appropriate protective measures.
Sexual dysfunction related to impotence due to intoxication	Encourage discontinuation of drug use and entry into treatment program. Discuss problem with spouse.
Sleep-pattern disturbance related to REM (rapid-eye movement) deprivation, CNS stimulation, or insomnia during withdrawal	Encourage discontinuation of drug use and entry into treatment program. Encourage exercise program.
Social isolation related to loss of job and family contacts	Encourage discontinuation of drug use and entry into treatment program.
Knowledge deficit related to drug abuse	Provide factual information concerning risks of drug abuse with respect to physical and mental health and ability to function effectively.
	Provide a positive role model by personal example.
	Exercise rigorous control over hospital drugs (in accordance with institutional policies) to prevent diversion into recreational and abusive use.
	Provide preventative drug abuse education in cooperation with school nurses, other health care professionals, teachers, and social workers.
	Help client understand personal and situational factors contributing to the pattern of abuse.
	Provide support and encouragement for dealing with the problem. Establish a supportive relationship with the client and convey respect rather than condemnation.
	Provide information about treatment programs, individual counseling or psychotherapy, couple's therapy, family therapy, or group therapy as appropriate. Encourage the client to begin addressing the problem.

2. Present a balanced view. This means, among other things, avoiding stereotypes (such as the depraved junkie) and admitting the positive sides (like "fun," "sociability") of drug use.
3. Avoid scare tactics. Sensational accounts conflict with the firsthand experiences of the audience. Most young people have used one or more psychotropic drugs for social purposes; most of the rest have talked to those who indulge. Therefore, it pays to present the facts as they exist without overstatement.
4. Avoid trying to defend the laws, especially the inconsistencies from state to state.
5. Do not neglect discussion of the drugs of abuse accepted by society: alcohol, nicotine, and caffeine.
6. When discussing the research literature relating to adverse effects, acknowledge the uncertainties that exist. Several factors contribute to the apparent and real contradictions in studies of drugs: variations in route, dosage, and dosage form; and matters of experimental design, such as the subject sample and adequacy of controls. Sometimes several reviewers of a given body of drug research literature can reach contradictory conclusions.
7. Urge parents to know the telltale signs of drug use (Table 10–8).
8. Know how to distinguish casual use from abuse by focusing on whether the use of the drug is resulting in impaired functioning.
9. Remember and urge others to understand that drug abuse is symptomatic of underlying problems, as well as a problem in its own right. Organic, psychological, and interpersonal factors must all be appreciated and addressed.

Case Study: Irrational Drug Utilization

An elderly female client, E. P., told the community health nurse she didn't believe in taking drugs "for every little thing" but later revealed that she took aspirin nightly to fall asleep, used cough syrup (with codeine) to "soothe" her throat when she had a cold or when she was singing with the choir, and even gave her 4-year-old grandson aspirin every time he cried because "he must be in pain." Thus, the woman was reinforcing not only her own drug-taking behavior but also the future drug-taking behavior of her grandson.

1. Are E. P.'s drug use habits better characterized as drug abuse or drug misuse?
2. If you were the nurse in this case, what steps would you now take to deal with E. P.'s misconceptions about the usefulness of drugs?

Answers appear at the end of the book.

Recommended Readings

Abruzzi W: Drug-induced psychosis. *Intern J Addictions* 1977;1212:183–193.

Bakdah D: Essentials the nurse should know about chemical dependency. *J Psychiatr Nurs* 1978;16(10):33–37.

Blum K: *Handbook of Abused Drugs.* New York, Gardner Press Inc, 1984.

Casselman G: Breaking the cycle of abuse. *Can Nurse* 1980;76(10):30–33.

Dupont RI, Goldstein A, O'Donnell J (eds): *Handbook on Drug Abuse.* Washington DC, National Institute on Drug Abuse, 1979.

Finley B: Primary and secondary prevention of substance abuse in nurses. *Occup Health Nurs* 1982;30(11):14–18.

Fitzpatrick E: Primary nursing: Treatment that works for the hospitalized drug dependent client. *Can Nurse* 1980;76(10):29–30.

Fulton K: Drug abuse among nurses: What nursing management can do! *Superv Nurse* 1981;12(1):18–20.

Hinson RE, Siegel S: Nonpharmacological bases of drug tolerance and dependence. *J Psychosom Res* 1982;26(5):495–503.

Jaffe JH: Drug addiction and drug abuse, in Gilman AG, Goodman LS, Gilman A (eds): *The Pharmacological Basis of Therapeutics,* ed 6. New York, Macmillan, 1980, pp. 535–584.

Khantzion E, McKenna J: Acute toxic and withdrawal reactions associated with drug use and abuse. *Ann Intern Med* 1979;90:361–372.

Krasnegor NA (ed): *Behavioral Analysis and Treatment of Substance Abuse.* National Institute on Drug Abuse Research Monograph, GPO No 017-024-00939-3, 1979, p 25.

Leporati NC, Chychula LH: How you can really help the drug-abusing patient. *Nursing (Horsham)* 1982;12(6):46–49.

Lettieri DJ, Sayers M, Pearson HW (eds): *Theories on Drug Abuse: Selected Contemporary Perspectives.* National Institute on Drug Abuse Research Monograph. 1980, p 30.

Milkman H, Sunderwith S: Addictive process. *J Psychoactive Drugs* 1982;14(3):177–192.

Pradhan SN, Dutta SN (eds): *Drug Abuse: Clinical and Basic Aspects.* St Louis, CV Mosby Co, 1977.

Ray OS: *Drugs, Society, and Human Behavior,* ed 3. St. Louis, CV Mosby, 1978.

Williams A: Primary care of parenteral substance abusers. *Nurse Pract* 1986;11(6):17–37.

Yowell S et al: Working with drug abuse patients in the ER. *Am J Nurs* 1977;77:82–85.

UNIT III

Drugs and the Central Nervous System

PART B

Arousal, Sleep, and Drugs

CHAPTER 11

Introduction to Sleep and Arousal

Certain drugs produce overall changes in the level of brain activity. Some such drugs (anesthetics, hypnotics, or analeptics) produce these widespread effects by interacting physically with cell membranes, and, without selectivity, alter the activity of neurons throughout the brain. Other drugs achieve somewhat similar results by influencing the systems within the brain that ordinarily regulate the level of brain activity. Thus, the amphetamine-like stimulants can activate brain arousal systems while antiadrenergic drugs can depress these same neural networks. The ability of these drugs to produce broad effects on the arousal of the brain is recognized by use of such slang terms as *uppers, downers,* and *getting high.*

This unit focuses on the drugs, depressant and stimulant, that produce changes in the overall activity level of the brain and drugs used to treat pathological conditions of brain arousal. This chapter introduces concepts that help to explain the mechanisms, clinical applications, and adverse effects of such drugs: electroencephalography, the brain systems that regulate arousal, and sleep.

Electroencephalography

The electroencephalogram (EEG) is the most sensitive and clinically useful measure of brain function and has become even more valuable with the advent of computerized techniques. It is a useful index of brain activity for describing states of arousal as well as the disturbances of cortical electrical activity that occur in epilepsy (see Chapter 23). The EEG is a recording of spontaneous voltage changes in the cerebral cortex as measured at two different sites. Sixteen or 32 electrodes may be attached to the scalp providing measurement of electrical activity over much of the cortical surface. A given electrode will pick up electrical activity from a circular area of the cortex up to 4 cm in diameter and to a depth of 3 mm. Action potentials have little influence on the EEG since these rapid discharges tend to cancel out in the population of millions of neurons that lie within range of a given electrode.The EEG measures primarily the excitatory and inhibitory postsynaptic potentials — the electrical discharges produced by the action of neurotransmitters on the dendrites of cortical neurons. Each line of an EEG recording measures fluctuations over time in the voltage difference between two electrodes. Thus, the EEG is a summation of the dendritic potentials of cortical neurons in the vicinity of the electrodes.

The most casual inspection of an EEG tracing reveals fluctuations in electrical potentials that appear as spontaneous waves, called brain waves. These waves vary in amplitude, frequency, and shape. Analysis of frequency of brain waves provides the most useful information. Brain wave frequencies from 0 to 4 Hz (hertz, or cycles per second) are designated as **delta activity;** frequencies from 4 to 8 Hz are called **theta activity;** frequencies from 8 to 12 Hz are designated **alpha activity;** and frequencies in excess of 12 Hz are known as **beta activity.** The simplest kind of frequency analysis is a qualitative description of an EEG in terms of the predominance of one or another of these frequencies.

Some rather reliable correlations occur between measured EEG frequencies and the age and behavioral state of a client. Delta waves, the slowest frequency range, predominate throughout infancy. They are also seen in adults during stage 4 of nondreaming sleep and in coma, whether induced by drugs or trauma. Delta waves in the awake adult may signify organic brain pathology.

Theta waves are the predominant frequency during childhood. In adults they occur mainly in delirium or in transitional states as a person is falling asleep or awakening. Nurses may observe theta waves in the EEG from the parietal and temporal regions of the brain in adults who are in emotional distress. Individuals who awaken slowly in the morning, struggling through their morning routine in a stuporous state, are people who experience an extended period of transitional theta waves.

Alpha waves are recorded symmetrically from the postcentral regions of the brain in most normal adults, interspersed with beta waves. Alpha activity is the predominant frequency in the awake but relaxed adult whose eyes are closed. When the eyes are opened, alpha waves give way to asynchronous beta waves. Alpha waves may occur continuously while a person is engaged in a relaxation or meditation technique. Alpha waves are typical when the attention of an individual has an internal focus. Alpha waves often slow down when clients undergo metabolic changes such as occur in anoxia or hypoglycemia.

Beta waves are most readily recorded from the precentral portion of the brain. Beta activity occurs when the individual is reacting to or interpreting sensory inputs. Beta activity is indicative of an alert, activated cortex. Beta activity predominates in some people who are tense and anxious.

The EEG is an effective aid in diagnosis when used in conjunction with other diagnostic techniques such as neurological, psychological, cognitive, and motor tests. However, negative EEG results have little meaning because of the limitations inherent in measurement of the EEG. For example, only a fraction of the mass of the cortex is close enough to the surface electrodes to influence the recording, and therefore deep-lying abnormalities are often not picked up by an EEG evaluation. The most obvious and consistently useful application of the EEG is in diagnosis of epilepsy (Chapter 23).

Brain Systems Regulating the EEG

Two brain systems, the diffuse thalamic system and the reticular activating system, share control of the cortical electrical activity that the EEG depicts. The diffuse thalamic system (DTS) is associated with the thalamus. It generates synchronous brain-wave patterns ranging in frequency from 0 to 12 Hz (encompassing the delta, theta, and alpha ranges). The reticular activating system, associated with the pontine and midbrain reticular formation, produces cerebral beta-wave activity.

Diffuse Thalamic System

The thalamus serves as the pacemaker for rhythmic waves of depolarization that sweep across the cortex. The thalami are a pair of egg-shaped structures that lie near the center of the brain, each composed of many nuclei. Some thalamic nuclei relay electrical signals conveying sensory information — touch, pain, vision, and hearing. Other nuclei give rise to nonspecific projections that travel to the associative regions of the cerebral cortex. Five of the eight major groups of nuclei contribute directly or indirectly to the diffuse thalamic system (Figure 9–5, p. 131). The pace set by the thalamic pacemaker determines the state of consciousness of the individual. Activity in the alpha range is associated with consciousness, activity in the delta range with unconsciousness, and activity in the intermediate theta range with semiconscious states.

Reticular Activating System

The reticular activating system (RAS) consists of the reticular formation of the brainstem and its projections to the cerebral cortex. The reticular formation is a dense, medially lying core of nerve cells that extends from the caudal medulla, through the brainstem to the thalamus (Figure 9–3, p. 130). Along its entire course it is surrounded by the tracts and nuclei of the sensory and motor systems and receives collateral inputs from all sensory modalities.

The RAS is a general alarm system for the brain that alerts it to the presence of environmental stimuli of potential importance to the individual's well-being. The RAS acts on the cerebral cortex to externalize attention when events in the environment require immediate concern. The behavioral response produced by RAS activity is the **orienting response,** in which the individual assumes a defensive posture, with attention riveted on the surroundings, eyes scanning the environment for danger. Injury to the RAS results in a diminished awareness of the environment. RAS activity is diminished by hypnotic drugs or anesthetics, which block transmission of impulses in the reticular formation.

In contrast to the DTS, which alters the frequency of its discharges over the course of the day within the delta, theta, and alpha ranges, the RAS produces only beta activity, but continuously varies the amount of beta activity it produces, based on the extent and significance of environmental stimuli. When the RAS is activated, the beta activity that it generates in the cerebral cortex is superimposed on whatever rhythmic activity is being produced by the DTS. When the quantity of RAS-generated beta activity in the EEG is considerable, the beta activity masks the underlying DTS-generated pattern under visual inspection of the EEG tracing, but presence of the underlying frequency can be established by electronic analysis using band-pass filters.

Control of Arousal

The DTS and the RAS together regulate the activity of the brain in a relationship that is both cooperative and competitive. The DTS maintains consciousness by activating neural groups within the cortex to produce a continuity of mental events. If the pace set by the DTS drops below about 5–7 Hz, the individual lapses into unconsciousness. The DTS provides an internal driving force for neural activity for generation of goal-directed behaviors. In opposition to the internalizing influence of the DTS is the externalizing influence of the RAS. Activation of the RAS shifts attention from internal control to more immediate necessities of contending with environmental events. Under RAS control, brain activity is organized toward generation of stimulus-controlled and drive-related behaviors.

The combined influences of the DTS and RAS thus determine the mode of operation of the brain, the behavioral state of the individual, and the EEG pattern. This relationship can be better appreciated by considering four permutations (Table 11–1). DTS activity in the delta range paired with RAS inactivity occurs in nondreaming sleep, and visual inspection of an EEG tracing reveals principally delta waves. DTS activity in the delta range paired with RAS activity occurs during dreaming sleep; the observed EEG frequency would be beta. An increase in the DTS pace into the alpha range activates consciousness. Paired with RAS inactivity, the result is a conscious, relaxed state, with mental activity internalized; predominantly alpha activity is observed in the EEG. DTS activity in the alpha range paired with RAS activity occurs when an individual is in an awake, alert, externalized, stimulus-processing state. The dominant EEG frequency in this case would be beta. Normal balance between the two arousal systems is maintained by interconnecting pathways. If the balance between the two systems is disrupted, psychopathological conditions such as attention deficit disorder may result.

Table 11–1
Behavioral States and Observed EEG Frequencies in Relation to Activity of the Two Arousal Systems

DTS pace (Hz)	RAS activity	Observed EEG frequency	Behavioral state
3	Inactive	Delta	Nondreaming sleep
3	Active	Beta	Dreaming sleep
10	Inactive	Alpha	Awake, relaxed, internalized
10	Active	Beta	Awake, externalized, stimulus-processing

Sleep and Dreaming

Sleep States and Stages

Sleep is a time when the individual's consciousness is suspended. It should allow for restoration of physical and mental well-being and should occur at periodic intervals. The need for rest and sleep varies greatly from one person to another and depends on age and activity. Recent studies have demonstrated that 6–8 hours of sleep each night are required for adults. Newborn infants and babies up to 4 months of age generally sleep an average of 15–16 hours in each 24. Toddlers require about 10–14 hours each day. Adolescents require more sleep because of the rapid growth they are undergoing, but they rarely get enough sleep and may think they require less. *Nurses need to be aware of individual sleep requirements and sleep cycles and how these are influenced by the changing health states of clients.*

Each person has internal rhythms that guide the bodily functions. Rhythms like the sleep-wake cycle that repeat once every 24 hours are called **diurnal rhythms.** If a diurnal rhythm is controlled by the daily light-dark cycle, it is said to be a **circadian rhythm.** The sleep-wake cycle is both diurnal and circadian. Rhythms vary from person to person. For example, some people are most alert in the morning, whereas others are most alert at midafternoon or in the evening.

A nurse observing a patient in sleep would notice a decrease in the tone of the musculoskeletal system as well as a decrease in heart rate, respiration, blood pressure, and body temperature. The patient's basal metabolic rate is also lowered and as a consequence, less urine is formed. Because the body is recumbent, there is an increase in the flow of blood to the brain, but the brain uses less oxygen than when awake.

Sleep consists of two quite different, though interrelated, states — dreaming and nondreaming sleep. Dreaming sleep is also known as paradoxical sleep, desynchronized sleep, and rapid eye movement (REM) sleep. Nondreaming sleep is divided into four stages. The sleeper progresses from the waking state through the stages in a predictable nightly pattern (Figure 11–1). Stages 1 and 3 are brief transitional stages. Stage 1 is the stage of drowsiness that occurs as a person is falling to sleep. It is debatable whether it even constitutes a sleep stage since persons in this stage respond to calling of their names. Stage 1 is characterized by a predominance of theta activity. After a few minutes in this stage, the sleeper progresses to stage 2.

Stage 2 of nondreaming sleep is the stage in which the largest portion of the night is spent. From stage 2, the sleeper periodically progresses into dreaming sleep or stage 4 nondreaming sleep. Each episode of dreaming or stage 4 sleep begins and ends in stage 2. In stage 2, the EEG exhibits two kinds of distinctive features: sleep spindles (bursts of 13–15 Hz activity) and K complexes. Stage 3 occurs as a brief transition into stage 4, or delta, sleep. Delta waves (high-voltage waves, typically about 2.5–3 Hz)

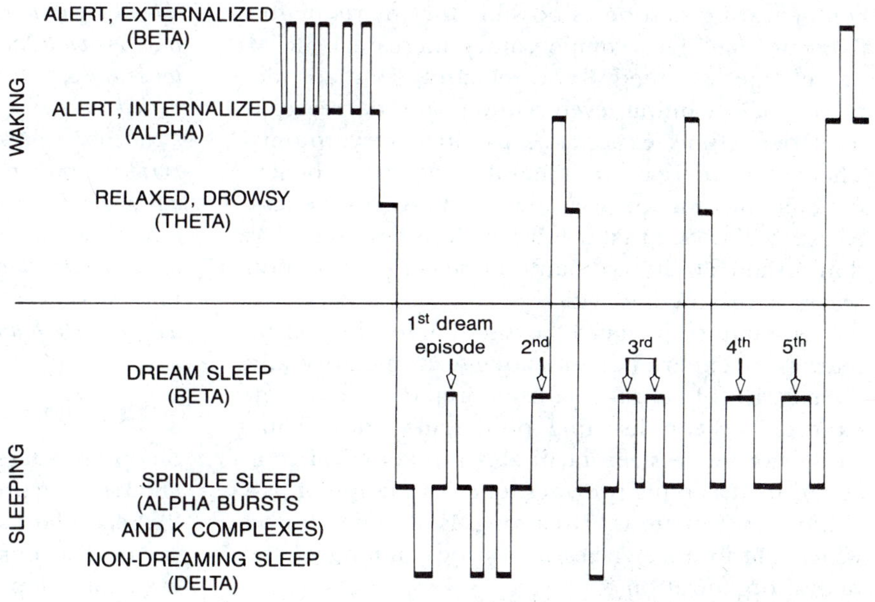

Figure 11–1
A typical pattern of stage shifts during the course of a night. From A. K. Swonger and L. L. Constantine, *Drugs and Therapy,* 2d ed. Boston: Little, Brown, 1983.

first appear in stage 3, and then become more evident in stage 4.

Stage 4 episodes occur near the beginning of the night, but the first dream episode normally occurs no sooner than 90 minutes after sleep begins. The frequency and the duration of dreaming increases toward morning. Slow-wave sleep and dreaming sleep have distinct functions in maintenance of health.

The Function of Slow-Wave Sleep

Slow-wave sleep appears to be controlled largely by the activity of the raphé system and appears to provide for physical restoration and answers the need that is manifested as physical tiredness. More slow-wave sleep is needed after strenuous physical exercise or when catabolism (breakdown of tissue) has been increased. Athletes experience more slow-wave sleep than nonathletes. The rate of synthesis of macromolecules (anabolism) increases during slow-wave sleep, as does proliferation and keratinization of skin cells. These correlations point to a role for slow-wave sleep in physical rejuvenation.

The Function of Dream Sleep

Dreaming sleep is triggered by a nucleus of the reticular formation and is accompanied by beta activity in the EEG, rapid eye movements, deep relaxation of postural muscle, penile erections in males, elevated pulse and respiratory rates, and characteristic pontine-geniculate-occipital (PGO) waves that provide the visual images of dreams.

The importance of dreaming is evident from the fact that the brain carefully guards total dream time, compensating as soon as possible for any reduction from normal. This compensatory increase in REM percentage is called **REM rebound.** Humans deprived of dreaming, even without any decrease in total sleep time, experience psychiatric symptoms. There is an increase in irritability, defensive behavior, feelings of persecution, and aggressiveness. Nurses will notice that the dream-deprived client has diminished ability to maintain selective attention and goal-oriented activities.

Dreaming appears to be essential for the consolidation of experience into long-term memory and the clearing of neural circuits in preparation for new experiences and learning of the next day. Thus, while slow-wave sleep facilitates physiological rejuvenation, dreaming provides for rejuvenation of psychological functions. Dreaming is a time during which the brain engages in reprogramming of the neural organization.

The time required for dreaming varies in direct relation to the magnitude of the challenges and requirements for change that confront the person. For example, requirements for dreaming may change with life circumstances. Periods of emotional stress, difficult learning, or increased intellectual activity are accompanied by an increase in REM percentage. Withdrawal from alcohol, barbiturates, or narcotics is accompanied by markedly increased REM percentage although total sleep time is sharply curtailed. Infants, whose life stresses and learning requirements are very high, not only sleep more than children or adults, but also have a much higher REM percentage. REM percentage stabilizes at about 20% by age 3 or 4, and then changes little over the course of a lifetime, while total sleep time continues to decline with aging. When compared to short or normal sleepers, long sleepers experience the same amount of nondreaming sleep but more dream time, suggesting that differences in requirements for dreaming account for differences in total sleep time.

Given the importance of dreaming to psychological functioning and mental health, the potential for drugs to suppress dreaming should be considered when using medications. It is of particular concern that REM suppression is produced by most sedative-hypnotics, since these drugs are most often employed for alleviation of insomnia. The use of sedative-hypnotics is often accompanied by a reduction in total dream time in spite of the increase in total sleep time. Whenever possible, preference should be given to the benzodiazepine hypnotics, since these drugs do not suppress dreaming.

Nurses should be sensitive to the importance of sleep, and particularly dreaming, to the health of individuals and should try to minimize drug and nondrug factors that may interfere with this important physiological process. In hospital settings, patients are often allowed to sleep for only short periods of time. Sleep may be disturbed by environmental factors (noise, temperature extremes), lack of opportunity to perform presleep rituals (bathing, reading, prayer), lack of daily exercise, nutritional needs, digestive disorders, pain, fear, anxiety, or breathing difficulties. Good nursing management dictates that procedures and medications should be arranged to allow the individual as much time as possible for adequate sleep and dreaming.

Sleep Disorders

Sleep disorders may be primary or secondary to psychiatric, organic, or behavioral problems (Table 11–2). Secondary sleep disturbances may occur with bipolar disorder, schizophrenia, anxiety states, and especially depression. In people with major depres-

Table 11–2
Sleep and Arousal Disorders

Diagnostic category	Type[a]	Incidence	Sex ratio	Drug treatments
Insomnias			F > M	Hypnotics, sleep-aids, or L-tryptophan
Psychophysiological[b]	P	+/−	?	As above
Associated with sleep apneas[c]	P	++	M > F	Imipramine
Associated with nocturnal myoclonus or akathisias	P	?	M = F	Diazepam
Drug-induced[d]	S	+	?	Eliminate drug.
Associated with psychiatric disorders[e]	S	+	F > M	Various
Associated with medical conditions[f]	S	+	?	Various
Excessive somnolence				
Excessive daytime sleepiness				
Associated with insomnia[g]	P or S	++	F > M	Determined by type of insomnia
Associated with insufficient sleep	P	+/−	?	None
Narcolepsy	P	−	M > F	Stimulants
Sleep drunkenness	P	−	M > F	None
Hypersomnia				
Psychophysiological hypersomnia[b]	P	+/−	?	None
Idiopathic hypersomnolence	P	−	?	Methysergide
Intermittent hypersomnias				
Kleine-Levin syndrome	P	−	M > F	None
Menstruation-associated	P	−	F	None
Infectious conditions[h]	S	−	M = F	Antimicrobials
Mixed				
Drug-induced[i]	S	+	?	Adjust dosage.
Disorders of the sleep-wake cycle				
Transient[j]	P	+/−	M = F	None
Persistent[k]	P	−	M = F	None
Parasomnias				
Stage 4-related				
Sleepwalking and night terrors	P	−	M > F	Diazepam
Functional enuresis	P	+	M > F	Imipramine
REM-related				
Nightmares	P	+/−	M = F	None
Other[l]	P	Varies	Varies	Various

Key: +, common; ++, very common; −, rare; +/−, rarely of clinical significance but probably common in the overall population.
[a]P, primary; S, secondary.
[b]Stress-related.
[c]Includes central apneas (failure of the medullary respiratory center), upper airway apneas (occlusion), and mixed apneas (combining both).
[d]Withdrawal from sedative-hypnotics or narcotics, or use of stimulants.
[e]Psychiatric disorders commonly associated with insomnia incude mania, depression, acute psychotic states, anxiety disorders, personality disorders, and drug dependence.
[f]Hyperthyroidism, chronic renal insufficiency, and epilepsy, for example.
[g]This is, after all, the usual chief complaint in insomnia.
[h]Trypanosomiasis (sleeping sickness), for example.
[i]Excessive use of depressants or rebound depression after chronic use of stimulants.
[j]Includes jet lag and work-schedule shifts.
[k]Sleep phase syndromes and nondiurnal sleep cycles.
[l]Bruxism, head-banging, painful erections, seizures, and asthma, for example.

sion, sleep is commonly fragmented, but some depressed persons sleep excessively during bouts of depression. Persons with bipolar disorder tend to sleep more while depressed and less during manic episodes. Acute psychotic episodes are usually accompanied by insomnia and a lack of REM rebound after deprivation, but in chronic schizophrenia, sleep patterns are surprisingly normal. Organic problems that often produce sleep disturbances include epilepsy, thyroid dysfunction, and chronic renal insufficiency.

Insomnias and anxiety disorders may be considered overlapping diagnostic categories. The most common type of insomnia, though not clinically most important, is insomnia related to stress, referred to as **psychophysiological insomnia.** Almost everyone has experienced at least occasional episodes of psychophysiological insomnia. Insomnia becomes a medical problem only when it occurs frequently.

Primary sleep disorders include insomnia, excessive somnolence, disorders of the sleep-wake cycle, and parasomnias. Insomnia is by far the most common sleep disorder for which people (women more often than men; see Figure 11–2) seek clinical attention. Primary insomnia includes conditions associated with sleep apneas, nocturnal myoclonus, or akathisias. **Sleep apneas** are episodes of suspended respiration during sleep. When hypoxia builds up to a sufficient level, respiration begins again, but the irregular, gasping breaths awaken the sleeper. This form of insomnia cannot be treated with the usual hypnotic drugs because such drugs suppress respiration and increase incidences of sleep apnea. A dreaded form of sleep apnea is the **sudden infant death syndrome** (SIDS). Many individuals exhibit myoclonic contractions while falling asleep; for some, these contractions are strong enough to cause awakening. Benzodiazepines are especially useful in this kind of insomnia because of their ability to relax skeletal muscles.

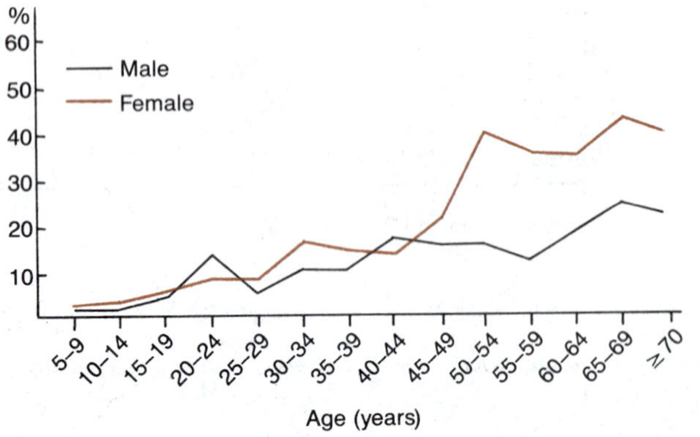

Figure 11–2
Prevalence of insomnia by age and sex. Modified from F. Cirignotta et al, Insomnia: an epidemiological survey. *Clin. Neuropharmacol. 8*:S41–S54, 1985. Raven Press, Publishers/New York.

Drug-induced insomnias can occur with use of stimulants or during withdrawal from sedative-hypnotics or narcotics. Caffeine use in the form of coffee, cola, tea, or cocoa is probably the most common drug cause of insomnia. Elimination of the causative drug is the preferred treatment when insomnia is drug-induced.

Insomnia can occur either at the beginning of the night (**initial insomnia**) or during the latter half (**early morning awakenings**). Initial insomnia requires a short-acting hypnotic that will induce sleep. Difficulty getting to sleep is often due to anxiety or stress. When the problem is awakening in the early hours of the morning, treatment requires an intermediate-acting agent that will sustain sleep. Early morning awakenings are often associated with aging and with depression.

Excessive somnolence encompasses two distinct kinds of problems: **hypersomnias,** in which individuals sleep more than a normal amount of time, and **excessive daytime sleepiness,** in which drowsiness occurs during the day. Hypersomnia can occur with stress, anxiety, or depression, trypanosomiasis, or as an intermittent phenomenon associated with menstruation or Kleine-Levin syndrome. Excessive daytime sleepiness is most commonly a direct result of insomnia or insufficient sleep.

One distinctive form of excessive daytime sleepiness is **narcolepsy.** The four characteristics of narcolepsy are short, irresistible sleep attacks, cataplexy (sudden loss of muscle tone), sleep paralysis, and hypnagogic hallucinations (vivid dreams before loss of consciousness). The latter two symptoms are less frequent and are not necessary to diagnose narcolepsy. Narcolepsy is treatable with amphetamine-like stimulants (Chapter 14).

Disorders of the sleep-wake cycle include the common, transient disruptions of the sleep cycle that accompany modern jet travel (**jet lag**) and rare persistent disorders of the cycle involving rhythms that are irregular or other than 24 hours in length. Parasomnias are disorders accompanying sleep, such as night terrors, enuresis, and sleepwalking (which occur during slow-wave sleep) and nightmares (which occur during REM).

Recommended Readings

Borkovec TD: Insomnia. *J Consult Clin Psychol* 1982; 50:880–895.

Gillin JC, Mendelson WB, Sitaram N, Wyatt RJ: The neuropharmacology of sleep and wakefulness. *Annu Rev Pharmacol Toxicol* 1978;18:563–579.

Hartmann EL: *The Functions of Sleep.* New Haven, Conn Yale University Press, 1977.

Hauri P: *The Sleep Disorders.* Kalamazoo, Mich, The Upjohn Co, 1977.

Jouvet M: Neuropharmacology of the sleep-waking cycle, in Iversen LL et al (eds): *Handbook of Psychopharmacology,* 8. New York, Plenum Press, 1977.

Quan SF, Bamforn CR, Beutler LE: Sleep disturbances in the elderly. *Geriatrics* 1984;39(9):42–47.

Siedel WF, Dement WC: Sleepiness in insomnia: Evaluation and treatment. *Sleep* 1982(5, Suppl 2):S182–S190.

Walsleben J: Sleep disorders. *Am J Nurs* 1982;82(6):936–940.

Weitzman ED: Sleep and its disorders. *Annu Rev Neurosci* 1981; 4:381–417.

Zarcone VP Jr: Diagnosis and treatment of excessive daytime sleepiness. *Clin Neuropharmacol* 1977;2:87–97.

CHAPTER 12

Sedative-Hypnotics and Sleep-Aids

The sedative-hypnotics are one of the oldest, largest, and most thoroughly studied of drug classes. Although other names have been employed for this drug class, such as **soporifics** and **somnifacients,** the name sedative-hypnotics is more apt because it draws attention to the ability of these drugs to produce varying degrees of depression of the central nervous system depending on the dose employed. Sedative-hypnotics produce generalized depression of cellular activity in many organ systems, but especially the CNS. **Sedation,** the mildest depression, is a decrease in arousal state without loss of consciousness. Sedating doses are most likely to be used during the day. Sedative-hypnotics are less often used for sedative purposes than they were before the advent of anxiolytics (see Chapter 19), drugs that alleviate anxiety without as much general depression.

At somewhat higher doses, sedative-hypnotic drugs produce a hypnotic effect — that is, they induce sleep. The term **hypnotic** as employed in pharmacology is not related to hypnosis or the hypnotic trance encountered in clinical psychology or psychiatry. In pharmacology, a hypnotic drug is simply one that can induce a state of sleep that more or less resembles natural sleep. Treatment of insomnia is presently the most common clinical application for sedative-hypnotics.

At still higher doses, sedative-hypnotic drugs can produce an anesthetic coma. Of the drugs in this class, only the ultrashort-acting barbiturates are employed as anesthetics because longer-acting sedative-hypnotics are less effective than inhalation agents (see Chapter 16) in providing extended surgical anesthesia, depressing vital functions to a greater extent. The ultimate depressant effect of sedative-hypnotics is death, which results from depression of vital centers of the medulla oblongata. So the sequence of depressant effects from least to greatest is sedation, sleep, coma, death.

The sedative-hypnotics available today are a somewhat homogeneous class; much of what is true of one member of the class is true for the class as a whole. Therefore, this chapter begins with the common characteristics of the class before turning to special features that differentiate specific agents from the group.

The General Pharmacology of Sedative-Hypnotics

Mechanisms and Effects Sedative-hypnotics are general depressants of cellular function. The electrical activity of nerve cells and all types of muscle cells is depressed by these drugs. There is a general reduction of oxygen consumption by cells and an inhibition of energy-storing processes after administration of a sedative-hypnotic. Although various peripheral tissues are affected by sedative-hypnotics, the CNS is particularly sensitive.

Within the CNS, the synapse is the site of action of sedative-hypnotics; conduction of nerve impulses along nerve axons is not altered. Sedative-hypnotics produce CNS depression by a combination of two actions on neurotransmission: an increase in inhibitory postsynaptic potentials and a decrease in excitatory postsynaptic potentials. The increase in inhibitory postsynaptic potentials is due to the interaction of these drugs with gamma-aminobutyric acid (GABA), the major inhibitory transmitter of the brain. The effect of depressants on GABA binding is known as **positive cooperativity.** Barbiturates, for example, bind to a modulatory protein that is part of the GABA receptor complex (Figure 12–1). The affinity of GABA receptors for GABA is then increased, which leads to more inhibitory postsynaptic potentials. Barbiturates also enhance GABA synthesis.

The other effect of sedative-hypnotics — the suppression of excitatory transmitter influences — is a less specific effect that is caused by an interaction with cell membranes. Depressants dissolve in cell membranes to cause a decrease in viscosity. This physical change in the membrane inhibits the opening of calcium channels in response to action potentials that reach the nerve terminal. Less calcium flows into the nerve terminal each time the neuron depolarizes. Since calcium is required for neurotransmitter release, the amount of transmitter released per action potential is diminished, resulting in fewer excitatory postsynaptic potentials.

All regions and systems of the brain are depressed by sedative-hypnotics at high doses, but some brain regions are more vulnerable, being depressed sooner and at lower doses. Since the synapse is the site of action of sedative-hypnotics, brain sys-

Figure 12–1
Neurochemical mechanisms of barbiturates. (1) Barbiturates do not affect the conduction process. Rather, barbiturates cause fluidization of cell membranes, reducing calcium influx (2) in response to action potentials (AP). The result is reduced turnover of excitatory transmitters and fewer excitatory postsynaptic potentials (EPSP) (3). Barbiturates have more specific interactions with transmission of gamma-aminobutyric acid (GABA), increasing GABA synthesis (4) and facilitating GABA-binding to postsynaptic receptors (5). The result is increased inhibitory postsynaptic potentials (PSP). From A. K. Swonger and L. L. Constantine, *Drugs and Therapy,* 2d ed. Boston: Little, Brown, 1983.

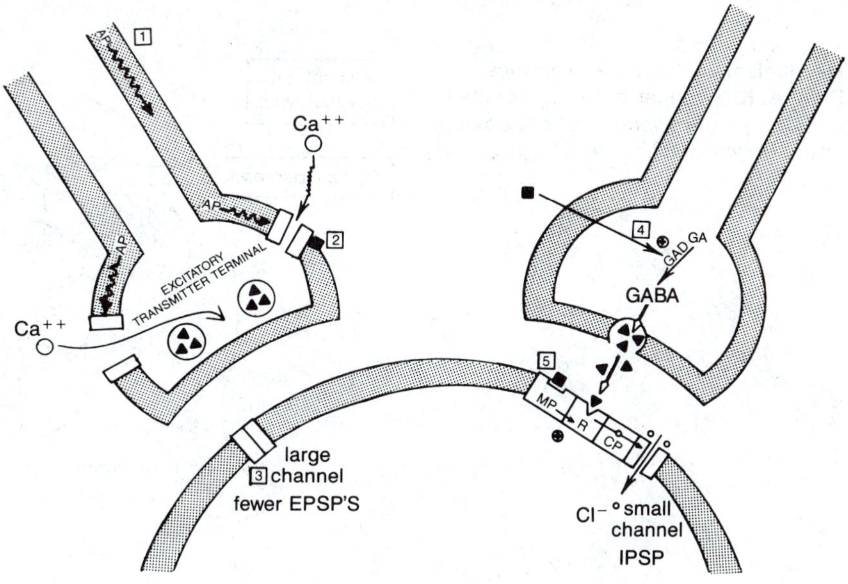

tems that are highly complex, with many synapses and many short-axoned neurons, tend to be most affected (Figure 12–2). Two such systems are the **reticular activating system** and the **punishment system.** Suppression of the reticular activating system results in reduced responsivity to arousal stimuli — one facet of sedation. Suppression of the punishment system contributes to the antianxiety effect of these drugs as well as to the likelihood that these drugs will be abused. The diffuse thalamic system is also sensitive to the action of sedative-hypnotics, exhibiting a dose-dependent decrease in its firing rate that ultimately contributes to the loss of consciousness produced by hypnotic or anesthetic doses of these drugs. Barbiturates and the related piperidinediones have somewhat greater effect on subcortical centers than on the cerebral cortex, while aldehydes, bromides, alcohol, and ethchlorvynol produce more suppression of the cerebral cortex than of subcortical centers.

Effects on Sleep The effects of sedative-hypnotics on sleep are complex. The most obvious effects are to **decrease latency to onset of sleep** and to **increase sleep duration.** Short-acting drugs are most effective in reducing latency to onset (helping the user get to sleep initially) but intermediate- or long-acting agents are most effective in sustaining and prolonging sleep.

In addition to these desirable effects on the quantity of sleep, sedative-hypnotics can have undesirable influences on the quality of sleep by altering the balance between dreaming and nondreaming sleep. The nature of the influence depends on the frequency with which the drug is employed. When a nonbenzodiazepine sedative-hypnotic is used for the first time or infrequently, the percentage of sleep time spent in dreaming sleep may drop from 20% to only 5%. Sedative-hypnotics that produce this effect are said to be REM suppressants. If the sedative-hypnotic is used for one night only, rapid eye movement sleep will exhibit a compensatory increase on the following night, an example of REM rebound. Thus, the acute effect of most sedative-hypnotics on the sleep pattern is **REM suppression** followed by **REM rebound** the next night.

With chronic use of a REM suppressant medication, REM suppression occurs until tolerance develops after about 2 weeks (Figure 12–3). If use of the drug continues beyond 2 weeks, REM percentage returns to the normal value of about 20%. However, tolerance to the beneficial effects of sedative-hypnotics on sleep duration and onset also occurs within about 2 weeks. After an extended period of use, withdrawal of a REM-suppressant sedative-hypnotic will result in REM elevation during the period of rebound hyperexcitability. If the amount of drug used or the duration of use is such that withdrawal results in a severe abstinence syndrome, REM percentage may rise to fully 100% of sleep time (although total sleep time is usually sharply reduced). Thus, the chronic effects of sedative-hypnotics on the sleep pattern consist of REM suppression, followed by tolerance to REM suppression, followed by REM eleva-

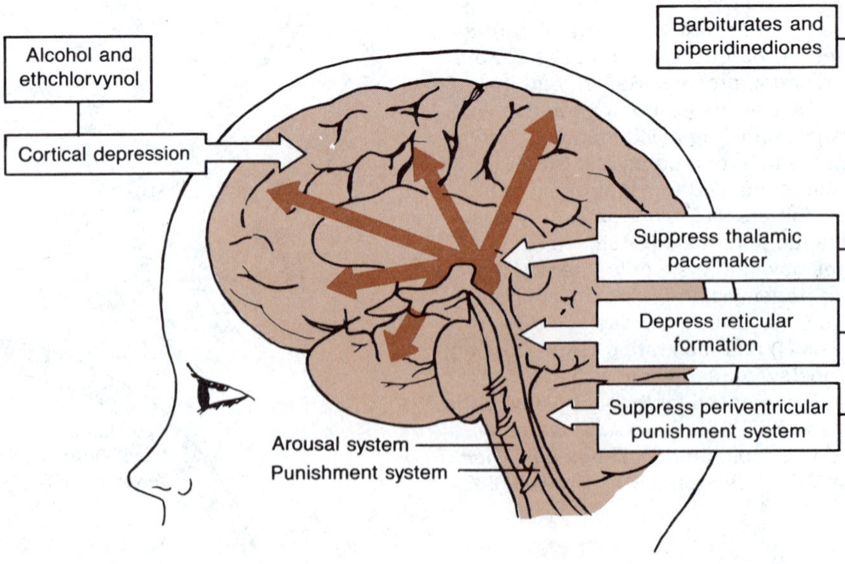

Figure 12–2
Mechanisms of sedative-hypnotics. From A. K. Swonger and L. L. Constantine, *Drugs and Therapy,* 2d ed. Boston: Little, Brown, 1983.

Figure 12–3
REM deprivation and recovery. Modified from P. Hauri, *The Sleep Disorders.* Kalamazoo, Mich.: The Upjohn Company, 1977.

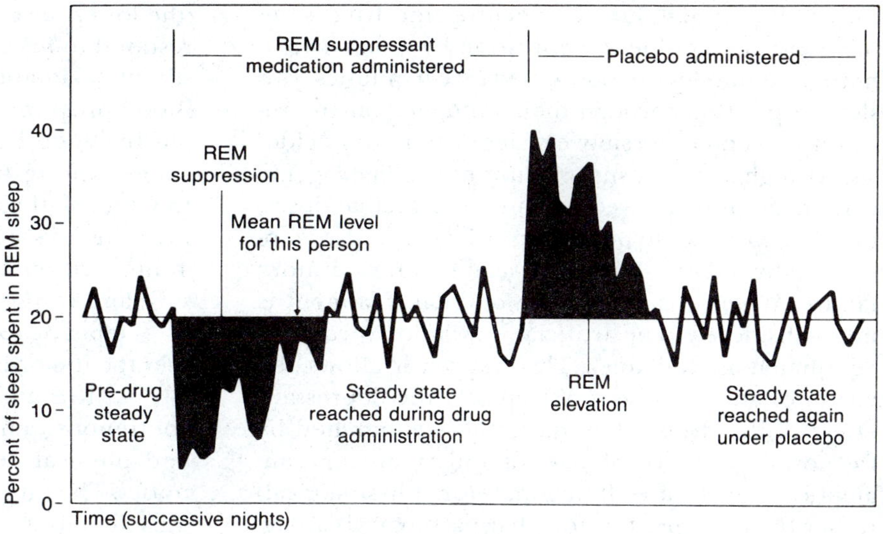

tion during drug withdrawal. Ultimately, REM percentage will return to normal 2–3 weeks after discontinuation of the sedative-hypnotic.

REM suppression occurs with most sedative-hypnotics, including alcohol. Two groups of sedatives that do not share these effects are chloral derivatives and benzodiazepines. Neither of these groups suppress REM sleep or cause REM elevation during withdrawal. Benzodiazepines do have a suppressant influence on slow-wave sleep and can cause vivid dreams and nightmares.

Some sedative-hypnotics cause relatively high incidence of **idiosyncratic reactions of excitation.** This effect, more common in the young than in the old, occurs commonly with barbiturates, alcohol, and benzodiazepines. The mechanism underlying such reactions is not understood. These idiosyncratic reactions may contribute to overdose, since users who have taken their nightly dose might become confused, forget that they have taken their medication or simply decide that they need more, and take a second or third dose. This phenomenon has been labeled "drug automatism." To what extent it actually contributes to overdoses is a matter of controversy. *To avoid this potential hazard, nurses should advise clients not to keep hypnotics at bedside.*

A user of sedatives may at times awaken with a residual concentration of the drug in the body. This is more likely with intermediate-acting drugs than with short-acting ones, and virtually inevitable with long-acting drugs. The residual drug may cause **depression in the morning.** The drug user may experience intoxication and feelings of euphoria and great energy but impaired performance and judgment. There is some risk that accidental injury may result because of impaired judgment or coordination. *If an intermediate or long-acting hypnotic is ordered for a client who must be up and alert in the morning, the nurse should call this to the attention of the physician and negotiate for a shorter-acting hypnotic if possible. Nurses need also to counsel clients concerning appropriate use of sedatives. When intermediate- or long-acting ones are ordered, clients should be advised not to plan to perform tasks that require judgment and accuracy in the morning.*

Short-acting sedative-hypnotics, though relatively unlikely to cause residual morning depression, are more likely than intermediate-acting drugs to cause two other kinds of problems. Short-acting sedative-hypnotics may actually increase the incidence of **early-morning awakenings** because, by morning, the user has entered the period of rebound hyperexcitability. For the same reason, short-acting drugs are also more likely than longer-acting agents to cause feelings of **anxiety** during the following day.

Effects on Respiration At moderate to high doses, vital centers of the medulla are suppressed by the action of sedative-hypnotics. The respiratory center is the first of the vital centers to be dangerously depressed, except with piperidinedione sedative-hypnotics, which may cause vasomotor collapse before respiratory arrest.

Normally, respiration is maintained by three drives: (1) the neurogenic drive, which is generated by the spontaneous rhythmicity within the respiratory center of the medulla, (2) the hypoxic drive, involving the influence of the carotid body chemoreceptors on the medulla, and (3) the hypercapnic drive, related to pH and levels of carbon dioxide in the cerebral spinal fluid. The neurogenic drive is the one most susceptible to depression by sedative-hypnotics. At moderate doses, sedative-hypnotics can slow respiration through their influence on the respiratory center, possibly causing respiratory acidosis. At higher doses, suppression of the neurogenic drive may cause labored respiration. At lethal doses, the hypoxic and hypercapnic drives are also suppressed by sedative-hypnotics, leading to respiratory failure. When this occurs, the optimal treatment is now considered to be artificial ventilation (provided equipment is available). This approach allows the victim of an overdose to "sleep off" the depressant effect of the drug, while the drug is eliminated by the normal pathways of inactivation. At one time, analeptics, which are functional (or physiological) rather than competitive (or pharmacological) antagonists of sedative-hypnotics, were widely used to counteract excessive doses of sedative-hypnotics. In current practice, analeptics are seldom used for treatment of sedative-hypnotic overdoses because of the risk of convulsions. Administration of high concentrations of oxygen is ill-advised for patients with labored respiration resulting from sedative-hypnotic overdosage because this tactic will eliminate the hypoxic drive, possibly producing respiratory arrest.

Intoxication, Tolerance, Dependence, and Abuse Although both glutethimide (Doriden) and methaqualone (Quaalude) were initially marketed with claims that they were nonaddictive, the claims ultimately proved false. All true sedative-hypnotics presently known are liable to be abused. The sleep aids discussed at the end of this chapter have little abuse liability but are not true sedative-hypnotics since they are unable to induce sleep. Among the true sedative-hypnotics, benzodiazepines are least liable to abuse. Other sedative-hypnotics are about equal to one another in their abuse liability. Barbiturate and nonbarbiturate sedative-hypnotics, including alcohol, exhibit cross-tolerance and freely substitute for one another in suppressing symptoms of withdrawal following chronic use. For example, a barbiturate could be used by an alcoholic both to maintain dependence and to postpone the onset of withdrawal.

All sedative-hypnotics have the capacity to induce **intoxication,** resembling that caused by alcohol. Signs of intoxication include highly changeable moods, disinhibition of sexual or aggressive impulses, irritability, talkativeness, slurred speech, incoordination, unsteady gait, impairment of attention or memory, and poor judgment or functioning. The extent of intoxication can be assessed according to the following four **grades of intoxication:** In grade 1 (the lowest level of intoxication), the client does not respond to his or her name, but responds to painful stimuli. Gag and deep tendon reflexes are present. Blood pressure and respirations are normal and stable. In Grade 2, the client no longer responds to pain stimuli and respirations are now slow but adequate. In Grade 3, the deep tendon reflex is lost and blood pressure is now low though stable. Finally, in Grade 4 intoxication, the gag reflex is lost and blood pressure and respirations are unstable.

Dependence does not necessarily follow from therapeutic or limited social use of sedative-hypnotics, but it is an inevitable consequence of repeated, continuous, immoderate use. Both psychological and physical dependence occur with sedative-hypnotics. The physical dependence associated with sedative-hypnotics is a very serious medical problem. Discontinuation of the chronic use of any sedative-hypnotic precipitates a **withdrawal syndrome** that begins within 24 hours after discontinuing the drug, reaches peak intensity between 48 and 72 hours following the last dose, and subsides slowly over the course of one week or more. The intensity of withdrawal symptoms is directly related to the severity of physical dependence — the duration of drug use and the dosage level being employed during the period immediately preceding drug discontinuation. The syndrome resembles closely that seen in alcohol dependence. The client may exhibit any or all of the following symptoms: anxiety, involuntary muscle twitches and tremors, muscular weakness, dizziness, nausea, vomiting, insomnia, weight loss, orthostatic hypotension, illusions, delusions, hallucinations, paranoia, delirium, and convulsive seizures. Some even die. The risk of death during withdrawal from alcohol, barbiturates, or other nonbenzodiazepine sedative-hypnotics is considerably greater than in narcotic withdrawal.

All sedative-hypnotics produce **tolerance.** With barbiturates and several of the other sedative-hypnotics, two independent mechanisms contribute to the development of tolerance: drug-disposition tolerance and pharmacodynamic tolerance. **Drug-disposition tolerance** results from an increase in the capacity of liver enzymes to dispose of the sedative-hypnotic agent. Drug-disposition tolerance not only increases the metabolism of the sedative-hypnotic itself but can also result in increased metabolism of certain other drugs administered concurrently. **Pharmacodynamic tolerance** is a brain phenomenon, involving a compensatory adjustment in the neurochemistry of the brain in response to chronic presence of the drug. Gradually the brain becomes hyperexcitable. The drug effect then results in a level of depression that is less than would occur in a person whose brain neurochemistry is normal. Discontinuation of the depressant drug at this point unmasks the hyperexcitability state, producing symptoms of withdrawal. Tolerance to sedative-hypnotics develops rapidly but is completely reversible. Sedative-hypnotics are widely used and abused. Barbiturates remain among the most frequent causes of drug fatalities, both accidental and suicidal.

Clinical Indications Sedative-hypnotics are indicated for short-term management of insomnia. Benzodiazepines can be employed up to 3 to 5 weeks on a chronic basis, while nonbenzodiazepine sedative-hypnotics are limited to 2 weeks of chronic use. Sedative-hypnotics may also be employed indefinitely for insomnia if used infrequently, as needed. Individuals having only difficulty falling asleep should be prescribed short-acting agents since these act promptly and result in minimal residual depression in the morning. Individuals who awake frequently in the early morning require intermediate-acting agents. If the client has both difficulty getting to sleep and difficulty sustaining sleep, flurazepam (Dalmane) or barbiturate mixtures such as Tuinal can be used effectively.

Sedative-hypnotics continue to be used occasionally as daytime sedatives for anxiety. Barbiturates, for example, may be used in low doses to relieve anxiety or for mild hypertension related to nervousness. Barbiturates are also used as preanesthetics. They are often administered the night before surgery and again just before the patient is taken to the operating room. Ultrashort-acting barbiturates are discussed in Chapter 16 as intravenous anesthetics and long-acting barbiturates in Chapter 23 as antiepileptics.

Adverse Effects and Contraindications The characteristic adverse effects of the sedative-hypnotic class fall mainly into five categories: (1) excess depression, (2) paradoxical excitation, (3) REM suppression, (4) hypersensitivity reactions, and (5) tolerance and dependence. Tolerance and dependence, which most constrain the use of these drugs, are discussed above.

Nursing Observations for Use of Sedative-Hypnotics for Insomnia

THERAPEUTIC GOAL	Adequate sleep and rest.
PREADMINISTRATION ASSESSMENT	
Baseline Data	Observe for excess daytime sleepiness; verbal complaints of being unable to sleep or "up all night"; irritability, or fatigue. Evaluate vital signs, respiration during sleep, and motor activity during sleep. Look for possible organic causes if insomnia is atypical for the individual.
Contraindications/ Precautions	Allergy to drug or related drugs, impaired liver function, latent porphyria, and respiratory distress. Precautions: history of drug abuse, impaired renal function, seizure disorders, pregnancy, lactation, hyperthyroidism, diabetes mellitus, or severe anemia. Use cautiously in elderly or debilitated adults and in children.
Potential Interactions	Check current drug regimens for CNS depressants, neuromuscular blockers, MAO inhibitors, and drugs metabolized by liver microsomal enzymes.
EVALUATION OF DRUG RESPONSE	
For Therapeutic Benefit	Monitor sleep time, daytime alertness, and verbal reports of extent to which client feels rested.
For Adverse Effects	Monitor for tolerance and dependence, excess depression, residual depression in the morning, paradoxical excitation, REM deprivation, and allergic reactions.
For Drug Interactions	Monitor for additive CNS depression and alteration in the metabolism of other drugs.
For Compliance	Evaluate the client's compliance with all facets of the therapeutic regimen by careful observation, interviewing, and review of progress. Report compliance problems to the physician and act as client-advocate when changes in the therapeutic regimen seem indicated.

Excess depression encompasses a host of possibilities. Somnolence (prolonged sleepiness) is the single most common adverse response to sedative-hypnotics. Other manifestations of excess depression include confusion, ataxia, loss of equilibrium, psychiatric depression, lethargy, weakness, hypoventilation, apnea, lack of concentration, and impaired cognition.

Paradoxical excitation can be manifested as agitation, anxiety, excitement, or nervousness. Disinhibition of sexual and aggressive impulses may occur. Some clients complain of nightmares or insomnia; others have hallucinations. They may also exhibit motor symptoms, such as hyperkinesia. Benzodiazepines sometimes induce paradoxical rage reactions. Some individuals experience excitatory reactions regularly when given barbiturates or benzodiazepines. Ethchlorvynol (Placidyl) and chloral derivatives are said to produce fewer responses of paradoxical excitation than other sedative-hypnotic agents and can be used to good effect in individuals prone to such reactions.

REM suppression occurs with all sedative-hypnotics except those in two groups: the benzodiazepines and the chloral derivatives. Tolerance develops to the REM suppressant action of sedative-hypnotics, but only when tolerance has also developed to the beneficial effects of the drugs on sleep

Nursing Diagnoses and Interventions for Use of Sedative-Hypnotics for Insomnia

Nursing Diagnoses	*Related Interventions*
TO ENHANCE DRUG BENEFITS OR REDUCE DRUG REQUIREMENTS	
Activity intolerance related to excess daytime sleepiness secondary to insomnia or residual drug depression; Alterations in thought processes related to sleep deprivation; Ineffective individual coping related to somnolence and irritability secondary to insomnia; Increased risk of injury: somnolence related to insomnia or excess depression from the drug; Sensory-perceptual alterations related to sleep deprivation; Sexual dysfunction related to fatigue due to insomnia; Sleep-pattern disturbance related to insomnia or REM deprivation caused by hypnotic	Provide comfort measures such as positioning the bed or arranging covers to suit the patient's preferences. Provide an environment conducive to rest and sleep by ensuring adequate ventilation, comfortable temperature, quiet, and the patient's preferred level of nighttime lighting. Ease stresses by visiting; minimize nighttime awakenings for medical procedures or drug administration; plan administrations of stimulant drugs so as not to interfere with sleep. Restrict use of caffeine. Allow time and opportunity for patient's bedtime rituals; provide sedation if indicated; select drug with most appropriate duration of action; use smallest dose.
TO ENSURE SAFE AND EFFICACIOUS DRUG USE	
Knowledge deficit related to drug regimen	Teach the client about the type of insomnia and the therapeutic plan for addressing the problem. Explain to clients that sedative-hypnotics do not have indefinite effectiveness when used on a regular basis, which means that sleeping pills are useful mainly for temporary sleep disturbances that result from some transient circumstance or recurrent but infrequent insomnia; chronic, frequent insomnia must be addressed mainly by implementation of nondrug measures. When using hypnotics that suppress REM sleep, explain to clients that the drug may leave them feeling less well rested even when it increases total sleep time. Provide client with a list of other adverse effects and drug interactions for each drug in the regimen and explain what to do if any of these occur.

latency and duration. Those agents that cause REM suppression necessarily produce REM rebound after acute use and REM elevation during withdrawal following chronic use.

Hypersensitivity reactions are not common with sedative-hypnotics but can at times be severe. Some clients develop angioderma, a condition in which swelling occurs in the mucous membranes of the lips, mouth, tongue, or other areas of the face and viscera. Usually the first indication that something is amiss is a prickly sensation in one area. As time elapses, the area becomes swollen. Others receiving barbiturates may develop skin rashes or exfoliative dermatitis of allergic origin. Skin rashes may spread widely over the trunk and limbs. *Nurses need to remember that people allergic to one barbiturate will likely be allergic to all others but can usually be safely placed on another agent from a different chemical group.*

Benzodiazepines also cause skin rashes or pruritus in some people. Ethchlorvynl can cause skin rash, urticaria, and rare reactions of thrombocytopenia and cholestatic jaundice. Skin rashes occur as well with chloral derivatives, piperidinediones, and other sedative-hypnotics. Known allergy to a given agent is a contraindication for its use.

Drug Interactions The interactions of sedative-hypnotics fall mainly into three categories: (1) additive CNS depression with other depressant drugs, (2) increased metabolism of certain other drugs due to sedative-hypnotic induction of liver microsomal enzymes, and (3) inhibition of metabolic degradation of a sedative-hypnotic by drugs that inhibit relevant liver enzymes. Additive CNS depression is the single most widely encountered of all drug interactions in clinical practice. Sedative-hypnotics produce depressant effects on the brain that are at least additive, and sometimes supraadditive, with all other classes of depressant agents, including alcohol, antihistamines, neuroleptics, antianxiety drugs, antiadrenergic antihypertensive agents, narcotics, and tertiary tricyclic antidepressants.

Induction of liver enzymes occurs with all sedative-hypnotics except for the benzodiazepines. Induction is an increase in the metabolic capacity of liver enzymes. Induction usually takes place after 3–5 days of daily use of the drug; when the drug is discontinued, activity of liver enzymes returns to normal in about the same time. Induction accounts for the drug-disposition component of tolerance produced by sedative-hypnotic drugs and for significant drug interactions. Although metabolism of many different kinds of drugs can be hastened after subchronic administration of an inducer, the extent of the effect is clinically significant only for drugs that have a rather narrow therapeutic index — drugs for which small changes in blood levels can result in substantial alterations in efficacy or toxicity. Induction of liver enzymes produced by sedative-hypnotics significantly increases metabolism of oral anticoagulants, glucocorticoids, and estrogens. Persons taking oral anticoagulants may require dosage adjustments when a sedative-hypnotic is added to the regimen or discontinued. There have been instances of pregnancies occurring in women using oral contraceptives concurrently with an inducer of liver enzymes. *The nurse should recommend that an alternative contraceptive method be considered when chronic use of an inducer of liver enzymes is required.*

Some drugs inhibit the metabolism of sedative-hypnotics, increasing risks of excess depression unless dosage adjustments are made. Sodium valproate (Depakene) and chloramphenicol have been reported to slow the metabolism of barbiturates. Phenytoin (Dilantin) has variable effects on barbiturate metabolism. Monoamine oxidase inhibitors slow the metabolism of barbiturates and prolong their action accordingly.

A unique interaction is the effect of barbiturates on absorption of griseofulvin (Fulvicin). Absorption of griseofulvin decreases after oral administration if barbiturates are being used concurrently. Use of griseofulvin and barbiturates together should be avoided.

Important Nursing Implications for Sedative-Hypnotics

- ☐ Advise clients receiving sedative-hypnotics that driving an automobile or operating heavy machinery could be dangerous while using the drug.
- ☐ Educate clients about the abuse likelihood of sedative-hypnotics. Avoid unnecessary administration of hypnotics when ordered to be taken as needed.
- ☐ Advocate that clients not be prescribed a sedative-hypnotic for periods in excess of their maximum time of effectiveness.
- ☐ Withdraw clients gradually after prolonged treatment with a sedative-hypnotic.
- ☐ Assess clients for occurrence of excess depression. Warn clients about the additive depressant effects when two or more CNS depressant drugs are employed concurrently. Evaluate the contribution of depressant drugs to instances of psychiatric depression.

- ☐ Observe clients for evidence of idiosyncratic excitation in response to sedative-hypnotic administration. Note that this reaction is especially likely when clients are in pain.
- ☐ Advise clients not to keep hypnotic drugs at bedside and to store them safely out of the reach of children.
- ☐ Teach clients to recognize allergic reactions and skin eruptions that can occur with sedative-hypnotic agents.

Early Sedative-Hypnotics

Bromides

Bromides, though still available, are seldom prescribed as sedatives because of their severe toxic effects. They are excreted very slowly and can accumulate in the body, causing intoxication to be unusually persistent. Intoxication begins with drowsiness, dizziness, impaired memory, and irritability. In severe cases, clients become delirious and develop hallucinations, delusions, mania, lethargy, and ultimately coma. Acetylcarbromal, a drug still available but seldom used, is a ureide that acts by releasing bromide. Bromides are readily excreted in breast milk and have caused depression and brominism in nursing infants. The adult dose for acetylcarbromal (Paxarel) is 250–500 mg PO, 2 or 3 times daily for sedative purposes.

Chloral Derivatives

Chloral derivatives include chloral hydrate (Noctec) and triclofos. Chloral hydrate was introduced into medicine in 1869, and its early use was in the management of psychiatric patients. Triclofos has been withdrawn from clinical use.

Mechanisms and Effects Chloral hydrate produces less depression of respiration or reflexes than barbiturates and less hangover or residual depression than intermediate-acting sedative-hypnotics (Table 12–1). Paradoxical excitation, tolerance, cumulative effects, and hypersensitivity reactions are rare. A distinct advantage of chloral hydrate is the fact that it does not suppress REM sleep.

Pharmacokinetics Chloral hydrate is a prodrug metabolized to trichloroethanol, an active metabolite. Trichloroethanol has a half-life of 8–10 hours and is inactivated by metabolism to trichloroacetic acid.

Clinical Indications Although chloral hydrate is still available, its use has sharply declined since the introduction of barbiturates. Chloral hydrate is rapid-acting. It is more useful for inducing sleep than for sustaining it although it has been employed for frequent nocturnal awakenings as well. Occasionally it is used as a preanesthetic or postanesthetic medication or to obtain EEG sleep recordings.

Adverse Effects and Contraindications A major drawback of chloral hydrate is that it produces considerable gastric irritation, as well as nausea and vomiting. *To reduce this effect, nurses should advise clients to take chloral hydrate capsules with a full glass of water.* Its irritant effect on mucous membranes can be additive with that produced by alcohol. Once widely used for management of delirium tremens, it has been replaced by chlordiazepoxide (Librium) for that application. Chloral hydrate may cause a mild sensation of dysgeusia. Chloral hydrate will appear in breast milk when used by women who are nursing.

Abuse liability is comparable to that of barbiturates. Although the drug is detoxified in the liver and eliminated by the kidneys, it can be safely used when there is moderate impairment of either organ. Chloral hydrate is contraindicated when there is marked hepatic or renal impairment.

Drug Interactions Chloral hydrate produces additive CNS depression with any other CNS depressant. Chloral hydrate has produced a mild degree of hypoprothrombinemia, which can be additive to that produced by oral anticoagulants. Use of chloral hydrate concurrently with furosemide (Lasix) has caused clients to experience a hemodynamic reaction characterized by vasodilation, diaphoresis, flushing, hypotension, and tachycardia.

Preparations and Administration *Nurses should warn clients for whom chloral hydrate syrups have been prescribed that they have an unpleasant taste and odor, which can be minimized by chilling the syrup before ingestion.*

Chloral Hydrate (Noctec and generic formulations)
Capsules, syrup, elixir, suppositories
Recommended Doses: For adults, 250 mg, tid after meals for sedation or 500–1,000 mg at bedtime for insomnia. For children, 25 mg/kg (maximum of 500 mg) for sedation and 50 mg/kg (maximum of 1g) for insomnia.

Paraldehyde (Paral)

Paraldehyde has been available as a sedative-hypnotic for more than a century. It survives despite its disadvantages because of some limited beneficial qualities. Paraldehyde is a clear, colorless liquid.

Table 12–1
Comparison of Attributes of Sedative-Hypnotics

	Benzodiazepines			Barbiturates				
Attribute	**Triazolam**	**Temazepam**	**Flurazepam**	**Short-acting**	**Intermediate-acting**	**Piperidinediones**	**Ethchlorvynol**	**Chloral derivatives**
Sleep effects								
Acute effectiveness as sleep inducer	++	++	++	++	0	++	++	++
Acute effectiveness as sleep sustainer	0	+	++	~0	++	0	0	++
Effectiveness after 2 weeks	+	++	++	0	0	0	0	0
Acute REM suppression	0	0	0	++	++	++	++	0
Elevated REM during withdrawal	0	0	0	++	++	++	++	0
Suppression of slow-wave sleep	++	++	++	+/–	+/–	+/–	+	+
Abuse potential								
Psychological dependence	+	+/–	+/–	++	++	++	++	++
Physical dependence	+	+/–	+/–	++	++	++	++	++
Induction of liver enzymes	0	0	0	++	++	++	++	++
Suicide potential	0	0	0	++	++	++	++	++
Adverse Effects								
Residual depression	0	+	++	+	++	+	+	++
Increased early morning awakenings	++	+	0	+	0	+	+	0
Paradoxical excitation	++	++	++	++	++	++	+	++
Acute intoxication	0	0	0	+	+	++	+	+

Key: 0, does not produce indicated effect; +/–, equivocal tendency toward effect; +, moderate tendency to produce effect; ++, strong likelihood or severity of effect.

Clinical Indications Use of paraldehyde today is largely restricted to institutional settings. Its major use is in controlling delirium tremens or other psychiatric states characterized by excitation. It can be used as an emergency treatment for convulsive states such as eclampsia, status epilepticus, or tetanus.

Adverse Effects and Contraindications The major disadvantage of paraldehyde is its unpleasant, burning, and pervasive odor. Exhalation of paraldehyde from a single treated individual may impart an odor to an entire room. *Patients who have received paraldehyde should remain in bed and they should not smoke. The room should be well ventilated to control the strong odor, which remains on the patient's breath for hours.*

Like chloral derivatives, paraldehyde is irritating to mucous membranes. Paraldehyde crosses the placental barrier and can cause respiratory depression in the fetus, or in the newborn if given in conjunction with labor. Paraldehyde causes additive

CNS depression with other depressants. Metabolism of paraldehyde is inhibited by disulfiram (Antabuse).

Preparations and Administration Paraldehyde liquid can be administered orally or rectally. The injection solution is for intramuscular or intravenous use. *Paraldehyde solutions, once exposed to air, light, or heat, liberate acetaldehyde, which oxidizes to acetic acid and smells like vinegar. Paraldehyde can cause decomposition of plastic materials, resulting in the production of toxic compounds.* When taken orally or administered rectally, the drug may produce ataxia and dizziness. Users can develop erythematous skin rash or become confused and excited. Intramuscular administration is often accompanied by transient pain at the site of injection. When the drug is given intravenously, the depression of the CNS is usually preceded by a brief period of excitement and coughing. Bronchial secretions may also be increased.

Paraldehyde (Paral and generic formulations)
Liquid, injection solution
Recommended doses: For insomnia, 4–8 ml, orally, in a capsule or dissolved in milk or juice to mask the disagreeable taste; 5 ml IM; or 3–5 ml IV diluted in several volumes of physiological saline, injected slowly.

Barbiturates

History and Sources Until recently, barbiturates were the most widely used sedative-hypnotics. They have been thoroughly studied and their actions and side effects are typical of the class.

Barbituric acid was synthesized in 1864 by Adolph von Baeyer, by the condensation of urea and malonic acid. The first hypnotic barbiturate, barbital, was employed therapeutically in 1903 by Emil Fischer. Barbital has not survived in medicine, but phenobarbital, introduced in 1912, remains one of the most important drugs available to medicine. In all, more than 2,500 barbiturates have been developed and some 50 marketed at one time or another. About a dozen barbiturates find use in current clinical practice.

Mechanisms and Effects Barbiturates are subclassified on the basis of duration of action: long-acting, intermediate-acting, short-acting, and ultrashort-acting. The long-acting group, including phenobarbital, mephobarbital, and metharbital, is employed chiefly in epilepsy, and will be discussed in Chapter 23. Latency to onset is 1 hour or more for the long-acting drugs; duration of effect is 10–14 hours. Ultrashort-acting barbiturates are employed as intravenous anesthetics to facilitate initial induction of anesthesia or to augment the effect of low potency anesthetics such as nitrous oxide. These agents are discussed in Chapter 16. Short-acting and intermediate-acting barbiturates are indicated for short-term or infrequent alleviation of insomnia. They also find use as preanesthetic sedatives.

Intermediate-acting barbiturates are useful as sleep sustainers, for individuals who experience frequent morning awakenings but who have no difficulty getting to sleep initially. Latency to onset is about 45–60 minutes; duration is 6–10 hours. An intermediate-acting barbiturate will produce substantial residual depression the morning after use as a hypnotic.

Short-acting barbiturates are used as sleep inducers. Latency to onset is about 15–30 minutes, and duration is typically 3–6 hours. Short-acting barbiturates produce little residual depression the morning after use for hypnotic purposes. Pentobarbital is frequently used prior to induction to general anesthesia, as an adjunct in manipulation or diagnostic procedures, and for emergency control of acute convulsive states.

Adverse Effects and Contraindications In addition to the adverse effects shared with other sedative-hypnotic agents discussed earlier in the chapter, barbiturates on rare occasions cause blood dyscrasias, including agranulocytosis and thrombocytopenia. *Nurses need to ask clients to report symptoms such as sore throat, nosebleed, petechiae, or easy bruising.* Liver damage and megaloblastic anemia have occurred after long-term use of barbiturates. The features of barbiturates are compared with those of other sedative-hypnotics in Table 12–1.

Known hypersensitivity to barbiturates is a specific contraindication. Since barbiturates are excreted in part unchanged by the kidneys, lower doses are required in clients with renal impairment. Elderly clients exhibit increased sensitivity to barbiturates necessitating use of lower doses. Depressant drugs may aggravate the cognitive impairment of chronic organic brain syndrome.

Preparations and Administration Amobarbital (Amytal), aprobarbital (Alurate), butabarbital (Butisol), and talbutal (Lotusate) are intermediate acting barbiturates. Amobarbital is the most widely encountered. As a street drug, amobarbital is known as "blue heaven." *For intramuscular administration, nurses should select a large muscle mass, usually the gluteus maxi-*

mus, and inject the drug deeply. Superficial injections are painful and may cause sloughing or the formation of sterile abscess. No more than 5 ml should be injected in any one site.

Patients who receive amobarbital intravenously require special monitoring. Onset of action occurs within 5 minutes. If the drug dosage is too large, or if it is administered too quickly, the patient's respirations may become depressed. Apnea and hypotension can occur. Therefore, nurses need to take the patient's blood pressure, pulse, and respiration during the period of injection and for several hours after the drug has been administered.

The short-acting barbiturates include pentobarbital and secobarbital. Pentobarbital has the street name "yellow jackets" and secobarbital the street name "red devil." *Patients receiving secobarbital intravenously must be monitored closely for evidence of respiratory depression or a fall in blood pressure. There should be equipment at bedside that can be used to maintain a patent airway in the event of laryngospasm. If the drug is to be administered intramuscularly, the nurse should inject the material deep into the muscle mass, making sure to aspirate prior to injecting the drug to be certain the needle is not in a blood vessel. The nurse needs to monitor the client for 20–30 minutes after injection to be certain that the response is not too severe.*

While pentobarbital is frequently administered orally, it can be given parenterally as well. *If a pentobarbital solution is cloudy or has a precipitate, it should not be used. Parenteral solutions of pentobarbital are highly alkaline; therefore, any extravasation may cause necrosis. As with other barbiturates, nurses should closely monitor the patient's respiration, blood pressure, and pulse during the instillation of drug; the necessary equipment for artificial respiration should be immediately available.*

INTERMEDIATE-ACTING BARBITURATES

Amobarbital (Amytal)
Tablets, capsules, powder, elixir
Recommended Doses: For adults, 15–120 mg PO, 2–4 times daily, for sedation; 100–200 mg at bedtime, for hypnosis, 30–60 minutes before bedtime on an empty stomach to speed absorption. For sedation of children, no more than 2 mg/kg, 3 times daily. Intravenous infusion rates should not exceed 1 ml/minute.

Aprobarbital (Alurate)
Elixir
Recommended Doses: In adults, 40 mg PO, tid for sedation; 40–160 mg at bedtime for insomnia.

Butabarbital (Butazem, Butisol, Butal, Butalan, Sarisol, Soduben, and generic formulations)
Capsules, tablets, powder, elixir
Recommended Doses: For adults, 15–30 mg PO, 3 or 4 times daily for sedation; 50–100 mg at bedtime for insomnia. In children 7.5–30 mg for sedation.

Talbutal (Lotusate)
Tablets
Recommended Doses: For adults, 120 mg PO at bedtime for insomnia.

SHORT-ACTING BARBITURATES

Secobarbital (Seconal and generic formulations)
Capsules, tablets, powder, elixir
Recommended Doses: In adults, 30–50 mg PO for sedation; 100–200 mg for insomnia; 200–300 mg for preanesthetic apprehensiveness. In children, 6 mg/kg/day in 3 divided doses for sedation; 50–100 mg for preoperative applications.

Pentobarbital (Nembutal and generic formulations)
Capsules, tablets, powder, elixir
Recommended Doses: For adults, 30 mg PO, 3 or 4 times daily, for sedation; 100 mg at bedtime for insomnia. In children, 8–30 mg depending on age, weight, for sedation.

Benzodiazepine Hypnotics

The benzodiazepines are the most distinctive sedative-hypnotics and in recent years have become the most widely prescribed in this class. Three benzodiazepines, flurazepam, (Dalmane), temazepam (Restoril), and triazolam (Halcion), are marketed expressly as hypnotics. Two new hypnotic benzodiazepines, nitrazepam and quazepam, currently have investigational status. Two other benzodiazepines, lorazepam (Ativan) and clorazepate (Tranxene), though marketed primarily as antianxiety agents, are used occasionally as hypnotics. Lorazepam, clorazepate, and other anxiolytic benzodiazepines are discussed in Chapter 19.

Mechanism and Effects Benzodiazepines present a number of special features, some positive, some negative. On balance, the positive features outweigh the negative characteristics for most clients (Table 12–1). The benzodiazepines are the only sedative-hypnotics that have demonstrated effectiveness beyond 14 consecutive nights of use. Triazolam has been demonstrated to be effective for at least 3 weeks, flurazepam for at least 4 weeks, and temazepam for at least 5 weeks. The benzodiazepines have the advantage of not interfering with dreaming. However, benzodiazepines have the unique adverse effect of suppressing stage 4 (slow-wave) sleep, causing some clients to experience sleep disturbances such as vivid nightmares.

Pharmacokinetics Flurazepam, temazepam, and triazolam are interchangeable except for differences in duration of action. Flurazepam has a duration of action equivalent to long-acting barbiturates although its onset of action is as rapid as short-acting barbiturates. It is rapidly absorbed from the gastrointestinal tract after oral administration, producing onset of sleep in 15–45 minutes. The parent compound is rapidly metabolized to an active metabolite, which has an extended half-life of 47–100 hours. Thus, the maximum effect will develop only after about three consecutive nightly doses. Temazepam does not produce an active metabolite and thus has a shorter action. Its half-life is about 10 hours, so that residual morning depression is minimal. Triazolam, a short-acting hypnotic, has a half-life of 2–5 hours, no active metabolite, and no accumulation of drug when used nightly; therefore it is least likely to result in complaints of residual depression.

Clinical Indications The long action of flurazepam makes it useful for both inducing and sustaining sleep, but there may be a considerable degree of residual depression in the morning. Temazepam is equivalent to an intermediate-acting barbiturate and is useful both for inducing and sustaining sleep. Triazolam is effective as a sleep inducer but not as a sleep sustainer.

Adverse Effects and Contraindications Paradoxical reactions of excitation to benzodiazepines, though infrequent, may take the form of rage reactions. Like other sedative-hypnotics, benzodiazepines can produce excess depression. The incidence of residual depression, the morning after use of a benzodiazepine, depends on the benzodiazepine selected. Residual depression is a common problem with flurazepam, uncommon with temazepam, and nonexistent with triazolam. However, there is some indication that tolerance and dependence may develop more quickly with short-acting than with long-acting benzodiazepines, and clients may complain that triazolam increases early morning awakenings and anxiety the next day. Use of short-acting agents is also more likely to be associated with insomnia during the period of drug withdrawal.

Benzodiazepines can cause mild neurological symptoms. Some clients may complain of dizziness and lightheadedness, ataxia, or a tendency to fall. Others may develop psychiatric symptoms such as nervousness, apprehensiveness, lethargy, or disorientation, or gastrointestinal symptoms such as nausea, vomiting, diarrhea, constipation, cramps, or heartburn. Rare adverse effects with benzodiazepines include hypersensitivity reactions (skin rash or pruritus), hematological reactions (leukopenia, granulocytopenia), and cholestatic jaundice. Benzodiazepines are contraindicated in clients with narrow angle glaucoma or prostatic hypertrophy. Because of potential adverse effects on the fetus, benzodiazepines should not be used during pregnancy. Nursing mothers should not use benzodiazepines because they are excreted in breast milk and adversely affect the infant.

Like other sedative-hypnotics, benzodiazepines possess abuse liability and are classified as schedule IV controlled substances. Because of the widespread use of benzodiazepines, the number of individuals developing abuse problems has been substantial. Nevertheless, abuse liability is less than that of barbiturates or other nonbenzodiazepine sedative-hypnotics. Dependence develops only when benzodiazepines are used for longer than the indicated duration of effectiveness (3–5 weeks when used nightly) or in excessive doses.

Drug Interactions Benzodiazepine overdose is rarely fatal, so that benzodiazepines are said to be virtually suicide-proof. However, like other sedative-hypnotics, benzodiazepines produce additive CNS depression with other depressant drugs. *Nurses should warn clients not to combine benzodiazepines with alcohol, antihistamines, or antidepressant drugs because the interactive effects impair both mental and physical performance and can result in coma or death.* Benzodiazepines do not, however, induce liver enzymes, which dispenses with one type of interaction that occurs with nonbenzodiazepine hypnotics.

Preparations and Administration

Flurazepam (Dalmane)
Capsules
Recommended Doses: For adults, 15 or 30 mg PO at bedtime for insomnia. For elderly or debilitated clients, 15 mg.

Temazepam (Restoril)
Capsules
Recommended Doses: For adults, 30 mg PO at bedtime for insomnia. For elderly or debilitated clients, 15 mg.

Triazolam (Halcion)
Tablets

Recommended Doses: For adults, 0.25–0.5 mg PO for insomnia. For elderly or debilitated clients, 0.125–0.25 mg for insomnia.

Other Sedative-Hypnotics

Piperidinediones

Mechanisms and Effects Although nonbarbiturates, the drugs in the piperidinedione group resemble barbiturates both in chemical structure and in pharmacology. Glutethimide (Doriden), introduced in 1954, and methyprylon (Noludar), introduced in 1955, produce effects barely distinguishable from those of secobarbital. Piperidinediones have a duration of action and latency to onset equivalent to that of the short-acting barbiturates.

Adverse Effects and Contraindications Compared to barbiturates, cardiovascular depression is greater for these substances in relation to the degree of respiratory depression. With other sedative-hypnotics, if the patient is breathing without mechanical support, vasomotor collapse is unlikely to occur, but with piperidinediones, circulatory collapse may precede respiratory failure. *In cases of overdose in which the drug is known to be a piperidinedione or if the identity of the agent is in question, it is important that blood pressure as well as respiration be monitored.*

Acute intoxication is more frequent because absorption of these drugs is irregular, and serious blood dyscrasias (thrombocytopenic purpura, aplastic anemia, or leukemia) have occurred in response to both glutethimide and methyprylon. Allergic reactions to glutethimide include exfoliative dermatitis in addition to rash and urticaria. Both drugs rarely result in intermittent porphyria. During withdrawal, some clients may develop hallucinations or convulsions. Therefore clients should be gradually withdrawn from these drugs over a period of several days. Since piperidinediones offer no distinctive advantages and several characteristic disadvantages, there is little justification for their continued use.

Some clients may complain of numbness of the extremities. Others may develop a skin rash; if the drug is discontinued, the rash will disappear within 2–3 days. Rarely, clients complain of gastric irritation and nausea or dry mouth.

Piperidinediones readily cross the placental barrier and should be avoided during pregnancy since they may cause fetal dependence. *Nurses working in newborn nurseries need to be cognizant of the potential effects of these drugs on neonates and to look for signs of CNS depression or withdrawal symptoms.*

Preparations and Administration

Glutethimide (Doriden and generic formulations)
Capsules, tablets
Recommended Dose: For adults, 250–500 mg PO at bedtime for insomnia.

Methyprylon (Noludar)
Capsules, tablets
Recommended Dose: For adults, 200–400 mg PO at bedtime for insomnia.

Ethchlorvynol (Placidyl)

Although a number of tertiary alcohols have been found to be potent CNS depressants, only ethchlorvynol is marketed for clinical use.

Mechanisms and Effects Ethchlorvynol is a short-acting agent capable of inducing sleep in about 15 minutes after oral administration. Ethchlorvynol is the sedative-hypnotic most like alcohol in its effects. Ethchlorvynol has an abuse liability comparable to barbiturates and alcohol.

Pharmacokinetics Ethchlorvynol is inactivated mainly by liver metabolism and has a half-life of 10–25 hours.

Clinical Indications Ethchlorvynol is indicated for short-term hypnotic therapy.

Adverse Effects and Contraindications Ethchlorvynol suppresses REM sleep and slightly suppresses slow-wave sleep and may produce excess depression and changes in behavior. *Clients may show evidence of giddiness, ataxia, and muscular weakness or complain of hangover.* Some clients develop idiosyncratic excitation (ranging from mild excitation to hysteria and delirium) or hypersensitivity reactions (urticaria, and rarely thrombocytopenia or cholestatic jaundice). Ethchlorvynol is said to cause paradoxical excitatory reactions less frequently than other sedative-hypnotics.

Ethchlorvynol is contraindicated for use in clients with porphyria or in women during the first or second trimester of pregnancy. Neurological reactions, such as dizziness, diplopia, and nystagmus, have been reported. Nausea and vomiting occur occasionally but can be controlled by giving ethchlorvynol with food. Administration with food also helps to prevent excess depression, which can be due to unusually rapid absorption on an empty stomach. Ethchlorvynol leaves a mild, mint-like aftertaste.

Drug Interactions Ethchlorvynol should not be administered to clients receiving MAO inhibitors or tricyclic antidepressants, since these combinations can result in marked excitation and delirium.

Preparations and Administration *When clients have been taking ethchlorvynol for an extended period of time, they are apt to develop withdrawal symptoms when the drug is discontinued, such as anxiety, tremors, slowed speech, irritability, hallucinations, or memory loss. Withdrawal symptoms can be minimized by gradual discontinuation of the drug over several days.*

Ethchlorvynol (Placidyl)
Capsules
Recommended Doses: In adults, 500 mg PO at bedtime for insomnia. Doses as high as 1,000 mg may be required. For elderly clients, smaller doses are required. Not effective if taken at bedtime as a sleep sustainer, but 100–200 mg may be taken upon awakening during the night, to aid in reinstituting sleep.

Ethinamate (Valmid)

Ethinamate, a carbamate sedative-hypnotic, is a short-acting agent, indicated for short-term control of insomnia. It is inactivated mainly by hydroxylation in the liver. Side effects include nausea and vomiting and hypersensitivity reactions, such as rash, fever, or thrombocytopenia. Ethinamate may produce idiosyncratic excitation and excess depression. Ethinamate (Valmid) is marketed in capsules. The recommended dose for insomnia is 500 or 1,000 mg before retiring.

Some clients develop gastrointestinal disturbances when this drug is used, others develop skin rash. Safe use during pregnancy and lactation has not been established. If depression or suicidal tendencies are exhibited, the nurse should advocate use of a different drug.

Methaqualone

Methaqualone is a sedative-hypnotic that closely resembles the barbiturates in its actions but also has antihistaminic activity and antitussive properties. Methaqualone was a popular street drug known as the "love drug." Its purported aphrodisiac properties reflect only the disinhibition of sexual impulses characteristic of all sedative-hypnotic drugs. Abuse of methaqualone reached nearly epidemic proportions in the United States in 1972–1973 and again in the early 1980s. Methaqualone has been withdrawn from clinical practice.

Sleep-Aids

The currently available nonprescription sleep-aids contain antihistamines that possess sedative properties. The pharmacology of these and other antihistaminic agents is discussed in detail in Chapter 50. Antihistamines are a group of substances commonly used for allergies and in cold remedies. Although some newer antihistamines (such as chlorpheniramine and phenindamine) produce little if any sedation and may even be mildly stimulating, the classic antihistamines are sedatives. Tolerance to the sedative effects tends to develop with continued use. A few of the most sedative antihistamines have found use as over-the-counter sleep-aids. Currently, there are three employed in sleep-aids: diphenhydramine in Sominex Formula 2, doxylamine in Unisom, and pyrilamine in most of the remaining formulas (Sominex Formula 1, Nytol, Sleep-Eze, and others). These sleep-aids have the distinct advantages of low abuse potential and no physical dependence, but they are only modestly effective.

Case Study: Barbiturate Intoxication

G. N., a married 22-year-old Caucasian man, was brought to an emergency room at 10 PM by a friend, who stated that G. N. had taken secobarbital. G. N. was cyanotic and in moderate respiratory distress. Vital signs were recorded as blood pressure 110/75, temperature 96.8° F, pulse 90, and respirations 12. G. N. was unresponsive to pain or verbal stimuli. Gag reflex and deep tendon reflexes were absent. A blood test indicated pH 7.18 (normal: 7.31–7.41), P_{CO_2} 60 mm Hg (normal: 41–51 mm Hg), and P_{O_2} 30 mm Hg (normal: 35–40 mm Hg). The serum secobarbital level was 2.3 mg/100 ml (toxic level: 0.7–2.0 mg/100 ml; lethal level: 2.0–3.0 mg/100 ml). The diagnosis was stage IV barbiturate intoxication.

G. N. was intubated and suctioned, which removed food and particles. He was then placed on intermittent positive pressure breathing, which resulted in improvement in the color of the skin. An intravenous infusion was begun with 5% dextrose in water at 125 ml/hour. Gastric lavage was conducted with a sodium sulfite solution. The client regained consciousness after 20 hours, and all vital signs and blood values were normal.

After the acute medical emergency had been managed successfully, one of the nurses became responsible for interviewing G. N. concerning his recreational use of sedative-hypnotics. G. N. persisted in explaining to the nurse that when he was under the influence of hypnotics he was actually more alert. However, the nurse discovered from conversation with G. N.'s wife that he tended to become aggressive and abusive when using these drugs. Moreover, when intoxicated, G. N. experienced memory and attention impairments, which had resulted in self-injury on two occasions. The overdose had occurred because he was unable to recall taking the pills and had taken additional ones. Through her discussions with G. N. and his wife, the nurse recognized that his use of the hypnotic drug was motivated by his need to belong, to be close to family and friends, and to be accepted by them. He felt more relaxed when using the drug and thought that he was better accepted as a result. What he did not realize was that his mood changes, irritability, and argumentativeness under the influence of the drug were actually tending to drive away the very people whose acceptance he wanted. Once these elements had been identified, the nurse was able to suggest alternate solutions to problems of anxiety and concerns about acceptance other than continued use of the drugs.

1. Which of the vital signs were abnormal? Explain each value.
2. Which of the values from the blood test were abnormal? Explain each value.
3. What observations indicated grade IV intoxication?
4. Why wasn't naloxone or an analeptic administered? Why wasn't dialysis performed?
5. What nursing diagnoses would relate to the nurse's findings?

Answers appear at the end of the book.

Recommended Readings

Dubnick B et al: The separation of 3H-benzodiazepine binding sites in the brain and of benzodiazepine pharmacological properties. *Pharmacol Biochem Behav* 1983;18:311–318.

Erman MK: Insomnia: Treatment approaches. *Drug Ther* 1984;14(8):103ff.

Gary NE, Tresnewsky O: Clinical aspects of drug intoxication: Barbiturates and a potpourri of other sedatives, hypnotics, and tranquilizers. *Heart Lung* 1983;12:122–127.

Harris E: Sedative-hypnotic drugs. *Am J Nurs* 1981;81(7):1329–1334.

Heel RC et al: Temazepam: A review of its pharmacological properties and therapeutic efficacy as an hypnotic. *Drugs* 1981;21:321–340.

Ho IK, Harris RA: Mechanism of action of barbiturates. *Annu Rev Pharmacol Toxicol* 1981;21:83–111.

Kales A et al: Rebound insomnia and rebound anxiety: A review. *Pharmacology* 1983;26:121–137.

Kroboth PD, Juhl RP: Triazolam. *Drug Intelligence and Clinical Pharmacy* 1983;17:495–500.

Lader M, Lugaresi E, Richardson RG (eds): The benzodiazepines and insomnia. *Clin Neuropharm* 1985;8(Suppl. 1).

Lader MH, Petursson H: Long-term effects of benzodiazepines. *Neuropharmacology* 1983;22:527–533.

Mar DD: Short- and long-acting benzodiazepines. *Am J Nurs* 1981;81:2200–2201.

Mendelson WB: *The Use and Misuse of Sleeping Pills: A Clinical Guide.* New York, Plenum Press, 1980.

Millman RP, Weaver TE: Broken sleep. *Am J Nurs* 1986; 86(2):146–150.

Nicholson AN: The use of short- and long-acting hypnotics in clinical medicine. *Br J Clin Pharmacol* 1981;11:615–695.

Nicoll R: Selective actions of barbiturates on synaptic transmission, in Lipton MA et al. (eds): *Psychopharmacology: A Generation of Progress.* New York, Raven Press, 1978.

Olsen RW: Drug interactions at the GABA receptor-ionophore complex. *Annu Rev Pharmacol Toxicol* 1982;22:245–247.

Rickels K: Clinical trials of hypnotics. *J Clin Psychopharmacol* 1983;3:133–139.

Simon C: Benzodiazepine hypnotics for insomnia. *AM J Nurs* 1983;83(9):1330–1332.

Wincor MZ: Insomnia and the new benzodiazepines. *Clin Pharm* 1982;1:425–432.

CHAPTER 13

Alcohol: The Nonprescription Sedative-Hypnotic

Alcohol: The Social Drug

Alcohol (ethyl alcohol) enjoys a unique position in the pharmacological repertoire of human society. Although its therapeutic value is quite limited, the consequences of its social use are profound. It is the most frequently self-administered drug, and the associated abuse problems are enormous.

The alcohol in alcoholic beverages results from **fermentation.** Fermentation is an enzymatic process carried out by yeasts that use sugar as a substrate to produce ethanol and carbon dioxide. Fermentation is initiated by adding an appropriate yeast to a mulch of any fruit, grain, or starchy plant. Fermentation is a self-limiting phenomenon because yeasts that catalyze the formation of alcohol tolerate concentrations of alcohol only to about 15%, after which the yeast dies and fermentation stops.

Types of Alcoholic Beverages

The use of alcohol from fermentation dates back into the recesses of early history. Fermented honey, called mead, may be the oldest form of alcoholic beverage. Berry wines and fermented grains were used as early as 6400 B.C.

Wines derived from grapes first appeared around 300 or 400 B.C. White wines are made from white grapes or from red grapes that have had their skins removed. Red wines are prepared from red grapes by leaving the skins in the mulch during fermentation. A rosé is produced by removing the skins after a few days of fermentation to produce a pinkish color. Most wines have an alcohol content of about 15%, but dessert wines, such as port and madeira, are fortified with brandy to increase alcohol content to about 20%. Carbonated wines, such as champagne and sparkling burgundy, are made by bottling the wine before fermentation is complete so that some of the carbon dioxide produced during fermentation is trapped in the bottle. Portugal, Italy, France, and Spain are major wine producers. Approximately 88% of wine produced in the United States is made in California and most of the rest in New York State.

Beer is made from barley by malting, a process that softens the grain by steeping it in water until it sprouts. The barley is then dried slowly to kill the sprout without denaturing its enzymes, which gradually convert the starch of the grain into sugar. Later, yeast is added to the filtered mulch to initiate fermentation, and hops, the dried blossoms of the female hop plant, are added for flavor. The usual alcohol concentration in beer is about 4.5%. Draft beer, typically sold in kegs, is beer that has not been pasteurized, so fermentation may continue after packaging. Beer sold in cans and bottles must be pasteurized so that the containers will not explode. Lager beer is stored briefly before packaging and malt liquor for longer periods. Malt liquor has less carbonation but more alcohol (typically 5.5–7.5%) and more calories. Ale is made with a yeast that rises to the top of the mulch and at a higher temperature with more malt and hops to produce a stronger flavor.

Spirits, also called hard liquors, are prepared by distillation. The distinctive tastes of the various forms of liquor are the result of volatile flavorings derived from the grain that is used, flavorings that are added after distillation, or flavor picked up from the barrels in which the liquor is aged or stored. Whiskey is made mainly from corn, scotch from malted barley, rum from fermenting molasses, and schnapps from fermenting potatoes. Vodka is pure alcohol diluted only with water. Vodka filtered through juniper berries produces gin. The alcohol content of spirits is defined by its **proof.** The proof number is twice the percent of alcohol, so that absolute alcohol is 200 proof. Eighty proof liquors contain 40% alcohol.

Incidence of Alcohol Use and Alcohol-Related Problems

The extent of alcohol use and beverage preferences vary from country to country (Figure 13–1). France has the highest per capita consumption of alcohol. Argentina, Chile, Italy, and West Germany also have high rates of alcohol consumption. The United States, Canada, England, Sweden, and Peru have alcohol consumption rates in the middle range; Mexico and Finland have low rates of alcohol consumption. In England, West Germany, Canada, and Mexico, beer is the preferred alcoholic beverage. Wine is the chief source of alcohol intake in Italy, France, Chile, and Argentina. In Scandinavian countries and in Central America, most alcohol is consumed in the form of spirits. In the United States, 49% of alcohol is consumed as beer, 39% as spirits, and 12% as wine.

In the United States, alcohol consumption varies by race, ethnicity, religion, age, and geographical location. Alcohol consumption is higher in whites than blacks, in Catholics, Jews and nonreligious individuals than in Protestants, and in younger than older individuals. Alcohol consumption is more prevalent in urban than in rural areas and in the larger cities. College-educated individuals drink more on the average than those with less education. California, New Jersey, New Hampshire, New York, and Rhode Island lead in the amount of alcohol consumed and the incidence of alcohol-related problems. Americans spend more than $40 billion annually in order to drink 34 gallons of beer and nearly 3 gallons each of wine and spirits per adult. This statistic underestimates the true rate of consumption of drinkers because 25% of men and 40% of women describe themselves as abstainers. In reality, alcohol users average about 4.5 ounces of alcohol each day, or the equivalent of three mixed drinks. One-half of all alcohol consumed yearly is by just 11% of users.

Alcoholic liver disease (cirrhosis) is now the seventh leading cause of death in the United States. In urban areas it is the third leading cause of death for people between ages 25 and 65. Approximately 80% of cases of liver cirrhosis are alcohol-related. There is a strong correlation between per capita alcohol consumption and incidence of liver cirrhosis for various countries. Cirrhosis is just one of many alcohol-related problems and social costs. For example, it has been estimated that alcohol is involved in at least 50% of homicides (either the slayer or the victim), 33% of suicides (as a precipitating factor), at least 50% of automobile fatalities, 30% of home accidents, 15% of occupational accidents, more than 50% of instances of psychiatric depression, and 60% of all hospitalizations (although the role of alcohol is often unappreciated by the physician or the patient).

The high frequency of alcohol-related vehicular accidents has resulted in carefully defined legal limits for the level of blood alcohol permissible while operating a motor vehicle. Few states have similar laws for other drugs. Most states have adopted a stan-

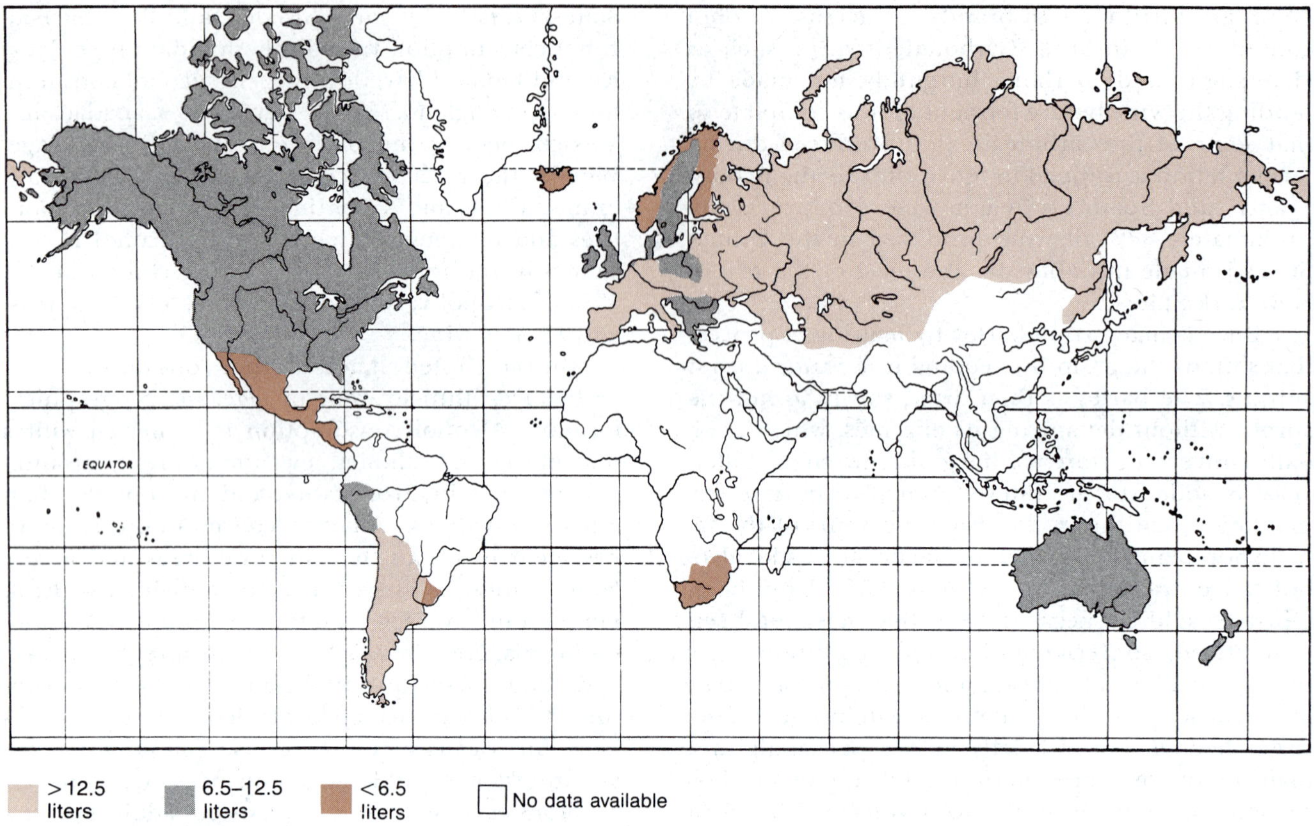

Figure 13–1
Per capita consumption rates (based on numbers of persons 15 years or older) of alcohol (in liters of absolute alcohol) by country.

dard of 0.10% (100 mg%, or 100 milligrams of alcohol per 100 milliliters of blood) as the legal limit (Figure 13–2). Automobile fatalities associated with alcohol consumption involve teenagers to a disproportionate extent, and comparative evidence makes it abundantly clear that states with lower minimum drinking ages lose more teenagers to automobile accidents each year than do states with a higher drinking age.

Acute Pharmacology of Alcohol

Mechanisms and Effects In most respects, the psychotropic effects of alcohol are not unlike those of other sedative-hypnotic substances. Clients experience a general and dose-dependent depression of the central nervous system that begins with mild sedation and, if imbibing continues, escalates to anesthesia, coma, and death (Figure 13–2). The "stimulation" ascribed to alcohol is a popular misconception; effects such as increased activity, laughter, and loud speech after alcohol ingestion actually result from suppression of areas of the brain normally responsible for inhibiting such behaviors (the punishment system). As with other sedative-hypnotics, there is a euphoriant effect with alcohol, but despite the increased confidence and assertiveness, motor and mental skills are almost universally impaired. *Nurses should warn clients about the dangers of excess alcohol consumption and use of alcohol with other drugs. The depressant action of alcohol is additive to that of other CNS depressants (narcotics, anxiolytics, hypnotics, antihistamines).* Typically libido is increased, but sexual functioning is impaired when alcohol is used in large amounts.

The reticular formation is particularly susceptible to alcohol because of its multisynaptic structure. There is a slowing of brain-wave frequencies and a release of the cortex from the integrating control of subcortical centers. Thought flows freely but is disordered and haphazard. The frontal lobe of the cerebral cortex is affected by alcohol blood levels as low as 0.01 to 0.1%. As a result, individuals who have

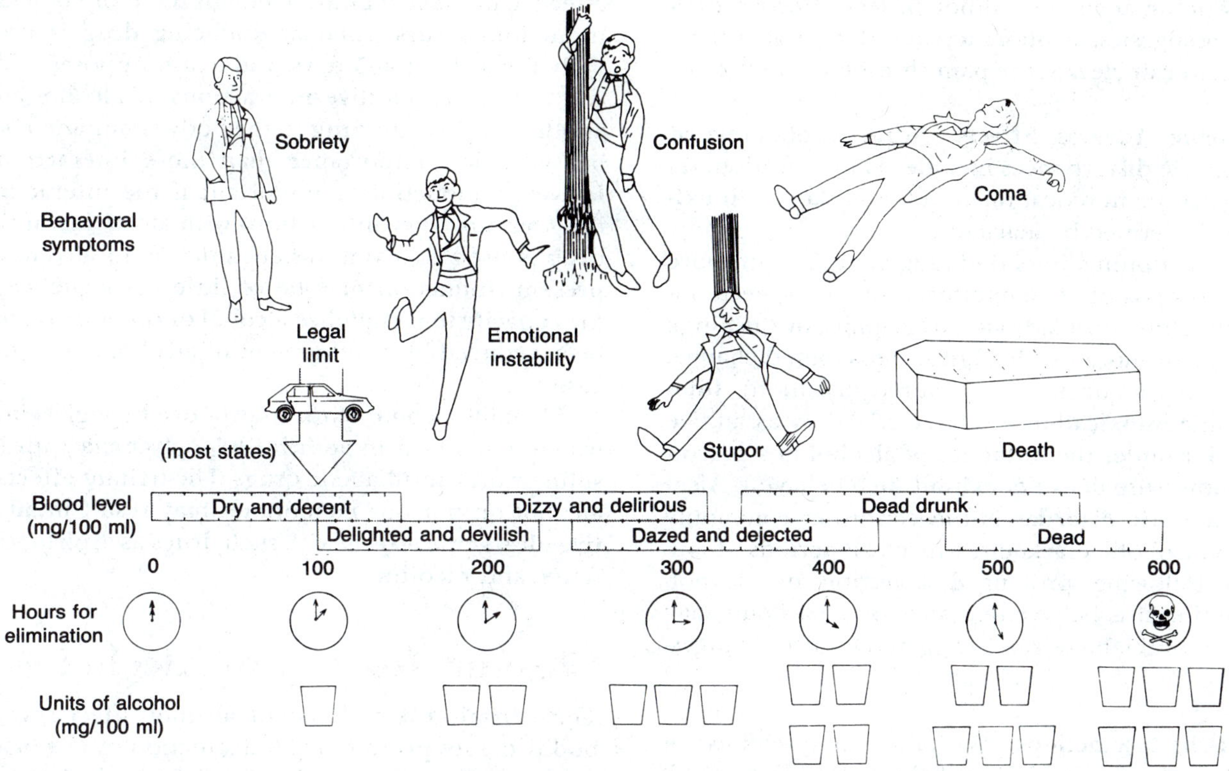

Figure 13–2
Stages of alcohol intoxication. A shot of liquor, two glasses of wine, or two cans of beer constitutes a unit of alcohol. From A. K. Swonger and L. L. Constantine, *Drugs and Therapy,* 2d ed. Boston: Little, Brown, 1983.

had even small amounts of alcohol experience exhilaration, expansiveness, impaired judgment, loquacity, and poor attention. Other cortical regions are depressed at blood levels between 0.1 and 0.3%, resulting in dulled sensibilities and an inability to move with normal coordination (ataxia) and power (apraxia). Speech becomes slurred, perception is distorted, and double vision (diplopia) may develop. The cerebellum responds to blood levels in the 0.1–0.3% range, resulting in disequilibrium.

The medulla oblongata is relatively insensitive to alcohol, but the fatal effects of alcohol ultimately stem from depression of the vital centers of the medulla by high concentrations. Blood levels of about 0.4% are necessary before depression of medullary centers becomes noticeable; levels of 0.55% are typically lethal. In the United States, fatalities due to alcohol overdose are about 300 per year, a small number in view of the number of alcohol users. The low risk of fatality from acute ingestion of alcohol is one of the few advantages of alcohol over other sedative-hypnotics.

The neurochemical basis for the effect of alcohol is poorly understood. Present evidence suggests that alcohol alters cell membrane function and thus neurotransmitter mechanisms. Turnover of norepinephrine increases while turnover of acetylcholine decreases. The cardiovascular system is affected very little at low doses. Clients who take moderate doses of alcohol will have vasodilation, resulting in flushing, warming of the skin, and heat loss. One study reported that light to moderate users of alcohol have a lower risk of heart attacks than nondrinkers due to the hypotensive effect of alcohol.

Clinical Indications Ethyl alcohol has few therapeutic applications. It is useful in treating toxicity caused by other alcohols, such as isopropanol or methanol. The few other clinical applications relate to local effects of alcohol on the skin, not to its systemic or CNS effects. At concentrations approaching 70%, alcohol is an effective bactericidal agent; higher concentrations, such as 90%, are less effective. Nurses often find alcohol useful in sponging clients with high fever or bathing the skin of bedridden clients to prevent bedsores (decubiti). Besides its use as a sedative, alcohol may be self-administered as a hypnotic or analgesic. Although less effective than other analgesics, alcohol increases detachment from pain and can elevate the pain threshold about 40%.

Acute Adverse Effects Acute alcohol-related psychiatric disturbances include (1) intoxication, (2) idiosyncratic intoxication, and (3) blackouts. **Intoxication** is defined by maladaptive behavior (fighting, poor functioning, impaired judgment); one or more physical signs of alcohol effects (slurred speech, incoordination, unsteady gait, nystagmus, or flushing); and one or more psychological signs (mood change, irritability, loquacity, or impaired attention). **Idiosyncratic intoxication** is characterized by assaultive behavior under the influence of alcohol in a person who otherwise does not exhibit such behavior. **Alcohol amnestic disorder** is the condition commonly called alcoholic blackouts, which are periods of amnesia following prolonged ingestion of alcohol. Some theorists believe that alcoholic blackouts may be temporal lobe seizures triggered by alcohol ingestion.

Drug Interactions With the widespread use of alcohol, there is a high probability that clients will have interactions between alcohol and other drugs. Interactions (excluding the one with disulfiram) fall into five categories: (1) additive CNS depression, (2) competition for degradative enzymes, (3) induction of liver enzymes, (4) additive hypoglycemia, and (5) additive ulcergenic actions.

The most common type of interaction involving alcohol is an **additive depressant effect** with other CNS depressants. The effect of alcohol is always at least additive with other depressants, including other sedative-hypnotics, anxiolytics, antipsychotic drugs, antidepressants that have sedative properties, lithium, narcotics, anticholinergics, antihistamines, and antiadrenergic drugs.

Some sedative-hypnotics, notably barbiturates, chloral hydrate, and meprobamate, interact with alcohol by a second mechanism as well. Alcohol and these sedative-hypnotics **compete for the same degradative enzymes.** When alcohol and one of these drugs are simultaneously present in the body, each will slow the other's metabolism, so that their combined effect is greater than the sum of their individual actions. This is called the "1 + 1 = 3" effect.

When used chronically, alcohol interacts with certain other drugs by causing **induction of liver microsomal enzymes.** When the liver microsomal enzyme system has to metabolize alcohol for more than a few days at a time, it increases its capacity to metabolize alcohol. This increase in metabolic capacity carries over to certain other drugs, which will be less effective because they are metabolized more quickly. Induction occurs when an inducing drug is used daily for at least 4–5 days. Induction opposes additive and supra-additive interactions of alcohol and another depressant drug in the body simultaneously but is of less importance than those interactions. However, induction is important if the interacting drug has no other interactions with alcohol or if the drug is used at a time when little or no alcohol is present. Induction may be of little consequence if the capacity to metabolize alcohol or other drugs has been reduced by development of alcoholic liver disease.

Finally, alcohol tends to produce hypoglycemia, which may result in **additive hypoglycemia** with insulin or oral antidiabetic drugs. The irritant effect of alcohol on mucous membranes may result in **additive ulcergenic effects** with such drugs as aspirin, caffeine, and nicotine.

Chronic Toxicity of Alcohol

The chronic toxic effects of alcohol affect several bodily tissues profoundly. A distinction can be made between effects that result directly from alcohol consumption and those that are secondary to the nutritional deficiencies that frequently accompany alcoholism. Some examples of tissue toxicity, such as fatty liver, may involve both factors.

Primary Toxic Effects

The primary toxic effects related directly to alcohol and its metabolites can be clustered into three groups: (1) effects related to alcohol itself, (2) effects related to the acetaldehyde metabolite of alcohol, and (3) effects related to excessive hydrogen formation from alcohol metabolism (Figure 13–3).

Alimentary Irritation Due to Alcohol Itself

People who drink large quantities of alcohol often develop esophagitis. By stimulating secretion of salivary fluids in the mouth and gastric acid in the stomach, alcohol precipitates or aggravates peptic ulcers. Chronic gastritis, which occurs in one-third of all alcoholics, is due to the irritant action of alcohol on the stomach lining. Alcohol may also contribute to acute and chronic pancreatitis.

Toxicity of Alcohol Metabolites

The adverse effects of alcohol after its absorption result from its metabolism in the body. After absorption from the intestines, alcohol is rapidly extracted from the blood by the liver. In the liver,

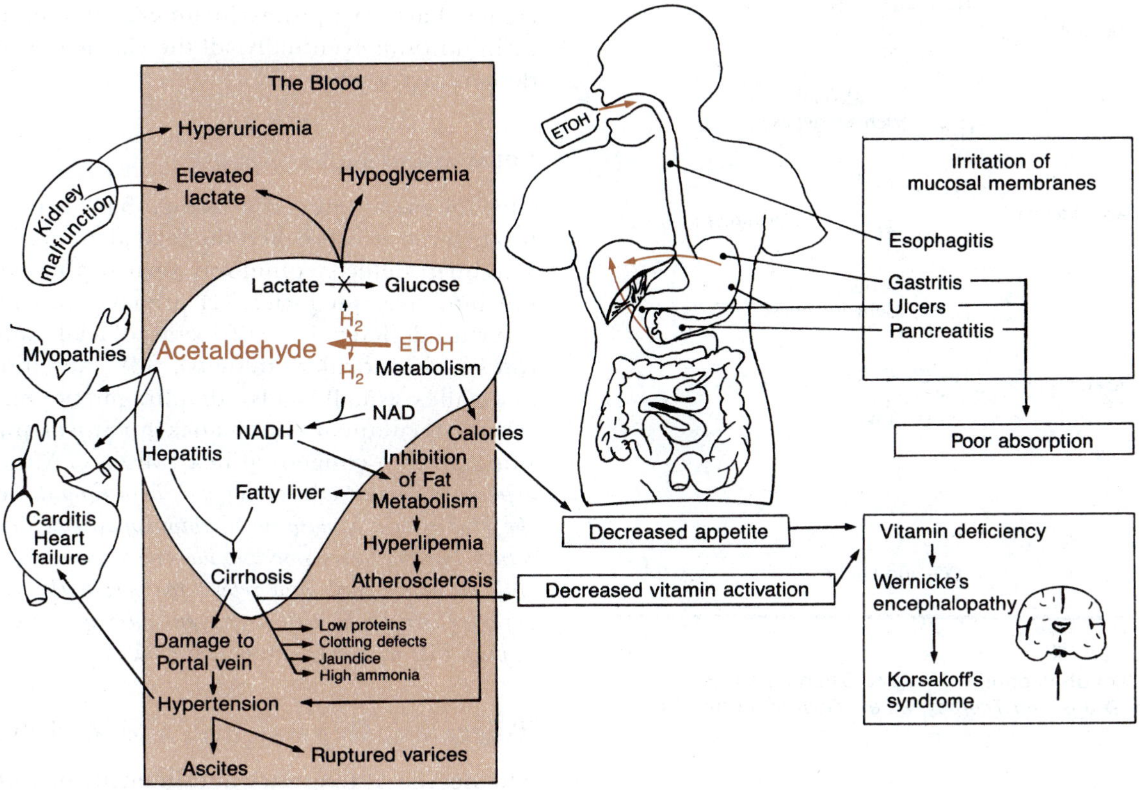

Figure 13–3
Tissue toxicities associated with chronic alcohol ingestion.

alcohol is converted to acetaldehyde by the action of the enzyme alcohol dehydrogenase (Figure 13–4). Hydrogen released in this reaction is used for converting the nucleotide nicotinamide adenine dinucleotide (NAD, a cellular energy intermediary) to its reduced form, NADH. Acetaldehyde is subsequently converted to acetic acid by the enzyme aldehyde dehydrogenase, providing additional hydrogen for reduction of NAD. Toxic consequences can result from both the formation of acetaldehyde and excessive conversion of NAD to NADH.

Chronic toxicities related to acetaldehyde include **skeletal myopathies** such as tremor, carditis, and liver inflammation (**hepatitis**). Formation of excessive NADH is toxic because the usual sources of hydrogen for reduction of NAD are fats and lactate. When high levels of NADH are formed from alcohol metabolism, the body has no need to metabolize lactate or fat. Inhibition of lactate metabolism leads to hypoglycemia and kidney malfunction. Diminished metabolism of fat leads to accumulation of lipids in the blood and liver, resulting in **hyperlipemia** (a risk factor in atherosclerosis and hypertension) and **fatty liver** (a frequent prelude to hepatitis and **cirrhosis**).

Hepatitis is an inflammatory condition in which the liver is enlarged due to infiltration of leukocytes and lymphocytes. Fatty liver, hepatitis, and even the earliest phase of cirrhosis are reversible if alcohol consumption is discontinued. However, if alcohol consumption continues, cirrhosis becomes irreversible. In its most advanced stage, cirrhosis is not only irreversible but progresses inevitably to death.

Cirrhosis involves the excessive production of **collagen,** a protein that is an essential constituent of connective tissue and one of the most abundant substances in the body. Overproduction of collagen literally splits apart the liver into nodular islands of cells. Blood flow is impeded and cells begin to die. As cirrhosis progresses, the liver capsule becomes firm to the touch and nodules appear. Gradually the liver shrinks in size and becomes finely nodular. The final stage of fatal liver injury is preceded by more limited impairments such as reduced production of serum proteins, clotting defects, jaundice, high am-

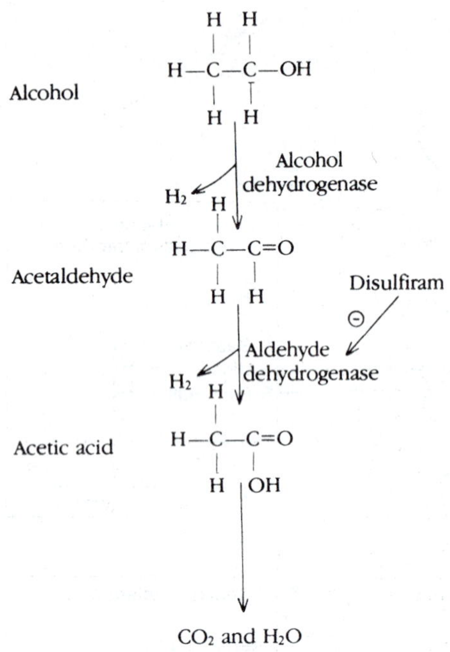

Figure 13–4
Metabolism of alcohol. From A. K. Swonger and L. L. Constantine, *Drugs and Therapy,* 2d ed. Boston: Little, Brown, 1983.

monia levels in the blood, hypertension, and decreased ability to activate vitamins. Nursing assessment during early stages of cirrhosis often reveals a client who has increased susceptibility to infection and bleeding tendencies.

Secondary Toxic Effects Related to Vitamin Deficiencies

Alcohol supplies a readily usable source of energy for the body. An alcoholic may obtain one-half or more of his or her caloric intake from alcoholic beverages. Such a diet is sadly lacking in vitamins. Vitamins that are ingested may be poorly absorbed because of gastritis and poorly activated because of hepatitis. As a result, alcoholics frequently develop vitamin deficiency diseases, such as anemia, nicotinic acid deficiency encephalopathy, and Wernicke's encephalopathy, a neurological disease. **Wernicke's encephalopathy** first affects limited brain regions (the mammillary bodies of the hypothalamus) but may later entail diffuse degeneration of cortical tissue. Wernicke's encephalopathy is associated with a behavioral syndrome called **Korsakoff's psychosis** (dementia associated with alcoholism). The mammillary bodies lie along the Papez circuit, which is instrumental in consolidation of short-term memory into long-term storage, so that a characteristic feature of Wernicke's encephalopathy is memory deficiency. Early symptoms include confabulation and disinhibition; eventually, all the classic symptoms of dementia are present.

Fetal Alcohol Syndrome

Alcohol use by pregnant women has been linked to teratogenic effects called the fetal alcohol syndrome. The birth defects commonly seen in this syndrome fall into five categories: (1) prenatal and postnatal growth deficiencies, (2) craniofacial anomalies (ptosis, intraocular deficits), (3) musculoskeletal anomalies (small nails, diaphragmatic malformations), (4) cutaneous anomalies (hirsutism, pigmentation), and (5) congential heart disease. *Nurses should explain to women who are or may be pregnant the risks to the fetus associated with consumption of alcohol during pregnancy. Further, nurses need to identify women whose unborn children are at risk and report the observations to health care personnel who will be present during delivery so that appropriate measures can be anticipated.*

Tolerance, Dependence, and Withdrawal

The degree of tolerance and intensity of withdrawal with alcohol use depend on the amount and duration of drinking. Tolerance to alcohol is less than occurs with many drugs of abuse, for example, narcotics, amphetamines, or psychedelics. Tolerance to alcohol is mostly the pharmacodynamic type, involving adjustments in the neurochemistry of the brain toward hyperexcitability. Inactivation of alcohol occurs almost entirely by metabolism rather than excretion of the unchanged drug, but increases in the metabolism of alcohol due to induction of liver enzymes contributes only about 20% to overall tolerance. Moreover, this drug-disposition component of tolerance may be inconsequential in the long-time drinker if liver disease has begun.

Alcohol abuse involves both psychological and physical dependence. Psychological dependence can vary from mild to strong. The person who is highly dependent on alcohol often drinks in situations other than social settings, such as when alone, on the job, or in school, and becomes obsessed with obtaining and using alcoholic beverages.

In its mildest form, the withdrawal syndrome contributes to the **hangover** experienced the morning after intoxication. In its moderate form, alcohol withdrawal is characterized by a coarse tremor of the hands, tongue, and eyelids, and one or more of the following: nausea, vomiting, malaise, tachycardia, sweating, hypertension, orthostatic hypotension, anxiety, depression, or irritability. Some individuals experience hallucinations — **alcohol hallucinosis** — during withdrawal. The most intense form of alcohol withdrawal is **delirium tremens** (or **withdrawal delirium**), which includes delirium and autonomic hyperactivity in addition to other symptoms of alcohol withdrawal.

Pharmacological Aspects of the Treatment of Alcoholism

Treatment of alcoholism is a long and often unsuccessful process involving social and psychological factors more than pharmacological ones. A review of these factors and the various kinds of treatment programs for alcohol-troubled individuals is beyond the scope of this book. Here we consider only two limited topics relating to treatment of alcohol problems: acute treatment of alcohol withdrawal and the use of disulfiram (Antabuse) in the treatment of alcoholism.

Treatment of Alcohol Withdrawal

Individuals who come to an emergency room or other health care facility with symptoms of alcohol withdrawal are generally treated in accordance with a set of guidelines established by that facility. A typical treatment protocol is discussed in this section, but it may differ in some respects from that required

Nursing Observations for Alcoholism and Treatment with Disulfiram

THERAPEUTIC GOAL	Detoxification and curtailment or elimination of alcohol use.
PREADMINISTRATION ASSESSMENT	
Baseline Data	Observe client for frequent or inappropriate use of alcohol or use of alcohol to an extent that is detrimental to the client's physical or psychological health or ability to function. Question family members concerning changes in the client that may indicate a problem. Evaluate cardiovascular, liver, neurological, gastrointestinal, and motor functions. Evaluate nutritional status. Look for ascites. Obtain an ECG and chest x-ray. Note the client's gait, presence of tremors, repeated lapses of memory, or slurred speech. Obtain laboratory tests including complete blood cell counts, urinalysis, serum enzymology, serum cholesterol, lactic acid levels, blood glucose levels, serum pH, hematocrit, hemoglobin, and electrolytes.
EVALUATION OF DRUG RESPONSE	
For Therapeutic Benefit	Diminished consumption of alcohol and improved ability to cope with life stresses without dependence on drugs.
For Adverse Effects of Disulfiram	Monitor for skin rashes, acneiform eruptions. Question client about presence of fatigue, lassitude, tremor, restlessness, headache, impotence, metallic taste, or gastrointestinal disturbances.
For Drug Interactions	Monitor for interactions of alcohol, including additive or supraadditive CNS depression, increased metabolism of certain other drugs, additive hypoglycemia, additive ulcergenic influence, and alcohol-disulfiram reactions. When disulfiram is used, in addition to the interaction with alcohol, monitor for interactions with metronidazole (Flagyl), isoniazid (Isoniazid), and certain other antimicrobial agents.
For Dietary Interactions	Monitor for nutritional deficiencies if there is heavy alcohol consumption. Monitor for ingestion of disguised forms of alcohol when disulfiram is being used.
For Compliance	Evaluate client's compliance with all facets of the therapeutic regimen by careful observation, interviewing, and review of progress. Report compliance problems to the physician and act as client-advocate when changes in the therapeutic regimen seem indicated.

at a particular facility. The protocol involves three steps: (1) history taking, (2) physical examination, and (3) treatment and disposition.

The history taking proceeds rapidly, often in conjunction with the physical examination or treatment, depending on the severity of withdrawal at initial presentation. The clinician seeks to establish the following: (1) the quantity and type of beverage recently ingested, (2) the duration and frequency of drinking during the latest bout, (3) the patient's attitude toward the drinking behavior, (4) the presence of medical complications, (5) history of any treatment for drinking, (6) history of psychiatric treatment, and (7) the course and severity of previous withdrawal episodes. The client and anyone who has accompanied the client to the facility are sources of information.

The nurse conducting the physical examination should take vital signs every 4 hours for 24 hours. The nurse also should conduct blood tests, including purified protein and prothrombin determinations, a complete blood cell count, measurements of blood urea nitrogen, fasting blood sugar, electrolytes, and a liver profile. A chest x-ray and electrocardiogram should also be obtained.

Most clients undergoing alcohol withdrawal are dehydrated, but a minority may be overhydrated. Administration of fluids as needed will correct dehydration in most cases and is safer than forcing fluids, since the condition of those clients who enter the emergency room in an overhydrated condition would be aggravated by forcing fluids. Although forcing fluids is the practice at some institutions, it is inadvisable and should be reserved for clients in whom dehydration has been definitely established and is severe.

Chlordiazepoxide (Librium), 50 mg, is usually given orally to suppress withdrawal symptoms. Diazepam (Valium) is used instead of or in addition to chlordiazepoxide if seizures are present or appear imminent. Thiamine (vitamin B_1) and multivitamins may be given to correct potential vitamin deficiency, but they have little effect on the acute withdrawal condition. An antacid may be administered for epigastric distress. Acetaminophen (Tylenol) may be given for headache; however, aspirin should be avoided because it irritates the gastrointestinal mucosa and increases seizure liability. Neuroleptics are avoided because they, too, increase seizure liability, but if delirium is pronounced and not corrected by chlordiazepoxide, thioridazine (Mellaril) is preferable to other neuroleptics.

All clients undergoing severe alcohol withdrawal should be hospitalized, but the reality imposed by the costs of hospitalization require the application of established criteria (Table 13–1) to determine which individuals should be admitted. A typical protocol for those not admitted would be 1–2 hours of observation after treatment with chlordiazepoxide, and a 3–6 day supply of the drug on release. Mild cases of alcohol withdrawal are sometimes dealt with more appropriately and effectively in social detoxification centers than in medical facilities.

Table 13–1
Guidelines for Determining Admission of Emergency Room Patients with Alcohol Withdrawal

Admission is indicated if the patient meets any one of the following criteria:
Active infectious disease
Temperature above 101° F or below 95°F
Alcohol-induced disorder (hepatitis, pancreatitis)
Significant metabolic problem (acidosis, hypoglycemia)
Congestive heart failure, dysrhythmia, or significant hypotension
Active gastrointestinal bleeding, significant vomiting, or significant dehydration
Significant degree of anemia
Alcoholic myopathy
Disulfiram reaction
Hallucinations or delirium
History of recent convulsions
Fluctuating levels of consciousness
Severe depression or contemplation of suicide
Lack of satisfactory care as an outpatient

Disulfiram (Antabuse)

Mechanisms and Effects Disulfiram is an inhibitor of the enzyme aldehyde dehydrogenase. As noted earlier, alcohol is first converted into acetaldehyde and hydrogen, both toxic products. In the second metabolic step, the enzyme aldehyde dehydrogenase converts acetaldehyde to acetic acid, a normal bodily substance that can be readily disposed of. Thus, the inhibition of aldehyde dehydrogenase by disulfiram interrupts alcohol metabolism at its most toxic step. If alcohol is ingested by the client who is taking disulfiram, acetaldehyde levels build up, causing the **disulfiram reaction,** which is an acetaldehyde syndrome. The symptoms of the disulfiram reaction, including severe nausea and vomiting, are so unpleasant that the drug is used as a deterrent to alcohol use: the client taking disulfiram refrains from taking alcohol in order to avoid the reaction.

Nursing Diagnoses and Interventions for Alcoholism

Nursing Diagnoses	*Related Interventions*
Alteration in family processes related to marital discord or inability to perform role functions	Refer for family or marital counseling.
Alteration in nutrition: intake less than required related to anorexia, impaired absorption, and impaired vitamin activation	Provide supplements of thiamine and other vitamins. Encourage eating well-balanced meals. Teach client the importance of good nutrition.
Anxiety related to loss of control and withdrawal	Provide detoxification; encourage entry into alcohol treatment program; discuss with client and family factors contributing to anxiety and its control.
Dehydration related to vomiting	Correct fluid and electrolyte disturbances; encourage fluid intake.
Impaired social interaction related to intoxication	Encourage client to stop using alcohol and enter a treatment progam.
Increased risk of injury related to impaired judgment and coordination	Provide safety measures; urge client not to drive after drinking; encourage family members to resist giving client car keys when client is "under the influence."
Ineffective individual coping: denial, anger, and inability to manage life stresses	Encourage discontinuation of alcohol use and entry into treatment program. Provide emotional support to family.
Potential for violence related to idiosyncratic intoxication or disinhibition of aggressive impulses	Provide necessary measures to ensure protection of public and staff; teach family members protective measures and encourage their participation in Alanon for support and counseling.
Sensory-perceptual alterations: mental distortions related to intoxication; hallucinations related to acute toxic psychosis; delirium during withdrawal	Provide chlordiazepoxide (Librium) for withdrawal; provide supportive care or antipsychotic drugs for toxic psychosis; provide emotional support to family members as well as physical care to client.
Sexual dysfunction related to impotence and inebriation	Encourage discontinuation of alcohol use and entry into treatment program.
Sleep-pattern disturbance related to deprivation of rapid eye movement (REM) sleep and insomnia during withdrawal	Encourage discontinuation of alcohol; assist client and family to reestablish healthful sleep patterns.
Social isolation related to loss of job and family contacts	Encourage discontinuation of alcohol use and entry into treatment program; provide client with entrance into appropriate social service agencies.
Knowledge deficit related to drug use	Explain the nature of alcohol abuse and dependence and the associated risks to medical and mental health and relationships.
	Encourage the client to enter into an alcohol treatment program.
	If disulfiram (Antabuse) is to be employed, warn client to avoid even minute quantities of alcohol and disguised forms of alcohol. Teach the side effects of disulfiram and the need to refrain from alcohol consumption for at least 2–3 weeks after discontinuing disulfiram.

Pharmacokinetics After oral administration, disulfiram is rapidly and completely absorbed. About 12 hours is required for full development of disulfiram inhibition of aldehyde dehydrogenase. About 1–2 weeks is required after the use of disulfiram is terminated for the activity of aldehyde dehydrogenase to return to normal. *Nurses should warn clients that the reaction to alcohol may occur as long as 2 weeks after disulfiram is discontinued.* There is a strong possibility of a severe disulfiram reaction if alcohol is ingested within 6 days after the use of disulfiram is terminated and a moderate reaction within 7–10 days after use is terminated.

Clinical Indications Disulfiram is used in alcohol treatment programs on the rationale that it can help to crystallize the alcohol troubled person's commitment to give up drinking. It is argued that with disulfiram use the decision not to drink needs to be made only once a day, when the medication is taken, and not every time a drink is offered. Since the disulfiram reaction is potentially fatal, the clients who are to receive the drug must be carefully selected. When disulfiram is used to enforce sobriety in uncommitted subjects — a common arrangement in plea-bargaining situations and in military judicial proceedings — the incidence of disulfiram reactions is high. Some clients mistakenly believe they can ingest small amounts of alcohol while taking disulfiram. Others discover the possibility of stimulating acetaldehyde activity by megadoses of vitamin C. Since the use of disulfiram is not without significant risks, it should be reserved for clients who are committed to abstinence and who feel they can support that commitment with disulfiram.

Adverse Effects Symptoms of a disulfiram reaction begin within 5–10 minutes after ingestion of alcohol. Marked vasodilation, flushing, warm skin, hot face, and pulsating headache, are followed by nausea and copious vomiting. Clients may complain of dizziness, blurred vision, heart palpitations, breathing difficulties, chest pain, and confusion. Thirst results from loss of fluid in vomiting. Severe hypotension may develop. The syndrome typically lasts from 30 minutes to several hours, but it may be fatal. *Before initiating treatment with disulfiram, nurses need to warn clients of the adverse consequences of ingesting alcohol while using disulfiram. They also need to warn clients using disulfiram to avoid disguised forms of alcohol, such as sauces, fermented vinegar, cough syrups, tinctures, and spirits (the last two are dosage forms in which alcohol acts as a vehicle). Even alcohol rubs or aftershave lotions can cause toxicity. Clients should be taught to read all labels to see what various products contain.*

It should be emphasized that the disulfiram reaction is in reality a disulfiram-alcohol interaction which occurs as a result of alcohol ingestion by a person taking disulfiram. Disulfiram reactions do not occur when the drug is used by itself, and this fact is the basis for its use in treatment programs. By itself, disulfiram is largely innocuous, although some clients may have allergic reactions, such as skin rash, acneiform eruptions, or urticaria. Other uncommon side effects include fatigue, lassitude, tremor, restlessness, headache, impotence, metallic taste, and gastrointestinal disturbances. Most of the minor side effects disappear or diminish with continued use of disulfiram.

Drug Interactions Disulfiram may interact with other drugs as well as alcohol. It may precipitate phenytoin intoxication in clients receiving that drug. In combination with metronidazole (Flagyl) or isoniazid (Nydrazid) or by itself in high doses, disulfiram has been observed to cause psychotic reactions. The excitatory component of the action of marihuana is enhanced by disulfiram. Disulfiram decreases plasma clearance and enhances pharmacological activity of diazepam and chlordiazepoxide, but some of the other benzodiazepines, including oxazepam (Serax), alprazolam (Xanax), and lorazepam (Ativan), can be used safely without interaction with disulfiram. Doses of oral anticoagulants frequently require adjustment when disulfiram therapy is initiated or discontinued. A variety of other drugs produce disulfiram-like interactions with alcohol (Table 13–2).

Table 13–2
Drugs Capable of Producing a Disulfiram-like Interaction with Alcohol

acetohexamide (Dymelor)
cefamandole (Mandol)
cefoperazone (Cefobid)
chloramphenicol (Chloromycetin)
chlorpropamide (Diabinese)
griseofulvin
metronidazole (Flagyl)
moxalactam (Moxam)
procarbazine (Matulane)
quinacrine (Atabrine)
tolazamide (Tolinase)
tolazoline (Priscoline)
tolbutamide (Orinase)

Preparations and Administration Treatment can be continued until the client is judged to be fully recovered. *Nurses should encourage clients receiving disulfiram to carry identification stating that they are using the drug and giving the names and telephone numbers of the consulting physicians.*

Disulfiram (Antabuse)
Tablets
Recommended Doses: For inhibition of aldehyde dehydrogenase in adults, 500 mg maximum daily, in a single dose for the first 1–2 weeks. Thereafter, a daily dose of 125–500 mg (250 mg is typical).

Case Study: Alcohol-Troubled Person

C. S., a 55-year-old economist, was brought to a hospital emergency room at noon by his 19-year-old son. C. S. was in a state of agitation. His son indicated that the father had an alcohol problem, that he had been drunk the night before, and that he began acting "crazy" that morning.

C. S. was hostile to the staff, muttered to himself continuously and appeared confused and somewhat delirious. His blood pressure was below normal and he complained of dizziness, nausea, and anxiety.

The staff first obtained a drinking history. The son provided the following information: the drinking problem had existed for at least 5 years. His father drank whiskey every morning. The amount was not known to the son since the father was very secretive about the drinking. The whiskey was kept "hidden" in the basement and the father "took the old newspapers down to the basement" several times each evening. The son did not know if there were any related medical problems, previous treatment, or history of withdrawal delirium. There was no other family source of information since the wife was an institutionalized psychiatric patient in late stages of Alzheimer's disease.

A call to the family physician revealed that the drinking problem was of long standing. The client had refused to undertake counseling, psychiatric treatment, or any other alcohol treatment program.

C. S.'s health had been good most of his life, but a physical examination a year ago revealed adult-onset diabetes mellitus and early indications of congestive heart failure. His medication regimen upon admission was NPH insulin 25 units every morning and regular insulin according to a sliding scale based on the early evening urine test. The son indicated that he thought his father took his insulin injection regularly. C. S. had no history of seizures or other drug prescriptions and did not use nonprescription medications often.

The staff ordered a complete array of physical tests for evaluation of withdrawal from alcohol. Urinalysis revealed presence of acidosis and significant dehydration. Blood tests revealed a conspicuously low blood sugar, reduced hematocrit, and prolonged prothrombin time. The ECG was normal. There was no evidence of significant infection and other test values were normal. Based on these results, C. S. was given a diagnosis of alcohol withdrawal delirium and hypoglycemia due to interaction of alcohol with insulin.

1. What immediate treatment should be provided for C. S.?
2. Should C. S. be admitted, or can he be treated satisfactorily as an outpatient?
3. What is the likely mechanism for each abnormal laboratory result?
4. How did the alcohol contribute to hypoglycemia? What are the symptoms of hypoglycemia?
5. What steps would you recommend for long-term resolution of C. S.'s problem?

Answers appear at the end of the book.

Recommended Readings

Burgess KE: Cerebral depressants. *Nursing* 1985;15(8):46–53.

Deitrich RA, Spuhler K: Genetics of alcoholism and alcohol actions, in Smart RG et al (eds): *Research Advances in Alcohol and Drug Problems.* New York, Plenum Press, 1984, pp 47–98.

Ellingboe J: Effects of alcohol on neurochemical processes, in Lipton MA et al (eds): *Psychopharmacology: A Generation of Progress.* New York, Raven Press, 1978.

Estes N, DiJulio K: *Nursing Diagnosis of the Alcoholic Patient.* St Louis, CV Mosby, 1980.

Feinberg JF: The Wernicke-Korsakoff syndrome. *Am Fam Physician* 1980;22(5):129–133.

Greenblatt DJ, Shader RI: Treatment of the alcohol withdrawal syndrome, in Shader RI (ed): *Manual of Psychiatric Therapeutics.* Boston, Little Brown & Co, 1975.

Lundwall L, Baekeland F: Disulfiram treatment in alcoholism: A review, in Klein DF, Gittelman-Klein R (eds): *Progress in Psychiatric Drug Treatment.* New York, Brunner/Mazel, 1975.

Majchrowicz E, Noble E (eds): *The Biochemistry and Pharmacology of Ethanol.* New York, Plenum Press, 1979.

Mello NK: Alcoholism and the behavioral pharmacology of alcohol: 1967–1977, in Lipton MA et al (eds): *Psychopharmacology: A Generation of Progress.* New York, Raven Press, 1978.

Mendelson JH, Mello NH (eds): *The Diagnosis and Treatment of Alcoholism.* New York, McGraw-Hill Book Co, 1984.

Myers RD: Psychopharmacology of alcohol. *Annu Rev Pharmacol* 1978;18:125–144.

Pattison EM, Kaufman E (eds): *Encyclopedic Handbook of Alcoholism.* New York, Gardner Press Inc, 1982.

Rubin E, Lieber CS: Alcoholism, alcohol, and drugs, in Klein DF, Gittelman-Klein R (eds): *Progress in Psychiatric Drug Treatment.* New York, Brunner/Mazel, 1975.

Toutant C, Lippmann S: Fetal alcohol syndrome. *Am Fam Physician* 1980;22(1):113–117.

Willoughby A: *The Alcohol-Troubled Person.* Chicago, Nelson-Hall, 1979.

CHAPTER 14

Stimulants

Stimulants of the central nervous system, also known as *psychostimulants,* are a heterogeneous assortment of agents that vary in mechanisms of action, chemical structure, likelihood of abuse and potency. In contrast to the sedative-hypnotics, it would be of little use to begin with the general properties of this class, since the subgroups of stimulants bear little in common with one another. We will consider the stimulants in four groups: (1) a group defined by a mechanism of action (the catecholamine-releasing stimulants), (2) a group of structurally related agents (the xanthines), (3) drugs that produce convulsions (the analeptics), and (4) cocaine, a distinctive drug.

Stimulants as a class have become less important as therapeutic agents in the last few decades. Several former therapeutic applications of the class have been discarded and some of the remaining applications are controversial. For example, stimulants have been used for weight reduction but have dubious value. The use of convulsant doses of analeptics (such as pentylenetetrazol) as shock therapy for depression has disappeared. In treatment of parkinsonism, stimulants have been replaced by levodopa and dopamine agonists (see Chapter 22). The limited value of stimulants for depression (because of rebound depression) is now fully appreciated. Routine use of stimulants in attention deficit disorder is coming under increasing criticism and researchers are helping to define better which children are most likely to benefit from such therapy. The use of analeptics to treat overdoses of respiratory depressants (such as barbiturates) has been replaced by the Scandinavian method that relies on mechanical support of respiration and maintenance of other vital functions. Few significant therapeutic indications remain.

The major applications of stimulants remaining are the treatment of narcolepsy, selected cases of attention deficit disorder, combination therapies for severe cases of epilepsy (when a stimulant may be required to counteract excessive depression caused by antiepileptic agents), and, rarely, acute treatment of drug-induced respiratory depression. Beyond these legitimate applications there is widespread licit and illicit self-administration of stimulants, notably caffeine, cocaine, nicotine, amphetamine, and methamphetamine (Desoxyn), and the excessive use of stimulants as diet aids. Thus, the shifting roles of stimulants dictate that this chapter be concerned with drug abuse as well as drug therapy. Because of the expanding roles of nurses as health care providers (for example, as counselors or client advocates in community, industrial, or school environments), it is increasingly important that they be able to identify, assess, and plan strategies to combat drug abuse.

Catecholamine-Releasing Stimulants and Other Anorexics

Mechanisms and Effects Catecholamine-releasing stimulants release norepinephrine from nerve terminals (Figure 14–1) in the sympathetic nervous system as well as in the brain, so that some

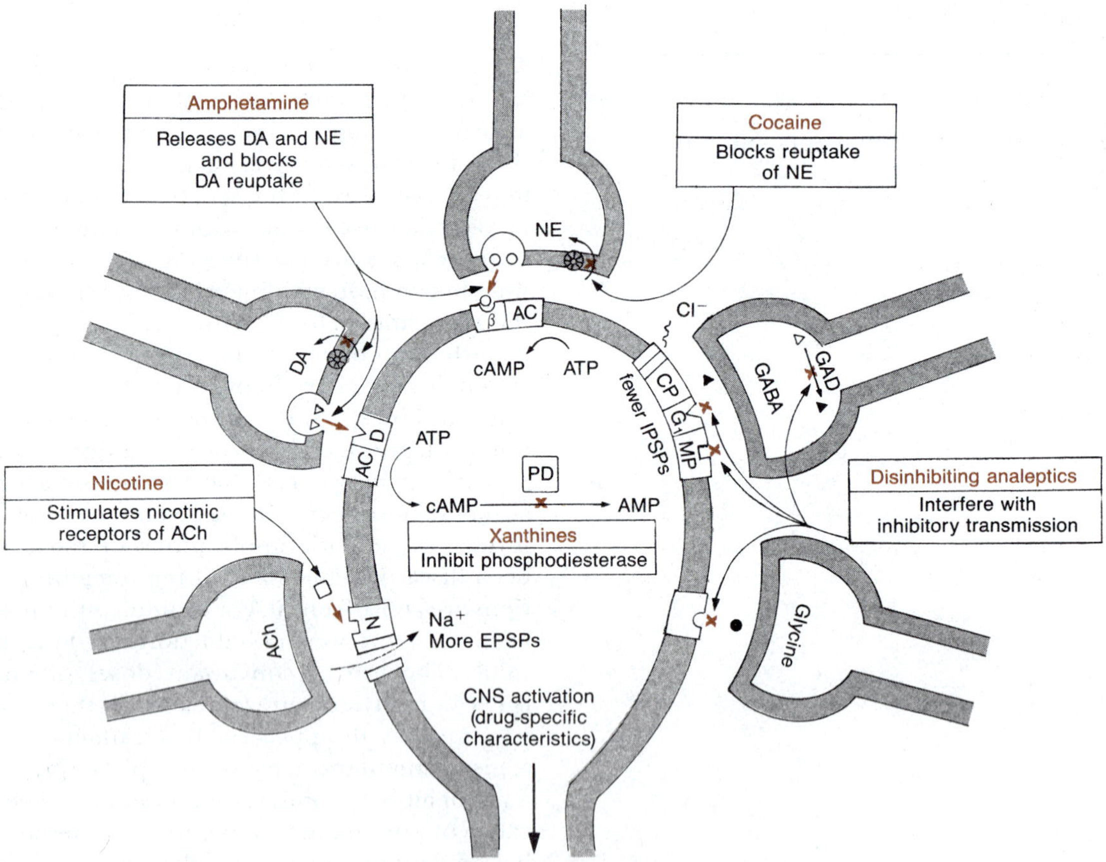

Figure 14–1
Neurochemical mechanisms of stimulants. AC, adenyl cyclase; ACh, acetylcholine; AMP, adenosine monophosphate; ATP, adenosine triphosphate; cAMP, cyclic adenosine monophosphate; β, β-adrenergic receptor; D, dopamine receptor; DA, dopamine; EPSP, excitatory postsynaptic potential; GABA, gamma-aminobutyric acid; G_1, GABA receptor, type 1; GAD, glutamic acid decarboxylase; IPSP, inhibitory postsynaptic potential; MP, modulatory protein; NE, norepinephrine; PD, phosphodiesterase.

of the drugs discussed here for their effects on the central nervous system are also discussed in Chapter 28 as indirect-acting sympathomimetics. These stimulants also promote release of dopamine and epinephrine, which together with norepinephrine, constitute the catecholamines. Among the catecholamine-releasing drugs, some such as tyramine are much more potent in effecting release from peripheral noradrenergic neurons, while others such as methylphenidate (Ritalin) are more active centrally.

Amphetamine is the best known catecholamine-releasing stimulant and the prototype of the class; other agents in the group are often designated amphetamine-like stimulants. Amphetamine exists as two forms: a dextrorotatary (D) isomer and a levorotatary (L) isomer. The two molecules are identical except that in three-dimensional configuration one is the mirror image of the other (Figure 14–2). The dextro isomer is about three times more active a stimulant as the levo isomer, but the levo isomer is slightly more potent in releasing peripheral norepinephrine. Amphetamine also blocks the reuptake of catecholamines after their release. In the brain, the dextro isomer is about 10 times more potent than the levo isomer in blocking reuptake of norepinephrine, but the two block reuptake of dopamine equally. Benzedrine consists of an equal (or racemic) mixture of the two isomers (thus DL-amphetamine). Dexedrine, by contrast, is the purified dextro isomer.

The usual effects of amphetamines include increased motor activity, euphoria, mood elevation, sleeplessness, agitation, and tremors. Perceptions may be enhanced and the individual may be able to perform physical feats that were not possible before. The client may experience an increased ability to concentrate which, combined with "feeling good," increases self-confidence. As long as the level of difficulty of the task is low, there may be enhancement of both the client's mental and physical abilities. However, performance of complex mental or physical tasks is impaired. Large doses or prolonged use of amphetamines can lead to psychotic reactions, resembling schizophrenia. Stimulants can mask fatigue, and prolonged use is associated with a rebound depression. *Nurses should advise clients that use of stimulants can lead to impaired performance in hazardous tasks, such as driving an automobile.*

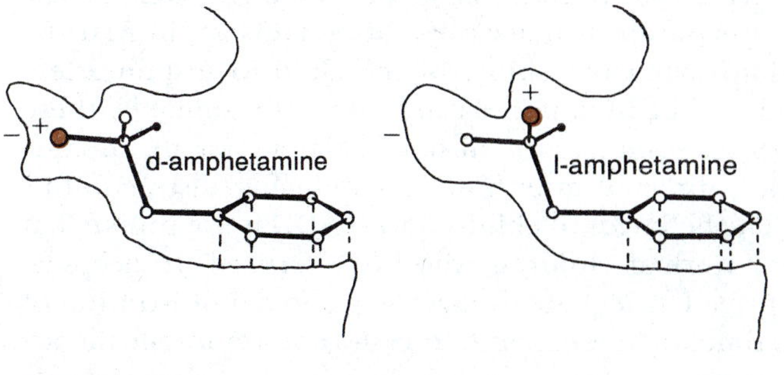

Figure 14–2
Stereospecificity of receptors for amphetamine. The dextrorotatary isomer (left) is better able than the levorotatary isomer (right) to activate the brain receptors responsible for CNS stimulation.

Amphetamine-like drugs postpone the need for sleep but not indefinitely. After the exhilarating effect of the drug has worn off, the user will require a prolonged period of rest. In addition to reducing total sleep time, amphetamines alter the percentage of sleep time spent dreaming, reducing it to one-half of normal. The waking brain wave pattern is also altered, shifting toward the higher (beta) frequencies. Amphetamine increases the firing rate of reticular neurons, which in turn activates the cerebral cortex. The increase in activity produced by amphetamine is related to a subcortical site of action.

Methylphenidate is an amphetamine-like stimulant of potency intermediate between that of caffeine and amphetamine. It has a greater selectivity for the CNS than amphetamine, producing fewer adverse reactions related to the sympathetic nervous system. Doses that produce substantial CNS stimulation have little effect on blood pressure. Pemoline (Cylert) is a CNS stimulant with a distinctive structure but a pharmacology similar to amphetamine and methylphenidate. It produces substantially less effect on the sympathetic nervous system than does either amphetamine or methylphenidate and may act by releasing dopamine rather than norepinephrine.

Most currently available anorexics are also amphetamine-like stimulants. One, mazindol (Mazenor), is an imidazoline derivative; two, phenmetrazine (Preludin) and phendimetrazine (Bontril), are morpholines; one, benzocaine (Anbesol), a local anesthetic; and the remaining agents are phenylethylamines directly related to amphetamine. They include fenfluramine (Pondimin), phentermine (Ionamin), chlorphentermine (Pre-Sate), clortermine (Voranil), benzphetamine (Didrex), diethylpropion (Tenuate), and phenylpropanolamine (Dexatrim). Although fenfluramine is structurally related to amphetamine, its pharmacology is substantially different; it releases serotonin and has a depressant effect.

Pharmacokinetics After oral administration, amphetamine-like stimulants are well absorbed. Onset of action begins within 15 minutes, and peak activity typically occurs in 2–4 hours. Therapeutic plasma concentrations of amphetamine itself range from 5 to 10 μg/100 ml. Amphetamine is inactivated by liver metabolism and renal excretion. The extent of renal excretion is pH dependent since amphetamine is a weak organic base. The elimination half-life of amphetamine can be as little as 7 hours if the urine is acidified or as much as 34 hours if the urine is alkalinized. Any drug a person may take that alkalinizes urine (such as acetazolamide or sodium bicarbonate) will increase the effects of amphetamine. Drugs that acidify the urine (such as ammonium chloride or ascorbic acid) will reduce effects of amphetamines. *Nurses need to learn what drugs clients are taking (prescribed or otherwise) and alert the physician, so that adjustments can be made in the regimen.*

Clinical Indications The approved therapeutic applications of amphetamine-like stimulants are narcolepsy, attention deficit disorder, and short-term weight reduction in exogenous obesity. **Narcolepsy** is a condition in which an individual falls asleep spontaneously many times a day — perhaps 10, 20, even 50 times. The condition is rather rare, affecting only about 0.07% of the population of the United States. Symptoms also include cataplexy, sleep paralysis, and hypnagogic hallucinations. The usefulness of amphetamine in preventing the sleep attacks of narcolepsy was first noted in 1935. Amphetamine-like stimulants have been found to be quite effective in allowing the narcoleptic client to function almost normally.

Attention deficit disorder (ADD), formerly called hyperkinetic syndrome or hyperactivity in children, is a childhood pattern characterized by impulsivity, elevated motor activity, short attention span and distractibility, explosive irritability, and often, but not always, hyperactivity. It may lead to problems in cognitive skills and learning. Development of reading, writing, and arithmetic skills may be delayed and parents may complain of disobedience. The criteria for ADD with hyperactivity (Table 14–1) include inattention, impulsivity, and hyperactivity and other criteria defining age of onset, duration, and exclusions. ADD usually disappears as the child approaches adolescence but occasionally persists into adulthood (the **residual type**). ADD and specific learning disabilities are overlapping diagnostic categories; both are subsumed under the label of **minimal brain dysfunction** (MBD). MBD is sometimes due to anoxia or injury occurring to a fetus during the mother's pregnancy or to an infant during birth.

About 4% of all grade school children are diagnosed as having ADD, boys far more commonly than girls. Drug treatment is not indicated in every instance. Clinical studies indicate that the children most likely to benefit from stimulant medication are those with (1) clear motor abnormalities, such as choreiform movements, tremors, or observable hyperkinetic symptoms, (2) a history of hyperactivity that extends back to infancy or preschool years, (3) sensory motor impairments, (4) defects of visual memory, (5) attention spans less than 25% of normal in timed visual or auditory tasks, (6) significant learning deficiencies or rank in the lower 25% of their class, or (7) electroencephalographic abnormalities.

Table 14–1
Criteria for Attention Deficit Disorder with Hyperactivity

Inattention (three or more of the following):
- Failure to complete projects
- Poor listening ability
- Distractibility
- Difficulty in concentrating

Impulsivity (three or more of the following):
- Acts before thinking
- Excessive shifting among activities
- Difficulty in organizing work
- Excessive need for supervision
- Frequent calling out in class
- Difficulty in waiting turn

Hyperactivity (two or more of the following):
- Runs or climbs about excessively
- Difficulty in sitting still
- Excessive sleep movements

Onset before age 7

Duration at least 6 months

Not secondary to schizophrenia, an affective disorder, or to mental retardation

Amphetamine was first reported to be effective in reducing activity of hyperactive children in 1939. Since the stimulant properties of amphetamine were already recognized, its action in ADD was described as paradoxical. Although the effect is sometimes described as "tranquilizing" or "calming," such a characterization is inaccurate. Stimulants act in ADD by improving the ability of the child to sustain attention, not by any sedating effect. Presumably, these drugs stimulate the diffuse thalamic system, enhancing directed attention and reducing distractibility. The behavior of children with ADD is not unlike that of normal children who are overtired or sleep-deprived. Adequate dream sleep and administration of stimulants both serve to restore norepinephrine activity.

Comparative studies suggest that methylphenidate (Ritalin) may be marginally more effective than amphetamine in ADD. However, amphetamine has two advantages over methylphenidate: it is less expensive and its absorption is not affected by food, allowing it to be taken with meals. Pemoline (Cylert) is perhaps slightly less effective than the other two stimulants used for ADD, but has fewer adverse effects related to the sympathetic nervous system.

Catecholamine-releasing stimulants are often used as **anorexics** (also called anorexiants, anorectics, or anorexigenics). Amphetamine itself is available by prescription as a diet aid (Obetrol). Over 90% of the 6,000 pounds of amphetamines produced annually are used for this purpose. A number of weaker drugs of similar mechanism are also available as prescription anorexics and two drugs, phenylpropanolamine (Appedrine, Dexatrim) and benzocaine (Ayds, Slim-Line), are available as nonprescription diet aids. Americans spend over $200 million dollars annually for nonprescription diet aids alone.

The evidence from controlled studies indicates that stimulants do work to help individuals lose weight, but only marginally. After 4–6 weeks of use, tolerance develops to the appetite-suppressing effect of stimulants. Moreover, weight lost with the aid of an appetite suppressant is almost always rapidly regained when the drug is discontinued. By contrast, weight loss achieved by behavioral techniques involving altered eating habits is sustained for longer periods of time. Thus, it would appear that the overall contribution of drugs to dietary regulation and weight loss is trivial at best. Therefore, in any responsible weight reduction program, anorexics will be prescribed only as short-term adjuncts in a regimen of weight reduction based on caloric restriction and exercise. When amphetamine is used as an anorexic, it should be taken about one-half hour to an hour before meals.

Adverse Effects and Contraindications Amphetamine-like stimulants may either increase or lower blood pressure. *Therefore, clients should be taught to monitor their blood pressure and report any changes. Nurses should pay particular attention to complaints of palpitations.* Amphetamine-like drugs are contraindicated in clients who have a history of hypersensitivity to sympathomimetic amines, hyperthyroidism, hypertension, angina pectoris, or other cardiovascular disorders and in children under 3 years of age.

Amphetamine-like stimulants may overstimulate clients, causing them to be talkative, restless, agitated, and nervous. Symptoms such as dizziness or headache may indicate that the dose is too high and should be reported immediately to the physician (usually the drug dosage will be reduced). Signs of psychological dependence are an indication that the drug should be discontinued.

Some clients may experience dry mouth and unpleasant taste. *To counter these problems, nurses should suggest rinsing the mouth with clear water, especially after eating. Clients should also increase their fluid intake and be meticulous in daily oral hygiene since the decrease or absence of saliva encourages demineralization of tooth enamel and mucosal erosion. Nurses should also advise the client to combat decreased bowel function by increasing daily intake of roughage, fruits and vegetables, and, if necessary, using a mild laxative.*

Excessive sweating, chills, elevated temperature, fatigue, and difficulty voiding are all indications of adverse response to the drug. Mothers who breastfeed should not take amphetamines, since these drugs are secreted in breast milk and will have a deleterious effect on the infant. Males may complain of impotence, gynecomastia, or altered libido.

Adverse effects of amphetamine-like stimulants in children relate primarily to the cardiovascular system, CNS, and gastrointestinal system. Amphetamines can cause elevated blood pressure and palpitations and dangerous cardiac dysrhythmias. *Nurses should teach parents to monitor children for hypertension or cardiac dysrhythmias.* The characteristic CNS symptoms are psychiatric or neurological manifestations of overstimulation. *Parents need to be taught to observe the child for increased restlessness, anxiety, insomnia, or euphoria and to be attentive to a child's complaints about feeling "funny" (usually meaning dizzy) or having tremors or headaches.* A few children may develop psychotic episodes or attacks of Gilles de la Tourette's syndrome.

Methylphenidate lowers the seizure threshold (amphetamine does not), and must be used with caution in epileptic children. *Nurses need to alert parents of children with epilepsy to this potential side effect and parents should keep a careful record of seizure occurrences so that the children's physicians can determine whether the seizures are being precipitated by the medication or by something else.*

As with adults, children may develop alimentary reactions to stimulants, such as dry mouth, dysgeusia, diarrhea, and constipation. Anorexia is an inevitable response. Amphetamine-like stimulants reduce the average growth in children by 10–30%. *Nurses should encourage parents to record their child's height and weight 2 or 3 times weekly.* If the drug regimen is discontinued during the summer months, children experience a rebound acceleration in growth rate 15–65% above normal. The accelerated growth rate subsides within 2 to 3 months.

Allergic reactions to amphetamine are rare and limited to **urticaria** (hives). Allergic reactions to methylphenidate are more varied and include urticaria, exfoliative dermatitis, erythema multiforme, thrombocytopenic purpura (an abnormal decrease in platelets), drug fever, and arthralgia. *Nurses should be certain that clients have platelet and blood cell counts conducted periodically during prolonged treatment with methylphenidate. Allergic reactions to pemoline (Cylert) include skin rashes and elevated serum enzyme levels, indicating liver injury. Liver function should be evaluated prior to initiating pemoline therapy and periodically during treatment as a precaution.*

Gastric lavage or an emetic may be used for amphetamine overdose. The physician may order barbiturates for their sedative effects, but these should be administered with caution. Physicians may order drugs to acidify the urine to enhance the renal excretion of amphetamines.

The adverse effects of amphetamine-like anorexics are the same as those of amphetamine, although the incidence and severity is somewhat less. Fenfluramine (Pondimin), however, is distinctive; it may aggravate psychiatric depression and prolongs bleeding time.

Abuse of Amphetamine-like Stimulants Amphetamines have been widely abused virtually since their discovery. As early as the 1930s college students used them to study for exams. Stimulants were employed by both sides in World War II to aid soldiers in maintaining alertness for extended periods of time. As early as 1938, the potential for amphetamine-induced toxic psychosis was evident. In the 1950s, the pop song "Who put the benzedrine in Mrs. Murphy's Ovaltine?" captured the spirit of fun that America was having with amphetamines. Until the 1960s, stimulants used for recreational purposes were usually obtained legally by prescription or over the counter (generally in the form of nasal inhalers), and amphetamines were widely prescribed for a variety of medical conditions.

In the mid-1960s, abuse of stimulants shifted from oral to intravenous use, from weaker to more potent forms (such as methamphetamine), and from conventional sources (which were gradually coming under stricter federal regulation) to the black market. Oral use was one thing: 5 mg of amphetamine taken orally produced subjective effects akin to a cup of strong coffee, providing an enhanced ability to maintain concentration for monotonous tasks and to fend off fatigue. Ten milligrams or more produced a distinct euphoria of gradual onset that might persist for several hours.

Intravenous amphetamines were another matter entirely. Immediately following IV injection of amphetamine, a user experiences a "rush," "flash," or "splash"—an abrupt awakening, a jolt of alertness accompanied by intense pleasurable sensations described as a "full-body orgasm." The new mode of amphetamine abuse of the 1960s became the *run and crash* pattern, in which users would embark on several days of intense drug use ended by development of complete tolerance to the stimulant.

The principal dangers of amphetamine abuse are chronic toxicity and violent behavior. Acute toxicity is less likely, although overdosage can occur. The rare instances of toxic psychosis associated with oral use became an epidemic with intravenous injection of amphetamines. A full-blown toxic psychosis resembles schizophrenia. The user becomes extremely hyperactive, experiences auditory hallucinations, and engages in compulsive, stereotypical behaviors, such as sorting and re-sorting, disassembling devices, repetitious acts, and effusive talking. Memory becomes hazy; the user may become paranoid and even brutally and senselessly violent. Drug users of the 1960s knew that "speed kills" and that "meth is death." The potential causes of death from abuse of stimulants are hepatitis, infection, cardiovascular damage, and violence.

Amphetamines produce severe psychological dependence, especially when used intravenously; recidivism is said to be particularly high among abusers of stimulants. Amphetamines do not produce a true physical dependence in the sense of an adaptive adjustment in the neurochemistry of the brain. The effect of chronic use is better understood as an exhaustion phenomenon, a progressive depletion of the catecholamine neurotransmitters. The recovery phase is likewise not a true withdrawal syndrome but a period when neurotransmitter stores are gradually replenished. The rebound phase following discontinuation of stimulants has substantial psychological and physical manifestations, including fatigue, depression, suicidal thoughts, increased appetite, disturbed sleep, and increased rapid eye movement (REM) sleep. Rebound symptoms generally subside in 3–7 days.

Next to androgens, stimulants are probably the class of drugs most abused by athletes seeking to increase athletic performance. Concerned with abuse of performance-enhancing drugs, the National Collegiate Athletic Association (NCAA) is implementing random blood testing of athletes in championship-level events.

Drug Interactions Haloperidol (Haldol) and other neuroleptics as well as lithium tend to antagonize the stimulatory effects of amphetamine-like drugs. Tricyclic antidepressants and monoamine oxidase (MAO) inhibitors can greatly potentiate the effects of stimulants when used with them. The use of amphetamine-like stimulants in individuals receiving a MAO inhibitor is dangerous because of the risk of hypertensive crisis due to catecholamine release in conjunction with diminished ability to metabolize the amines.

Stimulants may counteract the action of antihypertensive medications to some extent because of their hypertensive action and the depressant effect of sedative-hypnotics due to CNS stimulation. *Nurses who work with diabetic clients should inform them that insulin requirements may be altered because of the anorexic effect of the stimulant.*

Amphetamines may interefere with diagnostic tests. They can elevate plasma corticosteroids, especially the evening values, decrease fasting blood glucose, and can increase urinary epinephrine secretion.

Methylphenidate inhibits the metabolism of certain drugs, including coumarin anticoagulants, tricyclic antidepressants, phenylbutazone (Azolid), and several antiepileptic agents — phenytoin (Dilantin), primidone (Mysoline), and phenobarbital.

Fenfluramine (Pondimin) has several drug interactions not shared by other anorexics, including potentiation of antihypertensive medications (such as diuretics or antiadrenergic medications), additive CNS depression with other depressants, an additive hypoglycemia with other hypoglycemic agents (such as insulin and sulfonylureas), and an additive prolongation of bleeding time with anticoagulants. *If fenfluramine therapy is initiated, monitoring of blood pressure in clients on antihypertensive medication, and glucose levels in diabetics should be intensified. Nurses should also warn diabetic clients who are taking fenfluramine of possible hypoglycemic responses.*

Preparations and Administration The amphetamines currently available include racemic amphetamine sulfate, dextroamphetamine sulfate (Dexedrine), a resin complex of amphetamine and dextroamphetamine (Biphetamine), various mixtures of salts of amphetamine and dextroamphetamine (Obetrol, Delcobese), and methamphetamine (Desoxyn, Methampex). Amphetamine products should be stored at room temperature unless otherwise directed by the manufacturer. On the street, Benzedrine is known as "bennies," "hearts," or "peaches"; Dexedrine tablets as "oranges" or "footballs"; and Dexedrine spansule capsules as "wake-ups" or "lid-proppers." Methamphetamine (Desoxyn) is known as "speed."

AMPHETAMINE-LIKE STIMULANTS

Amphetamine (racemic, generic formulations)
Tablets
Recommended Doses: Same as for Dextroamphetamine.

Dextroamphetamine (Dexedrine, Dexampex, Ferndex, Oxydess, Spancap, generic formulations)
Capsules, tablets, sustained release capsules, elixir
Recommended Doses: For children ages 3–5, 2.5 mg PO daily initially, increased by increments of 2.5 mg/day at weekly intervals until an adequate response is achieved. For children over age 5, 5 mg, once or twice daily initially, increased in increments of 5 mg/day at weekly intervals until optimal response is obtained. The usual upper limit is 40 mg/day. Sustained release dosage forms are always used on a once-a-day basis. *Nurses should advise clients to take the last dose of amphetamine-like drugs at least 6 hours before retiring. If the client still complains of difficulty falling asleep, the time of administration may have to be adjusted or the dosage decreased. If the medication is in sustained release form, it should be taken early in the day (10–14 hours before bedtime).*

Methylphenidate (Ritalin)
Tablets, sustained release tablets
Recommended doses: For attention deficit disorder in children over age 6, 5 mg PO, bid initially, increased to a maximum of 60 mg/day in 1–3 divided doses. Methylphenidate is not approved for use in children under 6 years of age. *The nurse should instruct parents (and the child if appropriate) to take the first daily dose of methylphenidate 45–60 minutes before breakfast and subsequent doses 45–60 minutes before lunch and/or dinner. The last dose should generally be taken before 6:00 P.M. so as not to interfere with sleep. Sustained release tablets are taken in the morning.*

Pemoline (Cylert)
Tablets (scored)
Recommended doses: For attention deficit disorder in children, 37.5 mg/day in a single morning dose initially, increased gradually (at 1-week intervals) in increments of 18.75 mg to a maximum of 112.5 mg/day. The usual range of daily maintenance doses is 56.25–75 mg/day. Pemoline produces clinical improvement after approximately 2–3 weeks.

PRESCRIPTION ANOREXICS

Approximately 20 million prescriptions are written yearly for these agents.

Benzphetamine (Didrex)
Tablets
Recommended Doses: 25–50 mg orally once daily initially, increased if required to 25–50 mg, 1–3 times daily.

Chlorphentermine (Pre-Sate)
Tablets
Recommended Doses: 65 mg orally once a day after breakfast

Clortermine (Voranil)
Tablets
Recommended Doses: 50 mg orally once a day use in the morning

Diethylpropion (Tenuate, Tepanil)
Sustained release tablets
Recommended Doses: 25 mg orally, 3 times daily, 1 hour before meals and in midevening if required to overcome night hunger.

Fenfluramine (Pondimin)
Tablets
Recommended Doses: 20 mg orally, 3 times daily, 30–60 minutes before meals initially, increased if required at weekly intervals by 20 mg/day to a maximum of 40 mg, 3 times daily.

Mazindol (Mazanor, Sanorex)
Tablets
Recommended Doses: 1 mg orally, 3 times daily, 1 hour before meals, or 2 mg once daily, an hour before lunch.

Phendimetrazine (Plegine, others)
Capsules, tablets, sustained release capsule
Recommended Doses: 35 mg orally, 2 or 3 times daily, 1 hour before meals; or 1 sustained release capsule, once per day in the morning.

Phenmetrazine (Preludin)
Tablets, sustained release tablets
Recommended Doses: 50–75 mg orally maximum daily.

Phentermine (Ionamin, Phentrol, Adipex, Obestin, Obermine, Obephen, Tora, Parmine)
Capsules, tablets, sustained-release capsules
Recommended Doses: 8 mg orally, 3 times daily, ½ hour before meals, or 15–37.5 mg as a single morning dose.

Two anorexics are available without prescription: benzocaine (Ayds, Slim-Line) and phenylpropanolamine (Dexatrim and many others). Benzocaine is a local anesthetic. When applied topically to the mouth and tongue in the form of candy or gum, it decreases the client's ability to detect sweetness and helps to reduce craving for sweets. Benzocaine appears to have low toxicity when employed in this manner. The general pharmacology of benzocaine is discussed in Chapter 17.

Phenylpropanolamine is an indirect-acting sympathomimetic with significant peripheral actions mediated by both alpha- and beta-adrenergic receptors. It is also employed as a nasal decongestant and is marketed for this purpose in combination cold remedies. Because of the prevalence of phenylpropanolamine in a wide variety of over-the-counter remedies, there is a real risk of inadvertent overdose if several medications are being used. *Nurse should advise clients who are using preparations that contain phenylpropanolamine about other products that contain it, so that they do not take more than 50 mg at any one time nor a total daily dose exceeding 75 mg.* Adverse effects are similar in kind though less frequent or severe than those of amphetamine. Phenylpropanolamine should be stored in tight, light-resistant containers.

NONPRESCRIPTION ANOREXICS

Benzocaine (Ayds Appetite Suppressant or Slim-Line)
Candy, gum
Recommended Doses: 5–15 mg orally prior to food consumption up to a maximum of 45 mg/day.

Phenylpropanolamine
Capsules and tablets (Diadax, Diet Gard, Westrim, Resolution II Half-Strength), timed release capsules (Dexatrim, Dietac, Resolution I Maximum, Unitrol, Acutrim, Westrim), precision release tablet (Acutrim), combinations with caffeine (Prolamine, Dexadar, Dietac, Dexatrim, Resolution I, Dex-A-Diet Original Formula), combinations with fiber extracts (Fluidex), grapefruit extract (Grapefruit Diet Plan with Diadax), or vitamins (Appedrine, Trendex, Dexatrim Plus Vitamins, Vita-Slim).
Recommended Doses: For the immediate release forms, 25 mg orally, 3 times each day. For the timed release formulations, 1 capsule daily in the morning.

Important Nursing Implications for Amphetamine-like Stimulants

- ☐ Caution clients and family members about the danger of abuse of amphetamine-like stimulants.
- ☐ Explain to clients that use of stimulants does not reduce the body's requirements for rest.
- ☐ Advise clients who use stimulants chronically for medical purposes to maintain thorough oral hygiene and to rinse the mouth frequently to prevent drying of mucous membranes.
- ☐ Monitor clients receiving stimulants for hypertension or dysrhythmias.
- ☐ Monitor the height and weight of children who are receiving stimulants for attention deficit disorder. Provide drug-free intervals to allow near-normal growth to occur.
- ☐ Warn female clients who are breast-feeding that amphetamine excreted in the milk could have harmful effects on the infant.
- ☐ Advise diabetic clients that use of amphetamine-like stimulants could alter their requirements for insulin or oral hypoglycemic drugs.

- ☐ Advise clients to avoid abrupt withdrawal of amphetamine-like drugs after chronic use to prevent rebound depression.
- ☐ Administer amphetamine-like stimulants 30–60 minutes before meals when they are employed as anorexics.
- ☐ Administer the last dose of amphetamine-like stimulants no later than 4:00 P.M. in children with attention deficit disorder to avoid insomnia.
- ☐ Do not overlook other components of a comprehensive treatment plan (psychological support, remedial training, family therapy, environmental manipulation) when stimulants are employed in ADD. Family interventions include educating parents about the nature of ADD, encouraging increased structuring of the home environment, improving the parent-child relationship, dealing with complicating problems in the family, and removing any family resistance to improvement. In less severe cases, environmental manipulation should be considered first. The child might do better in a school environment that is less distracting because of low noise level, a subdued visual environment, and smaller class size.

Cocaine

History and Sources Cocaine is a constituent in the leaves of the coca plant which grows in the highlands of the Andes Mountains of South America. The leaves have been chewed and sucked by native Peruvians for at least 50 centuries, but coca leaves contain only up to 2% cocaine, and chewing provides slow absorption and only one-half the blood levels produced by inhaling the drug ("snorting" it). Because coca leaves do not retain their potency very well during transport from the distant South American growing fields, recreational use in Europe and the United States was limited until the middle of the nineteenth century, when cocaine was isolated from the plant. Freud was an early proponent of the use of cocaine, and the fictional character Sherlock Holmes attributed his magnificent powers of deduction to its use. Cocaine, a white powder, is smuggled into the United States, often through Miami, from distribution points in Colombia. It is sold under names such as "coke," "snow," "gold dust," and "lady." Often, it is diluted with procaine, lidocaine, amphetamine, or other chemicals. The cocaine sold on the street is typically 10–15% pure. However, a highly purified and deadly form of cocaine, called "crack," appeared in East Coast cities in 1986 and rapidly spread throughout the country.

Mechanisms and Effects Like amphetamine, cocaine elevates free catecholamine concentrations in the synapse, but by a distinctive mechanism. Cocaine prevents reuptake of norepinephrine into presynaptic cells and weakly inhibits monoamine oxidase. Cocaine also acts as local anesthetic and is structurally related to procaine (Novocain) and lidocaine (Xylocaine), two drugs widely employed as local anesthetics (see Chapter 17). The stimulant effect of cocaine may relate in part to the local anesthetic mechanism, since procaine reportedly produces similar subjective effects but does not block norepinephrine reuptake. Animals will self-administer procaine and lidocaine as readily as cocaine.

The effects of cocaine are almost as strong as those of amphetamine, but its duration of action is much shorter. Amphetamine effects typically last about 1–4 hours; a typical cocaine effect after "snorting" is only 5–15 minutes.

Routes of Utilization The route by which cocaine is utilized is all important in defining the risks involved. Four routes are employed: oral, intranasal, smoking, and intravenous (Table 14–2). Most commonly, cocaine is taken intranasally, by snorting the powder up into the nose, directly onto the nasal mucosa, where it can be rapidly absorbed. Euphoria occurs while the plasma concentrations of the drug are rising, not during peak concentration. A hazard of repeated intranasal use is perforation of the septum that separates the nostrils. The snorter may also have to contend with a perpetually runny nose. The severity of psychological dependence and rebound depression is initially minimal when cocaine is used by the intranasal or oral routes, but after two or more years of regular intranasal use, drug craving may become intense and there is also a tendency to graduate to intravenous use or smoking.

When cocaine is used intravenously or smoked, the severity of psychological dependence may disrupt psychological health and social functioning. Risks of overdose and toxic psychoses are much higher when cocaine is used by these routes. Rebound depression may be severe, to the extent of true anguish, after cocaine injection. The temptation is to stave off the depressive phase by injecting more cocaine. When the supply is gone, some users resort to narcotics to take the edge off the depression. For smoking, cocaine is converted from its usual form as a hydrochloride salt to the free base, or alkaloid form, which is considerably more heat-stabile. Smoking cocaine is often referred to as "free-basing." Both

Table 14–2
Cocaine Effects in Relation to Route of Administration

Form of drug and drug effects	Route of administration: Oral	Intranasal	Smoked	Intravenous
Form	Hydrochloride	Hydrochloride	Free base or paste	Hydrochloride
Time to peak plasma concentration (minutes)	60–80	60–80	15–20	<5
Rebound depression	+/−	+/−	++	++
Severity of drug craving	+/−	+	++	++
Risk of local tissue damage at site of administration	0	+	++	0
Risk of toxic psychosis or death from overdose	+	+	++	++

Key: 0, no effect; +/−, equivocal effect; +, mild to moderate effect; ++, intense or frequent effect.

"crack" and cocaine paste, an intermediate product in the manufacture of cocaine hydrochloride in South America, can be smoked. Lung damage is a special hazard associated with smoking cocaine, resulting from constriction of pulmonary blood vessels.

Hazards of Cocaine Abuse Physical dependence seldom occurs with cocaine, although recently physical dependence and subsequent withdrawal symptoms have been described following chronic cocaine use by the inhalation or intravenous routes. The symptoms of cocaine withdrawal include lethargy, somnolence, psychomotor retardation, depression, irritability, nausea, and vomiting. Tolerance develops to the anorexic, convulsant, cardiac, and respiratory effects of cocaine with chronic use. The pleasant subjective effects of cocaine disappear following a single dose more rapidly than the decline in blood concentrations, indicating occurrence of **acute tolerance.** Chronic use is associated with an increase in the sensitivity of the CNS to cocaine. At high doses, death can result from convulsions or from cardiac arrest. Cocaine overdoses in the United States averaged approximately 50 per year during the 1970s, but climbed to over 200 in 1981 and more than 700 in 1985. Cocaine now ranks among the top causes of drug fatalities. Cardiac arrest is a consequence of the local anesthetic action of cocaine, which leads to severe myocardial depression at toxic doses. Severe psychological dependence associated with intravenous injection or smoking of cocaine is often difficult to overcome. Imipramine and bromocriptine have been used successfully as adjuncts to psychotherapy in treatment of cocaine abusers.

Cocaine intoxication is characterized by psychological symptoms of restlessness, elation, talkativeness, grandiosity, anxiety, hypervigilance, and confusion. Physical symptoms include tachycardia, chills or fever, mydriasis, exophthalmos, elevated blood pressure, nausea, and vomiting. Diazepam (Valium) or a barbiturate is the treatment of choice. Delirium and convulsions may occur in severe cases, possibly followed by coma and then death. The cocaine toxic psychosis resembles that caused by amphetamines. Irritability, nervousness, suspiciousness, paranoia, mania, hallucinations, inability to concentrate, lapses of attention, and continuous fatigue are typical features. Chronic use of cocaine may result in substantial weight loss due to anorexia.

Xanthines

History and Sources Caffeine, theophylline, and theobromine are three closely related derivatives of xanthine and all occur naturally in various plants that are widely distributed throughout the world. Caffeine is found in coffee beans. Tea leaves contain caffeine and theophylline, while cocoa contains theobromine and caffeine. The nuts of the tree *Cola acuminata,* which provide an extract used in cola-flavored drinks, also contain caffeine.

Coffee is made from the beans of the coffee plant. The earliest recorded use of coffee is found in Arabian records dating from about AD 900. Originally, the beans were chewed or steeped in hot water, but the Arabs learned that the green beans of the plant could be roasted and ground before steeping to improve the flavor, aroma, and color. Coffee was brought to Europe early in the seventeenth century and around the middle of the century, coffeehouses sprang up in England and on the continent. Consumption of coffee became a focal point in the gender conflicts of the day, some women railing against the men who would "trifle away their time, scald their Chops, and spend their Money, all for a little base, black, thick, nasty bitter stinking, nauseous Puddle water." Other women were conniving to ensure themselves equal access to the beverage, leading Johann Sebastian Bach, in 1734, to write the Coffee Cantata on the topic.

Commercial coffee roasting began in New York City in 1790, and Maxwell House became the first blended coffee in 1892. Most coffee imported into the United States until recent years was the *arabica* variety from Latin America, especially Brazil and Colombia, but now more than half is the cheaper African variety (*robusta*) which can be used for making instant coffee. Coffee ranks second, only behind oil, as an international trade item. The big increase in the price of coffee in the 1950s reduced per capita consumption of coffee in the United States from the high of 20 pounds per person in 1946 to about 11 pounds per person in 1981. Current annual consumption of coffee in the United States is about 1 billion kg, which provides 7 million kg of caffeine. Almost 20% of coffee consumed currently is decaffeinated; the caffeine extracted from the coffee is used in making soft drinks. A cup of brewed coffee contains 80–150 mg of caffeine, instant coffee 85–100 mg, and decaffeinated coffee 2–4 mg.

The history of tea is only a little older than coffee. It is cited as a medicine in writings from as early as AD 350 and as a beverage in 780. Tea is made from the leaves of the tea tree, *Camellia sinensis.* The use of *ch'a,* as it was known in China, was confined to East Asia until its importation into Europe by the Dutch East India Company in 1610. Britain profited from the tea trade and by the end of the seventeenth century, tea had become firmly entrenched as the national beverage of England. Tea came to the English colonies in America in trade for cotton and tobacco. In 1765 and again in 1767, Parliament levied a tax on tea sold to the colonies, a tax that "fanned the fires that lit the musket that fired the shot heard round the world." The dispute altered beverage consumption on both sides of the Atlantic, since drinking tea became patriotic for the British and unthinkable for the colonists. America turned to coffee. In 1981 Americans drank just 0.8 pound of tea per person while their counterparts in England drank 10 times that quantity per person.

Today, most tea is grown in Sri Lanka, India, and Indonesia. Only the smallest, outermost leaves of each bud are used for tea. The leaves are dried, rolled, and allowed to oxidize by storage in a cold, damp site. In the process, the leaves change from green to bright red-brown. American teas are made from the oxidized leaves, while the tea sold in Chinese restaurants in America is made from the green leaves, and oolong tea is made from partially oxidized leaves. Both tea bags and iced tea originated in 1904; instant tea originated in the 1950s. The caffeine content in a cup of tea depends on both the brand and how long it is steeped. A weak cup of tea provides 18–45 mg of caffeine, medium tea 48–78 mg, and strong tea 70–107 mg.

Tea (and to a lesser extent coffee) also contains tannin, which may combine with certain drugs in the gastrointestinal tract, thus impairing their absorption. Analgesics, neuroleptics, and antihistamines are especially affected by tannin binding. Addition of cream or lemon to the tea or coffee substantially reduces this effect since these additives combine with tannins. *Clients should be told not to take medications with coffee or tea.*

Theobroma cacao provides the beans from which cocoa and chocolate are made. This tree was already cultivated by the Aztecs when the Spanish encountered their civilization. Cortez brought samples of cocoa from Mexico when he returned to Spain in 1528. By the seventeenth century chocolate was added to coffee and tea on the menus of European coffeehouses. In 1828, the Dutch introduced the process of removing much of the fat (called cocoa butter) from the chocolate liquor to make chocolate powder. In 1847, sugar, cocoa butter, and chocolate powder were mixed to make the first chocolate bars and in 1876 milk chocolate was developed by the Swiss by adding milk solids. The major active ingredient in chocolate is theobromine. A cup of cocoa contains about 200 mg of theobromine and 5–40 mg of caffeine.

The original cola beverage, Coca-Cola, was formulated with caramel, fruit flavorings, phosphoric acid, caffeine, and a secret ingredient called Merchandise No. 5, containing an extract of coca leaves and cola beans. The cocaine content of the coca leaves was and still is removed prior to preparation of the extract. Modern cola beverages contain not more than 0.2 mg/ml of caffeine, or about 34–52 mg per 12-oz can. In 1981 the FDA revised its regulation regarding cola beverages so that they no longer need contain any caffeine. Colas make up about 55% of the soft-drink market and Dr. Pepper-type beverages, which also contain caffeine, another 6%. Per capita consumption of soft-drinks has risen sharply in recent decades.

Mechanisms and Effects Of the three common xanthine derivatives, caffeine has the greatest potency as a CNS stimulant but the least potency in stimulating the heart and dilating coronary blood vessels, relaxing smooth muscles, and diuresis (Table 14–3). Caffeine impairs glucose tolerance in diabetic individuals. The use of xanthines has been linked to anxiety, increased risk of heart attacks, and pancreatic cancer. There are some tentative indications that caffeine consumption during pregnancy may present hazards to the fetus.

The symptoms of caffeine intoxication include restlessness, nervousness, insomnia, diuresis, muscle twitching, rambling flow of thought, cardiac dysrhythmias, psychomotor agitation, and periods of inexhaustibility. Such symptoms can develop from as little as 250 mg of caffeine, or about 2 cups of coffee in rapid succession. Heavy doses of caffeine (1,000 mg, or 7–10 cups of coffee) can produce restlessness and excitement progressing to mild delirium in some people. Clients may complain of sensory disturbances, such as ringing in the ears and trembling, yet not associate the symptoms with too much coffee. Caffeine intoxication is easily misdiagnosed by professionals and victims alike as psychoneurotic anxiety. *Nurses should routinely assess caffeine intake of clients as a part of the drug history and inform those using more than about 300 mg daily about the role of xanthines in anxiety as well as other health hazards.*

The cerebral cortex and the medulla are among the brain regions stimulated by caffeine. The cortical action probably accounts for the subjective effects of the drug, including the feeling of increased alertness, increased speed and efficiency in motor tasks, and enhancement of intellectual processes. The medullary stimulation produced by caffeine can be of therapeutic value in reversing drug-induced depression of respiration.

Although the neurochemical basis for xanthine stimulation is not known for certain, a likely possibility is its inhibition of the enzyme phosphodiesterase (see Figure 14–1). Phosphodiesterase catalyzes the breakdown of an important nucleotide, adenosine 3′,5′-cyclic monophosphate (cAMP). Many of the effects of catecholamine neurotransmitters are mediated through receptors that are linked to adenylate cyclase, the enzyme that forms cAMP. Xanthines therefore enhance the effects of receptor activation by catecholamine transmitters. The effect of xanthines on muscle tissue relates to their ability to increase permeability of the sarcoplasmic reticulum to calcium. Xanthines also compete with and inhibit adenosine receptors, leading to dilation of coronary and peripheral blood vessels except those in the cerebrum, which are constricted.

Xanthines are encountered in a limited range of therapeutic formulations in addition to the natural sources. Caffeine is marketed in nonprescription tablets and capsules to aid in maintaining wakeful-

Table 14–3
Relative Potency of Xanthines in Producing Various Pharmacological Effects

Systemic effect	Caffeine	Theophylline	Theobromine
CNS stimulation	+++	++	+
Cardiac stimulation	+	+++	++
Diuresis	+	+++	++
Muscle			
Vasodilation	+	+++	++
Vasoconstriction of cerebral vessels	+	+++	++
Visceral smooth muscle relaxation	+	+++	++
Skeletal muscle stimulation	+++	++	+

Key: least potent (+), most potent (+++).

ness and mental alertness. Caffeine is also found in combination with ergotamine (Cafergot) for use in migraine headaches (see Chapter 26). Theophylline is important medically as a bronchodilator (Primatene) (see Chapter 52) and is sometimes used in diuretic combinations (Chapter 43). Theobromine is marketed for use (but without established value) in arteriosclerosis under the brand name Athemol.

Caffeine

Caffeine (No Doz) is marketed as an aid in staying awake and restoring mental alertness. It has been used in the treatment of neonatal apnea and topically for atopic dermatitis, but these are not established indications.

Pharmacokinetics After oral administration, caffeine is 99% absorbed, reaching peak plasma levels in 15–45 minutes. Therapeutic plasma concentrations are 6–13 μg/ml, toxicity occurs when levels exceed about 20 μg/ml, and fatal concentrations are in excess of 100 μg/ml. Caffeine is inactivated by liver metabolism with an average half-life of 3.5 hours. Metabolism is slowed and the half-life prolonged by liver disease, concurrent use of cimetidine (Tagamet), use of oral contraceptives, during pregnancy, and in neonates.

Adverse Effects and Contraindications Adverse effects of caffeine include excess CNS stimulation, gastrointestinal irritation (nausea, pain, diarrhea, vomiting), cardiac stimulation, and diuresis. Caffeine use may result in restlessness, nervousness, insomnia, tremor, lightheadedness, scotoma (blind spots), and tinnitus. Excessive use of caffeine can produce a syndrome, caffeinism, resembling an anxiety neurosis, characterized by tremulousness, muscle twitches, irritability, sensory disturbances, flushing, diuresis, rapid pulse and respiration, gastrointestinal disturbances, and dysrhythmias. *Assessment of caffeine utilization should be conducted routinely in clients presenting with problems of anxiety.* Caffeine is an irritant to the gastrointestinal mucosa and potentially ulcergenic. *Clients with a tendency toward ulcers should be advised to refrain from use of caffeinated beverages or to drink them only with meals, to diminish the irritant effect on the stomach.*

Discontinuation of caffeine after prolonged use leads to characteristic withdrawal symptoms. *Clients should be warned that they may experience a vascular-type headache, anxiety, muscle tension, and impaired concentration.* Ingestion of coffee or tea within one hour after meals impairs absorption of iron and can contribute to iron deficiency. Long-term use of caffeinated beverages has been associated with cancer of the pancreas and increased risk of heart attacks. In addition, women with fibrocystic disease of the breast have been reported to improve after discontinuation of all caffeinated beverages.

Preparations and Administration *A nursing assessment of a client's caffeine intake should include total daily intake from all sources (summarized in Table 14–4). A short-acting barbiturate should be on hand to counteract possible excess stimulation when caffeine is used for drug poisoning.*

Caffeine

Tablets (No Doz, Tirend, Vivarin, and generic formulations), timed release capsules (Caffedrine and generic formulations), citrated caffeine tablets (caffeine and an equal amount of citric acid), tablets of caffeine with dextrose (Quick Pep), injection solution (caffeine and an equal amount of sodium benzoate), candy or mints (sold over the counter in truck stops along frequently traveled highways), combinations of caffeine with ergotamine for treatment of migraine headaches (Cafergot; see Chapter 26), combination formulations containing caffeine for analgesia (such as

Table 14–4
Sources of Xanthines

Source	Amount of Xanthine
Coffee, 1 cup	
brewed coffee	80–140 mg of caffeine
instant coffee	66–100 mg of caffeine
decaffeinated coffee	2–4 mg of caffeine
Tea, 1 cup	
leaf	30–75 mg of caffeine, and theophylline
bagged	42–100 mg of caffeine, and theophylline
Colas, 12 oz can	25–55 mg
Cocoa, 1 cup	5–50 mg and 200 mg of theobromine
Chocolate bar	25 mg of caffeine, and theobromine
APC combinations	32–66 mg of caffeine per tablet
OTC stimulants	100–200 mg of caffeine per tablet
Cafergot	100 mg of caffeine per tablet
Bronchodilators	50–500 mg of theophylline or 100–500 mg of aminophylline per tablet

Anacin and Excedrin) or colds (such as Triaminicin Tablets, Coldran Tablets, and Sinexin Capsules)

Recommended Doses: For maintaining alertness, 100–200 mg orally every 4 hours, as required. The drug is not recommended for use in children. For treatment of adults, who are in cardiovascular failure associated with poisoning by depressant drugs, 500 mg IM (or IV for emergencies); for children 8 mg/kg IM to a maximum of 500 mg. Intramuscular injections can be repeated after 4 hours.

Nicotine and Tobacco

History and Sources Tobacco, cultivated in the New World before the age of the explorers, was presented to Columbus by the natives of San Salvador upon his discovery of the New World in 1492. By the middle of the sixteenth century, tobacco was being touted as a medicinal for curing headaches, colds, abscesses, and sores, and the plant was being imported into Portugal from Brazil. A French ambassador to Portugal, Jean Nicot, became enamored with tobacco when he encountered it in Lisbon, and brought it back to France. The plant, called *Nicotiana,* was named for him. The Queen of France, Catherine de Medicis, found relief from her migraine headaches from use of tobacco, and tobacco accordingly became very popular among the French. The two major species of *Nicotiana* are *Nicotiana tobacum,* which is large-leafed and of superior quality, and *Nicotiana rustica,* which is small-leafed and inferior. Until 1612 the large-leafed species was grown only in South America, giving the Spanish a monopoly on quality tobacco. In 1612 John Rolfe, the leader of the English colony in Virginia, obtained seeds of *Nicotiana tobacum* and established that species as a major crop in Virginia, which became "the tobacco colony" as tobacco became a major New World export.

The eighteenth century was the great age of snuff (tobacco powder), which replaced smoking as the main form of usage. The Queen of England (nicknamed "Snuffy Charlotte") and Napoleon in France led the way. Snuff was inserted into the nose or placed in the buccal pouch between the cheek and gum. Tobacco was of major economic importance in the colonies when the Revolutionary War broke out. The fateful landing of Cornwallis in Virginia in 1780 was aimed at destroying the tobacco plantations but ended the war instead. By 1800 Americans preferred chewing tobacco, and spittoons and cuspidors became customary accommodations. When Civil War broke out in 1860, only 7 of 348 tobacco factories in Virginia were making tobacco for smoking; the rest made snuff or chewing tobacco.

Meanwhile, cigarettes became popular in Europe; by the middle of the nineteenth century their use was widespread. After the Civil War, cigarettes were being made in the United States, but cigars were more popular. As World War I approached, Chesterfields were launched (in 1912), followed by Camels (in 1913), and Lucky Strike (in 1916), and the cigarette market began to grow. Filters were introduced in 1954 (on Winstons). Nowadays, some 5 trillion cigarettes are smoked worldwide each year. The value of tobacco ranks fifth among crops, and the federal government collects some $3 billion in tobacco tax yearly. The United States is the foremost grower and exporter of tobacco. There are currently about 65 million smokers in the United States, comprising 34% of all adults — about 39% of men and 29% of women. The percentage of men who smoke has declined from a high of 53% in the mid-1950s while the percentage of women who smoke, especially young women, increased throughout the 1950s and 1960s to stabilize in 1970 at the current level of about 30%. The number of cigarettes smoked per user has continued to rise.

Mechanisms and Effects The psychoactive ingredient in tobacco was isolated by French chemists in 1828, and given the name **nicotine.** Nicotine belongs to a large and diverse class of drugs known as analeptics, drugs that produce convulsions at sufficient doses and is one of the most frequently self-administered drugs in the world. Nicotine has widespread effects on the peripheral nervous system, stimulating both sympathetic and parasympathetic ganglia. At toxic concentrations, there is a persistent suppression of autonomic activity due to a depolarizing blockade at ganglia. The adrenal medulla and the neuromuscular junctions of the somatic nervous system exhibit a similar biphasic response.

The stimulatory effect of nicotine on the brain is due to its agonistic activity at nicotinic cholinergic receptors (see Figure 14–1). At high doses, nicotine produces tremors and then convulsions. Although the site of action of nicotine in the CNS has not been firmly established, indications from behavioral studies suggest that the diffuse thalamic system and limbic structures are involved. Performance of tasks requiring attention is enhanced by nicotine.

The excitation occurring after nicotine administration is followed by CNS depression. During the excitatory phase, respiration is quickened. During the subsequent depression, respiration is inhibited, which may lead to death after ingestion of toxic quantities of nicotine. In cigarette smoking, acute adverse effects (including nausea, especially for novice smokers, and reduced physical endurance) are related principally to nicotine and carbon monoxide.

Adverse Effects of Tobacco The chronic toxic effects of cigarette smoking (Figure 14–3) are related only in part to nicotine. Some 270 distinct compounds have been indentified in cigarette smoke, of which 15 are known to cause cancer. Among the other more toxic substances are carbon monoxide, nicotine, tar, acrolein, hydrogen cyanide, nitric oxide, nitrogen dioxide, cresols, amphenols, acetaldehyde, acetone, acetonitrite, acryl nitrate, ammonia, benzene, DDT, and butylamine.

Nitrosamines and other carcinogens in cigarette smoke are implicated in lung cancer. Tobacco constituents suppress the activity of the hair-like cilia of the lungs. By thus interfering with the removal of carcinogen-containing smoke particles (tar), microorganisms, and other foreign substances such as dust, pollens, and soot, tobacco promotes lung cancer and bronchitis. Lung cancer is the most common type of cancer; at least 85% of cases of lung cancer are a direct result of cigarette smoking. Other forms of cancer whose incidence correlates with tobacco smoking are cancer of the lips, tongue, mouth, larynx, bladder, and kidney. Cancer of the mouth and pharynx is also associated with chewing tobacco, in direct proportion to the amount and duration of use. Tobacco smoking results in significant levels of carbon monoxide in the blood and a consequent reduction in oxygen-carrying capacity of hemoglobin. Emphysema has been linked to an oxidant in smoke which acts on a lung enzyme called elastase (see Chapter 52 for details of this mechanism). Smoke decreases the flexibility of the alveoli, interfering with exchange of carbon dioxide and oxygen. Production of phlegm is increased and the diameter of the airways is decreased by the action of irritants in cigarette smoke.

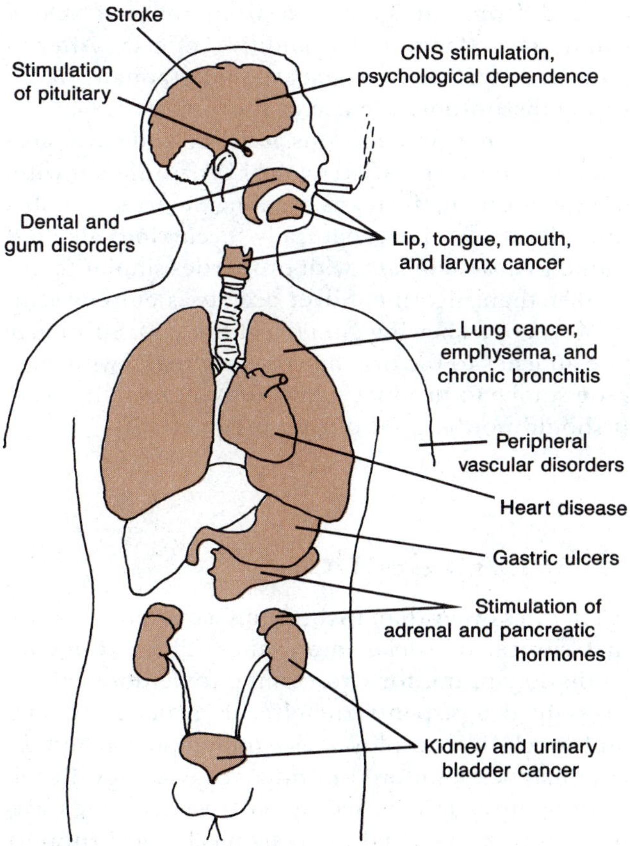

Figure 14–3
Adverse effects of smoking tobacco.

Nicotine is probably the main component of tobacco that contributes to cardiac disease, peripheral vascular disorders, cerebrovascular disease (stroke), and ulcers that frequently accompany long-term tobacco use. Cigarette smoking lowers the levels of high-density lipoproteins (HDL), which correlates with an increased risk of atherosclerosis, leading to heart disease and cerebrovascular disease. Nicotine stimulates the heart, increasing both heart rate and blood pressure after each cigarette. The increase in heart rate produced by smoking is less in regular smokers than in nonsmokers, indicating a partial tolerance to this effect; but the increase in systolic and diastolic pressure is the same in smokers and nonsmokers. Nicotine stimulates release of glucagon, which elevates blood glucose, which then stimulates release of insulin. The physiological responses to smoking a cigarette can be likened to a dose of stress.

Approximately one-third of fires are kindled by cigarettes; fires result in 8,000 deaths, 70,000 hospitalizations, and 2 million burns each year in the United States. Tobacco use contributes in all to more than 300,000 deaths per year. Smoking increases the probability of dying of lung cancer by elevenfold, other respiratory disorders by fourfold, other cancers twofold, and other causes twofold. Each cigarette smoked decreases average life expectancy by about 12 minutes; two packs per day reduces the remaining years of life by 20% at age 35 and by 34% at age 65. Cigarette smoking is the chief preventable cause of death in our society according to the surgeon general of the United States. Smoking by pregnant women after the fourth month of pregnancy is dangerous to the health and even the life of the fetus. Nicotine passes freely into breast milk and can have detrimental effects on nursing infants.

Both tolerance and dependence develop with tobacco smoking. Nicotine dependence is both physiological and psychological, and abstinence is marked by indications of withdrawal, including restlessness, inability to concentrate, and irritability. Other withdrawal symptoms include a craving for tobacco, anxiety, headache, drowsiness, and gastrointestinal disturbances.

The social stigma for the smoker increases with each passing year. The warnings on cigarette packages sold in the United States are becoming more and more explicit about the health risks involved, although American cigarettes are sold to Third World nations without such warnings. Increasing concern for possible adverse consequences for nonsmokers exposed passively to tobacco smoke will continue to constrain the opportunities for the smoker to pursue the habit conveniently. The data concerning the extent of danger to nonsmokers is not yet conclusive. For smokers who wish to quit, the task is often a difficult one, and recidivism is high. *The nurse may wish to consider recommending psychological treatment programs or use of a pharmacological adjunct for helping clients quit.* One comparative study showed that when nicotine gum was employed, 38% of individuals still abstained one year after smoking while 14% of subjects who received only psychotherapy were abstinent. However, it should be recognized that those using nicotine gum are spared further toxicity from components of tobacco smoke other than nicotine, but not nicotine itself.

Smoking Deterrents Drugs available for use as smoking deterrents are nicotine, silver acetate, and lobeline. Only nicotine is FDA certified as both safe and effective. **Nicotine** is provided in the form of a resin complex containing nicotine bound to an ion exchange resin in a chewing gum base. This preparation is indicated as a temporary aid for the cigarette smoker to give up smoking while participating in a behavioral modification program under medical supervision. Nicotine gum has been found to be most effective for smokers who have a high level of nicotine intake (smoking more than 15 cigarettes per day) and thus a severe physical dependence.

Nicotine gum is contraindicated for use during pregnancy. Nicotine use during the final trimester of pregnancy can impair fetal breathing movements and decrease placental perfusion. It is thought to play a perpetuating role in hypertension and ulcers and should thus be used with caution in individuals with such conditions. Nicotine stimulates release of catecholamines from the adrenal medulla, which may aggravate pheochromocytoma, hyperthyroidism, or insulin-dependent diabetes mellitus, and can aggravate esophagitis and oral or pharyngeal inflammations. Nicotine gum should be used with caution in individuals with dental difficulties that could be aggravated by chewing gum.

Tobacco smoking induces liver enzymes, increasing the metabolism of a variety of drugs, such as diazepam (Valium), xanthines, imipramine (Tofranil), pentazocine (Talacen, Talwen), furosemide (generic, Lasix), and propoxyphene (Darvon). During cessation of smoking, the response to such medications may increase as the rate of metabolism by the liver decreases. The pressor effect of nicotine is potentiated by concurrent administration of a beta-blocker such as propranolol (Inderal). Nicotine increases the levels of circulating adrenal hormones (catecholamines and corticosteroids), so therapy with these substances may need to be altered when nicotine gum is utilized or when smoking is discontinued.

Nicotine resin complex (Nicorette) is available as a gum containing 2 mg of nicotine per square. The dosage must be individualized, but most clients can be treated effectively with 10 pieces of the gum each day during the first month. The maximum daily dosage is 30 pieces. The candidate for nicotine therapy must agree to discontinue smoking completely during treatment with nicotine; otherwise, nicotine derived from the gum and from tobacco smoke could have dangerously additive effects. After 3 months of treatment, clients should gradually or abruptly discontinue the use of the gum.

Two other preparations, **lobeline** and **silver acetate,** have been classified by the FDA as safe but without established efficacy as smoking deterrents. Lobeline (Bantron) is a naturally occurring alkaloid found in *Lobelia inflata,* with properties similar to but weaker than nicotine. Silver acetate is employed in the form of a chewing gum (Healthbreak). Silver acetate attaches to the oral mucosa and reacts with cigarette smoke to produce an unpleasant metallic taste. It should not be used during pregnancy.

Other Analeptics

Analeptics other than nicotine are currently of minimal clinical or social importance. These drugs include doxapram, for overcoming toxic doses of depressant drugs; pentylenetetrazol, a diagnostic aid; and strychnine, employed as a rodent poison and occasionally encountered in human toxicology. Respiratory depression caused by sedative-hypnotic overdoses is best managed today by mechanical support for ventilation. A risk with the use of analeptics as antagonists of drug-induced respiratory depression is that convulsions may occur in some individuals, even before adequate respiratory stimulation has been achieved.

Doxapram (Dopram) is currently the analeptic of choice for those rare instances when any analeptic is employed because it provides a marginally superior ratio of respiratory stimulation to convulsant activity. Adverse CNS reactions to doxapram include headache, dizziness, apprehensiveness, disorientation, pupillary dilation, hyperactivity, clonus, increased reflexes, and convulsions. *An ultrashort-acting barbiturate should be at hand in case excessive CNS stimulation develops.* Other adverse effects are burning sensations in the genitalia or perineum, cough or dyspnea, laryngospasm or bronchospasm, a decrease in hemoglobin, phlebitis, dysrhythmias, nausea, vomiting, diarrhea, urinary retention, and spontaneous voiding.

Pentylenetetrazol (Metrazol) produces a diffuse stimulation throughout the CNS by interfering with binding of gamma-aminobutyric acid to its receptors (see Figure 14–1). It was formerly used as a respiratory stimulant, as an alternative to electroconvulsant shock therapy, and to increase mental alertness in elderly clients with dementia, but its efficacy for any of these applications is doubtful. Pentylenetetrazol has been useful in a screening test for new antiepileptic drugs since drugs that antagonize pentylenetetrazol-induced convulsions in mice tend to be useful clinically in petit mal epilepsy. Pentylenetetrazol has also been employed as a diagnostic aid in epilepsy.

Strychnine is occasionally encountered by children who find a container of rodent poison, as an occasional lacing agent for illicit drugs, and recently as a performance-enhancing agent for athletes competing in long-distance foot or bicycle races. Strychnine is a naturally occurring alkaloid found in nux vomica, the seeds of a tree found in India (*Strychnos nux-vomica*). Strychnine interferes with inhibitory influences exerted by glycine on nerve cells in the spinal cord (see Figure 14–1). Strychnine poisoning is treated by rapid intravenous administration of a short-acting barbiturate or a centrally acting muscle relaxant, such as mephenesin (Torserol), but strychnine acts so quickly that death often occurs before medical intervention can be initiated. Stomach lavage soon after ingestion of strychnine is best accomplished with potassium permanganate solution.

Preparations and Administration

Doxapram (Dopram)
Injection solution
Recommended Doses: For excess depression due to sedative-hypnotic overdose, 2.0 mg/kg initially, repeated in 5 minutes and every 1 or 2 hours until the patient regains consciousness. To hasten recovery of consciousness postanesthetically, 0.5–1.0 mg/kg as a single IV injection.

Case Study: Attention Deficit Disorder

B. T. was a 30-year-old divorcee and mother of M. T., a 6-year-old boy. She was asked to have M. T. evaluated because of poor work in school, short attention span, and impulsive behavior. At the clinic, M. T. was evaluated by the nurse, who noted that he was unable to sit still for more than a few seconds at a time. He seemed to be full of energy and highly distractible. After the nurse had completed her evaluation, M. T. was seen by the physician, who conducted a physical examination and an EEG evaluation with pentylenetetrazole (Metrazol) administration and strobe light stimulation. This test indicated that M. T. had a low threshold for seizure discharge activity. The physician observed that M. T. exhibited clear hyperkinetic symptoms. In a visual memory task, M. T. tested at 15% of the normal value for his age.

In the meantime, B. T. revealed to the nurse that she had been just like her son when she was younger. She had done poorly in school. The only time she was truly able to slow down was when she drank a lot of coffee or, in her early twenties, when she took amphetamines. She had married at 19, was divorced at 20, got pregnant at 23, married the baby's father when the pregnancy was apparent, and divorced again at 25. She had since had a string of three live-in boyfriends. She had changed jobs seven times in the last three years. The nurse discussed with B. T. the nature of attention deficit disorder and the possibility of residual symptoms in adulthood.

Ultimately, both B. T. and M. T. were prescribed methylphenidate (Ritalin). The nurse instructed them to take their medication 45–60 minutes before breakfast, lunch, and dinner. She also told them that the last dose should not be taken after 6:00 PM to prevent interference with sleep, but since they always had dinner by 6:00 PM, this would not pose a problem. B. T. was taught to keep a weight chart for both her son and herself as a guard against excessive weight loss due to the anorexic effect of methylphenidate. The nurse discussed with B. T. the behavior therapy programs and adjustments of the home environment that might aid in M. T.'s response. Before they left, the nurse took a blood sample from each client for a complete blood cell count. With B. T.'s permission, the nurse contacted the nurse at M. T.'s school to discuss the boy's situation and to establish a working relationship.

Both clients responded well to the therapeutic regimen. M. T. began doing better in school and his behavior improved. B. T. was able to improve her planning and her persistence in activities and relationships.

1. What would be the appropriate diagnosis for M. T.? For B. T.?
2. What observations suggest that M. T. is an appropriate candidate for methylphenidate therapy?
3. How might B. T.'s heavy use of coffee relate to her condition?
4. Why did the nurse take a blood sample for blood cell counts?

Answers appear at the end of the book.

Recommended Readings

Amphetamine-Like Stimulants

Angrist B, Sathananthan G, Wilk S, Gershon S: Amphetamine psychosis: Behavioral and biochemical aspects. *J Psychiatr Res* 1974;11:13–23.

Burgess KE: Understanding the spectrum of cerebral stimulants. *Nursing* 1985;15(7):50–56.

Goetz C, Kramer J, Weiner WJ: Pharmacology of minimal brain dysfunction. *Clin Neuropharm* 1978;3:185–201.

Gualtieri CT, Ondrusek MG, Finley C: Attention deficit disorders in adults. *Clin Neuropharm* 1985;8(4):343–356.

Huber CJ, Dalldorf JS: Minimal brain dysfunction syndrome. *Nurs Clin North Am* 1980;15(1):51–69.

Iversen LL, Iversen SD, Snyder SH (eds): *Handbook of Psychopharmacology.* New York, Plenum, 1978, Vol. 11: *Stimulants.*

Roth B: *Narcolepsy and Hypersomnia.* New York, Karger, 1980.

Satterfield JH et al: Physiological studies of the hyperkinetic child: I, in Klein DF, Gittelman-Klein R (eds): *Progress in Psychiatric Drug Treatment.* New York, Brunner/Mazel, 1975.

Smith DE (ed): *Amphetamine Use, Misuse, and Abuse.* Boston, GK Hall, 1979.

Stunkard AJ (ed): *Obesity.* Philadelphia, WB Saunders, 1980.

Zarcone VP Jr: Diagnosis and treatment of excessive daytime sleepiness. *Clin Neuropharm* 1977;2:87–97.

Cocaine

Gawin FH, Kleber HD: Cocaine abuse treatment. Open pilot trial with desipramine and lithium carbonate. *Arch Gen Psychiatry* 1984;41:903–909.

Holland DJ: Cocaine use and toxicity. *J Emerg Nurs* 1982;8(4):166–169.

Grabowski J (ed): *Cocaine: Pharmacology, Effects and Treatment of Abuse.* National Institute on Drug Abuse Research Monograph, US Dept of Health and Human Services Publication No (ADM) 84-1326, 1984.

Mule SJ: *Cocaine: Chemical, Biological, Clinical, Social, and Treatment Aspects.* Cleveland, CRC Press, 1976.

Van Dyke D, et al: Cocaine and lidocaine have similar psychological effects after intranasal application. *Life Sci* 1979;24:271–274.

Nicotine and Tobacco

Benowitz NL, Jacob P III: Daily intake of nicotine during cigarette smoking. *Clin Pharmacol Ther* 1984;35:499–504.

Correa P et al: Passive smoking and lung cancer. *Lancet* 1983;2:595–596.

Goldberg SR, Spealman RD, Goldberg DM: Persistent behavior at high rates maintained by intravenous self-administration of nicotine. *Science* 1981;214:573–575.

Hughes JR et al: Effect of nicotine on the tobacco withdrawal syndrome. *Psychopharmacology* 1984;83:82–87.

Jaffe JH, Jarvik ME: Tobacco use disorder, in Lipton MA et al (eds): *Psychopharmacology: A Generation of Progress.* New York, Raven Press, 1978.

Jarvik ME, Schneider NG: Degree of addiction and effectiveness of nicotine gum therapy for smoking. *Am J Psychiatry* 1984;141:790–791.

Krasnegor NA (ed): *Cigarette Smoking as a Dependence Process.* National Institute on Drug Abuse Research Monograph (GPO No. 017-024-0895-9, 1979, p 23.

Pinney JS (ed): *Health Consequences of Smoking for Women: A Report of the Surgeon General.* Bethesda, Md, Office on Smoking and Health, 1980.

Xanthines

Gilbert RM: Caffeine as a drug of abuse, in Gibbins RJ et al (eds): *Research Advances in Alcohol and Drug Problems, III.* New York, Plenum Press, 1984, pp 49–176.

Greden JF: Caffeinism and caffeine withdrawal, in Lowinson JH and Ruiz P (eds): *Substance Abuse: Clinical Problems and Perspectives.* Baltimore, Williams & Wilkins Co, 1981, pp 274–286.

Hallal JC: Caffeine: Is it hazardous to your patients' health? *Am J Nurs* 1986;86(4):422–425.

Pilette W: Caffeine: Psychiatric grounds for concern. *J Psychosoc Nurs Ment Health Serv* 1983;21(8):19–24.

CHAPTER 15
Psychedelic Drugs

The drugs discussed in this chapter have been called psychedelics, hallucinogens, illusinogens, psychotomimetics, psychotogens, fantasticas, and phantasticants, each name emphasizing a particular characteristic of the class. The term **hallucinogen** refers to the ability of these drugs to produce hallucinations. **Illusinogen** is slightly more accurate, since most users experience illusions (distorted sensory representations in response to real world stimuli) more than hallucinations (sensorial impressions with no source in reality). Although the visual modality is most affected, the bizarre sensory distortions may involve other senses or cross-modality (synesthetic) experiences, such as the one described by Albert Hoffmann, the discoverer of LSD, from his early experiences with the drug: "A remarkable feature was the manner in which all acoustic perceptions (e.g., the noise of a passing car) were transformed into optical effects, every sound causing a corresponding colored hallucination constantly changing in shape and color like pictures in a kaleidoscope."

The term **psychotomimetic** reflects the early interest in these drugs as a possible means of inducing psychoses experimentally, but the effects do not closely resemble natural psychoses. The amphetamine toxic psychosis is more similar to schizophrenia. Although members of this class of compounds may precipitate psychotic episodes, this result is not common enough to justify the name **psychotogens.** Aldous Huxley used the term **fantasticas,** and others have called them **phantasticants.** These names reflect the historical use of psychedelic-containing plants, mushrooms, and concoctions to explore the nature of reality by altering the processes of the human mind. The name **psychedelics** (literally "mind manifesting"), emphasizing the ability of these drugs to alter consciousness, is perhaps closest to neutral in its connotations.

The various psychedelics can be divided into four subgroups:

Group A: Substituted indole alkylamines
- lysergic acid diethylamide (LSD)
- bufotenin
- psilocybin
- psilocin
- dimethyltryptamine (DMT)

Group B: Substituted phenylalkylamines
- mescaline
- 2, 5 dimethyl-4-ethylamphetamine (STP, DOM)
- methoxymethylene-dioxyamphetamine (MMDA)
- paramethoxyamphetamine (PMA)

Group C: Phenylcyclohexyl derivatives
- phencyclidine (PCP)

Group D: Miscellaneous anticholinergic
- cannabis (marihuana, tetrahydrocannabinol)
- benzilic acid ester derivatives (Ditran)
- belladonna alkaloids

In pharmacological activity, groups A and B are very similar, while groups C and D differ substantially both from A and B and from each other. Drugs in groups A and B exhibit cross-tolerance and may even be subjectively indistinguishable. An individual who develops tolerance to an agent in group A or B is not tolerant to agents in groups C or D. This chapter emphasizes the three most widely encountered psychedelics, LSD, PCP, and marihuana.

LSD

History and Sources Lysergic acid diethylamide (LSD) is a newcomer among psychedelics. The two names most closely linked to its history are Albert Hoffman and Timothy Leary. LSD was discovered in 1938 by Hoffman, a chemist at Sandoz Pharmaceuticals. During the course of experiments in 1943, Hoffman accidentally absorbed a small amount of the drug through the skin of his fingers and soon experienced restlessness, dizziness, and what he called "extreme activity of imagination": "As I lay in a dazed condition with my eyes closed (I experienced daylight as disagreeably bright) there surged upon me an uninterrupted stream of fantastic images of extraordinary plasticity and vividness and accompanied by an intense, kaleidoscope-like play of colors."

Hoffman suspected that the effects were due to the drug with which he was experimenting and intentionally ingested a small amount of the agent 3 days later. After 40 minutes, Hoffman was overwhelmed by the same effects.

After Hoffman's experiences, the history of LSD was uneventful until 1960–1961, when two scientists at Harvard University, Timothy Leary and Richard Alpert, began experiments, first with psilocybin and then LSD, using graduate students and later undergraduates. At first the experiments were rigorously controlled and medically supervised, but Leary and Alpert became lax, performing the experiments at home and eliminating medical controls. Dismissed from Harvard in 1963, Leary became the guru of the psychedelic generation. Alpert became a guru of another sort, changing his name to Baba Ram Dass and turning to meditation. LSD flourished during the 1960s, but in 1967 reports of chromosomal damage reputedly caused by LSD and the arrest of Leary on drug charges marked the beginning of the end of the LSD era.

Mechanisms and Effects (See Figure 15–1.) LSD produces continuous beta activity by stimulation of the reticular formation; this activity can be seen in an electroencephalogram. LSD disrupts the functioning of the serotonin-rich pathways of the raphé system, acting on autoreceptors on raphé neuron cell bodies to depress their activity. LSD also acts as an antagonist at certain other serotonin receptors in the brain. The effects of LSD — dehabituation (ordinary objects or events are experienced as extraordinary), insomnia, and enhanced flow of sensory signals to the cortex — resemble the effects of serotonin depletion and prior depletion of brain serotonin potentiates LSD. Thus, LSD effects are a combination of amphetamine-like and antiserotonin actions. The former effect increases the flow of sensory signals along the neural pathways of the brainstem while the latter effect breaks down the gating function that normally regulates such flow. The result is a sensory overload, causing intensified perceptions, a feeling of full wakefulness, cross-sensory experiences, illusions, and hallucinations.

LSD is among the most potent drugs known, requiring only about 300 micrograms in an adult to produce dramatic effects on brain function. The altered perceptions, which begin about 45 minutes

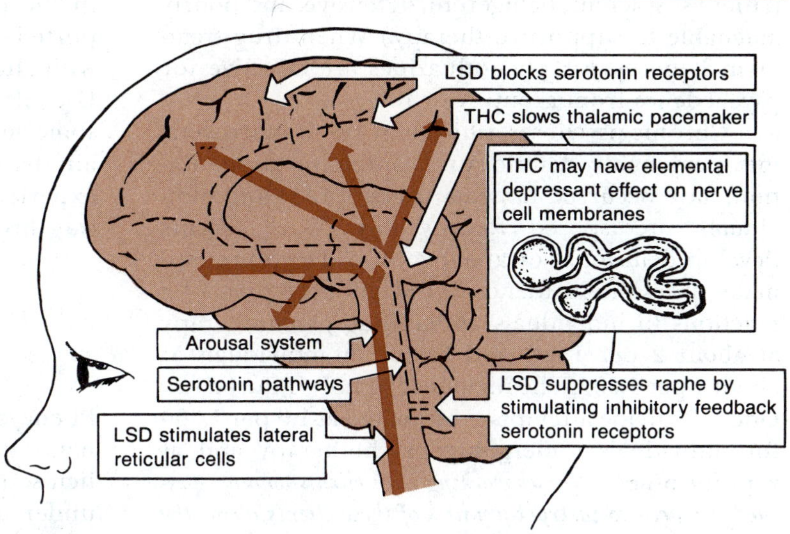

Figure 15–1
Mechanisms of the psychedelics lysergic acid diethylamide (LSD) and tetrahydrocannabinol (THC). From A. K. Swonger and L. L. Constantine, *Drugs and Therapy*, 2nd ed. Boston: Little, Brown, 1983.

after ingestion, may last as long as 18–24 hours. The subject who feels secure in the altered state may perceive the environment as unusually meaningful and beautiful and may experience an extraordinary degree of harmony between self and the environment, with a diminished capacity to distinguish the two. Sensory distortions, particularly of vision, may occupy the subject's attention. Nurses would notice that the individual is unable to maintain a conversation and is distracted frequently and easily. The individual's mood changes readily from gaiety to gravity; purposive behavior is disrupted and sleep is delayed.

The subjective and behavioral effects of psychedelic drugs depend more on influences of **mental set** and **environmental setting** than do the effects of other drugs. Mental set refers to the psychological state of the individual at the time the drug is taken. Health care professionals have noted that individuals whose lives are in turmoil or those with weak egos or unusual degrees of repressed anxiety or self-recrimination are likely to have negative or even frightening experiences. Those with well-established personality structures and positive self-concepts are more likely to have positive experiences, profoundly moving, and even mystical experiences of oneness with the universe. Similarly, a warm, supportive environment will encourage a positive experience, while a threatening or depersonalized setting, such as a laboratory, or panic-provoking circumstances, such as being given the drug without one's knowledge, frequently produce negative reactions, sometimes to the point of suicide. Perhaps the most widely publicized episode in the last category was the 1953 suicide of a biochemist, Dr. Frank Olson, less than 2 weeks after LSD was slipped into his after-dinner drink without his knowledge, by operatives of the Central Intelligence Agency as an experiment. Dr. Olson had a panic reaction, was taken to New York City Hospital for psychiatric care, and jumped out of a tenth story window. It was not until 1975 that the episode was uncovered and the circumstances clarified to the distraught family.

Adverse Effects The major risk with LSD is not the much publicized but unsubstantiated possibility of chromosomal damage, but the possibility of acute or chronic toxic psychoses. An acute psychotic episode, **hallucinogen hallucinosis,** will usually last no longer than 24 hours and will be characterized by (1) perceptual changes (intensification of perceptions, depersonalization, illusions, and hallucinations, (2) physical symptoms (dilation of the pupils, tachycardia, sweating, tremors, incoordination, palpitations, or blurred vision), and (3) maladaptive behaviors (marked anxiety or depression, fear of going crazy, paranoid ideation, impaired judgment or functioning). Nurses working with a client who is having a toxic psychosis should try to establish a supportive, empathic relationship. Friends or family should be called on to provide emotional support, especially if there is no prior relationship between the client and the medical personnel.

Individuals on LSD tend to be sensitive to positive or negative demeanor or suggestions by those around them, so it is often possible to provide the needed support through nondrug therapy. (This is in distinct contrast to PCP, which often makes the patient suspicious, belligerent, defensive, and poorly amenable to supportive therapy.) When drug treatment is necessary, phenothiazines are effective for psychedelics from group A or B.

Chronic psychoses, which may result in irreversible personality deterioration and institutionalization, have occurred in heavy users of LSD and individuals predisposed to psychosis. Such clients develop delusional or affective disorders. One estimate places the incidence of LSD-induced psychotic reactions in individuals undergoing psychotherapy at about 2 per 1,000 and for other individuals at about 1 per 1,000. The incidence of LSD-induced suicides or suicide attempts is estimated at 1.6 per 1,000 for individuals undergoing psychotherapy and at zero for others. *Nurses working with clients who use psychedelics need to instruct families of these clients about the signs and symptoms that might indicate an individual is considering suicide.*

Another troublesome aspect of LSD is the oft-reported phenomenon of flashback. A flashback is a spontaneous recurrence of an LSD experience days, weeks, or months later, even though the drug has long since been eliminated from the body. Frequency and circumstances in which flashbacks occur are largely unpredictable. One study indicated that they are most likely to occur while the former LSD user is experiencing psychological stress, falling asleep, using other drugs (especially stimulants), driving an automobile, or in stimulating situations, such as a rock concert. Flashbacks are most likely to occur in younger drug users. Most often, the flashbacks are perceived as threatening, but sometimes as pleasurable. The incidence of flashback reactions diminishes with time if the individual refrains from use of psychoactive drugs.

Physical dependence does not occur with LSD and psychological dependence is weak, but tolerance is of a distinctly high order, although short-lived. "Tripping on acid" on consecutive days is not possible because tolerance is close to complete for 1–3 days after using the drug. Chronic toxic effects on body tissues have not been observed, with the exception of the brain itself (flashback or chronic toxic psychosis). Thus, the important risks to be aware of with LSD are toxic psychosis, impaired judgment leading to accidental injury, and suicide attempts.

Experimental Uses There are no important, established therapeutic uses for psychedelics. A number of uses have been explored experimentally, mostly outside the United States. These include use in alcoholism and autism, in the terminally ill, and in conjunction with psychotherapy for certain clients when repression or denial is a central element in the pathological state. Some programs have reported favorable results, but no more than occurs with alternative treatment approaches in each case. Use of LSD in treatment of alcoholism has been somewhat more extensive in Canada and Great Britain than in the United States. Typically, a single LSD experience is induced in clients approximately midway through an extensive program of psychotherapy.

PCP

Phencyclidine (PCP) use has emerged as one of the major drug problems involving young people and illicit sources. The drug is widely available and is sold under a variety of names; "angel dust," "crystal," "peace weed," "horse tranqs," "sheets," and "tic tac" are some of the more common names. The usual dosage form involves spraying PCP onto mint, oregano, parsley, or marihuana for smoking. In the last case, the combination product is called "crystal joints" or "supergrass." Because of its bad street reputation, PCP may be "passed off" as cocaine, marihuana, LSD, or mescaline.

A typical PCP intoxication, or trip, lasts 4–6 hours, but episodes lasting as long as 72 hours occur. Users have a marked decrease in sensory experiences. Touch, pain, and temperature sensations are all acutely diminished. Users often withdraw into a state of apathy marked by depression, depersonalization, and anxiety; paranoia is a frequent component. Characteristic peripheral actions, which may be an aid in differential diagnosis, include profuse sweating, elevated blood pressure, flushing, numbness, and double vision. Another characteristic is an oscillation of the eyeball (vertical or horizontal nystagmus); pupil size, however, is unaffected.

The first priority in treating PCP overdoses is monitoring and maintenance of vital functions. The most common cause of death is extreme hypertension; therefore, a short-acting antihypertensive drug may be required for control of blood pressure. Diazepam (Valium) may be given to control muscle spasms or seizures. Drug elimination may be facilitated by acidification of the urine, gastric intubation, or both. Because of paranoia and withdrawal, clients having "bad trips" caused by PCP are often unresponsive to supportive psychotherapy. Depressants, such as phenothiazines and barbiturates, can aggravate the sensory isolation and withdrawal, but haloperidol (Haldol) is sometimes employed for control of psychotic symptoms. Placing the client in a quiet, dimly lit room may be helpful. Physical restraint may be required for violent behavior.

Other True Psychedelics

Other than LSD, **dimethyltryptamine** (DMT) is the best-known drug among the substituted indoles. The subjective effects are similar to those of LSD but of shorter duration, usually only 1–2 hours. **Psilocybin** and **psilocin** are found in mushrooms such as the *Psilocybe mexicana* and *Stropharia cubensis.* Mushrooms containing these hallucinogens grow in the northwestern United States and in Central America as well as other parts of the world. **Bufotenin** is found in *Amanita muscaria,* in secretions of the skin and parotid glands of toads, and in the seeds of the *Piptadenia peregrina,* a tree found in Haiti and Venezuela. **Lysergic acid amide,** a chemical related to LSD, is found in the seeds of the morning glory (*ololiluqui*). **Harmine,** another indole psychedelic, is a commonly used laboratory drug and a constituent of a Middle Eastern plant, *Peganium harmala.*

Phenylethylamine derivatives (group B) cause marked pupillary dilation and are more likely to induce nausea and vomiting than the tryptamine derivatives, reflecting their relatively greater autonomic activity. Paranoid and aggressive responses also are more likely with this group, and sensory effects are said to be especially vivid. Blood pressure may soar because of activation of the sympathetic nervous system. Psychedelic reactions may be long-lasting — up to 72 hours. **Mescaline** is found in the peyote cactus (*Lophophora williamsii*), a plant common in the southwestern United States and Mexico. **Peyote** has been used for centuries by certain Indian tribes for religious purposes, and this use is sanctioned by U.S. federal law.

The benzilic acid ester derivatives (group D) are extremely potent central anticholinergic compounds. Large doses of the more familiar anticholinergic drugs, the belladonna alkaloids, can produce psychic manifestations, characterized by confusion, dizziness, delirium, hallucinations, and memory distortions. The benzilic acid ester derivatives, of which the most familiar is Ditran, a combination of two such derivatives, produce marked CNS as well as autonomic nervous system effects. Users have elevated blood pressure, increased heart rate, pupillary dilation, confusion, and inability to focus attention. Some users exhibit delirium, experience distortions of time and space or hallucinations, and lose contact with reality.

Cannabis

History and Sources The recorded history of use of the *Cannabis sativa* plant dates back to 2737 BC, when it was listed as a sedative in a Chinese compendium of medicines. From China, use spread to India and Pakistan, where the drug is still widely employed. From there, cannabis spread westward into Asia Minor and North Africa. Cannabis may have first reached Europe in the backpacks of the retreating Napoleonic armies after an unsuccessful campaign in North Africa at the beginning of the nineteenth century. By 1830 cannabis had been added to opium, tea, coffee, cocoa, and tobacco as recreational items for nineteenth-century Europeans. Cannabis went largely unnoticed in the United States until the late 1920s. The federal government began regulating marihuana in 1937 when it passed the Marihuana Tax Act, which placed taxes on cultivation, sale, distribution, and purchase of marihuana.

Marihuana use rose slowly but steadily through the 1950s and 1960s. In the late 1960s and early 1970s, law enforcement agencies intensified efforts to control marihuana trafficking and use. In 1973 alone nearly a half million Americans were arrested on marihuana related charges. A gradual relaxation of the laws pertaining to possession of marihuana began in the mid-1970s, along with a sharp decline in resources devoted to enforcement of marihuana laws, though fewer than a dozen states have decriminalized possession thus far.

The cannabis plant is used in two forms. *Marihuana* is the dried, chopped-up parts of the plant. *Hashish* is the more potent gum-like resin from the plant. Cannabis exists in male and female varieties (Figure 15–2). The male plant is much less active. Street names of marihuana include "smoke," "weed," "pot," "grass," and "Mary Jane." Marihuana cigarettes are called "joints" or "reefers."

Cannabis potency varies. Assessment of the extent of drug influence that an individual experiences must therefore take into account not only the frequency of use but also the nature of the product being employed. Concentration of active ingredients differs from one plant part to another. Roots, seeds, and large stems have little or no activity; leaves have more. The flowering tops, or bracts, of the female plant and the plant resin are most potent. Marihuana from which seeds and stems have been removed is more potent, while marihuana low in bracts is weak. Other factors influencing marihuana potency include genetics, climate, and the time it is picked in relation to the growing season. Generally, marihuana grown near the equator, where the season is long, and picked late in the season is strongest. Marihuana potency also varies from year to year.

Mechanisms and Effects The cannabis plant contains several active substances. The main one

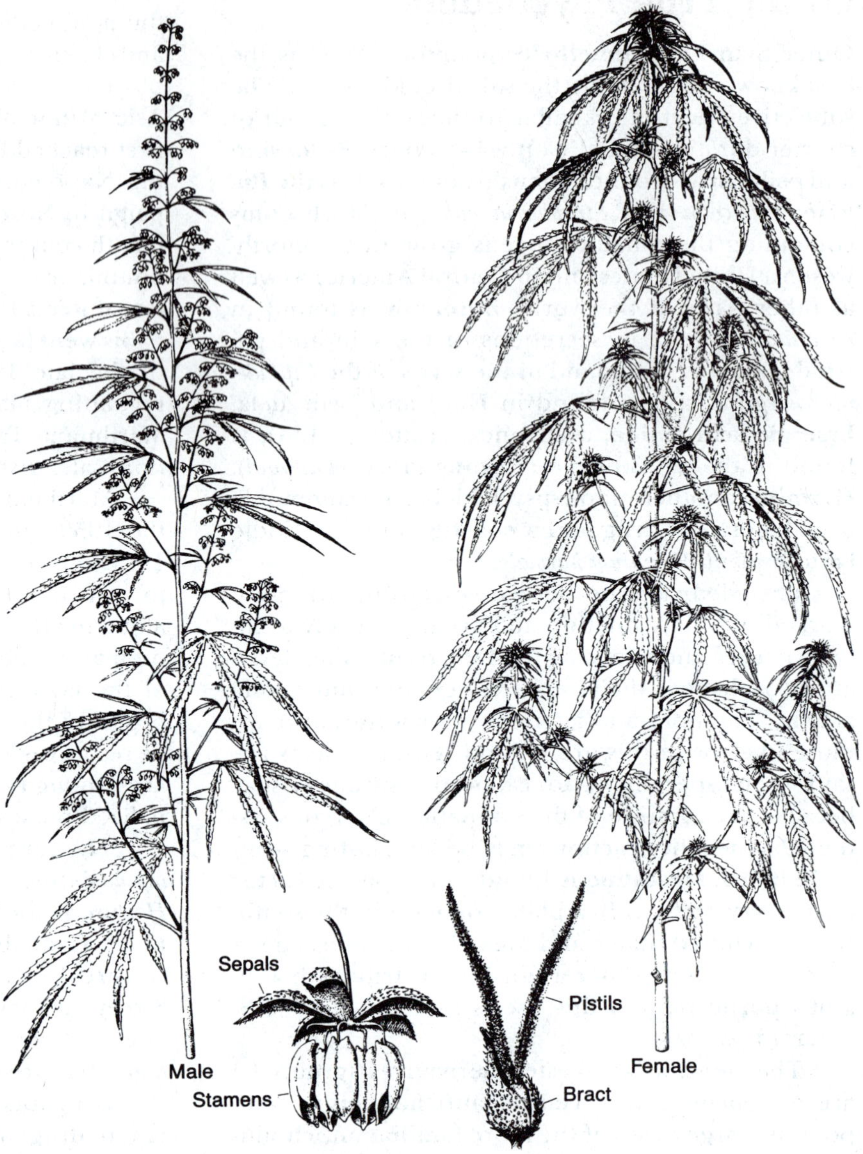

Figure 15–2
Hemp (*Cannabis sativa*) is a common weed in many parts of the world, where it is used as a medicine, an intoxicant, and a source of fiber. It is classified as a dioecious plant, that is, the male reproductive parts are on one individual (left) and the female parts are on another (right). Details of the two types of flower are shown at bottom. The active substances in the drug are contained in a sticky yellow resin that covers the flower clusters and top leaves of the female plant when it is ripe. Modified from L. Grinspoon, Marihuana. *Sci. Am. 221:* 17–25, 1969. © 1969 by Scientific American, Inc. All rights reserved.

contributing to subjective effects in humans is called Δ^9-THC (or by another system of nomenclature, Δ^1-THC). Two other active components are Δ^8-THC (Δ^6-THC) and cannabinol. Another ingredient, cannabidiol, has an antagonistic action, diminishing the psychic effects.

Cannabis has anticholinergic properties that contribute to some of its effects. Memory impairment, for example, is probably an anticholinergic action on the hippocampus (see Figure 15–1). The euphoriant effect may relate to another cholinergic brain area, the septal region (or "pleasure center"), which increases its firing rate in response to cannabis. Another aspect of the effect of marihuana is a low-level anesthetic action, related to marihuana's ability to increase fluidization of cell membranes, which impairs neural function.

Some pharmacologists classify cannabis and its major active constituent, tetrahydrocannabinol (THC), as a sedative rather than a psychedelic. Like sedatives and unlike LSD, cannabis prolongs barbiturate sleeping time; however, unlike sedatives, cannabis prolongs amphetamine-induced stimulation as does LSD. Cannabis produces classic psychedelic effects, such as intensification of perceptions and sensations of slowed time, but, like the sedatives, it causes dose-dependent apathy, ataxia, and somnolence. Thus cannabis does not fit perfectly into either group, but rather shares some properties with each. The one drug in the pharmacological arsenal most like cannabis is nitrous oxide ("laughing gas").

Cannabis produces sedation, ataxia, euphoria, intensification of perceptions, slowing of time, and sensory distortions. Maladaptive behaviors may occur, such as anxiety, suspiciousness, paranoid ideation, or impaired judgment or functioning. Appetite is increased and dryness of mouth occurs. Spontaneous activity generally decreases, hypothermia occurs, and corneal reflex is suppressed. Heart rate is quickened, which may be experienced as palpitations. A drooping of the eyelids (ptosis) and conjunctival swelling are characteristic signs of cannabis intoxication.

Adverse Effects Marihuana use causes apathy; adolescents who use the drug during school hours or during study time are likely to be poorly motivated toward school work. Marihuana also lowers testosterone levels in males and causes leukopenia. Heavy use of marihuana by adolescent males may result in breast enlargement. Marihuana smoke is more carcinogenic than tobacco smoke on a per cigarette basis. Marihuana may promote fetal abnormalities when used by women during pregnancy.

The issue of tolerance to cannabis is complex. The peripheral effects (on heart rate, for example) undergo normal tolerance with habitual marihuana use, but the psychic effects undergo a reverse or negative tolerance, so that regular users require smaller doses to "get high" than do occasional users. Factors that may contribute to negative tolerance include (1) more efficient extraction of THC by experienced users (by inhaling deeper and holding the drug longer in the lungs), (2) learned cooperation with the drug's effect by getting "in the mood," (3) tolerance to the depressant effects of marihuana without tolerance to the euphoric effect, (4) accumulation of marihuana in the body with daily use because of its high lipid solubility and extended half-life, and (5) chronic changes in the brain that increase sensitivity to the drug.

There is no physical dependence or withdrawal syndrome with chronic use of cannabis. Psychological dependence occurs in some users in much the same way that a percentage of alcohol users become dependent. Acute toxic psychosis (a delusional syndrome) is rare with marihuana but may occur with hashish. The number of active marihuana users in the United States (those employing the drug during the most recent 30-day period) is probably about 15–20 million.

Medical Uses of THC THC has two established medical uses. The most valuable use is for reducing nausea associated with cancer chemotherapy. THC is as good or better for this purpose than the conventional drug, prochlorperazine (Compazine). THC became commercially available as an antinausea agent in 1985 as dronabinol (Marinol). Marihuana and THC have been used for treating glaucoma that is refractory to the conventional first choice drug, pilocarpine.

Case Study: Bad Trip

E. P. was a 26-year-old white male living in a small apartment with several others in the inner city. He was well known to the street clinic, having come in on several previous occasions for help. E. P.'s father had left his mother when E. P. was still a child. His mother died when he was 12 and he lived with his grandparents until he finished high school. E. P. began using alcohol and marihuana in high school. After high school he married and had one child, but was left by his wife when he began using psychedelics frequently. He then moved into the neighborhood where he now resides. He continued use of LSD for several months while taking odd jobs and burglarizing apartments. One day, E. P. bought some STP from a dealer and experienced an acute psychotic reaction to the drug. When E. P. came to the clinic for help, he was extremely dysphoric, stating over and over again that he felt as if his mind were falling apart. He was hallucinating and confused. He stated that he wanted to kill himself.

The physician at the clinic examined E. P. and observed that his pupils were dilated, his pulse and blood pressure were elevated, and respiration was normal. There was no evidence of nystagmus or ptosis. The physician learned that E. P. believed the drug he was on was STP; the physician knew that this drug was readily available at that time. E. P.'s previous visits had not indicated use of depressants or narcotics. The physician administered 25 mg of chlorpromazine, IM, and spoke reassuringly with E. P.

1. What drug has the street name STP? How is it classified?

2. Which of the observations from the physical assessment suggest that the drug responsible for E. P.'s reaction was indeed STP or a related psychedelic rather than PCP, a barbiturate, or a narcotic?
3. Was chlorpromazine administration an appropriate response to E. P.'s condition? Chlorpromazine would be contraindicated if the toxic psychosis were due to what other street drugs?
4. The physician knew that, in the long run, treating the repeated episodes of toxic responses to drugs was not going to solve E. P.'s problem. What approach would you consider most likely to have a positive effect in moving E. P. toward more permanent resolution of his drug problem?

Answers appear at the end of the book.

Recommended Readings

LSD

Martin WR, Sloan, JW: Pharmacology and classification of LSD-like hallucinogens, in Martin WR (ed): *Drug Addiction.* Berlin, Springer-Verlag, 1977, vol II: *Amphetamine, Psychotogen, and Marihuana Dependence (Handbuch der Experimentellen Pharmakologie Vol 45. pt 2).*

Sankar DVS (ed): *LSD — A Total Study.* Westbury, NY, PJD Publishers Ltd, 1975.

Vardy MM, Kay SR: LSD psychosis or LSD-induced schizophrenia? *Arch Gen Psychiatry* 1983;40:877–883.

Marihuana

Branda MC, Szara S (eds): *Pharmacology of Marijuana.* New York, Raven Press, 1976.

Fehr KO, Kalant H (eds): *Cannabis and Health Hazards.* Toronto, The Addiction Research Foundation, 1983.

Harris LS: Cannabis: A review of progress. In Lipton MA et al (eds): *Psychopharmacology: A Generation of Progress.* New York, Raven Press, 1978.

Jones RT: Cannabis and health. *Annu Rev Med* 1983; 34:247–258.

Kandel, DB: Marijuana users in young adulthood. *Arch Gen Psychiatry* 1984;41:200–209.

Perez-Reyes et al: Comparison of effects of marihuana cigarettes of three different potencies. *Clin Pharmacol Ther* 1982;31:617–624.

Peterson RC (ed): *Marijuana Research Findings.* National Institute on Drug Abuse Research Monograph, 1980, p 31.

Phencyclidine

Balster RL, Chait LD: The behavioral pharmacology of phencyclidine. *Clin Toxicol* 1976;9:513–528.

Kamenka J-M, Domino EF, Geneste P (eds): *Phencyclidine and Related Arylcyclohexylamines: Present and Future Applications.* Ann Arbor, Mich, NPP Books, 1983.

McCoy S, Rice M, McFadden K: PCP intoxication: Psychiatric issues of nursing care. *J Psychiatr Nurs* 1981;19:17–23.

Peterson RC, Stillman RC (eds): *Phencyclidine (PCP) abuse: An appraisal.* National Institute on Drug Abuse Research Monograph GPO No. 017-024-00785-4, 1978, p 21.

Other Psychedelics

Efron DH, Holmstedt B, Kline NS (eds): *Ethnopharmacologic Search for Psychoactive Drugs.* Public Health Service Publication No 1645, 1967.

Schnoll SH et al: Street PCP scene: Issues on synthesis and contamination. *J Psychedelic Drugs* 1980;12(3–4):229–233.

UNIT III

Drugs and the Central Nervous System

PART C

Anesthesia and Anesthetics

CHAPTER 16

General Anesthetics and Adjunctives

Mechanisms of Anesthetic Action

General anesthesia is a reversible depression of the nervous system employed to alleviate sensitivity to pain during surgical procedures. Modern anesthesia dates from the middle of the nineteenth century, when the anesthetic potential of ether was dramatically demonstrated by William T. Morton at Massachusetts General Hospital (see the box on page 229). Prior to Morton's demonstration, surgery had been a terrifying and painful undertaking, although even in ancient times efforts were made to spare the victim excruciating pain. The ancient Egyptians employed narcotics and the ancient Chinese utilized hashish. The Assyrians used asphyxiation by strangulation. Such techniques generally failed to produce an adequate level of anesthesia. Morton's demonstration of ether anesthesia in 1846 was followed by successful use of chloroform in England in 1847. Colton introduced nitrous oxide in 1844 for dental surgery and revived its use in the 1860s. Ether, chloroform, and nitrous oxide remained the trio of anesthetics until well into the twentieth century. Ethylene was added after 1923, cyclopropane and barbiturates in the 1930s. The most widely used general anesthetic of today, halothane (Fluothane), is a relative newcomer, added in the early 1960s.

Although the mechanisms of general anesthetics are not fully elucidated, some aspects of their action are known. The lipid solubility of anesthetics is important to their efficacy, since there is a near perfect correlation between anesthetic potency and lipid solubility. In the brain, general anesthetics are con-

The Emergence of Modern Anesthesia

Before the advent of general anesthetics, surgery was a horrifying event in which haste was as much an objective as achieving the anatomical adjustment. In 1776 in England, ether was discovered by Joseph Priestley, who described its effects as "an highly pleasurable thrilling." Nitrous oxide was discovered in 1799 by Humphrey Davy who noted its ability to inhibit pain sensations. Although Davy suggested the use of nitrous oxide for surgical procedures, the idea was not acted upon until 1842. In the early nineteenth century, Faraday published a report (1818) describing ether analgesia in animals, and Hickman (1824) introduced the notion of "suspended animation" based on studies of the influence of carbon dioxide and hypoxia on animals.

In 1842 Crawford W. Long, a physician of Jefferson, Georgia, used ether on several occasions in his surgical practice but did not publish his experience with the drug. At about the same time a traveling chemist named Colton was touring the New England states giving demonstrations of the effects of nitrous oxide, called *laughing gas.* He organized grand demonstrations in which nitrous oxide was administered to volunteers from the audience. Strong men were hired to occupy the front rows in the event that a recipient of the gas should become rowdy.

In one such demonstration in 1844 at Hartford, Connecticut, a dentist named Horace Wells was in attendance. A drug clerk by the name of Cooley was administered nitrous oxide and became confused and belligerent. He jumped from the platform to fight with one of the strong men hired by Colton, but the strong man promptly fled with Cooley in pursuit. Cooley, however, tripped over a chair and, stunned, he came to his senses. In the excitement, Cooley had not noticed that he had gashed his leg quite severely in his fall and was surprised to observe that he felt no pain from the wound. Wells was standing nearby and questioned Cooley regarding the lack of pain sensitivity. The next day, Wells, with the aid of Colton, had one of his teeth extracted by an assistant under nitrous oxide anesthesia. After the procedure, Wells declared that this method would usher in "a new era in tooth-pulling!" Wells continued to use nitrous oxide in his dental practice, and in January 1845 he traveled to Massachusetts General Hospital in Boston to demonstrate his discovery. Unfortunately for Wells, the procedure failed. The patient came out of anesthesia before the surgery was complete, screaming in pain. Wells was ridiculed and, eclipsed by later events, finally committed suicide in despair.

Anesthesia was established as a recognized medical procedure by William T. G. Morton. Morton was a dentist who had worked with Wells, developing an interest not only in use of nitrous oxide but also

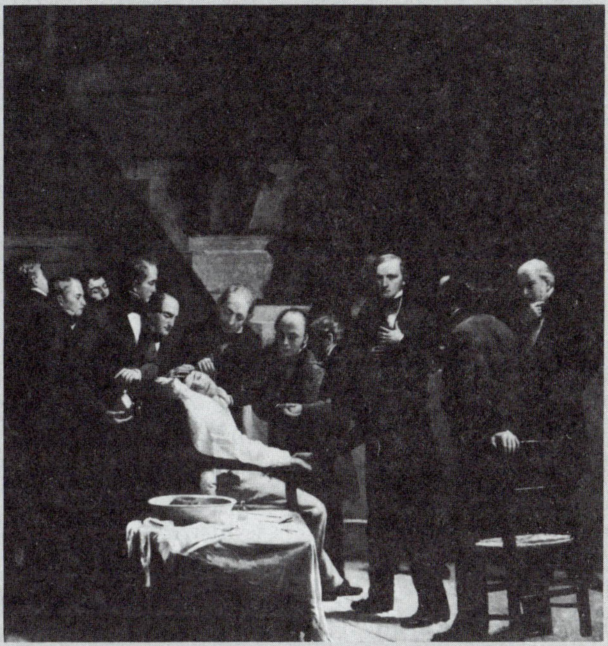

First demonstration of ether anesthesia by W. T. Morton in Ether Dome, Massachusetts General Hospital, Boston, October 16, 1846. Painting by Robert Hinckley. Used courtesy of the Boston Medical Library in The Francis A. Countway Library of Medicine.

ether. He entered Harvard Medical School as a medical student and continued his dental practice to help pay his expenses. Morton practiced with ether on various animals, his pet dog, and even himself, and ultimately employed the drug to extract a tooth. Finally, confident of his method, he requested and received permission to publically demonstrate his discovery in a surgical procedure to the faculty and students of the medical school. The date was October 16, 1846.

A roomful of doubtful and skeptical spectators had gathered in the operating room (now memorialized as "ether dome") in Massachusetts General Hospital to watch what they imagined would be the debunking of the preposterous claim of a presumptuous second year medical student. The patient, Gilbert Abbott, was brought in, and the surgeon, Dr. Warren, waited with the scalpel. At the appointed time, Morton still had not arrived. Fifteen more minutes passed and Dr. Warren grew impatient and irritated. Finally, he turned to the gallery saying, "As Dr. Morton has not arrived, I presume he is otherwise engaged." He then picked up his scalpel while the strong men stood ready to hold down the patient in accordance with accepted practice. Just then, Morton entered, having just completed the apparatus for administering the ether. Dr. Warren stepped back and, pointing to the patient, stated sarcastically,

(continued)

"Well, sir, your patient is ready." Surrounded by a silent and unsympathetic audience, Morton went to work and in a few minutes the patient lay quietly unconscious. Morton glanced up at the surgeon, saying, "Dr. Warren, *your* patient is ready."

The operation was performed with no sign of pain while the strong men stood idly by. At the end of the procedure, Dr. Warren turned to the incredulous audience and said, "Gentlemen, this is no humbug," and an eminent visiting surgeon in the audience, Dr. Bigelow, observed, "I have seen something today that will go around the world." And indeed it did. Within a few years, anesthesia became a worldwide medical practice.

The epitaph (furnished by Bigelow) over Morton's grave in Mt. Auburn Cemetery in Cambridge, Massachusetts, reads as follows:

William T. G. Morton
Inventor and Revealer of Anesthetic Inhalation
Before Whom, in All Time, Surgery Was Agony.
By Whom Pain in Surgery Was Averted and Annulled.
Since Whom Science Has Control of Pain.

centrated in the lipid-rich membranes of neurons (Figure 16–1). As the anesthetic dissolves in the membrane, it changes the membrane's physical characteristics, altering fluidity, volume, or both, which inhibits the opening of sodium channels. Since opening of sodium channels is instrumental in the ability of neurons to depolarize, anesthetics reversibly suppress the electrical excitability of neurons throughout the brain. The result is anesthetic coma.

Pharmacokinetics

Anesthesia requires that concentrations of the anesthetic in the central nervous system reach a critical level. Anesthetics given by inhalation pass from the alveoli of the lungs into the blood of pulmonary capillaries by passive diffusion and are then transported to all tissues. Concentrations of anesthetic build up rapidly in the brain because the brain is highly vascularized and because anesthetics dissolve readily in the lipid membranes of nerve cells. By controlling the concentration of anesthetic that is inhaled, the anesthesiologist can regulate the concentration of anesthetic in the brain, and thus the depth of anesthesia. Later, when administration of the anesthetic is discontinued, anesthetics are eliminated from the body mainly unchanged in exhaled air. As blood levels of the anesthetic decline, the molecules of anesthetic in brain tissue passively diffuse into the blood, ultimately reaching the lungs for elimination.

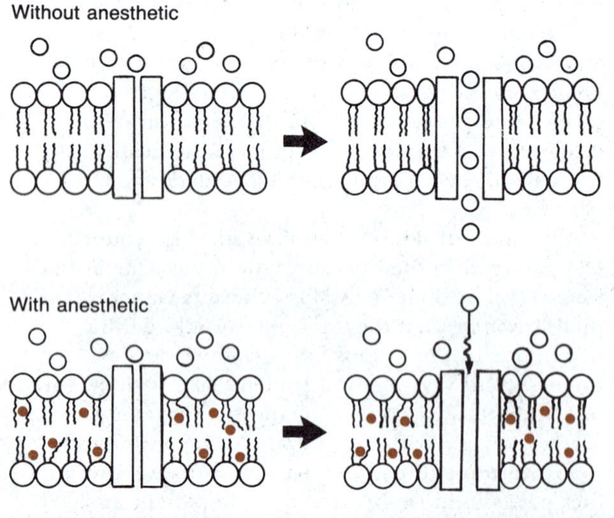

Figure 16–1
Mechanism of general anesthesia. In the absence of anesthesia (top), ion channels in cell membranes open freely in response to stimulation by nerve impulses; influx of ions then perpetuates the wave of excitation. When an anesthetic is administered (bottom), the molecules of anesthetic dissolve in the cell membrane and prevent the channels from opening, inhibiting excitability.

Stages of Anesthesia

Anesthesia is a dose-dependent phenomenon; the depth of anesthesia is determined by the concentration of anesthetic in the brain. As anesthesia deepens, the anesthetized individual passes through recognizable states (Figure 16–2). The stages of anesthesia were originally defined for ether by Guedel (Table 16–1). Other general anesthetics differ from ether with respect to which stages occur and how long each stage lasts, but the effects during a given stage are similar regardless of the drug being employed. The stages of anesthesia are best indicated by changes in respiration, pulse rate, blood pressure, reflexes, pupil size, and eye movements.

Stage I extends from the beginning of anesthesia to loss of consciousness. During this stage, analgesia occurs. Since the patient remains conscious, he or she can verbally report on the depth of anesthesia.

Stage II is marked by irregular respiration and delirium. The patient is unconscious but exhibits involuntary activity, frequently of an agitated and ex-

Figure 16–2
The cortical EEG pattern (in a cat) representative of each stage of anesthesia. Reproduced with permission, from Winter, W., Effects of Drugs on the Electrical Activity of the Brain: Anesthetics. *Ann. Rev. Pharmacol. Toxicol. 16:* 413–426, 1976. ©1976 by Annual Reviews Inc.

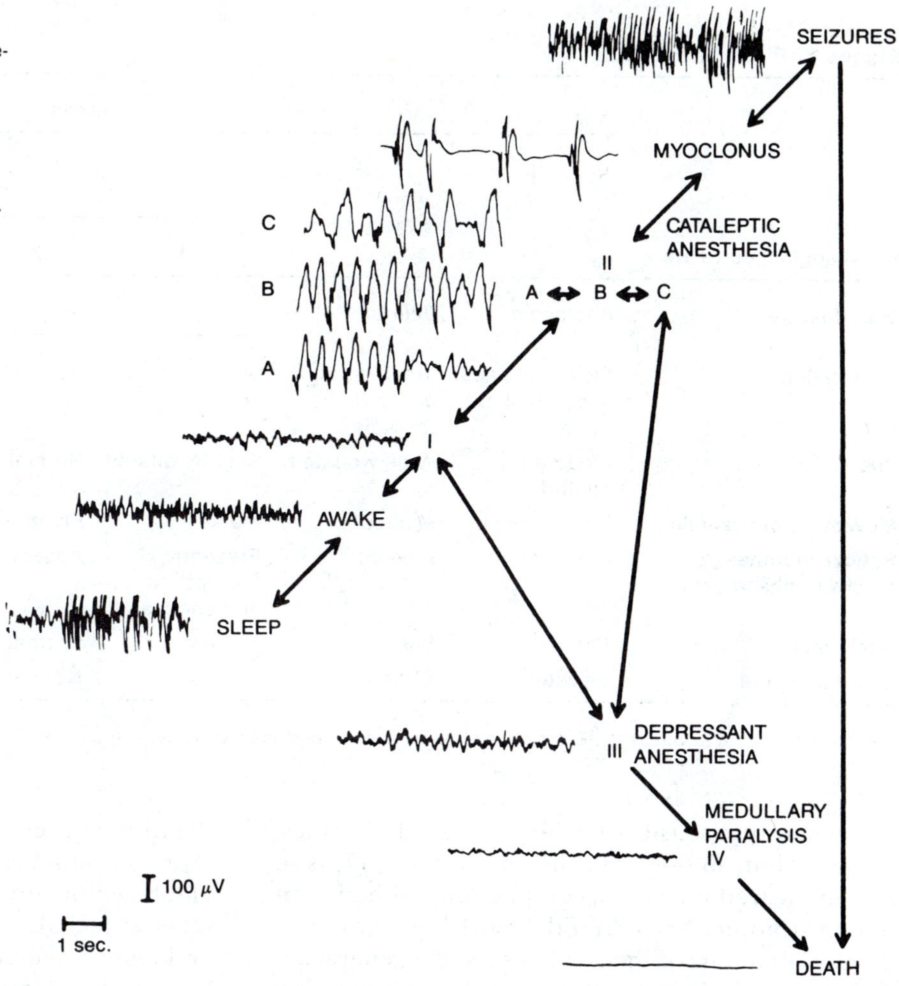

cited nature, with shouting and laughing or possibly urination, defecation, or vomiting. Stage II is a problem stage and is kept to a minimum. A revision of the Guedel stages of anesthesia proposed by Winter in 1976 divides stage II into three substages: IIA, IIB, and IIC. Stage IIA is characterized by hallucinations but no amnesia, Stage IIB by hallucinations and amnesia, Stage IIC by catalepsy and amnesia. Stage IIC is the anesthetic state produced by dissociative anesthetics such as ketamine, enflurane, and nitrous oxide.

Stage III is the stage of anesthesia in which most surgical procedures are conducted. Respiratory irregularities disappear, and the eyelid and conjunctival reflexes are absent. Stage III is subdivided into four planes. In the first, breathing becomes regular, but the eyeballs continue to move. In the second plane, the eyes become fixed and dilated, and respiration is regular. In the third plane, some skeletal muscle relaxation occurs, but respiration is still regular. In the fourth plane, there is complete paralysis of the diaphragm, labored breathing, and loss of the corneal reflex. Plane 2 is generally used for surgical procedures and plane 3 for incisions and sewing.

In **stage IV,** the toxic stage, medullary paralysis occurs. The respiratory and vasomotor centers are depressed, leading to respiratory failure and hypotension. Medullary control of the heart is also absent.

The Ideal Anesthetic

The ideal anesthetic should be capable of producing four effects: (1) unconsciousness, (2) analgesia, (3) relaxation of skeletal muscles, and (4) depression of reflexes. It should also possess the following pharmacodynamic properties: (1) rapid induction, (2) rapid recovery following the surgical procedure, (3) pleasant, nonirritating, and nontoxic effects, (4) a high therapeutic index, (5) lack of cardiovascular effects

Table 16–1
Stages of Ether Anesthesia

	Stages						
	I	II	III Plane				IV
Physiological correlate			1	2	3	4	
Main feature	Analgesia	Delirium	Surgical Stage				Medullary Paralysis
Respiration	Slow and deep; abdominal and thoracic	Irregular; abdominal and thoracic	Slow and regular	Normal	Deep; abdominal	Shallow; abdominal	Paralysis
Pupil size	Moderately dilated	Widely dilated	Slightly dilated	Normal	Dilated	Widely dilated	Entirely dilated
Movement of eyeballs	Voluntary	Marked	Marked	Fixed	Converged	Absent	Absent
Reflexes (corneal, conjunctival, pharyngeal)	Present	Present	Present (except conjunctival)	Absent	Absent	Absent	Absent
Pusle rate	Fast	Fast	Normal	Normal	Fast	Feeble	Absent
Blood pressure	Elevated	Elevated	Normal	Normal	Falling	Falling	Low

Source: Adapted from Guedel, A. E. *Inhalation Anesthesia: A Fundamental Guide,* 2nd ed. New York: Macmillan, 1951.

and inability to sensitize the heart to catecholamines, (6) nonflammability and nonexplosiveness, (7) ease of administration, and (8) compatibility with oxygen administration. No currently available anesthetic produces all four of the ideal effects of a general anesthetic to an adequate degree, much less possessing the ideal spectrum of pharmacodynamic properties. Therefore, other drugs are employed in conjunction with anesthetics to provide the desirable effects not furnished by the anesthetic itself to achieve a **balanced anesthesia.** Drugs employed in conjunction with anesthesia are called **preanesthetics** when given before anesthesia, or **adjunctives** when given with or during anesthesia.

General Anesthetics

General anesthetics are divided into three groups based on their mode of administration and their physical form: inhalation agents that are volatile liquids, inhalation agents that are gaseous, and intravenous agents. Characteristics of the inhalation agents are compared in Table 16–2.

Inhalation Agents — Volatile Liquids

The volatile liquid anesthetics include ethyl ether, chloroform, halothane (Fluothane), methoxyflurane (Penthrane), enflurane (Ethrane), and isoflurane (Forane). Ethyl ether and chloroform are no longer employed in clinical practice, but both of these, and ether especially, are important to the history of general anesthesia. Ether is included here because of its historical importance, but some instructors may elect to omit discussion of it.

Ethyl Ether

Ethyl ether (also called diethyl ether or, simply, ether) was the first general anesthetic and the most widely used in clinical practice for 100 years after its introduction. Ether anesthesia proceeds through all four stages. Ether is called a *complete anesthetic* because it can produce a full stage IV anesthesia without oxygen deprivation. An advantage of ether is the lack of significant cardiac effects prior to respiratory arrest, giving ether a margin of safety with respect to cardiac toxicity. There is little decrease in blood pressure, even when the myocardium is finally depressed, because ether stimulates compensatory release of catecholamines. In stage III, ether produces a level of relaxation of skeletal muscles and uterine smooth muscle that is entirely adequate for surgical procedures. The relaxant effect on skeletal muscles is additive with that produced by curare and other neuromuscular blockers. Ether causes little or no liver impairment and is inexpensive.

In spite of the positive features, ether is no

Table 16–2
Comparison of Inhalation Agents

Drug	Induction	MAC[a] (%)	Useful properties: Muscle relaxation	Useful properties: Analgesia	Adverse effects: Cardiovascular effects	Adverse effects: Other
Inhalation agents—volatile liquids						
Ethyl ether	Slow	1.92	Excellent	Excellent	Minimal	Nausea and vomiting during recovery; irritation of respiratory tract
Halothane	Rapid	0.77	Fair	Poor	Hypotension; sensitizes heart to catecholamines	Hepatitis
Methoxyflurane	Slow	0.16	Good	Excellent	Hypotension	Renal impairment
Enflurane	Rapid	1.68	Good	Excellent	Hypotension; sensitizes heart to catecholamines	Hypothermia and shivering, renal impairment
Isoflurane	Rapid	1.3	Good	Excellent	Minimal	Hyperthermia; respiratory depression
Inhalation agents—gaseous						
Nitrous oxide	Very rapid	101%	None	Good	Minimal	Hypoxemia: use with 20% oxygen
Cyclopropane	Very rapid	9.2	Good	Good	Minimal hypotension due to compensatory sympathoadrenal activation; sensitizes heart to catecholamines	Nausea, vomiting, headache, and delirium during emergence
Ethylene	Rapid	—	Poor	Poor	Minimal	Hypoxia

[a]Minimum alveolar concentration (at 1 atmosphere pressure) that prevents response to a pain stimulus in 50% of subjects.

longer used because of significant disadvantages. Most important, ether is irritating to the respiratory tract, which results in a reflexive stimulation of respiratory secretions. As a result, atropine was frequently required in conjunction with ether anesthesia to inhibit respiratory secretory activity.

Another disadvantage of ether is that stage II, the problem stage, is especially prominent. Simultaneous or initial administration of another anesthetic with ether was often required as a means of hastening induction to reduce stage II of anesthesia. Use of ether for surgery was also associated with considerable nausea and vomiting during the period of recovery. Ether is also flammable and explosive, necessitating care in handling, although the safety record with ether was excellent in the last few decades of its use.

Halothane (Fluothane, Generic)

Mechanisms and Effects Halothane, a widely used and potent anesthetic, is a nonflammable halogenated hydrocarbon ($CF_3CHClBr$) that can be administered safely with oxygen and with nitrous oxide. Induction and recovery are rapid, with little or no stage II. Clients given halothane anesthesia rarely develop nausea and vomiting. In addition, halothane does not irritate the respiratory tract and therefore causes no increase in a patient's bronchial secretions or salivation. Pharyngeal and laryngeal reflexes are suppressed by halothane. Halothane causes bronchodilation, a positive feature for anesthesia, especially in asthmatic individuals.

Adverse Effects and Contraindications With deep anesthesia, halothane may cause hypoxia and acidosis from respiratory depression. At concentrations in excess of 2%, halothane depresses the myocardium and the medullary cardiac center, which results in hypotension and reduced force of contraction in the heart and may cause sinoatrial nodal bradycardia and other cardiac dysrhythmias. Halothane also sensitizes the myocardium to the action of the catecholamines — norepinephrine and epinephrine. Administration of sympathomimetic pressor agents during halothane anesthesia may result in cardiac dysrhythmias. Halothane is not an effective analgesic and produces only a fair degree of muscle relaxation. Both analgesics and neuromuscular blockers are often employed as adjunctives with halothane.

Hepatic dysfunction and necrosis has occurred after halothane anesthesia, but it is not clear that halothane at normal dosage levels produces hepatic toxicity with greater frequency than other anesthetics. Exposure to high concentrations of halothane or repeated exposure to normal anesthetic concentrations has been related to occurrence of a hypersensitivity reaction that leads to hepatic damage. Individuals who exhibit signs of allergic sensitivity (fever, anorexia, prolonged nausea or vomiting, or jaundice) following halothane anesthesia should not be given the drug again.

Administration Halothane is usually employed in conjunction with nitrous oxide and a skeletal muscle relaxant. Nitrous oxide hastens induction, reduces the concentration of halothane required for surgical anesthesia, provides improved analgesia, and reduces the risks of halothane toxicity by lowering the dose of halothane required. A concentration of 0.5–1.5% of halothane is employed for maintenance of anesthesia.

Methoxyflurane (Penthrane)

Mechanisms and Effects Methoxyflurane is another halogenated hydrocarbon ($CHCl_2CF_2$-OCH_3), like halothane, that is nonflammable. It is a clear and colorless liquid that possesses a characteristic fruity odor. Methoxyflurane is the most potent of the general anesthetics currently available. It produces stages I–IV of anesthesia.

Nursing Observations for General Anesthesia

THERAPEUTIC GOAL	Preanesthetic comfort; unconsciousness, analgesia, areflexia, and muscle relaxation during surgery; postanesthetic recovery of vital functions, organ system functions, and wound healing.
PREADMINISTRATION ASSESSMENT	
Baseline Data	Observe patient in the preoperative phase for indications of undue tension. Observe in the postoperative phase for recovery of vital signs, airway clearance, and return of normal bladder and intestinal function. Evaluate condition of incision wound, vital signs, and patency of airways. Obtain laboratory tests as required by the specific surgical procedure.
EVALUATION OF DRUG RESPONSE	
During Anesthesia	The stages and planes of anesthesia are determined by monitoring level of consciousness, analgesia, depth and quality of respiration, reflexes, eye movements, pupillary diameter, and blood pressure.
For Adverse Effects	Monitor vital signs and urinary and intestinal function.
For Drug Interactions	Monitor for additive CNS depression or neuromuscular blockade postoperatively from residual anesthetic and postanesthetic medications.
For Dietary Interactions	Monitor for nutritional deficiency due to elevated requirements associated with wound healing and decreased intake due to anorexia, nausea, vomiting, or restrictions.
For Compliance	Evaluate patient compliance with all facets of the therapeutic regimen by careful observation, interviewing, and review of progress. Report compliance problems to the physician and act as patient-advocate when changes in the therapeutic regimen seem indicated.

Methoxyflurane is indicated for full surgical anesthesia, usually with oxygen and nitrous oxide, when the anticipated duration of anesthesia is 4 hours or less. It is also indicated at lower concentration for light levels of anesthesia. Methoxyflurane provides good analgesia but only poor skeletal muscle relaxation when used alone in low concentrations. Skeletal muscle relaxants are therefore often employed concomitantly. During recovery from methoxyflurane anesthesia, analgesia and drowsiness may persist after consciousness is regained, reducing the need for analgesics.

Adverse Effects and Contraindications When used alone, methoxyflurane induces anesthesia only slowly. Nitrous oxide (in oxygen) or thiopental (Pentothal) is often used to improve the rate of induction and to reduce the dose of methoxyflurane, which minimizes the risk of adverse reactions. Methoxyflurane causes appreciable respiratory depression in moderate to high concentrations; thus, respiratory assistance may be required to prevent respiratory acidosis. Cardiovascular depression can also occur at high concentrations.

Methoxyflurane can produce hepatic dysfunction and necrosis due to release of fluoride ion, but bronchoconstriction and laryngospasms do not typically occur. Occasionally, methoxyflurane triggers malignant hyperthermia, for which dantrolene is used in prophylaxis and treatment.

Administration Methoxyflurane (Penthrane) is given in concentrations up to 2% for induction of anesthesia, and at 0.1–0.2% for maintenance.

Enflurane (Ethrane)

Mechanisms and Effects Enflurane (Ethrane) is another potent and nonflammable halogenated hydrocarbon (CHF_2OCF_2CHFCl) resembling halothane. Enflurane provides rapid induction and recovery but does not produce significant respiratory depression until deep anesthesia is achieved. Muscle relaxation produced by enflurane is better than with halothane, but skeletal muscle relaxants are usually required to provide adequate paralysis. The level of anesthesia produced by enflurane has a tendency to change abruptly, resulting in difficulty controlling anesthesia and maintaining adequate respiration.

Adverse Effects and Contraindications Enflurane stimulates salivary and tracheobronchial secretions to a mild extent, but the effect is not excessive. Cardiovascular effects are minimal until deep anesthesia is achieved, then hypotension occurs. Cardiac rhythm is stable, and significant bradycardia is not observed. Like methoxyflurane, enflurane releases fluoride ions, which can result in hepatotoxicity and malignant hyperthermia. Enflurane is sometimes employed to provide analgesia for vaginal deliveries or with other anesthetics for cesarean section. However, high concentrations of enflurane should be avoided since these can cause uterine relaxation and bleeding.

Administration Enflurane is administered in concentrations of 2–4.5% for induction (which requires 7–10 minutes) and at 0.5–3% for maintenance.

Isoflurane (Forane)

Mechanisms and Effects Isoflurane is an isomer of enflurane and a potent anesthetic. It produces rapid induction and recovery. It is a good skeletal muscle relaxant, requiring supplementation with only small doses of neuromuscular blockers, and is effective in suppressing pharyngeal and laryngeal reflexes without stimulating respiratory secretions to a significant extent. Isoflurane is mildly pungent, which limits the rate at which it can be administered, but induction can be achieved in 7–10 minutes.

Adverse Effects and Contraindications Isoflurane causes considerable respiratory depression, requiring close monitoring of respiratory function. Mechanical support may be required when isoflurane is used alone. If nitrous oxide is employed concurrently, the concentration of isoflurane can be reduced, with the result that respiratory depression is minimal. When respiration is maintained at a level sufficient to ensure a normal arterial P_{CO_2}, cardiac output remains normal although stroke volume is diminished and rate compensatorily increased. Isoflurane does not sensitize the heart to catecholamines. Malignant hyperthermia has occurred in response to isoflurane anesthesia as with other general anesthetics.

Administration Isoflurane is administered for induction at concentrations of 1.5–3%. For maintenance, concentrations of 1.0–2.5% can sustain anesthesia when nitrous oxide is used concomitantly.

Inhalation Agents — Gases

Nitrous Oxide

Mechanisms and Effects Nitrous oxide (also known as "laughing gas") is a widely used general anesthetic. Because of its low potency, it is usually employed in combination with another anesthetic, a narcotic analgesic, and a skeletal muscle relaxant to achieve balanced anesthesia. When used alone, 65–70% nitrous oxide and 30–35% oxygen produces only a minimal degree of anesthesia, but good analgesia is nevertheless obtained. In fact, nitrous oxide can produce measurable analgesia at concentrations as low as 20–30%. When used in anesthetic combinations, nitrous oxide permits use of lesser concentrations of primary anesthetics such as halothane or methoxyflurane because of its excellent analgesic properties. Thus, overall cardiac depression is less when the balanced anesthesia approach is employed.

Pharmacological effects of nitrous oxide are not profound. There is no appreciable skeletal muscle relaxation, respiratory minute volume is slightly increased, and used alone, nitrous oxide has little effect on cardiac function. If used with halothane or methoxyflurane, however, it may add slightly to the depression of cardiac output, cardiac rate, and arterial pressure. Nitrous oxide does not sensitize the heart to catecholamines.

Adverse Effects and Contraindications Adverse reactions to nitrous oxide occur only if hypoxemia ensues — the major risk in using this drug. *Nitrous oxide should not be administered in less than 20% oxygen.* If the oxygen concentration is not adequate, confusion, convulsions, or permanent brain damage can result.

Nitrous oxide is usually pleasant and nonirritating, although vomiting may occur after high concentrations. Malignant hyperthermia can occur, as with other anesthetics, and is treated with dantrolene, a centrally acting muscle relaxant.

Administration Nitrous oxide is nonflammable and comes in blue cylinders.

Cyclopropane

Mechanisms and Effects Cyclopropane is capable of producing complete anesthesia. During induction, there is very little stage II excitation, but during recovery the patient may demonstrate excitation. Induction can be achieved in 1–2 minutes with this anesthetic.

Cyclopropane produces adequate skeletal muscle relaxation when used in concentrations that produce full surgical anesthesia. When cyclopropane is used for light anesthesia, a skeletal muscle relaxant, such as succinylcholine (Anectine) or curare, is used adjunctively to promote adequate skeletal muscle relaxation.

The major advantage of cyclopropane is that it does not cause a reduction in blood pressure; arterial pressure is either maintained or slightly increased due to sympathoadrenal activation. Like other anesthetics, the direct effect of cyclopropane on the myocardium is a depressant influence, but this is more than offset by the increase in circulating catecholamines. Cyclopropane is especially useful for anesthesia when hemorrhage or mild shock is present. Cyclopropane is thus the anesthetic of choice for patients with modestly compromised cardiovascular function.

Adverse Effects and Contraindications Patients may develop nausea and vomiting and complain of headaches. Administration of a narcotic analgesic prior to recovery will substantially reduce excitation during recovery. Cyclopropane strongly depresses the medullary respiratory center. When used to achieve full surgical anesthesia, ventilatory assistance is required, especially when narcotic analgesics are used concurrently. Cyclopropane should not be used in asthmatic patients because it can cause bronchospasm.

When cyclopropane is discontinued, rebound hypotension is sometimes observed. The elevation in circulating sympathetic amines produced by cyclopropane can cause transient hyperglycemia.

Like halothane, cyclopropane sensitizes the heart to catecholamines. Nurses may encounter clients who develop cardiac dysrhythmias because of this sensitization and the increased levels of catecholamines. They may observe ectopic beats, AV block, bigeminy rhythms, and other ventricular tachydysrhythmias. Heart rate may be slightly decreased by cyclopropane through reflexive vagal action. This effect is accentuated when morphine is used concurrently, since morphine also triggers vagal reflex activity.

Administration A major drawback with cyclopropane is its flammability and explosiveness. When cyclopropane is employed, precautions must be taken to prevent static. Electrocautery cannot be employed when the anesthetic is cyclopropane. Cyclopropane is supplied in orange cylinders.

Ethylene

Ethylene is the least used of the gaseous inhalation agents. Its chief limitations are its extreme flammability and its unpleasant odor. It provides rapid onset and recovery, adequate analgesia, but poor muscle relaxation. It does not cause significant bronchospasm or laryngospasm, and nausea and vomiting during recovery is minimal. Adverse effects occur only if hypoxemia has resulted from inadequate oxygenation. Ethylene is supplied in red cylinders

Nursing Diagnoses and Interventions for General Anesthesia

Nursing Diagnoses	*Related Interventions*
TO ENHANCE SUCCESSFUL ANESTHESIA	
Activity intolerance in the postoperative period related to pain, fatigue, and need for tissue repair	Provide ample rest and restrict activities as required.
Alteration in comfort: pain related to the surgical procedure	Provide comfort measures and analgesia as required.
Alteration in nutrition: intake less than requirements related to elevated requirements for wound healing and decreased intake due to anorexia, nausea, vomiting, or restrictions	Provide nutritional support as required. Encourage food intake that the client can tolerate in quantities acceptable to the client.
Anxiety in the preoperative period related to anticipation of surgery and uncertain outcome	Be present when the physician explains the anesthetic and surgical procedures to the patient so that you will be able to clear up any questions later; encourage patient to discuss the procedure, express feelings, and ask questions; provide diversions; keep patient active in self-care; provide comfort measures for preoperative insomnia or tension; provide analgesia as indicated; note the patient's emotional state during preoperative care; minimize irritative stimuli.
Potential for infection during the postoperative period related to incision	Provide proper care for the incision wound and teach the patient how to care for it upon discharge.
Self-care deficits related to limited mobility and pain	Provide grooming requirements and other needs for patient. Encourage grooming activities.
TO MINIMIZE DRUG SIDE EFFECTS OR INTERACTIONS	
Alteration in bowel elimination: constipation related to pain, immobility, and suppression of peristalsis by the anesthetic	Monitor intestinal function; observe for abdominal distention; provide exercise as appropriate to stimulate bowel function; notify physician if bowel movement is unduly delayed so that an intestinal stimulant or catheterization can be ordered.
Alteration in respiratory function in the immediate postoperative period related to residual anesthetic or narcotic depression, pain, and immobility	Unless otherwise instructed, position the patient on his or her side with the head flat on the bed without a pillow to minimize aspiration; monitor respiration and other vital signs at intervals of no more than 15 minutes until all vital signs are stabilized; report any deviations; ensure that airways are kept clear; have patient breath deeply, sigh, and cough to facilitate clearance of mucus.
Increased risk of injury related to postanesthetic depression or excitation	Provide necessary safety measures such as attaching bed rails. Stay with patient if excitation occurs.
TO ENSURE SAFE AND EFFICACIOUIS DRUG USE	
Knowledge deficit related to drug regimen	After the presurgical visit from the physician, encourage patient to ask questions and provide explanations about the surgical and anesthetic procedures. Initiate teaching during the preoperative phase of techniques required during the postoperative phase.

and is given in concentrations of 80% with 20% oxygen.

Intravenous Anesthetics

Ultrashort-acting Barbiturates

Barbiturates having especially short duration of activity and rapid onset of action are used effectively for inducing anesthesia by the intravenous route. The three agents employed in this manner are thiopental (Pentothal), thiamylal (Surital), and methohexital (Brevital).

Mechanisms and Effects The most frequent use of ultrashort-acting barbiturates is to hasten induction, after which the patient is maintained on an inhalation anesthetic. Ultrashort-acting barbiturates may be used with nitrous oxide for minor surgery, producing anesthesia within seconds and allowing complete control over the depth of anesthesia. Barbiturates are seldom used alone for anesthesia because they provide little analgesia and little skeletal muscle relaxation. Recovery is slow because drug elimination depends on metabolism, unlike the inhalation agents, which are breathed off. Emergence occurs as these drugs redistribute into fatty tissue, in which they are highly soluble. Metabolism occurs at a rate of about 15% per hour.

Adverse Effects and Contraindications Barbiturates cause depression of the vital centers of the medulla: first the respiratory center, then the vasomotor center, and finally the cardiac center. Ventilatory support may be required and respiratory acidosis is a risk. *Nurses should make certain that resuscitation equipment, an endotracheal tube, suction, and oxygen are on hand when barbiturates are employed for anesthesia.* Laryngospasms may occur but can be controlled with atropine. Barbiturates may further impair compromised circulatory function in patients in shock, but hepatic and renal toxicity do not occur with acute use. Barbiturates may cause increased sensitivity to cold, resulting in shivering, twitches, or tremors. *This reaction can be controlled by keeping the patient warm.*

Preparations and Administration *Barbiturate solutions must be freshly prepared. Solutions with a precipitate should be discarded. Extravasation during injection of ultrashort-acting barbiturates may cause local pain, which can be minimized by application of heat to enhance perfusion or by topical application of 1% procaine.*

Thiopental (Pentothal)
Preloaded syringes, vials with diluent, kits, rectal suspension
Recommended Doses: For induction of anesthesia in adults, 50–75 mg (2 or 3 ml of a 2.5% solution) at 20–40 second intervals.

Thiamylal (Surital)
Vials or ampules
Recommended Doses: For induction of anesthesia, 1.0 ml of a 2.5% solution injected every 5 seconds.

Methohexital (Brevital)
Vials or ampuls with diluent
Recommended Doses: For induction, 1% solution injected at about 1 ml per 5 seconds.

Etomidate (Amidate)

Etomidate is a nonbarbiturate sedative-hypnotic that can be employed as an aid in induction of anesthesia. It is short-acting and appears to be a GABA-mimetic agent. Etomidate produces minimal respiratory depression at the doses employed for induction but often causes myoclonic responses to pain in about one-third of treated individuals. It has little effect on cardiovascular parameters, such as myocardial metabolism, cardiac output, or peripheral circulation, and reduces cerebral blood flow, making it useful for neurosurgery in patients with increased intracranial pressure. Transient venous pain occurs in 20% of patients immediately following injection.

Etomidate (Amidate)
Injection solution
Recommended Doses: For induction of anesthesia in adults or children over 10, 0.2–0.6 mg/kg. 0.3 mg/kg injected over 30–60 seconds is typical.

Dissociative Anesthetics

Mechanisms and Effects Ketamine (Ketalar, Ketaject) and phencyclidine (Sernyl) are closely related anesthetics with a mechanism that is quite distinct from that of other anesthetics. They produce a dissociative anesthesia (stage IIC in Figure 16–2) in which the patient is cataleptic (unresponsive to surroundings or to painful stimuli). After recovery from anesthesia, the patient is amnesic for the period of the cataleptic state.

Phencyclidine is not used in human medicine but is employed in veterinary practice and is encountered as a drug of abuse (see Chapter 15). Ketamine is a rapid-acting anesthetic, providing anesthesia in 5–10 minutes after IV injection or 10–20 minutes after IM injections. Ketamine-induced anesthesia provides excellent analgesia but increased skeletal muscle tone. Respiratory depression is minimal, and laryngeal and pharyngeal reflexes are not activated. Respiratory secretions, blood pressure, and heart rate are increased.

Clinical Indications Ketamine is indicated for use alone only in surgical or diagnostic procedures that do not require skeletal muscle relaxation. It can also be employed to hasten induction when an inhalation agent is employed for surgery or to supplement nitrous oxide anesthesia.

Adverse Effects and Contraindications A distinct disadvantage of ketamine is the occurrence of emergence reactions in approximately 12% of treated individuals, including vivid, unpleasant dreams, delirium, vivid imagery, hallucinations, confusion, excitement, and irrational behavior. Reactions of this type occur *less* frequently in children under age 15 and in the elderly. Young and middle-age adults are most susceptible. The incidence of emergence phenomena can be reduced by concurrent IV administration of diazepam (Valium) and reduced doses of ketamine. Short- or ultrashort-acting barbiturates are used to terminate emergence reactions. *Allowing the patient to emerge gradually from ketamine anesthesia in a quiet environment with minimal tactile stimulation helps to reduce emergence symptoms. If psychic effects occur, the nurse should provide a calm environment and reassurance and the patient should not be left unattended. Family members should be enlisted to aid in providing reassurance.*

Ketamine is contraindicated in patients for whom an elevation in blood pressure could be dangerous (those with coronary artery disease, stroke, severe hypertension, or hyperthyroidism). It should be used cautiously in those with convulsive disorders, psychosis, or mild hypertension.

Adverse effects include elevated blood pressure and rate, diplopia, nystagmus, elevated intraocular pressure, catatonia, anorexia, nausea, vomiting, pain at the site of injection, and the psychiatric emergence phenomena described above. Ketamine increases salivation. *An anticholinergic should be administered preanesthetically to prevent this effect.*

Preparations and Administration

Ketamine (Ketaject, Ketalar)
Injection solution
Recommended Doses: 1.0–4.5 mg/kg, initially. Surgical anesthesia lasting 5–10 minutes requires an average of 2.0 mg/kg. *Ketamine should not be mixed in a syringe with a barbiturate because a precipitate will form.*

Opioid (Narcotic) Anesthetics

Three potent opioids are marketed for use as primary anesthetics or adjuncts to anesthesia: fentanyl (Sublimaze), alfentanyl (Alfenta), and sufentanil (Sufenta), Fentanyl is most often used in a combination (marketed as Innovar) with droperidol (Inapsine), a butyrophenone neuroleptic related to haloperidol. Potent neuroleptics induce **catalepsy** while potent narcotics induce a somewhat similar state called **catatonia.** In both states, immobility occurs, accompanied by a loss of sensation. Muscle tension is elevated in catatonia but not in catalepsy.

Innovar can be used alone to produce tranquilization and anesthesia for surgical and diagnostic procedures. It can also be used as a preanesthetic medication to facilitate induction or as an adjunct to help maintain general or regional anesthesia. The action of droperidol lasts for 3–6 hours and may persist well into recovery. Fentanyl, by contrast, exerts its analgesic effect for only 30 minutes. Since both drugs are CNS depressants, ventilatory support may be required during recovery. *Oxygen resuscitation equipment, suction, and an endotracheal tube should be on hand when Innovar is used.* Approximately 1% of patients receiving droperidol experience extrapyramidal side effects typical of neuroleptics. Innovar is contraindicated in patients with Parkinson's disease.

Sufentanil is a narcotic analgesic closely related to fentanyl, but 5–7 times more potent. Introduced in 1984, this agent is indicated as an adjunct for maintenance of analgesia in balanced anesthesia (usually with nitrous oxide or oxygen) or, in conjunction with 100% oxygen, as a primary anesthetic. Alfentanyl, an agent of similar pharmacology, was introduced at the end of 1986. In recent years, these potent narcotics have been employed increasingly as primary anesthetics in patients with cardiovascular disease because narcotics produce minimal cardiac depression and minimal compensatory sympathetic activation. Narcotics thus produce fewer unfavorable hemodynamic changes than do conventional general anesthetics.

Adverse reactions to opioid anesthetics include hypotension (in 5–10% of patients) and hypertension, bradycardia, and chest wall rigidity (each in about 3% of individuals). Opioid anesthetics also cause respiratory depression, and extended postoperative ventilatory support may be required. A respirator and an opioid antagonist, such as naloxone, should be available when any of these are used.

Fentanyl and Droperidol (Innovar)
Injection solution
Recommended Doses: Varies by application; see package insert.

Alfentanil (Alfenta)
Injection solution
Recommended Doses: As an adjunct to anesthesia, 8–50 μg/kg IV initially up to a maximum total dose of 75 μg/kg. As a primary anesthetic, 130–245 μg/kg IV for induction.

Sufentanil (Sufenta)
Ampuls containing sufentanil base
Recommended Doses: For use in balanced anesthesia, 1–2 μg/kg for minor surgical procedures and 2–8 μg/kg for more complicated surgery. For use as the primary anesthetic, 8–30 μg/kg.

Preanesthetic and Adjunctive Medications

Preanesthetic medications are used for a number of purposes. Barbiturates, anxiolytics, or phenothiazines are often administered before surgery to reduce anxiety, since excessive anxiety and fearfulness may activate central and autonomic stress reactions, which may alter the effect of the anesthetic. Use of sedative-hypnotics or tranquilizers may also help to smooth induction and diminish resistance to anesthesia. Promethazine (Phenergan) and propiomazine (Largon) are phenothiazines expressly indicated for use in conjunction with anesthesia. Pentobarbital and secobarbital are the most widely used barbiturates for this purpose. Midazolam (Versed), a benzodiazepine marketed in 1986, is used by intramuscular or intravenous injection as a preoperative sedative. *As a safety measure, siderails should always be raised following administration of preanesthetic depressants.*

Frequently, narcotics are used for their analgesic or depressant effects. Some anesthetics, such as nitrous oxide, have good analgesic properties, while others, such as halothane, are poor analgesics. Narcotics may be used before, during, and after surgery to promote analgesia. Morphine and meperidine are most widely employed for this purpose.

Antimuscarinic drugs, notably atropine and scopolamine, are used to inhibit respiratory and salivary secretions. These drugs also block reflexive cardiac slowing by inhibiting vagal effects on the heart. Other drugs may be ordered in anticipation of possible adverse reactions; antihistamines and antiemetics are often ordered during recovery to prevent nausea and vomiting.

During the period of anesthesia, skeletal muscle relaxants, such as curare or succinylcholine, are used to inhibit laryngospasms and to relax the skeletal musculature (see Chapter 29). Vasopressors may also be required if blood pressure is reduced by the action of the anesthetic, but sympathomimetic agents should be avoided if the anesthetic sensitizes the heart to catecholamines. Preanesthetic drugs may be readministered during the surgical procedure to reinforce desirable effects as required.

Prior to giving preanesthetic medications, nurses need to assess the patient by measuring pulse rate, respiration,

Table 16–3
Drugs That May Complicate Surgery, Anesthesia, or Postoperative Recovery

Type of drug	Type of complication
Antiarrhythmic drugs	Some may increase neuromuscular blockade
Antibiotics	Some antibiotics may predispose patients to renal insufficiency
	Some (especially aminoglycosides) increase neuromuscular blockade
	Some may combine unfavorably with anesthetic agents to produce untoward effects
Anticoagulants	May cause hemorrhage because of lack of hemostasis during surgery
Anticonvulsant drugs	May induce liver enzymes, hastening the metabolism of the anesthetic agent
Antihypertensive agents	May result in precipitous lowering of blood pressure following anesthesia
Aspirin	Hyperventilation and shortness of breath
	Hemorrhage
	Disturbance of acid-base balance
	Hypoglycemia in clients who have diabetes
Corticosteroids	May effectively block the body's response to shock and stress
	May decrease adrenal cortical function
Diuretics	Can cause disturbances in electrolyte balance postoperatively
	May cause hypotension
	Thiazide diuretics may lead to potassium retention
Insulin	May cause clients to have hypoglycemia during the periods when receiving nothing by mouth if not receiving intravenous fluids with glucose
MAO inhibitors	May lead to hypertensive crisis if sympathomimetic drugs are given during anesthesia
Narcotics	May lead to respiratory depression, increasing risk of respiratory failure
Propranolol	May cause cardiac depression
Sympathomimetics	Increased risk of catecholamine-induced dysrhythmias with certain anesthetics

blood pressure, and temperature. The patient's psychological status also needs to be noted. All preparation for surgery, including voiding, should be completed before medications are given. Patients typically receive the initial NPO (not by oral route) preoperative medications 1–2 hours prior to anesthesia.

Postanesthetic Medication and Nursing Care

Recovery from anesthesia is gradual because of the time required for elimination of the anesthetic from the brain. After surgery, patients are usually returned to the recovery room, where they remain until they are awake enough to give their name, age, and date of birth, and vital signs are stable. The patient's responses are compared with the baseline data obtained presurgically. The patient is placed on his or her side with the head tipped forward to prevent the tongue from falling backward and saliva and mucus from obstructing the airway. Nurses should watch patients for signs of hypoxia.

Rapid, shallow breathing, noisy snoring, or gasping respirations, thready pulse, increased restlessness, and confusion are symptoms that should be reported immediately. Also, patients may develop laryngospasm as a side effect of the anesthetic. If the patient produces a "crowing" sound, becomes restless, develops stridor (a high-pitched respiratory sound), or becomes cyanotic, the nurse should administer oxygen immediately and have the anesthesiologist called. An endotracheal tube is necessary to assure a patent airway and controlled respiration. Patients should be observed for hemorrhage. A drop in blood pressure or increase in pulse or respiration could indicate bleeding.

Once the patient has awakened, the nurse should encourage coughing and deep breathing at regular intervals, repeating the lessons learned during the preoperative period. Nurses need to closely monitor the client's renal functions to assure that fluid and electrolyte balance are maintained and to avoid overhydration or underhydration.

As the anesthetic wears off, the patient becomes aware of pain. An analgesic may be ordered and administered either intravenously, subcutaneously, or intramuscularly. The drugs commonly used to counteract postoperative pain can cause depression of vital centers; nurses therefore need to monitor blood pressure, pulse, and respirations prior to administering such drugs. Also, before giving pain medication, nurses should check patients for painful pressure points and should reposition them periodically to relieve discomfort, increase circulation, and improve respiratory function. The nurse also needs to check for distention of the abdomen and urinary bladder. A distended bladder is very painful and compounds the normal pain that follows a surgical procedure where tissues and organs have been manipulated and stretched. If the abdomen is distended, inserting a rectal tube or doing a Harris flush may relieve the gas pains and minimize the need for narcotics.

Nausea and vomiting are common occurrences postoperatively. Again, the nurse can expect a higher incidence following the use of certain anesthetics (cyclopropane and ether) and at certain levels of anesthesia. Nurses can expect the physician to order an antiemetic drug or small doses of sedatives or both to relieve nausea and vomiting. Nurses should check patients for hypotension and prolonged effects of the anesthesia.

Case Study: Surgical Procedure

S. M., a 45-year-old woman, required a left radical mastectomy. The night prior to surgery, she was given meprobamate orally and atropine intramuscularly. During the surgical procedure, she was given halothane-oxygen, nitrous oxide, meperidine, curare, and atropine. During postoperative recovery, S. M. had orders for ampicillin, 500 mg PO every 6 hours, meperidine, 100 mg PO every 3–4 hours PRN for pain, and acetaminophen, 650 mg PO every 4 hours as needed for fever.

The recovery room nurse had begun preparing for S. M.'s arrival even before the surgical procedure was completed. She had determined what equipment would be required and had placed it in the cubicle reserved for S. M. She checked the availability of emergency drugs and the operation of emergency equipment in the room. When S. M. arrived, she was semiconscious and was receiving positive pressure ventilatory support. The nurse checked vital signs. Blood pressure was 105/70. She checked the airways and found these clear. An intravenous line was already in place. The nurse inspected the incision site.

Over the next hour, S. M. gradually became more alert, responded to her name, and vital signs stabilized. Respiratory support was discontinued. The nurse turned S. M. onto her left side and talked with her in order to orient her to her surroundings. S. M. was covered with a blanket to protect her from postanesthetic hypothermia. The nurse helped S. M. perform the deep breathing and coughing exercises that she had learned during the preoperative period and gave S. M. her first oral dose of ampicillin. After another hour, S. M. complained of pain. Since S. M.'s blood pressure was still low, the nurse checked S. M. for signs of hypovolemia (elevated pulse, thirst, decreased urinary output, or clammy skin) and checked the time interval since the last administration of narcotic before providing the meperidine. S. M. was now fully oriented and exhibited no complications. The intravenous line was running according to schedule. S. M. was transferred to the intensive care unit. The nurse accompanied her to the new unit and discussed her status with the nurse there.

1. What is the likely reason for each drug given during the preoperative, operative, and postoperative phases?
2. Why was postoperative hypothermia anticipated in this case?
3. Why was the nurse concerned about administering meperidine while S. M. was still somewhat hypotensive?

Answers appear at the end of the book.

Recommended Readings

Bortnowski PM: Psychic disturbances traced to ketamine anesthesia. *Nurses' Drug Alert* 1978;2(12):141.

Davis AB: The development of anesthesia. *Am Scientist* 1982;70:522.

Eger EI II: *Anesthetic Uptake and Action.* Baltimore, Williams & Wilkins Co, 1974.

Eger EI II: Isoflurane: A review. *Anesthesiology* 1981;55:559–576.

Fink BR: *Progress in Anesthesiology.* New York, Raven Press, vol. 1 (1975), vol. 2 (1980): *Molecular Mechanisms of Anesthesia.*

Gronert GA: Malignant hyperthermia. *Anesthesiology* 1980;53:395–423.

Lichtiger M, Moya F (eds): *Introduction to the Practice of Anesthesia.* New York, Harper & Row, 1978.

Marshall BE, Wyche MQ: Hypoxemia during and after anesthesia. *Anesthesiology* 1972;37:178–209.

Price HL: Neuroleptic agents in anesthesia. *Am Fam Physician* 1973;8(4):222–224.

Roth SH: Physical mechanisms of anesthesia. *Annu Rev Pharmacol Toxicol* 1979;19:159–178.

Smith BJ: Safeguarding your patient after anesthesia. *Nursing* 1978;8(10):52–56.

Smith NT, Miller RD, Corbascio AN (eds): *Drug Interactions in Anesthesia.* Philadelphia, Lea & Febiger, 1981.

Zink J, Sasyniuk BI, Dresel PE: Halothane-epinephrine-induced cardiac arrhythmias and the role of heart rate. *Anesthesiology* 1975;43:548–555.

CHAPTER 17

Local Anesthetics

In medieval times, ice was applied directly to a pain source in order to kill sensations; the term **freezing** is still used by dentists and clients to describe the effect of local anesthetics. Clinical use of local anesthesia began in 1884 when Köller, an associate of Freud, introduced cocaine as a local anesthetic into ophthalmology. Its use spread rapidly after Köller's initial successes. Cocaine was introduced into dental practice in the same year and by 1885, the potential of local anesthesia for producing nerve block and spinal anesthesia was established. Twenty years after the introduction of cocaine, procaine (Novocain) gained widespread clinical acceptance. Procaine offered advantages over cocaine because of the variety of routes by which it could be administered safely. Lidocaine (Xylocaine and others) was introduced in 1948 and replaced procaine as the standard of comparison among local anesthetics.

A local anesthetic is a drug that blocks pain in a portion of the body without producing unconsciousness. Local anesthetics offer both advantages and disadvantages when compared with general anesthesia. With local anesthesia (topical, regional, epidural, or spinal), the patient remains awake and can provide important indications of physiological status. Systemic effects and toxicity are usually minimal. There is no appreciable effect on metabolism or liver and kidney function, no sensitization of the heart to norepinephrine, and no hypotensive action. Local anesthetics are not flammable or explosive. There are, however, significant drawbacks to local anesthesia. The effect of local anesthetics is variable because of peculiarities of application, so that occasionally the drug fails to produce adequate anesthesia. Although systemic toxicity is normally minimal, neurological and cardiac complications can occur if systemic absorption is excessive. The risk of systemic absorption varies greatly according to the route of administration. Spinal anesthesia produces the largest field of anesthesia that can be achieved using local anesthesia but provides the greatest risk of systemic toxicity.

The pharmacology of local anesthetics is also touched upon in other chapters. Some local anesthetic agents (benzocaine, butamben, cyclomethycaine, dimethisoquin, diperodon, dyclonine, hexylcaine, and pramoxine) are employed only by topical application to the skin and are discussed in Chapter 53. Benoxinate and proparacaine are employed only as ophthalmic anesthetics and are considered in Chapter 54. This chapter considers the general pharmacology of local anesthetics, methods for their application, and the specific agents that are appropriate for use by injection or on mucous membranes.

Pharmacology of Local Anesthetics

Mechanism of Action Local anesthetics represent the exception among drugs that act on the nervous system. While nearly every other kind of nervous system drug acts at synapses to alter neurotransmission, local anesthetics inhibit nerve impulse generation and conduction. Local anesthetics prevent the opening of sodium channels in the nerve cell axon. The rapid depolarization (phase zero) that occurs in the normal cell at the initiation of an action potential is the result of rapid influx of sodium through sodium channels that are momentarily opened. This influx of sodium ions into a nerve cell produces an inward electrical current that draws calcium ions off their binding sites on adjacent channels (Figure 17–1). The removal of the calcium ions opens the adjacent channels, permitting influx of sodium through these pores as well. The process is then repeated in the next segment of the membrane. The opening of sodium channels and the related depolarization passes in this manner like a wave along the length of the axon. When the local anesthetic is introduced into this process, the drug substitutes for calcium at the binding sites. The local anesthetic is less easily drawn from the binding sites than is calcium. The channels that are blocked by local anesthetic fail to participate normally in the process of propagation, and the action potential is arrested.

The locus of action of local anesthetics is on the inner surface of the cell membrane. Pharmacological activity of local anesthetics therefore depends on their ability to reach the cell interior. Local anes-

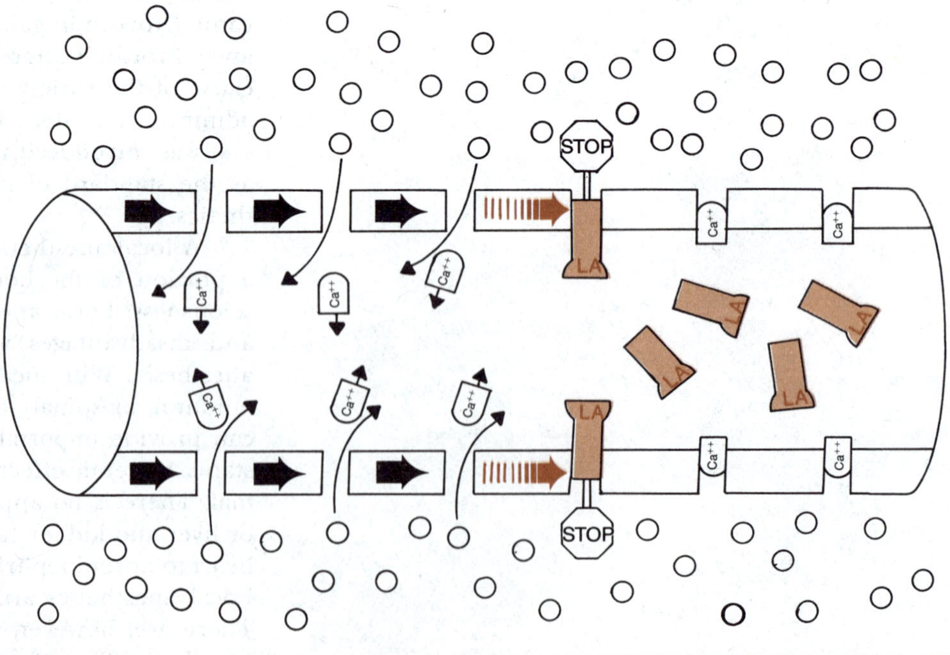

Figure 17–1
Mechanism of local anesthesia. Sodium ions enter the cell through channels, attracted by the negatively charged internal environment. The inward current of positive charges draws calcium ions away from adjacent ion channels, allowing influx of sodium ions through the next neural segment. As the process repeats, the signal is propagated down the axon. Propagation is blocked, however, by presence of molecules of local anesthetic, which bind tightly to the calcium-binding sites.

thetics that have poor lipid solubility can reach the binding sites only by passage through sodium channels that are momentarily open as a result of nerve cell activity. The extent of blockade produced by such local anesthetics therefore depends on the level of activity of a nerve cell. Highly active cells will be affected more quickly and to a greater extent than cells with low activity. Thus, the action of local anesthetics of low lipid solubility is said to exhibit **frequency dependence.** Local anesthetics that are highly lipid soluble are not especially affected by this phenomenon.

Small-diameter nerve fibers are more susceptible to the action of local anesthetics than are larger ones. Fortunately, pain fibers are among the smallest of nerve fibers. Following application of a local anesthetic, pain sensations disappear first, followed by sensations of cold, warmth, touch, or pressure. Muscle reflexes are readily depressed by local anesthetics because the gamma-motor neuron fibers that supply muscle spindle organs for reflexive activity are small. The duration of action is proportional to the time the drug remains in contact with the nerve fiber. Higher doses increase duration of the drug's action but also increase the probability of diffusion from the site of administration, placing clients at risk for increased toxicity.

Pharmacokinetics In contrast to the desirability of rapid absorption for most drugs, the ideal local anesthetic is one that remains in place at the site of application. All available local anesthetics are weak bases. Local anesthetics contain a tertiary nitrogen atom and ionize by conversion to the quaternary ammonium cation form. At physiological pH, only about 5–20% of a local anesthetic exists in the unionized form. This fraction is important because the ionized portion cannot diffuse through connective tissue to reach its site of action at nerve fibers.

The ionized form of a local anesthetic is poorly soluble. Therefore, local anesthetics are normally furnished as hydrochloride salts, which are not only more soluble but also more stable. The hydrochloride salt solutions are somewhat acidic, which increases ionization and decreases absorption.

The rate of absorption of a local anesthetic is an important determinant of systemic toxicity and depends on the drug's dosage, concentration, route of application, and degree of perfusion at the site of application. After absorption into the systemic circulation, a local anesthetic distributes broadly but is found in highest concentrations in tissues with high levels of perfusion: the heart, brain, liver, and lungs. Local anesthetics cross the placental barrier, the fetal/maternal ratio being determined by the dissociation constant of the drug, lipid solubility, and the extent of protein binding.

Inactivation of systemically absorbed local anesthetics of the ester-type (procaine, chlorprocaine, tetracaine) is achieved by hydrolysis of the ester linkage by plasma esterase and cholinesterase. The amide type of local anesthetic including lidocaine (Xylocaine), prilocaine, mepivacaine (Carbocaine, Isocaine), dibucaine (Nupercaine), bipulvacaine (Marcaine, Sensorcaine), and etidocaine (Duranest), are metabolized in the liver. A small fraction of absorbed local anesthetic is excreted unchanged in the urine. Local anesthetics have onsets of action ranging from 1 to 15 minutes and durations of action ranging from 0.25–0.5 hours for procaine to 3–7 hours for etidocaine with epinephrine.

Clinical Uses and Routes of Application Local anesthetics are used to prevent pain resulting from minor procedures, such as surgery of the eye, nose, and throat, dental procedures, removal of small growths, and suturing of minor lacerations. They may be used in diagnostic procedures, in labor and delivery, or applied topically to skin or mucous membranes to relieve pain and itching.

Important in any discussion of local anesthetics is the variety of routes and techniques used to administer them. The choice of method is dictated by exigencies of the clinical situation, and the method of administration in turn dictates the choice of a suitable agent. Local anesthetics are often classified on the basis of their mode of application.

Surface or **topical** anesthesia is carried out by applying the drug directly to the skin or to a mucous membrane by swabbing, spraying, or liquid instillation. This technique is widely practiced in surgery of the eye, ear, nose, or throat and commonly uses benzocaine, dibucaine, tetracaine, hexylcaine, benoxinate, butylaminobenzoate, and butacaine (see Chapters 53 and 54). Surface anesthesia provides the smallest field of anesthesia but the least risk of systemic toxicity. It is useful for alleviating pruritis associated with dermatoses (such as poison ivy), burns (including sunburn), minor injuries (such as abrasions, ulcerations, and lacerations), and fissured nipples occurring postpartum. Creams and ointments containing local anesthetics can also be applied topically to mucous membranes to relieve itching, such as that associated with pruritus ani or pruritus vulvae, or pain following removal of hemorrhoids. Local anesthetics may be applied as drops to the eye to facilitate ophthalmological procedures. Local anesthetics in the form of a spray are applied to the lar-

Nursing Observations for Local Anesthesia

THERAPEUTIC GOAL	Anesthesia without loss of consciousness.
PREADMINISTRATION ASSESSMENT	
Baseline Data	Evaluate vital signs, reflexes, orientation, sensation, motor function, respiratory sounds, bowel sounds, urinary output and continence, skin perfusion and temperature, and ECG.
Contraindications/ Precautions	Neurological or cardiovascular disorders, allergies to the drug being considered or structurally related drugs.
Potential Interactions	Check current drug regimen for CNS depressants, sulfonamides, and pressor drugs.
EVALUATION OF DRUG RESPONSE	
For Therapeutic Benefit	Monitor loss of sensitivity to pain.
For Adverse Effects	Monitor for allergic reactions and neurological and cardiovascular toxicity. Monitor for return of sensation and function.
For Drug Interactions	Monitor for inhibition of sulfonamide antibiotics by local anesthetics in the ester group. Monitor for additive CNS depression when local anesthetics are used with other CNS depressants. If the local anesthetic preparation contains epinephrine, observe for intensified hypertensive effects from epinephrine if the patient is using antidepressants.
For Compliance	Evaluate patient's compliance with all facets of the therapeutic regimen by careful observation, interviewing, and review of progress. Report compliance problems to the physician and act as patient-advocate when changes in the therapeutic regimen seem indicated.

ynx and trachea to facilitate endotracheal intubation or to the gastrointestinal or genitourinary tracts to facilitate introduction of instruments or to relieve pain.

Infiltration anesthesia is the injection of an agent into a circumscribed area of tissue in which superficial surgery is to take place to anesthetize local nerve endings. Application of local anesthetics by infiltration is most likely to be used to anesthetize the abdominal wall. A somewhat similar technique is **block** anesthesia, in which the local anesthetic is injected next to nerve fibers innervating a particular area. Block anesthesia can be either field block or regional nerve block. In **field block** anesthesia, often used for skin grafts or tumors, afferent nerves feeding the surgical field are anesthetized by application of the drug to an area surrounding, or just beneath, the site of incision. Field block is familiar to many people because of its frequent use for dental work. It is also used for minor surgical procedures involving the face, scalp, neck, larynx, and extremities. In **regional nerve block,** afferent fiber bundles are anesthetized some distance from the surgical site; as a result, the entire region innervated by the nerve bundle loses sensation. Field block is most likely to be employed for abdominal surgery. Procaine, lidocaine, and hexylcaine are important drugs for infiltration anesthesia and block anesthesia. Concentrations of local anesthetics required for infiltration anesthesia (0.5–1.0% lidocaine, for example) are less than those required for nerve block (1.5–2.0% lidocaine).

When the local anesthetic is applied to the space immediately outside the spinal sheaths, called **epidural** or **caudal** anesthesia, the spinal nerves are blocked. Epidural anesthesia may be used for surgical procedures involving the upper or lower abdomen or pelvis. It is most often employed for cesarean section. When local anesthetics are employed during delivery, the drug may enter the mother's circulation and cross the placental barrier, leading to depression in the infant. Epidural administration is technically difficult; errors in administration may result in inadequate anesthesia or excessive toxicity. Epidural administration may involve a single injection or continuous or repeated injections performed through an intact cannula. Procaine, lidocaine, prilocaine, piperocaine, tetracaine, and mepivacine are popular drugs for this method of delivery. Concentrations of 1–1.5% lidocaine are appropriate for caudal anesthesia.

Spinal anesthesia provides the largest field of anesthesia that can be achieved with local anesthetics. Spinal anesthesia is the injection of a local anesthetic into the subarachnoid space that separates the spinal cord from its covering sheaths, blocking nerve roots carrying afferent impulses into the spinal cord. There is more risk of toxicity with spinal anesthesia than with caudal anesthesia because the drug has access to the vital centers of the brain stem. A special problem associated with spinal anesthesia is postspinal headache, occurring in about 10% of cases. *Keeping the patient flat on the back for 6–12 hours after spinal anesthesia reduces likelihood of headache.* Spinal anesthesia is preferred to general anesthesia for clients with asthma or emphysema and for emergency surgery in patients who have recently eaten. Spinal anesthesia is contraindicated when clients have infections of the central nervous system or who are severely hypotensive. Relative contraindications include hypertension, coronary artery disease, and congestive heart failure.

High spinal anesthesia employs a solution of specific gravity equal to, or less than, that of the cerebral spinal fluid. For administration, the patient is placed in the Trendelenburg position with head sharply flexed. High spinal anesthesia is required for surgical procedures involving the upper extremities and trunk. In practice, it is seldom used. **Low spinal anesthesia** produces *saddle block* and the patient is placed in the flat, or Fowler position, for administration. In this instance, the anesthetic solution must have a specific gravity that is greater than that of cerebral spinal fluid. Saddle block results in loss of sensation in the perineum, buttocks, and thighs and is sometimes employed for obstetric surgery. Spinal anesthesia may involve a single injection (single-shot spinal anesthesia) or repeated applications via an in-place catheter throughout the surgical procedure (fractional spinal anesthesia). Tetracaine, dibucaine, procaine, and piperocaine are the anesthetics most widely used. High spinal anesthesia requires higher concentrations of drug (5% lidocaine, for example) than is required for low spinal anesthesia (1.5% lidocaine) or for other applications.

Adverse Effects and Contraindications The toxicity of local anesthetics is closely tied to variables that influence their rate of absorption from the site of injection. Rapid absorption and systemic distribution from a site of application increases systemic toxicity as well as decreasing the duration of effective anesthesia.

Adverse effects of local anesthetics cluster into three categories. CNS reactions, cardiac toxicity, and allergic reactions. Toxic response to local anesthetics has been dubbed the "caine reaction," since the names of all of the injectable local anesthetics end in "caine." The caine reaction exhibits three distinctive stages, depending on severity, that sometimes occur sequentially in severe toxicity (Table 17–1). The first stage is the stage of initial stimulation characterized by behavioral and neurological indications of excitement (see Table 17–1). *Nurses may be able to reduce the*

Table 17–1
Staging of Local Anesthetic Toxicity

Stage	CNS	CVS	Respiration
Stage I: Initial stimulation	Restlessness, apprehensiveness, tinnitus, dizziness, blurred vision, nausea, vomiting, chills, twitches, tremor, sudden headache	Bradycardia, hypertension and pallor, or hypotension and flushing	Increased tidal volume and respiratory rate
Stage II: Advanced stimulation	Tonic and clonic convulsions	Increased heart rate and blood pressure	Dyspnea, rapid irregular respiration, cyanosis
Stage III: Depression	Muscle paralysis, depression of reflexes, coma, death	Cardiac arrest, circulatory collapse, death	Respiratory failure, extreme cyanosis, death

Nursing Diagnoses and Interventions for Local Anesthesia

Nursing Diagnoses	*Related Interventions*
TO ENHANCE DRUG BENEFITS OR REDUCE DRUG REQUIREMENTS	
Alteration in comfort: pain related to injection or incomplete anesthesia	Provide comfort measures and analgesia.
Fear related to the procedure	Provide emotional support and encouragement; explain procedures.
TO MINIMIZE DRUG SIDE EFFECTS OR INTERACTIONS	
Activity intolerance related to diminished mobility	Provide rest as required; monitor for return of function; help patient to change positions; provide skin care to guard against bedsores.
Alteration in cardiac output related to cardiac toxicity of local anesthetics	Monitor blood pressure, pulse and rhythm and report any significant changes to the physician; keep patient confined to bed after spinal anesthesia while orthostatic hypotension is present.
Sensory-perceptual alterations related to suppression of somatosensory impulses	Monitor return of sensation; warn patient about risk of injury due to inability to feel pain in affected area.
TO ENSURE SAFE AND EFFICACIOUS DRUG USE	
Knowledge deficit related to drug regimen	Teach patient about the nature of the procedure including necessary preparations and recovery.
	Advise patient about potential adverse effects and enlist their aid in identifying their occurrence.

incidence of headache that occur in this stage by encouraging clients to maintain good hydration. A tight abdominal binder may also provide relief from headaches.

In the second stage, stimulation is more severe. Some patients may have a seizure resembling those seen in grand mal epilepsy. The third stage of local anesthetic toxicity is characterized by CNS and cardiovascular depression, which can be fatal in the absence of successful medical intervention. Local anesthetics result in approximately 50 deaths per year in the United States.

Some clients develop delayed neurologic symptoms such as transient nerve palsies about 2 weeks after spinal anesthesia. *The nurse should advise clients of this possibility and instruct them to report such occurrences to the physician.*

The other major type of adverse reaction to local anesthetics is the dose-independent hypersensitivity reactions. These can take the form of cutaneous lesions such as urticaria, pruritus, erythema, or angioneurotic edema. Other individuals may experience allergic reactions such as sneezing, drug fever, excessive sweating, syncope, or anaphylactoid reactions. Allergic reactions can also occur to a paraben (such as methylparaben) or a sulfite present as a preservative in some local anesthetic preparations. *A careful drug history should be taken prior to administration of any local anesthetic to ascertain drug sensitivities.*

Drug Interactions Mixtures of a quick-acting local anesthetic and a slow-acting anesthetic are sometimes employed to provide quick but long-lasting anesthesia. Such mixtures provide toxicity that is at least additive and sometimes more than additive.

The depressant effects of local anesthetics on the CNS can be additive with those produced by sedative-hypnotics. When local anesthetics are applied topically, heavy metal-containing antiseptics should not be used to disinfect the skin, since local anesthetics can interact with such metals, resulting in ionization of both the metal and the local anesthetic.

Local anesthetics in the ester group (procaine, chloroprocaine, and tetracaine) inhibit the action of sulfonamide antimicrobial agents.

Another type of interaction involving local anesthetic preparations relates to the pressor substance, epinephrine, incorporated into many such formulations. Pressor amines must be used with great caution in clients receiving MAO inhibitors, tricyclic antidepressants, or ergot-type oxytocics.

Local Anesthetic Agents

Amide-type Local Anesthetics

Lidocaine

Lidocaine is the standard of comparison for local anesthetics. It is the drug of choice for infiltration anesthesia and a versatile agent that can be applied by almost any of the routes of administration of local anesthetics (Table 17–2). The action of lidocaine is immediate in onset and typically lasts from 1 to 2 hours.

Nurses will have occasion to administer lidocaine for rapid control of ventricular dysrhythmias that occur during myocardial infarction. It is also used during cardiac surgery, cardiac catheterization, and for clients who have acute myocardial infarction induced by digitalis intoxication (see Chapter 38).

Lidocaine, like procaine, has low toxicity. However, lidocaine is chemically dissimilar from procaine, and there is no cross-sensitivity between the two. Lidocaine is an amide-type local anesthetic, metabolized by the liver, and its toxicity is therefore elevated in individuals with impaired hepatic function. *In taking the patient's history, it is important for nurses to note any hypersensitivity to amide-type local anesthetics or lidocaine injection.* Cardiac effects of lidocaine are pronounced when toxic levels occur. When administered too rapidly or in large doses, hypotension and convulsions may occur. Lidocaine is often administered with epinephrine to delay its rate of absorption. *Special care must be taken when lidocaine is used in clients who are elderly, in respiratory depression or shock, or who have myasthenia gravis. Nurses need to pay particular attention to complaints of drowsiness or sleepiness and any*

Table 17–2
Indications and Durations of Action (Hours) of Local Anesthetics

Drug	Spinal	Epidural	Infiltrative	Infiltrative with epinephrine	Topical to mucous membranes	Topical to skin	Topical to eye
Amides							
Lidocaine	0.5–1.5	1–3	0.5–1.0	2–6	0.5–1.0	Yes	No
Dibucaine	1.25–3.0	No	3–4	6	No	2–4	No
Bupivacaine	1.25–2.5	3–5	2–4	3–7	No	No	No
Etidocaine	No	3–5	2–3	3–7	No	No	No
Mepivacaine	0.5–1.5	1–3	0.75–1.5	2–6	No	No	No
Prilocaine	No	1–3	0.5–1.5	2–6	No	No	No
Esters							
Procaine	No	0.5–1.5	0.25–0.5	0.5–1.5	No	No	No
Chloroprocaine	No	0.5–1.5	0.25–0.5	0.5–1.5	No	No	No
Tetracaine	1.25–2.5	3–5	2–3	No	0.5–1.0	Yes	0.25–0.33
Benzocaine	No	No	No	No	1–2	Yes	No
Butamben picrate	No	No	No	No	No	0.5–1.0	No
Cocaine	No	No	No	No	0.5–2.0	No	No
Proparacaine	No	No	No	No	No	No	0.25–0.33
Benoxinate	No	No	No	No	No	No	0.25–0.33
Miscellaneous							
Dyclonine	No	No	No	No	No	<1.0	No
Pramoxine	No	No	No	No	Yes	No	No
Dimethisoquin	No	No	No	No	No	Yes	No
Diperodon	No	No	No	No	Yes	No	No

increased restlessness, irritability, apprehensiveness, or difficulty in speaking, breathing, or swallowing.

Preparations and Administration

Lidocaine (Xylocaine, Dilocaine, Nervocaine, Ultracaine)
Injection solutions, injection solutions with epinephrine, injection solution with dextrose (for saddle block anesthesia), injection solution with glucose for spinal anesthesia.
Recommended Doses: For infiltration, 0.5–1.0%; for nerve block, 1–2% (depending on the diameter of the nerve to be blocked); for epidural or caudal applications, 1–3%; for saddle block, 1.5% (with dextrose); for retrobulbar or transtracheal injection, 4%; for high spinal anesthesia, 5% (with glucose). *Lidocaine solutions for spinal or epidural anesthesia must not contain preservatives or epinephrine and must be specifically labeled for IV use.*

Other Amide-type Local Anesthetics

Dibucaine is about 5 times as potent as lidocaine. It has a very long action, up to 3–4 hours after infiltration injection even without epinephrine. Dibucaine can be employed for spinal anesthesia, infiltration, or topically to the skin. Dibucaine is seldom used topically because of its high level of toxicity; tissue sloughing has occurred after subcutaneous injections of dibucaine. Nurses are most likely to encounter dibucaine employed topically for the relief of pain and itching caused by hemorrhoids, nonpoisonous insect bites, sunburn, and minor burns and cuts. *Nurses should warn clients not to use dibucaine around the eyes and to discontinue its use if there is any irritation. Dibucaine precipitates in solutions that are even mildly alkaline. It is therefore recommended that syringes and needles used for dibucaine be rinsed in mildly acidified distilled water. Solutions of dibucaine that are discolored should be discarded.* Bupivacaine, mepivacaine, etidocaine, and prilocaine are other potent and long-lasting amide-type anesthetics. Mepivacaine has a vasoconstrictor action. Etidocaine may occasionally produce motor block that outlasts sensory block when employed for caudal anesthesia. Prilocaine can produce methemoglobinemia, and therefore is seldom employed.

Preparations and Administration

Bupivacaine (Marcaine, Sensorcaine, and generic formulations)
Injection solutions with or without epinephrine, for infiltration, caudal or epidural block, peripheral nerve block, retrobulbar block, sympathetic block, and dental block.

Dibucaine (Nupercaine)
Solutions for isobaric spinal anesthesia, for hypobaric spinal anesthesia, and for low spinal anesthesia.

Etidocaine (Duranest)
Injection solutions with epinephrine, for caudal anesthesia. Etidocaine is not used for spinal anesthesia.

Mepivacaine (Carbocaine, Isocaine)
Injection solutions for dental procedures, or with levonordefrin, a vasoconstrictor, for dental use.

Prilocaine (Citanest)
Injection solutions with or without epinephrine, in dental cartridges.

Ester-type Local Anesthetics

Procaine (Novocain), one of the oldest local anesthetics, has a short duration of action, just 15–30 minutes after infiltration or up to 1.5 hours if administered with epinephrine. Because of its extremely low toxicity, procaine is used routinely. While procaine is ineffective as a topical agent, it is useful for infiltration, peripheral nerve block, and spinal anesthesia. It is relatively nontoxic but is fairly likely to cause allergic reactions.

Procaine exhibits a unique drug interaction: the principal metabolite of procaine, para-aminobenzoic acid, antagonizes sulfonamide antimicrobial drugs and other folic acid inhibitors. For this reason, *procaine and sulfonamides should not be used concurrently and nurses should question any order to do so. Because procaine forms a precipitant with heavy metal ions, nurses should avoid use of topical antiseptics containing heavy metals before or with procaine. Procaine should be used with care in debilitated or elderly patients.*

Procaine should be used with caution for producing paracervical block during obstetrical delivery. It is important to monitor the fetal heart rate before, during, and after the use of procaine for evidence of fetal distress. Fetal bradycardia may indicate the presence of high concentrations of procaine which, in turn, can lead to fetal acidosis. A pregnant woman who has toxemia may also be at risk if procaine is used and will need constant monitoring. Nursing responsibilities in these situations include both observing clients and instituting corrective measures to counter adverse effects.

Chlorprocaine (Nesacaine) is related to procaine but is metabolized more rapidly. Tetracaine (Pontocaine) is a versatile local anesthetic that can be injected or applied topically to the skin, mucous membranes, or the eye. Tetracaine is about 10 times more potent and 6 times longer acting than procaine. Tetracaine has a vasodepressor action. A number of ester-type local anesthetics are marketed for topical use only. Benzocaine is employed on the skin or mucous membranes, butamben picrate on the skin, hexylcaine and cocaine on mucosal membranes, and proparacaine and benoxinate as ophthalmic preparations. These agents are discussed in Chapters 53 and 54.

Preparations and Administration

Procaine (Novocain, generic)
Solutions. If a vasoconstrictor effect is desired, 0.5–1.0 ml of a 1:1,000 epinephrine solution can be added to each 100 ml of procaine solution to achieve a 1:200,000 or 1:100,000 concentration of the pressor drug. *Procaine solutions containing a precipitate should be discarded.*

Chlorprocaine (Nesacaine)
Solutions

Tetracaine (Pontocaine)
Solutions. Solutions with dextrose for spinal anesthesia, topical creams and ointments (see Chapter 53), ophthalmic solutions and ointments (see Chapter 54).

Important Nursing Implications for Local Anesthetics

- ☐ Carefully check the patient's medication history for any evidence of allergic reactions to local anesthetics before administering a drug in this group.
- ☐ Avoid use of local anesthetics in patients who are in respiratory distress or shock or those who have myasthenia gravis.
- ☐ Clients are usually confined to bed for 6–8 hours following spinal or saddle block anesthesia. Ensure that clients shift position frequently during this period (the effect of the anesthetic blocks discomfort that normally motivates people to readjust their position before circulatory or nerve damage occurs). Advise these clients not to ambulate until sensory and motor functions have recovered completely.
- ☐ Know the indications of "caine" toxicity and how to determine which stage of toxicity the client is exhibiting.
- ☐ Ensure that clients maintain good hydration after spinal anesthesia to minimize occurrence of headache and other neurological reactions to local anesthetics.
- ☐ When local anesthetics are to be injected, make certain to have oxygen and an anticonvulsant drug at hand.
- ☐ Before injecting a local anesthetic, take a baseline pulse and blood pressure measurement.
- ☐ Lidocaine preparations that contain epinephrine must never be given intravenously.
- ☐ Implications related to use of local anesthetics as antidysrhythmic drugs are presented in Chapter 38.

Case Study: History of Allergic Reaction to a Local Anesthetic

Nurses need to recognize that clients may not make clear distinctions between names of anesthetics. In one instance, M. B., a 43-year-old female patient who was to receive procaine hydrochloride just happened to mention to the nurse that she hoped she would not have trouble "like the last time." Upon further questioning the client, the nurse learned that M. B. had been given novocain when she had a tooth extracted and had become dizzy and had developed blurred vision and hypotension. However, M. B. stated that she felt it would likely be different this time since the drug was different. The nurse explained to M. B. that the drug to be used was the same as the one used before. She explained about generic and trade names for drugs. Next, the nurse learned the name of the client's dentist and called to obtain further information concerning her reaction. She learned that M. B. had experienced urticaria and other manifestations of allergy. The total history of the client's experience was reported to the physician, who then selected a different type of local anesthetic for M. B.

1. What is the relationship between procaine and novocain?
2. What local anesthetic might the physician have chosen as an alternative which would be unlikely to exhibit cross-sensitivity with procaine?

Answers appear at the end of the book.

Recommended Readings

Adriani J, Naraghi M: Pharmacological principles of regional pain relief. *Annu Rev Pharmacol Toxicol* 1977;17:223–242.

Baida MR: Nursing care in the use of local anesthetics. *AORN J* 1978;28:855.

Covino BG: Comparative clinical pharmacology of local anesthetics. *Anesthesiology* 1971;35(2):158–167.

Covino BG, Vassallo HG: *Local Anesthetics: Mechanisms of Action and Clinical Use.* New York, Grune & Stratton Inc, 1976.

DeJong RH: Toxic effects of local anesthetics. *JAMA* 1978;239:1166–1168.

Greene NM: *Physiology of Spinal Anesthesia,* ed 3. Baltimore, Williams & Wilkins Co, 1981.

Lefevre M: Obstetric anesthesia. *Am Fam Physician* 1983;27(6):146–154.

Nicolls ET, Corke BC, Ostheimer GW: Epidural anesthesia for the woman in labor. *AM J Nurs* 1981;81:1826–1830.

Ritchie JM, Greengard P: On the mode of action of local anesthetics. *Annu Rev Pharmacol* 1966;6:405–430.

Strichartz GR (ed): *Handbook of Experimental Pharmacology.* Berlin, Springer-Verlag, 1985: *Local Anesthesia.*

UNIT III

Drugs and the Central Nervous System

PART D
Drug Treatment of Psychiatric Disorders

CHAPTER 18

Antipsychotic Drugs

Classification of Psychoses

Excluding drug-induced psychoses and organic brain disorders, there are three categories of psychoses listed in the *Diagnostic and Statistical Manual of the American Psychiatric Association (DSM-III):* schizophrenia, paranoid disorders, and other psychotic disorders. **Schizophrenia** is the most widely employed diagnosis for first admissions to mental hospitals.

Schizophrenia

Schizophrenia is diagnosed when a psychiatric profile meets five conditions (Table 18–1). The foremost condition is the presence of one or more overt symptoms, including delusions, hallucinations, incoherence, affective disturbances, catatonia, and disorganized behavior. It is not necessary and is unlikely that one person exhibit all these symptoms. The delusions of schizophrenia generally involve absurd beliefs, such as being controlled by forces or being capable of supernatural powers (such as telepathy). Often, the delusions are grandiose, religious, or nihilistic in nature. The hallucinations in schizophrenia are characteristically auditory, usually experienced as hearing one or more voices. Incoherence is a marked loosening of associations in which thinking becomes highly illogical. Common affective disturbances include blunted or flat affect, extreme ambivalence, or affective incongruity. Catatonia is a state of elevated muscle tone and rigid posture.

To be diagnosed as schizophrenic, the client must also exhibit certain criteria that rule out other diagnoses. There must be a noticeable deterioration

Table 18–1
Diagnostic Criteria for Schizophrenia

At least one of the following symptoms during a phase of the illness:
Delusions (bizarre or grandiose ideas)
Auditory hallucinations
Incoherence
Blunted, flat, or inappropriate affect
Catatonia or grossly disorganized behavior
Deterioration of previous level of functioning
Duration of at least 6 months
Onset before age 45 years
Exclusions:
No preceding depressive or manic episode of extended duration
Not secondary to organic brain syndrome or mental retardation

in the client's level of functioning in work, social relations, and self-care. The condition must have lasted at least 6 months and must have begun before age 45. And there must be no preceding depression, mania, organic brain syndrome, or mental retardation. *Nurses should learn the prodromal symptoms of schizophrenia (see Table 18–2), so as to recognize clients who are exhibiting the potential for schizophrenia. This knowledge is especially important for nurses who work independently, who are often in a position to note clients with symptoms of schizophrenia before others do.*

Schizophrenia is an episodic condition. Some individuals experience recurrent acute episodes (commonly referred to as nervous breakdowns) separated by periods of more or less normal functioning. Even in chronic schizophrenia, acute periods may alternate with periods of relative remission. Because of its episodic character, antipsychotic drugs are employed in three distinct manners for schizophrenia. First, a neuroleptic may be employed for the duration of an **acute** episode and withdrawn a few months after remission of symptoms. Second, clients subject to repeated acute episodes may be given **maintenance** doses, usually one-third to one-fifth the dose used in acute or chronic schizophrenia. This treatment has proved enormously successful in reducing the frequency and severity of subsequent episodes with minimal risk of adverse effects. Third, clients with **chronic** schizophrenia may be given neuroleptics for years on end as a means of providing relief of symptoms.

Table 18–2
Prodromal (or Residual) Symptoms of Schizophrenia

Social isolation or withdrawal
Impaired functioning
Peculiar behavior
Impaired personal hygiene
Flat or inappropriate affect
Digressive, overelaborate speech
Bizarre ideation
Recurrent illusions, delusions, or hallucinations

Neurobiological Theories of Schizophrenia

Most researchers now concede that organic factors are preeminent in the etiology of schizophrenia, at least to the extent of creating a predisposition or vulnerability to schizophrenia. Nonorganic factors are nevertheless important, most obviously in acute reactive psychosis. The once popular view that schizophrenia could be traced to contradictory messages conveyed from parent to child is now largely in disrepute. The nature of the organic alterations culminating in schizophrenia has yet to be clearly established. The three theories currently under consideration are the dopamine hypothesis, the transmethylation hypothesis, and the autoimmune hypothesis.

At present, the **dopamine hypothesis** is the strongest one. This view asserts that an elevation in dopamine activity accompanies schizophrenia and is responsible for some of the symptoms of the disorder, including catatonia, aggression, and paranoia. The main evidence for the dopamine hypothesis is pharmacological. Virtually all drugs that alleviate symptoms of schizophrenia interfere with dopamine activity, either by blocking dopamine receptors or by depleting the transmitter from storage vesicles. Conversely, drugs that elevate dopamine activity (levodopa or amphetamine) can generate schizoid symptoms. There is little doubt that dopamine is implicated in the pathogenesis of schizophrenia but it is doubtful that alterations in dopamine represent the fundamental etiology of schizophrenia, since dopamine-blocking drugs suppress some of the symptoms of schizophrenia but do not eliminate others. Thus, the dopamine hypothesis is simply a valuable piece of a largely unsolved puzzle.

The **transmethylation hypothesis** was proposed some 30 years ago by Osmond and Smythies. It notes the structural similarities between catecholamine neurotransmitters and certain psychedelics (such as mescaline) and suggests that an error in brain metabolism may lead to production of endogenous psychotomimetic substances (transmethylated catecholamines). Thus far, the theory remains an appealing speculation, since no evidence of synthesis or accumulation of such substances has been found.

The **autoimmune hypothesis,** first proposed by Heath in 1954, suggests that antibodies react to antigens in neurons of the nucleus accumbens septi. Fluorescent antibodies were found to accumulate in this brain region in schizophrenics. Efforts to confirm these findings have been unsuccessful, so that the hypothesis remains unsubstantiated.

Paranoid Disorders

There are four classifications of paranoid disorders — paranoia, shared paranoia, acute paranoia, and atypical paranoia — and six diagnostic criteria (Table 18–3). The essential symptom is persistent delusions with persecutory or jealous content. Paranoid disorders are considerably less common and more limited in the range of symptoms than schizophrenia. There are usually no affective or behavioral disturbances, except those relating to the delusions, and hallucinations are rare. The symptoms must last at least 1 week. Depression, mania, and organic brain syndrome must be excluded. The subclassification **shared paranoid disorder** (*folie à deux*) is a delusional syndrome shared by two people who are in close relationship.

Other Psychotic Disorders

The third group of psychotic disorders includes schizophreniform disorder, brief reactive psychosis, schizoaffective disorder, and atypical psychosis. The first two disorders are distinguished in part by duration. **Schizophreniform disorder** meets all the criteria of schizophrenia except that its duration is more than 2 weeks but less than 6 months. **Brief reactive psychosis** designates psychotic conditions of more than a few hours, but less than 2 weeks that follow an identifiable calamity that could evoke signs of distress in almost anyone. **Schizoaffective disorder** applies when a client exhibits symptoms of schizophrenia along with pronounced symptoms of mania or depression, where it is unclear that either the psychosis or the affective symptoms came first. This diagnosis should be avoided, because it encourages overindulgence in multiple-drug regimens. *Atypical psychosis* refers to psychotic conditions that do not meet the criteria for any of the specific categories.

Table 18–3
Diagnostic Criteria for Paranoid Disorders

Persistent delusions with persecutory or jealous content
No affective, associative, or behavioral disturbance except in relation to the delusional system
No prominent hallucinations
Duration at least 1 week
Exclusions:
No preceding depression, manic-depressive syndrome of extended duration, or organic brain syndrome

Antipsychotic Drugs

The terms **antipsychotic, neuroleptic,** and **major tranquilizer** are used interchangeably for the group of agents that calm agitated subjects and lessen reactions to emotional stimuli with little overall effect on consciousness. This class of drugs is distinct from the sedative-hypnotics (which alter emotional reactivity only at doses that significantly depress consciousness) and from the anxiolytics or minor tranquilizers. It is unfortunate that the term *tranquilizer* has been used to describe both the neuroleptics and the anxiolytics, since these two classes of drugs differ in almost every conceivable respect. The main use of neuroleptics is in treatment of psychoses, especially schizophrenia.

With the introduction of the first phenothiazine derivative in 1954, antipsychotic drugs, particularly chlorpromazine (Thorazine), have been among the most studied and most prescribed drugs. The year after the introduction of chlorpromazine was the first in which the trend toward an increasing population in psychiatric hospitals was reversed (Figure 18–1). Since institutionalization has been found to be the single strongest negative variable determining the prognosis in schizophrenic patients, the ability of neuroleptics to facilitate return to the community environment, sometimes as productive and contributing workers, is no small matter and perhaps the greatest benefit conferred by the medication.

There is a great similarity among the drugs currently used as antipsychotic medications, especially in efficacy. The principal distinctions among agents relates to likelihood and severity of particular adverse effects.

Mechanisms and Effects The neuroleptic syndrome comprises the gross behavioral effects of antipsychotic drugs. Clients may exhibit slowing of motor activity, decreased emotionality, indifference to stimuli, and diminished ability to perform tasks requiring motor coordination. At high doses, the body becomes rigidly fixed, an effect known as **catalepsy.**

The neuroleptic activity of antipsychotic drugs is related to a central reduction in dopaminergic activity (Figure 18–2). The ascending reticular activating system is depressed, and there is a related decrease in cortical release of acetylcholine. In contrast

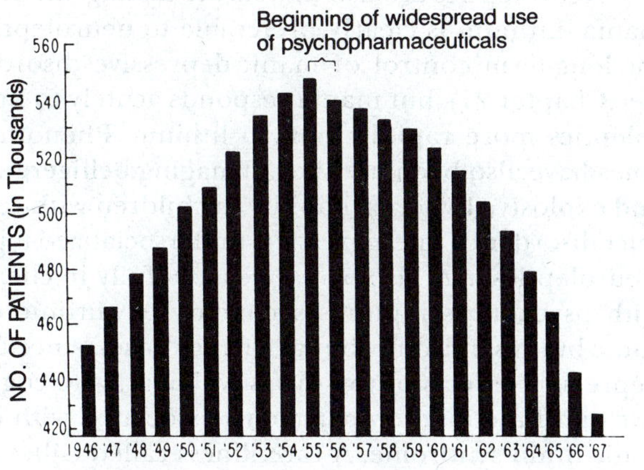

Figure 18–1
Number of resident patients in state and local government mental hospitals in the United States (based on U.S. Public Health Service figures), 1946–1967. Modified from N. Kline, Presidential Address. In E. Efron (Ed.), *Psychopharmacology: A Review of Progress, 1957–1967*. Washington, D.C.: U.S. Government Printing Office, 1968.

to barbiturates, neuroleptics depress the arousal caused by sensory stimulation but not that of direct electrical stimulation of the reticular formation (barbiturates depress arousal produced by either technique). Antipsychotic agents do not markedly cloud consciousness at normal therapeutic doses, and apathetic and withdrawn clients may even become more alert and responsive to communication. Clients who are hostile, hyperactive, violent and panic stricken become quieter and calmer and experience fewer thought disturbances, hallucinations, and delusions.

Antipsychotic potency is related to the ability of neuroleptics to block dopamine receptors. The ratio of blocking effects on dopamine versus norepinephrine receptors for a given drug can be ascertained by means of behavioral tests or receptor-binding studies. Butyrophenones and piperazine neuroleptics have substantially greater specificity for dopamine receptors than do other phenothiazines. Some neuroleptics, such as the diphenylbutylamines, are completely specific for dopamine receptors, being devoid of antiadrenergic and anticholinergic sedative and autonomic side effects.

There are five identified dopamine pathways in the brain, and each accounts for an effect of antipsychotic drugs. The mesolimbic dopamine pathway is probably involved in the antipsychotic efficacy of neuroleptics. The nigrostriatal dopamine pathway is implicated in the extrapyramidal side effects. The mesocortical pathway is probably involved in the sedative action of neuroleptics, and the hypothalamic-hypophyseal and incertohypothalamic pathways are responsible for the neuroendocrine side effects caused by neuroleptics. Of the two principal classes of dopamine receptors, the D_2 type appear to be more important for both schizophrenia and the extrapyramidal side effects of antipsychotic drugs, since the drugs with greatest affinity at the D_2-receptors also have greatest clinical potency in both respects.

The conventional view that relates the antipsychotic activity of neuroleptics to their ability to block dopamine receptors fails to account for the observed delay in clinical efficacy. It requires 3 weeks or more of neuroleptic treatment to ameliorate psychotic symptoms, but blockade of dopamine receptors is an

Figure 18–2
Mechanisms of neuroleptics. NE, norepinephrine; DA, dopamine; MAO, monoamine oxidase; CPZ, chlorpromazine; RAS, reticular activating system. From A. K. Swonger and L. L. Constantine, *Drugs and Therapy*, 2nd ed. Boston: Little, Brown, 1983.

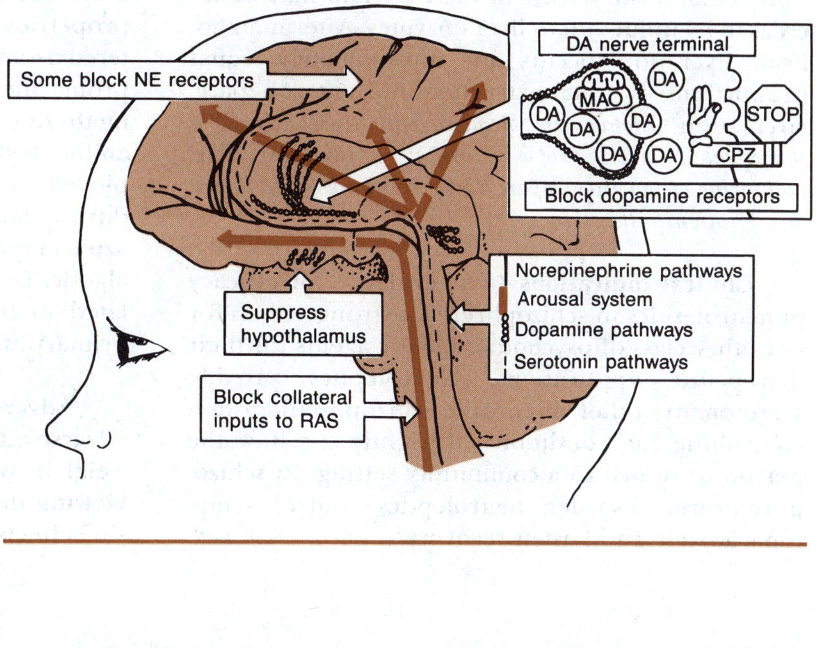

immediate biochemical effect. To explain the delay in clinical efficacy, it is necessary to look at adaptive adjustments that occur with chronic use. The immediate effect of a neuroleptic, the blocking of postsynaptic and presynaptic dopamine receptors, triggers a compensatory increase in synthesis and release of dopamine. These short-term compensatory changes largely offset the blocking action of the neuroleptics during the first 2–3 weeks. After 2–3 weeks of treatment, the compensatory mechanisms begin to undergo adaptation, and turnover and synthesis of dopamine return to normal. Long-term adaptations to the primary effect of neuroleptics also occur — postsynaptic and presynaptic receptors become supersensitive, but they do not offset the primary effect as effectively as did the compensatory responses during the first few weeks. Thus, with the disappearance of the compensatory responses, the primary effect becomes more apparent.

Pharmacokinetics Antipsychotic drugs can be administered orally, intramuscularly, or intravenously. After oral administration, absorption is variable, with peak plasma levels occurring in 2–4 hours: liquids provide the most reliable absorption, followed by conventional tablets, and then controlled release preparations. Bioavailability after intramuscular injection is 4–10 times that of oral administration.

Neuroleptics are widely distributed in the body with concentrations in the cerebrospinal fluid exceeding plasma levels. The neuroleptics are lipophilic agents, accumulating in lipid-rich tissues, including the brain and lungs. In the blood, neuroleptics are highly bound to plasma proteins, generally in excess of 90%.

Neuroleptics are 99% metabolized before excretion. Metabolism occurs in the liver and may be increased by induction of liver enzymes. After metabolism, excretion occurs in approximately equal proportions by renal extraction and enterohepatic circulation. *Metabolism of neuroleptics proceeds at a slower rate in elderly people, necessitating lower doses. Phenothiazine metabolites impart a harmless pink to red-brown discoloration to the urine.*

Clinical Indications The evidence for efficacy of neuroleptics in schizophrenia is stronger than for any other class of psychotherapeutic agents for their therapeutic applications. Neuroleptics provide symptomatic relief in chronic schizophrenia, often controlling the condition sufficiently to allow the person to return to a community setting. In schizophreniform disorder, neuroleptics control symptoms acutely and hasten recovery.

Neuroleptics are useful in acute management of mania. Lithium is clearly preferable to neuroleptics for long-term control of manic-depressive disorder (see Chapter 21), but mania responds acutely to neuroleptics more rapidly than to lithium. Phenothiazines have also been used for managing belligerence and explosive hyperexcitability in children with conduct disorder of the aggressive, undersocialized type. Neuroleptics may also be used successfully in clients with psychotic symptoms secondary to chronic organic brain syndrome, but at smaller doses, since the depressant effects of the drugs will aggravate cognitive and functional impairments associated with organic brain syndrome. A rare illness called Gilles de la Tourette's syndrome is treated with haloperidol (Haldol) or pimozide (Orap) (see Chapter 22).

Neuroleptics are frequently employed in the short-term treatment of **dysthymic disorder,** in which agitation, anxiety, or tension is a marked component. Alternative treatments include anxiolytics or antidepressants. Small doses of neuroleptics are sometimes also employed as a placebo-like therapy in generalized anxiety disorders as an alternative to potentially addictive anxiolytics. For a client who is likely to abuse drugs or who insists on drug treatment beyond the time limit of anxiolytic effectiveness, low-dose neuroleptic treatment is a reasonable approach.

Several neuroleptics, most notably prochlorperazine (Compazine), are used for conditions entirely unrelated to psychiatric disorders. For example, prochlorperazine is used to suppress nausea and vomiting associated with cancer chemotherapy or with motion sickness; its antipruritic action suppresses severe itching. Dosages for these purposes are at the low end of the dosage range. Promethazine, trimeprazine, and methdilazine are phenothiazine agents marketed for their antihistaminergic properties. Phenothiazines that may be administered as antiemetics include chlorpromazine, triflupromazine, perphenazine, prochlorperazine, promethazine, and thiethylperazine. Propiomazine, an aminoalkyl phenothiazine, is also sometimes employed as a parenteral sedative, preoperatively or during surgery. Methotrimeprazine is a phenothiazine employed as a centrally acting nonnarcotic analgesic. Droperidol, a butyrophenone derivative related to haloperidol, is used (with fentanyl) as a primary anesthetic or adjunct to general anesthesia.

Adverse Effects and Contraindications The adverse effects of neuroleptics are severe enough to weigh heavily in risk-benefit considerations when reviewing therapeutic options. The range of possible side effects is similar for the individual neuroleptics,

Nursing Observations for Neuroleptic Therapy of Schizophrenia

THERAPEUTIC GOAL	Suppression of florid symptoms of schizophrenia.
PREADMINISTRATION ASSESSMENT	
Baseline Data	Observe extent of delusions, hallucinations, incoherence, bizarre ideation, blunted or flat affect, catatonia, disorganized behavior, peculiar behavior, social isolation or withdrawal, and deterioration of functioning. Evaluate orientation, reflexes, muscle tone, hand steadiness, vital signs, tissue perfusion, abdominal and liver function, respiratory sounds, and visual function. Obtain laboratory tests including complete blood cell counts and urinalysis.
Contraindications	Seizure disorders, cardiovascular disease, hypotension, chronic obstructive pulmonary disease, bone marrow depression, hepatic failure, glaucoma, peptic ulcers, pregnancy, lactation, or allergies to phenothiazines or other antipsychotic drugs.
Potential Interactions	CNS depressants, anticholinergics, hypotensive agents, or lithium.
EVALUATION OF DRUG RESPONSE	
During Dosage Adjustment	Monitor alleviation of target symptoms and occurrence of adverse effects.
For Therapeutic Benefit	Monitor alleviation of target symptoms.
For Adverse Effects	Monitor for excess sedation, orthostatic hypotension, anticholinergic side effects, allergic reactions, bone marrow suppression, skin rash, jaundice, indication of seizure activity, appetite changes, sexual dysfunctions, photosensitivity, impaired temperature regulation, acute dystonias, akathisias, pseudoparkinsonian symptoms, and tardive dyskinesias.
For Drug Interactions	Monitor for additive CNS depression, additive hypotension, additive anticholinergic effects, and increased lithium toxicity.
For Dietary Interactions	Monitor for changes in appetite; provide riboflavin supplement (2–5 mg/day).
For Complicance	Evaluate client's compliance with all facets of the therapeutic regimen by careful observation, interviewing, and review of progress. Report compliance problems to the physician and act as client-advocate when changes in the therapeutic regimen seem indicated.

but the frequency and severity with which the various side effects occur differ from drug to drug, providing one basis for selecting a particular drug for a particular client. Most adverse effects of neuroleptics are reversible with dosage adjustment or discontinuation of the drug.

Adverse reactions to neuroleptics can be grouped into three clusters (Table 18-4): (1) "early" side effects, which generally occur soon after initiation of therapy, (2) continuing side effects, equally likely at all stages of therapy, and (3) multifaceted extrapyramidal side effects, of which three forms occur early in treatment and one late in treatment.

Early Side Effects. The early side effects of neuroleptics fall into four categories: anticholinergic side effects, sedation, orthostatic hypotension, and blood cell disorders. The **anticholinergic side effects** are a cluster of autonomic and CNS symptoms, including dryness of the mouth, blurred vision, constipation, and urinary retention. *Nurses should explain to clients that dryness of mouth can be alleviated by frequent sips of water, chewing sugarless gum, or frequent rinsing of the mouth with warm water. Good oral hygiene needs to be maintained to prevent candidal overgrowth. Nurses should carefully monitor hospital patients receiving neuroleptics for dietary intake, bowel elimination patterns, and the intake-output ratios for indications of constipation or urinary retention. Increasing dietary fiber and fluid intake may help to overcome neuroleptic-induced constipation.* Generally, neuroleptic drugs with the most intensive anticholinergic properties produce fewer early extrapyramidal side effects, a fact consistent with the efficacy of anticholinergic drugs such as benztropine (Cogentin) in both organic and drug-induced parkinsonism. There is some evidence, however, that anticholinergic

Table 18–4
Time of Maximal Risk of Various Neuroleptic Side Effects

Type of side effect	Period of maximal risk
Early	
Anticholinergic	First few weeks; tolerance develops
Sedation	First few weeks; tolerance develops
Orthostatic hypotension	First few weeks; tolerance develops
Blood cell disorders	
Dyscrasias	4–12 weeks
Allergies	1–8 weeks
Continuing	
Lowered seizure threshold	Any time
Hypothalamic	Any time
Extrapyramidal	
Acute dystonic reactions	1–5 days
Pseudoparkinsonism	5–30 days
Akathisias	5–60 days
Tardive dyskinesias	After months or years

properties have a negative effect on antipsychotic potency, which is also consistent with the observed interaction of benztropine with neuroleptic therapy.

The **sedation** produced by neuroleptics is due to the combination of anticholinergic, antidopaminergic, and antiadrenergic actions. All three of these transmitters are involved in CNS arousal.

Orthostatic hypotension caused by neuroleptics is due to central and peripheral antinoradrenergic actions that dilate blood vessels, and direct depressant effect on the heart. Tachycardia occurs because of the anticholinergic action of neuroleptics but also as a reflex reaction to falling blood pressure. *Elastic stockings may help to reduce the influence of orthostatic hypotension by preventing pooling of blood in the extremities. Clients should be advised to shift from a recumbent to an upright position gradually, to dangle the legs over the side of the bed before initial ambulation after drug administration, and to avoid extremes of heat, such as hot showers, baths, or prolonged exposure to sunshine.* Tolerance develops to the orthostatic hypotension after several weeks of chronic treatment.

Two types of blood cell disorders, **blood dyscrasias** and **allergies,** are occasionally observed in clients receiving neuroleptic medication. Leukopenia (a drop in the number of white blood cells, particularly granulocytes) may occur suddenly, usually between the fourth and twelfth weeks of treatment. *Nurses should warn clients to report any evidence of upper respiratory infection and a complete blood cell count should be ordered.* Fortunately, severe agranulocytosis occurs in only 1 in 10,000 individuals receiving neuroleptics. *Early signs of agranulocytosis include sore mouth, throat, or gums, elevated fever, and upper respiratory tract infections.*

Allergies occur in a wide variety of manifestations with the use of neuroleptics. The mildest and most common form of allergy is skin rash, occurring in about 5% of clients receiving chlorpromazine. Contact dermatitis may occur from contact of the drug with the skin surface. *Clients should be warned against spilling concentrates of neuroleptics on the skin. Should skin contact occur, the area should be washed well with soap and water.*

Allergic jaundice is a more severe allergic reaction and occurs most commonly in women between the second and fourth weeks of treatment. Early symptoms include marked increase in temperature, upper abdominal pain, nausea, diarrhea, skin rash, and yellowing of the skin, mucous membranes, and sclera (whites of the eyes).

Another allergic reaction, **photosensitivity,** has two manifestations: susceptibility to sunburn and pigmentary retinopathy. *Protective clothing and sunglasses are important aids in preventing photosensitivity reactions.* Pigmentary retinopathy may be particularly pronounced when high doses of thioridazine are used. Allergies generally occur within the first 8 weeks of treatment and abate when the drug is discontinued. Cross-sensitivity is likely to occur between two neuroleptics from the same chemical group, but not between agents from differing groups.

Continuing Side Effects. Some of the CNS side effects of neuroleptics can be characterized as continuing side effects because they do not undergo tolerance. Many of the neuroleptics **lower the seizure threshold.** Seizures occur in about 0.5–1% of individuals treated with neuroleptics. *When a neuroleptic is to be used in a seizure-prone client (in epilepsy or delirium tremens, for example), the drug selected should have minimal effect on the seizure threshold (molindone or thioridazine).*

Suppression of the hypothalamic-pituitary axis by neuroleptics results in another cluster of adverse effects. Neuroleptics suppress the temperature-regulating mechanism, so that a client who is taking a neuroleptic is more than usually susceptible to cold exposure or heat exhaustion. This loss of temperature-regulating ability is called **poikilothermy.** *Nurses need to warn clients to avoid extremes of temperature, since heat stroke or cold exposure could result. Injury can also*

Nursing Diagnoses and Interventions for Neuroleptic Therapy of Schizophrenia

Nursing Diagnoses	*Related Interventions*
TO ENHANCE DRUG BENEFITS OR REDUCE DRUG REQUIREMENTS	
Alteration in thought processes: delusions and bizarre ideation; Anxiety related to diminished ability to cope; Impaired social interactions related to withdrawal, paranoia, and peculiar behavior; Impaired verbal communications related to incoherence and poverty of thought	Provide emotional support and encouragement and psychotherapy as indicated. Confer with close family members, identifying apparent onset of changed behavior and any prior therapy. Determine if the client has been taking drugs which could contribute to altered behavior.
Impaired home maintenance management related to impaired judgment and inability to function effectively	Advise clients and their families about social services that are available; help families identify when clients are best served by inpatient or outpatient status.
Violence to self or others due to combativeness, paranoia, and delusions	Maintain vigilance when working with combative individuals. Provide appropriate protective measures to prevent client self-injury.
TO MINIMIZE DRUG SIDE EFFECTS OR INTERACTIONS	
Alteration in oral mucous membranes, urinary elimination, and bowel elimination related to anticholinergic properties of antipsychotic drugs	Encourage good oral hygiene; provide frequent rinses, gum, or hard candy to relieve dryness of mouth; maintain high fiber intake to minimize constipation and high fluid intake to counter urinary or bowel problems.
Increased risk of injury related to sedative, hypotensive, and extrapyramidal effects, suppression of conditioned avoidance responses, and photosensitivity	Warn clients receiving antipsychotic drugs not to drive or operate dangerous equipment, to make position changes slowly, to avoid extremes of heat or cold (hot showers or sunlight), to avoid prolonged standing in one place; to wear elastic stockings for orthostatic hypotension, and to use heating pads with caution. Provide safety measures, such as bed rails.
Sensory perceptual alterations related to drug-induced retinopathy	Warn client to protect the eyes and skin from exposure to sunlight with sunglasses and adequate clothing; schedule periodic assessment of visual function.
TO ENSURE SAFE AND EFFICACIOUIS DRUG USE	
Knowledge deficit related to drug regimen	Explain the nature of the disorder and the rationale for drug treatment to responsible family members and the client (to the extent of client's ability to comprehend).
	Provide client or responsible family member with a list of adverse effects and drug interactions for each drug in the regimen and explain what to do if any of these occur.
	Advise clients who are not institutionalized to wear medical identification tags or bracelets indicating the diagnosis and drug regimen.

occur with use of hot water bottles or heating pads and they should not be used. Clients and family members need to be taught the symptoms of heat stroke, such as redness, hot, dry skin, dilated pupils, dyspnea, a strong, bounding pulse, and markedly elevated body temperature. To lower body temperature, cold, moist cloths should be placed on the temples, neck, axilla, and groin, and cold, wet cloths or ice should be packed around the body. A physician should be called immediately.

Appetite is often altered by neuroleptics; most drugs increase appetite, but some (such as haloperidol) will suppress it. *Diabetic or prediabetic clients who are on long-term therapy with high doses of neuroleptics need special monitoring to avoid losing control of the diabetes from dietary deficiencies. Urine and blood glucose tests should be scheduled regularly to monitor sugar content. If sugar becomes elevated, the dosage of hypoglycemic medication may have to be adjusted or a different neuroleptic employed.*

Secretion of pituitary hormones regulated by dopamine is altered by neuroleptic therapy. Growth hormone-releasing factor secreted in the infundibular region of the hypothalamus, under the influence of dopaminergic neurons, is suppressed by neuroleptics; consequently, release of growth hormone from the pituitary is diminished. When neuroleptics are used in children, drug "holidays" (interruptions in the therapeutic regimen) must be provided to minimize stunting of growth.

Neuroleptics also affect **reproductive functioning.** Prolactin secretion, which stimulates lactation in the female, is inversely related to dopamine activity because the release of prolactin inhibitory factor is regulated by dopaminergic neurons. The stimulatory effect of dopamine-blocking drugs on prolactin release causes **pseudolactation.** Tolerance does not develop to the prolactin-releasing action of neuroleptics. Other effects include **anovulation** in women and **impotence** and **retrograde ejaculation** in men. Antiadrenergic neuroleptics, such as chlorpromazine, also suppress secretion of adrenocorticotropic hormone and antidiuretic hormone. A premenopausal woman may erroneously suspect pregnancy because of the amenorrhea produced by the drug therapy. *It is important to perform a thorough endocrine assessment both prior to and after initiation of neuroleptic therapy.*

Extrapyramidal Side Effects. Four types of extrapyramidal side effects occur with the use of antipsychotic drugs: pseudoparkinsonism, akathisias, acute dystonias, and tardive dyskinesias. The period of greatest risk of **pseudoparkinsonism** is between 5 and 30 days after initiating treatment. The symptoms of neuroleptic-induced parkinsonism are muscle rigidity, tremors, and akinesias. Pseudoparkinsonism occurs in 10–20% of individuals depending on the neuroleptic selected. **Akathisia** is a condition of motor restlessness that is easily mistaken for agitation. It develops in 10–20% of neuroleptic-treated individuals, most commonly after 5–60 days of treatment. **Acute dystonic reactions** appear as facial grimacing or muscle spasms, involving the tongue, face, neck, and back. These generally appear during the first 5 days. The incidence is from 2% to 10% of patients treated with neuroleptics, depending on the agent selected for treatment.

Tardive dyskinesias are late-occurring and persistent side effects. Tardive dyskinesias first appear as gnawing, curling, or twisting (vermicular) movements of the tongue. Full-blown dyskinesias may involve abnormal movements of the head, neck, and extremities in addition to tongue movements. The risk that tardive dyskinesia will develop increases with the duration of treatment as well as with dosage. The incidence varies from 15% to 45% depending on the agent employed in neuroleptic therapy. Tardive dyskinesias are particularly undesirable adverse effects because therapeutic response options are severely limited and the disorders may be persistent and even irreversible.

Anticholinergic drugs or amantadine are useful in treating the tremor and rigidity of pseudoparkinsonism and acute dystonic reactions, but they aggravate and sometimes trigger tardive dyskinesias. It is usually best not to employ anticholinergic drugs prophylactically. Benzodiazepines are probably the most useful drug group for alleviating akathisias. Dopamine-depleting drugs have some usefulness for managing tardive dyskinesias. (The appearance and treatment of these four types of drug-induced extrapyramidal side effects are further discussed in Chapter 22.)

Contraindications A specific contraindication for use of phenothiazines is in alcohol withdrawal, since the likelihood of seizures is increased, and neuroleptics in general have not proved useful. In elderly clients with chronic organic brain syndrome, neuroleptics may increase cognitive impairment and confusion. *Nurses may be able to assess these changes by questioning those most closely associated with elderly clients about possible regressive behaviors.* Autonomic side effects, such as hypotension and urinary retention, are often more serious in these clients. Therefore, blood pressure and fluid intake and output should be monitored. On the other hand, the fact that neuroleptics interfere less with cognitive functioning than do sedative-hypnotics is an advantage for their use in elderly clients. Thioridazine (Mellaril) may have special advantages in geriatric care because of its comparatively low incidence of extrapyramidal problems.

Pregnant women who must take an antipsychotic drug during pregnancy should discontinue the drug 1–2 weeks before delivery to avoid problems such as jaundice, prolonged extrapyramidal symptoms, and hyperreflexia. Discontinuation requires a scheduled reduction in dosage over a period of several weeks. *Nurses should establish a timetable complete with dosage requirements to help clients adhere to the protocol.*

Interactions with Other Drugs and Laboratory Tests Although neuroleptics inhibit the effectiveness of **antidepressants** and may increase pathologic states, they are too often used in combination with tricyclic antidepressants. Etrafon and Triavil are combination formulations containing perphenazine (a neuroleptic) and amitriptyline (an antidepressant). Clinical trials have failed to document a value for this combination, even in the dubious schizoaffective classification.

Combinations of **two or more neuroleptics** are frequently employed in particularly difficult cases, but controlled clinical trials have failed to indicate that such combinations enjoy any superiority over single-drug treatments. This negative evidence, together with risks related to uncertainties about drug interactions and dosage parameters in drug combinations, appears to argue against this approach.

Anxiolytics may be added adjunctively to the regimen of a psychotic client. Again there is no evidence that the addition of an anxiolytic lessens the client's psychosis. However, short-term administration of anxiolytics can alleviate akathisias and any anxiety that may be present. The value of alleviating these symptoms must be weighed against the costs of complicating the drug regimen and additional adverse effects.

The most common unplanned interaction of neuroleptics is **additive CNS depression,** which can occur with any two depressant drugs used concomitantly. Additive depression has been observed in particular when neuroleptics have been employed with alcohol, barbiturates, anesthetics, and narcotics. Many neuroleptics not only have anticholinergic properties but the potential for **additive anticholinergic effects** when used with other anticholinergic agents, including most antidepressants, many antiparkinsonian drugs, some narcotics, and belladonna alkaloids. *The nurse should instruct clients not to take any nonprescription medications without first consulting the physician who has prescribed the neuroleptic.*

Lithium in combination with several of the neuroleptics has resulted in severe neurotoxicity, which has been reported specifically with chlorpromazine, thioridazine, and haloperidol, but presumably applies to other neuroleptics as well. While this interaction is not common, nurses should note in their drug history whether or not clients have been taking lithium.

Phenothiazines have been reported to cause an increase in plasma concentrations of the **beta-blockers,** propranolol and metoprolol. These beta-blockers also elevate plasma levels of the phenothiazine being employed. Antipsychotic drugs diminish the antihypertensive effectiveness of **guanethidine** (Ismelin) by blocking its uptake into noradrenergic nerve terminals where it produces its depleting action on neurotransmitter stores. **Sympathomimetics** should not be used in combination with neuroleptics that have alpha-blocking properties, since this results in potentially dangerous cardiac stimulation without the balancing alpha-adrenergic effects of the sympathomimetic agents.

Antidiarrheal mixtures and antacids that contain **aluminum salts** reduce absorption of phenothiazines. *When it is necessary for a client who is receiving a phenothiazine to use an antacid, the medication should be given at least 1 hour, but preferably 2 hours, before the phenothiazines.* **Caffeine** has also been reported to interact chemically with neuroleptics in the gut to inhibit their absorption.

Neuroleptics have been reported to alter plasma concentrations of **phenytoin** (Dilantin) in either direction. More generally, neuroleptics may increase requirements for **antiepileptic medications,** since they tend to lower the seizure threshold. Phenothiazines have been reported to aggravate the neuromuscular blocking action of **polypeptide antibiotics. Methyldopa** (Aldomet) and haloperidol in combination are said to produce psychiatric reactions, including disorientation, irritability, or assaultiveness.

The antiemetic effect of neuroleptics may mask toxic effects of other drugs that clients are taking, making it difficult to diagnose those conditions whose primary symptoms are nausea and vomiting.

Neuroleptics produce alterations in certain laboratory tests. Phenothiazines impart a pink to red-brown color to the urine. False positives have been reported on pregnancy tests. Alterations in liver function tests may occur even in the absence of clinical signs of liver toxicity. Increases in protein-bound iodine can also occur when neuroleptics are being used. Phenothiazines and thioxanthines can interfere with bilirubin tests, resulting in false positive reactions. Chlorpromazine has the potential for interfering with the Coomb's test, producing false positive results.

Administration of Neuroleptics The typical pattern of administration of neuroleptics is an initial low daily dosage of one agent, which is gradually increased until a therapeutic response is obtained or significant side effects develop. If a client is uncooperative and combative, however, rapid neuroleptization is required, and the drug is initially given intramuscularly; oral administration usually can be instituted later in the treatment sequence.

The effective dose of neuroleptics varies considerably from individual to individual. Therefore, dosages need to be flexible and in accord with the client's response and any side effects. Clients should be monitored closely, but judgments should not be made too hastily. A therapeutic response may occur only after a few weeks or months of treatment at an adequate dosage. A client who is refractory to one agent may respond to another.

Therapeutic effectiveness is judged in terms of amelioration of target symptoms. The various symptoms frequently accompanying schizophrenia respond differentially to neuroleptics both in degree and time course. It has been noted that florid symptoms, such as combativeness or hallucinations, are more likely to respond than are negative symptoms, such as poor insight or memory, poverty of speech, affective blunting, and poor hygiene. In general, symptoms such as hyperreactivity and hostility respond relatively quickly (in 1–2 weeks); affective changes occur with moderate rapidity (in 2–6 weeks); and cognitive and perceptual changes occur only slowly (in 2–3 months).

If the client improves substantially in response to neuroleptic treatment, the question ultimately arises as to whether and when treatment should be curtailed or terminated. Relapse occurs with great frequency in both inpatients and outpatients who have been withdrawn from neuroleptic medication, but the side effects of these drugs are severe enough in many cases to encourage a reduction in dosage or cessation of drug treatment. Generally, a considerable reduction in dosage can be accomplished during the maintenance phase — to about one-fifth or one-third of the dosage used during the acute phase. *When neuroleptic therapy is to be discontinued, or if a sharp dosage reduction is to be effected, the dosage reduction should be gradual to minimize the possibility of recurrence of symptoms, onset of severe gastrointestinal disturbances, or the development of tardive dyskinesias.*

Maintenance drugs can and should be prescribed on a once-a-day basis. *Clients should be advised to schedule such administration for bedtime so that the peak period of sedation occurs during sleep.* Many studies have indicated that outpatients frequently do not comply with medication instructions. This is especially true with neuroleptics, because these drugs have negative reinforcement properties (as shown by self-administration studies in animals), produce annoying adverse effects, and are usually employed in individuals who are generally less dependable. However, clients tend to comply more readily if asked to take fewer different pills fewer times per day. Outpatients who repeatedly exhibit poor compliance can be placed on long-lasting dosage forms of fluphenazine (Prolixin) — the enanthate and decanoate esters. These oil emulsions are injected intramuscularly or subcutaneously, in 1 ml volumes. The therapeutic effects last 1–3 weeks for fluphenazine enanthate and up to 4 weeks for fluphenazine decanoate.

Maintenance treatment with neuroleptics generally continues for at least 6 months after an acute schizophrenic episode. Then, if conditions appear favorable, gradual discontinuation of drug treatment may be effected, with the understanding that resumption of treatment may be indicated later.

Important Nursing Implications for Antipsychotic Drugs

☐ Prior to initiation of therapy with a neuroleptic, ensure a thorough physical examination of the client, including complete blood cell analysis, liver function tests, urinalysis, an electroencephalogram, and ocular examination. Reevaluation should be undertaken at frequent intervals during treatment.

☐ Prior to initiating drug therapy with neuroleptics, take a thorough drug history of the client. Record any incidents of drug hypersensitivity. It is important to interview those closest to the client if the client is sufficiently disturbed that he or she cannot recount an accurate history.

☐ Inspire the client's confidence and willingness to share information about response to therapy by being compassionate and accurate in observations, evaluation, and judgments.

☐ Warn clients not to drive, operate dangerous machinery, or perform other tasks requiring mental alertness while using antipsychotic drugs.

☐ Monitor the blood pressure of clients while standing and lying down to assess the extent of orthostatic hypotension. Clients experiencing orthostatic hypotension should be warned not to stand for long periods, to avoid standing up quickly, and to avoid exposure to hot showers or sunlight.

- ☐ Monitor for indications of urinary retention and avoid use of neuroleptics if the client has a history of urinary hesitancy or retention.
- ☐ Avoid allowing neuroleptic concentrates to contact the skin, eyes, or clothing of the client. When preparing injectable or liquid forms, use rubber gloves. Avoid subcutaneous injections because of the high risk of allergic skin reactions.
- ☐ Assess client regularly for indications of developing extrapyramidal symptoms. Nurses should confer with persons closely connected to the client about changes in motor function and behavior resulting from therapy.
- ☐ Assess the client's skin and eyes for indications of allergic reactions, such as retinopathy, jaundice, or abnormal pigmentation of the skin when the client is exposed to sunlight. Advise clients to wear adequate protective clothing and sunglasses to minimize photosensitivity reactions.
- ☐ Observe client for signs of agranulocytosis such as sore throat, persistent fever, or malaise.
- ☐ Assess the client's endocrine system for drug-induced endocrine changes, including menstrual irregularity and breast engorgement in women and impotency and gynecomastia in men.
- ☐ Maintain a list of all medications that the client currently takes and check this for potential interactions.
- ☐ Stress to clients the importance of adhering to drug regimens, and remind them that sudden discontinuation may result in withdrawal symptoms.
- ☐ Observe inpatients to make certain that oral drugs have been swallowed and not hoarded. Severely depressed clients may hoard pills for a future suicide attempt. It may be advisable to give the client liquid preparations, because these permit better control over drug taking and may also improve compliance.
- ☐ Warn clients that it is harmful to share their drugs with others.
- ☐ Encourage clients to wear an identification bracelet indicating diagnosis, drugs the client takes, and whom to contact should the individual seek care elsewhere or be admitted to an emergency room for treatment.

Families of Neuroleptics

Distinguishing features among the various groups of neuroleptics as regards selective therapeutic spectra have been exaggerated by the advertising of pharmaceutical manufacturers. Among the antipsychotic drugs, no one drug or group of drugs is clearly superior to any other in efficacy at therapeutically equivalent doses (Table 18–5). Many researches consider the dopamine-blocking action of neuroleptic drugs to be the crucial characteristic for efficacy and any norepinephrine-blocking action to contribute only to the autonomic and sedative side effects. If one accepts this viewpoint, the neuroleptic of choice might be one with the highest ratio of antidopamine to antinorepinephrine properties. Clinical studies have failed to substantiate the superiority of neuroleptics

Table 18–5
Equivalent Dose and Daily Oral Adult Dosage Range

Drug	Equivalent dose[a]	Adult daily oral dosage range (mg)
Phenothiazines, aliphatic		
Chlorpromazine	100	30–1,000
Promazine	200	40–1,000
Triflupromazine	25	60–150
Phenothiazines, piperidine		
Thioridazine	100	150–800
Mesoridazine	50	30–400
Piperacetazine	10	20–160
Phenothiazines, piperazine		
Prochlorperazine	15	15–150
Perphenazine	10	12–64
Fluphenazine	2	0.5–20
Trifluoperazine	5	2–40
Acetophenazine	20	60–120
Carphenazine	25	25–400
Butyrophenone		
Haloperidol	2	1–15
Thioxanthenes		
Chlorprothixene	100	75–600
Thiothixene	5	6–60
Dihydroindolone		
Molindone	10	15–225
Dibenzoxazepine		
Loxapine	10	20–250

[a]Dose equivalent to 100 mg of chlorpromazine.

that have high dopamine specificity. Representatives of various subgroups, including chlorpromazine, perphenazine, prochlorperazine, triflupromazine, thioridazine, haloperidol, and thiothixene, have, generally, produced comparable results in clinical studies. There is some indication that thioridazine may be more effective in less severe cases and less effective in more severe cases than other neuroleptics. Although there are limited differences in overall efficacy in populations of psychotic patients, a given client may respond better to one agent than another.

The butyrophenones and piperazines have greater specificity for dopamine receptors than the older aliphatic phenothiazines, but are more likely to cause extrapyramidal reactions. Extrapyramidal symptoms were once regarded as inseparable from therapeutic effectiveness; however, the newer atypical neuroleptics provide substantial efficacy with little risk of such reactions.

There are distinct differences in the incidence of side effects of the various neuroleptics (Table 18–6). Side effects may interact with a component of the

Table 18–6
Side Effects of Various Neuroleptics

	Early side effects				Continuing		
Drug	Anticholinergic	Sedation	Orthostatic hypotension	Blood cell disorders	Lowered seizure threshold	Hypothalamic	Extrapyramidal
Phenothiazines, aliphatic							
Chlorpromazine	++	+++	+++	++	+++	++	++
Promazine	+++	++	++	++	+++	++	++
Triflupromazine	+++	+++	++	++	+++	++	++
Phenothiazines, piperidine							
Thioridazine	+++	+++	+++	+	+	++	+
Mesoridazine	++	+++	++	+	+	++	+
Piperacetazine	++	++	++	+	+	++	++
Phenothiazines, piperazine							
Prochlorperazine	+	++	+	++	+	++	+++
Perphenazine	++	+	+	++	+	++	+++
Fluphenazine	+	+	+	++	+	++	+++
Trifluoperazine	+	+	+	++	+	++	+++
Acetophenazine	++	++	+	++	+	++	+++
Carphenazine	+	++	+	++	+	++	+++
Butyrophenone							
Haloperidol	0	+	+	+	++	+++	+++
Thioxanthenes							
Chlorprothixene	++	+++	+++	++	+++	++	++
Thiothixene	+	+	+	++	++	++	+++
Dihydroindolone							
Molindone	++	++	+	+	0/+	+	++
Dibenzoxazepine							
Loxapine	+	++	+	++	++	+	+++
Dibenzodiazepines							
Clozapine (experimental)	+++	++	+++	++	+	0/+	0
Benzamides							
Sulpiride	+	0/+	+	0/+		++	+

psychosis itself or with concurrent medical difficulties of the individual. A drug selection is made to minimize the potential for these negative interactions. Thus, while the alternative neuroleptics are pharmacologically equivalent in their primary therapeutic action, at times they may be clinically distinguished by their respective patterns of side effects.

The phenothiazine class has three subgroups: the aminoalkyls (or aliphatics), the piperazines, and the piperadines.

Aminoalkyl Phenothiazines

Chlorpromazine (Thorazine), the first phenothiazine employed clinically, is an **aminoalkyl phenothiazine.** Promazine (Sparine) and triflupromazine (Vesprin) are others in this group used for treatment of psychoses. Promazine is less effective than other neuroleptics in treating psychoses. The aminoalkyls produce considerable sedation and hypotension and some intellectual impairment. They predispose to seizures and increase spike-and-burst activity in the EEG. On the other hand, extrapyramidal side effects are of moderate intensity and frequency. The high level of sedation with this group has led to their effective use in agitated rather than withdrawn schizophrenic patients. Chlorpromazine is frequently used in toxic psychoses induced by drugs (LSD, mescaline, or amphetamine).

Preparations and Administration

Chlorpromazine (Thorazine, Promapar, Thor-Prom, generic formulations, etc.)
Tablets, spansule capsules, syrup, concentrates (*should be prepared in one-half glass of juice, milk, or water immediately prior to use*), suppositories, injection solutions
Recommended Doses: For initial oral treatment of anxiety, agitation, tension, or for psychosis in adult outpatients, 10 mg, 3 or 4 times daily or 25 mg, 2 or 3 times daily. For more rapid control, 25 mg may be given IM and repeated, if necessary, in 1 hour. For hospitalized adult psychiatric patients (agitated, manic, or disturbed), 25 mg orally, 3 times daily initially, gradually titrated upward to a maximum of 400 mg daily. For more immediate control of acute situations, 25 mg IM followed by 25–50 mg per hour. Intramuscular doses can be gradually increased over several days up to 400 mg every 4–6 hours for very severe cases. For nausea and vomiting or in psychiatric outpatients under age 13, 0.25 mg/lb (0.5 mg/kg) orally every 4–6 hours as needed, or 0.5 mg/lb rectally every 6–8 hours. The intramuscular dose is 0.25 mg/lb every 6–8 hours, up to 40 mg/day for children under age 5 and 75 mg/day in children 6–12. For hospitalized psychiatric patients, doses are titrated upward gradually from a recommended initial dose of 50–100 mg daily (or 200 mg daily in older children).

Promazine (Sparine and generic formulations)
Tablets, syrup, concentrate, injection solutions
Recommended Doses: For severely agitated adult patients, 50–150 mg IM initially; once control is obtained, 10–200 mg orally or IM at 4–6 hour intervals. Total daily doses should not exceed 1,000 mg. For acute psychotic episodes in children over 12, 10–25 mg given orally at 4–6 hour intervals.

Triflupromazine (Vesprin)
Suspension, injection solutions (*When the drug is in solution, its color may range from clear to light amber. Darker solutions should not be used.*)
Recommended Doses: For adults with psychotic disorders, 100 mg orally initially, increased up to 150 mg/day; or 60 mg IM, up to 150 mg/day. For outpatients, 30 mg, up to 150 mg/day. For children, 2 mg/kg up to 150 mg/day orally in divided doses; or 0.2–0.25 mg/kg IM up to 10 mg/day. Triflupromazine is not recommended for children under 2.5 years of age. *Nurses need to take special precaution not to confuse this drug with trifluoperazine.*

Piperazine Phenothiazines

The piperazine phenothiazines cause less sedation, less impairment of performance in motor and cognitive tasks, considerably less hypotension, and fewer skin reactions. Extrapyramidal effects, particularly the acute dystonic reactions, are a greater problem than for the aminoalkyls. Members of this subgroup are prochlorperazine (Compazine), trifluoperazine (Stelazine), fluphenazine (Prolixin, Permitil), perphenazine (Trilafon), carphenazine (Proketazine), and acetophenazine (Tindal). The piperazines have less effect on the seizure threshold than aminoalkyls. The lack of sedative side effects has led to the use of piperazines in dull, withdrawn, or apathetic schizophrenic clients. In neurotic clients, perphenazine has been found useful and preferable to chlorpromazine. Piperazines are particularly effective in suppressing vomiting brought on by drugs or pathological conditions.

Prochlorperazine is seldom used in psychiatry because of the severity of extrapyramidal side effects, but it is the phenothiazine most likely to be employed (at relatively low doses) for nonpsychiatric applications, such as motion sickness and preanesthetic apprehensiveness.

Preparations and Administration Most piperazine phenothiazines are marketed in short-acting dosage forms. However, prolixin is available in two long-acting esterified forms (**prolixin enanthate** and **prolixin decanoate**) for intramuscular or subcutaneous injection. These dosage forms provide an extended antipsychotic action with an onset about 24–72 hours after injection and a duration of 1–3 weeks for the enanthate ester and up to 4 weeks for the decanoate ester.

Acetophenazine (Tindal)
Tablets
Recommended Doses: For outpatients, 20 mg orally, 2–4 times daily. For hospitalized patients, 80–120 mg/day PO. Doses as high as 400–600 mg/day have been employed in severely schizophrenic individuals.

Carphenazine (Proketazine)
Tablets
Recommended Doses: 12.5–25 mg orally, 2 or 3 times daily, increased gradually to a maximum of 100 mg/day.

Fluphenazine (Prolixin, Permitil)
Tablets, timed release tablets, concentrate, elixir, injection solution, long-acting depot formulations (prolixin enanthate and prolixin decanoate)
Recommended Doses: 0.5–10 mg orally initially in divided doses at 6–8 hour intervals, gradually titrated to individual requirements. More than 3 mg is seldom required, but doses as high as 40 mg are employed in extreme cases. The initial intramuscular dose for adults is 1.25, at 6–8 hour intervals, to a maximum of 2.5–10 mg daily. *Injections of this drug often cause acute and difficult-to-control extrapyramidal symptoms. Elderly and debilitated clients are particularly at risk.* When using the long-acting esterified forms by intramuscular or subcutaneous injection, 12.5–25 mg is employed initially and adjusted to a maximum of 100 mg per injection in accordance with response. The esters are employed only after initial dosage titration has been conducted with the shorter-acting forms of fluphenazine. Caution must be exercised in switching individuals to the longer-acting forms; lower total dosage should be employed initially until the extent of the response is determined.

Perphenazine (Trilafon)
Tablets, repeat-action tablets, concentrate, injection solution, combination tablets with amitriptyline (Triavil and Etrafon)
Recommended Doses: For moderately disturbed psychotic clients, 4–8 mg orally, 3 times daily initially (or 8–16 mg of the repeat-action form twice daily). For hospitalized psychotic patients, 8–16 mg PO, 2–4 times daily (or 8–32 mg of the repeat-action form twice daily). When a rapid action is required, 5 mg by deep IM injection, repeated at 6 hour intervals. *When the drug is administered IM, it should be given deep into the upper outer quadrant of the buttocks. The client should be in a recumbent position, and the nurse should advise the client to remain in a recumbent position for at least 1 hour after the injection. The pulse and blood pressure need to be monitored since perphenazine can cause hypotension. Also, clients need to be assessed for possible tachycardia and bradycardia. Clients can usually be placed on oral medication within 24–48 hours.*

Prochlorperazine (Compazine, Chlorazine, and generic formulations)
Tablets, sustained release capsules, suppositories, syrup, concentrate, injection solution
Recommended Doses: For mild psychiatric disturbances, 5–10 mg PO 3 or 4 times daily, gradually increased for optimum response, which can occur in some individuals with 50–75 mg/day PO, but in most cases with 100–150 mg/day. For more rapid control of severely disturbed adult patients, 10–20 mg by deep IM injection (into the upper outer quadrant of the buttock) repeated if necessary at intervals of 2–4 hours. Not recommended for children under 2 years of age or under 20 lb. For children ages 2–12, 2.5 mg, orally or rectally, 2 or 3 times daily up to 10 mg initially, increased to a maximum of 20 mg daily for children between 2 and 5 years or 25 mg for children 6–12.

Trifluoperazine (Stelazine, Suprazine, and generic formulations)
Tablets, concentrate, injection solution
Recommended Doses: For adult outpatients, 1–2 mg orally, twice daily, up to 4 mg/day. For hospitalized patients, oral doses of 2–5 mg daily. The usual IM dose in adults is 1–2 mg by deep IM injection, every 4–6 hours as needed. For children 6–12, 1 mg orally, initially once or twice daily; after titration, oral doses for children should seldom exceed 15 mg/day.

Piperidine Phenothiazines

The piperidine phenothiazines include two agents: thioridazine (Mellaril) and mesoridazine (Serentil). Thioridazine is currently the most widely used of all neuroleptics. Thioridazine produces little jaundice or rash and few extrapyramidal symptoms, but pseudolactation, inhibition of ejaculation, and pigmentary retinopathy are frequent adverse effects. Thioridazine is employed in withdrawn and hypoactive schizophrenic subjects, autistic children, dysthymic disorder, delirium tremens, positive spike pattern syndrome, and conduct disorders in children marked by explosive aggressiveness.

Preparations and Administration

Thioridazine (Mellaril, Millazine, and generic formulations)
Tablets, concentrate, oral suspension

Recommended Doses: For psychosis in adults, 50–100 mg orally, initially 3 times daily, increased in increments up to 800 mg/day. For agitation, anxiety, marked depression with anxiety, sleep disturbances, and fears in geriatric clients, 25 mg, 3 times daily up to a maximum of 200 mg/day is typical. For children ages 2–12, 0.5–3 mg/kg/day. A typical starting dose for moderate disturbances is 10 mg, 2 or 3 times daily.

Mesoridazine (Serentil)
Tablets, concentrate in alcohol, injection solution
Recommended Doses: 50 mg orally initially 3 times daily; gradually adjusted to about 100–400 mg/day. For IM administration, 25 mg initially, repeated at 30–60 minute intervals as required.

Butyrophenones

The butyrophenones are closely related to the phenothiazines in structure. Haloperidol (Haldol), the prototype of this group, is a more specific blocker of dopamine receptors than are any of the phenothiazines. The extrapyramidal effects of haloperidol are especially severe. *Thus, clients need to be assessed carefully for extrapyramidal reactions when haloperidol is employed.* In contrast to chlorpromazine, butyrophenones depress rather than stimulate appetite and produce hypothermia rather than poikilothermy. There are some indications that haloperidol has teratogenic effects. *When the client is a female outpatient, it should be ascertained if she is pregnant or contemplating a pregnancy; if so, the risk of birth defects should be discussed with the client.* Like chlorpromazine, haloperidol predisposes to seizures but to a lesser extent. The butyrophenones produce minimal early side effects (sedation, orthostatic hypotension, or anticholinergic effects).

Butyrophenones have been used experimentally to suppress withdrawal symptoms associated with chronic narcotic use. Schizophrenia that is resistant to other neuroleptic medications may respond favorably to the more potent butyrophenones. Haloperidol is one of the best neuroleptics for treatment of acute mania, and is usually the agent chosen for tranquilizing combative psychiatric patients. In children, it is used in severe behavioral problems (marked by combativeness and explosive hyperexcitability), in hyperactivity and associated conduct disorders, and in Gilles de la Tourette's syndrome (Chapter 22).

Preparations and Administration

Haloperidol (Haldol)
Tablets, concentrate, injection solution, long-acting depot formulation (haloperidol decanoate)
Recommended Doses: In adults, 0.5–5 mg orally, initially 2 or 3 times daily, then titrated to individual client needs. For prompt control of agitated patients, 2–5 mg intramuscularly, repeated as often as every 30–60 minutes if required; however, a dosage interval of 6–8 hours is often adequate. For children 3–12 years of age, 0.5 mg/day orally initially, increased by increments of 0.5 mg at intervals of 5–7 days up to a maximum of 6 mg/day. Haloperidol concentrate should not be employed with tea or coffee, since this can result in a precipitate in the gastrointestinal tract and lack of absorption. Haloperidol decanoate is given intramuscularly at doses 10–15 times the daily oral dose at intervals of 4 weeks.

Thioxanthenes

The thioxanthenes resemble the phenothiazines structurally and pharmacologically. In side effects, chlorprothixene (Taractan) most closely resembles the thioridazine while thiothixene (Navane) resembles the piperazine phenothiazines. Chlorprothixene has been reported to be effective in schizophrenia with a prominent depressive component. Although the overall responsiveness of schizophrenia to chlorprothixene is reportedly less than to chlorpromazine or haloperidol, some cases refractory to other drugs may respond to chlorprothixene. Thiothixene (Navane) has been used effectively in schizophrenia and appears to be as effective as the phenothiazines.

Preparations and Administration

Chlorprothixene (Taractan)
Tablets, concentrate, injection solution
Recommended Doses: For adults, 25–50 mg orally initially, 3 or 4 times daily to a maximum of 600 mg daily. For children over age 6 and elderly or debilitated clients, 10–25 mg orally, 3 or 4 times daily. The initial IM dose for adults and children over 12 is 25–50 mg, up to 3 or 4 times daily.

Thiothixene (Navane)
Capsules, concentrate, injection solution
Recommended Doses: 2 mg orally initially, 3 times daily, increased gradually up to 60 mg/day. Doses of 20–30 mg/day are usually optimal. The usual IM dose is 4 mg, up to 2–4 times daily as required.

Dihydroindolones

Molindone (Moban) is a dihydroindolone structurally unrelated to the phenothiazines, butyrophenones, or thioxanthenes. Molindone has an average liability with respect to sedation, anticholinergic effects, and extrapyramidal reactions. Advantages of molindone include a relatively low incidence of orthostatic hypotension, minimal effect on the seizure threshold, and no influence on the ratio of lithium distribution between intracellular and extracellular compartments. Molindone has been reported to cause resumption of menses in women experiencing amenorrhea at the time of initiation of the drug.

Preparations and Administration

Molindone (Moban)
Tablets, concentrate
Recommended Doses: For adults, 50–75 mg/day orally initially, increased in 3–4 days up to 100 mg/day and then individualized up to a maximum of 225 mg/day. For maintenance therapy of mild psychotic conditions, 5–15 mg, 3 or 4 times daily; moderate cases may require 10–25 mg, 3 or 4 times daily; and severe cases up to 225 mg daily.

Dibenzoxazepines

Loxapine (Loxitane) is another chemically distinctive neuroleptic. Its pattern of side effects resembles that of piperazine phenothiazines (such as prochlorperazine or fluphenazine), which is a rather high risk of extrapyramidal reactions and a relatively low incidence of early side effects. It has no distinctive advantages over other neuroleptics.

Preparations and Administration

Loxapine (Loxitane)
Capsules, concentrate, injection solution
Recommended Doses: For adults, 10 mg orally initially, twice daily, or 50 mg/day for severely disturbed patients. The usual range after titration is 60–100 mg/day and the maximum recommended dose is 250 mg/day. Maintenance therapy is usually conducted within the range of 20–60 mg/day. For prompt control of acutely agitated patients, 12.5–50 mg IM at intervals of 4–6 hours.

Atypical Neuroleptics

For most neuroleptics, therapeutic benefit in psychoses goes hand-in-hand with extrapyramidal side effects. A few neuroleptics that provide a degree of dissociation of efficacy from extrapyramidal side effects are referred to as **atypical** neuroleptics to distinguish them from **classical** neuroleptics, such as chlorpromazine and haloperidol. Among the marketed neuroleptics, thioridazine provides the greatest degree of efficacy in relation to risk of extrapyramidal reactions. In neuroleptic research, agents have been developed that extend this characteristic further. **Sulpiride** and **clozapine** are two atypical neuroleptics currently undergoing evaluation for possible clinical use. Sulpiride does not exhibit significant anticholinergic activity, yet is remarkably lacking in extrapyramidal effects. Experimental evidence with these drugs indicates that the dissociation of antipsychotic efficacy from extrapyramidal effects is due to their relative selectivity for dopamine receptors in the limbic system (nucleus accumbens, specifically) versus dopamine receptors in the corpus striatum.

Case Study: Acute Schizophrenic Episode

H. L., an unmarried 29-year-old man, had been employed as a postman for several years when he exhibited a sudden deterioration in behavior after 2 nights of total insomnia. He became extremely talkative, scurried about aimlessly, and became violent toward his father. After threatening to kill himself, he was admitted for acute care in a psychiatric ward.

H. L. could not remember the events that led to his hospitalization. He heard voices ordering him about and broke out laughing from time to time without apparent reason. H. L. was thin and disheveled, sometimes wearing his shirt and pants inside out. He was sometimes seen rolling about in his bed, assuming odd postures and sticking out his tongue. When interviewed by a member of the nursing staff, he demanded to see her credentials. He was noticeably anxious, paced about, and exhibited symptoms of depression. However, he was oriented as to person, time, and place.

The psychiatrist made a diagnosis of acute psychotic episode with secondary anxiety and depression and ordered chlorpromazine, 100 mg PO every 4 hours and 100 mg IM every 4 hours as required for agitation. The nursing staff gave H. L. the first oral dose of chlorpromazine; they then worked initially to calm and reassure him to avoid if possible the necessity of IM administration of the antipsychotic drug, which might have increased hostility and distrust. One nurse talked with H. L. and gathered his history: H. L. is one of three children whose mother was domineering, hypercritical, and nervous and whose father maintained a considerable detachment from the family. H. L. indicated that his mother had a nervous breakdown, his father was alcoholic, and one of his sisters had nervous problems as well.

During the first few days that H. L. was in the ward, the nurses focused on helping H. L. with his personal hygiene, providing emotional support and encouragement, and utilizing nursing interventions to counter the adverse effects of medication. For example, H. L. was given ample fluids throughout his waking hours to minimize dryness of mouth and constipation. He was warned not to change position rapidly, advised to dangle his feet from the side of the bed before arising in the morning and was aided in getting to the bathroom. The nursing staff monitored intake and output, frequency of bowel and urinary elimination, blood pressure (standing and prone), and weight. The nurses checked each day for indications of changes in muscle tone or presence of tremor or abnormal movements.

After 4 days, H. L. began to exhibit signs of improvement. He assumed increasing responsibility for his own hygiene and no longer exhibited bizarre behaviors or noticeable anxiety. He continued, however, to show signs of depression, including expressions of hopelessness and a sad countenance.

On the sixth day of neuroleptic therapy, H. L. began to exhibit intense motor restlessness, insomnia, and somatic discomfort. He complained of feeling bugs under his skin. One of the nurses reported these occurrences to the psychiatrist, who ordered the addition of diazepam (Valium) to the regimen. The symptoms subsided with this change in medication.

One week later, the psychiatrist discontinued diazepam and substituted a neuroleptic less likely to cause depression than the chlorpromazine; the change resulted in a gradual improvement in H. L.'s mood. One week after this, H. L. was discharged with a prescription for a single daily dose of the new neuroleptic. H. L. returned to work and was seen monthly for the next 6 months, after which the medication was discontinued.

1. Which of the criteria for schizophrenia does H. L. meet?
2. What evidence is there of a genetic influence in H. L.'s psychiatric condition? What evidence is there of interpersonal influences?
3. What were the nurses guarding against in advising H. L. not to change position rapidly and in helping him to the bathroom? By intake and output monitoring? By monitoring frequency of bowel and urinary elimination? By checking motor function?
4. How would you characterize the symptoms exhibited by H. L. after 6 days of neuroleptic therapy? Why was diazepam given instead of levodopa or an anticholinergic drug?
5. What antipsychotic drug might the psychiatrist have chosen as an alternative to chlorpromazine that would be less sedating?
6. Why was diazepam discontinued although it had apparently worked well controlling the adverse effect of chlorpromazine?
7. Why was H. L. continued on a neuroleptic for 6 months if he was essentially symptom-free at the time of discharge?
8. Why would the psychiatrist have H. L. take the maintenance neuroleptic once a day rather than every 4 hours as he did in the hospital?

Answers appear at the end of the book.

Recommended Readings

Baldessarini RJ: *Chemotherapy in Psychiatry,* ed 2. Cambridge, Mass, Harvard University Press, 1985.

Baldessarini RJ, Katz B, Cotton P: Dissimilar dosing with high-potency and low-potency neuroleptics. *Am J Psychiatry* 1984;141:748–752.

Cattabeni F et al (eds): *Advances in Biochemical Psychopharmacology.* New York, Raven Press, 1980, vol 24: *Long-term Effects of Neuroleptics.*

Coyle JT, Enna SJ (eds): *Neuroleptics: Neurochemical, Behavioral, and Clinical Perspectives.* New York, Raven Press, 1983.

Diamond JM, Santos AB: Unusual complications of antipsychotic drugs. *Am Fam Physician* 1982;26(4):153–157.

Donaldson SR, Gelenberg AJ, Baldessarini RJ: The pharmacological treatment of schizophrenia: A progress report. *Schizophr Bull* 1983;9:504–527.

Harris E: Antipsychotic medications. *Am J Nurs* 1981;81:1316–1323.

Harris E: Extrapyramidal side effects of antipsychotic medications. *Am J Nurs* 1981;81:1324–1328.

Harvey S: Role of the medicine nurse on the psychiatric team. *Psychiatr Nurs* 1982;20:16–17.

Hasan MK, Mooney RP: Once-a-day drug regimen for psychiatric patients. *Am Fam Physician* 1981;24(4):123–125.

Itil TM, Soldatos C: Epileptogenic side effects of psychotropic drugs. *JAMA* 1980;244:1460–1463.

Iversen LL et al. (eds): *Handbook of Psychopharmacology.* New York, Plenum, 1978, vol 10: *Neuroleptics and Schizophrenia.*

Rivera-Calimlim L, Hershey L: Neuroleptic concentrations and clinical response. *Annu Rev Pharmacol Toxicol* 1984;24:361–386.

Swonger A: The neural basis of psychotropic drug effects. *Hosp Formulary* 1977;12(11):800–807.

Wilson H, Kneisl CR: *Psychiatric Nursing.* Menlo Park, Ca, Addison-Wesley, 1983.

CHAPTER 19

Antianxiety Drugs

The Nature of Anxiety

Anxiety is a psychophysiological state at the core of which are subjective feelings of heightened tension, apprehensiveness, and uneasiness. It is distinguished from fear by the absence of a specific and appropriate circumstance responsible for the feeling. Anxiety exerts powerful influences on the body as well as the psyche and is associated with specific behavioral, autonomic, and motor correlates (Table 19–1). Autonomic correlates of anxiety arise from the activation of the hypothalamic-pituitary axis and are brought about by overstimulation of the adrenal glands and the sympathetic and parasympathetic branches of the autonomic nervous system. The motor symptoms, such as shakiness, tremor, and elevated muscle tension, involve the extrapyramidal motor system. The multifaceted nature of anxiety means that clients seek help for a variety of different reasons. Complaints may relate to the subjective state of tension or to one or more somatic symptoms, such as insomnia, headache, high blood pressure, or ulcers. Medical interventions may center on either the psychological state or on somatic manifestations.

When Is Anxiety Pathological?

Since anxiety is a universal human experience, the initial challenge facing health care professionals is to determine whether or not a given instance of anxiety warrants treatment at all. A certain amount of anxiety goes along with fulfilling needs, coping, and personal growth, but excessive anxiety is emotionally painful and disabling. Anxiety is considered patho-

Table 19–1
Symptoms of Anxiety

Subjective	Worry, apprehensiveness, rumination, edginess, tension
Behavioral	Hypervigilance, distractibility, insomnia, irritability, impatience, inability to relax, exaggerated self-consciousness, excessive need for reassurance
Motor	Shakiness, jumpiness, trembling, tremor, elevated tonus, fatigability, muscle aches, furrowed brow, fidgeting, restlessness, headaches
Autonomic	Increased heart rate, increased blood pressure, sweating, cold and moist palms, dizziness, upset stomach, diarrhea, frequent urination, flushing pallor, dry mouth, headaches

Table 19–2
Conditions Frequently Resulting in Secondary Anxiety

Somatic disorders	Drug-induced
Angina pectoris	Amphetamine-like stimulants
Bronchial asthma	Antihypertensive drugs
Cancer	Antituberculosis drugs
Hypertension	Belladonna alkaloids
Hyperthyroidism	Caffeine
Myocardial infarction	Cocaine
Neurodermatitis	Corticosteroids
Parathyroid disease	Indomethacin
Paroxysmal atrial tachycardia	Insulin
Pheochromocytoma	Levodopa
Ulcerative colitis	MAO inhibitors
	Narcotic withdrawal
Psychiatric disorders	Sedative-hypnotic withdrawal
Affective disorders	Succinimides
Drug dependence	Sulfonylureas
Hysteria	Sympathomimetics
Psychotic disorders	Thyroid hormones
Sleep disturbances	Tolazoline
	Tricyclic antidepressants

logical when the client is in obvious mental discomfort and is unresponsive to psychotherapeutic intervention or environmental manipulations to alleviate hyperactivity, intense fearfulness, excessive inhibition, or withdrawal. In such circumstances, drug treatment may reduce excessive anxiety to tolerable levels and possibly facilitate nondrug treatments or medical improvement.

Primary Versus Secondary Anxiety

Anxiety that occurs in various medical and psychiatric disorders or with use of certain drugs is **secondary anxiety** (Table 19–2). When anxiety is not caused by drug use or another disorder, it is **primary anxiety.** Primary anxiety is a clearer indication for antianxiety medication than is secondary anxiety. *When anxiety is secondary to drug use or another medical condition, treatment of the underlying disorder is given preference over use of an anxiolytic.* However, anxiolytics may be used in treating anxiety that is secondary to untreatable medical conditions or for short-term symptomatic relief of severe secondary anxiety. In assessing anxiety, evidence should be noted that might indicate presence of an organic cause: angina pectoris, bronchial asthma, hyperthyroidism, paroxysmal atrial tachycardia, sedative-hypnotic or narcotic withdrawal, or excessive use of caffeine.

Acute, Delayed, Episodic, or Chronic Anxiety

The terms *acute, delayed, episodic,* and *chronic* characterize the time course of anxiety — its duration, recurrence, and the latency between occurrence of a precipitating event and clinical manifestations. These characteristics in turn relate to practical matters including responsiveness to drug therapy, drug selection, and schedule of administration.

The terms *acute* and *delayed* are applicable mainly to **posttraumatic stress disorders** (Table 19–3), also called **reactive** anxiety. A delayed reaction of stress (at least 6 months after the causative episode) may be acute or chronic, once it develops. Acute posttraumatic stress disorder can be effectively managed with antianxiety drugs. Usually a regular schedule of drug utilization for a few days or a few weeks is appropriate for reactive anxiety. An antianxiety drug having a relatively long duration of action might be selected to provide a nearly continuous level of antianxiety action.

The majority of anxiety disorders seen in clinical practice are chronic ones that include chronic posttraumatic stress reactions, **generalized anxiety disorder** (a designation used only for adults), and **overanxious disorder** (a designation used mainly for children and adolescents). In the latter two conditions, anxiety may be considered to be *trait* rather than reactive. The usefulness of antianxiety drugs in chronic anxiety disorders is severely limited by the

Table 19–3
Diagnostic Categories of Anxiety Disorders and Corresponding Treatments

Disorder	Treatment correlates
Phobic disorders (or phobic neuroses)	Desensitization and other modes of psychotherapy (with or without adjunctive barbiturates); MAO inhibitors; imipramine for panic attacks
Agoraphobia with panic attacks	
Agoraphobia without panic attacks	
Social phobia	
Simple phobia	
Anxiety states (or anxiety neuroses)	
Panic disorder	Imipramine or alprazolam
Generalized anxiety disorder	Anxiolytics (effectiveness is limited to 3 or 4 months or longer if taken infrequently as needed)
Obsessive compulsive disorder	Anxiolytics (effective only in milder cases)
Posttraumatic stress disorder	
Acute	Anxiolytics (up to 3 or 4 months)
Chronic	Anxiolytics (effectiveness is limited to 3 or 4 months of daily use)
Atypical anxiety disorder	Case specific
Anxiety disorders of childhood or adolescence	
Separation anxiety disorder	Imipramine
Avoidant disorder of childhood or adolescence	Avoid depressants
Overanxious disorder	Anxiolytics (effectiveness is limited to 3 or 4 months)

tolerance that develops to their effectiveness within 2–3 months for benzodiazepines, and even sooner when meprobamate or phenobarbital are employed. It is the long-term use of anxiolytic drugs in chronic anxiety disorders that has drawn the most pointed criticism about current health care practice. Chronic anxiety can be treated effectively with drugs only when it is **situational anxiety,** occurring from time to time in response to particular life circumstances. Situational anxiety is most effectively treated with flexible regimens that provide for infrequent self-administration of a short-acting antianxiety drug as needed.

Phobias and **panic disorder** in adults, and **separation anxiety** in children are **episodic** conditions. Panic disorder and separation anxiety appear to be related in origin since adults who experience panic reactions are likely to have experienced separation anxiety as children. Panic reactions are characterized by periods of apprehensiveness (at least three episodes in 3 weeks) with at least four of the following symptoms: (1) dyspnea (irregular respiration), (2) palpitations, (3) chest pain, (4) sensations of choking or smothering, (5) dizziness, (6) feelings of unreality, (7) paresthesias (tingling in hands or feet), (8) hot or cold flashes, (9) sweating, (10) faintness, (11) trembling or shaking, and (12) fear of dying, going crazy, or losing control. Panic disorder and separation anxiety do not respond well to antianxiety drugs but respond dramatically to imipramine (Tofranil), a tricyclic antidepressant (see Chapter 20). Phobias (in which anxiety is focused on a particular object or situation) respond best to monoamine oxidase inhibitors or psychotherapeutic interventions such as desensitization therapy.

Nondrug Measures for Anxiety

Alternatives to drugs should not be neglected in managing clients with anxiety. Appropriate interventions by the staff psychologist or by nursing personnel may reduce anxiety and eliminate the need for drugs. The staff psychologist might employ psychotherapy to improve capacity to cope, desensitization techniques for anxiety related to phobias, or relaxation therapy. Nursing measures that minimize stress-provoking conditions in the environment and that provide comfort can often be employed instead of anxiolytic medication, to decrease the amount or frequency of anxiolytic drugs, or to enhance the efficacy of the drug regimen. One means of reducing stress and encouraging trust is through the use of touch, which communicates caring, support, and empathy and helps to establish rapport. Other measures that may reduce anxiety levels for hospitalized patients include adjusting the room temperature to fit the patient's needs and physical condition; providing warm fluids, fruit juices, or light snacks; changing the patient's position, tightening the bottom linen on the bed, adjusting the bed, dimming lights, or reducing noise; and limiting visiting time for visitors who stress the patient.

Anxiolytics

The actions and side effects of the anxiolytics (also called antianxiety drugs or minor tranquilizers) bear a close resemblance to those of the sedative-hypnotics (see Chapter 12) but have little in common with the antipsychotic drugs (or major tranquilizers, see

Chapter 18), with which they have shared the ambiguous designation *tranquilizer.* Anxiolytics are daytime sedatives with a greater than typical separation between doses that suppress anxiety and aggressiveness and doses that produce general depression. Currently, drugs in the benzodiazepine family are the foremost anxiolytics.

Benzodiazepines

The benzodiazepines include eight structurally related compounds marketed primarily for anxiety as well as three others including flurazepam (Dalmane), temazepam (Restoril), and triazolam (Halcion), marketed mainly as hypnotics (see Chapter 12), one, clonazepam (Clonopin), marketed for use in epilepsy (see Chapter 23), and one (midazolam) used only by injection to produce preoperative sedation. The eight that are employed for anxiety are diazepam (Valium), chlordiazepoxide (Librium, A-Poxide, and others), clorazepate (Tranxene, Azene), oxazepam (Serax), lorazepam (Ativan), prazepam (Verstran), alprazolam (Xanax), and halazepam (Paxipam). By and large, the eight benzodiazepines employed for anxiety are rather similar to one another in effects and side effects, differing mainly in duration of action.

Mechanisms and Effects Some of the neurochemical alterations contributing to the action of benzodiazepines have been established. Benzodiazepine receptors are modulatory proteins associated with GABA-receptor complexes. Through these receptors, benzodiazepines increase the affinity of GABA for its postsynaptic receptors, facilitating GABA neurotransmission (Figure 19–1). Recent work has suggested that there are at least two kinds of benzodiazepine receptors, called BZ_1 and BZ_2. The two types have different distributions in the brain: receptors in the cerebellum are all BZ_2, but the majority in the limbic system are BZ_1. They also have different binding preferences: most benzodiazepines bind to both types of receptors, but halazepam (Paxipam) and quazepam bind mainly to the BZ_1 receptors. Facilitation of GABA transmission results in decreased turnover of several other transmitters because of the role of GABA as an inhibitory transmitter. Many of the behavioral effects result from these secondary neurochemical actions. Benzodiazepines also have an inhibitory effect on phosphodiesterase, the enzyme that destroys cyclic adenosine monophosphate (see Chapter 9) and can mimic the effects of glycine and block dopamine reuptake.

The benzodiazepines produce an unusual EEG effect in which both slow-wave and fast-wave activity are increased while middle-range frequencies are diminished. They also slow electrical activity recorded from the septal region, amygdala, and hippocampus — three structures of the limbic system. This preferential effect on the limbic system (Figure 19–2) may be the main feature that distinguishes anxiolytics from sedative-hypnotic drugs.

The most striking behavioral effect of benzodiazepines is their ability to release behavior from inhibitory restraint by suppressing the punishment system (which suppresses behaviors in response to

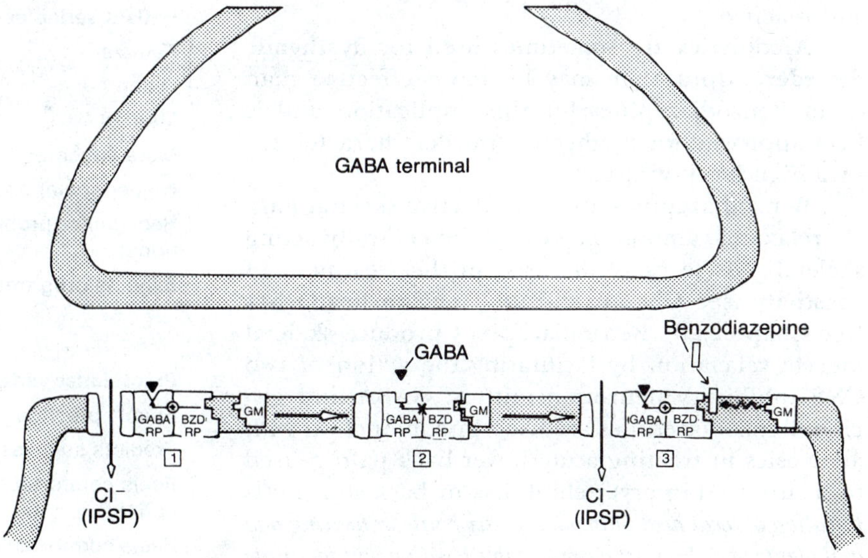

Figure 19–1
The neurochemical mechanism of benzodiazepine action. (1) The benzodiazepine recognition protein (BZD-RP) is a modulator of binding of gamma-aminobutyric acid (GABA) to type 1 GABA receptors. (2) Introduction of GABA-modulin (GM) prevents this. (3) Administration of a benzodiazepine blocks access of GM to the modulatory protein, thus facilitating GABA binding. From A. K. Swonger and L. L. Constantine, *Drugs and Therapy,* 2nd ed. Boston: Little, Brown, 1983.

Figure 19–2

Mechanisms of anxiolytics. Gamma-aminobutyric acid (GABA), monoamine oxidase (MAO), periventricular system (PVS), reticular activating system (RAS). From A. K. Swonger and L. L. Constantine, *Drugs and Therapy*, 2nd ed. Boston: Little, Brown, 1983.

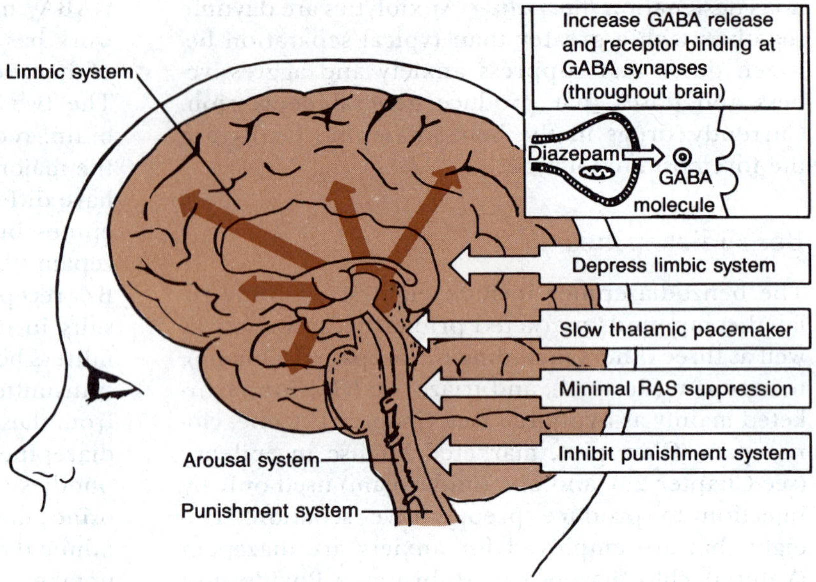

negative reinforcement). The punishment system is a brain region particularly vulnerable to the depressant action of any of the sedative-hypnotics, but especially the anxiolytics.

Clinical Indications Approximately 100 million prescriptions per year are written in the United States for the treatment of anxiety. One in every six adults is a recipient of antianxiety medication. Eighty percent of these prescriptions call for a benzodiazepine. A number of variables have been noted to correlate with the responsiveness of anxiety to benzodiazepines (Table 19–4), suggesting that antianxiety medication should be used selectively for severe anxiety, particularly where the anxiety is acute and reactive.

Anxiolytics are sometimes used for **dysthymic disorder.** Alprazolam may be more effective than other benzodiazepines for this application and is FDA approved for dysthymic disorder characterized by a high level of anxiety.

Benzodiazepines are also effective skeletal muscle relaxants, among the best of the centrally acting skeletal muscle relaxants used in the treatment of **spasticity** (see Chapter 22) and **tension headaches** (see Chapter 26). Benzodiazepines produce skeletal muscle relaxation by facilitating the action of two CNS inhibitory neurotransmitters: GABA and glycine. Benzodiazepines are used in conjunction with analgesics in treating acute lower back pain caused by a ruptured intervertebral disk or back strain. *Application of local heat with a hot water bottle or heating pad and plenty of bed rest in a comfortable position will facilitate the effectiveness of drug treatment of lower back pain.*

Diazepam (Valium) and clonazepam (Clonopin) are used acutely as anticonvulsants in **seizure states** and chronically in treatment regimens for certain forms of **epilepsy** and **myoclonus** (Chapter 23). Chlordiazepoxide (Librium) is used in detoxification of individuals from **alcohol dependence** (see Chapter 13). Various benzodiazepines have been used in the treatment of parasomnias, such as **sleep-walking** and

Table 19–4

Variables Predicting Responsiveness to Benzodiazepines

Patient variables	**Illness variables**
Female	Acute
Older	Reactive
Married	Few previous drugs
More educated	Good previous drug response
Higher social class	High severity if generalized anxiety
Recognizes problem is emotional	Low severity if obsessive-compulsive
Expects drug treatment	Many somatic symptoms
Practitioner variables	**Treatment variables**
Family practice	Occurrence of sedation
Predicts success	Short duration
Feels comfortable with patient	
Feels comfortable prescribing drugs	

night terrors, that are related to stage IV of non-dreaming sleep (see Chapter 11).

In hospital settings, diazepam is often employed for alleviation of **preoperative apprehensiveness** or just prior to anesthesia to facilitate induction. Benzodiazepines are employed frequently during **labor and delivery** and may reduce the need for analgesics. However, it has been noted that diazepam, at least, crosses the placental barrier and accumulates in the fetal circulation in concentrations higher than in the mother. The result may be lethargy, hypothermia, and respiratory depression in the newborn.

Adverse Effects and Contraindications The adverse effects of benzodiazepines are generally fewer in number, less frequent, and less severe than for most classes of drugs that act on the central nervous system (Table 19–5). As with all CNS depressants, there is risk of **excess depression** with benzodiazepines, especially if a benzodiazepine is employed in combination with other prescribed or self-administered depressant drugs. When assessing depression in clients who are receiving benzodiazepines, it is important to distinguish between depression caused by the drug and depression due to environmental factors such as interrupted sleep, pain, or fear of the hospital environment. Signs of excess depression include sedation, confusion, lethargy, ataxia, drowsiness, fatigue, somnolence, muscle weakness, nystagmus, and disorientation. Since these effects occur in a dose-dependent fashion, a reduction of dose or discontinuation of the medication should be considered when signs of excess depression are evident. *The client who is receiving benzodiazepine medication should be instructed to avoid driving or operating potentially dangerous tools, appliances, or equipment.*

Reactions of **paradoxical excitation** to benzodiazepines occur as commonly as with sedative-hypnotics and take the form of restlessness, agitation, or even rage. Explosions of temper that occur with min-

Nursing Observations for Antianxiety Drug Therapy

THERAPEUTIC GOAL	Increased ability to cope with stress, reduced exposure to stress-provoking circumstances, and management of stress-related physiological problems.
PREADMINISTRATION ASSESSMENT	
Baseline Data	Observe extent of anxiety symptoms: expressions of worry, tension, edginess, rumination, apprehensiveness; behaviors such as insomnia, distractibility, impatience, inability to relax, exaggerated self-consciousness, excessive need for reassurance; motor manifestations such as jumpiness, tremor, elevated muscle tone, furrowed brow, restlessness; or autonomic symptoms such as increased heart rate or blood pressure, diaphoresis, cold and moist palms, urinary frequency, flushing, or pallor. Obtain complete blood cells counts and hepatic function tests before initiating drug therapy.
Contraindications/ Precautions	Psychosis, renal or hepatic failure, narrow-angle glaucoma, respiratory distress, pregnancy, lactation, or allergy to the drug.
Potential Interactions	CNS depressants, MAO inhibitors, antacids, and tobacco.
EVALUATION OF DRUG RESPONSE	
For Therapeutic Benefit	Monitor subjective, behavioral, motor, and autonomic manifestations of anxiety.
For Adverse Effects	Monitor for excess depression, paradoxical excitation, night-terrors or other sleep disturbances, sexual impairments, blood cell dyscrasias, urinary retention, gastrointestinal irritation, and overuse.
For Drug Interactions	Monitor for additive CNS depression with other depressant drugs, especially alcohol.
For Compliance	Evaluate client's compliance with all facets of the therapeutic regimen by careful observation, interviewing, and review of progress. Report compliance problems or overcompliance to the physician and act as client-advocate when changes in the therapeutic regimen seem indicated.

Table 19–5
Adverse Effects of Benzodiazepines

Excess depression	Sedation, confusion, lethargy, ataxia, drowsiness, fatigue, somnolence, muscle weakness, nystagmus, disorientation
Paradoxical excitation	Restlessness, agitation, rage
Sleep disturbances	Stage IV suppression (but no REM suppression), vivid dreams, nightmares
Sexual and reproductive functioning	Decreased libido, menstrual irregularities, fetal abnormalities if used during first trimester of pregnancy, excreted in mother's milk with potentially adverse consequences for infant
Blood cell disorders	Occasional dyscrasias or allergic reactions
Abuse liability	Psychological dependence, tolerance, and physical dependence (when used at excessive doses or for too long a time period)
Other	Gastrointestinal disturbances, urinary retention, aggravation of narrow angle glaucoma

imal provocation may indicate paradoxical excitation, suggesting the need for a change in dose or drug selection. There is a risk that clients who experience paradoxical excitation will accidentally repeat dosing. *Nurses should instruct clients not to keep the drug at bedside to avoid repeating the dose in confusion if awakened.*

Benzodiazepines do not suppress dream sleep as do most sedative-hypnotics, but they do cause other types of **sleep disturbances,** such as vivid dreaming and nightmares (REM anxiety attacks), because they suppress stage IV of nondreaming sleep. The significance of stage IV suppression is less well established than the effects of dream suppression. Suppression of stage IV by benzodiazepines is used to good effect in treating parasomnias that occur characteristically during this stage (sleep-walking and night terrors).

Benzodiazepines frequently alter **sexual and reproductive functioning.** Successful participation in sexual relationships is important for both physiological and emotional well-being of men and women and can influence compliance with drug regimens. Clients who experience changes in libido after receiving benzodiazepines tend to discontinue the drug. *If a nurse suspects that a client has a problem with sexual functioning but will not discuss it, the suspected difficulty should be reported to the physician, so that a more accurate assessment may be made and an alternative drug choice prescribed.*

Women receiving benzodiazepines may experience menstrual irregularities. In particular, sexually active women who are in their reproductive years may have difficulty adjusting to irregularity, since there is also concern about potential pregnancy. *It is important, then, that women be alerted to the possibility of menstrual irregularity prior to beginning medication, and that questions relating to menstrual function be included in the nursing assessment.* If the client is undergoing menopause, menstrual irregularity may reflect that physiological stage rather than being an adverse effect of medication, so that once again proper assessment requires careful comparison of the client's current condition with an appropriate predrug history.

Benzodiazepines increase the risk of congenital birth defects. *Female clients should be questioned about plans concerning pregnancy.* Mothers who are nursing infants should not use benzodiazepines because they are excreted in the mother's milk and will have adverse effects on the infant.

A small number of clients receiving benzodiazepines experience skin irritation, persistent sore throat, fever, or malaise, which may reflect drug-induced **blood cell disorders** (allergies or leukopenia). *In taking a history, nurses should record incidence of skin rashes and flu-like symptoms since it may be important later to know whether the symptoms appeared before or after the initiation of the medication. Clients should be queried about ease of bruising — an indication of an impairment of the clotting mechanism.*

Benzodiazepines may cause **urinary retention** and should be used with caution in clients with renal impairment. *Clients should be alerted to the potential problem and taught to monitor fluid intake and output when benzodiazepines are used. Clients should be shown how to measure fluid that is a part of solid foods they eat so that an accurate assessment can be obtained.* When urinary retention occurs, urine that is produced often has a peculiar musty odor. *Clients should be questioned about changes they have noted in urinary frequency, odor, or color. Clients should also be asked about pressure in the region of the urinary bladder and if voiding is frequent but in small amounts.* The latter could well indicate that urine excreted is in fact overflow, one of the important signs of urinary retention.

Minor **gastrointestinal disturbances** are common with benzodiazepine administration. *Taking the drug with or shortly after meals or snacks may reduce gastrointestinal discomfort.* Benzodiazepines are contraindicated in **acute narrow angle glaucoma** because they aggravate this condition.

Abuse Liability Benzodiazepines are less likely to be abused than alcohol or other sedative-hypnotics, but with some 100 million prescriptions being written yearly, the number of abusers is substantial. When these drugs are used properly, the severity of psychological dependence seldom exceeds habituation. When used in excessive daily doses or for periods beyond 3–4 months of chronic, daily use, psychological dependence may become marked and may be accompanied by frank physical dependence. Moreover, controlled clinical trials have failed to demonstrate that benzodiazepines maintain effectiveness in alleviating anxiety when used on a daily basis beyond 3–4 months. Therefore, the use of benzodiazepines for anxiety should be limited to 3–4 months of daily doses or infrequent use as needed for longer periods of time. Clients should be instructed not to increase dose or frequency of administration without prior approval of the physician.

In long-term treatment with benzodiazepines, clients may develop physical dependence even at low doses. The withdrawal syndrome associated with abrupt withdrawal from benzodiazepines is qualitatively similar to that associated with sedative-hypnotics, but is somewhat slower to develop (2–12 days after drug elimination versus 8–72 hours with alcohol and other sedative-hypnotics) and a little longer in duration (9–14 days versus 5–10 with sedative-hypnotics). Benzodiazepines should be discontinued slowly if the client has been receiving the drug for a long period of time.

The risk of overdose with benzodiazepines is very low; they are virtually suicide proof. However, depressant effects of benzodiazepines are additive to those of other depressants such as alcohol and narcotics. Combined effects can be fatal even though no one drug is present in lethal amounts. Symptoms of benzodiazepine overdose are confusion, delirium, somnolence, impaired reflexes, and ultimately, coma. Treatment is supportive and symptomatic.

Drug Interactions The most important drug interaction of benzodiazepines is additive CNS depression with other depressant drugs. This risk exists whenever benzodiazepines are used concurrently with sedative-hypnotics, narcotics, antipsychotic drugs, anticholinergics, antihistamines, antihypertensive medications, antidepressants, or anesthetics.

Regular smoking of tobacco and use of anxiogenic drugs, including caffeine, cocaine, sympathomimetics, and levodopa decrease the effectiveness of anxiolytics. Cimetidine (Tagamet) taken concurrently with a benzodiazepine will increase the risk of excess depression.

Variations among the Benzodiazepines For the most part, differences within the benzodiazepine class are subtle. Diazepam (Valium) is less sedating than chlordiazepoxide (Librium) in most clients. The antiepileptic properties of diazepam exceed those of other benzodiazepines except clonazepam, a drug introduced expressly for use in epilepsy (see Chapter 23). The overall effectiveness of diazepam and chlordiazepoxide is equivalent, but diazepam may be preferable to chlordiazepoxide for dysthymic disorder and anxiety accompanied by insomnia or motor symptoms, while chlordiazepoxide may be more effective in reactive anxiety. Alprazolam (Xanax) appears to have greater effectiveness in dysthymic disorder than do other benzodiazepines. Chlordiazepoxide may be more effective than diazepam in treating alcohol withdrawal. Chlordiazepoxide is used in combination preparations for ulcers (Librax).

Oxazepam (Serax) and alprazolam are short-acting (Table 19–6) because they are inactivated fairly rapidly, without formation of active metabolites. These short-acting drugs are good choices for as-needed treatment of situational anxiety. Clorazepate (Tranxene), halazepam (Paxipam), and prazepam (Centrax) have active metabolites with long half-lives giving them extended durations of action. Generally a long half-life is advantageous if the drug is being used in a fixed regimen. Clorazepate is typically taken once per day while diazepam is usually taken three times per day (or once a day in the form of a spansule capsule).

Table 19–6
Comparisons of Benzodiazepines

Drug	Equivalent dose	Plasma half-life (Hr)[a]
Alprazolam	0.5	12
Chlordiazepoxide	10	8–28
Clorazepate	7	30–100
Diazepam	5	20–42
Halazepam	20	14
Lorazepam	1	12–15
Oxazepam	15	10–14
Prazepam	10	30–100

[a]For drug or active metabolite.

Nursing Diagnoses and Interventions for Antianxiety Drug Therapy

Nursing Diagnoses	*Related Interventions*
TO ENHANCE DRUG BENEFITS OR REDUCE DRUG REQUIREMENTS	
Impaired social relationships related to irritability, impatience, and inability to relax; Ineffective individual coping related to excessive anxiety; Ineffective individual coping: inability to manage or avoid stressors; Sleep pattern disturbance related to excessive stress	Provide emotional support and encouragement; provide comfort measures; teach nondrug measures for coping with stress such as relaxation techniques, exercise, and planned periods of quiet; consider referral for psychotherapy.
TO MINIMIZE DRUG SIDE EFFECTS OR INTERACTIONS	
Risk of injury related to CNS depression	Warn client to avoid driving or other hazardous tasks for a few hours after taking a benzodiazepine
TO ENSURE SAFE AND EFFICACIOUS DRUG USE	
Knowledge deficit related to drug regimen	Teach client about the nature of the anxiety disorder, the limitations in usefulness of drug therapy, and the importance of nondrug measures in controlling anxiety. Provide client with a list of adverse effects and drug interactions for each drug in the regimen and explain what to do if any of these occur.

Preparations and Administration Use of benzodiazepines should adhere to established time limits for daily use (not to exceed 3–4 months) and maximum daily doses. Doses and dosage schedules should be individualized. When possible, *as-needed regimens* should be employed in preference to fixed daily schedules. Dosage levels may need to be reduced considerably in clients who are elderly, debilitated, or experiencing liver or renal impairment.

Intravenous administration of diazepam often causes local irritation and pain, and may result in phlebitis. Injections should be made close to the insertion site and given slowly, not over 5 mg per minute. Vital signs should be monitored and resuscitation equipment should be available. Nurses should observe the patient for any signs of phlebitis and report them immediately to the physician. Intramuscular injection of diazepam results in slow and erratic absorption. *When intramuscular injection is required, diazepam should be injected in the deltoid muscle to maximize absorption.*

Chlordiazepoxide is prepared for intramuscular injection by using the diluent provided by the manufacturer. It should be prepared just prior to administration and unused solution should be discarded. Intramuscular injections should be deep and slow.

Alprazolam (Xanax)
Tablets
Recommended Doses: 0.25–0.5 mg PO, initially 3 times daily.

Chlordiazepoxide (Librium, A-poxide, SK-Lygen, Sereen, Murcil, Lipoxide, Reposans, and generic formulations)
Capsules (as the hydrochloride salt), tablets, powder for reconstitution and injection
Recommended Doses: For mild to moderate anxiety, 5–10 mg PO, 3 or 4 times daily. For more severe anxiety conditions, 20–25 mg, 3 or 4 times daily. For alcohol withdrawal, 50–100 mg initially. The first dose is often given parenterally.

Clorazepate (Tranxene)
Capsules, tablets, slow release tablets
Recommended Doses: For anxiety, 30 mg/day PO typically with a range of 15–60 mg/day, not to exceed 90 mg/day. The daily dose can be taken in 3 adminstrations using conventional tablets or capsules or as a single slow release tablet.

Diazepam (Valium)
Tablets, sustained release capsules, injection solution
Recommended Doses: For anxiety, 2–10 mg, 2–4 times daily.

Halazepam (Paxipam)
Tablets
Recommended Doses: For anxiety, 20–40 mg PO, initially 3 or 4 times daily.

Lorazepam (Ativan)
Tablets, injection solution
Recommended Doses: For anxiety, 2–3 mg/day PO, initially in 2 or 3 divided doses.

Oxazepam (Serax)
Capsules, tablets
Recommended Doses: For mild to moderate anxiety, 10–15 mg PO, 3 or 4 times daily.

Prazepam (Centrax)
Capsules, tablets
Recommended Doses: For anxiety, 30 mg/day PO typically in divided doses. The dosage range is 20–60 mg/day or 10–15 mg/day in elderly or debilitated clients.

Other Drugs Used for Anxiety Disorders

The main alternatives to the use of benzodiazepines in anxiety disorders are phenobarbital, propanediols, and diphenylmethane antihistamines (Table 19–7). In addition, a new drug having a distinctive profile, buspirone (Buspar), was approved at the end of 1986. Phenobarbital and the propanediols are less satisfactory choices for a number of reasons: (1) considerable general depression occurs at doses that suppress anxiety; (2) tolerance develops sooner than with benzodiazepines, restricting the useful period of chronic daily administration to no more than two weeks; (3) abuse potential is substantially greater (daily intake levels that produce dependence are only two- or threefold the upper end of the normal therapeutic dosage range while the corresponding ratio for benzodiazepines is about six- to eightfold for short-term use); (4) the risk of overdose is far greater (these drugs have a low therapeutic index — the lethal dose is only a few times the therapeutic dose); (5) the frequency of intoxication is great; and (6) they suppress dreaming sleep. The pharmacology of phenobarbital is discussed in detail in Chapter 23.

Propanediols

The propanediol used for anxiety is meprobamate (Equanil, Miltown, and generics). Prior to the advent of the benzodiazepines, it was the preeminent medication for anxiety. Meprobamate is only marginally more selective for anxiety than are the barbiturates and it shares all of the risks of overdosage and abuse liability of that group.

Table 19–7
Comparisons among Antianxiety and Sedative Drugs

Characteristic	Phenobarbital	Propanediol carbamates	Benzodiazepines	Diphenylmethane antihistamines	Buspirone
Effectiveness					
Antianxiety potency	+++	+++	+++	+	+++
Selectivity for anxiety	0	+	++	0	+++
Duration of action	+++	++	++	+	+
Period of usefulness in daily regimens	2 weeks	2 weeks	3 months	indefinite	undetermined
Muscle relaxation	+	+++	+++	0	0
Antiepileptic	+++	++	+++	0	0
Abuse potential					
Psychological dependence	++	+++	+	0	0
Physical dependence	++	+++	+	0	0
Suicide potential	++	+++	0	++	?
Adverse effects					
Acute intoxication	+	++	0	0	0
REM suppression	++	++	0	++	?
Stage IV suppression	0	0	++	0	?

Clinical Indications Meprobamate remains a widely prescribed drug. Although indicated for short-term relief of anxiety, its use has shifted somewhat toward hypnotic applications. Effectiveness beyond 4 months of daily use has not been established. Propanediols have skeletal muscle relaxant properties similar to the benzodiazepines. Meprobamate is also available in a combination preparation (Equagesic) that is marketed for tension headaches.

Adverse Effects and Contraindications The propanediols are contraindicated in acute intermittent porphyria and during pregnancy (especially the first trimester) because these drugs will pass the placental barrier and have been linked to increased risk of congenital malformations. Meprobamate is metabolized by the liver and excreted by the kidney and must be used cautiously in individuals with either hepatic or renal impairment.

Prolonged use of meprobamate may result in psychological and even physical dependence. The higher the dose employed, the greater the risk. The risk of withdrawal symptoms can be minimized by gradual discontinuation of the drug over a period of 1–2 weeks. The risk of acute intoxication is a problem with meprobamate. *When meprobamate is prescribed for individuals who are suicide prone, drug administration should be carefully supervised since clients have been known to accumulate tablets of meprobamate for suicide attempts.*

Meprobamate may cause drowsiness and other signs of excess depression. Older individuals are especially prone to such effects, particularly when meprobamate therapy is first initiated. For that reason, smaller doses are often used at first in elderly persons, and then gradually increased. *Nurses should advise clients to avoid use of alcohol in conjunction with meprobamate.* These two drugs have a supra-additive effect with each other because they compete for the same degratory enzymes and slow each other's metabolism. Allergic reactions such as skin rash and jaundice occur occasionally with meprobamate. *The nurse should inspect the skin and sclerae for indications of jaundice. The nurse should also inspect the skin for rashes and ask the client about pruritus.* With long-term use, liver impairment or blood cell disorders may occur. Periodic blood cell counts and liver function tests should be instituted.

Preparations and Administration

Meprobamate (Equanil, Miltown, Neuramate, SK-Bamate, Meprospan, Mepriam, Sedabamate, Tranmep, and generic formulations)
Tablets, capsules, sustained release capsules
Recommended Doses: For anxiety in adults, 1,200–1,600 mg PO daily in 3 or 4 divided doses. The maximum recommended daily dose for adults is 2,400 mg. For children 6–12 years of age, 100–200 mg PO, 2 or 3 times daily.

Diphenylmethane Antihistamines

Diphenylmethane antihistamines used for anxiety include hydroxyzine (Atarax, Vistaril) and diphenhydramine (Benadryl). These antihistaminic drugs produce considerable drowsiness and sedation, which is true of many of the antihistamines (see Chapter 50). The depressant effect of antihistamines is largely on subcortical centers; they have little effect on the cerebrum. When compared to benzodiazepines, the diphenylmethane antihistamines are safer, but they are also substantially less effective. They lack selectivity for anxiety, do not possess skeletal muscle relaxant properties, and are not sufficiently potent to represent an adequate treatment for the more refractory cases of anxiety. On the other hand, the antihistamines do not produce either psychological or physical dependence, tolerance, or acute intoxication. Because there is no tolerance development, they can be used for indefinite periods of time. They do have potential for use in suicides and are REM suppressants. They are often used for short-term alleviation of anxiety and stress, for example, in preoperative and postoperative applications. Side effects are minimal, but additive CNS depression occurs with other CNS depressants. The usual route of administration of hydroxyzine is oral; IM administration is reserved for emergencies.

Because of the marginal effectiveness of hydroxyzine in anxiety, its use for extended treatment of mild anxiety lies in the gray area between placebo therapy and true pharmacological intervention. Given the abuse potential of antianxiety drugs and the tendency of individuals to overmedicate for anxiety, use of hydroxyzine can be an attractive alternative to conventional anxiolytics. A physician who believes that drug treatment is not warranted in a given case but who suspects that it will be sought by the client until obtained, may wish to employ hydroxyzine as a safe, semi-placebo therapy.

Buspirone (Buspar)

Buspirone is a newly developed anxiolytic that is structurally unrelated to benzodiazepines, propanediols, diphenylmethane antihistamines, tricyclic antidepressants, or phenothiazines.

Mechanisms and Effects Buspirone is characterized as *anxioselective* because of its relative specificity in alleviating anxiety without many of the other effects of benzodiazepines. For example, buspirone lacks anticonvulsant and skeletal muscle relaxant properties, is less sedative than benzodiazepines, and does not appear to produce physical or psychological dependence. Higher than therapeutic doses of buspirone have been reported to produce dysphoria rather than euphoria. It has no direct effect on the GABA receptor complex (where benzodiazepines work), though it may activate it indirectly.

Pharmacokinetics Buspirone is readily absorbed after oral administration but undergoes extensive first pass extraction. Less than 1% of an administered dose is excreted unchanged, since the bulk of the drug is metabolized in the liver with the metabolites being excreted in the urine. The elimination half-life of buspirone is approximately 2.6 hours.

Clinical Indications Buspirone was approved for clinical use in late 1986. In clinical trials, buspirone was equally effective as diazepam in treatment of generalized anxiety disorders. In one study, buspirone was superior to diazepam in alleviating cognitive and interpersonal symptoms of anxiety but less effective in alleviating somatic symptoms. Buspirone is also reportedly superior to diazepam in alleviating anxiety-related depression. The antianxiety effects of buspirone are not observed until after one to two weeks of use, so it is not useful for clients requiring an immediate anxiolytic action or those requiring "as-needed" regimens for situational anxiety.

Adverse Effects and Contraindications The side effects most frequently observed with buspirone are dizziness, nervousness, and headache, each occurring in approximately 10% of clients. Significant sedation does not occur at normal therapeutic doses (20 mg/day) but may occur at higher doses.

Preparations and Administration

Buspirone (Buspar)
Tablets
Recommended Doses: For anxiety, 15–30 mg/day.

Important Nursing Implications for Antianxiety Drugs

- ☐ Observe clients carefully for indications of excessive anxiety, such as changes in behavior (argumentativeness or irritability), motor symptoms (tremor or increased muscle tone), or autonomic symptoms (gastric hyperacidity).
- ☐ The client's drug history should always include all prescription and nonprescription medications being taken and an evaluation of alcohol, nicotine, and caffeine consumption. The client should be advised to avoid alcohol consumption and not to exceed 300 mg of caffeine ingestion per day (see Chapter 14 for concentrations of caffeine in various sources).
- ☐ Take special care when anxiolytics are used to exhibit optimism about the likelihood of improvement and the efficacy of prescribed medications. If there is reason to doubt the value of the regimen, such concerns should be shared with the physician, not with the client or client's family.
- ☐ Observe clients for indications of adverse reactions to antianxiety medication and institute nursing measures to counter these adverse reactions as appropriate. Watch especially for evidences of excess depression, especially when anxiolytics are employed concurrently with other CNS depressants.
- ☐ Advocate changes in drug regimens when antianxiety drugs have been prescribed for regular daily use for time intervals that exceed their demonstrated periods of effectiveness.
- ☐ Whenever possible, employ nursing measures to comfort the client and to reduce stress in lieu of or to facilitate anxiolytic medication.
- ☐ Emphasize that clients not share medications with other individuals. Nurses working in outpatient settings should keep a careful record of the client's treatment and examine this record when the client returns to the clinic for frequency of requests for antianxiety drugs. Conversations with family members or friends of the client can also be useful in eliciting information concerning compliance, drug sharing, or drug dependency or abuse.
- ☐ Avoid abrupt withdrawal of antianxiety medications after prolonged periods of treatment. Be alert to evidence of withdrawal symptoms, which would indicate that withdrawal of drug has been too rapid.
- ☐ Monitor changes in blood cell counts when clients are receiving benzodiazepines for extended periods of time.
- ☐ Refrain from giving antianxiety medications to women who are pregnant or who are breast-feeding.
- ☐ Use lower doses of antianxiety drugs in elderly or debilitated clients.

- ☐ Instruct clients not to exceed the prescribed drug dose; to avoid nonprescription depressants, such as alcohol, while using benzodiazepines; and to keep these and all other medications out of the reach of children.
- ☐ Record family observations concerning client response on the client's care plan and transmit such findings to the health team.

Case Study: Posttraumatic Stress Disorder

T. P. was a 37-year-old married Vietnam veteran who had been recently laid off from his factory job. While looking for new employment, he watched a lot of television, including several retrospectives on the Vietnam War. This triggered memories of his combat experiences, including two incidents in which he had shot Vietcong guerrillas at point blank range, another occasion when he had been forced to kill a guerrilla in hand-to-hand combat, and several situations in which he had seen fellow soldiers killed by enemy fire. T. P. had learned to cope reasonably well with the requirements of combat and had adjusted to civilian life after only a brief period of being at loose ends. After returning from Vietnam, he had completed college, married, and had two young children. T. P. and his wife had a good marriage with only the normal complement of difficulties. As a result of the loss of his job and the television reminders of memories that he thought he had laid to rest, T. P. began to experience intense anxiety and nightmares. He awoke one night from a vivid nightmare in which he was reliving the incident of hand-to-hand combat. On another occasion while working in his yard, he heard explosions from a nearby construction site and jumped into the bushes, thinking that the explosions were enemy fire. With his wife's encouragement, T. P. sought help at a mental health clinic. T. P. was prescribed diazepam, 3 times daily, and entered into intensive psychotherapy. He responded well and the diazepam was discontinued after three weeks. T. P. continued less intensive psychotherapy for 4 months, at which time he and the psychotherapist decided he had no need to continue.

1. Is this case of posttraumatic stress disorder best classified as acute, chronic, or delayed?
2. What factors contributed to its occurrence?
3. Do you think that drug therapy was warranted in this instance? Was diazepam a reasonable selection? What other drugs might have been selected?
4. Why was diazepam discontinued after 3 weeks?

Answers appear at the end of the book.

Case Study: Generalized Anxiety Disorder

R. S., a 40-year-old married woman with three teenage children, came to the mental health clinic complaining of tension, nervousness, and difficulty coping with her problems. Among her list of problems were the usual difficulties associated with raising adolescents, a rather unsupportive spouse, and early indications of menopause. R. S. had no outstanding medical problems. Her vital signs were normal except that her blood pressure reading of 130/90 qualified her as borderline hypertensive. The physician prescribed diazepam, 2 mg, 3 times a day, for anxiety and referred R. S. to the psychiatric nurse for client counseling.

The nurse talked with R. S. about her problems and explained that antianxiety drugs are effective only for a limited period of time, after which tolerance develops to the antianxiety action. Thus, it would be necessary for R. S. to seek other ways of handling anxiety over the long term. The nurse talked with R. S. about relaxation therapy, counseling groups where she might explore and discuss her feelings, breathing techniques, meditation programs, and adjustments that could be made to reduce stressors. She asked about R. S.'s use of coffee, tea, and cola, and after assessing her total daily caffeine intake, suggested that R. S. gradually decrease her use of these beverages.

In addition, the nurse taught R. S. what she would need to know about the use of diazepam. For example, the nurse warned R. S. that while the drug might alleviate her anxiety, it might also result in feelings of fatigue, which could impair R. S.'s ability to drive her car safely. She told her that her ovulatory cycle, already irregular because of the early stages of menopause, might become more irregular. R. S. was also told that diazepam might cause her to experience vivid dreams or nightmares. The nurse also instructed R. S. not to take alcohol, antacids, or other nonprescription drugs while employing diazepam. The nurse suggested that if R. S. felt any gastrointestinal irritation from the drug, she should take each dose with food. Finally, the nurse advised R. S. to go to her physician for evaluation and possible treatment of her high blood pressure.

1. What are the apparent factors contributing to anxiety for R. S.?
2. What is the relationship between anxiety and high blood pressure?
3. How reasonable was the decision to prescribe diazepam for this client? How long should the physician allow R. S. to continue use of diazepam?
4. Why did the nurse inquire about use of caffeinated beverages by R. S.?
5. Why should R. S. avoid alcohol, antacids, and other nonprescription drugs while using diazepam?

Answers appear at the end of the book.

Recommended Readings

Ameer B, Greenblatt DJ: Lorazepam: Review of its clinical pharmacological properties and therapeutic uses. *Drugs* 1981;21:161–200.

Anderson G: Benzodiazepines. *Nurse Pract* 1980;47(1):50–51.

Bellantuono C et al: Benzodiazepines: Clinical pharmacology and therapeutic uses. *Drugs* 1980;19:195–219.

Costa E, Greengard P (eds): *Mechanisms of action of benzodiazepines.* New York, Raven Press, 1975.

Greenblatt DJ, Shader RI, Abernethy DR: Current status of benzodiazepines. *N Engl J Med* 1983;309:354–358, 410–416.

Greenblatt DJ, Shader RI: Prazepam and lorazepam: Two new benzodiazepines. *N Engl J Med* 1978;299:1342–1344.

Hollister LE et al: Long-term use of diazepam. *JAMA* 1981;246(14):1568–1570.

Kanto JH: Use of benzodiazepines during pregnancy, labour, and lactation, with particular reference to pharmacokinetic considerations. *Drugs* 1982;23(5):354–380.

Mackinnon GL, Parker WA: Benzodiazepine withdrawal syndrome: A literature review and evaluation. *Am J Drug Alcohol Abuse* 1982;9:19–33.

Malick JB, Enna SJ, Yamamura HI: *Anxiolytics: Neurochemical, Behavioral, and Clinical Perspectives.* New York, Raven, 1983.

Marks J: *The Benzodiazepines: Use, Overuse, Misuse, Abuse.* Baltimore, University Park Press, 1978.

Raskin M et al: Panic and generalized anxiety disorders: Developmental antecedents and precipitants. *Arch Gen Psychiatry* 1982;39:687–689.

Rickels K: Benzodiazepines in the treatment of anxiety. *Am J Psychother* 1982;36(3):358–370.

Sheehan DV: Current views on the treatment of panic and phobic disorders. *Drug Ther* 1982;7(10):74.

Skolnick P, Paul SM: Benzodiazepine receptors in the central nervous system. *Int Rev Neurobiol* 1982;23:103–140.

Study RE, Barker JL: Cellular mechanisms of benzodiazepine action. *JAMA* 1982;247:2147–2151.

Usdin E et al (eds): *Pharmacology of Benzodiazepines.* London, MacMillan Press Ltd, 1982.

White S, Williamson K: What to watch for with minor tranquilizers. *RN* 1979;11:57–59.

Wilson H, Kneisl CR: *Psychiatric Nursing.* Menlo Park, Ca, Addison-Wesley, 1983.

CHAPTER 20

Antidepressants

Diagnostic Classifications of Depression

Depression, like anxiety, occurs both as a natural component of psychological processes and as a pathological condition. As a normal, functional process, depression provides protection for the nervous system in the face of adverse circumstances for which there is no effective coping response. The grief reaction experienced following loss of a loved one is an example of a normal depressive reaction that generally follows predictable stages (protest, despair, detachment). As a pathological process, depression may occur as a primary affective disorder, a drug reaction, or an element in a wide variety of medical problems. The line between normal or pathological depression is a fine one, depending on the etiology, severity, and duration of the condition. As in the treatment of anxiety, the choice should be made carefully whether or not to use drug therapy. "Benign neglect" is often the preferred treatment in mild, reactive depression.

Unipolar Depression

Unipolar affective disorders are characterized by a depressive mood, loss of interest in activities, and lack of pleasure in previously satisfying activities (Table 20–1). Physiological symptoms may include changes in sleep time, dream time, REM latency, and decreased turnover rates of biogenic amines (serotonin and norepinephrine) as evidenced by decreased urinary or cerebrospinal fluid output of transmitter metabolites. It is among the most com-

Table 20–1
Unipolar Versus Bipolar Affective Disorders

Characteristics	Unipolar	Bipolar	
Essential features	Depressive mood; pervasive loss of interest or pleasure	Alternating episodes of manic and depressive moods	
Incidence			
Frequency	Common	Much less common	
Sex ratio	Females more than males	No sex difference	
Familial history	Sometimes present	Often present	
Physiological correlates			
		Manic phase:	*Depressive phase:*
Nocturnal EEG (usual)	↓Sleep time ↓REM % ↓REM latency	↓Sleep time ↓REM % ↑REM latency	↓Sleep time ↑REM % ↓REM latency
Transmitter metabolites	↓MHPG or 5-HIAA	↑MHPG	↓MHPG
Prognosis			
Spontaneous remission	Likely	Unlikely	
Recurrent episodes	Second episode: 75% Third episode: 50%	Almost always many episodes	
Drug effectiveness	Tricyclics much more effective than lithium	Lithium much more effective than tricyclics	
Subtypes	Major depression vs. dysthymic disorder	Manic-depressive disorder vs. cyclothymic personality	
	Endogenous vs. reactive	Bipolar I vs. bipolar II	
	Melancholia	Acute or recurrent mania (rare)	
	Atypical depression	Atypical bipolar disorder (includes bipolar II)	
	Serotonin vs. norepinephrine type		

mon psychiatric disorders and about twice as common in females as in males. A familial history is sometimes present but is by no means a consistent feature. Spontaneous remissions are commonplace and recurrence is by no means inevitable. About 25% of individuals who experience a unipolar depressive episode never have a second episode, and 50% do not have a third one. There is little overlap between the drugs that have proved useful in bipolar disorder (mainly lithium) and those that are effective in unipolar depression.

Primary Versus Secondary Depression

Unipolar depression is primary when it occurs independent of other disorders or when the affective disturbance is the major presenting dysfunction. Unipolar depression is secondary when it is related to another psychiatric disorder outside the affective category, an organic disorder, or drug use. The variety of medical disorders and conditions that can result in secondary depression is extensive (Table 20–2). It is also possible for these conditions to aggravate or compound preexisting primary depression.

Major Depression Versus Dysthymic Disorder

The American Psychiatric Association's *Diagnostic and Statistical Manual* of Mental Disorders, Third Edition (DSM-III) recognizes three categories of unipolar affective disorders; **major depression, dysthymic disorder** (formally depressive neurosis), and **atypical depression.** The criteria for major depression are the dysphoric mood itself and the circumstantial symptoms (Table 20–3). The dysphoric mood is characterized by feelings of sadness, hopelessness, and morbidness. The mood disturbance must be prominent (though not necessarily the dominant symptom), and persistent, not shifting frequently to anxiety or anger. The second criterion requires the occurrence of at least four circumstantial symptoms nearly every day for at least 2 weeks (see Table 20–3). Some clients with major depression exhibit psy-

Table 20–2
Conditions in Which Depression Is Often Secondary

Psychiatric
Organic brain syndrome
Schizophrenia
Obsessive compulsive disorder
Generalized anxiety disorder
Panic disorder
Drug dependence
Sexual deviances
Organic
Metabolic: hypoglycemia, potassium or calcium depletion, elevated blood urea nitrogen, hepatic dysfunction
Endocrine: hypothyroidism, diabetes mellitus, hyperthyroidism, Addison's disease, hypoglycemia, hepatic dysfunction
CNS: mental retardation, tumors, Parkinson's disease, multiple sclerosis, Alzheimer's disease, cerebral vascular insufficiency
Miscellaneous: anemia, carcinoma, systemic lupus erythematosus, infectious diseases, congestive heart failure, porphyria
Drug-induced
Alcohol
Other sedative-hypnotics
Antipsychotics
Anxiolytics
Antihistamines
Narcotic analgesics
Anticholinergics
Antihypertensives
Digitalis
Estrogen preparations
Immunosuppressives
Corticosteroids (withdrawal)
Stimulants (withdrawal)

chomotor agitation, while others exhibit psychomotor retardation, which is an important consideration in drug selection. Since many of the antidepressants exhibit approximately equivalent efficacy in depression, the selection of a particular drug is often based on matching it with the psychomotor activity level of the depressed individual. Antidepressants with significant sedative potential (the tertiary amines) are used in agitated individuals, while nonsedative drugs (the secondary amines) are used for clients with pronounced psychomotor retardation or marked social withdrawal.

With dysthymic disorder, the depressive symptoms are less severe or persistent but are present most or all the time for at least 2 years (possibly separated by periods of normal mood lasting days, weeks, or even a few months). The list of circumstantial symptoms is expanded (see Table 20–3).

Susceptibility to major depression or dysthymic disorder is correlated with sex and age. Among the adult population in the United States and Europe, 18–23% of females and 8–11% of males have experienced at least one major depressive episode. Major depression severe enough to require hospitalization occurs in 6% of adult females and 3% of adult males during the course of a lifetime. Dysthymic disorder is also more common in adult women than in adult men, but equally common in children of both sexes, suggesting that either sex hormone differences or societal sex-role stereotyping may be a factor in predisposing to depression.

Major depression and dysthymic disorder differ markedly in pharmacotherapeutic responsiveness, with antidepressants clearly indicated for use in major depression but less effective than either anxiolytics or neuroleptics in dysthymic disorder. Dysthymic disorder is not consistently responsive to any drug treatment. The two conditions also differ with respect to several physiological correlates: barbiturate sleep threshold, insulin responsiveness, and sensitivity of the stress response (see Table 20–3).

Endogenous Versus Exogenous (Reactive) Depression

The endogenous versus exogenous (or reactive) dichotomy, applied mainly to major depression, refers to the presumed etiology and characteristic symptoms of depression and carries implications for prognosis (Table 20–4). However, it should be observed that the distinction between endogenous and exogenous depression has been more useful as a theoretical concept than in clinical practice, since there is considerable variation in the application of these terms by various clinicians. Endogenous depression arises from within the individual, presumably at the organic level of organization, while exogenous, or reactive, depression is triggered by an obvious, identifiable precipitant at the psychological or interpersonal level. The presence of a precipitant, however, does not exclude the possibility of an endogenous contribution or "predisposition." The level of impairment and prominence of somatic symptoms is generally greater in endogenous depression. Even if the etiology in a given case can be clearly ascribed to one level or another, the manifestations of depression will affect organic, psychological, and interpersonal levels of organization that contribute to psychological health.

Exogenous (reactive) depression is usually experienced by the client as comprehensible and appropriate in view of the precipitating circumstances. The client knows why he or she is depressed. In en-

Table 20–3
Major Depression Versus Dysthymic Disorder

Criteria	Major depression	Dysthymic disorder
Dysphoric mood		
Severity	Great	Less severe
Duration	At least 2 weeks	At least 2 years
Persistence	Nearly continuous	May be intermittent
Circumstantial symptoms	*At least four:* Appetite or weight changes; Sleep disturbances; Psychomotor agitation or retardation; Apathy; Lethargy; Low self-esteem; Cognitive impairment; Thoughts of death or suicide, or suicide attempts	*At least three:* Any of those listed under Major Depression *or* Decreased productivity; Social withdrawal; Irritability; Nonresponsiveness to rewards; Pessimism or brooding; Frequent crying
Physiological correlates		
Barbiturate sleep threshold	Lowered	Elevated
Insulin responsiveness	Resistant	Normal
Stress response	Depressed	Normal
Pharmacological responsiveness	Antidepressants clearly superior to other choices	No consistently effective drug treatments; anxiolytics = neuroleptics > antidepressants

Table 20–4
Endogenous Versus Reactive Depression

Characteristic	Endogenous	Reactive
Etiology		
Onset	Gradual	Sudden
Precipitant	No or yes	Yes
Manifestations		
Somatic symptoms	Many	Few
Subjective impression	Not appropriate	Appropriate
Impairment of functioning	Great	Mild
Responsiveness		
Duration	Prolonged	Often brief
Spontaneous remission	Low	High
Environmental responsiveness	Low	High
Tricyclic responsiveness	High	Low-moderate
MAO inhibitor responsiveness	Low-moderate	High

dogenous depression, the client does not understand the cause of the depression and feels helpless to correct it. Exogenous depression is more responsive to serendipitous improvements in life circumstances and exhibits a fairly high rate of spontaneous remission. It is also more responsive to psychotherapeutic intervention, especially supportive therapy. Endogenous depression, however, exhibits greater responsiveness to tricyclic antidepressant drug therapy. About 20% of cases of major depression are endogenous and about 80% are exogenous.

Other Characterizations of Depression

Melancholia is a form of major depression in which there is a marked anhedonia, loss of pleasure in all or most activities and a lack of responsiveness to rewards. In addition, at least three of the following characteristics must be present: a depressed mood distinct from a normal grief reaction, a regular worsening of depression in the morning, early morning awakenings, marked psychomotor agitation or retardation, anorexia and weight loss, and excessive or inappropriate feelings of guilt. Melancholia lies at the severe end of the spectrum of depressive states.

Some individuals suffering from unipolar depression do not meet the criteria for either major depression or dysthymic disorder. DSM-III provides the category, **atypical depression,** for such instances. This label could be employed, for example, when a case of depression meets the criteria for dysthymic disorder except that the intermittent periods of normal mood exceed 2 months. Sometimes the term *atypical depression* is used to designate a distinctive form of depression consisting of recurrent short-lived depressive episodes that result from injuries to self-esteem (after rejection in a romantic relationship, for example), with lethargy, fatigue, hypersomnia, chronic anxiety, overeating and weight gain, and phobias. There is some indication that MAO inhibitors may be especially useful in this form of depression.

Neurochemical Theories of Depression

The Norepinephrine Hypothesis

The norepinephrine hypothesis of affective disorders asserts that mania and depression are related to disturbances in the availability of norepinephrine to its postsynaptic receptors (Table 20–5). The concentrations are postulated to be subnormal in depression and excessive in mania (the opposite of depression). Cerebrospinal fluid (CSF) levels of the norepinephrine metabolite 3-methoxy-4-hydroxyphenylglycoaldehyde (MHPG) are considered to be a good index of norepinephrine activity (turnover) in the brain. The CSF levels of MHPG are frequently low in depressed clients but increase after spontaneous or drug-induced recovery. The CSF levels of MHPG are high during mania and low during depression in manic-depressive disorder.

The strongest evidence for the norepinephrine hypothesis is from pharmacological observations: that is, most of the drugs that alleviate depression interact with norepinephrine to increase the availability of the neurotransmitter in the synapse, whereas drugs that deplete this amine or block its access to postsynaptic receptors tend to produce psychiatric depression. Each of the groups of drugs traditionally employed in depression increase free norepinephrine one way or another. Tricyclic antidepressants block the reuptake of the transmitter, MAO inhibitors prevent its breakdown by the enzyme MAO, and amphetamine-like stimulants promote release of norepinephrine. Some of the new generation of atypical antidepressants (see below) block presynaptic receptors, reducing feedback reg-

Table 20–5
Neurochemical Theories of Depression

Theory	Depression	Mania
Norepinephrine	Low	High
Permissive	Low 5-HT and low NE	Low 5-HT and high NE
Two-disease	NE type: low NE; 5-HT type: low 5-HT	No specification
Down-regulation	Supersensitive NE receptors	Subsensitive NE receptors

Key: NE, norepinephrine; 5-HT, 5-hydroxytryptamine (serotonin).

ulation of norepinephrine synthesis and release, thus allowing synaptic concentrations of the neurotransmitter to increase. Drugs that deplete norepinephrine, such as reserpine, α-methylparatyrosine, and guanethidine, and drugs that block norepinephrine receptors, such as phenoxybenzamine and propranolol, tend to cause depression.

However, a number of observations seem to run counter to the norepinephrine hypothesis: (1) Both the tricyclic antidepressants and the MAO inhibitors require about 10 days to 3 weeks of administration before clinical effectiveness is observed, but the respective biochemical alterations in norepinephrine reuptake or degradation occur immediately in laboratory animals. (2) Some drugs among the new atypical antidepressants do not have identified interactions with norepinephrine synapses. (3) The relative efficacy of a series of tricyclic antidepressants does not correlate well with potency in blocking reuptake. And (4), long-term use of tricyclic antidepressants leads to down-regulation, or subsensitivity, of postsynaptic norepinephrine receptors. This last observation has even led some researchers to reverse the norepinephrine hypothesis and argue for the **down-regulation** hypothesis, which suggests that depression is related to hypersensitivity of norepinephrine receptors and is relieved by drugs that reverse this receptor state. However, it is difficult to reconcile the down-regulation hypothesis with established clinical and pharmacological observations.

The Permissive Theory

According to the permissive theory, insufficient serotonin activity has a destabilizing effect on mood, predisposing to either depression or mania (Table 20–5). In this view, the actual outcome, mania or depression, is determined by norepinephrine. Thus, depression occurs when both serotonin and norepinephrine are low; mania occurs when serotonin is low and norepinephrine is high.

This theory is useful in explaining why a few depressed clients respond to the serotonin precursor 5-hydroxytryptophan (5-HTP). It also helps to explain the effectiveness of certain tricyclic antidepressants that act more on serotonin reuptake than norepinephrine reuptake and some of the atypical antidepressants that affect serotonin reuptake exclusively. And it has been observed that some depressed clients exhibit a significantly reduced serotonin turnover rate in the brain, as measured by accumulation of the serotonin metabolite 5-hydroxyindoleacetic acid (5-HIAA) in the CSF following probenecid treatment. The permissive theory also offers possibilities for explaining the mechanism of lithium by relating it to the serotonin system. But the theory falls short in its failure to account for why so few depressed clients respond to 5-HTP. The two-disease theory attempts to rectify this shortcoming.

The Two-Disease Theory

The two-disease theory postulates that depression occurs as a result of either low norepinephrine *or* low serotonin, and that there are therefore two types of depression, the norepinephrine-type and the serotonin-type (Table 20–5). This theory is designed to explain the variable responsiveness of depressed persons to 5-HTP. Studies of serotonin turnover rates using CSF samples appear to support the contention of two distinct populations of depressed clients, one group with clearly depressed serotonin turnover rates, the other (presumably having the norepinephrine-type of depression) with serotonin turnover rates comparable to control subjects. Additional supporting evidence comes from studies indicating that clients with low serotonin turnover (determined by measurement of 5-HIAA levels in the CSF after administering probenecid (Benemid)) respond better to tricyclics that are potent in blocking the reuptake of serotonin. On the other hand, clients responding to tricyclics that selectively block norepinephrine reuptake exhibit normal or high pretreatment values for 5-HIAA in the CSF, but low turnover of norepinephrine (based on urinary MHPG levels). Unfortunately, the probenecid method for determining serotonin turnover in the brain does not lend itself to routine application in the evaluation of clients. Considerable effort (thus far without success) has been directed toward trying to define clinical distinctions or diagnostic predictors of 5-HTP responsiveness that would support the idea of two neurochemical types of depression.

Tricyclic Antidepressants

The group of agents known as antidepressants began their clinical history in the late 1950s with the nearly simultaneous introduction of the tricyclic antidepressants and the MAO inhibitors. Recent years have seen the addition of agents called *second generation* antidepressants.

The chemical structures and the spectrum of side effects of the tricyclic antidepressants closely resemble the phenothiazine neuroleptics (Table 20–6). The tricyclic antidepressants can be usefully divided into two subgroups: the tertiary amines and the secondary amines. The tertiary amines have a relatively greater effect on serotonin than on norepinephrine

Table 20–6
Adverse Effects of Tricyclic Antidepressants

Clinical features	Anticholinergic	Cardiovascular	Allergies and dyscrasias	Psychiatric and neurological	Endocrine
Symptoms	Blurred vision Mydriasis Acute glaucoma Dryness of mouth Sweating Constipation Urinary retention Paralytic ileus Tachycardia Dysmnesia Mental confusion	Orthostatic hypotension Heart block Dysrhythmias	Cholestatic jaundice Skin rashes Agranulocytosis	Sedation (especially with tertiary amines) Drowsiness Excess stimulation Mood switch Tremors Epileptiform seizures Peripheral neuropathies Mild pseudoparkinsonism	Galactorrhea Amenorrhea Loss of libido Weight gain
Incidence	Common	Common	Rare	Common	Common
Period of risk	Early	Early	Early	Throughout	Throughout
Clinical response options	Tolerance occurs	Tolerance occurs	Interrupt treatment; symptoms may or may not recur with resumption	Adjust dose	Adjust dose

reuptake, while the reverse is true of the secondary amines. Consequently, the tertiary amines are more sedative (an effect attributable to elevations in serotonin). However, tertiary amines are converted to active secondary amines, thus producing serotonin reuptake blockade followed by norepinephrine reuptake blockade due to the metabolite.

Mechanisms of Action The conventional view of the mechanism of tricyclic antidepressants attributes clinical efficacy to the ability of these drugs to block the reuptake of norepinephrine or serotonin. This interpretation of the mechanism of action of tricyclics would appear to fit well with the neurochemical hypotheses of depression discussed above. Blockade of reuptake would elevate the levels of free norepinephrine or serotonin in the synapse, increasing postsynaptic receptor activation. The problem with this straightforward view is that there is no correlation between the times of occurrence of the two effects; blockade of reuptake occurs almost immediately, but the clinical efficacy requires 10 days–3 weeks of regular drug administration. This discrepancy has yet to be resolved satisfactorily. One revised view emphasizes the dynamic nature of adaptive neural mechanisms when a drug is used chronically. Accordingly, the immediate effect of tricyclics, blockade of reuptake, is largely offset by compensatory reductions in norepinephrine (or serotonin) release, mediated by presynaptic receptors. With continued use of the antidepressant, the compensatory reduction in release undergoes tolerance, but the primary effect (blockade of reuptake) persists. Long-term adaptations (such as down-regulation of postsynaptic receptors) begin to set in after weeks of tricyclic administration but less completely offset the primary action of the antidepressant. The composite effect, after 3 weeks or more of treatment, is a neural system stabilized against depression, with less sensitive postsynaptic receptors, but more free norepinephrine to act on those receptors.

The competing hypothesis to explain the discrepant observations of tricyclic action, the down-regulation hypothesis, postulates that depression is related to an excess of noradrenergic functional activity. Tricyclic therapy is seen as desensitizing postsynaptic receptors. This view is diametrically opposed to the norepinephrine hypothesis. For the time being, our understanding of the mechanism of antidepressants remains incomplete.

Pharmacokinetics Tricyclic antidepressants are well absorbed from the gastrointestinal tract after oral administration and reach peak plasma concentrations within 2–4 hours after administration. However, tricyclic antidepressants undergo a significant first-pass extraction by the liver. The extent of both first-pass extraction and the rate of metabolism exhibit a high degree of variability from one individual to another, resulting in a poor correlation between the dose administered and the resultant plasma concentration (bioavailability). On the other hand, there is a good correlation between plasma concentrations and therapeutic responsiveness (Table 20–7), since most tricyclics exhibit a **therapeutic window** of effective serum concentrations, above or below which clinical efficacy falls off sharply. Thus, variability in responsiveness to tricyclic antidepressants is largely caused by pharmacokinetic factors rather than pharmacodynamic factors. For all of these reasons, doses of tricyclic antidepressants must be titrated to meet the needs of the individual client in order to optimize clinical response, and ideally, doses should be titrated initially against measured serum concentrations. Later, the dose of a tricyclic should be individualized to the needs of the specific client based on clinical response.

In the blood, tricyclic antidepressants are highly bound to plasma proteins, in excess of 90%, are distributed widely throughout the body, and undergo enterohepatic cycling as well as renal excretion. The half-lives of tricyclics vary from 8 hours for amoxapine (Asendin) to 54–198 hours for protriptyline (Vivactil). Tricyclics are ideally given in 3 or 4 divided doses, an approach usually employed for hospitalized patients when compliance can be assured. However, once-a-day administration at bedtime helps to improve compliance for outpatients. Accumulation of tricyclics occur because of the long half-lives; steady-state concentrations may not be achieved for up to 10 days with some of the agents (Table 20–7). Therefore, dosage adjustments should not be undertaken more frequently than every 4 days. Tricyclic antidepressants must be used cautiously and at reduced doses (if at all) in clients with impaired renal or hepatic function.

Clinical Indications Antidepressants are employed in **major depression** and are superior to other drug treatments for this condition. The greatest success has been with endogenous depression. Reactive and episodic depressions are less successfully treated with drugs. Antidepressants are also used in dysthymic disorder, but with less success overall than alternative drug treatments. In severe depression, drug therapy may be used adjunctively

Table 20–7
Pharmacokinetic Parameters of Antidepressants

Drug	Therapeutic plasma level (ng/mL)	Half-life (hours)	Time to reach steady state (days)
Tertiary amines			
Amitriptyline	125–250[a]	17–40	4–10
Imipramine	150–300[a]	6–24	2–5
Trimipramine	180[a]	7–30	2–6
Doxepin	150–250[a]	8–36	2–8
Secondary amines			
Nortriptyline	50–150	15–93	4–19
Protriptyline	115–300	54–198	10
Desipramine	150–300	12–76	2–11
Amoxapine	200–400	8–30	2–7
Second generation antidepressants			
Maprotiline	200–300[a]	27–58	6–10
Trazodone	?	4–9	3–7
Bupropion	50–100	10–21	?

[a]Includes active metabolite.

Nursing Observations for Antidepressant Therapy of Depression

THERAPEUTIC GOAL	Alleviation of depression and associated behavioral and physiological symptoms.
PREADMINISTRATION ASSESSMENT	
Baseline Data	Observe extent of dysphoric mood, appetite or weight changes, sleep disturbances, psychomotor agitation or retardation, apathy, lethargy, low self-esteem, alterations in thought processes, talk of suicide, social withdrawal, decreased effectiveness, lack of responsiveness to rewards, lack of interest in activities, irritability, pessimism or brooding, and frequent crying. Evaluate neurological functioning, vital signs, ECG, perfusion, heart sounds, renal output, and abdomen. Examine eyes for glaucoma and disturbances of visual function. Check for organic causes of depression (see Table 20–2). Obtain laboratory tests, including complete blood cells counts and liver enzymes.
Contraindications/ Precautions	Cardiovascular disease, hepatic or renal failure, glaucoma, prostatic hypertrophy, urinary retention, pheochromocytoma, hyperthyroidism, pregnancy, lactation, or allergic reactions to tricyclics, phenothiazines, or tartrazine (found in certain products).
Potential Interactions	Check current regimen for stimulants, sympathomimetics, antidysrhythmic, and anticholinergic drugs.
EVALUATION OF DRUG RESPONSE	
During Dosage Adjustment	Monitor serum concentrations of the tricyclic antidepressant.
For Therapeutic Benefit	Alleviation of depression and depressive symptomatology.
For Adverse Effects	With tricyclic drugs, monitor for neurological responses (sedation, drowsiness, excess stimulation, mood switch, tremors, seizures, peripheral neuropathies, and pseudoparkinsonism); cardiovascular side effects (orthostatic hypotension, tachycardia, heart block, dysrhythmias); allergic reactions (jaundice, rash, or agranulocytosis); anticholinergic symptoms (blurred vision, dilated pupils, glaucoma, dryness of mouth, sweating, constipation, urinary retention, paralytic ileus, and mental confusion); and endocrine changes (galactorrhea, amenorrhea, loss of libido, and weight gain). With MAO inhibitors, monitor for orthostatic hypotension, excess stimulation, hypomania, headache, memory impairment, weakness, changes in visual function, liver dysfunction, and gastrointestinal irritation.
For Drug Interactions	Monitor additive CNS depression when tertiary amines are employed. With all tricyclics, watch for additive anticholinergic effects, potentiation of direct-acting sympathomimetic drugs, and alterations in tricyclic metabolism by tobacco smoke, methylphenidate (Ritalin), phenothiazines, and disulfiram (Antabuse). Look for potentiation of cardiovascular effects of tricyclic antidepressants by quinidine and procainamide and alterations in blood pressure control by antihypertensive drugs when tricyclics are added. Observe for supra-additive effects when two or more drugs from different antidepressant classes are combined. Monitor for potentiation of drugs such as barbiturates, meperidine, and cocaine by MAO inhibitors. Monitor for diminished efficacy of antidepressants when depressant drugs are employed, including oral contraceptives.
For Dietary Interactions	Monitor for ingestion of tyramine-containing foods when MAO inhibitors are employed.
For Compliance	Evaluate client compliance with all facets of the therapeutic regimen by careful observation, interviewing, and review of progress. Report compliance problems to the physician and act as client-advocate when changes in the therapeutic regimen seem indicated.

to electroconvulsant shock, but this increases the hazards of therapy.

In general efficacy, tricyclic antidepressants elicit significantly more positive responses in major depression than do placebo or psychotherapy alone, although the margin of difference is not great. Approximately one-fourth of those not responsive to psychotherapy or placebo alone respond to the antidepressant therapy. About 70% of severely depressed inpatients respond to antidepressant medication as against a 50% spontaneous recovery rate. Overall, drug treatment benefits a smaller percentage of severely depressed patients than electroconvulsant therapy, and the response to electroconvulsant therapy is considerably more rapid. However, it entails greater risks of debilitating effects on brain function. Tricyclic antidepressants appear to be useful in decreasing the risk of recurrent major depressive episodes when employed in small maintenance doses.

Selection of a particular tricyclic antidepressant is seldom based on efficacy, since the available drugs are generally comparable in generating a clinical response. The main considerations are past response and the likelihood of side effects (Table 20-8), especially sedation. The sedative antidepressants are utilized in agitated patients, while the nonsedative drugs are used in patients who exhibit psychomotor retardation. Protriptyline (Vivactil) may actually be activating rather than sedating and is especially useful in apathetic and withdrawn patients.

Three classes of drugs have been employed in **dysthymic disorder,** partly because no one has proved to be consistently effective. Tricyclic antidepressants, neuroleptics (usually thioridazine (Mellaril) or thiothixene (Navane)), and anxiolytics (diazepam (Valium), chlordiazepoxide (Librium), or alprazolam (Xanax)) are all commonly used. Anxiolytics are perhaps the most effective medications for dysthymic disorder, especially if the treatment period is to be brief and the condition has been long-term but mild — the usual case. Neuroleptics appear most effective when dysthymic disorder is severe and of recent origin. Tricyclic antidepressants are the

Table 20-8
Pharmacologic Properties and Adverse Effects of Antidepressants

	Reuptake block		Release		Major adverse effects		
Drug	**NE**	**5HT**	**NE**	**DA**	**Anticholinergic**	**Sedation**	**Orthostatic hypotension**
Tertiary amines							
Amitriptyline	+[a]	++++	0	0	++++	+++	++
Imipramine	+++[a]	+++	0	0	++	++	+++
Trimipramine	+	++	0	0	++	+++	++
Doxepin	+	+++	0	0	++	+++	++
Secondary amines							
Nortriptyline	++	+++	0	0	++	++	+
Protriptyline	+++	+	0	0	+++	+/−	+
Desipramine	++++	0	0	0	+	+/−	+
Amoxapine	+++	++	0	0	+	++	+
Second-generation antidepressants							
Maprotiline	++	+	0	0	+	++	+
Trazodone	0	+++	0	0	+	+	++
Nomifensine	++	+	0	++	0	0	0
Bupropion	+/−	0	0	+	0	+	0
Stimulants							
Amphetamine	0	0	+++	+++	0	0	0

Key: ++++ greatest degree; +++ high degree; ++ moderate degree; + slight degree; +/− slight or not at all; 0 not at all.

[a]Includes effect of secondary amine metabolites.

least effective of the three classes in dysthymic disorder.

Some of the tricyclic antidepressants have additional approved indications as well as unlabeled uses. Amitriptyline (Elavil and others) and imipramine (Tofranil and others) have been used as adjuncts to narcotic analgesic therapy for **chronic pain.** These agents potentiate the effect of narcotics permitting use of smaller doses and a longer period of effective therapy. Amitriptyline has been used for prophylaxis against **migraine** and exhibits an efficacy comparable to methysergide (Sansert). Imipramine has been used in treating functional enuresis (see Chapter 43) and is highly effective in **panic disorder, panic reactions associated with agoraphobia,** and **separation anxiety** in children (see Chapter 19).

Tricyclic antidepressants, especially protriptyline, have been used effectively in treatment of insomnia caused by **sleep apneas.** Traditional sleeping pills (sedative-hypnotics) cannot be used for this particular type of insomnia because they further depress the respiratory center. Doxepine (Adapin, Sinequan) is indicated for treatment of the **depressive phase of manic-depressive disorder,** as an adjunct to lithium therapy.

Adverse Effects and Contraindications The adverse effects of tricyclic antidepressants are many and varied (Table 20–6). Like the phenothiazines, the tricyclics possess both anticholinergic and antihistaminergic properties. Clients suffering from the **anticholinergic side effects** complain of too much sedation, dryness of mouth, mydriasis (dilation of pupils), and blurred vision. Clients may exhibit tachycardia, impaired memory, and mental confusion. Others complain of excessive sweating, constipation, and urinary retention. *Constipation caused by tricyclic antidepressants can be treated using a high-fiber diet, increased fluid intake, or, if necessary, a stool softener. Nurses should advise clients to report any difficulty with urination. Nurses should monitor the intake-output ratio of hospitalized clients and palpate for indications of bladder distention. Nonhospitalized clients and/or family members need to be taught to monitor for bladder distention.*

Dry mouth also occurs and becomes a factor in noncompliance because of the annoyance. It promotes erosion and shrinkage of gums and demineralization of tooth enamel. Speech and chewing and swallowing of food become difficult. Nurses may observe other indications of dry mouth such as crusting of the oral mucosa, continuous tongue and lip movements to lubricate the mouth, or a rough tongue surface. *Nurses should teach clients to compensate for dry mouth by chewing sugarless gum, rinsing the mouth with warm water, using a saliva substitute, increasing noncaloric fluid intake, and avoiding irritating foods.* Use of fluoride toothpaste helps to prevent demineralization.

Because of these anticholinergic effects, tricyclic antidepressants must be used with caution in individuals with a history of glaucoma, and those receiving other anticholinergic drugs for any purpose. *Nurses need to monitor clients for evidence of changes in vision. In particular, clients with a history of glaucoma should be monitored closely for occurrence of headache, halos, eye pain, dilated pupils, or nausea. Those with angle-closure glaucoma are extremely sensitive to tricyclic drugs and even small doses may precipitate an attack. Clients with glaucoma who are also receiving antidepressants should seek the supervision of an opthalmologist.*

Tricyclics with the weakest anticholinergic properties (Table 20–8) are preferred for individuals especially susceptible to anticholinergic toxicity. *Nurses should advise clients that anticholinergic side effects such as constipation usually diminish after a few weeks of treatment; this knowledge will help clients persist with therapy.*

Cardiovascular side effects of tricyclic antidepressants include orthostatic hypotension, flushing, nasal congestion, heart block, syncope, myocardial infarction, precipitation of congestive heart failure, stroke, hypertensive episodes, and arrhythmias. *Nurses should obtain an ECG recording prior to initiating therapy with tricyclics and periodically during treatment. They should check pulse rate and blood pressure frequently and teach outpatients to check and record their own pulse and blood pressure. Because of the potential for orthostatic hypotension, clients should be advised to avoid standing up quickly or taking excessively hot showers or baths. Dangling the feet over the side of the bed before initial ambulation in the morning will reduce the likelihood of fainting. Elderly individuals and clients with a history of cardiovascular disease require especially close monitoring for cardiovascular side effects. Hyperthyroid individuals and those receiving thyroid hormone supplements are especially subject to cardiovascular toxicity of tricyclics. Tricyclic antidepressants should be discontinued as long before elective surgery as is practical.*

Psychiatric and neurological side effects are among the most common. With the tertiary amines, sedation, drowsiness, or fatigue is especially frequent and problematic. *Nurses need to monitor closely clients who are receiving tricyclics for indications of changes in mental status. They should advise clients to refrain from use of alcohol and other depressant drugs, because of the potential for interaction with the sedative effect of the medication and the contribution that depressant drugs make to the depressive syndrome. It is important to remind clients that drowsiness and blurred vision caused by these drugs may* *impair ability to operate an automobile or performance of other hazardous tasks. If daytime sedation or dizziness presents a problem, the entire daily dose of most tricyclics can be administered at bedtime.*

Tricyclic antidepressants may cause confusion, impaired ability to concentrate, hallucinations, delusions, disorientation, anxiety, nervousness, agitation, panic, or mania. Schizophrenic or paranoid individuals may exhibit intensification of adverse symptoms under the influence of tricyclic medication. Mood switches can be triggered in manic-depressive individuals (from depression to hypomania or mania). Anxiety and agitation may also be intensified in clients with these disorders.

Suicide attempts are higher among depressed individuals than any other population of psychiatric clients. Suicide liability increases when therapy is initiated with tricyclic antidepressants. Therefore, client monitoring and supportive therapy should be intensified when drug therapy is begun. *Tricyclic antidepressants should be prescribed in small amounts to reduce the risk of intentional overdoses with the intent of suicide, especially during the initial phase of treatment.*

Like neuroleptics and narcotics, tricyclic antidepressants **lower the seizure threshold.** *Caution should be observed in administering these drugs to individuals with a history of seizures or those undergoing withdrawal from alcohol or other sedative-hypnotics.* Potential **adverse motor reactions** to tricyclic antidepressants include incoordination, weakness, motor hyperactivity, ataxia, akathisias, pseudoparkinsonism, and tardive dyskinesias. The incidence and severity of motor reactions is much less than occurs with neuroleptics. Other neurological symptoms include numbness, tingling, paresthesias, speech block, tinnitus, insomnia, nightmares, and dysarthria. Tricyclic antidepressants cause increased beta-wave and slow-wave activity on the EEG, and reduced alpha waves.

Allergic reactions to tricyclic antidepressants include skin rash, pruritus, urticaria, petechiae, photosensitivity, edema, vasculitis, and drug fever. *Clients should be advised to avoid intensive exposure to sunlight because of possible photosensitivity.* Cross-sensitivity among the various tricyclics is routinely observed. *Use of tricyclic antidepressants is contraindicated in individuals with a known hypersensitivity to any of the tricyclic compounds.* Alopecia occurs rarely with tricyclics. Some antidepressant products (Tofranil and Janimine, for example) contain tartrazine, a dye to which some individuals are allergic. Tartrazine sensitivity is most often encountered in individuals allergic to aspirin.

The **blood dyscrasias** that can occur in response to administration of tricyclics include agranulocytosis, eosinophilia, thrombocytopenia, and leukopenia. Agranulocytosis is most common in elderly women and during the second month of treatment. *The presence of petechiae, purpura, persistent sore throat or fever, easy bruising, and unusual bleeding is an indication that the client needs further testing to rule out dyscrasias. For clients at risk, baseline leukocyte counts should be obtained prior to initiation of a tricyclic antidepressant to be followed by periodic monitoring during therapy.*

Endocrine side effects of tricyclics are especially prominent in aspects of sexual functioning. Gynecomastia, testicular swelling, and impotence may occur in males; amenorrhea, galactorrhea, and breast enlargement in women. Decreased or (rarely) increased libido also occurs. *Nurses should ask clients about any changes in libido or reproductive function. Such information is often most readily obtained from discussions with the spouse.* Tricyclic antidepressants may cause alterations in blood sugar levels in either direction, thereby complicating management of diabetic clients. *Nurses should carefully monitor diabetic clients when tricyclic therapy is either initiated or discontinued and clients should be instructed in self-assessment for needed adjustments in antidiabetic medication.* Rarely, antidiuretic hormone secretion increases.

Adverse gastrointestinal effects of tricyclics include nausea, vomiting, anorexia, diarrhea, constipation, flatulence, epigastric distress, abdominal cramps, dysgeusia, dysphagia, stomatitis, black tongue, glossitis, or parotid swelling. *Nurses should advise clients to administer tricyclic antidepressants with or immediately after food to reduce gastric irritation.* Hepatitis and jaundice occur rarely. *A baseline evaluation of liver function should be conducted before initiation of therapy.* Both weight loss and weight gain can occur when tricyclic therapy is initiated.

Treatment of overdoses of tricyclic antidepressants is symptomatic and supportive, requiring removal of any residual drug from the stomach and maintenance of vital functions. Anticonvulsant or antidysrhythmic medication may be required. Physostigmine may be used to alleviate anticholinergic toxicity.

Drug Interactions Tricyclic antidepressants with sedative properties (see Table 20–8) will produce additive CNS depression with other **depressant drugs,** including alcohol, barbiturates, benzodiazepines, and narcotics.

Since tricyclic antidepressants interfere with neuronal uptake of norepinephrine and other **sympathetic amines,** the action of direct-acting amines (such as epinephrine) is potentiated. On the other hand, the action of indirect-acting agents (such as ephedrine or amphetamine) is diminished since these agents depend on uptake into nerve terminals

Nursing Diagnoses and Interventions for Antidepressant Therapy of Depression

Nursing Diagnoses	*Related Interventions*
TO ENHANCE DRUG BENEFITS OR REDUCE DRUG REQUIREMENTS	
Alteration in nutrition: intake either more or less than requirements related to nervous eating or anorexia	Provide nutrition guidance. Teach clients to keep a record of nutritional intake to use as a teaching tool.
Alterations in thought processes: negative cognitive set leading to polarized thinking, overgeneralization, and arbitrary inference; Disturbance of self-concept related to feelings of failure or worthlessness; Grieving due to personal loss	Provide emotional support and encouragement, psychotherapy, and drug therapy. Encourage client to discuss feelings.
Diversional activity deficit or sexual dysfunction related to anhedonia	Consider referral to a sex therapist.
Impaired social interactions related to alienation and constant complaining	Teach client and family methods of altering client's behavior.
Ineffective individual coping: anger related to low self-esteem or rejection; Powerlessness if depression is endogenous	Work with client and family on effective coping strategies.
Impaired home maintenance related to apathy and fatigue	Help family identify social services or temporary role adjustments to provide home maintenance.
Increased risk of injury related to apathy, negative affect, and depressant effects of tertiary amines	Provide appropriate safety measures and warn clients not to drive or to employ heavy machinery when experiencing sedation.
Ineffective family coping related to marital discord and role conflicts secondary to client's chronic depression	Encourage involvement in marital or family therapy.
Self-care deficit: impaired grooming	Provide help with personal hygiene, especially during early treatment of acute depressive episodes.
Sleep pattern disturbance: insomnia or hypersomnia secondary to depression	Provide environment conducive to maintaining a regular sleep pattern; provide hypnotics sparingly.
Violence to self related to feelings of hopelessness and loneliness	Be vigilant for indications of suicide intentions; intensify supportive therapy during initiation of tricyclic antidepressant therapy. Teach significant family members to watch for danger signs.
TO MINIMIZE DRUG SIDE EFFECTS OR INTERACTIONS	
Alteration in bowel movements: constipation related to lack of activity or use of tricyclics	Encourage client to increase activity; provide high fiber diet and increased fluid intake.
Alteration in cardiac output: orthostatic hypotension, tachycardia, and dysrhythmias related to tricyclic drugs	Monitor the ECG periodically; warn clients not to alter position quickly, to avoid hot showers or sunlight, or long periods of standing; suggest use of elastic hosiery.
Alteration in comfort: gastrointestinal irritation from antidepressant drugs	Instruct the client to take antidepressant medications with meals.
Alteration in oral mucous membranes: dryness related to tricyclic antidepressants	Advise client to increase oral hygiene and to take frequent sips of water or ice chips, hard candy, gum, or a saliva substitute.

Sensory-perceptual alterations related to hallucinations, excess stimulation, or blurred vision by antidepressants	Report incidence to physician for change in the drug prescription.
TO ENSURE SAFE AND EFFICACIOUS DRUG USE	
Knowledge deficit related to drug regimen	Teach clients about the nature of their disorder and the rationale for the treatment regimen.
	Explain to clients that therapeutic benefit with antidepressants frequently requires 2–4 weeks. Many of the adverse effects, on the other hand, are most intense at the beginning of therapy and gradually diminish. Encourage clients to continue with the drug regimen during this period of minimum benefit and maximum side effects.
	Provide client with a list of adverse effects and drug interactions for each drug in the regimen and explain what to do if any of these occur.
	When MAO inhibitors are employed, explain the drug-diet interactions.

to produce their releasing action. Many over-the-counter medications contain sympathetic amines, including anorexics and cold, cough, and allergy preparations containing decongestants. *The nurse should instruct clients who are receiving antidepressant medication not to use nonprescription drugs without first consulting the physician. Clients who suffer from allergies and carry epinephrine to counteract severe allergic reactions will need to be warned that effects of epinephrine are greatly increased in the presence of a tricyclic antidepressant, which could result in cardiac dysrhythmias.*

Tricyclic antidepressants may alter the efficacy of **antihypertensive drug regimens** because of blockade of norepinephrine reuptake. Blood pressure should be monitored when antidepressant therapy is begun, and dosages of antihypertensive medications adjusted accordingly. Procainamide and quinidine may increase the cardiovascular effects of tricyclic antidepressants. The combination of tricyclic antidepressants and reserpine should be avoided because reserpine aggravates depression and the combination can result in an initial stimulatory effect on blood pressure and brain function. The action of beta-adrenergic blocking agents is antagonized by tricyclic antidepressants.

Hepatic metabolism of tricyclic antidepressants is inhibited by several drugs: methylphenidate (Ritalin), phenothiazines, disulfiram (Antabuse), and probably cimetidine (Tagamet). On the other hand, tobacco smoking increases metabolism of tricyclics.

The combination of tricyclic antidepressants with **antidepressants from other groups** (MAO inhibitors or amphetamine-like stimulants) results in a supra-additive action. Such combinations can be used effectively and safely if appropriate adjustments are made to allow for the synergistic action. In practice, use of such combinations has often resulted in excess stimulation, hypertensive episodes, hyperpyretic crisis, convulsions, and death. When transferring a patient from MAO inhibitor therapy to tricyclic therapy, a minimum of 14 days must be allowed between discontinuation of the MAO inhibitor and initiation of tricyclic treatment to avoid synergy.

Preparations and Administration A few principles of administration are applicable to all tricyclic antidepressant compounds. Tricyclic antidepressants exhibit considerable variability in dosage requirements from client to client. Dosage must be individualized to meet the needs of each client, initially by titration against serum concentrations, later against clinical response and occurrence of side effects. When minor side effects develop, dosage reduction should be attempted; serious adverse reactions require discontinuation of the drug. Lower than standard doses are recommended for adolescents, elderly individuals, and outpatients. For example, elderly clients should receive doses one-fourth those given to young adults at the lower end of the range and one-half at the upper end of the range.

Initially, doses are usually small and divided, typically three times daily. Parenteral dosing is employed initially only for individuals unwilling or unable to receive oral medication. The dosage is gradually increased based on plasma levels or on efficacy and side effects. If sedation poses a problem, all or most of the daily allotment can be given at bedtime. A single nighttime dose is usually given in maintenance applications. From 2 weeks to 30 days of treatment may be required before full therapeutic benefit is achieved. Discontinuation of tricyclic antidepressants should be conducted gradually whenever possible. Abrupt discontinuation has been associated with nausea, vomiting, headache, chills, muscle aches, anxiety, akathisias, and malaise. *The nurse should advise clients not to discontinue antidepressant medication without advice of the physician.* Individuals experiencing an acute depressive episode, without a history of frequent recurrence, may recover completely and be withdrawn from medication after as little as 4–6 weeks. Others may require maintenance therapy or even full doses for the rest of their lives.

TERTIARY TRICYCLICS

Amitriptyline (Elavil, Amitril, Emitrip, Endep, and generic formulations)
Tablets, injection solution
Recommended Doses: For outpatients, 75 mg/day PO initially, in divided doses (usually 3), increased up to 150 mg/day. For inpatients, 100 mg/day PO initially, increased up to 300 mg if required. For elderly and adolescent individuals, 10 mg, 3 times daily. Injection solution is for IM administration only, initially 20–30 mg, 4 times daily.

Doxepin (Adapin, Sinequan)
Capsules, oral concentrate
Recommended Doses: For mild to moderate anxiety or depression, 25 mg, 3 times daily. The maximum recommended daily dose is 150 mg. The entire dose can be given at bedtime to improve compliance and to alleviate daytime sedative effects. For severe anxiety or depression, 50 mg initially, 3 times daily, increased up to 300 mg/day. Not recommended for children under 12.

Imipramine (Tofranil, Janimine, SK-Pramine, Tipramine, and generic formulations)
Tablets, injection solution

Imipramine Pamoate (Tofranil-PM)
Capsules
Recommended Doses: For outpatients, 75 mg/day PO initially, in divided doses, increased up to 200 mg/day. For inpatients, 100–150 mg/day PO initially, in divided doses, increased up to 300 mg/-day. For elderly and adolescent individuals, 30–40 mg/day PO initially, not to exceed 100 mg/day.

Trimipramine (Surmontil)
Capsules
Recommended Doses: For outpatients, 75 mg/day PO initially, increased up to 200 mg/day. For inpatients, 100 mg/day PO, up to a maximum of 300 mg/day. For adolescent and elderly clients, 50 mg/day PO initially, up to a maximum of 100 mg/day. For maintenance therapy, 50–150 mg/day PO. Not recommended for use in children.

SECONDARY TRICYCLICS

Amoxapine (Asendin)
Tablets
Recommended Doses: For depression in adults, 50 mg PO initially, 2 or 3 times daily, up to a maximum of 300 mg/day. For elderly clients, 25 mg PO initially, 2 or 3 times daily, up to a maximum of 300 mg/day. Not recommended for children under 16.

Desipramine (Norpramin, Pertofrane)
Tablets, capsules
Recommended Doses: For adults, 75–200 mg/day PO in divided doses, increased up to 300 mg/day. For geriatric and adolescent clients, 25–100 mg/day PO initially, up to 150 mg/day maximum. Not recommended for children.

Nortriptyline (Aventyl, Pamelor)
Capsules, oral liquid or solution
Recommended Doses: For adults, 25 mg PO initially, 3 or 4 times daily, up to 100 mg/day. For elderly and adolescent clients, 30–50 mg/day PO in divided doses. Not recommended for children.

Protriptyline (Vivactil)
Tablets
Recommended Doses: For adults, 15–40 mg/day PO initially, in 3 or 4 divided doses, increased gradually up to 60 mg/day. Increases should be made in the morning dose. For adolescent or geriatric clients, 5 mg PO initially, 3 times a day, increased gradually to 20 mg/day. Not recommended for use in children.

Second Generation (Atypical) Antidepressants

Second generation (atypical) antidepressants emerged in the 1980s. Many of the drugs in this group are still under development, but three are now marketed and a fourth (nomifensine) was marketed briefly in 1985–1986 before being withdrawn. Most of these drugs are unrelated to the tricyclics in structure and differ in one or more pharmacological actions. Two of them, maprotiline (Ludiomil) and mianserin, are tetracyclic compounds. Several block reuptake of serotonin selectively with little or no effect on norepinephrine. Some, like trazodone (Desyrel), have effects similar to the tricyclics on reuptake of norepinephrine or serotonin but are devoid of anticholinergic activity. One of them, mianserin, acts on presynaptic receptors rather than on the reuptake mechanism and lacks anticholinergic properties. Caroxazone is a newly developed MAO inhibitor that is much shorter-acting than conventional MAO inhibitors and devoid of anticholinergic, antihistaminergic, or antiserotonergic effects. Alprazolam (Xanax) is a benzodiazepine, discussed in Chapter 19, that appears to have value in dysthymic disorder as well as in anxiety. Bupropion (Wellbutrin) poses the greatest puzzle currently, having none of the conventional activities associated with antidepressants yet exhibiting substantial clinical efficacy.

Tetracyclic Antidepressants

The tetracyclic antidepressants include maprotiline and mianserin. Maprotiline has been available for clinical use since 1981; mianserin is currently in clinical trials. Maprotiline was the first of the second generation antidepressants to reach the market but is the least distinctive from the conventional tricyclics.

Maprotiline (Ludiomil)

The pharmacology of maprotiline generally parallels that of the secondary amines in the tricyclic family (Table 20–8) and presents a rather favorable balance between clinical responsiveness and adverse effects.

Clinical Indications Maprotiline is indicated for use not only in major depression, but also in dysthymic and bipolar disorders. Therapeutic response usually occurs in 2–3 weeks but may occur as early as 3–7 days after commencing therapy.

Adverse Effects and Contraindications Although less sedative than tertiary tricyclics, maprotiline is more so than protriptyline or desipramine. Drowsiness is reported in about 16% of treated individuals and weakness in 5%. *Nurses should make certain that clients receiving maprotiline have been advised not to perform hazardous tasks and to refrain from use of alcohol while taking maprotiline.* The incidence of anticholinergic side effects is less with maprotiline than with most tricyclics; dry mouth is reported in about 22% of individuals, constipation in 6%, and blurred vision in only 4%. *Maprotiline should be used with caution in individuals with a history of glaucoma (especially the angle-closure type) or urinary retention.*

Maprotiline, like the tricyclic compounds, can cause neurological impairments, including dizziness, tremors, insomnia, nervousness, and anxiety. The seizure threshold is lowered more by this compound than by tricyclic antidepressants, necessitating cautious use in individuals prone to seizure.

Drug Interactions Cardiovascular effects have occurred infrequently with maprotiline, but the antihypertensive activity of guanethidine (Ismelin) and other hypotensive medications may be antagonized by maprotiline in a manner similar to that observed with tricyclics. Clients who are hyperthyroid or receiving thyroid supplements and elderly individuals need to be monitored closely for adverse cardiovascular responses. Maprotiline should not be administered concurrently with MAO inhibitors.

Preparations and Administration

Maprotiline (Ludiomil)
Tablets
Recommended Doses: For mild to moderate depression, 75 mg/day orally, initially, in a single administration or divided. The initial dose should not be increased in less than 2 weeks, at which time the dose can be gradually increased in increments of 25 mg/day to a maximum of 225 mg/day. For severe depression, 100 mg/day orally initially, increased to a maximum of 300 mg/day. Recommended maintenance doses are 75–150 mg/day. For elderly clients, 50 to 75 mg/day for acute applications. Maprotiline is not recommended for individuals under 18 years of age.

Mianserin

Mianserin is a tetracyclic compound first prepared in 1966 that has distinctive behavior effects but EEG effects similar to amitriptyline. In a large multicenter study in Italy, mianserin exhibited antidepressant activity comparable to that of imipramine and amitriptyline, but a virtual absence of significant short-term side effects except for a modest degree of sedation. In particular, mianserin appears to lack anticholinergic and cardiotoxic properties. However, a relatively high incidence of liver problems has been associated with use of this drug. It is not sympathomimetic and does not inhibit MAO. Mianserin acts as an antagonist at presynaptic alpha-2 noradrenergic receptors that regulate release of norepinephrine from presynaptic terminals, thus freeing the terminal from the normal negative feedback constraints on transmitter release. Clinical studies are underway in the United States and mianserin (Bolvidon) is already marketed in England, Scandinavia, and central Europe.

Selective Inhibitors of Serotonin Reuptake

Several drugs that selectively block serotonin reuptake with little or no effect on norepinephrine are under study and one, trazodone, became available in the United States in 1982. Fluoxetine, fluvoxamine, zimelidine, citolopram, and viloxazine are agents in this group under investigation. Zimelidine has only slight anticholinergic properties and less cardiotoxicity than the traditional antidepressants, but agitation, sweating, and finger tremor have been reported as side effects. Fluoxetine and fluvoxamine are more selective than zimelidine. Fluvoxamine is under study in Europe and fluoxetine in the United States. Preliminary studies with fluvoxamine suggest that it is well tolerated, producing drowsiness and only very weak anticholinergic responses. Fluoxetine (Prozac) produced mixed results in a small clinical trial. Both fluvoxamine and fluoxetine may cause symptoms of anxiety, agitation, motor restlessness, racing thoughts, pressured speech, assertiveness, and apprehensiveness in some individuals, necessitating concurrent administration of anxiolytic medication.

Trazodone (Desyrel)

Trazodone (Desyrel), introduced into clinical practice in 1982, is structurally dissimilar from the tricyclic antidepressants.

Clinical Indications Indications for trazodone are major depression, with or without associated anxiety. Trazodone is comparable in efficacy with amitriptyline and imipramine.

Pharmacokinetics Trazodone is well absorbed after oral administration resulting in peak plasma levels in about 1 hour. Absorption is slightly increased in extent but slowed when the drug is taken with food, so that peak plasma levels are reduced and occur after about 2 hours. Trazodone is inactivated by liver metabolism in a biphasic pattern with an initial half-life of about 4.5 hours and a terminal half-life of about 7.5 hours.

Adverse Effects and Contraindications The incidence of anticholinergic effects with trazodone is very low as is the cardiotoxicity. The risk of overdose is lower for trazodone than for most other antidepressants, contributing to its great popularity for clinical use. Nevertheless, trazodone can produce neurological and psychiatric adverse effects, including drowsiness, fatigue, weakness, impaired memory, incoordination, anger, hostility, nightmares, hallucinations, delusions, confusion, disorientation, lightheadedness, excitement, dizziness, tremors, paresthesias, numbness, akathisias, impaired speech, and grand mal seizures. Depressant effects are additive with those produced by other CNS depressants.

Endocrine effects have included increased or decreased libido, impotence, priapism, or retrograde ejaculation in males, and early or missed menses in females. Gastrointestinal effects are uncommon but include nausea, dry mouth, hypersalivation, dysgeusia, diarrhea, constipation, and flatulence. Trazodone should be taken with or shortly after meals to minimize gastrointestinal disturbances. Hematological reactions to trazodone may include anemia, leukopenia, and neutropenia. Alterations in liver function tests have occurred occasionally, urinary frequency and retention have been reported, and appetite and weight changes have occurred in both directions.

Drug Interactions Trazodone is substantially hypotensive, necessitating a reduction in dose of most antihypertensive medications being used for hypertension. An exception is clonidine, the action of which may be antagonized by trazodone and concurrent use of clonidine and trazodone should be avoided. Trazodone has been reported to increase serum concentrations of concurrently administered digoxin or phenytoin.

Preparations and Administration Approximately one-half of treated individuals respond within 1 week of treatment and three-fourths within 2 weeks.

Trazodone (Desyrel)
Tablets
Recommended Doses: 150 mg/day PO initially, increased by increments of 50 mg/day at intervals of 3–4 days. Outpatients should not receive more than 400 mg/day and inpatients not more than 600 mg/day. Doses in excess of about 200 mg/day should be divided, but the major portion of the daily dose may be taken at bedtime to minimize daytime sedation.

Bupropion (Wellbutrin)

Bupropion is a second generation antidepressant approved for clinical use late in 1985. Bupropion is structurally similar to amphetamine but its mechanism of action is unknown. It blocks reuptake of norepinephrine and serotonin only very weakly, does not inhibit MAO, and lacks anticholinergic activity. It does not release biogenic amines from nerve terminals like amphetamine, but does have weak dopaminergic activity. One study reported that bupropion promotes down-regulation of beta-noradrenergic receptors in the manner of other antidepressants, but this was disputed by a later study.

Bupropion is readily absorbed after oral administration, reaching peak plasma levels in one to three hours. It is 82–88% bound to plasma proteins in the serum and freely crosses the placental and blood-brain barriers. It is inactivated almost exclusively by liver metabolism; the metabolites are excreted in the urine with a half-life of about 10–21 hours.

Based on large, multicenter studies, bupropion in doses of 300–750 mg/day appears to be clearly superior to placebo and comparable to imipramine (Tofranil) and amitriptyline (Elavil) in efficacy. Sedation, cardiotoxicity, anticholinergic effects, and antihistaminergic effects all appear to be minimal. The most frequent adverse effects are weight loss, dry mouth, and dizziness, but neurological reactions (increased motor activity, tremor, agitation, excitement, insomnia, and blurred vision), nausea, vomiting, constipation, urticaria, pruritus, and tachycardia occur uncommonly. The most significant adverse effect is a reduction in the seizure threshold and precipitation of seizures with a frequency comparable to that of imipramine. The risk of seizures is compounded when bupropion is administered in conjunction with lithium or neuroleptics. Bupropion counteracts depressant effects of concurrently administered alcohol and benzodiazepines.

Preparations and Administration

Bupropion (Wellbutrin)
Tablets
Recommended Doses: 150–600 mg PO, 3 divided doses.

Monoamine Oxidase (MAO) Inhibitors

Only three antidepressant MAO inhibitors are currently available: isocarboxazid (Marplan), phenelzine (Nardil), and tranylcypromine (Parnate). Tranylcypromine has been successfully employed in reactive and psychoneurotic depressions as well as in involutional melancholia (an especially severe form of depression). Phenelzine has been employed alone or with chlordiazepoxide (Librium) in various psychoneuroses with favorable results. In contrast to the tricyclics, MAO inhibitors produce more favorable results in mild, reactive, and atypical depressions. MAO inhibitors are reserved for cases of depression unresponsive to other medications because of the severity of drug-drug and drug-diet interactions associated with these agents. One exception is the treatment of atypical depression triggered by rejection and characterized by brief recurrent depressive episodes that include lethargy, fatigue, hypersomnia, overeating, and chronic anxiety. MAO inhibitors exhibit a preferential efficacy in this disorder.

Mechanism of Action MAO is a complex enzyme system, existing in multiple forms, and in the brain as well as the periphery. Inhibition of MAO decreases the rate of metabolism of endogenously produced or exogenously administered norepinephrine, dopamine, epinephrine, and serotonin, as well as numerous drugs and dietary tyramine. The most widely accepted nomenclature recognizes two types of MAO associated with sympathetic nerve terminals: Type A (about 15%) and Type B (about 85%). Type A acts preferentially on serotonin, norepinephrine, and epinephrine, and is especially sensitive to inhibition by tranylcypromine and phenelzine. Tranylcypromine protects serotonin more than norepinephrine, but phenelzine protects norepinephrine more than serotonin. Type B acts preferentially on certain other amines, such as benzylamine, 2-phenylethylamine, and tryptamine, and is especially sensitive to inhibition by pargyline. MAO inhibitors are well absorbed after oral administration and, in the case of tranylcypromine, excreted within 24 hours. However, the action exerted by the inhibitors on MAO is irreversible. After discontinuation of phenelzine or isocarboxazid, effects persist 1–2 weeks until the body can replace the existing, inactivated MAO with newly synthesized enzyme. Recovery from the effects of tranylcypromine is a little more rapid, occurring in 3–5 days. Tranylcypromine has a weak amphetamine-like activity as well as its primary action as an MAO inhibitor and may produce euphoria. Instances of self-administration in excess of prescribed doses have been reported in individuals with a history of drug abuse. Under such circumstances, withdrawal symptoms may occur when the agent is discontinued that include restlessness, anxiety, depression, confusion, hallucinations, headaches, weakness, and diarrhea.

Adverse Effects and Contraindications Apart from the drug-drug and drug-diet interactions, the adverse effects of MAO inhibitors are no worse and perhaps less than for most psychotropic drugs. The most common adverse reaction is **orthostatic hypotension,** sometimes resulting in episodes of fainting, syncope, falling, or disturbances in cardiac rate or rhythm. *Nurses should caution clients against sudden standing from a prone or sitting position. The use of elastic stockings may help to reduce the severity of orthostatic hypotension. Baseline measurements of blood pressure should be determined before initiating therapy. Clients who exhibit evidence of cardiovascular disorders or respiratory difficulties should be evaluated further since the use of MAO inhibitors is contraindicated in these instances. The nurse should monitor client blood pressure and pulse rate for tachycardia and other arrhythmias. If there is a history of cardiovascular* *disease, an ECG is advisable before instituting therapy. Persons with a history of angina pectoris should be monitored carefully for signs of further cardiac problems.*

Excess stimulation (hyperactivity, hyperreflexia, muscle twitches, hypomania, mania, jitteriness, confusion, insomnia, anxiety, agitation, and akathisias) is another commonplace response. Hypomania is the most common adverse psychiatric response, but clients may complain of other neurological effects, such as dizziness, vertigo, headache, memory impairment, and weakness.

Gastrointestinal symptoms such as constipation, nausea, diarrhea, anorexia, weight loss, and abdominal pain sometimes occur. *Clients should have their weight checked prior to instituting drug therapy, and biweekly checks of weight should ensue once therapy has been started.*

Minor skin irritations or rashes are sometimes reported. Rare adverse effects include chills, urinary incontinence or retention, black tongue, photosensitivity, and sexual disturbances. Visual problems such as glaucoma, nystagmus, and alterations in color perception or visual field occur occasionally (changes in red-green perception are often the first sign of ocular toxicity). MAO inhibitors lower the seizure threshold and should be used cautiously in epileptic clients. Reversible jaundice, hepatitis, and fatal progressive necrotizing hepatocellular damage have occurred very rarely with the currently available MAO inhibitors (hepatic damage was a common problem with some previously employed drugs in this class). The hepatic effects of MAO inhibitors may resemble viral hepatitis. *Periodic liver function tests are advised for clients receiving MAO inhibitors. Nurses should instruct clients to report immediately any darkening of urine, pale stools, yellowing of the skin, yellowing of the sclera, or pruritus.*

Phenelzine has been reported to have carcinogenic potential based on animal studies. *Women should be questioned concerning possible or potential pregnancy, since MAO inhibitors cross the placental barrier and may be teratogenic. In addition these drugs may be secreted in breast milk, and clients with nursing infants should be so advised.*

Table 20–9
Tyramine-Containing Foods

Cheeses
- Blue[a]
- Boursault[c]
- Brick, natural[b]
- Brie[a]
- Camember[c]
- Cheddar[c]
- Cottage[a]
- Emmenthaler[c]
- Gouda[a]
- Gruyere[a]
- Mozzarella[b]
- Parmesan[b]
- Provolone[a]
- Romano[c]
- Roquefort[b]
- Stilton[c]

Alcoholic beverages
- Beer and ale[a]
- Wines
  - Chianti[b]
  - Sherry[a]

Dairy products[a]
- Sour cream
- Yogurt

Fish and meats
- Beef liver[a]
- Bologna[b]
- Caviar[a]
- Chicken liver[a]
- Dried fish[a]
- Game meat[a]
- Herring, pickled or salted[b]
- Pepperoni[b]
- Salami[b]
- Tenderizer sauce[a]

Fruits[a]
- Bananas
- Figs, canned (overripe)
- Raisins

Vegetables
- Avocados (especially overripe)[a]
- Broad pea pods[a]
- Soy sauce[a]
- Yeast extracts[b]

[a]3–25 µg tyramine per gram of food.
[b]25–500 µg tyramine per gram of food.
[c]Over 500 µg tyramine per gram of food.

Drug-Diet Interactions of MAO Inhibitors Many foods (Table 20–9) contain the amine tyramine, which elevates blood pressure and is broken down by MAO. The interaction of MAO inhibitors with tyramine-containing foods is one of the most important examples of a drug-diet interaction. The effect of tyramine in the normal person is slight and transient because it is rapidly metabolized by liver and platelet MAO. In the individual taking an MAO inhibitor, the effect of tyramine on blood pressure is greatly potentiated, and a hypertensive crisis may occur. *Clients receiving MAO inhibitors must rigorously avoid ingestion of tyramine-containing foods (the nurse should provide a list similar to Table 20–9 to aid in this endeavor). In their assessment, nurses need to learn the nature of any special diets clients may be following and confer with a dietician concerning appropriate food replacements to avoid potential problems. For example, clients who require a potassium-rich diet may rely upon bananas as the major source of potassium, but bananas contain tyramine, which interacts with MAO inhibitors.* Since many tyramine-containing foods are found in combination foods, such as casseroles, even the most reliable of clients may occasionally fail to avoid drug-diet interactions. *The nurse or the client (if reliable) should have a rapid-acting alpha-blocking agent, such as phentolamine (Regitine), on hand in case hypertensive crisis does occur.*

MAO inhibitors also potentiate the hypertensive effects of other pressor substances encountered in the diet. *Nurses should advise clients to avoid caffeine-containing foods and beverages (chocolate, cola, coffee, tea) and fava beans (which contain phenylethylamine).*

Drug-Drug Interactions of MAO Inhibitors Many drugs are metabolized by MAO, including barbiturates, cocaine and meperidine (Demerol). Any drug metabolized by MAO will have a prolonged and intensified activity in the presence of MAO inhibition. MAO inhibitors greatly potentiate the activity of indirect-acting sympathomimetic agents, such as amphetamine, ephedrine, most anorexics, and many nasal decongestants. In a client taking ephedrine, for example, the MAO inhibitor combined with ephedrine could produce a marked elevation in blood pressure. The client could also develop fever, convulsions, and coma. *Clients should confer with their physicians for replacement agents that will not interact with the MAO inhibitor and consult the physician or a pharmacist before taking any over-the-counter preparations for coughs, colds, congestion, or allergic reactions.*

Direct-acting sympathomimetics, such as dopamine, epinephrine, and norepinephrine; antihypertensives such as methyldopa; antiparkinsonian agents such as levodopa; tricyclic antidepressants such as imipramine and desipramine; and the serotonin precursor tryptophan are also potentiated by MAO inhibitors. For example, the antihypertensives, reserpine and guanethidine (Ismelin), cause release of norepinephrine, which can result in profound hypertension in clients receiving MAO inhibitors. The potentiating effect of MAO inhibitors on various other drugs may persist up to two weeks after the last dose of the MAO inhibitor. MAO inhibitors should be discontinued for at least 2 weeks prior to elective surgery because they increase the risk of catecholamine-induced dysrhythmias that can occur during general anesthesia. MAO inhibitors also produce a hypoglycemic effect that is modest in its own right but can be additive with the action of insulin or oral hypoglycemic agents.

Preparations and Administration *Doses are titrated to the requirements of the individual client based on the improvement in depression or the occurrence of adverse effects. Accurate assessment of client response by the nurse is especially important during the period of dosage adjustment.* Therapeutic benefit ordinarily occurs within 2–21 days after initiation of treatment. *Indications of a positive clinical response include an improvement in mood, energy and interest level, sleep pattern, level of physical activity, appetite, or an improvement in somatic complaints.* If no response is observed by the third week, it is unlikely that the individual will respond to higher doses, but adverse effects become increasingly likely. For clients who have been receiving elevated doses for an extended period of time, drug withdrawal should be accomplished by gradually reducing the dose to maintenance levels before discontinuation. *Because of the risk of insomnia occurring as a side effect of MAO inhibitors, these drugs are usually not administered in the evening.*

Isocarboxazid (Marplan)
Tablets
Recommended Doses: 30 mg/day PO initially, in one or more administrations. For maintenance therapy, 10–20 mg PO daily, or less.

Phenelzine (Nardil)
Tablets
Recommended Doses: 15 mg PO initially, 3 times daily, increased to the range of 60–90 mg/day fairly rapidly. Clinical response may require as much as 4 weeks at a dose of at least 60 mg. For maintenance therapy, 15 mg PO daily or every other day.

Tranylcypromine (Parnate)
Tablets
Recommended Doses: 20 mg/day PO initially (10 mg in the morning and 10 mg in the afternoon), increased after 2 weeks in increments of 10 mg/day at intervals of 1–3 weeks. For maintenance therapy, 10–20 mg/day PO.

Use of Stimulants in Depression

Catecholamine-releasing stimulants such as amphetamine and methylphenidate (Ritalin) are occasionally used as antidepressants, although there are several limitations to their use. Stimulants produce a reliable antidepressant action that is much more rapid in its development than that generated by other antidepressant medications. Elevation in mood can be achieved acutely within one hour after oral administration. The principal concern is that rebound depression invariably follows as a result of depletion of amine stores. A second serious concern is the risk of psychological dependence. These limitations restrict the use of stimulants to the short-term treatment (up to 1–2 weeks) of reactive depression or the interim treatment of suicidal patients while initiating therapy with a conventional agent. The pharmacology of the stimulants is discussed in Chapter 14.

Important Nursing Implications for Antidepressants

- ☐ Complete a nursing history and assessment before drug therapy is instituted. Investigate the possibility of allergic responses, alcoholism, or schizophrenia.
- ☐ Clients who have glaucoma, a history of cardiovascular disorders, prostatic hypertrophy, or urinary retention usually should not be given

tricyclic drugs; if they are administered, take particular precautions so as to prevent adverse side effects.

- ☐ Observe for adverse effects of antidepressant medications such as excess depression, mood switches in clients with bipolar disorders, orthostatic hypotension, endocrine disturbances, anticholinergic effects, and extrapyramidal disorders.
- ☐ Monitor depressed clients closely during initiation of drug therapy for indications of suicide, since attempts at suicide increase during this period.
- ☐ Make accurate recordings of clinical responses and side effects during the early phase of treatment and report these to the physician for appropriate adjustments in the dose.
- ☐ Avoid use of antidepressants during pregnancy because of risks to the fetus.
- ☐ Monitor for drug interactions when antidepressants are employed, including additive CNS depression with tertiary amine tricyclic drugs, excess stimulation from concurrent use of multiple antidepressants, potentiation of sympathomimetic amines and thyroid hormones, requirements for increased doses of antiepileptic drugs, and additive hypotensive, dysrhythmic, or anticholinergic effects.
- ☐ When MAO inhibitors are employed, review other drugs the client may be taking and observe for potentiation of drugs such as barbiturates, meperidine, or cocaine, and for interactions with dietary tyramine.

Case Study: Depression

C. R., a 43-year-old white father of four, had been troubled by gradually deepening depression over a 6 week period. C. R. was finally coaxed by his wife into seeking help. When C. R. was seen initially by the clinic's psychiatric nurse, he complained of feeling tired, dejected, without energy, having no appetite, and losing 10 pounds in the last 6 weeks. He had become bored with his job, did not want to spend time with his family, and generally felt "rather useless." C. R. had been waking up early in the morning, unable to get back to sleep, thinking about how miserably his life seemed to be going. He stated that he did not know why he was so depressed and could cite no outstanding problem or setback in his life other than the depression itself. C. R. exhibited no signs of agitation or anxiety. The nurse asked C. R. about his use of alcohol and nonprescription drugs, learning that C. R. was a "social drinker," occasionally used Tylenol for headaches, but used no other drugs.

The physician ordered complete blood cell counts, serum glucose determination, urinalysis, and thyroid function tests. All results were within normal limits. The physician decided to prescribe a tricyclic antidepressant, and based on the nurse's earlier assessment of symptoms, selected protriptyline, 10 mg PO, tid. The nurse discussed with C. R. the potential adverse effects and drug interactions of protriptyline and advised him to suspend even occasional use of alcohol during this period of treatment.

After 1 week, C. R. returned for evaluation, complaining that he felt no better. In addition, he had difficulty with urination, often feeling that he had not completely voided. The nurse explained to C. R. that urinary retention was a common side effect of the drug he was using but that it usually diminished with continued use. The nurse further advised C. R. that the benefits of his drug regimen might not be apparent until after 2–4 weeks of treatment.

The nurse took a blood sample for measurement of protriptyline levels, which revealed a concentration of 150 mg/mL (therapeutic range: 115–210 mg/mL). After 2 more weeks on the medication, C. R.'s mood improved, he felt more energetic, his interest in work and family increased, and his insomnia relented.

1. What would be an appropriate diagnosis for C. R.? How many of the criteria for this condition does C. R.'s case meet?
2. Would you suspect that C. R.'s depression is endogenous or reactive?
3. Why did the nurse inquire about C. R.'s use of alcohol?
4. What was the physician looking for when ordering complete blood cell counts? Urinalysis? Serum glucose determination? Thyroid function tests?
5. What aspects of the nurse's assessment might have led the physician to prescribe protriptyline rather than, say, imipramine?
6. What are the adverse effects that you would expect the nurse to discuss with C. R.?
7. Why did the nurse take a blood sample for measurement of the protriptyline level?

Answers appear at the end of the book.

Recommended Readings

Costa E, Racagni, G (eds): *Typical and Atypical Antidepressants. (Advances in Biochemical Psychopharmology. Vol. 31 & 32).* New York, Raven Press, 1982.

DeGennaro MD et al: Antidepressant drug therapy. *Am J Nurs* 1981;81:1304–1310.

Enna SJ, Malick JB, Richelson E: *Antidepressants: Neurochemical, Behavioral, and Clinical Perspectives.* New York, Raven Press, 1981.

Feighner JP: The new generation of antidepressants. *J Clin Psychiatry* 1983;44(11):49–55.

Harris B: Drugs and depression. *Am J Nurs* 1986;86(3): 292–293.

Harris E: Antidepressants: Old drugs, new uses. *Am J Nurs* 1981;81:1308–1310.

Hollister LE: Current antidepressant drugs: Clinical use. *Drugs* 1981;22:129–152.

Hollister LE: Depression: The delicate art of lifting it with drug Rx. *Mod Med* 1982;50(1):110.

Kupfer DJ, Detre TP: Tricyclic and monoamine-oxidase inhibitor antidepressants: Clinical use, in Iversen LL et al (eds): *Handbook of Psychopharmacology,* 14. New York, Plenum Press, 1978.

Lasater MG: Nursing care of the patient with a tricyclic antidepressant overdose. *Crit Care Nurse* 1984;4(4):28.

Lippman S: Antidepressant pharmacotherapy. *Am Fam Physician* 1983;25(6):145–153.

McDaniel KD: Clinical pharmacology of monoamine oxidase inhibitors. *Clin Neuropharm* 1986;9(3):207–234.

Van Praag HM: Amine hypotheses of affective disorders, in Iversen LL et al (eds): *Handbook of Psychopharmacology,* 13. New York, Plenum Press, 1978.

Wilson H, Kneisl CR: *Psychiatric Nursing,* Menlo Park, Ca, Addison-Wesley, 1983.

CHAPTER 21

Antimanic Drugs

Bipolar Disorders

Since mania almost never occurs except as a facet of bipolar disorder (or manic-depressive disorder), evidence of the occurrence of manic episodes is tantamount to a diagnosis of bipolar disorder. During mania, the individual is highly energetic and mood is elevated. The person may be either irritable or euphoric. The high energy level is reflected in behavioral changes, such as talkativeness, continuous activity, and racing from one idea and one project to another. If mania is evident, the only other criteria that must be met for diagnosis of bipolar disorder (Table 21–1) are that the duration of behavioral disturbances exceed 1 week and the condition not be secondary to another condition such as schizophrenia, intoxication, or organic brain syndrome.

Five diagnostic categories are employed in defining the condition: bipolar I, currently manic; bipolar I, currently depressed; bipolar I, mixed (when manic and depressive episodes coexist); bipolar II (atypical bipolar disorder); and cyclothymic personality (Figure 21–1). In bipolar I, both manic and depressive episodes reach full intensity. In bipolar II, depressive episodes reach full intensity but manic periods are of only modest intensity (called hypomanic episodes). Bipolar II is easily mistaken for recurrent major depression. In cyclothymic personality (Table 21–2) neither the manic nor the depressive episodes reach full intensity (Figure 21–1). Cyclothymic personality is diagnosed more commonly in women than in men, but other biopolar disorders are equally common in men and women, occurring in about 0.4–1.2% of the adult population.

Table 21-1
Criteria for a Manic Episode

Mood disturbance:	
	Elevated, expansive, or irritable mood
Behavioral symptoms (at least three):	
	Increased activity (e.g., physical, social, occupational, sexual)
	Pressure to keep talking
	Flight of ideas
	Grandiosity
	Decreased need for sleep
	Distractibility
	Risk-seeking behaviors (reckless driving, buying sprees, sexual indiscretions)
Duration:	
	At least 1 week
Exclusions:	
	Does not meet criteria for schizophrenia: No mood-incongruent delusions or hallucinations; No bizarre behavior
	Not superimposed on schizophrenia, paranoia, or schizophreniform disorder
	Not secondary to organic brain syndrome
	Not secondary to substance intoxication

The genetic contribution to bipolar disorder is stronger than for any other psychiatric disorder. Although bipolar disorder is attributed to organic factors more than psychological factors, a childhood pattern is frequently noted in the life history of persons with this disorder: during the first year of life, a highly nurturing mother, supportive environment, and low demands; then in the second year, an abrupt change to increased requirements for self-sufficiency, often triggered by displacement by a younger sibling.

Lithium is the principal drug therapy for bipolar disorder. In addition, **neuroleptics** may be employed initially because the effectiveness of lithium occurs only after several days of administration. Typically, lithium and a neuroleptic are begun together and the neuroleptic is discontinued after a week or so when lithium begins to exert its influence. In recent years, **carbamazepine** (Tegretol) (see Chapter 23) has been used successfully in bipolar disorder although without approval of the U.S. Food and Drug Administration. One study reported that 12 of 22 individuals treated with carbamazepine responded, including several whose condition was previously resistant to lithium. The response rate was higher for clients who were manic at the beginning of treatment than in those who were depressed at the beginning of treatment.

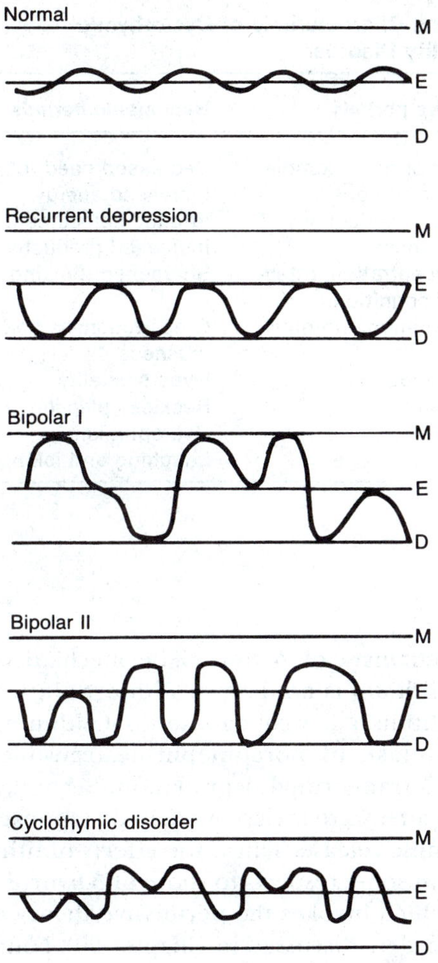

Figure 21-1
Depiction of five affective conditions. In bipolar I, mood ranges from full manic (M) to full depressive (D) episodes. In bipolar II, depressive episodes are full-fledged, but mood elevation does not exceed hypomania. In cyclothymic disorder, neither manic nor depressive episodes are full-blown. E = euthymia (normal mood).

Lithium

Lithium salts have been used successfully in mania and in bipolar disorder since 1954 and are generally superior to other drug treatments, including neuroleptics, antidepressants, or sedatives. Lithium is an invaluable prophylactic agent for preventing manic-depressive cycles. The principal effect of lithium is in the manic phase; hence, lithium is often classified as an antimanic agent. However, amelioraton of the manic phase of bipolar disorder leads secondarily to less severe depression. Prolonged use of lithium promotes a leveling of mood, and further mood cycles are aborted.

Table 21–2
Symptoms Characteristic of Cyclothymic Personality Disorder

Depressive periods	Hypomanic periods
Insomnia or hypersomnia	Decreased need for sleep
Lethargy or fatigue	Increased energy
Feelings of inadequacy	Inflated self-esteem
Ineffectiveness	Increased productivity
Poor concentration, attention, and cognition	Sharpened thinking
Social isolation and quietness	Gregariousness and garrulousness
Loss of libido	Hypersexuality
Anhedonia	Reckless pleasure-seeking
Pessimism	Overoptimism
Crying	Laughing and joking

Mechanism of Action The mechanism of action of lithium is not known with certainty. Four effects of lithium may contribute. First, lithium accelerates reuptake of norepinephrine, causing a shift toward intraneuronal degradation. Second, lithium inhibits adenylate cyclase-mediated responses to catecholamine release. Third, the effects of lithium are similar in some respects to those of 5-hydroxytryptophan (which invokes the permissive theory of affective disorders discussed in Chapter 20). Fourth (and perhaps most important), lithium ions can substitute for sodium ions during an action potential, but once inside the cell, lithium is not pumped out by the sodium pump (Figure 21–2). Instead, it exchanges with sodium via the countertransport mechanism. The sodium that enters into this exchange stimulates the electrogenic sodium-potassium pump, causing the cell to become hyperpolarized.

Pharmacokinetics Lithium is rapidly absorbed from the gastrointestinal tract but usually takes from 1 to 2 weeks to become therapeutically effective. This delay may be related to lithium's slow rate of passage across cellular membranes into intracellular spaces. Absorption is complete within 8 hours after administration and is not altered by concurrent ingestion of food. The volume of distribution of lithium is approximately equal to total body water, indicating that this ion readily distributes through all tissues, though the steady-state concentration of lithium in cerebral spinal fluid (CSF) is only about 40–50% of serum concentrations. Therapeutic plasma concentrations are in the range of 0.6–1.4 mEq/L; most clients respond best in the range of 0.8–1.2 mEq/L. *Clients receiving lithium should have routine checks of serum lithium to ascertain that therapy is being conducted safely and effectively.*

Lithium is eliminated almost entirely by renal excretion, with negligible amounts appearing in other bodily excretions, including sweat, feces, and breast milk. In renal failure, lithium doses must be reduced in proportion to the severity of the renal deficit. Lithium removal from the plasma follows a biphasic pattern, with a half-life of 4–6 hours during initial distribution and an elimination half-life of 7–20 hours. Steady-state concentrations of lithium in the body are achieved after about 5 days of administration.

Lithium clearance depends entirely on glomerular filtration rate; lithium clearance is maintained at 20–30% of creatinine clearance. *Nurses should advise clients to maintain adequate salt and fluid intake to avoid dehydration and undue retention of lithium in the body.* The plasma half-life is prolonged in elderly patients and younger individuals with impaired renal function. *Elderly clients normally receive reduced doses of lithium and require special monitoring to prevent toxicity because their ability to excrete lithium tends to be decreased.*

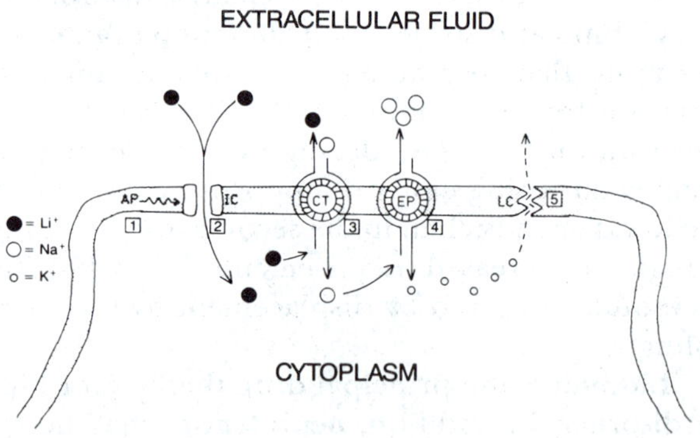

Figure 21–2
The ion distribution theory of lithium action. (1) The arrival of an action potential (AP) allows (2) an influx of ions, such as lithium and sodium, through ion channels (IC). (3) The countertransport mechanism (CT), which ordinarily exchanges sodium for sodium, now exchanges lithium for sodium. The sodium that enters the cell in this exchange is (4) expelled from the cell by the exchange pump (EP), in exchange for potassium ion. The exchange pump is electrogenic because some of the potassium brought in is able to (5) leak back out through the leakage channel (LC); but sodium expelled cannot leak back in because of its larger hydrated radius. Therefore, stimulation of the sodium pump leads to hyperpolarization of the cell. From A. K. Swonger and L. L. Constantine, *Drugs and Therapy,* 2nd ed. Boston: Little, Brown, 1983.

Clinical Indications Lithium is indicated prophylactically to reduce the frequency and intensity of mood cycles. Lithium has also been tried in depression and schizoaffective disorders, but neither application has been established by clinical tests, although the latter has been described as promising. Lithium may sometimes appear to be effective in depression when instances of bipolar II are misdiagnosed as recurrent major depression.

Lithium is often useful in treating chronic maladaptive behavioral patterns (exaggerated resistance to authority, truancy, poor work history) when they are secondary to manic-depressive mood swings. Lithium has also been successful for a variety of conditions secondary to manic-depressive mood swings, including hysterical personality, narcissistic personality disorder, attention deficit disorder, alcoholism and other forms of drug abuse, aggressive psychopathology, premenstrual tension syndrome, cluster headaches, and cyclical migraine headaches.

Adverse Effects and Contraindications Lithium produces many side effects (Table 21–3) and there are occasional fatalities from lithium toxicity.

Table 21–3
Adverse Effects of Lithium

Organ system	Symptoms	Frequency and period of maximal risk	Clinical responses
Neurological and psychiatric	Somnolence, fatigue, lethargy, slurred speech, aphasia, anesthesia of skin, blurred vision, tinnitus, dizziness, ataxia, giddiness, confusion, blackouts, stupor, coma, convulsions	Common, late	Reduce dose Spread medication over 24 hours
Neuromuscular	Tremor, weakness, fasciculations, twitching, clonic movements, choreoathetotic movements, dysarthria	Common, late	Reduce dose Spread medication over 24 hours Propranolol for tremor
Gastrointestinal	Nausea, vomiting, diarrhea, abdominal pain, anorexia, weight loss	Common, early	Adaptation may occur Spread medication over 24 hours
Cardiovascular	T-wave abnormality in ECG, dysrhythmias, hypotension, circulatory collapse	Common, throughout	Avoid drugs with additive cardiovascular effects (e.g., quinidine, tricyclics, neuroleptics)
Renal	Nephrogenic diabetes insipidus, polyuria, dehydration, xerostomia, thirst or (conversely) edema	Common early; rarely, late	Thiazide diuretic (paradoxical use in diabetes insipidus)
Endocrine	Hypothyroidism	Early or late	Reversible; lower dose or treat with thyroid hormone
Skin	Acneiform eruptions, folliculitis	Early	Interrupt treatment, then resume (skin reactions may or may not recur)

However, adverse reactions are seldom encountered at plasma serum concentrations below 1.5 mEq/L of blood. Mild to moderate toxicity is observed between about 1.5 and 2.0 mEq/L, moderate to severe adverse reactions between about 2.0 and 2.5 mEq/L, and life-threatening toxicity between 2.5 and 3.0 mEq/L. Fatal plasma concentrations are thus only about 2 times the upper level of therapeutic plasma concentrations.

The side effects are frequently divided into two types: early side effects, which dissipate after a few days, and side effects that occur throughout treatment. Early side effects include tremor, nausea, vomiting, diarrhea, and dry mouth. Diarrhea occurs in nearly every client sooner or later. Central nervous system side effects that may occur throughout therapy are blackouts, stupor, vertigo, ataxia, fatigue, headache, and slurred speech. *The nurse should advise clients that neurological side effects of lithium may impair ability to perform hazardous tasks such as driving an automobile. They should also caution clients to report immediately fatigue, blackouts, or stumbling gait.* Lithium does not have significant sedative or excitatory effects overall.

Nursing Observations for Lithium Therapy

THERAPEUTIC GOAL	Suppression of acute manic episodes; prevention of subsequent episodes of mania or depression.
PREADMINISTRATION ASSESSMENT	
Baseline Data	Observe extent of elevated, expansive, or irritable mood; increased activity, pressure to keep talking, flight of ideas, grandiosity, alterations in sleep patterns, distractibility, and risk-taking behaviors. Evaluate neurological function (brain scan and EEG), endocrine function (thyroid, pancreatic, and adrenal cortical), cardiovascular function, renal and hepatic function, and gastrointestinal function.
Contraindications/ Precautions	Renal impairment, pregnancy, and lactation. Safety for use in children under 12 is not established.
Potential Interactions	Check current drug regimen for interacting drugs: sodium depletors, certain neuroleptics, antithyroid drugs, neuromuscular blockers, urinary alkalinizers, and sympathomimetics.
EVALUATION OF DRUG RESPONSE	
During Dosage Adjustment	Monitor serum lithium concentrations: 1.0–1.2 mEq/L initially; 0.6–1.0 mEq/L for maintenance. The appropriate time to draw a blood sample for lithium levels is 10–12 hours after the last dose (typically between 7:00 and 9:00 AM after a 9:00 PM dose the night before).
For Therapeutic Benefit	Monitor stabilization of mood.
For Adverse Effects	Evaluate neurological and psychiatric status; neuromuscular, gastrointestinal, cardiovascular, renal, and thyroid functions, as well as skin integrity (see Table 21–3 for details).
For Drug Interactions	Evaluate for lithium toxicity with diuretics that deplete sodium and with certain neuroleptics. Watch for reduced lithium serum levels with urinary alkalinizers but increased lithium serum levels with thiazide diuretics. Observe for additive neurological impairment with other psychotropic drugs, additive antithyroid influence with antithyroid drugs, antagonism of the pressor effect of sympathomimetics, and potentiation of neuromuscular blockers when lithium is employed.
For Dietary Interactions	Evaluate amount of sodium in the daily diet for possible interaction with lithium therapy.
For Compliance	Evaluate client's compliance with all facets of the therapeutic regimen by careful observation, interviewing, and review of progress. Report compliance problems to the physician and act as client-advocate when changes in the therapeutic regimen seem indicated.

Weight change, hypotension, cardiac dysrhythmias, and nephrogenic diabetes insipidus may occur at any point during therapy. *The nurse should monitor client pulse and blood pressure prior to initiation of therapy, to provide baseline data against which to evaluate client responses once therapy has been instituted. The nurse should advise clients to be alert for occurrence of an increased output of dilute urine, accompanied by thirst. Elderly clients are especially liable to develop polydipsia and polyuria; these symptoms may disappear and reappear at unpredictable intervals and may necessitate dosage reduction. The nurse should teach clients to measure urine specific gravity, maintain a daily weight chart, and check for edema.*

Tremor, a common side effect of lithium at the usual therapeutic plasma concentrations, can be controlled with administration of the beta-blocker propranolol (Inderal, Inderide) at doses of 30–120 mg/day. Tremor and other motor symptoms, such as hyperactivity, ataxia, and aphasia, can also often be reduced by administering the medication over the full 24 hours of the day or by dosage reduction. Hypersensitivity reactions may occur early in treatment and may or may not recur when treatment is interrupted and resumed.

Lithium intoxication is characterized by drowsiness, slurred speech, and muscle spasms, which may persist for several days of elevated lithium levels before more serious symptoms set in. If it is left untreated, coma and death may result. *The nurse should immediately report occurrence of any of these symptoms to the physician.* Treatment of lithium intoxication consists of administration of sodium chloride (sodium antagonizes the action of lithium), alkalinization of the urine to hasten excretion, supportive measures as in barbiturate poisoning, and dialysis as a last resort. The ratio of lithium concentrations within blood cells and in the serum (the intracellular to extracellular ratio) can be used to predict toxicity; the ratio falls just prior to toxic levels of lithium, then rises sharply in the toxic zone.

Lithium use is absolutely contraindicated in myasthenia gravis (lithium decreases release of acetylcholine); in leukemia (lithium lowers white blood cell counts); in children under age 12; during the first trimester of pregnancy (lithium can cause cardiac defects in the fetus during this period); and during breast-feeding (lithium concentrations in breast milk approximate 30–100% of serum levels). *Because lithium is contraindicated during pregnancy, nurses should advise premenopausal women to use contraceptive measures while receiving lithium therapy. If a client becomes pregnant while taking lithium, the nurse should explain to her the risk of the drug therapy to the fetus. If lithium therapy is continued, serum lithium levels need to be monitored closely to prevent toxicity. Renal clearance of lithium increases during pregnancy but reverts to lower than normal for a period after delivery, often necessitating dosage reduction.* Relative contraindications for lithium use include organic brain syndrome (lithium may worsen dementia); myocardial infarction and dysrhythmias (lithium may trigger or aggravate dyrhythmias), and psoriasis or acne (lithium may worsen these skin conditions).

Interactions with the Diet, Other Drugs, and Laboratory Tests Lithium interacts with dietary sodium. Sodium competes with lithium, reducing both its effectiveness and its toxicity. Sodium depletion has the opposite effect. *Clients should avoid irregular sodium intake and maintain a steady low level of sodium chloride ingestion. Drugs that deplete bodily sodium, notably the diuretics, may intensify lithium toxicity. In addition, clients should be advised that many prescription and over-the-counter drugs provide sodium loads that can decrease the efficacy of lithium.*

Because the onset of lithium's action is delayed until a threshold tissue concentration is achieved, neuroleptics are frequently employed in conjunction with lithium in the interim for acute control of manic episodes. Haloperidol (Haldol) or molindone (Moban) is preferred because these drugs exhibit substantial efficacy and have minimal effect on lithium distribution and toxicity. Phenothiazines by contrast can substantially alter the distribution of lithium between intracellular and extracellular fluid compartments. Some phenothiazines double the ratio of distribution of lithium, thus inviting toxicity.

Drugs that alter the rate of lithium excretion by the kidneys also alter plasma concentrations of the antimanic agent. **Urinary alkalinizers** (such as carbonic anhydrase inhibitors, absorbable and "nonabsorbable" antacids), caffeine and other **xanthines,** and **osmotic diuretics** increase lithium excretion. **Thiazide diuretics,** on the other hand, decrease lithium clearance by the kidneys. It is not clear what the effect is of high-ceiling or potassium-sparing diuretics on lithium clearance.

Neurological impairment caused by lithium appears to be additive with the CNS effects of other psychotropic drugs (haloperidol (Haldol), chlorpromazine (Thorazine), thioridazine (Mellaril), phenytoin (Dilantin), and carbamazepine (Tegretol)) as well as with therapeutic agents (such as methyldopa (Aldomet), tetacycline, and mazindol (Mazanor, Sanorex)) and sometimes leads to an outright encephalopathic syndrome. Lithium prolongs the effects of **neuromuscular blocking agents** (both depolarizing and nondepolarizing types) and has a thyroid-suppressing action that is synergistic with that of **iodide.** Lithium also reduces the pressor effect of **sympathomimetic amines.**

Nursing Diagnoses and Interventions for Lithium Therapy of Bipolar Disorder

Nursing Diagnoses	*Related Interventions*
TO ENHANCE DRUG BENEFITS OR REDUCE DRUG REQUIREMENTS	
Alterations in thought processes: flights of ideas and distractibility during mania; poor concentration, attention, and cognition during depression; Disturbance in self-concept: inflated self-esteem or feelings of inadequacy; Impaired social interactions: inflated self-esteem, hostility, and manipulative behavior during mania; social isolation and withdrawal during depression; Impaired verbal communication: pressure to keep talking during mania; Potential for violence to others related to poor control of behavior; Sexual dysfunction: hypersexuality during mania; loss of libido during depression	Advise clients to avoid caffeinated beverages since these aggravate mania. Emphasize the importance of keeping follow-up appointments. Maintain a supportive and optimistic approach to clients. Institute suicide precautions.
Noncompliance due to desire to recapture manic high	Remind clients of the importance of strict adherence and compliance with the therapeutic regimen. Periodically monitor lithium serum concentrations for evidence of noncompliance or need for dosage adjustment.
Sleep-pattern disturbance: decreased need for sleep during manic episodes; insomnia or hypersomnia during depression	Discuss methods of facilitating sleep such as bedtime rituals.
TO MINIMIZE DRUG SIDE EFFECTS OR INTERACTIONS	
Alterations in cardiac output: dysrhythmias and hypotension related to lithium	Periodically monitor cardiovascular function (with ECG). Teach clients to avoid rapid changes in position, hot showers or sunlight, and prolonged standing.
Alterations in comfort: gastrointestinal irritation related to lithium	Advise clients to take lithium with or immediately after meals and to report continued diarrhea or constipation.
Fluid volume deficit: polyuria and thirst related to lithium	Teach clients to maintain a weight chart, to monitor urinary output, to measure urine specific gravity periodically; and to check wrists, ankles, and tibiae for edema. Advise clients to report any difficulty with voiding and to maintain a high level of fluid intake.
TO ENSURE SAFE AND EFFICACIOUS DRUG USE	
Knowledge deficit related to drug regimen	Teach clients about the lifelong nature of bipolar disorder, the rationale for the therapeutic regimen, and the need to maintain lithium therapy even after symptoms are no longer apparent. Advise clients not to switch brands of lithium without consulting the physician. Provide client with a list of adverse effects and drug interactions for each drug in the regimen and explain what to do if any of these occur. Explain the relationship between lithium activity and dietary sodium and instruct clients to maintain a constant level of sodium intake so as to avoid fluctuations in lithium action. Instruct clients to wear a medical alert tag or bracelet indicating the diagnosis and medication regimen.

Preparations and Administration Before initiating lithium therapy, a thorough clinical and laboratory evaluation must be conducted to rule out underlying organic disorders to which mania or depression might be secondary and to assess the client's ability to tolerate lithium therapy. Tests of CNS and endocrine function are paramount. Evaluation of the CNS may include electroencephalography, a brain scan, a computerized tomographic scan, a brain biopsy, or a lumbar puncture (to measure transmitter metabolites). Endocrine evaluation is important because disorders of the thyroid, adrenal cortex, or pancreas may produce symptoms that mimic or aggravate mania or depression and because lithium may have a significant impact on thyroid function. Other tissues frequently adversely affected by lithium (Table 21–3) are the cardiovascular system, kidney, liver, and gastrointestinal tract. Examination of these systems prior to initiation of lithium treatment provides both a means of predicting susceptibility to lithium toxicity and a baseline for later quantification of such toxicity. A standard workup would include an electrocardiogram, blood pressure measurement, and a complete blood count for assessment of cardiovascular function; serum enzyme measurement for evaluation of liver function; and analysis of blood urea nitrogen, electrolytes, urinalysis, creatinine clearance, and urine osmolarity for kidney function evaluation. Lithium is available in carbonate and citrate salts; the efficacy of the salts is entirely attributable to the lithium cation.

The nurse should advise clients that if they change their brand of lithium they may require hospitalization for readjustment of dosage because of product differences that affect the bioavailability of lithium. Blood samples for determination of lithium serum levels are drawn immediately prior to the next lithium dose (8–12 hours after the preceding dose). Hospitalization is normally required during the period of dosage adjustment to facilitate collection of blood samples.

In contrast to the once-a-day dosing often employed for other psychotropics, division of doses is essential in lithium therapy. Lithium is absorbed rapidly into the bloodstream, with serum concentrations peaking in 2–4 hours. Toxic reactions set in at blood concentrations above approximately 2.0 mEq/L. Lithium is excreted rapidly, and serum levels may fall by one-half in 1 day. To maintain effective tissue concentrations without excessive serum levels, several doses daily are required. *Lithium should be taken with or immediately after food or milk to minimize gastrointestinal disturbances. Lithium products should be stored at temperatures between 15° and 30°C (59° and 86°F) and protected from light and moisture.*

Maintenance medication with lithium prevents recurrence of either manic or depressive episodes rather than simply modifying symptoms. However, medication must continue indefinitely. Even after years of use, a single missed dose may precipitate recurrence of mania. For this reason, and because toxic levels are very close to therapeutic levels, close adherence to dosage regimens and close medical supervision are required. *The nurse should frequently reinforce the need to adhere to the established regimen and not to omit or alter doses.*

Clients' compliance with lithium regimens is not always good for a number of reasons. Some clients enjoy their manic episodes and may discontinue therapy to regain the elevated mood and high energy level that characterize periods of mania. Other clients begin to believe that medication is no longer necessary when they have been free of significant mood swings for a period of time.

Lithium

Capsules (Eskalith, Lithonate, and generic formulations), tablets (Eskalith, Lithane, Lithotabs, and generic formulations), slow release tablets (Lithobid) controlled release tablets (Eskalith), syrup as the citrate salt (Cibalith and generic)

Recommended Doses: Loading doses: 900 mg/day typically, adjusted thereafter to 900–3,600 mg/day until the condition is brought under control. A plasma concentration range of 0.9–1.2 mEq/L of blood is optimal during this initial phase. Maintenance doses: must be individualized to achieve plasma concentrations in the range of 0.5–1.0 mEq/L; 300 mg, 3 or 4 times daily is typical. When a slow release form is employed, the same total daily dose is required but may be divided into 2 or 3 administrations.

Important Nursing Implications for Lithium

- ☐ Prior to initiating lithium therapy, take the client's history and conduct a nursing assessment. Include in the history questions about any other drugs the client may be taking, any prior health problems, significant current problems, and any evidence of contraindications or cautions for use of lithium.
- ☐ Make sure that clients and family members know how to recognize adverse responses to lithium and what to do if any of these occur.
- ☐ Provide clients who are receiving lithium with a typed list of prescription and over-the-counter drugs that may interact with lithium.
- ☐ Teach clients that any factors that influence sodium concentrations in the body, including changes in dietary sodium intake and occur-

rence of vomiting or diarrhea, will alter the effects of lithium.

- ☐ Educate clients and family about lithium to promote client compliance. Include information about the nature of manic-depressive disorders, the approximate length of time required for obvious clinical improvement to occur (5–10 days), and the importance of not omitting or altering doses.
- ☐ Be certain that follow-up appointments are scheduled and kept so that the effectiveness of the therapeutic plan can be evaluated and any problems addressed. Give clients the name and telephone number of the person to contact should they have problems or should family members note behavioral changes or physical changes that appear to be contrary to expectations.
- ☐ Be supportive and serve as client-advocate when threats to the client's well-being are noted, such as too little attention being paid to possible adverse effects or interactions.

Case Study: Bipolar Affective Disorder

R. K., a 53-year-old white man, was referred to a mental health facility for treatment of mania. The current manic episode was his fourth, the first having occurred about 18 months before. The nurse who assessed R. K. observed hyperactivity, irritability, flight of ideas, pressure of speech, and distractibility. Therapy was instituted with chlorpromazine, 100 mg PO tid, and lithium, 600 mg PO tid. R. K. responded almost immediately to this regimen. On the third day, the lithium dose was reduced to 300 mg PO tid. After 1 week, chlorpromazine was discontinued and R. K. remained stable on the lithium regimen. A blood sample indicated a serum lithium concentration of 0.9 mEq/L (therapeutic maintenance range: 0.6–12. mEq/L). R. K. was discharged 1 week later with instructions to continue lithium therapy at the established level.

R. K. returned biweekly for the first month, during which time he experienced no adverse effect from the lithium except for mild thirst and a slight tremor. He then failed to keep his next appointment and was not seen again in the clinic until 8 weeks later, when he was again referred during a manic episode. His serum lithium concentration was determined at 0.1 mEq/L, and R. K. admitted that he had reduced his use of lithium to once a day to increase his energy level while working on an important project at work. The previous lithium regimen was reinstated and the manic symptoms remitted after 3 days.

1. What was the likelihood that the mood swings that R. K. experienced would stop spontaneously even if no drug treatment was instituted?
2. Would it have been safer to administer molindone (Moban) instead of chlorpromazine with lithium? Why?
3. Why was the dose of lithium reduced after 2 days?
4. Why was chlorpromazine discontinued after 1 week?
5. Does the occurrence of thirst and tremor indicate that the dose of lithium was excessive? If R. K. experienced more severe adverse effects, what could be done?
6. Was it surprising that R. K. would discontinue use of lithium when he had responded so well to therapy and was experiencing few adverse effects?
7. Why did R. K. respond quickly to the chlorpromazine and lithium combination when initially treated but only after 3 days when lithium alone was given during the later episode?

Answers appear at the end of the book.

Recommended Readings

Gever LN: monitoring lithium to detect toxicity. *Nursing* 1982;12(5):110–112.

Harris E: Lithium. *Am J Nurs* 1981;81(7):1310–1315.

Jann MW et al: Alternative drug therapies for mania: A literature review. *Drug Intell Clin Pharm* 1984;18:577–589.

Jefferson JW: Lithium carbonate-induced hypothyroidism: Its many faces. *JAMA* 1979;242:271–272.

Johnson FN: *Handbook of Lithium Therapy.* Baltimore, University Park Press, 1980.

Ostrow DG, Davis JM: Laboratory measurements in the clinical use of lithium. *Clin Neuropharm* 1982;5(3): 317–336.

Prien RP: Lithium in the treatment of affective disorders. *Clin Neuropharm* 1978;3:113–132.

Rosenberg JM, Kirschenbaum HL: Lithium. *RN* 1981; 44:44–46.

Tosteson DC: Lithium and mania. *Sci Am* 1981;244(4): 164–174.

Wilson H, Kneisl CR: *Psychiatric Nursing.* Menlo Park, Ca, Addison-Wesley, 1983.

UNIT III

Drugs and the Central Nervous System

PART E

Drug Treatment of Neurological Disorders

CHAPTER 22

Motor Disorders and Drugs

Motor **regulation** is the control of movement and tone of the skeletal muscles. Nearly all of what we call *behavior* is composed of sequences of motor activity. The **pyramidal** and **extrapyramidal** systems contribute most directly to the regulation of motor activity, ultimately influencing the alpha- and gamma-motor neurons of the cranial nerves and somatic spinal nerves, which then project the signals to the striated skeletal muscles.

Brain Systems Regulating Motor Activity

The **pyramidal system,** which controls voluntary behavior, is a well-defined fiber tract that originates in the motor strip of the cerebral cortex and extends without break through the midbrain and brainstem down to the α-motor neurons of the cranial nerve nuclei and spinal cord. Fibers of the pyramidal system arise from the motor strip, located in the back of the frontal lobe, and cross as they descend at the level of the medulla, so that control of muscles on the right side of the body resides in the left hemisphere and vice versa. The pyramidal tracts conduct impulses rapidly and initiate voluntary movements. Pyramidal signals also reach the corpus striatum and cerebellum, allowing coordination of pyramidal and extrapyramidal influences. The relative simplicity of the pyramidal system and the small number of synapses involved in transmitting impulses along the pyramidal pathway make this system relatively resistant to disruption by either disease or drugs.

The **extrapyramidal motor system** is, by contrast, a diffusely distributed network of brain regions and nuclei that are richly interconnected and organized for subconcious regulation of the muscles. The components of the extrapyramidal system include two major brain regions, the cerebellum and the corpus striatum, and several nuclei and pathways of the subthalamus, midbrain, pons, and medulla.

The Cerebellum

The cerebellum, which lies at the back of the brainstem, organizes muscle contractions into useful sequences. The afferents (inputs) to the cerebellum (mainly proprioceptive signals) come from the brainstem and spinal cord by way of three bridges, called the **cerebellar peduncles,** which connect the cerebellum to the brainstem. The cerebellar cortex is more homogeneous in its cellular structure than most brain regions, and the small variety of synapses and neurotransmitters makes it minimally vulnerable to disruption by drugs or diseases. The classical clinical indication of cerebellar dysfunction is ataxia, which occurs when large doses of depressant drugs are employed, usually only after most higher brain functions have been significantly depressed.

The Corpus Striatum

The corpus striatum, the highest level of organization of the extrapyramidal motor system, consists of three bilateral nuclear pairs: the caudate, globus pallidus, and putamen. These nuclei together with the amygdala of the limbic system are frequently referred to as the **basal ganglia** because of their location deep in the base of the telecephalon. The term *corpus striatum* refers to the striated appearance of this region caused by the myelinated fibers of the pyramidal system passing through and interdigitating with the grayish neurons of the corpus striatum.

Acetylcholine synthesis and degradation are unusually high in the caudate, and the corpus striatum is also rich in dopamine and serotonin. Acetylcholine is generally associated with neurons that are intrinsic to the corpus striatum. Most of the dopamine in the corpus striatum is found in nerve terminals of cells originating in the substantia nigra, an extrapyramidal nucleus of the midbrain. The serotonin is found in nerve terminals of cells arising in the raphé nuclei of the pons. Drugs that affect any of these three neurotransmitters can provoke or alleviate extrapyramidal disorders. Most of the disorders and drugs discussed in this chapter are related to alterations in the corpus striatum rather than the cerebellum or pyramidal system.

The corpus striatum receives inputs chiefly from the vestibular system and proprioceptive receptors of the muscles, joints, and tendons and uses these to regulate posture, stabilize movement, and produce associated movements (swinging the arms while walking, for example). There are many interconnections between the corpus striatum, cerebellum, and vestibular system, by way of extrapyramidal relay nuclei of the brainstem and subthalamus.

Organic Extrapyramidal Disorders and Related Drugs

The symptoms of extrapyramidal disorders include hyperkinesias, hypokinesias, and dystonias, which occur in various forms and combinations (Table 22–1). The drug treatment of motor disorders, summarized in Table 22–2, is largely limited to alleviating these motor symptoms.

Parkinsonism and Antiparkinsonian Drugs

Parkinsonism is a clinical syndrome related to dysfunction of the corpus striatum. The classic triad of symptoms of parkinsonism consists of **muscle rigidity, akinesias, and tremors.** Muscle rigidity and akinesias cause (1) postural changes (trunk and head are thrust forward, changing the center of gravity and to compensate, clients flex their knees, hips, neck, and elbows [Figure 22–1]); (2) the characteristic **diplomat's expression** or **masked facies;** (3) difficulty in chewing and swallowing food; and (4) the **cogwheel motion** (observed when a client is asked to bend the arm). Other movement abnormalities include involuntary tremor, pill-rolling motions of the hands, shuffling gait, trembling of the voluntary muscles, and absence of reflex arm swinging. The tremor of clients with parkinsonism includes both a **resting tremor** and an **action tremor.** Tremors are aggravated by emotional stress and fatique and tend to disappear during sleep.

The autonomic nervous system is also affected. Clients tend to have increased salivation, lacrimation, seborrhea (one observes increased oiliness of the skin), excessive perspiraton, constipation, incontinence, and decreased sexual function. Because of the poor control of muscles to the mouth, clients often drool, and are unable to swallow as before. While some older clients become mentally confused and suffer memory loss, intelligence is not impaired in most people with Parkinson's disease.

The neurochemical basis of parkinsonism is understood in part (Figure 22–2). At autopsy, a defi-

Table 22–1
Clinical Symptoms of Motor Disorder Syndromes

Pathologic syndromes

Clinical symptoms	**Infections**	Encephalitis	Neurosyphilis	Chorea gravidarum	Sydenham's chorea (St. Vitus' Dance)	Cerebrovascular lesions	CNS tumors	**Metabolic disorders**	Tay-Sachs disease	Hypoglycemia, hyperthyroidism, or elevated sympathetic tone	**Drug-induced disorders**	Heavy-metal or gas toxicities	Neuroleptic side effects	Stimulants, sympathomimetics, tricyclics, and lithium	Hypnotic or opiate intoxication	Hypnotic or opiate withdrawal
Hyperkinesias																
Choreas		•		•	•	•										
Athetosis		•	•			•			•							
Ballismus		•				•										
Tardive dyskinesias													•			
Dystonic movements		•	•			•										
Tremor:																
Alternating		•	•			•	•			•		•	•	•		•
Intention																
Myoclonus		•		•		•	•									
Akathisias		•											•			
Tics, habit rhythmias, hysterical movements																
Fasciculations																
Hypokinesias																
Akinesias		•											•			
Ataxias			•												•	
Weakness or paralysis										•					•	
Dystonias																
Hypertonias:																
Myotonia																
Rigidity		•	•			•							•			
Spasticity						•	•									
Hypotonia																

Clinical symptoms	**Degenerative disorders**	Huntington's disease	Wilson's disease	Double athetosis	Torsion dystonia	Spasmodic torticollis	Parkinsonism	Creutzfeldt's disease	Essential myoclonias	Myoclonic epilepsy	Cerebellar disorders	**Functional disorders**	**Multiple sclerosis**	**Peripheral neuromuscular disorders**	Muscular atrophies	Myasthenia gravis	Muscular dystrophies	Myotonic syndromes
Hyperkinesias																		
Choreas		•	•															
Athetosis			•	•														
Ballismus																		
Tardive dyskinesias																		
Dystonic movements			•	•	•	•												
Tremor:																		
Alternating				•			•											
Intention											•		•					
Myoclonus		•	•		•	•			•	•	•		•		•			
Akathisias																		
Tics, habit rhythmias, hysterical movements												•						
Fasciculations															•			
Hypokinesias																		
Akinesias		•					•	•										
Ataxias											•		•					
Weakness or paralysis													•		•	•	•	•
Dystonias																		
Hypertonias:																		
Myotonia																		•
Rigidity		•	•	•	•	•	•	•										
Spasticity													•					
Hypotonia											•				•	•	•	

ciency of dopamine in the corpus striatum is found in the brains of people with parkinsonism. A deficiency of dopamine leads to excessive activity of cholinergic interneurons, excessive release of acetylcholine, and excessive inhibition of output neurons that leave the corpus striatum. Thus, the neurochemical imbalance deprives the individual of the stabilizing and regulating influences of the corpus striatum on muscles, resulting in symptoms of tremor, rigidity, and weakness.

Etiology of parkinsonism is varied, and some elements of treatment will differ based on etiology. One type of parkinsonism follows attacks of encephalitis. This form of the disease is very rare in people born after 1930, and it is now believed that most cases resulted (either immediately or after a variable latency period) from contact with a β-encephalitis virus that was extant in the United States in the late 1920s. Other causes of parkinsonism include carbon monoxide or heavy metal neurotoxicity, neuro-

Table 22–2
Drug Management of Motor Symptoms

Symptom	Origin	Drug treatments
Hyperkinesias		
Choreas and athetosis	EP	Neuroleptics, tetrabenazine, sedatives, and anti-inflammatory drugs (if due to infection)
Ballismus	EP	Neuroleptics, tetrabenazine
Tardive dyskinesias	EP	Neuroleptics, tetrabenazine, α-methyltyrosine
Dystonic movements	EP	Spasmolytics
Tremor		
Resting	EP	Levodopa, dopamine agonists
Action	EP	Propranolol, anticholinergics
Intention	CB	None
Myoclonus	SC,EP,C	Clonazepam, L-5-hydroxytryptophan
Akathisias	EP	Benzodiazepines, anticholinergics
Tics, habit rhythmias, hysterical movements	C	Haloperidol or pimozide for Gilles de la Tourette's syndrome; benzodiazepines for other tics
Fasciculations	SC	None
Hypokinesias		
Akinesias	EP	Levodopa or dopamine agonists for parkinsonian akinesias
Ataxias	CB	None
Weakness or paralysis	Various	Neostigmine for myasthenia gravis
Dystonias		
Hypertonias		
Myotonia	M	Quinine, quinidine, procaine, or phenytoin
Rigidity	EP	Spasmolytics, anticholinergics, antiepileptics
Spasticity	C	Spasmolytics, antiepileptics
Hypotonia	Various	None

Key: C, cortical; CB, cerebellar; EP, extrapyramidal; M, muscle; SC, spinal cord.

syphilis, cerebrovascular disorders (arteriosclerosis, thrombosis, embolism, or hemorrhage), tumors, and degenerative disease of the corpus striatum (paralysis agitans). In mid-1982 and again in late 1983, more than 500 cases of parkinsonism developed on the West Coast as a result of exposure of individuals to a black-market "designer" drug called MPTP (1-methyl-4-phenyl-4-propionoxypiperidine), which was sold to unsuspecting drug abusers as heroin. A parkinsonian-like condition, called pseudoparkinsonism, can be induced by neuroleptics or, less commonly, antidepressants. Often the cause of parkinsonism for a particular client is not identified, in which case the condition is called idiopathic parkinsonism.

Two pharmacological approaches have proved effective in parkinsonism. The first, discovered some 100 years ago by Ordenstein, is the use of anticholin-

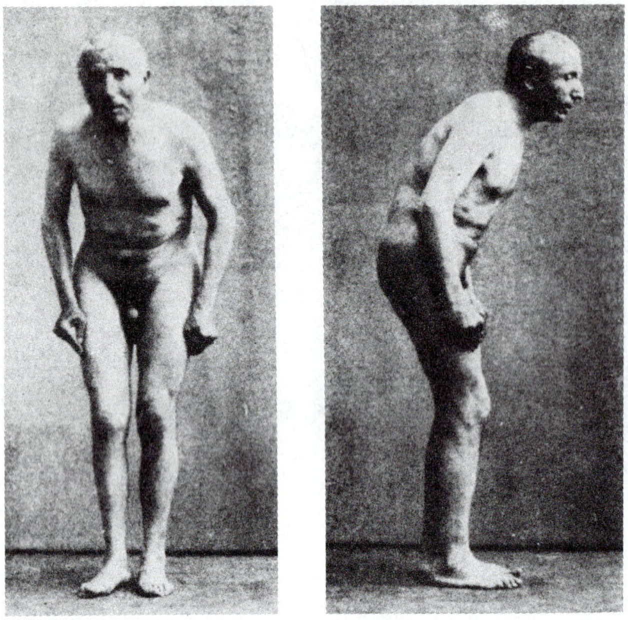

Figure 22-1
Bent posture of Parkinson's disease.

ergic drugs of the belladonna type to alleviate the excess of acetylcholine. A newer approach is the use of the dopamine precursor, levodopa, or dopamine agonists that treat the relative deficiency in dopamine in the corpus striatum of parkinsonian patients.

Anticholinergics

Mechanisms and Effects Anticholinergic drugs work in parkinsonism by reducing excessive cholinergic activity in the corpus striatum. The anticholinergic drugs reduce severity of the action tremor and rigidity by about 20% but have little effect on akinesias or resting tremor. Anticholinergics currently used in parkinsonism are procyclidine (Kemadrin), trihexyphenidyl (Artane, Tremin), benztropine (Cogentin), biperiden (Akineton), orphenadrine (Disipal), ethopropazine (Parsidol), and diphenhydramine (Benadryl). Ethopropazine is a phenothiazine derivative and like other phenothiazines has anticholinergic properties. It is less effective than other drugs in the group, results in a high incidence of adverse reactions, may aggravate symptoms, and may

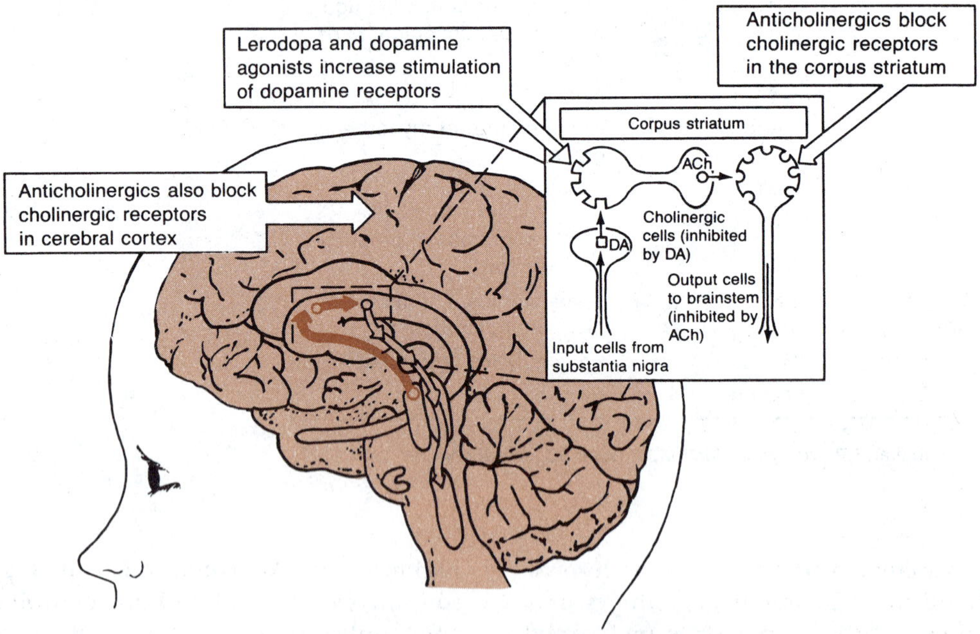

Figure 22-2
Mechanisms of antiparkinsonian agents. A deficiency in the nigrostiatal dopamine (DA) pathway in parkinsonism permits cholinergic cells in the corpus striatum to become overactive, suppressing outputs from the corpus striatum to the brainstem. Levodopa alleviates this by elevating dopamine, thus increasing inhibition of the cholinergic cells. From A. K. Swonger and L. L. Constantine, *Drugs and Therapy,* 2nd ed. Boston: Little, Brown, 1983.

cause undesirable behavioral disturbances. (Diphenhydramine is better known as an antihistamine than an anticholinergic agent.)

Pharmacokinetics Although the naturally occurring belladonna alkaloids (atropine and scopolamine) are active in alleviating parkinsonian symptoms, their high level of peripheral activity results in frequent peripheral anticholinergic side effects such as tachycardia, urinary retention, and constipation. The belladonna alkaloids have been replaced for use in parkinsonism by synthetic anticholinergics that more readily penetrate the blood-brain barrier, providing a higher ratio of central to peripheral activity.

Clinical Indications Anticholinergic drugs exert their modest therapeutic benefit in all forms of parkinsonism, including neuroleptic-induced pseudoparkinsonism. The anticholinergic agents are often employed in combinations with dopaminergic drugs since the two classes of antiparkinsonian agents tend to be effective with respect to different aspects of the disorder.

Adverse Effects and Contraindications The numerous adverse effects of anticholinergic drugs have been described as the **anticholinergic syndrome.** This syndrome includes both central and peripheral reactions. *Prior to giving anticholinergic agents, the nurse needs to determine if the client has any prior history of adverse reactions to anticholinergic medications.*

Cardiovascular manifestations include tachycardia, palpitations, postural hypotension, and flushing. *Nurses must be vigilant for adverse reactions in clients who have cardiac disease or chronic respiratory ailments such as asthma.* Visual components of the anticholinergic syndrome include blurred vision, diplopia, mydriasis, and an increase in intraocular pressure. *Clients with glaucoma should usually not receive these agents, but if it is necessary both client and family need to be fully aware of the signs and symptoms that indicate the drug should be withheld.*

Gastrointestinal and genitourinary symptoms are common. Among these symptoms are dry mouth, nausea, vomiting, epigastric distress, paralytic ileus (common with parkinsonism), urinary retention, urinary hesitancy, dysuria, and constipation (which can lead to fecal impaction). *Nurses need to note any complaints that could indicate gastrointestinal or genitourinary problems, such as pain suggesting obstruction of the gastrointestinal tract, jaundice, difficulty voiding, or a gray stool color suggestive of biliary obstruction. Clients need to be taught to monitor their urinary output, bowel elimination, and fluid intake, and to maintain bulk in the diet to prevent constipation.*

Some individuals experience muscle weakness, elevated body temperature, sweating, disorientation, or lightheadedness. Anticholinergics must be used with caution in hot weather, especially in the elderly, because of the potential for heat prostration and even fatal hyperthermia. Some clients develop memory impairment, agitation, depression, hallucinations, delusions, delirium, paranoia, or outright psychosis. Anticholinergic drugs produce a pronounced slowing of brain waves with a concomitant clouding of consciousness and can precipitate or aggravate tardive dyskinesias when employed for drug-induced parkinsonism. Since elderly people are especially vulnerable to adverse anticholinergic effects, dosages must be very carefully titrated for such clients.

Ethopropazine (Parsidol), a phenothiazine derivative, is the only one of the anticholinergics used in parkinsonism with significant unique side effects. It can produce many of the adverse reactions typical of phenothiazines, such as increased likelihood of seizure, hematological reactions, abnormal pigmentation of the cornea, lens, retina, or skin, endocrine disturbances, and allergic jaundice.

Drug Interactions The anticholinergic effects of these drugs are additive with those of any concurrently administered drugs. Other widely used drugs with anticholinergic activity include many of the narcotic analgesics, phenothiazines and other neuroleptics, tricyclic antidepressants, some of the antidysrhythmics (such as quinidine), and certain antihistamines (especially the ethanolamine group). *The nurse should advise clients to avoid use of nonprescription medications, since many of these contain anticholinergic constituents. The client who feels an urgent need to use such products should consult the physician, nurse, or pharmacist about potential interaction with the anticholinergic medication.*

The depressant effect of anticholinergics is additive with depression caused by any other central nervous system depressants. *The nurse should advise clients to avoid concurrent use of alcohol or other CNS depressants.*

Anticholinergic drugs delay gastric emptying time, which can delay the absorption of concurrently administered drugs and decrease total absorption of drugs that are degraded in the stomach. They also decrease intestinal motility, thus increasing absorption of drugs such as digoxin (Lanoxin) that benefit from a prolonged intestinal transit time, and decreasing absorption of drugs such as phenothiazines or haloperidol (Haldol) that are substantially metabolized in the intestines.

Preparations and Administration *Clients may take anticholinergic drugs before or after meals, depending on their reaction. Elderly clients or those who salivate excessively may prefer to take the drug after meals. If the client experiences dryness of the mouth, he or she may prefer to take it with meals. Drug-induced dryness of mouth can be relieved by chewing sugarless gum, eating hard candy, or taking frequent sips of water.*

Benztropine (Cogentin)
Tablets, injection solution
Recommended Doses: 1 or 2 mg/day PO typically for organic parkinsonism, but doses range from 0.5 to 6 mg/day. For drug-induced extrapyramidal disorders, 1–4 mg once or twice daily.

Biperiden (Akineton)
Tablets, injection solution
Recommended Doses: For organic parkinsonism, 2 mg PO 3 or 4 times daily; for drug-induced extrapyramidal symptoms, 2 mg PO 1–3 times daily, or by slow intravenous infusion.

Diphenhydramine (Benadryl)
Capsules, tablets, elixir
Recommended Doses: For parkinsonism, 25–50 mg orally, 3 or 4 times daily in adults; or 12.5–25 mg, 3 or 4 times daily in children. Doses should not exceed 400 mg daily in adults or 300 mg daily in children.

Ethopropazine (Parsidol)
Tablets
Recommended Doses: 50 mg PO initially, once or twice daily. The usual titrated dose is 100–400 mg PO daily for mild to moderate symptoms, or 500–600 mg daily for severe cases.

Orphenadrine (Disipal)
Tablets
Recommended Doses: 50 mg PO typically, tid after meals to decrease gastrointestinal upset, up to 250 mg tid.

Procyclidine (Kemadrin)
Tablets
Recommended Doses: For organic parkinsonism, 2.5 mg PO, tid, taken after meals to minimize gastrointestinal upset, and gradually increased if well tolerated to 5 mg, tid. For drug-induced parkinsonism, 2.5 mg initially, tid, increased in increments of 2.5 mg daily until a response is observed.

Trihexyphenidyl (Artane, Tremin, Aphen, Trihexane)
Tablets, sustained release capsule, elixir
Recommended Doses: 1–2 mg PO daily initially, increased by 2 mg increments at intervals of 3–5 days up to a dose of 6–10 mg for organic parkinsonism, or 5–15 mg for drug-induced parkinsonism.

Important Nursing Implications for Anticholinergic Drugs for Parkinson's Disease

- ☐ Check the client's medical history for contraindications for anticholinergic medications, such as glaucoma or obstructions of the pylorus, intestines, or urinary tract.
- ☐ Warn clients that anticholinergic drugs may cause drowsiness and mental confusion which could be dangerous if the client is driving an automobile or operating heavy equipment.
- ☐ Instruct clients to avoid use of other CNS depressants, including alcohol, to prevent additive CNS depression.
- ☐ Since anticholinergic drugs can cause orthostatic hypotension, warn clients to avoid rapid changes in position or prolonged periods of standing. Extreme heat, such as hot showers or sunlight, should also be avoided because anticholinergics diminish perspiration and predispose to heat exhaustion.
- ☐ Teach clients to expect dryness of mouth when using anticholinergic medications. They may be advised to use gum, hard candy, or frequent mouth rinses to alleviate dryness of mouth.
- ☐ Advise clients receiving anticholinergic drugs to have regular (yearly) ophthalmic evaulation as a precaution against drug-induced glaucoma.
- ☐ Teach clients to report signs of possible paralytic ileus, such as persistent constipation or abdominal distention.
- ☐ Since many clients taking these drugs are at home, provide them with literature that clearly indicates adverse effects and what to do about them.
- ☐ Check the client's current medications for other anticholinergic drugs and warn clients not to employ nonprescription drugs without checking with the physician to determine if they have anticholinergic effects. The combined influence of multiple anticholinergic medications can be serious anticholinergic toxicity.
- ☐ Give anticholinergic drugs with meals to minimize gastrointestinal upset.
- ☐ Have clients void prior to each dose of medication to minimize problems of urinary hesitancy or dysuria.

Levodopa

Mechanisms and Effects The newest treatment approach for parkinsonism, dating from 1961, is the use of agents that enhance dopamine activity in the brain. The first agent employed to achieve this effect was levodopa (L-dopa), the precursor of the neurotransmitter. Administered levodopa, like endogenous levodopa, is converted in the brain to dopamine. Levodopa is, in a sense, a kind of replacement therapy, since parkinsonian clients are deficient in brain dopamine. The drug is dramatically effective in alleviating akinesias and inhibiting the resting tremor of parkinsonism but less effective in blocking action tremors and rigidity (in contrast to anticholinergic therapy, which is most effective in reducing action tremors and rigidity). Therefore, a typical regimen for parkinsonism includes both levodopa and an anticholinergic compound.

Clinical Indications Levodopa is indicated for all forms of organic parkinsonism, including idiopathic, postencephalitic, arteriosclerotic, and parkinsonism caused by manganese, carbon monoxide, or other toxins. Levodopa is not useful in neuroleptic-induced pseudoparkinsonism because the beneficial effect on motor symptoms is accompanied by an aggravation of the psychotic condition for which the neuroleptic is being employed. Clients with advanced parkinsonism are less likely to respond to levodopa than are those in earlier stages. Significant improvement with levodopa may occur in 2–3 weeks after onset of therapy, or it may take 3–4 months or more. *Clients and families need to be informed of this variability at the outset so that unrealistic hopes may be avoided.* The effectiveness of levodopa tends to diminish gradually after 2–5 years of use, after which dopamine agonists may be added to the regimen to enhance efficacy of the drug.

Pharmacokinetics After oral administration, levodopa is absorbed from the small intestines, reaching peak plasma concentrations between 0.5 and 2 hours after administration. Drugs, such as anticholinergics, that delay gastric emptying time, delay not only the rate of absorption of levodopa, but also total bioavailability, since levodopa is degraded by gastric enzymes. Levodopa is substantially metabolized in the gastrointestinal tract and, after systemic absorption, is metabolized in peripheral nerve endings. Only about 1% reaches the brain without the benefit of coadministration of a peripheral decarboxylase inhibitor. The elimination half-life of levodopa is about 1–3 hours. It is eliminated mainly in the urine in the form of metabolites, especially dihydroxyphenylacetic acid (DOPAC) and homovanillic acid (HVA).

Use with Carbidopa Levodopa, rather than dopamine itself, is used in parkinsonism because unlike dopamine, it can cross the blood-brain barrier. Levodopa is converted to dopamine both outside the CNS (peripherally) and inside the CNS (centrally). Only the dopamine that is produced in the brain contributes to the relief of motor symptoms (Figure 22-3); peripheral conversion is undesirable, leading to orthostatic hypotension. The enzyme responsible for conversion of levodopa to dopamine is dopa decarboxylase, found both in the brain and in peripheral neural structures. One strategy for reducing pe-

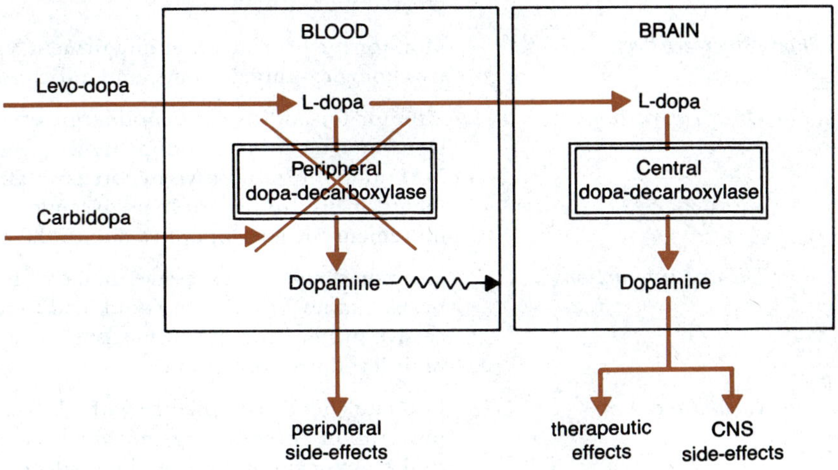

Figure 22–3
Schema illustrating the rationale for use of a peripheral decarboxylase inhibitor with levodopa to reduce peripheral side effects while increasing accumulation of the administered levodopa by the brain. From A. K. Swonger and L. L. Constantine, *Drugs and Therapy,* 2nd ed. Boston: Little, Brown, 1983.

ripheral conversion of levodopa to dopamine is the simultaneous administration of an inhibitor of the decarboxylase enzyme, such as carbidopa, that itself is unable to cross the blood-brain barrier. Carbidopa inhibits dopa decarboxylase in the periphery without affecting the corresponding enzyme in the brain. Levodopa and carbidopa are formulated in combination as Sinemet.

Adverse Effects and Contraindications Although the therapeutic benefit of levodopa is initially dramatic, the incidence of significant adverse effects is high. Among the most common of the adverse effects is occurrence of **choreiform or dystonic movements** (involuntary, adventitious movements that resemble those of Huntington's disease or the dyskinesias of long-term neuroleptic therapy). Anything less than optimal titration of dose is likely to result in motor symptoms. Early dyskinetic movements include muscle twitches and blepharospasm and indicate excessive dosing. Rarely, oculogyric crisis can develop.

Nursing Observations for Antiparkinsonian Drug Therapy

THERAPEUTIC GOAL	Improve mobility and strength and suppress tremors and rigidity.
PREADMINISTRATION ASSESSMENT	
Baseline Data	Observe extent of tremors, muscle weakness, muscle rigidity, or akinesia, difficulty walking or changing directions, shaky handwriting, monotone or muffled voice, increased salivation, lacrimation, seborrhea, incontinence, and difficulty chewing or swallowing; mental confusion and memory impairment may occur late in the progression of the disorder. Evaluate motor function (e.g., reflexes, gait, grip strength, amount of tremor), mental status, control of autonomic functions, vital signs, respiratory sounds, ECG, and bladder function. Obtain laboratory tests including complete blood cell counts, serum enzymes, and blood urea nitrogen before initiating drug therapy.
Contraindications/ Precautions	Cardiovascular disease, cardiac dysrhythmias, chronic obstructive pulmonary disease, glaucoma, peptic ulcers, psychosis, convulsive disorders, pregnancy, or lactation.
Potential Interactions	Check medication history for interacting drugs, including antihypertensives, anticholinergics, antidepressants, antipsychotic drugs, anxiolytics, oral hyperglycemics, antiepileptics, and vitamin B_6.
EVALUATION OF DRUG RESPONSE	
For Therapeutic Benefit	Monitor suppression of tremors and rigidity, increased muscle strength, and increased mobility.
For Adverse Effects	Monitor for liver or renal impairment, cardiovascular changes, neurological or psychological impairments, and anticholinergic side effects.
For Drug Interactions	Monitor for additive anticholinergic effects, additive CNS stimulation or depression, antagonism of levodopa by B_6 in multivitamins, potentiation of levodopa by MAO inhibitors, additive hypotensive effects with other drugs, increased requirement for insulin or oral hypoglycemics when levodopa is given, and increased requirement for antiepileptics due to the effect of levodopa on seizure threshold.
For Dietary Interactions	Monitor clients for excessive intake of foods rich in pyridoxine (lima beans, navy beans, kidney beans) that could lead to antagonism of levodopa. Observe for excessive protein content in meals, since amino acids derived from protein may inhibit levodopa absorption.
For Compliance	Evaluate client's compliance with all facets of the therapeutic regimen by careful observation, interviewing, and review of progress. Report compliance problems to the physician and act as client-advocate when changes in the therapeutic regimen seem indicated.

Levodopa is also likely to cause **nausea and vomiting** (in as many as 80% of individuals treated with the drug), dry mouth, dysphagia, and dysgeusia. *Nausea, vomiting, and anorexia can be lessened if clients are encouraged to take the drug with food or with antacids. Some clients may become constipated. To avoid this problem, nurses should encourage them to drink fairly large quantities of fluids and to include bulk foods in the diet.*

Other adverse responses include ataxia, increased action tremor, headache, dizziness, faintness, confusion, anxiety, agitation, increased libido, insomnia, nightmares, bruxism, hallucinations, delusions, fatigue, or depression. Depression may be severe to the extent of suicidal ideation. Any cognitive impairment may be increased by levodopa therapy. Levodopa is a potent suppressor of dreaming sleep, a fact that may be related to the psychological disturbances. *Nurses need to be prepared to offer the psychological support essential to counteract depression, discouragement, and hopelessness that clients may feel.*

Some clients exhibit a peculiar fluctuation in activity level (from hyperkinesia to bradykinesia) which has been termed the *on-off* phenomenon. Often a profound weakness develops within minutes and can last 1–3 hours. These cyclical exacerbations of parkinsonism often appear at the same time each day and may be due to excessive levodopa levels or may be precipitated by emotional stress. *To identify precipitating factors, clients and families should be encouraged to keep a record of on-off incidences (time of day, date, duration of the response, and any events connected with the incidences.*

Peripheral adverse effects are less frequent, especially when the combination of levodopa and carbidopa is employed. However, orthostatic hypotension, flushing, cardiac irregularities, and palpitations may occur. *Nurses should monitor blood pressure with clients in both supine and standing positions to facilitate detection of postural hypotension, and clients should be taught to avoid rapid changes of position.* Diarrhea, constipation, flatulence, skin rash, sweating, urinary incontinence, diplopia, loss of hair, priapism, hemolytic anemia, and agranulocytosis are additional peripheral side effects. *Clients should be informed of the possibility of voiding a pink-tinged urine which turns to dark black upon standing exposure to air. Perspiration may also be dark in color.*

Levodopa may cause blurred vision, dilated pupils, and aggravation of glaucoma. *Nurses need to monitor clients with wide angle glaucoma and teach clients to report any increase in headaches or other signs that glaucoma has worsened.* Levodopa can alter blood sugar levels in clients who are diabetic. *Nurses should advise such clients to intensify monitoring of blood glucose levels for possible alterations when levodopa therapy is initiated.*

Caution should be exercised when contemplating use of levodopa in clients with a history of myocardial infarction (because dopamine increases the strength of the heart's contractions), or peptic ulcer (upper gastrointestinal hemorrhage has been caused by levodopa), and in psychiatric clients. The safety of levodopa has not been established in pregnant or lactating women or children under age 12.

There are no known adverse effects of carbidopa independent of those attributable to potentiation of levodopa. Clients receiving carbidopa with levodopa (Sinemet) will be less likely to have cardiac dysrhythmias, nausea and vomiting, dizziness, or fainting.

Drug-Drug and Drug-Diet Interactions The therapeutic effect of levodopa is subject to antagonism by vitamin B_6 (pyridoxine). Oral doses of 10–25 mg of pyridoxine are sufficient to rapidly reverse the benefit of levodopa. *Clients need to be taught to avoid foods rich in pyridoxine (lima beans, navy beans, kidney beans, and fortified cereals), or excessive use of multivitamin preparations, which contain pyridoxine. Five milligrams or more per day of pyridoxine will reverse the effects of levodopa.* Pyridoxine has less tendency to reverse effects of levodopa given in combination with carbidopa. Reserpine (Serpasil), an antihypertensive medication, which depletes dopamine, and neuroleptics, which block dopamine receptors, may also interfere with the therapeutic benefits of levodopa.

Conversely, administration of levodopa together with anticholinergics is generally beneficial, since the two types of antiparkinsonian medications operate on different aspects of the condition. Also, anticholinergics tend to produce sedation, apathy, lethargy, or depression, while levodopa usually results in agitation, delirium, and increased excitation. Thus, the adverse effects of the two types of antiparkinsonian drugs tend to offset one another.

Postural hypotension produced by levodopa can be additive with that caused by antihypertensive medications, such as guanethidine (Ismelin), methyldopa (Aldomet), and diuretics. Administration of levodopa to individuals receiving monoamine oxidase inhibitors may result in hypertensive crisis due to inhibition of dopamine and norepinephrine metabolism. Combined administration of levodopa with direct- or indirect-acting sympathomimetics (see Chapter 28) causes excessive stimulation of the cardiovascular system as well.

Clients using levodopa should avoid large amounts of foods containing tyramine (which may neutralize the activity of levodopa), such as chocolate, aged cheeses, beer, or wine. Also, since amino acids compete with levodopa (itself an amino acid),

Nursing Diagnoses and Interventions for Antiparkinsonian Drug Therapy

Nursing Diagnoses	*Related Interventions*
TO ENHANCE DRUG BENEFITS OR REDUCE DRUG REQUIREMENTS	
Impaired physical mobility related to motor dysfunction or antiparkinsonian drug response	Help client to maintain muscle and joint function through physical therapy and proper drug therapy. Observe for "on-off" responses to levodopa. Teach clients to walk with a broad-based gait to improve balance and to practice marching to a rhythm to improve walking patterns and combat the tendency to shuffle.
Alteration in nutrition related to difficulty chewing and swallowing and need to avoid excess vitamin B_6	Ensure adequate nutrition but avoid vitamin preparations that contain pyridoxine and excessive intake of lima beans, navy beans, or kidney beans if levodopa is being used.
Increased risk of injury related to weakness or akinesia secondary to the disease process	Provide safety measures as required; warn clients not to perform dangerous tasks beyond their capabilities.
Ineffective airway clearance related to impaired ability to cough secondary to the disease process	Monitor for pulmonary congestion, instruct client to avoid contact with infected individuals, and teach deep coughing exercises.
Impaired home maintenance management related to immobility	Help the client remain as independent as possible. Teach clients to allow more time to accomplish tasks. Teach clients to simplify daily tasks (for example, wearing clothes that are easy to put on).
Alteration in family processes related to role adjustments; Grieving related to the nature of the disease; Ineffective individual coping: depression related to nature of the disease; Sexual dysfunction related to loss of libido or impotence	Provide emotional support and encouragement. Consider a referral of the client and family for psychological counseling.
Powerlessness related to inability to alter course of the disease	Encourage client to be self-directive in establishing health care and drug taking regimen.
Social isolation related to immobility and embarrassment	Encourage clients to socialize and to renew old contacts as they improve in response to drug therapy.
TO MINIMIZE DRUG SIDE EFFECTS OR INTERACTIONS	
Alteration in bowel function: constipation related to immobility and/or anticholinergic medications	Provide regular exercise commensurate with the client's capabilities; ensure adequate dietary fiber; monitor bowel elimination; give client laxatives or stool softeners.
Alteration in comfort related to headache or gastrointestinal irritation by drugs	Instruct client to take levodopa with food. Instruct client to report occurrence of headaches since these may indicate drug-induced glaucoma.
Alteration in oral mucous membranes related to dryness of mouth caused by anticholinergic medications	Advise client to intensify oral hygiene and to suck on ice chips or sugarless hard candies.
Alteration in thought processes related to effects of drugs	Observe for depression, psychotic symptoms, or delirium with levodopa, dopamine agonists, or anticholinergic drugs; advocate dosage adjustment if any of these occur. Ask families about behavioral changes.
Alteration in skin integrity: dryness related to anticholinergic drugs or oiliness and perspiration with levodopa	Suggest using skin moisturizers or increasing cleaning as required.

Alteration in urinary elimination: incontinence or retention caused by anticholinergic or dopamine agonist drugs	Ensure easy access to bathroom facilities; monitor intake-output. Have client void prior to each dose of medication.
Increased risk of injury related to orthostatic hypotension or neurological effects of drug therapy	Advise clients to change position slowly and to avoid very hot showers or hot sunlight. Adjust doses of antiparkinsonian drugs if psychotic symptoms, delirium, or euphoria occur.
TO ENSURE SAFE AND EFFICACIOUS DRUG USE	
Knowledge deficit related to drug regimen	Educate the client regarding the nature of the disorder and the rationale for the treatment regimen.
	Teach clients the physical exercises they can employ to increase strength and improve mobility as adverse symptoms improve.
	Provide client with a list of adverse effects and drug interactions for each drug in the regimen and explain what to do if any of these occur.

clients should avoid high protein meals. This competition from other amino acids for transport carriers in the intestinal tract and when crossing the blood-brain barrier contributes to the "on-off" phenomenon with levodopa.

Preparations and Administration Levodopa appears to be absorbed into fat depots from which it is released sporadically. *Clients who are obese tend to have more problems with regulation of drug dosage and nurses should teach them to observe their responses carefully and report any changes or adverse reactions. Nurses must monitor client vital signs, especially during the adjustment period, and teach families of clients who are at home to take and record blood pressure, pulse, and respiratory rate and rhythm. Levodopa should be given with food to reduce the incidence of gastrointestinal disturbances.* Therapeutic response may require as much as 6 months of treatment.

Carbidopa is available as a single agent (Lodosyn) for use when the doses of carbidopa and levodopa must be titrated separately. Usually, however, carbidopa is employed in combination with levodopa (Sinemet). Treatment with Sinemet should not be initiated sooner than 8 hours after discontinuing levodopa (single drug) formulations.

Levodopa (Dopar, Larodopa, and generic formulations)
Tablets, capsules
Recommended Doses: 0.5–1.0 g PO initially, in 2 or more divided doses daily. Doses must be titrated for each individual to optimize the balance between improvement and side effects. The dose may be gradually increased in increments of 0.75 g/day at intervals of 3–7 days, as tolerated. The maximum recommended dose is 8 g/day.

Levodopa/Carbidopa (Sinemet)
Tablets
Recommended Doses: One 10/100 tablet (10 mg levodopa and 100 mg carbidopa) or one 25/250 tablet PO, 3 times daily initially, increased by 1 tablet each day or every other day up to 6 tablets per day. If doses higher than about 500 mg daily of levodopa are required, the 25/250 tablet can be substituted and employed up to 4 times per day.

Dopamine Agonists

Two dopamine agonists are available for use in parkinsonism: amantadine (Symmetrel) and bromocriptine (Parlodel). Whereas levodopa produces its beneficial effects in parkinsonism indirectly by promoting formation of dopamine, amantadine and bromocriptine act directly on dopamine receptors. Amantadine is also employed as an antiviral agent (see Chapter 48).

Clinical Indications Neither amantadine nor bromocriptine provides as favorable an effect as levodopa in the initial therapy of early parkinsonism — amantadine because it is generally less effective and bromocriptine because the adverse effects are generally more pronounced. However, after several years of treatment with levodopa, parkinsonian clients often become refractory to the drug, possibly because degeneration of dopamine neurons has proceeded to the point where little enzyme remains for conversion of levodopa to dopamine. Addition of a dopamine agonist at this point frequently results in additional therapeutic benefit. Amantadine (but not levodopa or bromocriptine) can be used successfully in conjunction with neuroleptics for treatment of neuroleptic-induced pseudoparkinsonian symptoms. Evidence suggests that amantadine exerts a selective agonistic effect on dopamine receptors of the corpus striatum, with little action of receptors of the hypothalamus or limbic system. Thus, amantadine can reverse drug-induced parkinsonism without aggravating the psychotic condition for which the neuroleptic is being employed. Bromocriptine is recommended for use as an adjunct to levodopa therapy, to provide added benefit or to allow reduction of the dose of levodopa. The maximum effect of amantadine generally occurs in a few days to 1 week. However, the effectiveness sometimes wanes after 6–8 weeks of therapy.

Adverse Effects and Contraindications The central adverse effects of amantadine are depression, fatigue, hallucinations, confusion, ataxia, anxiety, dizziness, oculogyric crisis, seizures, and slurred speech. Clients who develop psychotic symptoms do so within a few days after therapy is initiated or after a dosage increase. Symptoms tend to subside when the drug is given in divided doses. Peripheral side effects of amantadine range from constipation, nausea, vomiting, anorexia, dry mouth, skin rash, orthostatic hypotension, edema, and visual disturbances, to convulsions, dyspnea, leukopenia, neutropenia, and congestive heart failure. Bromocriptine can cause nausea, blephorospasm, choreiform movements, drowsiness, ataxia, depression, hallucinations, confusion, insomnia, vomiting, abdominal discomfiture, orthostatic hypotension, and shortness of breath. Less commonly, bromocriptine has caused seizures, headaches, peripheral edema, nasal stuffiness, paresthesias, skin rash, urinary frequency, incontinence or retention, and exacerbation of Raynaud's syndrome.

Preparations and Administration

Amantadine (Symmetrel)
Capsules, syrup
Recommended Doses: For organic parkinsonism, 100 mg PO, twice daily (or 100 mg daily if there are serious associated medical problems), increased up to 400 mg daily as required to optimize benefit. For drug-induced extrapyramidal symptoms, 100 mg PO initially, twice daily, increased up to 300 mg PO daily as required for optimal response.

Bromocriptine (Parlodel)
Tablets, capsules
Recommended Doses: One-half of a 2.5 mg tablet initially, twice daily with meals, increased by 2.5 mg/day every 2–4 weeks until optimal response is achieved. When dosage reduction is indicated, the drug should be withdrawn gradually in increments of 2.5 mg/day.

Important Nursing Implications for Levodopa and Dopamine Agonists

- ☐ Review the client's medical history for contraindications for dopaminergic drugs, including epilepsy, psychosis, liver or renal impairment, cardiovascular disorders, endocrine diseases, glaucoma, peptic ulcers, or diabetes mellitus.
- ☐ Since levodopa and dopamine agonists can produce orthostatic hypotension, advise clients to make position changes slowly, dangle the feet before arising, and avoid prolonged standing or exposure to hot showers or sunlight.
- ☐ Warn clients to exercise caution when driving an automobile or operating heavy machinery while using levodopa or dopamine agonists because of risks of depression, confusion, hallucinations, and other neurological side effects that may impair functioning.
- ☐ Instruct clients to monitor and report abnormal movements.
- ☐ Advise clients to avoid use of nonprescription drugs, including vitamin preparations that contain pyridoxine, without consultation with the physician.
- ☐ Administer dopaminergic drugs with meals to minimize gastric irritation.
- ☐ Monitor vital signs when adjusting doses of dopaminergic agents.
- ☐ When dopamine agonists are discontinued, be aware that the dose will be gradually tapered since abrupt discontinuation may lead to acute aggravation of parkinsonian symptoms.

Huntington's Disease

Huntington's disease is an inherited organic extrapyramidal disorder. The condition is marked by occurrence of choreiform movements, which are involuntary motor tics. Clients exhibit abnormal, involuntary, purposeless movements of the tongue, extremities, and, sometimes, the trunk. Initially the movements may be limited, rapid twitching of the fingers or facial twitches. As the disease progresses, the jerking, twisting movements produce severe spasms of the face, tongue, neck, arms, trunk, and legs. Sudden flinging movements can result in clients injuring themselves or others. Among the most dangerous of the motor symptoms is difficulty in speaking and swallowing, which can lead to asphyxiation. While clients may remain at home in the early stages, they usually require institutionalization later on.

Huntington's disease begins between ages 37 and 47. In about 10% of cases, it begins prior to age 15. Dementia occurs in most patients, more often in cases of early onset. Behavioral symptoms include increased libido, catatonia, paranoia, and aggression. In some clients, behavioral changes, such as carelessness in personal hygiene, apathy, and irritability, are the first signs of Huntington's disease. Behavioral symptoms may precede motor manifestations by as much as a decade and are easily mistaken for schizophrenia. Both schizophrenia and Huntington's disease involve elevated dopaminergic activity in the brain, but Huntington's disease is genetically transmitted.

In Huntington's disease, there is degeneration of a gamma-aminobutyric acid pathway in the corpus striatum and substantia nigra. Atrophy is present throughout the brain, but is most pronounced in these regions. Huntington's disease is directly opposite to parkinsonism, involving excess dopamine activity, while parkinsonism entails a dopamine deficiency.

GABA-mimetic drug therapy is *not* useful in Huntington's disease. Apparently, when the GABA pathway degenerates, the GABA receptors in substantia nigra also degenerate. Current therapy for Huntington's disease involves depletion of dopamine or blockade of dopamine receptors. Reserpine (Serpasil) or the more rapid-acting tetrabenazine (Nitoman) can be used to deplete dopamine stores. These two closely related drugs prevent storage of dopamine (as well as norepinephrine and serotonin) in the vesicles of nerve terminals. Tetrabenazine is not marketed in the United States but may be obtained for experimental use in Huntington's disease. Doses of tetrabenazine that eliminate choreiform movements completely (25 mg, 3 times daily) often cause depression. To lessen side effects, it is often necessary to accept incomplete suppression of choreiform movements. Blockade of dopamine receptors can be achieved with neuroleptics; thioridazine (Mellaril) or haloperidol (Haldol) is most frequently selected. Neuroleptic therapy should be reserved for patients who are dangerously aggressive or severely ataxic.

Nursing care is oriented primarily toward safety of the client and assisting the client to remain independent as long as possible. The deterioration of mental functioning in the later stages of Huntington's disease causes unpredictable behavior in clients. As they lose sensation, they become susceptible to trauma, such as burns, and they often fall down. The psychological effects of the disease on families are devastating, causing fear and anxiety about genetic transmission to offspring. Recent research has identified genetic markers that allow individuals to know early in life whether or not they have inherited the condition.

Wilson's Disease

Wilson's disease (hepatolenticular degeneration) is a hereditary disease involving an error in copper metabolism which leads to copper deposits in many organs and tissues. In the CNS, this can result in degeneration of the corpus striatum, with the occurrence of tremors and choreas (especially "wing-beating"). Treatment involves chelating copper (with penicillamine or trientine) to enhance its excretion and a diet low in copper. Pyridoxine (vitamin B_6) is given as well. The use of penicillamine (Cuprimine) and trientine (Cuprid) as chelating agents is discussed in Chapter 57.

Clients who have Wilson's disease require low-copper diets. *Nurses should have the nutritionist review with clients a list of foods to avoid because of high concentrations of copper: for example, alcoholic beverages, chocolate, tea, organ meats, all shellfish, duck, goose, meat gelatin, dried lentils, molasses, mushrooms, nuts, dried beans, and bran products. The drinking water in the client's place of residence should be analyzed for copper content and if significant concentrations are found, the nurse should recommend using demineralized water.*

Hypertonias and Skeletal Muscle Relaxants

Dystonic movements are muscle spasms or contractures that can develop into full-fledged dystonias. Hypertonias are conditions of rigid muscle tone often associated with severe pain. When dystonic movements or hypertonias originate within the CNS, they are responsive to spasmolytic agents. The spasmolytic drugs currently marketed include 10 centrally acting skeletal muscle relaxants and a single direct-acting agent.

Mechanisms and Effects The centrally acting agents depress the interneuronal activity of the descending reticular formation or internuncial neurons within the spinal cord and can be divided into two groups: the first group acts primarily at the level of the brainstem and includes diazepam (Valium), meprobamate (Equanil), carisoprodol (Rela, Soma, Soprodol), cyclobenzaprine (Paraflex), and probably metaxalone (Skelaxin) and orphenadrine (Norflex); the second group acts primarily at the spinal cord level and includes methocarbamol (Delaxin, Robaxin), chlorzoxazone (Paraflex), chlorphenesin (Maolate), and probably baclofen (Lioreasal). The agents that act at the brainstem level generally have greater potential for producing depression.

One agent, dantrolene (Dantrium), is unique among the skeletal muscle relaxants in that its site of action is the skeletal muscle itself. Dantrolene inhibits the contractile elements of the skeletal muscle.

Clinical Indications The centrally acting skeletal muscle relaxants relieve the pain and discomfort associated with acute musculoskeletal conditions, such as sprains and arthritis. The suppression of spasticity may secondarily improve the client's ability to walk and to maintain balance and upright posture. Baclofen in particular is useful for spasticity associated with multiple sclerosis. Dantrolene is indicated for treating the spasticity of stroke, multiple sclerosis, spinal injuries, or cerebral palsies. Diazepam is the most widely used drug for alleviation of general muscle spasticity not associated with brain or nerve damage. Usually, therapeutic effectiveness may be seen in a few hours to a few weeks after initiation of muscle-relaxant therapy. The beneficial effects of dantrolene may not occur until one week or more after initiation of therapy.

Adverse Effects and Contraindications The most common adverse reactions to the centrally acting skeletal muscle relaxants are drowsiness, vertigo, ataxia, dizziness, headache, and psychiatric depression, or conversely, agitation, irritability, and insomnia. *Nurses should advise clients that use of muscle relaxants may impair ability to perform tasks requiring mental alertness, such as driving an automobile.* Allergic reactions may also occur. *If the client's urine becomes dark, the skin or sclera are yellowed, or pruritus develops, the drug should be discontinued.*

Some of the agents in the group have unique side effects: carisoprodol can cause hypotension, tachycardia, and hematological reactions; chlorphenesin can produce hematological reactions; cyclobenzaprine may cause blood dyscrasias and hepatic toxicity; chlorzoxazone has caused liver damage in a small number of treated individuals; methocarbamol may cause hypotension, bradycardia, and fainting; rarely, orphenadrine has caused aplastic anemia; and baclofen may cause nausea, constipation, urinary frequency, and hypotension. Carisoprodol has low incidence of toxicity, but drowsiness is a common side effect that may require a reduction in dosage.

When cyclobenzaprine is employed, clients should be warned to report unusual fatigue, unexplained fever, easy bruising or bleeding, and sore mouth or sore throat, since these could indicate presence of blood dyscrasias. If clients show signs of hepatotoxicity, such as abdominal pain, fever, nausea, dark urine, yellow skin or sclera, light-colored stools, or itchy skin, serial liver function tests should be ordered.

The principal adverse effect of dantrolene is muscle weakness, which may result in drooling or slurred speech, impaired ability to participate in physical therapy, or enuresis, diarrhea, nausea, and malaise. Sometimes insomnia and depression occur. Dantrolene may cause hepatitis and abnormal liver function and should be discontinued if either is revealed in tests. Hepatic problems are more common in women and in clients over age 35. Dantrolene also increases the incidence of benign and malignant mammary tumors and hepatic malignancies and should be used with caution in clients with impaired pulmonary function or cardiac disorders.

Skeletal muscle relaxants should not be used for more than 3 weeks at a time. When these drugs are discontinued after prolonged use, there is a risk of rebound spasticity, hallucinations, and other withdrawal symptoms. Withdrawal symptoms can be minimized by gradually tapering of the medication.

Drug Interactions Additive CNS depression is the principal drug interaction of centrally acting muscle relaxants. *Clients should be advised to refrain from using alcoholic beverages. Also, nurses should advise clients to check with the physician before purchasing over-the-counter drugs for any purpose. Antihistamines, for example, may produce additive depressant effects.*

Preparations and Administration

Baclofen (Lioresal)
Tablets
Recommended Doses: 5 mg PO 3 times daily initially, increased as required. The usual optimal dosage range after gradual adjustment is between 40 and 80 mg daily.

Carisoprodol (Rela, Soma, Soprodol, and generic formulations)
Tablets, combinations with aspirin (Soma Compound, Carisoprodol Compound); or aspirin and codeine (Soma Compound with Codeine)
Recommended Doses: 350 mg PO, 4 times daily. The drug is not recommended for children under age 12. For the combination products, 1 or 2 tab-

lets, 4 times daily. *Nurses should help the client schedule the drug so the last dose is taken at bedtime.*

Chlorphenesin (Maolate)
Tablets
Recommended Doses: 800 mg PO, 3 times daily.

Chlorzoxazone (Paraflex and generic formulations)
Tablets, combination tablets or capsules with acetaminophen (Paracet, Parafon, Polyflex, Zoxaphen, Chlorofon, Blanex, Flexaphen, Flexin, Lobac, Mus-Lax)
Recommended Doses: One or 2 tablets PO, 3 or 4 times daily. *Nurses should warn clients taking clorzoxazone that they may have some gastric distress. This can be relieved by taking the drug with meals or by crushing the tablets and mixing with food or liquid.*

Cyclobenzaprine (Flexeril)
Tablets
Recommended Doses: 10 mg PO, 3 times daily, not to exceed 60 mg/day.*Cyclobenzaprine should be taken with meals or milk to avoid gastrointestinal upset.*

Dantrolene (Dantrium)
Capsules, powder for reconstitution and injection
Recommended Doses: For chronic spasticity in adults, 25 mg orally, once daily initially; increased to 3 or 4 times daily; and then, in increments of 25 mg, to 100 mg 2 or 4 times daily, up to 400 mg daily. Doses higher than 400 mg daily are not recommended.

Diazepam (Valium)
Formulations: See Chapter 19
Recommended Doses: For spasticity, 5 mg PO twice daily initially, increased in 5 mg increments at 3-day intervals until spasticity is alleviated.

Meprobamate (Equanil)
Formulations: See Chapter 19
Recommended Doses: For spasticity, 400–1,200 mg PO daily.

Metaxalone (Skelaxin)
Tablets
Recommended Doses: For adults and children over 12, 800 mg PO, 3 or 4 times daily.

Methocarbamol (Delaxin, Robaxin, and generic)
Tablets, injection solution, combination tablets with aspirin
Recommended Doses: In adults, 1.5–4 g PO daily initially, in 4–6 divided doses. The maximum daily dose should not exceed 4 g.

Orphenadrine
Tablets (Marflex and generic), sustained release tablets (Norflex and generic), injection solution (Banflex, Flexoject, Flexon, K-Flex, Myolin, Norflex, O'Flex, X-Otag, and generic), combinations with aspirin and caffeine (Norgesic)
Recommended Doses: 75–200 mg PO daily; 100 mg both morning and evening is typical.

Important Nursing Implications for Skeletal Muscle Relaxants

- ☐ Warn clients to avoid driving and other activities requiring mental alertness, physical coordination, or judgment while employing these drugs.
- ☐ Clients should be advised to avoid other CNS depressant drugs while using centrally acting skeletal muscle relaxants because of the potential for additive CNS depression.
- ☐ Teach clients the indications of allergic reactions to muscle relaxants.
- ☐ Advise clients to avoid use of centrally acting skeletal muscle relaxants for more than 3 weeks.
- ☐ When centrally acting skeletal muscle relaxants are discontinued after long-term use, the dose should be tapered to minimize risk of rebound spasticity, hallucinations, and other withdrawal symptoms.
- ☐ Most drugs in this class are best taken with meals to minimize gastrointestinal side effects.

Drug-Induced Extrapyramidal Disorders

Extrapyramidal symptoms occur as side effects of drugs and as a component of withdrawal from sedative-hypnotics and narcotics. In alcoholism, for example, a rapid, coarse tremor develops involving the fingers, tongue, limbs, and head, most evident in the morning prior to alcohol ingestion and particularly severe in delirium tremens. Other drugs that can produce tremor include reserpine, methyldopa, and lithium. Extrapyramidal side effects are most often associated with two classes of psychotropic drugs: the neuroleptics and tricyclic antidepressants. The frequency and severity of side effects are greater with the neuroleptics than with the tricyclic antidepressants. Neuroleptic-induced extrapyramidal side effects are of four types: pseudoparkinsonism, acute dystonias, akathisias, and dyskinesias.

Pseudoparkinsonism

Drug-induced parkinsonism resembles organic parkinsonism; hence it is called **pseudoparkinsonism.** The same triad of symptoms occur as in organic parkinsonism; that is, tremor, rigidity, and akinesia. Severe reactions may take the form of catalepsy (Figure 22-4) or akinesia. Pseudoparkinsonism is a common

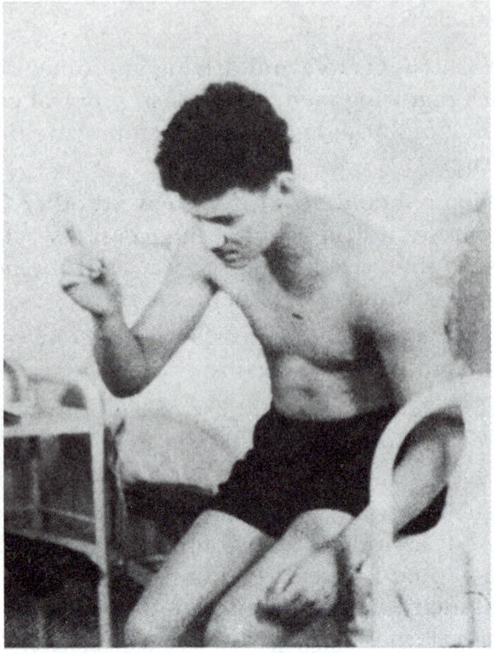

Figure 22–4
Prochlorperazine-induced catalepsy. From J. Delay and P. Deniker, Drug-induced extrapyramidal syndromes. *Handbook Clin. Neurol. 6:* 248–266, 1968. Reprinted by permission of the authors and Elsevier Science Publishers B. V., Amsterdam.

consequence of therapy for psychotic conditions, but can also occur in response to tricyclic antidepressants and methyldopa (Aldomet). The period of maximal risk is 5–30 days after the initiation of drug therapy.

When pseudoparkinsonism develops, there are several possible therapeutic responses (Table 22–3). The first choice when feasible is to lower the dosage of the offending drug, which may not be possible without the recurrence (or exacerbation) or symptoms for which the drug is being employed. The second option is to switch drug selection to a neuroleptic that produces fewer extrapyramidal reactions, for example, thioridazine (Mellaril). This also may not be feasible, for example, if a psychotic condition is severe, since the neuroleptics that produce the fewest extrapyramidal symptoms are generally the least efficacious. The third option is to add an antiparkinsonian agent, such as an anticholinergic drug or amantadine (Symmetrel). Levodopa (Laradopa) and bromocriptine (Parodel) cannot be used for this purpose because they antagonize the antipsychotic value of neuroleptics. Amantadine, however, appears to work against the extrapyramidal effects of neuroleptics without altering their actions in the hypothalamus or limbic system. Amantadine is as effective as the anticholinergic medications and produces fewer adverse effects. Anticholinergics are the least satisfactory option for dealing with pseudoparkinsonism because they mask the overt manifestations of drug-induced parkinsonism but do not prevent development of the underlying neural damage, and can aggravate symptoms of psychosis. It is seldom justifiable to employ antiparkinsonian agents prophylactically in anticipation of pseudoparkinsonian symptoms, because this practice will interfere with the ability to monitor the development of symptoms and make appropriate adjustments in drug dosages or selection.

Acute Dystonic Reactions

Acute dystonic reactions, such as facial grimaces, occur early in treatment, usually in the first 5 days. Severe examples include oculogyric crisis (Figure 22–5) and the bowed torso. Acute dystonias are self-limited, but they may be of such severity as to alarm the patient or family members. Rapid and gratifying alleviation of symptoms can be achieved by intravenous administration of a benzodiazepine, diphenhydramine (Benadryl), or an anticholinergic drug. When dystonic symptoms persist for more than a few

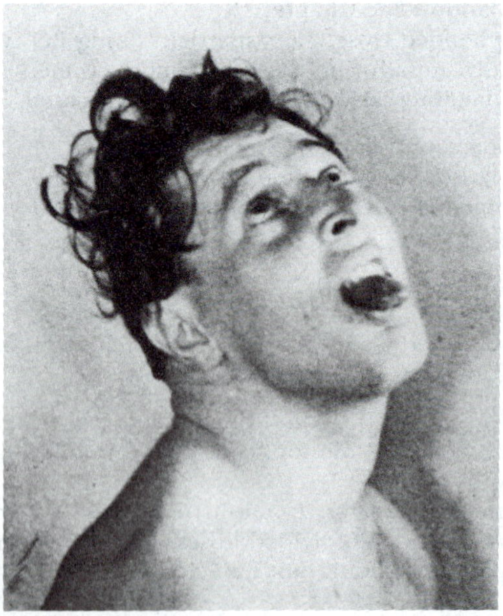

Figure 22–5
Neuroleptic-induced oculogyric crisis with torticollis and protrusion of the tongue. From J. Delay and P. Deniker, Drug-induced extrapyramidal syndromes. *Handbook Clin. Neurol. 6:* 248–266, 1968. Reprinted by permission of the authors and Elsevier Science Publishers B. V., Amsterdam.

Table 22–3
Treatment of Neuroleptic-Induced Extrapyramidal Side Effects

Type of side effect	Period of maximum risk	Treatments
Pseudoparkinsonism	5–30 days	Reduce dose of causative agent. Switch to drug with less risk of extrapyramidal symptoms. Add amantadine to regimen. Add a centrally active anticholinergic drug to the regimen.
Acute dystonias	1–5 days	Administer (IV) diazepam, diphenhydramine, or benztropine or another anticholinergic drug. Continue with oral therapy with same drugs as above.
Akathisias	1–60 days	Administer diazepam, diphenhydramine, or an anticholinergic. Lower dose or switch to a lower potency neuroleptic.
Dyskinesias		
Tardive	After months or years	Eliminate causative drug if possible. Hope for spontaneous remission after many months. Administer a dopamine-depleting drug: reserpine, tetrabenazine, or α-methyltyrosine. Elevate dose of neuroleptic to suppress symptoms temporarily.
Withdrawal-emergent	Upon discontinuation of the neuroleptic	Reinstitute neuroleptic and taper slowly. Wait for spontaneous abatement — these symptoms are self-limited.

days, oral therapy with the same drug can be substituted.

Akathisias

Akathisias are symptoms of motor restlessness. The patient cannot sit still or stand still and jumps or paces about continuously. Somatic discomfort is another component; the patient complains of "feeling bugs" or being on "pins and needles." Akathisias can be dismissed or mistaken for a worsening of schizophrenia, which can lead to erroneous management, such as raising the neuroleptic dose. The effectiveness of benzodiazepines, diphenhydramine, or anticholinergics for relieving akathisias has not been well demonstrated. Akathisias are most common during the first 2 months of neuroleptic treatment and usually disappear spontaneously without any specific drug therapy. Akathisias may become epidemic on a ward of patients receiving neuroleptics as patients react to each other's motor restlessness.

Dyskinesias

Dyskinesias can be either withdrawal-emergent or tardive (late-occurring) dyskinesias. **Withdrawal**

dyskinesias, which occur when neuroleptics are discontinued abruptly after extended use, are self-limiting in the manner of all withdrawal symptoms. No treatment is required, but if withdrawal dyskinesias cause alarm, the neuroleptic can be reinstituted and tapered gradually.

Tardive dyskinesias, on the other hand, develop after many months or even years of antipsychotic drug therapy. The symptoms of tardive dyskinesias appear to be opposite in their etiology from other neuroleptic-induced symptoms and are reminiscent of Huntington's disease. The earliest sign is usually a forward-backward or lateral movement of the tongue. Later, the tongue will protrude obviously or press against the inside of the cheek, in twisting, curling movements. Gnawing movements of the jaw, eyeblinking, and spasmodic grimacing are frequently observed. Tardive dyskinesias appear to be related to the supersensitivity of dopamine receptors caused by prolonged blockade by dopamine-blocking agents (namely the neuroleptics). When dyskinesias develop in the absence of discontinuation or a sharp dosage reduction of the neuroleptic, they can be assumed to be the tardive type. Tardive dyskinesias are persistent and sometimes irreversible, although recent clinical reports indicate that some improvement in severity of these extrapyramidal reactions may occur after extended periods free of the neuroleptic.

Unlike other kinds of neuroleptic-induced extrapyramidal reactions, tardive dyskinesias do not respond to and may actually be triggered or aggravated by antiparkinsonian drugs; hence, options for treatment are severely constrained. One option is to eliminate the causative agent and wait for spontaneous improvement in the severity of the symptoms, which leaves the client's psychosis untreated and superimposes withdrawal dyskinesias on the tardive dyskinesias. The second option is to institute treatment with drugs used in Huntington's disease that deplete dopamine by blocking its storage (reserpine or tetrabenazine) or its synthesis (α-methyltyrosine). These drugs are usually successful in alleviating symptoms of tardive dyskinesias. The third option is to increase the dose of the neuroleptic, which temporarily suppresses tardive dyskinesias but aggravates the problem over the long run.

Functional Motor Disorders

Both tremor and motor tics may arise as functional rather than organic or drug-induced disorders. Tremor of a more common or persistent nature occurs in generalized anxiety disorder and is coarse and irregular. Hysteria often entails tremor as well; it may be fine or coarse, limited or generalized, constant or paroxysmal.

About 75% of motor tics are classified as functional rather than organic, though it is possible that the distinction here between organic and functional will blur as understanding of etiology increases. A common form of functional tic is a burst of eye blinks. Other tics usually involve muscles of the face, especially the eyes and mouth, sometimes spreading to the trunk. Three-fourths of functional tics develop prior to age 30; the peak period of onset is ages 6–12.

Five categories of "stereotyped movement disorders" are designated in the *Diagnostic and Statistical Manual of the American Psychiatric Association, Third Edition* (DSM-III): transient tic disorder, chronic motor tic disorder, atypical tic disorder, and atypical stereotyped movement disorder. Gilles de la Tourette's syndrome is characterized by the occurrence of multiple motor and vocal tics, the latter frequently involving outbursts of obscenities (coprolalia) or involuntary repetition of a word or sentence just spoken by another person (echolalia). Drug therapy is important principally for this syndrome.

Haloperidol and Pimozide Therapy for Gilles de la Tourette's Syndrome

Haloperidol (Haldol) has been the drug of choice for Gilles de la Tourette's syndrome for about a decade. Pimozide (Orap) is reserved for patients who do not respond satisfactorily to haloperidol. Pimozide is employed only for individuals who are severely compromised in daily activities by the tics, not for situations where the tics present only a cosmetic problem. Haloperidol and especially pimozide are very potent neuroleptics with an elevated potential for producing the full range of severe extrapyramidal side effects. Thus the decision to use these drugs for Gilles de la Tourette's syndrome should not be made lightly. In addition, pimozide has caused cardiovascular changes (shown in the ECG as prolongation of the QT interval, for example) and even sudden death.

Like other neuroleptics, haloperidol and pimozide lower the seizure threshold. Clients with Gilles de la Tourette's syndrome who are also prone to seizures should be monitored with special care. Pimozide, but not haloperidol, has substantial anticholinergic properties and must be used with caution when other anticholinergic medications are being employed because of the potential for additive anticholinergic effects. Both of these neuroleptics are capable of producing additive depressant effects with other CNS depressants. Pimozide may cause headaches, depression or excitation, visual disturbances, decreased libido, postural hypotension or hypertension, weight changes, skin eruptions, and gastrointestinal disturbances. The full pharmacology of haloperidol is discussed in Chapter 18.

After oral administration, pimozide is only about 50% absorbed and is subject to considerable first-pass extraction. Peak plasma concentrations occur 6–8 hours after administration. Pimozide is metabolized in the liver and eliminated with a half-life of about 55 hours.

Unfortunately, data are generally lacking concerning the effects of this drug on children under age 12 in spite of the early age of onset (usually 2–15 years of age). Periodic attempts should be made to discontinue therapy with pimozide (or haloperidol) for the syndrome to see if the intensity of the tics has subsided.

Preparation and Administration

Pimozide (Orap)
Tablets
Recommended Doses: 1–2 mg daily initially, in divided doses, increased as required. Most clients receive less than 0.2 mg/kg/day or 10 mg/day, whichever is less. Doses should not exceed 0.3 mg/kg/day or 20 mg/day. Drug withdrawal should be gradual to minimize risk of withdrawal-emergent dyskinesias.

Case Study: Parkinson's Disease

R. J., a 62-year-old white man, is a long-time parkinsonian client being treated with some success with a combination of levodopa, carbidopa, and benztropine. However, R. J. recently came to the clinic because in the past few months he has begun to experience the return of his parkinsonian symptoms, including increasing weakness and tremor, and increased incidents of nausea, dizziness, and palpitations. The nurse asked R. J. about his compliance with the regimen, use of nonprescription drugs, and use of vitamins. R. J. insisted that he was continuing to comply with the prescribed regimen and used no nonprescription drugs or vitamins. The physician reviewed the findings, and before initiating additional drug therapy, ordered measurement of creatinine clearance. When normal results were returned, the physician added amantadine, 100 mg, PO, once daily. R. J. responded well to this new regimen.

1. What was the rationale for the original three-drug regimen?
2. What is the likely basis for the declining responsiveness of R. J. to the levodopa/carbidopa/benztropine regimen?
3. Why did the nurse ask about R. J.'s use of vitamins?
4. Why would the physician decide to add amantadine to the regimen?

Answers appear at the end of the book.

Case Study: Acute Dystonic Reaction

R. K., a 35-year-old Mexican-American man, was hospitalized in the state mental institution and diagnosed as schizophrenic. R. K. had a medical history of congestive heart failure secondary to diabetes mellitus of juvenile onset for which he took insulin, but not dependably. R. K. was placed on trifluoperazine (Stelazine), 15 mg, IM, tid, as well as digoxin and furosemide. On the second day of hospitalization, R. K. developed slurred speech, a propulsive gait, facial contortions, a gaze fixed upward and to the left, and inability to move his eyes. Trifluoperazine was discontinued and benztropine (Cogentin) was administered, 2 mg, IM. After the motor symptoms resolved, trifluoperazine was reinitiated at a dose of 4 mg, IM, tid.

1. What is the likely cause of the motor dysfunctions exhibited by R. K.?
2. Why was benztropine given?
3. If the acute dystonic reaction recurs at the lower dose of trifluoperazine, what drug might be substituted to reduce likelihood of extrapyramidal symptoms?

Answers appear at the end of the book.

Recommended Readings

Antiparkinsonian Drugs

Barbeau A: Use of L-dopa in Parkinson's disease: 20 year follow-up. *Trends Pharmacol Sci* 1981;1:297–299.

Boshes B: Sinemet and the treatment of parkinsonism. *Ann Intern Med* 1981;94(3):364–370.

Calne D et al: Advances in the neuropharmacology of parkinsonism. *Ann Intern Med* 1979;90(2):219–229.

Fischback F: Easing adjustment to Parkinson's disease. *Am J Nurs* 1978;78(1):66–69.

Gresh C: Helpful tips you can give your patient with Parkinson's disease. *Nursing* 1980;10(1)26–33.

Hahn K: Management of Parkinson's disease. *Nurse Pract* 1982;7(1):13–25,50.

Hardie RJ, Lees AJ, Stern GM: The controversial role of bromocriptine in Parkinson's disease. *Clin Neuropharm* 1985;8(2):150–155.

Hoehn MM: Bromocriptine and its use in parkinsonism. *J Am Geriatr Soc* 1981;29:251–258.

Hurtig I: Anticholinergics for Parkinson's disease. *Ann Neurol* 1980;7(5):495.

Parkes JD: Adverse effects of antiparkinsonian drugs. *Drugs* 1981;21(5):341–353.

Quinn NP: Antiparkinsonian drugs today. *Drugs* 1984; 28:236–262.

Riley T, Massey E: Managing the patient with Parkinson's disease. *Postgrad Med* 1980;68(3):85–89.

Simpson GM (ed): Identification and treatment of neuroleptic-induced extrapyramidal reactions. *Clin Neuropharm* 1983;6(Suppl 1).

Weiner M: Update on antiparkinsonian agents. *Geriatrics* 1982;37(9):81–91.

Yahr MD (ed): Parkinsonism: Current perspectives and new horizons. *Clin Neuropharm* 1986;9(Suppl 1).

Drug-Induced Extrapyramidal Disorders

Bickal T: A protocol for the diagnosis and treatment of extrapyramidal symptoms of neuroleptic drugs. *Nurs Pract* 1987;12(1):25–38.

Jewell JA: Tardive dyskinesias, the involuntary movement disorder that no one really understands. *Can Nurse* 1983;79:20–24.

Klawans H, Goetz C, Perlik S: Tardive dyskinesia: Review and update. *Am J Psychiatry* 1980;137:900–908.

Klawans HL, Goetz CG: Symposium on tardive dyskinesias. *Clin Neuropharm* 1983;6(2).

McAfee HA: Tardive dyskinesia. *Am J Nurs* 1978;788:395–397.

Rosal-Greif VLF: Drug-induced dyskinesias. *Am J Nurs* 1982;82(1):66–69.

Drugs for Huntington's Disease

Bird ED: Chemical pathology of Huntington's disease. *Annu Rev Pharmacol Toxicol* 1980;20:533–551.

Paulson GW: Huntington's disease. *Am Fam Physician* 1980;22(1):91–93.

Drug Therapy for Spasticity

Campbell EDR: Muscle relaxant drugs. *Practitioner* 1979;223:507–509.

Delisa JE, Little J: Managing spasticity. *Am Fam Physician* 1982;26(3):117–122.

Pinder RM et al.: Dantrolene sodium: A review of its pharmacological properties and therapeutic efficacy in spasticity. *Drugs* 1977;13:3–23.

Young RR, Delwaide PJ: Drug therapy: Spasticity (parts I & II). *N Engl J Med* 1981;304(1):28–33; 1981;304(2):96–99.

Drug Therapy for Tourette's Syndrome

Shapiro AK et al: Treatment of Gilles de la Tourette's syndrome with pimozide. *Am J Psychiatry* 1983;140:1183–1186.

CHAPTER 23

Antiepileptics

The Nature of Epilepsy

The term *epilepsy,* which is derived from a Greek word meaning *to seize,* encompasses a group of chronic disorders characterized by the occurrence of seizures. A **seizure** is an episode or attack in which there is a loss or disturbance of consciousness, sometimes accompanied by convulsions. Approximately 2 million Americans have epilepsy. Many are gainfully employed; others require prolonged hospitalization. Epilepsy does not generally shorten life, but neurological, psychiatric, or cognitive impairments can occur. Nevertheless, some of the greatest figures in history have been epileptics, including Alexander the Great, Julius Caesar, Mohammed, Peter the Great, Handel, Schiller, Mozart, Byron, Balzac, and Dostoevski.

Physiological Basis of Epilepsy

Epilepsy is related to the presence of a region of organic pathology in the brain, although in some cases, designated "idiopathic," the location of the pathological focus may not be apparent from the EEG because the focus lies too deep in the brain. The seizure focus may originate from congenital defects, cerebral trauma, ischemia caused by lesions in cerebral blood vessels or insufficiency of blood supply, tumors, infections, childhood illnesses, or hypoxia at birth. In grand mal epilepsy, the seizure focus lies within the cerebral cortex (Figure 23–1). In petit mal epilepsy, the seizure focus is subcortical, in the thalamus or midbrain (Figure 23–2). In positive spike pattern, the focus is in the thalamus or hypothala-

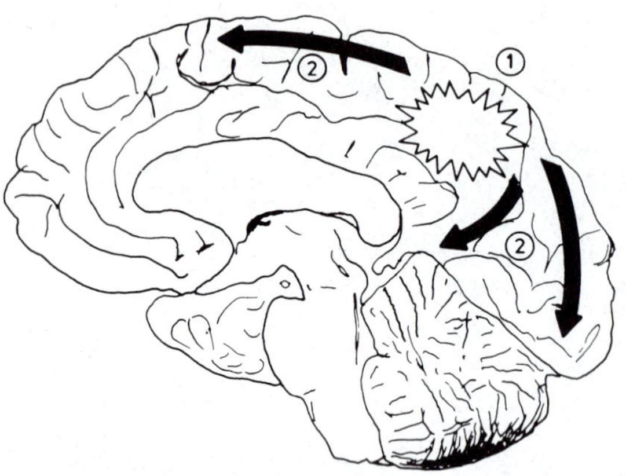

Figure 23–1
Pathogenesis of a grand mal seizure. A seizure focus (1) has developed as a result of localized damage due to organic causes such as hypoxia at birth or concussion. A reduction in cerebral inhibition permits the influence of the abnormal focal activity to spread (2) throughout the cortex. From A. K. Swonger and L. L. Constantine, *Drugs and Therapy*, 2nd ed. Boston: Little, Brown, 1983.

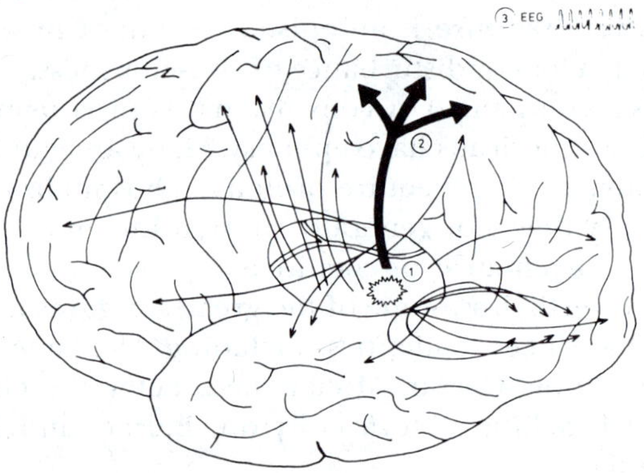

Figure 23–2
Pathogenesis of a petit mal seizure. In petit mal epilepsy, the seizure focus is subcortical (1). Abnormal discharges from the focus cause the diffuse thalamic projection system to produce (2) a characteristic 3 Hz spike-and-dome pattern of electrical activity (3) in the cortex. From A. K. Swonger and L. L. Constantine, *Drugs and Therapy*, 2nd ed. Boston: Little, Brown, 1983.

mus. Normally, the spread of electrical discharge from the seizure focus is prevented by cerebral inhibitory mechanisms. Seizures are initiated when physiological changes occur that facilitate the spread of paroxysmal discharges. Factors known to induce seizures are fatigue, emotional stress, hyperthermia, and changes in blood sugar levels, acidity, gas concentrations, electrolytes, or endocrine levels.

Types of Epilepsy

Grand Mal

Of the distinguishable forms of epilepsy, grand mal is the most common, occurring alone or in combination with other forms in 90% of cases. A grand mal attack is sometimes preceded by an **aura,** a vague premonitory symptom, of which gastric and visual sensations, paresthesias, or vertigo are the most common types. The aura is followed by convulsions during which the client loses consciousness. Convulsions may include either a tonic or clonic phase or both. When both occur, the tonic phase appears first and is short-lasting (about 3–15 seconds). Skeletal muscles tightly contract, the legs extend, arms cross over the chest, and the back arches. Respiration is impossible during this phase. In the clonic phase (clonus), the limbs flail about vigorously, and the person is at risk of concussion, injury to the limbs, or biting the tongue. Gradually, the clonic bursts subside into a restful coma. Slowly, the client regains consciousness and enters a period of postseizure depression. The interval between seizures may vary from a few minutes to years. When convulsive activity is continuous or when seizures come in rapid succession, the condition is known as **status epilepticus,** and can be fatal. Grand mal epilepsy is more common in males than females (Table 23–1).

Several less common forms of epilepsy are also characterized by occurrence of major (grand mal-like) seizures, but are distinguished by their etiologies (Table 23–1). The **petit mal variant** (not to be confused with petit mal epilepsy), also called Lennox-Gastaut syndrome, is associated in the electroencephalogram with a diffuse disturbance similar to petit mal in waveform, but slower. Neurological, psychiatric, and cognitive correlates are especially frequent in this form of epilepsy. **Infantile spasms** and **febrile convulsions** are two varieties that occur only in infants. In **focal seizures,** convulsive activity is limited to a particular part of the body, or to one side of the body. If an aura is present, its nature is often a clue to the location of the focus. When a seizure begins as a focal seizure and then gradually expands into a full grand mal convulsion, it is called a **Jacksonian seizure.**

Since many clients with epilepsy are at home, it is important for the nurse to teach their families how to care for them during a convulsion. *Nurses should instruct family members not to attempt to restrain the convulsing individual; instead, they should place a pillow or blanket under the head and loosen clothing that may be con-*

Table 23–1
Types of Epilepsy

Type of seizure	Age and sex correlates, seizure characteristics, and EEG correlates	Incidence of mental concomitants			
		Aura	Neuro-logical	Psychiatric	Cognitive
Grand mal	Onset: modal age groups 0–2 and 12–18 years; 59% males. Major convulsions and postseizure depression. Interval EEG may show spikes or may appear normal.	+	+	0	0
Petit mal variant	Onset: 65% before age 5; 95% before age 20; 58% males. Seizures may be mild (loss of posture, myoclonic jerks) or severe (major convulsions); seizures are frequent. Diffuse, spike and dome, <3 Hz.	0	+++	++	+++
Jacksonian and focal	Onset: 90% before age 10; 57% males. Frequency and type of seizure dependent on site and focus; partial convulsion. EEG shows localized abnormality.	++	+++	+	+
Febrile convulsions	Onset: before age 5. Triggered by fever; significant hereditary factor. Major convulsions.	0	+	0	0
Infantile spasms	Onset: by age 4; 65% boys. Major convulsions and progressive mental deterioration. Hypsarrhythmia.	0	++++	0	++
Petit mal (absences)	Onset: modal age is 5; 92% by age 15; 54% females. Syncope, loss of muscle tone, muscle fasciculations. 3 Hz spike and dome.	0	0	+	0
Psychomotor (temporal lobe) epilepsy	Onset: usually 10–30 years; 56% males. Blackouts. Interictal personality correlates.	+++	+	+++	+
Positive-spike pattern syndrome	Onset: modal age 12–18 years; 55% males. Major convulsions (55%); rage or tantrums (15%); syncope (30%); pain (20%).	+++	++	+++	+
Myoclonus	Isolated muscle contractions, combined with grand mal in 63% of cases. EEG often exhibits multiple spikes.	0	+	0	+

Key: 0, <8%; +, 8–17%; ++, 18–30%; +++, 31–50%, ++++, >50%.

stricting respiration or movement. A padded tongue depressor or other firm, soft object may be placed between the teeth to protect the tongue, but clenched teeth should not be forced apart. When the convulsion subsides, the client should be turned to the side to facilitate drainage of fluids from the respiratory tract. If the convulsing individual exhibits difficulty breathing, sustains injury, or experiences multiple convulsions in rapid succession, the family member should call for emergency help. Family members should be trained to make observations that will be relevant to later assessment by the nurse and physician, such as the type and distribution of movements, pupil size, seizure duration, and postseizure behavior of the client.

Petit Mal

Petit mal epilepsy differs considerably from grand mal. It is often referred to as **absence seizures** or **absences,** to further dissociate it from grand mal epilepsy and to reduce the stigma attached to use of the emotionally laden term *epilepsy.* In the EEG, particularly from the posterior frontal region of the brain, a pattern develops during petit mal seizures, called the **spike and dome.** This electrical disturbance is generated by the diffuse thalamic system under the influence of a seizure focus in the thalamus or midbrain. Petit mal epilepsy occurs mostly in children and slightly more frequently in girls than boys (see Table 23–1). Attacks are typically of short duration, from 5 to 15 seconds, and consist of syncope, or temporary cloudings of consciousness during which the individual may stare blankly or exhibit minor movements of the head or limbs. The individual is usually unaware of the attack and may become confused by the discontinuity of events. Psychiatric symptoms occur in 10% of petit mal clients, mainly in the category of behavioral problems.

Psychomotor Epilepsy

Psychomotor epilepsy is nearly synonymous with temporal lobe epilepsy since 90% of foci in the anterior temporal lobe produce the pattern of clinical presentation known as psychomotor epilepsy. This form of epilepsy is receiving increasing attention because of its association with psychopathological and even psychopathic behaviors. For example, an examination of individuals convicted of motiveless crimes indicated that some 70% had abnormal EEGs measured from temporal cortex. Psychomotor seizures are characterized by inappropriate activity that the client does not later recall. The acts may be innocuous, such as singing or undressing, or they may be violent and destructive. In 70% of cases of psychomotor epilepsy, grand mal is also present. Evidence of psychiatric disturbances is present between seizures in nearly 50% of clients with psychomotor epilepsy (or combined psychomotor and grand mal), three times the incidence of psychiatric concomitants in grand mal epilepsy. Typical psychiatric disturbances associated with psychomotor epilepsy include excessive daytime sleepiness, depression, suicidal tendencies, anxiety, hallucinations.

Auras are common in psychomotor epilepsy, with gastric auras occurring most often (in 11% of individuals). Other common types of aura in psychomotor epilepsy include déjà vu, visual, gustatory, auditory, or olfactory sensations, jamais vu, vertigo, nausea, paresthesia, or dream-like states. Psychomotor seizures have a great variety of common motor manifestations: incoordination, aggression, staring, groping, lip-smacking, swallowing, chewing, crying, laughing, shouting, screaming, confused talking, and undressing.

Another development in the understanding of epilepsy is the growing awareness that although **subictal** (or subseizure) varieties of temporal lobe epilepsy occur frequently, many are undiagnosed because of lack of hard signs (EEG findings may well be negative). One should suspect, however, that behavioral disturbances are secondary to subictal temporal lobe epilepsy when symptoms, such as explosive outbursts, appear to occur without provocation. Depression, hysterical symptoms, hallucinations, obsessional thinking, or anxiety are other behavior symptoms that may be linked to subictal states. Clues suggesting subictal psychomotor epilepsy are presence of the kinds of motor symptoms that occur during overt psychomotor seizures (see above), or frequent muscle fibrillations, twitchings, or involuntary uncoordinated movements of the extremities. When one or more of these signs of possible subictal temporal lobe epilepsy is present, a trial treatment with primidone (Mysoline), phenytoin (Dilantin), or phenobarbital may be initiated; an inferential diagnosis can then be made based on responsiveness of the behavioral symptoms to antiepileptic medication.

Positive Spike Pattern

Electroencephalographic evaluation of a client may identify the presence of positive spike pattern (see Table 23–1) characterized by the occurrence of 14 Hz and 6 Hz positive spikes. Psychiatric manifestations occur in 38% of clients and neurological correlates in 21%. Some clients have outbursts of intense rage; in other cases, affect may be severely blunted. Painful sensations are experienced by 20% of individuals with this syndrome and there may be autonomic dysfunctions and bodily aches as well as behavioral disorders. It is easy to attribute such symptoms to psychogenic origins if the positive spike pattern goes undetected.

Myoclonus

Myoclonus, a term of variable meaning to different clinicians, is the occurrence of isolated, involuntary muscular jerks of a clonic type (twitching movements, fasciculations, or contractions), occurring singly or in brief showers lasting 3–6 seconds. Myoclonias may be essential (primary) or secondary to a variety of neurological disorders, including encephalitis (acute and slow viral infections), encephalopathies, intoxications (mercury, methyl bromide, penicillin, imipramine, tetanus toxin), degenerative dementias, lipidoses (such as Tay-Sachs disease), and seizure disorders (infantile spasms or petit mal variant are sometimes classified as myoclonic epilepsies).

Nearly 30% of cases of essential myoclonias are unrelated to epilepsy or other extrapyramidal syndromes. In these cases, isolated clonic jerks (often associated with EEG spikes) are evoked by sensory stimuli and may be limited or generalized in distribution, rhythmic or dysrhythmic, or symmetrical or asymmetrical. Generally, the myoclonias of brainstem or spinal origin are rhythmic, while those originating in higher centers are dysrhythmic. The frequency of contractions increases in the morning, with fatigue and stress, and prior to the onset of menstruation. Among the essential myoclonias is paramyoclonus multiplex, a hereditary and progressive degenerative disorder.

Nocturnal myoclonus (fasciculations and jerks) occurs in virtually all normal people during stage 1 of slow-wave sleep. If such myoclonic episodes are too intense, the sleeper may be startled awake. Insomnia and excessive daytime sleepiness occur secondarily if such awakenings are frequent.

At least some forms of myoclonus are related to a deficiency of serotonin activity in the brain. A combination of the serotonin precursor, L-5-hydroxytryptophan, and carbidopa (a peripheral decarboxylase inhibitor) is often an effective treatment. Among the antiepileptics, only clonazepam (Clonopin) and valproic acid (Depakene) are notably effective in myoclonus.

EEG Diagnosis of Epilepsy

A number of reflections of epilepsy may occur in the EEG. In grand mal epilepsy, an electrode placed immediately above the focus will usually reveal a sharp, biphasic spike recurring at variable intervals (Figure 23–3). An abnormal slow wave may be seen instead, but this usually indicates the seizure focus is slightly removed from the electrode placement, either laterally or at a depth. Sometimes a *mirror* focus is found in the corresponding area of the opposite hemisphere, especially in temporal lobe epilepsy. If the focus lies so deep in the cortical tissue that it cannot be localized by means of the EEG, the epilepsy is *idiopathic* epilepsy, indicating an unknown cause.

The most dramatic and specific correlation between the EEG and a disease state is the occurrence of characteristic 3 Hz spike-and-dome discharges in petit mal. This complex consists of a sharp spike followed by a large-amplitude slow wave, which repeats with great regularity at a rate of 3 per second (Figure 23–4). The pattern may occur diffusely and symmetrically throughout the cortex, but it is particularly prominent in the posterior portion of the frontal lobe.

During a grand mal attack, an intense mixture of sharp spikes and high-amplitude theta or beta ac-

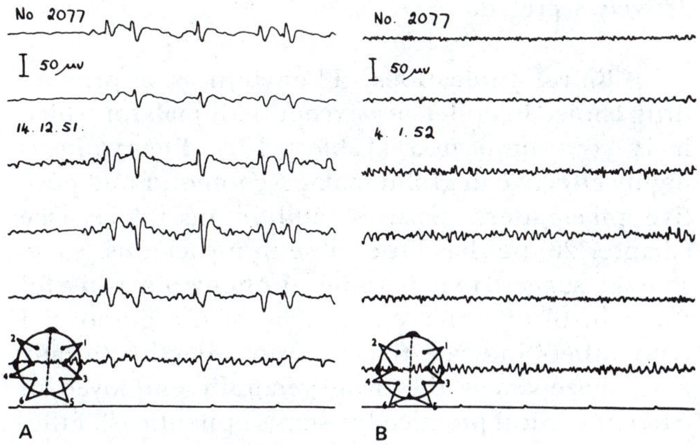

Figure 23–3
EEG tracing from six lead pairs showing focal discharges in a patient with a 32-year history of grand mal seizures. (A) Before treatment. (B) After treatment with phenytoin. From R. R. Hughes, *An Introduction to Clinical Electro-Encephalography,* Bristol, England: John Wright & Sons, Ltd., 1961.

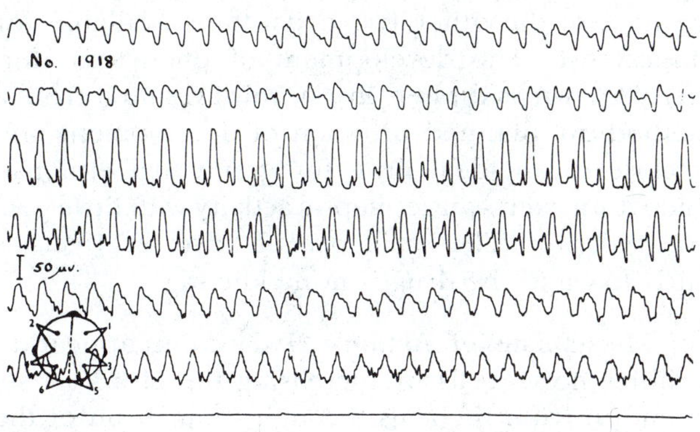

Figure 23–4
EEG tracing from six lead pairs showing typical petit mal spike-and-dome pattern. From R. R. Hughes, *An Introduction to Clinical Electro-Encephalography.* Bristol, England: John Wright & Sons, Ltd., 1961.

tivity can be observed that gradually subsides as the seizure concludes. The subsequent period of coma is accompanied by a markedly depressed (flat-line) EEG recording and the postictal depression by an EEG pattern consisting mainly of theta waves.

Antiepileptic Drugs Used Primarily for Major or Psychomotor Seizures

The term **anticonvulsant** should be used to denote a drug (such as diazepam, phenobarbital, or ultrashort-acting barbiturates) that is effective in terminating the drug-induced or epileptiform seizure itself, while the term **antiepileptic** should be used to denote an agent employed chronically to reduce the frequency of seizures in an epileptic. However, the term *anticonvulsant* is employed commonly for both categories of drugs. Medication with antiepileptic drugs is often a lifelong proposition, but seizure foci do undergo slow change over long periods of time, resulting in stabilization or deterioration. Some physicians will attempt to eliminate drug therapy after a period of 2–5 years without seizures.

There is no one drug of choice for epilepsy, since each drug is effective in only certain kinds of epilepsy. For grand mal epilepsy, the primary drug choices are phenytoin and phenobarbital.

Hydantoin Derivatives

Phenytoin (Dilantin, Diphenylan, Ditan, and generic formulations) is a hydantoin drug and is the best-studied, most widely employed, and least toxic of the group. Mephenytoin (Mesantoin) and ethotoin (Peganone) are the other two hydantoins available for clinical use. The development of phenytoin (formerly known as diphenylhydantoin) resulted from a methodical, planned program of development and is close to an ideal drug for grand mal epilepsy. Phenytoin exerts antiepileptic activity with little general sedation. The incidence of adverse effects is fairly low and the drug is nonaddicting.

Mechanism of Action Hydantoins appear to stabilize nerve cells by increasing the efflux of sodium ion from the cells through stimulation of the sodium pump (Figure 23–5), causing neuronal hyperpolarization. The increased stability of cortical neurons reduces the spread of abnormal discharges from the seizure focus to surrounding cortical areas.

Pharmacokinetics After oral administration, phenytoin is slowly absorbed from the small intestine. The various pharmaceutical preparations of phenytoin exhibit clear differences in rate and extent of absorption, so that alternative products are not bioequivalent. *The nurse should advise clients not to change from one phenytoin product to another.* Phenytoin is available in both prompt and extended dosage forms, the former typically requiring administration three times per day, the latter once per day. Phenytoin prompt produces peak plasma levels in about 2–3 hours and phenytoin extended in about 5–6 hours. Total absorption is greater per dosage unit for phenytoin prompt than for phenytoin extended. Absorption after IM administration of phenytoin is slow and unreliable, with peak plasma levels occurring typically after about 24 hours.

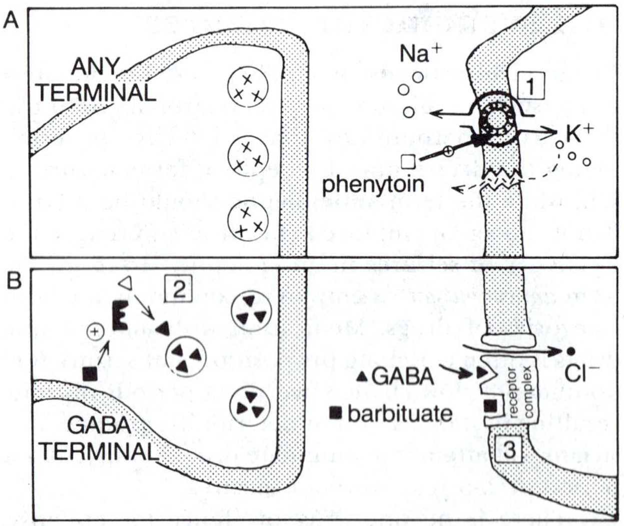

Figure 23–5
Neurochemical mechanisms of primary drug choices for grand mal epilepsy. (A) Phenytoin (Dilantin) stimulates the $NA^+ - K^+$ exchange pump to hyperpolarize nerve cells, increasing cortical inhibition. (B) Barbiturates facilitate synthesis and binding of GABA, increasing inhibitory neurotransmission. From A. K. Swonger and L. L. Constantine, *Drugs and Therapy,* 2nd ed. Boston: Little, Brown, 1983.

After absorption, phenytoin is highly bound (87–93%) to plasma proteins. Plasma concentrations correlate well with clinical efficacy. Concentrations below 5 μg/ml are not efficacious; levels of 5–10 μg/ml are efficacious in some clients; concentrations from 10 to 20 μg/ml are reliably effective; and levels of 30–50 μg/ml produce toxicity. The approximate fatal concentration of phenytoin is 100 μg/ml. For ethotoin, effective plasma concentrations are approximately 15–50 μg/ml.

Both phenytoin and ethotoin are metabolized in the liver in a reaction that follows zero order kinetics, which means that as the dose of one of these drugs is increased, the half-life becomes progressively longer. In addition, the rate of metabolism of hydantoins varies from one individual to another and is influenced by drug interactions. The result is that the half-life of phenytoin varies from as little as 8 to as much as 60 hours (even without the influence of drug interactions). Steady-state plasma concentrations typically occur after about 7–10 days of daily use of phenytoin. The half-life of ethotoin is shorter (about 3–9 hours) but similarly variable. Because of the high degree of variability in the pharmacokinetics of hydantoins, titration of dosage using serum level determinations is a requisite initial component of therapy. A small amount of phenytoin (about 1–5%) is excreted unchanged in the urine, being actively secreted.

Clinical Indications Phenytoin is a primary drug choice in epilepsies except petit mal, for which it is contraindicated (Table 23–2). Phenytoin is highly effective in grand mal, psychomotor and positive-spike-pattern seizures, and in neuralgias (see Chapter 26) but has little value in myoclonus. Some sources suggest that parenteral phenytoin is useful for control of status epilepticus of the grand mal type; others indicate that it is not effective (in any case, diazepam is the drug generally employed in current clinical practice for status epilepticus). Ethotoin is comparable in efficacy and adverse effects with phenytoin, but is shorter acting, requiring more frequent administration. Mephenytoin is more potent and more toxic than phenytoin and is reserved for clients with severe grand mal, psychomotor, focal, or Jacksonian seizures that are refractory to primary drug selections.

Table 23–2
Drug Spectra in the Treatment of Epilepsy

Type of drug	Type of seizure: Grand mal	Status epilepticus	Petit mal	Psycho-motor	Myoclonus	Infantile spasms
Hydantoins	++++	0	–	+++	+	0
Barbiturates	+++	++	+	++	+	0
Primidone	+++	0	+	++++	+++	+
Oxazolidones	–	–	++++	0	0	0
Succinimides	–	–	+++	0	0	0
Diazepam	+	++++	++	0	+++	+
Clonazepam	+	++++	+++	0	++++	++
Valproic acid	++	0	+++	++	+++	+

Key: +, efficacy in treatment; 0, no efficacy; –, contraindicated.

Adverse Effects and Contraindications The overall toxicity of phenytoin or ethotoin is low in comparison with that of most other antiepileptics and with that of psychotropic drugs in general. In comparison with phenobarbital, phenytoin has (1) the advantages of less sedation for a given level of efficacy and freedom from abuse potential, (2) more frequent hypersensitivity reactions, (3) a narrower spectrum of effectiveness (being contraindicated in petit mal), (4) more frequent side effects, especially hyperplasia of the gums, and (5) a higher incidence of teratogenicity when phenytoin is used during pregnancy. In the case of antiepileptic drugs, the risk of teratogenic effects on the fetus must be weighed against the risks of seizures in the mother for both the mother and the fetus. Use of phenytoin by women who are nursing also requires a careful weighing of risks and benefits.

Hyperplasia (overgrowth) and softening of the gums is the most common difficulty with phenytoin, occurring in about 20% of clients. It can be prevented or controlled in many cases by good oral hygiene, including increased brushing of the gums. *The nurse should advise clients to brush their teeth, daily or more frequently, with a soft toothbrush and to floss in order to remove dental plaque. If the client is a child, the parents should be instructed to brush and floss the child's teeth once daily up to ages 6–8.*

The next most common adverse effects of hydantoins are neurological or psychiatric signs of **excess depression:** ataxia, slurred speech, irritability, mental confusion, depression, or fatigue. These symptoms are dose related and may be lessened by a reduction of dosage. Motor disturbances which may occur include nystagmus, twitching, tremor, and transient hyperkinesias. Other neurological side effects include diplopia, dysarthria, headache, and psychotic disturbances. *The nurse should advise clients to avoid hazardous activities, such as driving during early therapy with phenytoin in particular.*

Gastrointestinal discomfort may occur with phenytoin, though it is not common or severe, because the drug is strongly alkaline. *Administration of phenytoin with or shortly after meals or with a half-glass of milk or water often helps to relieve nausea, vomiting, or diarrhea.* **Hematopoietic toxicity** occurs occasionally with hydantoins and can be fatal. Reactions have included thrombocytopenia, leukopenia, granulocytopenia, and pancytopenia. Megaloblastic anemia occurs occasionally, but responds well to administration of folic acid (folic acid supplements are recommended for clients receiving hydantoins). Lymphadenopathy occurs occasionally in response to hydantoins and requires temporary discontinuation of the medication. *Every effort should be made to substitute another antiepileptic for the hydantoin if lymphadenopathy occurs.*

Hydantoins can produce a full range of **dermatological eruptions.** Mild rashes are most common (usually of a morbilliform appearance, but sometimes urticarial or maculopapular). Photophobia can occur as well as serious and even fatal skin eruptions, such as toxic epidermal necrolysis, exfoliative dermatitis, lupus erythematosus, and erythema multiforme. *Hydantoins should be discontinued if any skin rash or eruption occurs and would not be recommended if the eruption is one of the more serious varieties.*

Hydantoins may cause or aggravate hyperglycemia by inhibiting release of insulin, so that dia-

Nursing Observations for Antiepileptic Drug Therapy

THERAPEUTIC GOAL	Eliminate seizures or, if that is not feasible, reduce their frequency and severity.
PREADMINISTRATION ASSESSMENT	
Baseline Data	Observe occurrences of syncope, muscle twitches, loss of muscle tone (petit mal); tonic or clonic convulsions (grand mal); episodes of bizarre behavior with subsequent amnesia (psychomotor). Evaluate the interval EEG for regions of abnormal spike or flat line patterns (grand mal); evaluate EEG for spike-and-dome pattern (petit mal); examine EEG for temporal lobe foci (psychomotor). Before instituting drug therapy, monitor neurological status (affect, orientation, reflexes, and EEG), vital signs, ECG, gastrointestinal function, and conditon of skin and mucosal membranes. Obtain laboratory tests including complete blood cell count, blood sugar, liver function tests, and urinalysis.
Contraindications/ Precautions	Hepatic or renal failure, hypotension, A-V block, bone marrow suppression, pregnancy, or lactation. Check medication history for drug allergies.
Potential Interactions	Check current medications for interacting drugs, including any other CNS depressants, inducers of liver enzymes, or drugs bound to plasma proteins.
EVALUATION OF DRUG RESPONSE	
During Dosage Adjustment	Monitor plasma levels for antiepileptic drugs with established therapeutic plasma concentrations.
For Therapeutic Benefit	Monitor changes in the incidence of seizures.
For Adverse Effects	Monitor for excess depression, allergic reactions, and other side effects specific for each antiepileptic drug (see individual drug discussions).
For Drug Interactions	Monitor for additive CNS depression, competition for plasma protein binding sites, altered metabolism of drugs due to induction of liver enzymes, and other drug-specific interactions (see drug discussions).
For Dietary Interactions	Monitor for vitamin deficiencies with phenytoin or primidone. Observe for general nutritional deficiency when particular drugs cause nausea, vomiting, or anorexia.
For Compliance	Evaluate client's compliance with all facets of the therapeutic regimen by careful observation, interviewing, and review of progress. Report compliance problems to the physician and act as client-advocate when changes in the therapeutic regimen seem indicated.

betic clients require special monitoring if phenytoin therapy is initiated. Hydantoins can also cause hepatitis, jaundice, hepatocellular degeneration, and fatal hepatocellular necrosis. *It is advisable to conduct liver function tests prior to initiating treatment with phenytoin and at monthly intervals during prolonged therapy.* Other adverse effects include alopecia, hirsutism, polyarteritis nodosa (Kussmaul's disease), pulmonary fibrosis, and acute pneumonitis. *The nurse should advise clients that phenytoin may impart a harmless pink or red-brown coloration to the urine.*

Drug-Drug and Drug-Diet Interactions Hydantoins exhibit a large variety of interactions with other drugs. Hydantoins **decrease the activity of other drugs** mainly through the induction of liver enzymes. Thus the metabolism of oral anticoagulants (such as dicumarol), antidysrhythmics (such as disopyramide (Norpace) or quinidine), corticosteroids, estrogens, and digitoxin are all increased by concurrent, chronic use of hydantoins. The effectiveness of oral contraceptives may be impaired, resulting in breakthrough bleeding or unanticipated pregnancy. Phenytoin also reportedly decreases intestinal absorption of furosemide.

Hydantoins **increase the activity of other drugs** mainly by competing for plasma protein binding sites. Thus, phenytoin will increase the anticoagulant action of warfarin by displacing it from inactive protein binding sites. Aspirin toxicity can also be increased in this manner. Phenytoin has been reported to increase the hypotensive effect of dopamine infusion, but no mechanism for this interaction has been established.

Drugs that **increase the action of hydantoins** include agents that inhibit liver metabolism of hydantoins, displace hydantoins from plasma protein binding sites, or have additive depressant effects. Coumarin anticoagulants, disulfiram (Antabuse), phenylbutazone (Azolid), dexamethasone, cimetidine, (Tagamet), isoniazid, sulfonamides and chloramphenicol (Chloromycetin) retard the metabolism of phenytoin. Aspirin and other salicylates displace phenytoin from plasma protein binding sites, increasing the free fraction and the pharmacological activity of the hydantoin. The depressant effects of other CNS depressants are potentially additive with those of hydantoins. *Clients should be warned to avoid use of alcohol in conjunction with antiepileptic medications.*

Drugs that **decrease the action of hydantoins** do so mainly by inducing their metabolism or impairing their absorption. Barbiturates, carbamazepine (Tegretol), and other inducers of liver enzymes speed the metabolism of phenytoin. Regular supplements of folic acid, which may be required in individuals receiving hydantoins, can also speed metabolism of phenytoin. Absorption of hydantoins can be impaired by concurrent administration of calcium supplements or salts, antacids (containing aluminum, magnesium, or calcium salts), oxacillin, or certain antineoplastic agents (vinblastine (Velban), cisplatin (Platinal), and bleomycin (Blenoxane)).

Drugs that lower the seizure threshold, such as tricyclic antidepressants, neuroleptics, and narcotics may **alter the dosage requirements for antiepileptic medications.** *Clients receiving these drugs should be monitored closely for signs of increasing seizure liability.* Phenytoin has been reported to interfere with the metapyrone and the dexamethasone tests of adrenal cortical functioning, as well as measurements of unbound T_4.

Clients who require prolonged therapy with phenytoin need adequate amounts of vitamin D, through vitamin D-rich foods in their diets, supplements, or sufficient exposure to sunlight. They should also have frequent checks for decreased levels of serum calcium, since phenytoin can contribute to demineralization of bone, resulting in rickets in children or osteomalacia in adults. The risk of vitamin D or calcium deficiency in conjunction with phenytoin therapy is especially great in clients who are inactive, have inadequate diets, lack exposure to sunlight, or receive additional antiepileptic medications. Black children are also especially susceptible.

Preparations and Administration The oral suspension should be thoroughly shaken before pouring to ensure uniform mixing. The importance of compliance needs to be especially emphasized when antiepileptic medications, such as phenytoin, are prescribed because the therapeutic benefit is essentially one of prophylaxis against subsequent seizures and is not readily apparent to the client. Clients should not alter the prescribed drug regimen nor purchase another drug brand when filling prescriptions, because phenytoin exhibits variable dissolution and absorption rates that result in significantly different serum levels and effectiveness from one brand to another. Phenytoin should be stored between 15 and 30°C (59–86°F).

The margin between therapeutic and toxic levels is very narrow when the drug is administered by IV injection. *Therefore the nurse needs to monitor blood pressure, pulse, and respirations and note evidence of central nervous system side effects, such as complaints of blurred or dimmed vision, drowsiness, dizziness, slurred speech, nystagmus, confusion, muscle twitching, hallucinations, or back and forth eye movements.* Phenytoin sodium generates a sodium load of 0.35 mEq per 100 mg capsule and 0.2 mEq per ml for the injectable form, which can be significant for clients on sodium-restricted diets for hypertension. Phenytoin is tapered slowly when discontinued over 1–3 months, using serum concentrations and EEG readings as guides, to minimize the risk of seizure recurrence. *Hydantoins are best taken with or shortly after food to minimize gastrointestinal irritation.*

Ethotoin (Peganone)
Tablets
Recommended Doses: For adults, 1,000 mg/day or less initially, in 4–6 divided oral doses. Based on response, this dose is usually increased gradually to a typical daily adult dosage of 2–3 g daily. For children, 750 mg/day initially. For maintenance in children, 500 mg to 1 g daily.

Mephenytoin (Mesantoin)
Tablets
Recommended doses: 50–100 mg/day PO initially, increased as required by increments of 50–100 mg/day at intervals of no less than 1 week. The typical maintenance level in adults is 200–600 mg/day and in children 100–400 mg/day.

Phenytoin (Dilantin, Ditan, and generic formulations)
Capsules, chewable tablets, extended action capsules, combination tablets with phenobarbital, oral suspensions, injection solution
Recommended Doses: For adults, 300 mg orally daily, in 3 doses if the prompt-acting dosage forms are employed or as a single daily dose when the extended action capsule is selected. For children, 5 mg/kg/day initially in 2 or 3 divided doses. Doses must be individualized for each client by

Nursing Diagnoses and Interventions for Antiepileptic Drug Therapy

Nursing Diagnoses	*Related Interventions*
TO ENHANCE DRUG BENEFITS OR REDUCE DRUG REQUIREMENTS	
Disturbance of self-concept related to interruption of developmental tasks	Provide emotional support, encouragement, and remedial help. Provide praise for tasks well done.
Fear related to anticipation of seizures	Explain the therapeutic plan; provide support and encouragement. Introduce to a peer group of successfully controlled seizure patients.
Increased risk of injury related to clonic convulsions	Teach clients to recognize warning signals of impending seizures and to lie down on something soft if possible: teach family members how to provide protection during convulsions. If present during a convulsion, place a pad under the head and a padded tongue blade between the teeth. Support the head and protect it from injury.
Social isolation related to fear of having a seizure in public	Provide emotional support and reassurance. Provide name of local support groups for people with epilepsy.
TO MINIMIZE DRUG SIDE EFFECTS OR INTERACTIONS	
Activity intolerance related to excess depression with antiepileptic medications	Advocate a reduction in the dosage of medication or addition of a stimulant to the regimen; provide adequate rest.
Alteration in bowel elimination: constipation with phenytoin (Dilantin)	Give phenytoin with food and plenty of water to minimize gastrointestinal disturbances. Encourage intake of fiber-rich foods.
Alteration in comfort: headache or joint pain from phenytoin	Provide analgesics for headache or arthralgia as required.
Alteration in nutrition related to nausea, vomiting, dysphagia, dysgeusia, or gingival hyperplasia from phenytoin; vitamin K deficiency with primidone	Provide nutritional information; supplement vitamins D, K, and folic acid when phenytoin is used chronically; advise client to take drug with meals to reduce GI upset; supplement vitamin K when primidone is employed.
Alteration of oral mucosal membranes related to gingival hyperplasia with phenytoin	Provide intensified oral hygiene; instruct client to use a soft toothbrush and to floss at least daily.
Alteration in thought processes: confusion related to phenytoin or other CNS depressants	Advocate reducing the doses of depressant medications; provide safety measures as indicated.
Impaired verbal communication related to slurred speech with phenytoin	Advocate a reduction in dosage of phenytoin. Teach clients methods of slowing speech to reduce slurring.
Sensory-perceptual alteration related to blurred or dimmed vision caused by phenytoin; hallucinations with phenytoin or succinimides	Warn clients about operating motor vehicles or dangerous machinery while drug effects are occurring.
Sleep pattern disturbance: REM suppression with phenobarbital	Explain that tolerance will occur to this effect with chronic use.
TO ENSURE SAFE AND EFFICACIOUS DRUG USE	
Knowledge deficit related to drug regimen	Explain the nature of the particular type of epilepsy, correcting misconceptions or partial information the client or family may have.

Explain the rationale for the therapeutic regimen.

Assure that the client and family understand how to administer the medications in accordance with the directions.

Provide client with a list of adverse effects and drug interactions for each drug in the regimen and explain what to do if any of these occur.

Advise female clients that adjustments in the regimen may be required if pregnancy occurs or is anticipated.

measurement of serum concentrations. Usually it is advantageous during the initial phase of treatment to employ the prompt-acting forms while doses are being adjusted. After an effective dosage level has been determined for the individual client, it is often convenient to give the full daily dose in a single administration using the slower-acting form. For clients who are elderly, debilitated, or those with liver damage, lower doses are required. *IV injection followed by a sterile saline flush through the same needle or catheter (to avoid local venous irritation caused by the alkalinity of phenytoin solution) is the preferred method of parenteral administration.* Addition to an IV infusate is not recommended because phenytoin is physically incompatible with most IV fluids and will form a precipitate. IM injection is also to be avoided because of erratic absorption. IV doses of 150–250 mg are employed for status epilepticus, with an additional 100–150 mg given 30 minutes later if required.

Barbiturates

Phenobarbital, the first antiepileptic with an acceptable level of toxicity, is still widely prescribed and is the other primary drug choice besides phenytoin for grand mal epilepsy. The overall incidence of side effects is slighly less than with phenytoin, teratogenicity is less, and phenobarbital is not contraindicated in any form of epilepsy. On the other hand, the abuse liability and greater degree of sedation are limiting features of the barbiturates. Tolerance creates a problem with respect to termination of drug treatment. Withdrawal of a client from barbiturate medication must be accomplished slowly, since seizure liability increases during sedative-hypnotic withdrawal. Antiepileptic potency is usually evident at doses that do not produce an unacceptable level of sedation. If higher dosages are required, phenobarbital can be given in combination with amphetamine, which has weak antiepileptic effects of its own, but more importantly, counters the sedative effect of the barbiturate.

Mechanisms and Effects The mechanism of the antiepileptic action of barbiturates is attributed to the effects of barbiturates on transmission that utilizes gamma-aminobutyric acid (GABA) (Figure 23–5). Only the long-acting barbiturates are appreciably useful in epilepsy because of the chronic nature of the illness. In any case, phenobarbital, mephobarbital (Mebaral), and metharbital (Gemonil) possess a special potency as antiepileptics because of the phenyl group that each of these long-acting barbiturates possesses. Mephobarbital is active in its own right as an antiepileptic, but is also metabolized in part to phenobarbital, which in this context is an active metabolite.

Clinical Indications Long-acting barbiturates are useful for long-term prophylactic therapy against focal seizures and generalized tonic, clonic, or tonic-clonic seizures of the grand mal type. They are less effective in myoclonus, petit mal seizures, and mixed types (grand mal with petit mal, grand mal with psychomotor epilepsy). Phenobarbital is also used for acute control of convulsive episodes caused by status epilepticus, eclampsia, meningitis, tetanus, or toxic reactions to local anesthetics or strychnine.

Adverse Effects and Contraindications Adverse reactions to barbiturates are discussed in detail in Chapter 12. The side effects fall into five categories: (1) excess depression, (2) tolerance and dependence, (3) suppression of dreaming sleep, (4) paradoxical excitation, and (5) allergic reactions. Skin rash develops in about 2% of individuals receiving phenobarbital and, rarely, fatal drug eruptions. *The use of bedrails may be advisable when phenobarbital is given to elderly clients or children because of the frequent incidence of paradoxical excitation. Nurses should warn clients that* *the depressant effects of barbiturates may impair performance of hazardous tasks. Nurses and family members should watch for signs of excess depression, such as ataxia, nystagmus, and somnolence. Nurses should also advise clients not to keep barbiturates at bedside because of the risk of taking the drug by mistake should they awaken during the night.*

Although barbiturates are considered less hazardous than phenytoin for use during pregnancy, they can nevertheless cause birth defects. Risks must be weighed against benefits in deciding whether or not to use antiepileptic medications during pregnancy. Possible teratogenicity of barbiturates is a special concern because oral contraception is less reliable when barbiturates are also being employed. *Nurses should so advise female clients of childbearing age.* Although hematological reactions are not common in response to barbiturates, individuals on prolonged therapy with these drugs should be advised to report immediately the occurrence of persistent fever, sore throat, easy bruising, mucosal bleeding, petechiae, jaundice, or rash.

Preparations and Administration *Phenobarbital solutions for injection are prepared by slowly mixing sterile water into an ampul containing phenobarbital powder and rotating the ampul to hasten dissolution. Solutions containing a precipitate should be discarded. Phenobarbital solutions should be used within 30 minutes of preparation. IM injections should be deep into a large muscle mass; after injections, vital signs should be closely monitored.*

Phenobarbital (Luminal, Barbita, Solfoton, PBR, and generic formulations)
Tablets, capsules, timed release capsules, drops, liquid, elixir, injection solutions, powder for reconstitution and injection
Recommended Doses: For epilepsy in adults, 50–100 mg PO, 2 or 3 times daily. The timed release form is taken in the morning and at bedtime, 65 mg each occasion. For children, 4–6 mg/kg/day initially for 7–10 days; adjusted to achieve a serum concentration of 10–15 μg/ml. The timed release form is not recommended for children under age 12. For alleviating convulsions, eclampsia, or status epilepticus, 200–300 mg IM or IV in adults or 3–5 mg/kg/dose (125 mg/m^2/dose) IM in infants or children. The dose can be repeated if required after 6 hours.

Mephobarbital (Mebaral)
Tablets
Recommended Doses: For epilepsy in adults, 400–600 mg PO daily. For children over age 5, 32–64 mg, 3 or 4 times per day; for children under age 5, 16–32 mg, 3 or 4 times daily. Treatment is initiated with small doses, which are later gradually increased.

Metharbital (Gemonil)
Tablets
Recommended Doses: For adults, 100 mg PO initially, 1–3 times daily. The recommended dose in children is 5–15 mg/kg/day. Dosages must be individualized in accordance with client response to obtain an optimal effect (doses of metharbital as high as 600–800 mg daily have been employed).

Primidone (Mysoline)

Primidone is a close relative of the barbiturates. It is a potent antiepileptic but is more likely to produce adverse effects than are phenobarbital or phenytoin. Although it is considered a secondary choice for grand mal and focal seizures, it has special usefulness in psychomotor epilepsy for which it is often employed as a first-line drug. It is useful in combinations with phenytoin or barbiturates for refractory cases of grand mal or focal epilepsy. Primidone has been used experimentally for control of essential tremor, an inherited extrapyramidal disorder.

Mechanism of Action and Pharmacokinetics The mechanism of action of primidone is not known. Primidone is active in its own right but also yields two active metabolites: phenobarbital (15–25% of total metabolism) and phenylethylmalonamide (PEMA) — the major metabolite. After administration orally, primidone is readily absorbed, reaching peak plasma levels in 0.5–9 hours (average 3.0 hours). Peak serum concentrations are achieved more rapidly upon initial administration than with repeated dosing. Primidone and PEMA are not substantially bound to plasma proteins. Primidone itself is inactivated with a half-life of 3–12 hours, but the active metabolites have half-lives of 1–2 days for PEMA and 2–6 days for phenobarbital. Accumulation of active metabolites occurs with chronic use; steady-state plasma concentrations may be achieved only after 7–10 days at a given dosage level. Monitoring of therapy requires measurements of phenobarbital as well as primidone. Therapeutic plasma concentrations are 5–12 μg/ml for primidone and 15–45 μg/ml for phenobarbital.

Adverse Effects and Contraindications The most common adverse reactions to primidone are indications of excessive **CNS depression,** such as ataxia and vertigo. These responses usually disappear with continued use of the drug or dosage reduction. *Clients should be advised that depressant effects of primidone may lead to impaired performance of hazardous tasks such as driving an automobile. Since the depressant effect of primidone is potentially additive with that of alcohol or* *other depressant drugs, clients should be cautioned against use of alcoholic beverages or over-the-counter medications without the approval of the physician.*

Primidone sometimes causes **gastrointestinal disturbances,** including nausea, anorexia, and vomiting. *The nurse should advise clients to take primidone with food if gastrointestinal upset occurs.* Primidone has also been noted to cause irritability, emotional disturbances, sexual impotency, headache, diplopia, and nystagmus. Rarely, mood changes and reactions of paranoia occur. **Allergic reactions** usually take the form of a morbilliform skin rash. *Primidone, like phenytoin, can cause a drug-induced folic acid deficiency leading to megaloblastic anemia. This disorder can be prevented or treated by folic acid supplements (about 15 mg daily).* Primidone should not be taken by nursing mothers. The drug appears in breast milk and has been noted to cause somnolence and drowsiness in newborn children. The effects of primidone use during pregnancy are not known except that neonatal hemorrhaging has been reported in newborns whose mothers were receiving primidone. *Pregnant women should receive vitamin K, 1–5 mg daily, for 1 month prior to delivery as prophylaxis against this effect.* Abrupt discontinuation of primidone results in a transient period of increased seizure liability.

Preparations and Administration

Primidone (Mysoline and generic formulations)
Tablets, oral suspension
Recommended Doses: For adults and children over 8 years of age, 100–125 mg PO at bedtime on days 1–3; 100–125 mg twice daily on days 4–6; 100–125 mg, tid on days 7–9; and maintenance therapy thereafter at a typical dose of 250 mg, 3 or 4 times daily. Doses must be individualized to achieve optimal results. The maximum recommended dose is 500 mg, 4 times daily. For children under 8, 50 mg at bedtime for 3 days; 50 mg twice daily for the next 3 days; 100 mg twice daily for 3 additional days; and maintenance therapy beginning with day 10 at doses of 125–250 mg, 3 times daily.

Carbamazepine (Tegretol)

Clinical Indications Carbamazepine is a potent antiepileptic agent that is reserved for treatment of cases refractory to first line drugs because of its substantial potential for severe adverse reactions. It is especially valuable for psychomotor seizures, generalized tonic-clonic seizures, and mixed seizure patterns but is ineffective in petit mal epilepsy. Carbamazepine has also exhibited exceptional efficacy for treatment of neuralgias (see Chapter 26). Carbamazepine has been used experimentally for treatment of manic-depressive disorder, alcohol withdrawal, and other psychiatric conditions, but there are no adequately controlled studies demonstrating that it has value in any of these disorders and it is not FDA-approved for these applications.

Pharmacokinetics Carbamazepine is well absorbed after oral administration, but plasma concentrations are variable (ranging from 0.5 to 25 μg/ml), with an inconsistent relationship to doses administered. Absorption of carbamazepine is enhanced when it is taken with food. In the blood, it is about 75% bound to plasma proteins. Concentrations in the cerebrospinal fluid reach about 22% of the serum level. Carbamazepine readily crosses the placental barrier and accumulates in fetal tissue. It is inactivated by liver metabolism and the metabolic products appear in the urine (75%) and in the feces (25%). The initial elimination half-life of 25–65 hours declines to 12–17 hours with repeated administrations.

Adverse Effects and Contraindications Common adverse reactions to carbamazepine are **CNS depression** (dizziness, drowsiness, confusion, fatigue, and unsteadiness) and mild **gastrointestinal disturbances** (nausea and vomiting). The latter problem can be alleviated somewhat by taking the drug with food. Less common CNS reactions include headache, visual hallucinations, speech disturbances, hyperkinesias, talkativeness, agitated depression, tinnitus, and paralysis. If neurological symptoms persist beyond the first week of therapy, dosage reduction should be initiated. *Clients should be warned that CNS depression due to carbamazepine may impair performance of hazardous tasks. Bedrails may be required for individuals exhibiting agitation.*

The limiting feature of carbamazepine is the occurrence of **hematological reactions,** including leukopenia, aplastic anemia, agranulocytosis, eosinophilia, leukocytosis, and thrombocytopenia. These hematological reactions can be fatal, so that early detection is extremely important. *Complete blood cell counts should be obtained before initiation of therapy with carbamazepine to provide a baseline for comparison. Blood cell evaluation should then be repeated at least weekly during the first three months of therapy and at least monthly thereafter. The nurse should advise clients to report any symptoms that might be indicative of hematological reactions, such as sore throat, easy bruising, ulcerations of the oral mucosa, petechial or purpuric hemorrhage, easy fatiguability, or pallor. The use of carbamazepine should be discontinued at the first sign of a blood cell disorder (e.g., erythrocyte count of* <4 *million/mm*^{3}*; hematocrit* $<32\%$*;*

hemoglobin <11 *gm/dl; leukocytes* $<4{,}000/mm^3$*; platelet count* $<100{,}000$ mm^3*; reticulocyte count* $<20{,}000$ mm^3*; or serum iron* >150 *μg/dl).*

Carbamazepine can cause **hepatic toxicity** as well, which can sometimes be fatal. Cholestatic and hepatocellular jaundice, hepatitis, and hepatic cellular necrosis also have occurred. Carbamazepine may impair renal function, resulting in renal failure, oliguria, urinary frequency, urinary retention, azotemia, proteinuria, glycosuria, or microscopic urinary deposits. *The nurse should monitor intake-output ratios and vital signs for indications of fluid retention, renal failure, or cardiovascular complications during the period of dosage adjustment when carbamazepine therapy is initiated.*

Potential **allergic reactions** to carbamazepine include pneumonitis or pneumonia, fever and chills, pruritus, skin rash, photosensitivity reactions, urticaria, erythema multiforme, erythema nodosum, purpura, exfoliative dermatitis, lupus erythematosus, alopecia, and alterations in pigmentation. *The nurse should advise clients to avoid excessive sunlight and to use an appropriate sunscreen agent because of the risk of photosensitivity. Clients should also be advised to report itching or hair loss.*

Potential **cardiovascular reactions** include congestive heart failure, edema, hypertension or hypotension, atrioventricular nodal block, and thrombophlebitis. *The client needs to be assessed for evidence of cardiac dysrhythmias, aggravation of coronary artery disease (complaints of chest pain or discomfort on exertion), edema, and congestive heart failure. Electrocardiograms should be obtained periodically throughout therapy with carbamazepine, particularly if the client's complaints suggest the presence or worsening of cardiovascular disease. Blood pressure and pulse rates should be recorded and clients or family members need to learn to monitor and report changes in these parameters.*

Carbamazepine can cause lens opacities, conjunctivitis, nystagmus, and diplopia. *A complete evaluation of visual function should be conducted prior to, and periodically during, carbamazepine therapy.* Osteomalacia and joint and muscle aches sometimes occur, as well as impotency. Withdrawal of carbamazepine may be associated with an elevated risk of seizures. Gradual withdrawal is preferred except when adverse reactions are severe.

Carbamazepine is contraindicated for use in individuals with a history of bone marrow depression or hypersensitivity to this drug or tricyclic antidepressants (to which it bears a structural resemblance).

Drug Interactions Carbamazepine should not be used in conjunction with **MAO inhibitors** or within 14 days after discontinuing them. Serum levels of carbamazepine may be increased to toxic levels by the macrolide antibiotics, **erythromycin** or **troleandomycin.** Carbamazepine is a classic **inducer of liver enzymes** and thereby speeds the metabolism of oral contraceptives, doxycycline (Vibramycin), warfarin (Coumadin), phenytoin (Dilantin), ethosuximide (Zarontin), or valproic acid (Depakene). Similarly, phenobarbital, phenytoin, and primidone can speed the metabolism of carbamazepine by induction of liver enzymes. By contrast, metabolism of carbamazepine is inhibited by **isoniazid** (Rifamate) and **propoxyphene** (Darvon). **Cimetidine** (Tagamet) also increases serum concentrations of carbamazepine. There have been occasional instances of carbamazepine increasing the toxicity of concurrently administered **lithium. Tests of thyroid function** may exhibit decreased values when carbamazepine is being administered.

Preparations and Administration

Carbamazepine (Tegretol)
Tablets, chewable tablets
Recommended Doses: For adults or children over age 12, 200 mg PO twice daily initially, increased gradually by 200 mg/day, with the daily dose divided into 3 or 4 administrations. Doses must be individualized to achieve maximal benefit with minimal risk. The usual maintenance requirement in clients over age 12 is 800 to 1,200 mg daily. The maximum recommended dose is 1,000 mg daily for children 12–15, and 1,200 mg daily for individuals over 15. For children 6–12, 100 mg twice daily initially, increased in increments of 100 mg daily, with the daily dose spread over 3 or 4 administrations as the dose increases. The typical maintenance dose in children ages 6–12 is 400–800 mg daily with a maximum of 1,000 mg.

Phenacemide (Phenurone)

Phenacemide is an antiepileptic medication reserved for severe cases of epilepsy that do not respond to first-line drugs. Its use is constrained by its ability to produce serious liver, renal, and hematological toxicity. Moreover, these toxic effects tend to be additive with similar toxicity produced by other antiepileptic medications. Psychic changes occur in a startling 17% of individuals treated with phenacemide. Particular care must be exercised in using phenacemide in individuals with a history of behavioral disorders, since psychoses and suicide attempts have resulted. Gastrointestinal disturbances such as anorexia and weight loss occur as well as drowsiness and dizziness that may impair performance of hazardous tasks. Some clients experience headache, insomnia, skin rashes, and occasionally jaundice. *Clients and family members should watch for and report signs of jaundice, such as yellow skin or sclera, petechiae, pruritus, or dark, amber urine. They should also be advised to report immediately if the client develops fever, sore mouth, sore throat, malaise, or skin rashes. Since blood dyscrasias occur occasionally in response to phenacemide, clients should report any unexplained bleeding.*

Phenacemide (Phenurone)
Tablets
Recommended Doses: For adults, 1.5 g/day in 3 divided doses initially. The total daily dose can be gradually increased as required by increasing the number of administrations rather than the dose per administration. The maximum recommended daily dose in adults is 3 g. For children 5–10 years of age, one-half the adult dose, on the same schedule. Because phenacemide produces severe toxic effects, dosage titration must be conducted carefully to determine the minimal effective dosage.

Antiepileptic Drugs Used Primarily for Petit Mal Seizures or Myoclonus

Oxazolidones

The oxazolidones (or oxazolidinediones) are used exclusively for petit mal epilepsy, and even for this condition, the severity of adverse effects limits their usefulness. The two drugs in this group currently available for clinical use are trimethadione (Tridione) and paramethadione (Paradione). Trimethadione, the first drug developed expressly for use in petit mal epilepsy, is still one of the most effective. Oxazolidones may work by stabilizing the thalamic pacemaker against the disruptive influence of a subcortical seizure focus.

Pharmacokinetics After oral administration, oxazolidones are rapidly absorbed. Both trimethadione and paramethadione are initially converted by the liver microsomal enzyme system to an active metabolite, dimethadione. Dimethadione is the chief elimination form, being excreted in the urine. The half-life of trimethadione is only 12–24 hours, but that of dimethadione is 6–13 days. Therapeutic benefit occurs with dimathadione serum concentrations of about 700 μg/ml. Oxazolidones may have to be administered for 1–4 weeks before therapeutic concentrations and benefits are achieved.

Adverse Effects and Contraindications *Because of the risk of **blood cell dyscrasias**, a complete blood cell evaluation should be conducted before initiating therapy with oxazolidones.* Hypoplastic anemia, pancytopenia, agranulocytosis, leukopenia, neutropenia, thrombocytopenia, eosinophilia, and even fatal aplastic anemia have been reported. Oxazolidones must be discontinued if there is a marked drop in blood cell count (for example, a neutrophil count of less than 2,500). Moderate neutropenia is not uncommon and does not require drug discontinuation, but monitoring should be intensified if the blood cell count approaches the critical level. *The nurse should instruct clients receiving an oxazolidone to report immediately symptoms of fever, sore throat, ulcerations of the oral mucosa, swollen glands, or joint pains.*

Fatal nephrosis with proteinuria has occurred with use of oxazolidones. Hepatitis has occurred, but only rarely. *Renal and hepatic function tests should be conducted prior to initiating oxazolidone therapy, and clients should immediately report signs of jaundice.* Gastrointestinal symptoms include nausea, vomiting, gastic distress, abdominal pain, anorexia, weight loss, and hiccoughs. *Oxazolidones may be taken with food to minimize gastrointestinal problems.*

Allergic reactions to oxazolidones include skin eruptions (acneiform or morbilliform rashes, erythema multiforme, exfoliative dermatitis), photophobia, lupus erythematosus, and lymphadenopathies. Previous hypersensitivity to oxazolidones is a specific contraindication for their use. Neurological reactions to long-term use of oxazolidones include a **myasthenia gravis-like syndrome** with symptoms such as muscle weakness and fatiguability. Oxazolidones should be discontinued at the first sign of symptoms of this syndrome. Other **neurological problems** include vertigo, malaise, drowsiness, fatigue, insomnia, personality changes, irritability, headaches, diplopia or paresthesias. Neurological disturbances can usually be eliminated by reduction of dosage. *Clients should be warned that occurrence of drowsiness and blurred vision with use of one of these drugs may impair driving ability.*

Oxazolidones can precipitate **grand mal seizures** and, if eliminated too abruptly, can increase petit mal seizures. The drug should therefore be withdrawn gradually. In the event of an allergic reaction or other serious adverse reaction, another antiepileptic medication should be substituted during the gradual elimination phase. Transitory increases in frequency of seizures have also been reported during the initial phase of treatment with oxazolidones. Oxazolidones should not be employed during pregnancy since their use has been linked to **fetal abnormalities.** The extent of excretion of oxazolidones in breast milk is not known.

Preparations and Administration Oxazolidones should be preserved in tightly closed containers at temperatures below 25° C.

Paramethadione (Paradione)
Capsules, oral solution
Recommended Doses: For adults with petit mal epilepsy, 900 mg/daily PO in 3 or 4 divided doses initially, increased by 300 mg daily at weekly intervals until the optimal therapeutic response is obtained to a maximum of 2.4 g/day. For children, 300–900 mg, which must be divided into 3 or 4 equal doses. *It may be necessary to dilute the alcohol solution of paramethadione when it is administered to children.*

Trimethadione (Tridione)
Capsules, chewable tablets, oral solution
Recommended Doses: Same as for paramethadione.

Succinimides

The succinimide derivatives, ethosuximide (Zarontin), methsuximide (Celontin), and phensuximide (Milontin), are used in petit mal. Ethosuximide has also been employed successfully in positive spike pattern. All produce drowsiness, but are somewhat less toxic overall than the oxazolidones. Succinimides suppress the 3 Hz spike-and-dome pattern and the associated lapses of consciousness associated with petit mal epilepsy. Of the three succinimides, ethosuximide has proved to have the most favorable balance of efficacy to toxicity. Methsuximide and phensuximide are indicated only for instances of petit mal refractory to other drug selections. Succinimides can be employed advantageously in combination with other drugs for petit mal epilepsy.

Pharmacokinetics Succinimides are well absorbed from the gastrointestinal tract. Peak plasma levels are achieved in 3–7 hours with ethosuximide. Succinimides are not significantly bound by plasma proteins. A fraction of the administered dose of succinimides is excreted unchanged, but most is metabolized in the liver to inactive metabolites before elimination. The plasma half-life for ethosuximide is 30 hours in children and 60 hours in adults. Therapeutic serum concentrations of ethosuximide are approximately 40–100 μg/ml.

Adverse Effects and Contraindications The most common adverse effects of succinimides are **gastrointestinal upset** (nausea, vomiting, cramps, diarrhea, anorexia, epigastric distress, constipation), fatigue, lethargy, headaches, and dizziness. *Succinimides may be taken with food or milk to lessen gastrointestinal symptoms.* Other **CNS side effects** of succinimides include drowsiness, ataxia, dizziness, irritability and nervousness, headache, euphoria, dream-like states, hyperactivity, and insomnia. Clients may become anxious and depressed with diminished ability to concentrate and may have auditory hallucinations and night terrors. Some become aggressive, paranoid, or suicidal, and libido is sometimes increased (such changes are most likely to occur in individuals with a prior history of emotional problems).

An uncommon but important side effect of succinimides is occurrence of **blood dyscrasias.** Eosinophilia, granulocytopenia, leukopenia, agranulocytosis, aplastic anemia, monocytosis, and pancytopenia have been reported. *Blood cell counts should be performed before initiating therapy and periodically during treatment. Clients should be advised to report signs of blood cell dyscrasias such as persistent fever, swollen glands, easy bruising, or oral bleeding.*

Allergic reactions to succinimides have included pruritus, urticaria, erythema multiforme, skin rashes, and systemic lupus erythematosus. *Before medication is initiated, nurses need to determine whether the client has a history of hypersensitivity to succinimides. Clients should be instructed to report skin eruptions to the nurse or physician.* Some succinimide products contain tartrazine, a preservative that can cause allergic reactions.

Other adverse effects of succinimides include grand mal seizures, urinary frequency, and renal damage. Phensuximide can cause hematuria and should be avoided in clients with acute intermittent porphyria. It also can cause a harmless pink, red, or red-brown discoloration of the urine. *Renal function tests should be obtained in all clients when succinimide therapy is contemplated, and clients should report immediately any change in urine output, which may be indicative of renal damage.*

Preparations and Administration

Ethosuximide (Zarontin)
Capsules, raspberry-flavored oral syrup
Recommended Doses: For children ages 3–6, 250 mg/day PO initially. For older children and adults, 500 mg/day, initially. The dose is then individualized to the optimum clinical response. The initial dose can be increased by 250 mg/day at intervals of 4–7 days to a maximum of 1.5 g/day.

Doses greater than 250 mg are divided into 2 or 3 equal doses each day.

Methsuximide (Celontin)
Capsules (with tartrazine as a preservative).
Recommended Doses: 300 mg/day PO initially, increased as required by increments of 300 mg/day at weekly intervals to a maximum of 1.2 g/day.

Phensuximide (Milontin)
Capsules
Recommended Doses: 1–3 g/day PO in 2 or 3 divided doses, irrespective of age.

Benzodiazepines in Epilepsy

Three of the benzodiazepines have applications in epilepsy: diazepam (Valium), clorazepate (Tranxene), and clonazepam (Clonopin). The detailed discussion of this family of drugs is found in Chapters 12 (as hypnotics) and 19 (in relation to anxiety).

Diazepam has not proved to be useful alone as a prophylactic agent in any form of epilepsy but is useful as an adjunct in combination regimens for petit mal epilepsy and grand mal epilepsy. The most important use of diazepam, however, is for acute control of seizures in progress. Diazepam is the drug of choice for status epilepticus and severe recurrent seizures. When treating a convulsing client, IV administration is preferred if practical; otherwise the injection is given by deep IM injection.

Clorazepate can be employed as an adjunct for treatment of partial seizures. This long-acting benzodiazepine provides sustained blood levels with administration 2 or 3 times daily. The full pharmacology of this drug is discussed in Chapter 19.

Preparations and Administration

Diazepam (Valium)
Oral dosage forms: See Chapter 19; injection solution
Recommended Doses: For adults, 5–10 mg initially, repeated at 10–15 minute intervals up to a maximum of 30 mg if necessary. For children over age 5, 1 mg every 2–5 minutes up to 10 mg. For children between 30 days and 5 years of age, 0.2–0.5 mg slowly every 2–5 minutes up to 5 mg. Diazepam therapy may be repeated at an interval of 2–4 hours if required.

Clorazepate (Tranxene)
Capsules, tablets
Recommended Doses: For adults or children over 12, 7.5 mg PO 3 times daily initially, increased by increments of up to 7.5 mg/day at intervals of 1 week to a maximum of 90 mg/day. For children ages 9–12, 7.5 mg PO twice daily initially, increased by increments of 7.5 mg/day at intervals of 1 week up to a maximum of 60 mg/day. Clorazepate is not recommended for children under 9 years of age.

Clonazepam (Clonopin)

Clonazepam is marketed exclusively for applications related to epilepsy and myoclonus. Clonazepam suppresses the 3 Hz spike-and-dome pattern characteristic of petit mal epilepsy as well as the associated syncope. After oral administration, clonazepam is rapidly absorbed, providing peak serum concentrations in 1–2 hours. Binding to plasma proteins is about 47% for clonazepam. Clonazepam is metabolized into at least five products which are excreted in the urine. The half-life for inactivation of clonazepam is about 20–40 hours. Efficacy is associated with plasma concentrations between 20–80 ng/ml of clonazepam.

Clinical Indications Clonazepam is effective alone or in combinations for petit mal and for petit mal variant (Lennox-Gestaut syndrome). In addition, clonazepam is considered the current drug of choice for treatment of myoclonus (Table 23–2). One drawback with clonazepam is that some tolerance may develop. About 30% of treated individuals require upward dosage adjustment after 3 months of clonazepam administration to maintain efficacy.

Adverse Effects and Contraindications Like other benzodiazepines, clonazepam causes **CNS depression.** Drowsiness occurs in about 50% of clients. *The nurse should warn clients that use of clonazepam may be associated with neurological symptoms, such as drowsiness and diplopia, that could impair driving ability.* Other **psychiatric and neurological side effects** of clonazepam include confusion, depression, forgetfulness, hysteria, hallucinations, insomnia, psychosis, suicide attempts, increased libido, nystagmus and other abnormal eye movements, slurred speech, tremor, vertigo, choreiform movements, and respiratory depression.

Clonazepam occasionally causes somatic side effects, such as alopecia or hirsutism, enuresis, nocturia, urinary retention, rhinorrhea, shortness of breath, palpitations, muscle weakness, and gastrointestinal disturbances. **Hepatic toxicity,** which occurs rarely, includes hepatomegaly and alterations in serum enzymes indicating liver dysfunction. *Liver function tests should be conducted initially and carried out periodically when clonazepam is utilized.* **Hematological reactions** such as anemia, leukopenia, thrombocytopenia, and eosinophilia have occasionally developed. *Thus, periodic blood cell evaluations should be con-*

ducted. **Allergic reactions** to clonazepam consist mainly of skin rash. Hypersensitivity to benzodiazepines is a contraindication for use of clonazepam. Abrupt withdrawal of clonazepam will increase **seizure liability.** *Nurses should stress to clients the importance of compliance and warn them not to discontinue clonazepam without the advice of their physicians. If the physician decides to change a client's medication, the transition should be made gradually, tapering the dose of the established medication while slowly instituting the new medication.*

Potential risks to the fetus from use of clonazepam by pregnant women have not been evaluated; however, women using clonazepam should not breast-feed. Both **psychological and physical dependence** are possibilities with benzodiazepines including clonazepam. *The nurse should observe for signs of overcompliance by keeping track of the client's utilization of clonazepam.*

Drug Interactions The CNS depressant effect of clonazepam is additive with that of other CNS depressants. The addition of clonazepam to an existing regimen for petit mal (such as a succinimide) will result in additive depressant influences. *The nurse should instruct clients not to employ alcohol and depressant over-the-counter medications with clonazepam.* Concurrent use of clonazepam and valproic acid (Depakene) has resulted in increased frequency of absence seizures, despite the fact that each of these medications alone is effective in petit mal epilepsy. Inducers of liver enzymes, such as phenytoin and phenobarbital, may reduce plasma levels of clonazepam.

Preparations and Administration

Clonazepam (Clonopin)
Tablets
Recommended Doses: For adults, not in excess of 1.5 mg/day PO in 3 divided doses initially, increased in increments of 0.5–1.0 mg/day at intervals of 3 days until optimal control of seizures is achieved. The maximum recommended maintenance dose is 20 mg/day PO. For infants and children up to 10 years of age, 0.01 and 0.03 mg/kg/day initially, not to exceed 0.05 mg/kg/day. The daily dose is given in 2 or preferably 3 divided doses. The initial dose may be increased in increments up to 0.25–0.5 mg/day at intervals of 3 days to a maximum of 0.1–0.3 mg/kg/day.

Valproic Acid

Valproic acid (Depakene) and its relatives, sodium valproate and divalproex sodium all yield valproic acid and may be considered pharmacologically equivalent. Valproic acid has a broad spectrum of usefulness (Table 23–2) but is probably not the best choice for any one form of epilepsy. Valproic acid elevates GABA levels, the likely basis for its action. The value of valproic acid is limited by frequent hepatic toxicity (in about 15–30% of those treated), occasionally leading to death.

Pharmacokinetics Valproic acid is rapidly absorbed, producing peak plasma levels in about 1–4 hours when the capsules are employed or in 15–120 minutes when the syrup is used. The dosage form containing divalproex, a coordination complex containing valproic acid, is enteric coated, which delays absorption about 1 hour. Administration of valproic acid with food slightly delays absorption but does not alter total absorption.

In the blood, valproic acid is highly bound (>90%) to plasma proteins. The therapeutic range of serum concentrations is about 50–100 μg/mL. Valproic acid crosses the placental barrier and accumulates in fetal tissue at levels higher than plasma concentrations. Inactivation of valproic acid is by liver glucoronidation, and the metabolite is excreted in the urine. The half-life for inactivation of valproic acid is about 6–16 hours (the lower values typically occur in individuals receiving other antiepileptic medications that are inducers of liver enzymes), but is extended in neonates (as high as 67 hours) and in individuals with impaired liver function (up to 25 hours).

Clinical Indications Valproic acid is indicated alone or in combination with other medications for treatment of petit mal epilepsy, complex seizures, and mixed types that include petit mal as a component. It has been employed investigationally in atypical absence seizures, myoclonus, grand mal epilepsy, and infantile spasms.

Adverse Effects and Contraindications The most common early side effects of valproic acid are **gastrointestinal symptoms,** including nausea, vomiting, indigestion, diarrhea, constipation, anorexia and weight loss, or conversely, increased appetite and weight gain. *Gastrointestinal symptoms can be reduced by use of the enteric coated tablets of divalproex sodium or by administration of other dosage forms with meals.*

CNS side effects of **excess depression** (sedation, psychiatric depression, ataxia, muscle weakness, nystagmus, diplopia, tremor, incoordination, dizziness, and coma) may occur and are additive with the depressant effects of other antiepileptic medications and other CNS depressants. *As with all other antiepileptic drugs, nurses should advise clients not to drive, operate other machinery, or perform potentially harzardous work re-*

quiring mental alertness and physical coordination after taking valproic acid. Epileptic clients should be advised to refrain from use of alcohol and should be cautioned about use of depressant over-the-counter medications, such as sleep aids. Administration of valproic acid at bedtime will help to minimize CNS depression during the waking hours. Valproic acid has also caused headache, insomnia, dysarthria, emotional instability, psychosis, aggression, and hyperactivity.

Valproic acid inhibits platelet aggregation, leading to an **increase in bleeding time.** It can also cause thrombocytopenia, further impairing the clotting mechanism. *Platelet count and bleeding time determinations should be conducted before initiating therapy with valproic acid. The nurse should instruct clients receiving this drug to report any indications of unusual bleeding, bruising, or purpura.* Less frequently, valproic acid may cause other blood cell dyscrasias, including leukopenia, eosinophilia, anemia, and pancytopenia. *Clients should be advised to tell their dentists that they are utilizing valproic acid prior to any kind of dental surgery, because of the increased risk of bleeding.*

Valproic acid can cause **endocrine problems** resulting in irregular menses or outright secondary amenorrhea, and alterations in thyroid function tests. Hyperglycemia and hyperammonemia are potential metabolic problems associated with use of valproic acid, so that diabetic clients need to intensify their monitoring of blood and urine glucose. Patients with preexisting nonketotic hyperglycinemia are at particular risk from valproate-induced hyperglycemia.

Of special concern with valproic acid derivatives is the risk of **hepatotoxicity.** Minor elevations in serum enzymes indicative of hepatic dysfunction are frequent and occur in a dose-related manner. Serious and fatal hepatotoxicity has occurred in a few individuals, usually during the first 6 months of treatment with valproic acid. *Liver function tests should be performed prior to initiating therapy with valproic acid and at frequent intervals during therapy, especially during the first 6 months.* Valproic acid is contraindicated for individuals with significant hepatic dysfunction.

Valproic acid use should be avoided if at all possible during pregnancy because of risk of teratogenicity. Valproic acid is excreted in breast milk at levels from 1 to 10% of serum concentrations, but it is not known if this level has an impact on the nursing infant.

Drug Interactions As with all antiepileptic medications, valproic acid has depressant influences on the brain which are potentially additive with those of other **CNS depressants.** *Epileptic clients should be advised to refrain from use of alcohol because it will interact with antiepileptic medications and increase seizure liability.*

Serum concentrations of **phenobarbital** should be monitored when valproic acid is employed with phenobarbital or phenobarbital prodrugs (primidone or mephobarbital). Valproic acid has been shown to raise serum concentrations of concurrently administered phenobarbital (and phenobarbital derived from metabolism of mephobarbital or primidone).

Valproic acid may interfere with the antiepileptic action of other antiepileptics. For example, breakthrough seizures have occurred when valproic acid has been used in conjunction with **phenytoin.** In some of these instances, phenytoin serum concentrations were depressed but in other cases phenytoin concentrations were elevated. Thus, the mechanism for this interaction remains unclear. Valproic acid and **clonazepam** used concurrently have been reported to increase the frequency of petit mal seizures.

The effect of valproic acid on bleeding time tends to enhance the anticoagulant effect of aspirin, warfarin, and other **anticoagulant drugs** not only because of the additive anticoagulant influences but also because these drugs compete for plasma protein binding sites. Valproic acid may also cause false positives in the **urine ketone test** and alter **thyroid function tests.**

Preparations and Administration *Depakene syrup should be kept out of the reach of children, since it is both attractive and flavorful.*

Valproic acid (Depakene)
Capsules, syrup (as the sodium salt), enteric coated tablets (Depakote) as a coordination complex, Divalproex sodium, that yields valproic acid
Recommended Doses: 15 mg/kg/day PO initially, increased by increments of 5–10 mg/kg/day at intervals of 1 week until control of seizures is achieved. The maximum recommended dose is 60 mg/kg/day PO. Doses exceeding 250 mg/day PO should be given in divided doses. Titration of dosage may be conducted against determinations of serum concentrations. The therapeutic range for serum levels of valproic acid is from 40–100 μg/ml in adults; from 50–200 μg/ml in children.

Important Nursing Implications for Antiepileptic Drugs

☐ Check the client's medication history for contraindications for each medication that is contemplated for use.

- ☐ When therapy with antiepileptic drugs is initiated, monitor plasma concentrations of the drug to ensure that the serum level achieved is within the established therapeutic range.
- ☐ Note indications of renal or hepatic impairment since these events will alter the response to antiepileptic medications.
- ☐ Teach clients the indications of allergic reactions that occur with each kind of antiepileptic medication they are receiving.
- ☐ Teach clients to monitor for and report occurrence of any of the adverse effects that occur with each medication.
- ☐ Warn clients to avoid driving an automobile or other activities requiring mental alertness while experiencing sedation or other neurological symptoms caused by antiepileptic medication.
- ☐ Advise clients to avoid use of alcohol or other CNS depressants that could add to the depressant influences of antiepileptic drugs.
- ☐ Explain to clients that antiepileptic medications are usually withdrawn slowly to prevent a rebound increase in incidence and severity of seizures.
- ☐ As with any other medication, clients need to be warned to keep their medications out of the reach of children. This is particularly important with antiepileptic medications since these drugs can produce death from overdose when inadvertently taken by children.
- ☐ Emphasize the importance of compliance since the therapeutic benefit (seizure prophylaxis) is not readily apparent to the client.
- ☐ Advise epileptic clients to obtain and wear medic alert tags specifying their condition and drug regimens.

Case Study: Grand Mal Epilepsy

L. R. was a 33-year-old white man brought by his wife to the emergency room of a general hospital in a state of coma. She stated that he had "an attack" during which his body had stiffened for about 5 or 10 seconds and then he slumped to the floor, shaking violently. On physical examination, L. R. appeared to be free of injury except for a small amount of blood in his saliva and on his lips. He appeared to have bitten his tongue and had urinated in his pants. After a few minutes in the emergency room, L. R. began to regain consciousness, but was disoriented and confused. His vital signs were unremarkable. After another 30 minutes, L. R. recognized his wife and knew where he was, although he did not recall what had happened nor why he was in the hospital.

The nurse learned from L. R. that these attacks had occurred from time to time over the past 4 years. Sometimes the attacks were at night and sometimes during the day. An EEG evaluation was ordered, but there was no identifiable abnormality; a brain scan was performed, but it was also negative. While in the hospital L. R. had another seizure. One nurse placed a padded tongue depressor between the teeth, and another gently but firmly held L. R.'s head on his pillow. Another nurse administered diazepam (Valium), 5 mg by deep intramuscular injection. The nurses also noted the characteristics of the seizure — a tonic-clonic major seizure — which they reported to the physician. L. R. was diagnosed as having grand mal epilepsy. The physician prescribed phenytoin (Dilantin), 100 mg tid, and a multivitamin.

The nurse explained to L. R. the nature of his disorder and the rationale for the drug regimen. The nurse also discussed with him the previous episodes of seizure and helped him to recognize that each of the episodes had occurred during a period of stress. She explained to L. R. the potential adverse effects of phenytoin as well as how to intensify oral hygiene measures to decrease the likelihood of gingival hyperplasia. A medical alert tag was made for him which he agreed to wear. The nurse spoke with L. R. and his wife about the difficulties they had experienced with the seizure episodes and how they planned to cope with the requirements of medication in the future.

After 3 days on this regimen, analysis of the serum concentration of phenytoin showed a value of 14 μg/ml, and L. R. was discharged. A week later, L. R. had another seizure. The physician then ordered the addition of phenobarbital, 15 mg PO, tid, and L. R. experienced no additional seizures.

1. Is it surprising that the EEG evaluation revealed no abnormality? Does it make sense that the physician would nevertheless diagnose grand mal epilepsy?
2. What circumstances besides stress are likely to precipitate seizures in seizure-prone individuals?

3. What was the nursing priority when L. R. went into seizure while in the hospital?
4. Why was diazepam given? Why was it given by intramuscular injection rather than orally or intravenously? Why deeply?
5. Why was a multivitamin given with phenytoin?
6. Why did the physician add phenobarbital to the regimen? Might he have simply increased the dose of phenytoin instead?
7. What adverse effect might be anticipated from the interaction of phenytoin and phenobarbital?

Answers appear at the end of the book.

Case Study: Petit Mal Epilepsy

At 7 years of age, Julia was observed by her teacher to have difficulty following instructions and keeping up with schoolwork. After attending a conference on organic problems that can contribute to learning disabilities, the teacher noticed that Julia exhibited some of the signs indicative of petit mal epilepsy: muscle twitches and periods of staring and unresponsiveness. The teacher referred Julia to the school nurse who found that Julia was normal for her age in sensory tests and mental ability. However, over the course of the hour, the nurse observed three episodes lasting about 10 seconds when Julia appeared to be in a trance. The nurse spoke to Julia's parents and referred them to a pediatrician who was experienced in the seizure disorders of childhood. The pediatrician's diagnosis of petit mal confirmed the suspicions of the teacher and nurse. Julia was begun on ethosuximide (Zarontin), 0.5 g daily, responded well, and was successfully managed on this medication until seventh grade.

At the beginning of seventh grade, Julia had made a favorable impression on her teachers although she was described as somewhat moody, withdrawn, and self-conscious. During the third quarter of that year, Julia's behavior and school work worsened. After several conflicts with teachers and other students, Julia was referred to the school nurse. The nurse reviewed Julia's medical history and noted the diagnosis of petit mal and the regimen of ethosuximide. In the assessment of Julia, the nurse noted that Julia's progression into puberty was about average for her age. The nurse asked Julia about her use of alcohol or other drugs, whether she was still taking her medication, and if she had any recurrence of seizures. After considerable coaxing, Julia revealed that she had secretly stopped taking the medication. She had noticed that when she brushed her hair in the morning she was losing it at an alarming rate, and she knew from what she had been told that this was probably a side effect of the drug. Julia was afraid of becoming bald and being ridiculed by her peers. The nurse discussed the compliance problem with Julia's physician and a change was made in the regimen.

1. What is the connection between petit mal epilepsy and learning disability?
2. Why did the nurse in the junior high school ask Julia about her use of alcohol or other drugs?
3. What are some of the reasons that compliance problems are especially common among adolescents?

Answers appear at the end of the book.

Recommended Readings

Brodoff AS: Intervening to stop status epilepticus. *Patient Care* 1983;17(17):153.

Brodoff AS: Keeping epilepsy under control. *Patient Care* 1983;17(17):107.

Browne TR: Valproic acid. *N Engl J Med* 1980;302:661–666.

Bruni J, Albright PS: The clinical pharmacology of antiepileptic drugs. *Clin Neuropharm* 1984;7(1):1–34.

Bruya MA et al: Epilepsy: A controllable disease — part 1: Classification and diagnosis. *Am J Nurs* 1976;76:388–392; part 2: Drug therapy and nursing care, 1976;76:393–397.

Dalessio DJ: Current concepts: Seizure disorders and pregnancy. *N Engl J Med* 1985;312:559–563.

Delgado-Escueta AV, Treiman DM, Walsh GO: The treatable epilepsies (parts I & II). *N Engl J Med* 1983; 308(26)1508–1514, 1576–1584.

Evans RW, Gualtieri CT: Carbamazepine: A neuropsychological and psychiatric profile. *Clin Neuropharm* 1985; 8(3):221–241.

Freeman JM: Febrile seizures: Consensus of significance, evaluation, and treatment. *Pediatrics* 1980;66:1009–1012.

Gever LN: Two forms of dilantin. *Nursing* 1981;11(9):78.

Gever LN: Your role in valproic acid therapy. *Nursing* 1982;12(6):104–106.

Glaser GH et al: *Antiepileptic Drugs: Mechanisms of Action.* New York, Raven, 1980.

Hawken M, Ozuna J: Practical aspects of anticonvulsant therapy. *Am J Nurs* 1979;79:1062–1068.

Ilvanainen M, Himberg J-J: Valproate and clonazepam in treatment of severe progressive myoclonus epilepsy. *Arch Neurol* 1982;39:236–238.

Koch-Weser J, Browne TR: Drug therapy: Clonazepam. *N Engl J Med* 1978;299:812–816.

Korberly BH et al: Ethotoin use in pediatric seizure patients. *Am J Dis Child* 1981;135:1139–1140.

Livingston S et al: Petit mal epilepsy. *Am Fam Physician* 1978;17(1):107–114.

Livingston S et al: Phenobarbital versus phenytoin for grand mal epilepsy. *Am Fam Physician* 1980;22(2):123–127.

Macdonald RL, McLean MJ: Cellular bases of barbiturate and phenytoin anticonvulsant drug action. *Epilepsia* 1982;23(Suppl 1):7–18.

MacDougall V: Teaching children and families about seizures. *Can Nurse* 1982;78(4):30–36.

Norman S, Browne T: Seizure disorders. *Am J Nurs* 1981;81(5):984–994.

Perucca E, Richens H: Drug interactions with phenytoin. *Drugs* 1981;21(2):120–137.

Thurston JH et al: Prognosis in childhood epilepsy: Additional follow-up of 148 children 15 to 23 years after withdrawal of anticonvulsant therapy. *N Engl J Med* 1982;306:831–836.

Trekas J: Managing epilepsy: Don't forget the patient. *Nursing* 1982;12(10):63–65.

Van Woert MH, Hwang EC: Biochemistry and pharmacology of myoclonus. *Clin Neuropharm* 1978;3:167–184.

Woodbury DM et al (eds): *Antiepileptic Drugs* ed 2. New York, Raven Press, 1982.

CHAPTER 24

Organic Brain Syndrome and Drugs

Organic Brain Syndrome

Although drug treatment for organic brain syndrome is still in its infancy, it is an area where much research is being done and where the nurse is likely to see important advances in the coming years. Organic brain syndromes are disorders of psychological or cognitive functioning caused by impairments of cerebral tissue. The term *organic brain syndrome* (OBS) designates a constellation of clinical signs and symptoms without specifying their etiologies. The manifestations of OBS are impairments in one or more of the following areas: (1) recent or remote memory and immediate recall, (2) attention, arousal, orientation, consciousness, and motivation, (3) intellectual functions such as comprehension, problem solving, learning, or judgment, (4) sensory or ideational perception, (5) psychological functioning, including affective state, anxiety, psychosis, or neurosis, and (6) neurological symptoms such as dizziness, faintness, headache, or anorexia. The psychological symptoms that occur in OBS can simulate a wide variety of functional disorders, including depression, schizophrenia, anxiety disorders, personality disorders, and conversion symptoms. Often individuals diagnosed as schizophrenics or primary depressives prove at autopsy to have had chronic OBS.

An accurate diagnosis of OBS is of utmost importance for several reasons. The psychiatric symptoms related to OBS do not respond as well to psychotherapy or medication as do true functional disorders; thus, therapeutic objectives will require modification if the psychological disturbances are in fact of organic origin. Conversely, individuals with dementia secondary to depression (**pseudodementia**) are likely to receive less vigorous and less effective treatment than if their condition is correctly identified (pseudodementia is reversible when the depression is resolved with antidepressants or psychotherapy). The psychiatric appraisal of clients with possible OBS should include a history of premorbid personality and mental status and tests of attention, language function, memory (including remote, recent, and immediate recall), perceptual functioning, and problem solving. Neurological testing should routinely include an EEG and computerized tomography scan. OBS is diagnosed when there is (1) a substantial degree of cognitive and memory impairment relative to the extent of behavioral change, or (2) presence of specific organic factors, such as pronounced EEG slowing, evidence of a cerebral mass, or a metabolic disturbance.

OBS comprises nearly 20% of initial admissions to mental hospitals, second only to schizophrenia. OBS classifications (Table 24–1) take into account three qualities: (1) global versus selective impairment, (2) reversible (or acute) versus irreversible (or chronic), and (3) senile versus presenile onset.

Global Versus Selective Organic Brain Syndrome

The two global forms of OBS are delirium and dementia. **Delirium** is a clouding of consciousness that disturbs the ability to sustain, shift, or focus attention and results in perceptual disturbances (illusions, hallucinations), disorientation, incoherent speech, insomnia or excessive daytime sleepiness, psychomotor agitation or retardation, memory impairment, and affective disturbances. Delirium is always of acute onset (over a few hours or a few days), most commonly caused by toxic or inflammatory conditions. The intensity of delirium often fluctuates, with lucid intervals occurring unpredictably.

Typical causes of delirium are systemic infections, hyperthermia, hypoglycemia or diabetes mellitus, myxedema, hypoxia or hypercapnia, fluid or electrolyte imbalances, nutritional (especially nicotinic acid or thiamine) deficiencies, substance intoxication or withdrawal (Table 24–2), hypertensive encephalopathy, hepatic or renal dysfunction, postoperative or postictal states, elevated intracranial pressure, diminished cerebral blood flow, meningitis, cerebral masses (abscesses, hematomas, or tumors), or head injury.

The delirious individual may be quiet (requiring little or no drug intervention), agitated (best managed with diazepam, 5–10 mg IV at 15 minute intervals as required), or restless and recalcitrant (controllable with 5–10 mg of haloperidol, 3–4 times per day as needed). Treatment of delirium focuses on identifying and eliminating the underlying organic cause.

Dementia affects an estimated 20% of people over age 80 but only 2% in their fifties. An estimated 5% of individuals over 65 (1.3 million) have severe dementia and another 15% (about 3 million) mild to moderate dementia. Dementia is defined as a loss of intellectual abilities that interferes with social or occupational functioning. Impairment occurs in memory and at least one of the following: abstract thinking, judgment, language ability, motor skills, object recognition, or impulse control. Consciousness is not clouded, which differentiates the condition from delirium. An estimated 20% of cases of dementia, usually cases of acute onset, are completely reversible. The causes of reversible dementia include endocrine disorders, vitamin deficiencies, hydrocephalus, brain masses, drug or heavy metal toxicities (Table 24–2), metabolic, fluid, or electrolyte imbalances, depression, and certain infections. The major irreversible forms are the primary degenerative dementias (notably Alzheimer's disease) and cerebral arteriosclerosis.

The circumscribed organic brain syndromes are less common than delirium and dementia and usually have identifiable causes, often drug use or head trauma. **Amnestic syndrome** is characterized by memory impairment, which may be retrograde or anterograde, but there is no clouding of the sensorium as in delirium. The most common cause of amnestic syndrome is thiamine deficiency, which is often associated with chronic use of alcohol. This condition is called **Wernicke's encephalopathy** and is characterized by damage to the mammillary bodies of the hypothalamus and behavioral symptoms known as **Korsakoff's syndrome** (see Chapter 13). The other principal causes of amnestic syndrome are head trauma, hypoxia, infarction, surgical intervention, or herpes simplex encephalitis. Acute drug-induced amnestic syndrome, commonly called blackouts, can occur with alcohol and other sedative-hypnotics.

Another kind of circumscribed OBS is **delusional syndrome,** in which delusions occur without the clouding of consciousness of delirium or the loss of intellectual skills of dementia. The acute toxic psychoses caused by stimulants (amphetamine or cocaine), psychedelics (LSD or cannabis) and certain other drugs (Table 24–2) are often delusional syndromes. Rarely, delusional syndromes occur by nondrug mechanisms, such as Huntington's disease, cerebral lesions of the nondominant hemisphere, or as interictal phenomena in temporal lobe epilepsy.

Table 24–1
Organic Brain Syndromes

Type	Typical Etiologies
I. Global cognitive impairment	
A. Delirium	Infections, metabolic disorders, blood gas imbalances, hypoglycemia, electrolyte imbalances, hepatic and renal disease, vitamin B_1 deficiency, postoperative states, intoxication with depressant drugs, withdrawal syndromes, head trauma, heavy metal poisoning
B. Dementias	
1. Primary degenerative dementias (68%)	
a. Presenile	Alzheimer's disease, Pick's disease
b. Senile	Senile dementia of the Alzheimer's type
2. Multi-infarct dementia (5%)	Cerebral arteriosclerosis
3. Pseudodementing depression (8%)	Primary depression
4. Vitamin B_{12} deficiency (5%)	Vitamin B_{12} deficiency
5. Other (14%)	Anemias (pernicious or folic acid deficiency), normal pressure hydrocephalus, CNS infections (neurosyphilis, Jakob-Creutzfeldt disease, fungal meningitis, viral encephalitis), brain trauma, (subdural hematoma, etc.), neurological diseases (progressive supranuclear palsy, hereditary palsies, Huntington's disease, multiple sclerosis, Parkinson's disease), extended hypothyroidism, incomplete recovery from severe anoxia, hypoglycemia or intoxication.
II. Selective impairments	
A. Amnestic syndrome	
1. Wernicke's/Korsakoff's syndrome	Vitamin B_1 deficiency secondary to alcohol abuse
2. Other	Damage to Papez circuit from heat trauma, surgery, hypoxia, infarction, or herpes simplex encephalitis
B. Organic hallucinosis	Alcohol, hallucinogens, sensory deprivation, seizure foci
C. Organic delusion syndrome	Amphetamines, cannabis, psychedelics, Huntington's chorea, temporal lobe epilepsy
D. Organic affective syndrome	Depressant drugs, thyroid disorders, adrenal cortical disorders, viral illnesses, carcinoma of the pancreas
E. Organic personality syndrome	
1. Frontal lobe syndrome	Neoplasms, head trauma, cerebrovascular disease causing structural damage to frontal lobes
2. Temporal lobe syndrome	Temporal lobe epilepsy, multiple sclerosis, Huntington's disease

Organic hallucinosis is most often a drug-induced condition. The toxic psychoses associated with hallucinogens or prolonged use of alcohol may take the form of an organic hallucinosis, occurring as persistent or recurrent hallucinations without clouding of consciousness, dementia, or underlying schizophrenia. Other conditions in which hallucinosis can occur include sensory deprivation (as in blindness, deafness, or sensory deprivation experiments), presence of seizure foci, or at the onset of sleep (hypnagogic hallucinations).

When affective disturbances (mania or depression) occur in response to organic disturbances without delirium or dementia, the condition is **organic affective syndrome.** This syndrome is usually a result of drug use or metabolic imbalances. Drug-induced depression is often associated with alcohol use, but can also be produced by other drugs such as anticholinergics, antiepileptics, antihistamines, antihypertensive agents (such as methyldopa, clonidine, reserpine, or guanethidine), anxiolytics, digitalis, estrogens (including oral contraceptives), immunosuppressives, narcotic analgesics, neuroleptics, sedative-hypnotics, or withdrawal from glucocorticoids or

Table 24–2
Drug Causes of Organic Brain Syndromes

Global organic brain syndromes		**Circumscribed organic brain syndromes**		
Delirium	*Dementia*	*Organic delusional syndrome*	*Organic amnestic syndrome*	*Organic affective syndrome*
Amphetamine-like stimulants	Aluminum	Amphetamine-like stimulants	Alcohol	Alcohol
Antidysrhythmic drugs	Arsenic	Antiepileptics	Barbiturates	Amphetamine-like stimulants
Antibiotics	Barbiturates	Antiparasitic drugs	Bromides	Antiarrhythmic drugs
Antiepileptic drugs	Bismuth	Antituberculosis drugs	Other sedative-hypnotics	Antibiotic drugs
Antihypertensive drugs	Bromides	Bromides		Anticholinergic drugs
Antineoplastic drugs	Lead	Corticosteroids	*Organic personality syndrome*	Antiepileptic drugs
Antiparasitic drugs	Manganese	Levodopa	Amphetamine-like stimulants	Antihistamines
Antipsychotic drugs	Mercury		Bromides	Antihypertensive drugs
Antituberculosis drugs	Thallium	*Hallucinosis*	Corticosteroids	Antineoplastic drugs
Antiviral drugs		Alcohol	Insulin	Antipsychotic drugs
Anxiolytics		Bromides		Anxiolytics
Belladonna alkaloids		Psychedelics		Bromides
Caffeine				Corticosteroids
Corticosteroids				Digitalis
Digitalis				Disulfiram
Diuretics				Estrogens
Insulin				Immunosuppressives
Levodopa				Levodopa
Lithium				Narcotic analgesics
Local anesthetics				Nonsteroidal anti-inflammatory drugs
MAO inhibitors				
Nonsteroidal anti-inflammatory drugs				
Salicylates				
Sedative-hypnotics				
Thyroid hormones				
Tricyclic antidepressants				

stimulants. Hypothyroidism, adrenocortical insufficiency, carcinoma of the pancreas, or viral illnesses can also lead to secondary depression. Mania is less likely to be secondary to organic factors, but may occur in hyperthyroidism or Cushing's syndrome. MAO inhibitors and analeptics have also caused manic episodes.

The diagnosis of **organic personality syndrome** is used for individuals who exhibit a marked change in personality due to a specific organic factor. The most common type of organic personality syndrome is the *frontal lobe syndrome,* which can occur with neoplasms or head trauma in the frontal lobes. In frontal lobe syndrome, either of two patterns may emerge: (1) emotional lability, impaired impulse control, poor social judgment, outbursts of temper or belligerence, sexual indiscretions, and bouts of crying, or (2) severe apathy, indifference, and loss of interest in activities. Another organic personality syndrome, which appears to involve the temporal lobes and is characterized by verbosity, religiosity, and sometimes aggressiveness, may occur in multiple sclerosis, Huntington's disease, or as an interictal phenomenon of temporal lobe epilepsy. Organic personality syndrome is sometimes drug-induced (Table 24–2).

Acute Versus Chronic Organic Brain Syndrome

OBS can be acute or chronic. The two designations carry substantially different implications (Table 24–3). When psychiatric or cognitive disturbances are of sudden onset because of organic disturbances, the condition is appropriately labeled acute OBS. **Acute OBS** has a generally positive prognosis: it is reversible if the underlying physiological cause is diagnosed and corrected quickly. Acute OBS is most frequently manifested as delirium, but dementia or one of the circumscribed organic brain syndromes can occur depending on the cause. The likely physiological precipitants of acute OBS include intoxication, drug withdrawal, metabolic or temperature imbalances, epilepsy, tumors, concussion, cardiovascular disorders, infections, inflammations, allergic reactions, elevated intracranial pressure, nutritional deficiencies, anemia, hypoxia, or endocrine disturbances.

Chronic OBS is an irreversible disorder characterized by progressive dementia. Intellectual deterioration occurs gradually. Chronic OBS begins with specific disturbances, such as memory loss and aphasia, and progresses to apathy, fragmentary utter-

Table 24–3
Comparison of Acute and Chronic Organic Brain Syndromes

Characteristic	Acute	Chronic
Causes	Intoxication, withdrawal, metabolic or temperature problems, epilepsy, tumor, concussion, cardiovascular disorders, infection, or allergic reactions	Senile brain disease, cerebral arteriosclerosis, degenerative brain diseases, Jakob-Creutzfeldt disease
DSM-III descriptive terms	Generalized: delirium, occasionally followed by dementia Circumscribed: amnestic syndrome, organic hallucinosis, organic affective syndrome, organic delusional syndrome, organic personality syndrome	Dementia, senile; dementia, presenile
Symptoms		
Intellect	Disorganized	Impoverished
Memory	Recent memory impaired in delirium or amnestic syndrome	Recent and/or remote memory impaired
Awareness	Confused, disoriented, attention deficiencies, perceptual disturbances	Relatively normal
Sleep-wake cycle	Often disturbed	Usually normal
Diagnosis and course		
Onset	Sudden	Insidious
Prognosis	Reversible	Irreversible
Resemblance to functional disorders	Easily distinguished by history of rapid onset	May mimic depression, anxiety, psychosis, or personality disorders
Treatment	Alleviate cause Diazepam for agitation or haloperidol (Haldol) for restlessness or recalcitrance	Pharmacotherapy to: control symptoms and improve cognitive functioning

ances, stupor, and finally complete muteness. Approximately two-thirds of cases of dementia are attributed to Alzheimer's disease. Another kind of irreversible dementia is that caused by multiple infarcts. **Multi-infarct dementia** is related to **arteriosclerosis,** a generic term covering several types of pathological changes in blood vessels in which accumulations of lipids cause a thickening of the blood vessel wall, narrowing of the vessel diameter, elevated blood pressure, and inadequate exchange of nutrients and wastes between the blood and tissues such as the brain. In multi-infarct dementia, deterioration in mental functioning tends to progress stepwise rather than as a continuous process, with some intellectual functions left relatively undamaged. There may also be focal neurological signs such as weakness in the limbs or reflexive asymmetries. All of these elements as well as examination of the brain upon autopsy suggest a series of infarcts, each resulting in a localized area of neural damage. The risk of arteriosclerosis is increased by diets high in cholesterol and saturated fats, lack of exercise, obesity, age, smoking tobacco, drinking alcohol, stress, androgens, diabetes, and hypertension and decreased by exercise, estrogens, and diets rich in polyunsaturated fats.

Other causes of irreversible dementia include neurological degenerative diseases such as Pick's disease, Friedreich's ataxia, multiple sclerosis, Huntington's disease, parkinsonism, progressive supranuclear palsy, and olivopontocerebellar atrophy. Infectious dementia occurs in Creutzfeldt-Jakob disease (which is probably caused by a slow virus, or prion) and subacute sclerosing panencephalitis (which can develop from herpes encephalitis or rarely from rubella virus vaccine).

Presenile Versus Senile Dementia

Dementia can arise in the senium or presenium. Overall, the incidence of dementia increases with age, but each form of dementia exhibits a characteristic age distribution with respect to onset (Figure 24–1). Pick's disease and Huntington's disease are classic presenile dementias, exhibiting age of onset peaks in the fourth, fifth, or sixth decades of life and declining abruptly in incidence thereafter. The term *Alzheimer's disease,* once reserved for dementias arising in the presenium, is now employed more generally for both senile and presenile dementias that lack specific etiologies.

Alzheimer's Disease

There is justifiable concern that the importance of Alzheimer's disease is likely to increase dramatically in the next 50 years for two reasons: the number of people in the upper age brackets is rising sharply, and other major causes of death (heart disease and cancer) appear likely to come under control sooner than Alzheimer's disease. Life expectancy may be further extended into the age range where incidence of Alzheimer's disease increases exponentially.

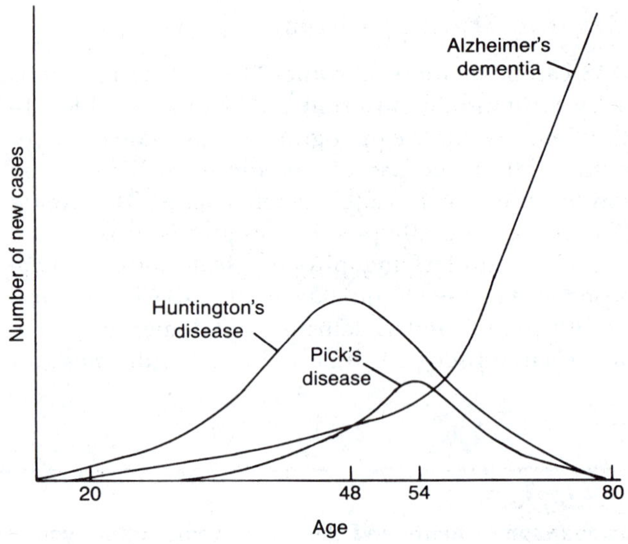

Figure 24–1
Schematic of frequency distribution for three progressive dementias. From L. L. Heston, Dementia of the Alzheimer type: a perspective from family studies. *Banbury Report 15:* 183–191, 1983. Reprinted by permission of the author and Cold Spring Harbor Laboratory, pub.

Although the causes of Alzheimer's disease remain unknown, a great deal has been learned in recent years about physiological changes in the brain that accompany aging in general and Alzheimer's disease in particular. At the level of gross brain morphology, aging is accompanied by diffuse changes (decrease in volume and weight of brain tissue), decreased glucose utilization, increased vascular resistance, reduced numbers of neurons in certain brain regions, and accumulation of lipofuscins.

At the level of the neuron, changes noted with aging are extensive (Figure 24–2). Damage to the DNA of neurons accumulates with successive exposures to radiation and free radicals. Transcription and translational mechanisms become increasingly faulty; nerve cells (like other cells) become increasingly resistant to insulin; transmitter synthesis is reduced; and morphologial changes occur in the effector elements (the axons and terminals) of the neuron. Several aspects of neurotransmission that are energy dependent, including maintenance of the resting potential, transmitter synthesis, and transmitter reuptake, are impaired in the aged neuron be-

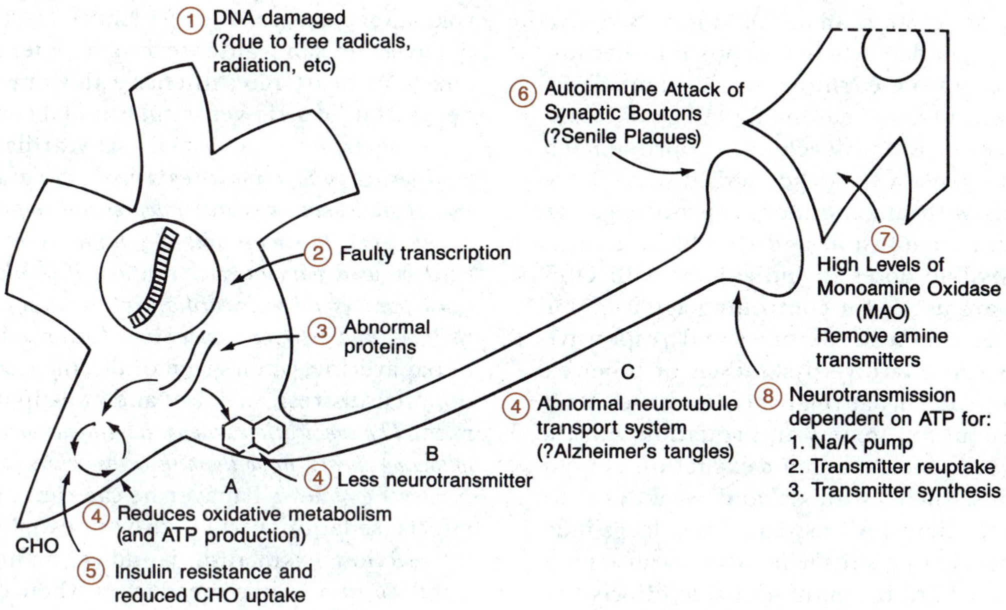

Figure 24–2
The aged neuron. From J. Yesavage, Pharmacotherapy of the aged central nervous system. *Clin. Neuropharmacol. 4:* 199–220, 1979. Reprinted by permission of Raven Press, New York.

cause of the decline in energy resources. The neurotubular transport system of the axons, responsible for delivery of substances between the nerve terminal and cell body, may undergo disorganization, leading to formation of so-called **Alzheimer's tangles,** a morphological feature of the brains of Alzheimer's victims upon postmortem examination. Another feature of brain tissue in Alzheimer's disease are **senile plaques** (amyloid-rich neuritic plaques) believed to evolve from degenerating cholinergic neurons.

Cholinergic neurons in the CNS are especially vulnerable and among the first to deteriorate in the progression toward severe dementia, especially the cholinergic pathways arising in the basal nucleus (of Meynert) that project to all regions of the cerebral cortex (Figure 9–12, page 141). Another neuronal population that declines significantly in Alzheimer's disease is the noradrenergic neurons of the locus ceruleus — part of the reward system.

There is no consistent evidence of a genetic abnormality in Alzheimer's clients, although in a small number of families, Alzheimer's disease appears to occur as an autosomal dominant condition or in association with Down's syndrome. Otherwise, individuals who are closely related to someone who has Alzheimer's disease have only a few-fold increase in likelihood of developing the condition, and this influence is observed mainly when the Alzheimer's disease is of early onset; much less so with late-onset dementia.

Alzheimer's clients consistently exhibit a diffuse, progressive, and symmetrical slowing of the EEG (correlating with the extent of cognitive impairment), reduced cerebral blood flow, and reduced oxygen and glucose utilization by cortical cells. Most of these alterations are also seen in other diseases that result in dementia.

One study has suggested a possible infectious origin for Alzheimer's disease, possibly a prion type of pathogen, which needs to be investigated further. Aluminum toxicity also has been thought to be a contributing factor, but it is doubtful that aluminum toxicity is involved in the vast majority of cases of Alzheimer's disease. Deferoxamine, an aluminum chelator, is being tested currently in clinical trials.

Drug Treatment of Organic Brain Syndrome

The objectives of drug therapy in chronic OBS are (1) to relieve the symptoms of psychiatric disturbances and (2) to improve cognitive functioning. Neuroleptics, especially thioridazine (Mellaril), are useful for emotional disturbances, anxiolytics for anxiety, and tricyclics for depression, all of which are administered at lower than usual doses. Sedative-hypnotics are avoided whenever possible because they tend to aggravate cognitive impairment. Tricyclic antidepressants are reasonably effective in secondary depression, which develops in approximately one-fourth of clients with Alzheimer's disease. However, tricyclics with anticholinergic properties can aggravate mental confusion and should be used at the lowest possible doses in individuals with OBS. Neuroleptics are useful for controlling agitation but tend to further diminish alertness and responsiveness and may cause tardive dyskinesias or other extrapyramidal problems at relatively low doses. Anxiolytics are useful for anxiety and agitation, but the incidence of paradoxical rage or excitation and adverse reactions, such as ataxia and weakness, are higher in these clients. All psychotropic drugs must be used cautiously in clients with OBS because paradoxical reactions are common and side effects that may be of little consequence in younger persons are often critical in older ones. Sometimes side effects develop in these clients at unusually low doses.

Five classes of drugs have been used to treat baseline cognitive impairment, but three of these classes exhibit little value. **Stimulants** (methylphenidate, pentylenetetrazole, and magnesium pemoline) have not demonstrated long-term effectiveness. **Vitamins, minerals, and hormones** have shown no evidence of value except for the use of vitamin B_{12} or nicotinic acid in dementias attributable specifically to the corresponding deficiency states.

Cerebral vasodilators (such as **papaverine**) provoke dangerous cardiovascular effects. For example, papaverine can cause severe hypotension, an increase in heart rate, intensive flushing of the face, depression of atrio-ventricular nodal conduction, ectopic beats, or paroxysmal tachycardia. *Prior to administering papaverine, clients need to be assessed for presence of glaucoma, myocardial depression, angina pectoris, or recent stroke. In clients with any of these problems, the drug must be used with extreme caution, if at all, since it can cause paroxysmal tachycardia, transient ventricular ectopic rhythms, and extreme hypotension.* Other adverse effects of papaverine, when given orally, include nausea, abdominal distress, malaise, and constipation or diarrhea. *The medication can be administered with meals, or following meals, or with milk or an antacid to reduce the incidence of nausea.* Papaverine can cause neurological effects (sedation, vertigo, drowsiness), hypersensitivity reactions (skin rash, jaundice, or hepatic eosinophilia), or vascular headaches when employed by either oral or parenteral routes. *Complaints of drowsiness or dry mouth and throat may indicate an adverse reaction; the nurse should monitor the client for changes in blood pressure, respiration, or cardiac function.* Hepatotoxicity sometimes occurs in response to papaverine, but it is reversible if identified quickly and the drug discontinued promptly. *Hepatic function tests should be conducted before the client begins receiving papaverine and periodically after drug therapy has begun. When papaverine is given parenterally, nurses need to establish baseline measurements of pulse, respiration, and blood pressure before administering the drug and should monitor these parameters*

Nursing Observations for Drug Therapy of Chronic Organic Brain Syndrome

THERAPEUTIC GOAL	(1) Control of psychiatric symptoms, and (2) improvement of cognitive functioning.
PREADMINISTRATION ASSESSMENT	
Baseline Data	Observe for impairments of judgment, affect, intellect, memory, arousal, orientation, and sensory perception. Evaluate neurological function (balance, appetite, orientation, arousal); EEG and CT scan. Evaluate client for any possible underlying organic or psychiatric factors that might be contributing, including endocrine problems, vitamin deficiency, depression, and cardiovascular disorders. Measure baseline vital signs before instituting therapy with dihydroergotoxine.
EVALUATION OF DRUG RESPONSE	
For Therapeutic Benefit	Note changes in psychiatric state or cognitive functioning.
For Compliance	Evaluate client compliance with all facets of the therapeutic regimen by careful observation, interviewing, and review of progress. Watch for possible hoarding of medicines. Report compliance problems to the physician and act as client-advocate when changes in the therapeutic regimen seem indicated.

Nursing Diagnoses and Interventions for Drug Therapy of Chronic Organic Brain Syndrome

Nursing Diagnoses	*Related Interventions*
TO ENHANCE DRUG BENEFITS OR REDUCE DRUG REQUIREMENTS	
Alteration in family processes related to diminished ability to maintain relationships and role functions Impaired home maintenance management related to dementia	Help the client remain independent as long as possible. Provide the client with stable routines and grooming. Encourage the family to interact with the individual. Help the client in participating with others as long as possible. Use the client's name; keep familiar objects around.
Increased risk of injury related to dementia or delirium	Provide safety measures as required.
Sensory-perceptual alterations related to diminished contact with reality	Provide a quiet environment.
TO ENSURE SAFE AND EFFICACIOUS DRUG USE	
Knowledge deficit related to drug regimen	Explain to the client the nature of the condition and the rationale for the medical regimen. Explanations should be in simple terms and tailored to the remaining level of intellectual capability. Provide clients and responsible family members with a list of adverse effects and drug interactions for each drug in the regimen and explain what to do if any of these occur.

routinely thereafter. All dosage forms of papaverine should be kept in tightly covered, light-resistant containers.

Preparations and Administration

Papaverine (numerous trade names)
Tablets, timed release capsules, liquid filled capsules, elixir, injection solutions
Recommended Doses: 60–300 mg orally, 1–5 times daily. *Clients should be told not to chew timed release capsules.* For IV or IM administration, 30–120 mg at 3-hour intervals as indicated.

The two most promising approaches for improvement of cognitive functioning in clients with OBS are the use of **stimulators of cerebral metabolism** and **precursors of transmitters** (levodopa, 5-hydroxytryptophan, and especially choline). **Dihydroergotoxine** (Hydergine), a combination of three ergot compounds (dihydroergocornine, dihydroergocristine, and dihydroergocryptine) is the only stimulator of cerebral metabolism currently available in the United States. Well-controlled studies support claims of the effectiveness of dihydroergotoxine based on both self-reports and assessments by clinical personnel. However, the extent of the benefit, though reproducible, is modest. Dihydroergotoxine has dopamine agonist properties, inhibits phosphodiesterase, stimulates cerebral metabolism, and has mild vasodilating activity, but the mechanism by which it improves cognitive functioning is uncertain. After oral administration of dihydroergotoxine, less than 50% of the dose reaches the systemic circulation. The mean biological half-life of the dihydrogenated ergot alkaloids is 3.5 hours. No serious adverse effects have been identified for this preparation. Transient nausea, heartburn, and sublingual irritation have been reported. Mild hypotenion and bradycardia can occur. *The nurse should establish baseline measurements of blood pressure and pulse and check these periodically when dihydroergotoxine is being used. Clients should be advised to change position slowly when standing up.*

The nurse should carefully instruct clients to keep sublingual tablets under the tongue until fully dissolved and not to eat, smoke, or drink anything until dissolution is complete. Dihydrogenated alkaloids should be protected from light, moisture, and heat (over 86°F). Beneficial results may not occur until after 3 or 4 weeks of treatment.

Preparations and Administration

Dihydroergotoxine (Hydergine, Circanol, Ergoloid, Gerigine, Spengine, Tri-Ergone, Trigot, and Deapril)
Tablets, sublingual tablets, oral liquid
Recommended Doses: 1 mg PO, tid.

An intriguing approach has been efforts to overcome the deficits in brain acetylcholine that occur in Alzheimer's disease, an approach that could be likened to the use of levodopa in parkinsonism. **Choline** and **lecithin** have been administered to clients with Alzheimer's disease in quantities sufficient to double plasma concentrations, but without benefit. Cholinesterase inhibitors and cholinomimetics are being tested currently. Studies to date suggest a slight benefit in some clients. Apparently, provision of acetylcholine precursors or mimics does not fully compensate for loss of functioning cholinergic nerve terminals. Choline and lecithin are available as nutritional products but have no established or approved therapeutic uses at present.

Case Study: Acute Exacerbation of Chronic Organic Brain Syndrome

M. S., a 76-year-old Caucasian female, was brought by her husband to a public clinic in a medium sized city while visiting in New England. The husband indicated that during the preceding 24 hours, M. S. had been extremely agitated and had been acting strangely. During the night, M. S. had slept poorly, tossing and turning, suffering frequent nightmares, and several times crying out in fright. She had also vomited three times during the night. M. S. appeared to hear imaginary voices, was not eating, and appeared restless. Vital signs were pulse 95, blood pressure 145–110, respirations 20, and temperature 100.2°F.

Since neither M. S. nor her husband were known to the health personnel at the clinic, the nurse interviewed the husband regarding his wife's normal behavior. M. S. was described as usually cooperative, pleasant, and subdued, although given to periods of depression. M. S. sometimes experienced mild impairment of recent memory and episodes of disorientation. Her husband described an example of her "totally forgetting that she was getting ready to go out shopping even though she had mentioned it several times a few minutes earlier." There was no indication of unusual stress in M. S.'s life at present.

M. S.'s husband indicated that she had a long history of using alcohol excessively, describing her as an alcoholic. She had been drinking heavily of late but not on the day she was brought to the hospital or the previous day. The husband gave a medication history for his wife as follows: "Sometimes uses aspirin for pain, takes a medication for high blood pressure and something for her problem with her memory, sometimes uses a sleeping pill, and sometimes takes vitamins." He said that she was not always good about taking her blood pressure medication but had been better in the last month.

The family physician was contacted for clarification of medications and diagnosed problems. He indicated that M. S. had a diagnosis of hypertension related to atherosclerosis and chronic organic brain syndrome secondary to generalized atherosclerosis and alcoholism. She was on a no-added-salt diet and was taking hydrochlorthiazide, 50 mg PO, daily, dihydroergotoxine (Hydergine), 1 mg tid, and a thiamine supplement. She also had a prescription for flurazepam (Dalmane), 30 mg PO as required, for insomnia. The physician confirmed that M. S. used alcohol excessively and had been advised that it would gradually aggravate her cardiovascular and mental problems.

M. S. was admitted to the unit for further evaluation and was given an orientation test. She appeared agitated during the testing but attempted to cooperate. She was unable to answer three of the ten questions used: where she was, what year it was, and the month of her birth. She exhibited diaphoresis and a coarse tremor of the hands and tongue. Blood tests were conducted, including electrolytes, oxygenation, blood cell counts, pH, and blood sugar levels; all values were within normal ranges except for a low serum potassium concentration. Measurement of alcohol and flurazepam failed to indicate significant concentrations of either substance in the blood. After 5 hours, M. S.'s degree of agitation had not lessened. Her condition was diagnosed as alcohol withdrawal delirium and acute exacerbation of chronic organic brain syndrome due to alcohol withdrawal and hypokalemia. Since there was no evidence of impending seizures, M. S. was prescribed chlordiazepoxide (Librium), 50 mg PO as needed, up to 300 mg/day, for 5 days, then 10 mg, 3 or 4 times daily for another 5 days; potassium chloride 15 mEq PO tid; continuation of the thiamine supplement, dihydroergotoxine, and thiazide diuretic. Withdrawal symptoms resolved quickly and the client's orientation gradually improved. M. S. was released after 5 days. She was instructed not to use alcohol or flurazepam while completing the regimen of chlordiazepoxide and advised to enter an alcohol treatment program.

1. What evidence in the case suggests alcohol withdrawal? Is an alternative diagnosis of acute alcohol toxic psychosis reasonable?
2. What is the likely cause of the hypokalemia referred to in the case? How does hypokalemia relate to organic brain syndrome?
3. Why does M. S. have a prescription for thiamine? (See Chapter 13.) Why does she have a prescription for dihydroergotoxine?
4. Could any of the drugs used by M. S. aggravate cognitive impairments of chronic organic brain syndrome?
5. What did the physician have in mind in ordering measurement of blood oxygenation? Blood cell count? Serum pH? Blood sugar levels?
6. Why was chlordiazepoxide given? Why was it given for 5 days, then 5 days at a reduced dose, then discontinued? (See Chapter 13.) Why was potassium chloride given?
7. Why was M. S. told not to take alcohol or flurazepam with chlordiazepoxide? (See Chapter 13.)

Answers appear at the end of the book.

Recommended Readings

Branconnier RJ, Cole JO: Effects of chronic papaverine administration on mild senile organic brain syndrome. *J Am Geriatr Soc* 1977;25:458–462.

Cook P, James I: Cerebral vasodilators. *N Engl J Med* 1981;305:1508–1513, 1560–1564.

Coyle JT et al: Alzheimer's disease: A disorder of cortical cholinergic innervation. *Science* 1983;219:1184–1190.

Fisman M: Clinical pharmacology of senile dementia. *Prog Neuropsychopharmacol* 1981;5(5–6):447–457.

Greenwald BS: Neurotransmitter deficits in Alzheimer's disease: Criteria for significance. *J Am Geriatr Soc* 1983;31:310–316.

Katzman R (ed): *Biological Aspects of Alzheimer's Disease.* Banbury Report 15. Cold Spring Harbor Laboratories, Cold Spring Harbor, NY, 1983.

Kolata G: Clues to Alzheimer's disease emerge. *Science* 1983;219:941–942.

Pricee DL: New perspectives on Alzheimer's disease. *Annu Rev Neurosci* 1986;9:489–512.

Prien, RF: *Chronic Organic Brain Syndrome.* GPO No 0-4820317 [189], 1972.

Shapira J, Schlesinger R, Cummings JL: Distinguishing dementias. *Am J Nurs* 1986;86(6):698–702.

Yesavage JA: Pharmacology of the aged central nervous system. *Clin Neuropharmacol* 1979;4:199–220.

Yesavage JA: Senile dementia: Combined pharmacologic and psychologic treatment. *J Am Geriatr Soc* 1981;29: 164–171.

CHAPTER 25

Analgesics

Neurophysiology of Pain

Pain Receptors

Pain is a component of somatosensory sensation. There are four modes of cutaneous sensation, served by four specific types of receptors: pain, by fine nerve endings; cold, by the bulbs of Krause; warmth, by Ruffini's corpuscles; and touch, by Pacini's and Meissner's corpuscles as well as nerve endings on hair follicles. Cutaneous afferents flow into the nervous system along two projection systems called the **epicritic** (or **lemniscal**) and the **protopathic** (or **spinothalamic**) systems. The protopathic system carries the afferents related to pain, temperature, and crude touch. The protopathic system includes a **neospinothalamic branch** and a **paleospinothalamic branch** (Figure 25–1). The neospinothalamic branch, providing the *informational component* of pain, is an express line from the spinal cord to the cerebral cortex that is little influenced by drugs because of the small number of intermediate synapses. The paleospinothalamic system, by contrast, is polysynaptic with many intermediate brainstem relay stations, where drugs (and endogenous regulators) can modify the flow of signals. The signals passing along the paleospinothalamic system ultimately reach the limbic system to provide the *affective component* of pain. These neuroanatomical characteristics of the pain pathways explain why narcotic analgesics alter the emotional response to pain more than its discrimination. After receiving an analgesic, a client is likely to say that the pain sensations are still felt, but they no longer hurt.

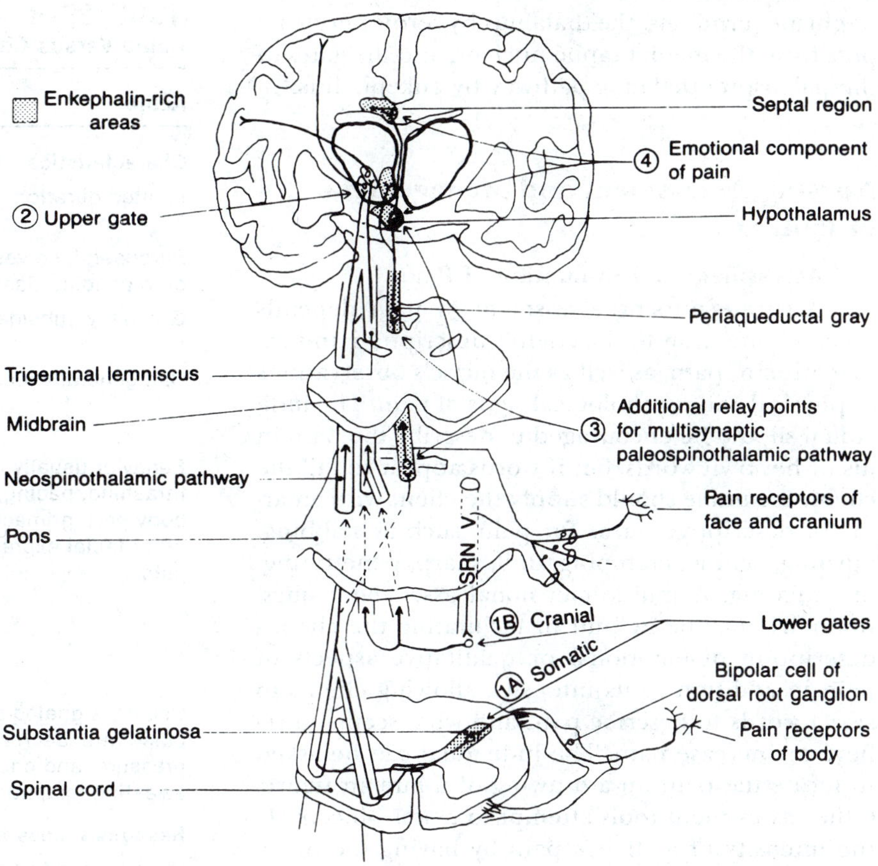

Figure 25–1
The pain pathways, illustrating the lower (1A and 1B) and upper (2) gates, where pain impulses are subject to modulation; additional relay points (3) of the paleospinothalamic pathway; and brain centers that contribute the affective quality to pain (4). From A. K. Swonger and L. L. Constantine, *Drugs and Therapy,* 2nd ed. Boston: Little, Brown, 1983.

Gating of Pain Signals

A pain signal originates in a peripheral receptor (free nerve ending) that acts as a transducer, converting physical or chemical stimuli into electrical impulses (action potentials) in the associated nerve fiber. An example of a chemical that can activate pain receptors is bradykinin, an autocoid released by injured cells. If the pain receptor is located below the cranium, the pain signal is carried by a long dendrite from a bipolar cell located in the dorsal root ganglion of the spinal cord (see Figure 25–1) into the gray matter of the spinal cord, where it reaches a region called the **substantia gelatinosa.** If the pain receptor is located in the cranium, the nerve impulse enters the brainstem along the fifth, seventh, or ninth cranial nerve to synapse in the spinal root and nucleus of the fifth cranial nerve (SRN-V), the brainstem analogue of substantia gelatinosa. Substantia gelatinosa and SRN-V serve as gates (the **lower gates**) where flow of pain signals can be regulated.

When pain signals succeed in passing through these gates, cells located in substantia gelatinosa or SRN-V next carry the signals upward to higher brain centers. Axons from cells in SRN-V travel in a pathway called the **trigeminal lemniscus;** fibers from the substantia gelatinosa travel in the spinothalamic pathway. Some of the pain impulses diverge into the multisynaptic paleospinothalamic pathway before reaching the limbic system. Other pain impulses take the express route to the thalamus, which serves as an **upper gate** for pain signals. From the thalamus, some of the pain signals are relayed to the somatosensory cortex in the parietal lobe.

When pain signals are persistent, the fraction of impulses allowed to pass through the various gates gradually declines. This phenomenon, called **habituation,** differs from **adaptation,** which occurs at the level of the pain receptors. Habituation is brought about by the action of peptide and amine transmitters that regulate the gates along the pain pathways. The lower gate for somatic pain sensations, substantia gelatinosa, is controlled by the peptide enkephalin and the amine serotonin. These transmitters control gating in substantia gelatinosa by regulating release of **substance P,** a peptide that conveys pain information. SRN-V is controlled by norepinephrine terminals, the thalamus by serotonergic inputs from the medial raphé nucleus, and the gates of the paleospinothalamic pathway by enkephalins.

Nursing Assessment and Management of Pain

Assessment and Evaluation of Pain

Accurate nursing assessment of pain depends on close attention to the client's description and explanation of pain, as well as the nurse's observations of physical and psychological signs of pain. The individual should be encouraged to describe the pain in his or her own words, but if words appear to fail the client, the nurse should supply the client with an array of descriptive terms for pain, such as stabbing, burning, aching, cramping, dull, sharp, penetrating, or radiating. A multidimensional assessment questionnaire may be helpful in facilitating the client's description of emotional or qualitative aspects of pain in addition to its intensity, allowing clients to select words to describe pain and what seems to relieve or increase pain. The individual can be asked to locate the pain on a drawing of a human figure. Other assessment tools attempt to assess objectively the intensity of a client's pain by having the nurse observe pain-related behaviors. After therapy has been instituted, these tools can be used again to assess the efficacy.

There are many different types of pain. **Superficial pain** is usually sharp and localized and occurs when surface structures are affected by painful stimuli. **Deep pain** occurs in tissues, such as muscles, periosteum, and viscera, and may arise directly from the site of the stimulus or may be poorly localized and perceived as a dull aching. **Referred pain** is felt at a site other than the area of stimulus. For example, in angina pectoris pain arises in the pericardium but is projected to the jaw, the arm, even the teeth.

Pain may also be acute or chronic. Usually **acute pain** occurs suddenly and is often sharp and unrelenting while it lasts, but eventually subsides. **Chronic pain** persists or recurs for an indefinite period of time and is refractory to treatment (examples are trigeminal neuralgia and arthritis). Chronic pain is exhausting, debilitating, and depressing; clients tend to become frustrated and ultimately develop adaptive behaviors. **Intractable pain** is chronic pain that resists antipain therapy and persists over long periods of time. There are important differences in response to drug treatment between acute and chronic pain (Table 25–1).

Table 25–1
Acute Versus Chronic Pain

Acute	Chronic
Characteristics	
Limited duration	Prolonged, generally lasting more than 6 months
Purposeful, serves as a sign of impending tissue damage	Serves no useful purpose
Gradually subsides	Often progresses in severity as pathology increases
Can generally localize pain	Localization imprecise; often pain is described as ache or soreness
Behavior usually restless, thrashing, pacing, rubbing body part, grimacing, and other facial expression of pain	Apt to be tired-looking, may or may not have facial expression of pain, often depressed. Suffering causes exhaustion of physical and mental capabilities. Pain becomes a central life focus. Accommodates behavior to pain.
Usually signaled by a rise in pulse rate, decrease in blood pressure, and onset of sweating (diaphoresis)	Often have complex history of surgical procedures and therapies and a history of dependence on medications.
Responsiveness to analgesics	
Usually readily responsive	Less responsive
Tolerance usually does not develop	Tolerance usually develops
Sedative effect of analgesic is an advantage	Sedative effect of analgesic is a disadvantage
Oral or parenteral routes	Usually oral route is employed
Standard doses can be used	Doses must be titrated to needs and level of tolerance of individual
Additional drugs are seldom required to manage pain	Additional drugs are often required to manage pain (tricyclic antidepressants or amphetamine)

Differences in Drug Therapy for Acute and Chronic Pain

Acute pain presents less difficulty than chronic pain for effective management. When pain is acute, the efficacy of analgesics is usually quite adequate to meet the needs of the client. The use of narcotics at doses that produce substantial sedation usually causes little difficulty when the requirements for pain relief are short-term. Often in these circumstances, the client is confined to bed or is under orders to rest, and thus benefits from the degree of sedation afforded by the analgesic drug. If the patient is hospitalized, the analgesic drug can be administered effectively by either oral or parenteral routes. Standardized doses can usually be employed since tolerance to the drug effect is not yet a factor and individual psychological factors related to pain sensitivity and response are not usually important at this stage. There is seldom any need to supplement the primary analgesic with other kinds of medications, and the drug can be repeated without concern for tolerance or dependence.

Chronic pain is more difficult to treat. The client may be expected or required to function, at least minimally, despite pain. Sedation caused by the analgesic may be detrimental to daily activity. Since the individual often is not hospitalized, administration of analgesics is largely limited to the oral route. It is not possible to depend on standardized doses because of individual variability in the intensity of pain, ability to tolerate pain, and pharmacological tolerance to the drug. The need for pain relief must be balanced against the risk that tolerance and dependence will develop if the drug selected for analgesia is a narcotic. It is often necessary to augment the action of the primary analgesic with one or more drugs from another category, as in the use of tricyclic antidepressants or amphetamine to potentiate the analgesic activity of narcotics.

Nursing Measures That Facilitate Analgesia

The management of pain by nondrug interventions is an important facet of nursing intervention. Nursing actions can help to relieve physical discomfort and also help the client feel cared for, both of which help to ease pain. These nursing actions can reduce the client's need for drugs. Attending to physical needs such as proper body position and alignment, providing general comfort measures, reducing the client's anxiety, and controlling environmental irritants are all important. Cutaneous stimulation by massage or applications of heat or cold can be useful in controlling some kinds of pain. Heat may relieve muscle spasm; cold may reduce swelling.

Biofeedback may be used as a nondrug technique to train an individual to control pain, muscle tension, and stress. Clients are taught relaxation, deep breathing, or other techniques to control tension or other biophysical parameters. Electromyography (EMG) feedback has been effective in relieving tension headache for example.

In the following sections, we will consider three classes of analgesic agents: narcotic analgesics, aspirin-like drugs, and phenothiazine analgesics.

Narcotic Analgesics and Antagonists

History and Sources The term *opium* is derived from the Greek word *opius* meaning "little juice," and is the term applied to the sap that can be collected from the unripened pods of the poppy plant, *Papaver somniferum.* Between the time when the petals drop from the seed pod and its ripening a week or so later, opium can be collected by placement of shallow cuts into, but not through, the seed pod. When these cuts are placed in the evening using a claw-shaped tool, sap oozes from the cuts during the night, oxidizing to a red-brown colored gummy resin, which is easily collected in the morning. Opium is one of the oldest drugs known to human beings. Written references to a *joy plant,* presumed to refer to the poppy plant, date back to 4000 BC. Opium was employed as a medicinal in both the Egyptian and Greek civilizations, and in Greece, at least, it was also utilized in opium cakes and candies for recreational purposes. The Arabs embraced the use of opium, as well as hashish, both for medicinal and social purposes, partly because the use of alcohol was strictly forbidden by the Koran. During the Dark Ages in Europe, the Arabs were in contact with the civilizations of the Far East and opium seeds were carried to China from North Africa by AD 600 or 700.

With the dawn of the Renaissance, opium was discovered by Europe, becoming a fixture in both European medicine and its social life. The phenomena of dependence and withdrawal were first recognized in the latter half of the sixteenth century. Toward the end of the seventeenth century, in England, Dr. Thomas Sydenham, the father of clinical medicine, developed laudanum, a compound containing opium, saffron, cinnamon, cloves, and Canary wine, a concoction he employed for nearly every disorder. Use of laudanum and opium continued to expand in England and on the continent through the next three centuries. In the early part of the nineteenth century, several English literary giants were addicted to opium, including De Quincey ("The Confessions of an English Opium-Eater"), Samuel Taylor Coleridge ("Kubla Khan"), and Elizabeth Barrett Browning. By the middle of the nineteenth century, opium dens flourished in England and the British East India Company had become the world's opium pusher.

In China, opium use developed in the seventeenth and eighteenth centuries, in part because of an unsuccessful attempt beginning in 1644 to eliminate smoking of tobacco. The Chinese people initially used opium to disguise their tobacco and then simply dropped the tobacco. In 1729 a law was passed in China forbidding the use of opium and providing for strangulation of opium shopowners. The British began smuggling opium into China from India, and in 1839 the Chinese attempted to close down trade with the British to suppress opium smuggling. This and the murder of a Chinese man by drunken British and American sailors touched off the first opium war, which was won by the British. After three years, the British reopened China to the opium trade and won the rights to Hong Kong. A second opium war in the 1850s reinforced the results of the first. British involvement in opium continued until 1913.

Until the turn of the nineteenth century, only crude preparations of the extract were available. In 1803 Frederich Sertürner, a young pharmacist's assistant in Germany, isolated the principal active ingredient of opium, which he named *morphium,* after Morpheus, the Greek god of dreams. Later, this name became *morphine,* which we use today. Sertürner's achievement was important not only in providing the first pure narcotic, but also as the first isolation of an alkaloid from a botanical source. With the development of the hypodermic needle in 1853, injection of morphine became possible. Morphine became a staple in the field hospitals of the wars of that era in America and Europe (American Civil War [1861–1865], the Prussian-Austrian War [1866], and the Franco-Prussian War [1870]) and morphine addiction became known as *soldier's disease.* By the end of the nineteenth century, narcotic addiction was estimated to involve 1% of the population in the United States, a fraction much higher than in more recent times. There were three distinct forms: smoking of opium, mainly among the Chinese who had been brought to this country as workers; the traditional oral use of opium, most often involving middle-aged whites, frequently women; and the injection of morphine. Much of this addiction was facilitated by physicians. Concern began to grow about opiate addiction, and in 1906, the Pure Food and Drugs Act required labeling of the kind and amounts of opiates in various formulations. Then, in 1914, the Harrison Narcotic Act removed opiates from the nonprescription market.

Heroin, the diacetylated form of morphine, was introduced commercially in 1898 as a nonaddictive substitute for codeine. Ten years passed before this assertion was proved false. Laboratory synthesis of morphine was achieved in 1952. In addition to morphine, codeine occurs as a natural constituent of opium. In recent years, dozens of synthetic and semisynthetic narcotics have been synthesized and studied. Nearly 20 narcotics are available for current clinical practice.

Mechanisms and Effects The effect of narcotic drugs on the central nervous system is known as **narcosis,** which is manifested by analgesia, change in mood, mental clouding, and impairment of mental and physical performance, especially in recently acquired and complex learning. The mood change effected by narcotics is variable and depends on the physical condition and drug experience of the individual. Clients in pain generally experience euphoria, partly as a result of the pain relief. The addict experiences euphoria, and the more powerful *rush* if the narcotic is taken intravenously rather than orally. Frequently, however, the first time social user may experience discomfort and dysphoria, related in part to the annoying gastrointestinal effects of the narcotic.

Although the overall effect of narcotics in humans is a depressant influence on the brain, there is an excitatory component as well. For example, children given codeine close to bedtime for suppression of cough sometimes exhibit restlessness and insomnia. In adults, narcotics lower the seizure threshold, an indication of impaired inhibitory mechanisms in the brain.

Narcotics suppress the affective component of pain. Narcotics act on relay centers along the pain pathway, including the substantia gelatinosa in the spinal cord and limbic centers in the paleospinothalamic pathway, which relay dull pain, especially from the viscera. The actual sensory threshold is unaffected, but the affective component is diminished. Analgesia produced by narcotics is additive with that produced by nonnarcotic analgesics. Narcotics act centrally, while the nonnarcotic drugs act largely at the level of the peripheral pain receptors. Analgesia produced by most narcotics typically begins 15–30 minutes after drug administration and lasts about 3–4 hours. Although drug manufacturers have succeeded in developing narcotic congeners that selectively duplicate the activity of narcotics on the cough center or on the gastrointestinal tract without the addiction liability or other brain effects of morphine, it has not yet proved possible to achieve the analgesic effect of a narcotic without the accompanying risk of dependence.

Narcotics depress two vital centers of the brainstem: the cough center and the respiratory center. The action of narcotics on the cough center has led to use of codeine and other narcotics in cough suppressant formulations. A synthetic narcotic congener, dextromethorphan, is an effective cough suppressant that lacks other kinds of narcotic activity and is nonaddicting (see Chapter 52).

In the respiratory center, narcotics initially depress responsiveness to carbon dioxide, eliminating the **hypercapnic drive** of respiration, so that respiration may become labored. At higher doses, the spontaneous rhythmicity of the respiratory neurons (the **neurogenic drive**) and the responsiveness of the respiratory center to hypoxia (the **hypoxic drive**) are also depressed, leading to respiratory arrest (the usual cause of death in cases of narcotic overdose). *Before administering a narcotic, the nurse needs to note the pulse rate and quality, and depth, rate, and rhythm of respiration. A respiration rate of 12 or less per minute may be a sign of toxicity, and the narcotic should be withheld.* Respiratory depression may be treated by artificially maintaining respiration or administering a specific narcotic antagonist (the usual practice). Use of a narcotic antagonist is a safe approach but may precipitate a severe withdrawal syndrome if the individual uses narcotics habitually.

The chemoreceptor trigger zone located in the medulla is stimulated by many narcotics, resulting in vomiting or feelings of nausea and dizziness, depending on the dosage and potency of the particular agents. Narcotics slow the EEG and, in particular, increase theta activity and the integrated amplitude.

Many of the narcotics cause orthostatic hypotension, primarily because of histamine release. In extreme circumstances, histamine release may be massive enough to cause anaphylactoid reactions. Certain smooth muscles are directly contracted by morphine, such as the smooth muscle of the gut and the pupils. The former effect leads to intestinal cramps; the latter effect produces the characteristic constricted pupil of the addict. *Nurses should check a client's pupils for constriction as a sign of toxicity. Pupillary size is best judged in a well-lighted room with the client facing away from the light source, rather than with a flashlight, because sudden light can cause immediate miosis.*

Narcotics have been used in medicine for their antidiarrheal action, but in recent years, narcotic congeners have been developed that are useful antidiarrheals with few or none of the other activities associated with morphine (see Chapter 51). Narcotics produce a flushing and warming of the skin that is related to dilation of cutaneous blood vessels.

Endogenous Morphine-Like Substances The mechanism of action of narcotic analgesics relates to an interaction with receptors normally acted on by endogenous morphine-like substances. The endogenous opiate receptor ligands are referred to collectively as **endorphins** and include two pentapeptides, called **met-enkephalin** and **leu-enkephalin,** and a protein called **beta-endorphin.** The receptors for these substances can be called **opiate receptors, endorphin receptors,** or **narcotic receptors** with equal propriety. The peptides, which are heavily concentrated along the pain pathways and in the substantia gelatinosa, periaqueductal gray, hypothalamus, and limbic system (see Figure 25–1) probably act as neurotransmitters. Their half-lives are short (about 2 minutes), and their analgesic potency is weak and short-lived as well. Beta-endorphin is found in highest concentration within the pituitary gland and is also localized in a descending pathway that influences the reward and punishment systems. The effects of beta-endorphin, including analgesia, euphoria, catatonia, and behavioral effects, are relatively enduring since the half-life of this small protein is about 4 hours.

There are several classes of opiate receptors, including mu (μ), kappa (κ), delta (Δ), and sigma (σ) receptors. Morphine and other narcotic agonists bind to and activate opiate receptors, while narcotic antagonists, such as naloxone, merely bind. Mu receptors provide the respiratory depression, euphoria, physical dependence, and supraspinal analgesia produced by narcotic agonists; kappa receptors provide spinal analgesia, miosis, and sedation; delta receptors provide the affective changes; and sigma receptors provide the paradoxical responses of dysphoria, hallucinations, and respiratory or vasomotor stimulation.

Opiate receptors exhibit adaptability. Chronic administration of opiate agonists such as morphine leads to down-regulation, brought about by reduced receptor-effector coupling, not by a reduced number of receptor sites. Conversely, narcotic antagonists administered chronically cause up-regulation, which is due to an increase in the number of receptor sites.

Clinical Indications Narcotic analgesics are indicated for relief of pain whenever nonnarcotic drugs are contraindicated or not sufficiently effective. As with most other effects of drugs, the analgesic action of narcotics is dose dependent. While the rule is to administer the smallest effective dose for the shortest time compatible with client needs, the health care professional needs to be especially careful not to provide so little drug as to be ineffective (often done from fear of causing addiction). The result is an anxious client in whom the stress of inordinate discomfort is in itself a threat to the client's health, safety and comfort needs. Clients feel the fullest effects of a narcotic if they receive the drug before the pain becomes intense.

Certain members of the narcotic family are also employed as antidiarrheal drugs (see Chapter 51) or cough suppressants (see Chapter 52).

Adverse Effects and Contraindications Adverse effects associated with acute use of narcotics are relatively mild. With chronic use, the limiting features are the risks of tolerance, dependence, and withdrawal, which are discussed below. Narcotics tend to **increase intracranial pressure,** which is ordinarily insignificant but may be problematic in patients with head injury, brain tumor, or other intracranial lesions. The **seizure threshold** is depressed by narcotics, increasing the risk of seizures in seizure-prone individuals.

Excess depression is a potential problem when narcotics are employed in high doses or in conjunction with other CNS depressants, including general anesthetics, sedative-hypnotics, antihistamines, neuroleptics, or tricyclic antidepressants that have sedative characteristics. *The nurse should monitor respiration for signs of slowing or apnea, and blood pressure for cardiovascular depression, cardiac arrest, or shock. A narcotic antagonist should be readily available whenever high doses of narcotics are employed.* Respiration is depressed by narcotics to a greater extent than cardiovascular function. Respiratory tidal volume may remain below normal for 4 hours after a normal therapeutic dose

Nursing Observations for Drug Therapy of Pain

THERAPEUTIC GOAL	Relief of pain.
PREADMINISTRATION ASSESSMENT	
Baseline Data	Evaluate subjective reports of extent of pain and behaviors (grimacing, moaning, clutching the painful site) indicative of unrelieved pain. Evaluate neurological status, vital signs, perfusion, gastrointestinal output and function, and skin color, integrity, and temperature. Check renal and liver function when long-term use of narcotics is anticipated. Check bleeding times when long-term use of nonnarcotic analgesics is anticipated.
Contraindications/ Precautions	For narcotics, head injury, increased intracranial pressure, chronic obstructive pulmonary disease, hypotension, convulsive disorders, Addison's disease, hepatic or renal failure, or pregnancy; for nonnarcotic analgesics, hemophilia, active bleeding, renal or hepatic failure, pregnancy, or lactation. Check medication history for evidence of allergies to narcotic or nonnarcotic analgesics or tartrazine.
Potential Interactions	Check current medications for interacting drugs, such as other depressants when narcotics are to be used, or drugs with ulcergenic or anticoagulant effects or a high level of binding to plasma proteins when nonnarcotic analgesics are to be used.
EVALUATION OF DRUG RESPONSE	
For Adverse Effects	With narcotic analgesics, monitor for respiratory depression, dysrhythmias, orthostatic hypotension, CNS depression, constipation, urinary retention, dry mouth, and allergic reactions; with nonnarcotic analgesics, monitor for gastrointestinal irritation, bleeding, or ulceration, hyperpnea, tinnitus, uric acid retention, and respiratory acidosis.
For Drug Interactions	With narcotic analgesics, monitor for additive CNS depression and additive hypotensive effects. With nonnarcotic analgesics, monitor for additive ulcergenic effects (with alcohol or caffeine), competition for plasma protein binding sites (shown by increased bleeding with oral anticoagulants, for example), and inhibition of renal excretion of organic acids (e.g., methotrexate).
For Compliance	Evaluate client's compliance with all facets of the therapeutic regimen by careful observation, interviewing, and review of progress. Report compliance problems to the physician and act as client-advocate when changes in the therapeutic regimen seem indicated.

of a narcotic. Other symptoms attributable to excess depression of neural function include delirium, disorientation, confusion, drowsiness, lethargy, impairment of performance of mental or motor tasks, and coma. The excitatory component of the action of narcotics may be manifested as agitation, hallucinations, or tremor. Other neurological side effects include headache, euphoria, dysphoria, and visual disturbances.

Gastrointestinal side effects of narcotics include anorexia, constipation, biliary tract spasm, and intestinal cramps. *The nurse should monitor the client's bowel pattern and bowel sounds and encourage attention to the defecation reflex. Inattention to the need to defecate contributes to the constipating effect of narcotics.* **Cardiovascular symptoms,** such as flushing, hypotension, tachycardia, palpitations, and syncope are mainly attributable to histamine release. Transient hypotension is likely to occur. *Clients who are ambulatory may feel lightheaded and dizzy.* Similar problems occur when a supine client assumes a head-up position because narcotics decrease the ability of the cardiovascular system to respond to gravitational shifts.

Narcotics can produce **urinary retention** and hesitancy, spasms of the ureter and vesical sphincters, and oliguria. Urinary retention and oliguria occur because narcotics dull perception of bladder stimuli. *The nurse should monitor intake-output ratio and pattern when potent narcotics are employed. When output seems inadequate, nurses need to palpate the lower abdomen for bladder distention.* With long-term use, narcotics produce impotency and decreased libido. **Allergic reactions** are uncommon and generally consist of mild skin eruptions. Anaphylactoid reactions can occur with intravenous injections of morphine because of histamine release.

Most narcotics suppress the cough and sigh reflexes, which may lead to impairments of respiratory function. *The nurse should encourage clients receiving narcotics to change position frequently, cough regularly (unless contraindicated by the patient's condition), and to breathe deeply.*

Narcotic Abuse The number of narcotic addicts in the United States varies from year to year depending on the extent of success of law enforcement and political efforts to control illegal narcotic traffic. The average age of abusers has steadily declined over the years; by 1969, it had declined to 22 years; by 1978 the modal age for onset of narcotic addiction was 11–20 years of age. Narcotic use has also spread to areas outside the traditional opiate center, New York City. Numerically, the heroin problem is not so great as that of alcohol, anxiolytics, tobacco, or even barbiturates. On the other hand, an estimated 1–2% of the narcotic addict population dies yearly from overdosage. Chronic use of narcotics is less likely to produce tissue damage than is chronic use of alcohol or tobacco, but neurological complications occur in about 3% of long-term addicts.

Opiate intoxication is quite unlike that produced by sedative-hypnotics. Opiate intoxication (the narcotic stupor) is defined in the *Diagnostic and Statistical Manual of the American Psychiatric Association, Third Edition* by five criteria: (1) recent use of an opioid, (2) pupillary constriction, (3) one or more psychological signs (euphoria, dysphoria, apathy, or psychomotor retardation), (4) one or more neurological signs (drowsiness, slurred speech, or impaired memory or attention), and (5) absence of an organic or psychiatric cause.

Tolerance, Dependence, and Withdrawal Tolerance develops to all effects of narcotics except those related to a direct action on smooth muscle (such as constipation and pupillary constriction) but does not necessarily develop uniformly to all actions at the same time. Although an increase in rate of metabolism of narcotics (drug-disposition tolerance) may account for a small part of overall tolerance, the most important factor is the adaptive changes in brain neurochemistry and receptor populations (pharmacodynamic tolerance). Although the full neurochemical basis for pharmacodynamic tolerance remains to be worked out, one important component during the initial stages is an increase in the turnover of dopamine in the corpus striatum. Later, after a few days of chronic morphine treatment, dopamine turnover returns to normal, but opiate receptors begin to exhibit subsensitivity and dopamine receptors become supersensitive.

Both psychological and physical dependence occur with chronic narcotic use. Dependence is such a characteristic occurrence with narcotics that the term *narcotic* as used by the legal profession has come to include many drugs that are unrelated to morphine but produce dependence. The degree of abuse potential within the narcotic group is related to the intensity of the euphoria produced by the agent, the intensity of withdrawal symptoms that follow its use, and its efficacy in suppressing withdrawal symptoms. The duration of treatment with the narcotic, the interval between doses, the total daily dose, and the personality of the client are all important factors in determining abuse liability. *Therefore, narcotic analgesics should always be given in the smallest amounts possible that provide an acceptable level of pain relief. Generally, the objective of analgesic therapy is to reduce pain to an acceptable level and not necessarily to eliminate it completely. Time limits for use of narcotics (established by individual facilities) should be adhered to faithfully.*

Should there be an abrupt cessation of narcotic administration when physical dependence exists, the abstinence syndrome will occur. The client becomes anxious, irritable, perspires profusely, yawns, and develops sneezing and watery eyes within 6 hours of the last dose. Within 14 hours, the pupils become dilated, clients complain of feeling cold, and have piloerection ("goose bumps"). There is tremulousness, muscle jerks, body aches, and insomnia or restless sleep; blood pressure, pulse rate, and body temperature rise. Within 36–48 hours, the client develops nausea, diarrhea, vomiting, and anorexia. There may be spontaneous ejaculation or orgasm. The severity, duration, and latency of the withdrawal syndrome depend on the average amount of drug used daily and the length of time used. Withdrawal from narcotics, while distinctly unpleasant, is less life-threatening than withdrawal from a sedative-hypnotic, because there is very little likelihood of convulsions.

Methadone Treatment Programs

Methadone has been employed both to wean and maintain narcotic addicts. For **weaning,** a dose of methadone is given that matches the intensity of the habit. One difficulty in assessing habit intensity is the highly variable quality of street narcotics. Such factors as frequency of use, duration of the habit, cost of the habit, and quality of illicit material generally found in the locale are taken into account. Once the habit has been stabilized for about 48 hours, the dose is reduced by 5–10 mg per day until withdrawal is complete. Methadone withdrawal symptoms are considerably milder than those accompanying morphine or heroin abstinence, although the symptoms may be more drawn out.

Clients who decline to enter a weaning program may be treated in a **methadone maintenance** program. In a maintenance program, the initial stabilization method is the same as used in weaning. One factor in determining dosage for maintenance is whether it is felt necessary to preclude the client from getting a "rush" from surreptitious use of street drugs; higher doses of methadone (50–100 mg) will prevent this. Lower doses (30–50 mg) do not block the action of street drugs, but they do eliminate drug craving. The maintenance program differs from the weaning program in that dosage is not reduced after the habit is stabilized.

Methadone maintenance programs have both advocates and detractors. On the plus side methadone does not produce the mood swings associated with heroin, because it is long-acting and has a prolonged plasma half-life (Figure 25–2). The duration of action of methadone when used acutely is about 4–6 hours, but it increases with daily use because of a cumulative effect due to the very long plasma half-life of 22–25 hours (Table 25–2). Thus, the addict adhering to a maintenance schedule of daily high-dose methadone administration cannot get the rush usually obtained by "shooting" heroin and is protected somewhat from the temptation to return to use of street drugs. Some addicts may be ready for detoxification after a period on methadone maintenance has helped them to reconstruct support systems, such as family ties and stable employment, which may have been destroyed in the addiction cycle.

On the negative side, risks of overdose with methadone are substantial and the addict remains completely dependent on continued drug usage with all the attendant risks. Outcome statistics suggest that few addicts who enter a maintenance program ultimately progress to a weaning program.

Typical criteria utilized in accepting applicants into a methadone maintenance program are (1) a minimal age of 18, or if the candidate is 16–18 years of age, guardian consent and at least two prior failures in a detoxification program, and (2) no history of dropping out of a maintenance program within the last 2 years (time period varies). During the first few months of participation in a program, the addict takes each dose under supervision. After several months in the program, this requirement may be relaxed to allow four or five of the seven weekly doses to be taken at home. Among the variables found to predict successful retention in a methadone maintenance program (as opposed to relapse to street drugs) are older age, better educated, employed, white, married, and few or no criminal convictions.

Specific Narcotic Drugs

Opium

Opium remains available for medical use and is employed mainly for its antidiarrheal activity. Synthetic congeners of narcotics with antidiarrheal activity that lack other narcotic effects are better selections for treatment of diarrhea (Chapter 51).

Preparations and Administration

Opium

Mixture of hydrochloride salts of opium alkaloids (Pantopon), with 20 mg of the preparation being equivalent to 15 mg of morphine; liquid preparation containing 10% opium in 19% alcohol (Opium Tincture); camphorated tincture of opium, each 5 ml equivalent of 2 mg of morphine (Paregoric); 12% paregoric with glycyrrhiza

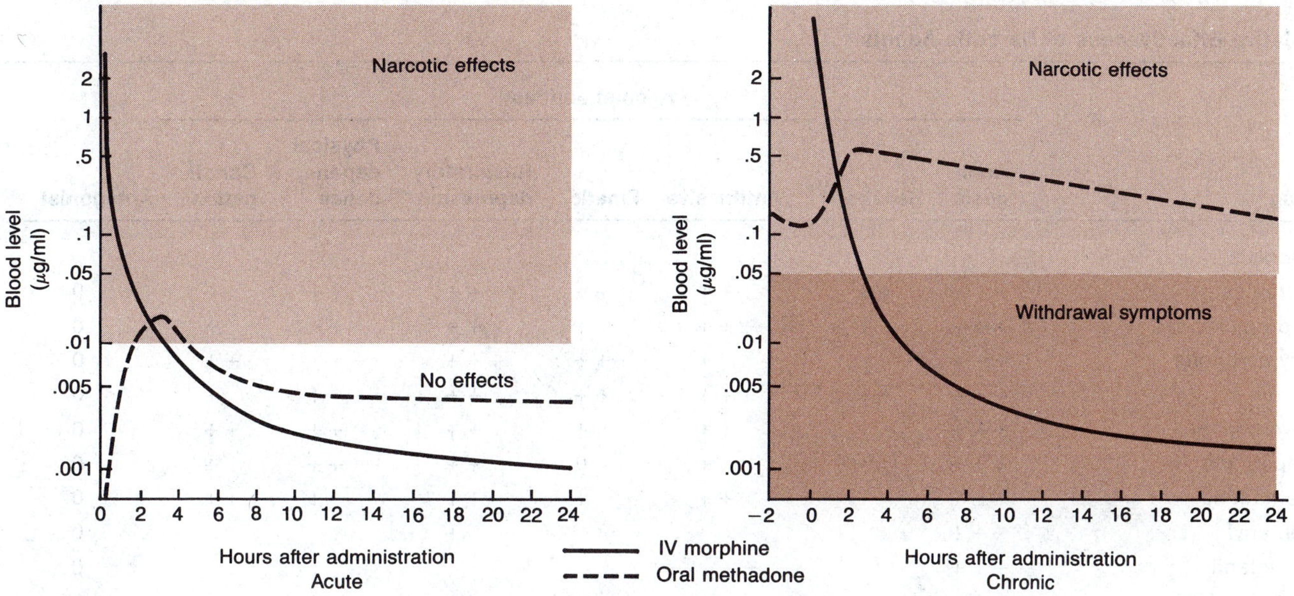

Figure 25–2
Narcotic blood levels of morphine and methadone. Acutely, oral methadone is slower to take effect and only slightly longer-acting than morphine. With chronic daily administration of 50–100 mg doses, methadone blood levels build up to produce a continuous, nearly stable, narcotic effect. From A. K. Swonger and L. L. Constantine, *Drugs and Therapy,* 2nd ed. Boston: Little, Brown, 1983.

fluid-extract, antimony potassium tartrate, and alcohol (Brown Mixture)

Morphine

Morphine is the major active alkaloid in opium and is generally considered to be the prototype of the narcotic analgesic class. It stimulates narcotic receptors of the mu and kappa types but has no effect on sigma receptors. It is a potent analgesic (see Table 25–2) but is limited by its rather poor oral effectiveness. Morphine is rarely given orally because oral doses required to achieve a given level of analgesia average six times greater than parenteral doses (Table 25–3). Oral administration is also less reliable, resulting in considerable individual variability in the fraction of the administered dose that is ultimately bioavailable. Morphine is a potent releaser of histamine and may cause hypersensitivity reactions. If the client has a history of hypersensitivity to opiates, morphine is contraindicated. As with other narcotics, morphine should not be employed in clients with increased intracranial pressure, convulsive disorders, acute alcoholism, acute bronchial asthma, chronic respiratory disease, severe respiratory depression, or pulmonary edema. The drug should be used with utmost caution and surveillance for clients who have prostatic hypertrophy, undiagnosed abdominal pain, pancreatitis, acute ulcerative colitis, or severe renal or liver insufficiency. Morphine remains a widely used in-hospital drug for parenteral injection and is encountered infrequently as an oral medication.

Preparations and Administration

Morphine
Injection solutions, soluble tablets, oral solutions, oral tablets, rectal suppositories
Recommended Doses: For pain in adults, 10 mg/70 kg SC or IM in adults is typical, but doses range from 5 mg/70 kg to 20 mg/70 kg. For children, doses range from 0.1 mg/kg to 0.2 mg/kg SC or IM. The usual adult IV dose is 4–10 mg injected slowly. Oral doses of 10–30 mg or rectal doses of 10–20 mg may be taken every 4 hours or as directed.

Codeine

Codeine is similar to morphine in its actions, equally effective as an antitussive, but less potent as an analgesic. Its potency as an antitussive is about one-half that of morphine, but it is only about one-fifth to one-tenth as potent as an analgesic and about

Table 25–2
Relative Effectiveness of Narcotic Agents

Drug	Agonist actions							
	Analgesia	Sedation	Antitussive	Emetic	Respiratory depression	Physical dependence	Constipation	Antagonist
Agonists								
Morphine	+++	++	+++	++	++	++	++	0
Hydromorphone	+++	+	+++	+	++	++	+	0
Oxymorphone	+++		+	+++	+++	+++	++	0
Heroin	+++	++	+++	++	++	+++	+	0
Levorphanol	+++	+	++	+	++	++	++	0
Meperidine	+++	+	+	0	++	++	+	0
Methadone	+++	+	++	+	++	+	++	0
Fentanyl	+++				+			0
Sufentanil	+++							0
Alphaprodine	+++	++		+	++	+	+	0
Oxycodone	+++	++	+++	++	++	++	++	0
Codeine	++	+	+++	+	+	+	+	0
Hydrocodone	++		+++			+		0
Propoxyphene	+	++		+	+	+		0
Agonist/antagonists								
Pentazocine	++				++	+		+
Nalbuphine	+++				++	+/−		++
Butorphanol	+++				+	+/−		+++
Antagonists								
Levallorphan	+				+	0		++
Naloxone	0	0	0	0	0	0	0	+++
Naltrexone	0	0	0	+	0	0	+	+++
Nonnarcotic congeners								
Dextromethorphan	0	0	+++	0	0	0	0	0
Diphenoxylate	0	+	0	+	+	+	++	0
Loperamide	0	0	0	+	0	0	++	0

one-tenth as potent as a respiratory depressant or emetic. This greater *relative* potency with respect to cough suppression made codeine the drug of choice for cough preparations until the introduction of dextromethorphan. Codeine continues to be marketed in many combination antitussive preparations. It is also widely used in the form of combination analgesics. It is found in combination with acetaminophen (Tylenol with Codeine) or aspirin (Emperin with Codeine); with acetaminophen and salicylamide (Codalan), or with butalbital (Fiorinal with codeine) for tension headaches. Tylenol with codeine is among the most widely prescribed drugs — ranking fourth in 1986. A major advantage of codeine over morphine is its greater oral effectiveness. The oral equivalent dose of codeine is only about 1.5 times its intramuscular dose, while the corresponding ratio for morphine is sixfold (see Table 25–3).

Clients should be discouraged from using codeine routinely for cough, since codeine can abolish the protective cough reflex. Productive cough should usually not be suppressed. Advising clients to avoid environmental irritants, such as smoke, dust, and fumes, may lessen the need for any cough suppressant.

Table 25-3
Pharmacokinetic Parameters of Narcotics

Drug	Route	Typical onset (minutes)	Typical peak effect (minutes)	Typical duration (hours)	Half-life (hours)	Equivalent dose (mg) IM	Equivalent dose (mg) Oral
Morphine	IM	20	60	5	2-3	10	60
Hydromorphone	IM	25	60	5	3-4	1.5	8
Oxymorphone	IM	10	60	5		1	6
Levorphanol	IM	45	90	6	4	2	4
Meperidine	IM	15	45	3	3-4	75	300
Methadone	IM	15	120	5	22-25	10	20
Fentanyl	IM	10	30	1-2	1.5-6	0.1	—
Sufentanil	IM	3		1	2.5	0.02	—
Alphaprodine	IV SC	1-2 2-30		1 1-20	2	45	—
Oxycodone	IM			5		15	30
Codeine	IM	25	1.5	5	3-4	130	200
Propoxyphene	PO	25	1.5	5	6-12	—	130
Pentazocine	PO	25	2	3	2-3	45	45
Nalbuphine	IM	15	60	5	5	10	—
Butorphanol	IM	10	45	4	3	2.5	—

Preparations and Administration

Codeine
Tablets, injection solution
Recommended Doses: For pain in adults, 15–60 mg every 4–6 hours; for cough in adults, 10–20 mg every 4–6 hours. For pain in children between 6 and 12 years of age, 0.5 mg/kg or 15 mg/m^2 (body surface area). For cough in children, 5–10 mg/kg every 4–6 hours. For children from 2–6 years of age, 2.5–5 mg every 4–6 hours.

Heroin

Heroin is diacetylmorphine and is prepared from morphine by a simple chemical reaction with acetic acid. It is classified as a semisynthetic drug. Since it is deacetylated in the brain, heroin acts simply as a carrier of morphine into the brain. Heroin crosses the blood-brain barrier more rapidly than morphine but is inactive until it is converted into morphine within the brain tissue. As a result of this increased delivery of drug to the brain, heroin produces less peripheral effect for a given level of central action. It is preferred by addicts for this very reason, since euphoria and analgesia are central effects, while the unpleasant intestinal cramps are peripherally mediated. On a weight basis, it is 2–3 times more potent than morphine and is a severe respiratory depressant.

Meperidine (Demerol)

Meperidine (also known by its international proprietary name of pethidine) is, next to morphine, the most widely used potent analgesic. It is well absorbed orally and equal to morphine as an analgesic. Meperidine is a synthetic narcotic, structurally related to diphenoxylate (Lomotil), loperamide (Imodium), and ethoheptazine (Zactane). The first two of these meperidine congeners are employed as antidiarrheal agents and possess low or no activity for other narcotic effects (see Chapter 51). Meperidine is indicated for relief of moderate to severe pain and as an analgesic adjunct to anesthesia.

Meperidine produces less gastrointestinal stimulation, less constipation, less sedation, and substantially less antitussive effect than morphine. However, meperidine is especially likely to cause orthostatic hypotension. *After meperidine administration, the nurse needs to observe clients for facial flushing, complaints of lightheadedness, and palpitation or evidence of bradycardia, tachycardia, or cardiovascular collapse. The nurse should pay particular attention to ambulatory clients since they are more likely to develop dizziness or faintness from a fall in blood pressure and are more prone to nausea and vomiting.* Some clients may develop a dry mouth, constipation, or biliary spasm. Others may develop urticaria, pruritus, or skin rashes.

Clients with a history of hypersensitivity to meperidine, convulsive disorders, acute abdominal conditions, increased intracranial pressure, or respiratory distress should not receive meperidine. Clients with head injury generally should not receive the drug because it is difficult to distinguish certain adverse effects of meperidine (headache, incoordination, and disorientation) from symptoms resulting from the injury itself.

Subcutaneous injection of meperidine is likely to result in local irritation; the IM route is preferred whenever multiple injections are given. Clients need to be warned of the painfulness of SC injections and special attention needs to be given to complaints of pain at the injection site. The IV route is used infrequently for administration of meperidine. *The high incidence of untoward reactions if meperidine is given IV suggests that facilities for administering oxygen and controlling respiration should be immediately available along with a narcotic antagonist.*

Preparations and Administration

Meperidine (Demerol, Pethadol, and generic formulations)
Injection solutions, tablets, syrup (*the syrup should be diluted before ingestion; undiluted it may cause a local anesthetic effect on the alimentary mucosa.*); combination formulations with acetaminohen (Demerol APAP), or with promethazine (Mepergan)
Recommended Doses: For analgesia in adults, 50–150 mg, IM, SC, or orally, every 3–4 hours as required. For analgesia in children, 0.5–0.8 mg/lb (1–1.8 mg/kg), up to the adult dose, IM, SC, or orally, every 3 or 4 hours. For preoperative purposes, 50–100 mg for adults or 0.5–1.0 mg/lb (1–2 mg/kg) for children IM or SC, 30–90 minutes before the beginning of anesthesia.

Methadone (Dolophine)

Methadone differs from other narcotics because of its long elimination half-life, resulting in a cumulative effect when the drug is taken daily. Used daily, methadone produces a relatively stable level of narcotic activity. Because of methadone accumulation, withdrawal symptoms may not occur until 36–72 hours after use is discontinued and may last 10–14 days. Also, because of drug accumulation, adjustment of dosage and lengthening of the between-dose interval may be required. In instances of methadone overdose, the depressant action of this narcotic may outlast the antagonistic action of a narcotic antagonist such as naloxone because of methadone's long half-life. The antagonist may have to be administered repeatedly.

Methadone is indicated for alleviation of severe pain and for use in methadone weaning and methadone maintenance programs as described earlier. Methadone produces a lower level of sedation and less risk of emesis or physical dependence than morphine, but is otherwise equivalent in activity. The incidence of adverse responses to methadone, such as orthostatic hypotension, sweating, constipation, drowsiness, gastrointestinal distress, and other transient side effects are often more pronounced in ambulatory clients. Methadone has a potency equivalent to morphine when injected but about 3 times that of morphine when taken orally.

Preparations and Administrations

Methadone (Dolophine and generic formulations)
Tablets, oral solution, dispersible tablets, injection solution
Recommended Doses: For analgesia in adults, 50–150 mg, IM, SC, or orally, every 3–4 hours as required. For analgesia in children, 0.5–0.8 mg/lb (1–1.8 mg/kg) up to the adult dose, IM, SC, or orally, at 3 or 4 hour intervals. For methadone maintenance, 30–100 mg PO daily.

Propoxyphene (Darvon)

Propoxyphene is the weakest of the narcotic agonists available for clinical practice. It provides less analgesic effectiveness than other narcotics but also less abuse liability. It is not constipating or antitussive, is minimally sedating or emetic, and produces little respiratory depression. The incidence of excitatory effects, such as tremulousness and restlessness, is greater for propoxyphene than for most other narcotics. Propoxyphene has been reported to increase the plasma levels of certain drugs by inhibiting their liver metabolism, such as phenobarbital, tricyclic antidepressants, and carbamazepine. The effectiveness of propoxyphene is decreased by drugs that induce liver enzymes, including tobacco. Propoxyphene has become a leading cause of drug-related fatalities in recent years. It is commonly abused and is often a factor in fatal overdoses, either alone or in combination with other drugs.

Propoxyphene can be advantageously combined with acetaminophen or aspirin to provide a combined analgesia approximately equivalent to a narcotic of intermediate analgesic effectiveness such as codeine. *Absorption of propoxyphene is somewhat delayed by presence of food in the stomach.*

Preparations and Administration

Propoxyphene (Darvon, Dolene, Doxaphene, Profene, SK-65, and generic formulations)
Capsules, combinations with acetaminophen (Darvocet, Dolene AP-65, SK-65 APAP, Wygesic), with aspirin (Darvon with A.S.A.), with aspirin and caffeine (Darvon Compound, Bexophene, Dolene Compound-65, Doxaphene Compound, SK-65 Compound)
Recommended Doses: For analgesia, 65 mg PO every 4 hours as needed.

Propoxyphene napsylate (Darvon-N)
Tablets, suspension, combinations with acetaminophen (Darvocet-N 50 + 100, Darvon-N 100), with aspirin (Darvon-N with A.S.A.)
Recommended Doses: For analgesia, 100 mg PO every 4 hours as needed.

Other Narcotic Agonists

Hydromorphone (dihydromorphinone, Dilaudid) is another semisynthetic narcotic, being derived, like heroin, from the naturally occurring alkaloid, morphine. It is some 5–10 times more potent than morphine as an analgesic and a respiratory depressant. It has less action on the pupil and is less emetic and less sedative.

Oxymorphone (Numorphan) is a potent analgesic but has a high liability for producing respiratory depression, emesis, and dependence. It is moderately constipating but relatively weak as an antitussive. It is about 10 times as potent as morphine on a weight basis.

Levorphanol (Levo-Dromoran) is another potent analgesic that produces only modest sedation and has low emetic potential, but is moderately active in other respects. Levorphanol is a levorotatory isomer; the corresponding dextrorotatory isomer, dextromethorphan, is an effective antitussive that lacks other narcotic actions (see Chapter 52).

Oxycodone closely resembles morphine in the extent of its various effects (see Table 25-2) but exhibits better oral effectiveness. It is twice as potent as morphine orally but 50% less effective after IM injection. Hydrocodone is a relatively weak analgesic but an effective antitussive. Hydrocodone and dihydrocodeine are marketed only in combinations.

Alphaprodine is unusual among the narcotics for its rapid but short analgesic effects. After SC injection, analgesia occurs in 2–30 minutes and lasts just 1–2 hours. After IV injection, the effect is seen in 1–2 minutes and lasts 30–90 minutes. Alphaprodine is indicated for use as an obstetric analgesic, for urological examination and procedures (especially cystoscopy), as an adjunct for surgery, and for dental procedures.

Fentanyl (Sublimaze) and sufentanil (Sufenta) are narcotics of exceptional potency (see Table 25-3) that are about 100 times as potent per weight than morphine. These two narcotics are employed mainly as adjuncts to anesthesia (general or regional), during the preoperative, induction, maintenance, or postoperative phases. They can also be employed as primary anesthetic agents with oxygen (see Chapter 16) in selected high-risk patients (such as those undergoing open heart surgery or major surgical procedures in the sitting position). Fentanyl is also available in a combination (Innovar) with droperidol, a potent neuroleptic, for use as a primary anesthetic or a preanesthetic adjunctive (Chapter 16).

Preparations and Administration

Alphaprodine (Nisentil)
Injection solution
Recommended Doses: 0.4–0.6 mg/kg IV or 0.4–1.2 mg/kg SC to a maximum of 30 mg IV or 60 mg SC. Low doses should be used initially.

Dihydrocodeine
Combinations with aspirin and caffeine (Synalgos-DC, Dihydrocodeine Compound Capsules, Sinodeine), or with acetaminophen and caffeine (Compal)

Fentanyl (Sublimaze)
Injection solution

Fentanyl/Droperidol (Innovar)
Injection solution

Hydrocodone
Combinations with acetaminophen (Lortab, Amacodone, Bancap, Co-Gesic, Damacet, Dolacet, Duradyne, Hycodaphen, Vicodin, Norcet, T-Gesic), with aspirin (Anexsia-D), or with aspirin and caffeine (Damason-P, Anodynos-DHC, Dia-Gesic)
Products containing hydrocodone may be taken with meals or food to reduce gastrointestinal irritation.

Hydromorphone (Dilaudid)
Tablets, injection solutions, suppository
Recommended Doses: 2 mg orally for moderate pain up to 4 mg for severe pain, every 4–6 hours; 3 mg rectally every 6–8 hours; or 2 mg SC or IM for moderate pain or 3–4 mg for severe pain every 4–6 hours as required.

Levorphanol (Levo-Dromoran)
Tablets, injection solution
Recommended Doses: For moderate to severe pain, 2 mg orally or SC initially.

Oxycodone (generic formulations)
Tablets, cherry flavored oral solution, combinations with acetaminophen (Percocet and Tylox), or with aspirin (Codoxy and Percodan)

Recommended Doses: For relief of moderate to severe pain in adults, 5 mg every 6 hours. *Administration of oxycodone with or after meals is recommended in order to minimize gastrointestinal irritation.* Oxycodone is not recommended for use in children.

Oxymorphone (Numorphan)
Injection solutions, suppository
Recommended Doses: 0.5 mg IV or 1–1.5 SC or IM at 4–6 hour intervals initially; or 5 mg rectally every 4–6 hours.

Sufentanil (Sufenta)
Injection solution

Important Nursing Implications for Narcotic Analgesics

- ☐ Evaluate the medical histories of clients for contraindications against use of narcotics, such as head injuries, elevated intracranial pressure, seizure disorders, and respiratory distress.
- ☐ Carefully evaluate the needs of clients for analgesia, remembering that uncontrolled pain negatively affects psychological health but that overuse of analgesics poses hazards as well. Check how often the drugs may be given, the time the last dosage was given, the prescribed route of administration, and validate the physician's orders.
- ☐ Implement appropriate comfort measures to reduce the need for analgesics
- ☐ Recognize that combinations of narcotic and nonnarcotic analgesics are often appropriate, providing additive efficacy but nonadditive liabilities.
- ☐ Teach clients to recognize adverse effects of narcotic analgesics such as excess depression, nausea and vomiting, constipation, urinary retention, orthostatic hypotension, suppression of the cough reflex, and signs of dependence.
- ☐ Warn clients to avoid hazardous tasks, such as driving an automobile, since narcotic analgesics may cause sedation, somnolence, and diminished performance.
- ☐ Implement appropriate nursing measures to counter adverse effects of analgesics when they occur.
- ☐ Advise clients to avoid use of other CNS depressants concurrently with narcotics to prevent additive CNS depression.
- ☐ Advocate changes in drug selection, frequency of doses, and route of administration when necessary to best meet the needs of clients.
- ☐ After long-term administration of narcotics, withdraw the drug gradually to prevent abstinence symptoms.

Mixed Narcotic Agonist/Antagonists

Four drugs marketed as analgesics have mixed narcotic agonist and antagonist properties: **pentazocine** (Talwin), **buprenorphine** (Buprenex), **nalbuphine** (Nubain), and **butorphanol** (Stadol).

Mechanisms and Effects These drugs can be designated as *partial agonists* or *partial antagonists* with equal accuracy. The major significance of the mixed character or these drugs is that they have limited abuse liability and are less likely to be diverted to use by narcotic addicts. If used by a person addicted to potent narcotic agonists, these drugs will act as antagonists, precipitating withdrawal. The maximum extent of effects that can be produced by these agents is limited by their low efficacy for the opiate receptor. Beyond a relatively modest concentration of the drug, no further activation of the narcotic receptor can be achieved.

Partial agonists have lower abuse liability than full narcotic agonists. Nevertheless, pentazocine has been abused in recent years in combination with tripelennamine, an antihistamine. Tablets of pentazocine and tripelennamine, usually in a 2 to 1 ratio, are dissolved and then injected intravenously, a form of abuse known as "T's and Blues" — T's for Talwin and Blues signifying the color of tripelennamine tablets. Naloxone has been added to one Talwin formulation to limit its abuse potential. The antagonist activities of the other mixed agonist/antagonists relative to pentazocine are 10 times greater for nalbuphine, 30 times for butorphanol, and 1,200 times for buprenorphine. Buprenorphine has antagonist activity equal to naloxone. Pentazocine is more of an agonist at kappa and sigma narcotic receptors but more of an antagonist at mu receptors.

Clinical Indications Pentazocine, buprenorphine, nalbuphine, and butorphanol are indicated for relief of moderate to severe pain and to provide supplemental analgesia in conjunction with general anesthesia.

Adverse Effects and Contraindications Overall, pentazocine has a somewhat higher incidence of adverse effects than propoxyphene, so that it is less widely used in spite of its exceptionally low abuse liability. Pentazocine and butorphanol (but not nalbuphine or buprenorphine) increase pulmonary artery pressure and systemic vascular resistance. These drugs should be avoided for individuals with cardiovascular disease or with respiratory conditions, such as bronchial asthma, obstructed respiration, cyanosis, limited respiratory reserve, or respiratory depression. All four of these agents appear to be safe for use during labor, but safety during earlier stages of pregnancy has not been established. Butorphanol is not recommended for use by nursing mothers, nor has safety been established for the other three partial agonists.

Preparations and Administration *IM injections are preferred to SC injections when multiple administrations of pentazocine are anticipated, since SC injection often causes irritation at the site of injection. IM sites should be rotated.*

Buprenorphine (Buprenex)
Injection solution
Recommended Doses: For clients over 13 years of age, 0.3 mg IM or slowly IV, every 6 hours as needed. Buprenorphine is compatible with saline, dextrose, and lactated Ringer's infusion solutions. Buprenorphine is also compatible with infusion solutions containing such drugs as scopolamine, haloperidol, and hydroxyzine, but is incompatible with diazepam and lorazepam.

Butorphanol (Stadol)
Injection solution
Recommended Doses: 2 mg IM or 1 mg IV, repeated every 3–4 hours as required.

Nalbuphine (Nubain)
Injection solution
Recommended Doses: 10 mg/70 kg (maximum 20 mg), SC, IM, or IV, repeated every 3–6 hours as required. The maximum recommended daily dose is 160 mg.

Pentazocine
Injection solution (Talwin), tablets with naloxone (Talwin NX), combination tablets with aspirin (Talwin Compound), or with acetaminophen (Talacen)
Recommended Doses: For pain in adults, 50 mg orally, every 3–4 hours initially, increased to 100 mg if necessary to a maximum daily dose of 600 mg; or 30 mg IM, SC, or IV, repeated every 3–4 hours. For clients in labor, a single 30 mg IM dose. Not recommended for children under age 12.

Narcotic Antagonists

Mechanisms and Effects **Naloxone** (Narcan), **levallorphan** (Lorfan), and **naltrexone** (Trexan) are narcotic antagonists, useful in terminating the activity of narcotic agonists. Naloxone and naltrexone are pure antagonists, while levallorphan has weak agonistic activity. Naloxone is an antagonist only at mu and kappa narcotic receptors; it does not bind effectively to the other types of narcotic receptors. Naloxone and levallorphan are effective only by parenteral administration. Naltrexone is effective orally and provides a longer duration of action than naloxone.

Clinical Indications Naloxone and levallorphan are indicated for achieving complete or partial reversal of narcotic depression, including respiratory depression in cases of opiate overdose. Naloxone is the drug of choice for this application because of its complete lack of agonist activity. It is also used to reverse narcotic effects in neonates born to narcotic-addicted women. Narcotic antagonists are effective against all drugs in the narcotic class but are ineffective in reversing respiratory or CNS depression caused by drugs in any other group. Naltrexone is indicated for use as an adjunct in maintaining the opioid-free status in detoxified former narcotic addicts.

Adverse Effects and Contraindications The principal adverse effect of narcotic antagonists is precipitation of abrupt withdrawal. When an antagonist is employed in an individual who is dependent on narcotics and who has acutely overdosed, the antagonist may trigger a withdrawal syndrome as well as reversing the acute overdose. Therefore, narcotic antagonists should be administered with caution to individuals known or suspected to be physically dependent on a narcotic, including neonates of addicted women. Clients who have responded well to naloxone must be closely monitored because naloxone is short-acting and may wear off before the action of a long-acting narcotic agonist.

Levallorphan has weak narcotic agonist activity. If there is any doubt whether respiratory depression is caused by a narcotic, naloxone should be used in preference to levallorphan, since levallorphan could aggravate the resiratory depression of other causes.

There have been reports of dose-related hepatic toxicity caused by naltrexone, although these responses occurred at doses approximately five times those recommended for use in promoting opioid-free status. As a precaution, it is recommended that naltrexone not be used in individuals with acute hepatitis or liver impairment and that liver function tests be conducted periodically while naltrexone is being employed.

Individuals receiving naltrexone will not benefit from normal therapeutic doses of narcotics administered for analgesic, antitussive, or antidiarrheal applications. If such effects are required in an emergency situation, higher than normal doses of narcotic agonists will be required and can overcome the competitive antagonism provided by naltrexone. *Individuals receiving naltrexone should carry an appropriate medic alert card.*

Preparations and Administration

Levallorphan (Lorfan)
Injection solution
Recommended Doses: For narcotic overdose in adults, 1 mg IV initially followed by 1 or 2 additional doses of 0.5 mg at 10–15 minute intervals. For alleviating neonatal respiratory depression, 0.05–0.1 mg, IM, SC, or (preferably) into the umbilical cord vein immediately after delivery.

Naloxone (Narcan)
Injection solution, neonatal injection solution
Recommended Doses: 0.01 mg/kg initially administered, IV, IM, or SC.

Naltrexone (Trexan)
Tablets
Recommended Doses: For maintenance of opioid-free state, 50 mg tablet every 24 hours, 100 mg every other day, or 150 mg every third day. Naltrexone therapy should not be initiated less than 7–10 days after termination of use of a short-acting narcotic substance.

Aspirin-like Analgesics/Antipyretics

A limited number of nonnarcotic drugs are available as alternatives to narcotics for relief of pain. By and large, the nonnarcotic analgesics are less effective than the potent narcotics, but have the distinct advantage of being nonaddictive. Moreover, for certain types of pain, nonnarcotic analgesics may actually be more effective than narcotics. Nevertheless, neurological and somatic side effects sometimes occur with aspirin-like drugs, and their occurrence must be weighed in the selection of an appropriate analgesic. Many of these agents share two additional therapeutic activities besides their analgesic potential, namely, an antipyretic and an anti-inflammatory effect. The common thread in these three seemingly diverse effects is the relationship of each to the family of endogenous autocoids known as the **prostaglandins.** The anti-inflammatory actions and applications of aspirin-like drugs are taken up in Chapter 45, where several drugs that are marketed only for inflammation are discussed. In the present chapter, only the analgesic and antipyretic actions and applications of aspirin-like drugs are discussed.

The Neurophysiology of Temperature Regulation

The body temperature of homo sapians is maintained within narrow limits (36°–38°C, 96.8°–100.4°F) despite wide fluctuations of environmental temperature. Maintenance of body temperature involves control of both heat production and heat loss. An increase of only 5°C may cause brain damage or heat stroke and the temperature-regulating function itself may be lost, further elevating temperature into the lethal range. The upper limit for survival is less than 10°C above normal.

A drop of 5°C also leads to impairment of the temperature-regulating function, and a 10°C drop results in complete loss of control. At 10°C below normal, human beings are highly susceptible to fatal disturbances of cardiac rhythm; otherwise, tissues other than the heart would be able to tolerate a further reduction, provided artificial means were available for rewarming. Heat production and conservation involve control of cutaneous vasoconstriction; metabolism of carbohydrate, fat, and protein; and shivering, muscle tension, and exercise or activity. Heat loss involves mainly cutaneous vasodilation, sweating, and an open body position.

About 20% of all neurons in the anterior hypothalamus are sensitive to temperature changes (Figure 25–3). Most respond to increases in temperature; about one-fourth respond to cooling. No markedly temperature-sensitive neurons have been found in other parts of the brain.

The anterior hypothalamus acts as a thermostat, the set point of which undergoes diurnal variations and may be displaced, for example, by pathogens, to produce fever. Prostaglandin production is involved in the elevation of the set point. The anterior hypothalamus also controls heat loss, and its stimulation results in panting, sweating, and vasodilation. Destruction of the anterior hypothalamus causes hyperthermia.

The posterior hypothalamic region controls heat conservation, and its stimulation provokes shivering and peripheral vasoconstriction. Destruction of the posterior hypothalamus results in loss of temperature regulation (poikilothermia) (not hypothermia as one might expect) due to interruption of fiber tracts from the anterior hypothalamus along with local neuronal damage.

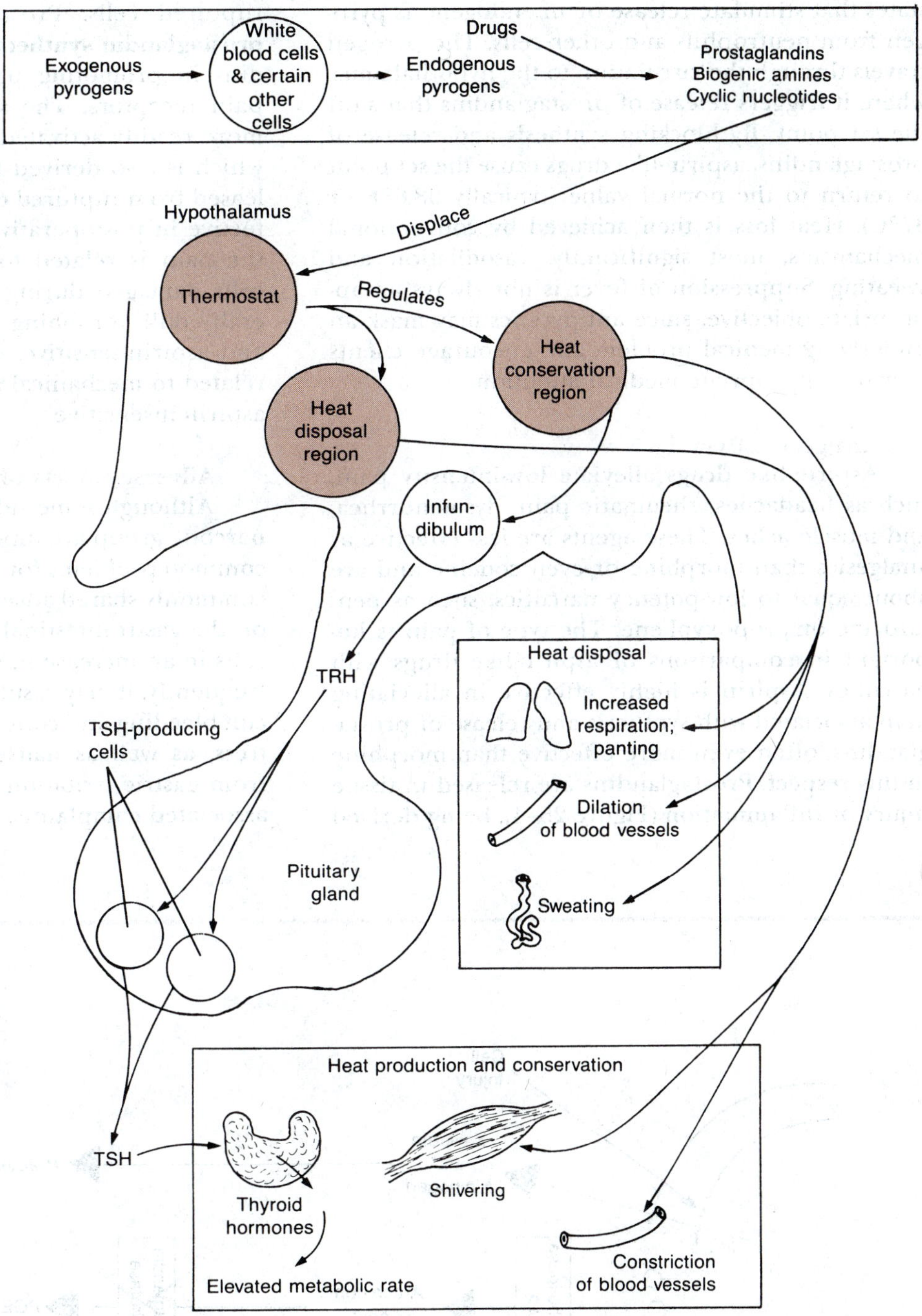

Figure 25–3
Temperature regulation by the hypothalamus. Exogenous pyrogens released by microbes can trigger release of an endogenous pyrogen from white blood cells or other cells. This endogenous pyrogen or pyrogenic drugs can displace the hypothalamic thermostat, resulting in fever. Antipyretic drugs reset the central thermostat, causing the hypothalamus to bring body temperature back to normal by increasing heat disposal.

Shared Pharmacological Properties of Aspirin-like Drugs

Antipyretic Effect

Aspirin-like drugs are effective in reducing elevated body temperature when it is caused by an alteration in the set point established by the hypothalamus. On the other hand, aspirin does not lower normal body temperature or correct hyperthermia caused by exposure to excessive environmental temperature, excessive heat production from exercise, or both. Hyperthermia related to an alteration in set point is called **fever.** A fever may result from infection, inflammation, allergic reactions, tissue damage, malignancies, toxins, dehydration, or other disease states that stimulate release of an endogenous pyrogen from neutrophils and other cells. The pyrogen travels through the circulation to the hypothalamus, where it triggers release of prostaglandins that shift the set point. By blocking synthesis and release of prostaglandins, aspirin-like drugs cause the set point to return to the normal value (typically 98.6°F or 37°C). Heat loss is then achieved by conventional mechanisms, most significantly, vasodilation and sweating. Suppression of fever is not always an appropriate objective, since antipyretics may mask an underlying medical problem and encourage clients to avoid appropriate medical attention.

Analgesic Effect

Aspirin-like drugs alleviate low-intensity pain, such as headaches, rheumatic pain, dysmenorrhea, and muscle aches. These agents are less effective as analgesics than morphine or even codeine and are about equal to low-potency narcotics, such as pentazocine or propoxyphene. The type of pain is important in comparisons of aspirin-like drugs with narcotics. Aspirin is highly effective in alleviating pain associated with synthesis and release of prostaglandins, often even more effective than morphine in this respect. Prostaglandins are released in tissue injury or inflammation (Figure 25–4), being derived from arachidonic acid released from membranes of ruptured cells. Prostaglandins are produced by **prostaglandin synthetase.** The action of prostaglandins in promoting pain sensations is to sensitize pain receptors. The sensitized receptors are then more readily activated by the autocoid, bradykinin, which is also derived from cellular constituents released from ruptured cells. Aspirin-like drugs are effective in postoperative pain, for example, because the pain is related to prostaglandin release from cells damaged during incision and stitching. Generally dull, throbbing pain is prostaglandin-related and aspirin-sensitive, while sharp, stabbing pain is related to mechanical activation of receptors and is aspirin-insensitive.

Adverse Effects of Aspirin-like Drugs

Although some side effects of drugs of the nonnarcotic group are unique to a given drug, some are common problems for the class as a whole. The most commonly shared adverse effect is an irritative effect on the gastrointestinal mucosa, which invariably results in an increase in gastrointestinal bleeding; less frequently, it may result in outright ulceration or occult bleeding and consequent anemia. Epigastric distress, as well as nausea and vomiting, may result from gastric irritation. Dyspnea and heartburn are associated complaints. The consistent association of

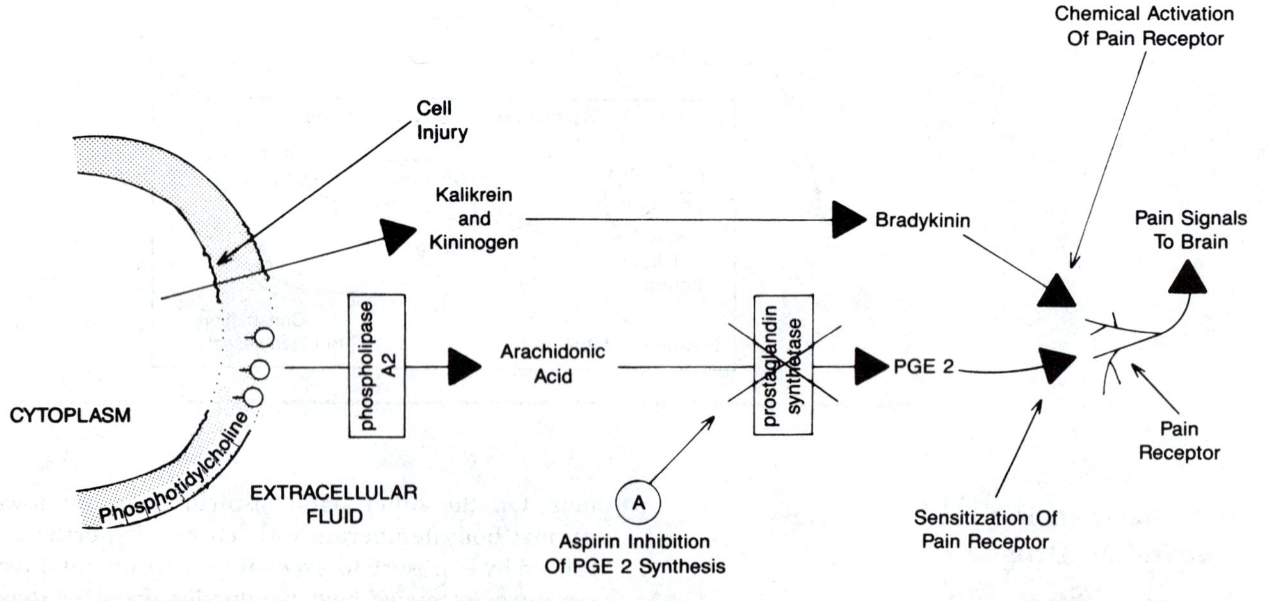

Figure 25–4
Mechanism of action of aspirin-like analgesics. PgE_2, prostaglandin E_2. From A. K. Swonger and L. L. Constantine, *Drugs and Therapy,* 2nd ed. Boston: Little, Brown, 1983.

Nursing Diagnoses and Interventions for Drug Therapy of Pain

Nursing Diagnoses	*Related Interventions*
TO ENHANCE DRUG BENEFITS OR REDUCE DRUG REQUIREMENTS	
Alterations in thought processes: depression related to pain	Provide emotional support and reassurance. Divert the client's attention to more pleasurable things. Speak in a calm voice and moderate tones to promote client's understanding.
Alterations in comfort: pain	Provide support, comfort measures, and analgesia as required.
TO MINIMIZE DRUG SIDE EFFECTS OR INTERACTIONS	
Alteration in bowel elimination: constipation related to use of narcotics	Maintain high fiber and fluid intake; increase exercise; administer laxatives if required.
Alteration in breathing pattern: hyperpnea with salicylates	If extreme, have client rebreathe air from a bag; administer 5% CO_2; correct pH imbalances.
Alteration in cardiac output: hypotension produced by narcotic analgesics	Avoid rapid changes in position. Dangle feet before arising. Avoid prolonged standing. Avoid hot showers or hot sun.
Alteration in comfort: pain from gastric irritation from nonnarcotic analgesics	Take nonnarcotic analgesics with food or a full glass of water; instruct the client to inform the physician or nurse if tarry stools, bleeding gums, petechiae, or nosebleeds are observed.
Increased risk of injury related to CNS depression and dizziness with narcotics	Provide safety measures and warn clients not to drive or operate dangerous equipment while these effects are present.
Ineffective airway clearance: cough suppression related to narcotics	Avoid narcotics when client has a productive cough; use narcotics least likely to suppress cough. Avoid narcotics in chronic obstructive pulmonary disease.
Ineffective individual coping related to insufficient control of pain or CNS depression from narcotics	Provide comfort measures and adjust analgesic regimens appropriately. Provide emotional support.
Ineffective individual coping related to CNS side effects of narcotics	Reduce dose of the narcotic; combine with other drugs that potentiate analgesia such as nonnarcotic analgesics, tricyclic antidepressants, or stimulants.
Potential sensory-perceptual alterations: tinnitus with salicylates	Reduce dose; treat salicylate toxicity.
TO ENSURE SAFE AND EFFICACIOUS DRUG USE	
Knowledge deficit related to drug regimen	Teach clients about the nature of the injury or disease that is responsible for pain.
	Explain the rationale for use of analgesic agents.
	Explain the importance of adhering to prescribed dosage schedules and the potential for serious adverse effects and diminished effectiveness of the drug with overuse.
	Provide client with a list of adverse effects and drug interactions for each drug in the regimen and explain what to do if any of these occur.
	Warn clients to keep analgesics safely out of the reach of children.

this side effect with the many varied drugs in the nonnarcotic analgesic class suggests that it is related in some way to prostaglandins. *Gastrointestinal irritation may be minimized by administering aspirin-like drugs with milk, food, an antacid, or a full glass of water. Chewing tablets before swallowing or crushing them and dissolving them in a suitable vehicle (such as orange juice or lemon juice) are other methods used to reduce the irritant effect on the gastric mucosa.*

Another shared adverse effect is an anticoagulant action caused by inhibition of platelet agglutination secondary to prostaglandin synthetase inhibition. Prostaglandin synthetase in platelets normally produces a substance called thromboxane A_2, which promotes platelet aggregation. Another adverse effect of aspirin-like drugs related to prostaglandins is an antifertility effect in males. Some aspirin-like drugs can be nephrotoxic, especially when abused, an effect possibly related to prostaglandins.

Salicylates

The salicylates include aspirin (acetylsalicylic acid), salsalate, sodium salicylate, sodium thiosalicylate, choline salicylate, magnesium salicylate, salicylamide, and diflunisal. Aspirin is the most often used by a wide margin.

Aspirin

Aspirin is the most potent inhibitor of prostaglandin synthetase among the salicylates. Aspirin is widely used as an analgesic and antipyretic and is an effective anti-inflammatory agent for acute rheumatic fever, rheumatoid arthritis (often in combination with gold compounds), psoriatic arthritis, osteoarthritis, gouty arthritis, bursitis, and ankylosing spondylitis. Doses of aspirin required for analgesic or antipyretic purposes (about 650 mg, repeated at intervals no less than 4 hours) are less than those required for anti-inflammatory purposes (typically 8 g daily in 1 g doses). Thus, aspirin toxicity is most problematic when the drug is employed for anti-inflammatory purposes, and the largest number of aspirin substitutes has been developed for that application (see Chapter 45).

Pharmacokinetics Aspirin is well absorbed after oral administration, although bioavailability of the enteric coated formulations is often erratic. Administration of aspirin with food slows the absorption of aspirin but does not reduce total absorption. Absorption of aspirin from rectal suppositories is slower and less reliable. Aspirin is hydrolyzed in part to salicylic acid during absorption. At low to moderate blood levels, it is highly bound to plasma proteins, in excess of 90%. However, as the dose increases, the percentage of drug that is bound to plasma proteins declines. Plasma concentrations in the range 100–150 μg/ml provide therapeutic results; levels around 200 μg/ml produce early signs of salicylism; and levels above 400 μg/ml result is severe toxicity. In the body, aspirin is hydrolyzed to salicylic acid with a half-life of about 15 minutes. Salicylic acid is inactivated both by metabolism and renal excretion with a half-life of about 2–3 hours. Renal excretion of salicylates is significantly influenced by urinary pH since these substances are weak organic acids. Alkalinization of urinary pH increases renal extraction and elimination.

Adverse Effects Aspirin has a stronger and longer-lasting effect on platelet aggregation than do other salicylates. A single analgesic dose of aspirin produces an irreversible **inhibition of platelet aggregation** that persists for the life of the platelet (about 8 days) and results in a prolongation of bleeding time. This effect of aspirin has been put to good use in reducing the risk in males of recurrent transient ischemic attacks or stroke caused by fibrin/platelet emboli. Aspirin has not been shown to be similarly useful in females or for treatment of completed strokes.

Aspirin use in children, for chickenpox or influenza, has been associated with occurrence of **Reye's syndrome,** a rare, acute life-threatening condition characterized by vomiting, lethargy, delirium, and coma leading to death (in 20–30% of cases) or brain damage. However, there is considerable controversy surrounding the evidence for this connection.

Large doses of aspirin may cause **hypoglycemia,** especially in children. *Aspirin administration should be scheduled at least 1 hour before exercise to minimize the risk that hypoglycemia will be additive with that associated with exercise.* Some individuals exhibit **allergic reactions** to aspirin. The most common one is an asthma-like bronchospasm. Other hypersensitivity reactions range from hives, rash, and rhinitis to fatal anaphylactic shock.

Drug Interactions Aspirin is highly bound to plasma albumin-binding sites. Consequently, it has an interaction of mutual potentiation with other drugs that are similarly highly bound to these sites, such as penicillin, valproic acid, methotrexate, triiodothyronine, sulfonamides, naproxen, thiopental, and phenytoin. Aspirin increases the anticoagulant effect of oral anticoagulants, such as warfarin, not only by displacing these drugs from plasma protein binding sites but also by its additive anticoagulant effects.

The analgesia produced by aspirin and narcotic analgesics is beneficially additive, and many preformulated combinations are available commercially. Aspirin inhibits the diuretic effect of spironolactone. Propranolol inhibits the anti-inflammatory efficacy of aspirin by competing for the relevant receptor sites. Doses of aspirin greater than 2 g/day have a hypoglycemic action that is potentially additive with that of oral hypoglycemic agents or insulin.

Although large doses of aspirin are uricosuric (promoting uric acid excretion in the urine), low to moderate doses antagonize the uricosuric effects of probenecid and sulfinpyrazone. Aspirin clearance is increased by corticosteroids and urinary alkalinizers (including absorbable antacids) and decreased by furosemide, and urinary acidifiers. Aspirin absorption may be impaired by concurrent administration of nonabsorbable antacids or activated charcoal.

Salicylate Toxicity Aspirin is one of the top five drugs in terms of frequency of drug-induced fatalities (about 200 annually). The fatal dose range is 10–30 g. Salicylate poisoning is especially common in children, accounting for 15% of all fatal poisonings in children under age 5. About 50,000 cases of aspirin poisoning (accidental or associated with suicide attempts) occur yearly; a few instances occur when aspirin is used for inflammation. The critical symptoms of salicylate poisoning fall into four categories: (1) vomiting, dehydration, and hyperthermia (an immediate threat to life), (2) tinnitus, mental confusion, delirium, and convulsions (another potentially fatal component), (3) bleeding, anemia, and lung damage (all related to the inhibition of platelet aggregation), and (4) acid-base imbalance. Hearing loss caused by aspirin overdose is usually reversible. The acid-base imbalance is initially triggered by stimulation of respiration (hyperpnea) due to an action of aspirin on the medullary respiratory center. Increased respiration causes excessive breathing-off of carbon dioxide, which raises plasma pH. Usually, alkalosis is adequately compensated by increased kidney excretion of alkalis, but this reduces blood buffering capacity and leaves the individual vulnerable to further acid-based problems.

Treatment of salicylate toxicity is based on removal of the drug (by stomach lavage, induced vomiting, or intravenous fluid replacement) and symptomatic treatment (correcting the pH with bicarbonate and stimulating synthesis of clotting factors with intravenous vitamin K).

The mental disturbances that occur in salicylate toxicity are sometimes called the **salicylate jag.** The syndrome may simulate alcohol inebriation and includes incoherent speech, delirium, hallucinations, garrulousness, lassitude, drowsiness, confusion, and apprehensiveness. Euphoria does not occur, however, and this may aid in differentiating salicylism from alcohol inebriation.

Preparations and Administration Aspirin is encountered in countless preparations — alone, buffered, enteric coated, and in combinations with narcotic analgesics and acetaminophen and in multidrug formulations for colds. In general, there is little evidence in the case of aspirin that formulation characteristics have much impact on ultimate effectiveness. Enteric-coated products in theory provide less gastric irritation, but absorption of aspirin from these products is more variable. Buffered products may provide less gastrointestinal irritation, but also provide a shorter duration of action due to alkalinization of the urine. Many aspirin products do not age well, developing a hard outer shell that resists dissolution when the product is ingested. *Therefore, nurses should advise clients not to stockpile aspirin products. Also, it is best to keep aspirin in an airtight container in a cool place because aspirin products decompose when subjected to moisture or extremes of temperature. Aspirin tablets with a vinegar smell (due to acetic acid) should be discarded.*

Other Salicylates

Salsalate, an ester, is hydrolyzed into two molecules of aspirin after absorption and in the intestines. It is not irritating to the gastric mucosa but otherwise shares the effects of aspirin. Sodium salicylate and salicylamide are both substantially less effective than aspirin. Sodium salicylate provides a sodium load of 6.25 mEq/g of drug. Salicylamide may cause drowsiness in addition to the common adverse effects of salicylates. Choline salicylate and magnesium salicylate are two salicylate products with fewer gastrointestinal adverse effects than aspirin. Magnesium salicylate is contraindicated in individuals with advanced renal failure.

Diflunisal, first marketed in 1982, is approved for use as an analgesic as well as for osteoarthritis. Its toxicity appears to be somewhat less than that of aspirin. The most frequently reported adverse effects of diflunisal are gastrointestinal reactions, including nausea, dyspepsia, pain, diarrhea, GI bleeding, and peptic ulceration. It produces neurological and allergic reactions similar to those that occur with aspirin. Diflunisal is 99% bound to plasma proteins in the blood and, like aspirin, it displaces various drugs from plasma protein binding sites. Its long duration of action permits twice daily administration but its onset of action is somewhat slower. A level of analgesia equivalent to that produced by 650 mg of aspirin requires 500 mg of diflunisal.

Preparations and Admiministration

Choline Salicylate (Arthropan)
Oral liquid, mint-flavored
Recommended Doses: For pain in adults or children over 12, 870 mg PO, repeated at 3 or 4 hour intervals up to 6 times daily.

Diflunisal (Dolobid)
Film coated tablets
Recommended Doses: For mild to moderate pain, 1,000 mg PO initially, followed by 500 mg at 8 or 12 hour intervals as required. Some clients respond adequately to one-half these recommended doses.

Magnesium salicylate (Doan's Pills, Durasal, Efficin, Magan, Mobidin, and MS-650)
Tablets
Recommended Doses: For adults or children over 12, 500–600 mg PO, 3 or 4 times daily, up to 3.6–4.8 g/day. It is not recommended for children under age 12.

Salicylamide (Uromide and generic formulations)
Tablets
Recommended Doses: For adults and children over 12, 325 to 650 mg PO, 3–4 times daily.

Salsalate (Disalcid, Artha-G, and Mono-Gesic)
Capsules, tablets
Recommended Doses: For adults, 3,000 mg/day PO in divided doses.

Sodium salicylate (Uracel 5 and generic formulations)
Tablets, enteric coated tablets
Recommended Doses: 325–650 mg PO every 4–8 hours.

Sodium thiosalicylate (numerous trade names)
Injection solution
Recommended Doses: For muscular pain, 50–100 mg IM on alternate days.

Acetaminophen

Acetaminophen belongs to the para-aminophenol family. The other principal member of this group, phenacetin, has been discontinued. Acetaminophen was first recognized as the active metabolite of phenacetin and of acetanilid, but is less toxic than either parent compound. Acetaminophen is second only to aspirin in frequency of use as a nonprescription analgesic, holding approximately a 30% market share. It is approximately equal to aspirin in analgesic and antipyretic effectiveness, but has only weak anti-inflammatory effects. It is indicated for use in relieving fever and mild to moderate pain and is valuable for individuals allergic to salicylates. The analgesic effect of acetaminophen is additive with that produced by narcotics and is potentiated by caffeine; thus it is frequently encountered in combinations with these agents. The ability of acetaminophen to inhibit prostaglandin synthetase within the CNS is equivalent to that of aspirin, but it has much less effect on the enzyme in the periphery. Hence, it has little anti-inflammatory action, produces little gastrointestinal irritation, and does not interfere with platelet aggregation.

Pharmacokinetics Acetaminophen is rapidly and almost fully absorbed, producing peak plasma concentrations in 30–120 minutes. Liquid formulations result in slightly faster absorption. Drugs that delay gastric emptying time, such as anticholinergics or narcotics, slow the rate but not the extent of acetaminophen absorption. Suppository forms produce variable absorption. In the blood, acetaminophen is bound to plasma proteins to an extent of only 20–50%. Therapeutic plasma concentrations are approximately 5–20 μg/ml. Acetaminophen is inactivated mainly (94%) by glucuronide and sulfate conjugation in the liver; the metabolites are eliminated by renal excretion. About 4% of the metabolism of acetaminophen is by the cytochrome P-450 oxidase system, which yields an hepatotoxic metabolite. This metabolite is normally detoxified by conjugation with liver glutathione, but when acetaminophen is used chronically, glutathione may become depleted, resulting in hepatic necrosis. The elimination half-life for acetaminophen is about 1–3.5 hours but is somewhat longer in neonates. Use of oral contraceptives has been reported to increase metabolism of acetaminophen and to decrease its half-life by as much as 20–30%.

Adverse Effects and Contraindications Acetaminophen produces little in the way of adverse effects when employed as directed. Some individuals exhibit allergic reactions to acetaminophen, such as skin rash, urticaria, or fever. Occurrence of such hypersensitivity reactions is a specific contraindication for further use of acetaminophen. Hypoglycemia, CNS depression, and CNS excitation occur occasionally. Prolonged use has been associated with hepatic and liver toxicity, and hematological reactions. In the last category, acetaminophen has caused uncommon instances of methemoglobinemia, hemolytic anemia, cyanosis, neutropenia, leukopenia, thrombocytopenia, and pancytopenia.

Hepatotoxicity may be manifested as jaundice; in overdose situations hepatic failure has occurred leading to encephalopathy, coma, and death. Individuals with a long history of alcohol consumption or poor nutrition are especially prone to acetaminophen-induced hepatotoxicity. *Hepatic function should be closely monitored during long-term therapy with acetaminophen.* Kidney necrosis has also occurred in overdoses. There are approximately 50 deaths yearly from acetaminophen overdose in the United States and United Kingdom. Acetaminophen poisoning has been divided into four stages: (1) nausea, vomiting, diaphoresis, and anorexia (12–24 hours), (2) an asymptomatic stage of rising serum enzymes (SGOT and SGPT), bilirubin, and prothrombin levels (24–48 hours), (3) peak hepatotoxic crisis (3–4 days), and (4) recovery (7–8 days).

Oral **N-acetylcysteine** (Mucomyst) has been employed as a specific antidote for acetaminophen toxicity but is not yet FDA approved in this capacity. N-acetylcysteine prevents or minimizes hepatic toxicity by supplying sulfhydryl groups that combine with the toxic acetaminophen metabolite in place of endogenous glutathione, which is depleted in acetaminophen overdose. N-acetylcysteine is employed only within 16 hours after ingestion of acetaminophen. It is given as a 5% solution in cola, grapefruit juice, orange juice, or water. The recommended loading dose is 140 mg/kg followed by maintenance doses of 70 mg/kg every 4 hours for 17 doses. N-acetylcysteine solutions should be employed within 1 hour after preparation. If the patient vomits within 1 hour after giving N-acetylcysteine, the dosage should be repeated. Activated charcoal may be used advantageously immediately after acetaminophen ingestion to minimize absorption of the drug.

Preparations and Administration

Acetaminophen (Tylenol, Valadol, Febrinol, Panadol, Datril, Tapanol, and generic formulations)

Tablets, capsules, chewable tablets, wafers, elixirs, oral liquid, oral solutions, suppositories, buffered effervescent granules (Bromo Seltzer); combinations with aspirin, salicylamide, or butalbital, with or without caffeine; various decongestant and antihistamine combinations for upper respiratory tract infections; various narcotics such as codeine, hydrocodone, dihydrocodeine, oxycodone, meperidine, propoxyphene, and pentazocine

Recommended Doses: For analgesia in adults, 300–650 mg every 4 hours. Doses up to 1,000 mg may be given up to 4 times daily for short periods of time. For children, up to 5 times daily: 0–3 months, 40 mg; 4–11 months, 80 mg; 1–2 years, 120 mg; 2–3 years, 160 mg; 4–5 years, 240 mg; 6–8 years, 320 mg; 9–10 years, 400 mg; 11–12 years, 480 mg; over 12, the adult dosage. Alternatively, doses for children can be calculated at 10 mg/kg/dose.

Mefenamic Acid (Ponstel)

Mefenamic acid belongs to the class of fenamates, and its relative, meclofenamate, is employed as a nonsteroidal anti-inflammatory agent (see Chapter 45). Mefenamic acid is somewhat more toxic than most other aspirin-like drugs, especially when use is extended. It is therefore approved only for relief of moderate pain for a period not to exceed 1 week of use. It has been used especially for relief of primary dysmenorrhea. Mefenamic acid is contraindicated for use in individuals with impaired renal function, ulceration or chronic inflammation of the gastrointestinal tract, or a history of allergic reactions to fenamates. *The nurse should advise clients receiving this drug to discontinue use if diarrhea, dark stools, hematemesis, ecchymoses, or rash occurs and to report such symptoms to the physician.* Mefenamic acid has been reported to cause false positives in the diazo tablet test of urinary bile. Insulin requirements in diabetic clients may have to be adjusted while mefenamic acid is being used. Mefenamic acid can cause dizziness and drowsiness. *Clients should be advised that performance of hazardous tasks, such as driving an automobile, may be impaired during use of this drug.*

Propionic Acid Derivatives

Three propionic acid derivatives are approved for use in mild to moderate pain or dysmenorrhea: ibuprofen (Motrin, Nuprin, Rufen, others), fenoprofen (Nalfon), and suprofen (Suprol). Ibuprofen and fenoprofen, as well as a fourth propionic acid derivative, naproxen, are approved for use as anti-inflammatory drugs in rheumatoid arthritis and related rheumatoid disorders. The pharmacology of propionic acid derivatives is covered in Chapter 45.

Important Nursing Implications for Aspirin-like Nonnarcotic Analgesics

- ☐ Observe clients (and teach clients to monitor themselves) for adverse effects of nonnarcotic analgesics, including indications of bleeding (dark stools, hematemesis, or ecchymoses), allergic reactions (rash), gastrointestinal irritation (diarrhea, nausea, epigastric distress), and antifertility effects in males.
- ☐ Observe clients for indications of nephrotoxicity or hepatotoxicity when nonnarcotic analgesics are used for extended periods of time.
- ☐ Teach clients that aspirin-like drugs are not as free of adverse effects as is often assumed.

- ☐ Make certain that clients understand the importance of not exceeding the maximum doses and frequencies of administration listed on the labels of drug containers.
- ☐ Advise clients of the importance of keeping nonnarcotic analgesic drugs out of the reach of children, especially if the tablet is sugar-coated or resembles candy in appearance.
- ☐ When clients self-administer aspirin, watch for alterations in the effects of other medications, especially those that are highly bound to plasma proteins and drugs that are ulcergenic or that inhibit blood coagulation.

Nonnarcotic, Centrally Acting Analgesic: Methotrimeprazine

Methotrimeprazine (Levoprome) is an analgesic that is unrelated in its pharmacology to either the narcotics or the aspirin-like drugs. This phenothiazine derivative produces sedation, a reduction in sensory impulses, an elevation in the pain threshold, and amnesia. Its analgesic effect is comparable in level to that produced by morphine or meperidine. It does not, however, suppress respiration significantly or alter the cough reflex. Its use is not associated with psychological or physical dependence. Methotrimeprazine has antihistaminic, antiadrenergic, and anticholinergic properties. It is indicated for relief of moderate to severe pain in nonambulatory patients, for obstetrical analgesia, or as a preanesthetic medication when respiratory depression must be avoided.

Pharmacokinetics Methotrimeprazine is given by IM injection only. After injection, it is absorbed rapidly, resulting in peak serum concentrations in 30–90 minutes and maximum analgesia in 20–40 minutes. Methotrimeprazine is inactivated mainly by liver metabolism.

Adverse Effects and Contraindications Adverse reactions seldom occur except when methotrimeprazine is used in high doses for extended periods. The most frequent problem is orthostatic hypotension, which can result in fainting, syncope, and weakness. *Clients should be kept supine for about 6–12 hours after injection of methotrimeprazine.* A small drop in blood pressure lasting from 4 to 6 hours is to be expected when methotrimeprazine is employed. Hypotensive effects of methotrimeprazine are additive with those produced by concurrently administered antihypertensive medications.

Other adverse effects include CNS depression (sedation, dizziness, weakness, slurred speech, and disorientation), nausea and vomiting, difficulty urinating, dry mouth, nasal congestion, and pain at the site of injection. CNS depression may be additive with that produced by other drugs. Anticholinergic effects of methotrimeprazine are potentially additive with those of atropine-like agents; caution should be exercised in using such drugs concurrently with methotrimeprazine. Allergic reactions, such as local inflammation and swelling sometimes occur. Jaundice and agranulocytosis has occurred only with long-term use of high doses. *When methotrimeprazine is employed for more than 30 days, blood cell counts and liver function tests should be conducted periodically.*

Preparations and Administration Methotrimeprazine should not be given by subcutaneous injection. *IM injections of methotrimeprazine should be deep into a large muscle mass. When giving multiple doses, the site of injection should be rotated to minimize local irritation. Methotrimeprazine should not be mixed in the same syringe with most drugs, but is compatible with either atropine or scopolamine.*

Methotrimeprazine (Levoprome)
Injection solution
Recommended Doses: For adults, 10–20 mg IM every 4–6 hours as required. Doses have ranged from 5–40 mg per dose. For elderly or debilitated clients who are likely to exhibit unusual sensitivity to phenothiazines, smaller doses of 5–10 mg should be given initially. For obstetrical analgesia, 15–20 mg during labor. For preanesthetic purposes, 2–20 mg, 45 minutes to 3 hours before surgery. In the postoperative period, small doses of 2.5–7.5 mg are recommended because of the potential for additive depression with residual anesthetic.

Case Study: Pain and Analgesia

M. B., a 27-year-old white man, was admitted to the emergency room of a general hospital 30 minutes after suffering a broken left arm in an automobile accident. He was in obvious pain, grimacing and vocalizing continuously. M. B. had no previous medical history. The nurse asked M. B. if he knew of any drug allergies that he had; he did not. He very rarely used nonprescription drugs but drank about one cup of coffee a day and two or three beers a week. Physical examination and x-rays revealed a break in the left radius. Blood tests were normal. M. B. was given 6 mg morphine by slow IV injection. After onset of analgesia, the bone was set. M. B. was transferred to the orthopedic unit with an order for bed rest, meperidine, 100 mg PO every 3 or 4 hours as needed for pain; or codeine, 30 mg, with acetaminophen, 600 mg PO every 3 or 4 hours as needed for less pain.

The nurse observed M. B.'s response to the first two doses of meperidine, noting that the pain relief appeared to be adequate. Before each scheduled dose of analgesic, the nurse assessed M. B. for signs of physical discomfort, such as grimacing, motor restlessness, sighing, verbal complaint of pain, and elevations in heart rate, blood pressure, or respiration. During the first day of hospitalization, the nurse administered meperidine every 3 or 4 hours. Between doses of analgesic, the nurse spent time talking with M. B. and making sure that he was comfortable. On the second day, M. B. exhibited lesser signs of pain; the nurse administered codeine with acetaminophen instead of meperidine. After another 24 hours, M. B. was discharged with a prescription for codeine with acetaminophen as required for pain, up to 7 days.

1. Since morphine was given initially, why wasn't it continued during M. B.'s recovery in the orthopedic unit?
2. Why is the analgesic switched to codeine with acetaminophen as soon as the severity of pain has declined sufficiently?
3. What is the reason for using acetaminophen in combination with codeine?

Answers appear at the end of the book.

Recommended Readings

Endorphins and Opiate Receptors

Huhman M: Endogenous opiates and pain. *Adv Nurs Sci* 1982;4(4):62–71.

Loh HH, Ross HH (eds): *Advances in Biochemical Psychopharmacology.* New York, Raven Press, 1979, Vol. 20: *Neurochemical Mechanisms of Opiates and Endorphins.*

Snyder SH, Childers SR: Opiate receptors and opiate peptides. *Annu Rev Neurosci* 1979;2:35–64.

West BZ: Understanding endorphins: Our natural pain relief system. *Nursing* 1981;11(2):50–53.

Wilson RW, Elmassian BJ: Endorphins. *Am J Nurs* 1981; 81(4):722–725.

Narcotic Analgesics and Antagonists

Alberico JG: Breaking the chronic pain cycle. *Am J Nurs* 1984;84:1222–1225.

DiGregorio GJ, Barbieri EJ: Pharmacologic management of pain. *Am Fam Physician* 1983;27(5):185–188.

DiGregorio GJ, Bukovinsky MA: Clonidine for narcotic withdrawal. *Am Fam Physician* 1981;24(3):203–204.

Foley KM: The practical use of narcotic analgesics. *Med Clin North Am* 1982;66(5):1091–1104.

Goodman CE: Pathophysiology of pain. *Arch Intern Med* 1983;143:527–530.

Heidrich G, Perry S: Helping the patient in pain. *Am J Nurs* 1982;82(12):1828–1833.

Mansky PA: Opiate: Human psychopharmacology, in Iversen LL et al (eds): *Handbook of Psychopharmacology,* 12. New York, Plenum Press, 1978, pp 95–185.

Mar DD: The narcotic analgesics. *Am J Nurs* 1981;81(7): 1364–1365.

Maxwell M: How to use methadone for the cancer patient's pain. *Am J Nurs* 1980;80(9):1606–1608.

McCaffery M: Patients shouldn't have to suffer: How to relieve pain with injectable narcotics. *Nursing* 1980; 10(10):34–39.

McCaffery M: How to relieve your patient's pain fast and effectively with oral analgesics. *Nursing* 1980;10(11): 58–63.

McGuire L, Dizard S: Managing pain in the young patient. *Nursing* 1982;12(8):52, 54–55.

McGuire L, Wright A: Continuous narcotic infusion — it's not just for cancer patients. *Nursing* 1984;14(12):50.

Miller RA: You can control cancer pain with drugs. *Nursing* 1982;12(6):50–58.

Panayotoff K: Managing pain in the elderly patient. *Nursing* 1982;12(8):53, 56–57.

Purtney RK: Pain consult. *Amer J Nurs* 1986;10(3):318.

Riordan CE, Kleber, HD: Rapid opiate detoxification with clonidine and naloxone. *Lancet* 1980;1:1079–1080.

Samuelsson B et al: Prostaglandins and thromboxanes. *Annu Rev Biochem* 1978;47:997–1029.

Showalter CV: T's and blues: Abuse of pentazocine and tripelennamine. *JAMA* 1980;244(1):1224–1225.

Washton AM, Resnick RB: Clonidine in opiate withdrawal: Review and appraisal of clinical findings. *Pharmacotherapy* 1981;1:140–146.

Wright Z: From IV to PO: titrating your patient's pain medication. *Nursing* 1981;11(7):39–43.

Zola EM, McLeod DC: Comparative effects and analgesic efficacy of the agonist-antagonist opioids. *Drug Intell Clin Pharm* 1983;17:411–417.

Nonnarcotic Analgesics

Beaver WT: Aspirin and acetaminophen as constituents of analgesic combinations. *Arch Intern Med* 1981;141(3): 293–300.

Curry R, Robinson J, Sughrue M: Acute renal failure after acetaminophen overdose. *Am J Nurs* 1982;82:1752.

Davies RO: Review of the animal and clinical pharmacology of diflunisal. *Pharmacotherapy* 1983;3:98–228.

Gever LN: A new treatment for a new problem — acetaminophen overdose. *Nursing* 1980;10(6):57.

Griffin JP: Fever — when to leave it alone. *Nursing* 1986; 16(2):58–61.

Hayes AH Jr: Therapeutic implications of drug interactions with acetaminophen and aspirin. *Arch Intern Med* 1981;141(3):301–304.

Langman MJS, Coggon D, Spiegelhalter D: Analgesic intake and the risk of acute upper gastrointestinal bleeding. *Am J Med* 1983;74(6A):79–82.

Levy G: Comparative pharmacokinetics of aspirin and acetaminophen. *Arch Intern Med* 1981;141:279–281.

Mar DD: The simple analgesics. *Am J Nurs* 1981;81(6): 1206–1208.

Mielke CH Jr: Influence of aspirin on platelets and the bleeding time. *Am J Med* 1983:74(6A):72–78.

Prescott LF: Treatment of severe acetaminophen poisoning with intravenous acetylcysteine. *Arch Intern Med* 1981;141(3):386–389.

Settipane GA: Adverse reactions to aspirin and related drugs. *Arch Intern Med* 1981;141:328–332.

Teitelbaum DT, Teitelbaum SB: Overdose: Handling aspirin and acetaminophen poisoning. *Consultant* 1983; 23(2):195–206.

Temple AR: Acute and chronic effects of aspirin toxicity and their treatment. *Arch Intern Med* 1981;141(3): 364–369.

CHAPTER 26

Drugs Used for Headaches

Headaches are very common and in many instances they can be effectively treated with nonnarcotic analgesics, such as aspirin and acetaminophen, that were discussed in the previous chapter. In this chapter, we consider certain kinds of headaches that often require other kinds of drug treatments.

Headaches and face pains arise from a wide variety of causes (Table 26–1), and so therapy takes many forms. Some headaches are associated with structural defects (tumors, hemorrhage, head injuries, meningitis, Paget's disease). Other headaches are allergic reactions to foods, pollens, or environmental allergens or are referred pains that originate in the teeth, ears, sinuses, or eyes. Glaucoma, eyestrain, and sinus headaches are common examples of referred headaches. Vascular and tension headaches are psychosomatic, because they are not associated with obvious organic or structural pathology but do not appear to be wholly psychogenic.

Although it might seem that the brain itself, with its vast array of neural elements, would be a likely source of pain sensations, pain does not in fact arise from brain tissue. The pain receptors that are found within the cranium are associated with the deep-lying, major trunks of cranial blood vessels and with the meninges, mainly the dura. Headaches occur from activation of one or both of these sets of receptors. Headaches that activate pain receptors associated with cranial blood vessels are called **vascular headaches.**

Table 26–1
Headaches: Classification, Age and Sex Correlates, and Treatments

Headache classification	Type	Age or sex correlates	Treatments other than analgesics
Vascular headaches			
Migraine	PS	Postpuberty; F>M	Prophylaxis: propranolol, methysergide, calcium channel blockers, antidepressants; rest, biofeedback (temperature) Acute: ergotamine, caffeine
Cluster	PS	>25; M>>F	Same as above; lithium; activity instead of rest
Drug-induced			
Caffeine withdrawal	OG	None	Caffeine or amphetamine
Alcohol "hangover"	OG	None	Oxygen
Vasodilators	OG	None	Adjust dose
Histamine	OG	None	Antihistamines
Other			
Allergies	OG	None	Antihistamines, pressors
Systemic infection	OG	None	Antihistamines, antibiotics
Hypoglycemia	OG	None	Dietary adjustments
Anoxia	OG	None	Oxygen
Postictal	OG	None	Oxygen
Hypertension[a]	OG	Adult	Antihypertensives
Cerebrovascular disease	OG	Adult	Anticoagulants, surgery
Muscle tension headaches	PS	None	Muscle relaxants, analgesics, rest, biofeedback (EMG)
Traction headaches			
Tumors	OG	None	Surgery, radiation
Hematoma or abscess	OG	Adults	Bed rest
Inflammatory headaches			
Meningitis	OG	None	Antibiotics
Subarachnoid hemorrhage	OG	Adults	Bed rest, hypotensives, surgery
Temporal arteritis	OG	>60; M>F	Steroids
Referred pain headaches			
Sinusitis	OG	None	Antihistamines, decongestants, rest, wet heat
Ophthalmologic	OG	None	Antiglaucoma drugs, glasses
Otologic	OG	None	Antibiotics, surgery
Dental	OG	None	Dental care
Ice-cream headache	OG	None	Eat cold foods slowly
Neuralgias			
Trigeminal	OG	Aged; F>M	Carbamazepine, phenytoin
Glossopharyngeal	OG	Aged; M>F	Carbamazepine, phenytoin
Psychogenic			
Conversion	PG	None	Psychotherapy
Hypochondriacal	PG	None	Psychotherapy
Delusional	PG	None	Antipsychotics

Key: OG, organogenic; PG, psychogenic; PS, psychosomatic.

[a]Includes hypertension due to pheochromacytoma, administration of pressor drugs, ingestion of tyramine in the diet, and essential hypertension.

Vascular Headaches

The pain receptors associated with cerebral blood vessels are free nerve endings that wrap around large blood vessels (Figure 26–1). These receptors become activated when the blood vessels are excessively dilated. Thus, the common element in the various types of vascular headaches is intensive dilation of cerebral blood vessels. Vasodilators can produce vascular headaches by directly dilating cranial blood vessels. For example, vasodilation of cranial blood vessels can occur in response to nitrites that are found in many processed meats, such as hot dogs. Experimentally, histamine produces the same effect. Although histamine is not employed as a drug, endogenous histamine is released in systemic infections and in allergic reactions of the immediate type. Caffeine is a cerebral vasoconstrictor; however, when use of caffeine is discontinued after heavy long-term use, a vascular headache may occur due to rebound vasodilation. When the brain is deprived of adequate glucose (as in hypoglycemia) or oxygen (in anoxia or after a major convulsion), blood vessels may dilate in an effort to overcome the deficiency, possibly resulting in headache. A vascular headache may occur following sexual orgasm as sympathetic tone subsides. Cerebrovascular accidents, including thrombosis and embolism of cerebral arteries, often result in localized headaches that correlate directly with the blood vessel that has been affected.

Hypertension can be associated with a vascular type of headache because elevated intravascular pressure may cause cerebral vessels to press outward against the surrounding pain receptors. Hypertension headaches occur equally often in men and women, are largely limited to adults, and increase in frequency with age. The pain is experienced as nonspecific or emanating from the occipital area and occurs suddenly, correlating with sudden increases in blood pressure. Physical or emotional stress and alcohol consumption are likely triggering factors. Treatment is based on correcting the hypertension with antihypertensive medications (see Chapter 39).

For most kinds of vascular headaches, the factor leading to excessive dilation of cerebral vessels is readily identified. Two kinds of vascular headaches pose a greater challenge: migraine and cluster headaches.

Migraine and Cluster Headaches

The term **migraine** has, unfortunately, been employed in two distinct ways. In most English-language medical literature, the term is used in a broad, inclusive sense to encompass both **classic** and **common** migraine. Non-English-language writers, on the other hand, employ *migraine* only for the classic variety and designate headaches of the common type as **nonmigrainous vascular headaches, cephalea vasomotoria,** or **common headache.** We employ the term in its broader sense, differentiating as required between classic and common varieties.

Migraine is characterized by brief, recurring headaches caused in part by emotional stress and accompanied by neurologic and gastrointestinal symptoms. Any of the following symptoms may occur: blurred vision, arcs or waves of color, tunnel vi-

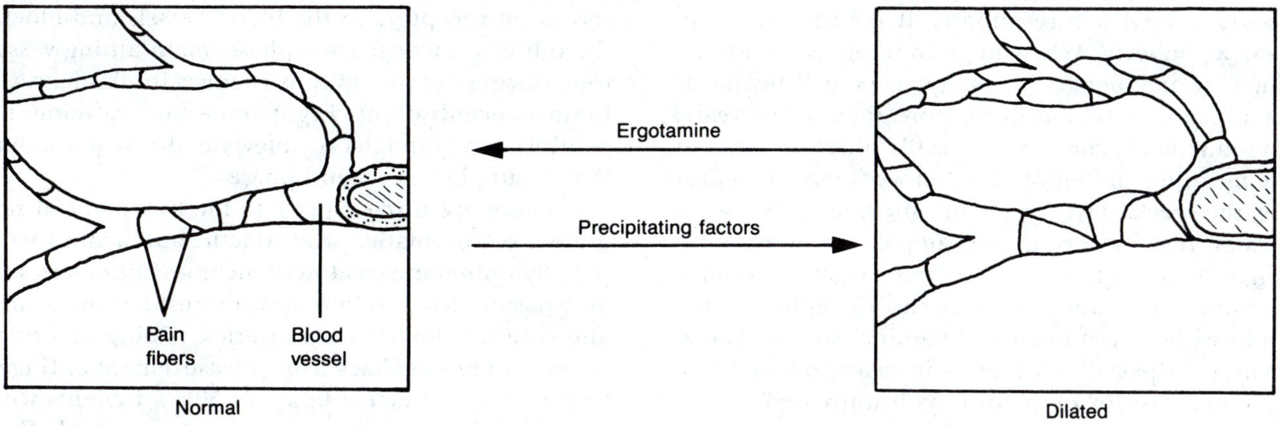

Figure 26–1
The pain of migraine is caused by pressure exerted by overly dilated cranial vessels (right) on surrounding pain receptors (free nerve endings). Ergotamine constricts cranial vessels, alleviating the pressure on the free nerve endings.

sion, temporary partial or complete blindness, scintillating scotomata (islands of blindness in the visual field), double vision, partial aphasia or other verbal disturbances, deafness, ataxia, nausea, or vertigo.

Visual prodromata (or preliminary symptoms) occur exclusively in classic migraine. Other prodromata occur in both types but are more prominent in the classic migraine. Classic migraine may be preceded by premonitory mood changes (either pleasant or unpleasant) and accompanied by nausea and vomiting. In classic migraine, the headache itself is usually on only one side of the head (hence the name *migraine,* meaning one-sided) and may vary in intensity from mild to severe. Prodromal visual symptoms are experienced unilaterally as well, on the side opposite to the subsequent headache. Attacks may occur in flurries, alternating between the left and right hemispheres. The frequency of classic migraine headaches increases for women during pregnancy.

In common migraine, headaches are often bilateral and dull, and nausea is less common and less severe. The pain is most often experienced as emanating from the temporal area of the cortex. The attacks are periodic, not clustered. The frequency of common migraine headaches decreases during pregnancy but increases during periods of life transition or stress, and premenstrually. *The nurse should try to help clients identify life circumstances that may be contributing to migraine headaches without implying that it is an entirely psychological condition.* Common migraine is among the most prevalent forms of headache, while classic migraine is comparatively rare, almost an oddity. Migraine headaches are about three times more common in women than in men.

Migraine headache may be experienced at any age between puberty and climacteric but usually begins in late adolescence or early adulthood. When it occurs (rarely) before puberty, it is likely to disappear at puberty. When migraine begins in adolescence, it may persist for many years; if it begins at menopause, it seldom lasts more than a few years. Migraine headaches are especially likely to occur in the morning and more often on weekends than during the week. Trigger factors include stress, withdrawal from stress (for example, on weekends), bright light or glare, hypoglycemia, cigarette smoke, tyramine-containing foods or chocolate, hot or humid weather, vasodilators, histamine, and hormonal changes, especially decreases in estrogens. A headache may last for hours or days if untreated.

Migraine tends to occur in persons having a personality profile marked by obsessive-compulsive tendencies, a great need for achievement, and neat, efficient, and perfectionistic inclinations. They may also exhibit a hypersensitivity to sensory stimuli and are more than normally likely to have allergies or epilepsy. They may be sexually maladjusted. Only a single rare subtype of migraine is linked to a specific gene, but a familial history of migraine is present in about 50% of cases.

Cluster headaches are diagnostically distinct from migraine headaches, but are treated similarly. Cluster headaches are unilateral severe pains occurring in and around the eyes that are accompanied by tearing, photophobia, a runny nose, and reddening of the eyes. The most common time of occurrence is shortly after falling asleep. Onset is usually abrupt and the headaches typically last from 20 to 120 minutes. Use of alcohol or lying down can be precipitating factors. The headaches occur in clusters (hence the name), with many of them occurring within a period of a few weeks and then none for weeks or months. Duodenal ulcers often accompany cluster headaches, supporting the theory that the condition is related to excess parasympathetic activity. Cluster headaches occur much more often in men than in women and usually begin after age 25 with no evidence of a familial component and no consistent personality profile.

The effectiveness of antiserotonin agents in treating migraine has highlighted the importance of serotonin levels in these headaches. Serotonin is a potent constrictor of cerebral arteries. Just before migraine attacks, serotonin is released from blood platelets, which triggers a **vasoconstrictor phase** that is associated with prodromal symptoms, including flash sensations, odd smells, and feelings of dread, but no pain. This phase lasts about 10 minutes and gives way to a compensatory **vasodilation phase** of severe pain lasting a few hours, days, or even a week. Methysergide is believed to act an an antagonist to serotonin receptors in the blood vessels and blocks the initial vasoconstrictor phase, maintaining vessel tone during the precipitous changes in plasma serotonin concentrations. Ergotamine and caffeine, by contrast, are thought to alleviate the vasodilation that occurs in the second phase.

There are three aspects to the treatment of migraine: symptomatic, prophylactic, and acute therapies. **Symptomatic treatment** includes antiemetics or antispasmodics to relieve gastrointestinal problems, and compression of scalp arteries, resting in a dark room, and **biofeedback** using measurement of finger temperature (effective in about 50% of clients with migraine) for pain. Psychotherapy has proved effective in only a small number of cases. The following sections describe the drugs employed for prophylaxis and for acute treatment respectively.

Drugs Used for Prophylaxis of Migraine

Specific prophylactic chemotherapy for migraine entails the use of antiserotonergic substances (methysergide, cyproheptadine, and pizotifen), beta-blockers, calcium channel blockers, alpha-2 agonists, the serotonin precursor L-tryptophan, tricyclic antidepressants of the tertiary amine group, and monoamine oxidase inhibitors (Table 26–2). Of these, the best known and most widely tested antimigraine drug is methysergide (Sansert).

Table 26–2
Drug Employed for Migraine

Drug	FDA-approved for use in migraine as of 1986
Acute treatment	
Ergot derivatives	
Ergotamine	Yes
Dihydroergotamine	Yes
Adjuncts for acute treatment	
Xanthines	
Caffeine	Yes
GI stimulant	
Metoclopramide	No
Prophylaxis	
Antiserotonergic agents	
Methysergide	Yes
Cyproheptadine	No
Pizotylline	No
Beta-blockers	
Propranolol	Yes
Atenolol	No
Labetolol	No
Metoprolol	No
Nadolol	No
Pindolol	No
Timolol	No
Alpha-2 agonist	
Clonidine	No
Calcium channel blockers	
Diltiazem	No
Flunarizine	No
Nifedipine	No
Nimodepine	No
Verapamil	No
Antidepressants	
Amitriptyline	No
Doxepin	No
Phenelzine	No
L-Tryptophan	No
Prophylaxis for cluster headaches only	
Lithium	No

Methysergide

Mechanisms and Effects Methysergide is a semisynthetic ergot derivative. Although lacking direct effects on blood vessels, it blocks the actions of serotonin, preventing the excessive vasoconstriction during the prodromal phase of migraine as well as the subsequent compensatory dilation.

Adverse Effects and Contraindications Methysergide is the most efficacious treatment currently available for prophylaxis against migraine, but causes many side effects, including heartburn, diarrhea, nausea, vomiting, and GI cramps. *Gatrointestinal distress from the drug can be minimized by taking it with meals or food. Gradual introduction of the medication also helps to minimize GI symptoms.* Because of its potential hazards, methysergide should be reserved for clients whose vascular headaches are frequent, severe, and uncontrollable by other means. The individual receiving methysergide needs close medical supervision while receiving the drug. CNS side effects include lightheadedness, nervousness, insomnia, euphoria, hallucinations, weakness, and a loss of appetite. Methysergide uncommonly causes neutropenia, eosinophilia, rashes, alopecia, and peripheral edema. A peculiar interaction of methysergide is a potentiation of the effects of phenothiazines, necessitating a reduction in dosage of the latter.

The most dangerous adverse effects of methysergide are associated with long-term use and include retroperitoneal **fibrosis,** pleuropulmonary fibrosis, and cardiac fibrosis. If one of these conditions occurs and the drug is quickly discontinued, regression almost always occurs. Thus monitoring for development of fibrosis is essential. Retroperitoneal fibrosis is manifested as general malaise, fatigue, weight loss, backache, urinary obstruction, low grade fever, polyuria, dysuria, oliguria, and vascular insufficiency to the lower limbs. *The nurse should advise clients receiving methysergide to report immediately any occurrence of coldness, numbness, or pain in the extremities; leg cramps from walking, or pain in the flank, chest, or girdle. The nurse should frequently auscultate major vessels for bruits, auscultate the heart and lungs, and check peripheral pulses.* Presence of retroperitoneal fibrosis can be confirmed by intravenous pyelography. Pleuropulmonary fibrosis should be suspected if the client shows signs of dyspnea, tightness of the chest, pleural effusion, or chest pain. The condition can be confirmed by x-ray examination. Cardiac fibrosis presents as cardiac murmurs or dyspnea. *Administration of methysergide should not be continued on a regular basis beyond 6 months.*

Preparations and Administration Therapeutic benefit develops after 1 or 2 days of use. If no effect occurs within 3 weeks, there is unlikely to be any response and the drug should be discontinued. After discontinuation, the effects of methysergide subside after 1–2 days. A drug-free interval of 3–4 weeks should be planned after every 6 months of treatment. When approaching a planned drug free period, doses of methysergide should be tapered gradually over a period of 2–3 weeks to avoid a rebound in incidence and severity of headaches, which is essentially a withdrawal phenomenon. Sansert contains tartrazine, a dye to which some individuals are allergic. The usual reaction to tartrazine is an asthma-like wheezing. Methysergide is not recommended for use in children.

Methysergide (Sansert)
Tablets
Recommended Doses: The recommended adult dosage is 4–8 mg PO daily, taken with meals.

Beta-blockers for Migraine

Propranolol (Inderal) is the only FDA-approved drug for migraine prophylaxis besides methysergide. This prototypical beta-adrenergic blocking agent exhibits efficacy roughly comparable to that of methysergide and is the current drug of choice for prophylaxis of migraine because of its low incidence of side effects compared with methysergide. Other beta-blocking agents, including atenolol (Tenormin), nadolol (Corgard), and timolol (Blocadren), have been used investigationally for migraine but have not yet received approval from the U.S. Food and Drug Administration. The efficacy of beta-blockers for prophylaxis against migraine does not appear to be due to blocking of either beta-1 or beta-2 receptors, since d-propranolol works as well in migraine as racemic propranolol yet lacks any beta-blocking properties. Both cardioselective and nonselective beta-blockers can be used successfully in migraine, but beta-blockers with intrinsic sympathomimetic activity (see Table 39–6) are ineffective.

Preparations and Administration

Propranolol (Inderal)
Formulations: See Chapter 39
Recommended Doses: For treatment of migraine, 80 mg/day PO, once daily initially, increased gradually. The usual effective dosage range for migraine is 160–240 mg/day PO. If no response is obtained within 4–6 weeks, propranolol should be discontinued.

Other Agents for Migraine Prophylaxis

Pizotylline (pizotifen, Sandomigran) is an antiserotonin agent widely employed in Europe and Australia that is not yet available in the United States. It is slightly less effective than methysergide but is devoid of most adverse effects. Other **antiserotonergic agents,** including cyproheptadine (Periactin), methdilazine (Tacaryl), and methylergol carbamide maleate (Lysenyl), have been tested clinically for use in migraine. Of these, only cyproheptadine is available in the United States and it is not FDA-approved for migraine. Its efficacy in migraine is less than that of methysergide, but it has been used successfully in treating cluster headaches. Cyproheptadine possesses antihistaminergic and anticholinergic properties as well as antiserotonergic effects (see Chapter 50).

Verapamil (Calan, Isoptin), a **calcium channel blocker,** has been studied, but not approved, for use in prophylaxis of migraine. Diltiazem (Cardizem) is employed in Europe for prophylaxis of migraine and nifedipine has undergone a successful clinical trial for migraine in France. Two calcium channel blockers, flunarizine and nimodepine, not yet available for routine clinical practice, are currently under study as antimigraine agents. Evidence suggests that the spasmolytic effect of calcium channel blockers protects against the initial vasospasm that occurs in the prodromal phase of migraine.

Clonidine (Catapres), an antihypertensive agent that stimulates alpha-2 noradrenergic receptors has been used unofficially for prophylaxis of migraine for more than a decade with mixed results. It has not fared as well in controlled clinical trials as many of the other agents mentioned here.

Three **antidepressant drugs,** amitriptyline (Elavil), doxepin (Sinequan), and phenelzine (Nardil), have been used experimentally for prophylaxis against vascular headaches, all yielding response rates comparable to that of methysergide. None are currently FDA-approved for use in migraine. The doses of amitriptyline employed for prevention of cluster or migraine headaches are 50–150 mg/day PO. **Lithium,** though not approved for use in vascular headaches, has been used successfully in doses of 600–900 mg/day PO for prevention of cluster headaches and cyclical migraine headache, but is said to aggravate most cases of migraine. **L-Tryptophan,** the precursor of serotonin and a drug sometimes classified as an antidepressant, is said to be moderately effective in migraine in doses of 500 mg or higher, taken orally, 4 times per day.

Drugs Used for Acute Relief of Migraine: Ergotamine and Dihydroergotamine

Mechanisms and Effects Ergotamine (Gynergen) and dihydroergotamine (D.H.E. 45) are alpha-adrenergic blocking agents that also act directly on vascular (as well as visceral) smooth muscle to produce vasoconstriction. The pharmacology of the two agents is equivalent; ergotamine is employed orally (the usual route) while dihydroergotamine is used by IM or IV injection. The effectiveness of these drugs in migraine is due to constriction of cranial blood vessels. Ergotamine is most effective if given early in an attack. Given more than 2 hours after the onset of an attack, it has little value. At least 70% of migraine headaches respond to ergotamine, but ergotamine may aggravate nausea and vomiting of migraine due to its stimulatory effect on visceral smooth muscle.

Pharmacokinetics Absorption of ergotamine is most reliable and rapid after inhalation of the aerosol preparation. Oral administration is unpredictable but usually adequate to relieve mild to moderate or incipient attacks, especially if administered early. Absorption from the buccal mucosa is especially poor, but sublingual absorption is rapid. Oral absorption is improved by concomitant administration of caffeine (which is present in many of the combination formulations). Peak plasma levels occur about 2 hours after oral administration; relief may not occur until after as much as 5 hours. Rectal suppositories containing ergotamine provide reliable absorption at a fairly constant rate. With IM injection, dihydroergotamine produces relief in about 15–30 minutes, lasting from 3–4 hours. Ergotamine is inactivated 90% by liver metabolism and the metabolites are eliminated in the bile. The plasma half-life of ergotamine is only about 2 hours, but it nevertheless exhibits cumulative effects because of tissue sequestration.

Clinical Indications Ergotamine is the drug of choice for acute relief of migraine attacks.

Adverse Effects and Ergotism Ergotamine produces few serious side effects when employed in a single, moderate dose. However, problems can arise when the drug is used frequently (such as daily). No more than 6 mg of ergotamine should be employed for a single migraine attack and no more than 10 mg total per week. In recent years, an increasingly common practice has been the use of ergotamine with metoclopramide (Reglan), an upper gastrointestinal tract stimulant that alleviates nausea and vomiting. The addition of metoclopramide allows successful treatment of migraine with smaller doses of ergotamine per administration, allowing more administrations per week for individuals who experience frequent attacks.

Side effects that occur at moderate doses include numbness and paresthesias of the fingers and toes, weakness in the legs, precordial (anginal) pain, pain in the muscles of the extremities, diarrhea, nausea, vomiting, localized edema, pruritus, and transient changes in heart rate. *Clients should be advised to report irregularities of heart beat or occurrence of*

Nursing Observations for Drugs Used for Headache Relief

THERAPEUTIC GOAL	Monitor frequency and severity of headaches.
PREADMINISTRATION ASSESSMENT	
Baseline Data	Evaluate verbal reports of head pain and behavioral expressions of pain such as grimacing, moaning, and irritability. Evaluate eyes, nose, and throat for signs of infection (inflammation or exudation) and neurological function. Take an EEG and CT scan if indicated. Dental and ophthalmological examinations should be conducted if the cause of the pain remains obscure. Obtain laboratory tests including complete blood cell count, blood glucose, and oxygenation.
Contraindications/ Precautions	Peripheral vascular disorders, ischemic heart disease, thrombophlebitis, renal or hepatic dysfunction, pregnancy, or hypertension.
EVALUATION OF DRUG RESPONSE	
For Adverse Effects and Drug Interactions	Monitor for side effects and drug interactions specific for each drug employed (see individual drug discussions).
For Compliance	Evaluate client's compliance with all facets of the therapeutic regimen by careful observation, interviewing, and review of progress. Report compliance problems to the physician and act as client-advocate when changes in the therapeutic regimen seem indicated.

nausea and vomiting. However, these symptoms are seldom severe enough to require discontinuation of the medication. Precordial pain is most likely to occur in susceptible individuals 5–10 minutes following IM injection of dihydroergotamine. Sublingual nitroglycerin may be required to provide relief. Chronic excessive use of ergotamine may result in vasospastic complications, usually involving the legs, resulting in cyanosis and burning pain or numbness. *Clients with peripheral vascular disease, severe hypertension, or ischemic heart disease should not take ergotamine. The nurse should instruct clients receiving ergotamine to report any weakness of the extremities, claudication, muscle pain, or cold or numb extremities (which may be warning signs of potential gangrene).* With excessive chronic use, there is a risk of both tolerance and dependence, necessitating higher doses to obtain relief from migraine headaches. *The nurse should emphasize the importance of not exceeding recommended doses of this drug.*

Acute overdose (egotism) is characterized by nausea, vomiting, diarrhea, and severe thirst, followed by confusion and coma. Residual sensory deficits involving somatosensory or visual sensations, may persist after acute intoxication. Treatment of ergotism requires prevention of further absorption of residual drug from the gastrointestinal system (by lavage or emesis, followed by activated charcoal and catharsis); supportive measures to maintain vital functions, and spasmolytic agents such as nitroglycerin or nitroprusside to relieve vasospasm. *Clients should be warned to keep ergotamine out of reach of children because fatal overdoses have occurred.*

Use of ergotamine is contraindicated in individuals with vasospastic peripheral vascular disorder, hypertension, sepsis, hepatic or renal disease, severe pruritus, or known hypersensitivity to ergot alkaloids. Ergotamine is contraindicated for use during pregnancy because it powerfully constricts uterine smooth muscle, with potentially harmful consequences to the fetus.

Drug Interactions The vasoconstrictor effect of ergotamine derivatives is additive with that of other pressor drugs. Use of pressor drugs, such as sympathomimetics, with ergotamine can result in dangerous hypertension. Troleandomycin (Tao), an antibiotic of the macrolide group, inhibits the metabolism of ergotamine and potentiates its effect. Oral nitroglycerin increases absorption and bioavailability of concurrently administered ergotamine.

Ergotamine is provided in combinations with caffeine for use in migraine headaches. In addition to promoting ergotamine absorption, caffeine has a constrictor effect of its own on cranial vessels.

Preparations and Administration *Sublingual tablets must remain under the tongue rather than in the buccal pouch, where absorption is very slow.* Rest and relaxation have a palliative effect for migraine. *The nurse should advise clients to lie down in a quiet, darkened room for at least 2 hours after taking medication for an acute migraine attack.*

Ergotamine (Gynergen, Ergomar, Ergostat, Wigrettes)
Tablets, sublingual tablets, aerosol for use in a medihaler; combinations with caffeine (Cafergot, Wigraine, Ercatab, and Cafetrate); combination suppository preparations (Cafergot, Wigraine, Migergot)
Recommended Doses: 2–6 tablets orally per attack, not to exceed 10 tablets weekly. One sublingual tablet at the first sign of attack and additional sublingual tablets at half-hour intervals up to 3 tablets per day and 10 mg (5 tablets) per week. One inhalation initially with the aerosol preparation, repeated at 5 minute intervals up to 6 inhalations per 24 hours or 15 inhalations per week. Two combination ergotamine and caffeine tablets are taken orally at the first sign of an attack, followed by 1 tablet every half-hour, as needed, to a maximum of 6 tablets per attack or 10 tablets per week. One combination suppository tablet inserted at the first sign of an attack, followed by a second 1 hour later, if needed. The maximum recommended dose for the suppository form is 2 tablets per attack, 5 tablets per week.

Dihydroergotamine Mesylate (D.H.E. 45)
Injection solution
Recommended Doses: 1 mg IM at the first sign of headache, repeated hourly to a maximum of 3 mg. For a more rapid effect, 1 mg IV, repeated once per attack, up to 6 mg/week.

Other Kinds of Drug-Responsive Headaches

Muscle Tension Headaches

Muscle tension headaches are psychosomatic because they are triggered by fatigue, emotional or physical stress, and sexual excitation. They are characterized by a dull, aching sensation, usually lasting 1–4 hours. These headaches are related to acute or chronic elevations in muscle tone, especially muscles of the neck and cranium. The pain is experienced bilaterally, especially in the occipital region. Onset is acute, most often in the late afternoon and evening. Tension headaches are equally common in males and females, occur at any age, and exhibit little familial trend. Individuals who are competitive, sensitive, and conscientious are at greatest risk.

Tension headaches are best treated pharmacologically with centrally acting skeletal muscle relax-

Nursing Diagnoses and Interventions for Drugs Used for Headache Relief

Nursing Diagnoses	*Related Interventions*
TO ENHANCE DRUG BENEFITS OR REDUCE DRUG REQUIREMENTS	
Alteration in comfort: pain of headache	Provide analgesics, muscle relaxants, or migraine drugs as indicated; provide comfort measures; teach biofeedback or relaxation techniques; when discontinuing methysergide, taper the doses to avoid rebound headaches.
Ineffective individual coping: irritability or depression related to pain	Provide emotional support and encouragement. Help the family develop strategies for coping with the client when headaches occur.
TO MINIMIZE DRUG SIDE EFFECTS OR INTERACTIONS	
Alteration in bowel elimination: diarrhea caused by methysergide or ergotamine	Have clients take methysergide with meals or snacks; introduce methysergide gradually.
Alteration in cardiac output from use of propranolol	Monitor client for signs of fluid retention, pulmonary congestion, or cyanosis and report any such symptoms to the physician at once.
Alteration in comfort: anginal pain from ergotamine	Administer sublingual nitroglycerin. Report episodes to physician for possible change in regimen.
Alterations in nutrition: intake less than requirements due to methysergide-induced anorexia	Provide nutritional support as indicated. Help client determine foods that are best tolerated.
Alteration in tissue perfusion related to methysergide-induced fibrosis or ergotamine-induced vasospasm	Instruct clients who receive methysergide to report any occurrence of coldness, pain, or numbness of the extremities, muscle cramps from walking, or pain in the flank, girdle or back; discontinue methysergide if these occur; instruct clients who receive ergotamine to report occurrence of weakness, coldness, or pain of the extremities, muscle pain, or claudication.
Ineffective breathing patterns: aggravation of asthma by propranolol	Report any symptoms of respiratory distress to the physician.
Potential for infection related to blood dyscrasias caused by carbamazepine or phenytoin used for neuralgias	Advise clients to report any episodes of persistent sore throat or fever. Conduct periodic blood cell counts during prolonged therapy.
TO ENSURE SAFE AND EFFICACIOUS DRUG USE	
Knowledge deficit related to drug regimen	Teach clients about the causes and characteristics of the type of headache from which they suffer. Explain the rationale for the therapeutic regimen prescribed. Teach clients employing ergotamine for acute relief of migraine headaches to take the drug as soon after onset of an attack as possible. Teach nondrug measures for combating particular types of headaches, such as relaxation techniques, dietary adjustments, avoidance of allergens, avoidance of fatigue and stress, and biofeedback. Provide client with a list of adverse effects and drug interactions for each drug in the regimen and explain what to do if any of these occur.

ants, such as diazepam or meprobamate, often in combination with analgesics. Equagesic, for example, is a combination of meprobamate with aspirin, marketed expressly for tension headaches. Another combination product marketed for this application is Fiorinal, which combines butalbital (a barbiturate) with aspirin and caffeine. Other combinations of centrally acting skeletal muscle relaxants and analgesics include methocarbamol and aspirin (Robaxisal is one example), carisoprodol and aspirin (Soma Compound, for example), chlorzoxazone and acetaminophen (Chlorzone, Paracet, Parafon, for example) and orphenadrine, aspirin, and caffeine (Norgesic). (These agents are described in Chapter 22.) Nondrug approaches have also proved valuable for treating tension headaches. Relaxation therapy and biofeedback using myoelectrical signals from the frontalis muscle of the forehead have been useful approaches.

Inflammatory Headaches

Inflammatory headaches may occur in association with meningitis, subarachnoid hemorrhage, temporal arteritis, or following pneumoencephalography. **Meningitis** is an inflammation of the meninges, caused by bacterial, viral, fungal or prion infections. The organisms most likely to cause bacterial meningitis in adults are *N. meningitidis* and *D. pneumoniae.* These bacteria are also frequent causes of meningitis in children, but *H. influenzae* is the most common cause (Table 26-3). Bacterial meningitis is treatable with appropriate antibacterial agents (Table 26-3). There are many potential viral and fungal causes of meningitis as well. Amphotericin B is the drug of choice for all forms of meningitis caused by fungal infections.

Temporal arteritis is an inflammation of the giant endothelial cells of the temporal artery, often occurring as an extension of aortitis. It is more common in men than women, usually occurs after age 60, and occurs exclusively in caucasians. The pain is experienced as severe and throbbing, emanating from the temple, jaw, or tongue, especially while eating. The individual may experience tenderness and redness of the scalp over the temporal artery. Attacks last for days or weeks; the condition may be continuous or episodic. Corticosteroids provide palliative relief, but no specific therapy exists.

Referred Pain Headaches

Disorders involving the eyes, sinuses, ears, or teeth may produce referred pain headaches. Sinus headaches occur in conjunction with sinusitis and constitutes one of the most common forms of recurrent headaches (see Chapter 55). They are treated with sinus preparations that typically contain a decongestant and an antihistamine. Wet heat, rest, and analgesics may also be helpful for sinus headaches. Other potential causes of referred pain headaches include dental problems (especially temporomandibular joint pain due to poor dental bite or grinding of teeth), otitis, ingestion of cold substances (as in the

Table 26-3
Antimicrobial Treatment of Bacterial Meningitis

Microbe	Incidence: Children	Incidence: Adults	Penicillin	Ampicillin	Cephalosporins	Sulfonamides	Tetracyclines	Chloramphenicol	Streptomycin	Erythromycin	Bacitracin
N. meningitidis	+++	+++++	✓✓	✓	✓	✓	✓	✓			
D. pneumoniae	++	++	✓✓	✓	✓	✓	✓	✓			
Streptococcus	+/−	+	✓✓	✓	✓	✓	✓	✓		✓	
Staphylococcus	+/−	+/−	✓✓	✓	✓	✓	✓			✓	✓
H. influenzae	++++	+/−		✓✓	✓	✓	✓	✓✓			
E. coli	+	+/−		✓✓	✓	✓	✓		✓		
Other	+	+									

Key: +/−, < 3%; +, 3-10%; ++ 10-19%; +++, 20-39%; ++++, 40-59%; +++++, 60-70%;
✓✓ indicates preferred drug choice; ✓ indicates effective drug.

"ice-cream headache"), and ocular problems, such as eye strain.

Neuralgias

Neuralgias are paroxysmal discharges of the cranial nerves that carry somatic sensory sensations from the face and skull to the brain. The most common neuralgias involve the trigeminal and glossopharyngeal nerves. Neuralgias are characteristically recurrent episodes of sharp, agonizing pain that may last days, weeks, or months, separated by similarly variable periods of complete relief. A critical diagnostic test for neuralgia is the presence of trigger zones on the surface of the face where light touch can excite the sharp, shooting pains. The prognosis for neuralgias is poor, since they tend to worsen with age and undermine psychological health and morale.

Trigeminal paroxysmal discharges usually arise from the descending nucleus of the nerve. The nucleus can be surgically destroyed, which may cure the neuralgia or produce an untreatable chronic burning sensation. Usual analgesics are notably ineffective. The most effective treatments are two antiepileptic agents, phenytoin (Dilantin) and carbamazepine (Tegretol). The former is tried first, since it is relatively free of serious side effects (see Chapter 23) but is effective in less than 50% of individuals. Carbamazepine is effective in 70% of cases and is considered almost a diagnostic test for neuralgia. It has many adverse effects, some of them quite serious, such as agranulocytosis, leukopenia, thrombocytopenia, and aplastic anemia. Frequent blood tests to monitor development of side effects are an integral part of carbamazipine therapy. The CNS side effects may include extrapyramidal reactions, dizziness, fatigue, and insomnia. Carbamazepine may also be indicated in glossopharyngeal neuralgias refractory to phenytoin. The complete pharmacology of carbamazepine was presented earlier, in Chapter 23.

Case Study: Migraine Headache

N. R., a 26-year-old female executive was brought to the emergency room of a hospital by a colleague after being found slumped on the floor of her office in distress and complaining of severe headache. Vital signs were blood pressure 155/90, pulse 105, and respirations 23. She was pale, disoriented, and kept her eyes closed except when being addressed. The nurse took a history from N. R., learning that she had experienced headaches about once a month during the past 2 years that had gradually become more severe. N. R. indicated that the headaches were usually preceded by a period of nausea, lightheadedness, and blindspots in her visual field. After a full examination, N. R. was diagnosed as having migraine headaches. The nurse discussed the nature of migraine with N. R., telling her that the medical team could help her, but that she would have to help herself as well. She reviewed N. R.'s medical history for evidence of any disorder that would be a contraindication for ergotamine therapy and the physician then prescribed ergotamine, 2 mg sublingually, to be taken at the first sign of an attack. The nurse instructed N. R. about the proper uses of sublingual tablets and the potential adverse effects that might occur and provided N. R. with a written summary of these instructions. Finally, the nurse explained to N. R. the role of stress and other factors in migraine occurrence and helped N. R. begin a diary to help identify relevant factors.

As a result, N. R. learned that the headaches generally occurred at the end of the work week, especially when the week had been a difficult and hectic one. She learned that she was likely to experience headaches the day after she consumed a lot of coffee or alcohol. She also found that getting extra sleep during especially stressful work periods helped to prevent attacks. N. R. learned that if she paid attention to warning signals, she was able to anticipate migraine attacks 1 or 2 hours before onset and that the severity of attacks could be diminished if she took ergotamine immediately and lay down in a dark, quiet room. Gradually, N. R. was able to reduce the frequency of attacks to about four or five per year and to reduce the average duration from 12 hours to 2 hours.

1. What characteristics suggest that N. R.'s headaches were migraine headaches and not due to some other cause?
2. What might the nurse have found in the medical history that would be a contraindication for use of ergotamine?
3. What is the reason for taking ergotamine quickly when there is indication of an impending migraine attack?
4. If N. R. had been less successful in reducing the incidence of attacks by nondrug measures, what drugs could have been prescribed for prophylaxis?

Answers appear at the end of the book.

Recommended Readings

Amery WK: Flunarizine, a calcium channel blocker: A new prophylactic drug in migraine. *Headache* 1983; 23:70–74.

Barrett-Griesemer P, Meisel S, Rate R: A guide to headaches and how to relieve their pain. *Nursing* 1981; 11(4):50–57.

Bruyn GW: The biochemical basis of migraine: A critique. *Clin Neuropharm* 1976;1:185–213.

Capildeo R, Rose FC: single-dose pizotifen, 1.5 mg nocte: A new approach in the prophylaxis of migraine. *Headache* 1982;22:272–275.

Couch JR, Hassanein RS: Amitriptyline in migraine prophylaxis. *Arch Neurol* 1979;36:695–699.

Diamond S et al: Long-term study of propranolol in the treatment of migraine. *Headache* 1982;22:268–271.

Forssman B, Lindblad CJ, Zbornikova V: Atenolol for migraine prophylaxis. *Headache* 1983;23:188–190.

Meyer JS, Hardenberg J: Clinical effectiveness of calcium entry blockers in prophylaxtic treatment of migraine and cluster headaches. *Headaches* 1983;23:266–277.

Peatfield R: Migraine: Current concepts of pathogenesis and treatment. *Drugs* 1983;26:364–371.

Peters BH, Fraim CJ, Masel BE: Comparison of 650 mg aspirin and 1000 mg acetaminophen with each other, and with placebo in moderately severe headache. *Am J Med* 1983;74(6A):36–42.

Saper JR: Migraine, part I: Classification and pathogenesis, *JAMA* 1978;239:2380–2383; part II: Treatment, 2480–2484.

Raskin: Pharmacology of migraine. *Annu Rev Pharmacol Toxicol* 1981;21:463–478.

Taylor JC et al: Long-term treatment of trigeminal neuralgia with carbamazepine. *Postgrad Med* 1981;57:16–18.

Tomson T et al: Carbamazepine therapy in trigeminal neuralgia: Clinical effects in relation to plasma concentrations. *Arch Neurol* 1980;37(11):699–703.

UNIT IV

Drugs and the Peripheral Nervous System

CHAPTER 27

Introduction to the Peripheral Nervous System

The influences of the central nervous system on behavior and visceral activity are transmitted to the skeletal muscles, organs, and glands by either the endocrine system or the peripheral nervous system. These systems are the subjects of this unit and the next. The synapses of the peripheral nervous system are especially vulnerable to drug influences because they are not protected (as are brain synapses) by the blood-brain barrier. The use of drugs to modify transmission at the various peripheral synapses is an important branch of pharmacotherapeutics.

Drugs modulate transmission in the peripheral nervous system and thereby alter the activity of one or more of the target tissues regulated by peripheral nervous system efferent nerve fibers. The drugs that affect transmission at autonomic synapses are discussed most fully in the chapters that deal with each major tissue that is innervated by the autonomic nervous system. Sympathetic agonists (or *sympathomimetics*) appear in later chapters pertaining to the eye, the respiratory system, and the cardiovascular system. *Sympatholytics* (drugs that block the receptors for norepinephrine) appear in chapters relating to the cardiovascular system and headaches. *Cholinomimetics* (drugs that mimic acetylcholine) are discussed in chapters pertaining to the eye, the heart, and the gastrointestinal system. And *cholinolytics* (drugs that block receptors for acetylcholine) appear in the chapters concerning the gastrointestinal system, the extrapyramidal system, toxicology, and the eye. This unit provides only a general overview of the use of autonomic drugs.

The peripheral nervous system has two major divisions: the somatic division (innervating skeletal muscles) and the autonomic nervous system (innervating the viscera, the heart, smooth muscle, and glands). Each of the two divisions has afferent nerves, carrying inputs into the brain, and efferent nerves, conveying brain influences to the periphery.

Drug influences on peripheral nerve impulses are almost always the result of effects on efferent rather than afferent pathways and on synapses (as in the CNS) rather than nerve impulse conduction along axons. Categories of peripheral nervous system drugs, therefore, are based on the categories of synapses in the efferent pathways, taking into account anatomical features, the identity of the synaptic transmitter, and receptor types.

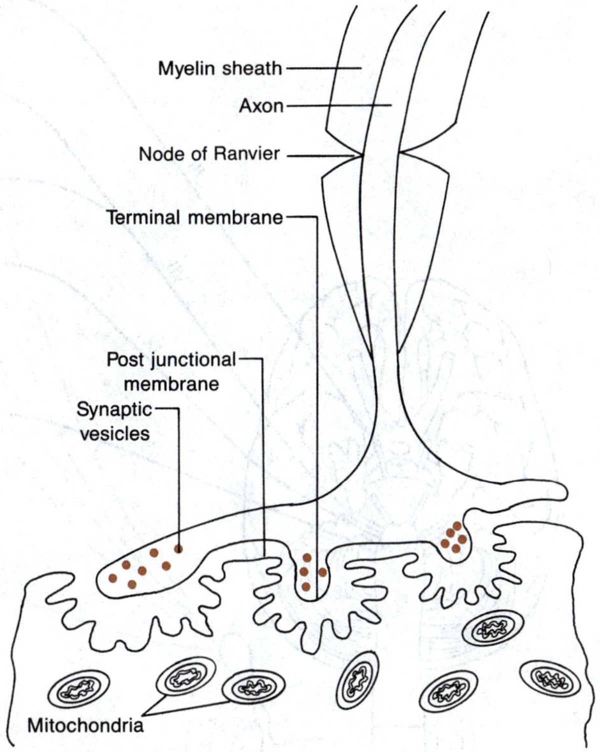

Figure 27–1
Neuromuscular junction

The Somatic Nervous System

The motor neurons of the somatic nervous system, which innervate the striated skeletal muscles, include alpha motor neurons, which cause contractions, and gamma motor neurons, which regulate muscle tone. The cell bodies of the somatic efferent nerves lie in the ventral horn of the gray matter of the spinal cord, and each one is innervated by hundreds of axons from the pyramidal and extrapyramidal systems of the CNS. The somatic efferents represent the final common pathway for all CNS influences on muscle activity.

The axons of somatic motor neurons extend without intermediate synapses to the striated muscles, where they form synaptic junctions with the end-plates of the skeletal muscles. The axons protrude from their myelin sheaths to form terminal feet that are recessed into the muscle fiber (Figure 27–1). The neuromuscular junction, the only kind of synapse in the somatic nervous system, is the principal peripheral target site for drug influences on muscle activity. The transmitter of the neuromuscular junction is acetylcholine.

Afferent neurons of the somatic nervous system make up the somatosensory and proprioceptive networks, carrying signals related to pain, pressure, skin temperature, and muscle position and movement. The afferent neurons are bipolar cells that propagate nerve impulses from the sensory receptors into the spinal cord. These afferent neurons are generally not affected by drugs.

The Autonomic Nervous System

The autonomic nervous system is divided into two branches, the sympathetic nervous system and the parasympathetic nervous system, which differ in their functions and their responses to drugs (Table 27–1). The functions of the two branches are often antagonistic, but together they maintain homeostasis. Both branches have intermediate synapses called ganglia (Figure 27–2). The axons that travel from the spinal cord or brainstem to the ganglia are called *preganglionic fibers;* those traveling from the ganglia to the target tissues are called *postganglionic fibers.* Autonomic efferents innervate the viscera, smooth muscles, cardiac muscle, and glands to regulate such functions as respiration, blood pressure, gastrointestinal activity, temperature, and metabolic functions. Overall, the two branches of the autonomic nervous system regulate the involuntary, vegetative functions that serve to maintain the internal physiological environment.

The Sympathetic Nervous System

Preganglionic cells of the sympathetic nervous system lie in the intermediolateral cell column of the spinal cord at thoracic and lumbar levels (from the first thoracic to the second or third lumbar segment). These cells are regulated by impulses from various

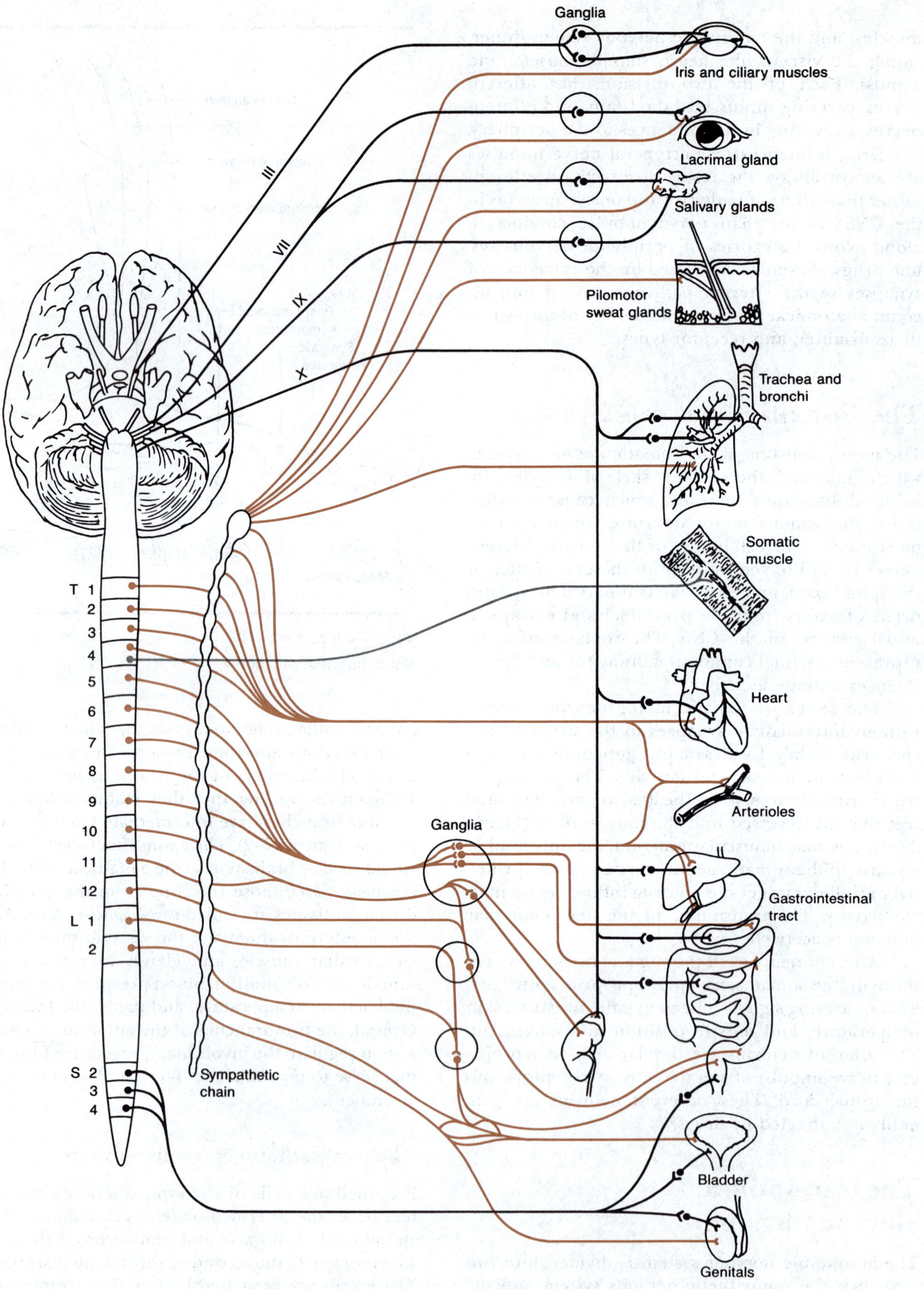
Ganglia
Iris and ciliary muscles
Lacrimal gland
Salivary glands
Pilomotor
sweat glands
Trachea and
bronchi
Somatic
muscle
Heart
Arterioles
Ganglia
Gastrointestinal
tract
Bladder
Genitals
III
VII
IX
X
T 1
2
3
4
5
6
7
8
9
10
11
12
L 1
2
S 2
3
4
Sympathetic
chain

Table 27–1
Contrasts Between the Sympathetic and Parasympathetic Branches of the Autonomic Nervous System

Characteristic	Sympathetic nervous system	Parasympathetic nervous system
Preganglionic fibers		
Level	Thoracolumbar	Craniosacral
Length	Short	Long
Ratio to postganglionic fibers	Typically 1:200	Usually 1:1
Ganglia		
Location	Close to the cord	Close to target tissues
Transmitter	Acetylcholine	Acetylcholine
Receptor type	Nicotinic	Nicotinic
Postganglionic fibers		
Length	Long	Short
Distribution	Diffuse	Limited
Postganglionic synapses		
Transmitter	Norepinephrine (most)	Acetylcholine
Receptor type	Alpha-adrenergic Beta-adrenergic	Muscarinic
Function	Mobilization of resources for coping with stress	Conservation of energy resources

parts of the brain, including sympathetic centers in the medulla (such as the vasomotor center), posterior and lateral nuclei of the hypothalamus, and portions of the limbic system and cerebral cortex. The preganglionic sympathetic fibers that extend outward from the spinal cord are small in diameter, slow-conducting, and project only a short distance to the sympathetic ganglia (Figure 27–3).

There are two major groups of sympathetic ganglia: (1) a paravertebral column, and (2) the prevertebral plexuses. The **paravertebral column** is a chain of 22 paired and interconnected ganglia that parallel the spinal cord, with 3 pairs of ganglia at cervical levels, 11 pairs at thoracic levels, and 4 each at lumbar and sacral levels. The uppermost thoracic ganglion, called the stellate ganglion, and the 3 cervical ganglia provide the cervical postganglionic sympathetic fibers that innervate the heart. The superior cervical ganglion also provides postganglionic sympathetic innervation to the eye and the salivary glands. The **prevertebral ganglia** make up the mesenteric neural plexuses that surround the aorta and its large branches in the abdomen. These ganglia innervate the stomach, intestines, colon, pancreas, liver, kidney, bladder, and external genitalia.

Preganglionic fibers of the sympathetic nervous system release acetylcholine. The postsynaptic receptors located on the dendrites and cell bodies of postganglionic neurons are classified as **nicotinic;** these receptors are stimulated by nicotinic agonists such as nicotine and blocked by ganglionic blockers such as hexamethonium. Some sympathetic ganglia also contain dopaminergic cells called **small intensely fluorescent (SIF)** cells, but their function is not fully established.

Postganglionic sympathetic axons are unmyelinated and even smaller in diameter than the preganglionic fibers; after passing through the gray rami, they proceed to various target tissues. Most postganglionic sympathetic fibers release norepinephrine. Exceptional postganglionic sympathetic terminals release acetylcholine, including fibers that innervate the sweat glands and certain blood vessels of skeletal muscles.

◄**Figure 27–2**
Autonomic nervous system schema showing principal ganglia

Figure 27–3
Detail of a sympathetic ganglion

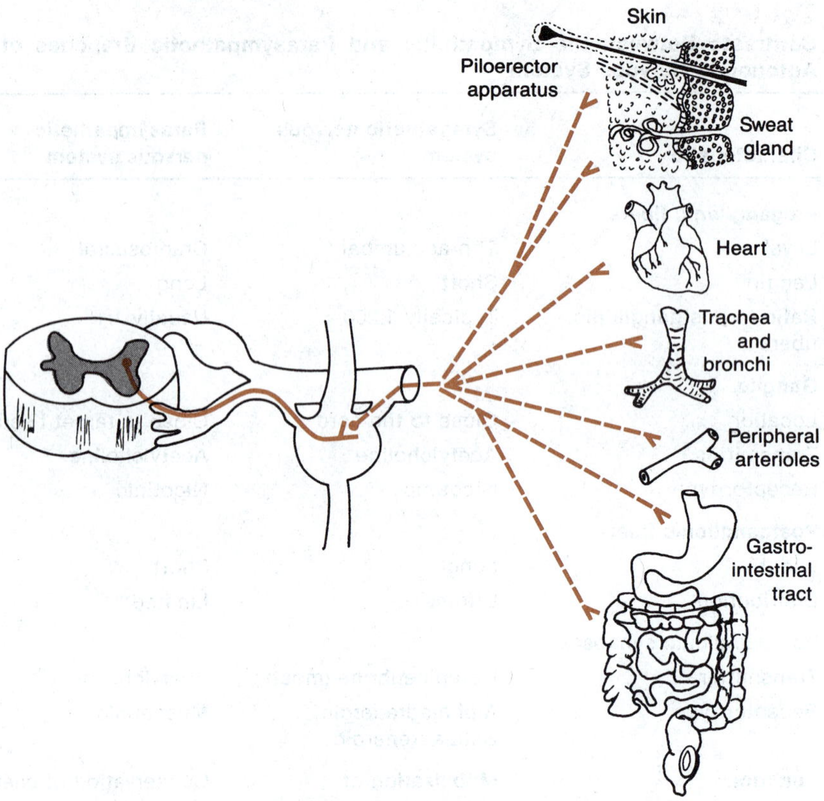

The secretory cells of the adrenal medulla are functionally equivalent in many respects to postganglionic sympathetic neurons and derive from the same embryological tissue. Like postganglionic sympathetic neurons, adrenal medullary cells are innervated directly by preganglionic sympathetic fibers that release acetylcholine. Adrenal medullary cells release epinephrine as well as norepinephrine. In stressful situations, the sympathetic nervous system and adrenal medulla function as a composite **sympathoadrenal axis.**

The sympathetic efferent nerves are distributed diffusely throughout the body. A given sympathetic nerve fiber can have a wide range of influence because the plexal system of sympathetic ganglia provides a great deal of interaction between individual sympathetic nerve projections. Moreover, in sympathetic ganglia, the ratio of presynaptic to postsynaptic fibers is typically 1:20, which means that a single activated presynaptic fiber can directly activate many postsynaptic neurons and indirectly activate others through collateral associations in the sympathetic plexuses. It is apparent that the sympathetic nervous system is organized to produce widespread physiological adjustments that prepare the body for coping with stress. These adjustments are termed the **fight or flight** reaction.

The Parasympathetic Nervous System

Parasympathetic nerves arise from the brainstem and the lowest, or sacral, portion of the spinal cord. Parasympathetic ganglia are either **cranial ganglia** or **terminal ganglia.** Most cranial preganglionic parasympathetic neurons lie in cranial nerve nuclei that form a column through the medulla. The remainder lie in the Edinger-Westphal nucleus in the midbrain. The preganglionic fibers exit from the brainstem in the third, seventh, ninth, and tenth cranial nerves. The third cranial nerve, the oculomotor nerve, extends to the ciliary ganglion; postganglionic fibers from the ciliary ganglion then innervate the sphincter of the iris and the ciliary body in the eye. The parasympathetic fibers of the seventh cranial nerve, the facial nerve, originate in the superior salivatory nucleus of the medulla and project to three cranial parasympathetic ganglia that send postganglionic fibers to the lacrimal gland, the nasopharyngeal blood vessels and glands, and the salivary glands. The ninth cranial nerve (the glossopharyngeal nerve) arises from the inferior salivatory nucleus of the medulla and projects to the otic ganglion, which then innervates the third salivary gland (the parotid gland). All of the postganglionic parasympathetic fibers are joined by postganglionic sympathetic fibers, traveling in mixed bundles to the target tissues.

The tenth cranial nerve, the vagus, arises from preganglionic parasympathetic cell bodies located in the dorsal motor nucleus of the vagus in the medulla. The vagus is the largest collection of parasympathetic fibers, innervating the entire thoracic and abdominal viscera: the heart, bronchi, spleen, stomach, intestines, and kidneys by way of terminal ganglia in these tissues. Tissues of the pelvic region receive parasympathetic innervation from sacral levels of the spinal cord. The second, third, and fourth sacral nerves join to form the pelvic nerve, which innervates the colon, bladder, and external genitalia via terminal ganglia.

Preganglionic parasympathetic fibers resemble their counterparts in the sympathetic nervous system, releasing acetylcholine. The postsynaptic receptors located on postganglionic cell bodies and dendrites are nicotinic. Parasympathetic and sympathetic ganglia are pharmacologically equivalent, responding to the same drug interventions in a like manner.

The parasympathetic nervous system has a less diffuse distribution than the sympathetic branch. Most parasympathetic ganglia are embedded within the target tissues, and the postganglionic fibers are short. At most parasympathetic ganglia, the ratio of preganglionic to postganglionic fibers is 1:1. Since the preganglionic fiber has already traveled most of the distance to the target tissue when it reaches the parasympathetic ganglion, there is little opportunity for it to produce effects that broadly affect other tissues.

Like preganglionic parasympathetic neurons, postganglionic parasympathetic neurons release acetylcholine, but the receptors at these synapses are **muscarinic.** These receptors exhibit affinities for agonist and antagonist drugs that differ sharply from the nicotinic receptors of ganglia. Drugs that block muscarinic receptors are called **antimuscarinic** drugs. The muscarinic receptors gained their name from the observation that the drug muscarine could mimic acetylcholine at these postganglionic synapses but not at ganglia.

The parasympathetic system is thus anatomically organized for discrete effects, target tissue by target tissue. From a functional point of view, the parasympathetic nervous system supports those activities that provide for conservation and storage of bodily resources and reproductive function, that is, **feeding and breeding.**

In the gut, there are large numbers of neurons, only some of which receive preganglionic parasympathetic or sympathetic inputs. These neurons are organized into two plexuses, the submucosal plexus (of Meissner) and the myenteric plexus (of Auerbach) that lie between the circular and longitudinal layers of smooth muscle. The ratio of preganglionic fibers to postganglionic cells in the myenteric plexuses is about 1:8,000. The partial independence of this **enteric nervous system** is illustrated by its intrinsic capacity for local, neurally mediated reflex activity; coordinated peristalsis continues to occur upon presentation of food to the gut even after complete denervation of autonomic inputs. Neurons in the gut release a variety of neurohormones, including various classic transmitters and peptide substances.

Summary of Autonomic Nervous System Physiology

Some key points to remember for study of autonomic drugs can be summarized as follows (Figure 27–4):

1. In the somatic division of the nervous system, the only type of peripheral synapse is the neuromuscular junction. It is cholinergic and exhibits drug sensitivities that are different from either muscarinic or nicotinic synapses, although closer to the latter than to the former.
2. Both branches of the autonomic division of the peripheral nervous system have intermediate synapses at ganglia as well as the postganglionic synapses at the target tissues.
3. Acetylcholine is the transmitter at all ganglia (both sympathetic and parasympathetic), and the receptors are classified as nicotinic.
4. Acetylcholine is also the transmitter at postganglionic parasympathetic synapses and at a few of the postganglionic sympathetic synapses (at sweat glands and a few blood vessels), but the receptors at these sites are classified as muscarinic.
5. Norepinephrine is the transmitter at most postganglionic sympathetic synapses.

The following summary of target tissue effects of peripheral nervous system impulses is provided to facilitate the study of autonomic drugs in Chapters 28 and 29. Table 27–2 should be read in conjunction with the following discussion.

Sympathetic influence on cardiovascular function is more profound than parasympathetic in-

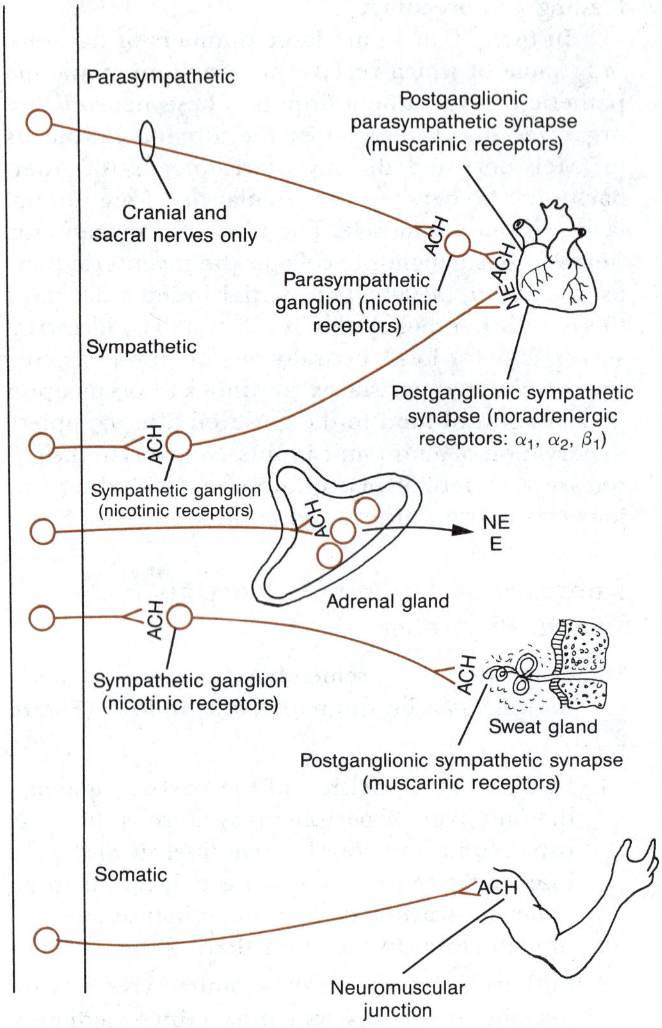

Figure 27-4
Somatic, sympathetic, and parasympathetic components of the peripheral nervous system showing transmitters released at each type of synapse: acetylcholine (ACh), epinephrine (E), norepinephrine (NE)

fluence, except in controlling heart rate. The overall effect of sympathoadrenal activation is to increase vasomotor tone, although vasodilation produced by the action of epinephrine can predominate in tissues, such as coronary and skeletal muscles, that are instrumental in generating "fight or flight" reactions. Parasympathetic fibers dilate blood vessels in the cerebrum and external genitalia. Sympathetic innervation of the heart produces a profound positive inotropic effect (increased contractility) and a lesser positive chronotropic effect (increased rate). Parasympathetic innervation has a profound influence on heart rate (slowing) and little effect on contractility.

In general, the activity of the viscera is suspended by sympathetic activation but stimulated by parasympathetic impulses. Thus sympathetic activity decreases intestinal motility and secretions, contracts gastrointestinal sphincters, inhibits the exocrine pancreas, and relaxes the gall bladder ducts. Parasympathetic activity relaxes alimentary sphincters and promotes digestive processes by increasing motility and secretions.

Other sympathoadrenal influences also contribute to the ability to cope with stress. Liver and skeletal muscle glycogenolysis is stimulated to promote availability of glucose in the blood to meet energy demands. Lipolysis is stimulated in fat cells to further increase available energy. The bronchial muscles relax to facilitate more rapid air flow through the airways. The pupils dilate to enhance visual acuity. The salivary glands are stimulated to produce a thick, viscous saliva more appropriate for frothing than digestion. In the skin, sweat glands are stimulated to facilitate heat dissipation, and the piloerector muscles are contracted to cause the hair to stand on end. In the nephrourinary system, micturition is inhibited and the kidney is induced to release renin to promote electrolyte retention. Thus the function of the sympathetic nervous system is to facilitate blood and air flow and the mobilization and exchange of materials and heat dissipation required during intense exertion.

Parasympathetic innervation opposes sympathetic activity not only in the alimentary system but also in the regulation of the eye and respiratory system. Parasympathetic impulses to the eye constrict the pupil and contract the ciliary muscle that controls the lens to produce accommodation for near vision. The lacrimal glands are stimulated to secrete tears by parasympathetic influence. In the respiratory system, parasympathetic influence contracts the bronchioles and stimulates bronchial and nasopharyngeal glands. Parasympathetic and sympathetic influences on sexual functioning are complementary rather than antagonistic. In the male, erection is parasympathetically mediated and ejaculation is sympathetically controlled.

The relatively limited distribution of parasympathetic innervation is reflected in the lack of parasympathetic fibers to the skin, skeletal muscle cells, fat tissue, and endocrine tissues. There is also a paucity of parasympathetic influence on the vasculature. Neither branch of the autonomic nervous system contributes to regulation of skeletal muscles, the province of the somatic nervous system.

Table 27–2
Autonomic Nervous System Regulation of Glands and Organs: Effects of Nerve Impulses from Each Branch

Effector system	Sympathoadrenal activity[a]	Parasympathetic activity
Eye		
Iris	Mydriasis (α_1)	Miosis
Ciliary muscle	No innervation	Accommodation for near vision
Aqueous humor		
Production	Decreased (β)	Little influence
Outflow	Increased (α)	Increased
Lacrimal glands	No innervation	Secretion
Cardiovascular system		
Heart		
Rate	Accelerated (β_1)	Slowed
Conduction velocity	Increased (β_1)	Decreased in atrioventricular node
Contractility	Increased (β_1)	Possibly slight decrease
Blood vessels		
Coronary	Dilated (β_2)	No innvervation
Skeletal muscles	Dilated (β_2; muscarinic)[c]	No innervation
Skin, mucosa, viscera	Constricted (α_1 and α_2)	Minimal innervation
Cerebral	Constricted (α_1 and α_2) or dilated (β_2)	Dilated
External genitalia	Constricted (α_1 and α_2) or dilated (β_2)	Dilated
Renal	Constricted (α_1 and α_2) or dilated (β_2)	No innervation
Respiratory system		
Bronchial smooth muscle	Relaxed (mainly β_2, slight β_1 contribution)	Contracted
Bronchial glands	Minimal or no innervation	Stimulation
Nasopharyngeal glands	No innervation	Stimulated
Alimentary system		
Salivary glands	Viscous secretion (α_1, β)	Watery secretion
Gastrointestinal tract		
Motility and tone	Decreased (α_2 and β_2)	Increased
Sphincters	Contracted	Relaxed
Secretions	Possibly decreased	Increased
Liver	Glycogenolysis (β_2) Gluconeogenesis (α) (lesser effect)	Glycogen synthesis
Splenic capsule	Contracted (α)	No innervation
Gall bladder ducts	Relaxation	Contraction
Pancreas (acini)	Inhibited (α)	Stimulated
Nephrourinary system		
Kidney	Renin release (β_2) Inhibition of renin release (α_2)	No innervation
Urinary bladder		
Detrusor	Relaxed (β_2)	Contracted
Trigone (internal sphincter)	Constricted (α_2)	Relaxed
External sphincter[b]	No innervation	No innervation
Ureter	Increased motility	Possibly increased

(continued)

Table 27-2

Autonomic Nervous System Regulation of Glands and Organs: Effects of Nerve Impulses from Each Branch *(continued)*

Effector system	Sympathoadrenal activity[a]	Parasympathetic activity
Endocrine system		
Pancreas (β-cells)	Inhibited (α_1); stimulated (β_2)	No innervation
Adrenal medulla	Stimulated (nicotinic)	No innervation
Pineal gland	Melatonin synthesis (β)	No innervation
Sexual function		
Uterus (pregnant)	Contraction (α_1 and α_2)	Minimal influence
Uterus (nonpregnant)	Relaxation (β_2)	Minimal influence
Erection	No influence	Stimulated
Ejaculation	Stimulated (α_1)	No influence
Skin		
Piloerector apparatus	Contracted (α_1)	No innveration
Sweat glands	Stimulated (muscarinic)	No innervation
Skeletal muscle		
Contraction[b]	No innervation[d]	No innervation
Glycogenolysis	Stimulated (β_2)	No innveration
Fat cells		
Lipolysis	Stimulated (α_1 and β_1)	No innervation

[a]Greek letters in parentheses indicate receptor type involved in the action. Refer to Chapter 28.

[b]Constricted by somatic nervous system impulses.

[c]Stimulated by somatic nervous system impulses.

[d]But epinephrine facilitates cholinergic transmission at the neuromuscular junction and increases contractility of skeletal muscle by a direct β_2-mediated effect.

Recommended Readings

Appenzeller O: *The Autonomic Nervous System: An Introduction to Basic and Clinical Concepts,* ed 3. Amsterdam, Elsevier/North Holland, 1982.

Day M: *Autonomic Pharmacology: Experimental and Clinical Aspects.* Edinburgh, Churchill Livingstone, 1979.

Carpenter MB, Sutin J: *Human Neuroanatomy,* ed 8. Baltimore, Williams & Wilkins Co, 1983.

Dalgas P: Understanding drugs that affect the autonomic nervous system. *Nursing* 1985;15(10):58–64.

Guyton AC: *Textbook of Medical Physiology,* ed 6. Philadelphia, WB Saunders, 1981.

Mountcastle VB (ed): *Medical Physiology,* ed 14. St Louis, CV Mosby, 1980.

CHAPTER 28

Adrenergic and Antiadrenergic Drugs

Drug Effects on Adrenergic Receptors

The pharmacology of adrenergic and antiadrenergic drugs is intimately related to the functions of the sympathetic nervous system and, more broadly, to the sympathoadrenal axis. Norepinephrine (noradrenaline) is released in the peripheral nervous system only from postganglionic sympathetic terminals. The vast majority of postganglionic sympathetic nerve endings release this transmitter, although a few — those innervating sweat glands and a fraction of skeletal muscle blood vessels — release acetylcholine. Adrenergic agonists are therefore referred to as sympathomimetics (that is, drugs that mimic the sympathetic transmitter) and adrenergic antagonists as sympatholytics (drugs that block sympathetic transmitters). Adrenergic agonists also mimic the actions of epinephrine released from the adrenal medulla.

Mechanisms of Noradrenergic Transmission

Cannon first reported in 1931 on an adrenaline-like substance released during sympathetic stimulation. Von Euler firmly established the identity of this substance as norepinephrine (or noradrenaline) in 1948. Norepinephrine transmission involves five sequential events: synthesis, storage, release, transmitter/receptor interactions, and inactivation (Figure 28–1).

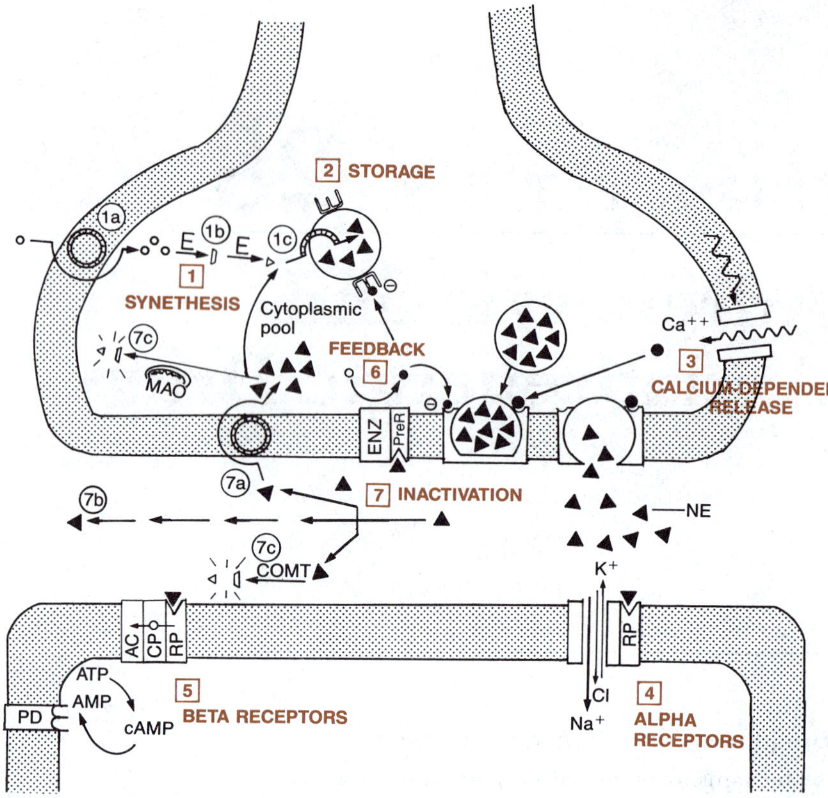

Figure 28–1
Noradrenergic synapse. (1) Production of norepinephrine (NE), including (1a) uptake of tyrosine, (1b) conversion of tyrosine to dihydroxyphenylalanine (dopa), (1c) conversion of dopa to dopamine, and (2) conversion of dopamine to norepinephrine and its storage in granules; (3) calcium-dependent release of NE; (4) interaction of NE with alpha receptor protein (RP); (5) interaction of NE with beta-receptor, which is linked via a coupling protein (CP) with adenylate cyclase (AC), an enzyme that catalyzes formation of cyclic adenosine monophosphate (cAMP) from adenosine triphosphate (ATP). Cyclic-AMP is later broken down to adenylate monophosphate (AMP) by the enzyme phosphodiesterase (PD); (6) feedback control of synthesis and release by action of NE on a presynaptic receptor (PreR); and (7) inactivation of NE by either (7a) reuptake, (7b) diffusion, or (7c) metabolism by catechol-O-methyl transferase (COMT) or monamine oxidase (MAO).

Synthesis and Storage of Norepinephrine

The synthesis of norepinephrine is a three-reaction sequence that begins with the amino acid **L-tyrosine.** Accumulated by sympathetic nerve terminals, this precursor of norepinephrine is converted to dihydroxyphenylalanine (**dopa**) by the enzyme **tyrosine hydroxylase.** The first step in the synthesis of norepinephrine is rate-limiting, which means that it determines the overall rate of formation. Tyrosine hydroxylase can be inhibited by a variety of drugs, including alpha-methylparatyrosine, which results in a gradual depletion of the transmitter. Norepinephrine exerts a competitive feedback inhibition on tyrosine hydroxylase which prevents an excess accumulation of norepinephrine.

The second step in synthesis of norepinephrine is the conversion of dopa to **dopamine,** which is carried out by the enzyme **1-aromatic amino acid decarboxylase.** Inhibition of this enzyme is frequently undertaken as a therapeutic measure in conjunction with levodopa therapy for parkinsonism (see Chapter 22).

The last step is the formation of norepinephrine itself by oxidation of dopamine by **dopamine-β-hydroxylase.** This enzyme is inhibited by disulfiram (Antabuse), which accounts for the vasodilation, hypotension, and lethargy that sometimes result when disulfiram is employed in alcohol treatment programs. The final step in synthesis of norepinephrine is linked to its storage.

Newly formed norepinephrine is stored in synaptic vesicles, which are abundant in the nerve terminals. Storage serves the dual purposes of protecting the transmitter from enzymatic degradation by cytoplasmic monoamine oxidase and providing uniform quantities of transmitter for subsequent release. The capacity of vesicles for storing norepinephrine can be impaired by certain drugs, notably reserpine, methyldopa, and tetrabenazine, which deplete norepinephrine by inhibiting its storage.

Release

Norepinephrine is released in response to the arrival of an action potential at postganglionic sympathetic nerve terminals. Calcium ions flow into the cell as a result of a momentary increase in membrane permeability. Calcium ions interact with transmitter-filled vesicles poised on the inner surface of the cellular membrane and provoke a fusion of the membrane of the vesicle with that of the cell, resulting in release of norepinephrine by exocytosis into the synaptic cleft.

Release of norepinephrine can also be initiated by certain drugs without depolarization of the nerve terminal. These drugs are called *indirect-acting sympathomimetics* (for example, tyramine) if their action is primarily peripheral, or *catecholamine-releasing stimulants* if they release norepinephrine within the brain. Amphetamine and other stimulants (such as methylphenidate (Ritalin) or diethylpropion (Tepanil)) act in this manner (see Chapter 14). A few drugs have the opposite effect, preventing norepinephrine release even when the nerve terminal is depolarized. Guanethidine (Ismelin), an antihypertensive agent, and bretylium (Bretylol), an antidysrhythmic drug, act in this way.

Interactions of Norepinephrine with Receptors

After release into the synapse, norepinephrine diffuses freely and will interact with norepinephrine receptors (sites that exhibit an affinity for its molecular configuration) on nearby postsynaptic and presynaptic membranes. Noradrenergic receptors, consisting of proteins embedded in the phospholipid mosaic that composes cell membranes, generate a physiological effect in response to the attachment of a molecule of norepinephrine. There are four classes of adrenergic receptors: α_1, α_2, β_1, and β_2. These classes are defined by differences in responses of the four types of receptors to various adrenergic agonists and antagonists. Each type of receptor is responsible for some of the physiological effects of norepinephrine or epinephrine. The classification of adrenergic receptors into four groups provides a conceptual framework for understanding most of the pharmacological effects of the various adrenergic and antiadrenergic drugs.

Postsynaptic adrenergic receptors mediate the effects of norepinephrine and epinephrine on effector organs. Presynaptic receptors (located on the cell membrane of presynaptic nerve terminals) exert a negative feedback influence on neurotransmission by suppressing both synthesis and release of norepinephrine. This mechanism tends to ensure that levels of transmitter within the synapse will be unable to build up excessively. Presynaptic receptors are predominantly, though not exclusively, α_2-receptors.

Inactivation

Released norepinephrine can be inactivated by any of three mechanisms: enzymatic degradation, dilution by diffusion, or reuptake by the presynaptic neuron. Two enzymes contribute to catabolism (degradation) of norepinephrine. One of these, monoamine oxidase (MAO), is associated with mitochondrial membranes. Inhibitors of MAO, such as tranylcypromine (Parnate) and isocarboxazid (Marplan), formerly occupied an important place in treatment of depression (see Chapter 20). The other enzyme capable of destroying norepinephrine, catechol-O-methyltransferase (COMT), has an extracellular location. There are no clinically important inhibitors of COMT, although tropolone has been used for this effect experimentally. Norepinephrine can be acted upon by its degradative enzymes singly or sequentially, providing three possible breakdown products.

Reuptake of norepinephrine into the presynaptic cell is accomplished by a high-affinity carrier protein that transports norepinephrine across the cell membrane from the extracellular fluid into the cytoplasm. Certain chemicals structurally related to norepinephrine can compete for this carrier, such as other amine transmitters (dopamine, serotonin), tricyclic antidepressants such as protriptyline (Vivactil), and cocaine. Inhibiting reuptake of norepinephrine within the brain may be the primary mechanism of the tricyclic antidepressants (see Chapter 20). The presence of norepinephrine in the synapse is prolonged if its reuptake is inhibited. A second carrier mechanism within the presynaptic neuron transports cytoplasmic norepinephrine into synaptic vesicles. This vesicular uptake mechanism provides storage of norepinephrine and is inhibited by a different set of drugs (reserpine (Serpasil), for example) from those that inhibit the cellular reuptake process.

Physiological Roles of Adrenergic Receptors

Each of the four classes of adrenergic receptors mediates a distinctive set of physiological effects (Table 28–1), although several effects are shared responsibilities. For example, cardiac stimulation is mediated mainly by β_1-receptors but entails a small contribution from β_2-receptors (the ratio of β_1-receptors to β_2-receptors in cardiac muscle is about 5:1). Bronchodilation is mainly a β_2-mediated effect, but there are one-fourth as many β_1- as β_2-receptors in bronchial smooth muscle. Vasoconstriction and uterine contraction entail activation of both α_1- and α_2-receptors; both α_1- and β_2-receptors contribute to postponing micturition; and both α_2- and β_2-receptors tend to decrease motility and tone in the intestines. Understanding the roles of the four kinds of adrenergic receptors will aid in understanding the therapeutic effects of the drugs that activate or block them.

Table 28–1
Physiological Roles of Adrenergic Receptors

α_1-receptors	Mixed or undetermined	α_2-receptors
CNS stimulation	Vasoconstriction (α_1 and α_2)	Relaxation of the gut
Lipolytic activity	Uterine contraction (α_1 and α_2)	↑Platelet adhesiveness
LH secretion	Drainage of aqueous humor (undetermined α)	Sedation
Ejaculation	Contraction of the splenic capsule (undetermined α)	Centrally mediated cardiovascular depression
Mydriasis		Inhibition of CNS reward system (locus coeruleus)
↓Insulin secretion		Anorexia (probably α_2)
↓Renin secretion		
Bladder trigone constricted		
Pilomotor erection		
Sweating		
Sparse, viscous saliva		

β_1-receptors	Mixed or undetermined	β_2-receptors
Lipolytic activity	Eosinopenia (undetermined β)	Bronchodilation ($\beta_2 >> \beta_1$)
Cerebral cortex — synaptic remodeling	Decreased formation of aqueous humor (undetermined β)	Vasodilation
Cardiac stimulation ($\beta_1 >> \beta_2$)	Melatonin synthesis (undetermined β)	Muscle and liver glycogenolysis
	Inhibition of histamine release by mast cells (undetermined β)	↑Renin secretion
		Insulin secretion
		Relaxation of the gut
		Bladder detrussor muscle relaxed
		Relaxation of the uterus
		Cerebellum — synaptic remodeling

Alpha-Receptors

The most important physiological influences of α_1-receptors from the point of view of clinical applications are (1) the pressor effect (increased blood pressure), (2) the centrally mediated stimulatory effect on motor activity and reflexes, and (3) dilation of the pupil. The α_1-agonists are used as pressor drugs (in certain hypotensive states and for decongestion), mydriatics, and CNS stimulants (Table 28–2).

Alpha-1-antagonists are useful for promoting peripheral blood flow in shock, for alleviating acute hypertensive states, for blocking exaggerated vasomotor effects of excessive catecholamines in pheochromocytoma, and for improving blood flow through spastic small vessels in peripheral vascular disorders. Most of the available alpha-blockers are not entirely selective (Table 28–3) and therefore cause adverse effects associated with blocking both α_1- and α_2-receptors (see Table 28–2).

Alpha-2-receptors contribute to vasoconstriction and uterine contraction and are responsible for the sparse viscous saliva associated with sympathetic activity. They also promote relaxation of the gut, increased platelet adhesiveness, and most of the α-receptor effects in the brain. This last category includes sedation, suppression of firing of neurons in the reward system, and a cardiodepressant action.

Alpha-2-agonists are employed exclusively for their ability to produce cardiovascular depression and hypotension through their centrally mediated hypotensive effect. This action is related to stimulation of α_2-receptors in the vasomotor and cardiac centers of the medulla oblongata. Clonidine (Catapres) acts by this mechanism to produce its antihypertensive benefit (see Chapter 39). It is likely that

Table 28–2
Therapeutic Uses and Adverse Effects of Alpha-Agonists and Antagonists

Drug class	Therapeutic uses	Adverse effects
α_1-Agonists	CNS stimulation Pressor effect Decongestion Mydriatic effect	Excess stimulation Anxiety Restlessness Apprehensiveness Pilomotor erection
α_1-Antagonists	Peripheral vascular disorders Pheochromocytoma Antihypertensive shock	Orthostatic hypotension Flushing Reflex tachycardia Pupillary constriction Inhibition of ejaculation Nasal stuffiness Fatigue Weakness Urinary frequency
α_2-Agonists	Centrally mediated anti-hypertensive effect	Sedation Dry mouth Withdrawal syndrome
α_2-Antagonists	Impotence in males of vascular or diabetic origin (experimental)	Gastrointestinal hyperactivity: cramps, nausea, vomiting, diarrhea, exacerbation of ulcers, gastritis Enhanced norepinephrine release (which results in side effects related to α_1 and β_1 stimulation)

methyldopa (Aldomet), another important antihypertensive medication, produces a metabolite in the brain that acts in the same manner as clonidine. There are some adverse effects related to stimulation of α_2-receptors (see Table 28–2).

Beta-Receptors

Beta-receptors are linked to adenylate cyclase and adenosine 3′:5′-cyclic phosphate (cyclic AMP) ultimately mediates all of the physiological results of beta-receptor activation. The activity of beta-receptors is influenced by a phospholipid methyltransferase modulatory protein and a guanosine triphosphate-sensitive modulatory protein, providing ample opportunity for subtle modulations of the receptor complex by various cellular substances. Thyroid hormone has a profound influence on beta-adrenergic receptors. In hyperthyroidism, the number of beta-receptors increases dramatically, and beta-blockers will alleviate many of the symptoms.

Beta-1-receptors are most important in regulating the heart and have a profound influence on contractility of the myocardium, providing the basis for the **positive inotropic** effect of cardiac sympathetic innervation. Beta-1-receptors also produce a positive chronotropic effect (increasing heart rate) and a positive dromotropic action (increasing impulse conduction). The only other significant peripheral effect known to be associated with β_1-receptors is a stimulation of lipolysis in fat cells — a calorigenic action. In the brain, noradrenergic receptors in the cerebral cortex are predominantly of the β_1 type.

Beta-1-agonists save lives by stimulating the heart during cardiac arrest or atrioventricular block, but excessive β_1-stimulation can lead to cardiac dysrhythmias, tachycardia, and other adverse effects (Table 28–4). Certain drugs, notably general anesthetics such as halothane, predispose the heart to dysrhythmias induced by adrenergic drugs through β_1-receptors.

Beta-adrenergic antagonists are usually employed for their ability to block β_1-receptors, but seven of the ten available for clinical practice currently are nonselective, blocking β_1- and β_2-receptors alike (Table 28–5). Beta-1-blockers are used to protect the heart from catecholamine-induced dysrhythmias and have limited value in other kinds of dysrhythmias. Beta-blockers are also among the foremost of the antianginal medications (Chapter 40) and are widely used in treatment of hypertension

Table 28–3
Selectivity of Alpha Agonists and Antagonists

Agonists	
Most selective for alpha-1	Phenylephrine (α_1)
	Methoxamine (α_1)
	Norepinephrine ($\alpha_1 > \alpha_2 > \beta_1$)
	Epinephrine ($\alpha_1 = \beta_1 > \alpha_2 = \beta_2$)
Mixed	Naphazoline ($\alpha_2 > \alpha_1 >> \beta$)
	Tetrahydrozoline ($\alpha_2 > \alpha_1 >> \beta$)
	Oxymetazoline ($\alpha_2 > \alpha_1 > \beta$)
	α-Methylnorepinephrine ($\alpha_2 > \alpha_1$)
Most selective for alpha-2	Clonidine ($\alpha_2 >> \alpha_1$)
	Azepexole (α_2)
Antagonists	
Most selective for alpha-1	Prazosin (α_1)
	Phenoxybenzamine ($\alpha_1 >> \alpha_2$)
	Clonidine (α_1 partial agonist)
Mixed	Phentolamine ($\alpha_1 = \alpha_2$)
Most selective for alpha-2	Tolazoline ($\alpha_2 > \alpha_1$)
	Dibenamine ($\alpha_2 > \alpha_1$)
	Yohimbine ($\alpha_2 >> \alpha_1$)

(Chapter 39). Propranolol (Inderal), a nonselective beta-blocker, is among the most widely used of all drugs. It is also approved by the U.S. Food and Drug Administration for use after acute stabilization of a myocardial infarction as a means of reducing mortality.

Adverse effects of beta-blockers associated with β_1-receptors occur with nonselective and selective agents alike, since all of the currently available drugs block at least the β_1-receptors (see Table 28–4). The nonselective agents produce additional side effects, such as bronchospasm, due to antagonism of β_2-receptors. The beta-blockers are compared in Chapter 39.

Beta-2-agonists (see Table 28–4) are important therapeutically for their ability to dilate the bronchioles. Several β_2-agonists are mainstays in treatment of bronchial asthma (see Chapter 52). Selective β_2-agonists can reduce resistance in the airways without cardiac stimulation, but nonselective β-agonists can produce cardiac dysrhythmias. Other clinical applications of β_2-stimulants are for peripheral vascular disorders and to delay premature labor.

Sympathomimetics

Structure/Activity Relationships

Sympathomimetic substances are derivatives of β-phenylethylamine (Figure 28–2). The β-phenylethylamine structure provides a number of potential sites (the amino group, the α-carbon, the β-carbon, or at the five open sites on the aromatic ring) for substituting various chemical groups. The kinds of substitution present in a given sympathetic amine determine its relative affinity for the various classes of adrenergic receptors, its ratio of central to peripheral activity, its ability to cause release of endogenous norepinephrine, and its duration of action. Hydroxyl (OH) groups in the 3 and 4 positions of the aromatic ring produce *catechol,* and the presence of an amine on the side chain results in substances called *catecholamines* (such as norepinephrine, epinephrine, and dopamine). Substitution at the β-carbon influences whether or not a given drug will cause release of endogenous norepinephrine (drugs with only a hydrogen here, such as tyramine and amphetamine, are potent releasers, but drugs with a hydroxyl group at the β-carbon have enhanced affinity for adrenergic receptors). The presence of a hydroxyl group in the β-position also limits the drug's ability to enter the central nervous system, because it lowers lipid solubility of the drug. Thus stimulation of CNS noradrenergic receptors must ordinarily be accomplished by indirect-acting drugs that release norepinephrine.

Substitutions at the α-carbon influence duration of action, while substitutions at either the α- or β-carbon position of β-phenylethylamine result in sub-

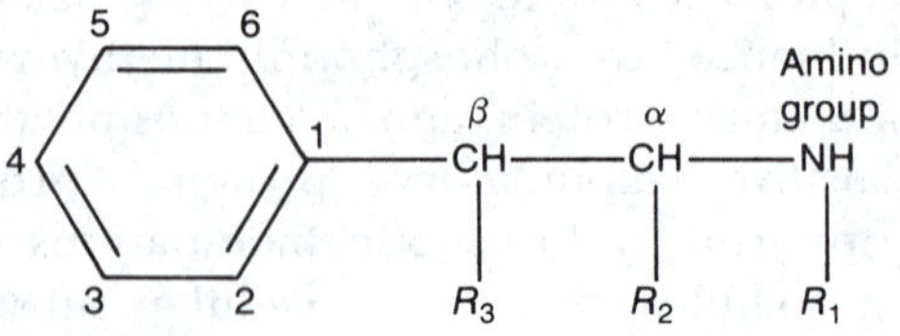

Figure 28–2
Beta-phenylethylamine, showing the sites where various substitutions occur in sympathomimetic drugs. Substitutions at R_1 influence affinity for the various classes of adrenergic receptors; substitutions at R_2 influence duration of action; substitutions at R_3 determine if the drug will be able to release endogenous norepinephrine; and substitutions at the 3 and 4 positions on the ring confer maximum potency.

Table 28–4
Therapeutic Uses and Adverse Effects of Beta-Agonists and Antagonists

Drug class	Therapeutic uses	Adverse effects
β_1-Agonists	Cardiac stimulation in arrest or atrioventricular block	Dysrhythmias Palpitations Angina (due to increased cardiac work)
β_1-Antagonists	Cardiac protection from excess catecholamines Antihypertensive Antianginal Antiarrhythmic Reduce mortality during recuperation from myocardial infarction	Heart block Congestive heart failure Reflex tachycardia Slight aggravation of asthma Withdrawal angina Psychiatric side effects Hallucinations Insomnia Nightmares Lassitude Dizziness Depression
β_2-Agonists	Bronchodilation Peripheral vascular disorders Delay premature labor	Angina (due to decreased coronary blood flow) Hypotension Tremor Vascular headaches Urinary retention
β_2-Antagonists	Migraine prophylaxis[a] Alleviate tremor	Pronounced aggravation of asthma Hypoglycemia Uterine contractions Gastrointestinal hyperactivity Nausea Vomiting Diarrhea

[a]Probably due to antiserotonergic properties of beta-blockers rather than to beta-blocking activity per se. Beta-blockers with intrinsic sympathomimetic activity are not effective against migraine.

stances that occur as optical isomers (dextro- and levorotatory forms). The two isomers usually differ in their ability to activate adrenergic receptors or to release norepinephrine. For example, the levorotatory isomers of norepinephrine and epinephrine are ten times more potent than the corresponding dextrorotatory isomers (which occur only in synthetic preparations).

Substitution in the amino group has the greatest influence on relative affinities for the four classes of adrenergic receptors. Selective α_2-agonist activity is conferred by elimination of the benzene ring entirely, replacing it with another kind of ring (such as the imidazoline ring found in naphazoline, tetrahydrozoline, oxymetazoline, and xylometazoline, the active ingredients in various over-the-counter eye drops or nasal sprays, and clonidine, an antihypertensive drug).

Endogenous Sympathetic Amines

The two endogenous sympathetic amines are epinephrine and norepinephrine. Epinephrine is the major amine secreted by the adrenal medulla, while norepinephrine is secreted by the adrenal gland to a lesser extent and from sympathetic nerve terminals. The two sympathoadrenal amines differ significantly in their influences on the different classes of adrenergic receptors (Table 28–6). Epinephrine is active at all classes of adrenergic receptors. Norepi-

Table 28–5
Selectivity of Beta-Agonists and Antagonists

Agonists	
Most selective for beta-1	Norepinephrine ($\alpha > \beta_1$)
	Dobutamine ($\beta_1 >> \beta_2 > \alpha$)
	Dopamine ($\beta_1 >> \beta_2 = \alpha$)
	Epinephrine ($\alpha_1 = \beta_1 > \alpha_2 = \beta_2$)
Mixed	Isoproterenol ($\beta_1 = \beta_2$)
	Ethylnorepinephrine ($\beta_1 = \beta_2 >> \alpha$)
	Mephentermine ($\beta_2 > \beta_1 > \alpha$)
	Nylidrin ($\beta_2 > \beta_1$)
	Isoxsuprine ($\beta_2 > \beta_1$)
	Isoetharine ($\beta_2 > \beta_1$)
Most selective for beta-2	Metaproterenol ($\beta_2 >> \beta_1$)
	Terbutaline ($\beta_2 >> \beta_1$)
	Albuterol (β_2)
	Salbutamol (β_2)
Antagonists	
Most selective for beta-1	Acebutolol ($\beta_1 >> \beta_2$)
	Betaxolol ($\beta_1 >> \beta_2$)
	Metoprolol ($\beta_1 >> \beta_2$)
Mixed	Atenolol ($\beta_1 > \beta_2$)
	Labetalol ($\beta_1 = \beta_2 = \alpha_1$)
	Nadolol ($\beta_1 = \beta_2$)
	Oxprenolol ($\beta_1 = \beta_2$)
	Pindolol ($\beta_1 = \beta_2$)
	Propranolol ($\beta_1 = \beta_2$)
	Timolol ($\beta_1 = \beta_2$)
Most selective for beta-2	Butoxamine (β_2) (not available for clinical use)

nephrine is active at α-receptors and β_1-receptors but not at β_2-receptors. Since epinephrine is an endocrine hormone while norepinephrine is mainly the postganglionic sympathetic transmitter, β_2-receptors are in effect endocrine receptors while the other classes of adrenergic receptors can be considered sympathetic receptors.

Epinephrine (Adrenaline)

Mechanisms and Effects Since epinephrine is active at all classes of adrenergic receptors, its pharmacology is the composite influences of α_1-, α_2-, β_1-, and β_2-adrenergic receptors. Epinephrine is not well absorbed into the brain, however, and therefore lacks substantial centrally mediated influences. It may cause apprehensiveness, restlessness, headache, and tremor, but these effects are at least partly due to peripheral vascular actions rather than direct effects on the brain.

Epinephrine influences blood pressure through each of the classes of receptors. In moderate to high doses, the dominant effect of epinephrine is increased blood pressure due to vasoconstriction mediated by α_1- and α_2-receptors in the vasculature. Alpha-agonists are used as nasal or ophthalmic decongestants because vasoconstriction can help shrink mucosal membranes that are swollen by dilated blood vessels. They can also increase vital capacity of respiration by a similar influence on the bronchial mucosa.

Stimulation of cardiac output mediated by β_1-receptors also contributes to the rise in blood pressure and results in systolic pressure rising to a greater extent than diastolic pressure. Stimulation of β_2-receptors produces vasodilation, a contrary influence on blood pressure. The β_2 effect has a somewhat mitigating influence on the overall pressor effect (increase in blood pressure) and prior administration of a β_2-antagonist will potentiate the pressor effect of epinephrine. Beta-2-receptors are somewhat more sensitive than other classes of adrenergic receptors, so that at low doses of epinephrine, vasodilation may occur without accompanying effects mediated by α- or β_1-receptors, resulting in a hypotensive effect.

The major site of vascular action of epinephrine is the small arterioles and precapillary sphincters, but larger arteries and veins also respond. Cutaneous blood flow is reduced most sharply. Renal blood flow also declines, but glomerular filtration is unaffected because the filtration fraction increases. On the other hand, blood flow through skeletal muscles increases and may even double. There is also a substantial increase in blood flow through the spleen and a small increase in cerebral blood flow. The increase in cerebral blood flow appears to be largely a passive response to the overall elevation in blood pressure. Coronary blood flow increases modestly in response to epinephrine but is due more to autoregulatory mechanisms (increased release of adenosine as cardiac work increases) and mechanical factors, such as increased duration of diastole (the phase of the cardiac cycle during which coronary blood flow can proceed), than to direct effects on sympathetic receptors. In fact, α-receptors predominate over β-receptors in the coronary vasculature. In vasospastic angina, hypersensitivity of coronary α-receptors results in a net decrease in coronary blood flow in response to sympathoadrenal activation, with consequent anginal attacks (see Chapter 40).

The direct **cardiac effects** of epinephrine, from activation of β_1-receptors, include an increase in myocardial contractility (positive inotropic action), an increase in rate of conductance of impulses (positive dromotropic action), and a slight initial increase in heart rate (positive chronotropic action). The systolic contraction is briefer and more powerful. Oxygen consumption by the heart is increased even more than cardiac work. In the intact physiological situation, heart rate may ultimately decrease even to the point of pronounced bradycardia due to compensatory vagal activity.

The effect of epinephrine on **visceral smooth muscle** in a given tissue depends on which type of adrenergic receptor predominates in that tissue. Generally, stimulatory effects of epinephrine are mediated by α_1-receptors while inhibitory influences are generated through β_2-receptors. Thus epinephrine constricts the trigone sphincter of the bladder, stimulates contractions in the vas deferens to promote ejaculation, contracts the piloerector muscles, and produces mydriasis by actions on α_1-receptors, but it also relaxes the detrussor muscle of the bladder, the uterus, and bronchial smooth muscle by an action on β_2-receptors.

Although **skeletal muscles** receive no sympathetic innervation except to skeletal muscle blood vessels, cholinergic transmission at the neuromuscular junction is facilitated by epinephrine through β_2-receptors, which explains why tremor is seen in anxiety states and hyperthyroidism and why propranolol (Inderal) is effective in alleviating such tremors.

In general, influences of sympathetic amines on **secretory glands** are less profound than are parasympathetic influences. Thus, bronchial glands are not affected and intestinal secretions are only slightly decreased if at all. The salivary glands are stimulated to produce a sparse, viscous saliva that is not useful for digestive purposes but which contributes to frothing at the mouth (perhaps of some value as a defense mechanism).

The dominant **metabolic effects** of epinephrine are calorigenic, providing mobilization of energy resources to meet the added demands of coping with stress. Epinephrine enhances glucagon release from the pancreas and inhibits insulin release (by an action on α-receptors of the pancreas, although there is a lesser tendency toward stimulation of insulin secretion that is controlled by β_2-receptors). Epinephrine has a biphasic effect on **potassium levels,** causing a brief period of hyperkalemia followed by a longer period of hypokalemia.

Epinephrine increases the total count of **white blood cells** (although it decreases eosinophils) and accelerates coagulation. Degranulation of **mast cells** (which contributes to allergic reactions such as asthma) is inhibited by epinephrine through an action on β-receptors.

Pharmacokinetics Epinephrine is not effective after oral administration because it is rapidly metabolized both in the gastrointestinal mucosa and in the liver. Epinephrine slows its own absorption after subcutaneous administration because of local vasoconstriction. *Injection of epinephrine into the extremities should be done with caution since its vasoconstrictor action can lead to gangrene. After subcutaneous administration, the nurse can promote more rapid absorption by application of heat or massage at the site of injection.* Intramuscular injection leads to quicker absorption. After absorption, epinephrine is rapidly metabolized in the liver and in other tissues. Metabolites are excreted mainly in the urine. Inhalation of epinephrine in concentrations of 10% provides mainly topical effects on the airways.

Clinical Indications Epinephrine is widely used for alpha- and beta-influences alike. The vasopressor effects of epinephrine are employed for alleviation of hypotensive states. It is useful topically as a nasal decongestant (Chapter 52); as an ophthalmic decongestant, mydriatic, or antiglaucoma agent (Chapter 54); to induce bronchodilation (Chapter 52); and as a topical hemostatic agent (Chapter 41). Administered subcutaneously, it is an effective treatment for status asthmaticus. Epinephrine remains the treatment of choice for anaphylactic shock and other severe allergic reactions to drugs or allergens (Chapter 50). Epinephrine is often used with local anesthetics so that its vasoconstrictor action can retard removal of the anesthetic from the site of application and its absorption into the systemic circulation (Chapter 17). Epinephrine is sometimes administered by direct intracardiac injection for its cardiac stimulatory properties in cardiac arrest.

Adverse Effects The most serious adverse effects are **cardiac dysrhythmias,** including ventricular tachycardia, extrasystoles, or fibrillation. These are particularly likely to occur in anesthetized patients. *Special care must be taken in calculating correct doses since toxicity and death can result from errors in administration. It is important to monitor vital signs during parenteral administration.* There is also a risk of **hypertension** when epinephrine is given. *Nurses should observe for hypertensive responses. Epinephrine should not be given to clients who have a history of heart disease, hypertension, or hyperthyroidism, or who are receiving cardiac glycosides. El-*

Table 28–6
Clinical Uses of Adrenergic Agonists

Drug	Receptor potencies				α-mediated			α_2-CNS mediated	α and β mediated	β_1-mediated	β_2-mediated		NE release in CNS	
	α_1	α_2	β_1	β_2	Decongestant	Mydriatic	Vasopressor	Antihypertensive	Glaucoma	Inotropism	Vasodilation	Bronchodilation	Anorexia	Stimulation
Natural catecholamines														
Epinephrine	+++	++	+++	++	✓	✓	✓		✓	✓		✓		
Norepinephrine	+++	++	++	0			✓			✓				
Primarily alpha-agonists														
Phenylephrine	++	0	0	0	✓	✓	✓							
Methoxamine	++	0	0	0	✓		✓							
Metaraminol	++	0	+/−	+	✓		✓							
Pseudoephedrine	++	?	+	+/−	✓									
Phenylpropanolamine	++	?	0	0	✓									
Naphazoline	++	+++	+	+	✓	✓								
Tetrahydrozoline	++	+++	+	+	✓	✓								
Oxymetazoline	++	+++	+	+	✓									
Xylometazoline	++	+++	+	+	✓									
Clonidine	+	+++	+	+				✓						
Primarily beta-agonists														
Isoproterenol	0	0	+++	+++						✓		✓		
Ethylnorepinephrine	+	?	+++	+++								✓		
Dobutamine	+/−	?	+++	+						✓				
Dopamine	−	?	+++	+						✓				
Nylidrin	0	0	+	++							✓			
Isoxsuprine	0	0	+	++							✓			

Isoetharine	0	0	++	+++							✓	
Metaproterenol	0	0	+	+++						✓		
Terbutaline	0	0	+	+++						✓		
Albuterol	0	0	0	+++						✓		
Salbutamol	0	0	0	+++						✓		
Primarily indirect-acting												
Ephedrine[a]	++	+	+	+	✓		✓		✓	✓		
Mephentermine[a]	+/−	?	+	++			✓		✓			
Amphetamine	Indirect[b]											✓
Hydroxyamphetamine	Indirect[b]				✓	✓	✓					
Methamphetamine	Indirect[b]						✓					✓
Methylphenidate	Indirect[b]											✓
Benzphetamine	Indirect[b]										✓	
Phentermine	Indirect[b]										✓	
Chlorphentermine	Indirect[b]										✓	
Fenfluramine	Indirect[b]										✓	
Diethylpropion	Indirect[b]										✓	
Phenmetrazine	Indirect[b]										✓	
Phendimetrazine	Indirect[b]										✓	
Dipivefrin	Epinephrine prodrug[c]							✓				

Key: +++, Highest potency; ++, moderate potency, +, low potency; +/−, little or no potency; 0, no potency; ?, not established.

[a]Substantial direct action as well.

[b]See norepinephrine

[c]See epinephrine

derly clients receiving epinephrine require careful monitoring.

Rapid intravenous injections or use of large doses by any route can cause cerebral and subarachnoid **hemorrhages.** *Epinephrine should be avoided in clients with a history of cerebral arteriosclerosis. Alpha-blockers or rapid-acting vasodilators, such as nitrates, are used to counteract excessive pressor effects of epinephrine.*

Epinephrine may cause pronounced **psychological and neurological reactions** secondary to the powerful cardiovascular influences. Clients may become weak, apprehensive, dizzy, anxious, or restless. They may experience tremors, vascular headache, or dyspnea. Adverse psychological and neurological reactions as well as exaggerated pressor responses are particularly likely in clients with anxiety disorders. *Use of epinephrine should therefore be avoided in agitated or anxious clients. Even seemingly small doses of epinephrine may cause some clients to become fearful and anxious. These effects, although not usually dangerous, may be disquieting.*

Even though epinephrine is frequently used by inhalation for asthma, its **inhibition of bronchial secretions** may make mucous plugs thicker and more difficult to remove. *Nurses need to observe clients for inhibition of bronchial secretions.*

Preparations and Administration Epinephrine is available in nasal sprays, respiratory inhalants, ophthalmic solutions, solutions for subcutaneous, intravenous, or intramuscular injection, and a sterile oil suspension for intramuscular injection. *The oil suspension has a prolonged duration of action and should not be repeated for at least 8 hours.*

In glaucoma, eyedrops containing epinephrine should be administered at night to avoid mydriasis and light sensitivity occurring during the day. Soft contact lenses should be removed before instilling epinephrine, since the lenses can be stained by the drug. Once the drops have been instilled in the eye, the lacrimal sac should be pressed gently for 1–2 minutes to minimize systemic absorption.

Nasal sprays are 1:1,000 aqueous solutions and are not sterile. *To administer nasal drops containing epinephrine, the client should be instructed to tip the head as far back as possible to keep the drug from dripping into the throat.*

Epinephrine is commonly used to relieve respiratory distress that results from bronchospasm and to provide rapid relief of hypersensitivity reactions to drugs or other allergens. Epinephrine solutions for inhalation are 1% (1:100) but can be diluted to 0.1% for use in a nebulizer. *When used for asthma, epinephrine should be administered at the first sign of bronchospasm. The mouth should be rinsed after inhalation to prevent swallowing of the medication.*

When used to counteract hypersensitivity, epinephrine is injected either intramuscularly or subcutaneously. Epinephrine for injection is a 1:1,000 sterile solution provided in ampuls or vials. The typical dose for hypotensive shock is 0.5 ml, which may be repeated every 5–15 minutes. *The nurse should be sure to aspirate (draw back on the syringe to assess location) before injecting epinephrine IM or SC since an inadvertent injection of the drug directly into the circulatory system could cause a severe hypertensive reaction. After injection, the rate of absorption can be enhanced by massage of the site of injection. If injections are to be repeated, the site should be rotated to decrease risk of necrosis. Nurses should avoid using the buttocks for IM injections because the anaerobic conditions caused by local vasoconstriction when epinephrine is injected favor growth of* Clostridium welchii, *which is often present in the feces and on the buttocks. Injection into the deltoid muscle is preferred.*

For intravenous infusion, 0.25–0.5 ml of a 1:10,000 solution is employed. *Care should be taken not to confuse 1:100, 1:1,000, and 1:10,000 solutions. Epinephrine solutions should be clear and colorless. If the solution develops a precipitate or becomes oxidized (acquiring a color that varies from pink to brown), it should be discarded. Ampuls of epinephrine should not be removed from cartons until they are to be used and should be protected from light at all times. These precautions should be taught to clients who may use the drug at home. After IV administration of epinephrine, blood pressure should be monitored until stabilized (5 minutes or longer).*

Epinephrine aqueous suspensions for relief of respiratory distress of asthmatic attacks are available in 1:200 (Sus-Phrine) and 1:400 (Asmolin) concentrations. The former is administered in doses of 0.1 to 0.3 ml SC in adults or 0.005 ml/kg SC in children. The latter is administered at 0.05–0.6 ml SC or IM. *Epinephrine suspensions should be thoroughly mixed before drawing a dose into a syringe.*

Important Nursing Implications for Epinephrine

- ☐ Question orders prescribing epinephrine if the client has a history of cerebral arteriosclerosis.
- ☐ Before administering epinephrine, inform clients that anxiety reactions may occur. Remain with the client after he or she has received an injection to help allay fear and anxiety.
- ☐ Always check and recheck doses and concentrations of epinephrine before injecting it.
- ☐ Observe asthmatic clients for indications of thickening of bronchial secretions.
- ☐ Question the client about any history of heart disease, hyperthyroidism, hypertension, and

use of digitalis for congestive heart failure before administering epinephrine.

- ☐ Administer ophthalmic drops containing epinephrine at night to avoid daytime mydriasis and light sensitivity. Instruct clients to remove soft contact lenses before instilling epinephrine drops and to gently press the lacrimal sac for 1–2 minutes after instilling the drops to minimize systemic absorption.
- ☐ Before giving intramuscular or subcutaneous injections of epinephrine, aspirate to establish that the tip of the needle is not in a blood vessel. Rotate the site when repeated injections are required. Massage injection sites to promote absorption. Avoid injecting epinephrine into the buttocks. Avoid injection into the extremities (ears, fingertips) where necrosis may result.
- ☐ Carefully follow all storage instructions for epinephrine and examine solutions for discoloration or precipitants before use.

Norepinephrine (Levophed)

Norepinephrine is also known as noradrenaline. The natural biological levorotatory isomer is sometimes called levarterenol. Norepinephrine is the neurotransmitter released by most postganglionic sympathetic nerve terminals.

Mechanisms and Effects Administered norepinephrine acts like increased sympathetic nerve impulses to alter the function of tissues innervated by the sympathetic branch of the autonomic nervous system. Norepinephrine is as potent as epinephrine in stimulating β_1-receptors, somewhat less potent at α-receptors, and almost devoid of activity at β_2-receptors. Therefore, norepinephrine does not dilate peripheral blood vessels and does not increase blood flow through vascular beds in skeletal muscle, the spleen, or the cerebrum in the manner of epinephrine. Norepinephrine also lacks significant ability to stimulate glycogenolysis or to dilate bronchial smooth muscles.

Like epinephrine, norepinephrine is not effective orally and does not cross the blood-brain barrier to a significant extent. Its absorption after subcutaneous administration is slow due to local vasoconstriction. Norepinephrine is metabolized rapidly after systemic absorption and less than 20% is excreted unchanged.

Clinical Indications Norepinephrine is used only for emergency treatment of acute hypotension and cardiac arrest. Norepinephrine is used to restore blood pressure and to control acute hypotensive states that may occur as a result of myocardial infarction or cardiac arrest. It is administered by slow intravenous infusion to elevate both systolic and diastolic pressures.

Adverse Effects and Contraindications Adverse reactions to norepinephrine are similar to epinephrine but less common and less severe. Anxiety, headache, apprehensiveness, and dypsnea occur occasionally. Vasoconstriction produced by norepinephrine reduces blood flow to the kidneys, spleen, skeletal muscles, and to the placenta of pregnant women. *When norepinephrine is used to maintain blood pressure, it should be accompanied by blood volume replacement; otherwise perfusion in the viscera and kidneys may be impaired.*

The elevation in blood pressure produced by norepinephrine may lead to reflex bradycardia. *Nurses should monitor pulse rate and instruct clients to report any chest pains immediately.*

Norepinephrine should not be used in pregnant women because of its ability to stimulate uterine contractions. It should not be used in clients with thromboses, since its constrictor effect can enlarge the area of ischemia. Use of norepinephrine can lead to peripheral ischemic reactions including intestinal, renal, or hepatic necrosis, myocardial ischemia, and gangrene in the extremities.

Preparations and Administration The pressor effect of norepinephrine dissipates in 1–2 minutes after infusion is terminated. *Like epinephrine, norepinephrine is oxidized by light.*

Norepinephrine (Levophed)
Injection solutions as norepinephrine bitartrate in tinted ampuls (equivalent to 0.1% norepinephrine)
Recommended Doses: The contents of one ampul (4 ml) are usually diluted in 1,000 ml of 5% dextrose for slow intravenous infusion at 2–3 ml/minute initially, tapered down to 0.5–1.0 ml/minute after a response is obtained.

Important Nursing Implications for Norepinephrine

- ☐ Provide adequate body fluid replacement when using norepinephrine for maintenance of blood pressure so that perfusion of the viscera and kidneys will remain adequate.
- ☐ Remember that a decline in urinary output may occur even when fluid replacement is adequate. Monitor blood pressure closely, record

fluid intake and output, and watch for other signs of poor tissue perfusion, such as tissue hypoxia and lactate acidosis. Nurses should periodically check skin color and temperature, acid-base balance, and cerebral function.

- ☐ Once a client is placed on norepinephrine, take the blood pressure every 2 minutes until a desired blood pressure is reached and then every 5 minutes. The client should never be left unattended, since the rate of flow needs to be monitored constantly. Observe for such symptoms as headache, palpitations, chest pain, blurred vision, or photophobia, which indicate excessive norepinephrine concentrations. Myocardial infarction or cerebral hemorrhage may result from excessive hypertension.
- ☐ Observe clients for bradycardia when administering norepinephrine. Any complaint of chest pain should suggest discontinuing the drug. Increased sweating or vomiting should be assessed immediately to ensure that the client is not having an adverse drug reaction.
- ☐ Discard solutions of norepinephrine that are discolored or that contain a precipitant.
- ☐ Norepinephrine is not compatible with whole blood or plasma infusions. A double-bottle setup should be used so that the intravenous fluids can be continued without interruption if norepinephrine infusion must be discontinued.
- ☐ Whenever possible, administer norepinephrine through a large vein, preferably an antecubital vein, to decrease the risk of necrosis of the underlying skin that can occur from prolonged vasoconstriction.
- ☐ Take care that the norepinephrine solution does not leak from the site of infusion into surrounding subcutaneous tissue, since this can cause necrosis and sloughing due to the powerful vasoconstrictor activity. If a leak does occur, the area of infiltration will appear hard, cold, and blanched. Infiltration of the tissue surrounding the site of infusion with a solution of phentolamine, an alpha-blocker, (5–10 mg in 5–10 ml of saline) will alleviate local vasoconstriction and impaired circulation.
- ☐ Have emergency drugs available (such as atropine for bradycardia and propranolol for cardiac arrhythmias) when a client is receiving norepinephrine in the event of cardiac abnormalities.

Alpha-Sympathomimetics

Alpha-agonists are used as pressors (in hypotension), nasal decongestants, and mydriatics. The use of phenylephrine, naphazoline, and tetrahydrozoline in ophthalmic preparations as mydriatics and ophthalmic decongestants is discussed in Chapter 54.

Pressor Agents

Phenylephrine (Neosynephrine), methoxamine (Vasoxyl), and metaraminol (Aramine) are pure α_1-agonists. They are used to raise blood pressure in hypotension (during anesthesia, for example) and are generally preferred to epinephrine or norepinephrine because they constrict blood vessels without any direct effect on the heart. This is particularly important in cardiogenic shock that accompanies myocardial infarction, because cardiac stimulation could seriously aggravate myocardial hypoxia already present. Pure α-agonists produce correspondingly more reflex bradycardia than is seen with epinephrine and norepinephrine, but this can be blocked with atropine if necessary. *The drugs in this group may promote headache and urinary frequency. Clients may experience pilomotor response or projectile vomiting. Clients with hyperthyroidism or hypertension or those receiving ergot alkaloids must be monitored very closely if one of these α-sympathomimetics is administered.*

Decongestants

A wide variety of α-agonists are employed as nasal and sinus decongestants. In addition to phenylephrine, metaraminol, and methoxamine, these include phenylpropanolamine, pseudoephedrine (Sudafed), phenylpropylmethylamine propylhexedrine, cyclopentamine, methylhexaneamine, and tuaminoheptane. These drugs generally have more effect on α_1- than α_2-receptors and tend to produce a mild CNS excitatory effect to the extent that they cross the blood-brain barrier. Naphazoline (Privine), tetrahydrozoline (Tyzine), xylometazoline (Otrivin), and oxymetazoline (Afrin) are another group of drugs used as nasal decongestants, but these agents have substantial α_2-agonist properties and tend to sedate or depress the CNS instead of stimulating it. Nasal decongestants are pressor agents and always pose a risk of increased hypertension. The hypertensive effect of nasal decongestants may be dangerously potentiated by MAO inhibitors; inhibitors of amine storage, such as reserpine (Serpasil) and guanethidine (Ismelin); and competitive inhibitors of uptake, such as tricyclic antidepressants or methyldopa (Aldomet). Beta-blockers also increase the pressor effect of nasal decongestants (by blocking any offsetting β_2-mediated vasodilatory activity the drug might have). Nasal decongestants are further discussed in Chapter 52.

Appropriate oral doses of pure α-agonists produce few adverse effects. *Mild gastrointestinal symptoms occur occasionally, but clients can alleviate such reactions by taking the drug with meals.* Tremor occurs occasionally. Signs of mild CNS stimulation include restlessness and insomnia. Cardiac symptoms such as palpitations occur only at extreme doses, but reflex bradycardia is common. Alpha-stimulants should be employed only with great caution in clients with heart block or bradycardia, and are contraindicated in clients with ischemic conditions, arteriosclerosis, or hypertension. Elderly clients and those with hyperthyroidism have exaggerated sensitivity to alpha-agonists. Topical ophthalmic solutions should not be employed in clients with narrow-angle glaucoma. The use of nasal decongestants should be limited to 7 days because of the risk of rebound nasal stuffiness after extended periods of use.

Nurses should determine if a client has any of the conditions, such as hypertension, hyperthyroidism, or diabetes mellitus, that make use of nasal decongestants hazardous. Nurses should teach clients what to look for in nasal decongestants that might aggravate health problems and not to exceed the maximum recommended daily doses of such drugs.

Selective α_2-Agonists

Selective α_2-agonists (clonidine, for example) with ability to cross the blood-brain barrier produce unique pharmacological activity. In the brain, α_2-agonists stimulate postsynaptic α_2-receptors in the vasomotor and cardiac centers that cause a decrease in vasomotor tone and a slowing of the heart. This cardiovascular depressant effect can be a useful therapeutic action in persons with essential hypertension. The pharmacology of clonidine (Catapres) and methyldopa (Aldomet) are discussed in Chapter 39.

Beta-Sympathomimetics

The available beta-sympathomimetics include nonselective agents that act on β_1- and β_2-receptors alike (isoproterenol, ethylnorepinephrine), relatively selective β_1-agonists (dobutamine and dopamine), and selective β_2-agonists (nylidrin, isoxsuprine, isoetharine, metaproterenol, terbutaline, albuterol, bitolterol, and salbutamol).

Isoproterenol (Isuprel)

Isoproterenol (isopropylnorepinephrine) is a catecholamine that acts exclusively on β-receptors and is equally active at β_1- and β_2-receptors. It thus has a powerful inotropic effect on the heart, improves atrioventricular conduction, relaxes bronchial smooth muscle, and dilates peripheral blood vessels. It also shares the metabolic effects of epinephrine in stimulating glycogenolysis and lipolysis, although the hyperglycemic effect is less than that of epinephrine because isoproterenol stimulates insulin release via β-receptors.

Pharmacokinetics Isoproterenol is not well absorbed when administered orally or sublingually, but parenteral injections and inhalation result in reliable effects. Isoproterenol is metabolized mainly by COMT in the liver and other tissues because it is a poor substrate for MAO. Its action, although longer than that of the natural catecholamines, is still rather brief.

Clinical Indications Isoproterenol has been used as a **bronchodilator** in asthma and other respiratory disorders characterized by constricted airways, but it is being replaced by selective β_2-agonists that lack its profound stimulatory effect on the heart. Prolonged or excessive use of isoproterenol as a bronchodilator is associated with tolerance to the therapeutic effect and rebound brochospasm if the drug is discontinued abruptly.

Isoproterenol is useful as a **cardiac stimulant** in heart block, in cardiogenic shock after myocardial infarction, or in septicemic shock. Its use in heart block derives from its positive effect on atrioventricular conduction. In shock, isoproterenol has the dual benefits of stimulating cardiac output and improving peripheral blood flow in ischemic tissues.

Adverse Effects and Contraindications The adverse effects of isoproterenol are mainly related to cardiac stimulation. Thus palpitations, tachycardias, and cardiac dysrhythmias are the main concerns. Isoproterenol should be used only with extreme caution in clients receiving cardiac glycosides since they increase liability toward catecholamine-induced dysrhythmias. Anginal pain may result from increased coronary oxygen consumption and decreased coronary blood flow. Headache and flushing of the skin can occur from dilation of cerebral and cutaneous blood vessels respectively. Propranolol may be employed to counter toxicity of isoproterenol. Isoproterenol should not be administered concurrently with epinephrine since both drugs stimulate the heart and together could precipitate cardiac dysrhythmias.

Preparations and Administration Aerosols and injectable solutions are the only dosage forms of isoproterenol that provide reliable effects. Prolonged use of sublingual tablets can cause damage to teeth. *Electrocardiographic monitoring should be established before initiating intravenous administration of isoproterenol. An isoproterenol infusion should be slowed or discontinued if premature beats occur or if heart rate exceeds 110 beats per minute. Isoproterenol solutions are oxidized by light exposure and should be stored in light-resistant containers. Solutions that are discolored or that contain precipitants should be discarded.*

Isoproterenol (Isuprel, Dispos-a-Med, Vapo-Iso, Aerolone, Norisodrine, Medihaler-Iso, and generic formulations). Inhalation solutions, inhalation aerosols, insufflation powder, injection solutions

Recommended Doses: For relief of dyspnea, 1–2 inhalations, the second inhalation taken 2–5 minutes after the first if relief is not evident. *The nurse should instruct the client to rinse the mouth after inhalation to prevent swallowing of the medication.* The usual parenteral dose is 0.01–0.02 mg IV of a 1:50,000 solution prepared by diluting 1 ml of the 1:5,000 commercial formulation to 10 ml with saline or 5% dextrose injection solutions.

Dopamine (Intropin) and Dobutamine (Dobutrex)

Dopamine and dobutamine are catecholamines that stimulate β_1-receptors to a greater extent than other classes of adrenergic receptors.

Clinical Indications Dopamine and dobutamine are useful in clinical circumstances requiring an inotropic effect without substantial changes in peripheral resistance or heart rate. Dopamine and dobutamine are used for short-term inotropic support to correct hemodynamic imbalances of shock due to septicemia, myocardial infarction, open heart surgery, congestive heart failure, renal failure, or trauma. If hypovolemia is present, restoration of fluid volume should precede administration of these cardiac stimulants. Dopamine and dobutamine improve renal perfusion and can help bring urine production back to normal in oliguric clients, providing that the degree of deterioration in function of the vital organs is not profound. Therapy is usually successful when urine flow exceeds 0.3 ml/minute but is occasionally successful even in more severe cases of impaired renal function.

Adverse Effects and Contraindications Cardiac stimulants can cause palpitations, serious dysrhythmias (ectopic beats, tachycardia), and angina and should not be administered in clients with preexisting tachydysrhythmias or ventricular fibrillation. Dobutamine increases atrioventricular conduction and will increase risk of ventricular tachydysrhythmias in clients with preexisting atrial flutter or fibrillation. Because of the vasoconstrictor effects of these drugs, caution should be exercised in using them in clients with a history of occlusive disorders, such as embolism, angina, arteriosclerosis, Raynaud's disease, Buerger's disease, frostbite, or diabetic endarteritis. *Changes in skin color or temperature may indicate compromised peripheral circulation. Clients with preexisting hypertension should be closely monitored for evidence of an excessive pressor response; clients should also be monitored for palpitations or ectopic beats.*

Anginal pain and dyspnea are other potential adverse reactions to inotropic drugs. Hypotension is another potential side effect with dopamine in particular. Less frequent side effects of dopamine and dobutamine include nausea, headache, pilomotor erection, azotemia, elevated blood pressure, and bradycardia.

Drug Interactions The actions of both dopamine and dobutamine are greatly potentiated by MAO inhibitors and somewhat potentiated by tricyclic antidepressants. Potassium depletion associated with use of diuretics augments the inotropic effects of dopamine. Halothane and cyclopropane sensitize the heart to catecholamine-induced dysrhythmias. Concurrent use of dopamine and dobutamine with oxytocic drugs in the postpartum period has been associated with severe and prolonged hypertension.

Preparations and Administration *The client should be monitored by ECG whenever these drugs are employed. Dopamine and dobutamine are oxidized by light. Discolored solutions should be discarded. As with norepinephrine, care must be exercised to avoid extravasation at the site of infusion, which can result in necrosis and sloughing of dermal tissue. Installation of phentolamine (Regitine) will help to minimize this risk.*

Dopamine (Intropin)
Injection solutions
Recommended Doses: For shock, 2–5 μg/kg/minute initially by an intravenous catheter or syringe after dilution, increased up to 20–50 μg/kg/minute in severe cases.

Dobutamine (Dobutrex)
Powder for reconstitution and further dilution
Recommended Doses: 2.5–10 μg/kg/minute by IV infusion.

Important Nursing Implications for Dopamine and Dobutamine.

☐ Monitor the client for indications of angina. Observe the client's position, since often clients will attempt to position themselves to relieve anginal pain, especially if the client has not previously experienced angina. Anginal pain does not always start in the chest: it can appear initially in the throat, neck, and jaws. Monitor clients for dyspnea; clients may not mention it, assuming it is caused by the problem that resulted in the need for drug therapy in the first place.

- ☐ Observe for symptoms of hypotension, such as faintness, lightheadedness, or weakness, and monitor for any obvious lowering in blood pressure.
- ☐ Monitor the client's ECG whenever dobutamine or dopamine is to be administered.
- ☐ Do not administer solutions of dopamine or dobutamine that are discolored.

Selective β_2-Sympathomimetics

In recent years, a number of drugs have been developed with selective agonist activity at β_2-receptors that provide a means of producing bronchodilation or peripheral vasodilation without appreciable cardiac stimulation. Those currently marketed in the United States as bronchodilators are metaproterenol (Metaprel, Alupent), terbutaline (Brethine, Bricanyl), albuterol (Proventil, Ventolin), bitolterol (Tornalate), and isoetharine (Dispos-a-Med, Bronkosol, and Bronkometer). Others in use in Europe include salbutamol, fenoterol, ritodrine, quinterenol, and soterenol. The pharmacology of these drugs is discussed in Chapter 52. The two employed as peripheral vasodilators are isoxsuprine and nylidrin, two drugs with greater β_2- than β_1-effects.

Clinical Indications Isoxsuprine and nylidrin dilate blood vessels primarily within skeletal muscles, but they are designated as "possibly effective" for relief of symptoms of cerebrovascular insufficiency and treatment of peripheral vascular disorders, such as Raynaud's disease, Buerger's disease, arteriosclerosis obliterans, and thromboangiitis obliterans. The value of β_2-agonists is due to both their spasmolytic and dilating effects. Isoxsuprine has also been used for its spasmolytic action to delay premature labor and in treatment of menstrual cramps.

Adverse Effects and Contraindications Adverse effects from oral isoxsuprine or nylidrin are uncommon but can include hypotension, reflex tachycardia, gastrointestinal symptoms (nausea, vomiting, cramps), dizziness, and rash.

Preparations and Administration Isoxsuprine can be given orally or by intramuscular injection. *If the client is expected to inject the drug without assistance, the nurse will need to teach the client how to perform the procedure as well as alerting the client to the possibility of developing hypotension with reflex tachycardia when this route is employed.*

Isoxsuprine (Vasodilan, Vasoprine, and generic formulations)
Tablets, injection solution
Recommended Doses: 10–20 mg orally tid or qid. The intramuscular dose is 5–10 mg bid or tid.

Nylidrin (Arlidin and generic formulations)
Tablets
Recommended Doses: 3–12 mg orally tid or qid.

Indirect-Acting Sympathetic Amines

Direct-acting sympathetic amines generally do not cross the blood-brain barrier to an appreciable extent. Absence of a hydroxyl group in the β-carbon position of phenylethylamine decreases the affinity of compounds for adrenergic receptors but increases their ability to enter the brain and their ability to release endogenous norepinephrine. Thus central noradrenergic actions are most efficiently produced by indirect-acting agents that release brain stores of norepinephrine. Amphetamine is the prototype drug of this type and others are often designated *amphetamine-like agents.* Indirect-acting sympathetic amines are most widely used as **anorexics** and **CNS stimulants.** Amphetamine itself has been discontinued as an anorexic, but it is used at times as a stimulant for treatment of narcolepsy, attention deficit disorder, and interim treatment of depression (see Chapter 14). Methylphenidate (Ritalin) and methamphetamine (Methedrine, Desoxyn) have similar efficacy. Methamphetamine and hydroxyamphetamine (Peredrine) are also used as **indirect-acting vasopressors.**

Anorexics that release norepinephrine centrally include phentermine (Ionamin, Wilpowr), benzphetamine (Didrex), chlorphentermine (Pre-sate), fenfluramine (Pondimin), phendimetrazine (Plegine), phenmetrazine (Preludin), and diethylpropion (Tenuate, Tepanil). The pharmacology of these drugs is discussed in Chapters 14 and 44.

Ephedrine and mephentermine are drugs that can act both directly and indirectly to activate adrenergic receptors. Ephedrine finds widespread use as a decongestant, pressor agent, bronchodilator, and less commonly as a cardiac stimulant. Mephentermine is used as a pressor agent, nasal decongestant, cardiac stimulator, and occasionally to produce CNS stimulation.

Dipivefrin is an epinephrine lipophilic prodrug that penetrates into the anterior chamber of the eye better than the more polar epinephrine after topical installation in the eye. It is converted by deesterification into epinephrine and pivalic acid within the eye. The pharmacology of this drug is discussed in Chapter 54.

Sympatholytics

Alpha-Blockers

Adrenergic antagonists are inherently selective with respect to α-receptors versus β-receptors. Within the category of α-receptors, some bind largely to α_1-receptors (phenoxybenzamine, prazosin), some exclusively to α_2-receptors (yohimbine), and some to both kinds of α-receptors (phentolamine, tolazoline). Blockers of α_2-receptors are being used experimentally in men for treatment of erectile impotence associated with vascular problems (see Chapter 35). Alpha-1-blockers are used mainly for acute or chronic antihypertensive effects or as diagnostic aids. Phenoxybenzamine (Dibenzyline) forms a strong covalent bond with α_1-receptors; its effect is irreversible and noncompetitive. Phentolamine (Regitine) and tolazoline (Priscoline) produce only a transient and competitive antagonism at α-receptors.

The pharmacology of blockers always depends on the physiological condition at the time of administration. A blocker does not activate the receptors to which it attaches; instead, it denies endogenous or exogenous agonists access to the receptor. In the presence of an alpha-blocker, the effect of epinephrine on blood pressure is converted from a pressor effect to a depressor effect because the ability of epinephrine to produce vasodilation via β_2-receptors is no longer outweighed by α-mediated vasoconstrictor activity. On the other hand, norepinephrine, which does not act on β_2-receptors, will exhibit only a diminished hypertensive effect in the presence of an α-blocker.

The action of an α-blocker depends on the extent to which the sympathoadrenal system is being utilized at the time the drug is administered. A relaxed, recumbent, healthy subject with normal fluid volume will exhibit little change in overall blood pressure or blood flow to specific tissues when administered an α-blocker. The same subject will exhibit a sharp drop in blood pressure upon standing up — the classic indication of orthostatic hypotension. Vasomotor sympathetic activity is increased by hypovolemia, rest, and cold temperature, so these conditions increase the effect of α-blockers. Drugs from other classes that produce orthostatic hypotension with compensatory sympathoadrenal activation (anesthetics, vasodilators, narcotics, antidepressants) also generate conditions in which the action of α-blockers will be magnified.

Like other peripheral vasodilators, α-blockers themselves tend to produce a compensatory increase in sympathetic activity as the body seeks to reestablish blood pressure. Release of norepinephrine from sympathetic nerve terminals increases because nerve impulses become more frequent and because presynaptic α_2-receptors that normally exert a limiting influence on norepinephrine release may be inhibited if the α-blocker is nonselective. The presence of the α-blocker prevents expression of this increased sympathetic activity on α-receptors in the blood vessels and elsewhere but does not protect the heart from exaggerated sympathetic activation via the coronary β_1-receptors. Thus, reflex tachycardia can be a problem with α-blockers. *In assessing a client's response to an alpha-blocker, nurses need to monitor blood pressure and pulse rate, and to ask clients about palpitations or "fluttery" sensations in the chest and under what circumstances these occur. Improvement in peripheral circulation can be confirmed by warmth and color in affected areas.*

Changes in blood pressure are the most obvious influence of α-blockers, but other α-mediated adrenergic effects are also inhibited. In the presence of an alpha-blocker, the usually predominant inhibitory action of epinephrine on insulin secretion is blocked, permitting the lesser beta-mediated stimulatory effect to come to the fore. The normal hyperglycemic effect of epinephrine is eliminated as glycogenolysis is effectively offset by insulin-activated glucose uptake by peripheral tissues.

Alpha-blockers can have significant activity on the CNS. Clients receiving alpha-blockers may experience sedation, depression, fatigue, and weakness as well as hyperventilation, vertigo, paresthesias, motor excitability, and occasionally convulsions. *Nurses need to question clients receiving alpha-blockers about any increase in weakness, fatigue, or lethargy that has developed since the alpha-blocker therapy began.* Inhibition of alpha-mediated mydriasis results in pronounced miosis in response to alpha-blockers. Pilomotor erection and adrenergic components of salivation and sweating are inhibited. Pituitary secretion of luteinizing hormone is suppressed and ejaculatory impotence and priapism can occur in males. *Impotence is a sensitive issue for males and may go unreported unless the nurse is skillful in guiding the client to reveal this information. Precise information should be provided in advance of therapy concerning possible effects on sexual functioning so that the role of the drug in producing such changes will be recognized by the client. If the client is married, the nurse may find that information concerning alterations in sexual functioning are obtained most readily from the wife.*

Urinary frequency and incontinence may occur due to loss of control of the trigone sphincter. *This adverse effect often contributes to noncompliance, since clients may discontinue the drug rather than suffer discomfort and embarrassment.* A small degree of gastrointestinal hyperactivity (nausea, vomiting, diarrhea, cramps) is sometimes evident. *If the client has peptic ulcer or gastritis, the problem may well be aggravated by the alpha-blocker.*

Phenoxybenzamine (Dibenzyline)

Mechanisms and Effects Phenoxybenzamine, a β-haloethylamine, is a potent alpha-blocker that produces a long-lasting, irreversible, and noncompetitive effect. Phenoxybenzamine is 100 times more active in blocking α_1- than α_2-receptors. It has no intrinsic adrenergic agonistic activity but can cause indirect activation of β-receptors because of its ability to increase norepinephrine turnover. Phenoxybenzamine is also a potent antihistaminic, comparable to drugs used clinically for that activity and has weaker anticholinergic and antiserotonergic effects as well.

Pharmacokinetics The half-life of phenoxybenzamine is approximately 24 hours, so a single dose can produce effects lasting 3 or 4 days. Phenoxybenzamine is active after oral administration or by injection, but oral administration is associated with erratic absorption and activity.

Clinical Indications Phenoxybenzamine is indicated for presurgical control of hypertensive episodes related to pheochromocytoma, a condition in which there is excess production and secretion of catecholamines from adrenal or adrenal-like tumors. It is designated as "possibly effective" in vasospastic diseases of peripheral blood vessels, such as Raynaud's syndrome or frostbite sequelae.

Adverse Effects and Contraindications Phenoxybenzamine causes adverse effects typical of alpha-blockers. Nasal congestion, pupillary constriction, ejaculatory impotence, orthostatic hypotension, and reflex tachycardia are common. Orthostatic hypotension decreases with therapy. *Clients receiving phenoxybenzamine should be advised to avoid rapid changes in posture such as standing up abruptly, especially if dizziness is experienced, and to dangle the legs over the side of the bed several minutes before arising. Use of elastic stockings can help by reducing gravitational blood flow. Nurses should inform clients that both alcohol and excessive physical exercise can aggravate postural hypotension. If faintness does occur, clients should be taught to sit or lie down with the head lowered.*

Gastrointestinal hyperactivity is usually mild. *Administration of phenoxybenzamine with milk, with meals, or in divided doses will reduce gastrointestinal symptoms.* Sedation, weakness, somnolence, and depression are typical CNS symptoms. Alpha-blockers should be used with extreme caution if at all in patients with coronary or cerebral vascular insufficiency or impaired renal function. Overdose with phenoxybenzamine is treated with norepinephrine.

Drug Interactions Patients should avoid concurrent use of drugs that cause vasodilation, such as alcohol, narcotics (morphine, meperidine (Demerol)), antidepressants, and neuroleptics, since these will augment the hypotensive effect of alpha-blockers. *Nurses need to be certain that clients understand that the vasodilating effects of alcohol can promote postural hypotension, mental confusion, and incoordination.*

Preparations and Doses *During the period of dosage adjustment, blood pressure and pulse should be monitored with the client in both recumbent and standing positions. The dosage needs to be adjusted until symptomatic relief or objective improvement is obtained without the client acquiring troublesome side effects. Nurses need to evaluate clients for the degree of vasodilation achieved, which means examining skin warmth and color and changes in peripheral pulses.*

Phenoxybenzamine (Dibenzyline)
Capsules, injection solution (by special arrangements with the manufacturer)
Recommended Doses: 10 mg orally, once daily. Doses must be individually adjusted based on relief of symptoms. After adjustment, the usual range of doses is 20–60 mg daily. The client's response to the drug should be monitored for at least 4 days before the dosage is increased. Each increment must be maintained for at least 4 days to achieve the full effect because the long half-life of phenoxybenzamine results in accumulation for nearly 1 week.

Imidazolines

Mechanisms and Effects Two related imidazoline derivatives, tolazoline (Priscoline) and phentolamine (Regitine), have alpha-blocking activity. These drugs are pharmacologically less specific than phenoxybenzamine, possessing considerable intrinsic sympathomimetic activity, parasympathomimetic activity, histaminic activity, and antiserotonergic activity. Their alpha-blocking effects are only moderate in potency and short in duration. Phentolamine has more alpha-blocking activity in relation to its other neurochemical activities than tolazoline. In the case of tolazoline, the net effect on blood pressure is usually an elevation due to cardiac stimulation, but both agents decrease peripheral resistance. The imidazolines have relatively greater effects on α_2-receptors than does phenoxybenzamine, causing elevated release of endogenous norepinephrine and contributing to the sympathomimetic activity of the drugs. Tolazoline and phentolamine cause mydriasis rather than miosis, indicating the substantial sympathomimetic characteristics of these drugs. Parasympathomimetic activity is expressed in the stimulation of respiratory, lacrimal, salivary, and intestinal secretions, the increase in intestinal motility, and the profuse sweating produced by both of these medications.

Pharmacokinetics Tolazoline is well absorbed after oral administration, but phentolamine must be given in a relatively high dose when given orally because of limited absorption. Tolazoline is excreted rapidly by the kidneys, but phentolamine is mostly metabolized before renal elimination. Each of the two drugs has a brief half-life.

Clinical Indications Phentolamine is indicated for control of hypertensive episodes associated with pheochromocytoma and has also been used as an aid in diagnosing the condition. Phentolamine has also been used successfully to inhibit dermal necrosis and sloughing caused by potent pressor agents, such as norepinephrine, when extravasation occurs with intravenous infusions. For this purpose, phentolamine is kept available during all norepinephrine infusions and is instilled directly onto the tissue surrounding the site of cannulation in the event of extravasation. Tolazoline is possibly effective for treatment of peripheral vasospastic disorders, such as Raynaud's disease, Buerger's disease, acrocyanosis, arteriosclerosis, gangrene, endarteritis, sequelae of frostbite, thrombophlebitis, or scleroderma. Imidazolines can also be used in therapy for clonidine (Catapres) overdose.

Adverse Effects and Contraindications Side effects are generally mild but numerous. Phentolamine causes orthostatic hypotension. *Patients should be advised to sit or lie down if faintness occurs.* Reflex sympathetic compensation leads to tachycardia and potentially to dysrhythmias and angina. Other adverse reactions include nasal stuffiness, weakness, flushing, and gastrointestinal hyperexcitability (nausea, vomiting, diarrhea, exacerbations of peptic ulcer, or epigastric distress). Tolazoline has a wider variety of side effects due to its greater sympathomimetic, parasympathomimetic, and histaminergic actions. Sympathomimetic side effects include pilomotor erection, hypertension (which can be marked), apprehensiveness, anginal pain, confusion and hallucinations. Parasympathetic and histaminergic activity adds to the gastrointestinal hyperexcitability attributable to the alpha-blocking property, resulting in a substantial liability toward activation of peptic ulcers. Tolazoline inhibits aldehyde dehydrogenase and can thus cause disulfiram-like reactions if alcohol is ingested concurrently.

Preparations and Administration

Phentolamine (Regitine)
Tablets, powder with diluent for reconstitution and injection
Recommended Doses: For control of pheochromocytoma, 50 mg orally, 4–6 times daily. For diagnosis of pheochromocytoma, 5 mg (1 ml in children), IV, in the resting, supine patient; blood pressure is recorded at 30-second intervals for 3 minutes and 60-second intervals for 7 more minutes. During the 24 hours preceding the test, hypotensive medications including sedatives, narcotics, and vasodilators, are withheld. Pheochromocytoma is indicated by a drop in systolic pressure of more than 35 mm Hg and in diastolic blood pressure of more than 25 mm Hg.

Tolazoline (Priscoline, Vasodil, and generic formulations)
Tablets, long-acting tablets, injection solution
Recommended Doses: For peripheral vascular disorders, 25 mg orally initially, 4–6 times daily (or the long-acting 80 mg form every 12 hours), individualized thereafter for each client. The parenteral dose is 10–50 mg qid, SC, IV, or IM. *During parenteral administration, the patient should be recumbent and should be monitored closely for signs of excessive hypotension (tachycardia, flushing, or cutaneous warmth).*

Prazosin (Minipress)

Mechanisms and Effects Prazosin is an antihypertensive drug and selective alpha-blocker that acts exclusively on α_1-receptors. Its lack of activity at α_2-receptors is advantageous because it minimizes the potential for enhanced release of endogenous norepinephrine. Nevertheless, as with all peripheral vasodilators, compensatory sympathoadrenal activation does occur in response to the hypotensive effect and a modest degree of tachycardia can occur. Prazosin produces dilation in both venous and arterial vessels. Venous return (preload) decreases leading to a small reduction in cardiac output. Afterload also declines, possibly resulting in pooling of blood in the extremities.

Clinical Indications Prazosin is indicated for treatment of hypertension, often in conjunction with a diuretic. The full pharmacology of prazosin is discussed in Chapter 39.

Adverse Effects and Contraindications Prazosin shares many of the adverse effects of other alpha-blockers: gastrointestinal hyperactivity (vomiting, diarrhea, abdominal discomfiture or pain), orthostatic hypotension (with possible edema or syncope), urinary frequency and incontinence, ejaculatory impotence, nasal congestion, dry mouth, and CNS depression. Other adverse effects include rash, pruritus, dyspnea, tinnitus, vertigo, blurred vision, reddened sclera, nasal stuffiness, paresthesias, and nervousness.

Important Nursing Implications for Alpha-Blockers

- ☐ Most clients will take alpha-blockers at home and will need special instructions concerning what to do if untoward effects develop. Establish a plan for client follow-up and for reporting untoward effects.
- ☐ Question the client to ascertain whether symptoms of a "cold" or "allergy" correspond to the period during which the client has been taking the alpha-blocker, since nasal stuffiness is a frequent adverse effect.
- ☐ Ask clients about increased fatigue or weakness that may have developed since therapy with the alpha-blocker was initiated.
- ☐ Instruct clients to report any sensations of palpitations.
- ☐ Encourage male clients and their partners to report any alterations in sexual performance resulting from administration of alpha-blockers.
- ☐ If urinary frequency or urgency occurs, ask the client about frequency of voiding and amount of fluid intake, and when voiding occurs most often (day or night) to distinguish between urinary problems of neurological origin and those secondary to cardiovascular disease or drug therapy.
- ☐ Assess clients for symptoms of gastric irritation, usually described by clients as a burning or gnawing sensation in the stomach. If a client has diarrhea, determine where there is an unusual odor, or if mucus or blood is present in the stool in large quantities.
- ☐ Teach clients to avoid rapid changes in position, such as standing up abruptly. Instruct clients to avoid prolonged standing, extremes of heat (such as hot showers or excessive exposure to the sun), or excessive exercise. Teach clients to sit or lie down and to lower the head if dizziness or faintness is experienced. Teach the client self-assessment of blood pressure. Advise clients to use elastic stockings and to put them on while supine, with feet elevated.
- ☐ Ensure that clients understand the importance of complying with the regimen.
- ☐ Advise clients to avoid use of alcohol, since it aggravates orthostatic hypotension caused by alpha-blockers.

Beta-Blockers

Beta-adrenergic blockers are among the most important therapeutic drug classes. There are currently nine drugs in clinical use from this family and a tenth approved by the FDA but not marketed. The original beta-blocker in clinical practice, propranolol (Inderal), is the drug with the greatest variety of clinical uses. Most beta-blockers are indicated for treatment of essential hypertension. The complete pharmacology of beta-blockers is therefore addressed in Chapter 39. Propranolol is also approved for use in migraine, angina pectoris (see Chapter 40), hypertropic subaortic stenosis, and reducing the risk of reinfarction after the acute phase of myocardial infarction. Nadolol is approved for use in angina pectoris as well as hypertension; and timolol, levobunolol, and betaxolol are approved for use in glaucoma (see Chapter 54). Metoprolol, atenolol, acebutolol, and betaxolol are said to be cardioselective; that is, they block β_1-receptors without blocking β_2-receptors. These drugs have the advantage of having no adverse effects related to β_2-receptor antagonism, such as aggravation of asthma and hypoglycemia. Cardioselective drugs may produce a slight aggravation of asthma because of the presence of some β_1-receptors in bronchial smooth muscle. Pindolol, oxprenolol, and acebutolol possess intrinsic sympathomimetic activity as well as beta-blocking properties. Another difference among the agents is the frequency of dosage: propranolol must be given 2 or 3 times daily; metoprolol, timolol, and pindolol twice daily; and nadolol and atenolol once daily. Propranolol has a potent quinidine-like local anesthetic (or membrane-stabilizing) effect; oxprenolol, labetalol, pindolol, and metoprolol produce this action to a lesser extent, and other beta-blockers not at all.

Shock

Three classes of drugs discussed in this chapter are used in the treatment of shock, and one class can contribute to its occurrence. **Shock** is a pathological state characterized by marked hypotension, decreased venous return, and decreased cardiac output. Common types of shock include (1) **cardiogenic shock** caused by cardiac arrest (see Chapter 37); (2) **hypovolemic shock,** caused by hemorrhage, burns, or dehydration (see Chapter 42); (3) **endotoxic** (or septic) **shock,** usually caused by gram-negative bacteria, but less commonly by gram-positive organisms; (4) **neurogenic shock,** caused by damage to or pharmacological blockade of sympathetic efferents to blood vessels; (5) and **anaphylactic shock,** caused by histamine release in type 1 allergic reactions (see Chapter 50). The last three of these shock etiologies (sepsis, neurovasodepression, and anaphylaxis) all produce a relative hypovolemia by promoting pooling or sequestration of blood in one body fluid compartment at the expense of the other compartments.

Regardless of the etiology, certain features are common in all cases of shock. Hypotension and diminished cardiac output trigger compensatory release of catecholamines, which produce peripheral vasoconstriction in order to shunt blood flow to the most vital organs — the heart and the brain. This results in a marked impairment of perfusion of viscero-cutaneous tissues, leading to hypoxia, ischemia, and reduced availability of nutrients to these tissues. The skin becomes cool and pale and may develop a grayish tinge as a result of stasis of blood in the capillaries. As tissue hypoxia proceeds, perfusion of the kidneys is drastically reduced and viscero-cutaneous tissues are obliged to rely on anaerobic metabolism. The lactic acid produced as the end-product of anaerobic metabolism accumulates because of the poor tissue perfusion, resulting in metabolic acidosis. Respiration increases in response to CO_2 accumulation, but this usually does not fully compensate for the metabolic acidosis. If the shock sequence reaches the stage of severe lactic acidosis, it tends to become self-perpetuating without vigorous clinical intervention, and death may ensue from respiratory distress or vasomotor collapse.

Certain clients are especially vulnerable to shock. These include clients with myocardial infarction, dehydration, infection, trauma (physical or emotional), and recent surgery. How long a client is in shock is important to his or her survival. *Astute nursing observations and accurate assessments are important in early detection of shock or impending shock and require understanding of the signs and symptoms of shock, such as a decrease in urinary output below 30 ml per hour.* When shock is prolonged, renal damage results. If a client develops anuria, it is an indication that the shock condition is severe. Urinary specific gravity, a measure of osmolarity, is another important indicator. Urine sodium concentration falls and osmolarity increases just prior to a reduction in the volume of urine.

Clients in shock appear restless and anxious in the early stages and may "feel funny" but are unable to be more specific. The client's level of consciousness, drowsiness, and disorientation must be assessed. Gradually, as shock progresses, the client becomes apathetic, although he or she may be more aware of the environment than is apparent.

Signs and symptoms of shock change depending on the client's stage of shock and the effectiveness of his or her compensatory mechanisms. *Nurses should evaluate arterial pressure, skin color, respiratory function, renal function, presence of sweating and whether the client has hot, dry skin, a thready pulse, intense thirst, rapid respiration, restlessness, or, by contrast, torpor or apathy.*

Treatment of Shock

The most vital step in treating shock other than cardiogenic shock is fluid administration, especially if the patient is hypovolemic. This measure increases blood flow through congested areas, dilutes serum catecholamines responsible for tachycardia and tissue ischemia, improves myocardial function, reduces risks of intravascular clotting, and improves cellular metabolism. The amount of fluid administered is determined by monitoring the response via blood pressure, heart rate, and urinary output. Fluid replacement may also help to correct acid-base and electrolyte imbalances. Another useful measure is administration of oxygen to reverse tissue hypoxia and decrease hyperventilation.

Drugs used in shock are varied. **Antibiotics** are used in septic shock to treat the underlying disorder but are also used as prophylaxis against infectious complications in other forms of shock. **Inotropic agents** (β_1-agonists such as dopamine) are most useful in cardiogenic shock but may be employed whenever cardiac output is inadequate. Dopamine is most often the first inotropic drug chosen for use in shock because it increases contractility of the myocardium while at the same time causing vasodilation of the renal and mesenteric veins. Dopamine increases the rate of glomerular filtration and the excretion of sodium. *Nurses need to monitor urinary output hourly for clients given dopamine. A decrease in output following an initial increase may indicate impaired renal blood flow from the vasoconstrictor effect of the drug. Nurses need to observe and report decreases in pulse pressure that occur dispropor-*

tionately to a rise in diastolic pressure as this may indicate too much vasoconstriction. With large doses of dopamine, there may be a decrease in renal blood flow and decreased urinary output. If this occurs, the dosage will need to be decreased.

Somewhat paradoxically, both vasopressors and vasodilators are used in management of shock. **Vasopressors** (α-agonists) help to raise blood pressure but are potentially dangerous because they can aggravate ischemia in viscero-cutaneous tissue, an important element in the pathology of shock. Their use must be limited to shock conditions in which ischemia and lactic acidosis is minimal, as a means of restoring coronary and cerebral blood flow. Although **vasodilators** (alpha-blockers) may appear to be of little use in shock because they can aggravate the already dangerously severe hypotension, they are an invaluable aid in improving perfusion of ischemic tissues. However, vasodilators must not be administered until after blood pressure has been substantially restored by fluid administration.

Corticosteroids are sometimes employed in shock to normalize permeability of cell and capillary membranes. After recovery of normal hemodynamics, **diuretics** can be administered to restore adequate urine output. In prolonged shock, an **anticoagulant** (heparin) may be required to reduce the risk or treat the occurrence of intravascular hypercoagulability.

The goals of nursing therapy for shock are to correct the underlying cause of shock, maintain maximum oxygenation of the tissues, and to increase tissue perfusion. Unnecessary moving of the individual can be detrimental to recovery. When caring for the patient in shock, nursing activities should be conducted quietly and calmly to allay fears and anxieties. The nurse should explain all therapy measures to the patient; the explanations need not be long but should be enough to reassure the person of the appropriateness of the therapy being used.

Meticulous aseptic technique must be maintained at all times since anyone in shock has an impaired immune system and is especially susceptible to infection.

Case Study: Shock

Mrs. R., a 72-year-old Caucasian, was brought to the emergency room by her daughter. She was disoriented and complained of abdominal pains and dysuria. The daughter said that her mother had a recent history of urinary tract infections and had experienced a recurrence of similar symptoms (pain on urination, flu-like symptoms) during the past 5 days. That morning, the mother had been unable to talk coherently.

In the emergency room the nurse checked vital signs: blood pressure was 75/50, pulse 115/minute, oral temperature 101°F, respirations 36/minute. The patient's skin was cold to the touch, pale, and lacking in turgor. Chest auscultations revealed no indication of pulmonary congestion. Mrs. R. was noted to be of normal height and only slightly overweight. The nurse concluded from assessment that the client exhibited hyperventilation, tachycardia, and delirium and was a likely candidate for septic shock.

The physician was notified immediately and started an IV infusion of 5% dextrose in water, allowing it to run rapidly. A unit of plasma was also ordered. Oxygen was administered to improve oxygenation. Laboratory tests were initiated to determine complete blood cell count and hemoglobin. A urine sample was obtained for culture.

In the meantime, the nurse reviewed Mrs. R.'s medical history and found that she had been previously treated for a urinary tract infection with sulfisoxazole (Gantrisin). The client was begun on gentamicin (Garamycin), an antibiotic. After blood pressure was elevated by volume expansion to 100/70, Mrs. R. was given an infusion of phentolamine (Regitine), an alpha-blocker, IV, over 5 minutes.

1. What observations support the nurse's assessment of probable septic shock?
2. Why did the physician order infusion of fluids?
3. Since the patient is obviously hypotensive, why wasn't an order given for a pressor drug such as phenylephrine?
4. Why was an alpha-blocker given?
5. Why did the physician wait until after fluid administration had produced some improvement in blood pressure before giving phentolamine?
6. Why was phentolamine given slowly?

Answers appear at the end of the book.

Recommended Readings

Ahlquist RP: A study of adrenotropic receptors. *Am J Physiol* 1948;153:586–600.

Barrows JJ: Shock demands drugs. *Nursing* 1982;12(2):34–41.

Empey DW, Medder KT: Nasal decongestants. *Drugs* 1981;21:438–443.

Lefkowitz RJ: Direct binding studies of adrenergic receptors: Biochemical, physiological, and clinical implications. *Ann Intern Med* 1979;91:450–458.

Lefkowitz RJ, Caron MG, Stiles GL: Mechanisms of membrane receptor regulation. Biochemical, physiological, and clinical insights derived from studies of the adrenergic receptors. *N Engl J Med* 1984;310:1570–1579.

Johnson GP, Johnson BC: Beta blockers. *Am J Nurs* 1983;83:1034–1043.

Moyer JH et al: Vasopressor agents in shock. *Am J Nurs* 1975;75:620–625.

Perry AG, Potter PA: *Shock: Comprehensive Nursing Management,* ed 2. St Louis, CV Mosby, 1985.

Ram C: Clinical application of beta adrenergic blocking drugs: A growing spectrum. *Heart Lung* 1979;8:116–123.

Rice V: Shock management, Part II: Pharmacologic intervention. *Crit Care Nurse* 1985;5(1):42–57.

Rivera-Calimlim L: A short review of adrenergic drug therapy. *Nurses' Drug Alert* 1981;5:25–27.

Rosenberg J, Kirschenbaum H: Alpha-adrenergic blockers. *RN* 1983;13:46–47.

Smith-Collins A: Dubutamine, a new inotropic agent. *Nursing* 1980;10(3):62–66.

Szekeres L (ed): *Adrenergic Activators and Inhibitors. Handbook of Experimental Pharmacology.* vol 54, Pts. 1 & 2. Berlin, Springer-Verlag, 1980, 1981.

CHAPTER 29

Cholinergic and Anticholinergic Drugs

Acetylcholine (ACH) is released from preganglionic parasympathetic terminals, from postganglionic parasympathetic nerve endings, from somatic efferents at the neuromuscular synapses, and from a minority of postganglionic sympathetic terminals. From the point of view of pharmacology, these cholinergic synapses are classified into three categories: **nicotinic** receptors (cholinergic receptors at both sympathetic and parasympathetic ganglia), **muscarinic** sites (cholinergic receptors at all postganglionic parasympathetic synapses and the small number of cholinergic postganglionic sympathetic synapses), and **neuromuscular** synapses of the somatic nervous system. Most cholinomimetic drugs are rather nonselective, mimicking the effects of acetylcholine at all types of cholinergic synapses, although some choline esters (such as methacholine) are more specific. By contrast, cholinergic blockers are usually specific for one type of cholinergic synapse or another and are classified as antimuscarinic drugs, antinicotinic drugs (ganglionic blockers), or neuromuscular blockers.

Cholinergic Transmission

Five stages occur in cholinergic transmission (Figure 29–1): synthesis, storage, release, transmitter/receptor interactions, and inactivation. The synthesis of ACH occurs in a single step: acetylation of choline. Choline is actively accumulated by cholinergic nerve terminals from the extracellular fluid, much of it being derived from breakdown of previously released ACH. Acetylation occurs within the cytoplasm and requires acetylcoenzyme A as a donor of the ace-

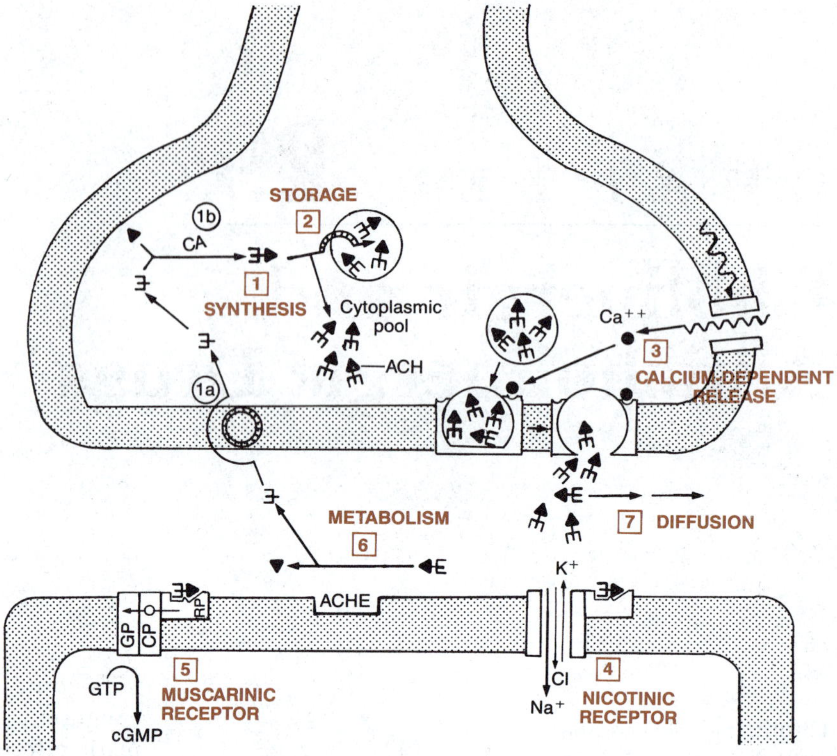

Figure 29–1
Cholinergic synapse. (1) Synthesis of acetylcholine (ACH), including (1a) choline uptake and (1b) acetylation of choline by choline acetylase (CA); (2) storage in vesicles; (3) calcium-dependent release; (4) interaction with a nicotinic receptor); (5) interaction with a muscarinic receptor linked by a coupling protein (CP) with guanadyl cyclase (GC), which catalyzes formation of cyclic-guanadyl monophosphate (cGMP) from guanadyl triphosphate (GTP); and (6) hydrolysis of ACH by acetylcholinesterase (ACHE).

tate group. Acetylcoenzyme A is readily available since it is an intermediate in the metabolism of glucose. Acetylation of choline is catalyzed by the enzyme choline acetyltransferase.

Within the nerve terminal, ACH is mainly sequestered in storage vesicles, although some remains in the cytoplasm. Small amounts of ACH are periodically released spontaneously but most ACH remains stored within the synaptic vesicles until released by arrival of a nerve impulse. Under the influence of calcium (which enters during nerve cell depolarization), the ACH-containing vesicles fuse with the presynaptic cell membrane and release their complement of ACH by exocytosis into the synapse.

After release, ACH diffuses freely through the extracellular fluid and interacts with the postsynaptic cholinergic receptors. After activation, the receptor becomes refractory for a brief period during which it is not susceptible to further activation. Thus, termination of the effect does not necessarily require removal of ACH from the synapse. A subsequent regenerative process reactivates the receptor.

In the meantime, released ACH undergoes inactivation by diffusion and metabolic degradation. Enzymatic destruction of ACH is especially important because ACH cannot be taken up by presynaptic terminals. Enzymatic degradation of ACH is carried out by two broad categories of cholinesterases: **acetylcholinesterase** (ACHE) and **pseudocholinesterase.** A number of drugs increase ACH levels by inhibiting ACHE. Most ACHE activity is localized on the surface of postsynaptic nerve cell membranes.

Although ACH itself activates all types of cholinergic receptors, the drug muscarine stimulates only one type (muscarinic), while the drug nicotine stimulates another type (nicotinic). Additional drugs, mainly antagonists, have been developed with specificity for one or the other class of cholinergic receptors. Neuromuscular receptors, classified in some textbooks with the ganglionic receptors as nicotinic, are sufficiently distinctive in drug affinities to warrant separate consideration. ACH given as a drug can stimulate all types of cholinergic receptors innervated by cholinergic neurons of the peripheral nervous system, but it can also produce direct effects on vascular smooth muscle through muscarinic-type receptors that are not associated with peripheral nervous system terminals.

Nicotinic Receptors

Nicotinic receptors consist of circular clusters of protein subunits. The nicotinic receptor is simpler in design than many of the receptor complexes for neurotransmitters and hormones because it serves as both a receptor and an effector that influences the target cell. ACH binds directly to the receptors, causing them to dilate and create sodium channels. The resultant influx of sodium causes a rapid excitatory postsynaptic potential that promotes depolarization of the postsynaptic cells.

Since peripheral nicotinic receptors are located in the efferent projection pathways of both the sympathetic and parasympathetic systems, a complete disruption of transmission at autonomic ganglia by blockade of nicotinic receptors will eliminate all autonomic regulation of tissue function. The effect on specific tissues depends on the predominance of sympathetic versus parasympathetic influences in that tissue. For example, in the vasculature, where sympathetic tone is more influential than parasympathetic activity, the effect of nicotinic antagonists is vasodilation of both arterioles and veins, while the effect of nicotinic agonists is constriction. Cardiac output usually declines when nicotinic receptors are blocked because of the loss of sympathetic tone that normally enhances contractility. On the other hand, parasympathetic influence is dominant in heart rate, intestinal motility, activity of salivary glands, and bladder tone, so that nicotinic antagonists cause tachycardia, constipation, dry mouth, and urinary retention. In the eye, parasympathetic inputs are stronger than sympathetic influences, so blockade of nicotinic receptors causes mydriasis and cycloplegia (paralysis of accommodation).

Nicotinic receptors have the unusual characteristic of being subject to two distinct kinds of blockade: the competitive kind of blockade that occurs at all types of receptors and the depolarization blockade that occurs uniquely at nicotinic and neuromuscular receptors. Depolarization blockage involves a failure of the receptor to regenerate to the excitable state after initial activation.

Muscarinic Receptors

The most direct effect of activating muscarinic receptors is the production of arachidonic acid and lysophospholipids from membrane phospholipids (phosphatidylinositol and polyphosphoinositides). Arachidonic acid is converted to hydroperoxide metabolites, which stimulate formation of guanasine 3′:5′ cyclic phosphate (cyclic GMP), which then serves as a second messenger in carrying out the cellular effects. One frequent end result of activating muscarinic receptors is a slow change in the cell's polarity. In some tissues the effect is a slow depolarization; in others a slow hyperpolarization.

At the tissue level, the physiological effects associated with muscarinic receptors are largely the same as the influences of the parasympathetic nervous system, with the addition of the small number of sympathetic effects (sweating and dilation of blood vessels in skeletal muscles) that are produced by cholinergic postganglionic sympathetic fibers. Thus, the principal effects associated with activation of muscarinic receptors occur in the (1) eye (miosis and accommodation for near vision), (2) exocrine glands (lacrimation, sweating, salivation; and stimulation of bronchial, nasopharyngeal, pancreatic, and gastrointestinal secretions), (3) visceral smooth muscle (contraction of bronchial smooth muscle, detrussor muscle, and gall bladder ducts; increased intestinal motility and tone), and (4) cardiac tissue (decreased automaticity, and decreased conduction velocity in the atrioventricular node). The vasculature is little affected overall, but dilation is produced by muscarinic receptors in certain vascular beds (for example, in the cerebrum or skeletal muscle). Despite little cholinergic innervation of most vascular beds, whether parasympathetic or sympathetic, muscarinic receptors are found in virtually all vascular smooth muscle and promote dilation when acetylcholine or other choline esters are administered systemically.

Neuromuscular Receptors

Neuromuscular cholinergic receptors resemble nicotinic receptors physiologically but exhibit some differences pharmacologically. These receptors, located on the external surface of the postjunctional membrane, increase permeability of the muscle fiber to sodium and potassium ions. The result is a localized excitatory postsynaptic potential (EPSP). If sufficient, the EPSP triggers an action potential that spreads along the nerve fiber, stimulating contraction. If neuromuscular receptors are persistently understimulated, whether because of pharmacological blockade or denervation, they gradually become supersensitive.

Drugs that activate cholinergic receptors at the neuromuscular junction cause muscle twitches, elevated muscle tone, and increased force of contraction of skeletal muscle. Antagonists or lack of adequate agonist activity result in flaccidity, weakness, and paralysis.

Cholinomimetics

For conditions such as glaucoma, urinary retention, or intestinal atony, stimulation of postganglionic parasympathetic sites (muscarinic sites) is of therapeutic value. For clients with myasthenia gravis, the stimulation of cholinergic receptors at the neuromuscular junction is beneficial. Stimulation of cholinergic receptors can be achieved in three ways: (1) by direct receptor activation using a cholinergic agonist; (2) by release of endogenous ACH; and (3) by inhibition of the normal metabolic degradation of ACH by cholinesterase, allowing accumulation of endogenous ACH. Drugs that act directly on cholinergic receptors are either choline esters like ACH itself or alkaloids from botanical sources.

Direct-Acting Cholinergic Stimulants

Choline Esters

Mechanisms and Effects ACH itself has little therapeutic value because it is rapidly hydrolyzed by acetylcholinesterase and by pseudocholinesterase. In addition, ACH lacks selectivity, stimulating muscarinic, nicotinic, and neuromuscular receptors in all tissues (Table 29–1). Its only unique characteristic is its inability, as a polar compound, to penetrate the blood-brain barrier. After intravenous administration, ACH produces a pronounced slowing of heart rate or even a transient cessation of the cardiac beat and a marked drop in blood pressure due to widespread vasodilation. The action typically lasts less than 1 minute.

Table 29–1
Comparative Action of Various Cholinomimetics and Cholinolytics

Class	Drug	Muscarinic actions: Heart	Muscarinic actions: Visceral smooth muscle	Muscarinic actions: Eye	Muscarinic actions: Glands	Muscarinic actions: Vascular smooth muscle	Nicotinic action	Neuromuscular action	CNS action
Choline esters	Acetylcholine	++	++	+	++	+++	+	+++	0
	Bethanechol	0	+++	++	+	+/0	0	0	0
	Carbechol	+	+++	++	++	+/0	+++	+++	0
	Methacholine	+++	++	+	+	+++	+	0	0
Cholinomimetic alkaloids	Muscarine	+++	++	++	++	+++	0	0	++
	Pilocarpine	+	++	+++	++	+	+	0	++
Cholinesterase inhibitors	Quaternary ammonium compounds	+++	+++	+++	+++	0	+++	+++	0
	Physostigmine	+++	+++	+++	+++	0	+++	+++	+++
	Organophosphates	+++	+++	+++	+++	0	+++	+++	+++
Antimuscarinics	Atropine	x x	x x	x x	x x x	++	0	0	x x
	Others	x x	x x	x x	x x x	0	0	0	x x
Ganglionic blockers	Trimethaphan	0	0	0	0	0	x x x	0	0
Neuromuscular blockers									
Nondepolarizing	Curare	0	0	0	0	0	x	x x x	0
Depolarizing	Succinylcholine	0	0	0	0	0	++	x x x	0

Key: +++, maximum agonist action; ++, moderate agonist action; +, slight agonist action; +/0, little or no effect; 0, no effect; x, slight antagonist action, xx, moderate antagonist action; xxx, maximum antagonist action.

Several analogues of ACH have been developed, including bethanechol (Urecholine), carbachol (Miostat), and methacholine (Mecolyl). They are resistant to breakdown by acetylcholinesterase (especially bethanechol and carbachol) and thus have a much longer duration of action than ACH. **Bethanechol** exhibits considerable preference for muscarinic sites over nicotinic or neuromuscular receptors. Moreover, bethanechol has relatively little effect on muscarinic receptors of vascular or cardiac smooth muscle, exerting its effect mainly on visceral smooth muscle. It stimulates micturition and gastrointestinal peristalsis and as a result has proven useful for improving the tone of the urinary bladder and motility in the intestinal tract after surgery.

Carbachol is unique among the choline esters because its effect is partly due to release of endogenous ACH, which results in a substantial degree of nicotinic as well as neuromuscular activity. For this reason, clinical use of carbachol is now limited to treatment of glaucoma. Cholinomimetics produce a transient rise in intraocular pressure followed by a more prolonged decrease. Carbachol produces less miosis but more headache than pilocarpine (the most widely used cholinomimetic). Clients may develop a sudden resistance to the drug.

Methacholine differs from both bethanechol and carbachol in its greater tendency for activating the muscarinic receptors of the cardiovascular system. Methacoline duplicates all of the cardiovascular effects of ACH itself but is about 200 times more potent and many times longer acting. Methacholine mimics the vasodilatory effect of ACH on vascular beds throughout the circulatory system. It produces a negative chronotropic effect (slows the heart rate) on the sinoatrial node equivalent to that produced by ACH. It mimics the negative dromotropic action by which ACH slows the rate of conduction, shortens the duration of action potentials, and shortens the refractory period in the atrium and atrioventricular node, thereby tending to perpetuate atrial flutter or fibrillation and to produce A-V block. Finally, methacholine, like AHC, produces a modest negative inotropic effect.

Pharmacokinetics Choline esters other than ACH are employed orally for most systemic purposes but may be injected subcutaneously. Toxicity is increased and selectivity of action is diminished if choline esters are used intramuscularly or intravenously. Carbachol and ACH are also applied topically to the eye.

Clinical Indications Acetylcholine intraocular solution is used to produce a rapid, complete, and short-lasting miosis for surgical procedures involving cataracts, iridectomy, or the anterior chamber of the eye. Acetylcholine is not useful for other therapeutic purposes because of its excessively rapid hydrolysis. Bethanechol is used postoperatively and postpartum for nonobstructive urinary retention and neurogenic atony of the urinary bladder with retention (see Chapter 43). Methacholine was once employed in the treatment of paroxysmal atrial tachycardia, but it is seldom used for this purpose any more because the intensity of its effect tends to be unpredictable. Fast-acting cholinesterase inhibitors, such as edrophonium (Tensilon), are used instead to slow A-V nodal conduction so that most of the rapid atrial beats during paroxysms of atrial tachycardia die out at the A-V node and are unable to reach the ventricular conductile elements. This is called "slowing the ventricular response rate." Methacholine was reintroduced into clinical practice in 1986 as a diagnostic aid for asthma. Carbachol is employed only topically as a secondary choice for treatment of glaucoma (see Chapter 54). Clinical uses of cholinomimetics are summarized in Table 29–2.

Table 29–2
Uses of Cholinomimetic Drugs

Drug class	Uses (therapeutic, social, commercial, military)
Choline esters	Glaucoma
	Chronic open-angle
	Acute narrow-angle
	Ophthalmoscopic examination:
	To counteract mydriatics
	Urinary retention
	Neurogenic atony of the bladder
Nicotinic Agonists	Aid in discontinuing use of tobacco
	Stimulation (from use of tobacco)
Cholinesterase Inhibitors	Glaucoma
	Myasthenia gravis
	Maintenance therapy
	Diagnosis
	Antagonism of neuromuscular blockers
	Bladder atony
	Insecticides
	Chemical warfare

Adverse Effects and Contraindications Adverse effects of choline esters are exaggerations of parasympathetically mediated physiological activities. The choline esters cause symptoms of **gastrointestinal hyperactivity,** including nausea, vomiting, epigastric distress, abdominal cramps, belching, diarrhea, and flatulence. Some clients experience substernal pain and pressure. *Because of the likelihood of vomiting, subcutaneous injections of bethanechol are best given about 2 hours prior to ingestion of food. Because of the stimulatory effects on intestinal motility, these drugs are contraindicated for clients with intestinal obstruction.*

Peptic ulcers can be activated or aggravated. *Therefore, any complaint of gnawing, aching, burning, or dull epigastric pain should be investigated. If an ulcer is being aggravated, the pain is usually located in the left epigastric area, usually appears 1–2 hours after eating, and is often relieved by the ingestion of food. Before administering a choline ester, the nurse should determine whether the client has a history of peptic ulcer or any inflammatory condition of the gastrointestinal tract. If a client is taking antacids, the nurse should ask about epigastric distress.*

Because of the stimulatory effect of cholinomimetics on the bladder and urinary tract, clients may complain of sensations of **tightness in the bladder.** *Cholinomimetics should not be administered to clients with urinary obstructions such as those caused by prostate enlargement or stones.* Rupture of the bladder might result. The **activity of exocrine glands** is also consistently enhanced; thus, clients tend to sweat profusely and may exhibit increased salivation and lacrimation. Fainting, headache, flushing, transient heart block, complete cardiac arrest, or atrial fibrillation can be signs of precipitous **hypotension.** Clients with hyperthyroidism are particularly vulnerable to the cardiovascular complications of cholinomimetics. Those with a history of latent or active asthma may develop **asthmatic attacks.** Some clients suffer **visual effects** including miosis, impaired accommodation, or, more typically, inability to see clearly at a distance. *When muscarinic agonists are in use, nurses need to monitor blood pressure and observe clients for early signs of cholinergic toxicity, such as salivation, sweating, flushing, and abdominal cramps.*

When severe adverse reactions occur, atropine is an effective antagonist of the muscarinic effects of cholinomimetics. A syringe of atropine, 0.6 mg, for SC or IM injection, should be available in the event of a severe adverse reaction. Ganglionic blockers may also be employed to block nicotinic effects of carbachol, and curare can be employed for neuromuscular influences. Epinephrine may also be used as a "physiological" antagonist, since sympathetic influences on many organ systems oppose parasympathetic influences.

Drug Interactions *Nurses who administer systemic cholinomimetic agents need to give special attention to the possibility of drug interactions.* Choline esters may antagonize the actions of quinidine and procainamide, and some cholinomimetic drugs are potentiated by cholinesterase inhibitors. Clients who are taking a ganglionic blocking agent may have a critical fall in blood pressure if given a cholinomimetic agent as well. *Nurses need to teach clients how to identify drugs that have the potential for interacting with prescribed cholinomimetics.* Carbachol, which is used only topically, has no established food or drug interactions.

Preparations and Administration *Acetylcholine chloride intraocular solutions should not be prepared until immediately prior to use since aqueous solutions are unstable. Solutions not used should be discarded immediately.*

When bethanechol is used for clients with urinary problems, nurses need to be certain clients are placed on intake and output monitoring. When it is used for gastrointestinal atony, nurses need to monitor for bowel sounds. Bethanechol is discussed further in Chapter 43.

Acetylcholine Chloride (Miochol)
Intraocular solution
Recommended Doses: For miosis, 0.5–2.0 ml.

Bethanechol (Urecholine, Uralax, Duvoid, Mictrol, Myotonachol, Vesicholine)
Tablets, injection solution
Recommended Doses: 10–50 mg orally, 2–4 times a day, up to 120 mg daily; or 5–10 mg SC initially, repeated at 15- to 30-minute intervals until a satisfactory response is obtained or until disturbing side effects occur. Doses as low as 2.5 mg SC may be effective, but doses as high as 10 mg are sometimes required.

Carbachol (Miostat)
Ophthalmic injection solution, ophthalmic topical solutions
Recommended Doses: For instillation into the anterior chamber to produce miosis before or after securing sutures during ocular surgery, 1 or 2 drops. For topical application to the eye in glaucoma, 1 or 2 drops instilled into the eyes 2 or 3 times daily. Usually it is necessary to add a wetting agent (benzalkonium) to carbachol solutions in order to achieve adequate corneal penetration.

Methacholine (Provocholine)
Powder for reconstitution and nebulization
Recommended Doses: An ascending series of concentrations are employed. At each concentration, the subject is administered 5 breaths by nebulizer.

Cholinomimetic Alkaloids

Three natural alkaloids have cholinomimetic actions that are largely muscarinic: **pilocarpine, are-**

choline, and **muscarine.** The last of these is especially selective for muscarinic receptors, and the drug has lent its name to this class of receptors. Muscarine is found in certain species of mushrooms, including *Amanita muscaria.* Arecholine is found in betel nuts, which have been used for thousands of years by natives of the East Indies for their euphoriant effect. Pilocarpine is extracted from the leaflets of the genus *Pilocarpus* that grows in South America. All three drugs are valuable research drugs, but only pilocarpine is used in therapeutic practice. The cholinomimetic alkaloids differ from the choline esters in having a much greater effect on the central nervous system.

Mechanisms and Effects Pilocarpine acts directly on muscarinic receptors; those controlling the sweat glands are especially sensitive. The drug also has unexplained effects on the cardiovascular system. Normally, it produces a slight and brief hypotensive action somewhat like that produced by bethanechol or carbachol. Muscarinic blockers prevent this effect, but nicotinic blockers taken concurrently convert pilocarpine's action to a pressor effect that can be antagonized by alpha-adrenergic blockers.

Applied to the eye, it causes effects like the choline esters: miosis, impaired accommodation, and a transient rise in intraocular pressure, followed by a persistent drop in intraocular pressure. Injected subcutaneously, pilocarpine causes effects similar to choline esters, but the degree of stimulation of sweating is remarkable, and individuals have been observed to lose 3 liters of sweat following a single injection. Gastric, salivary, pancreatic, and nasopharyngeal glands are stimulated, blood pressure drops, and the heart slows. In contrast to choline esters, which have little central nervous system activity, the cholinomimetic alkaloids cause a CNS activation that resembles activity of the reticular system, producing beta-waves in the electroencephalogram, orienting reactions, and externalization of attention. In extreme doses, as in mushroom poisoning, adverse psychological reactions may include hallucinations, delirium, restlessness, ataxia, and irritability.

Clinical Indications Pilocarpine is used topically for treatment of glaucoma. Pilocarpine is the drug preferred for treating and maintaining therapy of open-angle glaucoma, because it generally controls intraocular pressure with relatively few undesirable effects.

Adverse Effects and Contraindications Long-acting miotics such as pilocarpine may cause pupillary block, local irritation and burning, vascular congestion, and a forward movement of the lens of the eye. Pilocarpine can increase the risk of hemorrhage during ocular surgery.

Preparations and Administration In the form of drops, pilocarpine is applied 6 times daily for glaucoma, but the miotic effect tends to be longer in duration (up to a day) and the fixation of the lens shorter in duration (up to 2 hours) than the effect on intraocular pressure. The use of pilocarpine for glaucoma is discussed in detail in Chapter 54.

Pilocarpine
Ophthalmic solutions (usually as the hydrochloride salt, less commonly as the nitrate); combinations with epinephrine; long-acting ocular therapeutic system (Ocusert) described in Chapter 54

Indirect-Acting Cholinomimetics

Cholinesterase inhibitors can stimulate cholinergic receptors indirectly by preventing the breakdown of endogenous ACH by acetylcholinesterase (ACHE). Their pharmacology is essentially that of endogenous ACH. Cholinesterase inhibitors enhance activity at all classes of cholinergic receptors where there is associated cholinergic innervation: muscarinic sites receiving postganglionic parasympathetic innervation, nicotinic sites receiving preganglionic parasympathetic or sympathetic fibers, and neuromuscular receptors receiving somatic efferents. Cholinergic receptors in most vascular beds are little affected by cholinesterase inhibitors unless ACH accumulates systemically.

Reversible and Irreversible Cholinesterase Inhibitors

Cholinesterase inhibitors can be either reversible or irreversible inhibitors, depending on duration of action. The distinction has some implications for the treatment of overdose, but the general pharmacology of the two groups is qualitatively similar.

The original and prototype drug among the **reversible cholinesterase inhibitors** is physostigmine (Eserine), a naturally occurring alkaloid obtained from the Calabar (or ordeal) bean, the seed of a perennial plant of West Africa. Physostigmine was first isolated in pure form in 1864 and was introduced into medicine in 1877 for treatment of glaucoma. In the 1920s, the mechanism of action of physostigmine was determined and additional chemicals of similar activity were developed. The reversible cholinesterase inhibitors used in medicine today are quaternary ammonium derivatives: neostigmine (Prostigmin), pyridostigmine (Mestinon, Regonol), edrophonium (Tensilon), demecarium (Humorsol), and ambenonium (Mytelase). Another related agent, carbaryl, finds use as an insecticide.

The **irreversible cholinesterase inhibitors** are **organophosphates.** Many of these compounds are commercially important as insecticides and have become, as a result, important to clinical toxicology. Parathion, for example, is a widely employed agricultural insecticide that has caused numerous accidental poisonings, usually as a result of dermal or pulmonary absorption. Other organophosphate insecticides include o-ethyl o-(4-nitrophenyl) phenylphosphonothioate (EPN), malathion, and octamethyl pyrophosphoramide (OMPA). Parathion and OMPA are inert until converted into active metabolites in the body. Organophosphate inhibitors of cholinesterase have limited use in medicine, but two of them, isoflurophate and echothiophate, are useful in cases of glaucoma that are refractory to conventional drug treatments. Several organophosphate cholinesterase inhibitors of exceptional potency have been developed for use in chemical warfare. These so-called nerve gases, including tabun, sarin, and soman, are among the most potent toxins known.

Mechanisms and Effects Cholinesterase has two binding sites involved in ACH metabolism (Figure 29–2). The anionic site binds the ACH while the esteratic site donates electrons to hydrolyze the ACH into acetate and choline. When ACH is the substrate, hydrolysis occurs rapidly, yielding acetic acid, choline, and regenerated ACHE. Inhibitors of ACHE bind at one or both sites to prevent ACHE from operating on ACH. Reversible inhibitors, such as physostigmine, attach at both sites and are themselves slowly hydrolyzed. Edrophonium is hydrolyzed nearly as rapidly as ACH itself and as a result has a short duration of action. Irreversible inhibitors, the organophosphates, bind at the anionic site only and dissociate from the ACHE at a negligible rate. Cholinesterase activity returns only after the inactivated ACHE is replaced by synthesis of new enzyme.

The effects of cholinesterase inhibitors attributable to inhibition of ACHE include effects at all classes of cholinergic receptors that receive neural innervation. Physiological activities stimulated by muscarinic receptors are consistently enhanced. The secretory glands are stimulated, smooth muscle fibers are constricted (in the bronchioles, uterus, bladder, and intestine), the pupil of the eye is constricted, and heart rate slows. Nicotinic and neuromuscular transmission are initially enhanced, but at sufficiently high doses of cholinesterase inhibitors, stimulation may give way to depolarization blockade when ACH accumulates to a critical level. The quaternary ammonium compounds do not effectively cross the blood-brain barrier and have minimal CNS

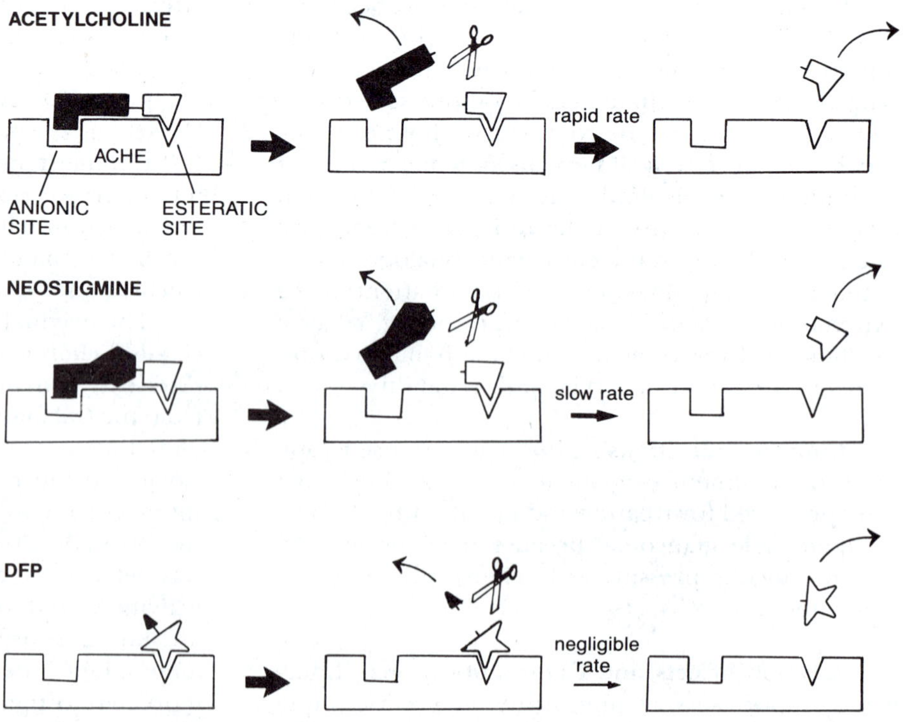

Figure 29–2
Interactions of acetylcholinesterase (ACHE) with the natural substate, acetylcholine (top), a reversible inhibitor, neostigmine (middle), and an irreversible inhibitor, DFP (bottom). Acetylcholine is readily hydrolyzed by ACHE and quickly dissociates, regenerating the enzyme. Neostigmine is hydrolyzed in a manner similar to acetylcholine but dissociates only slowly. DFP binds to the esteratic pocket rather than the anionic pocket and dissociates from the enzyme at a negligible rate.

activity. Physostigmine and the organophosphates, on the other hand, have substantial CNS effects.

Many of the cholinesterase inhibitors exert direct agonist effects on cholinergic receptors in addition to elevating ACH availability in the various cholinergic synapses. Physostigmine is an exception, acting virtually exclusively through inhibition of cholinesterase.

Pharmacokinetics Most of the reversible cholinesterase inhibitors do not penetrate cell membranes effectively. They are, therefore, poorly absorbed after oral administration, requiring doses many times the parenterally effective doses. They also do not cross the blood-brain barrier and thus have no significant CNS influences. By contrast physostigmine and especially the organophosphates are well absorbed from the intestines. Organophosphates have high lipid solubility and thus cross the blood-brain barrier and are well absorbed by all routes, including through the skin after dermal contact and through the lungs after inhalation of mist or dust.

Clinical Indications Cholinesterase inhibitors are useful clinically for certain diseases related to the eye, the intestinal tract and the bladder, the neuromuscular junction, the heart, and for antagonism of certain other drugs (Table 29-2). Anticholinesterase drugs constrict the pupil of the eye by stimulating the sphincter muscle of the iris, an effect that may last up to one day. The ciliary muscle is also stimulated, causing a spasm of accommodation; focus becomes fixed for near vision. This effect typically subsides more rapidly than the miosis, disappearing in just a few hours. Cholinesterase inhibitors stimulate outflow of aqueous humor, lowering intraocular pressure, and are indicated for use in **glaucoma** because of the favorable effect on intraocular pressure. They are helpful primarily in management of chronic open-angle glaucoma, alone or in combination with cholinomimetics such as pilocarpine. Cholinesterase inhibitors employed in glaucoma include both reversible agents (physostigmine and demecarium) and irreversible agents (echothiophate and isoflurophate). The latter agents have the advantage of longer duration of action and less frequent administration (once or twice daily), but are used only when glaucoma cannot be controlled by other agents because of risks of cataracts and neurotoxicity. The use of these drugs in treatment of glaucoma is discussed more fully in Chapter 54.

Cholinesterase inhibitors stimulate secretory activity throughout the gastrointestinal system and motility in the small and large intestines and the bowel especially. The intestinal effects involve activation of nicotinic receptors of parasympathetic ganglia as well as muscarinic receptors at postganglionic parasympathetic synapses. Neostigmine is the most widely employed of the drugs for this purpose.

Cholinesterase inhibitors are the mainstays of treatment of **myasthenia gravis,** a disease involving autoimmune attack on cholinergic receptors of the neuromuscular synapses, characterized by weakness and fatigability of the skeletal muscles. The strength of initial contraction of skeletal muscles is often normal in myasthenia gravis, but activity cannot be sustained for more than very brief periods. Cholinesterase inhibitors improve the response to tetanic stimulation and strengthen muscle activity in persons with myasthenia gravis. These effects do not occur in normal subjects, in whom cholinesterase inhibitors diminish the response to tetanic stimulation and cause muscle weakness and fasciculations. Cholinesterase inhibitors can also cause muscle weakness in clients with myasthenia gravis if the dose is excessive. Thus, it is apparent that optimal muscle activity requires sufficient but not excessive ACH. When ACH activity is deficient, receptors are understimulated; when it is excessive, depolarization blockade results. Titration of dose is therefore always required when treatment is initiated for myasthenia gravis.

Other clinical uses of cholinesterase inhibitors include treatment of anticholinergic toxicity and termination of curarization after anesthesia (see Drug Interactions).

Adverse Effects and Contraindications The adverse effects of anticholinesterase agents are predictable. Those related to excess muscarinic activity include gastrointestinal hyperactivity (nausea, vomiting, diarrhea, cramps), stimulation of exocrine glands (increased salivation and drooling, bronchial secretions, lacrimation, and diaphoresis), and ocular effects (miosis and spasms of accommodation). Ocular symptoms, including pain, brow ache, and miosis, are often the first signs of toxicity. Muscarinic effects can be countered by administration of atropine. *The nurse should keep atropine at hand whenever cholinesterase inhibitors are employed. In the event of severe adverse reactions or overdose, nurses should initiate artificial respiration without delay. Since many clients receiving cholinesterase inhibitors will be at home, family members need to be taught artificial respiration and when to use it.*

Blood pressure reacts highly variably to administration of cholinesterase inhibitors. Hypertensive reactions can occur as a result of stimulation of sympathetic ganglia, while hypotensive reactions and bradycardia may result from activation of muscarinic influences. Neuromuscular toxicity is manifested as fasciculations, twitches, weakness, and muscle cramps. CNS toxicity occurs only with the organophosphates and physostigmine. Symptoms include confusion, ataxia, slurred speech, and respiratory paralysis. In fatal overdoses, death usually occurs from respiratory arrest or secondary cardiovascular complications from respiratory distress, due to either central depression of the respiratory center of paralysis of respiratory muscles.

Drug Interactions Cholinesterase inhibitors have significant drug interactions. The effect of cholinesterase inhibitors opposes that of curare at the neuromuscular junction. Curare can be used to alleviate toxicity of cholinesterase inhibitors such as muscle twitches, cramps, or paralysis. Conversely, short-acting cholinesterase inhibitors, such as edrophonium (Tensilon), find use in terminating the effects of competitive neuromuscular blockers at the end of a surgical procedure (a decurarizing effect). Cholinesterase inhibitors can also antagonize drugs of other classes that produce curare-like effects on the neuromuscular junction: for example, aminoglycoside antibiotics, quinidine, and propranolol. On the other hand, cholinesterase inhibitors do not antagonize depolarizing neuromuscular blockers (such as succinylcholine (Anectine), decamethonium (Syncurine), or benzoquinonium) but in fact prolong the blockade produced by such drugs. For example, hexafluorenium (Mylaxen) has been used in conjunction with succinylcholine to prolong the duration of muscle relaxation from about 5 minutes to about 20–30 minutes and to eliminate succinylcholine-induced muscle fasciculations. Two milligrams of hexafluorenium are given for each milligram of succinylcholine employed.

Cholinesterase inhibitors can also be employed to good benefit when intoxication occurs from use of anticholinergic drugs (such as many neuroleptics, most antidepressants, and many antihistamines) or from ingesting certain plants. Physostigmine is an effective antidote for such symptoms. Since many of the symptoms of the anticholinergic syndrome are of CNS origin, physostigmine, which crosses the blood-brain barrier, is preferable to the quaternary ammonium compounds, which do not enter the brain. *When a cholinesterase inhibitor is used to reverse anticholinergic toxicity, the nurse should carefully monitor the state of consciousness of the client for recurrence of symptoms, since the effects of short-acting anticholinesterase drugs such as physostigmine may wear off before the toxicity of anticholinergic substances, causing the client to lapse into delirium and coma after initial improvement.*

Preparations and Administration The drugs used for treatment of myasthenia gravis are neostigmine, pyridostigmine, and ambenonium. After initial dosage titration, most patients will learn to adjust doses in relation to changing requirements. Among the factors that alter dosage requirements are changes in physical activity level, emotional stress, infections, menstruation, and the exacerbations and remissions that are inherent in the disease itself.

Dosage titration can be conducted using either an oral method or a more rapid intravenous procedure. In each method, a series of increasing doses of a cholinesterase inhibitor is administered at appropriate intervals (1 hour or more is required between doses in the oral method; a few minutes in the intravenous test). After each dose, strength is tested in various muscle groups by grip strength and vital capacity of respiration. Neostigmine and pyridostigmine are usually employed as the test agents. The procedure continues until the optimal dosage is determined.

Lack of improvement in myasthenia gravis can result from either underdosage or overdosage. Overdosage may cause cholinergic crisis characterized by increasing muscle weakness and difficult respiration. Increasing the dosage of neostigmine in a cholinergic crisis could have serious consequences. When the client is in myasthenia crisis, however, there may be need for more intensive anticholinesterase treatment. Edrophonium (Tensilon) may be administered to differentiate between the two states. If the client is in cholinergic crisis, he or she should be promptly withdrawn from the drug, and atropine should be used to eliminate or reduce the gastrointestinal side effects or other muscarinic reactions. If muscle strength improves after edrophonium has been administered, it indicates that the client has received inadequate medication rather than too much. When edrophonium is used, there should always be provisions for endotracheal intubation and oxygen.

Endrophonium, the shortest-acting cholinesterase inhibitor, is also used as a diagnostic test for differentiating cases of myasthenia gravis from similarly appearing neuromuscular diseases. Myasthenia gravis is the only neuromuscular disorder that responds to cholinesterase inhibition. Edrophonium has also largely supplanted methacholine for use in terminating attacks of paroxysmal supraventricular tachycardia.

Ambenonium (Mytelase)
Tablets
Recommended Doses: For myasthenia gravis, 15–200 mg PO daily in divided doses at intervals of 3–6 hours.

Edrophonium (Tensilon)
Injection Solution
Recommended Doses: For curare antagonism, 10 mg IV, slowly over 30–45 seconds, repeated as necessary up to 40 mg.

Neostigmine (Prostigmin and generic formulations)
Tablets, injection solutions
Recommended Doses: For myasthenia gravis, 15–375 mg/day PO, in divided doses at intervals of 2–3 hours. For myasthenia crisis, 0.5 mg, SC or IM, when clients have difficulty swallowing and breathing. For prevention and treatment of postoperative distention of the bladder and urinary retention, 1 ml of a 1:4,000 solution (for prophylaxis) or a 1:2,000 solution (for treatment), SC or IM.

Pyridostigmine (Mestinon and Regonol)
Tablets, syrup, sustained release tablet, injection solution
Recommended Doses: For myasthenia gravis, 60–1,500 mg/day PO (600 mg/day is average) in divided doses at intervals of 3–6 hours. Sustained release tablets should be employed only at bedtime. For myasthenia crisis or supplementation of the oral dose, one-thirtieth the client's established oral dose.

Cholinesterase Reactivators

Organophosphate inhibitors of acetylcholinesterase normally dissociate from the enzyme at negligible rates if at all. The rate of dissociation can sometimes be substantially increased by administration of a cholinesterase reactivator, thus providing antidotal therapy for toxicity caused by organophosphates encountered as insecticides or in chemical warfare. The prototype drug of this family is **pralidoxime** (Protopam and generic), also called **2-PAM.** Pralidoxime increases the rate of hydrolysis of organophosphate-cholinesterase complexes more than a million times. Newer entries into the group, available in Europe, are even more effective and include obidoxime (Toxogonin), trimedoxime, and diacetyl monoxime.

The effectiveness of cholinesterase reactivators depends on how rapidly they are given following absorption of the organophosphate agent. The complex formed between organophosphates and acetylcholinesterase undergoes a process called "aging" in which the bonds (relatively stable under the best of circumstances) become increasingly stable over the course of the first few minutes to hours.

Pralidoxime is not helpful in reversing toxicity caused by reversible cholinesterase inhibitors and are contraindicated for use in overdoses involving physostigmine or quaternary ammonium cholinesterase inhibitors because it has a weak anticholinesterase action of its own.

Treatment for organophosphate poisoning is conducted in the hospital. In addition to atropine and pralidoxime, equipment for artificial respiration, tracheostomy, gastric lavage, and electrocardiographic monitoring should be on hand. Oxygen and an anticonvulsant such as diazepam (Valium) or sodium thiopental (Pentothal) should also be available. During treatment, the nurse should closely monitor the client for changes in muscle strength, incidence of muscle twitches, adequacy of respiration, changes in mental status, or heart rate.

Drugs Altering ACH Release

The action of carbachol (Miostat) is partly related to release of acetylcholine from endogenous stores, in addition to its direct effects on cholinergic receptors. The drug **guanidine** acts exclusively by altering release of ACH, apparently increasing the amount of ACH released in response to each action potential.

Clinical Indications Guanidine is indicated for treatment of muscle weakness associated with the myasthenic syndrome of Eaton-Lambert, but is not used in myasthenia gravis.

Adverse Effects and Contraindications Guanidine is more toxic than cholinesterase inhibitors. The major problem is bone marrow suppression, which can cause anemia, leukopenia, and thrombocytopenia. Clients with symptoms of leukopenia typically complain of sore throat and persistent fever. Gastrointestinal symptoms include anorexia, nausea, diarrhea, and abdominal cramps. A variety of other adverse effects occurring with guanidine are not typical of cholinomimetics. These include skin eruptions (rash, folliculitis, purpura, petechiae) and dry skin; impaired renal function, including creatinine retention, chronic interstitial nephritis, and renal tubular necrosis; and cardiac dysrhythmias, including tachycardia, palpitations, and atrial fibrillation. Neurological side effects that clients are likely to complain about include paresthesias, nervousness, irritability, lightheadedness, and tremor. The client may develop an ataxic gait or appear moody or mentally confused, and there may be incidents of hallucinations and other psychotic symptoms.

Preparations and Administration

Guanidine
Tablets
Recommended Doses: 10–15 mg/kg/day PO initially in 3 or 4 divided doses, gradually raised as required to a maximum of 35 mg/kg/day.

Ganglionic Stimulants

Nicotine is a nearly unique cholinomimetic because of its selective agonist action on nicotinic receptors of autonomic ganglia and the CNS. Another natural alkaloid, lobeline (Bantron), has a similar activity spectrum but is less potent. At high doses nicotine can produce a depolarization blockade at ganglia, but at doses derived from smoking tobacco, both sympathetic and parasympathetic ganglia are stimulated. Cardiovascular effects (vasoconstriction, hypertension, and tachycardia) result from stimulation of sympathetic ganglia. Stimulation of parasympathetic ganglia causes gastrointestinal effects such as inhibition of hunger contractions, stimulation of motility in the colon, and increased tone and motility in the intestines. Nicotine also stimulates nicotinic receptors of the adrenal medulla, promoting release of adrenal catecholamines. Neuromuscular cholinergic receptors and several kinds of sensory receptors, including stretch receptors, pain receptors, temperature receptors, and chemoreceptors of the carotid bodies, are also activated by nicotine. The full pharmacology of nicotine, with emphasis on abuse liability of tobacco and chronic toxic effects of tobacco smoking, is discussed in Chapter 14.

Anticholinergics

Cholinergic antagonists, which are generally more selective than cholinomimetic drugs, include drugs in three groups: (1) antimuscarinic agents, (2) ganglionic blockers (antinicotinic drugs), and (3) neuromuscular blockers.

Antimuscarinic Drugs

Antimuscarinic drugs have a long history. Two of the drugs in this family, atropine and scopolamine, occur naturally in a number of plants, the best known of which is the belladonna plant (Atropa belladonna). These two natural alkaloids are thus often described as **belladonna alkaloids.** Other botanical sources of atropine and scopolamine include Jimson weed, stinkweed, thorn-apple, devil's apple, and henbane. Atropine was first purified from belladonna in 1831. Currently, atropine and scopolamine have been joined by numerous semisynthetic and synthetic antimuscarinic agents. Atropine continues to be considered the prototype of the class.

Mechanisms and Effects The two natural belladonna alkaloids exhibit a great degree of specificity for muscarinic receptors. Atropine has very little effect on nicotinic receptors and produces only a slight degree of neuromuscular blockade at even extremely high doses. Semisynthetic and synthetic antimuscarinic drugs that are quaternary ammonium compounds exhibit somewhat less specificity, producing varying degrees of nicotinic as well as muscarinic blockade. At very high doses, selectivity is still less absolute, and receptors for norepinephrine, histamine, and serotonin may be blocked as well as the muscarinic receptors.

The muscarinic receptors of various tissues are not equally sensitive to blockade by antimuscarinic drugs. Inhibitory effects occur in a predictable sequence as the dose of an antimuscarinic agent is gradually increased (Table 29–3). Inhibition of sweating, salivation, and bronchial secretions occurs most readily. Ocular effects (mydriasis, cycloplegia) and tachycardia occur next most readily, followed by inhibition of parasympathetic control of the bladder and intestines. Gastric secretions and motility are altered only at high doses of antimuscarinic drugs. The blockade of muscarinic receptors by atropine and related drugs is competitive in nature and can be overcome by elevating the concentration of ACH or other choline agonists in the vicinity of the receptor.

Antimuscarinic drugs affect both the central nervous system and the peripheral nervous system to varying degrees. Quaternary ammonium antimuscarinic drugs are essentially devoid of CNS activity, being unable to cross the blood-brain barrier. On the other hand, agents, such as benztropine (Cogentin), that are selected for use in parkinsonism are especially active in the CNS. Scopolamine has a higher central to peripheral ratio of activity than atropine. The CNS effects of antimuscarinic agents include se-

Table 29–3
Sequence of Antimuscarinic Effects

Low doses	Inhibition of salivation
	Inhibition of sweating
	Inhibition of bronchial secretions
Moderately low doses	Pupillary dilation
	Cycloplegia
	Tachycardia
Moderately high doses	Urinary retention
	Diminished intestinal tone and motility
High doses	Inhibition of motility and initial phase of gastric secretions

dation, somnolence, euphoria, amnesia, mental confusion, and suppression of dreaming sleep. Antimuscarinic drugs suppress tremor and nausea by effects on the brain.

Pharmacokinetics Belladonna alkaloids are rapidly absorbed after oral administration or from mucosal membrane surfaces. After topical application to the eye, significant systemic absorption may occur (there have been reports of severe anticholinergic reactions in children after topical application). The quaternary ammonium drugs in this family are more poorly absorbed. Typically only 10–25% of an orally administered dose reaches the blood. As noted above, the quaternary ammonium compounds do not distribute to the brain. Atropine is eliminated by renal excretion, but scopolamine is metabolized prior to renal elimination. Atropine appears in small amounts in breast milk.

Clinical Indications Clinical uses for antimuscarinic drugs are many and varied (Table 29–4). Antimuscarinic drugs were at one time widely employed in management of peptic ulcers. However, significant suppression of gastric secretions occurs only at high doses (see Table 29–3), so that it is impossible to obtain therapeutic benefit without wide-ranging adverse effects. Effects such as dryness of mouth, visual disturbances, and urinary retention always precede suppression of gastric secretions and motility. Furthermore, antimuscarinic drugs are specifically contraindicated in the many cases of peptic ulcer accompanied by pyloric obstruction because these drugs inhibit the opening of the pylorus, aggravating obstruction, and further delaying gastric emptying. The development of cimetidine, a specific antagonist at H_2-histamine receptors, contributed to the disuse of antimuscarinic drugs for ulcers.

Antimuscarinic agents (especially atropine) are frequently used as **adjunctives in general anesthesia,** suppressing the excessive salivation and bronchial secretions that often accompany general anesthesia. Reflex bradycardia from vagal activation is likewise suppressed. Antimuscarinic drugs are often said to produce "areflexia" because of this ability to inhibit both the bronchial secretory and the cardiac reflex.

Antimuscarinic drugs are used to treat **spasticity** of the intestines or the urinary bladder. Large doses are required, but can effectively reduce intestinal hypermotility or urinary frequency. Antimuscarinic drugs have been less successful for treatment of irritable colon, Salmonella dysenteries, ulcerative colitis, or regional enteritis. Urinary frequency can be reduced by antimuscarinic medications in conditions such as spastic paraplegia or functional enuresis in children, but no long-term benefit is derived. Oxybutynin chloride is an antimuscarinic agent marketed as a urinary tract antispasmodic. It is indicated for decreasing urinary frequency for clients with uninhibited or reflex neurogenic bladder.

Antimuscarinic drugs can be used successfully for conditions involving hypersecretion of exocrine glands and can suppress excessive salivation associated with heavy-metal poisoning or parkinsonism. Excess pancreatic secretions can also be suppressed. Antimuscarinic drugs are incorporated into some combination preparations for their ability to dry respiratory and nasopharyngeal secretions in the **common cold.**

Ophthalmological uses of antimuscarinic drugs are among the most important applications for this

Table 29–4
Therapeutic Uses of Cholinolytics

Drug class	Therapeutic uses
Antimuscarinics	Peptic ulcer (secondary choice)
	Antispasmodic
	Irritable bowel syndrome
	Ulcerative colitis
	Biliary spasms
	Urinary frequency or urgency
	Adjunct to anesthesia
	Parkinsonism
	Bronchial asthma (secondary choice)
	Motion sickness
	Bradycardia
	To produce mydriasis or cycloplegia
	Antagonism of cholinesterase inhibitors
Ganglionic blockers	Acute hypertensive crisis
	Induction of hypotensive states for surgery
Neuromuscular blockers	Adjunct to anesthesia
	Facilitation of tracheal intubation
	Protection from trauma during electroconvulsant shock therapy
	Facilitation of artifical respiration
	Diagnosis of myasthenia gravis

class. These drugs are widely used for inducing **mydriasis** and **cycloplegia** (paralysis of accommodation) to aid in the examination of the retina and optic disc. Antimuscarinic drugs can be used in alternation with miotics to break or prevent formation of adhesions between the lens and iris. Cycloplegia cannot be produced without mydriasis, but mydriasis can be produced alone by use of short-acting quaternary ammonium muscarinic blockers, such as cyclopentolate (Cyclogyl) or tropicamide (Mydriacyl). *Nurses should know that antimuscarinic drugs can dangerously increase intraocular pressure in clients with narrow-angle glaucoma, though it has little effect on intraocular pressure in clients with open-angle glaucoma or in normal eyes.*

The main cardiovascular effect of antimuscarinic drugs is tachycardia. Tachycardia is most evident in young individuals in whom vagal tone on the heart is substantial. Antimuscarinic drugs find use in severe **bradycardia** caused by excess vagal tone as in hypothermia, toxic sedation, or acute myocardial infarction, but there is a risk that uncontrollable tachydysrhythmias may develop. Antimuscarinic drugs can also reduce atrioventricular block when it is related to increased vagal tone. Atropine blocks vascular effects of choline esters but paradoxically may itself cause vasodilation and flushing at elevated doses.

Antimuscarinic drugs produce bronchial dilation as well as the suppression of respiratory secretions. Atropine is more effective than scopolamine as a bronchodilator and is especially good in relieving constriction due to cholinomimetics. Drugs of this family are less effective than β_2-agonists in asthma but appear to have comparable efficacy in alleviating airway constriction in chronic bronchitis. But long-term administration in chronic obstructive lung disease may produce negative effects due to inhibition of respiratory secretion.

Effects of antimuscarinic agents on the CNS can be put to therapeutic benefit in parkinsonism and motion sickness. Anticholinergics suppress the movement tremor and muscle rigidity of **parkinsonism** but have little impact on the muscle weakness or impaired mobility. Often anticholinergics are employed in combination with levodopa in parkinsonism (see Chapter 22) because of the differing benefits afforded by the two treatment approaches. Antimuscarinic drugs are also widely employed for alleviation of **extrapyramidal side effects** caused by neuroleptics. Antimuscarinic drugs find use for prophylaxis against **motion sickness** and are sometimes used for their sedative and amnesic properties to alleviate symptoms of **labor.**

Adverse Effects and Contraindications Antimuscarinic drugs produce a group of adverse effects that are collectively designated the **anticholinergic syndrome** (Table 29–5). Children and elderly people may react to even small doses of the drug. In fact, severe reactions have been observed in children after topical administration of anticholinergics to the eye, and fatalities have occurred with as little as 10 mg of atropine or scopolamine systemically. The earliest indicators of toxicity are dry mouth, inhibition of sweating (hence temperature elevation), and slight bradycardia. Clients may become either drowsy or agitated and excited. *Nurses need to be especially aware of this phenomenon if the client is receiving these drugs preoperatively, since the drug-induced agitation, added to already stressful circumstances, can have serious repercussions.*

Table 29–5
The Anticholinergic Syndrome

Organ system	Symptoms
CNS	Anxiety, agitation, restlessness, twitching, myoclonic contraction, hyperreflexia, amnesia, hallucinations, clouding of the sensorium, delirium, mania, impaired speech, impaired gait, seizures, coma, respiratory failure, circulatory collapse
Eyes	Mydriasis, photophobia, cycloplegia
Cardiovascular system	Tachycardia, vasodilation, weak pulse
Visceral smooth muscle	Urinary retention, decreased gastrointestinal motility
Exocrine glands	Decreased salivation, decreased nasopharangeal secretions, difficulty talking or swallowing, decreased sweating, hyperpyrexia, decreased bronchial secretions
Skin	Flushing, rash, desquamation
Memory aid for learning anticholinergic effects	
Dry as a bone:	Inhibition of secretions
Red as a beet:	Flushing related to absence of sweating
Hot as a hare:	Temperature elevation from absence of sweating
Blind as a bat:	Cycloplegia and mydriasis
Mad as a hatter:	Mental confusion, delirium

While dry mouth may be considered desirable during surgery, it may become a problem if it persists into the postoperative period. *Clients need to be forewarned and nurses should advise them that the problem can be alleviated by chewing gum, sucking hard candy, or taking frequent small sips of fluid. Some clients also complain of loss of taste and dysphagia. For some clients, the dryness of the mouth contributes to problems with speech.*

When clients are started on antimuscarinic agents, the normal tone and motility of smooth muscles are reduced in the gastrointestinal system, resulting in constipation, and in the urinary bladder, resulting in urinary retention. *Nurses need to note the amount and frequency of voiding to determine if there is urinary retention. In addition, nurses should ask clients whether they feel the bladder is being emptied and should palpate the area of the urinary bladder to check for distention or other evidence of urine retention. Nurses should monitor clients for bowel sounds and ask whether bowel movements occur regularly to determine if constipation is evident. Clients should be encouraged to include high-fiber foods in the diet and should be provided with a list of appropriate foods. If the problem is not countered by adjustments in diet and fluid intake, a stool softener or mild cathartic agent may have to be prescribed by the physician.*

Antimuscarinic agents produce marked dilation of the pupils (mydriasis) and paralysis of the ciliary muscles (cycloplegia). Thus the pupils do not respond to light, and the eye is unable to focus on near objects, causing blurred vision. *The discomfort of photophobia due to dilation of pupils may be alleviated somewhat by wearing sunglasses or reducing environmental light. Clients should be warned to avoid driving or other activities that require visual accuracy. Older clients need to be observed for increased intraocular pressure.*

While clinical doses of atropine do not produce marked changes in behavior, those who are especially sensitive to the drug and those given excessive doses may become restless and irritable or euphoric. Headache and fatigue occur commonly. *Clients need to be warned to avoid hazardous activities such as driving a car if they become drowsy or dizzy.*

Some anticholinergic agents contain tartrazine as a preservative. Clients who are allergic to aspirin may develop allergic responses to anticholinergic formulations containing this substance. *Nurses need to be certain to question clients about possible allergic responses to aspirin; those who are allergic should be advised to avoid taking products containing tartrazine. Clients should be advised to notify the physician immediately if they develop rash, flushing, or eye pain.*

Full toxicity is evident when tachycardia is profound, the pulse is weak, vision is very blurred, the skin is flushed, and body temperature is elevated. *The nurse should monitor the pulse of the patient when antimuscarinic drugs are initiated to guard against excessive tachycardia. When working with children and infants, nurses need to be especially alert for symptoms of atropine poisoning.* Heat prostration can occur when atropine-like drugs are given during hot weather. *The nurse should warn clients to avoid vigorous exercise or extremes of heat.* With marked anticholinergic toxicity, the client is likely to exhibit ataxia, delirium, excitement, hallucinations, and ultimately coma.

Specific contraindications for use of antimuscarinic drugs include narrow-angle glaucoma, pyloric obstruction, hypersensitivity to anticholinergic drugs, bradycardia, paralytic ileus, severe ulcerative colitis, hepatitis, obstructive uropathy, myasthenia gravis, and toxemia of pregnancy.

Drug Interactions A variety of drugs that are not specifically classified as antimuscarinic nevertheless block muscarinic receptors (Table 29–6). Tricyclic antidepressants, most neuroleptics, and meperidine are potent anticholinergics. Among the many antihistamine drugs (H_1-histamine blockers) with substantial anticholinergic activity are diphenhydramine (Benadryl), dimenhydrinate (Dramamine), and chlorpheniramine (Chlor-Trimeton). The anticholinergic properties of various drugs are additive. Toxic manifestations occur as a result of the additive influences of several such drugs more frequently than to a single anticholinergic agent. Thus the anticholinergic syndrome may occur even when no one drug is present in unusual quantity. The plants that are sources of belladonna alkaloids can also cause anticholinergic toxicity. MAO inhibitors block the metabolism of antimuscarinic drugs, potentiating their effects.

Antimuscarinic agents are useful for alleviating toxicity associated with excess stimulation of muscarinic receptors. Thus atropine finds use in alleviat-

Table 29–6
Drugs and Plants that Can Contribute to Anticholinergic Toxicity

Drugs	Plants
Antihistamines	Bittersweet
Antimuscarinic drugs	Black henbane
Antiparkinsonian drugs	Deadly nightshade
Belladonna alkaloids	Jimson weed
Neuroleptics	Jerusalem cherry
Tricyclic antidepressants	Potato leaves, sprouts, or tubers

ing symptoms of poisoning involving mushrooms, such as *Amanita muscaria,* and in antagonizing the muscarinic activity of cholinesterase inhibitors.

Antacids inhibit the absorption of anticholinergics and should not be used concurrently with oral anticholinergic drugs. Anticholinergics prolong gastric emptying time, which can slow absorption of many drugs.

Preparations and Administration A large variety of antimuscarinic preparations are available for use as gastrointestinal antispasmodics, including numerous combination preparations with sedatives such as phenobarbital, butabarbital, amobarbital, meprobamate, thiopropazate, hydroxyzine, prochlorperazine, or chlordiazepoxide. *When antimuscarinic drugs are taken orally for gastrointestinal problems, they are usually taken 30 minutes before mealtime.*

Quaternary ammonium blockers of muscarinic receptors offer no advantage over belladonna alkaloids, notwithstanding their frequent selection. Because they block nicotinic receptors, additional adverse effects (such as impotency) can occur.

Anticholinergic agents marketed for use in parkinsonism are discussed in Chapter 22. Included in this group are cycrimine HCl (Pagitane), procyclidine (Kemadrin), trihexyphenidyl HCl (Artane, Tremin, generic), benztropine (Cogentin) biperiden (Akineton), ethopropazine HCl (Parsidol), orphenadrine HCl (Disipal), chlorphenoxamine HCl (Phenoxene), and diphenhydramine (Benadryl). Ophthalmic preparations of antimuscarinic agents, which include solutions and ointments containing atropine, homatropine, cyclopentolate (Cyclogyl), and tropicamide (Mydriacyl), are discussed in Chapter 54.

BELLADONNA ALKALOIDS

Atropine
Tablets as the sulfate salt, injection solutions
Recommended Doses: For spastic conditions of the gastrointestinal tract in adults, 0.4–0.6 mg.

Belladonna
Tablets, tincture
Recommended Doses: For adults, one 15 mg tablet or 0.6–1.0 ml of the tincture, 3 times daily PO.

L-Hyoscyamine (Levsin, Anaspaz, Levamine, Cysto-Spaz)
Tablets, capsules, drops, elixir, injection solution
Recommended Doses: For adults, 0.125–0.25 mg 3 or 4 times daily, orally or sublingually; or 0.25–0.5 mg SC, IM, or IV, 3 or 4 times daily.

Levorotatory alkaloids of belladonna (Bellafoline)
Tablets, injection solution
Recommended Doses: For adults, 0.25–0.5 mg tid.

Scopolamine hydrobromide (Hyoscine HBr)
Tablets, injection solutions
Recommended Doses: 0.4–0.8 mg orally or 0.3–0.6 mg parenterally in adults. Doses in children are adjusted by weight.

QUATERNARY AMMONIUM COMPOUNDS

Anisotropine (Anisotropine and Valpin)
Tablets
Recommended Doses: 50 mg PO tid.

Clidinium (Quarzan)
Tablets
Recommended Doses: For adults, 2.5–5.0 mg PO 3 or 4 times daily, before meals and at bedtime.

Dicyclomine (Bentyl, Antispas, Dibent, Dicen, Dilomine, Nospaz, Or-Tyl, Spasmoject, generic)
Capsules, tablets, syrup, injection solution
Recommended Doses: For adults, 10–20 mg PO, 3 or 4 times daily. For children, 10 mg PO, 3 or 4 times daily. For infants, 5 mg of syrup PO, 3 or 4 times daily.

Glycopyrrolate (Robinul, Glycobarb, generic)
Tablets
Recommended Doses: For acute ulcer therapy in adults, 1 mg PO tid or 2 mg 2 or 3 times daily. For maintenance, 1 mg PO bid.

Hexocyclium (Tral)
Tablets, timed release tablets
Recommended Doses: For adults, 25 mg PO 4 times daily or 50 mg PO timed release tablet daily.

Isopropamide (Darbid)
Tablets
Recommended Doses: For adults, 5–10 mg PO twice daily.

Mepenzolate (Cantil)
Tablets
Recommended Doses: For adults, 25–50 mg PO 4 times daily, before meals and at bedtime.

Methantheline (Banthine)
Tablets
Recommended Doses: For adults, 50–100 mg PO every six hours. For children, 12.5–50 mg PO qid. For infants, 12.5–25 mg PO qid. For neonates, 12.5 mg PO, 2 or 3 times daily.

Methscopolamine (Pamine)
Tablets
Recommended Doses: 2.5 mg PO 30 minutes before meals, and 2.5–5.0 mg PO at bedtime.

Oxybutynin (Ditropan)
Tablets, syrup
Recommended Doses: For urinary tract spasms in adults, 5 mg PO, 2 or 3 times daily. For children, 5 mg PO twice daily.

Oxyphencyclimine
Tablets
Recommended Doses: For adults, 10 mg PO two times daily, in the morning and at bedtime.

Oxyphenonium (Antrenyl)
Tablets
Recommended Doses: For adults, 10 mg PO qid.

Propantheline (Pro-Banthine, Norpanth, Ropanth, SK-Propantheline, generic)
Tablets
Recommended Doses: For adults, 15 mg PO 30 minutes before meals and 30 mg at bedtime.

Trihexethyl (Pathilon)
Tablets, sustained release tablets, injection solution
Recommended Doses: 25–50 mg PO, 3 or 4 times daily, before meals and at bedtime.

Important Nursing Implications for Antimuscarinic Drugs

- ☐ Advise clients about methods of countering the most common side effects of anticholinergic drugs: dry mouth, constipation, and urinary retention.
- ☐ Warn clients to avoid excessive exercise or exposure to the sun since inhibition of sweating caused by antimuscarinic drugs makes them susceptible to heat prostration.
- ☐ Advise clients to chew gum, suck on hard candy, take frequent sips of fluid, and increase oral hygiene if dry mouth poses a problem.
- ☐ Assess bladder function prior to administering antimuscarinic drug. After administration, monitor amount and frequency of voiding to determine if urinary retention is occurring. Palpate for bladder or bowel distention and monitor bowel sounds. Increasing dietary fiber or fluid intake or use of a stool softener may help to alleviate constipation.
- ☐ Advise clients to wear sunglasses to protect the eyes, because antimuscarinic drugs cause mydriasis.
- ☐ Warn clients to avoid driving and other activities that require mental alertness or visual acuity.
- ☐ Question clients about any history of allergy to anticholinergic drugs and instruct clients to report any occurrence of skin eruptions.
- ☐ Monitor for signs of cholinergic toxicity: tachycardia, hot, dry, flushed skin, fever, changes in respiratory rate, and mental confusion.
- ☐ Observe clients, especially children and elderly individuals, for behavioral changes, such as agitation, delirium, or excitement.
- ☐ Do not administer antimuscarinic drugs to clients with narrow-angle glaucoma, asthma, myasthenia gravis, renal or hepatic disease, gastrointestinal or urinary obstructions, or ulcerative colitis.

Ganglionic Blockers

Mechanisms and Effects Ganglionic blockers are highly nonspecific drugs that act as competitive, nondepolarizing blockers at the nicotinic receptors of autonomic ganglia. Transmission of impulses from preganglionic fibers to postganglionic fibers is blocked by these drugs. Both sympathetic and parasympathetic transmission are inhibited. The net influence on each tissue depends on the relative amount of sympathetic versus parasympathetic innervation exerted on the tissue.

With blood pressure, sympathetic innervation is the dominant influence, and ganglionic blockers produce hypotension. The extent of hypotensive response to a given dose of a ganglionic blocker depends on preexisting sympathetic tone. A recumbent client will usually experience little change in blood pressure, but a client who is standing is likely to experience a sharp drop in pressure. Thus, ganglionic blockers produce a true postural hypotension. Heart rate is controlled mainly by vagal tone, and ganglionic blockers produce tachycardia in proportion to preexisting vagal tone.

Other effects produced by ganglionic blockers related to inhibition of transmission at parasympathetic ganglia include decreased exocrine secretions and smooth muscle motility. Perspiration, salivation, gastric secretions, and pancreatic secretions are all diminished. Intestinal motility is reduced and urinary retention occurs. Gastric emptying time is greatly prolonged. In the eye, mydriasis and cycloplegia occur because of inhibition of the preponderant parasympathetic regulation. Impotency occurs in males with ganglionic blockade as a result of sympathetic inhibition.

Pharmacokinetics When taken orally, ganglionic blockers are absorbed only to a limited and variable extent. They complicate their own absorption as well as that of other drugs by greatly prolonging gastric emptying time. Reduced intestinal motility also impairs absorption. Of the two ganglionic blockers that remain on the market, mecamylamine (Inversine) is employed orally and trimethaphan (Arfonad) by intravenous injection or infusion. After absorption, ganglionic blockers distribute only within the extracellular fluid. Mecamylamine is excreted largely unchanged by the kidneys, but the slow rate of renal extraction makes mecamylamine a relatively long-acting ganglionic blocker.

Clinical Indications Ganglionic blockers have been replaced for chronic use in essential hypertension because of the broad range and severity of their adverse effects. In current clinical practice, ganglionic blockers are employed mainly for acute, emergency treatment of **hypertensive crisis.** Ganglionic blockers may be infused intravenously to rapidly lower dangerously elevated pressure to normal. Ganglionic blockers are also useful for **inducing hypotension** in preparation for surgery. Ganglionic blockers have been used as well in the management of **autonomic hyperreflexia,** which occurs in injuries of the upper spinal cord.

Adverse Effects and Contraindications Adverse effects of ganglionic blockers are extensions of their primary actions. Arteriolar and venous dilation caused by these agents results in orthostatic hypotension. *Nurses should warn clients that changes in position should be made slowly.* Tachycardia occurs due to vagal inhibition.

Urinary retention, constipation, or even paralytic ileus may occur as a result of inhibiting parasympathetic influence on smooth muscles of the viscera. *Nurses should monitor the clients for early signs of paralytic ileus: constipation, abdominal distention, and decreased bowel sounds. Clients who have cerebral or renal insufficiency, or an obstruction of the urethra (such as occurs with prostatic hypertrophy), also need to be monitored for urinary retention.* Bulk-forming laxatives should not be used, but stool softeners and mild saline laxatives can reduce constipation. Impotence, anorexia, abdominal discomfort, a bitter taste, and dry skin are other side effects. *Dry mouth, which occurs due to inhibition of exocrine secretions, can be alleviated by having the client chew gum, suck on hard candy, or take frequent sips of fluid. Dental caries related to reduced flow of saliva can be reduced by meticulous oral hygiene.*

Visual side effects include cycloplegia, mydriasis, and conjunctival suffusion. Other side effects clients may experience are fatigue and sedation, tremors, delusions, and hallucinations. *Nurses need to monitor client behavior and to ask a responsible family member to help in this task to assure that behavioral symptoms are reported.* Clients with glaucoma, coronary insufficiency, or a recent myocardial infarction should not receive ganglionic blockers.

Preparations and Administration Only two ganglionic blockers remain on the market in the United States. *Mecamylamine should be administered in consistent relation to mealtime. It is usually best to take the drug after meals since the presence of food in the stomach and intestines promotes a more even absorption and a less abrupt effect on blood pressure.* It may be desirable to employ smaller doses in the morning when blood pressure is relatively low and larger doses in the late afternoon or evening. Seasonal variations in average blood pressure may also result in a need for dosage adjustments. Smaller doses are often required in the summer than in the winter.

Evaluation of the effect of ganglionic blockers is based on blood pressure measured while the client is in an erect position. Since clients will generally be taking these drugs at home, it is advisable to teach them and a responsible family member how to take blood pressure readings and how to adjust the drug dosage based on these readings. Nurses need to teach such clients how to keep an accurate record of blood pressure readings and changes in drug dosage.

Mecamylamine (Inversine)
Tablets
Recommended Doses: For essential hypertension, 2.5 mg, bid, initially.

Trimethaphan (Arfonad)
Injection Solution
Recommended Doses: For hypertensive crisis or induction of hypotension for surgical procedures, 0.1% infused IV in 5% dextrose.

Neuromuscular Blockers

Nueromuscular blockers have only a relatively short history in medicine, dating back to 1932, but the prototype drug, curare, has a long history of use among the tribes of South American Indians as an arrow poison. For centuries, curare-tipped arrows were used for hunting game, but preparation of curare was a carefully guarded secret known only to the tribal witch doctors. Early European explorers became interested in this mysterious chemical and its secret botanical sources, but it was not until the nineteenth century that the plant was determined to be a South American variety of *Strychnos,* which contains curariform alkaloids. The site of action of curare was demonstrated to be the neuromuscular junction by Claude Bernard in a classic set of experiments in the 1850s. The name "curare" designates the various natural alkaloids with neuromuscular blocking properties obtained from *Strychnos.* The most abundant of these alkaloids is *d*-tubocurarine.

In the last 15 years, a variety of semisynthetic and synthetic agents have joined *d*-tubocurarine as neuromuscular blockers for clinical applications. The drugs fall into two distinct groups based on mechanism of action (Table 29-7). One group, in-

Table 29–7
Comparisons Between Competitive and Depolarizing Blockers

	Competitive	Depolarizing
Example drugs	*d*-Tubocurarine Gallamine Metocurine Pancuronium Atracurium Vecuronium	Succinylcholine Decamethonium
Effect on neuromuscular transmission	Competitive blockade of ACH receptors	Persistent depolarization
Initial muscle activation	No	Yes
Interaction with previous dose of *d*-Tubocurarine	Cumulative effect	Antagonistic
Interaction with cholinesterase inhibitor	Antagonized	Potentiated

cluding *d*-tubocurarine, comprises the competitive (or stabilizing) blockers. The other group, of which succinylcholine is the prototype, consists of the depolarizing blockers.

Mechanisms and Effects **Competitive neuromuscular blockers,** such as *d*-tubocurarine, compete with ACH for the receptor sites of the neuromuscular junction. The effect of **competitive blockers** depends on the relative concentrations of blocker and transmitter at the neuromuscular junction. As the dose of blocker is increased, the magnitude and duration of excitatory postsynaptic potentials on the motor end-plate progressively decline. The result is progressive paralysis. Small muscles with high rates of activity, such as those in the fingers, eyes, and jaw, exhibit paralysis soonest and at lowest doses. Long muscles of the limbs are the next most sensitive, and respiratory muscles develop problems last. *Thus, nursing assessment of residual neuromuscular blockade in the recovery room should include questions concerning changes in vision or ability to use the fingers, to talk, or to chew. The intercostal muscles are paralyzed before the diaphragmatic muscles, so that the nurse needs to note if the patient's respiration has become more diaphragmatic, which occurs just prior to complete respiratory failure.* The extent of neuromuscular blockade is dependent on acid-base balance, electrolyte concentrations, and preexisting neuromuscular disease.

Depolarizing blockers, such as succinylcholine (Anectine), have a quite different mechanism of action that results in distinct clinical implications. Depolarizing agents have small, flexible structures not unlike that of ACH itself. They occupy and activate the cholinergic receptors of the neuromuscular junction, but the effects differ from that produced by ACH by their greater persistence. The motor endplate and the immediately adjacent sacroplasmic membrane of the skeletal muscle is locked in a depolarized state. Clients exhibit transient muscle activation (twitches and fasciculations) prior to paralysis. Depolarizing blockers paralyze the muscle of the neck and limbs first, then the muscles of the face, jaw, tongue, pharynx, and larynx; the respiratory muscles are affected last.

Curariform agents can cause varying degrees of hypotension as a result of a weak antagonistic action at autonomic ganglia. Pancuronium (Pavulon) and metocurine (Metubine) are less hypotensive than *d*-tubocurarine. However, pancuronium has a vagolytic action that can lead to tachycardia or, when used in conjunction with fentanyl (Innovar or Sublimase) or sufentanil (Sufenta), which cause bradycardia, can offset the cardiac slowing caused by anesthesia. Succinylcholine, in contrast to the competitive blockers, stimulates nicotinic receptors in the manner of nicotine. Blood pressure may rise accordingly. At extremely high doses, succinylcholine can produce a depolarizing blockade at ganglia as well as at the neuromuscular junction.

d-Tubucararine is likely to cause histamine release, as are metocurine, atracurium (Tracrium), pancuronium, and succinylcholine to a lesser degree. As a result, clients may develop bronchospasm, hypotension, and wheals. Other drugs in this family, such as vecuronium (Norcuron), do not cause signifi-

Table 29–8
Comparison of Neuromuscular Blockers

Generic name	Trade name	Duration	Histamine release	Blood pressure effect
Competitive type				
Atracurium	Tracrium	Intermediate	Less likely	Decrease
Gallamine	Flaxedil	Long	Less likely	Decrease
Metocurine	Metubine	Long	Most likely	Slight decrease
Pancuronium	Pavulon	Long	Less likely	Slight decrease
d-Tubocurarine	—	Long	Most likely	Decrease
Vecuronium	Norcuron	Intermediate	Least likely	Decrease
Depolarizing type				
Decamethonium	Syncurine	Long	Less likely	?
Succinylcholine	Anectine	Short	Less likely	Increase

cant histamine release at usual doses. Comparisons among the neuromuscular blockers are summarized in Table 29–8.

Pharmacokinetics *d*-Tubocurarine is not absorbed after oral administration to any extent, which is the reason that primitive people could safely eat meat from animals killed by curare-tipped arrows. Absorption is rapid after injection by any parenteral route. Paralysis produced by a single dose of *d*-tubocurarine typically lasts about 20 minutes, although some muscle weakness may be detectable for as long as 4 hours. The half-life of curare, however, is sufficiently long so that cumulative activity occurs if administration of the drug is repeated sooner than 24 hours. Curare is excreted in the urine and in the bile, both changed and unchanged. Renal insufficiency results in prolonged activity. Other competitive neuromuscular blockers with a duration of action similar to that of curare include metocurine, gallamine (Flaxadil), and pancuronium, although pancuronium is eliminated mainly by hydroxylation and gallamine entirely by renal excretion. Atracurium and vecuronium are shorter-acting than curare but longer-acting than the depolarizing blocker succinylcholine. Atracurium and vecuronium are therefore characterized as intermediate-acting neuromuscular blockers. The duration of action of atracurium or vecuronium is about one-third to one-half that of curare. Recovery from atracurium is 95% complete after 60 minutes. *d*-Tubocurarine does not cross the blood-brain or placental barriers.

Among the depolarizing blockers, succinylcholine usually has a much shorter action, reaching its peak in only 3 minutes and dissipating in 5 minutes. The brevity of action of the drug is due to rapid metabolism by pseudocholinesterase. Some patients have deficiencies in this enzyme due to genetic anomalies, nutritional deficiencies, or hepatic disease. Such patients will have a greatly prolonged apneic response to succinylcholine. For this reason, artificial respiration should always be at hand when succinylcholine is employed. Decamethonium (Syncurine) has a duration of activity similar to that of the competitive neuromuscular antagonists and is eliminated by renal excretion.

Clinical Indications Neuromuscular blockers have one major and several minor clinical indications (Table 29–4). The major use is to induce skeletal muscle relaxation as an aid in conducting abdominal surgery. This use of neuromuscular blockers as adjuncts to anesthesia is discussed in Chapter 16. The minor uses of neuromuscular blockers include facilitation of endotracheal intubation, induction of muscle paralysis in patients being administered electroconvulsant shock, control of tetanus, and muscle relaxation for orthopedic procedures.

Adverse Effects and Contraindications Because of the short-term nature of use of these drugs, adverse reactions are infrequent. The three concerns when neuromuscular blockers are employed are **prolonged apnea, cardiovascular collapse,** and effects caused by **histamine release.** Apnea is an exaggeration of the therapeutic effect. When the drug is succinylcholine, prolonged apnea may be a true idiosyncratic reaction due to pseudocholinesterase deficiency. In other cases, prolonged respiratory effects may be caused by drug interactions. Treatment of respiratory paralysis caused by neuromuscular blockers is undertaken with positive-pressure artificial respiration and oxygen. Epinephrine and antihistamines are employed for relief of symptoms associated with histamine release.

Usually, curariform agents are used in conjunction with general anesthesia; thus few patients experience the subjective effects of curare. When curare is used in conscious patients, the effects are distinctively unpleasant. Dizziness and flushing are followed by visual disturbances (diplopia, ptosis), weakness of muscles in the jaw, head, neck, and limbs, shortness of breath, and increased auditory acuity for low-frequency sounds.

Neuromuscular blockers are highly potent drugs, capable of causing respiratory failure and death if they are used without adequate precautions or by inadequately trained personnel. Obviously, clients who have myasthenia gravis or those who have liver, kidney, or respiratory disorders should be monitored closely when these drugs are administered. Special care should be taken when the drugs are given to elderly or debilitated people.

Drug Interactions Neuromuscular blockers interact with a variety of drugs with potentially severe clinical effects. The interactions of the two types of neuromuscular blockers are quite different, sometimes even opposite from one another (Table 29-7). The competitive neuromuscular blockers can be antagonized effectively by drugs that elevate concentrations of acetylcholine in the neuromuscular junction, namely the cholinesterase inhibitors. Short-acting cholinesterase inhibitors, like edrophonium (Tensilon) and neostigmine (Prostigmin), are used for this purpose.

A substantial number of drugs can **potentiate neuromuscular blocking effects of curariform agents** or produce recurarization if administered shortly after effects of a competitive blocker have worn off. Most important in this category are general anesthetics, certain antibiotics, and diuretics. Among the **general anesthetics,** additive neuromuscular blockade occurs with halothane, methoxyflurane, enflurane, and cyclopropane. Doses of competitive blockers must be sharply reduced (to one-half or less) when employed in conjunction with these anesthetics. Several antibiotics have weak neuromuscular blocking activity in their own right that is additive with that caused by curariform agents. Aminoglycosides, such as streptomycin, are especially likely to cause additive neuromuscular blockade, which also occurs with polymyxins, colistin, clindamycin, and lincomycin. **Hypokalemia** impairs neuromuscular transmission. Drugs that cause hypokalemia therefore increase effects of competitive neuromuscular blockers. Potassium-depleting **diuretics** (thiazides and high-ceiling agents) are the most important examples of drugs interacting with curariform agents in this manner. **Local anesthetics** and **antidysrhythmic drugs** with local anesthetic properties such as propranolol (Inderal), quinidine, and procainamide (Pronestyl) also enhance neuromuscular blockade. **Centrally acting skeletal muscle relaxants** (such as benzodiazepines, meprobamate, and opiates) produce additive effects with the peripherally acting neuromuscular blockers. Neuromuscular blockade is also enhanced by calcium and magnesium salts. *The nurse should carefully monitor respiratory function of postoperative patients given drugs known to have the potential for producing recurarization.*

Cholinesterase inhibitors do not antagonize depolarizing neuromuscular blockers like succinylcholine. In fact, one cholinesterase inhibitor, hexafluorenium, is marketed for use with succinylcholine to increase its duration of action by inhibiting its metabolism.

Preparations and Administration *All injections of neuromuscular blockers must be made by the physician. Artificial respiration equipment and oxygen should be on hand.*

COMPETITIVE BLOCKERS

Atracurium (Tracrium)
Injection solution
Recommended Doses: 0.4–0.5 mg/kg by intravenous bolus, initially. Doses of 0.08–0.10 mg/kg are recommended for maintenance of neuromuscular blockade during surgery.

Gallamine (Flaxedil)
Injection solutions
Recommended Doses: 1 mg/kg initially.

Metocurine (Metubine)
Injection solution
Recommended Doses: The average initial dose is approximately 2 mg.

Pancuronium (Pavulon)
Injection solutions
Recommended Doses: Initial intravenous doses range from 0.04 to 0.1 mg/kg.

d-Tubocurarine
Injection solution
Recommended Doses: 6–9 mg (40–60 units) at the time of surgical incision by slow IV injection over 1.0–1.5 minutes or IM. Repeat injections of 3–4.5 mg are given as required to maintain skeletal muscle relaxation. Solutions of *d*-tubocurarine that are more than slightly discolored should be discarded. *d*-Tubucararine is unstable in basic solutions.

Vecuronium (Norcuron)
Injection solution with preservative-free sterile water for use as the diluent
Recommended Doses: 0.08–0.10 mg/kg, by IV bolus injection initially. The effect lasts about 25–30 minutes and can be extended by subsequent administration of maintenance doses of 0.010–0.015 mg/kg at 25–30 minute intervals.

DEPOLARIZING BLOCKERS

Decamethonium (Syncurine)
Injection solution
Recommended Doses: 2.0–2.5 mg initially.

Succinylcholine (Anectine, Quelicin, Sucostrin, and Sux-Cert)
Injection solutions, powder for preparing infusions
Recommended Doses: In adults, 25–75 mg, IV or, less commonly IM. *Intramuscular injections should be made deeply, ideally in the deltoid muscle.* An initial test dose of 10 mg provides a determination of sensitivity to the drug. In children and infants, 1–2 mg typically. *Succinylcholine breaks down spontaneously in basic solutions and therefore should not be mixed with basic drugs. Refrigeration of the drug is required. Only freshly prepared solutions should be employed.*

Important Nursing Implications for Neuromuscular Blockers

- ☐ Ensure availability of equipment for intubation, artificial respiration, and administration of oxygen before administering a neuromuscular blocker. Ensure that an appropriate antagonist, such as edrophonium, is on hand before giving a competitive neuromuscular blocker.
- ☐ Measure serum electrolytes before administering a competitive neuromuscular blocker, since their effects are potentiated by hypokalemia or hypermagnesia.
- ☐ Evaluate renal function before administering a neuromuscular blocker since diminished renal excretion of the drug could dangerously potentiate its effect.
- ☐ Monitor vital signs during administration of the drug.
- ☐ Evaluate sensitivity to succinylcholine before using a full dose of this drug, since some clients have a genetic deficiency in pseudocholinesterase, the enzyme that metabolizes succinylcholine.
- ☐ Evaluate drugs given postoperatively to patients who have received a neuromuscular blocker for potential interactions.
- ☐ Avoid the histamine-releasing neuromuscular blockers in clients with a history of immediate hypersensitivity reactions.

Case Study: Myasthenia Gravis

F. B., a married woman of 37, developed a drooping eyelid and muscular weakness that she interpreted as a ministroke. Although she knew no one her age who had suffered a stroke, she had read that they could occur in people as young as 25, and stroke had been diagnosed in some of her older friends with similar symptoms. A nurse friend suggested that F. B. report her changes to her physician. F. B. had hypertension during her pregnancy the year before, and at first the physician thought that possibly F. B.'s blood pressure was elevated. However, the physician insisted that F. B. have a complete physical examination and further tests to check all the possibilities. When F. B. arrived for the physical examination, the nurse friend accompanied her and pointed out to the physician other observations she had made, such as F. B.'s increasing fatigue, even to the point of finding it difficult to comb her hair. A series of studies revealed that F. B. had myasthenia gravis.

Neostigmine (Prostigmin) was ordered to counteract the symptoms of fatigue and weakness. An optimal dose was determined by an intravenous procedure based on measurement of changes in F. B.'s grip strength. The nurse who had encouraged F. B. to go to the physician agreed to monitor her friend for any adverse side effects, since F. B.'s spouse was often away on business trips. The nurse monitored F. B. for adverse effects, such as abdominal cramping that might be caused by the increased peristalsis or diarrhea. The nurse checked F. B. for complaints of nausea, vomiting, and increased salivation or mucus and questioned her about any changes in urinary habits since urinary frequency is an adverse response to the drug. The nurse assisted F. B. in adjusting her dosage as suited her physical requirements. F. B. learned to watch for runny nose, pupillary constriction, indications of bronchoconstriction, behavioral changes, or muscle twitchings and weakness, which might reflect excessive cholinergic activity.

In addition, the nurse worked with F. B. to decrease stress where possible since the effectiveness of drug therapy can vary with the level of emotional as well as physical exertion. The nurse assisted F. B. in coordinating the amount and frequency of medication with her menstrual cycle. Together, they determined when F. B. typically felt most stressed and increased the dosage of medication accordingly. The nurse also cautioned F. B. to be certain to note when she was experiencing infections because infections usually require medication adjustment.

While F. B.'s disease was not far advanced at this time, the nurse made certain to include in her assessment any observation that the muscular weakness had spread to muscles of the face. She checked F. B. for any difficulty in chewing and listened carefully for any evidence that F. B. had difficulty talking. The nurse checked for problems with swallowing and noted any difficulty F. B. may have had walking or using her arms. She had F. B. keep a written record of events so that she could note whether the handwriting changed, which might indicate additional muscle involvement and progression of the disease to report to the physician.

In addition, the nurse worked out a chart system with F. B. that would enable her to remember to take her medication and to record it, which helped to ensure that F. B. was taking the medication as recommended. She also explained symptoms of overdosage to F. B. and Mr. B. and printed these out on a card.

F. B. was provided with a list of drugs to be avoided because of their potential for increasing muscular weakness. For example, she was told to avoid the antibiotics streptomycin, kanamycin, neomycin, and gentamicin in the event of an infection. Since anyone with myasthenia gravis is particularly sensitive to respiratory depressants such as sedatives, hypnotics, and morphine-like opiates, F. B. was told to avoid use of these drugs. She was also advised to wear a Medic Alert bracelet to facilitate proper management in case of a crisis or accident. F. B. also had to avoid quinine tonic drinks since these, too, can cause muscle weakness. Fortunately, F. B. did not have any medical condition that might have necessitated her taking diuretics, so hypokalemia was not an immediate concern.

Because F. B. was at home, the physician ordered special equipment such as a hand respirator (Ambu bag), a suction machine, and plastic oral airway. The nurse spent time with Mr. and Mrs. B. assuring that they understood and could use the equipment should this become necessary.

1. Which of the presenting symptoms at the time of initial evaluation were suggestive of myasthenia gravis? Why wasn't it immediately evident to the nurse and physician that F. B. was suffering from myasthenia gravis?
2. What kind of a drug is neostigmine? In the event of overdose, what medical intervention would be required?
3. What advantage does the intravenous titration method have over the oral method when the initial dose of a cholinesterase inhibitor is being determined?
4. Why was the nurse concerned about observing F. B. for vomiting, increased salivation, or excessive mucus? What hazard might these occurrences pose for F. B.?
5. Why is it fortunate that F. B. does not require a diuretic? How do diuretics interact with myasthenia gravis and its treatment?

Answers appear at the end of the book.

Recommended Readings

Antimuscarinic Agents

Adami H-O et al: Cimetidine or propantheline combined with antacid therapy for short-term treatment of duodenal ulcer. *Digest Dis Sci* 1982;27:388–393.

Brimblecombe RW: *Drug Actions on Cholinergic Systems.* Baltimore, University Park Press, 1974.

Gever LN: Anticholinergics. *Nursing* 1984;14(9):64–65.

Shader R, Greenblatt D: Belladonna alkaloids and synthetic anticholinergics: Uses and toxicity, in Shader RI (ed): *Psychiatric Complications of Medical Drugs.* New York, Raven Ps, 1972, pp 103–172.

Cholinomimetics

Barry L: The patient with myasthenia gravis really needs you. *Nursing* 1982;12(7):50–53.

Brumback RA: The neuromuscular junction. Part II: Myasthenia gravis. *Am Fam Physician* 1981;23(2):126–133.

DiPalma J: Pharmacology of myasthenia gravis. *Am Fam Physician* 1980;22(4):158–159.

Drachman DB: The biology of myasthenia gravis. *Annu Rev Neurosci* 1981;4:195–225.

Gever L: Cholinergics. *Nursing* 1984;14(5):41.

Grob D (ed): Myasthenia gravis: pathophysiology and management. *Ann NY Acad Sci* 1981;371:1–902.

Ganglionic Blockers and Stimulating Agents

Kharkevich DA (ed): *Pharmacology of Ganglionic Transmission.* Berlin, Springer-Verlag, 1980.

Miletick DJ, Ivankovich AD: Cardiovascular effects of ganglionic blocking drugs. *Int Anesthesiol Clin* 1978;16:151–170.

Salem MR: Therapeutic uses of ganglionic blocking drugs. *Int Anesthesiol Clin* 1978;16:171–200.

Neuromuscular Blockers

Argov Z, Mastaglia, FL: Disorders of neuromuscular transmission caused by drugs. *N Engl J Med* 1979;301:409–413.

Brumback RA: The neuromuscular junction. Part I: Physiology and the effects of drugs and toxins. *Am Fam Physician* 1981;23(1):188–192.

Conner CS: Atracurium and vecuronium: Two unique neuromuscular blocking agents. *Drug Intell Clin Pharm* 1984;18:714–716.

Fambrough D: Control of acetylcholine receptors in skeletal muscle. *Physiol Rev* 1979;59:165–227.

Feldman S: Neuromuscular blocking drugs, in Churchill-Davidson HC, Wylie WD (eds): *A Practice of Anaesthesia,* ed 5. Chicago, Year Book Medical Publishers Inc, 1984, pp 722–734.

Whittaker M: Plasma cholinesterase variants and the anaesthetist. *Anaesthesia* 1980;35:174–197.

UNIT V

Drugs and the Endocrine System

CHAPTER 30

Introduction to Endocrine Pharmacology and the Pituitary Gland

Some Basic Principles of Endocrinology

The processes of the body are regulated by two major control systems: the nervous system and the endocrine system. The nervous system, as we saw in Units III and IV, broadly regulates the organs, glands, and musculature on a moment-to-moment basis and is capable of altering the activity of any of these tissues in a fraction of a second. By contrast, the endocrine system is generally concerned with the metabolic functions of cells, including the rate of uptake of substances into cells and the rate of biochemical reactions. Although some endocrine responses occur within seconds, many are slow in onset (requiring hours or days) and long in duration.

The principal organs and glands of endocrine function are illustrated in Figure 30–1. The **pituitary gland,** located at the base of the brain, provides the main coordination between the nervous system and the endocrine system. The **thyroid** and **parathyroid** complex is situated in the neck and secretes four hormones: two involved in control of metabolic rate and two involved in calcium homeostatis. The **adrenal gland,** located above the kidneys, encompasses two distinct endocrine tissues: the adrenal medulla and the adrenal cortex. The adrenal medulla secretes catecholamines, which are functionally related to the sympathetic nervous system. The adrenal cortex, as well as the gonads (testes in men and ovaries in women), secrete steroids. The endocrine portion of the **pancreas,** called the islets of Langerhans, secretes four hormones, most importantly insulin and glucagon. The thymus and pineal glands currently

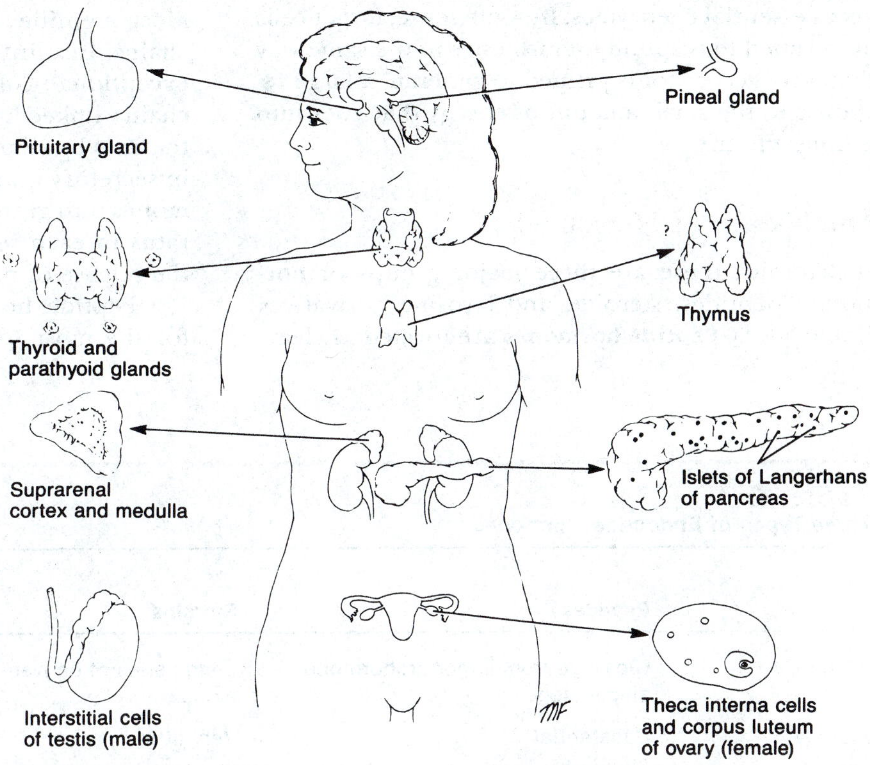

Figure 30–1
Endocrine glands. From B. L. Bullock and P. P. Rosendahl, *Pathophysiology: Adaptations and Alterations in Function*, © 1984 by Barbara L. Bullock and Pearl Rosendahl. Reprinted by permission of Little, Brown and Company.

have little importance for pharmacology. In addition to these major endocrine tissues, the brain, heart, kidneys, and gastrointestinal tissues have endocrine functions as well as their primary organ functions.

Information transfer in the endocrine system occurs through the release and action of chemical messengers called **hormones.** Hormones are produced mainly by specialized cells that are grouped together in the ductless glands of the endocrine system. Hormones are secreted in response to various signals — nervous system signals, changes in blood concentrations of the substances regulated by hormones, or changes in levels of other hormones. The process by which the release of a hormone is regulated by the substance it controls is known as **negative feedback** (Figure 30–2).

The general hormones of the endocrine system are released into the circulation and dispersed widely throughout the body. Not all tissues respond to the action of all hormones, however. Hormones control specific activities of target tissues. The presence of receptors for the hormone determines the target tissue's susceptibility to the regulatory influence of a particular hormone. Hormones are active in minute concentrations and do not supply energy or material in quantities sufficient to account

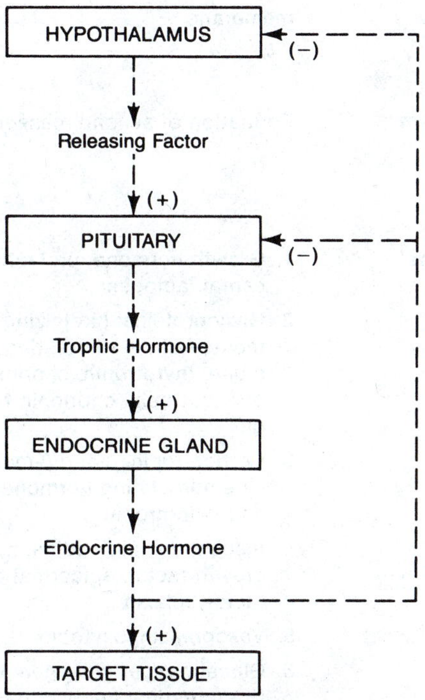

Figure 30–2
The concept of negative feedback in control of endocrine substances.

for the magnitude of their effects. Nor do hormones act as essential coenzymes. In some sense, target cells are primed to respond to hormones in the same way that a cocked pistol is primed to generate a large response to the small amount of energy that goes into pulling the trigger.

The Nature of Hormones

Structurally, there are three major groups of hormones: peptides, steroids, and tyrosine derivatives (Table 30–1). **Peptide hormones** are formed as cleavage products from larger peptide prohormones. Most peptide hormones are single polypeptide chains. Insulin and the glycoprotein hormones are exceptional, consisting in each case of two peptide chains linked together. Peptide hormones are synthesized by ribosomes and stored in large quantities in secretory granules. The packaging of peptide hormones into granules is carried out by the Golgi apparatus in each secretory cell. Calcium is involved in the release of most peptide hormones.

Peptide hormones are rather large molecules for the most part and therefore are effectively ex-

Table 30–1
Three Types of Endocrine Hormones

	Peptides	Steroids	Tyrosine derivatives
Synthesis	Cleavage from larger prohormone in single step	Long series of conversions	2–3 steps
Storage	Substantial quantities	Very little	Substantial quantities
Peripheral transformations to active substances	No	Yes	No
Receptor location	Plasma cell membrane	Cytoplasm	Plasma cell membrane (norepinephrine and epinephrine); Nucleus (thyroxine and triiodothyronine)
Mechanism	Formation of second messenger	Activation of genome	Formation of second messenger (norepinephrine and epinephrine) Activation of genome (thyroxine and thiiodothyronine)
Subgroups	1. Growth hormone, prolactin, placental lactogen 2. Glycoproteins: luteinizing hormone, follicle-stimulating hormone, thyrotropin, chorionic gonadotropin, chorionic thyrotropin 3. Corticotropin, α-and β-melanocyte stimulating hormones, β- and γ-lipotropin 4. Insulin, somatomedins, nerve growth factor, epidermal growth factor, relaxin 5. Vasopressin, oxytocin 6. Glucagon, gut glucagon, vasoactive intestinal peptide, gastric inhibitory polypeptide 7. Gastrin, cholecystikinin (pancreozymin)	1. Glucocorticoids 2. Mineralocorticoids 3. Androgens 4. Estrogens 5. Progestins 6. Calcitriol	1. Thyroid hormones 2. Catecholamines

cluded from the interior of cells. They therefore must act on receptors on the exterior surface of the plasma cell membrane. These receptors are often linked to adenylate cyclase which catalyzes formation of adenosine 3′:5′ cyclic phosphate. The cyclic AMP formed as a result of hormone/receptor interaction acts as a *second messenger,* conveying the influences of the hormone to the cell interior.

The **steroid hormones** include the glucocorticoids, mineralocorticoids, and weak androgens produced by the adrenal cortex; testosterone produced by the testes; estrogens and progestins produced by the ovaries; and calcitriol, the active form of vitamin D, synthesized by the kidney. Steroids are unusual because their synthesis from glycerol requires elaborate sequences of reactions and because these hormones are not stored before release. They are also unusual in acting on receptors located in the cytoplasm of the target tissue cells. Unlike the peptide hormones, which are relatively large molecules, the steroids, being smaller, can pass through cell membranes to reach intracellular receptor sites. A steroid-receptor complex forms in the cytoplasm and then moves into the nucleus to interact with nuclear proteins that govern activity of the genetic material of the cell. The cytoplasmic receptors are expended in the process and must be replenished in order to restore full sensitivity to further steroid activation. Within the nucleus, the steroids activate the cell's own genes to increase synthesis of specific ribonucleic acid (RNA) and protein molecules. Thus steroids have the unique capacity to alter the way in which each type of target cell expresses its genetic potential. This explains why steroids can produce such a variety of regulatory effects on different target tissues.

Hormone derivatives of tyrosine include the principal thyroid hormones and the catecholamines of the adrenal medulla. The thyroid hormones are noteworthy for their long half-life and their site of action — the nucleus of target cells. Their mechanism resembles somewhat that of steroids since both result in genome activation. But the thyroid hormones act not by way of cytoplasmic receptors, but directly within the nucleus. The catecholamines, by contrast, resemble the peptide transmitters in that they act extracellulary through the stimulation of adenylate cyclase.

Feedback Control of Endocrine Activity

The principle of feedback in the endocrine system can be seen in the regulation of blood glucose by insulin. Release of insulin into the blood is stimulated by glucose. Insulin in turn reduces blood glucose, in part by promoting its uptake into muscle cells. When levels of glucose decline during fasting, insulin secretion is minimal. After ingestion of glucose in the form of a meal or snack, blood glucose levels rise and insulin release increases to stimulate uptake of glucose into tissue cells until blood glucose levels return to normal. This kind of feedback mechanism, called **negative feedback,** tends to maintain a homeostasis in the concentration of the controlled substance.

Because of feedback control, therapy for endocrine disorders must take into account the impact of an intervention on the entire feedback system as well as on individual elements of the system. Doses used to supplement deficient endogenous production often must exceed the difference between the pretreatment level of the hormone and normal values, because when that amount is given it will usually further suppress endogenous production. For example, when synthetic corticosteroids are administered, any remaining endogenous production of steroids is suppressed by feedback inhibition. Withdrawal symptoms may follow long-term therapy with hormones if endogenous production of the hormone, suppressed during therapy, does not rebound quickly. This problem occurs most often with glucocorticoids, since these are the hormones most often used for other than replacement purposes.

Sometimes feedback effects reach beyond the domain of the hormone itself. For example, when testosterone is given to males, the hormone causes feedback suppression not only of luteinizing hormone, which normally promotes endogenous testosterone secretion, but also of follicle-stimulating hormone, which normally stimulates spermatogenesis and maintains testicular morphology. The result is inhibition of spermatogenesis and gonadal atrophy.

Disorders of the Endocrine System

There are two basic types of endocrine disorders: overproduction and underproduction of a given hormone. Within these general categories are many subtle variations of derangements that lead to similar symptomatologies. In some cases, distinguishing the cause is necessary for proper treatment. A variety of tests of endocrine function can help in diagnosis. To begin with, blood or urine levels of the hormone and its metabolites can be measured. However, a better indication of how well a given endocrine gland is functioning is to test its responsiveness to an appropriate stimulus. Examples include the glucose tolerance test, thyroid suppression test, and stress response. Special tests can measure activities unique to particular glands — for example, thyroid uptake of iodide. Glands that manufacture hormones also tend to show changes in their structure if their function is disturbed for any period of time. Unusual demands on endocrine glands can cause compensatory hyperplasia. For example, certain diseases of the kidney may result in large concentrations of calcium ions being excreted in the urine. The body's effort to compensate for this loss results in a hyperplasia of the parathyroid glands, since these glands play an important role in regulating blood levels of calcium.

The Anterior Pituitary

The pituitary gland has been called the master gland of the endocrine system because it regulates several other endocrine glands. It is the major interface between the nervous system and the endocrine system. Neural signals from the hypothalamus influence pituitary function and through it the thyroid gland, the adrenal cortex, the kidney, the gonads, and many other target tissues, both endocrine and other. The pituitary is situated adjacent to the hypothalamus, a portion of the brain involved in regulating the vital processes of the body. The hypothalamus exerts both neural and hormonal control over the pituitary (Figure 30–3). Structurally, the pituitary gland consists of two distinct endocrine glands: the epithelial anterior lobe and the smaller posterior lobe of neural origin.

The anterior pituitary in humans secretes six hormones of importance. Two of these are the gonadotropins — luteinizing hormone (LH) and follicle-stimulating hormone (FSH) — which regulate development, activity, and, in women, cyclical functioning of the gonads. Their release is controlled by a hypothalamic releasing factor called gonadotropin-releasing factor (GRF). Two other trophic hormones that control specific endocrine glands are corticotropin (ACTH), which regulates the adrenal

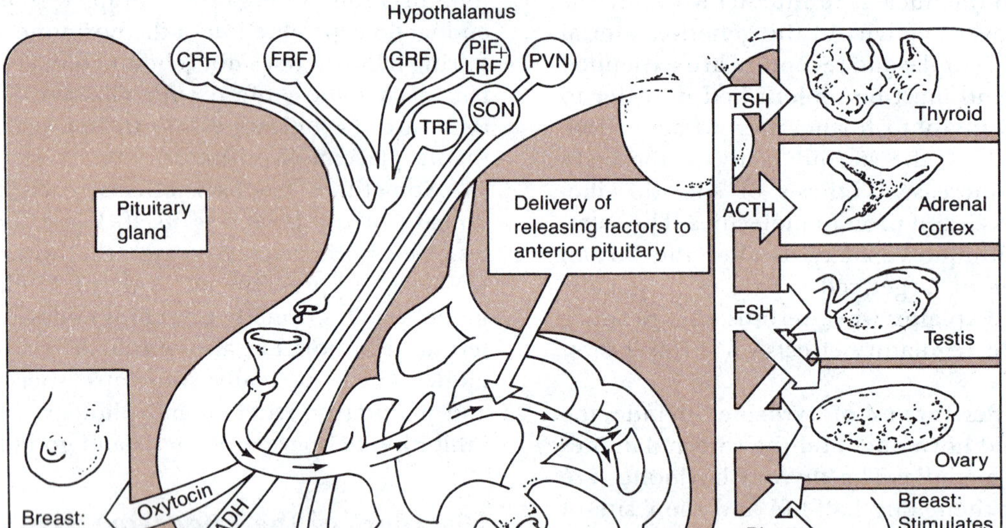

Figure 30–3
The hypothalamus and pituitary gland, showing the pituitary hormones: adrenocorticotropic hormone (ACTH); antidiuretic hormone (ADH); corticotropin releasing factor (CRF); follicle-stimulating hormone releasing factor (FRF); follicle stimulating hormone (FSH); growth hormone (GH); growth hormone releasing factor (GRF); luteinizing hormone (LH); luteinizing hormone releasing factor (LRF); prolactin inhibitory factor (PIF); prolactin (PL); paraventricular nucleus (PVN); supraoptic nucleus (SON); thyrotropin releasing factor (TRF); thyroid-stimulating hormone (TSH). Modified from A. K. Swonger: *Nursing Pharmacology.* Boston: Little, Brown, 1978.

cortex, and thyrotropin (TSH), which controls thyroid function. ACTH release from the pituitary is controlled by corticotropin-releasing factor (CRF) produced by the hypothalamus. TSH release is similarly regulated by thyrotropin-releasing factor (TRF) of the hypothalamus. The remaining two anterior pituitary hormones are prolactin and growth hormone, two polypeptides of related structure. Prolactin promotes production of milk by the mammary glands while growth hormone has significant and diverse anabolic influences on many target tissues. Prolactin release is regulated by a hypothalamic factor called prolactin inhibitory factor (PIF) and growth hormone by growth hormone releasing factor (GHRF). With the exception of growth hormone, the hormones of the anterior pituitary are discussed in subsequent chapters in connection with the systems they regulate: TSH in Chapter 31, ACTH in Chapter 32, prolactin and the gonadotropins in Chapters 34 and 35.

Pituitary Dwarfism and Growth Hormone

Pituitary dwarfism sometimes occurs in hypopituitarism, a deficiency of hormonal activity of the pituitary gland. The characteristics of hypopituitarism depend mainly on two factors: (1) whether the condition occurs in childhood or adulthood, and (2) whether the deficiency involves all anterior pituitary hormones (panhypopituitarism) or is selective for specific hormones. Pituitary dwarfism occurs when panhypopituitarism or selective growth hormone defiency occurs in children, but pituitary insufficiency accounts for less than 10% of all cases of dwarfism. Thus, other causes of growth impairment must be ruled out, including constitutional short stature, hypothyroidism, precocious puberty, diabetes mellitus, Cushing's syndrome, and Addison's disease. Pituitary dwarfism involving selective growth hormone deficiency is occasionally hereditary, but most instances of pituitary dwarfism are related to craniopharyngioma or have no demonstrable etiology. In pituitary dwarfism, body proportions are normal but diminutive, in contrast to the abnormal proportions seen in Down's syndrome. Treatment of pituitary dwarfism involves replacement therapy with growth hormone. If the growth hormone deficiency has occurred as a component of panhypopituitarism, cortisol and thyroid hormone replacement therapy is also instituted and gonadotropins may be required during adolescence to promote sexual maturation.

Growth Hormone

Growth hormone (GH) is the most abundant of the anterior pituitary hormones, comprising 10% of the total dry weight of the gland. GH exists in large and small forms; the former is probably a prohormone storage form, the latter the main form in plasma and more biologically active. The small form consists of a peptide chain with 191 amino acids and two internal disulfide bonds. Although there is some homology in GH structure across species, there is also considerable variability. Humans do not respond well to GH derived, for example, from cows.

Mechanisms and Effects GH promotes growth of all bodily tissues, except perhaps the eye and brain. The bones, muscle, skin, and viscera are all increased in mass by the action of GH. The heart, kidney, gonads, and thyroid and adrenal glands are all affected. Although the gonads are enlarged by GH, sexual maturation and development are not advanced.

The metabolic basis for the growth-promoting effect of GH has been amply studied. GH promotes a positive nitrogen balance and protein synthesis required for tissue expansion. The energy required for this anabolic (growth-promoting) activity is provided by lipid rather than carbohydrate metabolism. GH inhibits utilization of glucose, raising blood sugar levels and increasing bodily requirements for insulin. The mobilization of fat is perhaps the single most pronounced effect of GH.

The half-life of GH in serum is only about 20 minutes, but its effects are long-lasting. This is because many of the effects of GH are mediated by a family of plasma peptides called **somatomedins.** The somatomedins that have been isolated are structurally related to insulin. The somatomedins include nerve growth factor, epidermal growth factor, and others. GH causes accumulation of somatomedins in the serum, and these in turn promote anabolic effects — synthesis of DNA, RNA, and protein — in diverse tissues.

Growth hormone is synthesized in acidophilic cells of the pituitary and released under the influence of GH-releasing factor (GHRF) and GH-inhibitory factor (somatostatin). Release of GHRF is promoted by dopaminergic neurons of the hypothalamic-pituitary tract. Dopamine antagonists (such as antipsychotic drugs) have a growth-inhibiting effect. GH secretion is elevated during fasting or other hypoglycemic conditions, and during nondreaming sleep. It is secreted in high concentrations before and during puberty, especially in boys.

Clinical Indications Growth hormone and synthetic growth hormone (somatrem (Protropin)) are employed for treatment of pituitary dwarfism.

Adverse Effects and Contraindications Somatrem is contraindicated for use in clients with closed epiphyses, evidence of intracranial lesions, or sensitivity to benzyl alcohol (used as a preservative in somatrem). Approximately 30% of individuals treated with somatrem develop persistent antibodies to the hormone, but the antibodies seldom interfere with the response to therapy.

Somatrem occasionally induces a state of impaired glucose tolerance. *Nurses should advise parents of children receiving somatrem to watch for early indications of impaired glucose tolerance such as polyuria or weight loss.* Sometimes hypothyroidism develops during therapy with growth hormone and reduces the therapeutic response to the hormone. *Periodic evaluation of thyroid function should be conducted during somatrem therapy.*

Preparations and Administration Growth hormone extracted from cadavers, called somatropin, was available through 1985 in modest quantities for clinical applications. It was an expensive and scarce drug. The first individual treated with it grew 14 inches in a period of 7 years of treatment, finally reaching a height of 64 inches. Growth hormone synthesized by recombinant DNA technology, called somatrem, became available in January 1986. Somatrem is therapeutically equivalent to natural growth hormone. Because it is a protein, growth hormone must be stored under refrigeration, between 36° and 46°F (2°–8°C).

Somatrem (Protropin)
Powder for reconstitution in bacteriostatic water
Recommended Doses: Up to 0.1 mg/kg IM, 3 times per week.

Acromegaly and Gigantism

When pituitary secretion of GH is excessive, acromegaly and gigantism result. Usually the excessive activity of the anterior pituitary is triggered by presence of an adenoma (benign tumor), most commonly restricted to the acidophilic cells that secrete GH and prolactin. When GH excess occurs early in life, before the epiphyses have closed, there is a growth of bone in both length and width. Heights of more than 8 feet have occurred. Growth of the mandible causes protrusion of the jaw, overbite, and separation of the teeth, and facial features become coarse. In the hands and feet, the acral parts become broad and the digits enlarged. The term acromegaly refers to all of these features that are a consequence of excessive bone growth. Visceral complications include enlargement of the heart and kidneys, with possible hypertension. Skin is thickened, hirsutism may occur, and galactorrhea is often present because of concurrent involvement of prolactin.

Treatment of GH hypersecretion often involves surgery or radiation therapy directed at the pituitary. Another approach, paradoxically, has been the use of the dopamine agonist, bromocriptine (Parlodel). In normal individuals, dopamine agonists increase secretion of growth hormone. In pituitary gigantism, however, bromocriptine suppresses GH secretion by pituitary tumors. The drug is typically given in divided doses providing a daily total of 2.5–40 mg. Small doses are used initially to minimize side effects, which include nausea, vomiting, constipation, and occasionally hypotension. Bromocriptine is effective in suppressing GH secretion in 25% of cases, but withdrawal of the drug is associated with resurgence of GH secretion.

The Posterior Pituitary

The posterior pituitary releases two hormones, oxytocin and vasopressin (also known as antidiuretic hormone, or ADH). These hormones are synthesized within certain nuclei of the hypothalamus and transported by axonal flow from the hypothalamus to the posterior lobe of the pituitary, where they are stored and secreted. Secretion is regulated by nerve impulses arising in the same nuclei of the hypothalamus in which the hormones are synthesized.

Oxytocin stimulates uterine contraction and ejection of milk. Its release is initiated by uterine distention, vaginal distention, or suckling. Oxytocin also produces a transient fall in blood pressure caused by vasodilation. Oxytocin is used to induce labor at term and to treat postpartum hemorrhage or uterine atony. It is administered intravenously or intramuscularly. Available preparations are synthetic. Oxytocin is contraindicated in the first and second stages of labor because contractions may be too vigorous; fetal deaths have been reported when oxytocin was so used. Its use is discussed further in Chapter 34.

Vasopressin, or antidiuretic hormone (ADH), acts preeminently on the distal tubule of the nephron of the kidney, promoting permeability of the renal tubule epithelium to water and thereby diminishing excretion of water. Secretion of ADH is controlled by the hypothalamus, which has specialized osmoreceptors that monitor body hydration. The disease associated with ADH deficiency is **diabetes insipidus.** In this disease, large quantities of dilute urine are produced. Vasopressin is given intramuscularly or subcutaneously to alleviate diabetes insipidus. Vasopressin has weak oxytocic effects but is not used for this purpose. The most serious side effect of ADH is spasms of the coronary arteries. If the dose is excessive, water retention may become exaggerated. The role of ADH is discussed further in Chapter 43.

Case Study: Isolated Growth Hormone Deficiency

R. G., age 4 months, was brought to the pediatrician at the local clinic. Examination confirmed the mother's suspicion that the infant was showing signs of growth failure. Although there was no familial history of deficient pituitary function, the preliminary diagnosis of growth hormone deficiency was confirmed by measurement of plasma growth hormone concentrations by radioimmunoassay. Treatment with somatrem was initiated at 0.1 mg/kg IM, 3 times weekly. The nurse taught the parents of R. G. to reconstitute the powder in preparation for injections, to make sure that the solution was clear of particulate matter, and to inject the dosage properly to ensure that the solution reached muscle tissue. The nurse explained to the parents the importance of storing the powder between 36° and 46°F and of using reconstituted solution within 7 days. The parents were taught to mark on a calendar when the solution was reconstituted to assure accuracy. The nurse also instructed the parents to keep a daily record of the child's length and weight and to watch for and record any early symptoms of glucose intolerance, such as polyuria or weight loss. The parents were taught to keep track of the number of diaper changes and degree of wetness as a means of assessing urinary output. The nurse established a schedule with the parents for evaluation of therapy, including general assessment and evaluation of injection sites monthly at first and measurements of serum thyroxine and T_3 resin uptake at 6-month intervals.

1. Is it surprising that there was no familial history of dwarfism in this case? Why?
2. Why is it important to store growth hormone between 36° and 46°F?
3. Why did the nurse instruct the parents about symptoms of glucose intolerance?
4. Why did the nurse schedule periodic assessment of thyroid function?

Answers appear at the end of the book.

Recommended Readings

Daniels CA: A "little" boy — treatment with human growth hormone. *Nurs Times* 1980;76:1921–1922.

Frasier SD: Human pituitary growth hormone (hGH) therapy in growth hormone deficiency. *Endocr Rev* 1983;4: 155–170.

Hall MB: New heights for growth hormone-deficient children. *Nurse Pract* 1982;7(10):26–36.

Hintz RL, Rosenfeld RG: Clinical uses of synthetic growth hormone. *Hosp Pract* 1983;18(10):115.

Phillips LS, Vassilopoulou-Sellin R: Somatomedins. *N Engl J Med* 1980;302:371–380.

Salomon B: The hypothalamus and the pituitary gland: An overview. *Nurs Clin North Am* 1980;15(3):435–451.

Vale W et al: Regulatory peptides of the hypothalamus. *Annu Rev Physiol* 1977;39:473–527.

CHAPTER 31

Drugs Used for Thyroid and Parathyroid Disorders

The thyroid and parathyroid glands are located in the neck. The yellowish thyroid gland is a butterfly-shaped structure that wraps around the trachea. The four parathyroid glands appear as two pairs of small nodes, one pair at each lateral pole of the thyroid. The thyroid and parathyroid glands produce four hormones that are involved in two distinct regulatory activities. **Thyroxine** (T_4) and **triiodothyronine** (T_3), secreted by the thyroid gland, are involved in energy balance. The third thyroid hormone, **calcitonin,** and **parathyroid hormone** (PTH) are engaged in regulating calcium homeostasis. This chapter begins with consideration of the thyroid hormones related to energy metabolism and then, in the second section, turns to the hormones involved in regulation of calcium.

Regulation of Energy Metabolism: T_3 and T_4

Thyroid Hormones

Physiological Effects of Thyroid Hormones

The thyroid hormones stimulate oxidative metabolism, elevating basal metabolic rate and promoting growth and differentiation. The effects of thyroid hormones are observed in nearly every tissue. Metabolic activity in the heart, liver, kidney, skeletal muscles, nervous system tissue, and secretory organs of the skin is stimulated by thyroid hormones. The ovaries and uterus are rare exceptions, being unresponsive to thyroid hormones. It is believed that thyroid hormones bind to receptors within the nucleus of target cells to regulate protein synthesis in some manner that results in an increase in metabolic activity in the cell. T_3 is several times more active than T_4 because it binds more readily to the receptor sites in the nucleus. However, T_4 is converted in the liver into T_3, which is then returned to the blood. Much of the pharmacological activity associated with administered T_4 is due to the more active metabolite. Thyroid hormones promote lipolysis (breakdown of fat), carbohydrate utilization, protein synthesis, and oxygen consumption. At the organ system level, thyroid hormones increase cardiac output, possibly due to an increased cardiac sensitivity to catecholamines. Thyroid hormones must be present in early infancy for normal development of the cerebral cortex. Thyroid hormones promote excretion of water and electrolytes, help to generate heat in temperature regulation, and are required for the periodicity of the menstrual cycle.

Synthesis of Thyroid Hormones

Thyroid hormones are synthesized by enzymatic conversions of the tyrosine residues of a thyroid protein called thyroglobulin (Figure 31–1). This protein is abundant in the thyroid, representing a large portion of the mass of the thyroid. Synthesis occurs in five steps. First, the thyroid gland efficiently traps iodide from the circulation. The thyroid accumulates levels normally about 25 times that of the blood and, when stimulated, over 100 times the serum concentration. Second, after uptake, iodide is oxygenated by action of a peroxidase enzyme. In the third step, one or two of these oxygenated iodine atoms are then attached to each tyrosine residue of thyroglobulin to form monoiodotyrosyl (MIT) or diiodotyrosyl (DIT) moieties. Fourth, one of each of these, or two of the latter, are coupled together to form, respectively, triiodothyronine (T_3) or thyroxine (T_4) segments, still integrated within the thyroglobulin protein. Normally, more T_4 than T_3 is formed, by a 4:1 margin. However, if there is a deficiency of iodide, T_3 may be formed preferentially. This improves the efficiency of utilization of iodide not only because T_3 contains one less iodide atom per molecule but also because T_3 is about four times as active as T_4. Large amounts of T_3 and T_4 are stored in the form of constituents of thyroglobulin, providing a degree of insurance against short-term iodide deficiency.

The final step, release of T_3 and T_4, is brought about by the action of proteolytic enzymes that systematically break apart the thyroglobulin protein to release the T_3 or T_4 into the blood as cleavage products. The activity of the proteolytic enzymes, and thus the release of T_3 and T_4, can be stimulated by TSH or by long-acting thyroid stimulator (LATS), an immunoglobulin formed as a result of autoimmunity and responsible for many cases of hyperthyroidism.

The normal daily production of T_4 is about 70–90 μg. T_3 production is less, about 15–30 μg, and only about 20% of this comes from the thyroid. The remainder derives from peripheral conversion of T_4 to T_3 by partial deiodination.

Regulation of the Thyroid

The thyroid gland is regulated by thyrotropin (TSH) from the pituitary in three distinct ways. TSH stimulates secretion of thyroid hormones, increases iodide uptake and synthesis of thyroid hormone, and promotes hypertrophy, hyperplasia, and increased vascularity of the thyroid gland.

Release of TSH from the anterior pituitary is itself controlled by hypothalamic thyrotropin releasing hormone (TRH). The release of TRH from the pituitary is stimulated by activity of brain noradrenergic neurons but inhibited by dopaminergic activity. Feedback inhibition is exerted by thyroid hormones at the level of the pituitary and possibly in the hypothalamus as well.

There are several other stimulators of the thyroid, including prostaglandin E, a glycoprotein called chorionic thyrotropin secreted by the placenta during pregnancy, and a thyrotropin secreted by hydatidiform moles. Most important of the thyroid stimulators other than TSH is long-acting thyroid stimulator (LATS). The binding of this immunoglobulin to antigenic sites on the surface of thyroid follicular cells is a major cause of thyrotoxicosis.

Transport and Elimination of Thyroid Hormones

In the plasma, most T_3 and T_4 (about 99.5%) is bound by plasma proteins. The bound fraction is in equilibrium with free hormone and serves as the immediate source of resupply. Protein binding protects the bulk of the thyroid hormone from metabolism and excretion, providing thyroid hormone with an unusually long plasma half-life (6–7 days, normally). T_3 constitutes only about 5% of the total thyroid hormone in the circulation but makes up closer to 33% of the free fraction because it is less securely bound than T_4.

The major pathway of metabolism of thyroid hormones is deiodination in the liver. This accounts for about 80% of inactivation of T_3 and T_4. Most of the rest consists of conjugation in the liver with subsequent biliary excretion. Deiodination of T_4 initially produces T_3, and as much as 80% of T_3 may derive from this process.

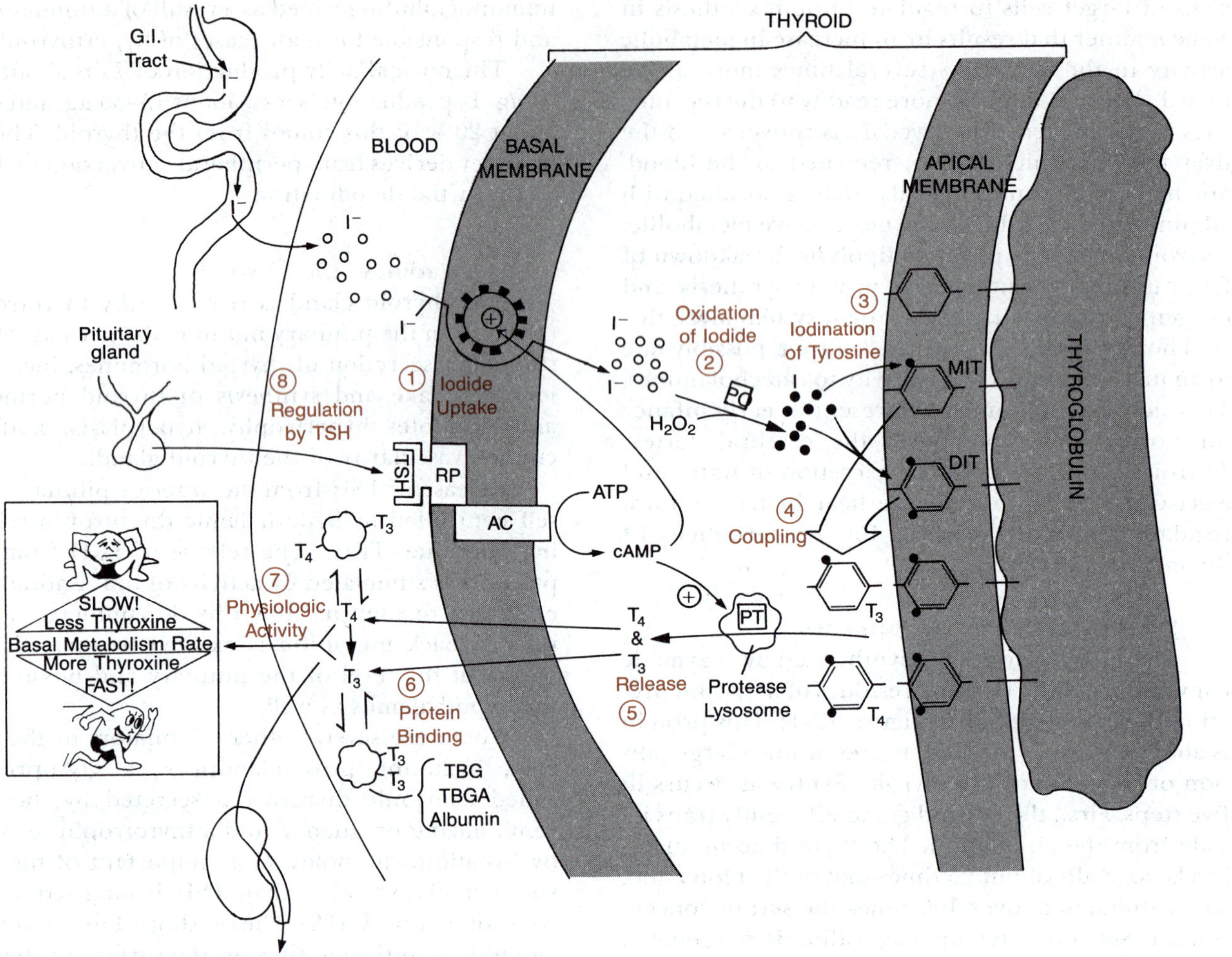

Figure 31–1

Physiology of the thyroid hormones. The thyroid gland takes up iodide (1), which is oxidized to iodine (2) by a peroxidase (PO) enzyme. Iodine is used for the iodination (3) of tyrosine residues of thyroglobulin, producing monoiodotyrosine (MIT) or diiodotyrosine (DIT). A DIT is coupled (4) with a MIT to form triiodothyronine (T_3) or with another DIT to form thyroxine (T_4). T_3 and T_4 can be severed from thyroglobulin by the action of the enzyme protease, and released into the blood (5). In the blood, thyroid hormones are reversibly bound (6) to the plasma protein thyroxine-binding globulin (TBG), thyroxine-binding prealbumin (TBPA), and albumin proteins. The unbound T_3 and T_4 fractions exert the physiological influence (7) on basal metabolic rate of tissue cells. TSH controls (8) the activity of the iodide uptake mechanism, the activity of the protease enzyme, and the growth of the thyroid over time.

Evaluation of Thyroid Function

The initial objective in evaluation of thyroid function is an estimate of free thyroid hormone; however, amounts of free T_3 and T_4 in the plasma are minute. Therefore, the usual first test of thyroid function, called **serum total thyroxine,** measures both free and bound T_4. This radioimmunoassay, and all others that measure total T_3 or T_4, give false positives when levels of thyroid-binding globulin (TBG) are unusually high or low, even though free thyroid hormone may be normal.

A serum total thyroxine test may be followed by a **T_3 resin uptake** test to resolve whether abnormal thyroxine levels indicate only an alteration in protein-binding sites or reflect instead a clinically significant decrease in free *and* bound thyroid hormone

Table 31–1
Results of Thyroid Function Tests in Relation to Various Thyroid Conditions

Physiological condition	Serum total T_4 test	T_3 resin uptake
Euthyroid (normal)	4.0–13.0 µg/100 ml	25–35% bound to resin (65–75% bound to plasma proteins)
Hyperthyroid	↑	↑
Euthyroid with thyroxine-binding globulin (TBG) ↑ by estrogen	↑	↓
Hypothyroid	↓	↓
Euthyroid with TBG ↓ by anabolic steroids or presence of a competitive ligand (such as phenytoin)	↓	↑

(Table 31–1). Low values in this test indicate a large number of unoccupied serum binding sites, which occurs in hypothyroidism or when TBG is elevated. High values indicate hyperthyroidism or reduced levels of TBG. The product of the results from a total serum thyroxine test and a T_3 resin uptake test is called the **free thyroxine index,** and provides a good indicator of thyroid status. Normal values range from about 0.75–2.5.

Still other tests help to determine the etiology when abnormal thyroid function is evident. **Serum thyroid-stimulating hormone** (TSH) can be measured by radioimmunoassay. In primary hypothyroidism, it is elevated due to reduced negative feedback; in secondary hypothyroidism, TSH is usually undetectable. If this test indicates secondary hypothyroidism, a **challenge dose of TRH** can be administered to determine further if the defect is hypothalamic or pituitary. If the defect is hypothalamic, the normally functioning pituitary should respond to TRH with a surge of TSH release. In primary hyperthyroidism, **thyroid scanning** can be used to characterize the nature of the structural abnormality. **Radioactive iodine uptake** is sometimes used to confirm a diagnosis of hyperthyroidism or to aid dosage determination when ^{131}I is going to be used as the treatment method in Graves' disease.

Various drugs can distort the results of tests employed to evaluate thyroid function (Table 31–2). *Whenever one or more laboratory tests of thyroid function is ordered, the nurse should review the client's medication regimen for drugs that might alter test results and inform both the physician and the laboratory when such drugs are being employed.*

Table 31–2
Drugs that May Alter Thyroid Function Tests

Thyroid function test	Drugs that decrease test values	Drugs that increase test values
Serum T_4	Anabolic steroids Androgens Antithyroid drugs Asparaginase Barbiturates Corticosteroids Danazol Diazepam Ethionamide Heparin Lithium Mitotane Nitroprusside Oxyphenbutazone Phenylbutazone Phenytoin Resorcinol Salicylates Sulfonylureas	Estrogens (including oral contraceptives) Fluorouracil Insulin Methadone Perphenazine Propranolol
T_3 resin uptake	Antithyroid drugs Estrogens (including oral contraceptives) Fluorouracil Lithium Methadone Perphenazine Resorcinol	Anabolic steroids Androgens Asparaginase Corticosteroids Danazol Heparin Oxyphenbutazone Phenylbutazone
Free thyroxine index	Antithyroid drugs Barbiturates Corticosteroids Diazepam Lithium Oxyphenbutazone Perphenazine Phenylbutazone Phenytoin Resorcinol	Estrogens Heparin Propranolol
Serum TSH	Corticosteriods Danazol	Antithyroid drugs Lithium Resorcinol

Hypothyroidism

Inadequate production of thyroid hormones is called **hypothyroidism,** or **myxedema** (Figure 31–2). Hypothyroidism is usually primary — due to a dys-

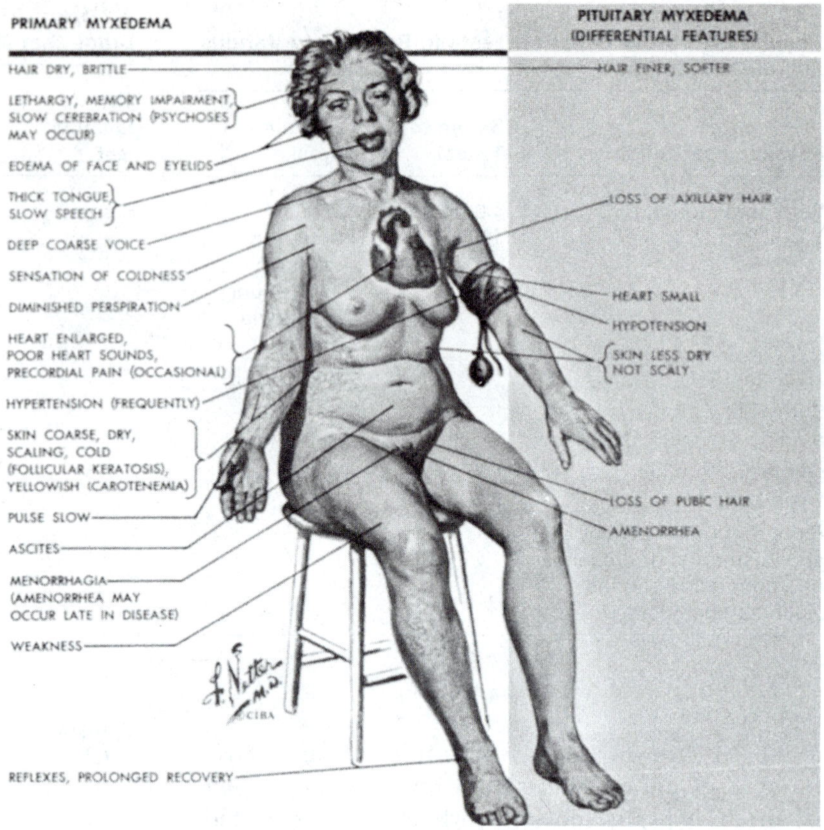

Figure 31–2
Clinical manifestations of myxedema. © Copyright 1969 CIBA-GEIGY Corporation. Reproduced, with permission, from *The CIBA Collection of Medical Illustrations* by Frank H. Netter, M.D. All rights reserved.

function of the thyroid gland itself. Secondary hypothyroidism occurs when the pituitary fails to produce adequate TSH, because of either hypopituitarism or inadequate TRH secretion by the hypothalamus.

A deficiency of thyroid hormone can occur at any age. Congenital deficiency results in cretinism. Cretinism is characterized by dwarfism. The individual has short extremities and is mentally lethargic and retarded. Respiratory distress, cyanosis, jaundice, a puffy and expressionless face, enlarged and protruding tongue, poor feeding, hypothermia, and umbilical hernia are common. Prompt identification and treatment is crucial for minimization of defects.

When thyroid deficiency occurs later in childhood, growth and development are impaired; in adolescence, short stature and precocious puberty may occur. Weakness and lethargy often result, and hypothyroid children tend to be inactive and overweight, and are often considered dull. *When juvenile hypothyroid clients begin thyroid replacement therapy, the nurse should alert both the client and the parents to the dramatic changes they can expect, such as rapid growth and weight loss, increased assertiveness, and shedding of hair. If the child is young, the nurse needs to teach parents safety measures to minimize dangers that occur as the child increases ambulation. Nurses should also work with parents of hypothyroid children to encourage maintenance of a nutritious diet.* In addition to abnormalities related to growth, children also suffer from the adult symptoms of hypothyroidism.

In classic adult hypothyroidism, there is loss of thyroid tissue, usually as a sequel to Hashimoto's thyroiditis or a therapeutic intervention for hyperthyroidism. Clients with mild hypothyroidism may exhibit subtle and insidious signs and symptoms that are often unrecognized as endocrine disorders. In severe cases, symptoms become obvious. The skin is cold, dry, and scaly, reflecting the low metabolic rate of secretory cells. The skin may also be pallid or carotenous due to carotene accumulation in the expanded subepidermal fatty tissue. The hair is coarse, thin, and brittle. The nails are thick but brittle. The voice is deepened, the tongue is thickened, and speech is impaired. Mental function is impaired as well, with a general slowing of cognitive activity, depression, lethargy, a lack of expression, and in extreme cases, frank psychosis. Heart rate is slowed and eyelids droop due to diminished sympathetic tone. Appetite is poor and body temperature is low because of the reduced basal metabolic rate. Gastrointestinal secretory activity is also reduced, causing constipation and distention. Anemia occurs in some cases. Menstrual bleeding is increased in some women.

The most common cause of hypothyroidism is **Hashimoto's thyroiditis.** This autoimmune disorder occurs much more commonly in women than men (8:1 ratio) and mainly in those 30–50 years of age. A familial history of the disorder is common. Many patients with this condition also have other autoimmune or endocrine disorders such as pernicious anemia, rheumatoid arthritis, adrenal insufficiency, hypoparathyroidism, or diabetes mellitus. In Hashimoto's thyroiditis, antibodies are formed against an exposed, antigenic component of the thyroid gland and extensive infiltration of the gland by white blood cells follows.

Thyroiditis can also occur as a temporary, subacute response to viral infection, marked by throat pain and enlarged thyroid tissue. Nonsteroidal anti-inflammatory drugs are indicated for subacute thyroiditis.

Thyroid Hormones as Drugs

Pharmacokinetics After oral administration, T_3 is better absorbed than T_4, being 95% absorbed within 4 hours after administration. Absorption of T_4 is not only less but is more variable. Absorption ranges from about 50% to 80% with T_4, with higher values likely when the drug is taken on an empty stomach. Both T_3 and T_4 are highly bound to plasma proteins.

There are important differences between T_3 and T_4 with respect to duration of action, since the activity of T_4 is mainly due to T_3 formed from deiodination of T_4 in the liver, kidneys, and other tissues. The half-life of T_4 is 6–7 days, while that of T_3 is less than 2 days.

Clinical Indications Thyroid hormone preparations are indicated for replacement therapy for hypothyroidism. The objective of therapy is to establish a normal level of thyroid hormone activity (called a euthyroid state). T_3 is preferred over T_4 during initiation of therapy because its more rapid inactivation permits quick adjustments if cardiac dysrhythmias occur during the early stages of replacement. But T_4 is preferred to T_3 for long-term replacement because the rapid inactivation of T_3 would necessitate administration 2 or 3 times per day, and even then standard replacement quantities would result in periods of functional hyperthyroidism 2–4 hours after each administration.

Adverse Effects and Contraindications The most significant adverse response to thyroid hormone is a risk of **cardiac dysrhythmias,** sometimes fatal, early in therapy. Thyroid medication should be used with caution if the person receiving it has a history of cardiovascular disease, since an increase in metabolic activity may place added demand on cardiac workload. This is more likely to occur when replacement is conducted with T_3 than with T_4 because of the more rapid action of T_3. *The nurse should be quick to note occurrence of chest pains. An increase in pulse rate during sleep is one of the first indicators of thyroid hormone toxicity. Children placed on thyroid hormone and thyroxin should have their pulse monitored both when they are asleep and in the morning before breakfast.* Thyroid hormones should also be used cautiously for clients with hypertension or diabetes mellitus.

Some women may report irregularities of the menstrual cycle. Increased bowel motility may cause a client to have diarrhea. Also there is a potential for development of anaphylactic reactions in response to thyroid hormones. Sudden profuse sweating, clammy skin, or pallor should be interpreted as symptoms that require immediate attention of a physician, and clients and their families need to know what to look for and what to do.

Drug-Drug and Drug-Diet Interactions With long-term thyroid hormone therapy, adrenocortical insufficiency may occur. Clients who are diabetic may require adjustments in **antidiabetic drug** regimens when thyroid hormone doses are increased or decreased because thyroid hormones increase appetite and cellular requirements for glucose.

Clients receiving **oral anticoagulants** may likewise require dosage adjustment in the period following initiation of thyroid hormone treatment. Thyroid hormones can potentiate anticoagulant effects of substances such as bishydroxycoumarin. *People receiving both of these kinds of drugs simultaneously should be monitored closely. If the client is a women, the nurse should ask whether menstrual flow is normal or recently excessive. The nurse should also inquire as to whether the client has a tendency to bleed when he or she has a minor injury.*

Cardiac glycosides and **lithium** may aggravate hypothyroidism and may increase requirements for thyroid hormone supplements. At the same time, it should be recognized that thyroid hormones increase the risk of dysrhythmias developing in response to cardiac glycosides.

Nursing Observations for Thyroid Hormone Therapy of Hypothyroidism

THERAPEUTIC GOAL	Restore normal or near-normal functioning by hormone replacement.
PREADMINISTRATION ASSESSMENT	
Baseline Data	Evaluate temperature, respiration, pulse, blood pressure, electrocardiogram, heart sounds, skin texture and perfusion, reflexes, affect, and orientation. Review laboratory tests of thryoid function and glucose levels in the urine and blood.
Contraindications/ Precautions	Check medical history for cardiovascular disorders.
Potential Interactions	Check current medication regimen for cardiac glycosides, anion exchange resins, oral anticoagulants, oral hypoglycemics, or insulin.
EVALUATION OF DRUG RESPONSE	
During Dosage Adjustment	Monitor temperature, respiration, pulse, blood pressure, glucose content of blood and urine, weight, and height (if the client is a child). Observe for angina, orthopnea, or dyspnea since too rapid replacement may result in cardiac distress.
For Therapeutic Benefit	Increased activity, improved mood and memory, and diminished edema can be expected to occur within 2 weeks. At home, the client should monitor and record pulse, weight, and height (if a child) on a daily basis.
For Adverse Effects	Monitor for diarrhea, menstrual irregularities, rash, anaphylactoid reactions, clammy skin, pallor, nervousness, insomnia, and hypoglycemia.
For Drug Interactions	Monitor clients who are begun on thyroid replacement therapy for increased bleeding with oral anticoagulants and increased cardiac toxicity with cardiac glycosides; observe clients who are also receiving insulin or oral hypoglycemics for evidence of a need to increase the dose of the antidiabetic drug when thyroid hormone doses are increased or a need to reduce the dose of antidiabetic drug when thyroid hormone doses are reduced.
For Dietary Interactions	Monitor for excessive ingestion of goitrogenic foods such as cabbage, turnips, rutabagas, peaches, pears, spinach, carrots, soybeans, kale, cauliflower, and brussel sprouts.
For Compliance	Evaluate client's compliance with all facets of the therapeutic regimen by careful observation, interviewing, and review of progress. Report compliance problems to the physician and act as client-advocate when changes in the therapeutic regimen seem indicated.

Thyroid hormones increase toxicity of **iodine,** so that even small amounts must be avoided during replacement therapy. *Clients must be taught to avoid use of iodinized salt as well as multivitamins, dentifrices, and other nonprescription medications (even topical ones) that contain iodine.*

People receiving thyroid hormone therapy should also be counseled on **diet,** to ensure that the selection of foods will accommodate their increased appetite and energy demands. Some specific foods are goitrogenic and may alter requirements for thyroid hormones if there is residual endogenous thyroid hormone production. Goitrogenic foods include cabbage, turnips, rutabagas, peaches, pears, spinach, carrots, soybeans, kale, kelp, iodized salt, cauliflower, and brussel sprouts.

Preparations and Administration Thyroid, USP consists of the dried and powdered thyroids of animals, usually pigs, compressed into tablets. The "USP" stands for **United States Pharmacopeia** and specifies an iodine content between 0.17% and 0.23%. The dosage formulations currently available are listed in Table 31–3. Thyroid, USP is inexpensive but variable in the proportion of T_3 to T_4, and therefore in its activity. *Thyroid, USP should be stored in light- and moisture-resistant containers.*

Thyroglobulin, USP (Proloid), is a purified ex-

Nursing Diagnoses and Interventions for Thyroid Drug Replacement Therapy for Hypothyroidism

Nursing Diagnoses	*Related Interventions*
TO ENHANCE DRUG BENEFITS OR REDUCE DRUG REQUIREMENTS	
Alteration in nutrition: intake exceeds reduced metabolic needs	Control caloric intake.
Activity intolerance related to fatigue and weakness	Encourage adequate rest and schedule rest periods during the day.
Altered bowel function: constipation related to decreased peristalsis	Minimize constipation with appropriate regimens of fluids, dietary bulk, exercise, and laxatives if necessary; avoid enemas.
Impaired skin integrity related to edema and diminished secretions	Minimize risk of skin irritation. Keep skin clean and well lubricated.
Alteration in comfort: cold intolerance	Keep environment comfortably warm; dress appropriately for the environment.
Decreased cardiac output	Monitor cardiac status and report any deficit to the physician.
Impaired social interactions related to depression and lethargy	Provide emotional support and reassurance. Avoid depressant drugs.
Impaired verbal communication related to enlarged tongue and mental depression	Encourage those who communicate with the client to take special care to understand the client's speech; consider referral for speech therapy.
TO MINIMIZE DRUG SIDE EFFECTS OR INTERACTIONS	
Alteration in cardiac output and tissue perfusion related to thyroid medication	Monitor for fluid accumulation and other signs of altered cardiac output and report these to the physician.
Alteration in comfort: heat intolerance and diaphoresis related to thyroid medication	Adjust environmental temperature or clothing.
Alteration in nutrition: intake less than metabolic requirements related to thyroid drugs	Provide balanced diet, and increase number of meals as required.
Altered bowel function: diarrhea related to increased peristalsis due to thyroid drugs	Adjust dietary bulk.
Potential for injury related to tremor	Utilize safety measures to prevent injury from falls or dropping of heavy objects.
TO ENSURE SAFE AND EFFICACIOUS DRUG USE	
Knowledge deficit related to drug regimen	Explain importance of lifelong continuance of replacement therapy even after normal thyroid activity is restored.
	Provide client with list of symptoms of hyper- and hypothyroidism to aid in recognizing need for dosage adjustment.
	Teach client to record and report any incidents of angina, shortness of breath, or difficulty breathing in response to thyroid hormone therapy.
	Explain the action of the drug and how it is to be taken.
	Explain the need to wear an identification tag or bracelet that indicates the drug regimen.

Table 31-3
Thyroid Hormone Preparations

Generic	Trade names	Dosage forms
Thyroid, USP (desiccated animal thyroid glands)	Various	Tablets: 16, 32, 65, 98, 130, 195, 260, and 325 mg Enteric coated tablets: 65 and 130 mg
	Thyroid strong	Tablets: 32, 65, 130, and 195 mg (50% stronger than thyroid, USP)
	Thyrar (bovine thyroid)	Tablets: 32, 65, and 130 mg
	S-P-T (pork thyroid in soybean oil)	Capsules: 65, 130, 195, and 325 mg
Thyroglobulin (2.5:1 ratio of T_4 to T_3)	Proloid	Tablets: 32, 65, 100, 130, and 200 mg
Levothyroxine sodium (synthetic T_4)	Levothroid, Synthroid	Tablets: 0.025, 0.05, 0.075, 0.1, 0.125, 0.15, 0.175, 0.2, 0.3 mg Injection: 200 or 500 µg/vial
Liothyronine sodium (synthetic T_3)	Cytomel, Cyronine, generic	Tablets: 5, 25, and 50 µg
Liotrix (4:1 mixture of synthetic T_4 and T_3)	Euthroid, Thyolar	Tablets: equivalent to 15, 30, 60, 120, or 180 mg of thyroid, USP

tract of thyroglobulin from thyroid glands of pigs, containing T_4 and T_3 in an approximate 2.5:1 ratio. Preparations are standardized by biological assay. It is about twice as expensive as thyroid, USP. The dose requirements are the same as thyroid, USP.

Both T_3 and T_4 are available as synthetics. Levothyroxine sodium (Synthroid, Levothroid, Syroxine) is the sodium salt of T_4. Compliance is readily monitored with this preparation using the radioimmune assay for thyroxine. Levothyroxine sodium is stable and has predictable content. Absorption is variable, however. *Thyroxine should be taken on an empty stomach to minimize variability of absorption. It is usually taken once daily before breakfast.*

Liothyronine sodium (Cytomel) is the sodium salt of T_3. It is stable and of reliable content but short-acting and expensive. Preparations containing T_4 have durations of about 3 weeks, while T_3 preparations last only 5–6 days. Since liothyronine is shorter acting than other thyroid preparations, care must be taken in switching patients from thyroxine to liothyronine or vice versa. *When switching from thyroxine to liothyronine, thyroxine is discontinued and liothyronine is begun at low doses, then gradually increased. When switching from liothyronine to another thyroid hormone preparation, the new preparation is begun several days before liothyronine is discontinued.*

Liotrix (Euthroid, Thyrolar) consists of a 4:1 mixture of T_4 to T_3 that resembles the natural proportions of the two hormones. This product is more expensive and there is no convincing evidence that the two hormones have differential value.

Doses of thyroid preparations can be adjusted on the basis of symptom alleviation or signs of hyperthyroidism. Serum levels of T_4 may also be monitored. Replacement therapy is usually begun on the low side, for example, with 50 μg per day of thyroxine. After 1–2 weeks, the dose is increased to 100 μg, and in another week or two to 150 μg. Adjustment is then made based on symptoms and serum tests. If, on the other hand, there appears to be significant risk of complications of hypothyroidism such as accumulations of pericardial or pleural effusions, a full replacement dose may be employed from the beginning. *A single daily dose, preferably before breakfast, optimizes the benefit and compliance.*

For cretinism, early recognition and treatment are essential. Typical doses of levothyroxine are 10 μg/kg during the first 6 months after birth, 8 μg/kg during the second 6 months, 6 μg/kg until age 5, and 5 μg/kg until age 10. Thyroxine and TSH are monitored in the serum. Indications of inadequate replacement in an infant include bradycardia, inactivity, constipation, and a hoarse cry.

Myxedema coma is treated with intravenous injections of levothyroxine (500 μg) or preferably liothyronine (100 μg) given as a bolus. Cortisol may be given additionally because of frequent concomitant adrenal cortical insufficiency. Maintenance doses of T_4 (50 μg/day, IV) or T_3 (20 μg/day, IV) are continued until oral replacement therapy can be initiated. Body temperature is low in myxedema coma but should be raised gradually to minimize the risk of dysrhythmias.

Thyroid, USP
Formulations: See Table 31-3.
Recommended Doses: For daily replacement, 2–3 g PO.

Thyroglobulin, USP (Proloid)
Formulations: See Table 31-3.
Recommended Doses: Same as for thyroid, USP.

Levothyroxine sodium (Synthroid, Levothroid, Syroxine)
Tablets, powder for injection.

Recommended Doses: For daily replacement, 100–300 μg PO. Injections are given (IM or IV, but not in infusion solutions) only in clients who cannot take substances by the enteral route for extended periods of time.

Liothyronine sodium (Cytomel)
Tablets
Recommended Doses: 5–25 μg/day PO initially; 25–100 μg/day PO maintenance.

Liotrix (Euthroid, Thyrolar)
Tablets (T_4 content and one-quarter as much T_3)
Recommended Doses: Based on thyroid, USP equivalents: 60 mg liotrix equals 1 grain thyroid, U.S.P.

Important Nursing Implications for Thyroid Hormones

- ☐ Maintenance doses of thyroid hormone are best taken once each day, before breakfast, on an empty stomach.
- ☐ Instruct clients not to change brands of thyroid hormone preparation without the physician's approval since the various products vary in content and effect.
- ☐ Doses of thyroid hormones in growing children may be higher than those in adults.
- ☐ During initiation of thyroid replacement therapy, observe clients carefully for symptoms of cardiac toxicity such as tachycardia or chest pain.
- ☐ Assess the pulse rate prior to administering each dose of thyroid hormone. The drug should generally be withheld if the pulse rate exceeds 100/minute.
- ☐ Instruct clients who may be taking thyroid hormone without medical supervision for obesity, depression, or other ailments that thyroid hormone preparations are dangerous and no longer considered appropriate for such uses.
- ☐ Instruct clients not to exceed prescribed dosage frequency or amount because of the possible complications that may accompany thyroid replacement therapy.
- ☐ Instruct parents of children receiving thyroid supplements to maintain a record of height as an indicator of thyroid hormone activity and to observe children closely for evidence of over-dosage.
- ☐ When caring for clients receiving thyroid medications at home, carefully monitor the individual's progress and involve the family as well to assure that all potential hazards are identified and reported immediately to the physician.
- ☐ Monitor clients receiving insulin or oral hypoglycemic agents and all children for evidence of hypoglycemic reactions, such as nervousness, irritability, difficulty sleeping, profuse sweating, fatigue, and hunger.
- ☐ Monitor clients receiving oral anticoagulants for evidence of increased bleeding when thyroid replacement therapy is undertaken.
- ☐ Advise clients to avoid both ingestion and topical use of iodine-containing nonprescription drugs, multivitamins, and dentifrices. Teach clients what to look for on the labels.
- ☐ Advise clients to avoid goitrogenic foods, such as cabbage, turnips, rutabagas, peaches, pears, spinach, carrots, soybeans, kale, kelp, iodized salt, cauliflower, and brussel sprouts.
- ☐ Stress the importance of compliance, since discontinuing the drug therapy will cause the condition to revert. As improvements occur, the individual may feel that medication is no longer essential. Clients need to realize that thyroid replacement therapy is a lifelong process.

Hyperthyroidism

Hyperthyroidism occurs when there is either an elevation of unbound T_4 and T_3 or, occasionally, an elevation in only T_3. An elevation in both will be revealed by elevated total serum T_4 and ^{131}I uptake. When only T_3 is elevated, diagnosis is more difficult, requiring a radioimmunoassay specifically for T_3.

The symptoms of hyperthyroidism are many and varied (Figure 31–3) and are all related to an increase in metabolic rate. The skin is warm, moist, and thin. Heart rate is rapid and pulse pressure is increased. A fine tremor is often present. Goiter (enlargement of the thyroid gland) and exophthalmos (bulging eyeballs) occur commonly. Severe cases may be accompanied by atrial fibrillation.

Because of rapid metabolism, the individual feels warm, sweats profusely, and has a voracious appetite but nevertheless experiences weight loss, muscle wasting, and weakness. Frequency of bowel movements is increased, with possible diarrhea. The psychiatric symptoms include nervousness, irritability, increased activity, emotional instability, insomnia, hypersensitivity to stimuli, and restlessness. Many, but not all, of the symptoms of hyperthyroidism seem to indicate excess sympathetic activity (Table 31–4) and are controllable by administration of

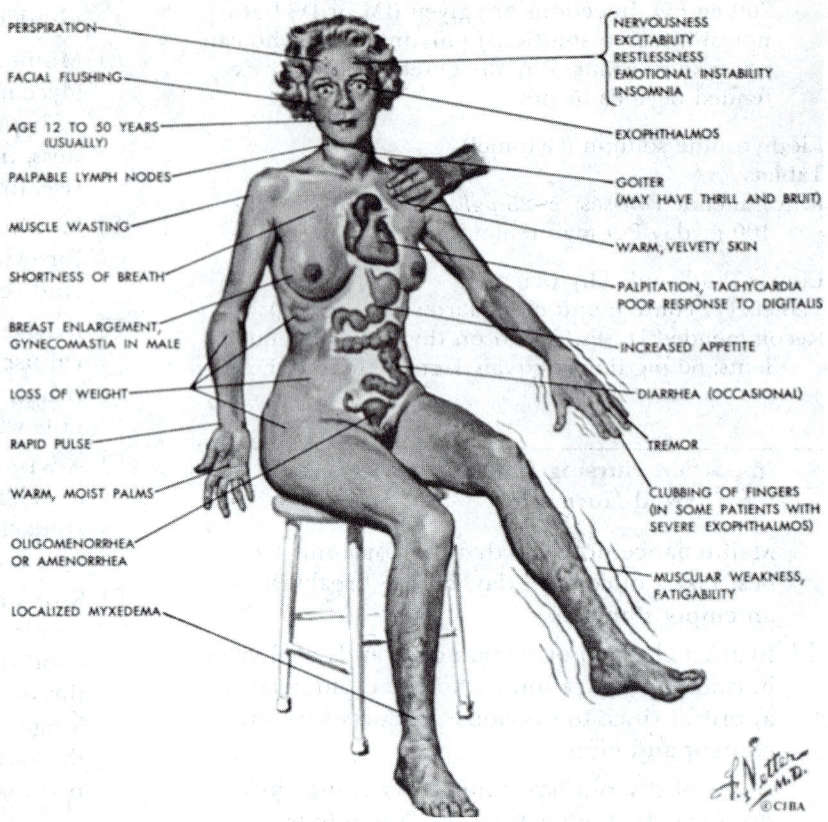

Figure 31–3
Clinical manifestations of hyperthyroidism. Similar symptoms can result from overly vigorous therapy with thyroid hormones. © Copyright 1969 CIBA-GEIGY Corporation. Reproduced, with permission, from *The CIBA Collection of Medical Illustrations* by Frank H. Netter, M.D. All right reserved.

Table 31–4
Symptoms of Hyperthyroidism

Related to adrenergic supersensitivity	Not related to adrenergic supersensitivity
Tachycardia	Increased oxygen consumption
Atrial fibrillation	Elevated appetite
Palpitations	Goiter
Tremor	Muscle wasting
Psychiatric symptoms	Exophthalmos
Diarrhea	Infiltrative dermopathy
Heat intolerance	
Sweating	
Stare	

beta-adrenergic blockers, such as propranolol (Inderal). Thyroid hormones are thought to increase sensitivity of adrenergic receptors to adrenergic hormones.

Hyperthyroidism may be caused by a diffuse goiter (Graves' disease), a multinodular goiter (Plummer's disease), a thyroid adenoma, subacute thyroiditis, or surreptitious self-administration of thyroid hormones (thyrotoxicosis factitia). Additional rare causes include secondary hyperthyroidism caused by a TSH-producing pituitary tumor, choriocarcinoma, or metastatic embryonal carcinoma of the testes. Most clients with Graves' disease have elevated serum levels of antibodies for the TSH receptor, either LATS or LATS-P.

Thyroid storm is an acute, life-threatening exacerbation of Graves' disease. Symptoms include fever, weakness, muscle wasting, mood lability, psychosis, hepatomegaly, and even coma. It occurs when untreated hyperthyroidism is acutely aggravated by infection, trauma, acidosis, stress, toxemia of pregnancy, thyroid surgery, irradiation, or as a rebound phenomenon when antithyroid drugs are discontinued. Treatment of thyroid storm includes administration of propranolol, propylthiouracil, iodine or iodide, and intravenous glucose; correction of dehydration, electrolyte imbalances, and hyperthermia; and digitalis, glucocorticoids, or antibiotics as required.

Goiter often occurs in association with hyperthyroidism but sometimes develops in hypothyroidism or without abnormal thyroid hormone activity (euthyroid goiter). **Endemic goiter** is caused by a deficiency in dietary iodide. If the deficiency is severe, hypothyroidism is seen as well as goiter, but when iodide deficiency is mild, the enlargement of the thyroid permits it to maintain normal hormone production. Provision of adequate dietary iodine alleviates the condition. Transient **euthyroid goiters** often occur during puberty, pregnancy, and menopause. They may occur in response to ingestion of goods containing goitrogens, such as turnips, or use of goitrogenic drugs, such as lithium or sulfonylureas.

Hyperthyroidism and associated goiter, if present, are treated in one of three ways: surgical removal of part of the thyroid, radioactive destruction of part of the thyroid by administration of ^{131}I, or use of antithyroid drugs.

Antithyroid Drugs

The antithyroid drugs include four groups of drugs: (1) thioamides including propylthiouracil, methimazole, and carbimazole; (2) monovalent anion inhibitors of iodide uptake, including thiocyanate and perchlorate; (3) iodide itself, in high concentrations; and (4) radioactive iodide, ^{131}I. In addition, certain drugs are useful for short-term alleviation of symptoms or complications of hyperthyroidism, most notably propranolol and to a lesser extent anxiolytics and vitamins.

Thioamides

Mechanisms and Effects Thioamides, such as propylthiouracil, inhibit formation of thyroid hormones by a combination of several mechanisms. They interfere with the incorporation of iodine into tyrosyl residues of thyroglobulin either by inhibiting the peroxidase enzyme or by reducing iodine that is ready for incorporation. In addition, thioamides inhibit coupling of monoiodinated and diiodinated tyrosyl residues. Propylthiouracil, but not other thioamides, may also inhibit peripheral conversion of T_4 to T_3 by deiodination. Clinical efficacy is observed only after thyroid stores of iodinated thyroglobulin are depleted, at which time circulating levels of thyroid hormones begin to decline.

Pharmacokinetics Thioamides are rapidly absorbed after oral administration, resulting in effective blood levels within 30 minutes. The half-life of propylthiouracil is about 2 hours and that of methimazole is 6–13 hours. A small dose of propylthiouracil is effective for only 2–3 hours and much larger doses last only 6–8 hours. The drugs and their metabolites are excreted mainly in the urine. Antithyroid drugs cross the placenta and are excreted in breast milk and can cause hypothyroidism in the fetus or neonate.

Clinical Indications Antithyroid drugs are used either as the sole mode of treatment for hyperthyroidism or as interim treatment for clients awaiting subtotal thyroidectomy or the full effects of radioiodine therapy. Clinical improvement is usually delayed a few days to a few weeks following initiation of antithyroid drug therapy. The length of the delay depends on the extent of the stores of preformed hormone, the turnover rate, and the completeness of inhibition by the antithyroid drug. After initial stabilization, treatment can continue with monthly or bimonthly assessments. Dosage adjustment is based on symptoms of hyper- or hypothyroidism and periodic measurement of total serum thyroxine. Individuals receiving too high a dosage of drug may complain of fatigue or weight gain. Symptoms of hypothyroidism indicate a need for dosage reduction and must sometimes be treated with short-term thyroid hormone supplements.

Some clients go into remission a few months after a euthyroid status has been achieved by drug therapy. Studies have suggested as few as 16% or as many as 50% may require no further drug treatment after a course of antithyroid drug therapy lasting 6 months to a year. These statistics are complicated by the possibility that remission and ultimately hypothyroidism may be the natural course of events in some cases of Graves' disease in the absence of treatment. Indications that remission has occurred include reduction in the size of the goiter, feedback suppression of endogenous thyroid activity (measured by ^{131}I uptake) when thyroid hormone is given, and complete absence of signs of hyperthyroidism when the smallest maintenance doses of propylthiouracil are employed. Most clients, and virtually all of those with Plummer's disease, ultimately require surgery or ^{131}I treatment.

Antithyroid drugs can be used to good effect to reduce the hazards of thyroid surgery. Common practice involves establishing a euthyroid state through drug therapy, followed by 7–10 days of iodide just prior to surgery to produce involution (shrinkage) and reduced vascularity of the thyroid gland. The physician may elect to take a patient off antithyroid medication for a period of time prior to surgery to reduce the potential of bleeding problems. *The nurse should reinforce the altered medication schedule by assuring that the client understands the need for the change.*

Nursing Observations for Antithyroid Drug Therapy of Hyperthyroidism

THERAPEUTIC GOAL	Restore normal thyroid function by reducing endogenous production of hormones.
PREADMINISTRATION ASSESSMENT	
Baseline Data	Observe extent of anxiety, nervousness, agitation, mood swings, talkativeness, and irritability; exopthalmos; tremor and increased tendon reflexes; tachycardia or other tachydysrhythmias; diarrhea, voracious appetite, weight loss, muscle wasting; warm, moist skin, diaphoresis. Evaluate pulse, blood pressure, heart sounds, respiration, ECG, skin texture, appetite, orientation, affect, and reflexes. If therapy with antithyroid drugs is anticipated, determine prothrombin time and obtain a complete blood cell count. Evaluate thyroid function and glucose levels in the blood and urine.
Contraindications/ Precautions	Determine if client is pregnant or nursing an infant.
Potential Interactions	Check medication history for use of oral anticoagulants, insulin, or an anion exchange resin.
EVALUATION OF DRUG RESPONSE	
During Dosage Adjustment	Monitor pulse, blood pressure, temperature, respiration, weight, and glucose levels in blood and urine. Question client regarding subjective changes.
For Therapeutic Benefit	Improvement in psychological symptoms, reduction in pulse rate, reduced appetite and weight gain, improvement in tremor and exophthalmos, and reduced diaphoresis can be expected in 3–8 weeks after initiation of antithyroid drug regimens. More immediate relief of mental symptoms, tachycardia, and tremor can be achieved in the interim by administration of propranolol.
For Exacerbation of the Condition	Evaluate symptoms for indications of intensification during stress or acute infections.
For Adverse Effects	Monitor T_3 and T_4 levels, neurological changes, prothrombin time, complete blood cell count, fever or sore throat, occurrence of skin rash, changes in weight, and fluid accumulation. Watch for symptoms of either hypothyroidism (excessive drug effect) or hyperthyroidism (insufficient control of the disorder).
For Drug Interactions	Monitor increased bleeding tendency with oral anticoagulants.
For Dietary Interactions	Monitor for excessive ingestion of goitrogenic foods resulting in symptoms of hypothyroidism.
For Compliance	Evaluate client's compliance with all facets of the therapeutic regimen by careful observation, interviewing, and review of progress. Report compliance problems to the physician and act as client-advocate when changes in the therapeutic regimen seem indicated.

Adverse Effects and Contraindications The most significant adverse effect of antithyroid drugs is **agranulocytosis.** The frequency of this adverse effect is approximately 1 in 500 or less. It occurs unpredictably, shortly after initiation of therapy or after many months. *Patients on thioamides should be advised to report immediately indications of agranulocytosis such as sore throat or persistent fever. Clients should be warned not to begin taking over-the-counter drugs in response to these symptoms on the assumption that they have a cold or other upper respiratory ailment.*

About 5% of clients receiving antithyroid drugs experience minor untoward effects, including dysarthria, urticaria, skin rash, paresthesia, headache, nausea, alopecia, or loss of hair pigmentation. **Hypoprothrombinemia** may occur. *The nurse should be alert for indications of hypoprothrombinemia such as purpura, ecchymoses, petechiae, or bleeding.* Individuals who have any underlying heart disease require close monitoring when given antithyroid medications. Complaints of shortness of breath, weakness, or tachycardia are signs of **cardiac insufficiency** that should be reported to a physician immediately.

Antithyroid drugs can cross the placental barrier, thereby causing **hypothyroidism in the fetus** that may extend into the early weeks of infancy. Therefore, while antithyroid drugs may be given during pregnancy, the amount of drug may need to be reduced. In fact, since many thyroid dysfunctions decrease during pregnancy, a physician may decide to eliminate the drug until 2 or 3 weeks after delivery. However, pregnant women who are or have been taking antithyroid drugs need close surveillance. Health care professionals who will be involved in the delivery of the baby should be made aware if a woman is continuing to receive antithyroid medication, since these drugs increase the potential for bleeding during delivery. Further, since antithyroid drugs are transmitted in breast milk and can cause hypothyroidism in infants, mothers who are receiving such drugs should not breast-feed their infants.

Preparations and Administration Two thioamides are available in the United States: propylthiouracil and methimazole (Tapazole). A third member of this family, carbimazole (Neomercazole) is available in Great Britain. *These drugs should be administered in a consistent relationship to mealtime since food will alter their absorption rates.*

Clients and families need to be told that antithyroid medication may not achieve immediate results. The amount of stored thyroid hormone present in the system varies from client to client. As the stores of hormone are depleted, symptoms of nervousness, anxiety, and abnormal sweating will gradually disappear. Observable changes can take from 3 days to 6 weeks after the onset of therapy. *Because of the delay in observable changes, many clients become discouraged. It is important to reassure such individuals continually, especially those at home.*

Propylthiouracil
Tablets
Recommended Doses: 100–150 mg orally, tid, initially. The dose is increased as required by increasing the number of daily doses rather than the amount given per dose.

Methimazole (Tapazole)
Tablets
Recommended Doses: 10–15 mg/day PO, in 2 or 3 divided doses. The dose is increased as required by increasing the number of daily doses rather than the amount given per dose.

Important Nursing Implications for Thioamides

- ☐ Teach clients to administer thioamides in consistent relation to mealtime each day.
- ☐ Withhold the drug if persistent fever, malaise, skin rash, or sore throat occurs and report the occurrence to the physician at once. Instruct clients who will be taking the drug at home to report such symptoms immediately.
- ☐ Inform the physician if the client has received radioactive iodide within the last 3–5 days before administering a thioamide.
- ☐ Urge the physician to reduce the dose of a thioamide or discontinue it altogether if the client becomes pregnant. Urge the physician to discontinue the thioamide at least 2 weeks prior to anticipated delivery.
- ☐ Advise women who are breast-feeding infants not to use thioamides.
- ☐ Advise clients that the therapeutic benefit of a thioamide may not occur until weeks or months after initiation of therapy.
- ☐ Teach clients how to monitor their progress by taking their own pulse daily, noting subjective symptoms, and keeping a record of weight changes.
- ☐ Instruct clients to adjust their caloric intake to match their changing caloric requirements.
- ☐ Arrange for complete blood cell counts at intervals of no more than 3 months during extended therapy with thioamides.
- ☐ Observe clients for symptoms of hypo- or hyperthyroidism that might occur as a result of inappropriate dosage.
- ☐ Watch for indications of bleeding (petechiae, purpura, bleeding of the gums), especially in clients also receiving oral anticoagulants.
- ☐ Instruct clients to avoid use of goitrogenic foods and over-the-counter medications containing iodide.
- ☐ Stress the importance of careful compliance with the prescribed regimen.

Monovalent Anions as Antithyroid Drugs

Thiocyanate and **perchlorate** (ClO_4^-) are monovalent anions that compete with iodide for the iodide uptake mechanism in the thyroid. These drugs are effective inhibitors of thyroid hormone production but are unacceptably toxic for most purposes, since they may produce aplastic anemia. Presence of thiocyanate in foods such as cabbage

Nursing Diagnoses and Interventions for Antithyroid Drug Therapy of Hyperthyroidism

Nursing Diagnoses	*Related Interventions*
TO ENHANCE DRUG BENEFITS OR REDUCE DRUG REQUIREMENTS	
Activity intolerance related to fatigue and muscle wasting in hyperthyroidism	Provide for adequate rest. Teach client the importance of ritual activities for sleep induction.
Alteration in cardiac output and tissue perfusion in hyperthyroidism	Monitor for fluid accumulation and other signs of altered cardiac output and report these to the physician.
Alteration in comfort: heat intolerance and diaphoresis in hyperthyroidism	Keep environment cool. Encourage client to wear light cotton clothing.
Alteration in nutrition: intake less than metabolic requirements in hyperthyroidism	Teach client to maintain a balanced diet and to increase number of meals as required.
Altered bowel function: diarrhea related to increased peristalsis in hyperthyroidism	Avoid bulk foods. Encourage adequate fluid intake to replace losses.
Impaired social interactions related to irritability and emotional instability in hyperthyroidism	Minimize stressful circumstances; avoid caffeine. Explain reasons for disturbed behavior to family and friends.
Potential for injury: corneal abrasions related to inability to close eyelids related to exopthalmos of hyperthyroidism	Teach the client to use methycellulose drops qid, to use protective glasses and a sleep mask, to exercise the ocular muscles, and to restrict sodium intake.
Potential for injury related to tremor of hyperthyroidism	Teach client to utilize safety measures to prevent injury from falls or dropping of heavy objects.
TO ENSURE SAFE AND EFFICACIOUS DRUG USE	
Knowledge deficit related to drug regimen	Teach the client the relationship between normal thyroid function and physical and mental well-being.
	Advise the client that benefits of antithyroid therapy may not be seen for several days or weeks.
	Instruct the client how to administer any antithyroid drugs appropriately.
	Provide the client with a list of the symptoms of hyper- and hypothyroidism.
	Instruct the clients receiving thioamides to report occurrence of persistent fever or sore throat.
	Instruct client about the importance of wearing a bracelet or other device that identifies the medical condition and drug regimen.

may contribute to endemic goiter if iodide intake is deficient.

Iodide/Iodine as Antithyroid Agents

Large doses of iodide produce a paradoxical inhibition of thyroid activity. Uptake of iodide is inhibited and iodination of tyrosyl residues is blocked. The gland itself shrinks and exhibits reduced vascularity. But iodide therapy fails to suppress thyroid function completely, and after a few weeks, thyroid activity returns to normal or may even increase. The most useful application of high-dose iodide therapy is for inducing involution of the thyroid gland in preparation for surgery.

Iodine, in a solution of potassium iodide, is sometimes ordered for clients to inhibit the synthesis and release of thyroid hormone. The dosage required is small and needs to be measured carefully, since one drop of saturated iodine solution contains 48 mg of iodine and one drop of strong iodine solution (Lugol's solution) contains 8 mg of iodine. (Some authorities suggest 6 mg daily is enough for the average client.)

Iodine solutions have a brassy taste and can cause a burning sensation in the mouth. *To alleviate the disagreeable taste and encourage compliance, nurses should suggest that the drug be diluted in water, orange juice, or chocolate milk. To decrease the sensation of burning in the mouth and possible discoloration or damage to tooth enamel, clients should use straws when drinking beverages in which iodine solutions have been dissolved.* Iodine solutions can also cause hypersalivation, which can be annoying. Some clients may be sensitive to the iodine and, in consequence, develop skin rashes. Others may develop diarrhea or gastric distress.

Radioactive Iodide in Hyperthyroidism

Clinical Indications Radioactive iodide (^{131}I) is used for both diagnostic and treatment purposes. Small doses given orally provide a useful technique for evaluating thyroid activity in hyperthyroidism. The rate of accumulation of the labeled iodide by the thyroid is monitored by placing a scanning device against the neck exterior to the thyroid gland. Higher doses of ^{131}I can be given orally or intravenously to produce destruction of part of the thyroid.

Adverse Effects and Contraindications Significant adverse reactions almost never occur when ^{131}I is employed in low doses for diagnostic purposes. On the other hand, adverse effects are common when higher doses are employed for destruction of thyroid tissue.

Clients should be advised that about 3 days after beginning therapy with ^{131}I, they can expect to have some tenderness and swelling of the neck. They will have a sore throat, they may have a cough, and they may experience pain when they swallow. Alerting the client to these likely reactions is important because these symptoms may resemble an upper respiratory tract infection. If not warned, the client might institute his or her own therapy, using over-the-counter drugs or leftover antibiotics. Some of the problems with swallowing can be alleviated by having the client lower the head on the chest when drinking or swallowing foods.

As time progresses, clients may develop nausea and vomiting, producing electrolyte imbalance. Their hematopoietic system and bone marrow may be depressed. As a consequence, blood cell production is reduced and there is a tendency to have immature erythrocytes released in the system. Lowered platelet count can result in hemorrhages in soft tissues. *Nurses need to assess clients carefully for easy bruising. They need to question clients concerning any changes in bowel habits or changes in the color of the stool. Any change should be reported immediately.*

Clients receiving ^{131}I therapy will have bone marrow depression, leaving them susceptible to infection. *Therefore, nurses must screen visitors to make sure the client is not exposed to infections. Utensils that the client uses should be kept clean, and the client should be encouraged to practice good personal hygiene.*

Some clients may undergo a thyroid crisis and should be observed carefully for signs of impending problems. *Nurses should monitor the patient's pulse rate as the patient sleeps as well as taking basal morning temperatures.* There may be a thinning of hair. *Nurses should reassure clients that loss of hair is temporary. Finally, clients need to be observed carefully for symptoms of hypothyroidism; any such symptoms should be reported immediately.*

Administration for Destruction of Thyroid Tissue Doses of radioactive iodine must be individualized for each patient based on uptake of a preliminary tracer dose. The dose is then determined so as to provide 7,000–10,000 rad/g of thyroid tissue. Even with careful dosage adjustment, there is a high risk that patients treated with ^{131}I will develop hypothyroidism either immediately or later in life. If, on the other hand, the dose is too small, hyperthyroidism may recur. When multiple treatments are required before control of the hyperthyroidism is achieved, there may be a long delay before relief is obtained from annoying clinical symptoms. *Radioactive iodide is not employed during pregnancy and is avoided in women under 40 because of unknown risks to offspring.*

Important Nursing Implications for ^{131}I

- ☐ Before initiating therapy, determine if the client has any history of sensitivity to administered iodine or iodine-rich foods such as shellfish. Ask the client if he or she has had any adverse reactions to previous medications or diagnostic tests where iodide was used.
- ☐ Delay the treatment regimen if the client has received any antithyroid medication within 2–3 days prior to the scheduled treatment. The nurse should alert the physician and other health team members.
- ☐ The nurse should explain any changes in plans to the client, particularly if the individual is receiving therapy for thyroid cancer. Some clients might otherwise interpret postponement of treatment as an indication that the disease has progressed beyond hope or that the condition does not really require treatment. In

either case the client might fail to keep the subsequent appointment.

- ☐ Withhold the scheduled treatment if the client is pregnant or nursing an infant.
- ☐ Institute measures for the protection of visitors and staff. Nurses need to know the specific activity of ^{131}I that is being excreted. If more than 30 mc is to be used for the client, the nurse needs to initiate precautionary measures to protect staff and visitors. Each institution has its own policy concerning the proper disposal of a patient's body wastes. It is important to use principles of time, distance, and shielding to decrease exposure of family, visitors, and hospital personnel. Nurses must keep at least a minimum distance from the patient and limit the amount of time they spend with the patient. It is important in these instances to explain these actions and to provide emotional support and reassurance during this difficult treatment. Nurses should also use a lead shield when caring for the patient.

Other Drugs in Hyperthyroidism

Propranolol (Inderal) alleviates those symptoms of hyperthyroidism attributable to elevated sensitivity to catecholamines (see Table 31–4). It is useful for interim management while awaiting effects of radioactive iodine or thioamides. The usual dose of propranolol for symptoms of hyperthyroidism is 20–40 mg, orally, qid. Antianxiety drugs may be useful temporarily to diminish the psychiatric manifestations. Vitamin supplements are appropriate in hyperthyroidism because rapid metabolic rate may lead to a functional deficiency of some vitamins.

Regulation of Calcium: Parathyroid Hormone and Calcitonin

The thyroid hormone calcitonin and parathyroid hormone are major contributors to calcium homeostasis, along with vitamin D (see Chapter 44). Many other hormones contribute less directly to calcium metabolism, including growth hormone, anabolic steroids, glucocorticoids, thyroid hormones, and pancreatic hormones.

Calcium Homeostasis

Calcium is the fifth most plentiful element in the body. It is important as a major constituent of bone and for nerve and muscle excitability, blood coagulation, cardiac function, and membrane structure. For these activities to be carried out successfully, the body must regulate the distribution and concentrations of calcium in the various compartments. It does so by regulating calcium entry through the intestines and exit through the kidneys, and by maintaining a large reserve of calcium in the skeletal tissue which can be used as a source for mobilization or a repository for excess calcium.

The skeleton contains 90% of all the bodily calcium. This large store is in equilibrium with soluble calcium of the extracellular fluid, which in turn exchanges calcium with the plasma. Bone is composed of calcium and phosphorus crystals embedded in a matrix of protein fibers (mainly collagen). Calcium and phosphorus provide strength while the protein provides flexibility. The outer layer of bone is composed of cortical bone, which is hard, while the bone interior is made up of porous trabecular bone. Two kinds of cells found in bone regulate the balance between soluble calcium and bone calcium: osteoblasts promote deposition of calcium to increase bone mass, and osteoclasts promote resorption of calcium from bone into blood.

Serum calcium is maintained at about 2.5 millimolar or 8.8–10.4 mg/100 ml. About 45% of the serum calcium is bound to serum proteins, 10% is complexed with anions (mainly citrate and phosphate), and the remainder is free, ionized calcium. This last fraction is the biologically active species. Until recently, only total serum calcium could be measured, but development of ion-specific electrodes has made feasible the measurement of serum ionized calcium.

Calcium is an essential dietary requirement. The recommended dietary allowance is 800 mg daily for children and adults, 1,200 mg for adolescents and women who are pregnant or lactating. Infants require 360 mg/day in the first 6 months; 540 mg in the second 6 months. The American diet provides anywhere from 200 to 2,500 mg per day, the major source being dairy products.

Calcium is absorbed mainly from the proximal portion of the small intestines by a carrier-mediated process. About one-third of ingested calcium is normally absorbed, yielding about 0.3–0.8 g, but the fraction absorbed is increased in calcium deficiency. Absorption of calcium is regulated principally by vitamin D, which promotes synthesis of the carrier proteins. Vitamin D deficiency results in impaired calcium absorption. Other causes of impaired calcium absorption include high levels of phytates, oxalate, or phosphate in the diet, chronic administration of glucocorticoids, diarrhea, malabsorption syndrome, or steatorrhea. Antiepileptic drugs, including phenobarbital, phenytoin (Dilantin), and primidone (Mysoline), and other inducers of liver enzymes increase liver metabolism of vitamin D and consequently may result in subnormal calcium levels.

Calcium is lost in small amounts in saliva, bile, sweat, pancreatic secretions, and breast milk, but renal excretion is the main form of elimination. Calcium is filtered and reabsorbed but not secreted. Reabsorption occurs throughout the length of the nephron and is stimulated by parathyroid hormone in the distal tubule and by vitamin D in the proximal tubule.

Cytoplasmic concentrations of calcium are very low because calcium is sequestered by the sacroplasmic reticulum and mitochondria. Calcium influx from the extracellular fluid and release from the sacroplasmic reticulum occur when nerve or muscle cells are electrically excited. Release of transmitters, hormones, or autocoids by all types of neurosecretory cells is dependent on this rapid rise in cytoplasmic calcium concentrations. Calcium influx also alters metabolic activities within cells by binding with calcium-sensitive regulatory proteins such as calmodulin and troponin. Calcium is needed for propagation of action potentials, regulation of sodium channels, and excitation-contraction coupling in muscles. Serum calcium levels are maintained most directly by parathyroid hormone, in concert with vitamin D, and by calcitonin.

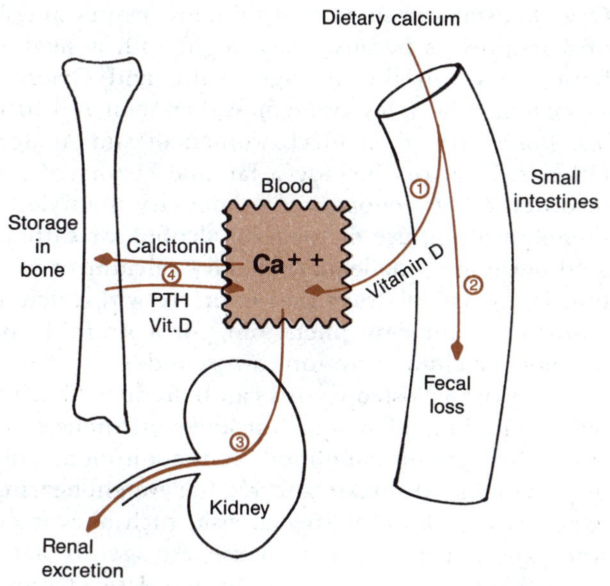

Figure 31–4
Causes of hypocalcemia. (1) Increased fecal loss of calcium in diarrhea or steatorrhea; (2) decreased absorption due to vitamin D deficiency or glucocorticoids; (3) increased renal excretion of calcium caused by diuretics, chronic renal failure, or hyperphosphatemia; and (4) decreased solubilization of calcium from bone in hypoparathyroidism or vitamin D deficiency.

Hypocalcemia and Osteoporosis

Hypocalcemia is diagnosed when total serum calcium falls below 8.8 mg/100 ml. The most prominent effect of hypocalcemia is tetany, which occurs at levels of calcium of 7 mg/100 ml or less. Clinical manifestations of tetany may include paresthesias, muscle twitches, hyperreflexia, laryngospasm, muscle cramps, and tetanic convulsions similar to grand mal epilepsy. Hypocalcemia can be due to deficiency of parathyroid hormone (PTH), vitamin D deficiency (low dietary intake, little exposure to sunlight, malabsorption, or increased vitamin D metabolism), hereditary vitamin D dependency, renal dysfunction (which impairs activation of vitamin D to calcitriol), magnesium depletion (which reduces PTH secretion), diuretic therapy, and acute pancreatitis (which causes calcium chelation to lipolytic products) (Figure 31–4). Hypoproteinemia is associated with a decrease in bound and total serum calcium but is asymptomatic because free ionized calcium is unchanged. Alkalosis causes an increase in calcium binding to serum protein and may cause symptoms of hypocalcemia even though total serum calcium concentrations are normal. Hypocalcemic tetany is treated by intravenous infusions of calcium salts such as calcium gluconate.

Chronic hypocalcemia is characterized by **osteomalacia** (softening of bone) and **osteoporosis** (loss of bony substance). Osteoporosis currently affects approximately 20 million Americans and that number can be expected to increase as the proportion of the population over 65 increases. Approximately 1.3 million osteoporosis-related fractures occur each year in the United States, mainly involving vertebral, femur, or pelvic bones. Nearly one-third of women and one-sixth of men who live until age 90 suffer at least one pelvic fracture. Many never fully recover and in 20% of instances, death ultimately results from complications of the injury.

Occurrence of osteoporosis is partly a function of aging. Hip fractures, which occur with equal frequency in men and women, are associated with a loss of both kinds of bone material, trabecular and cortical. Osteoporosis is also partly a function of a loss of estrogen production during and after menopause in women. Vertebral fractures occur with greatest frequency in postmenopausal women and are associated with loss of trabecular bone specifically. Women, especially women who are white or Oriental, small in stature, or thin, are at special risk of osteoporosis because they begin with a smaller bone mass. On the average, white and Oriental women have 30% less bone mass than men and 10% less bone mass than black women of similar age. Other risk factors include a familial history of the disorder, early menopause, a sedentary life-style or immobilization, use of tobacco, alcohol, or caffeinated beverages, inadequate dietary calcium or vitamin D, or use of drugs that interfere with calcium absorption (antacids, phenytoin, corticosteroids) or promote calcium excretion (furosemide).

The risk of osteoporosis can be reduced but requires a lifelong plan of action: adequate dietary calcium throughout childhood and adulthood, adequate vitamin D intake, and regular weight-bearing exercise. For those at special risk, such as women who experience early menopause, estrogen replacement therapy may also be indicated. Use of estrogens for osteoporosis is discussed in Chapter 34. Treatment of existing osteoporosis is more difficult than prevention. Calcium supplements do not promote an increase in bone mass in postmenopausal women. Likewise, vitamin D supplements do not increase bone mass and may actually result in increased calcium losses. Adequate intake of both of these micronutrients (1,000–1,500 mg of calcium; 300–400 units of vitamin D) should be assured, but higher quantities will not be beneficial. Estrogen replacement for treatment of existing osteoporosis is most beneficial if initiated soon after menopause and appears to be of little value in elderly clients.

Calcium Salts

Clinical Indications Oral calcium salts, such as calcium gluconate or calcium lactate, often in concert with vitamin D, are useful in treatment of acute hypocalcemia and for prevention of osteoporosis. Women should maintain a daily intake of 1,000–1,500 mg of elemental calcium. When dietary assessment indicates that less than this amount is being obtained from the diet, oral calcium supplements are indicated.

Adverse Effects Excess ingestion of calcium salts, especially if associated with ulcerative lesions, extensive use of dairy products, or ingestion of antacids, may result in hypercalcemia. The symptoms of hypercalcemia are discussed below.

Preparations and Administration Calcium gluconate is the treatment of choice for parenteral administration. Calcium chloride and calcium gluceptate are also available for injection but produce some irritation to veins along with burning or tingling sensations. Injections of calcium chloride also cause vasodilation. Calcium salts are usually not given intramuscularly or subcutaneously because of local irritation. When given intravenously, care must be taken to prevent extravasation.

Other calcium salts found in oral tablets are the chloride, carbonate, and phosphate compounds. Calcium phosphate has poor solubility but may be used when serum phosphate levels are also deficient. Calcium chloride is irritating to the gastrointestinal mucosa and should be administered in a suitable fluid, such as milk.

Calcium carbonate
Tablets, chewable tablets, chewy squares
Recommended Doses: For oral dietary supplementation, 500 mg to 2 g, 2–4 times daily.

Calcium chloride
Injection solution
Recommended Doses: For hypocalcemia, 500 mg to 1 g at intervals of 1–3 days by IV infusion at a rate not to exceed 1 ml/minute. For magnesium intoxication, 500 mg promptly. For hyperkalemia, adjust dosage by ECG monitoring.

Calcium gluceptate
Injection solution
Recommended Doses: For hypocalcemia, 2–5 ml IM or 5–20 ml IV.

Calcium gluconate (Kalcinate and generic)
Injection solution, tablets
Recommended Doses: For hypocalcemia in adults, 0.5–2.0 g (1–15 g daily) by IV infusion at 0.5 ml/minute. For children, 500 mg/kg/day by IV infusion in divided doses. For oral dietary supplementation, 500 mg to 2 g, 2–4 times daily.

Parathyroid Hormone

Parathyroid hormone is synthesized in the parathyroid glands. It consists of a polypeptide which is derived by cleavage from a larger prohormone. It is stored in secretory granules until released into the circulation, but the extent of storage is small. Parathyroid hormone is released in response to declining serum levels of calcium, and its effects seem designed to correct calcium deficits.

Mechanisms and Effects Parathyroid hormone has four principal actions: (1) it increases resorption of calcium from bone into the blood, (2) it stimulates renal reabsorption of calcium (and thus decreases excretion of calcium), (3) it decreases renal reabsorption of phosphate, and (4) it stimulates intestinal absorption of calcium by increasing renal activation of vitamin D. The effect of PTH on bone is related to formation of adenosine 3′:5′ cyclic phosphate and requires vitamin D for full expression. The renal effects are also mediated by cyclic AMP.

Hypoparathyroidism occurs when production of parathyroid hormone by the parathyroid glands is deficient. Hypoparathyroidism leads rapidly to hypocalcemia. The most common cause of hypoparathyroidism is damage to or removal of the parathyroid glands in conjunction with surgical removal of the thyroid tissue. Damage to the vessels supplying blood to the gland may also result in interference with glandular function. *Nurses need to be alert to symptoms of parathyroid crisis or parathyroid storm that may occur following such procedures.*

When symptoms indicate that clients have hypoparathyroidism, calcium balance must be restored. Calcium gluconate is often administered intravenously and should be given slowly. When the symptoms of tetany are not acute, the calcium may be administered orally as calcium lactate, calcium gluconate, or calcium chloride. *Nurses need to assess clients' response to calcium, having their plasma calcium levels measured every week or two.*

Clinical Indications Parathyroid hormone is seldom used chronically to counter hypoparathyroidism because individuals become unresponsive to the drug. The one significant application of parathyroid hormone is as a diagnostic aid in identifying causes of hypocalcemia.

Adverse Effects and Contraindications *Clients receiving PTH must be monitored closely, since elevated calcium levels in the blood can lead to renal or cardiac problems. Nurses also need to be aware that clients receiving this hormone may experience anorexia, vomiting, and diarrhea, which could, in turn, cause electrolyte imbalance. Nurses should report complaints of weakness immediately to the physician and to other members of the health team.*

Preparations and Administration Parathyroid hormone derived from bovine parathyroid glands is available as parathyroid injection, USP. It is standardized by bioassay, with one unit of activity defined as one-hundredth the amount required to raise calcium in plasma (in dogs) by 1 mg/100 ml within 16–18 hours. Parathyroid hormone must be given parenterally, usually subcutaneously or intravenously. The peak effect occurs about 18 hours after subcutaneous injection and lasts about 36 hours. *Prior to administration, a skin test should be performed to determine if the client is allergic to parathyroid hormone. If parathyroid hormone is given intravenously, epinephrine should be at bedside in case of anaphylaxis.*

Parathyroid Hormone
Injection solution

Hypercalcemia

Hypercalcemia is diagnosed when serum levels exceed 10.5 mg/100 ml. It is usually caused by excessive resorption of calcium from bone into the blood (osteolysis). This, in turn, could be due to hyperparathyroidism, malignancies (some tumors secrete PTH-like peptides), hyperthyroidism, excess vitamin D intake, or prolonged immobility during periods of rapid bone remodeling (young clients or those with Paget's disease). Excess calcium absorption is unlikely to occur solely because of excess ingestion of calcium salts. But presence of ulcerative lesions in the gastrointestinal tract combined with ingestion of extensive amounts of milk can result in the milk-alkali syndrome, characterized by hypercalcemia. Vitamin D intoxication results in hypercalcemia because of both excess resorption and excess absorption of calcium. Excess absorption also occurs in sarcoidosis. Asymptomatic hypercalcemia occurs when serum protein levels are elevated, providing increased binding sites for calcium. In Addison's disease or following removal of the adrenal glands, hypercalcemia occasionally occurs since sodium and water may be lost in excess of calcium. Thiazide diuretics do not stimulate calcium loss as much as they do water and sodium loss and may therefore cause hypercalcemia. Idiopathic infantile hypercalcemia is a condition of unknown etiology resembling vitamin D intoxication.

Clinical signs of hypercalcemia include constipation, anorexia, nausea, vomiting, abdominal pain, and ileus (intestinal obstruction). The kidney is perhaps most vulnerable to hypercalcemia. Pathological changes in the collecting ducts and distal tubules lead to impaired renal function, resulting in polyuria and polydipsia. Elevations of calcium above 12 mg/100 ml are associated with mental aberrations such as confusion, delirium, stupor, and coma. Muscle weakness and lethargy occur because the threshold for excitability of nerve and muscle cells is increased. Hypercalcemia in excess of 18 mg/100 ml may result in renal failure, shock, and death.

Treatment of hypercalcemia is based on correction of the underlying cause. In severe cases, immediate measures must also be taken to alleviate the calcium elevation. Volume expansion is often instituted in order to promote renal excretion of calcium. After correction of any volume depletion, isotonic saline is infused along with furosemide, if renal function is intact.

Less satisfactory measures for treating severe hypercalcemia include administration of calcium chelators or sodium phosphate. Chelators such as edetate disodium are seldom used because of the risk that ionized calcium levels will be reduced too rapidly. Sodium phosphate is also hazardous because it precipitates calcium as calcium phosphate salts. Dialysis is the current best choice for reducing serum calcium rapidly. Mithramycin, a cytotoxic antibiotic, is also effective, blocking calcium resorption at doses that are only one-tenth those used for anticancer applications of the drug. Glucocorticoids are effective in hypercalcemia related to vitamin D intoxication since glucocorticoids inhibit the hepatic step in activation of vitamin C. Calcitonin has been used experimentally for treatment of hypercalcemia, especially for Paget's disease.

Calcitonin

Calcitonin, also called thyrocalcitonin, is synthesized mainly in the parafollicular "C" cells of the thyroid, although it is also present in the parathyroid glands and thymus. Secretion of calcitonin is brought about by increasing serum calcium concentrations. Cyclic AMP may be involved as an intermediary in calcitonin release. Once released it has a short half-life of about 10 minutes.

Mechanisms and Effects Calcitonin decreases calcium levels, mainly by inhibiting resorption of calcium from bone into the blood. Calcitonin also increases excretion of calcium, phosphate, and sodium. When calcitonin secretion is deficient, hypercalcemia may result.

Clinical Indications Calcitonin is currently being used experimentally for treatment of hypercalcemia, especially Paget's disease. When employed in clients with Paget's disease, calcitonin reduces resorption of calcium from bone and lowers serum calcium by increasing excretion. However, calcitonin does not appear to promote long-term bone formation. Paget's disease clients with neurological lesions require longer therapy. They may have good responses initially but later relapse. Nurses need to check such people carefully, noting any evidences of change. When the client is at home, the family members need to report changes or side effects.

Calcitonin has also been used to treat idiopathic hypercalcemia of infancy, vitamin D intoxication, osteolytic bone metastases, and hyperphosphatemia.

Adverse Effects and Contraindications Calcitonin can cause hypocalcemia. *Therefore, nurses need to observe clients for signs of tetany. Nurses should be certain that parenteral calcium is available for administration for any person receiving calcitonin.* Nausea, vomiting, and diarrhea are not unusual and can be serious for people who are elderly. These symptoms can cause dehydration and electrolyte imbalance. Clients may also complain of flushing of the hands and face. When working with middle-aged female clients, it may be difficult to differentiate between the symptoms of drug side effects and those of menopause. Advising clients to keep a diary recording the incidence of these disturbances may help make the determination. Osteoporosis and pregnancy are contraindications for use of calcitonin.

Preparations and Administration *Since calcitonin is a protein, nurses should be certain that clients receive skin tests for allergy to the drug.* Salmon calcitonin is stored between 2° and 6° C; human calcitonin below 25° C and protected from light.

Human calcitonin (Cibacalcin)
Injection solution
Recommended Doses: For Paget's disease, 0.5 mg/day initially, up to 1.0 mg/day.

Salmon calcitonin (Calcimar)
Injection solution
Recommended Doses: 100 units/day.

Case Study: Thyroid Disorders

G. M. was a 23-year-old single female who initially sought help from a clinical psychologist for "emotional problems," including stormy fights with her boyfriend and her mother. After several sessions with this client, the clinical psychologist began to suspect that there might be an endocrine imbalance present as a contributing factor in the behavioral disturbances. G. M. was referred to a medical clinic where she was initially interviewed by the nurse. G. M. complained of feeling restless, nervous, and upset. She was often unable to get to sleep, sometimes not sleeping an entire night. She complained of being insatiably hungry and of losing weight. She reported frequently feeling warm.

The nurse conducted a physical examination of G. M. and recorded a rapid pulse, a fine tremor of the hand, increased tendon reflexes, a warm, moist quality of skin, and exophthalmos. G. M. was found to weigh 8 pounds less than the minimum desirable weight for her height. Other measurements were within normal limits. Based on her assessment, the nurse concluded that G. M. probably had hyperthyroidism.

G. M. was referred to the physician, who reviewed the nurse's findings and ordered thyroid function tests. The serum total T_4 and T_3 resin uptake test results were both higher than normal, verifying the diagnosis of hyperthyroidism.

The physician and the nurse explained to the client the alternative treatments employed for hyperthyroidism. With the client's concurrence and after establishing that the client was not pregnant or attempting to become pregnant, therapy was initiated with propylthiouracil at 300 mg/day. In addition, because of the presence of an alarming degree of tachycardia, propranolol (Inderal) was ordered for a period of two weeks at 20 mg, tid. The client was instructed to watch for and to report any symptoms of persistent sore throat or fever. The nurse also provided G. M. with a list of the symptoms of hyper- and hypothyroidism. The nurse advised G. M. to wear protective glasses, to use a sleep mask at night, and to restrict sodium intake. And she advised G. M. to explain the reason for her behavioral difficulties to her boyfriend and mother.

When G. M. was examined after 1 week of treatment, she reported that she felt less nervous, that her hand was steadier, and her heart was no longer pounding, but she complained that she had noticed no improvement in the appearance of her eyes or in her weight. The nurse reassured her, pointing out that results are not always seen in the first few days and sometimes not for a few weeks. By the third week, the client reported that she had begun to gain weight and that the bulging of her eyes had diminished.

When G. M. again reported for examination after 6 weeks, she complained of feeling tired and gaining weight. The nurse advised G. M. of methods to balance her caloric intake better with her changing requirements. The nurse inquired about G. M.'s use of depressant drugs, but G. M. seldom used alcohol and had not used a sleep aid during the last month, since her problems with insomnia had been alleviated. The nurse reported the new symptoms to the physician, who reduced the dose of propylthiouracil to 150 mg daily.

After 6 months of treatment with propylthiouracil, the physician discontinued the medication. The nurse intensified her monitoring of G. M.'s physical and mental status during this period. There was no recurrence of symptoms of hyperthyroidism.

G. M. stopped coming to the clinic 2 months after discontinuation of the medication regimen. After almost 3 years, she returned to the clinic reporting symptoms that she recognized from her previous client education as indicative of hyperthyroidism. In addition, she had discovered a lump in her neck and suspected goiter. After evaluation, the physician recommended a surgical procedure to determine the nature of the nodule. Prior to the scheduled surgical procedure, G. M. was given 0.3 ml of strong iodine solution, tid (providing 2.4 mg of iodine each dose) for a period of 1 week. During the surgical procedure, the nodule was found to be benign, but an adenoma was disovered in the parathyroids. The surgeon removed the thyroid and part of the parathyroids.

During recovery in the hospital, the drug order for G. M. was liothyronine sodium (Cytomel) tablets, 25 μg daily; calcium gluconate tablets, 1 g PO, tid; and ergocalciferol (Calciferol), 50,000 IU daily. In spite of this regimen, G. M. began to complain of tingling sensations in her feet and muscle cramps. The physician ordered measurement of serum total calcium (which turned out to be 8.3 mg/ml) and increased the order for calcium gluconate to 2 g, tid. This adjustment alleviated the paresthesias and cramps and raised the serum total calcium to within normal limits. Before releasing G. M., the physician switched her thyroid replacement regimen from liothyronine sodium to levothyroxine sodium (Synthroid), 0.1 mg PO, once daily, instructing the nursing staff to initiate the levothyroxine 3 days prior to discontinuation of the liothyronine. The nurse stressed to G. M. the importance of lifelong continuation of the regimen. She reviewed with G. M. the symptoms of hyper- and hypothyroidism.

When G. M. was next assessed, 10 days after release from the hospital, serum total calcium was within normal limits. She exhibited only slight symptoms of hypothyroidism. The physician increased her dose of levothyroxine sodium to 0.2 mg PO daily. When G. M. returned to the clinic after 1 month, she had begun to feel anxious, warm, and to lose weight. The physician reduced the dosage of levothyroxine sodium to 0.15 mg daily and G. M. showed no further indications of hyperthyroid or hypothyroid symptoms.

1. Which of the original complaints can be attributed to the hormonal imbalance, entirely or in part?
2. Why was it necessary to obtain results from both the serum total T_4 test and the T_3 resin uptake test in order to establish the diagnosis of hyperthyroidism?

3. Why did the nurse question the client regarding pregnancy before initiating treatment with propylthiouracil?
4. Why is propranolol sometimes used adjunctively in hyperthyroidism?
5. Is it surprising that some symptoms had improved after a week of therapy while other symptoms had not? Explain why?
6. What was the likely cause of the fatigue and weight gain after 6 weeks of treatment?
7. Why didn't G. M. again experience symptoms of hyperthyroidism when the medication was discontinued after 6 months?
8. Why was iodine administered for 1 week prior to the surgical procedure?
9. After removal of the thyroid and parathyroid tissue, why was replacement therapy initiated with T_3 rather than T_4? Why was T_4 later substituted? Why was T_4 initiated 3 days before discontinuing the T_3?
10. What was the rationale behind administration of calcium gluconate and ergocalciferol?
11. What was the likely cause of the cramps and paresthesias?
12. What was the likely cause of the symptoms of anxiety, warmth, and weight loss after the dose of levothyroxine sodium had been increased?

Answers appear at the end of the book.

Recommended Readings

Calcium Homeostasis and Related Hormones

Austin LA, Heath H: Calcitonin: Physiology and pathophysiology, *N Engl J Med* 1981;304(5):269–278.

Beil AV: Osteoporosis: How to avoid its crippling effects. *RN* 1986;49(8):14–17.

Doepfner WE: Pharmacologic effects of calcitonin. *Triangle* 1983;22:57–68.

Elliott GI, McKenzie, MW: Treatment of hypercalcemia. *Drug Intell Clin Pharm* 1983;17(1):12–22.

MacIntyre I: The physiological actions of calcitonin. *Triangle* 1983;22:69–74.

Spencer H: Osteoporosis: Goals of therapy. *Hosp Pract* 1982;17:131–138.

Thyroid Hormones

Balkin MS: A guide to thyroid function tests. *Emerg Med* 1983;15(3):116–122.

Brennan MD: Thyroid hormone. *Mayo Clin Proc* 1980;55:33–44.

Carlson HE, Hershman JM: The hypothalamic-pituitary-thyroid axis. *Med Clin North Am* 1975;59(5):1045–1053.

Cooper DS: Antithyroid drugs. *N Engl J Med* 1984;311:1353–1362.

Davidson B et al: Thiourea and cyanamide as inhibitors of thyroid peroxidase: The role of iodide. *Endocrinology* 1979;104:919–924.

Evangelisti J: Thyroid storm: A nursing crisis. *Heart Lung* 1983;12(2):184–193.

Evanier D: Look for these clues to thyrotoxicosis. *Patient Care* 1983;17:143–147.

Feck CM et al: Combination of potassium iodide and propranolol in preparation of patients with Graves' disease for thyroid surgery. *N Engl J Med* 1981;302:883–885.

Mackin JF et al: Thyroid storm and its management. *N Engl J Med* 1974;291:1396–1398.

McKenzie JM et al: Graves' disease. *Med Clin North Am* 1975;59(5):1177–1192.

McKenzie JM, Zakarija M: LATS in Graves' disease. *Rec Prog Horm Res* 1977;33:29–57.

McLaren EH, Alexander WD: Goitrogens. *Clin Endocrin Metab* 1979;8:129–144.

Oppenheimer JH: Thyroid hormone action at the cellular level. *Science* 1979;203:971–979.

Refetoff S: Thyroid hormone therapy. *Med Clin North Am* 1975;59(5):1147–1162.

Reynolds LR, Kotchen TA: Antithyroid drugs and radioactive iodine: Fifteen years experience with Graves' disease. *Arch Int Med* 1979;139:651–653.

Sterling K: Radioactive iodine therapy. *Med Clin North Am* 1975:59(5):1217–1220.

Wake M, Brensinger J: The nurse's role in hypothyroidism. *Nurs Clin North Am* 1980;15(3):453–467.

CHAPTER 32

Drugs Used for Disorders of the Adrenal Cortex

Corticosteroids are one of the groups of hormones produced by the adrenal gland. Like the pituitary glands, each adrenal gland consists of two distinct endocrine tissues — the pinkish inner portion called the adrenal medulla and the surrounding yellowish adrenal cortex. The two portions of the adrenal gland are functionally independent and controlled by different mechanisms. However, the two tissues share in the stress response, helping to prepare the body for physical exertion in response to an external challenge.

The adrenal medulla releases epinephrine and norepinephrine under the regulation of preganglionic sympathetic afferents. The adrenal medulla functions in coordination with the sympathetic nervous system, providing systemic fluctuations in catecholamine effects. Thus the pharmacology of the adrenal medulla is closely linked to the pharmacology of the sympathetic nervous system and is addressed in Chapter 28.

The adrenal cortex produces five classes of steroids belonging to two groups: the corticosteroids (glucocorticoids and mineralocorticoids) and the sex steroids (androgens, estrogens, and progestins). The sex steroids are taken up in Chapters 34 and 35 because of their relationship to sexual functioning. This chapter is concerned with the pharmacology of the corticosteroids.

The Adrenal Cortex

The corticosteroids are classified on the basis of their physiological activity into glucocorticoids and mineralocorticoids. The two types of corticosteroids differ in their site of production within the three layers of the adrenal cortex: the zona glomerulosa, zona fasciculata, and zona reticulata. The mineralocorticoids, mainly corticosterone and aldosterone, are synthesized and released by the zona glomerulosa; they exert significant direct influence only on the kidney, where they regulate reabsorption of electrolytes. The glucocorticoids are secreted from the zonae fasciculata and reticulata. They exert widespread influence expressed through many different target tissues. One effect of glucocorticoids, the suppression of the inflammatory mechanism, is discussed in depth in Chapter 45. In this chapter we consider the general physiology and pharmacology of corticosteroids.

Glucocorticoids

Glucocorticoids are synthesized under the impetus of the pituitary hormone adrenocorticotropic hormone (ACTH) and are secreted as they are synthesized. The most abundant glucocorticoid, cortisol, is secreted at a rate of 20 mg/day. In the plasma, cortisol is reversibly bound to two protein carriers: corticosteroid-binding globulin and an albumin protein. About 10% of the serum concentration of cortisol is unbound. The unusual characteristic of glucocorticoids as hormones is the diversity of effects that they produce in various target tissues.

Glucocorticoid Receptors

The basis for the diversity of action of glucocorticoids is the special mechanism by which they influence target cells, a mechanism that glucocorticoids share with all other steroids but not with nonsteroid hormones or transmitters. The receptors for glucocorticoids are small intracellular protein dimers, located in the cytoplasm of target cells. Only tissues that are susceptible to the influence of glucocorticoids contain these receptors. Glucocorticoids bind to these receptors to form a complex that is then translocated into the cell nucleus. There, the complex interacts with nonhistone proteins that control how a cell expresses its genetic potential through transcriptional and translational activity. The effect of glucocorticoids is therefore unique in each kind of cell, because they act by influencing the inherent genetically regulated synthetic activities of that cell type.

Physiological Roles

The glucocorticoids modify metabolism of proteins, carbohydrates, and fats, increase neural excitability, enhance work capacity of skeletal muscles, alter levels of all of the formed elements of the blood, and suppress the inflammatory response (Table 32–1). In addition, cortisol and other natural glucocorticoids have mineralocorticoid activity, promoting sodium reabsorption in the kidney, water retention, hypokalemia, and increased blood pressure. The common thread in these diverse effects is their relation to preparation for coping with stressful circumstances. Steroid production is controlled by ACTH, and ACTH is released in response to stress stimuli such as trauma, infection, extremes of temperature, surgical procedures, physical restraint, debilitating disease, threatening circumstances, and emotional strain. The steroids, along with the sympathetic nervous system and adrenal medullary hormones, tune the biochemistry and physiology of the body to facilitate behavioral responses that may be adequate to meet the stressful circumstances.

Metabolic effects of glucocorticoids seem to be designed to assure the availability of energy resources for the brain and skeletal muscles. To do this, glucocorticoids stimulate production of glucose, causing an immediate rise in blood glucose levels and, over a longer span of time, a replenishment of glycogen stores in the liver. The glucocorticoids inhibit utilization of glucose by peripheral tissues not crucially involved in stress responses, including fat, skin, and fibroblasts. Meanwhile, the energy resources required for gluconeogenesis are augmented by catabolism of protein and fat. Thus glucocorticoids act in concert with other hormones in regulating the balance between fat and carbohydrate utilization. Excessive protein catabolism due to excessive levels of glucocorticoids can lead to muscle wasting, osteoporosis (triggered by a breakdown of the protein matrix of bone), thinning of the skin, a negative nitrogen balance, and atrophy of lymphatic tissue.

A proper glucocorticoid balance is required for efficient **muscular activity.** Too little cortisol reduces the capacity of muscles for work, but too much cortisol causes muscle wasting. In the **central nervous system,** glucocorticoids not only increase availability of glucose to the brain but also stimulate neural excitability in some as yet undetermined manner.

Glucocorticoids alter levels of **blood cells.** Red blood cells increase in number probably because of a decrease in their rate of destruction when glucocorticoids are given. Neutrophils (polymorphonuclear leukocytes) also increase, apparently due to both increased bone marrow production and diminished removal from the blood. The concentration of all the remaining formed elements of the blood declines in response to glucocorticoids. Circulating lymphocytes are reduced 70% by a single dose of

Table 32–1
Effects of Corticosteroids

Primary physiological effects	Related symptoms if activity is excessive (Cushing's syndrome)	Related symptoms if activity is deficient (Addison's disease)
I. Glucocorticoid actions		
A. Metabolic		
1. Gluconeogenesis	Hyperglycemia	Hypoglycemia
	Neural excitability	Lethargy
	Insulin secretion	Muscle weakness
	Beta-cell exhaustion	
2. Protein catabolism	Muscle wasting	Impaired stress response
	Osteoporosis	
	Thinning of skin	
	Negative nitrogen balance	
	Atrophy of lymphatic tissue	
3. Fat catabolism	Loss of fat from extremities	Impaired stress response
	Fat redistribution	
	Buffalo hump	
	Pendulous abdomen	
	Moon face	
B. Skeletal muscle	Muscle wasting	Diminished work capacity
C. Central nervous system	Increased excitability	Apathy
	EEG activation	Depression
	Restlessness	Psychosis
	Anxiety	
	Insomnia	
	Schizoid symptoms	
D. Blood cells		
1. ↑RBC's	Polycythemia	Mild normochromic, normocytic anemia
2. ↑Neutrophils; ↓Lymphocytes, monocyte, basophils, platelets	Weakened inflammatory response	Increased lymph mass
	Decreased lymph mass	
	Poor wound healing	
	Weak immune response	
	Impaired clotting	
II. Mineralocortoicoid actions		
A. ↑Reabsorption of Na^+	Hypernatremia	Hyponatremia
	Hypervolemia	Hypovolemia
	Hypertension	Hypotension
	Hyperchlorhydria	Circulatory collapse
B. ↓Reabsorption of K^+	Hypokalemia	Hyperkalemia
C. ↓Reabsorption of H^+	Alkalosis	Acidosis

cortisol, with the T-lymphocytes especially affected. Monocytes may be reduced 90%.

Mineralocorticoids

Aldosterone is the principal endogenous mineralocorticoid; desoxycorticosterone, the next most potent mineralocorticoid prossesses only 1–3% of the mineralocorticoid activity of aldosterone. Mineralocorticoids act on the distal convoluted tubule of the nephron in the kidney to enhance reabsorption of sodium. Mineralocorticoids stimulate both the pumps that reabsorb sodium with chloride and those that exchange sodium for potassium or hydrogen. Therefore mineralocorticoids cause not only sodium retention (hypernatremia) but also potassium and hydrogen depletion (hypokalemic alkalosis). These electrolyte alterations lead to hypervolemia, edema, hypertension, and potentially congestive heart failure.

Secretion of aldosterone is controlled mainly by the concentration of serum potassium and the renin-angiotensin system. This system is discussed more fully in Chapter 43. In brief, a drop in plasma volume stimulates release of renin from the kidney. Renin stimulates liver conversion of angiotensinogen to angiotensin I, which enters the blood. Angiotensin I is converted to angiotensin II, which stimulates the synthesis of aldosterone by the zona glomerulosa of the adrenal cortex. Aldosterone stimulates sodium reabsorption and water retention to correct the hypovolemia. Aldosterone also helps to maintain potassium homeostasis and acid-base balance.

Pituitary Control of the Adrenal Gland: Adrenocorticotropic Hormone (ACTH)

Synthesis of glucocorticoids is regulated by the pituitary hormone adrenocorticotropic hormone (ACTH, or corticotropin). The release of weak androgens from the adrenals is also controlled by ACTH; however, release of the principal mineralocorticoid, aldosterone, is largely controlled by independent mechanisms, and only slightly stimulated by ACTH. ACTH is a polypeptide of 39 amino acids residues.

The adrenal cortex does not store preformed steroids, so the rate of release equals the rate of synthesis. Control of synthetic rate by ACTH thus effectively regulates the rate of secretion and biological activity. ACTH also maintains normal morphology of the adrenal gland. Removal of the pituitary (hypophysectomy) causes atrophy of the adrenal gland in animals. Prolonged excessive stimulation of the adrenals by ACTH causes adrenal hyperplasia and hypersecretory activity.

ACTH is synthesized in basophilic cells of the anterior pituitary. The rate of synthesis of ACTH is determined by hypothalamic regulatory influences and negative feedback control exerted by corticosteroids. The hypothalamic influence is conveyed by corticotropin releasing factor (CRF). Release of CRF (and hence ACTH and glucocorticoids) exhibits diurnal fluctuations and is sensitive to stress provoked by severe infection, surgery, parturition, cold, exercise, and emotional situations. The hormones of the adrenal-pituitary axis are elevated during the early daylight hours, decline during the day, and reach their nadir around midnight. This pattern is both diurnal (24-hour) and circadian (light-linked) and is secondary to the serotonin rhythm (sleep-wake cycle) of the brain.

Certain of the corticosteroids, notably cortisol (the most abundant in humans) and corticosterone, exert negative feedback control over ACTH and probably CRF release. Administration of high levels of glucocorticoids causes a reduction in secretion of ACTH, and as a result, atrophy of the adrenal cortex. On the other hand, adrenalectomy and Addison's disease (in which steroid production is deficient) are associated with elevations in both basal and stress-stimulated ACTH serum concentrations. Current evidence suggests that the negative feedback effect of corticosteroids occurs primarily at the level of the hypothalamus, but there may also be a direct suppressant effect at the level of the pituitary.

Adrenal Insufficiency, Corticosteroids, and ACTH

Adrenocortical insufficiency can be primary or secondary. Primary adrenocortical insufficiency may be chronic (Addison's disease) or acute (adrenal crisis). **Addison's disease** develops slowly and is progressive. The total incidence is about 4 per 100,000 people in the United States. Seventy percent of cases are due to atrophy of the adrenal cortex. The remaining 30% of cases are due to partial destruction of the adrenal cortex by neoplasm, granuloma (for example, in tuberculosis), amyloidosis, or inflammatory necrosis. Addison's disease is characterized by hypotension, hyponatremia, hyperkalemia, hypovolemia, and circulatory collapse due to inadequate mineralocorticoid activity. In addition, cortisol deficiency causes inhibition of carbohydrate formation, hypoglycemia due to decreased release of glucose from liver glycogen stores, severe insulin sensitivity, hypometabolism, decreased cold tolerance, and weakness. A third cluster of symptoms is due to elevated ACTH: increased pigmentation of skin, diffuse tanning, freckling, vitiligo (patches of depigmentation), and bluish-black discolorations of mucous membranes. Nonspecific symptoms include nausea, vomiting, anorexia, diarrhea, weight loss, dizziness, and syncope. Laboratory findings in Addison's disease include low serum sodium and glucose and elevated potassium and ACTH. Blood urea nitrogen is elevated. Hematocrit is elevated, but white blood cell count is reduced. Treatment consists of replacement therapy with a mixed glucocorticoid and mineralocorticoid such as hydrocortisone.

Adrenal crisis is primary adrenocortical insufficiency of sudden onset. It is characterized by profound weakness, fluctuating fever, pain in the abdomen, back, and legs, marked hypotension, extensive purpura and cyanosis, circulatory collapse, and renal shutdown. The usual causes are septicemia, trauma, surgical procedures, or hemorrhagic destruction of the adrenal gland. In the absence of replacement therapy, death occurs in 3 days to 2 weeks.

Secondary adrenocortical insufficiency is caused by inadequate pituitary secretion of ACTH. It occurs in panhypopituitarism as well as during and following treatment with glucocorticoids. Glucocorticoids suppress ACTH production and endogenous steroidogenesis. Since ACTH production is low in secondary adrenocortical insufficiency, skin pigmentation does not occur. Treatment is similar to that for Addison's disease.

Glucocorticoids

The most important clinical uses of glucocorticoids are as antiallergic drugs, in replacement therapy, in treatment of malignancies, and, most commonly, as anti-inflammatory drugs.

Mechanisms and Effects Glucocorticoids suppress all components of inflammation from the initial redness and fibrin deposition, through the edema and swelling, to the massing of leukocytes and their phagocytic activity, and finally including the reparative processes of capillary proliferation, fibroblast proliferation, and collagen deposition. The anti-inflammatory action occurs regardless of the cause of inflammation: heat, mechanical damage, caustics, infections, or allergens. Glucocorticoid therapy is palliative, alleviating pain, inconvenience, and perhaps secondary complications of inflammation, but not the underlying cause. The specific mechanisms by which glucocorticoids suppress inflammation include (1) stimulation of the migration of neutrophils, (2) suppression of the release of the lysosomal contents by neutrophils, (3) inhibition of formation of a macrophage activator of plasminogen, (4) inhibition of release of arachidonic acid, the precursor of prostaglandins, and (5) inhibition of fibroblasts.

The antiallergic effect of glucocorticoids in supressing cell-mediated (delayed) hypersensitivity reactions (type IV — see Chapter 46) is not a direct action on the immune system at all but an indirect effect caused by suppression of the inflammatory process. Lymphocytes of the immune system continue to identify antigens in the presence of glucocorticoids and to initiate reaction to them by secretion of lymphokines. One of the lymphokines, migration inhibitory factor (MIF), normally causes accumulation of macrophages in the vicinity of the antigen by suppressing their motility. The macrophages, functional units of the inflammatory process, then proceed to digest the antigen. Glucocorticoids inhibit the effect of MIF on macrophages, thus preventing their accumulating at the site of allergic reaction.

Glucocorticoids also exert an antiallergic effect in hypersensitivity reactions of the immediate type (type I) and the immune-complex type (type III). Glucocorticoids produce their palliative influence in the IgE-mediated type I reactions by inhibiting degranulation of mast cells.

When glucocorticoids are employed in clinical practice, matters of therapeutic goals, dose, dosage schedule, and duration of treatment are of paramount importance. Except in replacement therapy for adrenocortical insufficiency, the use of glucocorticoids is palliative and empiric; the goal is symptomatic relief. Because of the risks associated with glucocorticoids, however, the therapeutic objective usually is reduction in symptoms to a tolerable level, not their complete elimination.

Pharmacokinetics Most of the natural and synthetic steroids are well absorbed after oral administration. Intramuscular injection also provides good effect. Esters and suspensions injected intramuscularly can provide an extended action, and rapid effect can be achieved with intravenous administration of water-soluble preparations. Glucocorticoids are often applied topically to the skin or conjunctival sac, in which case significant absorption may result in systemic effects if the area of application is large.

Metabolism of steroids, both natural and synthetic, occurs in the liver and peripheral tissues. Liver metabolism accounts for perhaps 70% of inactivation. Steroid metabolites are largely excreted in the urine.

Clinical Indications The use of glucocorticoids to suppress inflammation is discussed in Chapter 45; topical application is discussed in Chapters 52–54. **Inflammatory disorders** for which glucocorticoids may be useful include arthritis, carditis, intestinal inflammations, renal disease, collagen diseases, ocular inflammations, skin disorders, and hepatitis. Glucocorticoids are invaluable in replacement therapy of **adrenocortical insufficiency,** whether it is Addison's disease, adrenal crisis, congential hyperplasia, or secondary adrenal insufficiency.

Glucocorticoids have some limited value in **al-**

Nursing Observations for Corticosteroid Therapy of Addison's Disease

THERAPEUTIC GOAL	Reestablish normal glucocorticoid and mineralocorticoid activity by replacement therapy.
PREADMINISTRATION ASSESSMENT	
Baseline Data	Observe extent of abnormal pigmentation or vitiligo, fainting or other symptoms of orthostatic hypotenstion, weight loss, activity intolerance, visual changes, gastrointestinal complaints, and vague signs of infection. Measure blood pressure (lying down, sitting, and standing), body temperature, pulse, heart sounds, edema, and peripheral perfusion; evaluate mental status and reflexes; skin integrity; bowel function (appetite, sounds, and stool consistency). Obtain laboratory tests including x-ray evaluation for reduced heart size, urinalysis, and blood urea nitrogen.
Contraindications/ Precautions	Congestive heart failure, hypertension, active infection, metastatic carcinoma, myasthenia gravis, hyperthryoidism, psychosis, epilepsy, diabetes, ulcers, osteoporosis, or glaucoma. Check medication history for evidence of allergic reactions to steroids or tartrazine (a coloring agent in certain preparations).
Possible Interactions	Check current medications for drugs that may interact with corticosteroids, including antidiabetic medications, cardiac glycosides, oral contraceptives, anticoagulants, and drugs influenced by induction of liver enzymes.
EVALUATION OF DRUG RESPONSE	
For Therapeutic Benefit	Check for stable blood pressure recordings. Evaluate fluid and electrolyte balance, blood glucose levels, appetite, increased energy level, and decreased pigmentation.
For Adverse Effects	Monitor blood pressure, intake-output, serum electrolytes, weight changes, and blood and urine glucose levels. Watch for evidence of poor wound healing or changes in fat distribution (moon face, pendulous abdomen, etc.). Observe for evidence (fuzzy tongue, fever, persistent colds) of masked infections. Question clients about signs of osteoporosis, such as backache. Conduct periodic blood cell counts for leukopenia. Evaluate emotional and mental state for changes.
For Drug Interactions	When glucocorticoids are used in replacement, monitor clients with diabetes for altered insulin or oral hypoglycemic requirements; warn women using oral contraceptives about possible loss of contraceptive action; observe for reduced effectiveness of phenytoin, phenobarbital, ephedrine, or rifampin due to induction of liver metabolism; check for reduced anticoagulant activity of oral anticoagulants or aspirin. When drugs with mineralocorticoid activity are employed, monitor for additive hypokalemia with diuretics and increased toxicity from cardiac glycosides.
For Dietary Interactions	Monitor fluid and electrolyte balance. Watch for signs of osteoporosis.
For Compliance	Evaluate client compliance with all facets of the therapeutic regimen by careful observation, interviewing, and review of progress. Report compliance problems to the physician and act as client-advocate when changes in the therapeutic regimen seem indicated.

lergies. The effect is not rapid enough to be of much benefit in severe hypersensitivity reactions such as anaphylaxis. Glucocorticoids are used adjunctively for short-lasting allergic reactions such as hay fever, serum sickness, urticaria, contact dermatitis, drug reactions, bee stings, or angioneurotic edema, but antihistamines are the preferred treatment in milder cases. Glucocorticoids are a last resort in severe bronchial asthma that does not respond to conventional drugs.

Glucocorticoids have some usefulness in treatment of **malignancies.** They can reduce cerebral edema associated with brain tumors, but not edema due to other causes, such as trauma or cerebral hemorrhage. Combination therapies including glucocorticoids are employed for acute lymphocytic leukemia and lymphomas. Glucocorticoids in such regimens decrease lymphatic mass. Glucocorticoids can be used in breast cancer to suppress ACTH release by negative feedback. Reduction of ACTH will reduce adrenal production of androgens that are precursors for tissue production of estrogens. The ultimate goal is to reduce the levels of estrogens because they stimulate breast cell proliferation.

Adverse Effects and Contraindications Toxicity from glucocorticoids is almost never seen with single doses or even in short courses of therapy, up to 2 or 3 weeks. Toxicity occurs with prolonged use of moderate to high doses and during subsequent drug withdrawal (Table 32–2).

Electrolyte imbalance and **cardiovascular complications** occur to the extent that the drug selected has excessive mineralocorticoid properties. *Clients receiving glucocorticoids with mineralocorticoid activity need to be evaluated repeatedly for increased sodium and fluid retention. Sodium retention is likely to be present if the client exhibits weight gain, increased extracellular fluid, and hypertension. Clients should be taught to weigh themselves daily at the same time each day, wearing the same amount of clothing, and using the same scale. If signs of fluid and salt retention are observed, the diet should be adjusted to provide low sodium and high potassium. Clients should be encouraged to consume foods high in potassium such as bananas and other fruits. Helping clients to identify which foods are low in sodium and what to look for on labels of canned or processed foods is important in encouraging clients to comply with the prescribed protocol. Serum electrolytes should be monitored and the client should be monitored for indications of hypocalcemia: muscle twitches, cramps, and spasms.* The newer synthetics provide complete separation of glucocorticoid from mineralocorticoid activity (Table 32–3).

Dietary adjustments should also be made if **glycosuria** occurs. Clients with diabetes may need to increase their insulin dose while receiving glucocorticoids. *Clients with a history of diabetes should monitor urine sugar levels daily when glucocorticoid therapy is initiated.* There is a risk that diabetes mellitus will develop with long-term therapy due to beta-cell exhaustion.

Steroids may cause **peptic ulceration** with prolonged use, but the evidence is not clear that they do. Antacid therapy should be instituted if ulcers appear to be developing, and caffeine, nicotine, alcohol, and aspirin should be avoided. *Because of increased secretion of gastric juices, clients should be encouraged to eat frequent but small meals. Bedtime snacks may also be helpful. Nurses need to alert clients to the signs of possible gastrointestinal bleeding that can result from steroid therapy. Occurrence of weakness, tarry stools, fatigue, or cold, clammy skin should be reported immediately. Also, to avoid problems of ulceration, clients should be advised to take glucocorticoids with food or milk.*

Muscle wasting is a potentially debilitating adverse effect caused by the negative nitrogen balance that prolonged use of glucocorticoids can produce. It is part of the Cushing's syndrome. *Nurses need to encourage clients to eat a diet high in protein to prevent the problem. They also need to alert clients to symptoms suggestive of negative nitrogen balance, such as muscle wasting and easy fatigability. The breakdown of proteins and conversion of the end-products to glucose may cause clients to exhibit symptoms similar to those experienced by diabetic clients.*

As an individual continues taking corticosteroids, there is usually a **change in the distribution of fat.** Fat deposits occur in the face, causing a "moon face." Fat also accumulates in the supraclavicular area in the back of the neck, creating a "buffalo hump," but there is a decrease in fat deposits in the lower extremities. This change in appearance often causes clients to become self-conscious, especially if they have been thin in the past. *It is very important, then, for the nurse to encourage clients not to discontinue therapy with the notion of reversing the changes. Any sudden change in the regimen could provoke symptoms of adrenal insufficiency.*

Ocular effects of extended glucocorticoid therapy include cataracts (posterior subcapsular) and increased intraocular pressure. *Caution is required when administering glucocorticoids to clients with a history of glaucoma.* Clients who have a history of ocular herpes simplex usually should not be placed on corticosteroids since there is a danger that this will result in corneal perforation.

Osteoporosis occurs for several reasons: the catabolic effect of glucocorticoids causes a reduction in the protein matrix of bones, glucocorticoids inhibit osteoblasts, and glucocorticoids inhibit hepatic activation of vitamin D (a steroid), which in turn is

Table 32–2
Adverse Effects of Prolonged Glucocorticoid Therapy

Excess glucocorticoid activity	Excess mineralocorticoid activity	Withdrawal
Carbohydrate metabolism	Electrolyte imbalance	Fever
Hyperglycemia	Hypernatremia	Myalgia
Glycosuria	Hypokalemia	Arthralgia
Diabetes mellitus	Alkalosis	Malaise
Blood cells	Hypervolemia	Depression
Lymphocytopenia	Hypercalcemia	Fatigue
Monocytopenia	Cardiovascular effect	Hypotension
Eosinopenia	Hypertension	Anorexia
Neutrophilia	Congestive heart failue	Nausea
Involution of lymph tissue		Vomiting
Ocular		
Increased intraocular pressure		
Cataracts		
Ulcers (possibly)		
Psychological dependence		
Growth suppression in children		
Suppression of pituitary/ardenal axis		
Cushing's syndrome		
Psychosis		
Irritability		
Susceptiblity to infection		
Easy bruisability		
Acne		
Redistribution of fat		
Moon face		
Buffalo hump		
Pendulous abdomen		
Striae		
Negative nitrogen balance		
Muscle wasting		
Osteoporosis		

required for calcium absorption. As calcium levels fall, parathyroid hormone is released, stimulating calcium resorption from bone. Glucocorticoid therapy is especially hazardous in postmenopausal women, since this population is already at risk of osteoporosis. Glucocorticoid use in children can cause growth suppression. Alternate-day therapy reduces this risk. *Clients should be encouraged to exercise to decrease the possible development of osteoporosis.*

Clients receiving adrenocorticosteroids have a tendency to increase the production of polymorphonuclear leukocytes (neutrophils), while decreasing basophils, eosinophils, lymphocytes, and monocytes. As a result, there is a decrease in lymphoid tissue mass and a lessening of the inflammatory and immunological responsiveness. Clients have an **elevated susceptibility to infection.** *Nurses need to monitor blood cell counts and to teach clients how to avoid unnecessary risks of infection. Personal hygiene is extremely important. If the person receiving a glucocorticoid is a child or is mentally impaired, the community health nurse will be in a crucial position for observing living habits and health measures and will be able to reinforce good habits and correct bad ones. The nurse can also involve the family in assuring that hygienic measures are maintained. Care must be taken to protect clients on glucocorticoids from contact with those who have infectious diseases.*

When clients receive steroids, they may develop

Table 32–3
Comparative Activities of Some Corticosteroids in Relation to Cortisol (Cortisol = 1)

Name of substance	Mineralocorticoid activity	Equivalent dose (mg) for mineralocorticoid activity	Glucocorticoid activity	Equivalent dose (mg) for glucocorticoid activity
Natural steroids				
Cortisol (hydrocortisone)	1	—	1	20
Cortisone	0.8	—	0.8	25
Corticosterone	15	—	0.35	—
11-Desoxycorticosterone	30	2	0	—
Aldosterone	3,000	—	0.3	—
Synthetic steroids				
Prednisone	0.6	—	3.5	5
Prednisolone	0.6	—	4.0	5
Methylprednisolone	0.5	—	5.0	4
Fluprednisolone	0	—	10.0	1.6
Triamcinolone	0	—	5.0	4
Paramethasone	0	—	10.0	2
Betamethasone	0	—	35.0	0.6
Dexamethasone	0	—	30.0	0.75
Fludrocortisone	125	0.1	10.0	—

infections without the usual warning signs of inflammation. Thus, a lesion may go untreated since the usual redness may not be present. Further, when steroids are given to reduce inflammation, clients may misinterpret the lessening of symptoms as evidence of cure and cease taking the medication once the desired result seems to have been obtained. *Part of the nursing assessment and diagnosis must include identification of the client's knowledge concerning the medication being taken, the possible side effects, and the rationale for continuing therapy once the most obvious symptoms have subsided.* Glucocorticoids often impair the body's ability to confine infections, so that infections frequently become systemic. This can pose particular problems for a client who must undergo surgery. In addition, people who have a history of tuberculosis should not be given glucocorticoids, since they can cause fulminating or disseminated tuberculosis.

Psychiatric disturbances may be severe, being expressed as manic-depressive or schizophrenic symptomatology. Clients often undergo wide changes in mood, ranging from euphoria to depression to psychosis. They may suffer insomnia, which in turn may cause behavioral changes, including depression or euphoria. *In this event, the regimen might be altered to avoid giving steroids in the evening. It is important for the individual and his or her family to report changes in behavior.*

Systemic administration of glucocorticoids (and occasionally even topical administration) may cause **suppression of the hypothalamic-pituitary-adrenal axis.** This results in a decrease or absence of secretion of ACTH, ultimately resulting in atrophy of the adrenal cortex. As a consequence, the client is no longer able to produce glucocorticoids in response to stress. Sudden withdrawal can produce adrenal insufficiency. In some instances, full adrenocortical function may never be regained. This is one of the major risks of extended treatment with glucocorticoids. The risk is reduced by low doses, brief courses of therapy, or alternate-day schedules of administration.

Female clients may develop **menstrual irregularities** when receiving glucocorticoids. This can be troublesome, especially to women who are sexually active or in the childbearing years, since such irregularity often results in concerns about pregnancy. When working with pregnant women, the benefits of using glucocorticoids must be weighed against the potential **harm of steroids to the fetus.** *In taking histories of female clients who are in their reproductive years, it is critical to determine the regularity of the woman's ovulatory cycle and the likelihood of existing pregnancy. If there is any question, the information must be shared with the physician and pharmacist on the health team. If the woman is pregnant and it is decided to proceed with the drug reg-*

imen, both the mother and the fetus must be monitored carefully for signs of distress. In addition, once the infant is born, the child should be observed for signs of hypoadrenalism.

Drug Interactions Corticosteroids can interact with other drugs in a number of ways (Table 32–4). Glucocorticoids are possibly ulcergenic. *Patients receiving glucocorticoids should be warned about use of ulcergenic drugs such as caffeine, nicotine, alcohol, and aspirin.* Inducers of liver enzymes increase metabolism of glucocorticoids and may necessitate an increase in the dose of the steroid.

Because glucocorticoids tend to cause hyperglycemia and glycosuria, it is often necessary to make dietary adjustments or increase dosages of antidiabetic drugs. *Diabetic clients should be advised to intensify monitoring of blood sugar during administration of glucocorticoids.*

Vaccines such as smallpox vaccine are more likely to cause neurological complications in clients on glucocorticoid therapy if steroid therapy is in excess of replacement levels. *Nurses should avoid giving immunizations to clients receiving glucocorticoids.*

Corticosteroids with mineralocorticoid activity may also reduce the effectiveness of diuretic therapy by stimulating retention of sodium, or increase toxicity of cardiac glycosides and amphotericin B by depleting potassium.

Preparations and Administration Glucocorticoid preparations are available as oral tablets; solutions, suspensions, or powders for intramuscular, intrasynovial, intralesional, and intravenous injections; implantable pellets; and as topical preparations including dermal creams, ointments, lotions, or aerosols, ophthalmic ointments and solutions, respiratory aerosols, dental pastes, enemas, and rectal foams (Table 32–5). The selection of a preparation is based on the required route of administration and the desired balance between glucocorticoid and mineralocorticoid activity (Table 32–3). In 1985 five glucocorticoid preparations were among the top 200 prescription drugs: Lidex (fluocinonide topical cream and ointment), Valisone (betamethasone valerate for topical application), prednisone (generic), Medrol (methylprednisolone tablets), and Kenalog (triamcinolone acetonide dermal ointment). Two other glucocorticoid-containing preparations among

Table 32–4
Interactions of Glucocorticoids

Result of interaction and mechanism	Example drugs
Increased glucocorticoid action	
Additive ulcergenic effect	Caffeine, alcohol, nicotine, aspirin, indomethacin, and other nonsteroidal anti-inflammatory drugs
Decreased glucocorticoid action	
Increased steroid metabolism	Inducers of liver enzymes such as phenytoin, phenobarbital, and rifampin
Inhibition of catabolic effect in muscles	Anabolic steroids
Reduced Effect of Interacting Drug	
Na^+ retention (only for steroids with mineralocorticoid activity)	Diuretics
Steroid-induced hyperglycemia and glycosuria	Oral hypoglycemics and insulin
Inhibition of vitamin D activation by liver	Vitamin D, calcium salts
Increased effect of interacting drug	
K^+ loss (only for steroids with mineralocorticoid activity)	Increased toxicity of cardiac glycosides, amphotericin B, and diuretics
Immunosuppression	Increased toxicity of certain vaccines (smallpox, for example)

Nursing Diagnoses and Interventions for Corticosteroid Therapy of Addison's Disease

Nursing Diagnosis	*Related Interventions*
TO ENHANCE DRUG BENEFITS OR REDUCE DRUG REQUIREMENTS	
Activity intolerance related to fatigue in Addison's disease	Discuss need for adequate periods of rest. Work with client to establish a schedule of activity and rest.
Disturbance in self-concept related to skin pigmentation and loss of axillary and pubic hair in Addison's disease	Explain changes to the client and suggest cosmetic measures for skin pigmentation.
Ineffective coping: impaired stress response in Addison's disease	Increase doses of glucocorticoids in stressful circumstances such as surgery or infection; minimize stress and exposure to infection.
Potential for injury because of postural hypotension in Addisons' disease	Teach client safety measures to prevent injuries such as rising slowly and sitting when feeling faint.
TO MINIMIZE DRUG SIDE EFFECTS OR INTERACTIONS	
Altered nutrition: intake less than requirements related to anorexia and nausea caused by corticosteroids	Advise the client to report such symptoms to the physician (especially if it interferes with taking the medication); an antinausea drug may be required.
Sensory/perceptual alterations from use of corticosteroids	Provide support and encourage to remain on the drug regimen.
Fluid volume excess or alteration in cardiac output related to mineralocorticoid activity of corticosteroids	Report indications immediately to the physician: requires adjustment of mineralocorticoid replacement or dietary intake of salt.
Ineffective coping with alterations in drug regimen	Changes in glucocorticoid regimens should usually be gradual.
TO ENSURE SAFE AND EFFICACIOUS DRUG USE	
Knowledge deficit related to drug regimen	Teach the client about the nature of Addison's disease and the lifelong requirement for replacement therapy.
	Be certain the client knows that corticosteroid therapy should not be discontinued without consultation with the physician and that abrupt discontinuation leads to withdrawal symptoms.
	Instruct the client in the proper administration of drug(s) employed for replacement.
	Instruct the client to maintain a high-protein diet with adequate levels of calcium. Ensure that the client understands any special restrictions prescribed by the physician with respect to sodium or potassium content in the diet.
	Advise the client to maintain a regular schedule of exercise.
	Advise the client that he or she has a diminished capacity to cope with stress and should avoid stressful situations and exposure to infection. Teach coping strategies for managing stress.
	Provide the client with a list of adverse effects and instructions for monitoring each of them.
	Provide the client with a list of drugs that may interact with corticosteroids (Table 32-6).
	Advise the client of the importance of wearing an identification bracelet or tag indicating the disorder and medication regimen.

Table 32–5
Preparations of Corticosteroids

		Dosage forms		
Generic name	**Trade names**	**Oral**	**Parenteral**	**Topical**
Glucocorticoids				
Cortisol (hydrocortisone)	Cortef Hydrocortone	5, 10, 20 mg tablets	25, 50 mg/ml suspension	0.125–2.5% cream 0.25, 2.5% ointment 0.125, 2.5% lotion 0.5%, 1.5% gel 0.5% aerosol 100 mg/60 ml enema 0.2% ophthalmic suspension
Cortisol acetate	Cortef Acetate Biosone Fernisone Cortil Acetate Hydrocortone Acetate		25, 50 mg/ml suspension	1, 2.5% ointment 15, 25 mg suppositories 10% rectal foam 2.5% ophthalmic suspension 1.5% ophthalmic ointment
Cortisol cypionate	Cortef	2 mg/ml suspension		
Cortisol sodium phosphate	Hydrocortone Phosphate		50 mg/ml	
Cortisol sodium succinate	Solu-Cortef		100, 250, 500, 1,000 mg powder	
Cortisone acetate	Cortone Acetate	5, 10, 25 mg tablets	25, 50 mg/ml suspension	1.5, 2.5% ophthalmic suspension
Beclomethasone dipropionate	Vanceril			10 mg inhaler
Betamethasone	Celestone	0.6 mg tablets 0.6 mg/5ml syrup	4 mg/ml	0.2% cream
Betamethasone benzoate	Benisone Flurobate			0.025% cream, gel, or lotion
Betamethasone dipropionate	Diprosonel			0.05% ointment, cream, or lotion 0.1% aerosol
Betamethasone sodium phosphate	Celestone Phosphate		4 mg/ml solution	
Betamethasone sodium phosphate and acetate	Celestone Soluspan		6 mg/ml suspension	
Betamethasone valerate	Valisone			0.01, 0.1% cream 0.1% ointment 0.1% lotion 0.15% aerosol

Table 32–5
Preparations of Corticosteroids (*continued*)

		Dosage forms		
Generic name	**Trade names**	**Oral**	**Parenteral**	**Topical**
Dexamethasone	Decadron Gammacorten Dexone Hexadrol	0.25, 0.5, 0.75, 1.5, 4.0 mg tablets; 0.5 mg/5ml elixir		0.04% cream 0.1% gel 0.01% topical aerosol 0.1% ophthalmic suspension
Dexamethasone acetate	Decodron-L.A.		8 mg/ml	
Dexamethasone sodium phosphate	Decadron Phosphate and others		4, 10, 24 mg/ml	0.1% cream 0.1% ophthalmic solution 0.05% ophthalmic ointment
Fluprednisolone	Alphadrol	1.5 mg tablet		
Methylprednisolone	Medrol	2, 4, 8, 16, 24, 32 mg tablets		
Methylprednisolone acetate	Depo-medrol and others		20, 40, 80 mg/ml tablets	
Methylprednisolone sodium succinate	Solu-medrol		40, 125, 500, 1000 mg/ml powder	
Paramethasone acetate	Haldrone	1, 2 mg tablets		
Prednisolone	Cortalone Delta-Cortef and others	1, 2.5, 5 mg tablets		
Prednisolone acetate	Meticortelone Acetate, Savacort, and others		25, 50, 100 mg/ml suspension	0.12, 1% ophthalmic suspension
Prednisolone acetate and sodium phosphate	Predalone and others		60, 80 mg/ml suspension	
Prednisolone sodium phosphate	Hydeltrasol and others		20 mg/ml solution	0.125, 0.5, 1% ophthalmic solution; 0.25% ophthalmic ointment
Prednisolone terbutate	Hydeltra-T.B.A. and others		20 mg/ml suspension	
Prednisone	Deltasone, Paracort, and others	1, 2.5, 5, 10, 20, 50 mg tablets		

(*continued*)

Table 32–5
Preparations of Corticosteroids (*continued*)

Generic name	Trade names	Dosage forms: Oral	Dosage forms: Parenteral	Dosage forms: Topical
Triamcinolone	Aristocort, Kenacort, and others	1, 2, 4, 8, 16 mg tablets; 2.4 mg/5 ml syrup		
Triamcinolone acetonide	Aristoderm, Kenalog, and others		10, 40 mg/ml suspensions	0.025, 0.1, 0.5% cream; 0.025, 0.5% ointment; 0.1% foam; 0.025, 0.1% lotion; 0.1% gel; 0.1% spray; 0.1% dental paste
Triamcinolone diacetate	Aristocort Diacetate and others		25, 40 mg/ml suspension	
Triamcinolone hexacetonide	Aristospan		5, 20 mg/ml suspension	
Topical only				
Clobetasol	Temovate			0.05% cream or ointment
Desonide	Tridesilon			0.05% cream or ointment
Desoximetasone	Topicort			0.25% cream
Flumethasone pivalate	Locorten			0.25% cream
Fluocinolone acetonide	Fluonid; Synalar			0.01, 0.025, 0.2% cream; 0.025% ointment; 0.01% solution
Flucocinonide	Lidex; Topsynget			0.05% cream, gel, or ointment
Fluorometholone	Oxylone			0.025% cream; 0.1% ophthalmic suspension
Flurandrenolide	Cordran			0.025, 0.05% cream or ointment; 0.05% lotion; 4 μg/cm² tape
Halcinonide	Halog			0.025, 0.1% cream; 0.1% ointment; 0.1% solution
Medrysone	Medrocort and others			1% ophthalmic suspension

Table 32–5
Preparations of Corticosteroids (*continued*)

		Dosage forms		
Generic name	**Trade names**	**Oral**	**Parenteral**	**Topical**
Mineralocorticoids				
Desoxycorticosterone acetate	DOCA Acetate Percorten Acetate		5 mg/ml in oil; 125 mg pellets	
Desoxycorticosterone pivalate	Percorten Pivalate		25 mg/ml repository suspension	
Fludrocortisone acetate	Florinef Acetate	0.1 mg tablets		

the top 200 prescription drugs were Cortisporin and Neo-Synalar, topical creams containing hydrocortisone and antibiotics. *Oral doses are best taken at mealtime or with a snack to reduce gastric irritation. Single daily doses are best given in the morning to mimic the natural diurnal rhythm.*

When intramuscular injections are indicated, the nurse should place the needle deep in the outer upper quadrant of the buttock so as to prevent local atrophy. The deltoid muscle should be avoided for intramuscular injections. Subcutaneous injection is not recommended for glucocorticoids because dermal suppression and pseudoatrophy may occur. Hydrocortisone sodium succinate is sometimes given by intra-articular injection or soft tissue injection.

Hydrocortisone may also be administered rectally in the form of a retention enema. *In this case, the nurse needs to encourage the client to retain the fluid for at least 30 minutes following instillation to assure absorption of the drug through the rectal mucosa. When clients receive the drug in the form of a suppository, the suppository should be inserted well above the anal sphincter and against the wall of the rectum. If the client is to provide self-care, it is important for the nurse to teach him or her proper methods of inserting the suppository and to avoid defecation for at least 30 minutes after insertion.*

For adrenal crisis, 100 mg of a water-soluble hydrocortisone ester is injected intravenously and followed by an intravenous infusion at a rate of 100 mg over 2–8 hours. The other three insufficiency conditions of the adrenal cortex are treated with maintenance therapy, typically starting at about 20–40 mg/day of hydrocortisone, taken orally. A 30 mg dose might be parceled out as 20 mg in the morning and 10 mg in the afternoon to mimic more closely the natural diurnal rhythm. Night doses should be avoided to prevent insomnia. Mineralocorticoid replacement is usually required as well. Fludrocortisone acetate (0.1–0.3 mg daily) is most often employed.

Important Nursing Implications for Glucocorticoids

☐ Avoid use of glucocorticoids in clients who have a history of psychiatric problems, peptic ulcer, diabetes, tuberculosis, glomerulonephritis, osteoporosis, myasthenia gravis, or uncontrolled infections.

☐ Avoid use of glucocorticoids during pregnancy because of possible teratogenicity. Inform female clients who are pregnant that self-administration of glucocorticoids, even topically, can be hazardous to the fetus.

☐ Because a moderate level of glucocorticoid activity is the normal physiological state of affairs, acute or subacute administration of glucocorticoids (up to about 10 days), even in moderately high doses, is not likely to cause serious adverse effects. For that reason, it is justifiable and often even critically important to rapidly administer a glucocorticoid at a dose within the normal range in a crisis where a steroid deficiency is probable, before diagnostic procedures have fully delineated the patient's status. Short courses of glucocorticoids can likewise be employed when appropriate for conditions that may not be life-threatening or disabling.

☐ Long-term treatment (in excess of about 10 days) of clients with glucocorticoids in amounts exceeding what may be required for replacement therapy is fraught with the danger of debilitating or even fatal adverse effects. The level of danger is an interaction between duration and dose as well as predictable and unpredictable factors related to the client's constitution. When administration is to be long-term, administer the smallest dose that provides adequate response. Since therapy with glucocorticoids is empirical, this will require dosage titration. If the condition is not life-threatening, the initial dose should be small and gradually increased to achieve a minimally acceptable benefit. In life-threatening conditions, dosage adjustment may begin with an initially high dose that is as certain as possible to provide the life-sustaining effect. Duration of treatment should be as brief as is possible.

- ☐ In times of stress such as illness or emotional trauma, clients may need to increase the amount of drug they take. Clients receiving glucocorticoids need to be helped to understand that under such circumstances dosage alteration is appropriate. Teach clients how to regulate the dosage of drug to meet their particular needs.
- ☐ Educate the client about the critical importance of compliance with dosing instructions when glucocorticoids are being employed. When clients are required to take corticosteroids over an extended period of time, they need constant encouragement to comply with the drug regimen.
- ☐ If the individual has been receiving corticosteroid therapy for a period of time prior to the nurse's first contact with the client, it is important to obtain the background history and, where possible, discuss the client's progress to date with other health team members, the client, and the family. Nurses must identify each team member's perception of the client's progress, as well as the progress as indicated on the individual's health record, in order to make accurate judgments.
- ☐ Oral doses are best taken with meals to minimize gastrointestinal irritation. Single daily doses should be taken in the morning to mimic the natural diurnal rhythm.
- ☐ Family members and clients need to be taught how to give parenteral preparations intramuscularly in the event that the individual cannot take the drug orally. For example, nausea and vomiting from whatever cause would interfere with bioavailability of an orally administered drug, necessitating parenteral injection. Should the client require parenteral administration of drug over an extended period of time, both the client and family members should be taught to rotate the injection sites to avoid atrophy at the site of administration. They should also be taught to avoid the deltoid muscle and not to administer the drug subcutaneously. If parenteral injection is to be routine for a period of time, the nurse should periodically check to ensure that sites are being rotated and that the medication is being properly administered.
- ☐ Teach clients how to recognize the adverse effects of glucocorticoids, including fluid retention, electrolyte imbalances, peptic ulcerations, muscle wasting, osteoporosis, menstrual irregularities, ocular problems, susceptibility to infection, and psychiatric disturbances. Teach clients how to minimize the risk of these effects and what to do if an adverse effect develops.
- ☐ Provide clients with a list of drugs that interact with corticosteroids and explain the potential untoward interactions. Give a copy of the list to a responsible family member. Clients should be taught to inquire about any drugs being prescribed by persons other than the physician who has been following the progress of steroid therapy. If the client is elderly or has visual impairment, the names of drugs should be clearly printed out in large letters so that there can be no mistaking drug identity.
- ☐ If discontinuation is required after extended use of glucocorticoids, monitor clients carefully during the period when doses are being tapered for signs of adrenocortical insufficiency. Teach clients the importance of slow withdrawal once it has been determined that the original purpose for which the drug was prescribed has been achieved. Carefully explain the symptoms of rebound and encourage the client to report them if they occur. The usual rate of withdrawal is 2.5 mg of prednisone (or an equivalent amount of another steroid) every 4–10 days. If withdrawal symptoms appear, the previous dose is reinstituted for 7 days before continuing withdrawal.
- ☐ Encourage clients receiving steroid therapy to wear identification indicating what drugs they have been taking so that in the event of stress caused by accident or surgery, the health team would be aware of the potential problems.

Mineralocorticoids

Clinical Indications Aldosterone deficiency is seldom seen in secondary adrenal insufficiency, since ACTH has little impact on the zona glomerulosa. However, mineralocorticoid deficiency is an important part of Addison's disease and adrenal crisis. In fact, mineralocorticoid deficiency, not the glucocorticoid deficiency, contributes the life-threatening character to adrenal crises. Dehydration, hypotension, and small heart size that occur in advanced Addison's disease as well as peripheral vascular collapse and renal failure in adrenal crisis are all attributable to deficient mineralocorticoid activity. When high doses of natural glucocorticoids (cortisol or cortisone) are used for primary adrenal insufficiency, it is not always necessary to employ a mineralocorticoid as well since these natural glucocorticoids also possess weak mineralocorticoid activity. In other cases, a mineralocorticoid will need to be added to the regimen because the glucocorticoid selected fails to provide sufficient mineralocorticoid activity.

Adverse Effects The only significant side effects of mineralocorticoids are caused by less than ideal dosage adjustment. Excessive doses lead to symptoms of hyperaldosteronism (hypertension, hypernatremia, hypokalemic alkalosis). *The client should be assessed periodically for blood pressure changes and evidence of edema. Serum electrolyte levels should be monitored periodically during mineralocorticoid therapy. Hypernatremia may be controlled by dietary adjustments in salt and hypokalemia with potassium chloride supplements.*

Preparations and Administration For maintenance therapy, the mineralocorticoid desoxycorticosterone acetate (Doca Acetate, Percoten), or more commonly, fludrocortisone acetate (Florinef) can be used in conjunction with a glucocorticoid. Mineralocorticoids are available as oral tablets, injectable oil suspension, or pellets. Preparations of these drugs are listed in Table 32–5. Fludrocortisone is useful orally and is thus more convenient than desoxycorticosterone for most applications.

ACTH as a Drug

Clinical Indications ACTH is used as a diagnostic agent for differentiating between the various causes of corticosteroid deficiency. When the deficiency is due to primary adrenocortical failure, ACTH administration will not elicit a surge in steroid production. When corticosteroid deficiency is due to pituitary insufficiency (secondary adrenocortical insufficiency), ACTH will elicit an elevation in steroid levels either acutely or with repeated doses.

ACTH is not widely used for therapy of secondary adrenocortical insufficiency for the simple reason that it is less convenient and more expensive than administration of the readily available steroids. The effects of ACTH are the combined effects of glucocorticoids, mineralocorticoids, and weak androgens. The pharmacological activity of ACTH is not equivalent to glucocorticoid therapy alone, because it promotes release of all three types of adrenal steroids, although mineralocorticoids only to a small extent.

Pharmacokinetics ACTH is readily absorbed after parenteral administration. It is usually given by intramuscular injection, less often by intravenous infusion. It has a half-life of about 15 minutes.

Adverse Effects ACTH toxicity consists of excess production of steroids with the predictable consequences. Rarely, hypersensitivity reactions are reported. *The nurse should note complaints of dizziness, nausea, or vomiting since these can be early signs of sensitivity to the drug that could progress to anaphylactic shock.* ACTH also has one extra-adrenal effect of clinical relevance: a stimulation of melanocytes, resulting in hyperpigmentation.

During administration of ACTH clients may complain of feeling very weak as a result of a decrease in muscle strength. Some clients may develop respiratory difficulties. *Therefore, nurses need to have mechanical support immediately available as a precaution. Clients who experience muscle weakness may find it very frightening and need to be reassured that with the termination of the drug administration, muscle strength will return to normal.*

Preparations and Administration ACTH (Corticotropin) is currently available in four kinds of preparations. *The repository preparation should be shaken well and, when given intramuscularly, injected deep into gluteal muscle. Corticotropin products except for cosyntropin are derived from food-source mammals, mainly hogs. Individuals sensitive to porcine proteins should not be given these products. Clients should be observed closely for 15 minutes following drug administration. If hypersensitivity is suspected, a skin test should be given prior to administration of the ACTH.*

Corticotropin
Injection solution (USP and Acthar), repository corticotropin injection (Acthar Gel, Cortigel, others), corticotropin zinc hydroxide suspension (Cor-

trophin-Zinc), cosyntropin (Cortrosyn), a synthetic peptide preparation consisting of the first 24 amino acid residues of ACTH

Recommended Doses: For diagnostic appraisal in adrenocorticoid insufficiency, 25 units of the sterile injection solution infused over 8 hours or 80 units given per day in 1–4 intramuscular or subcutaneous injections; or 40 units of repository corticotropin injection once a day, subcutaneously or intramuscularly; or corticotropin zinc hydroxide suspension, 40 units, once a day; or 0.25 mg of cosyntropin (equivalent to 25 units of ACTH), IM.

Hyperfunctioning of the Adrenal Cortex and Steroid Inhibitors

Conditions of hyperfunctioning can involve one or all of the classes of adrenal steroids (Table 32–6). Excessive adrenal androgens result in adrenal virilism; excessive glucocorticoid levels lead to Cushing's syndrome; and overproduction of aldosterone causes hyperaldosteronism. Since none of the natural steroids is absolutely selective in its activity, there is some overlap in characteristics of these three hyperfunctional conditions. The three physiological causes of excess adrenal activity are hyperplasias (caused by too much ACTH), adenomas, and adenocarcinomas. In addition, the symptoms of adrenal hyperfunctioning can be mimicked by adminstration of excessive amounts of the respective steroids.

Hyperaldosteronism

Primary hyperaldosteronism (Conn's syndrome) is almost always due to an adenoma in the zona glomerulosa of the adrenal cortex. Rarely, it is due to hyperplasia or carcinoma. Metabolic symptoms include hypernatremia, hypervolemia, hyperchlorhydria, hypokalemia, and metabolic alkalosis. Clinical signs are episodes of weakness and paralysis, tetany, and paresthesias. Primary aldosteronism is treated by tumor removal. Secondary hyperaldosteronism is caused by excess renin release from the kidney, and is a major, if not *the* major, factor in essential hypertension (see Chapter 43).

Cushing's Syndrome

Cushing's syndrome, the most common disorder of the adrenal glands, results from excessive levels of glucocorticoids. The causes are varied (Table 32–6). Cushing's syndrome may be due to hyperplasia, in

Table 32–6
Causes of Adrenal Hyperfunctioning

Cushing's syndrome (excess glucocorticoid activity)	Aldosteronism (excess mineralocorticoid activity)	Adrenal virilism (excess adrenal androgen activity)
I. ACTH-dependent hypersecretion (hyperplasia) A. Pituitary adenoma (Cushing's Disease) B. Ectopic ACTH-producing tumor C. ACTH administration II. ACTH-independent glucocorticoid excess A. Adenoma B. Adenocarcinoma C. Glucocorticoid administration	I. Tumor in zona glomerulosa: A. Adenoma B. Adenocarcinoma C. Hyperplasia II. Secondary A. Excess renin production	I. ACTH-dependent hypersecretion (hyperplasia) A. Pituitary adenoma B. Ectopic ACTH-producing tumor C. ACTH administration D. Congenital hyperplasias (Defective cortisol production) II. ACTH-independent hypersecretion A. Adenomas B. Adenocarcinomas C. Androgen administration

which case it is said to be ACTH-dependent. The term Cushing's disease is reserved for adrenal hyperplasia due specifically to a pituitary adenoma. Tumors in the adrenal cortex or chronic administration of high doses of glucocorticoids produce ACTH-independent Cushing's syndrome.

The clinical symptoms include redistribution of the fat pads, resulting in the "moon face," pendulous abdomen, buffalo hump, and purple abdominal striae (Figure 32–1). The skin becomes thin. Because of the anti-inflammatory action of glucocorticoids, there is poor wound healing and easy bruising. Other symptoms include hypertension (due to mineralocorticoid effects of cortisol), renal calculi, osteoporosis (due to vitamin D antagonism), glucose intolerance, and psychiatric disturbances resembling symptoms of schizophrenia. Since Cushing's syndrome may be accompanied by increased adrenal androgen secretion, there may be signs of virilism in women: menstrual irregularities, balding, hirsutism, and so forth. *Nurses should identify what medications a client has been taking since symptoms of adrenal hyperfunctioning can be mimicked by administration of excessive amounts of the respective steroids.*

Treatment of Cushing's syndrome is determined by the etiology but may entail bilateral adrenalectomy, surgical removal of adrenal or ectopic tumors, hypophysectomy, or inhibitors of steroid synthesis (metyrapone, mitotane, or aminoglutethimide). *People who have Cushing's syndrome need to be prepared for long-term therapy. This means that nursing plans must provide for early and sustained support of the client.*

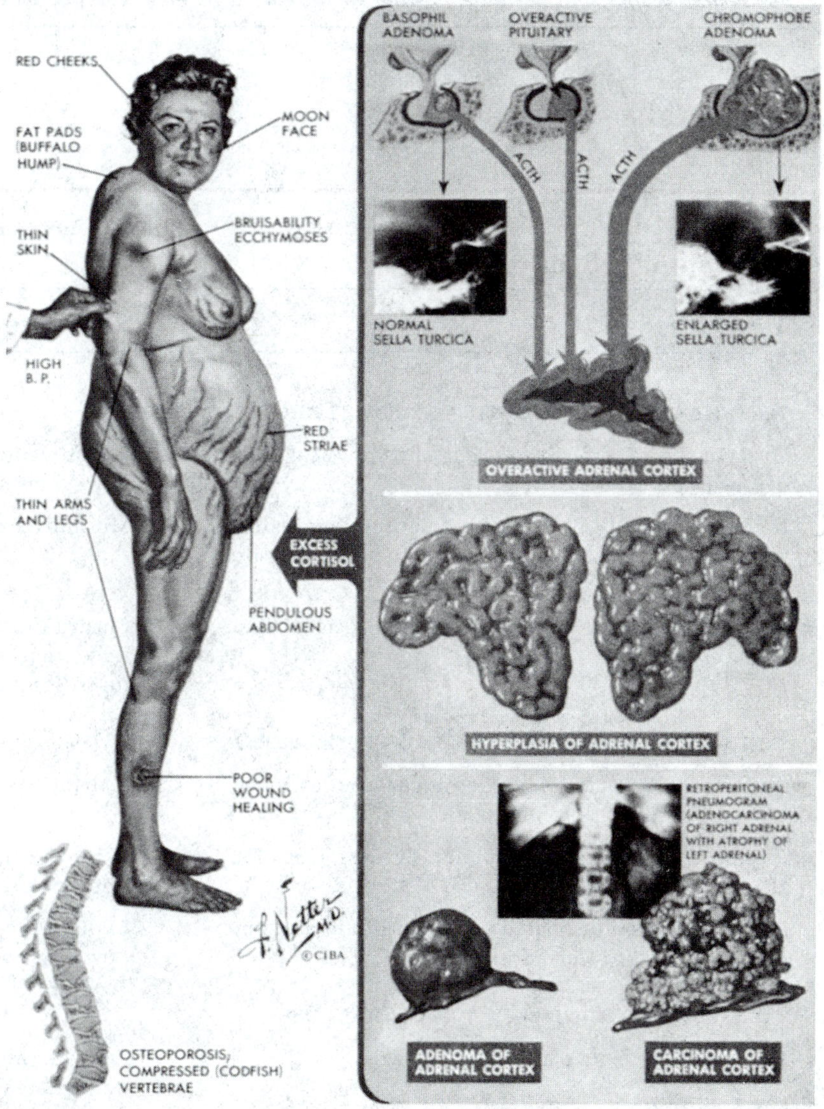

Figure 32–1
Clinical manifestations of Cushing's syndrome. Symptoms are similar whether they are caused by excess endogenous production or are drug induced.

Nursing Observations for Use of Steroid Inhibitors in Cushing's Syndrome

THERAPEUTIC GOAL	Reduction of corticosteroid activity to normal level by drug therapy with mitotane, metyrapone, trilostane, or aminoglutethimide.
PREADMINISTRATION ASSESSMENT	
Baseline Data	Observe for extent of fluid retention (swelling of hands, feet, or fingers), moon face, buffalo hump, pendulous abdomen, thin skin, abdominal striae, virilism, and menstrual irregularities in women, arrested growth in children. Evaluate blood pressure, x-rays for adrenal or pituitary tumors and renal calculi, urinalysis. Obtain laboratory tests including serum and urinary glucose levels, glucose tolerance test, plasma cortisol, urinary free cortisol, dexamethasone tests (low and high dose), ACTH levels, metyrapone test, and ACTH stimulation test.
EVALUATION OF DRUG RESPONSE	
For Therapeutic Benefit	Redetermine serum and blood glucose levels, glucose tolerance, plasma cortisol, and urinary free cortisol.
For Adverse Effects	Monitor for indications of adrenocortical insufficiency.

Nursing Diagnoses and Interventions for Use of Steroid Inhibitors in Cushing's Syndrome

Nursing Diagnoses	*Related Interventions*
TO ENHANCE DRUG BENEFITS OR REDUCE DRUG REQUIREMENTS	
Disturbance in self-concept related to physical changes of Cushing's disease	Provide emotional support and encouragement. Introduce client to peer support group if available.
Increased risk of infection due to anti-inflammatory and anti-allergic effects of glucocorticoids in Cushing's disease	Minimize exposure to infections.
Increased risk of injury due to osteoporosis in Cushing's disease	Ensure that diet provides adequate intake of calcium. Encourage adequate exercise for weight bearing structures (long bones) to prevent demineralization.
TO MINIMIZE DRUG SIDE EFFECTS OR INTERACTIONS	
Activity intolerance related to fatigue and lassitude caused by steroid inhibitors	Provide adequate periods of rest.
Impaired skin integrity related to dryness, loss of tissue, and edema from inhibition of steroids	Minimize risk of skin infection. Apply emollients to improve skin lubrication.
Sexual dysfunction related to loss of libido and amenorrhea related to steroid inhibition.	Explain the origin of the problem and provide support and encouragement.
TO ENSURE SAFE AND EFFICACIOUS DRUG USE	
Knowledge deficit related to drug regimen	Educate the client concerning the nature of the disorder and the need for surgical or drug intervention to correct the problem.

Inhibitors of Steroid Synthesis

Four drugs are available for inhibition of steroid synthesis: mitotane, metyrapone, aminoglutethimide, and trilostane. Mitotane is a relative of the insecticide DDT. It has cytotoxic effects on cells of the adrenal cortex and has been used for this effect in therapy for tumors of the adrenal cortex.

Metyropone (Metapirone) is an inhibitor of the 11-L-hydroxylation step in steroid synthesis that leads to production of cortisol and corticosterone. Its main use is as a diagnostic tool for differentiating the various causes of Cushing's syndrome. It has been employed for treatment of ACTH-independent adrenal tumors and hyperplasias caused by ectopic ACTH-producing tumors.

Aminoglutethimide (Cytraden) inhibits a much earlier step in steroidogenesis, the conversion of cholesterol to pregnenolone. It thus prevents formation of all classes of adrenal steroids. It is used in treatment of Cushing's syndrome. The major risk with use of aminoglutethimide is that suppression of steroidogenesis may be so complete as to bring about adrenocortical insufficiency, with symptoms of hypotension, drowsiness, and so forth. It may be necessary to institute glucocorticoid and mineralocorticoid replacement therapy. Hospitalization is required until a stable dosage regimen is established.

Trilostane (Modrastane) was introduced in 1985. It is a synthetic steroid that inhibits formation of glucocorticoids. Based on limited data, trilostane appears to be less likely to result in serious side effects than the other steroid inhibitors. The problems most commonly observed with use of trilostane are diarrhea and gastrointestinal irritation (each occurring in about 16–17% of clients), burning of nasal membranes (in about 8% of clients), and nausea, headache, and bloating or flatulence (each in about 4–5% of clients). Trilostane is teratogenic and therefore contraindicated in pregnancy. It is also contraindicated in clients with severe renal or hepatic dysfunction or adrenal insufficiency.

Aminoglutethimide (Cytraden)
Tablets
Recommended Doses: 250 mg qid, orally, initially. Plasma cortisol levels are monitored as the basis for dosage adjustment.

Metyrapone (Metopirone)
Tablets
Recommended Doses: For testing adrenal function, 750 mg every 4 hours for 6 doses in adults; 15 mg/kg every 4 hours for 6 doses in children.

Trilostane (Modrastane)
Capsules
Recommended Doses: 30 mg, 4 times daily initially, increased at intervals of 3–4 days up to 40 mg/day.

Case Study: Cushing's Syndrome

B. T., a 43-year-old single female was brought to the clinic by a friend because of bizarre behavior, including apparently carrying on conversations with voices that she heard. The nurse who examined her noted that her skin was red, her cheeks rounded, and her eyelids puffy. The client was obese about the thighs and buttocks, but thin in the extremities. She had several bruises and red striae on the abdomen and thighs. B. T. had no recent history of medical care. The nurse suspected Cushing's syndrome and referred the client to a physician.

Laboratory tests were ordered. Plasma and free cortisol levels were both elevated with absence of normal diurnal variations and plasma ACTH was depressed. Baseline urinary 17-hydroxysteroids were normal, but exhibited no suppression in low- or high-dose dexamethasone tests and no elevation after administration of metapirone. Administration of a test dose of ACTH caused an increase in urinary 17-hydroxysteroids. Based on these data, the physician concluded that B. T. most likely had Cushing's syndrome due to presence of an adenoma. Surgery was scheduled for B. T., the diagnosis was confirmed by inspection of the adrenal glands, and they were removed. After surgery, replacement therapy was instituted. The nurse educated the client with respect to the importance of exact compliance with the replacement regimen and the possible adverse effects should the dosage be either too small or too large.

1. Which of the physical signs observed by the examining nurse can be attributed to Cushing's syndrome?
2. How did each of the laboratory tests contribute to the ultimate diagnosis of an adenoma?
3. What were the alternatives to surgical intervention?
4. What symptoms should the client look for as indications of too little glucocorticoid activity? Too much glucocorticoid activity? Too little mineralocorticoid activity? Too much mineralocorticoid activity?

Answers appear at the end of the book.

Case Study: Addison's Disease

A. B., a 62-year-old married man, was admitted to the hospital because of weakness, fatigue, nausea, and vomiting. During physical examination, the nurse noted presence of black freckles over the neck and shoulders and bluish-black pigmentation of the mucous membranes of the areolas, lips, and rectum. Blood pressure was within normal limits (120/82) when measured while the patient was supine or sitting, but dropped markedly when A. B. stood up. Dizziness and sometimes syncope occurred during this maneuver. Body temperature was 98.8°F, pulse 86, and respirations 24. The patient's medication history indicated that he was not receiving diuretics or other prescription drugs and seldom self-administered nonprescription medications. A. B. employed alcohol only occasionally and used no other social drugs. The nurse made a provisional diagnosis of Addison's disease and reported her findings to the physician.

The physician, concurring with the nurse's assessment, ordered blood studies and x-ray evaluation. Laboratory findings from blood studies showed low serum sodium (118 mEq/L), elevated serum potassium (5.2 mEq/L), a low fasting blood sugar level (45 mg/100 ml), an elevated blood urea nitrogen (23 mg/100 ml), and a low white blood cell count. X-ray findings provided no evidence of renal or pulmonary tuberculosis. A single-dose metyrapone test was conducted: A. B. was given the drug (at a dose of 30 mg/kg) at midnight with a small amount of food. A plasma sample drawn at 8:00 AM the next day revealed no increase in 17-hydroxysteroids, a lower than normal level of cortisol, and high level of ACTH. It was concluded that A. B. had primary Addison's disease due to idiopathic atrophy of the adrenal cortex.

Therapy was initiated with hydrocortisone sodium succinate, 100 mg injected IV over 30 seconds, followed by 1 liter of 5% glucose in saline and another 100 mg of hydrocortisone sodium succinate infused over 2 hours. Hydrocortisone therapy was continued at 400 mg/day during stabilization of the condition. During this period, the nurse monitored daily weight, urine glucose, intake and output, serum electrolytes, and vital signs. The nurse instructed A. B. about Addison's disease, explaining the symptoms of Addisonian crisis, adverse effects of steroids, and the need for lifelong therapy. She taught A. B. the benefits of regular exercise and maintaining a high-protein diet. She explained to A. B. that replacement requirements for glucocorticoids might be increased during surgery, infection, or periods of stress. As the condition stabilized, oral replacement therapy was initiated and A. B. was discharged from the hospital on a regimen of 10 mg of prednisone in the morning and 5 mg in the afternoon, and 0.1 mg of fludrocortisone once daily.

1. Which of the physical symptoms at the time of initial presentation led the nurse to the provisional diagnosis of Addison's disease?
2. Why did the nurse inquire especially about whether A. B. was receiving diuretic therapy?
3. Which of the values from the blood evaluation were confirmatory of Addison's disease? Why do these abnormal values occur in Addison's disease?
4. Why was the physician concerned with checking for possible evidence of tuberculosis?
5. After administration of metyrapone, which measurement provided the basis for the conclusion that the Addison's disease was primary, not secondary?
6. Explain the basis for each of the points made by the nurse in instructing A. B. about his condition and therapeutic regimen.
7. Why was A. B. switched from the hydrocortisone ester to prednisone before discharge?
8. Why did the oral replacement regimen for A. B. provide a larger dose in the morning than in the afternoon?
9. Why was fludrocortisone given as well as prednisone?

Answers appear at the end of the book.

Recommended Readings

Baxter JD, Rousseau GG (eds): *Glucocorticoid Hormone Action.* New York, Springer-Verlag, 1979.

Cupps TR, Fauci AS: Corticosteroid-mediated immunoregulation in man. *Immunol Rev* 1982;65:133–154.

Dixon R, Christy N: On the various forms of corticosteroid withdrawal syndrome. *Am J Med* 1980;68:224–230.

Ganong WF et al.: ACTH and the regulation of adrenocortical secretion. *N Engl J Med* 1974;290:1006–1011.

Gill GN: Diagnosing and treating Cushing's syndrome. *Consultant* 1980;20:50.

Gotch PM: Teaching patients about adrenal corticosteroids. *Am J. Nurs* 1981;81:78–81.

Jones SG: Adrenal patient: Proceed with caution. Cushing's sydrome. *RN* 1982;45:66–68.

Lamb, C: Corticosteroid misuse and ill effects. *Patient Care* 1981;15:69–72.

LoDolce D et al: Alternate programs of steroid administration for patients on long-term therapy. *J Neurosurg Nurs* 1980;12:187–194.

Melby JC: Clinical pharmacology of systemic steroids. *Annu Rev Pharmacol Toxicol* 1977;17:511–527.

Streeten DHP: Corticosteroid therapy. 1. Pharmacologic properties and principles of corticosteroid use. *JAMA* 1975;232:944–947.

Vernoski B, Chernow B: Steroids: Use and abuse. *Crit Care Q* 1983;6(3):28.

CHAPTER 33

Drugs Used for Disorders of the Endocrine Pancreas

Regulation of Blood Glucose

The pancreas is a yellowish, elongated gland located transversely along the upper, posterior abdominal wall. It has the shape of a tadpole with its head end tucked into the bends of the duodenum and its tail extended horizontally behind the stomach. It is both an exocrine and an endocrine gland. The exocrine portion (discussed in chapter 51) constitutes 99% of the gland by mass and secretes large amounts of digestive enzymes and sodium bicarbonate into the duodenum. The endocrine portion of the pancreas consists of the islets of Langerhans, so named because they appear as small islands amid the comparatively expansive exocrine tissue (Figure 33–1). The islets contain four types of cells, the most important of which are the alpha-cells, which produce glucagon, and the beta-cells, which produce insulin. Beta-cells make up 70% of the islet mass while alpha-cells make up 20%.

Glucose Homeostasis

Under normal circumstances, blood glucose levels are tightly regulated to prevent undue loss of glucose in the urine while ensuring availability of energy to tissues such as the brain, kidney, retina, blood cells, and germinal epithelium of the gonads that are highly dependent on blood glucose. Normal blood glucose values in adults are about 80–90 mg/100 ml in the fasting state.

When the level of blood glucose is elevated — as, for example, after meals, when the level may rise to 120–140 mg/100 ml — the beta-cells release in-

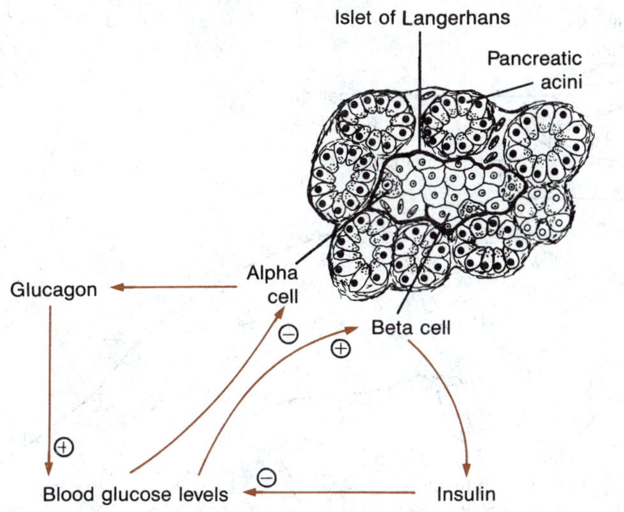

Figure 33–1
Double-feedback control of blood glucose levels. Elevated blood glucose levels stimulate the beta-cells to release insulin, which lowers blood glucose levels by promoting its uptake into tissue cells. Lowered blood glucose levels stimulate release of glucagon from alpha-cells, which raises blood glucose by stimulating release of glucose from storage in the liver.

sulin into the bloodstream. Insulin lowers blood glucose by promoting its uptake into tissue cells, where it is stored or utilized. As the levels of glucose decline, the impetus for insulin secretion dissipates, another example of a negative feedback relationship between a hormone and a regulated substance. Insulin is the only hormone known to reduce blood glucose levels. Blood glucose levels in excess of about 100 mg/100 ml are sufficient to stimulate the beta-cells to release insulin. Changes in the secretory rate of insulin from beta-cells occur very rapidly in response to fluctuations in blood glucose. Increase in insulin secretion can even occur in anticipation of rises in blood glucose because several gastrointestinal hormones (secretin, gastrin, gastric-inhibiting peptide, and pancreozymin-cholecystokinin) released during digestive activity stimulate insulin release.

When the level of blood glucose is depressed, the alpha cells release glucagon into the bloodstream. Its effects are generally opposite to those of insulin, and the factors that initiate its release are also opposite. Thus, while insulin is the hormone promoting fuel storage, glucagon is the hormone of fuel mobilization. Following a meal, insulin release and glucagon inhibition promote storage activities (Figure 33–1). During fasting, glucagon release and insulin inhibition provoke mobilization of fuels from storage depots.

Insulin

Insulin is a protein consisting of two amino acid chains connected by a pair of disulfide bridges. The longer chain (30 amino acid residues) extends beyond the shorter chain (21 amino acid residues) on both sides, partially enclosing it (Figure 33–2). Insulin is synthesized as part of a larger protein called preproinsulin, which is converted immediately to proinsulin by removal of a peptide segment. Proinsulin is then converted to insulin by removal of another peptide segment. The conversion of proinsulin to insulin is incomplete, and proinsulin may be found in small amounts in many commercial insulin preparations.

Actions of Insulin

The role of insulin is to promote the storage of fuel substances derived from dietary sources, primarily glucose in humans, but also amino acids, fatty acids, potassium, and magnesium. At the cellular level, the effect of insulin is a stimulation of glucose uptake, which is by carrier-mediated diffusion (Figure 33–2). Normal levels of insulin can increase facilitated diffusion of glucose fourfold, and high concentrations of insulin can increase glucose uptake another fivefold.

The action of insulin occurs mainly if not exclusively at the cell surface. The identified insulin receptor is a glycoprotein embedded in the plasma membrane, which, for all practical purposes, is completely specific for insulin. Effects of insulin are not imparted equally on all tissues. Insulin does not alter glucose transport in the brain, red or white blood cells, the parenchyma of the kidney, or the intestinal mucosa. These tissues have maximal capacity to accumulate glucose even in the absence of insulin because they are highly dependent on glucose for their high-level energy requirements. These tissues are, on the other hand, especially vulnerable to hypoglycemia. The muscles, adipose tissue, and liver are the three main targets of insulin activity.

In muscle tissue, insulin stimulates transport of glucose into the cells, where it is utilized for energy production via the glycolytic pathway and Krebs cycle, or stored as glycogen when there is no immediate requirement for energy. In adipose tissue, glucose uptake is also stimulated by insulin. The glucose taken up by fat cells is converted into triglycerides for storage as fat. Glucose uptake by fat and muscle cells in the absence of insulin is negligible.

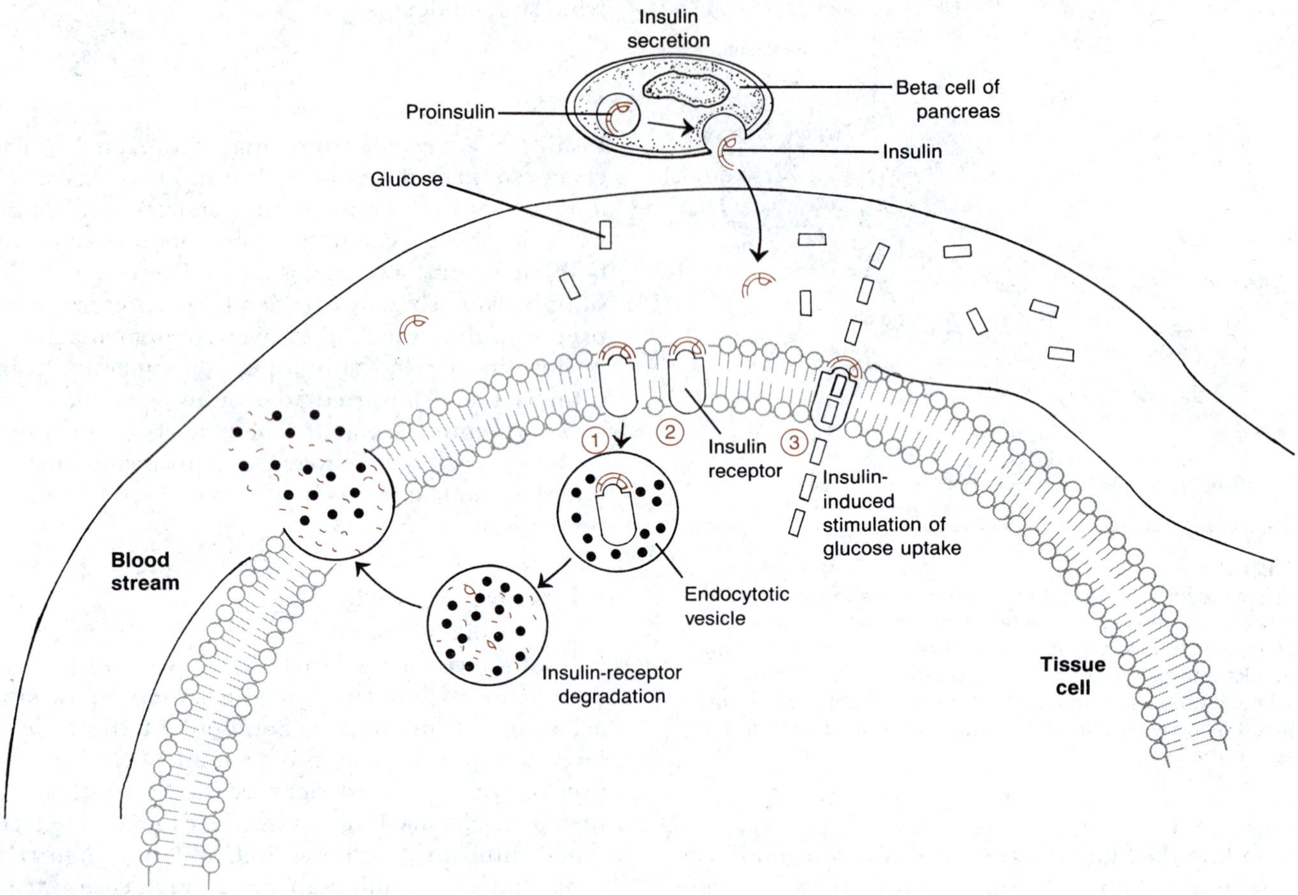

Figure 33–2
Life-cycle of insulin. Insulin is stored as proinsulin in the beta-cells of the pancreas until release into the blood. Upon attachment to an insulin receptor of a tissue cell, insulin stimulates glucose uptake. Later the insulin-receptor complex is incorporated into an endocytotic vesicle and degraded.

In the liver, the action of insulin is quite different. Liver cells do not require insulin for glucose uptake, since they are freely permeable to glucose as well as other hexoses. Nevertheless, insulin stimulates the ability of hepatic cells to form glycogen, the major storage form of glucose. This glycogen can later be utilized, when newly absorbed glucose is less available, to furnish the energy requirements of the organism. In the basal or fasting state, glucose is released from the liver at a steady rate of 2.0–3.5 mg/kg/minute. This continuous effusion of glucose sustains the organism, and especially those tissues that are crucially dependent on blood glucose for their energy requirements, during the period between meals. The glucose released by the liver is derived from glycogenolysis (hydrolysis of liver glycogen stores) and from gluconeogenesis (conversion of fat to glucose). Both glycogenolysis and gluconeogenesis are inhibited by the action of insulin when newly absorbed glucose is present in abundance.

In summary, insulin promotes the uptake and utilization of nutrients and their storage as glycogen and fats during periods of abundance following ingestion of foods. The stored energy resources can be utilized later to sustain the organism in times of nutrient scarcity.

Secretion, Distribution, and Elimination

Blood glucose level is the primary determinant of insulin secretion, but other factors are involved as well. For example, several other endocrine hormones elevate blood glucose (glucagon, cortisol, growth hormone, epinephrine, estrogens, and progesterone). When any one of these hormones is available in chronic excess, whether from endogenous or exogenous sources, the resultant hyperglycemia will act as a continuous stimulus for insulin production. This can lead to beta cell exhaustion and diabetes mellitus.

Neural impulses can also influence beta cell activity. Sympathetic amines can either stimulate insulin secretion through B_2-adrenergic receptors, or inhibit its release through α-receptors. Acetylcholine and the vagus nerve increase insulin release. These neural inputs appear to control basal insulin secretion and stress-mediated suppression. Certain drugs, most notably the sulfonylureas discussed later in this chapter, stimulate the beta-cells, while other drugs can inhibit or even damage the islet cells.

In the plasma and lymph, insulin circulates largely in an unbound form. Insulin is eliminated almost entirely by metabolism since it is reabsorbed by the renal tubules. A good deal of the metabolism occurs in the kidney as well as in the liver. Target tissues also inactivate insulin by incorporating absorbed insulin into vesicles that contain digestive enzymes.

Receptor Regulation

The tissue receptors for insulin undergo alterations in both number and sensitivity under certain circumstances. Such changes can often have clinical significance. Receptor changes can occur in either direction, resulting in increased responsiveness to insulin or resistance to insulin. Changes in insulin receptors may be adaptive responses related to alterations in availability of insulin, or they may be primary alterations independent of hormone levels. It is well established that chronic hyperinsulinism, whether experimentally induced or associated with excessive caloric intake and obesity, produces a "down-regulation" of insulin receptors. Obese clients with mild insulin resistance have a reduced number of insulin receptors while those with greater insulin resistance have a decrease in both receptor number and sensitivity. Cases of juvenile-onset obesity tend to exhibit mild insulin resistance while cases of adult-onset obesity entail more severe resistance. The reduction in the number of insulin receptors is brought about by a more rapid rate of receptor degradation.

In insulin-independent diabetes mellitus, change in insulin receptor populations may be a primary mechanism in the disorder and is certainly a factor to be reckoned with in the treatment process.

Glucagon

Glucagon is a small protein hormone consisting of a single chain of 29 amino acids, without disulfide bridges. It is structurally similar to the gastrointestinal hormone secretin. Glucagon release is stimulated most powerfully by declining serum glucose concentrations. Administration of glucose inhibits glucagon secretion. Glucose taken orally is more potent in suppressing glucagon release than glucose given intravenously, suggesting that gastrointestinal hormones may play a role. Secretin, the gastrointestinal hormone resembling glucagon in structure, has been noted to inhibit glucagon release. Fatty acids suppress glucagon secretion. Sympathetic nerve impulses stimulate glucagon release, and epinephrine and glucagon have similar effects on the liver. The effects of both hormones are mediated by cyclic AMP.

In the liver, glucagon stimulates glycogenolysis and gluconeogenesis, releasing sugar into the blood. As little as 1 μg/kg of glucagon can elevate blood glucose levels by 50% in a matter of minutes, so the effect is both rapid and potent. Glucagon also inhibits glycogen formation in muscles as well as the liver and stimulates lipolysis in adipose tissue. Glucagon release is also stimulated by exercise, infection, and trauma.

Glucagon is degraded in the liver, kidney, plasma, and by target tissue cells. Enzymatic destruction is by proteolysis. Its half-life is similar to that of insulin, about 3–6 minutes.

Diabetes Mellitus

Diabetes mellitus is an age-old disease. As long as 3,000 years ago the characteristic sweetness of the urine was recognized by its ability to attract ants. The name was given to the disorder by the first-century Greek physician, Arataeus, and suggests a "melting down of the flesh into urine." The islets of the pancreas were described by Langerhans while he was still a medical student in 1869, but it was not until the extraction of insulin from the islets and its physiological testing in 1921–1922 by Banting and Best that the significance of the islets and insulin was grasped. Within a year, insulin was being used to save the lives of diabetic patients. Currently, there are about 12 million diabetic patients in the United States and the number is increasing. Diabetic patients occupy 5–7% of all hospital beds. In the United States, diabetes is twice as common in women as in men, but in some other countries diabetes is more common in men than women.

Classification and Etiology

Diabetes is characterized by a fasting blood-glucose level of above 140 mg/100 ml in adults. The revised classification of diabetes mellitus produced by the

National Diabetes Data Group recognizes five subclasses of diabetes (Table 33–1): type I diabetes mellitus, type II diabetes mellitus, secondary diabetes, gestational diabetes, and impaired glucose tolerance.

About 10% of clients with primary diabetes have type I, or **insulin-dependent diabetes mellitus,** formerly called diabetes mellitus of juvenile onset or ketotic diabetes. Each of the older names is descriptive of a feature of the condition. It usually begins in youth, most commonly before age 20. It is characterized by a severe deficiency in production of insulin by the beta cells, and the risk of ketoacidosis (a manifestation of cellular glucose deprivation) is high. Apparently, in this type of diabetes, beta-cells are gradually destroyed by an autoimmune mechanism and insulin production is impaired or even lost entirely. Plasma concentrations of insulin are invariably subnormal. There is only a modest familial trend in the occurrence of type I diabetes. Obesity is not a contributing factor in insulin-dependent diabetes, and, in fact, these clients are generally lean due to "melt down" of tissue mass. Clients with type I diabetes are absolutely dependent on administration of exogenous insulin for their survival; prior to the discovery of insulin, this type of diabetes was rapidly fatal. Oral hypoglycemics are ineffective in type I diabetes.

Type II, or **noninsulin-dependent diabetes mellitus** differs in several respects from type I (Table 33–2). Of the 90% of diabetics who have type II diabetes, 80–90% are obese. The familial trend is much more evident than in type I and twin concordance is virtually absolute. The condition usually begins after age 30 or 40 (hence the former name "maturity-onset di-

Table 33–1
Classification of Diabetes

National diabetes data group classification	Type I: Insulin-dependent diabetes mellitus (IDDM)	Type II: Noninsulin-dependent diabetes mellitus (NIDDM)	Secondary diabetes	Gestational diabetes	Impaired glucose tolerance
Equivalent terminology	Juvenile-onset Youth onset Ketotic Brittle	Adult-onset Maturity-onset Nonketotic	Hyperglycemia secondary to pancreatic disease, endocrine disorders, drugs, chemicals, or genetic syndromes		Asymptomatic diabetes Chemical diabetes Borderline diabetes Latent diabetes, mild nonketotic
Proposed etiology	Autoimmune destruction of beta-cells	Insulin-resistant receptors	Various primary disorders		Mildly insulin-resistant receptors
Diet	Regular meal schedule Increased meal frequency Restrict simple sugars Limit fats Avoid fad diets Increase fiber No restriction on total carbohydrates	Limit calories Hypocaloric intake if obese Avoid simple sugars Limit fats Increase fiber	Dictated by underlying disorder	Avoid simple sugars Avoid weight gain	Limit caloric intake to avoid weight gain or promote weight loss if overweight
Insulin	Treatment of choice	Not usually indicated	Useful	Useful	Not usually indicated
Oral hypoglycemics	Not effective	Useful	Useful	Contraindicated	Not usually indicated

Table 33–2
Characteristics of Diabetes Mellitus

Characteristic	Type I Insulin-dependent	Type II Noninsulin-dependent
Age of onset	Usually before age 20	Usually after age 40
Onset	Abrupt	Insidious
Body type	Lean	Obese (90%)
Insulin release	Deficient	Variable
Histocompatibility (HLA) antigens for beta-cells	Present	Absent
Familial history	Occasionally	Often
Beta-cell morphology	Destruction	Hyperplasia
Occurrence of ketoacidosis	Common	Uncommon
Insulin administration required	Yes	Not usually
Oral hypoglycemics effective	No	Yes

abetes"), but some cases occur as early as age 10 (formerly called MODY, for maturity-onset diabetes in the young).

In type II diabetes, insulin function is initially normal and often remains normal into middle age. The diabetic condition develops insidiously. Type II diabetes mellitus is characterized by insulin resistance caused by a decrease in the number of insulin receptors. In the mild cases, the deficiency in the number of insulin receptors is generally the sole factor, since insulin secretion is normal. Insulin levels may even be above normal, and the beta-cells may exhibit hyperplasia as the pancreas attempts to overcome the hyperglycemia caused by deficient glucose uptake by adipose and muscle tissues. As the condition progresses, the beta-cells ultimately become exhausted and the level of synthesis and release of insulin declines. Thus in the severe cases, insulin resistance and inadequate insulin secretion combine to produce a more profound deficit in uptake of glucose by peripheral tissues. As a result, blood levels of glucose are inordinately elevated.

Milder cases, representing the early or latent stages of type II, are identified as a separate diagnostic category called **impaired glucose tolerance.** Impaired glucose tolerance is diagnosed when fasting blood sugar levels lie between those of normal people (<115 mg/100 ml in adults) and those of diabetics (>140 mg/100 mg in adults); it is also diagnosed when oral glucose tolerance test values similarly fall between those of normal people (<140 mg/ml at 2 hours and one earlier time point) and those of diabetics (>200 mg/100 ml).

Impaired glucose tolerance can usually be managed adequately by dietary restrictions alone. The overt cases, qualifying as type II, can usually be treated effectively with oral hypoglycemic agents. About 25–30% of the most severe cases require exogenous insulin. In type II diabetes mellitus, the level of disturbance seldom advances to the stage of ketoacidosis.

The cause of receptor resistance to insulin that leads to noninsulin-dependent diabetes has been identified in some individual cases and varies from case to case. Usually there is an actual decrease in the number of insulin receptors. Less commonly, insulin receptors and insulin are both normal, but their interaction fails to produce the normal increase in glucose uptake by cells, or an insulin antagonist is present in the circulation in unusual quantities.

Sometimes diabetes occurs as a consequence of some other medical problem and is designated **secondary diabetes.** For example, a chronic excess of glucocorticoids elevates blood glucose levels, stimulating and ultimately exhausting the beta cells. Certain chemicals, notably allocane and streptozotocin, damage the beta cells and induce diabetes. Diazoxide (Hyperstat, Proglycem), a drug often used to alleviate acute hypertensive states, produces a prompt, dose-dependent, and reversible suppression of insulin release from the pancreas. Other causes of secondary diabetes include diseases of the pancreas, some genetic syndromes, and pregnancy. This last cause of diabetes is given a separate designation in the new classification scheme: **gestational diabetes.** Gestational diabetes is first discovered during pregnancy and is typically transitory but recurrent during the pregnancy.

Complications of Diabetes Mellitus

Diabetes mellitus is a difficult disorder to manage effectively because it leads to long-term complications in a number of tissues in addition to the immediate problems of metabolic balance. The complications associated with diabetes mellitus affect blood vessels, the kidneys, eyes, mouth, nervous system, skin, immunological mechanisms, and gestation, in addition to the pancreas itself. In the pancreas, loss of beta-cells, fibrosis, and infiltration by lymphocytes often occur in type I diabetes. In type II, the number of islet cells is often normal or expanded, but hyaline deposits infiltrate between islet cells in 30% of clients.

Vascular diseases of both large and small vessels are characteristic of diabetes. Coronary atherosclerosis is five times more common among diabetics than in the population as a whole, and myocardial infarction is a common cause of death in diabetics. Cerebrovascular accidents are also more prevalent in people with diabetes. They are also more prone to peripheral vascular disorders, by a factor of 50 or 100 times. The usual manifestation is ischemic lesions and gangrene of the feet and lower extremities. Diabetes mellitus is responsible for more than 20,000 leg and foot amputations yearly.

In the microcirculation, thickening of the basement membrane leads to various consequences, among them renal failure and retinopathy. Renal failure is another major cause of death among those with diabetes, and diabetes is the second leading cause of blindness, resulting in 5,000 new cases of blindness annually. Diabetic retinopathy occurs as a result of microvascular thickening, microaneurysms, and microangiopathies. Cataracts are also likely to occur with diabetes.

Both the **peripheral and central nervous systems** undergo changes in long-term diabetes mellitus, leading to such complications as sensory loss or pain, muscle weakness and atrophy, paresthesias, movement disorders, loss of sexual functioning, bladder atony, nocturnal diarrhea, postural hypotension, and increased gastric emptying time. Sexual impotency in males is the most common indication of neurological deterioration, and diabetes is one of the most common causes of impotency. A neurogenic joint disease, called Charcot's joints, occurs as a result of increased joint torsion and leads to fractures and bone collapse, usually in the feet.

Skin lesions of diabetes occur in response to microvascular dysfunction and hyperlipidemia of diabetes. Skin turgor is poor and infections are more common (especially *Candida albicans*). Papules and dark spots may also appear on the skin. Females with diabetes have an increased risk of complications during pregnancy.

The tissues most prone to complications in diabetes — the retina, lens, nerves, and kidneys — have one property in common. None of them require insulin for uptake of glucose. Glucose is taken up freely by these cells at a rate that is determined only by the blood level of glucose. The diabetic individual, even if well-regulated, experiences periods of hyperglycemia. While cells of tissues such as the skeletal muscles are being starved of glucose due to inadequate insulin, cells in the retina, lens, kidneys, and nervous tissue are literally awash in glucose. When glucose levels in a cell are excessive, glucose is converted to sorbitol and other related polyols by the enzyme aldose reductase. Sorbitol does not penetrate cell membranes very rapidly and thus tends to accumulate within the cells in which it is synthesized. As a result of the build-up of sorbitol, the cytoplasm becomes hypertonic and draws water into the cell. Gradually the cell swells to the point that it is unable to function effectively, resulting in the familiar irreversible changes that lead to cataracts, retinal damage, corneal ulcerations, nephropathy, and neuropathies. Two **inhibitors of aldose reductase,** tolrestat (Alredase) and sorbinil, are currently in stage III clinical trials for prevention of cataracts, and evidence from animal studies already indicates their ability to prevent cataract formation in diabetic laboratory animals. These drugs hold out some real hope for progress in the management of diabetes mellitus.

The current clinical course for diabetes mellitus varies from rapid deterioration with repeated bouts of ketoacidosis and vascular complications to mild, nonprogressive glucose intolerance that may be adequately controlled by dietary adjustments with little significant impact on quality or length of life.

Metabolic Disorders in Diabetes Mellitus

Metabolic disturbances are the quintessence of uncontrolled diabetes and not uncommon in type I diabetes under the best of circumstances. Fluctuations in endogenous insulin production, changes in diet, increase or decrease in physical activity, and poor compliance with treatment regimens all contribute to the development of metabolic crises. One problem confronting the clinical team is that the diabetic client is prone to four distinct kinds of metabolic problems, any one of which can result in coma. Each of the four types requires a different clinical response. The response that is appropriate for one type of coma could be lethally inappropriate for another. Therefore, the nurse and other members of the health care team must be aware of the distinguishing features of the four severe metabolic disorders of diabetes (Table 33–3): ketoacidosis, hyperglycemic hyperosmolar nonketotic coma, lactic acidosis, and insulin shock (or hypoglycemic crisis).

Ketoacidosis occurs when the biochemical alterations characteristic of diabetes are particularly severe. When insulin insufficiency reaches critical proportions, muscle and fat cells are deprived of glucose for their energy requirements. Metabolism of lipids in adipose tissue and protein in muscle cells is accelerated to furnish energy but results in increased generation of the corresponding breakdown products: fatty acids and amino acids. Subsequent hepatic me-

Table 33–3
Metabolic Disturbances Associated with Diabetes

Characteristic	Insulin shock	Ketoacidotic coma	HHNK	Lactic acidosis
History				
Food intake	Acutely insufficient	Normal or excessive	Normal or excessive	Normal or excessive
Insulin	Excessive	Insufficient	Insufficient	Insufficient
Onset	Sudden (minutes–hours)	Gradual (hours–days)	Gradual (hours–days)	Gradual (hours–days)
Typical precipitants	Insulin injection	Illness or stress	Surgery, illness, stress	Hypotension, alcohol intoxication
Physical examination				
Physical signs	Tremor, nervousness, weakness	Nausea, vomiting, polyuria, polydipsia, polyphagia, headache	Polyuria, polydipsia, polyphagia	Polyuria, polydipsia, polyphagia
Mental status	Anxious, irritable, confused, comatose	Irritable, comatose	Seizures, stuporous	Stuporous, comatose
Skin and membranes	Cold, moist, pale	Dry, warm, flushed	Very dry	Dry, pale
Eyeballs	Normal	Soft	Very soft	Soft
Infection	Absent	Frequent	Frequent	Frequent
Temperature	Normal or hypothermic	Fever	Fever	Fever
Respiration	Normal	Hyperventilation, acetone breath	Normal	Hyperventilation
Blood pressure	Normal	Low	Low	Low
Pulse	Weak and rapid	Strong	Variable	Strong
Laboratory findings				
Urine glucose[a]	$0\text{–}2^+$	4^+	4^+	$0\text{–}2^+$
Urine acetone[a]	0	4^+	$0\text{–}1^+$	$0\text{–}2^+$
Blood glucose	<40 mg	300–800 mg	800–2,000 mg	80–200 mg
Serum ketones[a]	0	4^+	$0\text{–}2^+$	$0\text{–}2^+$
Blood CO_2	24–30	5–16	18–24	5–16
Serum lactic acid	Normal	Normal	Normal	High
Plasma pH	7.4	7.1–7.3	7.4	6.8–7.2
Prognosis	Rapid response to carbohydrate administration or glucagon	Gradual recovery (6–12 hours) after insulin injection	Not as good as ketoacidotic coma	Good response is likely to sodium bicarbonate or insulin as required

[a]Color chart "plus" scale: 0 = negative; 1 = minimal level; 4 = maximal level.

tabolism of these substances produces urea and ketones, respectively. Ketones in the blood form acidic ketone bodies, which cause hyperventilation and acidosis, and acetone, which is volatile and contributes a fruity odor to the breath. Coma ultimately results from the acidosis, and to a lesser extent cellular dehydration and electrolyte depletion. Insulin and intravenous fluids are the cornerstones of treatment.

In **hyperglycemic hyperosmolar nonketotic coma (HHNK),** cellular dehydration is the major factor in coma, while ketonuria is negligible and acidosis is absent. Cellular dehydration occurs in HHNK when water is drawn into the vascular compartment by the osmotic gradient created by extreme concentrations (800–2,000 mg/100 ml) of glucose. The typical complaint is constant thirst and dry skin. Treatment is initiated with intravenous saline to restore fluid volume. **Lactic acidosis** can occur in clients with diabetes as a complication of ketoacidosis or HHNK because hypotension that accompanies ketoacidosis or HHNK can result in relative hypoxia. In the absence of oxygen, lactic acid is the end-product of glucose metabolism.

Insulin shock is a reaction to extreme hypoglycemia. Insulin shock may be triggered by an overdose of insulin or by factors that acutely increase the effect of a normal dose, such as intense exercise, reduced carbohydrate intake, fluid or electrolyte imbalances due to vomiting or diarrhea, or a surge of endogenous insulin production. When hypoglycemia begins to develop, epinephrine and glucagon are released as the body attempts to forestall the drop in blood glucose. The epinephrine causes signs of sympathetic activation: sweating, tremor, headache, palpitations, and elevated blood pressure. If the blood glucose levels continue to drop, declining brain function produces symptoms of nervousness, confusion, anxiety, irritability, dullness, apathy, and agitation. Still further reductions in blood glucose lead to disorientation, impaired perception, altered states of consciousness, and ultimately coma or seizure. Treatment of insulin shock requires administration of a fast-acting carbohydrate source followed by a slower-acting carbohydrate source. Glucagon is occasionally employed for insulin shock.

Table 33–4

Drugs and Hormones that Cause False Positives in Fasting Blood Sugar of Glucose Tolerance Testing by Elevating Blood Sugar Levels

Class	Drugs
Antihypertensives	Clonidine, diazoxide
Antineoplastics	Alloxan, L-asparaginase, streptozocin
CNS drugs	Neuroleptics (including phenothiazines, haloperidol, and chlorprothixene), tricyclic antidepressants, lithium, phenytoin, levodopa
Diuretics	Thiazides and related diuretics, high-ceiling diuretics, triamterene
Hormones	Catecholamines, steroids (including glucocorticoids, mineralocorticoids, estrogens, and progestins), growth hormone, glucagon, and thyroid hormones (toxic levels only)
Miscellaneous	Indomethacin, isoniazid, niacin

Diagnostic Tests

Since the pathological features of diabetes are variable and not unique to the condition, diagnosis of diabetes ultimately depends on measurement of blood glucose levels. Presence of polyuria (>2 L per day), polydipsia, ketonuria, glycosuria, and sudden weight loss are indicative, but confirmation hinges on presence of at least one of two types of elevations of serum glucose concentrations: the fasting blood sugar and the glucose tolerance tests.

A **fasting blood sugar** determination is made early in the morning after at least 8 hours of fasting. Normal values are less than 115 mg/100 ml and typically 65–100 mg/100 ml. Values of 140 mg/100 ml or above on two or more occasions are diagnostic of diabetes. Intermediate values of greater than 115 but less than 140 mg/100 ml indicate glucose intolerance. Care must be taken in this test to avoid potential sources of error. The test is not valid during a complicating illness, pregnancy, or in the presence of drugs known to elevate blood sugar levels (Table 33–4). Only about 30–40% of diabetic clients can be diagnosed on the basis of fasting blood sugar, so the test is not exclusionary.

The **oral glucose tolerance test** is a functional test that measures the response of the pancreas to a glucose challenge. The test is performed in the morning after at least 3 days of normal physical activity and unrestricted diet containing at least 150 g of carbohydrate daily. The test is immediately preceded by 10–16 hours of fasting. The client must remain seated and not smoke during the test. A pretest blood sample is taken. The challenge dose of glucose (1.75 g/kg of ideal body weight up to 75 g) is given orally in no more than 5 minutes. Blood samples are then collected at 30-minute intervals for 2 hours. The usual curve exhibits a gradual rise over the first hour and a subsequent return to normal that is substantially complete in two hours (Figure 33–3). Diabetes is indicated when the 2-hour test and at least one other test value are in excess of 200 mg/100 ml. Normal values are less than 140 mg/100 ml; intermediate values are diagnostic of glucose intolerance. The glucose tolerance test is a more sensitive indicator of diabetes, especially in the early stages when fasting blood sugar is often normal. The test may provide false positives when administered to people experiencing unusual stress or employing drugs or hormones that alter blood glucose levels (Table 33–4).

Educating the Diabetic for Self-Care

Since persons with diabetes are typically expected to engage in self-care, it is critical that they understand diabetes mellitus, the importance of diet and exercise, and the interrelationship of these factors with

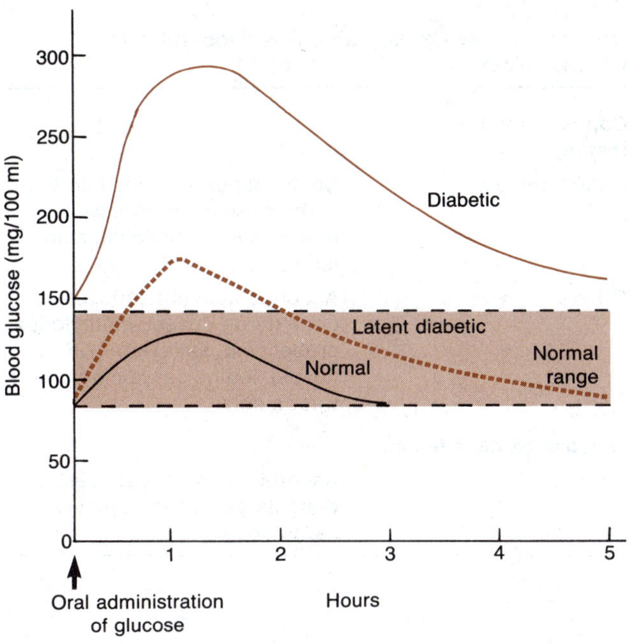

Figure 33–3
Example of blood glucose curves after administration of oral gluocse to a diabetic client, a latent diabetic, and a normal.

the drugs essential to controlling the hormonal problem. To this end, nurses must assess the client's ability to comprehend information necessary for full participation in self-care and identify appropriate family members who can be educated to assist in the management and observation process.

Teaching clients is a major component of nursing care for diabetic individuals. Normally the body adapts to changes that occur as a result of altered internal environments. The individual with diabetes lacks an essential component for adaptation. Consequently, a large part of teaching self-care revolves around encouraging diabetic clients to develop regularity in their daily routine and to identify those situations that can threaten to exacerbate symptoms. Clients with diabetes must be taught the essentials of a well-balanced diet, eating at regular intervals, regular sleeping habits, a routine of exercise, and a minimization of stress in their lives. To improve potential compliance with the prescribed regimen, it is essential that consideration be given to the individual's life-style and values.

Diet and Exercise in Diabetes Mellitus

The objectives and techniques of dietary management are substantially different in the two major forms of diabetes mellitus — insulin-dependent and noninsulin-dependent varieties (Table 33–1). The insulin-dependent diabetic is usually young and not obese. Reduction in caloric intake is not a factor, but regularity in the timing of meals and the amount of daily caloric intake is essential. The client needs to be taught that undereating poses as much threat as overeating. Adjustments of caloric intake in relation to unusual periods of exercise or exertion are appropriate, and a carbohydrate source should always be on hand in the event of impending hypoglycemic crisis.

In contrast, most noninsulin-dependent diabetics are obese; weight loss (and therefore reduction of caloric intake) is essential. A total caloric intake of 1,200 kcal from a balance of carbohydrates, proteins, and fats is a typical objective. In about one-third of type II diabetics, there is evidence of hyperlipemia, and special attention to reducing dietary fats is justified. The diet should be planned to provide adequate amounts of micronutrients. No change in frequency of meals or unusual day-to-day consistency is required.

Compliance is a major problem in restriction of diets, and every effort should be made to encourage compliance by providing techniques for varying the diet without defeating the objectives. Grouping foods into categories of equivalent foods is one such method. It is particularly important to take into consideration the client's ethnic, religious, and cultural background to assure that special foods important to the person are included in the diet to encourage compliance. Ultimately, success of the dietary program requires careful monitoring and continuing support, reinforcement, and education.

In recent years, there has been a distinct shift in the view of professionals concerning the role of exercise in management of diabetics. Physicians once worried that exercise might disrupt control of blood glucose levels. Now, however, the value of exercise in forestalling pathophysiological developments of chronic diabetes is recognized. In current practice, a regular program of exercise may actually be prescribed as part of the treatment plan. Diabetics have a high risk of vascular disturbances, and regular exercise has a beneficial effect in maintaining good cardiovascular function. Exercise programs, like dietary regimens, should be fitted to the interests of the client in order to promote compliance.

Self-monitoring

Because blood glucose levels fluctuate in response to changes in diet, exercise, or functioning of the pancreas, diabetic clients frequently must monitor their own levels in order to adjust their eating and insulin dosage. Blood glucose levels can be measured by testing either the urine or the blood. Blood testing provides a more accurate reflection of serum glucose concentration. Tests are conducted before meals or insulin injections. A drop of blood is placed on a test strip (Chemstrip bG, Dextrostix) and after a minute is washed off. The color of the strip is visually compared to a color chart or placed in a meter for a quantitative readout.

Urine tests are less reliable but more convenient. They operate on the principle that when serum concentrations of glucose exceed about 180 mg/ml, the capacity of the kidney to reabsorb glucose is exceeded, and the overflow spills out into the urine. Urine samples must be obtained by double voiding: the client should void completely and then 45–60 minutes later obtain a sample. The three sources of error in urine testing are (1) failure to empty the bladder completely in the first voiding (as, for example, in bladder atony or prostatic obstruction), (2) presence of drugs that alter the measurement, or (3) changes in renal threshold for glucose reabsorption. Urine samples should be periodically correlated with blood testing to avoid the latter problem. Two types of urine tests for glucose are available. The copper reduction test (Clinitest tablets, Benedict's solution) is based on the fact that glucose is a reducing sugar. The testing preparation contains cupric sulfate, which is converted to cuprous oxide, a colored substance. The intensity of the color can be compared to a chart to yield a fairly accurate determination. The test measures presence of any reducing substance in the urine, so that false positives may occur when drugs are employed that yield urinary metabolites that are reducing agents (Table 33–5).

A second test for urine glucose is the **glucose oxidase test** (TesTape, Diastix). The incidence of false positives from drug metabolites is very low (Table 33–5). The test is easier to perform than the copper reduction test, but the colors are more difficult to compare and the timing interval is crucial.

Special monitoring devices are available to aid the visually impaired client with urine testing. Uricator, for example, buzzes to indicate the level of sugar in the urine. There is another device that can be used to monitor blood glucose levels at designated times by the visually impaired client and read at a later time by a sighted person (nurse or family member). A "talking" blood glucose analyzer is also available. Acquainting clients with such devices and teaching the use of the devices to the client and family members often assures a level of independence not otherwise achievable and enhances the client's feelings of self-worth.

Table 33–5
Drugs that may Cause False Positives in Urine Glucose Testing

Copper reduction testing	
Antimicrobials	Cephalosporins, penicillin G (large doses), streptomycin, nitrofurantoin, nalidixic acid, isoniazid
Others	Ascorbic acid (megadoses), L-dopa (large doses), methyldopa, probenecid, salicylates (large doses), iodine-containing contrast media
Glucose oxidase testing	
Various	Ascorbic acid (megadoses), L-dopa (large doses), salicylates (large doses)

Nurses should also teach diabetics and their families to identify complications of diabetes. One example is examining the eyes for microaneurysms or hemorrhages (very small red spots in the sclera) and the skin for signs of infection. Some of the symptoms of diabetes may seem to disappear, leading clients and families to think that the problem has regressed completely. *Nurses need to carefully question both the client and family concerning changes that have been noted, however transiently, and both the client and the nurse should keep a record of such occurrences. Nurses should also educate diabetic clients and families to note and report neurological signs of change such as reduced proprioceptive or tactile sensitivity, impotence, or paresthesias.*

Insulin

History and Sources Insulin was discovered in the early 1920s with the isolation of the hormone and demonstration of its value in diabetes by Banting and Best. The first diabetic patient received insulin in January 1922, with dramatic results. The complete structure of insulin was determined by Banger and associates in the decade from 1945 to 1955.

Currently, there are five sources of insulin: pork pancreas, beef pancreas, pork-beef mixtures, human insulin derived from conversion of pork insulin, and human insulin synthesized through recombinant DNA technology. The human insulins are associated with a much lower incidence of allergic reaction.

Certain clients should definitely receive human insulin: clients with insulin resistance, insulin allergies, lipotrophy or lipohypertrophy, all type II diabetics receiving short-term insulin for periods of acute exacerbation (surgery, stress, infections), and pregnant diabetic clients. Theoretically, human insulin is the preferred preparation for all diabetics receiving insulin, but its high cost will ensure the continued use of nonhuman insulins for some time to come.

All insulin preparations are considerably purer today than a few years ago. The three manufacturers of insulin are Nordisk, Squibb-Novo, and Lilly. Human insulin produced by recombinant DNA technology by Lilly is virtually pure. All three manufacturers make products from animal sources with less than one part per million (1 ppm) contamination with proinsulin, the substance that is measured to determine levels of pancreatic impurities. Lilly has additional products at less than 10 ppm and Squibb-Nova at less than 25 ppm of proinsulin. It is not clear that the added level of purity of the purest preparations is of clinical significance or worth the added cost, except for clients who have exhibited allergic reactions to the less purified preparations.

Table 33–6
Factors that Alter Insulin Requirements in the Diabetic Client

The level of endogenous secretion of insulin and fluctuations therein
Dietary preferences and changes
Development of insulin antibodies
Changes in other carbohydrate-regulating hormones
Changes in extent of exercise or activity
Emotional stress
Pregnancy
Use of oral contraceptives
Menstruation
Administration of anesthetics
Use of the various other drugs that influence glucose levels
Presence of infection
Cigarette smoking
Alcohol consumption
Compliance with therapeutic regimens
Site and depth of injection
The concentration and type of insulin preparation

Mechanisms and Effects Insulin therapy for diabetes mellitus is replacement therapy designed to overcome the deficiency in endogenous insulin activity. The therapeutic goal is to move glucose across cell membranes to the energy-producing metabolic cycles within the cells.The immediate objectives of treatment are to prevent ketoacidosis or other severe metabolic aberrations and to control the symptoms of hyperglycemia. Long-term objectives are to minimize the risks of morbidity and mortality caused by the pathological complications of diabetes. In recent years, considerable progress has been made in providing more physiologic patterns of insulin availability. The more closely the blood chemistry of the person with diabetes resembles the normal state, the less the likelihood of long-term pathological complications such as vascular and ocular problems. Control of the diabetic condition is complicated by numerous factors that alter insulin levels, requirements, or effectiveness (Table 33–6).

The nurse must closely observe the client's response to therapy. If the dosage of drug is not enough in relation to the food intake or activity level, the client will exhibit increasing signs of failing energy production. If the amount of insulin is too much, rapid mobilization of glucose out of the blood and into the cells is equally hazardous.

Pharmacokinetics Insulin is always injected because oral administration would result in enzymatic destruction of the hormone in the gastrointestinal tract before absorption could occur. Because of local irritation and accumulation of fat caused by insulin when injected subcutaneously, it is necesary to rotate the site of administration, but rotating from one tissue to another (from the arm to the leg or abdomen) will alter the rate of absorption. A better practice is to rotate sites within one general anatomical area. Fat accumulation at a site of administration (lipodystrophy) can interfere with systemic absorption of insulin, or produce a delayed but sudden absorption. Rotation of the site of injection minimizes but does not completely prevent occurrence of lipodystrophy.

The principal difference among the various insulin preparations, and the major factor in choice of drug, is duration of action. There are six available types of insulin that fall into three categories with respect to onset of action: rapid, intermediate, and prolonged (Table 33–7). In the rapid-acting category are regular or crystalline-zinc solutions (Actrapid, Velosulin, Humulin, and Regular Insulin). These drugs have a rapid onset and short duration of action, and they are the only insulin preparations that may be injected intravenously. They are used for treatment of ketoacidosis and other acute hyperglycemic states. Prompt insulin zinc suspensions have a

Table 33–7
Preparations of Insulin

Characteristic type	Insulin preparations: Rapid		Intermediate		Long	
Preparation	Regular or crystalline zinc (insulin injection)	Prompt insulin zinc suspension (Semilente, Semitard)	Isophane insulin suspension (NPH insulin)	Slow insulin zinc suspension (Lente, Monotard, Lentard)	Protamine zinc insulin	Extended insulin zinc suspension (Ultralente, Ultratard)
Source	Beef, pork, beef-pork, human (converted pork), human (recombinant DNA)	Beef, pork, or beef-pork	Beef, pork, beef-pork, human (recombinant DNA)	Beef, pork, beef-pork, human (converted pork)	Beef, pork, or beef-pork	Beef or beef-pork
Protein modifier	None	None	Protamine	None	Protamine	None
Appearance	Clear solution	Cloudy suspension	Cloudy suspension	Cloudy suspension	Cloudy suspension	Cloudy suspension
Time of administration	15–20 minutes before meal (SC); any time for ketoacidosis (IV)	30–45 minutes before breakfast	1 hour before breakfast	1 hour before breakfast	1 hour before breakfast	1 hour before breakfast
Latency to onset (hours)	< 1	1–3	3–4	2–4	4–6	8
Peak effect (hours)	2–3	2–8	4–12	6.5–14.5	14–20	16–18
Time when hypoglycemia is most likely	Before lunch	Before lunch	Before dinner	Before dinner	Late night	Late night or early morning
Duration (hours)	5–7	12–16	24–28	24–28	30–36	36+
Time when glycosuria is most likely	At night	At night	Before lunch the next day.	Before lunch the next day.	At bedtime the next day.	At bedtime the next day.

similar rapid onset and short duration. Both types of rapid acting preparations are useful in combination with longer-acting preparations. The long-acting preparation provides a stable basal level of insulin availability and the short-acting preparations are used to fine-tune the response based on daily urine or blood tests.

The intermediate-acting preparations include isophane insulin suspension (NPH insulin, Insulatard, NPH Iletin, Protaphane, Humulin) and slow insulin zinc suspension (Lente, Lentard, Monotard). These preparations provide an effect in the general range of 18–24 hours. Most diabetes can be controlled with a single early morning injection of an intermediate-acting preparation. When intermediate-acting preparations are used, the most likely time of occurrence of hypoglycemic reactions is before dinner, during the peak action of the drug. Glycosuria is most likely to occur during the time of minimal drug effect, in the nighttime hours before the next morning injection. The usual starting dose is 10–20 units per day, given subcutaneously. The dosage is then individualized to the requirements of the client by incremental changes until urine and blood tests reveal a satisfactory response. Clients with frequent fluctuations in response often require the addition of a short-acting insulin preparation, which is taken either in combination with the morning injection, as indicated based on self-monitoring, or in divided morning (two-thirds) and late-afternoon (one-third) doses.

The long-acting preparations are protamine zinc insulin suspension (Protamine, Zinc and Iletin I) and extended insulin zinc suspension (Ultralente, Ultratard). The long-acting preparations are seldom used because stability in the client's response is difficult to achieve. These drugs are taken prior to breakfast, are most likely to cause hypoglycemia in the early morning hours before the next injection, and glycosuria at bedtime.

Clinical Indications Insulin preparations are indicated for treatment of all clients with type I diabetes mellitus and those with severe cases of type II diabetes. Intermediate- and long-actng preparations are indicated for daily maintenance while short-acting preparations are most useful for fine-tuning of therapy and for rapid reversal of ketoacidosis.

Adverse Effects and Contraindications Excessive insulin action leads to hypoglycemia and, in the extreme, the coma of insulin shock. *Families as well as clients need to be alerted to the signs and symptoms of im-*

Nursing Observations for Use of Hypoglycemic Drugs in Diabetes Mellitus

THERAPEUTIC GOAL	Maintain normal serum glucose levels (70–140 mg/100 ml) to avoid acute metabolic imbalances and minimize long-term complications related to hyperglycemia and hypoglycemia.
PREADMINISTRATION ASSESSMENT	
Baseline Data	Observe for and question clients about nausea, vomiting, polyuria, polydipsia, polyphagia or loss of appetite, headache, irritability, flushed skin (especially in the lower extremities), waxy skin, fever, hyperventilation, blurring of vision, soft eyeballs, strong pulse, or frequent infections (a female client with frequent episodes of vulvitus, for example). Observe for lethargy and fatigue in a previously energetic person or a "sweet" odor to the urine. Evaluate blood pressure, heart rate, ECG, tissue perfusion, peripheral pulses, edema, respiratory rate and sounds, bowel function and sounds, intake-output, orientation, affect, reflexes, peripheral touch sensitivity, and visual function. Check eyes for opacites or aneurysms. Obtain laboratory tests including fasting blood glucose levels, urinary glucose, pH, serum electrolytes, and glucose tolerance test.
Contraindications/ Precautions	Check medication history for allergies to porcine or bovine products.
Potential Interactions	Check current medications for interacting drugs including any drugs that cause hyper- or hypoglycemia or potassium depletion.
EVALUATION OF DRUG RESPONSE	
For Therapeutic Benefit	Blood and urinary sugar levels and subjective changes.
For Adverse Effects	Monitor blood sugar levels and occurrence of symptoms indicating hyper- or hypoglycemia.
For Drug Interactions	Determine if the client is using any drugs that give false positives in fasting blood sugar, glucose tolerance, or urine glucose testing. Monitor for additive hypoglycemic effects, opposing hyperglycemic effects, additive hypokalemia with potassium depletors, pharmacokinetic potentiation of oral hypoglycemic agents, and alcohol intolerance. See drug interactions sections under Insulin and Oral Hypoglycemics.
For Dietary Interactions	Monitor for symptoms of hyper- or hypoglycemia and potassium depletion.
For Compliance	Evaluate client's compliance with all facets of the therapeutic regimen by careful observation, interviewing, and review of progress. Report compliance problems to the physician and act as client-advocate when changes in the therapeutic regimen seem indicated.

Nursing Diagnoses and Interventions for Use of Hypoglycemic Drugs in Diabetes Mellitus

Nursing Diagnoses	*Related Interventions*
TO ENHANCE DRUG BENEFITS OR REDUCE DRUG REQUIREMENTS	
Alterations in tissue perfusion related to disturbed vasomotor tone caused by peripheral neuropathies	Monitor for edema and report any such problem to the physician for possible medication.
Increased risk of infections	Monitor closely for signs of infection and instruct client to report fever, swollen glands, or other signs
Impairment of skin integrity related to increased risk of fungal infections and pruritis associated with diabetes	Assess the condition of the skin and nails and provide intensified skin care as required. Teach good care of the feet.
Increased risk of injury related to somatosensory and visual defects secondary to paresthesias, peripheral neuropathies, and retinopathy	Ensure that adequate safety measures are provided to minimize risk of injuries. Teach clients how to recognize neuropathies and what to do about them.
Powerlessness, impaired self-concept, or ineffective coping related to diabetes mellitus	Provide support and encouragement, involve family members, and recommend appropriate support groups. Introduce clients to others who have made a successful adjustment to their health problem and who live independent, successful lives.
Sexual dysfunction (in males) related to impotence associated with diabetes mellitus	Provide emotional support and encourage understanding on the part of sexual partners. Consider referral to a professional sex counselor.
Noncompliance related to complexity of the regimen	Assume a positive approach and reinforce importance of client and family compliance with the therapeutic regimen. Assure that clients understand the nature of the health problem and the treatment rationale.

pending hypoglycemia, such as fatigue, headache, tremulousness, or drowsiness. Diabetic individuals should be taught to keep a record of incidents of hypoglycemia and the circumstances surrounding them to see if a pattern emerges that might suggest a need to alter the diet, modify living habits, or change the dosage of insulin. Clients need to be taught that hypoglycemia may occur because the dose of insulin was absolutely excessive or because the factors that influence responsivity to insulin made an otherwise normal dose relatively excessive. Severe hypoglycemic reactions are most likely to occur during physical exertion. *Diabetic clients prone to hypoglycemic reactions should be instructed to carry a carbohydrate source with them at all times, especially when involved in physical activity. Activity that overtires the client should be avoided.* Hypoglycemia is treated by administration of a soluble carbohydrate source, such as orange juice or sugar cubes, orally; or if the client is unconscious, by administration of dextrose intravenously.

Local allergic reactions occur in a few clients. The purer preparations available nowadays, especially those containing human insulin, are less likely to cause such reactions. When allergic reactions occur, the client is switched to a preparation derived from a different species than the one that caused the allergic response. In some individuals, allergic reactions are related to the zinc content. The usual manifestations of insulin allergies are mild, consisting of urticaria, pruritus, and redness in the area of injection. Antihistamines can be used to relieve symptoms of allergic reaction.

Drug Interactions Many drugs alter the action of insulin indirectly through their effects on blood glucose. The drugs listed in Table 33–4 that cause false positives in a glucose tolerance test are also drugs that reduce the effect of insulin. On the other hand, alcohol, oral hypoglycemic drugs, anabolic

TO MINIMIZE DRUG SIDE EFFECTS OR INTERACTIONS	
Alterations in nutrition: intake more than or less than body requirements	Provide instruction regarding the prescribed dietary regimen; teach client to carry a quick carbohydrate source when exercising. Provide medical support in the event of ketoacidosis, insulin shock, or other metabolic imbalances.
TO ENSURE SAFE AND EFFICACIOUS DRUG USE	
Knowledge deficit related to drug regimen	Educate client and family members about the nature of the disease and the need for lifelong dietary and drug management. Teach the client and a family member the early signs of hypo- and hyperglycemia, and what to do in each case. Teach the client the techniques for dietary and exercise management that minimize risk of metabolic imbalances. Instruct clients how to measure urinary and serum levels of glucose and how to adjust medications accordingly. Teach client how to correctly calculate drug doses, mix suspensions, sterilize equipment, rotate the site of injection, recognize adverse effects, and minimize drug interactions (see Nursing Implications of Insulin and Oral Hypoglycemics). Explain the relationship between duration of action and when the drug should be taken, when hypoglycemia is most likely, and when hyperglycemia is most likely. Advise the client to wear an identifying medical bracelet or tag indicating the disorder and drug regimen.

steroids, salicylates, fenfluramine, propoxyphene, guanethidine, propranolol and other beta-blockers, chlorpromazine, haloperidol, and MAO inhibitors can produce additive hypoglycemic effects with insulin. Oral hypoglycemic drugs are seldom used with insulin except in highly insulin-resistant clients.

Finally, insulin increases cellular uptake of potassium, as well as glucose and other nutrients, and can therefore reduce serum potassium. Low serum potassium increases the toxicity of cardiac glycosides. Therefore, clients receiving both insulin and digitalis must be monitored very carefully.

Preparations and Administration Insulin preparations are summarized in Table 33–7. Insulin doses are quantified as units of activity, one unit being the amount that will promote uptake or metabolism of 1.5 g of glucose. The amount of glucose obtained from the diet should be stabilized and matched with the dosage of insulin provided. Insulin preparations are marketed only in concentrations of 40 or 100 units/ml and in the next few years the 40 unit/ml concentration is scheduled to be discontinued.

Insulin preparations are stable for considerable periods of time at room temperature. *The vial in use should be kept at room temperature and any additional supply refrigerated and protected from strong light. The preparations that are suspensions should be mixed thoroughly by rotation and inversion before the dose is withdrawn. Shaking the preparation is ill-advised as it causes foaming.*

Care must be exercised in mixing of insulin preparations. The three insulin zinc suspensions (prompt, slow, and extended) can be mixed freely with each other in any ratio, but *not* with other preparations. Regular insulin can be mixed with Protamine, Zinc insulin, NPH insulin, or Lente, but the combinations are only briefly stable and the resultant effect is de-

Figure 33–4
Insulin injection sites.

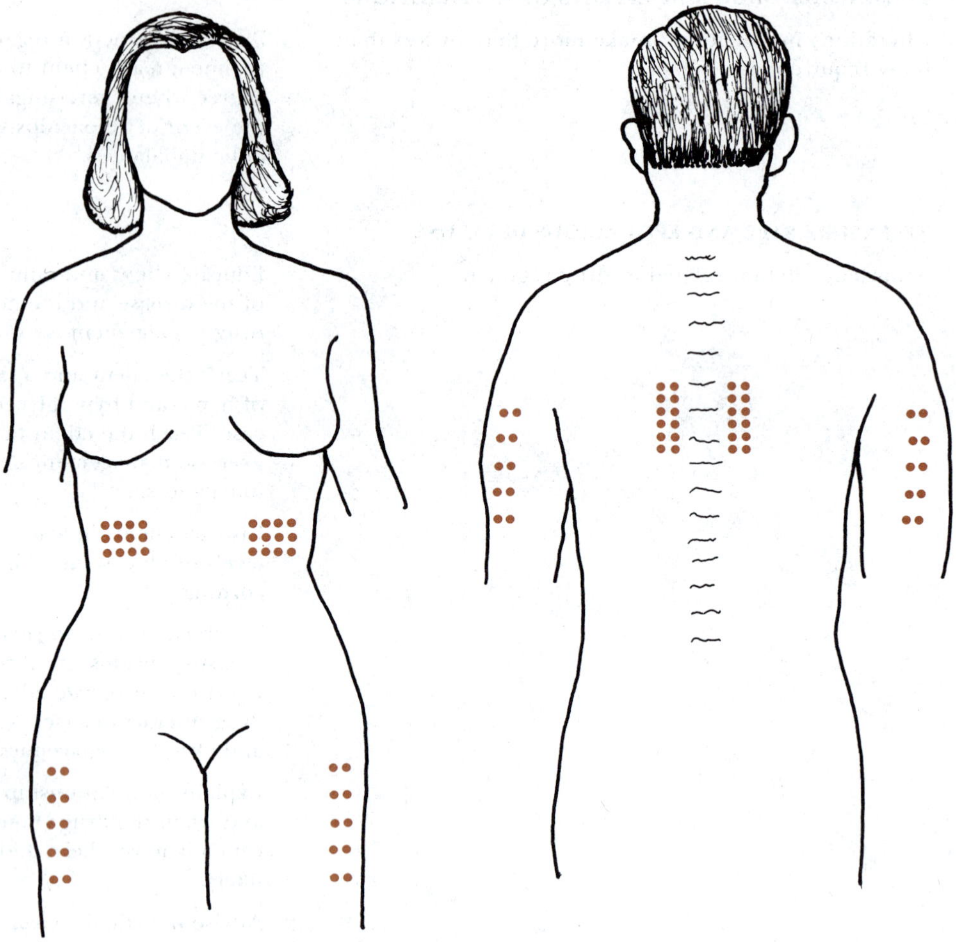

pendent on the ratios of the two preparations in the mixture. *When using regular insulin along with isophane (NPH) or crystalline-zinc insulin, clients should be taught to draw up the regular insulin first followed by the second type in the same syringe.*

The usual sites for injection are the upper lateral aspect of the thighs, the deltoid areas of the arms, the abdomen, or the upper back, lateral to the spinal cord (Figure 33–4).

Important Nursing Implications for Insulin Preparations

- ☐ Teach the client with diabetes to recognize the symptoms of hyperglycemia (such as thirst, flushed skin, fruity breath odor, polyuria) and hypoglycemia (fatigue, lassitude, irritability, hunger, nausea, headache, or tremors) and what to do when these occur. Mild hypoglycemia is usually controlled by ingesting a quick sugar source such as orange juice, soda, or hard candy. Mild hyperglycemia is controlled by an appropriate upward adjustment in the dose of insulin. In frank insulin shock, glucagon is sometimes given to counteract insulin overdosage.
- ☐ Make certain that the client understands the difference between rapid-, intermediate-, and slow-acting preparations and when hypo- and hyperglycemia are most likely to occur with each preparation being employed. Clients should not change from one form of insulin to another without medical supervision.
- ☐ Teach clients the importance of frequent self-monitoring and how to conduct urine and serum testing. Urine samples are usually obtained by the double-voiding method: the cli-

ent voids once 45–60 minutes before the scheduled insulin injection, then again immediately before the injection. The second sample is used for the measurement. Clients should be provided with a list of drugs that can alter the results of the two types of urine tests. Inform clients with special requirements about special monitoring devices that help to overcome deficits such as visual impairment.

- ☐ Instruct the client about proper storage of insulin preparations. Insulin preparations are stable indefinitely when protected from temperature extremes. Insulin can be stored up to 1 month at room temperature. If a supply is to be kept for longer than 1 month, it should be refrigerated, but not frozen. Advise clients to let the insulin come to room temperature (but without heating) before injection. Insulin suspensions should be rotated, not shaken, for at least 1 minute before drawing up a dose, to ensure homogeneity.
- ☐ Insulin should always be administered using an insulin syringe. These syringes vary slightly. Some devices have been marketed that will assist with measuring the dose by allowing the nurse to preset the insulin so that clients merely take the material from the refrigerator at the proper time and inject it. A device that requires presetting is not useful for persons who need to mix two forms of insulin.
- ☐ Disposable syringes and needles are convenient but costly. Persons with limited resources may be as well served by using reusable equipment that can be sterilized and stored after each usage. Instruct clients to use a container, with a lid, that can be boiled along with the needles and syringes. Insulin is a protein, and any contact with alcohol or similar substances can cause denaturation of the hormone. Therefore, teach clients that syringes and needles used for insulin injections need to be kept in sterile containers. They should not be stored in alcohol solutions between injections. Keeping at least one sterile needle on hand assists clients and families in meeting those emergency situations in which additional insulin may be required.
- ☐ Clients who are visually impaired need special care. Teach them about the special devices that help administer insulin and monitor glucose levels. There are, for example, syringe magnifiers that magnify calibrations on insulin syringes and make air bubbles easier to detect. One type of injection device has a braille letter taped to it that can be especially helpful for clients who have visual impairments. There is a needle guide that helps clients insert the needle into the rubber stopper without contaminating it.
- ☐ For clients who find injections intolerable, Medi-Jector II permits subcutaneous administration of insulin without a needle. The jet injection device is powered by compressed gas and can be adjusted to the client's skin sensitivity. The device shoots ultrafine pressurized streams of insulin through the skin, delivering doses that are accurate to within tenths of a unit of insulin activity. It can deliver 2–100 units of insulin per injection in increments of one-half unit. The injections are relatively painless.
- ☐ Teach clients how to calculate insulin doses accurately and how to measure doses precisely. Nurses should stress that minor variations in drawing up the solution could cause overdosage and hypoglycemic reactions. Bubbles should be carefully removed from the syringe before the fluid is injected. Also, clients should be cautioned always to check the label before drawing up the drug to be sure they are using insulin of the prescribed strength and not past its expiration date. If the client lacks ability to calculate dosage correctly, arrange for this function to be performed by another family member or a home health care nurse.
- ☐ When more than one form of insulin is to be employed, teach clients which forms can be mixed together. Regular insulin can be mixed with any other insulin; insulin zinc suspensions can be mixed only with each other or regular insulin. When mixing regular insulin with a modified insulin, the regular insulin is drawn up into the syringe first.
- ☐ Insulin is usually administered subcutaneously. The injection site must be rotated to avoid hypertrophy, irritation, and lipodystrophy. It is best to rotate sites within a given anatomical area to reduce variability in absorption. The sites for insulin injection are the upper arms, outer thighs, back, buttocks, and abdomen (excluding the midline). Absorption is most rapid from the abdomen and back, then the upper arm, followed by the thigh and buttocks. Teach clients how to chart injection sites on a diagram.

- ☐ The client and at least one family member should be taught and observed for correct administration technique. The injection site should not be rubbed. Clients should be informed that local reactions to injection, such as itching, swelling, or redness, are not uncommon and usually clear within 2 weeks.
- ☐ Teach clients to recognize indications of systemic allergic reactions to insulin preparations. If a client experiences an allergic reaction to an insulin product derived from beef or pork, a human insulin prepartion should be used instead.
- ☐ Provide clients with a list of drugs that may alter requirements for insulin, such as alcohol, oral contraceptives, steroids, thyroid hormones, growth hormone, and other (see Drug Interactions of Insulin).
- ☐ Educate the diabetic client about conditions that may alter insulin requirements, including changes in food intake, stress, infections, exercise, surgery, pregnancy, menstruation, or beginning or discontinuing use of other drugs.
- ☐ Some diabetic clients, called "brittle" diabetics, pose particular difficulties in management because of rapid swings between the extremes of hypoglycemia and glycosuria. Gaining control over such fluctuations is crucial to the success of therapy. Severe cases require an all-out effort to determine and control the causes of variability: (1) client self-monitoring can be intensified to provide an extensive series of measurements to try to pin down the pattern of fluctuations; (2) dietary restrictions, insulin administration, and stress-provoking circumstances can be more rigorously controlled; (3) more frequent injections of shorter-acting insulin preparations can be instituted for fine-tuning of blood glucose levels; or (4) total calories can be divided into more frequent but smaller meals.
- ☐ Profuse perspiration during sleep indicates a hypoglycemic reaction. Families should be taught to awaken the individual and give a soluble carbohydrate. Orange juice or some similar liquid at bedside every night will assure an immediate supply of carbohydrate. Family members need to understand that if a diabetic client awakens and requests orange juice or some similar food, they should receive the food quickly. After a hypoglycemic episode, the diabetic client should be monitored closely to be certain that there is no further reaction.

Oral Hypoglycemics (Sulfonylureas)

The sulfonylureas are the only class of orally effective antidiabetic drugs currently available. Formerly, a second class of drugs, the biguanides, were used for this purpose, but the prototype biguanide, phenformin, was withdrawn because of its tendency to produce lactic acidosis. The hypoglycemic effect of sulfonylureas was first recognized in 1957, and tolbutamide was ultimately introduced for use in diabetes mellitus. There are currently six sulfonylurea drugs available in the United States. Four are first-generation drugs: tolbutamide, acetohexamide, tolazamide, and chlorpropamide. These drugs differ mainly in duration of action and, to a minor degree, in the occurrence of certain side effects. Two second-generation drugs first became available in the United States in 1984 after several years of widespread use in Europe. In fact, 90% of clients in Europe receiving sulfonylureas are prescribed the second-generation drugs, glyburide or glipizide.

Mechanisms and Effects The sufonylureas stimulate the beta-cells of the pancreas and increase the release of endogenous insulin. This action does not require entrance of the drug into the beta cells, and it is thought that sulfonylureas may increase the sensitivity of the beta cells to their natural stimulus, glucose. The stimulatory effect of sulfonylureas on beta-cell secretory activity apparently does not persist with chronic administration, but extrapancreatic effects come into play. Sulfonylureas increase the binding of insulin to peripheral target tissues and increase the number of receptors for insulin, in effect reversing insulin resistance to some extent. Tolbutamide not only enhances uptake of glucose by peripheral tissues but also enhances other physiological effects of insulin such as the antilipolytic action and the stimulation of glycogen formation in the liver. Thus prolonged administration of oral hypoglycemics produces a reduction in serum glucose without a change in circulating insulin concentrations.

Pharmacokinetics The pharmacokinetic features of each drug are summarized in Table 33–8. One important point is that the sulfonylureas that are shorter-acting, such as tolbutamide and acetohexamide, must often be given more than once a day while the longer-acting agents, such as chlorpropamide (Diabinase), accumulate for the first few days when given just once a day. Thus chlorpropamide doses can be adjusted only quite slowly since it re-

Table 33–8
Comparisons Among Oral Hypoglycemic Agents

	Drug					
Characteristic	Tolbutamide	Acetahex-amide	Tolazamide	Chlorpro-pamide	Glyburide	Glipizide
Generation	First	First	First	First	Second	Second
Preparations	Orinase	Dymelor	Tolinase	Diabinase	DiaBeta	Glucotrol
Potency	+	++	+	+++	+++++	+++++
Typical daily dose	0.5–3 g	0.25–1.5 g	0.1–1.0 g	0.1–0.75 g	2.5–30 mg	2.5–40 mg
Number of doses daily	2 or 3	1 or 2	1 or 2	1	1 or 2	1 or 2
Onset (hours)	1	1	4–6	1	2–4	1–1.5
Half-life (hours)	5–6	1.6 parent compound; 5.3 active metabolite	7	30–36	biphasic: 3.2 and 10	3–4
Duration (hours)	6–12	10–24	10–20	30–72	10–24	6–24
Absorption	Rapid, complete	Rapid, complete	Slow	Well absorbed	Only 24%	Well absorbed
Metabolism in liver	100%	100%	100%	80%	100%	100%
Activity of metabolite	Inactive	More active	Less active	Inactive	Inactive	Inactive
Excreted via	Urine	Urine	Urine	Urine	Urine and bile	Urine
Protein binding	High	High	High	High	Low	Low

quires at least 3 days before the effects of a new dosage level can be assessed. The half-lives of the second-generation drugs are appropriate for once-a-day administration. The first-generation drugs are highly bound to plasma proteins and interact with other drugs that compete for these binding sites, but second-generation drugs are less polar, and hence not substantially bound by plasma proteins. Thus, second-generation drugs have the distinct advantage of one less type of drug interaction. The second-generation sulfonylureas are 50–200 times more potent, so that much lower doses are employed.

Clinical Indications There is considerable controversy about the appropriate use of sulfonylureas. It is widely agreed that sulfonylureas are never indicated as the sole medication for clients with insulin-dependent diabetes mellitus, because these clients have an absolute requirement for exogenous insulin. Among clients with type II diabetes mellitus, those requiring more than 40 units/day of insulin can seldom be adequately controlled with sulfonylureas. At the other end of the spectrum, clients with impaired glucose tolerance who can be adequately controlled with a combination of diet and exercise should not receive sulfonylureas. There is some controversial evidence that sulfonylureas may actually increase the risk of cardiovascular deaths and overall mortality relative to dietary regulation alone. For clients with insulin-independent diabetes mellitus of moderate severity, who would otherwise require up to 40 units of insulin per day, sulfonylureas can be substituted for insulin to control symptoms of hyperglycemia. However, even in this group, better control of serum glucose levels can be achieved with dietary restrictions and insulin. Treatment failures with sulfonylureas are commonplace and can occur from the very beginning of therapy (primary failures) or after a few months of temporary responsiveness (secondary failures). In addition, there is no evidence that oral hypoglycemics reduce the risk of pathological complications of diabetes. *Nurses should emphasize to clients that diet is critical to control diabetes mellitus and that oral hypoglycemics are not a substitute for appropriate diet.*

Those clients who respond adequately to sulfonylureas in most circumstances may require insulin injections (with human insulin) during critical periods of trauma, surgery, infection, or fever. *Transfer of clients from insulin to oral hypoglycemics is best accomplished by reducing the insulin dose 30–50%, while initiating oral therapy, followed by a gradual elimination of the insulin and concurrent dosage adjustment of the oral hypoglycemic.*

The fact that sulfonylureas appear to increase the number of insulin receptors has suggested another use of this class of drugs. Some clients with extreme resistance to insulin, who otherwise require extremely large doses of insulin, have been successfully treated with addition of sulfonylureas to an insulin regimen.

Adverse Effects and Contraindications The acute adverse effects of oral hypoglycemics are modest and uncommon. Adverse effects possible with any of the oral hypoglycemics include hematological reactions (leukopenia, agranulocytosis, thrombocytopenia, pancytopenia, and hemolytic anemia) in less than 1% of clients; skin reactions (rash, photosensitivity) in about 1% of clients; gastrointestinal disturbances (nausea, vomiting, hemorrhage) in about 1.5%; neurological symptoms (paresthesias, headache, tinnitus), and cholestatic jaundice in less than 0.5% in each case.

Hypoglycemic reactions can occur from an excessive action of sulfonylureas and can be mild to fatal. Typical indications of hypoglycemic reactions are hunger, fatigue, lassitude, irritability, tremors or tremulousness. When caused by long-acting drugs, carbohydrate treatment may have to be continued for hours. Many factors contribute to occurrence of hypoglycemic reactions, including drug interactions, alcohol ingestion, reduced food intake, heavy exercise, impaired renal or hepatic function (reducing drug elimination), or advanced age. Additive hypoglycemia occurs with all drugs that cause hypoglycemia. *Frequent serum glucose determination should be made to evaluate the need for dosage adjustments. Oral hypoglycemics should not be taken at bedtime because of the risk of nocturnal hypoglycemia. Oral hypoglycemic drugs should be taken at the same time each day so that stability of response can be achieved.*

Oral hypoglycemic agents sometimes cause fluid retention. *Nurses need to question clients about possible signs of edema such as swollen hands or fingers.* Sulfonylureas may cause skin eruptions and neurological reactions such as tinnitus and paresthesias. *Some individuals receiving sulfonylureas have been known to develop pounding headaches and, as a result, stop taking the medication.*

Drug Interactions Oral hypoglycemic drugs exhibit five kinds of drug interactions: (1) additive hypoglycemia, (2) decreased effectiveness of the sulfonylurea caused by concurrent use of hyperglycemic drugs, (3) pharmacokinetic potentiation by inhibitors of sulfonylurea metabolism, (4) pharmacokinetic potentiation by drugs that compete for plasma protein binding sites, and (5) disulfiram-like reactions with alcohol.

Additive hypoglycemia occurs with salicylates, beta-adrenergic blockers, monoamine oxidase inhibitors, alcohol, coumarin anticoagulants, guanethidine, probenecid, and anabolic steroids. Drugs with opposing hyperglycemic actions include thiazides, triamterene, and high-ceiling diuretics, catabolic steroids (which includes estrogens in birth control pills), phenytoin, thyroid hormones, L-asparaginase, epinephrine, glucagon, and diazoxide. *Female clients who have been using oral contraceptives should be advised to select another method of birth control while on oral sulfonylureas.* Sulfonylurea metabolism is inhibited by sulfonamides, chloramphenicol, phenylbutazone, and clofibrate. Drugs substantially bound to plasma protein binding sites include warfarin, salicylates, diazepam, phenytoin, phenobarbital, and other drugs listed in Table 4–6. *Clients should be instructed not to take any medication without consulting the physician who has prescribed the oral hypoglycemic drug.*

Some of the sulfonylureas can produce disulfiram reactions when alcohol is ingested. Such reactions occur most often with chlorpropamide and never with the second-generation drugs. In any case, use of alcohol complicates management of the diabetic client because of its hypoglycemic effect. *The nurse should advise diabetic clients to refrain from even moderate consumption of alcohol because of the potential for intense toxic reactions.*

Preparations and Administration The trade names, available strengths, and usual doses of sulfonylureas are listed in Table 33–8. Currently, chlorpropamide (Diabinase) is the most widely used, tolazamide (Tolinase) is second, and tolbutamide (Orinase) third. Each of these drugs is among the 200 most widely prescribed of all drugs. With the recent introduction of second-generation drugs, a shift in the market for these drugs is to be expected.

When the prescribed drug is a long-acting one, taken once per day, it is usually best to take it in the morning to minimize nocturnal hypoglycemia. If the drug is taken 2 or 3 times per day, administration shortly before meals will help to maximize postprandial insulin release. Taking the medications just prior to meals will also serve to reduce gastrointestinal irritation.

Important Nursing Implications for Oral Hypoglycemics

- ☐ When oral hypoglycemic drugs are employed, dietary management and weight reduction are usually at least as important as the drug regimen in achieving control of the diabetes. Therefore, stress to clients receiving these drugs the importance of good dietary regulation.
- ☐ Educate clients receiving these drugs about symptoms that are indicative of hypoglycemia (fatigue, irritability, hunger, nausea, tremors) or hyperglycemia (polyuria, thirst, flushing, fatigue, diarrhea or abdominal cramps, blurred vision, or a fruity breath odor). Instruct clients to have a quick glucose source available at all times, especially when exercising, to counter hypoglycemic reactions. Oral hypoglycemics should not be taken at night because of the risk of nocturnal hypoglycemia.
- ☐ Advise clients who are managed on oral hypoglycemic drugs that they may require insulin injections during periods of stress, injury, infection, or surgery.
- ☐ Caution clients receiving oral hypoglycemics against the use of alcohol because (1) alcohol causes additive hypoglycemia, and (2) some oral hypoglycemics inhibit the metabolism of alcohol (the disulfiram-like action).
- ☐ Provide clients with a list of drugs that interact with oral hypoglycemics and instruct them always to check with their physicians and pharmacists before taking any new medication.
- ☐ Advise client to take once-a-day preparations in the morning and bid or tid preparations before meals.
- ☐ When switching a client from insulin to oral hypoglycemic therapy, intensify monitoring of serum and urine glucose levels and gradually reduce the insulin dose while initiating the oral hypoglycemic.
- ☐ Oral hypoglycemics are not to be used during pregnancy.

Hypoglycemia

Abnormally low blood levels of glucose cause a predictable set of symptoms that become increasingly severe as blood levels decline. Symptoms of hypoglycemia often begin to appear at glucose blood levels of less than about 80 mg/100 ml, but the rate of decline is often as important as the absolute level. Plasma glucose levels below 50 mg/100 mg are diagnostic of hypoglycemia if associated with the characteristic signs and symptoms. The symptoms are relieved by ingestion of carbohydrate-rich foods.

Hypoglycemia has five main causes (Table 33–9). Hyperinsulinism is a common basis for the condition. Essentially equivalent is insulin shock caused by exogenous insulin. Another frequent cause of hypoglycemia is alcoholism. Alcohol inhibits gluconeogenesis, depresses appetite, and impairs absorption of nutrients. Fasting or starvation lead to hypoglycemia. Mild hypoglycemia can be exhibited on a frequent or even daily basis in some individuals — late in the afternoon or late at night — especially if a meal is missed. Such mild instances of hypoglycemia may have significant impact on psychological func-

Table 33–9
Causes of Hypoglycemia

Hormonal
Hyperinsulinism
Deficiency of hormones that elevate blood glucose: glucagon, epinephrine, growth hormone, glucocorticoids, thyroid hormones
Drug-induced
Drugs increasing glucose utilization
Insulin
Oral hypoglycemics
Drugs inhibiting glucose production
Alcohol, salicylates, haloperidol, chlorpromazine, propoxyphene, beta-blockers
Dietary
Fasting, starvation, crash diets, nutritionally deficient diets
Unusual glucose utilization
Exercise, fever, pregnancy, tumors
Inhibition of hepatic glucose output
Hereditary
Fructose, galactose, or leucine intolerance
Defective hepatic enzymes for gluconeogenesis or glycolysis
Acquired
Liver disease

tioning. Intense exertion, exercise, pregnancy can promote hypoglycemia.

Symptoms of hypoglycemia fall into two clusters. The first group are symptoms related to compensatory responses of the body, mainly epinephrine secretion. Epinephrine released in response to hypoglycemia causes tremulousness, flushing, faintness, palpitations, hunger, and nervousness. The second cluster of symptoms are neurological signs indicative of the brain being deprived of glucose: headache, confusion, visual disturbances, ataxia, weakness, aphasia, and ultimately coma or convulsions.

Treatment of hypoglycemia depends on the cause, the severity, and the time course of the condition. Acute, severe episodes require administration of oral glucose in conscious clients, intravenous glucose or glucagon in unconscious clients. Dosage adjustment of insulin or sulfonylureas is indicated when these agents are causative. Alcohol use should be curtailed or eliminated if possible. Daily or frequent episodes of hypoglycemia with undue impact on personality may be addressed through dietary alterations such as more frequent small meals.

Hyperglycemic Drugs

Glucagon is effective in treatment of severe insulin-induced hypoglycemia as an alternative when intravenous dextrose infusion is not immediately available. It is not effective in chronic hypoglycemia, such as in starvation, because liver glycogen stores have long since been depleted. Glucagon may be used intravenously, intramuscularly, or subcutaneously and usually produces a response within 20 minutes. Diabetic clients prone to severe hypoglycemic reactions should have glucagon on hand and family members should be trained in its administration. Nausea and vomiting are the most common adverse effects.

Preparations and Administration

Glucagon
Ampuls with separate vials of diluting solution, stable for 4–5 years without refrigeration.
Recommended Doses: 0.5–1 mg.

Another potent hyperglycemic drug is diazoxide. This nondiuretic thiazide is discussed in Chapter 37 as an antihypertensive. Diazoxide causes a hyperglycemic response lasting up to 8 hours. Its effect is achieved by an alpha-adrenergic receptor-mediated suppression of insulin release and a stimulation of peripheral glucose utilization. Diazoxide also increases serum lipid levels, uric acid levels, and chloride concentations.

Diazoxide is highly bound by plasma proteins (about 90%) and has an extended half-life (about 30 hours). Overdosage can cause severe hyperglycemia and even ketoacidosis or HHNK. This reaction can be alleviated by administration of insulin. Since diazoxide is long-acting, insulin adminstration may need to be repeated. Other adverse effects of diazoxide include hirsutism, sodium and fluid retention, gastrointestinal disturbances, tachycardia, uric acid retention, neutropenia, and thrombocytopenia.

The principal hyperglycemic use of this drug is for treatment of inoperable, insulin-releasing islet tumors, but it is contraindicated in functional hyperinsulinism (an excessive secretion of insulin in response to carbohydrate ingestion).

Diazoxide (Proglycem)
Capsules, oral suspension
Recommended Doses: For adults, 3–8 mg/kg, divided in 2 or 3 administrations.

Important Nursing Implications for Glucagon

- ☐ Routine treatment of hypoglycemic reactions to insulin or oral hypoglycemic drugs is administration of a quick-acting glucose source followed by a slower-acting glucose source. A family member should be taught proper administration of glucagon. Frequent hypoglycemic episodes may indicate the need to teach the client more about factors that contribute to hypoglycemia.
- ☐ Observe for hypersensitivity reactions to glucagon, since it is a protein.
- ☐ After reconstitution, glucagon is stable for 3 months if refrigerated and 24 hours at room temperature.
- ☐ When prepared for intravenous administration, glucagon is diluted in 5% dextrose solution. It is *incompatible* with saline, forming a precipitate. Glucagon is also *incompatible* with potassium or calcium salts.

Case Study: Diabetes Mellitus

E. S., a white man, 50 years old, was initially diagnosed for adult-onset diabetes based on presenting symptoms, a family history of the condition, a glucose tolerance test, and an exercise tolerance test. The physician instituted replacement therapy with a regimen of 40 units NPH insulin and 15 units of regular insulin every morning. Two weeks later, Humulin R was substituted for the regular insulin and Humulin N for NPH insulin because E. S. had developed a rash in response to the original drug regimen. At the time of initial diagnosis and institution of therapy, the nurse taught E. S. about the nature of diabetes, the role of diet and exercise in management of diabetes, and proper technique for administration of insulin.

After 1 year, E. S. reported to a health clinic at the urging of his wife because he was experiencing frequent headaches, fatigue, and confusion in the middle of the day. Assessment revealed that E. S. played handball 2 or 3 times weekly and was especially likely to experience the symptoms on those days. Urinalysis over the course of the day revealed glucose values averaging 4+ before breakfast, 0 before lunch, and 2–3 before dinner and at bedtime. E. S. acknowledged that he often deviated from his prescribed diet but did not use alcohol or tobacco. E. S. also revealed that he frequently experienced nausea and abdominal pain, rapid pulse, and flushed skin during the evening. The nurse concluded that the symptoms E. S. experienced were due to poor control of blood sugar levels, with hypoglycemia occurring at midday and hyperglycemia later in the day.

The physician, after conferring with the nurse, reduced the dose of Humulin R to 10 units and increased the dose of Humulin N to 50 units. The nurse enrolled E. S. in her teaching program for diabetic clients after finding that he remembered little of his original education on the subject. During one of the classes, E. S., who had never been treated with sulfonylureas, asked about "oral insulin" and wondered if he might substitute such a drug for his injections.

E. S. continued to be seen regularly in the clinic over the next decade. His ability to administer the medication accurately and to control his diet and exercise improved. The altered drug regimen provided reasonably good control of his blood sugar levels over the course of the day. E. S. learned to carry a quick sugar snack with him when he played handball to alleviate hypoglycemia. Over the course of the decade, he experienced only one episode of ketoacidosis (after forgetting his daily dose of insulin), for which he required hospitalization and received 200 units of Humulin R and 3 liters of half normal saline with sodium bicarbonate and potassium chloride. His blood chemistry was normalized within 4 hours.

After nearly 10 years of treatment for diabetes mellitus, E. S. began to exhibit characteristic complications of the disorder, including retinopathy, numbness and pain in the feet, and impotency. E. S. was well-educated about the possible complications of diabetes mellitus and sought appropriate medical help as these problems arose. With the help of an ophthalmologist (to whom the nurse had referred E. S.), adequate visual function was maintained. After 2 more years, it became necessary to amputate all of the toes of the left foot. Over the next 5 years, E. S. developed chronic renal failure. E. S. ultimately died at age 71 of diabetic complications.

1. Why did the physician prescribe two types of insulin for E. S.?
2. Why was Humulin substituted for the insulins of beef and pork origin when E. S. developed a rash?
3. What is the probable basis for the midday symptoms that brought E. S. to the clinic? What is the likely basis for the evening symptoms? Why is it plausible that E. S. experienced symptoms of both hypo- and hyperglycemia?
4. What is the significance of E. S.'s playing handball?
5. Why did the nurse inquire about use of alcohol and tobacco by the client?
6. What is the rationale for decreasing the dose of the prompt-acting insulin preparation while simultaneously increasing the dose of the intermediate-acting preparation?
7. What factors might have contributed to E. S.'s poor retention of his initial education regarding his condition and its management?
8. What would you tell E. S. in response to his question about use of oral hypoglycemics?
9. Why was Humulin R selected for treating the episode of ketoacidosis? Why were fluid, bicarbonate, and potassium chloride given?
10. How does the occurrence of complications of diabetes mellitus after 10 years of the disorder reflect on the medical care that E. S. was receiving?

Answers appear at the end of the book.

Recommended Readings

Askew GB: Oral hypoglycemic agents. *Nursing* 1975;5:45–50.

Bar RS: Factors that control insulin action at the receptor. *Am J Med* 1983;74(1A):18–30.

Blankenship GW, Skyler JS: Diabetic retinopathy: A general survey. *Diabetes Care* 1978;1(2):127–137.

Blevins DR: *The Diabetic and Nursing Care.* New York, McGraw-Hill Book Co, 1979.

Bliss M: *The Discovery of Insulin.* Chicago, University of Chicago Press, 1983.

Boyden TW: The proper place of oral hypoglycemics in diabetes management. *Drug Ther* 1978;8:66–77.

Bressler R, Galloway JA: The insulins: Pharmacology and uses. *Drug Ther* 1978;8:43–61.

Cavalier JP: Crucial decisions in diabetic emergencies. *RN* 1980;43:32–39.

Chambers JK: Save your diabetic patient from early kidney damage. *Nursing* 1983;13(5):58–63.

Christman C: Diabetes: new names, new test, new diet. *Nursing* 1987;17(1):34–42.

Dardick L, Rodney WM, Sakiyama R: Human insulin. *Am Fam Physician* 1984;29(6):204–206.

DeFronzo RA, Ferrannini E, Koivisto V: New concepts in the pathogenesis and treatment of noninsulin-dependent diabetes mellitus. *Am J Med* 1983;74(1A):52–81.

Essig M: Update your knowledge of oral antidiabetic agents. *Nursing* 1983;13(10):58–64.

Fletcher HP: The oral antidiabetic drugs: Pro and con. *Am J Nurs* 1976;76(4):596–599.

Fonville AM: Teaching patients to rotate injection sites. *Am J Nurs* 1978;78(5):880–883.

Galloway JA, Bressler R: Insulin treatment in diabetes. *Med Clin North Am* 1978;62(4):663–680.

Guthrie D: Helping the diabetic manage his self-care. *Nursing* 1980;10(2):57–64.

Guthrie D, Guthrie R: Diabetic ketoacidosis: Breaking the vicious cycle. *Nursing* 1981;11(6):54–61.

Haire-Joshu D: Diabetes: controlling the insulin balance. *Am J Nurs* 1986;86(11):1239–1258.

Hayter J: Fine points in diabetic care. *Am J Nurs* 1976; 76:594–599.

Herget M: For visually impaired diabetics. *Am J Nurs* 1983;83:1557–1560.

Home PD, Alberti, KG: The new insulins: Their characteristics and clinical indications. *Drugs* 1982;24(5): 401–413.

Jarett L et al: The chemical mediators of insulin action: Possible targets for postreceptor defects. *Am J Med* 1983;74(1A):31–37.

Kolterman DG, Prince MJ, Olefsky JM: Insulin resistance in noninsulin-dependent diabetes mellitus: Impact of sulfonylurea agents in vivo and in vitro. *Am J Med* 1982;74(1A):82–101.

Nemchick R: Diabetes today. Part 6: The new insulin in pumps: Tight control at a price, *RN* 1983;46:52–54.

Olefsky JM, Kolterman OG: Mechanisms of insulin resistance in obesity and noninsulin-dependent diabetes. *Am J Med* 1981;79:151–168.

Page M et al: Treatment of diabetic ketoacidosis. *N Engl J Med* 1976;294:1183.

Pelczynski L, Reilly A: Helping your diabetic patients help themselves: A plan for inpatient education. *Nursing* 1981;11(5)24–29.

Pendergast B: Glyburide and glipizide, second-generation oral sulfonylurea hypoglycemic agents. *Clin Pharm* 1984;3:473–485.

Poole D: Type II diabetes mellitus update: Diagnosis and management. *Nurse Pract* 1986;11(8):26–41.

Price MJ: Insulin and oral hypoglycemic agents. *Nurs Clin North Am* 1983;18(4):687–706.

Rancilio H: When a pregnant woman is diabetic: Postpartal care. *Am J Nurs* 1979;79(3):453–456.

Renshaw DC: Impotence in diabetics. *Dis Nerv System* 1975;36(7):369–371.

Rizza RA et al: Control of blood sugar in insulin-dependent diabetes: Comparison of an artificial endocrine pancreas, continuous subcutaneous insulin infusion, and intensified conventional insulin therapy. *N Engl J Med* 1980;303:1313–1318.

Robertson C: How to teach patients to monitor blood glucose. *RN* 1985;48(12):24–25.

Robertson C: When an insulin-dependent diabetic must be N.P.O. *Nursing* 1986;16(6):30–31.

Rodman M: Glyburide. *RN* 1984;84(8):76–78.

Schuler K: When a pregnant woman is diabetic: Antepartal care. *Am J Nurs* 1979;79(3):448–450.

Shen SW, Bressler R: Clinical pharmacology of oral antidiabetic agents. *N Engl J Med* 1977;296:493–497, 787–793.

Slater NL: Insulin reactions vs ketoacidosis: Guidelines for diagnosis and intervention. *Am J Nurs* 1978;78(5):875–877.

Steven D: Monitoring blood glucose at home. *Am J Nurs* 1981;81(11):2026–2027.

Surr C: Teaching patients to use the new blood glucose monitoring products. *Nursing* 1983;13:42–45.

Thatcher G: Insulin injections: the case against random rotation. *Amer J Nurs* 1985;9(6):690–692.

Walesky ME: Diabetic ketoacidosis. *Am J Nurs* 1978; 78(5):772–874.

Wilson DE: Excessive insulin therapy: Biochemical effects and clinical repercussions: Current concepts of counterregulation in type I diabetes. *Ann Intern Med* 1983;98(2):219.

Witty KT (ed): Retinopathy: Eye care for your diabetic patients. *Patient Care* 1978;12:174–196.

CHAPTER 34

Drugs Acting on the Female Reproductive System

Interactions of drugs with both sexual and reproductive function are commonplace. In females, drugs influence all aspects of the reproductive system, from ovulation and menstruation to conception, pregnancy, and lactation. Fortunately, the growing personal and social consciousness of women about their special concerns has increased discussion of women's health issues. Since so many nurses are women, the nursing profession has quite naturally led the way among health professionals toward a greater sensitivity and responsiveness to women's health care concerns.

Female Reproductive Function

The Female Cycle

The fundamental process in the female reproductive cycle is ovulation. Release of mature ova begins at menarche and continues until menopause. The female reproductive cycle (Figure 34–1) consists of the development and release of a mature ovum from the ovaries and the preparation of the endometrial wall of the uterus for implantation of the fertilized egg. Regulation of the 28-day ovulatory cycle involves the hypothalamus, pituitary, and the ovaries.

Gonadotropin releasing hormone (GnRH) is produced by the hypothalamus and transported to the anterior pituitary. There, GnRH stimulates synthesis and secretion of follicle-stimulating hormone (FSH) and luteinizing hormone (LH). In the first few days of each cycle, FSH and LH are released together. FSH stimulates the growth of the follicle (the ovum and its encasing cells) and LH provokes the ripening of the follicle. Under the influence of LH, the maturing follicle produces increasing amounts of estrogen from day 6 until just prior to midcycle. This period before ovulation is called the **proliferative phase** because during this period, the uterine wall, or endometrium, undergoes rapid proliferation in response to estrogen stimulation.

During the proliferative phase, the levels of FSH and LH initially decline and then surge to cause the release of the egg. The follicle, under the influence of FSH and LH, begins to secrete a peptide called *inhibin.* As early as day 7, inhibin secretion is sufficient to produce some feedback inhibition of FSH release. At the same time, the step-up in production of estrogen by the maturing follicle from day 6 up to midcycle increasingly inhibits FSH secretion, and, at first, even LH secretion. But as estrogen levels continue to rise, the feedback effect on LH secretion becomes positive until finally, at very high levels, estrogen sensitizes the pituitary to the stimulatory effects of GnRH, causing a sudden surge in both FSH and LH at midcycle. The ovaries respond to this surge by rupturing and expelling one of the ripening follicles into the fallopian tube. The ovum can be fertilized only during the brief period (probably at most 24 hours) following its expulsion but, since a few sperm cells may survive in the uterus for up to 72 hours, intercourse during the 3 days before ovulation can lead to fertilization.

After expulsion of the ovum, a small yellowish body, called the *corpus luteum,* forms within the ruptured follicle. Under the influence of FSH and LH, the corpus luteum begins to secrete progesterone and estrogen in increasing amounts during the latter half of the cycle, the **secretory phase.** These hormones stimulate swelling of the endometrial wall of the uterus and secretion of endometrial fluid in anticipation of fertilization and implantation. Endometrial fluid is rich in nutrients suitable for nourishing a fertilized ovum. If fertilization has not occurred, a fall-off in secretion of LH at around day 24 permits degeneration of the corpus luteum, causing a subsequent sharp drop in estrogen and progesterone production on about day 26. As a result, **menstruation** begins on day 28. Blood vessels supplying the endometrium become spastic, causing necrosis of the outer layers, and for the next 48 hours, these outer layers are sloughed and expelled by uterine contractions. About 70 ml of blood and serum are lost in the process. During this time, the uterus is protected from infection by a high concentration of leukocytes, which are lost with the blood, fluid, and necrotic tissue. After about 5 days, menstruation is complete and a new cycle of ovulation and endometrial proliferation is underway.

Gonadotropins are absent or nearly absent before puberty. At puberty, the hypothalamus begins to release GnRH. The age of onset of puberty varies from one individual to another, depending on such factors as genetics, health, nutrition, and geographical location. The changes that occur during puberty extend over a period of 2–4 years. Breast budding (thelarche) typically occurs first, followed by growth of pubic hair (pubarche), a spurt of growth (2.4–4.3 inches), feminization of body contours, onset of menstruation (menarche), growth of axillary hair, and further development of the breast. Ovulation during the first year or year-and-a-half following menarche is usually absent or irregular. Menstrual bleeding may be irregular as well.

Toward the end of the reproductive years, menopause occurs. The age of menopause is variable, but the late 40s is typical. Estrogen levels begin to decline, ovulation ceases to occur, and a year or two later, menstruation becomes irregular and ulti-

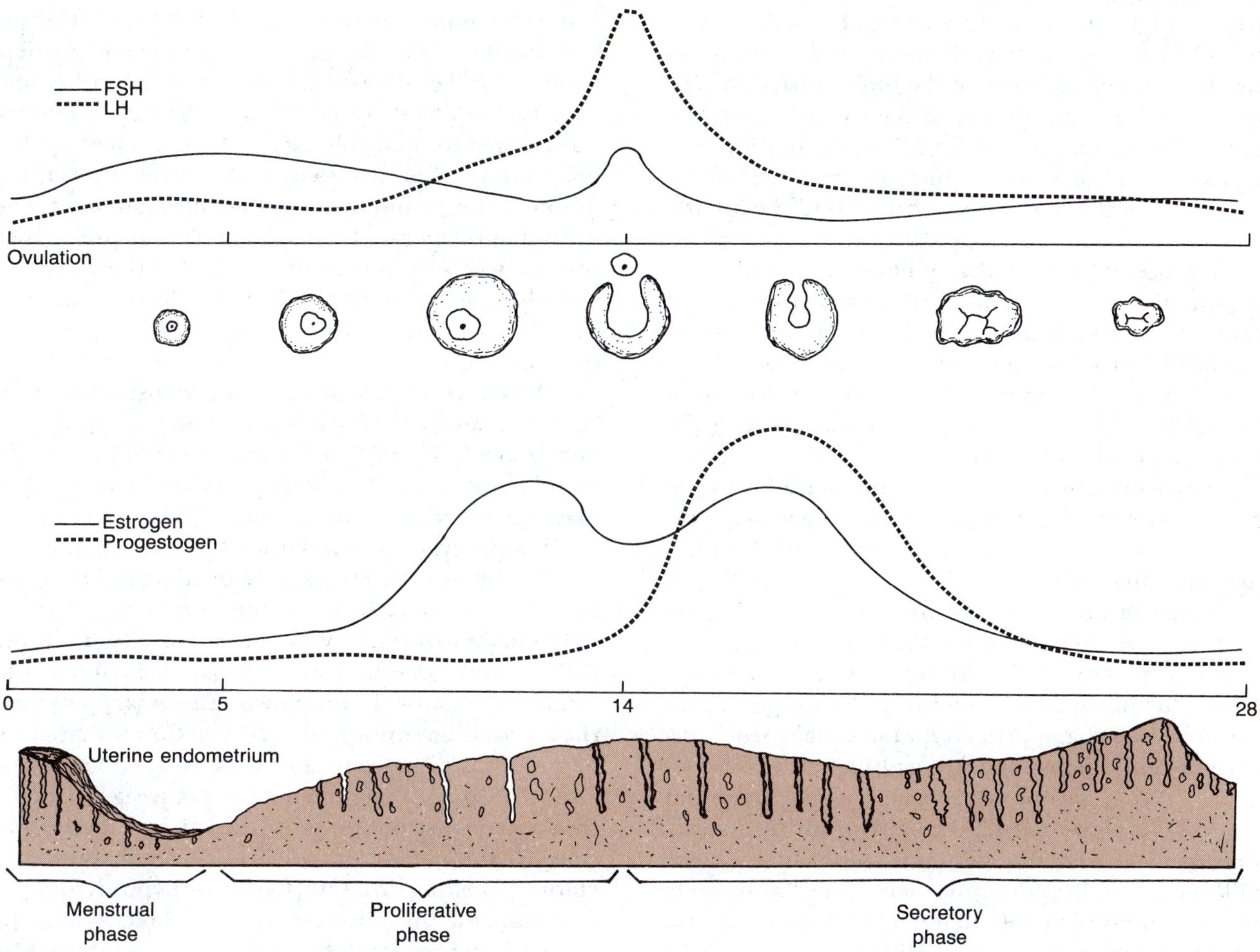

Figure 34–1
Changes in levels of gonadotropins, the ovaries, female sex hormone levels, and the uterus during the 28-day ovulatory cycle.

mately ceases. In some women, menopause is associated with dysmenorrhea, hormonal imbalances (producing symptoms such as hot flashes and excessive sweating), behavioral symptoms (including nervousness, irritability, and depression), changes in sleep patterns, headache, palpitations, genital atrophy, vaginitis, or osteoporosis.

Ovarian Hormones

The ovaries produce three classes of steroid hormones: estrogens, progestins, and androgens. These hormones are produced by both men and women, but estrogens and progestins are referred to as female sex hormones and androgens as male sex hormones because of differences in the quantities found in the two sexes. In women, secretion of the female sex hormones also occurs from the adrenals and the placenta. The female sex hormones not only control the endometrial cycle but also have important roles in development.

Estrogens are synthesized from cholesterol. The three major natural estrogens are estradiol, estrone, and estriol. Estradiol is produced from testosterone and is the major estrogen secreted by the ovaries. Estrone is made either from androstenedione or estradiol. There is free conversion between estradiol and estrone. The third natural estrogen, estriol, is synthesized from estrone.

Estrogen plays an important role in feminization. Estrogen secretion increases twentyfold at puberty and stimulates growth of the vagina, uterus, fallopian tubes, external genitalia, and female pattern of pubic hair (flat anterior border). It is one of the hormones responsible for breast development. Estrogens stimulate skeletal growth and broadening of the pelvis and promote early union of the epiphyses with the elongated bones of the limbs. Estrogens are weakly anabolic, producing a slight increase in protein synthesis, an increase in calcium retention and deposition in bone, and an increase in fat accumulation in subcutaneous regions and around the breasts and hips.

Estrogens have a weak mineralocorticoid activity, stimulating retention of sodium, chloride, and water. They also increase levels of serum proteins that bind thyroxine and corticosteroids. Coagulability of blood is increased by estrogens because of an elevation in factor V and prothrombin, and a decrease in activity of antithrombin.

Estrogens are secreted in small quantities by the adrenal cortex. During pregnancy, they are produced in massive amounts by the plancenta, at rates 300 times that of the ovaries.

Progesterone is synthesized from steroid precursors of testosterone. Its main role is to stimulate secretory activity in the fallopian tubes and in the uterus during the endometrial cycle. Progesterone transforms estrogen-primed endometrial tissue into secretory endometrium leading ultimately to desquamation. Progesterone also brings about the final stage of development of the milk-producing structures of the breast, though it does not actually cause milk secretion. Progesterone causes the rise in body temperature (about 1°F) that begins at midcycle and persists until menses. Although progesterone, like estrogens, has weak mineralocorticoid activity, it may actually decrease sodium reabsorption by competitively antagonizing the action of aldosterone, which is many times more potent. Progesterone, in contrast to estrogens and androgens, has a weak catabolic effect on protein synthesis. The role of progesterone is thus tissue differentiation more than tissue growth. Progesterone is secreted in extraordinary amounts during pregnancy and it is very important in providing the required physiological milieu.

Androgens, though less important in females than in males, do contribute to life-cycle changes in women. For example, they stimulate the more rapid growth, acne, and growth of hair in puberty, in women as well as men, and contribute in a subtle way to the changes accompanying menopause.

Disorders of the Female Reproductive Cycle

Infertility and Amenorrhea

Infertility is defined pragmatically as the absence of conception after 1 year of regular intercourse without use of contraceptives. About 15% of married couples in the United States are affected. Usually the cause of infertility can be identified; about 40–50% of cases involve male infertility and 50–60% of cases are of female etiology. Some instances involve multiple factors. In the female, infertility is most often due to tubal occlusion, preventing union of sperm and ovum in the fallopian tubes. The second most frequent cause is a hormonal imbalance resulting in ovarian dysfunction. Another nonhormonal cause of infertility is a hostile cervical environment (mucus erosion, infection, or presence of sperm antibodies).

Amenorrhea (the absence of menstruation) occurs as a normal physiological condition prior to menarche, following menopause, during pregnancy, and during at least the early period of lactation. **Primary amenorrhea** is an absence of menarche by age 18. It is generally accompanied by other signs of delayed puberty such as lack of pubic hair, breast development, or maturation of the genitalia. Anorexia nervosa, depression, severe illness, obesity, undernutrition, and genetic anomalies all contribute, but usually the cause is unknown. **Secondary amenorrhea** is an interruption of menstruation for a period of 6 months or more in the years between menarche and menopause; oligomenorrhea is irregular or infrequent menstruation, with less than 4 cycles per year. Hormonal factors are frequently involved, including Cushing's disease, hyper- or hypothyroidism, or failure of the pituitary-hypothalamic axis to release adequate gonadotropins. Stress and drugs (Table 34–1) can also be factors.

If amenorrhea is associated with specific underlying pathology, such as endometriosis, treatment is directed toward the causative disorder. In primary amenorrhea, if pregnancy is not desired, feminization can be achieved by administration of estrogens. Treatment of secondary amenorrhea is indicated only if pregnancy is desired and infertility is due to anovulation and amenorrhea. Ovulation can often be stimulated by use of human gonadotropins or antiestrogens. Pituitary **gonadotropins** can be obtained from the urine of postmenopausal women. Purified preparations include menotropins (Pergonal) and urofollitropin (Metrodin). These preparations contain both FSH and LH, but LH activity is insufficient to induce ovulation. Human chorionic gonadotropin (HCG), obtained from the urine of pregnant women, can likewise be given (10,000 IU, intramuscularly) at the appropriate time to stimulate ovulation. Pregnancy can be made possible in about 50% of women so treated, but hyperstimulation of the ovaries, resulting in enlargement of the ovaries, intraperitoneal bleeding, and multiple ovulation, is a real risk.

Table 34–1
Drug Effects on Female Sexual and Reproductive Functions

Drugs	Libido	Ovulation/ menstruation	Lactation	Masculinization
Androgens	0 or ↑	0	↓	↑
Antiestrogens				
Clomiphene	0	↑	0	0
Antihypertensives				
Methyldopa	0 or ↓	0	0	0
Reserpine	0 or ↓	0	0	0
Antiulcer drugs				
Anticholinergics	0	0	↓	0
Cimetidine	↑ or ↓	0	↑	0
Diuretics				
High ceiling	0	0	↓	0
Spironolactone	0	↓	0	0
Thiazides	0	0	↓	0
Estrogens/progestins	0 or ↓	↓	↓	↓
Glucocorticoids	0	↓	0	0
Gonadotropins				
HCG	0	↑	0	0
Menotropins	0	↑	0	0
Psychotropics				
Alcohol	0 or ↓	0	↓	0
Amphetamine	0 or ↓	0	0	0
Antipsychotics	0	↓	↑	0
Benzodiazepines	↓ or ↑	↓	0	0
Levodopa	0	0	↓	0
Narcotics	0	0	↑	0
Tricyclic antide-pressants	0 or ↓	↓	↑	0
Urinary tract spasmolytic				
Oxybutynin	0	0	↓	0
Vitamins				
B_6	0	0	↓	0

Key: 0: no effect; ↑:increased; ↓:decreased.

Because of the risks involved in treatment of infertility with gonadotropins, **antiestrogens** such as clomiphene (Clomid) are given first preference. Clomiphene and the related drugs nafoxidine and tamoxifen inhibit the feedback effect of estrogen on the pituitary, by which estrogen suppresses pituitary secretion of gonadotropins. Under the influence of clomiphen, the pituitary releases FSH and LH, leading to ovarian stimulation. Clomiphene permits induction of pregnancy in a high percentage of cases of infertility in which the pituitary-ovarian system is intact but dysfunctional. Use of clomiphene is indicated in many cases of secondary amenorrhea, Stein-Leventhal syndrome, and dysfunctional uterine bleeding. In large doses of 100–200 mg/day, there is a risk of ovarian cyst or enlargement, but this seldom occurs at doses of 50–75 mg daily. *Clomiphene increases the incidence of multiple births to about 8% and prospective parents should be advised of this possibility.* In addition, clomiphene may cause other adverse effects including vomiting, skin rashes, headaches, visual disturbances, breast enlargement, and hot flashes.

Clomiphene (Clomid)
Tablets
Recommended Doses: 50 mg/day for 5 days. If a menstrual cycle is in evidence, clomiphene is usually begun on the fifth day. The sequence can be repeated monthly.

Dysmenorrhea and Premenstrual Tension

Dysmenorrhea can be defined as pain associated with menstruation. It is a common disability often associated with work and school absences. Pain is most often experienced as lower abdominal cramps or backaches, but sometimes involves headache, nausea, and vomiting. Premenstrual tension is a frequent concomitant. Symptoms usually persist for about 2 days. Dysmenorrhea may be secondary to problems such as endometriosis, adenomyosis, or an especially tight cervical os; treatment consists of correction of the underlying problem if possible or symptomatic relief otherwise. The causes of primary dysmenorrhea are unknown and the treatment varied. Initial treatment might involve local heat to alleviate cramping. Drugs such as nonnarcotic analgesics, which are protaglandin inhibitors, can also reduce pain. Nonprescription preparations for treatment of dysmenorrhea typically contain a nonnarcotic analgesic and some combination of weak diuretics of dubious value, antihistamines in subeffective doses, caffeine, and plant extracts. It is doubtful that any of these preparations are better than an unadorned nonnarcotic analgesic like aspirin. Cramps associated with uterine spasms sometimes respond to sympathomimetics. Rest and regular exercise are also helpful. If these measures are inadequate, low-dose combination birth control pills can be used to suppress ovulation. It is not at all clear why suppression of ovulation alleviates pain of dysmenorrhea.

Premenstrual tension is characterized by nervousness, depression, emotional instability, irritability, fatigue, headaches, insomnia, anxiety, abdominal distention, edema, and breast tenderness. The syndrome is related to elevations in estrogen and progesterone. Estrogen has mineralocorticoid activity leading to fluid retention, pelvic congestion, bloating, weight gain, and edema. Estrogens also cause vasospasm just prior to onset of menstruation. Premenstrual tension is more common in younger women. Treatment of premenstrual tension involves control of fluid accumulation and relief of emotional symptoms. Limitation of dietary salt and administration of diuretics is helpful in the first respect. Diuretics such as thiazides are begun a day in advance of the usual monthly onset of the tension syndrome. Antianxiety drugs such as diazepam (Valium) can be used if required to reduce irritability.

Abnormal Uterine Bleeding

Abnormal uterine bleeding has a variety of manifestations and causes. Irritation, infection, and trauma to the skin of the vulva may contribute to bleeding. In women between 30 and 40, endometriosis may be a cause. In postmenopausal women, atrophic vaginitis often occurs with associated bleeding. Dysfunctional uterine bleeding occurs commonly in the early and late stages of the reproductive span, when ovulation is absent, since estrogen produced by the adrenals or taken as a drug stimulates the endometrium, unopposed by progesterone. Endometrial bleeding can also occur from irritation by intrauterine devices, endometrial carcinomas, disorders of blood coagulation, or use of estrogenic drugs. Women who are receiving anticoagulant therapy, thiazide diuretics, anticholinergic drugs, or drugs designed to depress the hypothalamus may likewise exhibit increased bleeding. *The client who mentions irregular menses and who experiences fatigue should be examined for possible anemia.*

Treatment of abnormal uterine bleeding depends on the cause. For dysfunctional uterine bleeding, treatment may include (1) assessment and correction of hematological status if bleeding is profuse, (2) elimination of the estrogen source if possible, and (3) stabilization of menses by cyclical administration of estrogen-progesterone therapy.

Leukorrhea

Leukorrhea is an abnormal, whitish vaginal discharge, usually indicative of infection of the lower reproductive tract. Leukorrhea should not be confused with normal surges in vaginal mucus such as those that occur during midcycle (to facilitate fertilization), following menses, during sexual arousal or intercourse, or after topical application of vaginal irritants. Leukorrhea is often accompanied by itching and irritation. The vagina is normally quite resistant to infection due to the low vaginal pH (3.8–4.2) that results from metabolic activity of the normal vaginal flora, especially *Lactobacillus acidophilus.* However, vaginal pH rises before menarche, after menopause, and during parturition. This change in pH, as well as such factors as poor hygiene, foreign bodies, venereal disease, pregnancy, tight-fitting underwear, immunosuppression, or disturbances of the normal vaginal flora can encourage infection.

The usual organisms responsible for leukorrhea are *Candida albicans, Trichomonas vaginalis, Gardnerella vaginalis,* or *Haemophilus.* The most effective method of treatment is specific antimicrobial therapy. Metronidazole (Flagyl) is employed for *Trichomonas vaginalis,* sulfa vaginal creams are useful for *Haemophilus,* and *Candida albicans* can be treated with nystatin (Mycostatin), candicidin (Vanobid), miconazole (Monistat), butoconazole (Femstat), or clotrimazole (Gyne-Lotrimin). These topical antimicrobial drugs are discussed in Chapter 53.

Douching, which serves no useful medical purpose under normal circumstances, may relieve itching and irritation associated with leukorrhea caused by infection. There is no evidence that commercial products provide more effective relief than simple home preparations such as vinegar (2 tablespoons) diluted in water (1 liter). *It is important in nursing assessment to learn why a woman is douching, since unpleasant odors or discharges may be significant indications of a disease process. Clients need to be taught that overzealous douching may disrupt the normal bacterial flora of the vagina and make the client more susceptible to infection.*

Endometriosis

Endometriosis is a condition in which endometrial tissue arises outside of the uterus, in abnormal locations. Typically, these sites lie within the pelvic cavity, for example, the uterine wall or ovaries, although endometriosis has been found on supporting structures of the pelvic floor and the rectum. Endometrial tissue can form nonfunctioning plaques or nodules, or it can develop as functioning tissue that responds to the ovarian hormonal cycle. The symptoms are highly variable but include pain (in the abdomen, back, or suprapubic or rectal areas), dysmenorrhea, urinary bleeding, infertility, and constipation.

Treatment depends on severity, the extent of infiltration into abdominal tissues, and the client's desire to have children. Hormonal therapy or pregnancy will inhibit endometriosis. Women who plan to become pregnant should be encouraged to do so quickly, but 30–40% of clients with endometriosis are infertile. Oral contraceptives not only suppress the endometriosis but may also facilitate conception after withdrawal, since the endometrial mass may not become active again. Some women are given progestin, a conservative treatment that promotes fibrosis and scarring of endometrial nodules. Some women are treated with methyltestosterone, 5 mg daily for 6 months, to relieve symptoms. The dosage is small enough that the women should not develop masculinization. Danizol, a synthetic estrogen derivative, may by employed. *All women receiving endocrine therapy need to be carefully monitored. Reports of amenorrhea or scant menstrual bleeding are indications that an adjustment in the medication is needed.* In more severe cases, surgical removal of endometrial masses can be conducted or, if no further children are desired, total hysterectomy and salpingo-oophorectomy.

Estrogens as Drugs

Estrogenic activity is found in a number of steroid compounds of natural origin as well as in nonsteroidal synthetic substances. The three major estrogenic hormones found in humans are rapidly metabolized and ineffective after oral administration, but various synthetic drugs have been produced that are effective orally. Some of the synthetic estrogens are structural modifications of the natural hormones (ethinyl estradiol, mestranol, conjugated estrogens, esterified estrogens, and sulfate esters), while others are nonsteroidal (chlorotrianisene, dienestrol, methallenestril, and, most important, diethylstilbestrol). The actions of estrogen derivatives and nonsteroidal estrogens mimic the effects of the endogenous estrogens. At equipotent doses, effectiveness and adverse effects are comparable for all agents.

Pharmacokinetics Estrogens in current use are, for the most part, rapidly absorbed from the gastrointestinal tract or even through the skin or mucosal membranes. Natural estrogens are metabolized in the liver too quickly to be effective after oral administration. However, esterified natural estrogens injected in oil solution are gradually absorbed and therefore effective over a long period. Synthetic estrogens such as ethinyl estradiol and diethylstilbestrol are effective orally because they are well absorbed and metabolized only slowly. After topical administration to the skin or mucous membranes, estrogens appear in the plasma occasionally at concentrations that will produce systemic effects.

The natural estrogen hormones circulate in plasma bound to globulin and albumin. Both the natural estrogens and derivatives are metabolized in the liver and the metabolites are rapidly excreted in the urine. Urinary levels of estrogen metabolites vary during the ovulatory cycle with peaks corresponding to the periods of peak estrogen secretion — one at midcycle and a smaller one during the luteal phase.

Clinical Indications Estrogens are or have been used in a wide range of clinical situations (Table 34–2). In combination with progestogens, estrogens are used in oral contraceptives (see page 559).

Estrogens are employed to alleviate severe symptoms of **menopause,** such as hot flashes, sweats, and chills; vaginal and vulval epithelial atrophy; insomnia; and possibly osteoporosis. This use of estro-

Table 34–2
Clinical Indications for Estrogens

Oral contraception
Combination pills (with progestins)
Morning-after pills
Severe symptoms of menopause
Postmenopausal osteoporosis
Dysmenorrhea (usually with progestins)
Failure of ovarian development
Cancers of the prostate (in males)
Cancers of the breast (in females)
Postpartum suppression of lactation
Acne

gens is controversial. Many women proceed through the menopausal years without undue strain; others are genuinely miserable. About 20% of menopausal women seek medical treatment. Estrogens provide direct and specific treatment for menopausal symptoms that relate to declining production of endogenous estrogen.

Estrogens may help to alleviate **dysmenorrhea.** Usually combinations of estrogens and progestins such as those used for oral contraception are employed to produce a natural monthly cycle. Dysmenorrhea caused by endometriosis can be controlled with estrogen therapy, but progestins are even more effective for this purpose. **Atrophic vaginitis,** atrophy of the vaginal wall often with associated infection and abnormal bleeding, responds to topical estrogen preparations — vaginal creams or suppositories.

Estrogens may be useful in certain conditions in which there is a **failure of ovarian development.** In Turner's syndrome, young girls exhibit dwarfism, congenital anomalies, and a lack of ovarian development. This condition is often diagnosed before puberty, permitting estrogen therapy to be instituted to mimic the normal changes of adolescence. Small doses of estrogens are given for a year or so, followed by larger doses in cyclical fashion to initiate menstrual events, a pattern much like natural development. Androgens may be used as well to stimulate growth. This therapeutic approach is successful in promoting breast development, maturation of the genitalia, growth of axillary and pubic hair, and the characteristic feminine changes in bone structure.

Estrogens have been employed in **cancers of the prostate and breast.** With respect to breast cancer, hormone therapy is reserved for clients for whom radiation therapy or surgery is not an option. Estrogen therapy is used only in women at least 5 years past menopause. Remissions, usually of 6 months to 1 year in duration, occur in 30–40% of this group.

Estrogens can be employed for **suppression of postpartum milk production.** They are more effective if given immediately after delivery than after lactation is underway. Estrogens are typically given for 5–7 days in full doses and tapered off over several days. Androgens are also used for this purpose.

Estrogens are a secondary drug choice for treatment of **acne** of puberty. Current understanding of acne indicates that androgens are most important in causing the skin blemishes. Tretinoin or antibiotics are preferred drug regimens. Estrogen is an alternative for young women. The administered estrogen suppresses the ovaries, reducing production of androgens. Use of estrogen therapy in males is limited by the feminizing effect of the drugs: suppression of testicular function, gynecomastia, and epiphyseal closure.

Estrogens have some limited value in **osteoporosis,** a condition in which bones are thin, weak, and translucent. Estrogens are effective in prophylaxis of osteoporosis following menopause, though calcium salts are safer and work as well in most cases. The benefit of estrogens in osteoporosis is short-lived: 9–14 months.

One former use of estrogens is currently in disrepute. Estrogens were formerly given during pregnancy in women prone to miscarriage, but both male and female offspring exposed to excessive estrogens in utero have increased risk of teratogenic effects.

Adverse Effects and Contraindications The most common adverse effect of estrogen therapy is nausea. It resembles the "morning sickness" of pregnancy, being most noticeable before breakfast. The nausea seldom interferes with eating, although elevated doses of estrogen may cause vomiting and diarrhea. Tolerance usually develops after 1–2 weeks. Beginning therapy with small doses may prevent nausea.

Estrogens should not be used in pregnancy, especially during the first trimester. Such use has been associated with teratogenic effects, as noted above. Estrogens are also contraindicated in clients with a history of thromboembolic disorders or estrogen dependent tumors. *Clients receiving estrogens should be taught how to conduct self-examination for breast tumors. Clients who have diabetes should be warned to watch for reappearance of sugar in the urine since estrogens can reduce glucose tolerance. Diabetic clients may need to increase the dosage of insulin or an oral hypoglycemic medication. Such clients should be instructed to keep a record of the number of incidents when glucosuria has occurred and extra insulin or oral hypoglycemic agent has been required.*

Other important adverse effects are discussed with oral contraceptives on pages 562–564.

Preparations and Administration Oral contraceptive preparations containing estrogen are described on pages 565–566 and in Table 34–4. Other estrogen preparations include oral estrogens, injectable forms, suppositories, transdermal adhesive strips, and vaginal creams (Table 34–3). For parenteral use, natural human estrogens serve well, while the esters of the human estrogens provide a prolonged action because of the reduced rate of absorption of these nonpolar compounds. *Injections should be given slowly and deeply.* The natural human estrogens are ineffective for oral use because of rapid metabolism. Premarin, a product containing esterified estrogens, is currently the market leader among es-

Table 34–3
Representative Estrogen Preparations

Generic drug	Dosage forms	Representative trade names
Parenteral		
Natural human estrogens:		
Estrone	Aqueous solution	Theelin aqueous
	Oil solution	Various
Estradiol	Pellets	Progynon
Estradiol esters	Cypionate	Depo-Estradiol cypionate
	Valerate	Delestrogen
Oral		
Natural human estrogens		
Estradiol	Tablets	Estrace
Estradiol/estrone/estriol	Tablets	Hormonin
Modified natural estrogens		
Conjugated estrogens	Tablets	Premarin
Esterified estrogens	Tablets	Menest, Evex, Estratab, Amnestrogen
Piperazine estrone sulfate (estropitate)	Tablets	Ogen
Ethinyl estradiol	Tablets	Estinyl
Nonsteroidal synthetic estrogens		
Chlorotrianisene	Capsules	Tace
Diethylstilbestrol	Tablets	Diethylstilbestrol, USP
Oral combinations for symptoms of menopause		
Diethylstilbestrol and methyltestosterone (an androgen)	Tablets	Tylosterone
Ethyl estradiol and methyltestosterone (an androgen)	Tablets	Gynetone
Conjugated estrogens and methyltestosterone (an androgen)	Tablets	Premarin with methyltestosterone
Conjugated estrogens and meprobamate (a sedative)	Tablets	Milprem
Esterified estrogens and chlordiazepoxide (an anxiolytic)	Tablets	Menrium
Vaginal creams		
Conjugated estrogens	Cream	Premarin vaginal cream
Dienestrol	Cream	Dienestrol, DV
Suppositories		
Diethylstilbestrol	Suppository	Diethylstilbestrol suppositories
Estrone	Suppository	Theelin
Dienestrol	Suppository	DV
Transdermal system		
Estradiol	Adhesive strip	Estraderm

trogen preparations exclusive of combinations for contraception, and by a wide margin. *Oral estrogens should be taken at mealtime to reduce nausea.* Treatment of symptoms of menopause usually consists of 3 weeks on estrogen replacement and 1 week off each month. Doses are adjusted to be sufficient to suppress the target symptoms but not so high as to cause withdrawal bleeding during the week off. Periodic attempts should be made to discontinue or taper estrogen therapy.

Typical starting doses for esterified or conjugated estrogens in treating symptoms of menopause are 0.625–1.25 mg daily. Ethinyl estradiol is the most active of the oral preparations. Starting daily doses of ethinyl estradiol for menopausal symptoms are 0.02–0.05 mg. Its close relative, mestranol, is employed in oral contraceptive combinations. Nonsteroid synthetic estrogens include chlorotrianisene and diethylstilbestrol. When the latter is used for symptoms of menopause, typical starting doses are 0.20–0.5 mg daily. When estrogens are employed for osteoporosis associated with menopause, concurrent administration of 1,500 mg of calcium daily allows smaller doses of estrogens to be used effectively (for example, 0.3 mg of esterified or conjugated estrogens).

Estrogens are found in combinations with methyltestosterone or sedatives for use in menopause. There is some evidence that symptoms of menopause are more completely alleviated when treatment includes small amounts of an androgen along with the estrogen. Some physicians elect to include a sedative in the treatment regimen.

Estrogens formulated as vaginal creams are useful for treatment of senile vaginitis and kraurosis vulvae. The transdermal system is useful for mild to severe symptoms associated with menopause, female hypogonadism, and atrophic conditions related to estrogen deficiency, such as atrophic vaginitis and kraurosis vulvae.

Important Nursing Implications for estrogens are discussed with oral contraceptives on pages 566–567.

Progestins as Drugs

Synthetic compounds with progestin activity were first prepared in the 1950s, permitting investigation of the role of progesterone and its therapeutic applications. All of the progestins currently available are steroid derivatives. Some are relatively similar in action to progesterone, while others possess substantial androgenic or estrogenic activity.

Pharmacokinetics As a drug, progesterone can be given in an oil solution by injection, but it is absorbed rapidly and inactivated quickly by the liver. After oral administration, progesterone is subject to first-pass extraction by the liver to a large extent, rendering it ineffective. Synthetic progestins are less quickly inactivated and are therefore used in preference to progesterone.

Clinical Indications Progestins are used most frequently in oral contraceptive preparations (see page 559). They are also used in cyclical therapy in conjunction with estrogens for stabilization of **dysfunctional uterine bleeding** patterns due to hormonal imbalance. Typically, dysfunctional uterine bleeding is caused by anovulation combined with an unopposed estrogen source. Cyclical therapy consists of a 28-day cycle. An estrogen is begun on day 1. A progestin is added orally at day 5 and continued until day 25, or alternatively, by depot injection on day 15. For clients not already on cyclic therapy, acute bleeding episodes may be alleviated by 10 days of treatment with a progestin or high-dose progestin-estrogen combinations. Withdrawal bleeding similar to normal menses should occur 3–7 days after withdrawal of drug treatment. Clients with recurrent episodes should be begun on cyclic therapy.

Progestins may alleviate **dysmenorrhea** when employed in combination with estrogens. The progestin is given with an estrogen from days 5 to 25 of the menstrual cycle, or added to the estrogen during the last 5 days. Symptoms of **premenstrual tension** are sometimes diminished by administration of a progestin during the last 7–10 days prior to menstruation.

Progestins and estrogen combinations are useful in **endometriosis.** They act to suppress the endometrial mass. Combination preparations marketed for this purpose are Enovid 10 mg (containing 150 μg of mestranol as the estrogenic component and 9.85 mg of norethynodrel as the progestin) and Enovid 5 mg (containing smaller amounts of the same two ingredients, 75 μg of mestranol and 5.0 mg norethynodrel, respectively). The progestin component is of more importance and sometimes medroxyprogesterone acetate is used alone, in doses of 2.5 mg daily for 2–3 weeks, followed by doses of 10–15 mg daily for indefinite periods. Progestins shrink or slow growth of **endometrial carcinomas** in about 50% of cases.

Progestins can be used instead of, or in addition to, estrogens in the immediate postpartum period for **suppression of lactation.** Progestins have also been used in this manner to alleviate breast engorgement.

Adverse Effects and Contraindications As with estrogen therapy, progestins can cause serious side effects; *nurses should be certain that clients know what these are.* Exposure of the fetus in utero to progestins has been associated with **congenital anomalies** including limb reduction and heart defects.

Progestins may cause a decrease in **glucose tolerance.** Diabetic clients need to pay particular attention to urine tests and report if it becomes necessary to increase doses of insulin or oral hypoglycemic agents.

Progestins are contraindicated in clients hypersensitive to progestins and in clients with a history of thromboembolic disorders or with known or suspected carcinoma of the breast or genital organs. Progestins should be discontinued if pregnancy occurs, in the event of a thrombotic disorder, during lactation, and if ophthalmological effects occur, such as sudden partial or complete loss of vision, diplopia, or migraine. *The nurse should encourage clients to report headaches immediately and should ask clients from time to time whether headaches are occurring. Nurses should also question clients about changes such as blurring of vision, partial loss of vision, diplopia, or dizziness.*

Progestins occasionally cause **depression,** mainly in clients with a history of depression. *Clients with a history of depression should be observed with special care when using progestins. Nurses can enlist the help of close family members for this purpose.* If depression occurs, discontinuing the drug may be the best course of action.

Occasionally **hypersensitivity reactions** occur, including cholestatic jaundice, rash, acneiform eruptions, or photosensitivity. *Clients should be advised to use a sunscreen lotion if photosensitivity occurs.* **Breakthrough bleeding,** spotting, and changes in menstrual flow are occasionally noted. Both **hirsutism** and **alopecia** are rarely reported. *Clients taking progestins should be examined for loss of hair.*

Progestins may produce **fluid retention.** Clients with conditions that might be affected by edema should be monitored. This includes clients with epilepsy, migraine, hypertension, asthma, congestive heart disease, or renal dysfunction. *The nurse should encourage clients receiving progestins to take their own blood pressure periodically since progestin therapy can cause a rise in blood pressure among susceptible people.* An elevation in blood pressure may be indicative of more serious consequences ahead and necessitate drug discontinuation or intensified monitoring. Clients with a history of liver disease or markedly impaired liver function should not receive progestins.

Preparations and Administration Progesterone is rapidly metabolized and causes painful irritation at the site of injection. The alternative for intramuscular use is hydroxyprogesterone caproate, which has a duration of action of 9–17 days. Synthetic progestins for oral use include medroxyprogesterone acetate, norethindrone, and norethindrone acetate. Other progestins are found in combinations with estrogenics for use as oral contraceptives. Medroxyprogesterone is currently the most widely prescribed progestin.

Progesterone (Progelan and others)
Oil and aqueous solutions
Recommended Doses: For dysfunctional uterine bleeding, 5–10 mg/day IM.

Hydroxyprogesterone caproate (Delalutin and others)
Oil emulsion
Recommended Doses: For amenorrhea or abnormal uterine bleeding, 375 mg IM one time followed after 21 days or after 4 days of desquamation by 28-day cyclical therapy consisting of 20 mg estradiol valerate on the first day, and 250 mg of hydroxyprogesterone caproate and 5 mg estradiol valerate on day 15.

Medroxyprogesterone (Provera)
Tablets
Recommended Doses: 5–10 mg daily, orally.

Norethindrone (Norlutin)
Norethindrone Acetate (Norlutate)
Tablets
Recommended Doses: For dysfunctional uterine bleeding, 5–20 mg PO per day of norethindrone; 2.5–10 mg per day of norethindrone acetate. For endometriosis, 10–30 mg PO per day of norethindrone; 5–15 mg per day of norethindrone acetate.

Oral Contraceptives

Since women often turn to nurses for information about birth control, it is important that the nurse be able to furnish accurate and current information that will help women make informed choices. *Before providing information, the nurse should conduct a nursing assessment. Age, cultural, moral, and religious beliefs need to be determined as well as what is aesthetically acceptable. The nurse should also determine what the client already knows about birth control.* Often people have vague ideas or misconceptions about birth control methods and do not realize that birth control practices can be individualized or that for some people certain methods of contraception might be contraindicated. Finally, the nurse should determine if there are risk factors that could complicate the choice of birth control method. For example, research has shown that women who smoke or who have a strong family history of breast cancer are at increased risk for developing breast and lung cancer from use of oral contraceptives. Clients who are receiving anticonvulsant drugs, chloramphenicol, tetracyclines, or tranquilizers may experience a decrease in effectiveness of oral contraceptives. *The nurse needs to conduct a careful drug history before clients are placed on contraceptive medicines and discuss potential drug interactions with them. Once a client has been placed on an oral contraceptive agent, the nurse must monitor closely for side effects and teach the client and family how to watch for the side effects as well.*

Each of the principal forms of birth control currently available — oral contraceptives, intrauterine devices, diaphragms, spermicidal foams, and condoms — has its advantages and disadvantages. The role of the nurse should be that of an information resource and guide, so that the woman or couple can select the method most suitable to their requirements. The nurse can also help to instruct persons in the proper use of birth control aids. In comparing alternative methods, "effectiveness" is defined as the ability of the method to deter pregnancy when used for one year.

Given the risks associated with use of oral contraceptives, some women or couples prefer alternative methods. An **intrauterine device** (IUD) is a small plastic or copper apparatus in the shape of a 7, T, Y, loop, or T-coil which is inserted in the uterus. Prevention of conception occurs because of mechanical effects on the wall of the uterus. One T-shaped IUD called Progestasert provides release of 38 mg of progesterone daily, which acts topically to inhibit implantation. In theory, IUDs are 97–99% effective, but in practice, they are only 90–95% effective because of errors in use. Adverse effects associated with IUDs include dysmenorrhea, uterine perforation, cramps, irregular bleeding, pelvic inflammatory disease, and heavy menses. IUDs are contraindicated in women with active pelvic infection, a small uterus, severe dysmenorrhea, or a history of ectopic pregnancy.

A **diaphragm** is a dome-shaped rubber cup that is inserted into the vagina over the cervix. It acts as a mechanical barrier to the passage of the sperm. It is used with a spermicidal jelly or cream that destroys sperm cells near the cervix. Effectiveness is 97% with proper use, but in practice is only about 83%. The device must be inserted properly within 1 hour of intercourse and kept in place for at least 6 hours after intercourse. There are no significant adverse effects except for rare allergic reactions to the spermicidal substances and no hazards to either sex partner or the offspring should conception occur. The available spermicides are nonoxynol and octoxynol. Nonoxynol is available as a foam (Dalkon Kit, Emko, Koromex) or gel (Koromex II-A). Octoxynol (Koromex II) is available as a cream or gel. Spermicidal foams or gels can also be used alone by placement in the vagina near the cervix, to be spread around by coital movement.

The **condom** is a sheath made of rubber or animal membrane fitted over the penis. It provides a physical barrier to passage of sperm cells into the vagina. While 97% effective in theory, actual effectiveness is 80–90%. There are no adverse effects. The condom also provides some protection against sexually transmitted infections.

The **rhythm method** is based upon abstinence from sexual intercourse during the fertile midcycle period. It is about 80% effective for women who have regular cycles if abstinence is maintained for at least 8 days each cycle. For many women who have irregular cycles, this method is totally unreliable.

The Combination Pill

It is an indication of the central place that oral contraceptives have assumed in our society that the most frequently used kind is often referred to simply as "the pill." There are three kinds of oral contraceptive pills; "the pill" is a combination of an estrogen and a progestin; the "mini-pill" contains only a progestin; and "the morning-after pill" contains only an estrogen.

Mechanisms and Effects The various combination oral contraceptives all contain both an estrogen and a progestin, although the identities of the two components vary (Table 34–4). The estrogen component in all currently marketed preparations is either ethinyl estradiol or mestranol and the quantity of the estrogenic substance ranges from 0.02 mg to 0.15 mg. The contraceptive effect of combination pills is due mainly to the estrogen. Estrogen produces a feedback suppression of FSH release by the pituitary gland, thus preventing ovulation almost invariably. Even if ovulation should occur, the condition of the endometrium that has been under the influence of an estrogen and a progestin since the beginning of the cycle is not suitable for implantation. Moreover, the hormonal balance is presumably not appropriate for the transport of spermatozoa to the egg or for the proper timing of delivery of a fertilized egg to the uterine wall. In practice, then, it is likely that contraception is achieved due to absence of several of the requirements for impregnation.

The role of progestins in contraception is less apparent. Progestins produce feedback suppression of the hypothalamic-pituitary axis but affect mainly LH. This in itself would lead to contraception by inhibiting growth of the expelled follicle, but in most

Table 34–4
Content and Activity of Oral Contraceptives

Estrogen (mcq)	Progestin (mq)	Androgenic activity	Trade names
Low Estrogen			
20 ethinyl estradiol	1 norethindrone (low)	Intermediate	Loestrin 1/20
20 ethinyl estradiol	0.3 norgestrel (intermediate)	Intermediate	Lo/Ovral
30 ethinyl estradiol	1.5 norethindrone (intermediate)	High	Loestrin 1.5/30
35 ethinyl estradiol	0.4 norethindrone (low)	Intermediate	Ovcon-35
35 ethinyl estradiol	0.5 norethindrone (low)	Intermediate	Brevicon, Modicon
35 ethinyl estradiol	1.0 norethindrone (low)	Intermediate	Ortho-Novum 1/35 Norinyl 1+35
50 mestranol	1.0 norethindrone (low)	Intermediate	Ortho-Novum 1/50 Norinyl 1+50
Intermediate Estrogen			
50 ethinyl estradiol	0.5 norethindrone (low)	Intermediate	Norlestrin 2.5/50
50 ethinyl estradiol	1.0 ethynodioldiacetate (high)	High	Demulen
50 ethinyl estradiol	1.0 norethindrone acetate (low)	Intermediate	Norlestrin 1/50
50 ethinyl estradiol	1.0 norethindrone (low)	Intermediate	Ovcon-50
80 mestranol	1.0 norethindrone (low)	Intermediate	Ortho-Novum 1/80 Norinyl 1+80
High Estrogen			
75 mestranol[a]	5.0 norethynodrel (intermediate)	None	Enovid 5 mg
100 mestranol	1.0 ethynodioldiacetate (high)	High	Ovulen
100 mestranol	2.0 norethindrone (intermediate)	High	Ortho-Novum 2mg Norinyl 2mg
100 mestranol	2.0 norethynodrel (low)	None	Enovid E

[a]High total estrogenic activity because norethynodrel has substantial estrogenic as well as progestin activity.

cases the follicle is not released because of the action of estrogen. Progesterone may contribute to the hostile environment for implantation. Clearly in the combination pill, estrogen alone is sufficient to produce contraception. The main role of progesterone is to ensure that withdrawal bleeding at the end of each cycle will be prompt, brief, and similar to normal menses.

The effectiveness of the combination pill is virtually 100% for preparations containing at least 0.05 mg of estrogen taken as directed. Even when the factor of noncompliance is included, actual use results in better than 99% protection. Combination pills with less than 0.05 mg of estrogen are still 98–99% effective. So the advantage of combination pills in comparison with alternative contraceptive methods is the high level of protection together with convenience. The disadvantage is the risk of adverse effects.

Nursing Observations Relating to Use of Oral Contraceptives

THERAPEUTIC GOAL	Contraception.
PREADMINISTRATION ASSESSMENT	
Baseline Data	Evaluate blood pressure, pulse, edema, perfusion, heart sounds, respiration (rate and sounds), and mental status. Conduct pelvic examination. Examine breasts and skin for lesions or growths. Obtain laboratory tests including Pap smear and urinalysis.
Contraindications/ Precautions	Personal or family history of breast cancer, personal history of thromboembolic disorders, estrogen-dependent tumors, coronary disease, abnormal uterine bleeding, osteoporosis, renal disease, or diabetes. Determine if there is any likelihood that the woman is currently pregnant or if she is breast-feeding an infant. Check medication history for evidence of allergic reaction to tartrazine (found in some formulations).
EVALUATION OF DRUG RESPONSE	
For Therapeutic Benefit	Monitor for indications of pregnancy.
For Adverse Effects	Monitor blood pressure, occurrence of breakthrough bleeding, edema, headache, changes in secondary sexual characteristics, breast tumors, and indications of thromboembolic disorders.
For Drug Interactions	Monitor for changes in glucose tolerance in clients receiving insulin or oral hypoglycemics; check for decrease in effectiveness of antihypertensive regimens; and monitor for need to increase doses of anticoagulants.
For Compliance	Evaluate client reliability in taking pills as scheduled.

Adverse Effects and Contraindications The use of oral contraceptives has been associated with a large variety of adverse effects, some major and some minor, some clearly established and some only possibly related to use of the pill, some common and some rare (Table 34–5). The adverse effects can be caused by either an excess or a deficiency of either of the hormones. Deficiencies can occur if the amount of either hormone given in the pill does not compensate adequately for the suppression of endogenous production when ovulation is prevented.

Most important of all is evidence indicating that women using combination pills have an increased liability toward **thrombophlebitis** and **thromboembolism** (primarily pulmonary embolism, cerebral thrombosis, coronary thrombosis, and myocardial infarct). These conditions are rare in women aged 15–35 who do not use birth control pills; risk is increased sixfold to tenfold with use of oral contraceptives. Current evidence implicates the estrogenic component; progestins do not appear to increase the risk of thromboembolic disorders. Women who have any history of intravascular clots should not use oral contraceptives. The risk of thromboembolism is greatest in women over 35, those with hypertension, and those who smoke cigarettes heavily (over 15 per day).

Nurses should question clients about early signs of thromboembolic disorders such as (1) pain or tenderness in the legs, especially the calves, (2) swelling of the legs, (3) redness or warmth of the calf of the leg, (4) weight gain, (5) sudden severe headaches, (6) chest pain, (7) shortness of breath, or (8) changes in vision. Such symptoms should be reported immediately and clients may be advised to stop taking the medication.

Use of oral contraceptives is associated with **hypertension** in about 5% of women. This is attributable to the mineralocorticoid activity of estrogens. *Before a client begins taking an oral contraceptive agent, the nurse should weigh her and take her blood pressure. These measurements can then be used as baseline data against which to measure future weight and blood pressure changes. Clients placed on estrogen therapy should be taught to monitor their own blood pressure, to record it, and report any elevation to the health professional.* Some clients receiving estrogen therapy may complain of weight gain. They should be assessed for cardiac disorders and to determine if the weight gain is the result of fluid

Table 34–5
Adverse Effects of Oral Contraceptives

Estrogen excess	Estrogen deficiency	Progestin excess	Progestin deficiency
Thromboembolism	Early or midcycle breakthrough bleeding	Tiredness	Late breakthrough bleeding
Thrombophlebitis	Increased spotting	Fatigue	Amenorrhea
Benign hepatic adenomas	Hypomenorrhea (decreased amount of flow)	Depression	Delayed menses
Pregnancy-like symptoms	Decreased libido	Hypomenorrhea (decreased duration of flow)	
Nausea		Hair loss	
Vomiting		Monilial vaginitis	
Breast tenderness		Breast regression	
Leg cramps		Cholestatic jaundice	
Uterine cramps		Androgenic activity	
Leukorrhea		Increased appetite	
Mineralocorticoid activity		Weight gain	
Hypertension		Acne	
Edema		Oily scalp	
Bloating		Hirsutism	
Migraine			

retention. Cyclic fluid retention may be effectively managed by decreasing the amounts of sodium in the diet or possibly by diuretics. *Because of the possibility of fluid retention, anyone with coronary artery disease, renal dysfunction, or cerebral vascular problems should be monitored especially closely.*

Estrogen has been shown to increase incidence of **carcinomas** of the breast, uterus, cervix, vagina, ovaries, liver, and pituitary glands in certain animals. In humans, the only established connection is that prolonged estrogen therapy in postmenopausal women increases incidence of endometrial carcinoma. No increased risk of any kind of cancer has to date been linked to use of oral contraceptives, but considering the long latent period for neoplastic disorders, evaluation of potential risk will continue. *Women using estrogenic preparations should be taught how to conduct self-examinations for breast tumors. Nurses should encourage clients to have periodic pap smears and examinations of pelvic organs and breasts.* Rare **benign hepatic adenomas** have been attributed to use of oral contraceptives and occasionally result in death.

The remaining side effects (Table 34–5) are less severe but generally more frequent. Achieving proper hormonal balance will minimize these symptoms. Combination pills containing low concentrations of the estrogenic component are least likely to cause symptoms related to estrogen excess but may cause bleeding irregularities related to estrogen deficiency. Since the life-threatening adverse effects are all associated with excess estrogen, estrogen is increased only cautiously to regularize minor bleeding. *Nevertheless, any woman receiving estrogen therapy should be instructed to report any unusual vaginal bleeding, changes in menstrual flow, spotting, or missed menstrual cycles.* Most preparations available now contain low progestin doses, so side effects related to progestin excess are uncommon. The progestins contained in oral contraceptives have varying degrees of estrogenic, antiestrogenic, and androgenic activity, as well as their progestational activity (Table 34–6). By careful drug selection (Table 34–7), the physician can balance hormonal requirements to eliminate most of these side effects.

Estrogens are poorly metabolized by those with impaired liver function. *Nurses should ask clients if they have had jaundice or indications of hepatic dysfunction such as dark urine, light-colored stools, pruritus, abdominal tenderness, or discoloration of the sclera. Clients should be encouraged to return after 3 months for an evaluation of blood glucose levels, triglycerides, serum enzymes, and to be checked for any evidence of liver pathology.*

Estrogens promote occurrence of **melasma** (freckling) when the skin is exposed to sunlight. *All*

Table 34–6
Activity of Progestins Used in Oral Contraceptives

Drug	Activities: Progestin	Estrogen	Antiestrogen	Androgen
Ethynodiol diacetate	+ +	+	+[a]	+ +
Norethindrone	+	+	+[a]	+ +
Norethindrone acetate	+	+	+ + +[a]	+ +
Norethynodrel	+	+ + +	0	0
Norgestrel	+ + +	0	+ + +	+ + +

Key: 0, no activity; +, slight activity; + +, moderate activity; + + +, substantial activity.
[a]Only at high doses.

clients receiving estrogen therapy should be cautioned against prolonged exposure to the sun or ultraviolet light.

The progestin component of oral contraceptives can cause fatigue and even **depression.** *Both clients and their families should be alerted to the potential for behavioral changes.*

Some women experience **nausea or vomiting** when using oral contraceptives. *The nurse should advise such clients that these symptoms usually subside after a few months of use. Nausea and vomiting may often be lessened by taking the pill at night with a light snack. If nausea or vomiting persist, a change in the product selection should be considered.*

Interactions with Drugs and Laboratory Tests Diabetic clients should be monitored for changes

Table 34–7
Oral Contraceptives

Progestin level	Estrogen level: Low	Medium	High
High		Demulen (8th) Ovral (3rd)(10th)	Ovulen
Medium	Loestrin 1.5/30 Lo/Ovral (1st)(6th)	Norlestrin 2.5/50	Norinyl 2 mg Ortho-Novum 2 mg Enovid - 5 mg
Low	Norinyl 1 + 50 Ortho-Novum 1/50 (2nd)(7th) Norinyl 1 + 35 Ortho-Novum 1/35 (4th)(5th) Ortho-Novum 10/11 (9th) Brevicon Modicon Ovcon - 35 Loestrin 1/20	Norinyl 1 + 80 Ortho-Novum 1/80 Ovcon - 50 Norlestrin 1/50	Enovid - E

Key: Numbers in parentheses indicate market rank in 1983. When two numbers appear after a product name, it appears twice in the top ten best sellers in different packaging formats.

in glucose tolerance and requirements for hypoglycemic medication when beginning use of estrogen-containing oral contraceptives. Use of tobacco increases the risk of thromboembolic disorders when oral contraceptives are employed. Inducers of liver enzymes may reduce the effectiveness of oral contraceptives to the point that they no longer suppress ovulation. These drugs include sedative-hypnotics, antiepileptic drugs, phenylbutazone, ampicillin, and rifampin.

Estrogens and progestins may interfere with laboratory measurements of prothrombin, factors VII–X, protein-bound iodine (PBI), serum triglycerides, and phospholipids. *If any of these tests are requested, the nurse should include a notation that the client is taking estrogens.*

Preparations and Administration In practice, the ten most widely prescribed oral contraceptives come from just three of the nine types of combinations shown in Table 34–7: low estrogen/low progestin, low estrogen/medium progestin, and medium estrogen/high progestin. Ortho-Novum and Ovral products dominate the market. A good starting point

Nursing Diagnoses and Interventions Relating to Use of Oral Contraceptives

Nursing Diagnoses	*Related Interventions*
TO ENHANCE DRUG BENEFITS OR REDUCE DRUG REQUIREMENTS	
Cognitive dissonance related to conflicting cultural, moral, or religious beliefs	Respect the right of the client to make a personal decision based on her own views. Teach methods of contraception that are consistent with the client's beliefs and personal concerns.
TO MINIMIZE DRUG SIDE EFFECTS OR INTERACTIONS	
Alterations in tissue perfusion	Instruct client to immediately report any tissue tenderness, pain, or swelling (especially in the thigh) since this might indicate a thrombophlebitis. Monitor for edema and advocate adjustments in the selection of oral contraceptive preparation if hormonal balance is not optimum.
Alterations in thought processes: depression or fatigue	Advocate a change to a preparation with less progestin activity.
Disturbance in self-concept related to side effects of oral contraceptives	Advocate adjustment in drug selection if woman is disturbed by androgenic effects such as weight gain, acne, oily skin, or hirsutism or estrogen-induced melasma.
Sexual dysfunction	Advocate adjustment in drug selection if menses are delayed or absent, if flow is greatly decreased, if breakthrough bleeding or spotting occurs repeatedly, if leukorrhea occurs, or if libido is excessively depressed.
TO ENSURE SAFE AND EFFICACIOUS DRUG USE	
Knowledge deficit related to drug regimen	Instruct clients to take oral contraceptives with meals if gastrointestinal problems occur. Educate client regarding the action of oral contraceptives and what to do in the event of missing one or more scheduled administrations. Provide a list of potential adverse effects, instructions as to what to do if any one occurs, and a list of drugs that may interact with oral contraceptives.

for therapy is a product low in estrogen and either low or intermediate in progestin activity.

Most oral contraceptive products are classified as *monophasic,* meaning that one kind of pill is taken during each of 21 days of the cycle followed by a 7-day period of taking no pill or an inert pill. The monophasic type of oral contraceptive provides a fixed amount of estrogen and progestin activity throughout the 21 days that the active pills are taken. Ortho-Novum 10/11-21 and Ortho-Novum 10/11-28 are classified as *biphasic* oral contraceptives (Table 34–8). These products provide a constant level of estrogenic activity throughout the 21 days of drug administration in each cycle, but half as much progestin activity during the first 10 days than during the final 11 days. Ortho-Novum 10/11-28, like many of the monophasic products, also provides 7 inert tablets to be taken during the hormone-free period. *Triphasic* oral contraceptives were introduced in 1986 (Table 34–8). Tri Norinyl and Ortho Novum 7/7/7 provide a constant level of estrogen activity throughout the 21 day period of hormone administration, but different patterns of progestin administration. Tri-Levien and Triphasil vary both the amount of estrogen and progestin during the three phases.

Important Nursing Implications for Estrogens, Progestins, and Combination Oral Contraceptives

- ☐ Encourage clients to read all labels and package inserts that come with the oral contraceptives and to seek answers to any questions from the nurse, pharmacist, or physician.
- ☐ Help clients develop methods of remembering to take their medication each day. Establishing a routine such as taking the pill at bedtime or with a specific meal, or recording the event on a calendar may be helpful.

Table 34–8
Biphasic and Triphasic Oral Contraceptives

Biphasic product	Phase one	Phase two
Ortho-Novum 10/11-21 or 10/11-28		
Phase duration	10 days	11 days
Estrogen	35 µg ethinyl estradiol	35 µg ethinyl estradiol
Progestin	0.5 mg norethindrone	1.0 mg norethindrone

Triphasic product	Phase one	Phase two	Phase three
Ortho-Novum 7/7/7			
Phase duration	7 days	7 days	7 days
Estrogen	35 µg ethinyl estradiol	35 µg ethinyl estradiol	35 µg ethinyl estradiol
Progestin	0.5 mg norethindrone	0.75 mg norethindrone	1.0 mg norethindrone
Tri-Levien-21, Tri-Levien-28, Triphasil-21, and Triphasil-28			
Phase duration	6 days	5 days	10 days
Estrogen	30 µg ethinyl estradiol	40 µg ethinyl estradiol	35 µg ethinyl estradiol
Progestin	0.05 mg levonorgestrel	0.075 mg levonorgestrel	0.125 mg levonorgestrel
Tri Norinyl			
Phase duration	7 days	9 days	5 days
Estrogen	35 µg ethinyl estradiol	35 µg ethinyl estradiol	35 µg ethinyl estradiol
Progestin	0.5 mg norethindrone	1.0 mg norethindrone	0.5 mg norethindrone

- ☐ Instruct the client how to compensate for missed administrations of an oral contraceptive. A single missed pill should be taken as soon as remembered. If two are missed, the client should double up on each of the next 2 days. If three or more are missed, the client should stop the sequence, wait 7 days from the first missed day, and begin a new cycle.
- ☐ For a client considering the use of oral contraceptives, determine if there is any family or personal history of cardiovascular disease, hypertension, thromboembolic disorders, liver dysfunction, diabetes, seizure disorders, or obesity.
- ☐ Teach clients the importance of reporting side effects of estrogens, progestins, and oral contraceptives such as changes in color of the skin or sclera, visual disturbances, depression, unusual bleeding tendencies, tenderness around a vein, or shortness of breath.
- ☐ Encourage women who wish to use an oral contraceptive to refrain from smoking cigarettes and explain the increased risk of thromboembolic disorders if smoking is continued.
- ☐ Teach the client to monitor weight and blood pressure and to conduct regular self-examination for breast tumors when using estrogens, progestins, or oral contraceptives.
- ☐ Warn diabetic clients that dosage adjustments may be required in their antidiabetic regimen when oral contraceptives are initiated.
- ☐ Instruct clients to terminate use of estrogens, progestins, or oral contraceptives if pregnancy is suspected or if two consecutive menses are missed.
- ☐ Teach clients using estradiol transdermal strips to apply the adhesive side to a clean dry area of skin on the trunk of the body, but not to the breasts. Teach clients to avoid the waistline and areas where the skin is irritated. Teach clients to rotate the site of application.

The Mini-Pill

The "mini-pill" contains no estrogen and only comparatively small amounts of progestins. It was introduced in order to eliminate the adverse effects associated with estrogen. The progesterone in a mini-pill is not necessarily sufficient to inhibit ovulation in all cases. However, the progestin reduces the chances of a union between sperm and egg and also interferes with implantation. The effectiveness of the mini-pill is about 97–98%. Side effects associated with the mini-pill are those listed under progesterone deficiency and estrogen deficiency in Table 34–5. Mini-pills currently available consist of 0.35 mg of norethindrone (Micronor and Nor-Q.D.) or norgestrel (Ovrette). Although free of the life-threatening adverse effects seen with combination pills, the mini-pills have not gained favor because of the frequent irregularity of bleeding and the less-than-complete protection.

The Morning-After Pill

The morning-after pill consists of a rather large dose therapy (25–50 mg/day for 5 days) with the estrogenic drug, diethylstilbestrol. Drug administration is begun preferably within 24 hours and not more than 72 hours after unprotected intercourse. This method is approved for use only in emergency situations, such as rape or incest, when there is maximum incentive to avoid pregnancy. Treatment is usually unpleasant, with nausea and vomiting the most common symptoms. Effectiveness is greater than 98%.

Therapeutic Uses of Drugs in Pregnancy, Birth, and Puerperium

Drugs to Treat Toxemia of Pregnancy

Toxemia of pregnancy encompasses preeclampsia and eclampsia. *Preeclampsia* is an acute hypertensive state with associated albuminuria and edema occurring between week 20 of pregnancy and week 1 postpartum. *Eclampsia* is coma or seizures occurring as a sequel. Preeclampsia occurs in 5–7% of pregnancies and is one of the two major causes (along with infection) of maternal and prenatal mortality. Preeclampsia is usually seen in first pregnancies. If untreated, preeclampsia often progresses to eclampsia.

A blood pressure of 140/90 together with edema or albuminuria is indicative of preeclampsia, even though pressures higher than 140/90 would not necessarily be diagnosed as hypertension in nonpregnant women. Blood pressures as low as 130/80 in the last trimester may indicate preeclampsia.

Treatment of toxemia of pregnancy is based on severity. In mild cases, bedrest may be sufficient. If the client does not respond well to bedrest, hospitalization is usually required. Conservative pharmacological intervention is initiated with a mild sedative.

If preeclampsia occurs after 34 or 35 weeks, labor may be induced.

In more severe cases, the first goal of treatment is preserving the life and health of the mother. Intravenous fluid therapy is established with a balanced salt solution containing dextrose. Magnesium sulfate may be used both to control and to prevent preeclampsia and eclampsia, but it should not be employed if there is any history of heart block or kidney impairment or if the woman is within 2 hours of delivery. Two to four grams of the salt is given by addition to the intravenous solution, with administration spread over 5–10 minutes until hyperreflexia is reduced. Magnesium infusion is continued at 1–2 g/hour by addition to the infusion fluid. *Serum levels of magnesium should be monitored. The nurse should monitor signs of magnesium toxicity including complaints of thirst or feeling hot all over, or loss of the patellar reflex.* Calcium gluconate (10–20 ml of a 10% solution) can be given as an antidote. If high blood pressure does not respond to the magnesium sulfate, hydralazine (Apresoline) can be infused at a concentration of 40 mg/1,000 ml.

The patient with full eclampsia is treated similarly except that diazepam in doses of 5 mg may be given to control seizures. *Clients receiving diazepam should be monitored by the nurse for hypotension and complaints of drowsiness or unusual fatigue.* After severe preeclampsia or eclampsia is stabilized, delivery is indicated, vaginally if possible or by cesarian section.

Drugs to Induce Labor

The smooth muscles of the uterus are stimulated by both sympathetic and parasympathetic activity, but autonomic drugs are not used to initiate labor because their effects are not specific to the uterus. The drugs employed to induce labor in obstetrical practice are oxytocin, ergot alkaloids, and certain prostaglandins.

Oxytocin (Pitocin, Syntocinon)

Oxytocin is one of the natural hormones secreted by the posterior pituitary. It is an octapeptide that contracts the uterus and stimulates milk ejection in response to suckling.

Mechanisms and Effects Oxytocin stimulates physiologically natural contractions by the pregnant uterus. The normal (nonpregnant) uterus is relatively insensitive to oxytocin. Endogenous oxytocin contributes to onset of labor, but in its absence, labor will occur anyway.

Clinical Indications Oxytocin is used to induce labor or, after delivery, to contract uterine muscle in order to reduce hemorrhage. It is also used to correct postpartum uterine atony or to produce therapeutic abortions after the first trimester. A nasal spray containing oxytocin is marketed for promoting initial letdown of milk.

Nursing Observations for Use of Drugs to Induce Labor

THERAPEUTIC GOAL	Induction of labor and delivery.
PREADMINISTRATION ASSESSMENT	
Baseline Data	Evaluate blood pressure, pulse, respiration, uterine tone and contractions, and neurological status.
Contraindications/ Precautions	Abnormalities of fetal position or presentation, fetal distress, sensitivity to the drug, severe toxemia, renal disease, or hypertension. Relative contraindications: first pregnancy in a woman over 35, several previous deliveries, a previous cesarean section, or previous difficult delivery.
Potential Interactions	Check medication chart for current use of sympathomimetic drugs.
EVALUATION OF DRUG RESPONSE	
For Therapeutic Benefit	Optimal response is 3 or 4 good contractions in 10 minutes.
For Adverse Effects	Monitor for uterine spasms, cold or clammy skin, anaphylactic reactions, fetal distress, cardiac dysrhythmias, edema, and changes in mental status, or gastrointestinal status.

Adverse Effects and Contraindications Use of oxytocin is contraindicated in the first stage of labor, in severe preeclampsia, in fetal distress, if the fetus has presented abnormally, or the mother is predisposed to uterine rupture. A history of hypersensitivity to the drug would also indicate that oxytocics should not be used.

Adverse effects do not usually occur in response to oxytocin at the doses employed to induce labor. However, once administration of oxytocin has begun, the patient must be monitored constantly to detect any evidence of overstimulation of the uterus. Even with proper administration and adequate supervision, a patient whose uterus is hypersensitive to oxytocin can develop hypertonic contractions. This can result in uterine tetany, uterine rupture, amniotic fluid embolism, or cervical laceration. In addition, there may be a decrease in the uteroplacental blood flow and hypoxia resulting from trauma to the fetus. *Thus nurses must monitor both mother and fetus to detect any changes that might signal distress to mother and baby.* An oxytocin-challenge test may be used to test the adequacy of fetal placental function in high-risk obstetrical patients. *Once a decision has been made to use oxytocin to induce labor, the nurse should check the patient and fetal heart rate or fetal monitor at least every 10 minutes. The nurse should record the frequency, length, and strength of the mother's contractions. Incidents that might suggest that the drug should be stopped are uterine spasm, a patient who becomes cold, clammy and sweaty (an indication of possible anaphylactic shock), cardiac irregularities, or vomiting and nausea. If uterine hyperactivity or fetal distress is evident, the drug should be discontinued and oxygen administered to the mother.*

Oxytocics may cause anoxia, asphyxia, and trauma in the fetus as a result of their vasoconstrictor and spasmogenic actions. Oxytocic drugs can cause antidiuretic effects and thus water intoxication and hypertension. Indications that this has occurred include anuria, edema, and complaints of headache, listlessness, or confusion. *The nurse should make observations of the patient's level of alertness, fluid intake and output ratios, and blood pressure.*

Preparations and Administration Oxytocin (Pitocin, Syntocinon) is digested by trypsin in the gastrointestinal tract and therefore is not effective orally. It can be given intravenously, intramuscularly, subcutaneously, intranasally, or buccally. Oxytocin should not be used simultaneously by more than one route, since this complicates the problem of controlling dosage. Slow intravenous infusion is most common. By this method, administration can be titrated to provide optimal uterine response (3–4 contractions per 10 minutes). Overdose can occur even with very low rates of infusion. Oxytocin has a short half-life of a few minutes, being rapidly removed by the liver and kidneys.

Oxytocin (Pitocin, Syntocinon, and generic formulations)
Injection solution, nasal spray
Recommended Doses: For induction of labor, 1 ml (10 units) added to a 1 liter bottle of infusion solution for infusion at 1–2 mu/min. For postpartum uterine bleeding, 10–40 units added to a nonhydrating infusion solution. For initial milk letdown, 1 spray into one or both nostrils 2–3 minutes before nursing or pumping of breasts.

Important Nursing Implications for Oxytocin

- ☐ Consider use of oxytocin only in a hospital with a physician at hand.
- ☐ Optimal uterine response is considered to be 3 or 4 good-quality contractions in 10 minutes.
- ☐ Carefully review the patient's history for any contraindications before giving oxytocin.
- ☐ Inform the patient at the outset of the rationale for using oxytocic agents and the signs and symptoms that all is going well or symptoms suggesting a need to alter the therapy.
- ☐ Monitor the fetal pulse rate and the mother's blood pressure and, if feasible, employ a fetal monitor whenever oxytocin is administered.
- ☐ Try to instill confidence in clients and encourage them to disclose how they feel physically and emotionally; this communication will help to determine how the therapy is progressing.
- ☐ Never leave the mother unattended by a qualified nurse.

Ergot Alkaloids

Mechanisms and Effects Ergot alkaloids, such as ergotamine, ergonovine (Ergotrate), and methylergonovine (Methergine), are effective stimulants of uterine motility. Ergotamine is also effective in constricting cerebral blood vessels that are overdistended during migraine headaches (see Chapter 26). Ergonovine and methylergonovine are more effective producing uterine contractions. These drugs are derived from the fungus *Claviceps purpurea,* the common ergot fungus that grows on rye and other grains.

Clinical Indications Ergot alkaloids have been used for many years to control postpartum bleeding. Ergonovine malleate is intended primarily for intramuscular injection in routine obstetric practice.

Nursing Diagnoses and Interventions for Use of Drugs to Induce Labor

Nursing Diagnoses	*Related Interventions*
TO MINIMIZE DRUG SIDE EFFECTS OR INTERACTIONS	
Alteration in comfort: pain related to uterine contractions and vaginal or cervical lacerations	Provide comfort measures such as a cold cloth on forehead, a tissue lubricant, or analgesia.
Increased potential for injury	Ensure that provision has been made for emergency surgical intervention.
Ineffective coping related to impaired mental state, pain, or fear	Provide support, encouragement, and reassurance. When permitted, encourage presence of the father of the infant.
Potential fluid volume excess related to antidiuretic activity of oxytocics	Monitor maternal blood pressure and pulse and fetal heart sounds at 15-minute intervals or less; adjust intravenous drip.
TO ENSURE SAFE AND EFFICACIOUS DRUG USE	
Knowledge deficit related to drug regimen	Advise clients not to consider self-administration of oxytocic drugs as means of attempting to terminate an unwanted pregnancy.
	Explain to clients who become impatient with normal labor why it is preferable not to hasten normal labor with oxytocic drugs.
	Explain to clients who require induction of labor the reason for the decision.
	Explain the reason for any monitoring procedures used during labor.
	Be certain the client knows what symptoms to report that may indicate a need to alter the rate of administration of oxytocic drugs.

When administered in this fashion, it produces a firm contraction of the uterine muscle within 6–15 minutes.

Adverse Effects and Contraindications Uterine contractions induced by ergot alkaloids may be painful. *Question clients after medication to ascertain the extent to which painful cramping has occurred. The nurse should feel the uterine muscle contract by placing the hand over the uterus, in order to determine if the uterus is responding as intended to the drug.* Some clients who have calcium deficiencies may fail to respond to the drug. *Laboratory reports or physical evidence indicating a calcium deficiency should alert the nurse to expect a diminished response.* If this occurs, the client may continue to have excessive uterine bleeding. *The nurse should monitor the amount of bleeding, the number of times pads need to be changed, the consistency of the bleeding, and the presence of clots as an indication of the response to ergonovine. The physician should be kept informed of all changes in the client's condition.*

Although side effects are minimal at doses used in obstetrics, ergot alkaloids can be toxic if the dose is excessive. Symptoms of ergot poisoning include vomiting, diarrhea, thirst, itching, coldness of the skin, tingling sensations in the extremities, tachycardia, weak pulse, confusion, and coma. Blood pressure may be elevated by ergot alkaloids, especially in those clients who have had regional anesthesia or who have had vasoconstrictor drugs prior to delivery. Feelings of coldness or numbness of the feet or legs, or muscle pain could indicate severe vasoconstriction which could potentially lead to gangrene of the extremities. Other symptoms of excessive dosage are headache, nausea, vomiting, diarrhea, and dizziness.

Preparations and Administration *Clients are usually expected to take the drug until uterine strength has returned to normal. If the client is at home, she needs to be taught how to administer the drug, how to determine when uterine strength has returned to normal, and how to recognize adverse reactions.*

Ergonovine (Ergotrate)
Tablets, injection solution
Recommended Doses: For controlling postpartum uterine bleeding, 0.2–0.3 mg, IM or IV. For promoting involution of the uterus, 0.2–0.4 mg orally, tid, until involution has progressed satisfactorily.

Methylergonovine (Methergine)
Tablets, injection solution
Recommended Doses: Same as for ergonovine.

Dinoprost Tromethamine

Mechanisms and Effects Dinoprost tromethamine is a salt of a naturally occurring prostaglandin that stimulates uterine contractions.

Clinical Indications Dinoprost is indicated for use in labor induction. Dinoprostone (Prostin E_2), a suppository form of dinoprost tromethamine, is used to stimulate uterine contractions in order to produce abortion in the second trimester of pregnancy, to induce labor when a client has an hydatidiform mole, or for treatment of a missed abortion (in which the fetus has died prior to the twentieth week of gestation but where the products of conception are retained in the uterus for 8 weeks or longer).

Adverse Effects and Contraindications *Before clients are given dinoprost, a careful history should be taken.* Women who have a history of asthma, or who have diabetes, glaucoma, or anemia need to be carefully monitored if they are given this drug. Women who have epilepsy, cardiovascular problems, or renal or hepatic disease are at special risk for untoward effects. Vaginitis, cervicitis, or endometriosis also increase risk of side effects. Dinoprost is specifically contraindicted for use in women who have acute pelvic inflammatory disease or a history of hypersensitivity to prostaglandins, cesarean section, hysterotomy, uterine fibroids, or cervical stenosis.

Vomiting, nausea, abdominal cramps, and uterine pain are common side effects. Other reported side effects include headache, flushing, coughing, wheezing, paresthesias, breast tenderness, hyperventilation, burning sensations around the eyes or breasts, urinary retention, hematuria, hypertension, and polydipsia. Severe reactions including convulsions, uterine rupture, and second-degree heart block have been reported.

Preparations and Administration *When administered to induce abortion, the client should be told that the fetus can be expected to be expelled between 20 and 48 hours after instillation. The nurse should also explain that if the client continues to bleed after the fetus and other tissues have been expelled, she may have had an incomplete abortion.* This is usually the result of retention of parts of the placenta or afterbirth and may require the administration of oxytocin (10–40 mg) or dinoprost, or dilation and evacuation of the uterus.

When dinoprost is instilled into the amniotic sac, 1 ml or more of amniotic fluid is removed and a transabdominal needle is inserted. If the amniotic fluid is clear, 40 mg (8 ml) of dinoprost is injected slowly. If the fluid is cloudy or tinged with blood, the drug should not be injected.

This preparation has also been approved for therapeutic abortions during the second trimester, by intramuscular injection or instillation of a vaginal suppository. *Suppositories should be stored at temperatures of −20° C (−4° F). Before insertion, the suppository should be warmed to room temperature. Clients should be in a supine position during insertion. They should remain supine for at least 10 minutes after administration.*

Dinopost
Injection solution, suppositories
Recommended Doses: For induction of labor, 40 mg instilled into the amniotic sac. For therapeutic abortion, 20 mg inserted as a suppository high in the vagina every 3–5 hours until abortion occurs.

Important Nursing Implications for Dinoprost

- ☐ It is important that both nurses and clients understand the fact that these compounds do not cause fetal death. It is possible for a client to deliver a live fetus. Clients should be made aware of this possibility prior to administration of dinoprost tromethamine or dinoprostone and they should receive counseling to help them cope with this possibility.
- ☐ Some nurses who oppose abortion may not wish to participate in the procedure. When possible, a nurse who opposes abortion should not be expected to participate. Those who do participate should not force their opinions on the

client. Once the abortion has been completed, nurses have an obligation to provide supportive nursing care for the client.

Drugs to Reduce Pain or Anxiety During Labor

Drugs used to diminish pain during delivery include narcotic analgesics, local anesthetics, and general anesthetics. All of these drugs pass freely across the placental barrier and can cause CNS depression in the fetus, complicating the birth process. When narcotics are used, naloxone should be available in case fetal respiration is unduly depressed. Diazepam is frequently used for sedation, but its use may be associated with hypothermia and low Apgar scores in the newborn. The current trend is toward less use of medications and better preparation for the process through courses teaching birthing technique (such as Lamaze).

Drugs to Suppress Lactation

Preparation for lactation involves a sequence of several hormones. Beginning in puberty, estrogen secretion promotes development of the breasts. The duct system expands, and fat is deposited to increase the size of the breasts. Progesterone stimulates growth of the lobules and alveoli. During pregnancy, estrogen and progesterone prepare the breast for secretion but suppress actual secretion of milk. After parturition, increased release of prolactin, along with the drop in estrogen and progesterone levels, stimulates milk secretion into the alveoli of the breast. The flow of milk from the breast is controlled by still another hormone — oxytocin. Oxytocin secretion by the posterior pituitary gland is stimulated by the suckling action of the baby. The milk normally begins to flow under the influence of this hormonal reflex within a half minute of initiation of suckling.

After parturition, if the mother does not wish to breast feed her infant, lactation can be suppressed by administration of estrogenic drugs or progestins for a period of about 4 days following delivery. Androgens have also been used effectively for this purpose. Suppression of lactation by this technique is most effective if instituted before lactation is established. Once lactation is established, low doses of estrogen or progestins, such as those found in oral contraceptives, may diminish lactation and increase the protein content of breast milk but are unlikely to suppress lactation entirely. Another drug used clinically for suppression of lactation is bromocriptine.

Bromocriptine (Parlodel)

Mechanisms and Effects Bromocriptine is a dopamine agonist that suppresses secretion of prolactin, usually triggering reinitiation of menses in 6–8 weeks and relieving galactorrhea in 8–12 weeks.

Clinical Indications Bromocriptine is indicated for relief of galactorrhea and associated amenorrhea caused by excessive prolactin. Bromocriptine can also be used as an alternative to estrogens, progestins, or androgens to suppress physiological lactation after parturition if breast-feeding is not desired. Bromocriptine is also used in parkinsonism (see Chapter 22) and has recently been found of some value in alleviating drug craving during initial treatment of cocaine addicts.

Pharmacokinetics An average of only 28% of an orally administered dose of bromocriptine is absorbed. In the serum, bromocriptine is 90–96% bound to plasma proteins. It is metabolized in the liver and excreted mainly in the bile.

Adverse Effects and Contraindications Adverse effects are common but usually mild. Nausea, vomiting, intestinal cramps, diarrhea, headache, dizziness, fatigue, lightheadedness, and nasal congestion are the symptoms usually reported. *The gastrointestinal symptoms are reduced if the drug is taken with meals.*

Postural hypotension is usually modest and asymptomatic but can rarely be severe. *The first dose should be taken while lying down and the client should be advised to refrain from sudden changes in position while using bromocriptine.* The hypotensive action of bromocriptine is additive with that produced by vasodilators, diuretics, and other hypotensive medications. Dizziness and lightheadedness are possible reactions.

Oral contraceptives should not be employed during bromocriptine therapy. Clients who are hypersensitive to ergot alkaloids should not take bromocriptine. Bromocriptine should not be taken during pregnancy.

Preparations and Administration

Bromocriptine (Parlodel)
Tablets as the mesylate salt
Recommended Doses: For amenorrhea/galactorrhea, 2.5 mg PO, bid or tid, with meals for a period not to exceed 6 months.

Adverse Effects of Drugs in Pregnancy, Birth, and Puerperium

Adverse Effects of Drugs on Gametes and Fertilization

Although seldom considered, significant drug effects may occur prior to fertilization. Some drugs accumulate in high concentrations in reproductive cells. For example, phenytoin (Dilantin), phenobarbital, and tetrahydrocannabinol have been noted to concentrate in the ovum. The blood flow to the ovaries is very high and increases during pregnancy, so drug delivery to the ovaries is substantial in most cases. The ultimate impact on the offspring when there has been drug accumulation in the ovum is not known, but it is known that phenytoin and phenobarbital alter steroid synthesis and metabolism. In the male, spermatogenesis can be affected by a variety of drugs, most notably antineoplastics, corticosteroids, and antimicrobials. Such effects are reversible but full recovery often requires 2 years or more. Men given methotrexate are warned to avoid fertilization during the period of treatment since chromosomal abnormalities have been noted in germ cell epithelium.

Following ovulation, the expelled ovum exists in the environment of the luminal secretions as it passes through the oviduct and fallopian tube into the uterus. Lipid soluble and acidic drugs are most likely to appear in the luminal fluid. After fertilization, the blastocyst is also exposed to the luminal fluid. It has been reported that nicotine, caffeine, DDT, isoniazid, and thiopental accumulate in uterine fluid during pregnancy at concentrations as much as 50% in excess of plasma levels, and these substances have been measured in preimplantation blastocysts in rabbits. The ultimate impact of the presence of drugs during these early stages of life is not yet established.

Adverse Effects of Drugs on the Fetus

After development of the placenta, drug entrance into the fetus occurs via placental transfer. The main mechanism is passive diffusion. Glucose and iron are transferred by facilitated diffusion and a few substances, such as vitamin B_{12} and certain amino acids, are transported actively. The transfer of highly lipid soluble drugs is determined mainly by maternal placental blood flow, while the transfer of substances that are highly ionized or poorly soluble in lipids is determined mainly by protein binding in the maternal plasma. As with all penetration barriers, small and nonpolar drugs pass the placental barrier more readily than large or polar molecules. Some drug metabolism is carried out by the placenta, but the rate of metabolism is far less per unit of tissue than in the maternal or fetal liver. Placental resistance to drug transfer is greater in the second trimester than in the first or third.

Once inside the fetus, drugs enter the portal circulation, but unlike the adult human, nearly 50% of portal blood bypasses the liver. Liver extraction is thus less complete. The fetal liver is capable of drug metabolism as early as the eighth week after gestation.

The fetal blood has far less capacity to bind drugs to plasma proteins. When a drug reaches equilibrium distribution between the maternal and fetal circulations, concentrations of free drug are equivalent but total concentrations in the fetus are less because of low plasma binding. Toxicity is dictated by the concentration of free drug.

Some drugs concentrate in specific fetal tissues to produce characteristic teratogenicity (fetal injury). For example, chloroquine and phenothiazines accumulate in the eye and cause visual anomalies. Phenytoin accumulates in the fetal liver, heart, kidney, and intestines.

The fetus is susceptible to adverse effects of drugs at every stage of development. During the first month or so, all the major organs are being formed, and effects of drugs are generally either lethal or benign. During the subsequent 2 months the detailed structures of tissues are being elaborated and the risk of birth defects is greatest. Teratisms associated with drug use in the second and third trimesters are generally predictable from the pharmacology of the drug in question (for example, depression with anesthetics or sedative-hypnotics). Unfortunately, the potentially harmful effects of many drugs on fetal development has been poorly studied. Lack of adverse effects in adult humans is no guarantee of safety to the fetus during pregnancy. The known effects of drugs on fetal development are listed in Table 34–9.

Important variables in teratogenicity include (1) duration of exposure, (2) amount of drug crossing the placenta, (3) the rate of drug transfer to the fetus, (4) the properties and effects of the drug, and (5) the stage of fetal development. The thalidomide tragedy of the early 1960s effectively dramatized the risk of drug-induced birth defects. Nevertheless, surveys indicate that most pregnant women consume many prescription and nonprescription drugs during

Table 34–9
Some Potential Teratogens

Drug	Teratism
Alcohol	Regular use during pregnancy is associated with a fetal alcohol syndrome and withdrawal symptoms at birth.
Androgens	Prolonged therapy with high doses during first 12 weeks causes masculinization of the female fetus.
Antiepileptics	Phenytoin (Dilantin) may cause cleft palate and congenital heart anomalies. Teratogenicity has also been reported for phenobarbital, trimethadione, and primidone. Risk of teratogenicity has to be weighed against risk to fetus if mother has a seizure during pregnancy. Antiepileptics also cause vitamin K deficiency in fetus.
Antimicrobials	Tetracyclines complex with calcium in the developing fetal skeleton. They should not be used from the middle to the end of pregnancy. Ototoxic antimicrobials, such as gentamicin, streptomycin, and kanamycin cross the placenta and may damage the fetal labyrinth. The fetal liver cannot metabolize chloramphenicol, and therefore its use in the mother can cause a "gray baby syndrome." Sulfonamides given near term may cause jaundice in the neonate, but when given earlier in pregnancy, the fetus is protected from this effect by placental metabolism of bilirubin. Other teratogenic antimicrobials include isoniazid, novobiocin, quinine, chloroquine, and nitrofurantoin.
Antineoplastics	Methotrexate, mercaptopurine, cytosine arabinoside, and others have been noted to cause teratogenic effects, most frequently when used during the first trimester.
Antithyroid drugs	Hypothyroidism in fetus.
Anxiolytics	No teratogenicity was found in a large study but some isolated reports. FDA requires warning that use of anxiolytics (meprobamate and benzodiazepines) during the first trimester of pregnancy may increase risk of congenital malformations.
Digitoxin	Harmful late in pregnancy.
Estrogens	Female offspring have higher risk of adenocarcinoma if exposed to estrogens in utero.
Glucocorticoids	Fetal abnormalities when given in large doses during pregnancy.
Iodide 131	Can destroy thyroid of fetus.
Magnesium sulfate	This drug, often used in preeclampsia, causes respiratory depression if used close to time of delivery.
Narcotics	Addiction in mother causes a withdrawal syndrome in the infant at birth. Use near the time of delivery causes difficulty in initiating respiration that can be alleviated by administering a narcotic antagonist to the infant.
Oral anticoagulants	Coumarins cross the placenta freely and may cause bleeding in the fetus. Coumarins given during the first trimester have been associated with fetal anomalies. Heparin can be used safely.
Oral hypoglycemics	Can cause profound hypoglycemia in the baby. Should not be used during pregnancy. Insulin can be used instead since it does not cross the placenta.
Oxidant drugs	May cause hemolysis if fetus has G6PD deficiency (see Chapter 41). Oxidant drugs include primaquine, nitrofurantoin, naphthalene, sulfonamides, chloramphenicol, and vitamin K.
Phenothiazines	Accumulate in the eye of the fetus and may cause retinopathy.
Piperazine antihistamines	Meclizine and cyclizine are teratogenic at least in animal studies.
Progesterone	Use by the mother during the first 12 weeks may be associated with congenital anomalies or masculinization of the female genitalia.
Propranolol	Can produce bradycardia, hypoglycemia, and growth retardation in the fetus.
Reserpine	Causes norepinephrine depletion leading to respiratory distress, lethargy, bradycardia, and nasal stuffiness.
Salicylates	Given late in pregnancy, salicylates may cause hypoprothrombinemia and fetal or neonatal hemorrhage. Salicylates compete with bilirubin for protein binding sites and may cause kernicterus.
Thiazide diuretics	Unknown risks. Thiazides cross the placenta and are not recommended for routine use in pregnancy.
Tobacco	Use during pregnancy is associated with decreased birthweight and increased spontaneous abortions.
Vaccines	Live vaccines should be avoided during pregnancy since fetal infection may occur.
Vitamin C	Megadoses may cause withdrawal scurvy in the infant at birth.

pregnancy, not to mention alcohol, nicotine, and caffeine. Less than half of pregnant women suspend use of alcohol or nicotine.

Because of the many uncertainties regarding drug effects during fertilization and pregnancy, prudence dictates conservative use of drugs during pregnancy and times of reproduction efforts. Women who are or may be pregnant should be warned to check the safety of all drugs with their physician or pharmacist before taking them. Any nursing assessment of women who are pregnant should include the drugs clients have been taking prior to pregnancy, during the period when pregnancy was uncertain, and after pregnancy was suspected. This assessment should include prescription medications, over-the-counter preparations, illicit drugs, and the recreational drugs — alcohol, nicotine, and caffeine.

Adverse Effects of Drugs on Lactation and the Nursing Infant

Breast-feeding has many positive benefits for the mother and infant alike. In the first few days of the puerperium, it stimulates uterine involution by triggering release of oxytocin. Breast milk has distinct nutritional advantages over formulas or cow's milk, and it provides immunoglobulins that afford some protection to the neonate. Moreover, breast-feeding ensures close physical contact between the mother and infant that promotes bonding. Because of these values, women inclined toward breast-feeding should be encouraged and provided with the health care support they need. Some physicians are far too prone to insist that nursing mothers wean their babies when medication is prescribed. Weaning should be considered only as a last alternative, and only if all of the following circumstances apply: (1) the medication is truly essential for the well-being of the mother, (2) there is no alternative medication that is safe for use while nursing, and (3) it is known or likely that the drug causes adverse effects in the infant, not merely that it appears in the milk in modest quantities. Drugs for which the level of risk to the nursing infant is at least tentatively established should generally be preferred over new drug entries of unknown liability for the infant.

Drugs appear in breast milk to different extents: some not at all, some in small amounts, and some in concentrations equal to or even higher than in the mother's serum. The factors determining the extent to which a drug will be present in the milk are the lipid solubility, pKa, molecular size, and protein binding of the drug, and the pH of the milk. Absorption into breast milk is by passive diffusion and therefore related to the concentration gradient. The fraction of a drug that is protein-bound does not contribute to the concentration gradient, but displacement by drugs that compete for plasma protein binding sites can increase the free fraction and elevate drug excretion in the milk.

The pH of milk is slightly less than that of plasma. Therefore, at equilibrium, the concentration of weak bases will be somewhat higher in the milk than in plasma; the concentration of weak acids will be lower in the milk than in plasma.

Whether the presence of the drug in the milk will be of clinical significance for the infant depends on several factors: (1) the amount of drug in the milk, (2) the amount of drug-containing milk ingested by the infant, (3) the extent of absorption of the drug by the infant, (4) the capacity of the infant's liver to metabolize drugs, (5) and the action of the drug on various infant tissues. The amount of drug ingested by the infant will be greatest for drugs used chronically by the mother and drugs taken acutely shortly before the infant's feeding. Some drugs are contraindicated during nursing (Table 34–10). If these must be used, nursing should usually be discontinued. Some drugs may be used if necessary but require close monitoring of the infant (Table 34–11). Some drugs are either present in small quantities of no apparent clinical significance or not excreted in the milk at all (Table 34–12).

Some drugs may alter formation of breast milk (Table 34–1) or its content. Atropine, alcohol, diuretics, levodopa, MAO inhibitors, and vitamin B_6, may inhibit lactation.

Some drugs cause either pseudolactation in women who are not breast-feeding or galactorrhea in those who are (Table 34–1). Release of the hormone prolactin is regulated predominantly by the hypothalamic hormone prolactin inhibitory factor (PLIF), which is itself regulated by the dopamine neurons in the hypothalamus. Some evidence suggests that PLIF may in fact be dopamine. Dopamine blocking drugs, namely the family of neuroleptic agents, increase release of prolactin to produce pseudolactation. Antidepressants and reserpine can have a similar effect. Galactorrhea can also result from use of oral contraceptives. Galactorrhea associated with amenorrhea sometimes occurs in females independent of drug influences due to excess prolactin secretion. This can be caused by a pituitary adenoma that stimulates prolactin output (Forbes-Albright syndrome) or excessive prolactin secretion following pregnancy (Chiari-Frommel syndrome). Galactorrhea has even been known to occur in males due to pituitary adenomas. Galactorrhea can occur in females due to breast stimulation or hypothyroidism.

Table 34–10
Drugs Contraindicated in Nursing Mothers

Drug class	Comment
Antimicrobials (some)	
Amantadine	Possible vomiting, urinary retention, skin rash.
Chloramphenicol	Infant's capacity to metabolize this drug is underdeveloped.
Metronidazole	Avoid breast-feeding for 3 days after a single dose.
Sulfonamides	Possible allergic skin reactions, jaundice, or hemolysis in G6PD-deficient infants.
Streptomycin	Accumulates in liver of infant.
Tetracyclines	Possible discoloration of teeth of infant.
Antineoplastics	Nursing should be discontinued.
Antithyroid drugs	May cause goiter or myxedema.
Atropine	May cause atropine intoxication.
Bromides	Cause rash and drowsiness.
Cathartics	Diarrhea in infant.
Cimetidine	Induces liver enzymes, suppresses gastric secretions, and stimulates the CNS in the infant.
Ergot alkaloids	Vomiting, diarrhea, weak pulse, unstable blood pressure in the infant.
Heavy metals	Mercury and lead poisoning can occur in infants if mother's milk is contaminated.
Iodides	May cause thyroid impairment in infant.
Narcotics	May cause addiction in infant.
Oral anticoagulants (especially phenindione)	Cause hypocoagulation in the infant.
Oral hypoglycemics	Tolbutamide achieves high concentration in milk; possible adverse effect on pancreas of infant.
Radioactive drugs	Contraindicted in nursing mothers.

Drugs and Female Sexuality

The stimuli that initiate female sexuality are similar to those that operate in males. Genital and psychic stimulation combine to initiate sexual arousal. The clitoris contains the largest concentration of sensitive end-organs in the female. Erectile tissue surrounding the vaginal entrance and extending to the clitoris responds to parasympathetic impulses in much the same way as does penile erectile tissue. Glands in the vaginal mucosa and beneath the labia minora secrete lubricating mucus. When the level of stimulation is sufficient, the orgasmic reflex is triggered.

Dysfunctions of female sexuality include inhibited sexual excitement, inhibited orgasm, and inhibited sexual desire. **Inhibited sexual excitement,** or frigidity, is usually due to psychological factors. It is characterized by a recurrent inhibition of sexual excitement during sexual interaction as evidenced by lack of lubrication and swelling responses. Marital discord accounts for 80% of cases. Other women experience sexual excitement but **inhibited orgasm.** Causes of inhibited orgasm include inadequate stimulation during foreplay, fear of "letting go," normal variability in responsiveness, and diabetes. **Inhibited sexual desire** can occur in women as a lifelong generalized inhibition due to traumatic events of childhood or adolescence, or rarely, due to abnormally low levels of testosterone. Inhibited sexual desire may occur situationally because of depression, boredom with one's sexual partner, or because of effects of drugs.

A few drugs produce alterations in libido in some women, including methyldopa (Aldomet), reserpine (Serpasil), tricyclic antidepressants, alcohol,

Table 34–11
Drugs Requiring Close Observation of Infant when Administered to Nursing Mothers

Drug	Comment
Alcohol	O.K. in small amounts; large amounts depress infant and inhibit lactation.
Antimicrobiols	
Cephalosporins, 3rd generation	Possible enterocolitis.
Erythromycin	Concentrated in milk. Possible jaundice.
Isoniazid	Concentration is the same in milk as in serum; monitor child for possible toxicity.
Kanamycin	Monitor child for toxicity.
Nalidixic acid	Possible hemolytic anemia.
Penicillin G or V	Possible hypersensitivity reactions.
Barbiturates	Induce liver enzymes in infant.
Benzodiazepines	Possible drowsiness.
Carbamazepine	Possible tiredness, vomiting, or poor suckling.
Chloral hydrate	Possible sedation in infant.
Decongestants	May decrease milk volume.
Diuretics (thiazides, high ceiling, spironolactone)	Avoid use during lactation; they decrease milk production and appear in milk.
Glucocorticoids	Growth suppression; suppression of infant's production of glucocorticoids; retarded sexual development.
Indomethacin	Convulsions reported in one breast-fed infant.
Lithium	Monitor child for lithium toxicity.
Meprobamate	Concentrated in milk 2 to 4× plasma level; monitor child for depressive effects.
Methyldopa	Possible depression of respirations, blood pressure, and alertness.
Minoxidil	Monitor for hypertrichosis.
Neuroleptics	May cause galactorrhea in mother; not present in significant amounts in milk.
Nicotine	Nicotine effects in infant occur if rate is greater than 20 cigarettes per day.
Oral contraceptives	Gynecomastia in male infants.
Phenytoin	One case of methemoglobinemia reported; induces liver enzymes.
Primidone	Somnolence or drowsiness may occur in infant.
Reserpine	Nasal stuffiness and lethargy in infant; galactorrhea in mother.
Salicylates	Cause bleeding tendency; mother should take after feedings, not before. Possible skin rash.
Vitamin D	Possible hypercalcemia in infant.

and amphetamines. Oral contraceptives cause a suppression of the midcycle surge in libido in many women. Benzodiazepines may cause changes in libido in either direction, the increased libido in some women being most likely related to disinhibition of repressed sexual desires. Cimetidine (Tagamet) has also been noted to cause variable alterations in libido. Small doses of androgenic substances in women may stimulate libido, while antiandrogens decrease libido.

Table 34–12
Drugs that Appear to Pose Little or No Risk When Used During Lactation

Some drugs excreted in human milk but without apparent clinical significance.		Some drugs not excreted in human milk
Acetaminophen	Meperidine	Amitriptyline
Ampicillin	Mesoridazine	Cephalosporins, first and second generation
Antihistamines	Morphine	Chloroquine
β_2-Agonists	Nitrofurantoin	Desipramine
Caffeine	Novobiocin	Dextroamphetamine
Codeine	Propranolol	Heparin
Colchicine	Propantheline	Imipramine
Digoxin	Quinidine	Oxacillin
Diphenhydramine	Quinine	Pentazocine
Guanethidine	Scopolamine	Phenylbutazone
Hydroxyphenbutazone	Thyroid hormones	
Insulin	Tolmetin	
Lidocaine	Tranylcypromine	
Mefenamic acid		

Case Study: Contraception with a Combination Oral Contraceptive

S. S., a 22-year-old, healthy female, had been taking a combination birth control pill for the last 6 months. During a routine visit to her gynecologist, S. S. complained to the nurse conducting the assessment of breakthrough bleeding, decreased menstrual flow, and decreased libido. The nurse asked S. S. when during the cycle the breakthrough bleeding occurred and S. S. indicated that it occurred within the first week or so after her period. The nurse noted that S. S. had been prescribed Norlestrin 2.5/50, a combination pill with a medium level of estrogenic activity and a medium level of progestin activity. She further noted that the progestin employed in Norlestrin, norethindrone, is one with moderate androgenic activity. The nurse reported her findings to the physician, and together they determined that S. S. might experience fewer adverse effects if her prescription was changed to Ortho-Novum 2 mg, a combination that exhibits high estrogen and medium progestin activity. S. S. responded well to this change in her regimen. The only further complaint on subsequent evaluations was concern about dark spots she had noted on her cheeks and arms.

One month S. S. missed taking the oral contraceptive for the first 3 days because she delayed in refilling her prescription. She called the nurse to inquire about what to do. S. S. told the nurse that she had on two earlier occasions missed taking the pill for "a day or two" near the end of her cycle and had not become pregnant. The nurse pointed out to her that the risk that ovulation will occur is greatest when the days missed are near the beginning of the cycle and increases with each day missed. The nurse told her that she should discard the first three pills from the container and take the remainder according to the normal schedule, ending the medication sequence on the same day that she would have had she not missed taking the pill for 3 days. She warned S. S. that she should employ a second method of contraception for the remainder of the month. She also reminded S. S. that if withdrawal bleeding did not occur, she should be suspicious of pregnancy and should discontinue use of the oral contraceptive until a definite determination could be made.

1. Adverse effects of combination oral contraceptives can be attributed to estrogen excess, estrogen deficiency, progestin excess, progestin deficiency, or excess androgenic activity from the progestin component. Which of these is the most likely factor in the complaints of S. S.? Explain.
2. What was the basis for the selection of Ortho-Novum 2 mg as an alternative preparation for S. S.?
3. Should the nurse have told S. S. to double up on the first few doses after missing 3 days? Should she have told S. S. to take all 21 pills, one each day, extending the end of the cycle 3 days?
4. Why did the nurse suggest using a second method of contraception? Why should S. S. discontinue using the pill if she suspects pregnancy?

Answers appear at the end of the book.

Case Study: Pregnancy and Postpartum

F. W. was a 25-year-old pregnant married woman, 5 feet 2 inches tall, weighing 115 pounds. When examined by the nurse and obstetrician during the first trimester of pregnancy, her blood pressure was 118/80 and all other parameters were normal. The nurse reviewed F. W.'s dietary habits and found that she maintained a well-balanced diet. The physician prescribed a prenatal vitamin for F. W. containing 250 mg of calcium, 60 mg of iron, 25 mg of zinc, 8,000 units of vitamin A, 400 units of vitamin D, 30 units vitamin E, 3 mg of B_1, 3.4 mg of B_2, 20 mg of B_3, 4 mg of B_6, 12 mg of B_{12}, 100 mg of vitamin C, 1 mg of folic acid, and trace concentrations of copper, iodine, and magnesium. The nurse advised F. W. to discontinue use of tobacco and alcohol during pregnancy; F. W. did refrain from use of alcohol but continued to smoke approximately 20 cigarettes per day throughout pregnancy.

During her fourth month of pregnancy, F. W. developed an abscess for which she sought treatment. The physician determined that the cause was *Pasteurella multocida* and, unaware that F. W. was pregnant, prescribed tetracycline.

During her twenty-seventh week of pregnancy, F. W. noticed that her fingers, wrists, ankles, and feet were swollen. She asked her pharmacist to recommend a nonprescription preparation that she might use to reduce the swelling, but he advised her that these symptoms might be an indication of a significant problem and that she should see her obstetrician. The obstetrician prescribed a thiazide diuretic and a low-salt diet. The nurse advised F. W. to increase her bedrest and to lie on her left side as much as possible. The swelling diminished somewhat following these measures.

During her thirty-sixth week of gestation, F. W. again began to experience swelling, and this time it was not responsive to increased bedrest. Her blood pressure was 150/85 and urinalysis revealed albuminuria. The nurse immediately reported these findings to the obstetrician, who arranged to have F. W. admitted to the hospital for preeclampsia. There she received magnesium sulfate and bedrest. Three days following admission, pelvic examination revealed that the cervix was soft, 4 cm dilated and approximately 50% effaced, and the head of the fetus engaged. Labor was induced by administration of a total of 10 milliunits of oxytocin administered by IV infusion. During labor F. W. was given 50 mg of meperidine by SC injection. After 4 hours of labor, F. W. gave birth to a 3 kg baby boy. At birth, the child did not spontaneously initiate respiration and the obstetrician administered 0.03 mg of naloxone, by IM injection. Seconds after administration of naloxone the infant began to breathe.

After delivery, the nursing staff closely monitored F. W. during recovery for signs of possible eclampsia, such as confusion, pain, or excessive bleeding. Blood pressure, pulse, and respirations were recorded several times daily. A complete blood cell count and urinalysis were conducted prior to discharge and all values were normal.

During hospitalization, the nurse discussed with F. W. the advantages of breast-feeding. F. W. had originally intended to bottle feed her child, but decided after conversations with the nurse to attempt breast-feeding. The nurse provided F. W. with a list of drugs that should not be employed during lactation. F. W. noted that use of oral contraceptives by a lactating mother may cause gynecomastia in a male infant and discussed alternative forms of birth control with the nurse.

1. In view of F. W.'s well-balanced diet, why did the physician prescribe a prenatal multivitamin?
2. What hazards are posed for the fetus if the mother employs tobacco or alcohol during pregnancy?
3. What risks are inherent in the use of tetracyclines during pregnancy?
4. Was the prescription of a thiazide diuretic for edema of pregnancy a reasonable approach? Why? Why did the nurse recommend bedrest and lying on the left side?
5. Which of the symptoms at 36 weeks of gestation were indicative of preeclampsia? What value was there in administering magnesium sulfate?
6. Why did the physician induce labor in this circumstance rather than allowing labor to develop naturally? How does oxytocin achieve this effect?
7. Why was naloxone administered to the infant immediately after birth?
8. Why was it important to continue to monitor F. W. closely after delivery?
9. What advantages might the nurse have cited for breast feeding? What should the nurse teach F. W. about use of drugs while breast-feeding?

Answers appear at the end of the book.

Recommended Readings

Aladin F: Interactions with oral contraceptives. *Continuing Practice* 1983;10(1):19–21.

Bartosch JC: Oral contraception: Selection and management. *Nurse Pract* 1983;8(5):56–63, 79.

Cefalo RC: Alcohol and birth defects — what every woman should know. *Drug Ther* 1983;13(4):179.

Cefalo RC: Drugs in pregnancy: Which to use and which to avoid. *Drug Ther* 1983;13(4):167.

Chan L, O'Malley BW: The mechanism of action of sex steroid hormones. *N Engl J Med* 1976;294:1322–1328.

Chapman JD: Dysmenorrhea: Changing concepts and therapies. *Mod Med* 1983;51(3):164.

Conner CS: Marijuana and alcohol use in pregnancy. *Drug Intell Clin Pharm* 1984;18:233–234.

Dickerson J: The pill: a closer look. *Am J Nurs* 1983;83:1392–1398.

Drill VA: Oral contraceptives: Relation to mammary cancer, benign breast lesions, and cervical cancer. *Annu Rev Pharmacol* 1975;15:367–385.

Findlay JWA: The distribution of some commonly used drugs in human breast milk. *Drug Metab Rev* 1983;14(4):653–684.

Gambrell RD Jr: Menopause: Benefits and risks of estrogen-progestogen replacement therapy. *Fertil Steril* 1982;37:457–474.

Hulka BS et al: Protection against endometrial carcinoma by combination-product oral contraceptives. *JAMA* 1982;247:475–477.

Iazzetta J: Low-dose oral contraceptives. *Continuing Practice* 1980;7(4):11–12.

Jordan VC: Biochemical pharmacology of antiestrogen action. *Pharmacol Rev* 1984;36:245–276.

Lawrence RA: *Breastfeeding: A guide for the medical profession* ed 2. St. Louis, CV Mosby, 1985.

Lindsay R et al: Long-term prevention of osteoporosis by estrogen. *Lancet* 1976;1:1038–1040.

Mann JI, Inman WHW: Oral contraceptives and death from myocardial infarction. *Br Med J* 1975;2:245–248.

Meade TW: Oral contraceptives: Clotting factors and thrombosis. *Am J Obstet Gynecol* 1982;142:758–761.

Mines A: Suppressing lactation in the non-nursing mother safely, comfortably, and knowledgeably. *Can Nurs* 1982;78(5):42–46.

Pearson L: Climacteric. *Am J Nurs* 1982;82(7):1098–1102.

Redmond MA: Couple-directed contraceptives counseling. *Can Nurse* 1982;78(8):38–39.

Siemens S, Brandzel RC: *Sexuality: Nursing assessment and intervention.* Philadelphia, JB Lippincott Co, 1982.

Stoehr GP, White J: Managing drug interactions with oral contraceptives. *J Obstet Gynecol Nurs* 1983;12(5):327–331.

Washington D: Helping the patient with vaginitis. *RN* 1984;47(9):63–69.

Weinstein MC: Estrogen use in postmenopausal women — costs, risks, benefits. *N Engl J Med* 1980;303(6):308–316.

Wentz AC: Assessment of estrogen and progestin therapy in gynecology and obstetrics. *Clin Obstet Gynecol* 1977;20(2):461–482.

Wicklund S: Special report: Drugs for two in pregnancy. *Am J Nurs* 1982;82(6):980–981.

Wicklund S: Special report: Drugs for two in lactation. *Am J Nurs* 1982;82(9):1428–1430.

Woods JS: Drug effects on human sexual behavior, in Woods NF (ed): *Human Sexuality in Health and Illness,* ed 3. St. Louis, CV Mosby, 1984.

Yen SS: Clinical applications of gonadotropin-releasing hormone and gonadotropin-releasing hormone analogs. *Fertil Steril* 1983;39:257–266.

Youngkin EQ, Miller LG: The triphasics: Insight for effective clinical use. *Nurse Pract* 1987;12(2):17–28.

CHAPTER 35

Drugs Acting on the Male Reproductive System

Male Reproductive Function

Spermatogenesis is the central event in the reproductive functioning of the male; the male sex act is the mechanism of delivery for the mature sperm cells. Spermatogenesis is closely linked to the activity of the male sex hormones. It occurs in the seminiferous tubules of the testes and is regulated by two hormones secreted by the anterior pituitary gland. **Follicle-stimulating hormone** (FSH) controls the initial production of spermatocytes; without FSH, spermatogenesis cannot occur. **Interstitial cell-stimulating hormone** (ICSH; known as luteinizing hormone (LH) in females) stimulates the interstitial cells of the testes to secrete testosterone. Sperm cells cannot mature without testosterone, so both anterior pituitary hormones are necessary to complete spermatogenesis. ICSH release is subject to feedback regulation by the sex hormones. Spermatogenesis normally begins between the ages of 10 and 13 years, at the onset of puberty.

Androgens

Androgens are produced in males in the testes and adrenals. Testosterone is the principal androgen in males and is secreted by the interstitial cells of the testes. The adrenal glands and the testes secrete small amounts of a variety of androgens, called 17-ketosteroids, which are less potent than testosterone. The adrenal glands produce about 10% of all androgens in the male, not enough to maintain masculine secondary sexual characteristics without the support of testicular androgens. Adult males produce about 2.5–11 mg of testosterone per day.

Androgens are responsible for the full set of changes that occur at puberty in males. Testosterone stimulates growth and darkening of the scrotum and penis; increased height, weight, and muscularization; and enlargement of the larynx (causing deepening of the voice). The skin becomes thick and oily under the influence of testosterone, but subcutaneous fat is lost. Changes in bodily hair occur: growth of pubic hair at the beginning of puberty, axillary hair and hair on the chest and limbs later, and finally growth of a beard, and in some individuals, recession of the hair line toward the end of puberty.

Testosterone also affects the testes themselves, not only after puberty but also in early fetal life. Testosterone secretion is somewhat elevated in utero and for a short time after birth, before dropping to low levels until puberty. Testosterone in this early stage of development is required for assumption of the male phenotype. Later, after puberty, testosterone is required for spermatogenesis and maturation of the sperm cells as they pass through the epididymis and vas deferens.

Testosterone is anabolic, which means that it produces a positive nitrogen balance, promoting tissue growth. The anabolic effect is more pronounced in those with low endogenous testosterone levels — women, boys, or hypogonadal men. Maximal doses of testosterone (25 mg/day) produce both anabolic effects and masculinization. Small doses (5 mg/day) produce little discernible masculinization but still produce one-half the anabolic action of higher doses. Synthetic anabolic steroids provide an even greater dissociation of these two actions, being 2–3 times more potent as anabolic agents than as androgens. Estrogens have anabolic effects qualitatively similar to those of testosterone, but less pronounced. Progesterone, by contrast, is weakly catabolic.

Testosterone is specifically responsible for the acne of puberty due to stimulation of sebaceous glands. Antiandrogens are currently being used to treat severe cases of acne. Estrogen is effective as well because of its feedback effect on the pituitary which ultimately leads to suppression of testosterone production by the ovaries or testes.

Sometimes secretion of androgens from the adrenal gland is excessive — a condition called **adrenal virilism.** It can be due to a congenital hyperplasia or it may be acquired. Acquired cases are due to adenomas, adenocarcinomas, or hyperplasias. It is more apparent when it occurs in women than in men. The symptoms include hirsutism, baldness, acne, deepening of the voice, increased muscularity, amenorrhea, clitoral hypertrophy, uterine atrophy, decreased breast size, and increased libido.

Disorders of the Male Reproductive System

The major disorders of male reproductive function include hypogonadism, precocious puberty, infertility, priapism, urethritis, scrotal masses, and tumors of the prostate gland and testes. The testes ordinarily conduct two functions: production of sperm in the seminiferous tubules and secretion of testosterone by the interstitial Leydig cells. **Hypogonadism** is a failure in either or both of these functions. Testosterone deficiency in the developing fetus results in the female phenotype while testosterone deficiency at puberty results in failure to develop the secondary male sexual characteristics. Hypogonadism can be caused genetically (for example, the presence of an extra X chromosome, called Klinefelter's syndrome) or by malnutrition, chronic disease, aging, renal failure, alcohol, lead poisoning, panhypopituitarism, or a specific deficiency in FSH and LH secretion. Boys with hypogonadism remain prepubescent until treated with gonadotropins (usually HCG) or testosterone.

Male **infertility** accounts for 40–50% of couples unable to conceive. It can be caused by impaired spermatogenesis (which occurs in hypogonadism, undescended testes, testicular atrophy, prolonged fever, exposure to radiation, heavy metal poisoning, or chronic use of glucocorticoids, testosterone, or marihuana), obstruction of the seminal tract (caused by vasectomy, congenital anomalies, or inflammations of the epididymis, prostate, urethra, seminal vesicles, or vas deferens), or inability to deliver the sperm into the vagina (which occurs in premature or retrograde ejaculation or impotence). The term *aspermia* is used to indicate an absence of ejaculate whereas *azoospermia* is an absence of sperm in the semen. Oligospermia is a condition of low sperm count; counts less than 20 million/ml decrease the likelihood of fertilization. Sperm cells may also exhibit diminished motility or viability.

Priapism is occurrence of painful, persistent erections associated with sexual urgency. It can be caused by drugs such as prazocin (Minipress) and trazodone (Desyrel), and with initiation of testosterone treatment for hypogonadism. Other causes include pelvic vascular thrombosis, leukemia, sickle cell disease, pelvic hematoma or neoplasm, or infections of the male genital tract. Infections of the male genital tract such as **urethritis, prostatitis,** and **epididymitis,** are most commonly due to gram-negative bacteria or sexually transmitted pathogens. Antimicrobial therapy is indicated. **Scrotal masses** may be due to inflammation of the epididymis (epididymitis) or testes (orchitis), trauma involving the scrotal contents, or testicular neoplasms. **Testicular tumors** are usually malignant and require orchiectomy. It is the most common type of solid tumor in males under 30. **Prostate tumors,** on the other hand, account for the majority of malignancies in men over 65. Prostate tumors are almost always adenocarcinomas. Prostatectomy or radiation therapy can cure many early and localized prostate cancers. More advanced prostate cancers can be managed by administration of high doses of estrogen.

Androgenic and Anabolic Drugs

Pharmacokinetics Testosterone injected in an oil solution or taken orally is well absorbed but metabolized so quickly by the liver as to be ineffective. Esters of testosterone, much less polar and more gradually metabolized, can be employed by intramuscular injection in oil. The propionate ester is gradually absorbed over 2–3 days; the cyprionate and enanthate esters over 1–2 weeks. Testosterone pellets are available for implantation and provide steady absorption for up to 6–8 months.

Once absorbed, testosterone is transported in the blood bound 99% to sex hormone-binding globulin (SHBG), which it shares with estradiol, and other plasma proteins (Figure 35–1). The small amount of free testosterone provides the physiological activity and exhibits a half-life of 10–20 minutes. Testosterone is metabolized mainly in the liver and ultimately is excreted in the urine (>90%) and in the bile. The esters of testosterone are eliminated in a similar fashion. The synaptic androgenic and anabolic steroids are metabolized more slowly. Be-

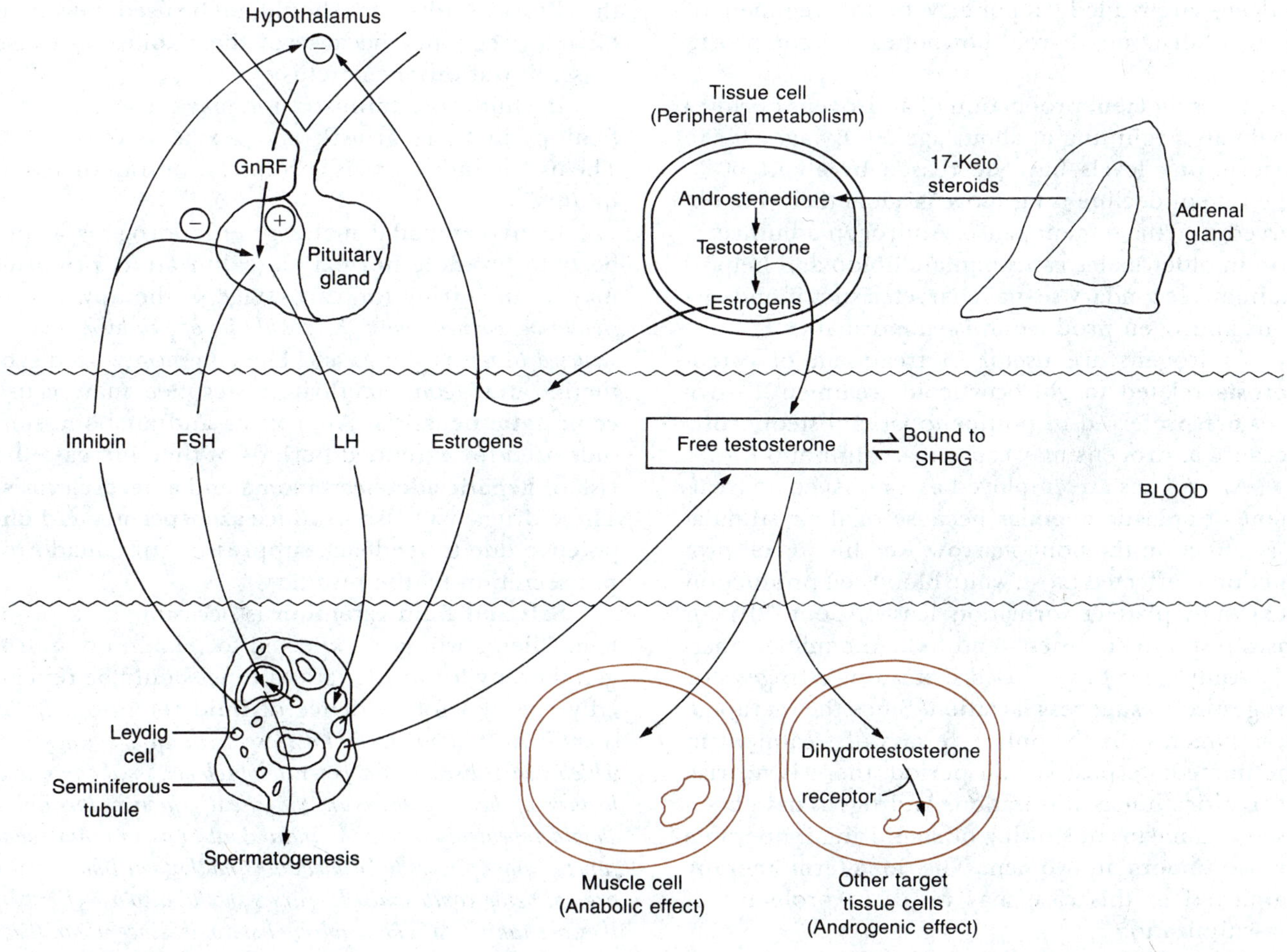

Figure 35–1

Mechanisms of anabolic and androgenic steroids: follicle stimulating hormone (FSH); gonadotropin releasing factor (Gn RF); luteinizing hormone (LH); sex hormone binding globulin (SHBG).

cause testosterone is inactivated mainly in the liver, clients who have severe liver damage should not receive the drug.

Clinical Indications Therapy with androgens is indicated mainly for hypogonadism in males, including eunuchism or eunuchoidism, postpuberal cryptorchidism, impotency due to inadequate androgen production, oligospermia, panhypopituitarism (together with other hormones), and delayed puberty. In females, androgens are used to inhibit lactation or to treat breast engorgement.

In **delayed puberty,** androgens are given in 4–6 month courses with similar periods of interrupted therapy. Smaller doses are used during the first year and full doses thereafter. If the deficiency of endogenous androgen production is complete, intramuscular dosage forms will be required; if endogenous production is present but insufficient, oral forms may be satisfactory. In panhypopituitarism in males, androgens are added at puberty to the regimen of growth hormone, thyroid hormone, and glucocorticoids.

In **aging men,** production of androgens declines gradually beginning at about age 50. By age 80–90, testosterone levels have decreased by about 60%. The rate of decline is far more gradual than that observed in female menopause. Androgen administration in older males can stimulate libido and help to maintain secondary sexual characteristics if endogenous androgen production is subnormal.

Androgens are useful in treatment of **osteoporosis** related to glucocorticoid treatment. Estrogens are preferred in postmenopausal osteoporosis because androgens may cause masculinization.

Androgens are employed as a nonspecific treatment of **aplastic anemias** because of their stimulatory effect on the bone marrow. Red blood cell production is effected most, white blood cell production next, and platelet formation least. About 50% of cases respond and these tend to be the milder ones.

Androgens can be used instead of estrogens or progestins to **suppress lactation.** Since the therapeutic regimen calls for only 1–5 days of treatment in the immediate postpartum period, there is no risk of significant masculinization. Androgens have been used as a means of slowing or stabilizing inoperable **breast tumors** in women. The long-term therapy employed in this case may result in problems of masculinization.

Anabolic steroids are synthetic drugs that produce somewhat more of the anabolic effects of testosterone than the androgenic effects. The specificity of action is incomplete, but some produce no discernible masculinization at doses that produce significant anabolic activity. Anabolic steroids are used to promote a **positive nitrogen balance** that will facilitate weight gain and tissue repair. They have been used during postoperative recuperation, chronic debilitating diseases, and in body-building programs for athletes. Anabolic steroids and androgenic agents should never be used without close supervision by a medically trained person. The National Collegiate Athletic Association (NCAA) is examining measures, such as random drug testing at championship events, aimed at eliminating use of anabolic steroids by athletes seeking to add muscle mass and weight.

Adverse Effects and Contraindications When used in women, **masculinization** may occur. Indications of this include acne, growth of facial hair, deepening of the voice, excessive body hair, increased musculature, balding, and hypertrophy of the clitoris. Androgens should not be used in women during pregnancy because of their ability to cause masculinization of the fetus.

In children, administration may cause major difficulties in bone growth and sexual development. The use of androgens is absolutely contraindicted in infants.

In hypogonadal males given androgens at puberty to promote normal masculinization, **priapism** may occur during the early stage of therapy. *Clients should be warned about the possibility of priapism and instructed to report if it occurs.* The commonly used synthetic androgen, methyltestosterone, may cause **cholestatic hepatitis.** Androgens and anabolic steroids used for extended periods of time increase the risk of **hepatic adenocarcinoma** and **atherosclerosis.** These drugs may also produce **azoospermia** and **impotence** due to feedback suppression of gonadotropin secretion by the pituitary.

Salt and fluid retention is occasionally a problem. Clients who are expected to remain on androgen therapy for any length of time should be repeatedly checked for evidence of fluid retention. *If the client has a history of renal disease, is in an age bracket in which heart disease is a potential problem, or if there is a history of heart disease in the client's family, the nurse should repeatedly assess the individual to assure that renal functioning appears to be adequate and that cardiac reserves are not being compromised. Nurses should also ask clients if they are taking ACTH or adrenal steroids, since use of these agents concomitantly with androgens can result in increased edema.*

Serum calcium, serum chloride, serum creatinine, blood glucose, hematocrit, serum potassium,

Nursing Observations for Male Hormone Therapy

THERAPEUTIC GOAL	Stimulation of sexual development in hypogonadal boys, maintenance of sexual potency in older males, palliative therapy of metastatic carcinomas in women, erythropoiesis in aplastic anemias, or more rapid recuperation from surgery.
PREADMINISTRATION ASSESSMENT	
Baseline Data	Evaluate blood pressure, pulse, heart sounds, respiration, neurological status, genitourinary function, size of prostate, hair distribution, and skin texture. Obtain laboratory tests including serum electrolytes (including calcium in women), coagulation, blood cells, and liver function.
Contraindications/ Precautions	Prostatic cancer or hypertrophy, breast cancer in a male, pregnancy, diabetes, hepatic or renal dysfunction, or coronary artery disese. Check for history of allergies to anabolic steroids or tartrazine (found in certain preparations).
Potential Interactions	Check medication history for interacting drugs including anticoagulants, hypoglycemic agents, and mineralocorticoids.
EVALUATION OF DRUG RESPONSE	
For Therapeutic Benefit	Changes in sexual function, tumor regression, increased erythropoiesis, increased tissue mass.
For Adverse Effects	Monitor increased libido, weight gain, edema and bloating, masculinization in females (growth of facial hair, deepening of voice, acne, clitoral hypertrophy, male pattern baldness), precocious sexual development in prepubertal boys, prostate enlargement in men, liver dysfunction, electrolyte imbalances, and hypoglycemia.
For Drug Interactions	Monitor for additive hypoglycemia when anabolic steroids are used together with insulin or oral hypoglycemics; potentiation of oral anticoagulants; additive fluid retention with agents having mineralocorticoid activity.
For Dietary Interactions	Monitor for increased dietary requirements to support anabolic activity.
For Effects on Laboratory Tests	Changes in thyroid function, glucose tolerance, and coagulation tests.
For Compliance	Evaluate client's compliance with all facets of the therapeutic regimen by careful observation, interviewing, and review of progress. Report compliance problems to the physician and act as client-advocate when changes in the therapeutic regimen seem indicated.

and plasma-bound iodide (PBI) may be increased. Serum samples to detect such changes and urine samples for measurement of 17-ketosteroids should be performed periodically to detect evidence of change. **Hypercalcemia** may occur, in which event the drug should be discontinued. Symptoms suggesting possible hypercalcemia include thirst, polyuria, weakness, or constipation.

Anabolic steroids may contain tartrazine, a substance to which some individuals are allergic. Such individuals are usually also allergic to aspirin. *The nursing assessment of clients who are to be given androgens should include a history concerning allergic responses to aspirin.*

Drug Interactions Androgens and anabolic steroids may increase the effect of oral anticoagulants by inhibiting their metabolism. *Clients receiving oral anticoagulants and androgens should be instructed to report any indications of bleeding.* Androgens may increase serum levels of phenylbutazone and oxyphenbutazone, necessitating dosage reduction when these nonsteroidal anti-inflammatory drugs are employed.

Anabolic steroids may lower blood glucose levels in diabetic clients, enhancing the hypoglycemic effects of oral hypoglycemic agents and insulin. *Nurses should caution these clients that they may be experiencing a hypoglycemic reaction if anabolic steroids make them feel shaky or irritable. Clients should report such reac-*

tions to their physician and may need to adjust the dose of insulin or oral hypoglycemic agent.

Preparations and Administration Testosterone is too short-acting for most purposes. Testosterone pellets provide extended activity but dosage regulation is less flexible with this method.

With methyltestosterone, absorption through the buccal mucosa is twice as efficient as gastrointestinal absorption. *Buccal tablets are placed in the upper or lower buccal pouch, between the cheek and gum. The client should be instructed not to chew or swallow the tablet or to eat, drink, or smoke until the tablet is fully absorbed (at least 60 minutes). Conscientious oral hygiene and rotation of the site of application within the buccal cavity will help to reduce the local irritation to the cheek or gums.*

Some clients will experience gastric irritation from anabolic steroids. *Advising clients to take their medication with food or after meals may decrease the extent of gastric irritation and promote client compliance with the prescribed regimen.*

ANDROGENIC STEROIDS

Testosterone
Aqueous suspension for injection, testosterone pellets (Oreton)
Recommended Doses: Two to six pellets implanted to provide 150–450 mg of testosterone per day for 3–4 months.

Testosterone enanthate (numerous tradenames)
Oil suspension for injection
Recommended Doses: 200 mg once every 2–4 weeks by deep IM injection.

Testosterone cyprionate (numerous tradenames)
Oil suspension for injection
Recommended Doses: 200 mg once every 2–4 weeks by deep IM injection.

Testosterone propionate (Testex and generic)
Oil suspension for injection, buccal tablets
Recommended Doses: 25 mg IM, 3 times weekly. Doses for buccal tablets are the same as for methyltestosterone.

Nursing Diagnoses and Interventions for Male Hormone Therapy

Nursing Diagnoses	*Related Interventions*
TO ENHANCE DRUG BENEFITS OR REDUCE DRUG REQUIREMENTS	
Alterations in self-concept in young males related to eunuchism or in older males related to loss of sexual potency	Provide support and encouragement required to cope with changes in sexual functioning
TO MINIMIZE DRUG SIDE EFFECTS OR INTERACTIONS	
Alterations in cardiac output caused by androgens	Monitor for edema and report any indications to the physician.
Alterations in self-concept in females related to masculinization	Provide support and encouragement required to cope with changes in sexual characteristics.
Sexual dysfunction related to disorder or to inappropriate use of anabolic steroids	Discourage use of anabolic steroids for body-building purposes; efficacy is not established, most athletic agencies disapprove of their use, and the practice poses hazards for the athlete.
TO ENSURE SAFE AND EFFICACIOUS DRUG USE	
Knowledge deficit related to drug regimen	Teach the client about the effects of the drug, rationale for its use, and proper administration. Provide the client with a list of side effects, precautions, and potential drug interactions. Advise against the use of anabolic steroids for body-building purposes.

Fluoxymesterone (Halotestin, Ora-Testryl, Android-F, and generic)
Tablets
Recommended Doses: For hypogonadism, delayed puberty, impotence due to testicular deficiency, male climacteric, or breast engorgement, 2–10 mg PO daily. Larger doses are required for inoperable carcinoma.

Methyltestosterone (numerous tradenames)
Tablets, capsules, timed release capsules, buccal tablets
Recommended Doses: For hypogonadism or male climacteric, 10–40 mg orally or 5–20 buccally. For suppression of lactation, 80 mg orally or 40 mg buccally daily for 3–5 days. For postpuberal cryptorchidism, 30 mg orally (or 15 mg buccally) daily. For palliative treatment of breast cancer, 200 mg daily orally or 100 mg buccally.

ANABOLIC STEROIDS

Ethylestrenol (Maxibolin)
Tablets
Recommended Doses: For mild catabolism in adults, 4 mg/day PO. For severe catabolism, 6–8 mg/day PO initially, reduced to 4 mg/day when improvement is discernible. For children, 1–3 mg/day PO (2 mg/day is typical). Discontinue use in children at least 6 months before chronologic age for bone maturation.

Methandrostenolone (Dianabol)
Tablets
Recommended Doses: For senile and postmenopausal osteoporosis, 5 mg/day PO initially; 2.5–5.0 mg/day maintenance.

Nandrolone decanoate
Oil suspension
Recommended Doses: For anemia of renal insufficiency, in women, 50–100 mg/week IM; in men, 100–200 mg/week IM; in children 2–13 years of age, 25–50 mg every 3–4 weeks IM.

Nandrolone phenpropionate (numerous tradenames)
Oil suspension
Recommended Doses: For metastatic breast cancer, 50–100 mg IM weekly.

Oxandrolone (Anavar)
Tablets
Recommended Doses: For weight gain, relief of bone pain in osteoporosis, or to offset protein catabolism, in adults, 2.5 mg PO, 2–4 times daily for 2–4 weeks; in children, 0.25 mg/kg/day PO.

Oxymetholone (Adroyd and Anadrol)
Tablets
Recommended Doses: For anemias, 1–5 mg/kg/day PO (1–2 mg/kg/day is usual) for at least 3–6 months.

Stanozolol (Winstrol)
Tablets
Recommended Doses: For hereditary angioedema, 2 mg PO tid, initially; reduced gradually after response to a maintenance dose of 2 mg/day.

Important Implications for Androgenic and Anabolic Steroids

- ☐ Review the client's history for conditions that are cautions for use of androgens, including prostatic hypertrophy, hypertension, cardiovascular or renal disease, acne, or allergies to aspirin.
- ☐ Androgens should not be given to women who are pregnant or lactating or to men who have cancer of the prostate or breast.
- ☐ Review the client's current medications for possible interacting drugs such as oral anticoagulants, antidiabetic medications, or phenylbutazone.
- ☐ Instruct clients receiving androgenic and anabolic steroids to monitor their blood pressure and weight and to restrict their dietary intake of sodium.
- ☐ Teach the client the symptoms that may indicate hypercalcemia.
- ☐ Fully apprise females taking androgenic agents of the possible virilizing influences of these drugs and caution them to report such symptoms immediately.
- ☐ Advise male clients that long-term use of androgenic and anabolic drugs may result in irreversible impotence.
- ☐ Instruct clients to watch for changes in color of the skin or sclera or occurrence of pruritus since these symptoms may indicate liver dysfunction resulting from androgen therapy.
- ☐ Warn individuals using anabolic steroids in body-building programs that there is a significant potential for adverse effects and that there is no substantial evidence that these drugs increase athletic performance.

Antiandrogenic Drugs

Antiandrogenic drugs are being developed for possible use in treatment of cancer of the prostate, virilization in women, precocious puberty in boys, acne, and as male contraceptives. Estrogens and progesterone are antiandrogenic but rather weakly so and without sufficient specificity. More specific agents are under development and one, cyproterone acetate, is available for clinical use. **Cyproterone acetate** is a potent antiandrogen but also possesses progestogenic properties and suppresses gonadotropin secretion by the pituitary. In animal studies, it has been shown capable of producing atrophy of tissues normally stimulated by androgens such as the seminal vesicles and prostate. At high doses, the Leydig cells are suppressed, inhibiting spermatogenesis. In humans, antiandrogens have been used in males with sexually deviant behavior patterns (paraphilias) as a kind of chemical castration. Loss of libido occurs, but gynecomastia does not. Cyproterone has been used with success in hirsutism and virilization in women, and in acne and baldness in men and women. It has also been used in precocious puberty, but there is a risk of suppressing the anabolic as well as the androgenic effects of testosterone, thus impairing growth. Cyproterone has shown promise in clinical trials for treatment of prostate carcinomas.

Male Contraceptives

As of yet, there are no satisfactory male contraceptives. The ideal drug would provide reversible but complete suppression of spermatogenesis without interfering with testosterone production. It would also be convenient and nontoxic. Antiandrogens inhibit spermatogenesis only at doses that markedly suppress testosterone secretion, inhibiting libido. Estrogens are effective because they suppress gonadotropin secretion, but both spermatogenesis and testosterone secretion is suppressed. Libido and potency are diministed and gynecomastia often occurs. Moderate to high doses of exogenous androgens suppress spermatogenesis by inhibiting gonadotropin release, but there is a potential for such side effects as jaundice, edema, and elevated blood cholesterol. The most promising possibility at this time is a combination of an androgen and a progestin. The progestin suppresses gonadotropin release and the androgen replaces endogenous androgen production. This combination can produce inhibition of spermatogenesis with minimal side effects. Treatment must be undertaken for several months before sterility occurs because of the lag time between sperm production and its delivery to the seminal vesicle.

Drugs and Male Sexuality

The sex act in males is initiated by excitatory stimuli of either a tactile or psychic nature. Specialized sensory end-organs are located in the glans penis, scrotum, other perineal areas, the vas deferens, testes, and prostate gland. When the combination of tactile and psychic stimuli is adequate, erection occurs. Stimulation of parasympathetic nerves causes dilation of arterioles, while inhibition of sympathetic nerves causes venous constriction in the erectile tissue of the penis, resulting in congestion of blood and erection. Lubrication is achieved by parasympathetically innervated glands of the urethra. Semen then forms in the urethra when peristaltic contractions of the testes, epididymis, and vas deferens expel sperm cells (spermatozoa) and the seminal vesicles and prostate gland secrete their fluids. Rhythmical impulses to the muscles encircling the base of the erect penis then cause waves of pressure to pass along the penis and eject the semen.

Disorders of male sexuality include inhibited sexual desire, erectile impotence, ejaculatory impotence, premature ejaculation, and sexual anhedonia. **Inhibited sexual desire** may be lifelong or short-term and is due to the same causes as in women: childhood emotional trauma, depression, boredom, use of drugs that suppress libido, or sexual repression. **Erectile impotence** is the inability to sustain an erection for a sufficient time to enable coitus. Since failure to sustain an erection occurs occasionally in many men, erectile dysfunction is considered present only if it occurs in 25% or more of sexual encounters. Physical factors are frequently involved, including diabetes mellitus, syphilis, dependence on alcohol, narcotics, or other drugs, hypopituitarism, hypothyroidism, spinal cord lesions, multiple sclerosis, stroke, aortic aneurysm, and sometimes prostatectomy or castration. Psychological factors are likely if erectile dysfunction is situational, but these may be superimposed on physical factors. Counseling may alleviate psychic factors. If hypopituitarism is the major factor, human chorionic gonadotropin and testosterone may be helpful.

Ejaculatory impotence, or inhibited orgasm, is usually psychogenic, but it can be secondary to diabetes mellitus, multiple sclerosis, or use of certain drugs. **Retrograde ejaculation** occurs in nearly all men who have had prostatectomies and may accompany use of amphetamine, antihypertensives, neuroleptics, and benzodiazepines. **Premature ejaculation** is defined as ejaculation sooner than desired or so quickly after intromission as to leave the female partner unsatisfied. Controlled stimulation or more frequent orgasms may ameliorate this difficulty. **Sexual anhedonia** is a rare condition in which erection and ejaculation occur normally but without pleasure during orgasm.

A variety of diseases are transmitted sexually (Appendix Table). Sexually transmitted diseases are the most common communicable diseases in the world, and the rate is increasing. The five age-old venereal diseases — syphilis, gonorrhea, chancroid, lymphogranuloma venereum, and granuloma inguinale — are no longer as prevalent as the more recently recognized entities: nonspecific urethritis, candidiasis, herpes, acquired immune deficiency syndrome (AIDS), chlamydial infections, trichomoniasis, lice, mites, and genital warts. Nevertheless, gonorrhea still afflicts 250 million and syphilis 50 million people annually around the world. In the United States, gonorrhea occurs in 3 million people annually and syphilis in about 0.4 million.

Drug Effects on Male Sexual Functioning

Yohimbine, an α_2-adrenergic blocking agent, has been employed successfully in treating erectile impotence in males, especially in instances associated with diabetes and vascular problems, but the drug has no FDA sanctioned indications. Yohimbine promotes erection by increasing penile blood inflow and decreasing penile blood outflow. It has no effect on libido. Its use is contraindicated in clients with renal disease or hypersensitivity to yohimbine. This drug should not be employed by clients receiving antidepressants because it has a stimulating action on mood. Yohimbine has a mild stimulatory influence on release of antidiuretic hormone and may therefore cause fluid retention and mild hypertension.

Yohimbine (Yocon, Yohimex, and generic formulations)
Tablets
Experimental Doses: For impotence, 5.4 mg PO, 3 times daily.

Many drugs adversely affect male sexual functioning (Table 35–1). Some drugs act on the central nervous system to alter libido; others impair autonomic regulation of the sex act per se. Central nervous system depressants, including alcohol, barbiturates, other sedative-hypnotics, and narcotics, tend to depress sexual function by depressing CNS centers. Narcotics depress libido as well as performance. Alcohol and sedatives may increase sexual interest as a result of disinhibition effects, but sexual performance is impaired. Anticholinergic drugs interfere with the parasympathetic aspects of sexual behavior (i.e., erection), while adrenergic blockers prevent sympathetic aspects (i.e., ejaculation). Certain neuroleptics, notably thioridazine and haloperidol, and tricyclic antidepressants may produce impotence.

Table 35–1
Drug Effects on Male Sexual Functioning

Drug	Libido	Erection	Ejaculation
Androgens	↑	↑	↓
Antiandrogens	↓	0	0
Anticoagulant			
Heparin	0	P	0
Antihypertensives			
Alpha-blockers	0	P	↓
Beta-blockers	↓	0	↓
Clonidine	0	↓	0
Ganglionic blockers	0	↓	↓
Guanethidine	0	P	↓
Hydralazine	0	P	0
Methyldopa	↓	0	↓
Reserpine	↓	0	↓
Antimicrobial drugs			
Metronidazole	↓	0	0
Antiulcer drugs			
Antimuscarinics	0	↓	↓
Cimetidine	↑↓	0	↓
Estrogens/progestins	↓	0	0
Psychotropics			
Alcohol	0↑	↓P	0
Amphetamine (acute)	0↑	0	0
Amphetamine (chronic)	↓	0	↓R
Antiepileptics			
Carbamazepine	0	↓	↓
Clonazepam	↑	0	0
Primidone	0	↓	↓
Succinimides	↑	0	0
Antihistamines	0	↓	0
Antipsychotics			
Chlorpromazine	↓	P	↓
Haloperidol	↓	0	↓R
Thioridazine	↓	P	↓R
Benzodiazepines	↑↓	0	↓R
Cannabis	↑↓	0↓P	0↓
Cocaine (acute)	0↑	0	↓
Cocaine (chronic)	↓	↓	↓
Fenfluramine	↑↓	0	↓
Levodopa	↑	0	0
Lithium	0	0↓	0
MAO inhibitors	0	0	↓
Narcotics (chronic)	↓	↓	↓
Trazodone	0↓	P	0
Tricyclic antidepressants	0↓	↓	0
Urinary tract spasmolytic			
Oxybutynin	0	0	↓

Key: 0 = no change; ↑ = increased; ↓= decreased; R = may cause retrograde ejaculation; P = may cause priapism.

Estrogen therapy in males (for prostate cancer) depresses libido. Androgens, on the other hand, stimulate sexual interest in both sexes. Testosterone also suppresses testicular function by feedback suppression of gonadotropins. Acutely, stimulants such as amphetamine, cocaine, and levodopa, and psychedelics such as lysergic acid diethylamide (LSD), mescaline, and marihuana enhance libido and perceived intensity of orgasm but may have stimulatory or inhibitory effects on sexual performance, including both erection and ejaculation. Parachlorophenylalanine, an experimental drug that depletes brain serotonin, reportedly stimulates libido. A variety of drugs produce priapism (Table 35-1) or gynecomastia (Table 35-2) in males.

Table 35-2
Drugs Causing Gynecomastia in Males

Androgens	Ethionamide
Anorexics	Griseofulvin
Antipsychotic drugs	Meprobamate
Bisulfan	Methyldopa
Cardiac glycosides	Narcotics
Chlortetracycline	Reserpine
Cimetidine	Spironolactone
Chorionic gonadotropin	Tricyclic antidepressants
Estrogens	Vitamin D_2

Case Study: Abuse of Anabolic Steroids

R. W. was a 21-year-old college student and member of the intercollegiate wrestling team. He came to the University Health Services because of symptoms of influenza. While he was being examined by the nurse, R. W. asked her if she knew anything about anabolic steroids: if they worked and if they caused any problems.

The nurse told R. W. that she had recently participated on a university committee reviewing the use of drugs by athletes and that anabolic steroids had been one of the problem areas discussed. She had therefore had a recent opportunity to review relevant literature concerning these drugs. She told R. W. that there is a lack of substantial evidence that anabolic steroids improve performance in athletic activities. These drugs do promote an increase in muscle mass, but only when employed in substantial doses over a period of time. She pointed out that when used in large enough doses and for periods of time sufficient to influence muscle mass, anabolic steroids produce a number of adverse effects. For example, in men these drugs can alter sexual and reproductive function. They interfere with formation of sperm cells and, if taken for long periods of time, may cause irreversible impotence. Anabolic steroids also tend to cause salt and water retention. Some of the synthetic anabolic agents can cause liver problems, such as jaundice. R. W. thanked the nurse for the information.

1. What is the policy of the NCAA regarding use of performance-enhancing drugs by athletes competing in intercollegiate sports?
2. What additional adverse effects occur when androgens are employed by women or prepubertal boys?

Answers appear at the end of the book.

Recommended Readings

Lamb DR: Anabolic steroids: How well do they work and how dangerous are they? *Am J Sports Med* 1984;12(1):31–38.

Lipsett MB: Use and abuse of androgens. *Consultant* 1980;20:146.

Marks R, Fuentes R, Rosenberg J: How drugs can change fertility. *RN* 1983;46:61–63.

Neumann F: Pharmacology and clinical use of antiandrogens: A short review. *Ir J Med Sci* 1982;15:61–70.

Pardridge WM et al: Androgens and sexual behavior. *Ann Intern Med* 1982;96:488–501.

Shahadi NT: Anabolic androgenic hormones. *Am J Med* 1977;62:546–548.

Siemens S, Brandzel RC: *Sexuality; Nursing assessment and intervention.* Philadelphia, JB Lippincott Co, 1982.

Smith MC: Drugs and sports. *US Pharmacist* 1977; (May): 75–76.

Wartofsky L: Guidelines for the treatment of hyperthyroidism. *Am Fam Physician* 1984;30(1):198–210.

Wilson JD, Griffin JE: Use and misuse of androgens. *Metabolism* 1980;29:1278–1295.

Woods JS: Drug effects on human sexual behavior, in Woods NF (ed): *Human Sexuality in health and illness,* ed 3. St Louis, CV Mosby, 1984.

Appendix
Sexually Transmitted Diseases

Condition	Cause	Predisposing factors	Symptoms	Treatment
Acquired immune deficiency syndrome (AIDS)	Exposure to AIDS virus	Frequent homosexual encounters among males in the United States Blood transfusions Haitian refugees Hemophilia A Parenteral drug abuse; use of volatile nitrites	T-cell immune deficiency	No cure or vaccine; zidovudine (AZT, Retrovir) to delay progression
Balanoposthitis/balanitis (if circumcised)	Often a complication of gonorrhea, syphilis, trichomoniasis, or candidiasis. Can be caused by tight prepuce. May be a drug eruption.	Diabetes mellitus	Inflammation of the glans penis and prepuce	Treat underlying cause
Candidiasis	*Candida albicans* (a yeast organism)	Use of oral contraceptives or broad-spectrum antibiotics; pregnancy; diabetes mellitus; pernicious anemia; corticosteroids; immunosuppressives	Vaginitis and vulvar pruritis; leukorrhea; males are usually asymptomatic carriers but may experience balanoposthitis	Female: Nystatin (14 days), clotrimazole (7 days), or miconazole (7 days) as vaginal gel, cream, or tablets. Male: Nystatin cream on prepuce.
Chancroid	*Hemophilus ducreyi* (a gram-negative bacillus)	None	Genital ulcers and swollen lymph nodes in groin	Sulfonamides (10–14 days)
Gonorrhea	*Neisseria gonorrhoeae*	None	Men: creamy yellow discharge; burning sensation on urination; lips of meatus red and swollen; epididymitis Women: often unnoticed; dysuria and vaginitis; salpingitis	Procaine penicillin G (one dose, 4.8 million units, IM); ampicillin and probenecid (3.5 g orally); or tetracycline (500 mg orally, qid for 5 days
Granuloma inguinale	*Donovania granulomatis* (gram-negative bacillus)	Mostly in tropical or subtropical areas	Red nodule progressing to granulomatous mass on penis, scrotum, groin, or thighs of males; vulva, vagina, or perineum of females; anus and buttocks in male homosexuals	Streptomycin or tetracyclines
Herpes simplex	Herpes simplex virus, mainly type 2	None	Painful, itchy lesions; flu-like symptoms; dysuria	Acyclovir for initial infections. No cure for recurrent infections. Lesions should be kept clean and normal saline applied twice daily
Lymphogranuloma venereum	Chlamydia	Mostly in tropical or subtropical areas	Genital lesions followed by lymphangitis	Tetracycline

(continued)

Sexually Transmitted Diseases (*continued*)

Condition	Cause	Predisposing factors	Symptoms	Treatment
Pediculosis	Phthrius pubis (crab lice)	None	Intense pruritus over pubic/genital area; lice ova on pubic hair	Gamma benzene hexachloride (Kwell) lotion, cream, or shampoo applied to pubic area; sterilize all sheets and towels
Proctitis	Rectal gonorrhea, candidiasis, syphilis, or genital warts	None	Inflammation of rectal mucosa; anal discharge	Treat underlying cause
Scabies	Sarcoptes scabieri (mites)	None	Intense pruritis in genital areas	Gamma benzene hexachloride (Kwell) or Crotamiton (Eurax) applied to entire body
Syphilis	*Treponema pallidum*	Promiscuous male homosexuals at greatest risk; congenital transmission from infected mother to fetus.	Stage I: painless red papules on genitals Stage II: skin rash, lymphangitis; flu-like symptoms Stage III: internal and external ulcerations, arthritis, cardiovascular syphilis; neurosyphilis	Penicillin G (600,000 units IM for 8–10 days) Benzathine penicillin G (Bicillin) (2.4 million units IM) Erythromycin (500 mg orally, qid for 20 days)
Trichomoniasis	Trichomonas (protozoa)	Gonorrhea	Women: vaginitis with vulvar pruritus; yellow-green frothy discharge; dysuria Males: asymptomatic carriers or urethral discharge; dysuria	Metronidazole (Flagyl) (250 mg orally tid) for 7–10 days
Urethritis — nongonococcal	*Chlamydia trachomatis;* ureaplasma urealyticum; others	None	Women: usually asymptomatic; occasionally, vaginal discharge, mild dysuria, pelvic pain, proctitis Men: mild dysuria, mucopurulent discharge, red meatus, proctitis	Tetracycline (500 mg orally qid) for 7–14 days
Vaginitis (nonspecific) (see also trichomonas and candidiasis)	*Haemophilus vaginalis* *Corynebacterium vaginalis* *Gardnerella vaginalis*	Frequent douching, poor hygiene, snug underwear, postmenopausal atrophy, pregnancy, diabetes mellitus	Leukorrhea	Metronidazole (Flagyl) Cephalosporins Ampicillin Tetracycline (oral for 5 days) Oxytetracycline (vaginal suppository, 7–14 days) Sulfonamides (topical) if due to *H. vaginalis*
Warts, genital	Papilloma virus	Poor hygiene	Soft, moist red swellings in moist areas such as subpreputial area, urethral meatus, shaft of penis, vulva, vaginal wall, cervix, perineum, perianal region, and rectum	25% podophyllum applied to warts

UNIT VI

Drugs and the Cardiovascular System

CHAPTER 36

Introduction to Cardiovascular Pharmacology

This unit covers six aspects of the physiology and pharmacology of the cardiovascular system. Chapter 36 reviews the physiology of normal cardiovascular functioning, a necessary foundation for understanding cardiovascular disorders and the role of drugs in their treatment. In Chapter 37, the **mechanical function** of cardiac muscle is reviewed, together with the disorder associated with impaired contractility (congestive heart failure) and the drugs used to enhance contractility (the cardiac glycosides). The **electrophysiological function** of the heart is next considered, along with dysrhythmias and antidysrhythmic drugs, in Chapter 38. The **hemodynamics** of the cardiovascular system — the integrated physiology of the heart, blood vessels, and regulatory systems — set the stage in Chapter 39 for examination of hypertension and antihypertensive drugs. Chapter 40 considers the **coronary blood supply** and the clinical characteristics and treatment of ischemic heart disease. Finally, in Chapter 41, the physiology of the blood, **hematology,** provides the background for studying coagulation and anticoagulant drugs as well as the red blood cells, anemia, and related drugs.

General Anatomy and Physiology of the Heart and Circulatory System

The Cycle of Blood Flow

The heart consists of two pumps. The right side of the heart pumps blood to the lungs, where the blood receives oxygen before returning to the left side of the heart. The left side of the heart pumps this oxygenated blood to the peripheral tissues via the systemic arteries. After supplying the tissues with oxygen and nutrients and collecting tissue waste products, the blood returns to the right side of the heart to begin the cycle anew.

Cardiac output is equal to stroke volume (the amount of blood ejected with each beat) times the heart rate (number of beats per minute). Ordinarily cardiac output is about 5,040 ml of blood per minute for adults. The output depends on venous return, cardiac rate, and strength of contraction.

The Cardiac Chambers

The heart has four chambers (Figure 36–1), the left and right atria and the left and right ventricles. The right atrium receives the systemic venous blood returning through the superior vena cava (from the upper extremities) and the inferior vena cava (from the lower extremities). It passes the blood along to the right ventricle during diastole (the period when the muscle is relaxed) and contracts to provide a final surge of ventricular filling. The tricuspid valves, lying between the right atrium and right ventricle, permit blood to flow from the atrium into the ventricle during atrial contraction (diastole) but prevent it from flowing back into the atrium during ventricular contraction (systole). The right ventricle contracts, pumping blood into the pulmonary arteries, left and right, through the open pulmonary valves, which then close at the end of the ventricular contraction (systole). After the blood has passed through the pulmonary capillary beds, it returns, freshly oxygenated, via the two left and two right pulmonary veins, to the left atrium. When the left atrium contracts, blood is forced through the mitral valve into the left ventricle. Contraction of the left ventricle forces the mitral valve closed (preventing backflow to the atrium) and pumps blood into the systemic arterial circulation through the aortic valve into the aorta.

The walls of the cardiac chambers consist of three layers: the epicardium, the myocardium, and the endocardium. The epicardium is a thin external membrane. It overlies the myocardium, a thick middle layer composed of muscle fibers that provide the mechanical function of the heart. The inner layer is

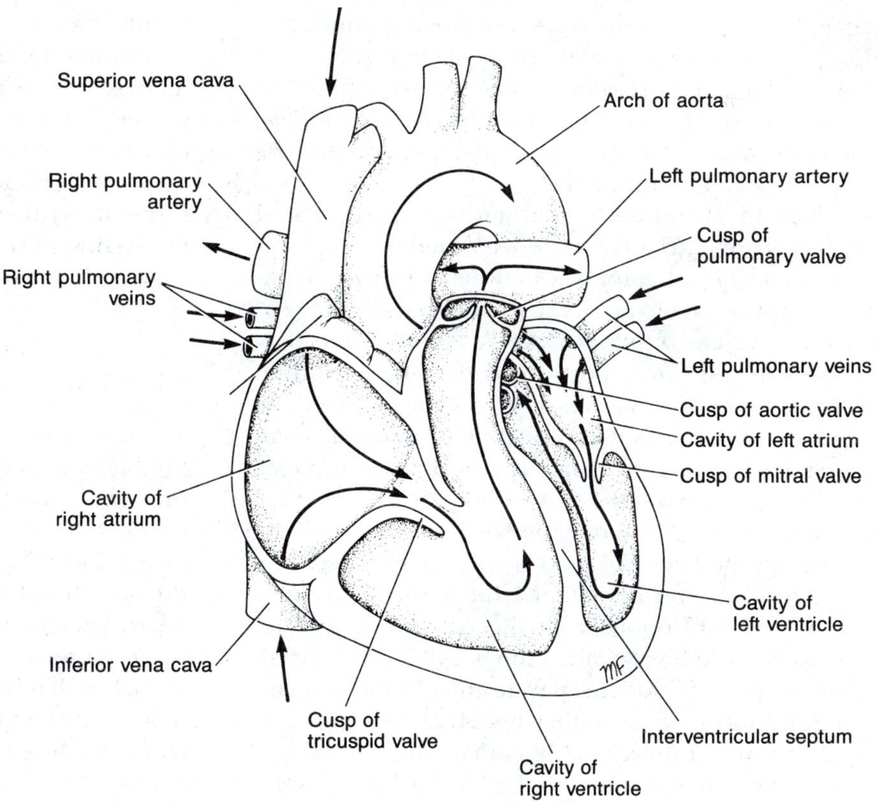

Figure 36–1
Anatomy of the heart and great vessels. Arrows show the direction of blood flow through the heart. From R. S. Snell, *Clinical and Functional Histology for Medical Students.* Boston: Little, Brown, 1984.

the endocardium, a thin, continuous sheath covering the four chambers and valves. The two atria are separated by a wall called the atrial septum, the two ventricles by the ventricular septum. Surrounding the heart is a fibrous sack, the pericardium, that protects the heart and secretes lubrication to minimize friction and facilitate heart movements.

Electrical Events of the Heart

The effectiveness of the heart as a pump depends on the extent to which it is able to coordinate the contractions of the four chambers. Coordination is achieved by a system that conducts electrical impulses to excite each chamber at just the right time. Each beat normally originates in the sinoauricular (or sinoatrial) node (**S-A node**), at the junction of the superior vena cava and right atrium because the cells of the S-A node have the highest rate of **automaticity** (spontaneous depolarization) of any cells within the heart. Thus, the S-A node is known as the pacemaker and initiates the beat in the normal heart by emitting an electrical impulse approximately 72 times per minute in the average adult. **Conduction** within the S-A node is slow, but once the electrical impulse has spread into the atrial muscle, it travels quickly along the muscle fibers. Cells of the cardiac muscle are connected in series to form long fibers. The resistance between adjacent cells in a fiber is unusually low, so excitatory potentials are spread rapidly along the fiber. For this reason, cardiac muscles function as a complex, unitary network, or *functional syncytium,* meaning that the muscle of a given chamber contracts as a single unit.

The atrial and ventricular muscles are separated by the atrioventricular node (**A-V node**), which restricts passage of impulses between the two chambers. Impulses from atrial muscle can pass to the ventricular muscle only over the A-V node, which is located in the lower portion of the atrial septum. Since the rate of conduction across the A-V node is slow, the impulse is delayed while the atrium completes its contraction. Once the impulse completes its passage across the A-V node, the excitation spreads very rapidly along the **His-Purkinje** network, activating the fibers of the ventricular muscle.

The His-Purkinje system, lying in the ventricular septum, is continuous with the A-V node. Special cardiac muscle fibers, called the bundle of His, originate in the A-V node, separate into branches, and extend down into the ventricles. Here they give rise to a network of Purkinje fibers that spread throughout the ventricular muscle. The His-Purkinje system provides for rapid relay of impulses from the A-V node to the ventricles, enabling the entire ventricular muscle to contract as a unit.

The A-V node is capable of generating impulses when the S-A node fails to function. However, when this occurs it generates only about 40–50 beats per minute, enough to sustain human life provided there is reduced physical activity. In the event of A-V nodal failure, lower pacemakers in the His-Purkinje system or in the ventricular muscle take over the task of forming impulses, but usually at rates too slow to sustain adequate tissue perfusion (30–40 beats per minute).

Sympathetic and Parasympathetic Influence

Although the heart functions up to a point as a self-contained system by generating its own impulses, it is regulated by both the parasympathetic and sympathetic nervous systems. Both heart rate and rhythm are controlled neurohormonally by the transmitters released from parasympathetic and sympathetic nerve terminals. Efferent fibers transmit impulses from the cardiac center in the medulla oblongata of the brain through sympathetic fibers that speed the heart rate and strengthen the force of contraction and through parasympathetic fibers of the vagal (tenth cranial) nerve that slow the heart. Norepinephrine released by sympathetic nerve endings also increases peripheral resistance to blood flow by its powerful vasoconstrictor activity. Acetylcholine released by the vagus nerve from terminals on the S-A node, A-V node, and bundle of His weakens the force of cardiac muscle contractions and lengthens the resting period of the heart muscle, in addition to slowing heart rate.

Circulatory System

The circulatory system distributes blood throughout the body. It is divided into two major networks: (1) the pulmonary circulation that receives blood pumped by the right heart and returns it to the left heart; and (2) the systemic circulation that receives the output of the left heart and returns it to the right heart. Each of the circulatory networks is organized in a pattern resembling a tree, with numerous branches that become successively smaller as they extend farther from the central vessels. Flow of blood from the heart to the peripheral capillary beds is provided by the arteries, while return of blood from the periphery to the heart is provided by the veins and by the lymphatic ducts.

The arterial side includes large, elastic arteries, smaller distributive arteries, arterioles, and finally the capillary beds. The arterioles provide the main control of peripheral resistance by constricting and relaxing their precapillary sphincters. The capillaries are the site of the essential exchange of nutrients, gases, and waste with tissue cells. The smallest vessels on the venous side are the venules, which receive blood from the capillaries and share the exchange function with the capillaries. The venules merge to form veins. By the time blood reaches the veins, the force imparted by the heart's contraction has declined to such an extent that blood flow here depends upon the contraction of neighboring muscles applying pressure to veins and forcing blood through them. The veins contain valves that prevent back flow and permit the blood to flow only toward the heart. Superficial veins drain by way of larger perforator veins into larger deep veins, which finally return blood to the heart via the pulmonary veins or vena cava.

The Role of Drug Therapy in Cardiovascular Disorders

The usefulness of drug therapy in treating cardiovascular disorders varies widely according to the disorder (Table 36–1). For some cardiovascular disorders,

Table 36–1
Overview of the Role of Drugs in Treatment of Cardiovascular Disorders

Disorder	Drug treatments
Generalized cardiovascular disorders	
Hypertension	
Essential	Antihypertensive agents (Chapter 39)
Secondary[a]	Specific by etiology
Orthostatic hypotension	Pressor drugs; mineralocorticoids, salt
Shock	Fluids; pressor drugs or conversely alpha-blockers (Chapter 28)
Syphilis of the cardiovascular system	Penicillin (Chapter 47)
Vascular Disorders	
Generalized arteriosclerosis	
Cerebral arteriosclerosis	Cerebral metabolic stimulants, etc. (Chapter 24)
Coronary arteriosclerosis	Antianginal drugs, etc. (Chapter 40)
Diabetic arteriosclerosis	Insulin, aldose reductase inhibitors, etc. (Chapter 33)
Hyperlipemia	Clofibrate; resins (Chapter 44)
Obliterative atherosclerotic disorders	
Aortic arch syndrome	Vasodilators, anticoagulants, corticosteroids — palliative only
Renal artery occlusion	None; surgically correctable
Splanchnic artery occulsion	None; often surgically correctable
Peripheral atherosclerosis	Eliminate tobacco; vasodilators dubiously effective
Spastic disorders	
Raynaud's phenomenon and disease	Eliminate tobacco: vasodilators, alpha-blockers, β_2-stimulants (Chapter 28)
Acrocyanosis[b]	Vasodilators (usually not required or effective)
Erythromelalgia[c]	Vasoconstrictors
Vasospastic angina	Certain antianginal drugs (Chapter 40)
Thromboembolic disorders	Anticoagulants (Chapter 41)
Inflammatory disorders	
Temporal arteritis	Corticosteroids (Chapter 45)
Aortitis	Corticosteroids (Chapter 45)
Valvular incompetence	
Varicose veins	Sclerosing therapy with sodium tetradecylsulfate
Aneurysms[d]	No specific drug treatment. Drugs as required for control of blood pressure
Fistulas[e]	None; surgery required.

(continued)

Table 36–1
Overview of the Role of Drugs in Treatment of Cardiovascular Disorders (*continued*)

Disorder	Drug treatments
Cardiac Disorders	
Congestive heart failure	Cardiac glycosides (Chapter 37)
Left heart failure	
Right heart failure	
Congenital heart disease	Few specific drug treatments
Promote closure of the ductus arteriosus	Indomethacin
Maintain patency of ductus arteriosus	Alprostadil
Cardiac dysrhythmias	Antidysrhythmic agents (Chapter 38)
Coronary artery disease	
Typical angina pectoris	Antianginal drugs (Chapter 40)
Myocardial infarction	Various (Chapter 40)
Myocardial disease	
Myocarditis	Corticosteroids (Chapter 45)
Cardiomyopathy	Eliminate toxic causes
Valvular heart disease	No specific drug treatments
Mitral valve disease	
Aortic valve disease	
Tricuspid valve disease	
Endocardial and pericardial disease	
Bacterial endocarditis	Antibacterial agents (Chapter 47)
Pericarditis	Anti-inflammatory drugs (Chapter 45)
Cardiac tamponade[f]	None; pericardiocentesis may be required

[a]Disorders such as those associated with pheochromocytoma, Cushing's disease, aldosteronism, hyperthyroidism, myxedema, renal vascular disease, unilateral renal disease, or bilateral renal parenchymal disease.

[b]Persistent, painless cyanosis of the skin of the extremities due to vasospasm of small vessels.

[c]Paroxysms of vasodilation accompanied by redness and burning pain sensation on the feet or hands.

[d]Localized dilation or longitudinal cleavage of an arterial vessel.

[e]Arterial-venous shunts.

[f]Effusion of fluid between the pericardium and heart to an extent that impairs cardiac function.

drug therapy represents the most important component of treatment. In this category are hypertension, congestive heart failure, coronary artery disease (including angina pectoris and myocardial infarction), dysrhythmias, and thromboembolic disorders. For some cardiovascular disorders, drugs have little or no importance in treatment. Thus, there is little in the way of primary drug therapies for renal or splanchnic artery occlusion, fistulas, cardiomyopathies, valvular diseases, congenital heart diseases, or cardiac tamponade, These conditions are generally dealt with by surgical interventions. Between these two extremes are the situations in which drugs aid nondrug approaches or in which drugs provide only modest or dubious benefit, or merely manage complications. Cerebral arteriosclerosis, peripheral atherosclerosis, acrocyanosis, varicose veins, aneurysms, and aortic arch syndrome fall into this category.

For some cardiovascular disorders, drug therapy entails use of therapeutic agents that are properly considered outside the domain of cardiovascular pharmacology. Cardiovascular disorders of infectious origin, such as syphilis of the cardiovascular system or bacterial endocarditis, are treated with antimicrobial agents (Chapter 47). Inflammatory disorders of the cardiovascular system, including temporal arteritis, aortitis, myocarditis, and pericarditis, are treated with the same kinds of drugs used in inflammatory disorders involving other bodily systems (Chapter 45). Autonomic drugs also find important applications in cardiovascular disorders: sympathomimetics are used in orthostatic hypotension, certain instances of shock, and erythromelalgia; sympatholytics are used in Raynaud's disease and some instances of shock; and antimuscarinic drugs in certain dysrhythmias and conditions of excess vagal tone. These drugs are covered in Unit IV, Drugs and the Peripheral Nervous System.

Recommended Readings

Andreoli K et al: *Comprehensive cardiac care: A text for nurses, physicians, and other health practitioners,* ed 5. St Louis, CV Mosby, 1983.

Berne R, Levy M: *Cardiovascular Physiology,* ed 4. St Louis, CV Mosby, 1981.

Goldberger E: *Textbook of Clinical Cardiology.* St Louis, CV Mosby, 1982.

Goldberger E: *Treatment of Cardiac Emergencies,* ed 4. St Louis, CV Mosby, 1985.

Hedges JR: Preload and afterload revisited. *J Emerg Nurs* 1983;9(5):262–267.

Underhill SL et al: *Cardiac Nursing.* Philadelphia, JB Lippincott Co, 1982.

CHAPTER 37

Cardiotonics

This chapter is concerned with the contractility of the heart. The heart acts as a pump to maintain flow of blood through the circulatory system. The pumping action of the heart is derived from the ability of the left and right ventricles to contract after filling with blood, thus forcing a flow of blood under pressure into the pulmonary or systemic arterial vessels. The contractility of the cardiac chambers is a direct function of the largest structural element of the heart — the cardiac muscle, or myocardium. In this chapter we will examine the physiological mechanisms underlying contractility of the myocardium, the disorders associated with impaired contractility, and the cardiotonics — drugs used to increase contractility in the failing heart.

Myocardial Contractility

Excitation-Contraction Coupling

The myocardium is composed of numerous cardiac muscle cells that have the shape of elongated fibers (Figure 37–1). The cells are attached to one another by interlocking disks that provide a pathway for conduction of electrical impulses between cells. Under the electron microscope, the interior structure of cardiac cells appears as a highly organized array of repeating units called *sarcomeres.* The sarcomere is the functional unit of the myocardium, providing contractile capability. At the center of each sarcomere is the dark A band where relatively thick myofilaments, composed of myosin, interdigitate with thinner filaments made of actin (Figure 37–1). The

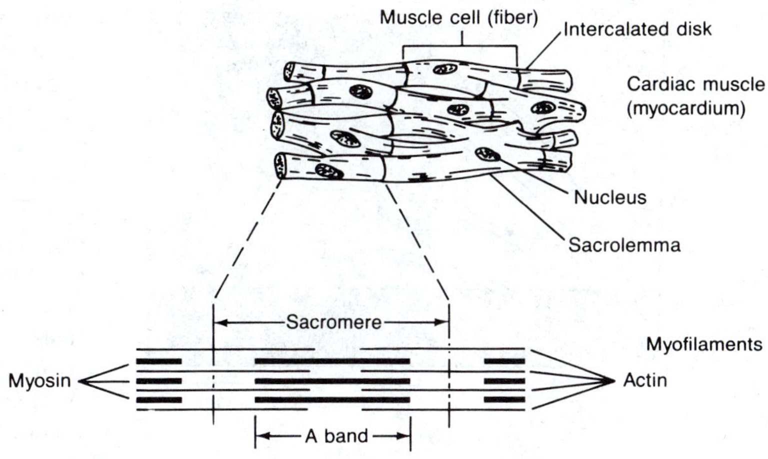

Figure 37–1
Ultrastructure of the myocardium.

myosin myofilaments possess small side chains called crossbridges which, under the influence of calcium, form crosslinks with the actin filaments. The formation of these crosslinks draws the actin fibers inward along the myosin fibers, causing the sarcomere to contract. Coordinated contraction of innumerable sarcomeres in millions of cardiac cells provides the powerful contractions of the cardiac muscle.

The impetus for contraction of the myocardium is electrical excitation. Each heart beat consists of a wave of depolarization spreading throughout the heart, initially by specialized conductile tissue and then from cell to cell within the myocardium. Since the mechanics and rhythm of the heart beat are considered in Chapter 36, the discussion here is limited to the events following the arrival of the electrical impulse at each myocardial cell. The arrival of a depolarizing electrical impulse produces a temporary increase in permeability of the plasma membrane to small ions, especially sodium (Na^+), potassium (K^+), and calcium (Ca^{++}). Rapid entry of sodium ions into myocardial cells is responsible for the reversal of the cell's electrical potential, called depolarization, and potassium efflux from the cells contributes to repolarization. Contraction, on the other hand, is initiated by the influx of calcium ions, which enter the cell more slowly through a set of pores called calcium channels. The amount of calcium that actually enters the cell is small but multiplies its influence by triggering release of calcium stored within the cell.

The calcium ions thus released into the cytoplasm rapidly bind to troponin, an enzyme that regulates the formation of crosslinks between the actin and myosin microfilaments. Adenosine 5′-triphosphate (ATP) serves as a coenzyme and the energy source. The formation of these links pulls the actin filaments inward along the myosin filaments to shorten the sarcomere. In the process, the chemical energy of ATP is converted to the mechanical energy of contraction. Subsequent relaxation of the muscle tissue and each individual sarcomere depends upon removal of free intracellular calcium by active transport out of the cell or into intracellular storage compartments. This active transport occurs by a carrier mechanism that exchanges intracellular calcium for extracellular sodium (which is later removed by the sodium-potassium exchange pump that maintains the resting potential).

Factors Regulating Cardiac Output

The healthy heart exhibits a remarkable ability to adjust its output in response to changing systemic requirements. The nervous system, endocrine substances, autacoids (locally acting hormones), and intrinsic cardiac relationships together regulate venous return, cardiac output, and arterial blood flow and distribution to meet the changing demands as the individual rests or exercises.

The principal mechanism influencing cardiac output that is intrinsic to the heart is the **Frank-Starling relationship,** or ventricular function curve. The Frank-Starling relationship states that the work performed during contraction of cardiac muscle is directly proportional to the degree of stretch of the myocardial fiber before contraction (Figure 37–2). Thus, the mechanical energy released during contraction depends on the length of the muscle fibers. The degree of stretch of the fibers is determined by the volume of the ventricle at the end of diastole, immediately before contraction. End-diastolic vol-

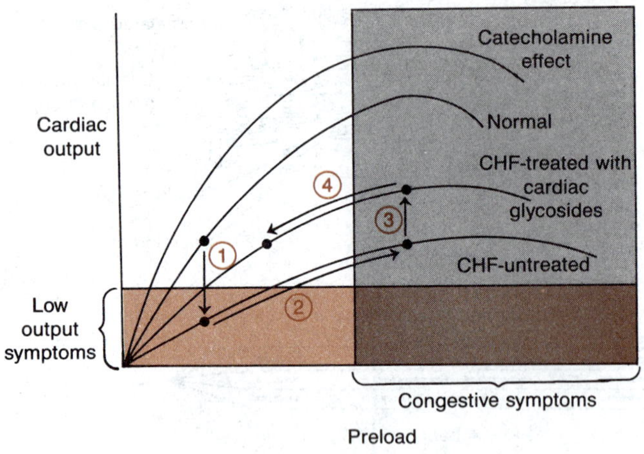

Figure 37–2
The Frank-Starling relationship between preload (initial stretch of cardiac fibers) and cardiac output for the normal heart and after administration of drugs in congestive heart failure (CHF). (1) Myocardial response curves shift downward with diminished contractility, resulting in low output; (2) preload rises in early CHF providing a compensatory increase in cardiac output but resulting in congestive symptoms; (3) cardiac glycosides cause a shift to a higher contractility curve; and (4) preload decreases as a result of treatment, resulting in alleviation of clinical symptoms.

ume, often referred to as the **preload,** is itself determined by the filling pressure. An elevated filling pressure increases the volume of blood that enters the ventricle and thus the degree of stretch of the ventricular fibers before contraction. Filling pressure is, in turn, determined mainly by venous pressure at the end of diastole and secondarily by the "kick," or surge, provided by atrial contraction. The Frank-Starling relationship indicates that within physiological limits, the heart adjusts its output in response to changes in venous return or preload, so that normally congestion of blood on the venous side of the circulatory tree is prevented and adequate arterial blood volume and flow is assured.

Catecholamines, such as norepinephrine and epinephrine, increase the force of contraction at a given preload (Figure 37–2). These neurohormones, released by postganglionic sympathetic fibers and by the adrenal medulla, play an important role in bringing about short-term adjustments in cardiac output.

Another factor that significantly influences cardiac performance is **afterload,** the resistance of the arteries to receiving the blood the heart pushes into them. Afterload acts as a force opposing the emptying of the ventricles. Factors that increase afterload decrease cardiac output while increasing cardiac work. Afterload is increased by hypertension or aortic stenosis and is decreased by arterial vasodilation. A persistent increase in afterload leads to congestive heart failure.

A final and profound influence on cardiac output is the adequacy of the **supply of energy** needed to power the work of the heart. The mechanical energy required for contraction is derived from chemical energy contained in molecules of ATP. Cardiac cells can generate little ATP without oxygen, so the heart has become very efficient in extracting oxygen from the blood — more efficient than any other tissue. As a result, however, the heart cannot readily meet extraordinary oxygen requirements by improving its extraction of oxygen. Therefore, the heart depends on coronary blood flow being adequate to meet its normal oxygen requirements as well as any unusual requirements. In coronary artery disease, the availability of oxygen may not equal oxygen demand in the heart, with the result that cardiac output diminishes. In addition, in the absence of sufficient blood supply, lactic acid, the waste product of anaerobic metabolism, accumulates and stimulates pain receptors in the vicinity of the heart to bring about angina pectoris. When the supply of energy for the work of the myocardium is inadequate, relief depends on improving energy production or decreasing cardiac work, or both.

Congestive Heart Failure

Congestive heart failure (CHF) is the failure of the myocardium to pump enough blood to meet systemic requirements, with the result that peripheral tissues become congested. The disease is a defect of the pump itself rather than of the vasculature; the contractility of the cardiac muscle is impaired, and thus the force of contraction of the myocardium in response to initial stretch is less than that of the normal heart (Figure 37–2). Stroke volume is reduced and emptying is incomplete.

In the early phase of the disease, compensatory mechanisms may prevent obvious clinical manifestations. For example, when end-diastolic pressure and preload begin to rise as a result of incomplete ventricular emptying, the Frank-Starling relationship comes into effect; the increase in ventricular filling produces an increase in the force of contraction, with the result that cardiac output tends to return toward normal. Ventricular hypertrophy may develop as a long-term compensatory response. In clients with long-standing systemic hypertension, for example, the ventricle must pump against increased afterload, the myocardium of the ventricle gradually hypertrophies, the heart pumps with greater force, and the rate is elevated. These elements may be present and affecting normal cardiac output for years before onset of cardiac failure. However, over time, the cardiac muscle can no longer function efficiently and symptoms of impairment occur.

Clinically, congestive heart failure is characterized by the abnormal retention of sodium and water that occurs when the kidneys attempt to compensate for the decreased cardiac output by increasing blood volume. Circulatory overload occurs as a result of the decreased cardiac output, the concomitant increased blood volume, and the increased venous return.

If the disease continues, the cardiac muscle is ultimately unable to increase its contractility enough to respond to escalating ventricular filling pressures. Cardiac output gradually declines and pulmonary or systemic congestion occurs retrograde to the ventricle that is failing. Clinical signs become increasingly evident during this phase. **Cardiogenic shock,** a severe decline in vascular tone and tissue perfusion, is the ultimate consequence of extreme heart failure. When heart failure advances to this extent, mortality rates are very high. When cardiogenic shock is mild, an increase in sympathetic nervous system activity may be sufficient to restore arterial pressure, resulting in **compensated shock.** Other times, the condition continues to deteriorate because of the tissue responses to poor perfusion (including elevated lactic acid production), progressing ultimately to irreversible shock.

The contractility of the myocardium can decline, leading to heart failure, as a result of any kind of myocardial disease or as a secondary disorder in a variety of clinical conditions. Intrinsic causes of heart failure include cardiomyopathy, myocardial infarction, myocarditis, ischemic heart disease, congenital heart defects, pericarditis, and cardiac dysrhythmias. Heart failure occurs as a secondary disorder in hypertension, pulmonary embolism, anemia, thyrotoxicosis, metabolic or respiratory acidosis, or volume overload. Drug toxicity can be an important contributing factor, especially in connection with volume overload. Among the agents that can contribute to volume expansion are steroids (androgens, estrogens, glucocorticoids), vasodilators, sympatholytic drugs, osmotic agents, and salicylates. Dietary factors, such as consuming excessive licorice or salt, may also contribute. Drugs that decrease contractility, such as beta-blockers, or that have cardiotoxic effects, such as alcohol or daunorubicin (Cerubidine), may also contribute to congestive heart failure.

Left and Right Heart Failure

In most instances of heart failure, one or the other of the two ventricles is primarily involved, although serious deterioration in the function of one ultimately leads to deterioration of the other. Both left and right heart failure involve *forward effects,* the consequence of reduced output of blood from the impaired ventricle, and *backward effects,* the consequence of congestion of blood behind the impaired chamber.

Left heart failure (LHF) occurs when the output of the left ventricle cannot keep up with pulmonary venous return. The most common causes of LHF are systemic hypertension and myocardial infarction, followed by aortic stenosis, aortic valve disease, mitral regurgitation, coronary artery disease, and cardiomyopathy. The backward manifestations of LHF begin with a damming up of blood retrograde to the left ventricle, with pooling first in the left atrium and then in the pulmonary veins and pulmonary capillary bed. Fluid is gradually forced into the interstitium surrounding the alveoli of the lungs, resulting in pulmonary edema, dyspnea (respiratory difficulty), basal rales, gasping or wheezing respiration, cough with frothy and often bloody sputum, hoarseness, and orthopnea (inability to breathe in a supine position) (Figure 37–3). At the same time, left ventricular output declines, resulting in forward effects of LHF. Body tissues become hypoxic, producing clinical symptoms of easy fatigability, dizziness, disorientation, confusion, or even coma. Hypertrophy of the myocardium and chamber dilation are frequent consequences of LHF.

Right heart failure (RHF) occurs when the output of the right ventricle cannot keep up with systemic venous return. The most common cause is LHF that has advanced to the point of significant pulmonary hypertension. The resulting chronic elevation in afterload of the right ventricle produces a strain that gradually impairs myocardial contractility. Other causes include chronic obstructive lung disease, mitral stenosis, pulmonary embolisms, tricuspid regurgitation, and congenital defects. The classic backward manifestation of RHF is systemic venous hypertension and edema, which can cause seepage of fluid into the peritoneal cavity (ascites) and distention of soft tissues, especially the spleen and liver. Forward manifestations of RHF are initially limited to poor pulmonary circulation, with

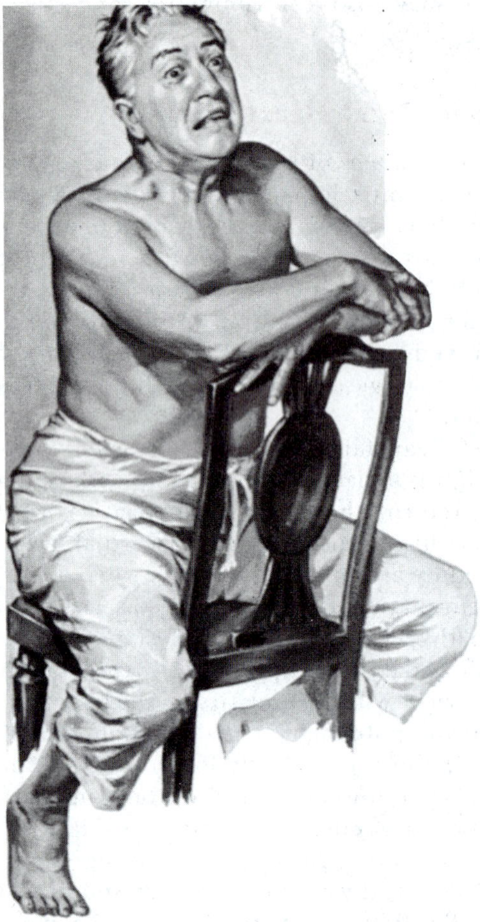

Figure 37–3
Typical clinical presentation of left heart failure. (© Copyright 1969 CIBA-GEIGY Corporation. Reproduced, with permission, from The CIBA Collection of Medical Illustrations by Frank H. Netter, M.D. All right reserved.)

consequent cyanosis, and lead ultimately to decreased venous return to the left heart and thus LHF.

Treatment of Congestive Heart Failure: General Considerations

The objectives for treatment of congestive heart failure are (1) to improve cardiac performance (contractility and output), (2) to reduce cardiac workload, and (3) to correct related impairments in organ function or fluid balance. In addition, if the congestive heart failure has developed acutely, as for example in conjunction with myocardial infarction, treatment aims to ensure optimum conditions for healing and to minimize the zone of infarction (see Chapter 40).

Improving Cardiac Performance

Cardiac performance can often be improved by **cardiac glycosides,** which increase the contractility of the heart. Cardiac glycosides are the mainstay of therapy for congestive heart failure. The clinical pharmacology of these important agents is discussed fully in the next section of this chapter.

If impaired cardiac performance is related in part to atrial dysrhythmias, correction of the dysrhythmia by cardioversion or administration of antidysrhythmic drugs will improve cardiac performance. In atrial tachycardia or flutter, for example, drugs are employed to reduce the ventricular response rate, and then conversion of atrial dysrhythmia is attempted by administration of drugs or direct current (cardioversion) or both.

Reducing Cardiac Workload

Cardiac workload can be reduced sometimes by alterations in life-style. Bedrest may be required for acute management. In mild cases, reducing physical activity, providing rest periods during the day, reducing stress-provoking circumstances, and controlling weight may provide sufficient improvement to allow the client to continue his or her normal activities. The degree of restriction of activities depends on the severity of the heart failure. Use of sedatives may be indicated when emotional stress is a contributing factor. *Nursing care is directed to providing physical and psychological rest to decrease demands on the heart. Clients must be helped to learn how to accommodate their life-styles to their new limitations. Some clients may be asymptomatic despite the anatomical and physiological changes that have occurred; they may be less inclined to adapt to recommended changes or to adhere to therapy. Clients may be classified according to the extent of cardiac compromise (Table 37–1).*

Table 37–1
Classification of Heart Disease

Classification	Cardiac status	Prognosis
1	Uncompromised	Good
2	Slightly compromised	Good with therapy
3	Moderately compromised	Fair with therapy
4	Severely compromised	Guarded despite therapy

Nursing management and evaluation should be based on the extent of rehabilitation and amount of activity the individual can logically be expected to achieve given his or her cardiac status.

Salt and water retention and edema are frequent factors in congestive heart failure. Although retention of salt and water helps to maintain systemic pressure in congestive heart failure, it also increases the work of the heart. Once cardiac output has begun to improve in response to treatment with cardiac gylcosides, a correction of fluid balance is indicated. Often some degree of correction occurs passively in response to bedrest and increased cardiac output. **Salt restriction** and diuretics can facilitate the process. Clients may be placed on a mildly restricted sodium diet (2 g of sodium daily), a moderately restrictive diet (1 g daily), or a severely restrictive diet (250–500 mg daily), depending on the severity of the problem. The usual American diet provides about 6–15 g of salt. Elimination of salt from the table and from cooking reduces salt intake to 3–4 g per day. Elimination of salty foods and avoidance of salt-containing drugs and food supplements achieves the remainder of the required reduction in daily salt intake. *Nurses need to teach clients about sodium content of foods and should warn clients that salt substitutes sometimes interfere with the drugs a client is taking or exacerbate a related problem. Clients should be encouraged to verify that the substitute they are considering is safe for them.*

Diuretics are employed in congestive heart failure whenever salt restriction alone is not sufficient to eliminate fluid excess. In mild congestive heart failure, thiazide diuretics, such as hydrochlorthiazide, are preferred. Potassium supplementation through dietary adjustments, ingestion of potassium salts, or concurrent use of potassium-sparing diuretics is usually required. In severe congestive heart failure, high-ceiling diuretics, such as furosemide (Lasix), are often required. Diuretics are discussed in Chapter 43.

A recent development in management of congestive heart failure is the addition of **vasodilators** to the treatment protocol. Congestive heart failure is characterized by an increase in preload (end-diastolic pressure) and usually afterload (end-systolic pressure). Thus, both venodilation, which reduces preload, and arteriolar dilation, which reduces afterload, are desirable interventions in congestive heart failure. In addition, certain vasodilators may enhance oxygen availability to the myocardium and thereby improve contractility of cardiac muscle fibers. Drugs such as nitroprusside, nitroglycerin, isosorbide, (Isordil), hydralazine (Apresoline), prazosin (Minipress), minoxidil (Loniten), and calcium channel blockers are employed. The pharmacology of these drugs is discussed in Chapters 39 and 40. Vasodilator therapy is especially indicated in congestive heart failure that is unresponsive to treatment with cardiac glycosides and diuretics.

Correcting Related Impairments

The third objective of therapy for congestive heart failure is to prevent or correct secondary deterioration in organ function. Foremost in this category is specific therapy for alleviation of **pulmonary edema.** Acute pulmonary edema may present as a medical emergency. The patient manifests extreme dyspnea, hyperpnea, tachypnea, pallor, cyanosis, apprehensiveness, and a feeling of suffocation. Rales and wheezing may be noted. Treatment of pulmonary edema is multifaceted. Morphine sulfate may be given to depress the respiratory center and to reduce apprehensiveness. Morphine sulfate also promotes pooling of fluid in peripheral venous vessels. Oxygen is frequently administered to alleviate hypoxia. The patient is positioned in an erect (high Fowler's) posture to allow pulmonary fluid to pool at the base of the lungs and to facilitate respiratory effort. Rotating tourniquets may be applied to three limbs at a time to reduce venous return. High-ceiling diuretics are given to promote fluid elimination and arterial vasodilators may be given to reduce afterload and improve cardiac output.

Cardiac Glycosides

History and Sources The cardiac glycosides, though among the oldest drugs in the pharmacological arsenal, are without equal in their effectiveness in treatment of heart failure. This family of drugs is derived from a variety of natural sources and various crude preparations have been used for thousands of years. The squill, or sea onion, contains a cardiac glycoside and was known as a medicinal in the early Egyptian civilization. The squill continued to be used in the Roman Empire as a heart tonic, diuretic, and rodent poison. The Chinese employed dried toad skin as a medicinal for many centuries, and it is now recognized as another source of cardiac glycosides. An arrow poison used by primitive tribes in Africa was identified in 1890 as containing a cardiac glycoside called ouabain.

Digitalis, the dried leaves of the foxglove plant, was known at least as early as AD 1250, when it was mentioned in written records of Welsh physicians.

The purple foxglove was given its botanical name *Digitalis purpurea* by Fuchsius in the sixteenth century. The first systematic study of digitalis was conducted by William Withering in 1785; he recognized its effectiveness in alleviating edema (called dropsy at the time) and its potent effect on the heart, though he did not appreciate the connection between the two actions. The value of digitalis in congestive heart failure has been recognized only in the present century.

Presently, *Digitalis purpurea* (the purple foxglove) and *Digitalis lanata* (the white foxglove) are cultivated in Europe and North America for production of cardiac glycosides. The dried leaves may still be used, but more commonly the active glycosides are employed in purified form. Digitoxin (Crystodigin, De-Tone, Purodigin) and digoxin (Lanoxin) are the two major glycoside constituents of foxglove and the principal cardiotonics in clinical practice. Ouabain is prepared by purification from the plant *Strophanthus gratus*.

Each cardiac glycoside consists of a steroid portion and a sugar portion. The steroid portion provides the pharmacological activity after the sugar portion is removed by hydrolysis and is similar in structure to the sex hormones, glucocorticoids, and bile acids; hence it is not surprising that chronic administration of cardiac glycosides can cause gynecomastia (development of the mammary glands) in male clients.

Mechanisms and Effects The pharmacodynamic activity of the various cardiac glycoside drugs can be considered to be identical, though their pharmacokinetic properties vary considerably. The actions of glycosides on cardiac function are both direct and indirect, toxic and therapeutic.

The direct actions of digitalis on the heart are twofold: (1) a positive inotropic action; and (2) negative chronotropic and negative dromotropic actions. (*Inotropic* means influencing muscular contractility; *chronotropic* means influencing the rate of contraction; *dromotropic* means influencing the conductivity of nerve fibers.) The **positive inotropic effect** is the major action that contributes to the treatment of congestive heart failure. Digitalis increases the contractility of the myocardium and therefore the force of the contraction. In the normal heart, digitalis produces little net influence on cardiac output because the enhanced contractility is effectively offset by increased systemic vascular resistance and a slight decrease in heart rate. In the failing heart, however, digitalis produces a profound enhancement of cardiac output. The ventricular chambers are able to develop more tension, eject more blood, and empty more completely. Since the chambers empty more completely, the filling pressure, or preload, is reduced, venous congestion is alleviated, and end-diastolic pressure declines.

Cardiac glycosides act on an enzyme called sodium-potassium ATPase (Na^+-K^+ATPase) which is found in the membrane of cardiac cells and which provides energy for the sodium-potassium pump. Digitalis renders the enzyme less active, diminishing sodium expulsion from cardiac muscle cells and increasing sodium concentration within the cells. The increase in intracellular sodium in turn increases calcium concentration, since free intracellular calcium is normally expelled from muscle cells in exchange for extracellular sodium. The increase in calcium concentration increases the force of myocardial contractions — the positive inotropic effect. This effect of digitalis is dose dependent since the greater the degree of inhibition of the Na^+-K^+ ATPase, the greater the rise in intracellular calcium and the greater the increase in contractility.

The other direct effects of digitalis on the myocardium, the negative chronotropic and dromotropic actions, are important for the secondary therapeutic use of digitalis: slowing of the ventricular response in atrial dysrhythmias. The negative chronotropic and dromotropic effects are also mainly responsible for the cardiotoxicity of digitalis. Digitalis slows heart rate (the **negative chronotropic effect**) by affecting automaticity (the rate at which cardiac cells spontaneously depolarize). At low to moderate doses, digitalis depresses automaticity in the S-A node indirectly, as a result of increased vagal activity, and therefore slows heart rate. At toxic doses, however, digitalis directly increases automaticity of all cardiac cells that exhibit spontaneous depolarization. As a result, digitalis is liable to induce tachycardia or fibrillation.

Digitalis decreases conduction velocity (the **negative dromotropic effect**) in a dose-dependent manner. Increasing doses slow and then finally block the passage of impulses through the A-V node. The negative dromotropic effect of digitalis provides its therapeutic benefit when it is used to reduce ventricular response rates in atrial tachydysrhythmias. The refractory period of cardiac tissue (the time when the cells are unresponsive to stimulation) is also affected by digitalis. In the A-V node, even small doses of digitalis prolong the refractory period, contributing to A-V block. At toxic doses, the refractory period in the ventricular myocardium is diminished, potentially provoking ventricular tachydysrhythmias.

The major indirect effect of digitalis on cardiac function is an increase in vagal activity. At low to moderate doses, this action slows the heart rate. Sympathetic impulses may be diminished reflexively by digitalis, as cardiac function and hemodynamics improve. At toxic levels, however, digitalis can increase sympathetic outflow by a mechanism that has yet to be established.

Pharmacokinetics Though similar in pharmacodynamic activity, digitoxin and digoxin differ considerably in pharmacokinetic characteristics (Table 37–2). After oral administration, digitoxin is absorbed almost completely (90–100%) because of its substantial lipid solubility. Absorption of digoxin is less complete and can be a source of problems because it depends on time of dosing in relation to meals, gastric emptying time, and the product formulation. Antibiotics (especially oral aminoglycosides), steroid-binding resins, antidiarrheal suspensions containing kaolin-pectin, sulfasalazine, aminosalicylic acid, and malabsorption syndrome can all significantly impair digoxin absorption. Tablets produced by different manufacturers vary widely in the extent and rate of absorption. *The nurse should instruct the client to be consistent about the taking of digoxin in relation to mealtime and not to switch brands.* The physician should generally specify the brand or source when digoxin is prescribed.

A major distinction between digoxin and digitoxin is that digoxin is excreted by the kidneys, whereas digitoxin is primarily metabolized in the liver. Changes in renal function greatly influence the effects of digoxin, while changes in hepatic function substantially modify the effects of digitoxin.

Another important difference is the comparative half-lives of the two major cardiac glycosides. Digoxin, with a half-life of 36 hours, has the advantage that toxic effects dissipate fairly rapidly after drug discontinuation; but, on the other hand, plasma concentrations are subject to greater fluctuations, especially if the client's compliance is sporadic. Digitoxin has a half-life of 5–7 days. A single missed dose of digitoxin has relatively little impact on therapeutic activity, but toxicity may persist for days after discontinuation. If the individual is to change from digoxin maintenance to digitoxin maintenance, the amount of digitalis available to the heart may be too small temporarily unless the dosage is adjusted. Conversely, transition from digitoxin to digoxin may cause digitalis toxicity if temporary adjustment in dosage is not made.

Metabolism of cardiac glycosides is significantly altered by the influence of the thyroid gland on overall basal metabolic rate. In hypothyroidism, doses of cardiac glycosides must be reduced. In hyperthyroidism, elevated doses are required.

Clinical Indications There are only two established uses for cardiac glycosides. The more important of the two is treatment of congestive heart failure. Digitalis is most effective in heart failure related to chronic overload from diseases such as hypertension, atherosclerosis, or valve lesions. The drug is of much less value when cardiac failure is secondary to thyrotoxicosis, hypoxia, advanced cardiomyopathy, or myocarditis due to infection or drugs. The secondary use of cardiac glycosides is for reducing the ventricular response rate during atrial tachydysrhythmias. Digitalis is indicated in most forms of atrial tachydysrhythmias, including atrial fibrillation, atrial flutter, and paroxysmal atrial tachycardia. Digitalis is effective by virtue of its ability to produce A-V block and thereby reduce ventricular response rates.

Adverse Effects and Contraindications The adverse effects of cardiac glycosides generally fall into five categories (Table 37–3): (1) cardiac toxicity,

Table 37–2
Comparative Pharmacokinetic Data for Digoxin and Digitoxin

Parameter	Digoxin	Digitoxin
Onset		
PO	1.5–6 hours	3–6 hours
IV	5–30 minutes	0.5–2 hours
Peak effect		
PO	4–6 hours	6–12 hours
IV	1.5–3 hours	4–8 hours
Half-life	36 hours	5–7 days
Gastrointestinal absorption		
Typical	75%	95%
Range	(40–90%)	(90–100%)
Major route of inactivation	Renal excretion	Hepatic metabolism
Plasma protein binding	25%	97%
Daily loading dose		
PO	1.25–3.0 mg	0.7–1.6 mg
IV	0.75–1.0 mg	1.0–1.6 mg
Daily maintenance dose (PO)	0.25–0.75 mg	0.05–0.2 mg
Effective plasma concentrations	0.8–1.6 ng/ml	14–26 ng/ml
Toxic plasma concentrations	> 2.4 ng/ml	> 34 ng/ml

Table 37–3
Digitalis Toxicity

Cardiovascular	Premature ventricular beats, tachydysrhythmias, A-V block, bradycardia
Gastrointestinal	Anorexia, nausea, vomiting, diarrhea
Neurological	Headache, neurological pain, fatigue, drowsiness, malaise, convulsions
Psychiatric	Digitalis delirium: disorientation, confusion, aphasia, delirium, hallucinations
	Visual illusions (white halos, yellow-green tinge; less commonly: red, brown, or blue tinge), diplopia, scotomata
Other	Skin rash, eosinophilia, gynecomastia in men

(2) gastrointestinal side effects, (3) neurological side effects, (4) psychiatric and perceptual side effects, and (5) other side effects. Of these, the cardiac effects are the most important.

Cardiac glycosides can produce a range of **dysrhythmias** that mimic virtually the full gamut of natural dysrhythmias. At the level of the S-A node, cardiac glycosides produce negative chronotropic and negative dromotropic effects. Sinus bradycardia occurs frequently and complete S-A block rarely. Atropine alleviates sinus bradycardia or block to the extent that it is related to elevated vagal activity. At toxic levels, cardiac glycosides may cause atrial tachydysrhythmias.

At the level of the A-V node, cardiac glycosides suppress conduction and prolong the refractory period. First degree A-V block, indicated by a prolongation of the P-R interval in the electrocardiogram, is

Nursing Observations For Use of Cardiotonics in Congestive Heart Failure

THERAPEUTIC GOAL	Reduce cardiac workload, improve cardiac performance, and correct related impairments in organ function or fluid balance.
PREADMINISTRATION ASSESSMENT	
Baseline Data	Observe for increased fatigue, shortness of breath upon exertion, fluid retention, hypotension, hypothermia, anorexia, dyspnea, orthopnea, and cyanosis. Evaluate blood pressure, pulse, ECG, chest x-rays, heart sound, peripheral pulses and perfusion, edema and ascites, respiratory rate and sounds, bowel sounds, urinary output, weight changes, neurological status, and vision. Obtain laboratory tests including liver and renal function and serum electrolytes.
Contraindications/ Precautions	Cardiac dysrhythmias, renal or hepatic insufficiency, pregnancy or lactation, electrolyte imbalances, or allergies to cardiac glycosides or tartrazine (found in some preparations).
Potential Interactions	Check medication chart for use of sympathomimetic or thyroid drugs.
EVALUATION OF DRUG RESPONSE	
During Dosage Adjustment	Monitor serum levels of the cardiotonic and monitor the ECG.
For Therapeutic Benefit	Diminished edema and congestion; reduced heart rate; increased tissue perfusion and oxygenation; and weight reduction. Continue to monitor for possible reemergence of congestive heart failure.
For Adverse Effects	Monitor for dysrhythmias, electrolyte imbalance, gastrointestinal irritation, neurological symptoms, and visual disturbances.
For Drug Interactions	Monitor for drug-induced hypo- or hyperkalemia, additive A-V block with antidysrhythmics, and drug-induced alterations in cardiotonic serum concentrations.
For Dietary Interactions	Monitor for dietary alterations in potassium intake that could increase or decrease the effect and toxicity of cardiotonics.
For Compliance	Evaluate client's compliance with all facets of the therapeutic regimen by careful observation, interviewing, and review of progress. Report compliance problems to the physician and act as client-advocate when changes in the therapeutic regimen seem indicated.

commonplace with digitalis. Higher levels of A-V block can occur, generally accompanied by ectopic "escape" beats originating in the bundle of His, producing a so-called junctional rhythm. A-V block is in part a direct effect of cardiac glycosides and in part a vagal influence.

Ventricular dysrhythmias also occur with digitalis toxicity. Premature ventricular beats are first to occur. These may become regular, perhaps alternating with normal beats to produce a bigeminy pattern (Figure 37–4B). In severe toxicity, ventricular tachycardia or fibrillation may ensue.

It is often difficult to diagnose dysrhythmias in digitalized clients. These clients are usually prime candidates for both digitalis-induced dysrhythmias and dysrhythmias related to the primary disease process, so that occurrence of dysrhythmias may or may not reflect digitalis toxicity. Electrocardiographic evidence together with observation of overt signs and symptoms can help distinguish the two. The ECG changes typical of a moderate level of cardiac glycoside activity include depression and shortening of the S-T segment, decrease in rate, and prolongation of the P-R interval (Figure 37–4A).

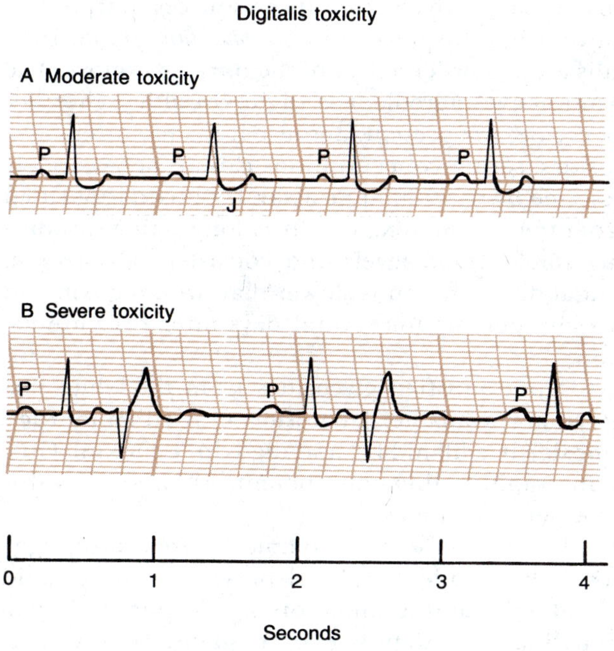

Figure 37–4
Digitalis toxicity. A. Moderate digitalis toxicity: depression of the J point and the S-T interval, decreased rate, prolonged P-R interval, and shortened Q-T interval. B. Severe digitalis toxicity: bigeminy rhythm due to ventricular extrasystoles, which could progress to complete A-V block, ventricular tachycardia, or ventricular fibrillation.

Digitalis-induced dysrhythmias almost always respond to appropriate treatment. Digitalis and diuretic therapy is immediately discontinued. If the dysrhythmia is severe, therapy with an antidysrhythmic agent is initiated. Phenytoin (Dilantin), potassium salts, and lidocaine (Xylocaine) are the most useful agents for digitalis-induced dysrhythmias. Phenytoin is employed for all types of digitalis-induced dysrhythmias; lidocaine for ventricular dysrhythmias only. Potassium ion directly antagonizes the effects of digitalis, decreasing its binding to the Na^+-K^+ ATPase and stimulating the activity of the enzyme. Potassium is beneficial, however, only if plasma concentrations of the ion are low or normal before administration of the potassium salt. Therefore, serum potassium concentration should be measured if use of potassium salts is contemplated. Atropine may be useful in alleviating A-V or S-A block in digitalis toxicity.

The noncardiac adverse effects of cardiac glycosides are not life-threatening or debilitating but may be seriously annoying for the client. **Gastrointestinal effects** are common and early manifestations of digitalis toxicity. Anorexia, nausea, and vomiting occur with all cardiac glycoside preparations but especially with the crude digitalis leaf. Diarrhea and abdominal discomfort are also frequent.

Neurological symptoms of cardiac glycosides include headache, neurological pain, fatigue, drowsiness, and malaise. Rarely, convulsions occur. Psychiatric and perceptual effects range from disorientation, confusion, and aphasia to delirium and hallucinations. The mental syndrome, known as **digitalis delirium,** is especially likely in elderly clients. A characteristic feature of cardiac glycosides is the occurrence of visual illusions. White halos are frequently perceived surrounding dark objects. Color vision may be disturbed so that a yellow and green tinge occurs over the visual field. Less commonly, the predominant hue may be red, brown, or blue. Double-vision (diplopia) or islands of blindness in the visual field (scotomata) are sometimes evident. The visual influences of digitalis can be observed in some of the paintings of Van Gogh, a long-time cardiac patient who was treated with cardiac glycosides.

Other adverse effects of cardiac glycosides include skin rash; while uncommon, it is an indication that the client is allergic to the drug, necessitating that other measures be sought to achieve the desired alteration of heart function. Eosinophilia (an excess of eosinophils, one of the classes of white blood cells) sometimes occurs and may be pronounced. Gynecomastia in males may also occur and is probably due to the steriod component of the glycoside structure.

Adverse effects and even severe toxicity are commonplace when cardiac glycosides are used. About 25% of hospitalized patients receiving cardiac glycosides experience toxicity. Toxicity can be caused by inappropriate initial dosage adjustment, overcompliance, changeover to a product with greater bioavailability, decrease in renal function (especially with digoxin), and potassium depletion. Serum potassium concentrations have a profound influence on the activity of digitalis; so any factor that alters potassium levels can affect digitalis therapy. Potassium depletion may be due to (1) concomitant use of potassium-depleting diurectics, (2) extensive loss of body fluids such as might result from vomiting, diarrhea, or certain surgical procedures, (3) inadequate dietary intake, (4) excessive mineralocorticoid activity, or (5) intravenous fluid therapy without adequate potassium concentrations. In practice, concurrent use of potassium-depleting diuretics without adequate potassium supplementation is the most common cause of digitalis toxicity. Serum potassium levels should be evaluated before initiating therapy with cardiac glycosides and periodically thereafter.

Digitalis is contraindicated in heart block (exept Stokes-Adams syndrome, where digitalis is used specifically to convert intermittent third-degree block to full third-degree block). Usually dosage reduction is required in myocardial infarction or myocarditis because of the elevated risk of dysrhythmias. Renal insufficiency greatly prolongs the presence of digoxin in the body; its effect on digitoxin is much less. Elderly clients are often more susceptible to digitalis toxicity and require reduced doses.

Drug Interactions A digoxin **antidote,** digoxin-immune antigen-binding fragments (FAB) (Digibind), was marketed in 1986 for therapy of digoxin toxicity. Digoxin-immune FAB consists of digoxin antibodies produced by sheep. Its use is indicated when serum digoxin concentrations exceed 10 ng/ml and it is administered by intravenous infusion over 30-minute periods. The principal precaution in using digoxin-immune FAB is that cardiac function may deteriorate due to reduction in digoxin support of cardiac output.

Quinidine (Duraquin) causes a significant increase in plasma concentrations of digoxin when the two drugs are given concurrently, possibly because it displaces digoxin from inactive tissue binding sites. The effects of digoxin are therefore increased by quinidine. Monitoring for digoxin toxicity should be intensified if quinidine is added to the regimen. Other drugs noted to increase digoxin levels include calcium channel blockers, anticholinergic drugs, erythromycin, and tetracycline.

Cardiac glycosides interact with any drug or dietary influence that alters potassium levels in the body fluids. Most notable among these influences is the effect of potassium-depleting diuretics. Amphotericin B, an antibiotic, also causes hypokalemia.

Antidysrhythmic agents that decrease A-V conduction enhance the depressant effect of cardiac glycosides on the A-V node, and elevate the risk of A-V block. On the other hand, the positive inotropic effect of cardiac glycosides is enhanced in the presence of calcium, epinephrine, ephedrine, and other agents.

Liver metabolism of digitoxin (but not digoxin) is significantly affected by drugs that are inducers of liver enzymes, including barbiturates, hydantoin derivatives (Dilantin), antihistamines, oral hypoglycemic agents, rifampin (Rifadin) and phenylbutazone (Azolid). Other pharmacokinetic interactions occur between digitalis and antacids, antidiarrheals, aminoglycosides, steroid-binding resins, laxatives, and thyroid hormone, as described in the earlier section pertaining to the pharmacokinetics of cardiac glycosides.

Preparations and Administration Cardiac glycosides are derived from three sources: purple foxglove, white foxglove, and *Strophanthus gratus.* Digitalis is the powdered leaf of the purple foxglove. The main active ingredient is digitoxin although other glycosides are present. Because it is a mixture of glycosides, serum concentrations cannot be accurately assessed by radioimmune assay. Digitoxin is purified from the purple foxglove. It is long-acting, producing stable blood levels and consistent absorption. Initial digitalization is slower than with digoxin and toxicity persists for several days after discontinuation.

Three purified glycosides from the white foxglove are available: lanatoside C (Cedilanid), deslanoside (Cedilanid-D), and digoxin (Lanoxin). Ouabain, rapid acting and potent, is used only for emergency treatment.

Digoxin is the most commonly used cardiac glycoside by a wide margin. It provides a more rapid initial onset and termination of effect upon discontinuation than digitoxin or digitalis. However, its plasma concentrations are less stable if compliance is sporadic. *Digoxin should be kept in airtight containers, protected from light. Parenteral solutions should not be used if discolored. Nurses need to caution patients being released from the hospital to keep their digoxin tablets in airtight opaque containers at home.*

Nursing Diagnoses and Interventions For Use of Cardiotonics in Congestive Heart Failure

Nursing Diagnoses	*Related Interventions*
TO ENHANCE DRUG BENEFITS OR REDUCE DRUG REQUIREMENTS	
Alteration in tissue perfusion and fluid volume related to venous congestion	Encourage client to lie on left side. Report symptoms to the physician for possible adjustment of the regimen.
Anxiety related to respiratory distress and impaired gas exchange; fear related to uncertain future	Provide support and encouragement to help client cope with the disorder and the treatment regimen. Stress the need to avoid circumstances that cause acute exacerbation such as episodes of rage, extremes of temperature, or heavy exercise.
Impaired gas exchange related to accumulation of fluid	Elevate head of bed. Administer oxygen.
Impaired home maintenance, self-care, and activity tolerance related to fatigue and breathlessness	Provide adequate rest periods. Encourage environment adjustments that ease requirements for exertion. Administer oxygen for acute breathlessness.
Sleep-rest disturbance related to nocturnal dyspnea and orthopnea	Minimize interruptions of sleep and promote a restful environment.
TO MINIMIZE DRUG SIDE EFFECTS OR INTERACTIONS	
Alteration in nutrition: intake less than requirements related to drug-induced nausea and anorexia	Provide any necessary nutritional support.
Alterations in urinary elimination when cardiotonic therapy is instituted	Provide bathroom facilities appropriate to the client's physical limitations and increased requirements.
TO ENSURE SAFE AND EFFICACIOUS DRUG USE	
Knowledge deficit related to drug regimen	Teach the client about the nature of the disease, the action of the drug, and importance of adhering to the medication schedule. Explain how to determine the correct dosage and the special importance of avoiding errors with cardiotonic drugs because of the low therapeutic index. Explain the importance of administering cardiotonic drugs at the same time each day, in consistent relation to meals, and not changing brands. Demonstrate to the client how to maintain a record of weight and pulse changes. Provide the client with a list of potential adverse effects and drug interactions and what to do if any of these occur. Explain any dietary or activity restrictions that are prescribed. Provide clients with a list of laboratory tests that may be altered by use of cardiotonic drugs.

When therapy with cardiac glycosides is initiated without any urgency for an immediate response, as in long-standing, mild heart failure, maintenance doses can be given from the beginning and the maximal effect will be achieved in approximately four half-lives (about 1 week for digoxin or 1 month for digitoxin). If, on the other hand, a more rapid response is desired, an initial **loading dose,** or **digitalizing dose,** is administered. The loading dose can be given orally or intravenously. An IV loading dose is given slowly over 10–20 minutes, and is often divided into two administrations, given 3 or 4 hours apart. The loading dose is given only once. **Maintenance doses** are given daily thereafter, and are gradually adjusted to achieve the desired therapeutic benefit and minimize the adverse effects. The maintenance dose is calculated so as to replace exactly the amount of drug lost daily by metabolism and renal excretion. The therapeutic ratio for cardiac glycosides is low, and toxicity frequently occurs in clinical practice, with sometimes fatal consequences. Frequent monitoring is essential.

All cardiac glycosides are highly poisonous. *Clients should be advised to follow regimens exactly, not to skip or double up on doses, to keep the drugs out of the reach of children, and to keep cardiac glycosides only in their original containers without other medications.*

Digitalis
Tablets, capsules
Recommended Doses: Loading dose, 1.2 g PO in several divided doses at 6-hour intervals. Maintenance doses, 100–200 mg/day PO typically, with extremes of 30–400 mg/day.

Mixtures of cardiac glycosides from purple foxglove (Digiglusin, Gitaligin)
Tablets
Recommended Doses: Loading dose (rapid), 2.5 mg PO followed by 0.75 mg every 6 hours until benefit or toxicity occurs. Loading dose (slow), 1.5 mg PO once daily for 4–6 days. Maintenance, 0.25–1.25 mg/day (0.5 mg is typical).

Digitoxin (Crystodigin, De-Tone, Purodigin)
Tablets, injection solution
Recommended Doses: Parenteral loading dose in adults, typically 1.2–1.6 mg IV. Rapid oral loading dose in adults, 0.6 mg initially, followed by 0.4 mg, then 0.2 mg at intervals of 4–6 hours. Slow oral loading dose in adults, 0.2 mg twice daily for 4 days. Adult maintenance range, 0.05–0.3 mg daily. Loading doses in children; premature and newborn, 0.022 mg/kg under 1 year of age, 0.045 mg/kg; 1–2 years of age, 0.04 mg/kg; over 2 years of age, 0.03 mg/kg. Maintenance doses in children, one-tenth the loading dose.

Lanatoside C (Cedilanid)
Tablets
Recommended Doses: Loading dose, typically 10 mg PO given over 3 days. Maintenance dose, typically 0.5–1.5 mg/day PO.

Deslanoside (Cedilanid-D)
Injection solution
Recommended Doses: Loading dose, typically 1.6 mg given in 1 or 2 doses, intravenously or intramuscularly. This preparation is not used for maintenance purposes.

Digoxin (Lanoxin)
Tablets, pediatric elixir, injection solution
Recommended Doses: Loading dose, 1–1.5 mg. Maintenance dose range, 0.125–0.5 mg PO, limited to 0.25 in the elderly. Doses in infants and children determined by weight.

Ouabain
Injection solution
Recommended Doses: 0.25–0.5 mg IV.

Important Nursing Implications for Cardiotonic Drugs

- ☐ Always take the patient's apical pulse rate prior to giving each dose of drug. If the pulse rate is below 60 beats per minute for an adult, or 110 beats per minute for a child, the drug should be temporarily withheld (unless orders indicate otherwise) and the physician notified. If the pulse rate suddenly increases, decreases, or if the patient develops an abnormal rhythm not present prior to beginning drug therapy, the patient should not receive the drug and the physician should be notified.
- ☐ Teach clients and families to monitor the client's pulse rate and rhythm prior to each dose of digitalis, digoxin, or digitoxin, and advise clients not to take the drug and to contact the physician if they note any changes. Note that *any* change in rate or rhythm can indicate digitalis toxicity.
- ☐ The margin between therapeutic and toxic levels of cardiac glycosides is very narrow. To assure the client's health and safety as well as appropriate response to drug therapy, obtain baseline electrocardiogram readings and serum electrolytes before digitalization begins and carefully monitor these parameters during drug therapy. Serum samples for measurement of digitalis concentrations should usually be taken 2 hours before the next daily oral dose.

- ☐ During the period of digitalization, monitor patients especially closely, noting changes in pulse rate, rhythm, and blood pressure, serum electrolytes, and the ECG. Digitalization doses in some patients differ little from toxic doses, making adverse reactions commonplace. The intake-output ratio should also be monitored carefully so that any reduction in renal excretion can be quickly identified.
- ☐ In preparing clients for discharge, instruct them to weigh themselves during the maintenance phase each day at the same time without variation in clothing and to report rapid weight gain to the physician. Maintenance doses are adjusted in relation to changes in body weight, venous pressure, heart rate, exercise tolerance, edema, serum electrolyte concentrations, ECG measurements, and signs of toxicity. Dosage adjustments may be required if antidysrhythmics are added to the regimen, if diarrhea or malabsorption occurs, if laxatives are taken, or if the brand or drug selection is changed.
- ☐ Be certain that clients have been carefully instructed about the importance of precise compliance when cardiac glycosides are employed. Instruct clients to take cardiac glycosides at the same time each day, in the same relation to meals, and not to change brands without consulting the physician.
- ☐ If clients complain of nausea and anorexia, instruct them to take their oral medications after meals. However, the nurse should be aware that complaints of nausea, vomiting, or anorexia are also early signs of digitalis toxicity and should be reported immediately to the physician. The drug should be withheld until the physician determines the course of action to be followed. Clients and their families also need to have this information since otherwise the symptoms might be overlooked.
- ☐ Teach clients to record any unusual cardiac sensations they may experience and report these to nurses and physicians so that appropriate medical responses can be made. Such sensations are often early signs of disturbances of the cardiac rhythm. The most common disturbance caused by digitalis is premature ventricular beats. Others are paroxysmal and nonparoxysmal nodal rhythms, atrioventricular dissociation, and paroxysmal atrial tachycardia. Excessive slowing of the pulse should alert the nurse to look for such problems. They indicate drug overdose which can lead to A-V block.
- ☐ Question clients concerning the presence of central nervous system side effects such as headaches or weakness of the extremities. Complaints of extreme fatigue, seeing abnormal colors, having blurred vision, flashing or flickering of lights, or changes in color perception should be investigated, since these, too, are symptoms of toxicity.
- ☐ Be alert for indications of behavioral changes. Since nurses tend to see clients on a continuing basis, they are the health care professionals most likely to notice such changes. The client's family ought to be questioned about such incidents and about evidence of disorientation or mental confusion in the client, since about half of such noncardiac symptoms precede adverse effects on the heart.
- ☐ When clients are receiving diuretics in addition to cardiac glycosides, decreased blood levels of potassium and calcium ions may result in adverse reactions. Teach these clients the importance of eating foods high in potassium and calcium. Subnormal levels of serum potassium increase the risk that digitalis-induced ectopic pacemakers can cause dysrhythmias.
- ☐ Advise clients about drugs that may interfere with cardiac glycosides. For example, antacids may decrease the absorption of digitalis glycosides, thereby decreasing the therapeutic effect of the drug. Corticosteroids can produce hypokalemia, thereby increasing the possibility of digitalis toxicity. Epinephrine or other adrenergic agents can produce additive positive inotropic effects that result in cardiac dysrhythmias. Thyroid preparations, anticonvulsant agents, antihistamines, barbiturates, and hypoglycemic agents increase client susceptibility to digitalis toxicity.
- ☐ Teach clients to report all drugs they take to physicians and nurses if they visit walk-in clinics where they are not known by the medical and nursing staff. Encourage them to discuss the drugs they take with their pharmacists so that the pharmacists can advise them about possible drug interactions.
- ☐ Instruct clients receiving cardiotonic drugs to wear an identifying bracelet indicating they have a heart problem and are taking medications.

Other Positive Inotropic Agents

Amrinone lactate (Inocor) is a nonglycosidic, noncatecholamine, positive inotropic agent introduced in 1984. An analogue of amrinone, milrinone, is currently undergoing clinical assessment and may provide a greater margin of safety and fewer adverse effects.

Mechanisms and Effects The structure of amrinone and its mode of action differ from both the cardiac glycosides and the catecholamines. It has no effect on the sodium-potassium ATPase that is acted upon by cardiac glycosides. Instead, amrinone enhances myocardial contractility by increasing levels of adenosine 3′:5′ cyclic phosphate (cyclic AMP) by inhibiting the enzyme (phosphodiesterase) that normally breaks down this substance. Cyclic AMP enhances cardiac contractility by speeding the penetration of calcium ions into the cells. Amrinone also dilates the vessels and thus reduces afterload and preload. Improvement in cardiac output occurs in most clients without signs of myocardial ischemia when amrinone is given.

Pharmacokinetics Amrinone is given only by intravenous injection. It has a volume of distribution of 1.2 liters/kg, a distribution half-life of about 5 minutes, and a peak effect in about 10 minutes. The elimination half-life of amrinone is about 3.6 hours. It is inactivated both by renal excretion and liver metabolism.

Clinical Indications Amrinone is indicated for short-term management of congestive heart failure when the client has not responded satisfactorily to digitalis, diuretics, or vasodilators. The inotropic effect of amrinone is fully additive to that of cardiac glycosides. Amrinone can be used in a digitalized client without resulting in digitalis toxicity.

Adverse Effects The most common adverse reactions to amrinone are thrombocytopenia, dysrhythmias, hypotension, nausea, and vomiting. None of these occur in more than 3% of clients. Allergic reactions have occurred with use of amrinone for periods of 2 weeks or more.

Preparations and Administration The drug can be administered as supplied or diluted with normal or half normal saline to a concentration of 1–3 mg/ml. Amrinone should not be prediluted with solutions containing dextrose, but it may be injected into a running dextrose infusion.

Amrinone (Inocor)
Injection solution
Recommended Doses: 0.75 mg/kg initially, given as an IV bolus over 2–3 minutes. For maintenance, 5–10 μg/kg/minute, or an additional bolus injection of 0.75 mg/kg, 30 minutes after the first injection. The total daily dose should not exceed 10 mg/kg.

Milrinone (Win–47203)
Investigational

Case Study: Congestive Heart Failure

J. D. was a 63-year-old, white married man who had been in good health all of his life. One night while lying in bed he experienced shortness of breath. He felt better when he stood up and took a few deep breaths. Upon lying down again, the symptoms returned. He soon learned that he could alleviate the breathlessness by propping himself up on extra pillows. Over the course of the next 2 weeks, J. D. felt progressively weaker, experienced breathlessness upon exertion, and noticed that his ankles were becoming swollen. One night, symptoms became so severe that J. D. found breathing difficult and painful. His wife called an ambulance and J. D. was admitted to the hospital. Physical examination revealed a heart rate of 96, a weak pulse, wheezes, rales, cyanosis, edema, and cardiomegaly. Blood tests revealed normal hemoglobin, slightly elevated white blood cell count, a slightly elevated blood urea nitrogen (BUN), and a slightly depressed serum potassium concentration. The physician ordered an intravenous infusion of 5% dextrose in water (at 50 ml/hour), 40 mg furosemide injected intravenously, and digoxin (Lanoxin), 0.5 mg immediately and every 4 hours for three doses, sodium restriction, and rotating tourniquets on three extremities. J. D. responded well to this regimen. His skin color was pink, rales had decreased, respiration was no longer painful, and edema was receding. The nurse demonstrated deep breathing and coughing exercises to J. D. to facilitate clearing of sputum from the lungs. J. D. was stabilized on an oral regimen of 0.5 mg of digoxin, once daily; 50 mg of hydrochlorthiazide, twice daily; and 24 mEq of potassium chloride syrup, twice daily. The nurse instructed J. D. about his condition, diet, and medication regimen prior to discharge.

Two weeks after his initial discharge, J. D. was readmitted to the hospital with complaints of lack of energy, weakness, impaired balance, nausea and poor appetite, and frequent diarrhea. Upon questioning by the nurse, J. D. also revealed having experienced visual disturbances, including white halos and a yellow-green tint. Physical examination indicated a respiratory rate of 19 per minute, pulse rate of 56 beats per minute, normal blood pressure, and normal temperature. There was no evidence of edema in the hands or feet or fluid congestion in the lungs. X-ray evaluation revealed no enlargement of the heart. J. D. was given an ECG, which showed occasional premature ventricular beats (with inversion of the QRS wave), a prolongation of the P-R interval, and depression of the S-T segment. Upon questioning, J. D. indicated that he had taken both the digoxin and the hydrochlorthiazide every day in accordance with his prescribed regimen but had stopped taking the potassium syrup because he did not like its bitter taste. The physician ordered immediate evaluation of serum electrolytes while the nurse prepared a syringe with lidocaine and another with phenytoin (Dilantin). The blood tests showed a serum potassium value of 2.1 mEq/l. The physician ordered intravenous fluids, a low-sodium diet, a cardiac monitor, and vital signs every 4 hours. Repeat serum electrolyte measurements after 12 hours indicated that serum potassium had increased to 4.0 mEq/l. After 24 hours, the heart rate had increased to 70 beats per minute, there were no longer any premature ventricular beats, balance and appetite had improved, and visual disturbances had cleared. After 5 days, J. D. was released. His daily regime was altered to allow him to take the potassium chloride supplement in the form of tablets.

J. D. had no further symptoms of congestive heart failure or digitalis toxicity until 2 years later when he again began to experience progressive weakness and dyspnea. After 3 days of these symptoms, J. D. was admitted to the hospital with symptoms of uncontrolled congestive heart failure. Furosemide (Lasix) was ordered immediately along with laboratory evaluation of J. D.'s serum digoxin level. This was found to be 0.18 ng/ml. J. D. indicated that he had continued to take his digoxin regularly and that he had not changed brands. He was, however, no longer taking the drug in the morning, taking it instead after lunch with a glass of cold milk. J. D. was stabilized in the hospital on his former regimen of digoxin, 0.5 mg daily. Given in the morning on an empty stomach, this dose was found to provide therapeutic serum concentrations. J. D. was released with instructions to take the digoxin in the morning on an empty stomach.

1. How did each of the original presenting symptoms contribute to a diagnosis of congestive heart failure?
2. What was the purpose of administering furosemide? The application of rotating tourniquets? The use of digoxin?
3. What is the mechanism behind the beneficial effect of digoxin?
4. What is the significance of the findings from the blood studies conducted when J. D. was first treated for congestive heart failure?
5. J. D. received a total of 2.0 mg of digoxin during the first day of treatment but only 0.5 mg each day thereafter. What was the reason for this discrepancy?
6. How did J. D.'s failure to take the prescribed potassium supplement contribute to the occurrence of digitalis toxicity? Why were lidocaine and phenytoin prepared for injection while the blood tests were being conducted?
7. Ultimately, J. D. recovered from the cardiotoxic effects of digitalis without the necessity of administering an antidysrhythmic agent. To what do you attribute the recovery?
8. What factors might have contributed to the inadequate serum concentrations of digoxin in spite of J. D.'s continuing to take the same daily dose that he had used for 2 years? Why did the nurse inquire as to whether J. D. had changed brands of digoxin?

Answers appear at the end of the book.

Recommended Readings

Albeit S et al: Recognizing digitalis toxicity. *Am J Nurs* 1977;77:1935–1943.

Baim D et al: Evaluation of a new bipyridine inotropic agent — milrinone — in patients with severe CHF. *N Engl J Med* 1983;309:748–756.

Brown DD, Spector R, Juhl RP: Drug interactions with digoxin. *Drugs* 1980;20:198–206.

Cavanaugh AL, Manconi RE: Drug interactions and digitalis toxicity. *Am J Nurs* 1980;80:2170–2171.

Cohen S: New concepts in understanding congestive heart failure. *Am J Nurs* 1981;81(2):357–380.

Farah AE et al: Positive inotropic agents. *Annu Rev Pharmacol Toxicol* 1984;24:275–328.

Goldberg PB: How do digitalis tolerance and toxicity change with age? *Geriatr Nurs* 1980;1:142–144.

Hovrath PT, DePew CC: Towards preventing digitalis toxicity. *Nurs Drug Alert* 1980;4:25.

Kirschenbaum M: Digitalis. *RN* 1981;81(11):69–71.

Kumpuris A, Raizner A, Luchi R: The role of serum digitalis levels in clinical practice. *Heart Lung* 1979;8:711–715.

McCauley K: Probing the ins and outs of congestive heart failure. *Nursing* 1982;12(11):60–66.

McCauley K, Burke K: Your detailed guide to drugs for congestive heart failure. *Nursing* 1984;14(5):47–50.

Meissner JE, Gever LN: Reducing the risks of digitalis toxicity. *Nursing* 1980;10:32–38.

Michaelson CR (ed): *Congestive Heart Failure* St Louis, CV Mosby Co, 1983.

Sloan RW: Digitalis glycosides. *Am Fam Physician* 1983;28(5):206–216.

Winslow EH: Digitalis *Am J Nurs* 1974;74:1062–1065.

CHAPTER 38

Antidysrhythmic Drugs

The clinical pharmacology of antidysrhythmic drugs is one of the more complex areas of pharmacology. Appropriate use of these agents depends on a sound understanding of normal and abnormal cardiac rhythm, the interaction between antidysrhythmic drugs and the electrophysiology of the heart, and the variety of adverse reactions and drug interactions of the antidysrhythmic agents. During the last decade, there has been considerable progress in classifying antidysrhythmic drugs, understanding their mechanisms, and developing new drugs. It appears likely that this will continue to be an area of rapid development in the near future. We begin this chapter with a review of the electrophysiology of the heart beat and the pathophysiology of dysrhythmias.

Electrophysiology of the Heart Beat

Resting and Action Potentials

In Chapter 37, we examined the mechanical events that culminate in contraction of the myocardium. Here we consider the corresponding electrical events. Like other electrically excitable cells, cardiac muscle cells exhibit a resting potential and, when appropriately stimulated, an action potential. The resting potential is the voltage differential that exists across the cell's membrane, called the **transmembrane potential.** Generally the inside of the typical cardiac muscle cell is about 80–90 millivolts (mV) more negative than the extracellular fluid. The resting potential is generated mainly by transport of sodium by the sodium-potassium pump. When a cardiac cell is excited, a series of shifts in the electrical potential of the cell occurs over about a half second as a result of transfers of ions across the membrane. The sequence of changes in transmembrane potential is called the **action potential** (Figure 38–1).

The action potential can be divided into five phases. In phase 0, the sodium channels in the cell's membrane open and sodium ions rush in, resulting in rapid depolarization. The property of **membrane responsiveness** reflects the availability of excitable sodium channels and therefore the ability of the cell to enter phase 0.

In phase 1, the sodium channels close, and chloride ions enter the cell, repolarizing it. In phase 2, the inward flow of negatively charged chloride ions is offset by the inward flow of positively charged calcium ions, creating a plateau. The phase 2 plateau is a feature of the action potential unique to cardiac muscle and Purkinje fibers; it does not occur in A-V or S-A nodal cells or in nerve cells. Calcium ions enter the cells through **calcium channels,** also called slow channels because they open more slowly than the sodium channels. The influx of calcium releases calcium stored within the cell. The overall increase in free calcium initiates contractile mechanisms discussed in Chapter 37.

In phase 3, repolarization is completed as potassium ions leave the cell. During phase 3, the sodium channels gradually recover from their activation during phase 0. Thus full membrane responsiveness is not reestablished until after the end of phase 3; many cardiac cells are refractory (unresponsive) to further activation until that point or beyond. The minimum interval between successive action potentials is called the **effective refractory period.** Phase 4 is the resting potential.

An action potential can be triggered in a resting cell either from without, by an impulse received from another cell, or from within, by spontaneous depolarization. Spontaneous depolarization occurs in many cardiac cells because the potential during phase 4 in these cells is unstable, gradually drifting upward toward the threshold potential (the level of partial depolarization at which the process of depolarization becomes self-perpetuating, leading to an action potential). Such repetitive, spontaneous depolarization during phase 4 is referred to as **automaticity.** Cells having the property of automaticity are found in the S-A node, elsewhere in the atrium, and in the His-Purkinje conductile elements, including the A-V node. In the normally functioning heart, the cells of the S-A node have the fastest automaticity and therefore determine the heart rate. The S-A node is often referred to as the **pacemaker.**

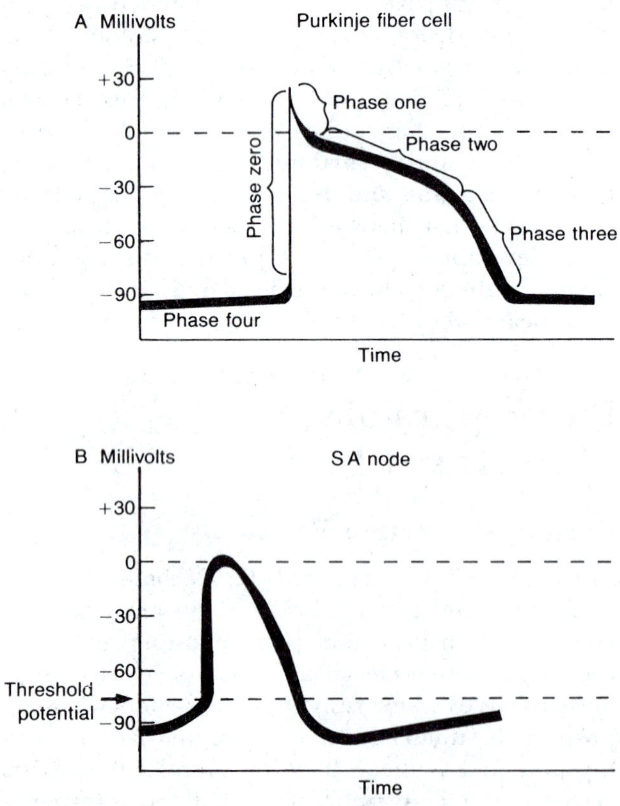

Figure 38–1
Typical action potentials in a Purkinje fiber cell (A) and in the S-A node (B).

Conductance

As we saw in Chapter 36, the heart is able to maintain coordinated pumping because it has evolved a specialized conduction system that carries the wave of depolarization throughout the cardiac musculature. Each beat begins with the spontaneous development of an action potential in the sinoatrial (S-A) node. Conduction within the S-A node is slow. Once the action potential has spread into the atrial muscle, it travels rapidly along the muscle fibers. The atrial and ventricular muscles are separated by the atrioventricular (A-V) node, which restricts passage of impulses between the two chambers. Impulses from atrial muscle can reach the ventricular muscle only by crossing the A-V node. The delay in conduction at the A-V node ensures that atrial contraction will be complete before ventricular contraction begins. After crossing the A-V node, the excitation spreads very rapidly along the His-Purkinje network, activating the fibers of the ventricular muscle. Depolarization of the musculature is immediately followed by contraction.

Electrocardiogram

The electrocardiogram (ECG) is a measure and graphic recording of the electrical events occurring during cardiac excitation. In the normal ECG (Figure 38–2), three characteristic waves occur during each beat: the P wave, the QRS complex, and the T wave. The P wave reflects atrial depolarization, the QRS complex the ventricular depolarization, and the T wave ventricular repolarization. Atrial repolarization is not usually observed because it is of lesser magnitude and is masked by the QRS complex. The Q wave marks the beginning of ventricular systole (contraction). Ventricular diastole (relaxation) accompanies the T wave, while atrial diastole occurs during the QRS complex, and atrial systole during the P wave. The P-R interval reflects the delay caused by the slow rate of conduction across the A-V node. The Q-T interval reflects the duration of the action potential in the ventricles and is generally a rough indication of the refractory period.

Autonomic Influences on Cardiac Electrical Events

Both parasympathetic and sympathetic nerve fibers act on the heart to modify the electrical events of the heart beat. The parasympathetic vagus nerve, acting mainly on the S-A and A-V nodes and conductile elements, decreases automaticity and slows A-V conduction. Heart rate is slowed as a result of the depressed rate of automaticity, the **negative chronotropic effect.** The P-R interval is increased as a result of the prolonged delay in passage of each impulse across the A-V node.

Sympathetic fibers innervate mainly the ventricular muscle and conducting elements. The major effect of sympathetic stimulation of the heart is to increase contractility, the **positive inotropic effect** (see Chapter 37). Norepinephrine increases the rate of conduction of impulses (the **positive dromotropic effect**) across the A-V node, increases the rate of automaticity (the **positive chronotropic effect**), and decreases the refractory period of most cardiac cells. Sympathetic nervous system activity may indirectly decrease heart rate in spite of the direct positive chronotropic influence because the rise in blood pressure may trigger vagal compensatory activity that slows the heart.

Summary: Electrophysiological Properties of the Heart

Four properties of cardiac tissue are crucial to the electrical activity of the heart: **membrane responsiveness** (the capacity of a cardiac cell to depolarize, or enter into phase 0 of the action potential), **effective**

Figure 38–2
A normal electrocardiogram (ECG) pattern. From A. K. Swonger: *Nursing Pharmacology.* Boston: Little, Brown, 1978.

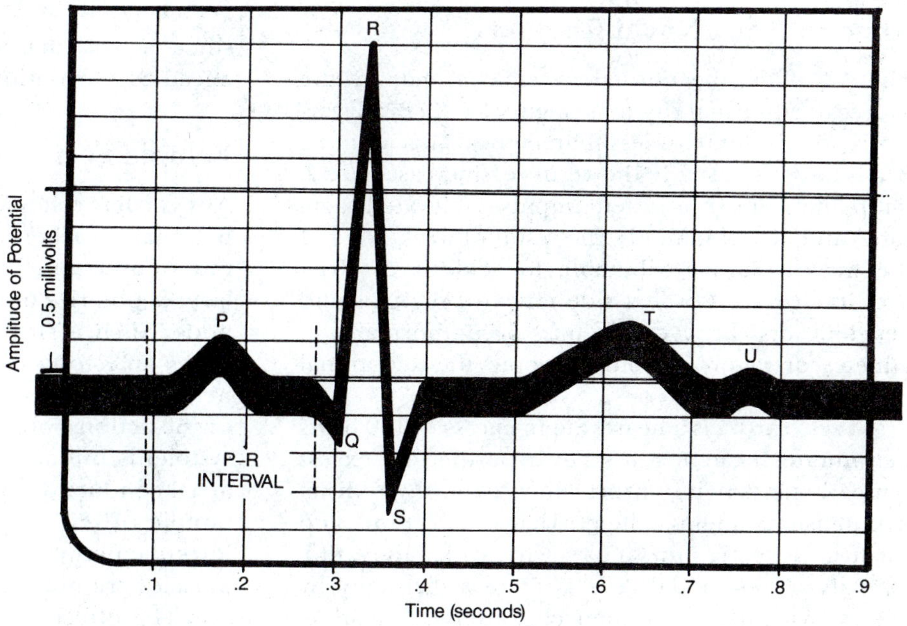

refractory period (the period during which the cell is unresponsive to stimuli, corresponding approximately to phase 3 of the action potential), **automaticity** (the ability to generate an impulse spontaneously, reflected as the slope of the action potential in phase 4), and **conductance** (the rate of spread of the action potential through the various elements in the pathway of conduction). Each of the four properties is reflected in the ECG, and the ECG can be used to evaluate changes in any of these parameters. Each is subject to modulation by autonomic nervous system influence. Further, these same four properties are also subject to pathological disturbances and modification by therapeutic agents, as discussed in the rest of the chapter.

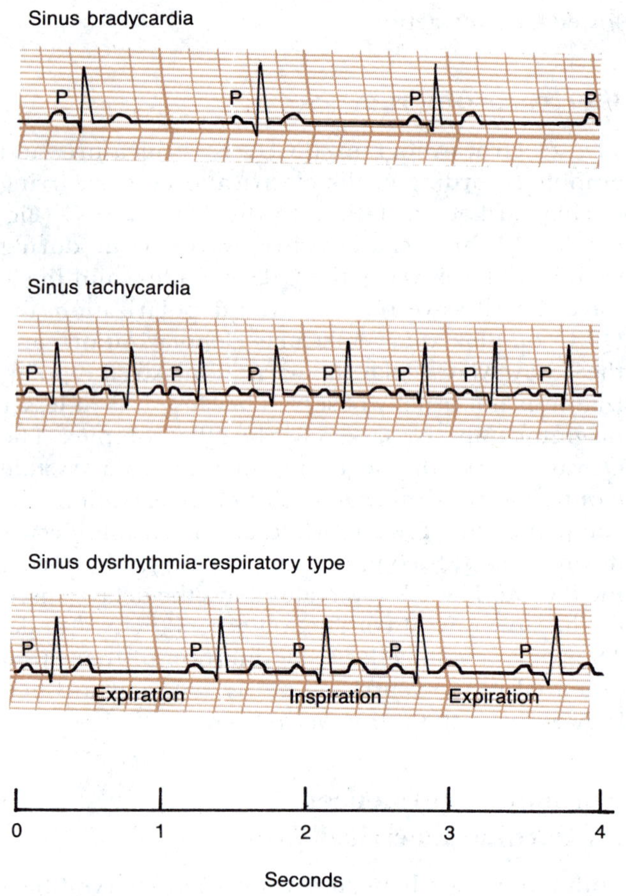

Figure 38–3
ECG patterns illustrating three atrial dysrhythmias.

Dysrhythmias

Disturbances of cardiac rhythm are called *dysrhythmias.* (An older term, *arrhythmias,* is somewhat less accurate since it means literally an absence of rhythm, which is usually not the case.) The heart normally beats approximately 70 times per minute for an adult at rest. However, heart rate and rhythm may be affected by respiration, body temperature, exercise, infections, cardiovascular disease, drugs, and concentrations of ions.

The dysrhythmias can be grouped into five broad categories: (1) abnormal S-A nodal rhythms, (2) ectopic foci, (3) reentrant cycles, (4) conduction blocks, and (5) ventricular preexcitation.

Abnormal S-A Nodal Rhythms

The S-A node, the normal pacemaker, may be the source of abnormal rhythms (Figure 38–3). **Bradycardia** is an atrial rate of less than 60 beats per minute. Bradycardia is usually the result of increased parasympathetic nervous system impulses (elevated vagal tone) and, less commonly, the result of weakening of the myocardium attributable to acidosis or drug toxicity. It can also be a side effect of digitalis and beta-blockers. Bradycardia may occur normally in athletes or vigorous young people in exceptional physical shape.

Tachycardia is a heart rate in excess of 100 beats per minute. It can be caused by hyperthermia, excess sympathetic activity, myocarditis, hyperthyroidism, hypotension, anemia, hemorrhage, infection, and cardiac ischemia. In sinus tachycardia, the automaticity of S-A nodal cells is increased usually by excess sympathetic influence. Caffeine, nicotine, marihuana, and antimuscarinic drugs also cause sinus tachycardia. Sinus tachycardia is often experienced as a sensation of a racing heart beat.

Ectopic Foci

Any cardiac cell that exhibits automaticity is a latent pacemaker. When a group of cells has an elevated rate of automaticity, they may occasionally or regularly depolarize at a rate faster than that of the S-A node. Such a site then becomes an **ectopic focus.** When an ectopic (or "out of place") focus fires while neighboring cells are in their resting state (phase 4 of the action potential), a premature beat (or extrasystole) is initiated. Ectopic foci can develop in the atrial conduction system, the atrial myocardium, the bundle of His, or the terminal bundles of the His-Purkinje network. The A-V node and the ventricular muscles are not sources of ectopic beats.

The effect of an ectopic focus depends on its location and the frequency with which it initiates

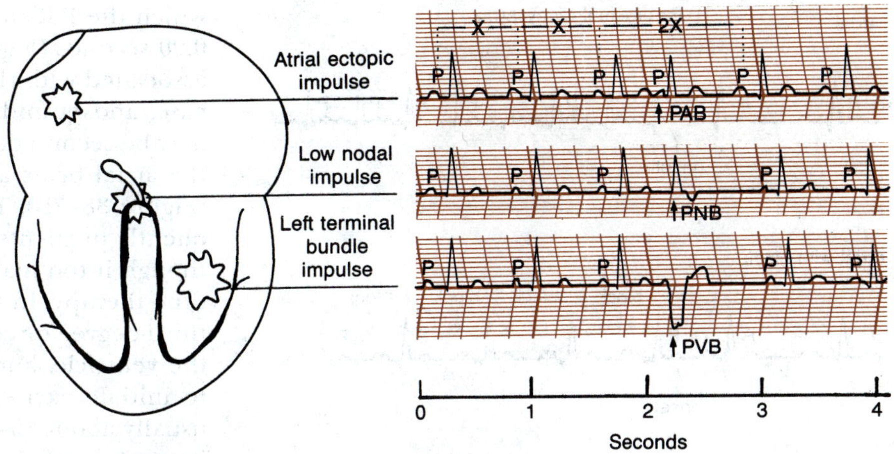

Figure 38–4
ECG patterns illustrating premature beats of atrial, nodal, and ventricular origin: premature atrial beat (PAB), premature nodal beat (PNB), premature ventricular beat (PVB).

beats (Figure 38–4). Occasional ectopic beats have little clinical significance regardless of the location of the ectopic focus, but they may herald paroxysmal tachycardias, flutter, and fibrillation. Ectopic beats are identified in the ECG by the premature occurrence of the spike and the subsequent compensatory pause before the next beat. Premature beats associated with the terminal His-Purkinje bundles are distinctive also because they produce an inversion of the QRS complex, which occurs because the impulse is traveling in the direction opposite to the usual.

When located in the atrium, an ectopic focus gives rise to **atrial ectopic tachycardia.** The most common causes of atrial ectopic tachycardia are hypokalemia, digitalis, alcohol consumption, myocarditis, and pericarditis. Ectopic foci located in the His bundle can give rise to **His bundle rhythms,** formerly called junctional rhythms. Junctional tachycardias are generally of short duration and nonparoxysmal. Persistent, rapidly firing ectopic foci located in the Purkinje system give rise to **ventricular tachycardia.** Ventricular paroxysmal tachycardia is considered serious because it is often a prelude to ventricular fibrillation. The usual causes are arteriosclerotic heart disease, coronary artery disease, and digitalis toxicity. Ventricular tachycardia can also occur in relation to reentry of excitatory electrical signals.

Reentry Dysrhythmias

Reentry dysrhythmias are abnormal cyclical patterns of depolarization in the musculature of the atria or ventricles, brought about by waves of depolarization that circle back along an abnormal pathway of conduction to a site already passed. If the impulse reaches a site that has completed its refractory period, it may stimulate a cyclical pattern of activation, sometimes called a **circus movement.** Three factors can contribute to development of circus movements: (1) the pathway of conduction may be abnormal, providing a means of reentry of the depolarization wave after the end of the refractory period; (2) conduction velocity may be unusually slow, so that potentially cyclical impulses reach sites that have had time to return to their resting state; or (3) the refractory period may be shortened. Digitalis increases the risk of circus movements by slowing conduction velocity, while norepinephrine does so by shortening the refractory period.

Rapid cycles of electrical activity established by circus movements sometimes occur as brief bursts, causing paroxysmal tachycardia (Figure 38–5). In the atrium, signal reentry occurs via the A-V node to produce **paroxysmal supraventricular tachycardia** (PST). During an acute attack, hypotension usually occurs, with feelings of faintness and dizziness. Rapid cycles in the atrium may also lead to **atrial flutter,** a wave pattern of 240–400 cycles per second, or more commonly **atrial fibrillation,** a pattern of 300–600 cycles per second (Figure 38–6). At these rates many of the cardiac cells are refractory while others are excitable. The result is a chaotic, uncoordinated quivering movement of the atrium. Some degree of A-V block occurs, so that the ventricles contract at a rapid rate, but less than the rate of the atrium.

In the ventricles, short-lasting reentry phenomena may cause **paroxysmal ventricular tachycardia.** More persistent circular wave patterns lead to **ventricular fibrillation** (Figure 38–6C), a rapid ventricular dysrhythmia in which contractions are chaotic and ineffective. Ventricular fibrillation results in

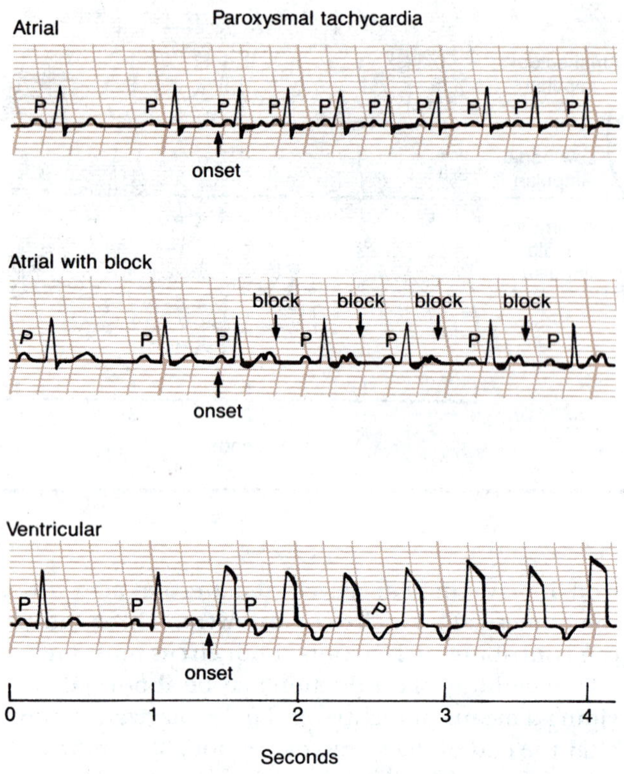

Figure 38–5
ECG patterns illustrating types of paroxysmal tachycardia: atrial paroxysmal tachycardia without and with A-V block and ventricular paroxysmal tachycardia.

death within minutes unless terminated quickly. Myocardial infarcts often lead to fibrillation and death. A strong electrical current applied to the ventricles for a brief interval can often abort fibrillation by producing a synchronous refractory period, following which coordinated activity may begin again. External cardiac massage may be used to maintain coronary blood supply until defibrillation is attempted.

Conduction Blocks

Conduction blocks prevent or partially prevent passage of action potentials along the conductile pathways. By far the most common type of block occurs at the A-V node, although blocks also occur in the Purkinje system or, infrequently, at the S-A node before the impulse reaches the atrial muscle. Blockage at the A-V node or within the ventricle is caused by ischemia, inflammation, compression of conductile tissue, gross changes in the electrolyte composition of the blood or tissue, or, in the case of A-V block, by excessive stimulation by the vagus nerve.

A-V block may be first-degree incomplete, in which the P-R interval is merely prolonged beyond 0.20 seconds (Figure 38–7A). This condition is often associated with rheumatic fever, coronary artery disease, and quinidine or digitalis therapy. A-V block may be second-degree incomplete, in which some of the atrial beats are not passed on to the ventricles (Figure 38–7B). This type of block occurs most frequently in clients with arteriosclerotic heart disease, though it too may be the result of digitalis or quinidine therapy. In the most severe form of A-V block, third-degree or complete, no impulses are passed to the ventricle, and a portion of the ventricle begins to initiate excitement at its own spontaneous rate, usually about 30–40 beats per minute. The ventricular and atrial rhythms then proceed independently (Figure 38–7C), a situation referred to as **ventricular escape.** The most common causes of third-degree heart block are rheumatic fever, fibrosis due to myocardial infarction, digitalis toxicity, and congenital abnormalities.

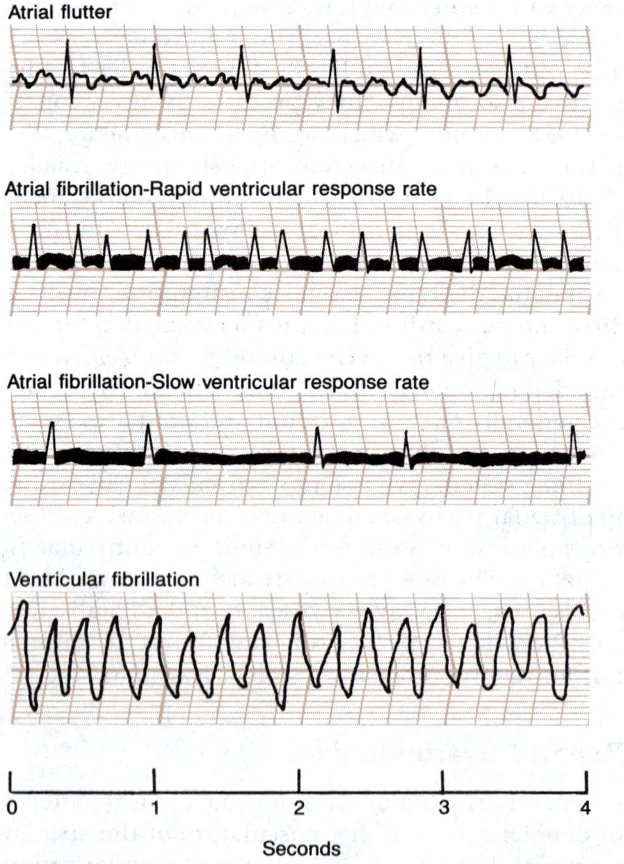

Figure 38–6
Electrocardiogram patterns illustrating flutter and fibrillation.

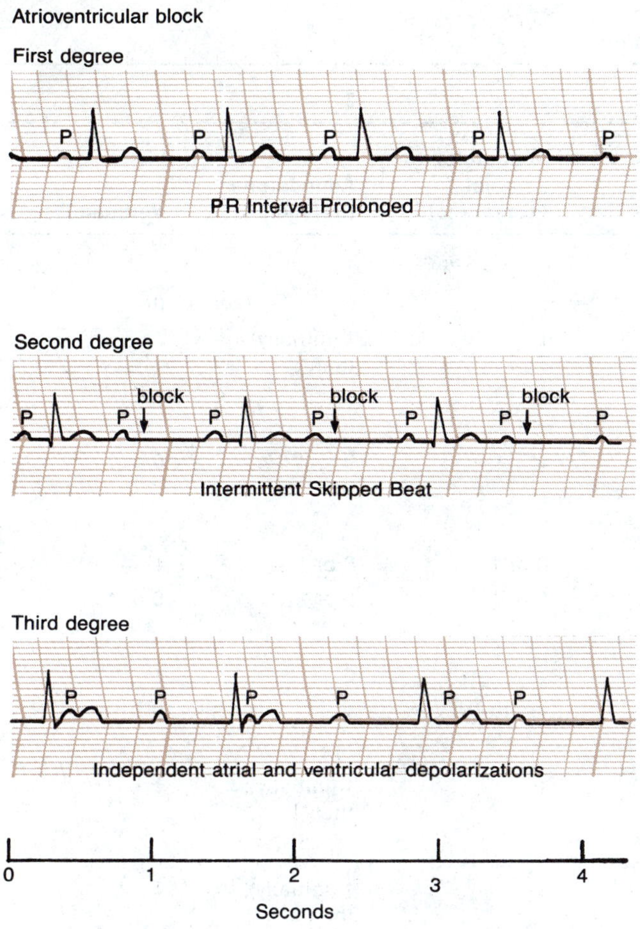

Figure 38–7
Atrioventricular block: first, second, and third degree.

A-V block may be complete but intermittent, a condition called *Stokes-Adams syndrome.* For 5–10 seconds after onset of sudden complete A-V block, no ventricular beats occur, then a ventricular pacemaker escapes, and ventricular contractions begin at the new rate. During the interval before a ventricular pacemaker escapes, the individual may faint or develop convulsions, regaining consciousness once the ventricular pacemaker takes over. Stokes-Adams syndrome can be more dangerous than complete A-V block because during an attack, ventricular escape might be delayed or not occur at all, and cardiac arrest might result. Stokes-Adams patients are sometimes treated with digitalis or quinidine to convert their condition to total A-V block.

Ventricular Preexcitation

The usual form of ventricular preexcitation is called the Wolff-Parkinson-White (WPW) syndrome. In this disorder, an abnormal conduction pathway exists between the atrium and one of the ventricles, in addition to the normal connection via the A-V node and His-Purkinje system. As a result, QRS waves are fusion complexes reflecting the combined influence of the two waves of activation. The P-R interval is typically short because the abnormal pathway provides less impulse delay than does the A-V node. WPW syndrome is asymptomatic unless, as often occurs, it is accompanied by paroxysmal supraventricular tachycardia. Treatment of WPW involves preventing episodes of paroxysmal supraventricular tachycardia or surgical interruption of the reentry pathway.

Antidysrhythmic Drugs

Antidysrhythmic drugs are used clinically to prevent or control disturbances of the normal cardiac rhythm. No single drug is effective in all types or instances of dysrhythmia. Antidysrhythmic drugs act to (1) alter the conduction velocity of the heart beat, (2) alter the membrane responsiveness of cardiac cells to stimuli, (3) shorten or lengthen the refractory period, or (4) alter the influence of catecholamines (norepinephrine and epinephrine) on the heart.

The antidysrhythmic drugs in current use have been classified into four groups based on clinical indications and mechanisms of action. Group 1 drugs are sodium channel blockers and thereby slow conduction and decrease membrane responsiveness. Group 2 are the beta-blockers, of which only three — propranolol (Inderal), acebutolol (Sectral), and esmolol (Brevibloc) — are approved for use in dysrhythmias. Group 3 drugs act primarily to prolong repolarization; bretylium (Bretylol) and amiodarone (Cordarone) are the group 3 drugs available for clinical use. Group 4 drugs are the calcium channel blockers, of which verapamil (Calan, Isoptin) is the only one currently approved for use in dysrhythmias. The effects of antidysrhythmic drugs on the electrophysiological properties of the heart, the ECG, autonomic regulation of the heart, contractility, and hemodynamics are summarized in Table 38–1 and the clinical effectiveness in various kinds of dysrhythmias in Table 38–2.

Group 1-A Drugs

Quinidine

History and Sources Quinidine is the dextrorotatary isomer of quinine. Both drugs are derived from a natural source, the bark of a Peruvian tree, *Cinchona officinatis.* The earliest written reference to use of an extract from the tree is found in a book

Table 38–1
Effects of Antidysrhythmic Drugs on Cardiovascular Functioning

Group	1A	1B and 1C	2	3	4
Example drugs	Quinidine Procainamide Disopyramide	Lidocaine Phenytoin Flecainide	Acebutolol Esmolol Propranolol	Amiodarone Bretylium	Verapamil
Electrophysiologic effects					
Membrane responsiveness	↓↓[a]	↓[a]	↓	0	0
Automaticity (chronotropic effect)	↓	0 or ↓	↓[a]	↑ (initially); then ↓	↓
Effective refractory period	↓ (A-V node); ↑ (ventricle)	↓	↓	↑[a]	↑[a]
Conductance (dromotropic effect)	↓[b]	0 (1B) ↓↓[a] (1C)	↓[a]	0	0 or ↓
ECG effects					
P-R interval	0 or ↑	0 or ↓	0 or ↑	0 or ↑	↑
Q-T interval	↑	0 or ↓	0 or ↓	0 or ↑	0 or ↑
Autonomic effects					
Vagal activity	↓	0	↓	0	↑[b]
Sympathetic activity	0	0	↓beta	↓	0
Contractility					
Inotropic effect	↓	0	↓[b]	↑ (initially); then ↓	↓
Hemodynamic effects					
Cardiac output	↓	0 or ↓	↓	↑ (initially); then ↓	↓
Blood pressure	↓	0 or ↓	↓	↓	↓
Peripheral vasomotor tone	↓[b]	0	0	↓	↓[b]

Key: 0, no change; ↓, small decrease; ↓↓, large decrease; ↑, small increase.

[a]Principal mechanism contributing to the main therapeutic application of the drug in dysrhythmias.

[b]Effects that contribute significantly to adverse clinical reactions, lesser therapeutic applications, or limitations.

written in 1633 by an Augustinian monk, in which use of the powdered bark for cure of fever is described. Both quinine and quinidine possess antipyretic (fever-suppressing) properties. According to legend, the Spanish viceroy of Peru obtained some of the remedy from Peruvian natives for use by his wife, the Countess Anna del Chinchon, and she was miraculously cured of her ailments. The countess's name was thereafter lent to both the tree and the extract, which became known as cinchona.

By 1639, the preparation was being shipped to Spain and thence to other European countries. After two centuries of use of the powder and extract, the active alkaloids, quinine and quinidine, were isolated in 1820. Quinidine was given its present name by Louis Pasteur in 1853. Throughout the eighteenth and nineteenth centuries, cinchona was used for treatment of malaria, and until the 1930s, quinine remained the only specific antimalarial drug. In 1749 the French physician Jean-Baptiste de Sénac reported the use of cinchona in atrial fibrillation, but this observation was forgotten until 1914, when the antidysrhythmic properties of quinine were rediscovered by a Dutch sea merchant, who demonstrated the drug's effect to a Viennese cardiologist. In 1918, W. Frey showed that quinidine was superior to quinine or cinchona as an antidysrhythmic. Since that time, quinidine has been a mainstay among antidysrhythmic drugs. Its mechanism was first elucidated in 1962 but continues to be clarified by current research.

Mechanisms and Effects Quinidine blocks the sodium channels that normally open to permit in-

Table 38–2
Effectiveness of Antidysrhythmic Drugs by Group

Group	1A	1B and 1C	2	3	4
Supraventricular dysrhythmias					
Premature beats	+++	0	++	0	+++
Conversion of flutter or fibrillation	++	0	+	0	++
Termination of paroxysmal tachycardia	+++	0	+++	0	+++
Prophylaxis	++++	0	++	0	++
Ventricular Dysrhythmias					
Premature beats	+++	++ to ++++[a]	+	+	0
Tachycardia	++ to ++++[b]	++ to ++++[a]	+ to +++[c]	+++	0
Digitalis-induced dysrhythmias	+	+++	++	0	0

Key: 0 = not effective; + = poorly effective; ++ = fairly effective; +++ = effective; ++++ = very effective.
[a]lidocaine or tocainide (++++); phenytoin (++).
[b]procainamide (++++); disopyramide (+++); quinidine (++).
[c]propranolol: +++ if dysrhythmia is catecholamine-related; otherwise only +.

flux of sodium during phase 0 of the action potential. The affinity of quinidine for sodium channels is much greater for activated than for inactivated channels. The action of quinidine is therefore greater on cells that are in use (depolarizing frequently) and is said to be "use dependent." By blocking sodium channels, quinidine (1) decreases membrane responsiveness, (2) decreases automaticity, especially in tissue exhibiting high rates of depolarization, (3) increases the duration of the action potential and thus slows conductance, and (4) prolongs the effective refractory period. The effect on automaticity accounts for the ability of quinidine to suppress premature beats caused by ectopic foci, but since the effect is use dependent, there is relatively little influence on the normal pacemaker firing at its usual rate. The prolongation of the effective refractory period helps in treating dysrhythmias due to reentry phenomena, but the effect on conductance may be harmful in such cases. The effects of quinidine are reflected in the ECG as increases in the P-R, QRS, and Q-T intervals.

The effectiveness of quinidine is enhanced by potassium and reduced by hypokalemia. *Therefore, nurses need to know the client's serum electrolyte levels, diet, and drug regimens in order to know if the serum potassium levels are sufficient to enhance the effectiveness of the drug.*

Quinidine also produces indirect effects through both branches of the autonomic nervous system. It possesses significant antimuscarinic (vagolytic) activity that may cause heart rate to increase in spite of the direct depressant effect of quinidine on automaticity. Quinidine also has an alpha-adrenergic blocking action that results in vasodilation and hypotension. The hypotension may trigger a compensatory stimulation of the heart via beta-adrenergic receptors. This together with the vagolytic action of quinidine accounts for the occasional paradoxical occurrence of ventricular dysrhythmias when quinidine is used. Quinidine can increase A-V conductance so that ventricular response rate to an abnormally fast sinus rhythm may accelerate. Digitalis is often administered before quinidine to reduce A-V conductance and prevent the adverse stimulation of quinidine on the A-V node.

Pharmacokinetics Quinidine sulfate (Cin-Quin, Quinora, Quinidex) is almost always given orally. It is rapidly absorbed, having an onset of action in about 0.5 hours and reaching peak concentrations in 1–1.5 hours. Quinidine gluconate (Quinaglute, Duraquin) and quinidine polygalacturonate (Cardioquin) are absorbed more slowly, reaching peak levels in about 3–4 hours.

In the blood, quinidine is about 60–80% bound to plasma proteins. In patients with low serum protein levels, such as those with liver disease, doses of quinidine may need to be reduced. Quinidine enters into erythrocytes, where it binds to hemoglobin, and freely enters most tissues with the exception of the brain. Therapeutic concentrations of quinidine are 3–6 μg/ml.

Quinidine is metabolized in the liver and the products are excreted in the urine. Less than 20% of the absorbed dose is excreted unchanged if liver and kidney function are normal. Excretion of unchanged quinidine is increased if the urine is acidic. Some quinidine metabolites appear to be cardioactive. The elimination half-life is about 6–7 hours. The large individual variations in absorption and elimination of quinidine make it advisable to titrate doses against plasma levels and against ECG recordings.

Clinical Indications Quinidine is useful acutely and chronically for a broad spectrum of dysrhythmias. Quinidine and other group 1-A drugs are favored for chronic prophylaxis aimed at preventing supraventricular dysrhythmias or suppressing ventricular premature beats. Quinidine is also used for acute treatment aimed at terminating paroxysmal supraventricular tachycardias, supraventricular premature beats, or atrial flutter or fibrillation. In current practice, quinidine is employed mainly as an adjunctive to direct current cardioversion (electroshock therapy) for atrial flutter and fibrillation. About one-third of patients given quinidine for 1–2 days prior to scheduled DC cardioversion convert to a normal sinus rhythm without DC shock. Quinidine is continued after cardioversion by the drug or by DC to minimize the risk of recurrence of the atrial dysrhythmia. Quinidine is useful, but not a first choice, in ventricular tachycardias or digitalis-induced dysrhythmias.

Adverse Effects and Contraindications The adverse effects of quinidine fall into six clusters: (1)

Nursing Observations for Use of Antidysrhythmic Drugs

THERAPEUTIC GOAL	Convert the dysrhythmia to a normal sinus rhythm.
PREADMINISTRATION ASSESSMENT	
Baseline Data	Observe extent of palpitations, sensations of fluttering or missed beats, chest pains, or fainting episodes. Evaluate blood pressure, pulse, ECG, heart sounds, peripheral perfusion, respiratory rate and sounds, bowel sounds and function, urine output, and neurological function. Obtain laboratory tests including liver and renal function and blood glucose levels.
Contraindications/ Precautions	Congestive heart failure, A-V block, hypotension, electrolyte imbalance, myasthenia gravis, renal or hepatic failure, or pregnancy or lactation. Check medication history for allergies to antidysrhythmic drugs or tartrazine (found in some formulations).
Potential Interactions	Check medication chart for interacting drugs including hypotensive agents, cardiac glycosides, or neuromuscular blockers.
EVALUATION OF DRUG RESPONSE	
During Dosage Adjustment	Monitor serum concentrations of the antidysrhythmic agent.
For Therapeutic Benefit	Monitor the ECG for recession of the dysrhythmia and normal sinus rhythm.
For Adverse Effects	Monitor for dysrhythmias, chest pain, changes in renal or hepatic function, congestive heart failure, allergic reactions, and other side effects specific to each drug.
For Drug Interactions	Monitor for additive A-V node depression with cardiac glycosides, additive hypotension with hypotensive agents, additive neuromuscular blockade with neuromuscular blockers, and other interactions specific for each drug.
For Dietary Interactions	Assess for reduced effect of quinidine when alkaline foods are ingested.
For Compliance	Evaluate client's compliance with all facets of the therapeutic regimen by careful observation, interviewing, and review of progress. Report compliance problems to the physician and act as client-advocate when changes in the therapeutic regimen seem indicated.

cinchonism, (2) neurological symptoms, (3) hypotension, (4) cardiotoxicity, (5) arterial embolisms, and (6) hypersensitivity reactions.

Cinchonism is a syndrome that occurs with quinidine and other cinchona alkaloids and is closely similar to salicylism. The symptoms include headache, flushing, fever, apprehensiveness, excitement, confusion, and delirium; hearing and vestibular impairments including tinnitus, decreased auditory acuity, and vertigo; visual impairments including blurred vision, disturbed color perception, photophobia, diplopia, night blindness, scotomata, and mydriasis; gastrointestinal symptoms such as nausea, vomiting, abdominal pain, and diarrhea; and hypoprothrombinemia and thrombocytopenia. *Petechial hemorrhages of the oral membranes are indications of thrombocytopenic purpura. The mouth should be examined frequently for oral bleeding. Clients should be instructed to report any alterations in auditory or visual function.*

Although quinidine does not readily penetrate the brain, **neurological and psychiatric symptoms** do occur. Other than the symptoms of cinchonism, psychiatric depression is the main central nervous system side effect.

Hypotension, attributable to vasodilation, can be severe when quinidine is employed. *When quinidine is initially given to hospitalized patients, blood pressure should be determined before administration and compared with values obtained prior to the cardiac event if available. If significant hypotension is noted, the nurse should withhold the drug until the physician is consulted. Norepinephrine should be available when quinidine is first employed in the event of excessive hypotension. The patient should be advised that syncope may occur. Patients should have continuous ECG monitoring and determinations of plasma quinidine levels when more than 2 g/day is being administered.*

One of the most troublesome problems with use of quinidine is the risk of **idiosyncratic ventricular tachycardia** or even fibrillation. Such reactions occur in about 4% of patients treated with quinidine during the acute phase of atrial fibrillation. In atrial fibrillation, second-degree A-V block limits the ventricular response. Quinidine may increase A-V conduction because of its vagolytic action, increasing the proportion of atrial waves that elicit ventricular responses, resulting in ventricular tachycardia. *Although idiosyncratic ventricular tachycardia is not a common reaction, the severity is such that it is usually wise to administer digitalis to patients before administering quinidine for conversion of atrial fibrillation.*

At elevated doses, quinidine may cause other forms of **cardiotoxicity** in relation to its primary mechanism of reducing excitability of cardiac tissue. S-A block, A-V block, or cardiac arrest are possibilities. *Monitoring of the ECG provides the best means of avoiding cardiotoxic reactions since they almost always occur when the QRS or Q-T intervals are unduly prolonged (by 25 to 50% or more). Electrocardiographic examination is also the surest means of detecting conduction blocks or ventricular tachycardia (signs of toxicity) or recurrence of atrial dysrhythmias (inadequate response). Pulse rate should be determined before administration, and the drug should be withheld if rate or rhythm has changed significantly.* Quinidine is contraindicated in patients with conduction defects and is seldom used in digitalis toxicity because of its ability to aggravate A-V block.

There is a risk of **arterial embolism** when cardioversion of atrial fibrillation is undertaken, whether with quinidine alone, or quinidine and DC shock. Thrombi have a tendency to form in a fibrillating atrium because the atrium is not contracting effectively. After conversion to a normal sinus rhythm, the thrombi may be dislodged and, after entering the systemic circulation, may become relodged in a peripheral artery. The sooner conversion is undertaken, the lower is the risk that embolism will occur. When cardioversion is undertaken as an elective procedure, oral anticoagulants may be administered prophylactically for a week or two prior to the procedure.

Allergic reactions occur uncommonly with quinidine. Skin rash is the usual manifestation. Rarely, asthma-like dyspnea, anaphylactic reactions, or fever may occur. Quinidine is contraindicated in patients who are hypersensitive to the drug.

Drug Interactions **Drugs that induce liver enzymes,** such as barbiturates and phenytoin (Dilantin), reduce the bioavailability of quinidine by speeding its metabolism and subsequent elimination. Often people with cardiovascular diseases have difficulty sleeping, especially elderly clients. As a consequence, physicians may prescribe hypnotics, and often these induce liver enzymes.

Alkalinization of the urine by drugs (such as thiazide diuretics, carbonic anhydrase inhibitors, sodium bicarbonate, or antacids) or alkaline-ash foods (such as milk, citrus fruits, or vegetables) increases the half-life of quinidine.

Quinidine has a weak curare-like neuromuscular blocking action. While usually of little importance, this effect may compound that of other neuromuscular blockers or decrease the effectiveness of cholinesterase inhibitors in use for myasthenia gravis. Cardiac depressant effects of quinidine may be increased by concurrent administration of other antidysrhythmic drugs, phenothiazines, or reserpine (Serpasil). Anticholinergic effects of quinidine are additive with other anticholinergic drugs.

Hypoprothrombinemia produced by quinidine may be additive to anticoagulant effects of warfarin (Coumadin) or aspirin. *Nurses should closely monitor clients who are receiving both anticoagulant therapy and quinidine for evidence of excessive bleeding tendencies, ease of bruising, or any other evidences of blood loss.* The hypotensive effect of quinidine may be additive to that of antihypertensive medications. Elevations in serum potassium increase the actions of quinidine. Quinidine increases serum concentrations of digitalis.

Quinidine interferes with certain drug and laboratory tests. For example, it interferes with 17-hydroxycorticosteroid tests when modifications of the Reddy, Jenkins, and Thorn procedures are used. *If a client is to have a urine test using any of these procedures, the laboratory should be informed that the client is receiving quinidine.*

Preparations and Administration Quinidine is given parenterally only when oral administration is

Nursing Diagnoses and Interventions for Use of Antidysrhythmic Drugs

Nursing Diagnoses	*Related Interventions*
TO ENHANCE DRUG BENEFITS OR REDUCE DRUG REQUIREMENTS	
Fear related to uncertain prognosis	Provide support and encouragement for coping with the disorder, interventions, and adverse effects.
TO MINIMIZE DRUG SIDE EFFECTS OR INTERACTIONS	
Alteration in bowel elimination related to diarrhea caused by antidysrhythmic drugs	Advise client to take the antidysrhythmic drug with meals if gastrointestinal irritation is excessive. Assess for signs of altered acid-base balance.
Alteration in cardiac output, fluid volume, and tissue perfusion related to administration of antidysrhythmic drugs	Report symptoms immediately to the physician so that dosage of the antidysrhythmic agent can be adjusted.
Potential for injury related to overdose of antidysrhythmic drugs	Closely monitor for adverse effects and serum concentrations of drug.
TO ENSURE SAFE AND EFFICACIOUS DRUG USE	
Knowledge deficit related to drug regimen	Teach the client about the nature of the disorder and the drug(s) prescribed for treatment. Make certain that the client understands the importance of maintaining the prescribed dosage amount and frequency. Help the client develop a system for keeping track of medication taken. Provide the client with a list of potential adverse effects and drug interactions for each drug in the regimen, and what to do if any of these occur. Advise the client not to take other drugs (even nonprescription ones) without consulting the physician who has prescribed the antidysrhythmic agent. Explain any dietary or activity restrictions included in the regimen. Advise the client to wear a bracelet or tag identifying the disorder and drug regimen. Discuss with the client how to manage persistent side effects such as constipation or hyperglycemia. Explain the importance of keeping follow-up appointments for reevaluation.

not feasible. *Quinidine is best taken on an empty stomach with a full glass of water to optimize absorption. However, if gastrointestinal irritation becomes troublesome, quinidine may be taken with meals to reduce this adverse effect.* The gluconate and polygalacturonate preparations are reported to produce less gastrointestinal irritation. Steady-state plasma concentrations are achieved in 1–5 days. Doses are titrated by measurement of serum levels (the therapeutic level is 2–7 μg/ml) and ECG monitoring.

Quinidine gluconate (Quinaglute, Duraquin)
Sustained release tablets
Recommended Doses: 268 mg PO are equivalent to 200 mg of quinidine sulfate.

Quinidine polygalacturonate (Cardioquin)
Tablets
Recommended Doses: 275 mg PO are equivalent to 200 mg of quinidine sulfate.

Quinidine sulfate (Cin-Quin, Quinora, Quinidex)
Capsules, tablets, sustained release capsule
Recommended Doses: 300–500 mg PO qid initially. Maintenance doses, 200–600 mg PO daily.

Important Nursing Implications for Quinidine

- ☐ Usually administer oral quinidine with a full glass of water on an empty stomach 1–2 hours after meals. Give with meals if nausea, vomiting, or diarrhea occur to a significant degree.
- ☐ Use a test dose if ordered by the physician to determine allergic sensitivity to quinidine.
- ☐ Monitor plasma concentrations of quinidine carefully. The therapeutic range of serum concentrations for quinidine is 3–6 μg/ml.
- ☐ During intravenous administration, monitor closely for indications of vasodilation or cardiac depression. Monitor the ECG for widening of the QRS complex, loss of P waves, or premature ventricular beats.
- ☐ Monitor serum electrolytes, blood cell counts, and intake-output during prolonged quinidine therapy.
- ☐ Monitor the ECG and pulse for indications of paradoxical ventricular tachydysrhythmias when quinidine is used for atrial dysrhythmias.
- ☐ Advise clients to report palpitations or faintness, which might indicate quinidine-induced ventricular dysrhythmia.
- ☐ Instruct clients to report indications of abnormal bleeding such as petechiae or bleeding of the gums. Observe for potentiation of bleeding effects of oral anticoagulants.
- ☐ Monitor for symptoms of thromboemboli when quinidine is used for cardioversion.
- ☐ Watch for adverse interactions of quinidine with cardiac glycosides. Quinidine increases plasma levels of digoxin. The two drugs also have additive depressant effects on A-V conduction.
- ☐ Do not use quinidine in clients with A-V block, congestive heart failure, myasthenia gravis, or hypotension.
- ☐ Observe for neurological deficits and sensory impairments indicative of cinchonism.

Procainamide (Pronestyl)

Like quinidine, procainamide is related to a previously known drug that was itself used to treat dysrhythmias — in this case procaine. In a comparative study of analogues of procaine, procainamide was found to possess superior antidysrhythmic properties.

Mechanisms and Effects The direct action of procainamide on cardiac cells is indistinguishable from that of quinidine. Like quinidine, it blocks sodium channels, thereby reducing membrane responsiveness, prolonging the refractory period and action potential, decreasing automaticity, and suppressing conductance. Procainamide does differ from quinidine in its effects on the heart that are mediated through the autonomic nervous system. Procainamide has much less anticholinergic activity than quinidine and as a result is less likely to cause idiosyncratic ventricular tachycardia when used for conversion of atrial fibrillation. Procainamide also lacks alpha-adrenergic blocking activity and hence produces less hypotension.

Pharmacokinetics Procainamide is well absorbed after oral administration, being taken up from the small intestine where the alkaline pH favors its absorption. Onset of action occurs in about 30 minutes and plasma concentrations peak in 45–75 minutes when capsules are employed. Absorption is slower with procainamide tablets. If administration is initiated while cardiac function is impaired (for example, following a myocardial infarction), absorption may be substantially altered by poor perfusion of the intestinal mucosa and the regimen may be rendered ineffective. Procainamide has a half-life of about 2.5–4.5 hours and a single dose is effective for about 3 hours. Sustained release preparations can provide effectiveness for up to 8 hours.

Procainamide is only modestly bound by plasma proteins (15–20%) and distributes rapidly throughout the body. Therapeutic plasma concentrations of procainamide are 4–8 μg/ml and toxicity occurs at concentrations above 16 μg/ml. It is eliminated by renal excretion (50–60%) and hepatic metabolism (40–50%), mainly N-acetylation.

Clinical Indications Procainamide is not generally used for chronic prophylaxis because of the frequency of significant side effects. Procainamide is useful for acute applications in conversion of atrial or ventricular dysrhythmias. Procainamide is especially effective in terminating ventricular premature beats and ventricular tachycardia. Procainamide is superior to quinidine in the latter application. In practice, lidocaine (Xylocaine) is generally given first preference for alleviation of ventricular dysrhythmias, but procainamide is a useful second-choice treatment. Procainamide is not as effective as alternative drugs for digitalis-induced dysrhythmias.

Procainamide is as effective as quinidine in terminating atrial tachycardia, flutter, or fibrillation. Like quinidine, it is more effective in atrial tachycardia than in converting flutter or fibrillation.

Procainamide produces much less hypotension than quinidine and can therefore be used successfully for dysrhythmias associated with anesthesia and surgery. However, the hypotensive effect of procainamide is additive with that of other hypotensive medications.

Adverse Effects and Contraindications Adverse effects of procainamide include (1) cardiotoxicity, (2) hypotension, (3) gastrointestinal symptoms, (4) neurological symptoms, and (5) hypersensitivity reactions. **Cardiotoxicity** resembles that produced by quinidine. Idiosyncratic ventricular tachycardia, though less common with procainamide, can occur paradoxically when atrial rate is slowed by procainamide. Excessive levels of procainamide, like quinidine, can suppress cardiac excitability to the extent that S-A or A-V block or even cardiac arrest occurs. In the case of procainamide, cardiotoxicity is not reliably preceded by lengthening of the Q-T interval. *Nevertheless, nurses should monitor the patient's ECG prior to any parenteral administration of procainamide.*

Procainamide is contraindicated in patients with severely damaged hearts or heart block. Increased atrial contraction can be enough to dislodge existing thrombi and result in pulmonary embolisms. *Nurses need to monitor patients who are receiving procainamide for symptoms of pulmonary emboli such as pleuritic chest pain and tachypnea.*

When procainamide is given by infusion, a blood pressure drop of greater than 15 mm Hg indicates an excessive rate of infusion. Infusion rate can usually be adjusted to avoid significant **hypotension.** *Good nursing management requires that phenylephrine, dopamine (Inotropin), or levarterenol be available for immediate use in the event of excessive hypotension. Patients should always be kept supine during procainamide infusions.*

When procainamide is administered orally, adverse **gastrointestinal reactions** include anorexia, nausea, vomiting, and diarrhea. Such reactions are more common with procainamide than with quinidine. **Neurological symptoms** induced by procainamide include confusion, hallucinations, irritability, nightmares, depression, and aggravation of myasthenia gravis.

The most troublesome of the side effects of procainamide are the **hypersensitivity reactions;** these substantially limit the usefulness of procainamide in clinical practice. Allergic reactions to procainamide often result in bone marrow suppression, leading to agranulocytosis, thrombocytopenia, or hemolytic anemia. Fatal infections may ensue. Skin rashes, fever, myalgias, and Raynaud's phenomena are additional allergic manifestations. *Before giving procainamide, nurses need to uncover any evidence of hypersensitivity to the drug. Patients hypersensitive to procaine and related drugs are also likely to be sensitive to procainamide and therefore should not receive this drug. During administration, the nurse should be alert for signs of allergic reactions to procainamide. Outpatients receiving procainamide should be advised to report any evidence of agranulocytosis, such as recurrent respiratory infections, sore throat, fever, malaise, joint and muscle pain, or unexplained bleeding or bruising. It is especially important to stress the need to report such symptoms because many clients would otherwise consider these to be signs of flu or a cold, and too minor to be of any significance. Family members need to be aware of these symptoms of harmful effects of the drug. Routine blood counts are advisable. If leukocyte counts indicate cellular depression, the drug should be discontinued.*

An allergic reaction to procainamide that occurs with alarming frequency when the drug is used chronically is a drug-induced **systemic lupus erythematosus-like syndrome.** Symptoms include arthralgia, pericarditis, pleuritic pain, fever, insomnia, and hepatomegaly. The syndrome is reversible when procainamide is discontinued. About 25% of patients on extended procainamide therapy experience this reaction within a year of treatment, and up to 70% of patients exhibit elevated antinuclear antibodies. *The nurse should be attentive for symptoms of the lupus syndrome in clients receiving chronic procainamide.* Clients who are slow acetylators (an inherited characteristic) may be at increased risk of developing the lupus-like syndrome.

Drug Interactions Procainamide, like quinidine, has weak neuromuscular blocking activity. This effect is additive with the neuromuscular blocking action of curare, neomycin, and drugs of like activity. *Clients known to have myasthenia gravis should not receive procainamide.* Procainamide tends to antagonize the efficacy of cholinergic agonists.

The hypotensive effect of procainamide can be additive to that of other hypotensive drugs, including diuretics. Cardiac depression produced by procainamide may be additive with other antidysrhythmic drugs or cardiac glycosides.

Administration of procainamide simultaneously with the H_2-blocker cimetidine results in reduced renal excretion of both procainamide and its principal metabolite. Dosage adjustment may be required.

Preparations and Administration Since the half-life of procainamide is short, frequent administration of tablets and capsules (other than sustained release capsules) would be required except that patients receiving procainamide generally have impaired cardiac function and possibly renal function as well. Thus, in many clients, administration of tablets or capsules 4 times per day suffices. Sustained release capsules may be given every 6 hours but are not recommended for initial therapy. *The ECG should be monitored daily during institution of oral therapy. If clients are placed on oral procainamide after discharge, the drug should be taken at equal intervals around the clock. It is important for the nurse to assist the client in establishing an appropriate protocol to assure that adequate drug levels will be maintained. Procainamide absorption is optimized by administration on an empty stomach with a full glass of water. However, if clients complain of gastrointestinal irritation, the drug should be administered with food.*

Procainamide (Pronestyl)
Tablets, capsules, sustained release capsules, injection solution
Recommended Doses: 3–6 g PO daily for chronic applications. For acute control of dysrhythmias, continuous intravenous infusion in 5% glucose or slow (over 1 minute) injections of 100 mg, repeated every 5 minutes until control is achieved. The full dose is never given in a single bolus.

Important Nursing Implications for Procainamide

- ☐ Carefully monitor the ECG, blood pressure, and flow rate of the drug during intravenous infusions of procainamide.
- ☐ Instruct clients to take oral procainamide on an empty stomach with a full glass of water.
- ☐ Before giving procainamide, check the medication history for any evidence of allergic reactions to procainamide, procaine, or structurally related drugs. After administration, observe the client for signs of allergic reaction.
- ☐ When procainamide is given by infusion, keep the client supine and watch for indications of excessive hypotension. Keep epinephrine on hand in the event of excessive hypotension.
- ☐ Periodically evaluate clients on long-term procainamide therapy for lupus erythematosus cells, antibody titers, blood cell counts, presence of fever, arthralgia, cough, or pleuritic pain, and renal and hepatic function since procainamide can cause a systemic lupus erythematosus-like reaction.
- ☐ Instruct clients and families to report frequent upper respiratory infections or other symptoms of blood dyscrasias. Obtain periodic complete blood cell counts.
- ☐ Store procainamide tablets at room temperature and injection solutions between 50–80° F.
- ☐ Do not employ procainamide in clients with A-V block, hepatic or renal dysfunction, or myasthenia gravis.

Disopyramide (Norpace)

Disopyramide phosphate was introduced into clinical practice in 1978 for oral use in the treatment of ventricular dysrhythmias.

Mechanisms and Effects Although chemically unrelated to quinidine or procainamide, disopyramide has effects on cardiac cells similar to those of the other group 1-A drugs. Automaticity is depressed, more in ectopic pacemakers than in normally firing S-A nodal cells. Disopyramide increases the effective refractory period in atrial and ventricular tissue but has less effect on the His-Purkinje system, so that conduction of impulses in the specialized conductile tissue is little affected. The P-R interval is consequently unaltered by disopyramide. Like quinidine, disopyramide has a vagolytic action, but it does not block adrenergic receptors.

Pharmacokinetics Disopyramide is about 90% absorbed after oral administration and first pass elimination is insignificant. The onset of action occurs in about 30 minutes and peak plasma levels are achieved in 1–2 hours. About 30% (20–60%) of the plasma concentration is protein bound at normal doses.

About 50% of an administered dose is excreted unchanged by the kidneys, the rest being metabolized by the liver. The elimination half-life is about 5–8 hours and the duration of action about 6 hours. The main metabolite is weakly active. Patients with impaired renal or liver function require correspondingly lower doses. *Urinary output should be measured and observed for any signs of change.*

Clinical Indications Disopyramide is approved only for use in ventricular dysrhythmias in adult patients. It is effective for suppression of premature ventricular beats and ventricular tachycardia, except those secondary to digitalis toxicity. It is used both acutely, for conversion of ventricular dysrhythmias, and for chronic prophylaxis after cardioversion. In Europe, disopyramide is also used for conversion of atrial dysrhythmias with success comparable to that obtained with other group 1-A drugs.

Adverse Effects and Contraindications Disopyramide has a significantly lower incidence of adverse effects than either quinidine or procainamide. Although cardiotoxicity is less of a problem than with quinidine or procainamide, it is important to monitor clients for **hypotension** and indications of **first-degree A-V block.** If significant hypotension occurs, the drug should be discontinued. *Clients taking the drug at home need to be taught how to monitor their own pressure and to keep accurate records as a baseline against which to measure change.*

The **anticholinergic effects** of this drug are greater than with quinidine or procainamide. *Nurses should question clients about the presence of dry mouth, constipation, urinary hesitancy, urgency, frequency, or retention, blurred vision, aggravation of glaucoma, or other classic anticholinergic symptoms.* Gastrointestinal symptoms such as nausea, vomiting, cramps, or diarrhea can occur, but are considerably less common than with quinidine or procainamide. Cardiotoxicity can occur as with other group 1-A drugs. Disopyramide causes an increase in peripheral resistance which results in a rise in blood pressure, despite a reduction in cardiac output.

Preparations and Administration

Disopyramide phosphate (Norpace)
Capsules
Recommended Doses: 100 or 150 mg PO, qid up to 800 mg daily. When rapid control is required, an initial loading dose of 300 mg PO is recommended except for patients with cardiomyopathies or possible cardiac decompensation. Smaller doses (such as 100 mg qid) are used in patients with renal or hepatic failure.

Important Nursing Implications for Disopyramide

- ☐ Monitor blood pressure and teach the client to monitor blood pressure for indications of excessive hypotension. Instruct clients to change positions slowly and to avoid hot showers, hot sunlight, and long periods of standing.
- ☐ Teach clients to report quickly indications of congestive heart failure such as dyspnea, orthopnea, edema, rales, cyanosis, or sudden weight gain. Provide clients with printed instructions concerning when and what to report. Be sure to use lay terms and to define medical terms.
- ☐ Periodically monitor the ECG for indications of cardiotoxicity: widening of the QRS complex, prolongation of the Q-T interval, or an excessive increase in the P-R interval.
- ☐ Periodically monitor serum potassium levels since hyperkalemia increases toxicity of disopyramide. Correct any potassium imbalances before instituting therapy.
- ☐ Monitor the client for evidence of anticholinergic side effects. Monitor intake and output for evidence of urinary retention.
- ☐ If clients experience dryness of mouth, suggest the use of frequent rinses, gum, or hard candies and avoidance of alcohol.
- ☐ Include responsible family members in observation of the client's responses, since the client may not report some side effects that he or she considers embarrassing. This is especially true if the client begins to show signs of mental confusion.
- ☐ Do not administer disopyramide to individuals with A-V block or allergies to disopyramide or who are in cardiogenic shock.
- ☐ Store disopyramide between 59–86°F in an airtight container.

Group 1-B and 1-C Drugs: Local Anesthetic Agents

Group 1-B drugs depress membrane responsiveness only slightly and hasten repolarization. For a number of years, lidocaine (Xylocaine), a local anesthetic, has been used effectively in treatment of ventricular dysrhythmias. Its usefulness is limited, however, by the fact that it must be administered parenterally. Lidocaine is widely used in emergency management of ventricular dysrhythmias that occur during cardiac surgery or following myocardial infarction. Its advantages for emergency application in coronary care units include its rapid action and quick elimination that permit fairly precise control by regulation of infusion rate. Recently, drugs related to lidocaine that can be given orally have been developed. Tocainide (Tonocard), introduced late in 1984, and mexiletine (Mexitil), introduced early in 1986, are drugs with electrophysiological properties very similar to those of lidocaine, but with good oral effectiveness. Tocainide is often referred to as "oral lidocaine."

Still more recently, three additional drugs, flecainide (Tambocor), encainide (Enkaid), and lorcainide, have been developed that are somewhat similar to lidocaine, though less so than tocainide. These three new agents are classified as Group 1-C drugs. Unlike group 1-B drugs, group 1-C drugs slow conduction — a negative dromotropic effect. Flecainide was marketed in early 1986; encainide is approved as an investigational drug; lorcainide is still in development.

Mechanisms and Effects The effects of group 1-B and 1-C drugs differ substantially from the effects of group 1-A drugs (Table 38–1). Their principal effect is to increase the outward flow of potassium, with the result that the excitability threshold of cardiac tissue is increased. Automaticity is little affected and effective refractory period is reduced. Conductance is usually not altered by group 1-B drugs but is significantly depressed by group 1-C drugs. Group 1-B drugs cause relatively little alteration of the ECG, but group 1-C drugs widen the QRS wave and prolong the P-R and Q-T intervals because of their affect on conduction velocity. In contrast to group 1-A drugs, group 1-B and 1-C drugs have no important indirect effects on autonomic innervation of the heart.

Pharmacokinetics After oral administration, lidocaine blood levels are usually very low due to extensive first pass metabolism; that is, most of the drug is metabolized on its first pass through the portal vein. Moreover, oral administration often causes substantial gastrointestinal discomfort. Therefore, lidocaine is given by intramuscular injection, intravenous bolus, or intravenous infusion. After intramuscular injection, absorption is nearly complete. In the plasma, lidocaine is 50% bound to protein. Elimination of lidocaine is by liver metabolism. The half-life for elimination is about 1–2 hours. The duration of action is very short after infusion is discontinued.

Tocainide and **mexiletine** are rapidly and almost completely (90 to 100%) absorbed after oral administration, reaching peak serum concentrations within 3.0 hours. Ingestion of food with tocainide or mexiletine administration slows but does not affect total absorption, and absorption of mexiletine is slowed by narcotics, atropine, and aluminum or magnesium hydroxides. First-pass extraction by the liver is negligible for either drug. Binding to plasma proteins is about 10–20% for tocainide and 50–60% for mexiletine. Both tocainide and mexiletine are inactivated by the liver with a half-life of 11–15 hours for tocainide and 10–12 hours for mexiletine.

Flecainide is almost completely absorbed after oral administration, reaching peak serum concentrations in about 3.0 hours. Absorption is not substantially affected by food or antacids and first-pass extraction is negligible. Binding to plasma proteins by flecainide is about 40%. Flecainide inactivation involves both renal excretion (30%) and biotransformation (70%). Its biological half-life is about 20 hours.

Absorption of **encainide** after oral administration is more erratic than for flecainide or tocainide. The drug that reaches the plasma is 90% bound to plasma proteins. Encainide is inactivated mainly by metabolism with a half-life of about 3.4 hours.

Dangerous drug accumulation can occur with any of these drugs if there is kidney or liver impairment. *The nurse should check the client's chart, question the client, and pay special attention to blood chemistries that might provide an indication of kidney or liver insufficiency. Use of any of the group 1-B or 1-C drugs in these circumstances would be contraindicated.*

Clinical Indications Lidocaine is used exclusively for acute management of ventricular dysrhythmias, including premature ventricular beats and ventricular tachycardia. It is very rapid in onset but has a short duration of action. It is useful for ventricular dysrhythmias triggered by cardiac manipulation during surgery, myocardial infarcts, or digitalis toxicity. Lidocaine is a drug with a limited spectrum of effectiveness, but it is the most important in-hospital drug for acute control of ventricular dysrhythmias.

Tocainide, mexiletine, and flecainide are indicated for suppression of documented or symptomatic ventricular dysrhythmias, including frequent premature ventricular beats and ventricular tachydysrhythmias. Encainide is in clinical trials for use in these same conditions. Flecainide should be used with caution because of its potential for producing paradoxical ventricular tachydysrhythmias.

Adverse Effects and Contraindications Lidocaine seldom produces significant cardiotoxicity because it is typically used for brief periods of time. Nevertheless, during intravenous infusion, the ECG should be continuously monitored for signs of **excess cardiac depression** such as prolongation of the P-R or QRS intervals. The principal toxic effects are on the central nervous system and include drowsiness, paresthesias, agitation, feelings of dissociation, blurred vision, tinnitus, and euphoria. Elevated doses may cause convulsions or respiratory arrest. Diazepam (Valium) should be available in the event of convulsions. Drowsiness is a common side effect, but since rest is an important part of therapy for those who have experienced a myocardial infarction, the drowsiness may, in fact, be beneficial. Dizziness, numbness of the lips and tongue, and distrubances of speech are all signs of lidocaine toxicity and indications that the drug should be discontinued.

The oral lidocaine-like drugs may cause significant cardiac and noncardiac toxicities. The group 1-B and 1-C drugs should not be employed in patients with second- or third-degree A-V block. *If the client's record indicates presence of Stokes-Adams syndrome or severe heart block, the nurse should withhold the medication until the order has been double-checked with the physician.* Caution must be exercised in using these drugs in clients with known heart failure, especially when a beta-blocker is also being employed. **Aggravation of pre-existing congestive heart failure** has been observed in about 5% of clients given flecainide.

A troublesome feature of the activity of tocainide, mexiletine, flecainide, and encainide is potential worsening of existing dysrhythmias or occurrence of new dysrhythmias is response to the drug. This action is referred to as a **prodysrhythmic effect.** Group 1-B drugs are less likely to cause such problems than group 1-C agents. The incidence of dysrhythmogenesis or exacerbation of existing dysrhythmias is estimated at 7% for flecainide and 11% for encainide, but only 1–2% for tocainide and mexiletine.

Hypersensitivity to amide-type local anesthetics is a specific contraindication for use of tocainide. *The nurse needs to assess clients for hypersensitivity to local anesthetics before administering lidocaine or tocainide. If there is evidence of hypersensitivity, use of lidocaine or tocainide is contraindicated and nurses should refrain from administering these drugs. Nurses should also check the client's past medication history to determine if he or she has had repeated or prolonged use of one of these drugs.*

The most common adverse reactions to tocainide are rash, headache, lightheadedness, nausea, paresthesias, and nervousness. There have been infrequent hematological reactions (leukopenia, thrombocytopenia, agranulocytosis) and pulmonary reactions (fibrosis, pneumonitis, pneumonia, or edema). *The nurse should advise patients receiving tocainide to report such symptoms as bruising, bleeding, sore throat, chills, fever, exertional dyspnea, cough, or wheezing.* The most common adverse effects of mexiletine are heartburn or nausea, diarrhea, tremor nervousness, lightheadedness, incoordination, changes in sleep patterns, visual disturbances, palpitations, chest pain, rash, and dyspnea.

Flecainide produces neurological side effects similar to those caused by tocainide: dizziness, lightheadedness, visual disturbances (such as blurred vision and spots in the visual field), headache, nausea, fatigue, and tremor. Other problems that have been noted in greater than 1% of clients are dyspnea, gastrointestinal disturbances, chest pains, and palpitations. In the limited clinical experience with encainide, neurological problems have been the most common adverse effects.

Preparations and Administration Lidocaine (Xylocaine) that is formulated for use in dysrhythmias is without epinephrine or preservatives, while that manufactured for use as a local anesthetic often contains one or both additional substances.

GROUP 1-B

Lidocaine
Injection solutions, prefilled syringes
Recommended Doses: Intravenous infusion at rates from 1 to 5 mg/minute. The therapeutic range of plasma concentrations is 1–5 mcg/ml. For intravenous injection, 1–2 mg/kg. For IM injection, 4–5 mg/kg (seldom utilized). *Injection into the deltoid muscle provides faster absorption than into the gluteus or lateral thigh.* Since the action of lidocaine is brief, repeated injections may be required.

Mexiletine (Mexitil)
Capsules
Recommended Doses: 200 mg PO every 8 hours. The total daily dose should not exceed 1,200 mg. Mexiletine should be given with food or an antacid.

Tocainide (Tonocard)
Film-coated tablets
Recommended Doses: 400 mg PO every 8 hours initially. Some patients have been treated with doses in excess of 2,400 mg/day PO. Individuals with impaired renal or hepatic function may be successfully treated with doses less than 1,200 mg/day PO.

GROUP 1-C

Encainide (Enkaid)
Investigational

Flecainide (Tambocor)
Tablets
Recommended Doses: 100 mg PO every 12 hours initially. The individual doses can be increased by 50 mg PO increments (to a maximum of 200 mg/dose) at intervals of 4 days until effective.

Lorcainide
Investigational

Important Nursing Implications for Local Anesthetic-Type Antidysrhythmic Drugs

- ☐ Never use lidocaine that contains preservatives or epinephrine for antidysrhythmic purposes.
- ☐ Determine whether the client has a history of allergies to local anesthetic drugs.
- ☐ During intravenous infusion of lidocaine, carefully monitor flow rate, the ECG, and blood pressure. Observe the ECG for prolongation of the P-R interval or QRS complex or aggravation of dysrhythmia. Use lidocaine cautiously if the client has prior hypotension, A-V block, congestive heart failure, renal or hepatic dysfunction, or during pregnancy.
- ☐ Assess clients for neurological side effects (such as dizziness, lightheadedness, confusion, paresthesias, blurred vision, headache) when any of the local anesthetic type of antidysrhythmic drugs are employed.
- ☐ Assess clients for evidence of bleeding tendencies when flecainide is employed.
- ☐ Be aware that elderly clients should receive lower doses.
- ☐ Give intramuscular injections of lidocaine in the deltoid muscle.
- ☐ Discard partially used containers of lidocaine for injection since these solutions contain no preservatives.

Phenytoin (Dilantin)

Phenytoin, a group 1-B drug as well as an antiepileptic agent used widely to control grand mal seizures, is often used clinically to control digitalis-induced ventricular dysrhythmias although it is not approved by the U.S. Food and Drug Administration as an antidysrhythmic drug.

Mechanisms and Effects The cardiac effects of phenytoin resemble those of lidocaine (Xylocaine). The principal effect is to increase potassium conductance, which tends to speed repolarization and to hyperpolarize cells, increasing the threshold for stimulation of cardiac cells. Phenytoin does not significantly alter normal automaticity but does significantly reduce digitalis-induced increases in automaticity. Like lidocaine, phenytoin has little effect on conduction of impulses and shortens the effective refractory period. Alterations in the ECG are minimal. Phenytoin has no peripheral interactions with the autonomic nervous system but can modify autonomic impulse traffic through its CNS actions.

Pharmacokinetics Absorption of phenytoin after oral administration or intramuscular injection is slow and variable, but intravenous injection provides rapid distribution. In the plasma, phenytoin is 70–95% bound to protein. The serum concentration required for control of dysrhythmias is typically 10–20 μg/ml, but this is altered if serum protein binding is reduced by hypoalbuminemia or competition with other drugs. Phenytoin is eliminated by liver hydroxylation and subsequent urinary or biliary excretion. The elimination half-life is 18–24 hours.

Clinical Indications Phenytoin is effective for control of ventricular dysrhythmias, especially those associated with digitalis toxicity. It is ineffective for atrial dysrhythmias, except when caused by digitalis overdose. Oral maintenance therapy with phenytoin may prevent further occurrence of dysrhythmia.

Adverse Effects and Contraindications Cardiotoxicity is uncommon with phenytoin, but heart block and bradycardia occur occasionally. Vasodilation and hypotension sometimes occur. Rapid intravenous administration has been observed to cause cardiac arrest. *Monitor the ECG during IV administration to avoid hypotension and bradycardia.* The risk of cardiotoxicity is increased when the client is elderly, alcoholic, or hypotensive and when he or she has diabetes mellitus, respiratory disorders, hepatic or renal dysfunction, or a pancreatic adenoma.

The most frequent adverse effects of phenytoin relate to the CNS. Drowsiness, ataxia, vertigo, nausea, tremors, nervousness, confusion, and nystagmus are prominent reactions. Adverse effects and drug interactions associated with chronic use of phenytoin are discussed in Chapter 23.

Preparations and Administration The vehicle furnished with phenytoin has a pH of 11 and will cause severe phlebitis if given by infusion; therefore phenytoin for dysrhythmias is given by slow intermittent intravenous injection. *Oral doses should be taken with milk, water, or meals to reduce gastric irritation by this alkaline drug.*

Phenytoin (Dilantin and generic)
Oral dosage forms (see Chapter 23), injection solution with special diluents for reconstitution.
Recommended Doses: For control of digitalis-induced dysrhythmias, 100 mg every 5 minutes until control is achieved to a maximum dose of 1,000 mg. Serum concentrations of greater than 20 μg/ml provide no additional efficacy. Oral doses, 100–200 mg tid typically.

Group 2 Drugs: The Beta-blockers

Currently, propranolol (Inderal), acebutolol (Sectral), and esmolol (Brevibloc) are the only beta-blockers approved as antidysrhythmic drugs. The overall pharmacology of beta-blockers is discussed in Chapter 39 in relation to their use as antihypertensive drugs. In this section, only their use as antidysrhythmic agents will be discussed.

Mechanisms and Effects The antidysrhythmic efficacy of propranolol is in large measure attributable to its beta-blocking properties but also involves direct effects on ionic currents. Like quinidine, propranolol depresses sodium influx, and like lidocaine, it increases potassium efflux. Propranolol blocks both β_1- and β_2-receptors. Acebutolol and esmolol block β_1-receptors (those involved in sympathetic regulation of the heart) but not β_2-receptors and lack the quinidine-like action of propranolol. Esmolol is ultra-short-acting.

Propranolol decreases automaticity of S-A nodal cells only when automaticity has been increased by adrenergic stimulation. Propranolol also decreases myocardial contractility, decreases conduction velocity of impulses, and prolongs the effective refractory period by its beta-blocking action. The quinidine-like direct action contributes to decreasing conduction velocity as well but tends to reduce refractory period. In the A-V node, the dominant influence on effective refractory period is the increase attributable to beta-blockade. This effect is the basis for the primary use of propranolol and other beta-blockers, to reduce ventricular response rates in supraventricular tachydysrhythmias. The increase in A-V node refractory period reduces the proportion of atrial impulses that are able to transverse the A-V node.

Pharmacokinetics The pharmacokinetics of propranolol and acebutolol are disturbingly variable. After oral administration, absorption is nearly complete, but extensive and unpredictable first-pass metabolism occurs, severely curtailing bioavailability. *Nurses should recognize that ingestion of beta-blockers with food reduces absorption but also reduces first-pass extraction.* About 30% of an orally administered dose of propranolol or 40% of a dose of acebutolol reaches the systemic circulation after first-pass extraction. After oral administration, propranolol is effective in about 30 minutes and persists for 3–6 hours. Acebutolol has a similar onset and a half-life of 3–4 hours. Onset of action occurs with propranolol in about 2 minutes following intravenous administration and peak effect occurs in about 5 minutes. The duration of action after intravenous injection is about 2–4 hours with propranolol. Cigarette smoking or use of other inducers of liver enzymes decreases bioavailability of propranolol. Propranolol is eliminated by hepatic metabolism. The therapeutic window of plasma concentrations is approximately 0.04–0.1 μg/ml. Esmolol is given only by intravenous injection or infusion and its effect lasts only 30 minutes.

Clinical Indications Propranolol is most successfully employed for limiting ventricular response rates in supraventricular dysrhythmias including atrial tachycardia, flutter, and fibrillation. It does so by increasing the refractory period of A-V nodal cells. Occasionally, propranolol also produces conversion of the atrial dysrhythmia to a normal sinus rhythm.

Propranolol is also used successfully for ventricular dysrhythmias related to excess catecholamine activity, such as occur in pheochromocytoma, hyperthyroidism, intense emotional states, or other conditions of sympathetic excess. Propranolol is effective in such conditions because it suppresses automaticity in ectopic foci stimulated by norepinephrine action. Propranolol may also be effective in ventricular dysrhythmias that are not obviously linked to catecholamine excess. Propranolol is less useful than other drugs for digitalis-induced dysrhythmias. Acebutolol is indicated only for management of ventricular premature beats. Esmolol is used for short-term treatment of supraventricular tachycardia.

Adverse Effects and Contraindications Adverse effects of beta-blockers are described more fully in Chapter 39. Cardiotoxic effects of propranolol can result from the suppression of sympathetic influence on the heart, which may be maintaining cardiac function. **Congestive heart failure** is therefore a risk when propranolol is employed, especially if there is a history of compromised heart function. **Bradycardia** is the most common cardiotoxic effect of propranolol and is especially likely in patients with Wolff-Parkinson-White syndrome or digitalis intoxication. Propranolol can also cause **A-V block** as an extension of its therapeutically useful effect on

A-V nodal conduction and refractory period. Propranolol often causes significant hypotension, which may lead to cardiovascular collapse. Sudden discontinuation of propranolol can aggravate **coronary artery insufficiency,** leading to anginal pain or even myocardial infarction. *Following chronic use of propranolol, withdrawal should be gradual (over about 2 weeks) to minimize risks of angina or infarction.*

Propranolol, but not acebutolol or esmolol, blocks β_2- as well as β_1-adrenergic receptors and therefore inhibits catecholamine-mediated bronchodilation. Propranolol should therefore not be given to patients with bronchial asthma. Propranolol inhibits physiological compensatory reactions to excess insulin and masks certain of the consequent symptoms of hypoglycemia (pulse rate and blood pressure elevation.) *Therefore diabetic patients should be monitored carefully for signs of hypoglycemia when given propranolol.*

Preparations and Administration During administration of propranolol for dysrhythmias, the ECG should be monitored closely.

Acebutolol (Sectral)
Capsules
Recommended Doses: For ventricular dysrhythmias, 400 mg PO initially in 2 divided doses, increased gradually until an optimal response is obtained (typically 600–1,200 mg/day PO).

Esmolol (Brevibloc)
Injection solution

Propranolol (Inderal)
Tablets, injection solution
Recommended Doses: For dysrhythmias, 10–30 mg PO, 3 or 4 times per day. For intravenous use, 1–3 mg at a rate of not more than 1 mg/minute, followed by a second dose after 2 or more minutes. Additional doses may be given at 4-hour intervals.

Group 3 Drugs

The clinically available group 3 drugs are bretylium (Bretylol) and amiodarone (Cordarone). Bretylium was employed in the 1950s as an antihypertensive, but was discontinued because tolerance develops rapidly. Bretylium was approved for use as an antidysrhythmic in 1978 and amiodarone in 1986. Both are indicated only for emergency use in ventricular dysrhythmias not responsive to other drugs.

Mechanisms and Effects Bretylium and amiodarone act both directly on cardiac tissue and indirectly by interaction with sympathetic nerve terminals. These group 3 drugs rapidly accumulate in sympathetic nerve endings, initially displace and release norepinephrine, and later inhibit release of norepinephrine in response to sympathetic impulses. The result is a noncompetitive inhibition of α- and β-adrenergic activity. The main effect of group 3 drugs on electrophysiological properties of cardiac tissue is to increase the effective refractory period and duration of action potentials in ventricular muscle, especially in compromised tissue. Group 3 drugs are thus able to disrupt ventricular dysrhythmias associated with reentry currents. Group 3 drugs have no significant effects on automaticity, the threshold of excitability, membrane responsiveness, or conduction. Thus, the unique quality of group 3 drugs is their ability to increase refractory period without affecting conduction rate. The Q-T interval is increased (reflecting the effect of these drugs on the refractory period), A-V conduction is somewhat slowed, and the P-R interval correspondingly prolonged.

Pharmacokinetics Bretylium is given only by intravenous or intramuscular injection or by intravenous infusion. Amiodarone is employed orally. After oral administration, amiodarone absorption is slow and variable, with bioavailability approximating 50%. The main route of inactivation is by excretion in the bile.

Clinical Indications Group 3 drugs are currently approved for treatment of life-threatening ventricular dysrhythmias. They are secondary choices for ventricular dysrhythmias that are not responsive to lidocaine or procainamide, or ventricular fibrillation not responsive to countershock.

Adverse Effects and Contraindications The major complication with bretylium therapy is **hypotension.** Inhibition of norepinephrine release from peripheral sympathetic terminals causes the vasodilation that leads to hypotension. Tolerance often develops to the hypotensive effect. *Patients should be kept in the supine position during use of bretylium to minimize hypotensive responses. The ECG and blood pressure should be monitored during drug administration. Bretylium should not be employed in patients who take digitalis.*

Adverse effects occur commonly with amiodarone, necessitating discontinuation of treatment in 7–18% of patients receiving 400 mg/day or higher doses. Common adverse reactions include neurological problems, gastrointestinal complaints, dermatological eruptions, or pulmonary inflammation or fibrosis. **Corneal microdeposits** occur in more than half of adults treated with amiodarone, leading to blurred vision and visual halos. Amiodarone also inhibits conversion of thyroxine to triiodothyronine, resulting in elevations in thyroxine and depletion of triiodothyronine. Since triiodothyronine is more active than thyroxine, **hypothyroidism** may occur. **Cardiovascular toxicity** includes bradycardia, congestive heart failure, and exacerbation of dysrhythmias. *The ECG and blood pressure should be monitored carefully during initial titration of dosage and during any subsequent adjustments in dosage.*

Drug Interactions The initial release of norepinephrine caused by bretylium may intensify toxicity of cardiac glycosides. Simultaneous use of bretylium with cardiac glycosides should therefore be avoided.

Amiodarone potentiates the effect of oral anticoagulants, necessitating a reduction in dose of the anticoagulant by one-third to one-half. Amiodarone increases serum levels of digoxin, necessitating a reduction in dosage of the cardiac glycoside by one-half. Amiodarone also increases serum levels of other antidysrhythmic drugs, including quinidine, procainamide, and phenytoin. Doses of these drugs should be reduced.

Bradycardia and A-V block produced by group 3 antidysrhythmic drugs can be additive with that caused by beta-blockers, calcium channel blockers, and other cardiosuppressant medications.

Preparations and Administration Commercial bretylium tosylate is diluted fivefold or more prior to intravenous infusion. *Intravenous doses are given slowly to prevent occurrence of nausea and vomiting.* The typical intramuscular dose is 5–10 mg/kg of undiluted solution, which can be repeated after 6–8 hours. *The site for intramuscular injections should be rotated when repeated administration is required to prevent necrosis or fibrosis.* Bretylium is seldom continued beyond 3–5 days before substituting another antidysrhythmic drug. *Bretylium is stored at room temperature (59–86° F).*

Because of the variability in absorption of amiodarone, amiodarone therapy should be undertaken only by physicians experienced in treatment of life-threatening dysrhythmias and with access to laboratory facilities for monitoring client response and adverse effects. Amiodarone is administered in divided doses with meals if the daily dose is 1,000 mg or greater or when gastrointestinal disturbances occur.

Bretylium tosylate (Bretylol)
Injection solution
Recommended Doses: 5–10 mg/kg infused over 10–30 minutes, or in emergency situations, 5 mg/kg of undiluted solution by intravenous injection repeated as indicated up to 30 mg/kg.

Amiodarone (Cordarone)
Tablets
Recommended Doses: Loading doses, 800–1,600 mg/day PO for 1–3 weeks, until therapeutic response is achieved; then, 600–800 mg for 1 month, and maintenance doses thereafter of typically 400 mg.

Group 4 Drugs: The Calcium Channel Blockers

Group 4 drugs consist of the calcium channel blockers. Verapamil is the only drug in this family currently approved for use in dysrhythmias. The overall pharmacology of this drug group is discussed in Chapter 40. In this section, we will consider only the use of verapamil as an antidysrhythmic drug.

Verapamil (Calan, Isoptin)

Mechanism and Effects Verapamil blocks calcium influx through calcium channels. Because calcium influx is essential for excitation-contraction coupling, verapamil decreases contractility (a negative inotropic effect). This means that verapamil should not be used in patients with compromised cardiac contractility. Calcium is also important for maintenance of smooth muscle tone in coronary and peripheral capillary sphincters, so verapamil also increases cardiac perfusion and peripheral vasodilation. The increased cardiac perfusion is beneficial when the ventricular response rate to atrial tachydysrhythmias is high, because rapid rates of ventricular contraction increase oxygen demand. Peripheral vasodilation, however, presents an unwanted action when verapamil is employed in cardiac dysrhythmias.

The major benefit of verapamil is an increase in the refractory period of the A-V node. This effect reduces ventricular response to an elevated atrial rate. Because of it, verapamil should not be used in patients with A-V block.

Pharmacokinetics Verapamil is given intravenously for antidysrhythmic purposes. Onset of action occurs in 1–5 minutes and lasts 10–20 minutes. Hypotensive effects follow a similar time course. Verapamil is 83–92% protein bound in plasma. The therapeutic range of plasma concentrations is 80–300 ng/ml. Verapamil is metabolized in the liver initially to an active metabolite, norverapamil. The metabolites of verapamil are excreted mainly in the urine and to a lesser extent in the bile. The elimination half-life is about 4 hours.

Clinical Indications Verapamil is effective in terminating paroxysmal supraventricular tachycardia and in chronic prophylaxis after conversion of this condition. Its efficacy is comparable to that of quinidine or propranolol in this respect. Verapamil is also effective in reducing ventricular response rates in atrial flutter or fibrillation.

Adverse Effects and Contraindications The general adverse effects of calcium channel blockers are discussed in Chapter 40. The major adverse cardiovascular effects of verapamil are vasodilation, negative inotropism, and S-A or A-V block. *Baseline evaluation of cardiac function should be established before administration of verapamil. Nurses should also teach clients how to take their own blood pressure routinely during verapamil therapy.* The hypotensive effect of verapamil may result in such symptoms as dizziness, headache, and peripheral edema. The negative inotropism may precipitate congestive heart failure and pulmonary edema. Verapamil should be used with caution in clients with compromised contractility. Verapamil should not be used in conditions involving A-V block.

Verapamil has the potential for additive depressant effects on A-V conduction and myocardial contractility with other antidysrhythmic drugs such as propranolol. *It is especially important to monitor clients and to teach clients and their families how to monitor for symptoms of negative inotropism when such combinations are employed.*

The most common noncardiovascular side effects are nausea and abdominal discomfort.

Preparations and Administration

Verapamil (Calan, Isoptin, generic)
Tablets, injection solution

Recommended Doses: For acute control of dysrhythmias, 10 mg IV by slow injection over 2 minutes or more. A second dose can be given after 10–30 minutes. For oral prophylaxis, 80 mg, tid or qid, to a daily total of 240–480 mg.

Important Nursing Implications for All Antidysrhythmic Drugs

- ☐ Before administering an antidysrhythmic drug, make baseline observations of pulse rate and blood pressure. Any irregularity of rhythm should be noted. If the ECG is being monitored, the recording should be carefully examined. The nurse should immediately report (1) widening of the QRS or Q-T intervals by more than 25%, (2) ectopic beats not previously observed, (3) a sudden increase in frequency of ectopic beats, (4) a significant change in heart rate, (5) disappearance of P waves, or (6) other obvious changes. Signs of hypotension (faintness, headache, lightheadedness, increasing peripheral edema) or decreased perfusion (cold extremities, low urinary output, confusion) should be noted and reported.
- ☐ Review the adverse effects of each drug being administered and watch for such symptoms. The client should be told about likely side effects and enlisted in monitoring for their occurrence.
- ☐ Teach the client the importance of precise compliance when antidysrhythmic drugs are used. Clients should be encouraged to discontinue use of caffeine-containing beverages, alcohol, and cigarettes.

Case Study: Ventricular Fibrillation

P. L. was a 56-year-old married man, admitted to the hospital emergency room at 2:00 PM with severe chest pain following several sets of tennis. In the emergency room, P. L. went into ventricular fibrillation, which the staff terminated by direct current cardioversion. P. L. was admitted to the coronary care unit. There the nurse obtained a history indicating that P. L. smoked about two packs of cigarettes a day and drank from four to six beers a day. P. L. had recently changed jobs. Vital signs were blood pressure 130/85, pulse 105 and irregular, temperature 99.8° F, and respirations 22/minute. Auscultation revealed no congestion of the lungs. Palpation revealed no obvious organomegaly. The physician ordered an ECG, which revealed premature ventricular beats (about 4/minute) and an anterior wall myocardial infarction of indeterminant age. P. L. was noticeably anxious about his condition. The physician ordered cardiac monitor, bedrest, a low-salt soft diet, diazepam (Valium) 5 mg orally every 4 hours as required for anxiety, and morphine sulfate 5–15 mg IV as required for pain.

At 9:30 PM on the day of admission, P. L. began to have more frequent premature ventricular beats (PVBs) (about 10/minute). Since lidocaine (Xylocaine) for frequent PVBs was a standing order in the coronary care unit at this hopital, the nurse injected 50 mg intravenously and began a lidocaine drip at 2.5 mg/minute. After 15 minutes, PVBs were no longer evident in the ECG.

Since P. L. exhibited a continuing tendency toward frequent PVBs over the next 2 weeks of hospitalization whenever lidocaine was discontinued, the physician began P. L. on tocainide (Tonocard), 400 mg every 8 hours, orally. The nurse told P. L. to notify the physician immediately if he experienced painful respiration, wheezing, cough, palpitations, tremor, bruising or bleeding, or persistent sore throat, fever, or chills. She also provided P. L. with a list of these potential adverse reactions as a reminder. She warned P. L. that he might experience dizziness or drowsiness and should exercise caution when driving his car. She told P. L. that he could take this medication with meals or a snack if he experienced nausea, vomiting, or diarrhea when taking the medication on an empty stomach, but that he should adhere closely to the required 8-hour interval between doses.

1. What factors may have contributed to P. L.'s initial episode of ventricular fibrillation?
2. Why was defibrillation conducted by DC cardioversion rather than with an antidysrhythmic agent?
3. Why was diazepam, as needed, ordered by the physician?
4. Was the nurse's decision to administer lidocaine an appropriate response to the frequent PVBs?
5. Why was P. L. stabilized on tocainide rather than lidocaine before discharge from the hospital?
6. Will the beneficial effect of tocainide be impaired if P. L. takes the medication with food?

Answers appear at end of the book.

Case Study: Cinchonism

D. S. was a 70-year-old white man who had been hospitalized for 1 week while receiving quinidine treatment for a cardiac dysrhythmia. The nurse noted that D. S., who was an avid reader, suddenly stopped reading the books or magazines he had brought with him to the hospital. When the nurse asked D. S. about an article in one of the magazines, she learned that he had not read it because "the words all ran together." Realizing that he had developed blurred vision and was possibly having an adverse reaction to quinidine, the nurse pursued with other questions. She learned that D. S. also had found that the light he used for reading hurt his eyes. The nurse noted that his pupils were dilated and as a result he was experiencing photophobia. Other inquiry revealed that although D. S. at first said he felt fine, he really did not feel well. He said he "felt vomity." The nurse found D. S.'s temperature was elevated. He began expressing considerable concern about his condition. The nurse recorded her observations and D. S.'s complaints, checked his chart for the result of blood studies and any other evidence that might indicate a problem, reviewed the literature in the ward library, and reported the findings to the physician. The nurse reviewed her findings with the members of the health team and it was concluded that D. S. was having an untoward response to quinidine therapy. The physician elected to discontinue the therapy. More serious problems were averted and, in time, D. S.'s symptoms disappeared.

1. Which of the observations made by the nurse led her to the conclusion that D. S. was experiencing cinchonism?
2. Analyze the activities of the nurse in this case using the steps of the nursing process.

Answers appear at the end of the book.

Recommended Readings

Akhtar M: Management of ventricular tachyarrhythmias. *JAMA* 1982;247:671–674.

Befeler B: Clinical pharmacology of the antiarrhythmic agent disopyramide phosphate (Norpace). *Heart Lung* 1980;9(3):475–487.

Bigger JT Jr et al: Quinidine and digoxin: An important drug interaction. *Drugs* 1982;24:229–239.

Budassi SA: Management of cardiopulmonary arrest. *Nurs Clin North Am* 1981;16(1):37–53.

Crumpley L: An overview of antiarrhythmic drug. *Crit Care Nurse* 1983;3(4):57–64.

Federman J, Vlietstra RE: Antiarrhythmic drug therapy. *Mayo Clin Proc* 1979;54:531–542.

Geyer LN: Giving procainamide safely. *Nursing* 1984; 14(5):116.

Johnson GP, Johnson BC: Beta blockers. *Am J Nurs* 1983; 83:1034–1043.

Moore LC: An on-the-spot guide to antihypertensive drugs. *Nursing* 1986;16(1):54–57.

Moses HW et al: Antiarrhythmic drugs. *J Clin Pharmacol* 1980;20:598–618.

Nademanee K et al: Advances in antiarrhythmic therapy: The role of newer antiarrhythmic drugs. *JAMA* 1982; 247:217–222.

Pepper GA: New antiarrhythmic drugs. *Nurse Pract* 1986;11(7):62–70.

Rossi LP, Antman EM: Calcium-channel blockers — new treatment. *Am J Nurs* 1983;83:382–387.

Sasyniuk BI, Ogilvie RI: Antiarrhythmic drugs: Electrophysiological and pharmacokinetic considerations. *Annu Rev Pharmacol Toxicol* 1975;15:131–155.

Sjogren E: Tocainide (Tonocard). *Crit Care Nurse* 1983; 3(6):12–13.

Sjogren E. Lidocaine HCL injection. *Crit Care Nurse* 1983;3(6):14–15.

Stanford JL, Felner JM, Arensburg D: Antiarrhythmic drug therapy. *Nursing* 1980;10:1288–1295.

Stewart S: Nadolol (Corgard). *Crit Care Nurse* 1983; 3(1):96.

Velebit V et al: Aggravation and provocation of ventricular arrhythmias by antiarrhythmic drugs. *Circulation* 1982;65:886–894.

Warner, HW: Therapy of common arrhythmia. *Med Clin North Am* 1974;58(5):995–1017.

CHAPTER 39

Antihypertensives

Hypertension is among the most prevalent medical disorders in the United States, affecting some 35 million individuals. Drugs are widely employed for their ability to control (but not cure) hypertension and its complications. An indication of the prominence of antihypertensive medications is the presence of more than 20 drugs used primarily for hypertension among the 200 most frequently prescribed drugs.

Determinants of Blood Pressure

Blood pressure is the result of a complex interaction between the cardiovascular, renal, autonomic, endocrine, and central nervous systems. Arterial blood pressure is the product of two major determinants (see Table 39–1): cardiac output and peripheral resistance. Cardiac output is in turn related to heart rate and stroke volume, and the latter of these is determined by the force of contraction of the myocardium. The autonomic nervous system plays a major role in regulating cardiac output. Peripheral resistance is influenced by body fluid volume, sympathetic tone, and the tone of the vascular smooth muscle. The functioning of the cardiovascular system is monitored by specialized sensing devices — the baroreceptors, chemoreceptors, and the renin-releasing cells of the kidneys. Information concerning blood pressure and concentration of blood gases, derived from baroreceptors and chemoreceptors, is conveyed to the brain. There it influences the cardiac and vasomotor centers of the medulla to determine sympathetic and vagal outputs that regulate

Table 39–1
Factors in Hypertension

Determinants of blood pressure	Related factors in hypertension	Related antihypertensive medications
Cardiac output		
Heart rate	Vagal destruction	Beta-blockers
Force of contraction (beta-receptors)	Excess sympathetic tone	Beta-blockers
Peripheral resistance		
Sympathetic tone (alpha-receptors)	Excess sympathetic tone	Centrally acting sympatholytics
		Drugs acting on postganglionic sympathetic nerve terminals
		Alpha-blockers
Other influences on vascular smooth muscle		Direct-acting vasodilators
Body fluid volume	Edema	Diuretics
Renin/angiotensin/aldosterone		Angiotensin-converting enzyme inhibitors

the heart and vasomotor tone. The juxtaglomerular cells of the kidney monitor and regulate blood sodium through endocrine and renal mechanisms.

Cardiac Output

Cardiac output is regulated by both intrinsic and extrinsic influences. The most important of the **intrinsic hemodynamic influences** is the Frank-Starling relationship, which states that the force of contraction of cardiac fibers increases in proportion to the degree of initial stretch. Initial stretch in the intact heart is a function of preload; that is, the more the chamber is filled, the more the muscle stretches. When preload is great, a greater force of contraction will be required to expel the large volume of blood and empty the chamber. The Frank-Starling law ensures that the force of contraction in a healthy heart will be sufficient to meet the demands imposed by any given preload.

The most important **extrinsic regulatory influences** on the heart are autonomic. Afferent fibers from the sympathetic nervous system innervate the ventricular wall, the conductile elements including the A-V node, the atrial wall, and least of all the S-A node. Release of norepinephrine from these sympathetic fibers has several effects, the most pronounced of which is to increase the force of contraction of the cardiac muscle (the positive inotropic effect). Sympathetic innervation also promotes an increase in conduction rate in the A-V node and Purkinje fibers, an increase in automaticity, and a decrease in the refractory period of the muscle cells. Increase in the automaticity of cells in the S-A node results in an increase in heart rate (the positive chronotropic effect). Sympathetic nerve terminals also influence blood supply to the heart itself by way of the coronary arteries. Norepinephrine causes a constriction of coronary arteries initially.

Parasympathetic influence on the heart is achieved through the vagal nerve. Vagal fibers terminate mainly in the S-A node, atrial muscle, and the A-V node. Acetylcholine released from the postganglionic parasympathetic terminals slows heart rate by its action on the S-A node (a negative chronotropic effect) and depresses conduction of impulses across the A-V node. Acetylcholine has little effect on force of contraction.

The principal brain area regulating cardiac output is the cardiac center of the medulla. One portion of this center (the dorsal motor nucleus of the vagus nerve) controls heart rate while an adjacent area regulates sympathetic influences on the heart.

Peripheral Resistance

Peripheral resistance is a function of vasomotor tone — the degree or constriction or dilation of blood vessels. The mechanics of regulation of vasomotor tone are directly attributable to the anatomy of blood vessels. The large arteries, such as the aorta, are elastic vessels, providing little resistance to blood flow. They stretch to receive the stroke volume of the heart and then rebound to their resting contour, which helps to push the blood along through the arterial system. The branches from the major arteries are called nutrient or distributing arteries because they function in the distribution of nutrients and gases to the organs and tissues. The nutrient arteries give rise to smaller branches called arterioles, which lead into the capillary beds. The arterioles are the chief determinants of peripheral resistance. The last segment of the arteriole, the precapillary sphincter, constricts or relaxes in response to autacoids (local hormones), sympathetic nervous system influences, and local changes in temperature, pH, or blood gases. Constriction of the arterioles increases peripheral resistance and raises arterial blood pressure, but it decreases capillary filtration pressure. Dilation of arterioles has the opposite effects.

Arterioles are composed of three layers: the tunica intima, the tunica media, and the tunica adventitia. The innermost layer, the tunica intima, provides a smooth coat that minimizes friction to blood passage. The outermost layer, the tunica adventitia, provides form and support. The middle layer, the tunica media, is the major determinant of peripheral resistance. It consists of vascular smooth muscle that contracts to constrict the diameter of the arterioles or relaxes to dilate the vessel.

The capillary beds and the venules comprise the exchange vessels and have quite different anatomical design. Their walls consist of endothelial cells surrounded by a basement membrane. The blood pressure in the capillaries is typically about 30 mm Hg and constitutes the single most important component of filtration pressure.

Venous blood pressure is only indirectly determined by cardiac output and is not normally pulsate. Blood moves through the venous circulation and lymphatic vessels due to pressures produced by skeletal, thoracic, and visceral muscle movements and valves that prevent backflow of blood. Under normal circumstances, about 75% of the blood is found in the venous circulation. Venous blood vessels are called capacitance vessels because they freely stretch to contain whatever blood is delivered to them. Venous return is an important factor in cardiac output in that it determines preload. Excessive pooling of blood in the capacitance vessels can contribute to **orthostatic hypotension.**

Autonomic regulation of peripheral resistance to blood flow is mediated almost exclusively by sympathetic innervation of arterioles. The parasympathetic nervous system has little influence over blood vessels except in a few vascular beds, such as in the salivary glands. Vasoconstriction is brought about by the action of norepinephrine on alpha-receptors, most strongly in skeletal muscles, skin, and the viscera; less so in the heart and lungs; and least of all in the cerebral cortex. Vasodilation can occur in response to epinephrine and is mediated by β_2-receptors. It occurs mainly in the heart and skeletal muscles.

The primary brain area involved in regulating autonomic influences on vasomotor tone is the **vasomotor center** of the medulla oblongata. It includes a pressor region and a depressor region. The medulla oblongata receives two kinds of information concerning cardiovascular function to aid in its regulatory role: blood pressure and concentrations of blood gases. **Baroreceptors,** pressure-sensitive organs located mainly in the carotid sinuses and aortic arch, measure blood pressure by responding to the degree of stretch in these elastic vessels and transmit this information to the medulla. **Chemoreceptors** found in the medulla itself monitor CO_2 (indirectly by measuring pH of the cerebral spinal fluid). Other chemoreceptors in the carotid and aortic bodies monitor oxygen in the arterial blood.

Hormonal influences on precapillary sphincters include both endocrine hormones and autacoids. Vasopressin, the main endocrine substance, has significant effects on peripheral resistance. A wide variety of autacoids are involved in autoregulation of blood flow to specific tissues. Renin, kinins, and prostaglandins have been implicated in regulation of renal blood flow. Kinins and prostaglandins are probably of similar importance in other tissues as well. Serotonin, histamine, kinins, and prostaglandins are involved in regulating local constrictor or dilatory responses that relate to clotting or inflammation.

Body Fluid Volume

A clear relationship exists between sodium retention and elevated blood pressure. Epidemiological studies show that groups of people with low sodium diets have a low incidence of hypertension, while groups with high sodium diets have a much higher incidence of hypertension. Renal control of sodium is critical to maintenance of normal blood pressure. The renin-angiotensin-aldosterone system, discussed in Chapter 43, is primarily responsible for maintaining sodium balance; activation of this system leads to sodium retention and fluid volume expansion. Correction of the fluid and sodium retention with diuretics lowers blood pressure.

In some clients with hypertension and edema, there is a clear increase in renin release by the kidney, with a consequent activation of the renin-angiotensin-aldosterone salt-retaining mechanism. In another group, renin production is "normal" to the extent that it is similar to that of normotensive individuals. In this group, however, normal renin production may be considered abnormal because renin release should be low when pressure is elevated. Thus, one significant factor contributing to excessive retention of fluids and salt may be an imbalance in the renin-angiotensin-aldosterone system.

Another hormone that may play a role in hypertension is atrial natriuretic factor (ANF). ANF normally plays an important role in preventing hypertension by reducing fluid volume when atrial pressure rises. ANF reduces fluid volume by (1) inhibiting secretion of renin and (2) direct effects on the renal nephron. Preliminary studies in spontaneously hypertensive animals suggest that ANF may become depleted during extended hypertension. Further research on ANF may ultimately lead to new treatments for hypertension.

Hypertension

Hypertension is probably the most common disorder of the cardiovascular system. When it is severe and persistent, it can cause extensive adverse effects on the tissues of the body, but especially on the heart, arteries, kidneys, and brain. Hypertension is defined as an elevation in systolic and/or diastolic blood pressure. For purposes of clinical diagnosis, specific ranges have been established to define hypertension in each age group (Table 39–2). Each incremental increase in diastolic blood pressure over 90 mm Hg further reduces life expectancy. Because diastolic pressure reflects peripheral resistance, it may be the more telling of the two blood pressure measurements in defining severity.

Essential hypertension is hypertension that is not determined to be secondary to an identifiable renal, endocrine, or other disorder. It accounts for 85–90% of all cases of hypertension. Essential hypertension is a multifactorial disorder, involving hereditary, environmental, dietary, cardiovascular, neurogenic, and hormonal factors. Individuals with established essential hypertension exhibit hypersensitivity to sympathetic stimuli, increased peripheral resistance to blood flow, resetting of carotid sinus baroreceptors, and increased sodium and water in arteriolar walls. Some exhibit sodium retention and edema, and some have definite elevations in renal renin secretion.

Epidemiological factors in hypertension include age, sex, race, weight, exercise, dietary sodium, dietary cholesterol, cigarette smoking, and atherosclerosis. Blood pressure in the overall population rises gradually with age, and the incidence of hypertension rises with it. In the United States there are about 35 million hypertensives (with blood pressure greater than 160/95 mm Hg), about 15% of the adult population. The incidence of hypertension in blacks is nearly twice that in whites, and the consequences appear to be more severe in blacks than whites. Obesity is a major risk factor and weight reduction often relieves hypertension. Cigarette smoking, excessive dietary salt, hyperglycemia, and hypercholesterolemia are other major risk factors. Diabetes mellitus is associated with vascular pathology that may culminate in atherosclerosis and hypertension.

Hypertension is itself a risk factor in atherosclerosis, cardiovascular disease, and overall mortality rates. Although there are no obvious pathological changes early in essential hypertension, if it persists, three symptoms develop: arteriosclerosis, kidney damage, and hypertrophy of the left ventricle. In some cases, another feature may be aneurysms associated with perforations of small vessels. Hypertension is a major risk factor in congestive heart failure, coronary artery disease, myocardial infarction, chronic renal failure, and cerebrovascular accidents.

Secondary hypertension is most often associated with bilateral renal parenchymal disease, and this type of secondary hypertension accounts for 5–10% of all cases of hypertension. Only about 1–2% of hypertensive individuals have high blood pressure secondary to such potentially curable disorders as pheochromocytoma, primary aldosteronism, Cushing's syndrome, hyperthyroidism, hypothyroidism, renal vascular disease, unilateral renal disease, or

Table 39–2
Diagnostic Criteria for Hypertension

Age group	Normal	Hypertensive
Infants (0–6)	80/40	> 90/60
Children (7–11)	100/60	> 120/80
Teenagers (12–19)	115/70	> 130/80
Young adults (20–45)	120/80	> 135/90
Middle-aged adults (45–65)	135/85	> 140/90
Elderly (over 65)	150/85	> 160/90

congenital constriction of the aorta. Some instances of secondary hypertension are drug-induced, as may occur with the use of oral contraceptives.

Often in hypertension, blood pressure is continuously elevated, but in **labile hypertension** there are periodic bouts of hypertension. **Systolic hypertension** is sometimes used to designate those cases of hypertension where diastolic pressure is normal but systolic pressure is elevated. It is most often seen in labile hypertensives or hypertension secondary to hyperthyroidism, aortic regurgitation, or aortic arteriosclerosis. It indicates hypertension due to increased cardiac output. The term **malignant hypertension** is used to designate instances of elevated blood pressure that are rapidly progressive and uncontrollable. This form of hypertension is associated with a high incidence of cerebral vascular accidents, congestive heart failure, encephalopathy, retinal hemorrhages, and renal failure.

General Considerations of Therapy

There is no cure for essential hypertension nor for most types of secondary hypertension. But it should be stressed that treatment of hypertension not only can lower blood pressure itself, but more important, it can substantially diminish or forestall the incidence of most if not all of the complications. Therefore, treatment of hypertension should be appropriately vigorous for the level of severity of the condition (Table 39–3).

As of yet, there is no evidence to indicate that drug therapy is warranted in people who have borderline hypertension with diastolic pressure between 85 and 94 mm Hg. For borderline hypertensive clients, every effort should be made to forestall development of hypertension through nondrug measures: restriction of dietary sodium, cholesterol, smoking, and excessive consumption of alcohol and coffee; weight control through exercise and diet; and discontinuing the use of oral contraceptives.

The decision whether or not to initiate drug therapy is difficult only for clients with mild hypertension (95–104 mm Hg). In such clients, nondrug measures may be explored first, but drug therapy should be initiated if the diastolic pressure does not shortly drop to less than 90 mm Hg. When cardiovascular or target tissue complications are present, drug therapy should be initiated without waiting to explore the effect of nondrug approaches. Risk factors should be assessed, including presence of hypercholesterolemia, diabetes, systolic pressure over 165, or the client's being male, black, or under 45. One often used guideline suggests that in the absence of cardiovascular or target tissue complications, drug therapy should be initiated immediately if diastolic pressure is between 90 and 95 when four risk factors are present; between 95 and 100 when three risk factors are present; or between 100 and 105 when two risk factors are present. Clients with mild hypertension may respond adequately to a single drug regimen, typically a diuretic or, less commonly, a beta-adrenergic blocker.

Numerous clinical studies have shown that only a small minority of all hypertensive clients receive treatment that even approximates optimal control of the condition, and only about 50% of hypertensive individuals have adequately controlled blood pressure. The problems encountered include selection of inappropriate drug combinations, failure to individ-

Table 39–3
Categories of Hypertension in Adults

Classification	Diastolic pressure	Systolic pressure	Treatment
Normal	75–84	120–125	None
Borderline hypertensive	85–94	126–139	Salt restriction, exercise, weight loss, relaxation, low cholesterol diet
Mildly hypertensive	95–104	140–159	Usually a single drug[a]
Moderately hypertensive	105–115	160–180	Drug combinations
Severely hypertensive	> 115	> 180	Drug combinations

[a]For mild hypertension, the decision whether or not to initiate drug therapy is based on where the diastolic pressure falls within the range and the presence or absence of risk factors such as being male, black, less than 45 years of age, or presence of systolic pressure over 165, target organ complications, cardiovascular complications, high blood cholesterol, or diabetes.

ualize dosage to optimize response or to minimize side effects, failure to adjust doses appropriately over time as the condition of the client changes, poor compliance, and inadequate monitoring or self-monitoring of blood pressure.

Antihypertensives

Antihypertensive drugs are a varied family of substances with several distinct sites of action (Figure 39–1 and Table 39–4) and different side effects. Diuretics and inhibitors of the renin-angiotensin system reduce body fluid volume. Beta-blockers reduce cardiac output. The three other major groups — centrally acting sympathomimetics, peripherally acting sympatholytics, and vasodilators — reduce peripheral resistance. Other classes used in special situations of hypertension include alpha-blockers, ganglionic blockers, and drugs that alter sensitivity of baroreceptors. All of these groups of drugs reduce peripheral resistance, directly or indirectly.

We will first consider the four classes of antihypertensive drugs that act directly to reduce the

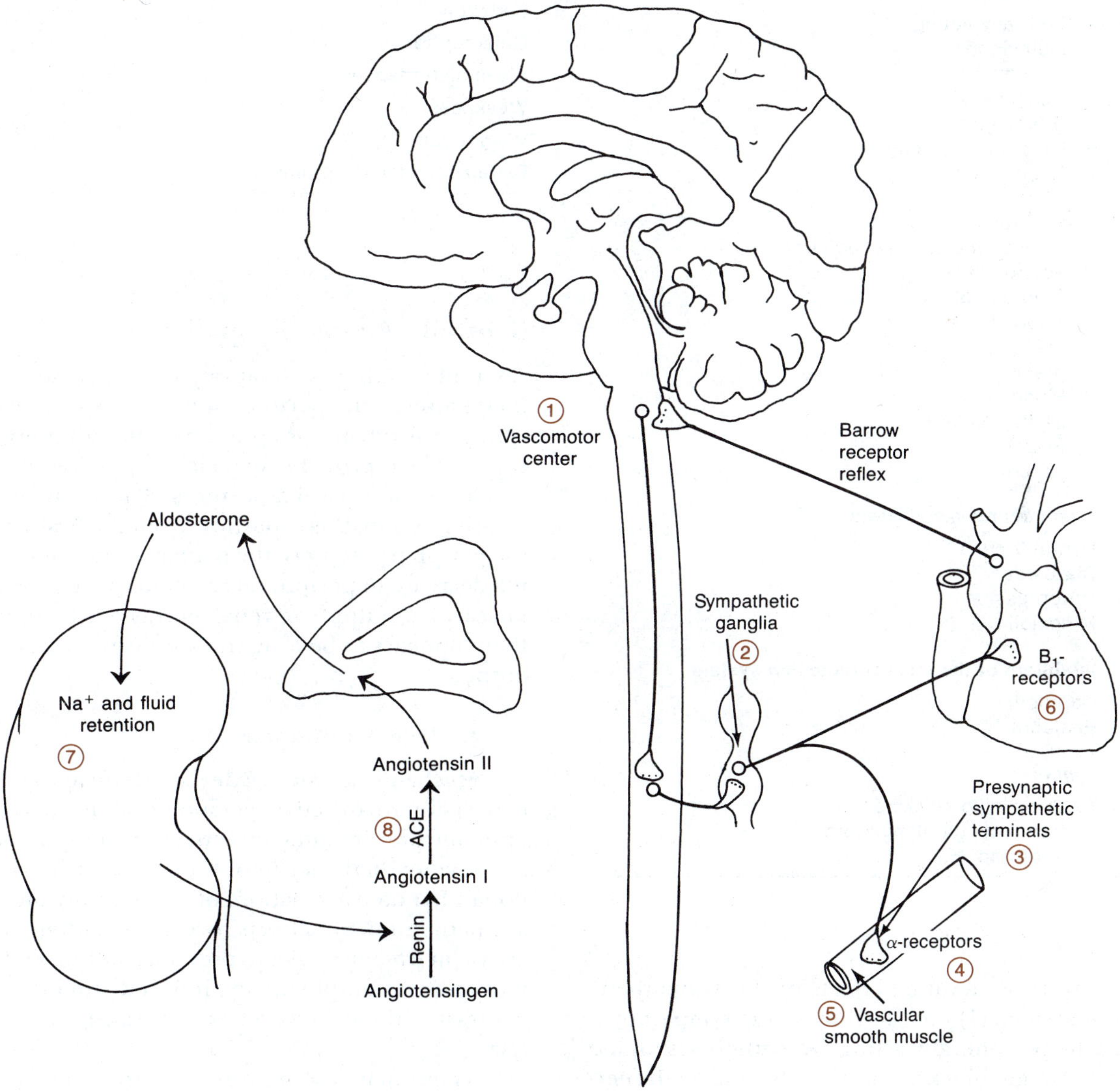

Figure 39–1
Sites of action of antihypertensive drugs.

Table 39–4
Classifications of Antihypertensive Drugs

I. Diuretics
- A. Thiazide and related
  - Hydrochlorthiazide
  - Many others (See Chapter 43)
- B. High-ceiling
  - Furosemide
  - Bumetanide
  - Ethacrynic acid
- C. Potassium-sparing
  - Amiloride
  - Triamterene
  - Spironolactone

II. Sympatholytics
- A. Centrally acting
  - Methyldopa
  - Clonidine
  - Guanabenz
  - Guanfacine
- B. Peripherally acting
  - Guanethidine
  - Guanadrel
  - Reserpine
  - Monoamine oxidase inhibitors
- C. Beta-blockers
  - Propranolol
  - Nadolol
  - Metoprolol
  - Atenolol
  - Pindolol
- D. Alpha-blockers
  - Prazosin
  - Others

III. Direct-acting vasodilators
- Hydralazine
- Diazoxide
- Nitroprusside
- Minoxidil

IV. Inhibitors of the renin-angiotensin system
- Captopril
- Enalapril

V. Others
- A. Ganglionic blockers
- B. Baroreceptor stimulators
  - Veratrum

blood pressure elevating effects of the sympathetic nervous system: (1) the centrally acting sympatholytics, (2) the peripherally acting sympatholytics (3) the beta-adrenergic blockers, and (4) the alpha-adrenergic blockers. These drugs share the potential for antiadrenergic side effects (Table 39–5).

Table 39–5
Antiadrenergic Side Effects

Peripheral
- Orthostatic hypotension
- Excess gastrointestinal activity
  - Nausea
  - Ulcers
  - Diarrhea
- Impotency
- Bladder and eye control problems
- Aggravation of asthma
- Vascular headaches

Central
- Sedation
- Galactorrhea
- Sleep disturbances
- Weakness
- Weight gain
- Extrapyramidal symptoms

Centrally Acting Sympatholytics

Centrally acting sympatholytics decrease sympathetic tone in the peripheral nervous system by activating central presynaptic alpha-noradrenergic receptors that provide feedback suppression of the vasomotor and cardiac centers. The result is a decrease in sympathetic outflow from the brainstem to the periphery. Acutely, the main hemodynamic effect is a decrease in peripheral resistance with little effect on cardiac output or renal perfusion. Chronically, there appears to be a significant decrease in cardiac output.

Methyldopa (Aldomet)

Mechanisms and Effects Methyldopa (after conversion to an active metabolite, alpha-methylnorepinephrine) imitates the effect of norepinephrine at α_2-sympathetic receptors. In addition to methyldopa's hypotensive action, other centrally mediated sympathomimetic effects occur, including an increase in dreaming sleep, pseudolactation, and a potentiation of amphetamine-induced stimulation. In contrast to these, however, is a consistent sedative effect.

There may also be one or more minor peripheral contributions to the overall sympatholytic action as well, for example a reduced resistance to blood flow in the renal vasculature. In this vascular bed, the active metabolite of methyldopa is a much weaker constrictor than the norepinephrine it displaces and thus may reduce sympathetic tone in the renal vasculature. Methyldopa has been frequently employed in renal hypertension.

Methyldopa does not impair the integrity of sympathetic neurons peripherally. As a result, sympathetic reflex activity remains largely intact, and orthostatic hypotension, exercise-induced hypotension, and other antiadrenergic side effects occur to a much lesser extent than with peripherally acting sympatholytics.

Pharmacokinetics Methyldopa is only about 25% absorbed after oral administration. There is evidence that some metabolism of methyldopa occurs in the intestinal mucosa itself since intravenous administration results in a substantially different pattern of metabolism. The peak effect of methyldopa occurs in 4–6 hours. Elimination of methyldopa is biphasic with a half-life of about 1.8 hours for the second phase. The duration of action of the drug is about 10–16 hours. Most of the elimination of methyldopa is by renal excretion. Therefore people with impaired renal function may respond to smaller doses of the drug. Elderly clients and those with advanced arteriosclerotic vascular disease may have hypersensitivity responses that can be avoided by using lower doses of the drug.

For intravenous use, the ethyl ester of methyldopa, called methyldopate, is employed. This drug is not necessarily equivalent to methyldopa, since less than half of the ester is converted to methyldopa and some of it is excreted unchanged. The ester can cause paradoxical hypertensive responses.

Clinical Indications The only major clinical indication is for treatment of essential hypertension, usually as a second step after use of a diuretic. It has been used to a limited extent in treatment of carcinoid disease.

Adverse Effects Methyldopa produces the full range of **antiadrenergic side effects** (Table 39–5). A frequent antiadrenergic side effect of methyldopa is sedation. This effect often diminishes with chronic use but may continue in some clients and result in lassitude, apathy, and somnolence. *The nurse, client, and family members should report signs of mental depression or decreased mental acuity. Clients should be warned that the sedative effects of the drug may increase the danger of such tasks as driving an automobile.*

Other adverse effects on the central nervous system include depression, nightmares, extrapyramidal reactions, paresthesias, vertigo, drug fever, and pseudolactation (in males as well as females). *The nurse should be alert to complaints of tingling sensations or numbness, or to changes in the client's gait or the presence of tremors. Such disturbances need to be reported immediately and the behavior or sensations compared with pretreatment status.* During the early phases of treatment, clients may complain of headaches or weakness. *Nurses should reassure clients that the symptoms will generally disappear as they continue taking the drug. However, the nurse should also be certain to reassess clients to be sure that these symptoms do not linger.*

Symptoms attributable to peripheral antiadrenergic effects are much less severe than with guanethidine or reserpine, but complaints of dry mouth, nasal stuffiness, gastrointestinal hyperactivity, orthostatic hypotension, exercise-induced hypotension, and impotence should be reported to the client's physician.

Reduction of blood pressure may reduce renal filtration pressure, resulting in **salt and water retention,** edema, and weight gain. *As a precautionary measure, nurses should encourage clients to limit sodium intake. If edema persists, the condition should be reported to the physician, who will most likely prescribe a diuretic.* Abrupt withdrawal of methyldopa may be associated with **rebound hypertension,** but less so than occurs with clonidine (Catapres).

Hypersensitivity reactions can occur with methyldopa. About 25% of clients on prolonged therapy at the usual therapeutic dose develop a positive direct Coombs' test indicative of presence of an immunoglobulin of the IgG class directed against red blood cells. Methyldopa acts as a hapten, attaching to red blood cells and causing them to be recognized as antigen. In about 1% of clients receiving methyldopa, the resultant **hemolytic anemia** is severe enough to require drug discontinuation. *Before initiating methyldopa therapy, a hematocrit, hemoglobin, or red cell count should be done to provide baseline data as well as to determine if the client has anemia. Once therapy is started, the nurse should check periodically for the presence of hemolytic anemia. Complaints by the client of feeling cold should prompt the nurse to further check the individual's hematocrit to determine if anemia is present.*

Methyldopa will cause false positives in tests for pheochromocytoma because of its close relation to the natural catecholamines.

Preparations and Administration *Dosage increases of methyldopa should be started in the evening to reduce the amount of sedation likely to occur. In this way,* *morning hypotension may be prevented while at the same time the afternoon blood pressure is controlled. When methyldopa is to be given along with other antihypertensive agents, the dosage needs to be gradually adjusted to ensure a smooth transition. Methyldopa should be stored at room temperature in an airtight container.*

Methyldopa (Aldomet)
Tablets, combination with hydrochlorthiazide (Aldoril)
Recommended Doses: 1,000 mg/day PO in 1–3 administrations.

Methyldopate Hydrochloride (Aldomet Ester Hydrochloride)
Injection solution
Recommended Doses: 500–1,000 mg by intravenous infusion, with doses adjusted to the requirements of the client.

Clonidine (Catapres) and Related Drugs

Clonidine has become an important antihypertensive drug since its introduction in the 1970s. Guanabenz (Wytensin), a drug of similar mechanism was marketed in 1982. Guanfacine (Tenex) was approved in 1986 and will be marketed in 1987.

Mechanisms and Effects The mechanism underlying the antihypertensive effect of clonidine and related drugs is similar to that of methyldopa. They stimulate alpha-2 adrenergic receptors in the vicinity of the cardiac and vasomotor centers of the brain. Vagal outflow increases, causing bradycardia and decreased cardiac output. Sympathetic outflow decreases, causing peripheral vasodilation and decreased resistance to blood flow.

The hypotensive effect of clonidine and related drugs is attributable to the combined influence of diminished peripheral resistance and bradycardia. As with methyldopa, peripheral sympathetic reflexes remain intact. Therefore, orthostatic hypotension is of modest severity, and exercise causes an appropriate increase in blood pressure. With clonidine, glomerular filtration rate is diminished and leads to sodium and fluid retention. Thus, clonidine is often used in combination with diuretic therapy. Renal blood flow is well maintained during clonidine hypotension and renin secretion is marginally diminished.

Pharmacokinetics Clonidine is about 75% absorbed after oral administration. Sixty percent is excreted by the kidneys unchanged. The remainder is metabolized in the liver and then excreted in the urine or feces. The half-life of clonidine is about 8.5 hours and its duration is typically 8 hours. Guanabenz is also 75% absorbed. It is metabolized before excretion and has a half-life of about 6 hours. Guanfacine is completely absorbed after oral administration. In the plasma, guanfacine is 80–90% bound. It is 30% excreted unchanged and 70% metabolized. Its half-life is 12–23 hours.

Clinical Indications Clonidine, guanabenz, and guanfacine are employed mainly as second-line drugs in treatment of hypertension. Clonidine has been used investigationally in migraine.

Adverse Effects and Contraindications Clonidine, guanabenz, and guanfacine tend to cause **dry mouth** and **sedation.** These reactions are both frequent and often severe. *Nurses should advise clients to avoid use of alcohol or other CNS depressants, since these may potentiate the sedative influence of clonidine and related drugs.* Peripheral antiadrenergic side effects, including impotency and orthostatic hypotension, are less pronounced than with guanethidine and reserpine. Clients may develop anorexia and malaise, and CNS symptoms including insomnia, restlessness, anxiety, vivid dreams, or nightmares. *If any one of these phenomena occur, nurses should question the client further to learn if any other antiadrenergic symptoms are present.* With clonidine, **sodium and fluid retention** often occur and tend to negate the therapeutic value unless diuretic therapy is instituted, but this is not a problem with guanabenz or guanfacine. Overall, the incidence and severity of side effects is greater with clonidine than with methyldopa. Guanabenz and especially guanfacine are better tolerated than either clonidine or methyldopa.

A particular problem with clonidine is **withdrawal hypertension,** which occurs when the drug is stopped abruptly, causing hypertensive crisis. Rebound hypertension occurs less often with guanabenz and guanfacine. *Clients should be taught that careful compliance is necessary to avoid withdrawal hypertension. Complaints of nervousness, headaches, insomnia, tremors, nausea, or abdominal pain should prompt the nurse to question if the client has missed a dose or stopped taking the drug altogether.* Gradual elimination of clonidine (over 2–4 days) avoids the problem. With guanfacine, rebound hypertension occurs more gradually, developing after 2–7 days. If hypertensive crisis occurs, alpha- and beta-blockers may be required to control the symptoms.

Nurses should note in the client's drug history if he or she is receiving tricyclic antidepressants. If so, clonidine should not be used since tricyclics render clonidine ineffective. Clonidine occasionally causes Raynaud's phenomenon. Clonidine is contraindicated for use in women who are pregnant or are contemplating pregnancy. *In their initial assessment of the client, nurses should determine the individual's age and intentions with respect to pregnancy.*

Preparations and Administration *Clonidine should be stored at room temperature in an airtight container.*

Clonidine (Catapres)
Tablets
Recommended Doses: 200 μg to 2 mg PO daily, typically in two administrations. Usually a larger portion is given at bedtime and a smaller portion around noon.

Guanabenz (Wytensin)
Tablets
Recommended Doses: 4 mg PO twice daily, initially, increased in increments of 4–8 mg per day every 1–2 weeks.

Guanfacine (Tenex)
Tablets
Recommended Doses: For hypertension in adults, 0.5–1.0 mg PO daily.

Peripherally Acting Sympatholytics

Peripherally acting sympatholytics act on peripheral nerve terminals. They are accumulated by noradrenergic nerve terminals and are stored in synaptic vesicles, displacing the natural transmitter. As a result, the blood pressure response to sympathetic nerve stimulation or indirect-acting sympathomimetics such as amphetamine is inhibited. The displaced norepinephrine may cause a transient rise in blood pressure when therapy is begun.

A drawback with chronic administration of peripherally acting sympatholytic agents is that postsynaptic adrenergic receptors become supersensitive, a classic response of receptors to chronic deficiency of transmitter. When adrenergic receptors are supersensitive, direct-acting sympathomimetics such as epinephrine will raise blood pressure more than usual. *Thus, nurses should advise clients who are receiving peripherally acting sympatholytics to avoid use of decongestants since these usually include or consist of sympathomimetic agents.*

Guanethidine (Ismelin) and Guanadrel (Hylorel)

Mechanisms and Effects Guanethidine and guanadrel not only displace norepinephrine from synaptic vesicles but also have a second action that is probably even more important: they inhibit the release of norepinephrine from presynaptic terminals. both actions result in vasodilation, decreased cardiac output, and a lowering of blood pressure. Guanadrel, a new agent, appears on the basis of limited studies to be pharmacologically equivalent to guanethidine, differing only in its pharmacokinetics.

Guanethidine causes a full set of sympatholytic actions. Blood pressure may be lowered for several days after a single dose. Pulse pressure and heart rate decline, resulting in decreased cardiac output. Systolic pressure is more affected when measured in the standing than in the supine position, and this is consistent with the substantial orthostatic and exercise hypotension observed in those who take the drug. Plasma renin is slightly decreased.

The reduction in blood pressure effected by guanethidine reduces glomerular filtration rate (GFR). As a result, fluid and sodium retention may occur, as with most nondiuretic antihypertensives. Renal blood flow is sometimes reduced slightly and this may contribute to a reduction in GFR.

Pharmacokinetics Guanethidine is absorbed rather poorly after oral administration; only 3–30% is absorbed. Absorption is fairly consistent in a given client. After absorption, guanethidine is sequestered in sympathetic nerve terminals and other sites of uptake. The portion remaining in the plasma is eliminated fairly rapidly by renal excretion.

Guanadrel has substantially different pharmacokinetic properties from guanethidine. It is readily absorbed after oral administration and has a rapid onset and short duration of action. A bedtime dose therefore produces less morning orthostatic hypotension than with guanethidine. On the other hand, guanadrel must be given 2–4 times per day.

Clinical Indications Guanethidine and guanadrel are used only in treatment of essential hypertension. They are reserve drugs for patients who do not respond adequately to diuretic, beta-blocker, methyldopa, or vasodilator therapy.

Adverse Effects and Contraindications Guanethidine and guanadrel can produce any of the side effects in the antiadrenergic cluster (Table 39–5). Common **antiadrenergic side effects** with guanethidine and guanadrel are sedation, weakness, urinary frequency, nocturia, gas pains, and diarrhea. *Because of the gastric stimulation produced by guanethidine and guanadrel, these drugs should be used cautiously in clients with a history of peptic ulcers. The client should be closely monitored by the nurse and family for signs of excessive mental depression. Nurses should advise clients to avoid using alcoholic beverages or other CNS depressants because of the potential for additive CNS depression with guanethidine.*

Initially, the effects of guanethidine may not stabilize for several weeks because of accumulation of the drug. Therefore, adverse effects may appear early on or after many days.

Another frequent problem with guanethidine or guanadrel is **orthostatic hypotension.** The problem is accentuated by warm weather, exercise, or use of alcohol. *Orthostatic hypotension is more severe in the morning, so clients need to be advised to arise slowly, gradually adjusting themselves to changes in position. Clients should be warned to avoid situations that commonly induce orthostatic hypotensive reactions: hot showers or baths, prolonged standing or sitting in one position, or standing up rapidly.*

Some clients develop increased smooth muscle activity resulting in **diarrhea.** This may be severe at times or even incapacitating. Unfortunately, the loss of fluid and electrolytes that accompanies severe diarrhea can produce the fainting or dizziness that clients have been warned about in relation to orthostatic hypotension. *When clients report episodes of fainting or dizziness, the nurse needs to assess the events carefully and report the findings to the physician so that it can be decided whether or not to discontinue the prescribed medication. Measurement of serum electrolytes may be indicated.*

Salt and water retention may occur with guanethidine and guanadrel. This leads to edema and weight gain and may diminish the therapeutic benefit if diuretic therapy is not employed concurrently. *Clients receiving guanethidine or guanadrel need to be encouraged to weigh themselves daily, since changes in weight may indicate water retention.* Guanethidine is contraindicated in pheochromocytoma.

Guanethidine may complicate pharmacological control of blood pressure during surgical procedures because of its long duration of action and its tendency to cause supersensitivity of sympathetic receptors. Therefore, patients undergoing elective surgery are sometimes withdrawn from guanethidine at least 2 weeks prior to surgery. Other physicians feel that this is an unnecessary and even hazardous precaution. *Nurses should impress upon clients who are receiving guanethidine or guanadrel that they should inform health care professionals that they are taking the drug, especially in the event of emergency surgery, since the preanesthetic and anesthetic agents may have to be given in reduced dosage to prevent harmful effects.*

A common problem for male clients is **inhibition of ejaculation** (without alteration in capacity for erection). This problem may cause men to discontinue the medication.

Drug Interactions Tricyclic antidepressants, indirect-acting symphtomimetics, certain neuroleptics (phenothiazines and thioxanthenes), and oral contraceptives may interfere with the efficacy of guanethidine by blocking its required uptake into sympathetic nerve terminals. Guanethidine increases sensitivity to sympathetic amines that act directly due to development of supersensitivity of adrenergic receptors when guanethidine is used chronically.

Preparations and Administration *Guanethidine and guanadrel are stored at room temperature in airtight containers.*

Guanethidine (Ismelin)
Tablets
Recommended Doses: 25–50 mg PO, once a day, individualized for each client.

Guanadrel (Hylorel)
Tablets
Recommended Doses: 10 mg PO daily initially, gradually adjusted upward to the range of 20–75 mg daily, given in 2–4 divided doses.

Rauwolfia Alkaloids

Reserpine and rauwolfia have been used throughout recorded history. Rauwolfia is derived from the plant *Rauwolfia serpentina,* a climbing shrub that grows in India, and reserpine is one of its active alkaloids. Reserpine was introduced in 1954 as an antipsychotic drug, at about the same time as chlorpromazine (Thorazine). It is no longer used for that purpose but has since been employed for its antihypertensive effects.

Mechanisms and Effects Reserpine reduces granular stores of catecholamines and serotonin in the brain, sympathetic nerve terminals, and the adrenal medulla. Depletion begins within 1 hour after administration and reaches maximal levels in about 24 hours. Reserpine appears to block the vesicular uptake of the norepinephrine precursor dopamine, preventing its conversion to norepinephrine and subsequent storage. Reserpine, unlike guanethidine, is not itself released and it may well be that it is irreversibly bound to the vesicular uptake mechanism. Recovery from the effect of reserpine occurs only when new vesicles are delivered to the nerve terminal from their site of synthesis in the cell body. As with guanethidine, chronic administration of reserpine results in development of postsynaptic receptor supersensitivity.

Reserpine gradually reduces blood pressure. A decline in cardiac output appears to be the major cause, although there may also be a reduction in peripheral resistance when clients lie down. The latter effect presumably contributes to the common occurrence of orthostatic hypotension. Bradycardia is another feature of reserpine-induced hypotension.

Reserpine causes a full range of central and peripheral antiadrenergic effects. Notable among these are sedation and indifference, depression, and gastrointestinal stimulation.

Pharmacokinetics Onset of action is slow with reserpine because depletion of existing stores of norepinephrine requires several days. The full therapeutic action occurs only after a week or more of treatment, and effects persist for several weeks after discontinuation. Absorption of reserpine after oral administration is affected by recent food ingestion. *Nurses should advise clients using this drug to adopt a uniform time of administration.* Reserpine is inactivated mainly by metabolism.

Clinical Indications Reserpine is used only for treatment of essential hypertension. Under the trade name of Ser-Ap-Es, a combination product containing hydrochlorthiazide and hydralazine in addition to reserpine, it is a widely prescribed antihypertensive. Reserpine is employed as a second step when hypertension is not controlled by a diuretic alone.

Adverse Effects Reserpine causes all of the **antiadrenergic side effects** (Table 39–5). Notable among these with reserpine are gastrointestinal stimulation including diarrhea, hypersecretion, ulcerations, nausea, anorexia, and hemorrhage). *Nurses need to tell clients that reserpine-containing preparations should be taken with meals, milk, or snacks to minimize gastrointestinal irritation. Reserpine should be avoided for clients with a history of peptic ulcers.*

Centrally mediated antiadrenergic side effects of reserpine include extrapyramidal symptoms, depressive episodes, nightmares, sedation, and weight gain. *The client, family, and nurse should be alert for indications of mental depression and should report any signs of despondency, early morning insomnia, loss of appetite, or other symptoms of depression to the physician, especially if the client has a prior history of depression.*

Orthostatic hypotension in response to reserpine use is pronounced and may be associated with nasal stuffiness, flushing, and vascular headaches. *The nurse needs to warn clients about circumstances that can provoke fainting and dizziness in individuals experiencing orthostatic hypotension: exposure to excessive heat (hot*

Nursing Observations for Use of Antihypertensive Drugs

THERAPEUTIC GOAL	Reduce diastolic blood pressure to less than 90 mm Hg.
PREADMINISTRATION ASSESSMENT	
Baseline Data	Evaluate blood pressure (sitting, standing, and lying), pulse, ECG, peripheral pulses, heart sounds, edema, respiratory rate and sounds, bowel sounds, and neurologic status. Obtain laboratory tests including serum electrolytes, liver function tests, serum lipids and uric acid, and urinalysis.
Contraindications/ Precautions	Check history for evidence of drug allergies or allergies to tartrazine (found in some formulations).
Potential Interactions	Assess current medications for interacting drugs, especially other hypotensive agents.
EVALUATION OF DRUG RESPONSE	
For Therapeutic Benefit	Daily blood pressure measurements.
For Adverse Effects	Monitor for congestive heart failure, symptoms of excess hypotension, antiadrenergic side effects, allergic reactions, and side effects specific to each drug.
For Drug Interactions	Monitor for additive hypotensive effects, additive antiadrenergic effects, supersensitivity to sympathomimetics, and drug interactions specific for each agent.
For Dietary Interactions	Monitor changes in salt intake for destabilization of therapy; monitor changes in dietary potassium if a diuretic is being used.
For Compliance	Evaluate client's compliance with all facets of the therapeutic regimen by careful observation, interviewing, and review of progress. Report compliance problems to the physician and act as client-advocate when changes in the therapeutic regimen seem indicated.

showers or baths, prolonged standing or sitting in one position, or rapid standing). Reserpine may cause fluid and electrolyte retention, resulting in edema. *Clients need to be monitored for clinical signs of fluid and electrolyte imbalance, particularly hyponatremia, hypochloremic alkalosis, and hypokalemia.* Reserpine has been reported in two studies to cause an increase in the incidence of breast cancer, but there is controversy concerning this finding.

Reserpine can cause **cardiac dysrhythmias** in clients who have been taking digitalis or quinidine. *Nurses caring for such clients need to observe them for symptoms indicating the presence of cardiac dysrhythmias and need to teach responsible family members what to watch for as well.*

Drug Interactions Hypotensive effects of reserpine are additive with those of other hypotensive drugs, including levodopa, methyldopa, diuretics, ganglionic blockers, guanethidine, and vasodilators. It antagonizes the effects of indirect-acting sympathomimetics such as amphetamine and has additive effects with other sympatholytic drugs such as beta-blockers. It should be used cautiously in combination with cardiac glycosides, quinidine, or theophylline since these combinations have resulted in occurrence of dysrhythmias. Reserpine will produce additive CNS depression with other depressant drugs. Reserpine antagonizes the gastric acid suppressing effects of anticholinergic drugs.

Preparations and Administration Reserpine is available both in the form of whole root Rauwolfia and as the pure drug. Three related rauwolfia alkaloids are deserpidine (Harmonyl), rescinnamine (Moderil, Cinnasil), and alseroxylon (Raufensin, Rauwiloid). Alseroxylon is a mixture of rauwolfia alkaloids. *Rauwolfia derivatives should be stored at room temperature in an airtight, light-resistant container. As with all hypotensive agents, nurses need to stress the importance of compliance with the prescribed regimen.*

Rauwolfia (Raudixin, Wolfina, Rauval, and others)
Tablets
Recommended Doses: 200–400 mg PO daily in 2 divided doses, morning and evening.

Reserpine (Serpasil, Hiserpia, Serpate, Sandril, and others)
Tablets, capsules, elixir, injection solution
Recommended Doses: 0.5 mg PO daily initially, reduced to 0.1–0.25 mg daily for maintenance.

Monoamine Oxidase (MAO) Inhibitors

MAO inhibitors have long been known to produce orthostatic hypotension when used for depression. The properties of this drug class are discussed more fully in Chapter 20, in relation to their use as antidepressants. One MAO inhibitor, pargyline HCl, is marketed for use in hypertension, but it is seldom used because of the broad range of drug-drug and drug-diet interactions associated with MAO inhibitors. *Educating and closely supervising the client are of utmost importance if pargyline is used because of the multitude of potential interactions with other drugs and dietary tyramine.*

Preparations and Administration

Pargyline (Eutonyl)
Tablets
Recommended Doses: 25 mg PO once a day, increased in increments of 10 mg up to 200 mg until a satisfactory response is achieved, which may require 4 days to 3 weeks for full efficacy.

Beta-Adrenergic Blockers

There are currently nine beta-adrenergic blockers on the market; all but betaxolol (an ophthalmic agent for glaucoma) are approved for use systemically as antihypertensive agents (Table 39–6). Propranolol (Inderal), the prototype of the class and the one that has been available for clinical use for some time, is approved for several other applications in addition to hypertension. Propranolol is discussed in Chapter 38 as an antidysrhythmic drug, in Chapter 40 as an antianginal drug, and in Chapter 26 as prophylaxis against migraine headaches. The general pharmacology of beta-blockers is also addressed in Chapter 28, in relation to the autonomic nervous system. The foremost clinical application of beta-blockers is for hypertension, and several of the available agents are currently approved only for that purpose. This section's discussion is limited to that application, but the full range of adverse effects and interactions are discussed.

The eight beta-blockers available for hypertension share the ability to block β_1-adrenergic receptors but differ in the extent of four other pharmacological activities: ability to block β_2-receptors, intrinsic sympathomimetic activity, a quinidine-like, local anesthetic action, and lipid solubility. Each of these properties influences adverse effects, contraindications, or additional indications of the drugs.

Mechanisms and Effects The effects of beta-blockers ultimately depend on the level of sympathetic activity at the time they are administered. For example, beta-receptor blockade has little effect on cardiac function in the resting, unstressed individual but has a profound effect when sympathetic tone is elevated, as in exercise, pheochromocytoma, stress,

Table 39–6
Comparative Properties of Beta-Adrenergic Blocking Drugs

Property	Acebutolol	Atenolol	Labetalol	Metoprolol	Nadolol	Oxprenolol	Pindolol	Propranolol	Timolol
Pharmacological actions									
β_1 blockade	Yes	Yes	Yes	Yes	Yes	Yes	Yes	Yes	Yes
β_2 blockade	No	No	Yes	No	Yes	Yes	Yes	Yes	Yes
α_1 blockade	No	No	Yes	No	No	No	No	No	No
Local anesthetic activity	0	0	+	+/−	0	+	+	++	0
Intrinsic sympathetic activity	+	0	0	0	0	++	+++	0	0
Pharmacokinetic properties									
Equivalent dose (propranolol = 1)	8.0	1.0	2.0	1.5	0.5	—	0.25	1.0	0.5
Half-life (hours)	3–4	6–8	6–8	3–4	20	2	3–4	3–5	4–5
Absolute bioavailability (%)	40	40	25	50	30	30	90	30	50
Lipid solubility	Low	Low	Moderate	Moderate	Low	Moderate	Moderate	High	Low
Approved applications									
Hypertension	Yes	Yes	Yes	Yes	Yes	Yes	Yes	Yes	Yes
Antidysrhythmic	Yes							Yes	
Angina pectoris					Yes			Yes	
Hypertrophic subaortic stenosis								Yes	
Pheochromocytoma								Yes	
Migraine prophylaxis								Yes	
After myocardial infarct								Yes	Yes
Glaucoma									Yes

or hypertension associated with excess sympathetic outflow. The reduction in cardiac output in these circumstances is a result of a decrease in both heart rate and contractility. Peripheral resistance to blood flow is slightly increased by beta-blockers as a compensatory response.

Another important factor determining the extent of changes in cardiac output and blood pressure in response to a beta-blocker is the **intrinsic sympathomimetic activity** of the drug itself. Among the approved agents, pindolol (Visken) has the most intrinsic sympathomimetic activity — it is a partial agonist. In the unstressed, normotensive individual, pindolol could actually increase cardiac output. Oxprenolol also has substantial intrinsic sympathomimetic activity while acebutolol (Sectral) has only a little. Beta-blockers that possess relatively high intrinsic sympathomimetic activity are useful for clients with mild bradycardia or compromised pulmonary function who might be adversely affected by a pure antagonist. These drugs are also useful in withdrawing clients from beta-blocker therapy.

The beta-blockers reduce renin secretion; this reduction is probably a significant factor in the antihypertensive effect of beta-blockers. Clients with elevated renin levels respond to low doses of beta-blockers, while those with low renin levels respond only to substantially higher doses.

Labetalol (Normodyne, Trandate) is unique among the beta-blockers in that it also blocks α_1-adrenergic receptors. This property contributes to the antihypertensive efficacy of labetalol. It has been effective in some hypertensive patients who have not been adequately responsive to selective beta-blockers and it acts more rapidly than the other drugs in its family.

Pharmacokinetics **Propranolol** (Inderal) is almost completely absorbed after oral administration but is subject to a very high level of first-pass extraction by the liver. Therefore, only about 30–40% reaches the systemic circulation. Differences in first-pass extraction and in sympathetic tone among individuals make dosage difficult to establish; hence, dosages must be titrated to the needs of each client. First-pass elimination is proportionately less at higher doses and decreases with chronic administration, a further complication in adjusting dosage. The half-life of propranolol is 2–3 hours initially but increases, because of reduced hepatic extraction, to about 4 hours. The propranolol that does reach the blood is 90–95% bound, another potential source of variability. Propranolol and other beta-blockers that have high lipid solubility are nearly entirely metabolized before excretion in the urine. Therefore, its half-life will be substantially prolonged in hepatic disease.

Labetalol is well absorbed, but like propranolol is subject to extensive first-pass extraction. Its absolute bioavailability is about 25%, but this can be increased by administration of the drug with food. Like propranolol, labetalol is metabolized before excretion, and its half-life is therefore altered more in hepatic disease than in renal failure.

Metoprolol (Lopressor) is well absorbed but subject to extensive first-pass extraction, so that only about 40% reaches the systemic circulation. The peak level is reached in about 90 minutes. Only about 10% of the drug is excreted unchanged, the rest being metabolized in the liver to largely inactive products. The half-life is about 3 hours. Metoprolol is only 13% bound in the serum to plasma proteins.

Pindolol (Visken) is rapidly and almost completely absorbed (95%) after oral administration. Its absorption is not significantly influenced by coadministration of food, and there is no significant first-pass effect. Pindolol is metabolized by the liver prior to renal elimination. Dosage adjustment may be required in patients with impaired liver function.

Nadolol (Corgard) also exhibits variability of dosage requirements. About 30% of the administered dose survives first-pass extraction to reach the systemic circulation. The peak concentration is achieved in 3–4 hours. There it is approximately 30% bound to plasma proteins. Nadolol (like other beta-blockers with low lipid solubility) is excreted largely unchanged in the urine; its half-life is therefore more altered by renal failure than by hepatic disease. It has a long half-life of 20–24 hours, permitting once-a-day administration. Accumulation of the drug occurs, with the plateau being reached in 6–9 days.

Fifty percent of an administered dose of **atenolol** (Tenormin) survives first-pass extraction to reach the systemic circulation. Peak levels occur in about 2–4 hours. Only about 10% of the serum concentration is bound to plasma proteins. The elimination half-life is about 6–9 hours and the duration of effect is about 24 hours. Atenolol is excreted unchanged in the urine.

Because of the variable absorption of beta-blockers, nurses need to work with clients to ensure consistency about the time of drug ingestion in relation to meals. The manufacturer of propranolol recommends taking the drug before meals and at bedtime, but consistency is a more important consideration. Dosage adjustment with beta-blockers requires careful monitoring of blood pressure during the initiation of therapy.

Adverse Effects and Contraindications **Heart failure** may occur, not only because of the depressant effect of beta-blockers on cardiac output, but also because beta-blockers, like all antihypertensives except diuretics, reduce glomerular filtration rate and excretion of sodium as they lower blood pressure. As a result, sodium may accumulate and edema may occur. However, cardiac failure occurs mainly when cardiac function has been previously compromised or other cardiac depressants (antidysrhythmics, local anesthetics, general anesthetics) are being employed concurrently. *At the first sign of heart failure, the nurse should conduct a quick assessment and contact the physician so that the client can be given digitalis or a diuretic or both. Clients and families need to be taught what changes to watch for. For most people taking propranolol, pulse rates will normally be lowered to what may seem to be an alarming extent. In monitoring a client's response to propranolol therapy, the nurse must often rely on changes other than pulse rate as indications of cardiac distress or adverse response to the drug.*

Beta-blockers may cause **withdrawal symptoms** if discontinued abruptly. There may be a sharp rebound in blood pressure to values in excess of those present prior to instituting drug treatment. Angina

Nursing Diagnoses and Interventions for Use of Antihypertensive Drugs

Nursing Diagnoses	*Related Interventions*
TO MINIMIZE DRUG SIDE EFFECTS OR INTERACTIONS	
Alterations in cardiac function: decreased cardiac output related to administration of beta-blockers or reflex cardiac stimulation with vasodilators	Monitor for changes in pulse that may indicate need to alter the drug regimen. Assess for dizziness or palpitations.
Alterations in tissue perfusion caused by antihypertensive medications	Teach client appropriate position and dietary adjustments and advocate adjustments in regimen if edema persists.
Increased risk of injury related to fainting or dizziness secondary to excess vasodilation	Advise client to make position changes slowly if orthostatic hypotension is apparent. In the hospital provide safety measures to protect client from dangerous falls. Discuss with client and family safety measures that can be taken at home.
Noncompliance related to lack of immediate health deficits in hypertension and unpleasant adverse effects of medication	Teach clients the relationship between hypertension and risks of coronary diseases, stroke, and overall mortality rates. Suggest appropriate nonprescription medications or comfort measures for dealing with adverse effects.
Sexual dysfunction related to impotence caused by sympatholytic drugs	Provide support and encouragement in dealing with sexual dysfunction or advocate adjustments in the regimen if continuing impotence interferes with compliance.
TO ENSURE SAFE AND EFFICACIOUS DRUG USE	
Knowledge deficit related to drug regimen	Teach clients about the nature of hypertension, its relationship to other health problems, and the role of drugs and diet in its management.
	Encourage clients to exercise, reduce excess weight, and to minimize stress.
	Teach clients how to monitor their blood pressure to determine if treatment is successful. Discourage clients from using coin-operated sphygmomanometers in shopping malls. These sphygmomanometers are not consistent or accurate.
	Instruct clients about the warning signs of cardiac disorders and stroke that may develop if hypertension is poorly controlled. Praise clients for compliance with prescribed regimen.
	Ensure that clients understand the dosage requirements and schedule of administration of each medication in relation to meals.
	Provide clients with a list of the adverse effects and drug interactions of each medication in the regimen and what to do if any of these occur.

can be aggravated during withdrawal to the extent that myocardial infarct becomes a serious threat. Since withdrawal responses can develop in as little as a few hours, compliance with drug regimens is of crucial importance. *Clients should be advised of the risks of abrupt discontinuation of beta-blockers or irregular compliance.* Sweating, nervousness, palpitations, trepidation, and anginal pain are early signs of angina-like attacks. When these occur, the physician should be notified and the drug should be immediately reinstituted.

Beta-blockers have significant **metabolic effects** pertaining to lipid and carbohydrate metabolism. Epinephrine mobilizes both fats and glucose mainly through beta-receptor actions. Beta-blockers tend to increase low-density lipoproteins and very-low-density lipoproteins, the levels of which correlate with development of atherosclerosis. Nonselective beta-blockers inhibit sympathetic stimulation of insulin release, but more important, they prevent the epinephrine-mediated hyperglycemic reaction to insulin excess. *Nurses need to alert people who are receiving insulin that they will have an increased risk of insulin shock if they are also receiving beta-blockers for hypertension. Such clients need to be taught to monitor themselves carefully for signs of hypoglycemia (sweating, hunger, fatigue). Nondiabetic clients should be warned to avoid prolonged fasting or crash diets while taking a beta-blocker.*

Ordinarily, β_2-receptors contribute to maintaining dilation of bronchioles. Nonselective beta-blockers **increase airway resistance,** an effect that is significant only in asthmatic patients. Highly selective blockers such as metoprolol are 50–100 times more specific for β_1-receptors than propranolol, yet even these drugs can cause respiratory distress in asthmatic clients when given in high doses. Propranolol, but not metoprolol, blocks the bronchodilatory action of isoproterenol, a beta-agonist.

Asthma or diabetes mellitus are thus relative contraindications for use of beta-blockers. Generally other antihypertensive medications should be selected for these clients. *The nurse should encourage asthmatic or diabetic clients always to carry identification indicating their medical condition and drug regimens.* Selective β_1-blockers reduce but do not eliminate the risks for each of these groups.

Uncommonly, beta-blockers **increase gastrointestinal activity** to the extent of causing nausea, vomiting, mild diarrhea, or constipation. *Taking the medication 1 hour after meals will relieve the distress. Stool softeners will relieve constipation.*

Also rare are **psychiatric symptoms** such as nightmares, hallucinations, insomnia, depression, or lassitude. It is often difficult to determine if fatigue is the result of the drug or the insomnia. Clients sometimes complain of short-term memory loss and a feeling of lightheadedness, of tingling sensations of the hands or a mottling of the skin, or intolerance to cold. *Such complaints need to be monitored and, if accompanied by other serious side effects, may mean that the client should be taken off propranolol.* **Allergic reactions** are seldom seen and when they occur are mild (rash or purpura).

Reduction in blood pressure produced by beta-blockers may cause lightheadedness and dizziness. *Clients should be advised to avoid driving or other potentially hazardous activities.*

Labetalol has unique alpha-blocking as well as beta-blocking properties and is therefore less likely to cause peripheral vascular symptoms, bradycardia, or congestive heart failure. On the other hand, it has side effects associated with its alpha-blocking action that are not shared by the other beta-blockers, including increased risk of orthostatic hypotension, sexual dysfunction, urinary retention, and nasal stuffiness. Orthostatic hypotension is most likely to occur 2 to 4 hours after administration of the drug.

Drug Interactions Beta-blockers that block β_2-receptors as well as β_1-receptors potentiate the pressor effects of epinephrine. This occurs because ordinarily the alpha-mediated pressor effect of epinephrine is slightly offset by its β_2-mediated vasodilatory action. β_2-blocking drugs block the vasodilatory effect, allowing the vasoconstrictor effect to be accentuated. For this reason, nonselective beta-blockers should not be used in alleviating symptoms of pheochromocytoma unless an alpha-receptor blocker is given first. Metoprolol, a selective β_1-blocker, does not potentiate the pressor effects of epinephrine.

Although beta-blockers may alleviate ectopic beats caused by cardiac glycosides, they enhance the suppression of A-V nodal conduction caused by glycosides, with the result that A-V block may occur.

Anaphylaxis can pose special problems for clients on beta-blockers, since the usual treatment for anaphylaxis, epinephrine, is ineffective in the presence of beta-blockers. Beta-blockers that act on β_2-receptors not only aggravate asthma, but also reduce the bronchodilating efficacy of beta-agonists or theophylline.

Diuretics and vasodilators may have additive hypotensive effects with beta-blockers. Activity of beta-blockers may also be increased by chlorpromazine, cimetidine, and oral contraceptives. On the other hand, cigarette smoking or use of salicylates or indomethacin may decrease the effectiveness of beta-blockers.

Preparations and Administration Inderal is one of the most widely prescribed of all drugs. Lopressor is the third most widely used nondiuretic antihypertensive and was the fifteenth most widely prescribed of all drugs in 1983. Tenormin is the fourth most widely used nondiuretic antihypertensive.

Acebutolol (Sectral)
Capsules
Recommended Doses: For hypertension, 400 mg/day PO in 1 or 2 doses. The optimum dose is usually between 400 and 800 mg daily, but may range from 200 mg to 1,200 mg daily.

Atenolol (Tenormin)
Tablets
Recommended Doses: 50 mg PO initially, once a day, increased to 100 mg, once a day.

Labetalol (Normodyne, Trandate)
Tablets, injection solution
Recommended Doses: 100 mg orally initially twice daily, alone or with a diuretic. The dose is then titrated against blood pressure (at 2–3 day intervals in increments of 100 mg/dose) until an adequate response is achieved. Maintenance doses are usually between 400 and 800 mg/day PO (in two divided doses), but 1,200–2,400 mg/day may be required for severe hypertension.

Metoprolol Tartrate (Lopressor)
Tablets
Recommended Doses: 50 mg PO bid initially. The usual maintenance range is 100–450 mg/day.

Nadolol (Corgard)
Tablets
Recommended Doses: 40 mg PO initially, once daily, increased in 40–80 mg increments up to 640 mg. The usual range is 80–320 mg PO.

Oxprenolol
FDA approved for hypertension, but not currently marketed.

Pindolol (Visken)
Tablets
Recommended Doses: 10 mg PO initially, bid, gradually adjusted upward at intervals of 2–3 weeks in increments of 10 mg/day to a maximum of 60 mg/day.

Propranolol (Inderal)
Tablets, combination with hydrochlorthiazide (Inderide)
Recommended Doses: 40 mg PO bid initially is typical, but dosage must be individualized by gradual titration. The dose is increased gradually up to a daily maximum of 640 mg. The usual range is 160 to 480 mg/day. The total daily dose is divided into 2 or 3 administrations.

Timolol (Blocadren)
Tablets
Recommended Doses: 10 mg PO initially, twice daily, alone or with a diuretic. Typical maintenance doses are 20–40 mg/day in 2 divided doses. The maximum recommended dose is 60 mg/day in 2 divided doses. Titration of the dose should be conducted at intervals no less than 7 days between increments.

Alpha-Adrenergic Blockers

Alpha-receptors play a major role in maintenance of vasomotor tone, so blocking these receptors would appear to be an attractive approach to alleviating high blood pressure. Also, alpha-blockers decrease levels of low-density lipoprotein (LDL) and very-low-density lipoprotein (VLDL), both of which substances correlate positively with development of atherosclerosis. This is in contrast to the tendency of beta-blockers to increase levels of these lipoproteins. However, two factors have limited the use of alpha-blockers. First, significant vasodilation brought about by alpha-blockers is generally associated with a reflex stimulation of the heart by way of beta-receptors, leading to tachycardia and palpitations. Second, alpha-receptors mediate a host of extracardiovascular functions that can be seriously compromised by alpha-blockers, producing unwanted side effects. The traditional alpha-blockers, such as **phenoxybenzamine, phentolamine,** and **tolazoline,** have been largely restricted to control of acute hypertensive states, such as the hypertensive crisis associated with the interaction of MAO inhibitors with tyramine and the hypertensive state associated with pheochromocytoma. These drugs are described in Chapter 28. Despite these effects, one drug with apparent alpha-blocking properties is used extensively in essential hypertension: prazosin. Another one, terazosin (Vasocard), currently has investigational status.

Prazosin (Minipress) and Terazosin (Vasocard)

Mechanisms and Effects Prazosin and terazosin are alpha-adrenergic blockers that exhibit unusual selectivity in two respects: they are selective for alpha-receptors associated with vascular smooth muscle, and they block postsynaptic receptors only, without significantly affecting presynaptic (α_2) receptors that regulate norepinephrine turnover. As a result, there is no increase in norepinephrine turnover and little reflexive effect on cardiac function.

Prazosin and terazosin reduce peripheral resistance to blood flow by dilating both arterioles and venuoles. Heart rate is only modestly increased, and renin release is not elevated.

Pharmacokinetics Prazosin is substantially extracted by first-pass elimination and only 5% of the administered dose reaches the systemic circulation. Peak plasma concentrations occur 2–3 hours after oral administration. Prazosin is highly bound in plasma (93%) and fully metabolized before elimination in the bile. Its half-life is about 3 hours.

Terazosin is readily absorbed after oral administration with peak plasma concentrations occurring after 1–2 hours.

Adverse Effects Because of the effect on venous capacitance, **orthostatic hypotension** is considerable and nurses must use special care when initiating therapy with prazosin. If full doses are employed initially, orthostatic hypotension may be severe enough to cause syncope, preceded by a rapid drop in heart rate. This response can be avoided by slowly instituting therapy with small doses. The first dose should be taken at bedtime.

The hypotensive effect of prazosin and terazosin promotes **salt and fluid retention,** which can counteract the effectiveness of the drug with chronic use, in as little as 4 days' time. For this reason, prazosin is usually employed as an add-on to a regimen including a diuretic or a beta-blocker.

The side effects of prazosin and terazosin attributable to **alpha-blocking effects** on non-vascular tissue include drowsiness, fatigability, and impotence. Other side effects are indicative of vasodilation, including headache, dizziness, and palpitations. Overall, the side effects are infrequent and mild, though nevertheless important to the client. Terazosin may possibly be tumorigenic.

Preparations and Administration *Each time the dose of prazosin is incrementally advanced, the first dose at the higher level should be given at bedtime to minimize the risk of syncope.*

Prazosin (Minipress)
Capsules
Recommended Doses: For hypertension, initially 1 mg PO, bid or tid. The usual therapeutic range of daily doses is 6–15 mg. The maximum daily dose is 40 mg in divided doses, 2 or 3 per day.

Terazosin (Vasocard)
Investigational

Vasodilators

In addition to prazosin, there are four vasodilators that act directly on smooth muscle and are marketed for hypertension. Two of these, hydralazine (Apresoline) and minoxidil (Loniten), are used chronically in essential hypertension, while the remaining two, nitroprusside (Nipride) and diazoxide (Hyperstat IV), are reserved for acute hypertensive emergencies. A fifth vasodilator, nitrendipine (Baypress), a type II calcium channel blocker, is currently undergoing clinical trials. The vasodilators reduce peripheral resistance by relaxing vascular smooth muscle. They act directly on the smooth muscle itself, not by way of receptors for norepinephrine or any other known transmitter.

Vasodilators are employed mainly in combination regimens for hypertension. They are seldom used alone because their primary effect on the vasculature triggers reflexive stimulation of heart rate and force of contraction, resulting in annoying side effects and more serious consequences such as angina, myocardial infarct, or congestive heart failure. All vasodilators increase sodium and fluid retention, as do other nondiuretic antihypertensives.

Hydralazine (Apresoline)

Mechanisms and Effects Hydralazine is a direct-acting vasodilator that produces greater effects on arterioles than on veins. It has no significant direct effects on systems other than the cardiovascular system.

Pharmacokinetics Hydralazine is well absorbed but subject to extensive but variable intestinal metabolism and first-pass elimination. Hydralazine is acetylated by the kidneys. People who are rapid acetylators (an inherited characteristic) extract the drug more rapidly, and only about 30% becomes bioavailable. Slow acetylators extract the drug less efficiently, so that 50% of the administered dose is bioavailable. If hydralazine is taken with food, first-pass extraction is reduced to some extent, increasing bioavailability. The effect of hydralazine develops slowly over 15–20 minutes after it becomes bioavailable and lasts about 2–4 hours. Its elimination half-life averages 3 hours. Less than 15% of serum hydralazine is excreted unchanged in the urine.

Adverse Effects When used alone, hydralazine produces a high incidence of adverse effects, caused by **vasodilation, reduced blood pressure, compensatory cardiac stimulation,** or **salt and water retention.** These effects include headache, anorexia, nausea, dizziness, sweating, flushing, nasal congestion, lacrimation, paresthesias, tremors, muscle cramps, conjunctivitis, palpitations, and edema. Gradual institution of therapy beginning at low doses may reduce the incidence and severity of adverse reactions. With chronic use, some tolerance may develop to many of the unpleasant effects. *The nurse should keep in mind that menopausal women may mistake these symptoms for those of menopause.*

Hydralazine is seldom employed except in combination with diuretics or beta-blockers. The combination sharply reduces adverse effects because smaller doses can be used and because beta-blockers prevent the reflex cardiac stimulation, and diuretics the edema.

Hydralazine has been known to cause **gastrointestinal bleeding.** *Nurses should ask the client whether there is evidence of bleeding — for example, black tarry stools or frank red blood in the stools. These events should be reported and the drug discontinued. However, if blood pressure has been substantially reduced as a result of hydralazine therapy, the drug will need to be withdrawn gradually.*

A reversible, drug-induced **lupus-like syndrome** occurs in 10–20% of clients receiving doses in excess of the maximum allowable dose of 400 mg. The syndrome occurs less commonly at doses below that level and mainly in slow acetylators, almost always caucasians. *Clients should have laboratory tests such as lupus erythematosus cell preparation, antinuclear antibody titers, and a complete blood count taken before and during treatment with hydralazine.*

Neuropathies occur occasionally with hydralazine and are attributable to a functional vitamin B_6 deficiency produced by the drug. A vitamin B_6 supplement of 25–100 mg should be employed prophylactically when hydralazine is used.

Preparations and Administration With chronic administration, some tolerance may develop, necessitating higher doses. *Hydralazine should be stored at room temperature in an airtight, light-resistant container.*

Hydralazine (Apresoline, Rolazine, Dralzine)
Tablets, injection solution
Recommended Doses: For oral administration, 10 mg initially, qid for 2–4 days, then 25 mg qid for the remainder of the first week. The dose is then increased to 50 mg qid and gradually adjusted to the lowest effective dose. The maximum daily dose is 400 mg. Parenteral administration in hospitalized patients who cannot take the drug orally, 20–40 mg IM or IV, repeated as necessary, for up to 1–2 days.

Minoxidil (Loniten)

Mechanisms and Effects Minoxidil resembles hydralazine in most respects but is more potent. It is orally effective and acts directly on vascular smooth muscle by blocking uptake of calcium into cells. It has more action on the arterioles than the veins.

Pharmacokinetics Minoxidil is 90% absorbed after oral administration, reaching peak serum concentrations in about 1 hour. It is 90% metabolized before renal excretion, with a half-life of 4.2 hours on average. The known metabolites are largely inactive.

Clinical Indications Minoxidil is indicated for moderate to severe hypertension because it is more effective than hydralazine. It should be used only in conjunction with diuretic and beta-blocker therapy, since the former will prevent minoxidil-induced edema and the latter will prevent reflex cardiac stimulation.

Adverse Effects and Contraindications As with hydralazine (Apresoline), **reflex stimulation of the heart** occurs as well as **salt and fluid retention.** Edema may be particularly troublesome and may lead to pericardial effusion. Clients receiving minoxidil should be periodically examined by echocardiography as a precaution against this effect. *Nurses need to monitor clients receiving minoxidil for salt and fluid retention, tachycardia, and evidence of congestive heart failure.* Because minoxidil increases heart rate, it can precipitate or worsen anginal attacks. *Clients need to be warned to report occurrence of chest pain, and nurses should question anginal clients about any change in requirements for nitroglycerin, numbers of anginal attacks, and circumstances of occurrence.* Another disturbing side effect is generalized **hypertrichosis:** excess hair growth over the shoulders, back, forearms, temples, and cheeks. Women are, naturally, more concerned with this side effect than men. *The nurse should reassure clients that hypertrichosis is reversible upon discontinuation of the medication.*

Preparations and Administration *Minoxidil should be stored at room temperature.*

Minoxidil (Loniten)
Tablets
Recommended Doses: In clients over 12, 5 PO mg initially, once per day. The maximum daily dose is 100 mg, in 1 or more administrations.

Diazoxide (Hyperstat IV)

Mechanisms and Effects Diazoxide is chemically related to the thiazide diuretics but differs in its pharmacological activity. Diazoxide is not a diuretic but exerts a powerful direct action on vascular smooth muscle, producing arteriolar dilation and a rapid reduction in blood pressure. The capacitance vessels (veins) are unaffected by diazoxide, and therefore postural hypotension seldom develops. Also, excessive hypotension seldom occurs because of the lack of venous effect.

Pharmacokinetics After intravenous bolus administration, diazoxide has a rapid onset of action, producing a maximal fall in blood pressure within 5 minutes. Blood pressure begins to increase at a fairly rapid rate in the first half-hour but more slowly thereafter, for up to 2–12 hours. Diazoxide is 90% bound to plasma proteins and may displace other bound drugs such as oral anticoagulants. Its elimination half-life is approximately 28 hours.

Clinical Indications Diazoxide is often considered the drug of choice for treatment of acute hypertensive crises because of its rapid effect and relative safety. It is also used effectively in control of malignant hypertension that is refractory to other regimens.

Adverse Effects Like other vasodilators, diazoxide causes marked **reflex cardiac stimulation,** which may result in anginal attacks or even infarction, and **hypervolemia**, which may precipitate congestive heart failure. *Close monitoring is important and any evidence of increased cardiac output or marked increase in heart rate should be reported. Sympathomimetics should be readily available for emergency use.* Diazoxide commonly causes salt retention, which in turn causes edema. This can be controlled by use of diuretics, but if the diuretic is a thiazide, the two drugs will have additive hyperuricemic and hyperglycemic effects. The **hyperglycemic** effect of diazoxide is caused by inhibition of insulin release from the pancreas. It is a transient effect and of no consequence except in clients who have diabetes or latent diabetes. *Such clients need to be warned of the potential hyperglycemic effect of diazoxide, and nurses should be prepared to increase dosages of insulin or oral hypoglycemic agents. In rare instances, individuals develop hyperglycemic coma; therefore, nurses need to observe for symptoms that may indicate impending problems.*

Diazoxide also causes uric acid retention (like other thiazides), but this is rarely a problem, since diazoxide is generally used only for brief periods. Other side effects include nausea, vomiting, and abdominal cramps. **Irritation** may occur at the site of administration, including burning sensations, and phlebitis. Diazoxide solutions are highly alkaline and can result in severe local pain and tissue damage. *Care must be taken to avoid extravasation.*

Preparations and Administration After injection, blood pressure should be monitored closely, for 5 minutes, and at 5-minute intervals for the first hour. In ambulatory clients, pressure should be measured while standing. Intravenous therapy should be limited to a few days. *Diazoxide should be stored at room temperature, protected from light.*

Diazoxide (Hyperstat IV)
Injection solution
Recommended Doses: 300 mg given as an intravenous bolus in 30 seconds or less. Slow injection may fail to produce an adequate response. Diazoxide can be repeated at intervals of 4–24 hours until oral antihypertensive therapy can be instituted.

Sodium Nitroprusside (Nipride)

Mechanisms and Effects Sodium nitroprusside is a powerful, direct-acting vasodilator that is useful for precise control of blood pressure by intravenous infusion. Nitroprusside differs from the other direct-acting vasodilators in its ability to relax both venous and arterial vessels. It is selective for vascular smooth muscle, having no effect on the visceral smooth muscle of the gastrointestinal tract or uterus. Like other vasodilators, nitroprusside causes reflex sympathetic activation; however, the special ability of nitroprusside to dilate veins reduces cardiac preload, which in turn decreases cardiac output. Thus, the predominant effect of sympathetic activation of the heart after nitroprusside is tachycardia, with no increase in cardiac output.

Pharmacokinetics The effects of nitroprusside occur rapidly after intravenous infusion is initiated and terminate quickly when it is halted. The half-life is only a few minutes. Adjustment of the infusion rate permits tight control of blood pressure.

Clinical Indications Nitroprusside is indicated for short-term control of high blood pressure by intravenous infusion in hospitalized patients. It is used in hypertensive emergencies and during surgery to control bleeding. It may also be useful as an adjunct to management of acute congestive heart failure.

Adverse Effects Adverse effects are insignificant with short-term use if the dose is titrated appropriately. The venous dilation produced by nitroprusside permits pooling of blood to occur in the extremities and is associated therefore with **orthostatic hypotension.** However, this is seldom of concern since nitroprusside is used only by intravenous infusion in nonambulatory clients. Renal blood flow and glomerular filtration rate are not adversely affected. Unlike other vasodilators, nitroprusside does not aggravate angina and, in fact, has a palliative effect.

Excessive vasodilation can result in headache, nausea, vomiting, sweating, palpitation, and apprehensiveness. *Complaints of headache, vomiting, dizziness, or palpitations should alert the nurse that blood pressure may be falling too rapidly. If the nurse observes the patient becoming listless, an increase in diaphoresis, cyanosis, or dyspnea, an adjustment in the flow rate of nitroprusside is indicated.*

Nitroprusside is metabolized to **cyanide** and then to **thiocyanate.** Cyanide toxicity almost never occurs. *However, the nurse should observe patients receiving nitroprusside for such symptoms as widely dilated pupils, imperceptible pulse rate, distant heart sounds, pink skin coloration, or impaired reflexes.* With prolonged nitroprusside therapy, thiocyanate may accumulate (it has a half-life of about 4 days) and produce symptoms such as weakness, hypoxia, tinnitus, muscle spasms, hypothyroidism, disorientation, and psychosis. *If thiocyanate-related symptoms occur, nitroprusside must be discontinued.*

Preparations and Administration *Solutions must be used within 4 hours of reconstitution and protected from light in the meantime. Fresh solutions have a faint brown color; change in color to red, blue, or green is an indication of decomposition.* Infusion should be controlled by an infusion pump or microdrip regulator to ensure precise control of flow rate. *Careful supervision and constant monitoring of blood pressure is required. Blood pressure should not be permitted to decline too rapidly. Care should be taken to avoid extravasation since the alkalinity of the solution can cause severe inflammation should it infiltrate into tissue.*

Nitroprusside (Nipride)
Powder (reddish brown) for reconstitution in water or 5% dextrose in water
Recommended Doses: The normal adult intravenous flow rate is 3 μg/kg/minute or about 200 μg/minute. The maximum rate of infusion is 800 μg/minute.

Nitrendipine (Baypress)

Mechanisms and Effects Nitrendipine is an investigational drug classified as a type II calcium channel blocker. It is structurally similar to nifedipine (Procardia), a calcium channel blocker discussed in Chapter 40 as an antianginal agent. Nitrendipine differs from type I calcium channel blockers because it has little effect on the electrophysiology of the heart at usual doses, but produces profound relaxation of peripheral vascular smooth muscle. Its action is mainly on arteriolar vessels.

Pharmacokinetics Nitrendipine is well absorbed after oral administration. The peak effect occurs approximately 4 hours after oral administration. The elimination half-life averages 8–11 hours, permitting effective therapy with 2 or 3 doses daily.

Clinical Indications Nitrendipine appears useful for lowering blood pressure in hypertensives, especially in cases where renin is not elevated.

Adverse Effects and Contraindications Nitrendipine is free of some of the side effects that occur with other antihypertensives, since it does not cause hypokalemia, hyperglycemia, or increases in serum uric acid or triglyceride levels. Its profile of adverse effects is similar to that of nifedipine. Vascular headache is the most frequently reported problem. Fatigue, edema, flushing, and palpitations may occur.

Nitrendipine (Baypress)
Investigational

Volume Depletors

Diuretics

Diuretics are the mainstay of treatment for hypertension. The details of their pharmacology and adverse effects are discussed in Chapter 43. Here, only their use in hypertension will be considered. Diuretics are usually the first step in treatment of hypertension, with additional drugs being added as required. Diuretics not only reduce hypertension themselves but also enhance the effectiveness of other antihypertensive drugs.

The mechanism of diuretics in lowering blood pressure is not fully determined. Both sodium depletion and decreased body fluid volume contribute, since replacement of fluids eliminated by diuretic therapy without replacement of sodium does not reverse the antihypertensive action.

When diuretic therapy is initiated, there is a decrease in cardiac output. With chronic administration, peripheral resistance decreases and cardiac output returns to normal. Depletion of sodium from vascular smooth muscle cells may contribute to the relaxation of blood vessels.

Most nondiuretic antihypertensive drugs cause sodium and fluid retention as blood pressure is lowered because a reduction in systemic blood pressure is associated with a diminished filtration by the kidney. Sodium and fluid retention can negate the primary effect of nondiuretic antihypertensives. Diuretics enhance the value of nondiuretic antihypertensives by preventing fluid and sodium accumulation.

Thiazides, high-ceiling diuretics, and spironolactone (Aldactone) have all been used in hypertension. Often a thiazide is used alone for mild hypertension or with nondiuretic antihypertensives to treat moderate to severe hypertension. High-ceiling diuretics are reserved for those cases not sufficiently responsive to thiazides.

Renin-Angiotensin-Aldosterone System Antagonists

The latest development in treatment of hypertension is the introduction of inhibitors of angiotensin-converting enzyme (ACE). The renin-angiotensin-aldosterone system is discussed in detail in Chapter 43. In brief, a decrease in sodium load in the tubule of the nephron, together with other stimuli, promotes release of renin in the kidney. Renin catalyzes conversion of angiotensinogen to angiotensin I, which is further converted by angiotensin converting enzyme to angiotensin II. Angiotensin II promotes secretion of aldosterone from the adrenal cortex, and aldosterone promotes sodium and fluid retention to correct the low sodium concentration that leads to renin release. Some cases of hypertension clearly involve a disturbance in this system as indicated by elevated renin levels. Even in hypertensive clients with normal renin activity, a depression of renin activity would be more physiologically appropriate given the presence of elevated salt and water concentrations. But it is not evident that renin is involved in all cases of hypertension.

Mechanisms and Effects The newly available ACE-inhibitors, captopril (Capoten) and enalapril (Vasotec), inhibit the formation of angiotensin II, thus suppressing the renin-angiotensin-aldosterone system. ACE-inhibitors thus block release of aldosterone and therefore reduce retention of sodium and fluid. In early clinical trials, results indicated that clients with both high and low initial renin plasma levels responded to treatment with an ACE-inhibitor. Although the effect of ACE-inhibitors on angiotensin is believed to be of primary importance, there may also be an effect related to the kallikrein-kinin-prostaglandin system (see Chapter 43).

Pharmacokinetics Captopril and enalapril are absorbed rapidly after oral administration, reaching peak plasma concentrations in 1 hour. Absorption of captopril is substantially reduced if taken with food, so it is recommended that it be given 1 hour before meals. The half-life of the two available ACE-inhibitors is less than 2 hours when renal function is normal. Renal extraction accounts for 75% of elimination, and renal insufficiency increases the magnitude and duration of effect.

Clinical Indications ACE-inhibitors are indicated for essential hypertension, but because of the potential for serious adverse effects, they are reserved for clients not adequately responsive to primary drug regimens. They are effective alone but should usually be combined with a thiazide diuretic for maximum benefit with least toxicity. When combined with thiazide diuretics, antihypertensive effects of ACE-inhibitors and thiazides are additive.

Adverse Effects The adverse effects shared by the two ACE-inhibitors are neurological symptoms, cardiovascular reactions, gastrointestinal irritation, hyperkalemia, cough and dyspnea, and skin reactions.

Neurological symptoms occurring in response to ACE-inhibitors include headache, dizziness, fatigue, paresthesias, insomnia, and dysgeusia (diminished taste sensitivity). **Cardiovascular side effects** with ACE-inhibitors, occurring in about 1% of clients, are excess hypotension and symptoms due to reflex sympathetic activation: tachycardia, angina, myocardial infarct, congestive heart failure, and Raynaud's phenomenon. **Gastrointestinal reactions** include nausea, vomiting, and diarrhea.

ACE-inhibitors may cause **potassium retention.** *Since many clients take the drug at home after they are discharged from the hospital, they need to be taught the indications of potassium retention. If ACE-inhibitors are employed in conjunction with a diuretic, potassium-sparing agents should be avoided. Nurses should advise clients receiving captopril to avoid foods that are especially rich in potassium.*

Allergic skin reactions, occurring during the first few weeks of therapy in about 10% of clients, consist of pruritus, rash, and urticaria, accompanied in some cases by fever and eosinophilia.

Captopril induces a **renal nephrotic syndrome** in 1–2% of clients, with resultant proteinuria. Renal insufficiency, polyuria, oliguria, increased urinary frequency, and renal failure have also been reported. Caution must be exercised in clients with preexisting renal dysfunctions, so urinary protein should be monitored during the first year of treatment. *Nurses need to monitor urinary function of clients receiving captopril and to teach self-monitoring to the clients.* Renal problems have not been observed with enalapril.

Blood cell disorders, including neutropenia and agranulocytosis, occur in about 0.3% of clients receiving captopril. Blood cell counts should be taken every 2 weeks during the first 3 months of therapy.

Drug Interactions The effects of ACE-inhibitors are potentially additive with those of spironolactone with respect to diuresis and potassium retention. Spironolactone should be discontinued and potassium levels restored to normal before an ACE-inhibitor is begun. Care must be exercised if clients are utilizing potassium supplements that hyperkalemia does not develop. Catopril causes false positives in the urine acetone test.

Preparations and Administration *Captopril tablets should be stored in an airtight, moisture-free container at 86° F or below. All doses of captopril should be taken 1 hour before meals.*

Captopril (Capoten)
Tablets
Recommended Doses: 25 mg PO initially, tid. After 1–2 weeks without satisfactory response, the dose can be increased to 50 mg, tid. After another 1–2 weeks, a thiazide diuretic should be added before further increasing the dose of captopril. If the response is still not satisfactory, further dosage increases can be effected up to 100 mg, tid, and later, to 150 mg, tid, as required.

Enalapril (Vasotec)
Tablets
Recommended Doses: For individuals not currently receiving a diuretic, 5 mg PO initially, once a day. The dose is adjusted according to response to a maximum of 40 mg/day. The usual dosage range is 10–40 mg/day.

Ganglionic Blockers

Ganglionic blockers have little remaining usefulness in hypertension. Drugs in this class block transmission between preganglionic and postganglionic neurons in both branches of the autonomic nervous system. Therefore, they are exceedingly nonspecific. All organ functions regulated by the autonomic nervous system are potentially altered. Both arteriolar and venous blood vessels are dilated, resulting in arterial hypotension and orthostatic hypotension respectively. Impotence, cycloplegia, tachycardia, dry mouth, and decreased gastrointestinal motility and secretions are additional problems. Hypothermia and inhibition of sweating also occur. The drugs remaining on the market from this family are mecamylamine hydrochloride (Inversine) and trimethaphan camsylate (Arfonad). Mecamylamine is marketed for essential hypertension but is almost never used. Trimethaphan is a rapid-acting drug indicated for immediate relief of hypertensive crisis, especially pulmonary hypertension, or for control of blood pressure during surgical procedures. Tachycardia and respiratory depression are important potential complications. Ganglionic blockers are discussed more fully in Chapter 29.

Trimethaphan Camsylate (Arfonad)
Infusion solution
Recommended Doses: Continuous intravenous infusion as a 0.1% solution in 5% dextrose or normal saline.

Combination Therapy for Hypertension

When essential hypertension is moderate to severe, it is often necessary to consider multiple drug regimens. Often two antihypertensive drugs having different mechanisms will produce a better response with fewer adverse effects than a single agent at a high dose. Nondiuretic antihypertensives generally produce salt and water retention, which can be prevented by concurrent use of a diuretic. Vasodilators cause reflex sympathetic stimulation of the heart, which can be alleviated by beta-blockers. There is, on the other hand, no rational basis for concurrent use of two antihypertensive drugs from the same pharmacological family. The most widely advocated approach in the United States is the so-called **step approach** (Table 39–7).

In this approach, the first step in treatment of hypertension is the administration of a thiazide diuretic. A high-ceiling diuretic might be used instead

Table 39–7
The Step Approach to Treatment of Essential Hypertension

STEP 1	Thiazide diuretic	
	or	High-ceiling diuretic if azotemia is present
STEP 2	Add	Beta-blocker[a]
	or	Other sympatholytic: Methyldopa, Clonidine, Reserpine
STEP 3	Add	Vasodilator: Prazosin[b], Hydralazine, Minoxidil
STEP 4	Add	Guanethidine[c]
		Clonidine[d]
		Phenoxybenzamine[e]

[a]Sometimes employed as step 1.
[b]Sometimes employed as step 2.
[c]Not if reserpine was used in step 2.
[d]Not if methyldopa was used in step 2.
[e]Only if a beta-blocker was used in step 2.

if azotemia is present. If after dosage adjustment, the diuretic does not provide an adequate response, the second step is to add a beta-blocker or a sympatholytic. In current practice, beta-blockers are more widely used. If a sympatholytic is selected, first preference goes to methyldopa. Clonidine or reserpine can be used if adverse reactions such as hemolytic anemia develop in response to methyldopa. In Europe, beta-blockers are often used as the first or only medication for hypertension.

If hypertension is still not adequately controlled in a two-drug regimen, a direct-acting vasodilator may be added in step 3. Prazosin, hydralazine, or minoxidil are employed in that order of preference. Occasionally prazosin is employed in step 2, without concurrent use of a beta-blocker or other sympatholytic. If hypertension remains refractory, a fourth drug may be added: guanethidine (Ismelin) (unless reserpine was selected in step 2), or phenoxybenzamine (Dibenzaline) if a beta-blocker was selected in step 2.

Important Nursing Implications for Antihypertensive Drugs

- ☐ Explain all studies, tests, procedures, medications, and anticipated responses to clients, using terminology they can understand. Ask the client to explain the medical problem and expected drug response to make sure he or she understands.
- ☐ Teach clients who have hypertension to schedule routine periods of rest and relaxation during the day in a quiet atmosphere. Encourage clients to engage in an appropriate program of exercise each day.
- ☐ Show clients how to measure their own blood pressure and how to keep a record of daily measurements. When the client is taking medication once a day, recordings should be taken before the daily dose. Regular monitoring of blood pressure will help the client and medical team identify if tolerance is occurring and if blood pressure control is no longer effective.
- ☐ Explain the importance of restricting dietary intake of salt and, when appropriate, increasing dietary potassium. Encourage clients to maintain a weight that is appropriate for their height and physique.
- ☐ Teach clients to weigh themselves daily and to keep a record of these determinations as an aid in identifying occurrences of edema. Teach clients to look for other signs of edema.
- ☐ Educate clients about the importance of maintaining continuous, uninterrupted therapy. When the regimen requires administration two or more times each day, the last dose should be taken before retiring to maintain blood pressure control through the night. Clients should be certain to maintain an adequate supply of medication, especially when traveling. Medication should not be discontinued without consultation with the physician. Abrupt discontinuation of medication could lead to rebound hypertension, especially when clonidine is part of the regimen.
- ☐ Be certain that clients understand the importance of continuing their medication regimen even though there may be no overt symptoms of hypertension or related health deficits.
- ☐ Teach clients the importance of common complaints such as weakness, fainting, nausea, or vomiting as indications of adverse reactions to antihypertensive medications. Instruct the client to lie down, elevate the legs and feet, and to put the head down on the knees when feeling dizzy. Clients should also flex their thigh muscles and wiggle their toes, thereby decreasing the pool of blood in the lower extremities and increasing the flow of blood to the brain. Teach clients to rise slowly from a supine position and to sit for a minute before standing.
- ☐ Teach clients to avoid hot baths, excessive heat, and alcohol and to warm up and cool down when exercising. Vasodilation resulting from these activities could cause fainting. Instruct clients to avoid standing in one place, especially during the first hour after taking medication. Standing causes blood to pool within the vessels of the legs, draining blood from the brain and other vital organs, possibly resulting in fainting. If the client must stand, he or she should move the legs and flex the leg muscles.
- ☐ Advise clients to elevate the head of the bed if headache occurs or if insomnia occurs.
- ☐ Warn clients taking antihypertensive drugs not to drive within 2 hours after taking the drug because of the potential for CNS depression. Monitor clients for evidences of psychiatric depression since many antihypertensive drugs can contribute to depression.
- ☐ Instruct clients not to employ any over-the-counter medications without first consulting the physician who has prescribed the antihypertensive regimen.

- ☐ Encourage clients to eat a diet high in fiber to avoid constipation. If this measure proves insufficient, a stool softener may be necessary. However, gastrointestinal symptoms should not go unheeded since they may be indicative of serious bowel problems as well.
- ☐ Advise clients using sympatholytic drugs that sexual dysfunction is a potential side effect. Assess clients given these drugs to determine if they have ceased taking the medication in order to avoid the problem.
- ☐ Advise clients about drug-specific adverse effects and interactions for each medication prescribed (see individual drug discussions).
- ☐ Instruct clients concerning the storage requirements for each medication prescribed.
- ☐ Advise clients to wear a medical identification tag or bracelet or to carry a wallet card stating the medical diagnosis and drug regimen.

Case Study: Essential Hypertension

R. H., a 6-foot-tall, 185 lb, black man of 50, kept insisting his blood pressure of 140/120 was perfectly normal since he had had the same pressure for several years and "nothing had happened." R. H. experienced headaches periodically for which he took aspirin, but because of his macho self-image, he did not care to discuss the occurrence of the headaches or precipitating factors. The client had consistently refused to seek medical assistance and the only health care management the nurse was at first able to institute was to encourage him to reduce intake of alcohol, eliminate tea and coffee from his diet, reduce sodium content, and limit his intake of food high in saturated fats and cholesterol.

About 90% of people who have hypertension have no identifiable cause (essential or primary hypertension). This was the pattern of events that the nurse identified with R. H. From discussing his family history, it appeared that his problem was due, at least in part, to heredity. Restricting sodium in his diet tended to contain his pressure to the range 140/100 to 140/120. R. H. exercised and also did hard physical work. All these elements helped R. H. to maintain a normal weight. In assessing R. H., the nurse determined that most of the risk factors could be limited. The major problem was going to be to get R. H. to seek the medical help he needed.

In collaboration with Mrs. H., the nurse encouraged R. H. to submit to routine measurement of his blood pressure. Mrs. H. was taught how to take the blood pressure and to record this along with incidents of headache and circumstances under which these occurred. The nurse taught Mrs. H. about dietary adjustments that would help control blood pressure and encouraged her to have R. H. submit to urinalysis, blood chemistry tests, and electrocardiography. The routine measurements served as baseline data against which to determine the effectiveness of dietary therapy as well as that of drug therapy when they finally were able to persuade R. H. to submit to a medical follow-up. The nurse and Mrs. H. encouraged the client to respond to this threat to his health in a way that allowed him to retain a positive self-concept. In discussions with the client, it was evident that getting him to seek medical assistance was going to be difficult. R. H. repeatedly proclaimed the uselessness of chemicals, stating that they are rarely of any value to one's health. Also, R. H. demonstrated repeatedly that he did not wish to be found in error.

In working with R. H., the nurse's knowledge of his religious denomination was particularly helpful, since the particular religious group preaches abstinence from alcohol, tea, and coffee as well as healthful living through diet and exercise. This information helped the nurse convince R. H. not only to change his diet but also eventually to seek medical assistance. In time (several months in fact) and after much gentle persuasion, R. H. finally admitted to having a "touch of high blood pressure" and was willing to seek professional help and to accept the need for medication. Because of the steps already taken to reduce his blood pressure by dietary adjustments, R. H.'s high blood pressure responded satisfactorily to a regimen of hydrochlorothiazide, 50 mg PO once daily. The nurse and Mrs. H. kept count of the number of pills that R. H. used each week and the nurse and physician closely monitored R. H. for his blood pressure response and changes in serum electrolytes.

1. What risk factors for hypertension were present in R. H.'s case?
2. What is the relationship between headaches and hypertension?
3. If, as R. H. insisted, there were no observable consequences from his high blood pressure, why was it important for him to seek medical treatment?

4. What additional drugs might have been added to the regimen if R. H.'s blood pressure had not responded to hydrochlorothiazide alone?
5. What was the purpose of keeping track of the pills consumed by R. H.?
6. What was the value of continuing to monitor blood pressure and electrolytes after the initial satisfactory response?

Answers appear at the end of the book.

Recommended Readings

Clark AB et al: A nurse's clinician's role in the management of hypertension. *Arch Intern Med* 1976;136:903–904.

Daniels LL: What influences adherence to hypertensive therapy. *Nurs Forum* 1979;18:231–245.

Finnerty FA: The nurse and care of the hypertensive patient. *Ann Intern Med* 1976;84:746.

Frishman WH: *Clinical Pharmacology of the Beta-adrenoceptor Blocking Drugs.* New York, Appleton-Century-Crofts, 1980.

Geyskes, GG, Boer P, Mees EJD: Clonidine withdrawal: Mechanism and frequency of rebound hypertension. *Br J Clin Pharm* 1979;7:55–62.

Hansson L, Werko L: Beta adrenergic blockade in hypertension. *Am Heart J* 1977;93:394–402.

Hartshorn JC: What to do when the patient's in hypertensive crisis. *Nursing* 1980;10(7):36–45.

Hill M: Helping the hypertensive patient control sodium intake. *Am J Nurs* 1979;79(5):906–909.

Hill MH, Foster SB: Seeking and finding all those patients with high blood pressure. *Nursing* 1982;12(2):72–75.

Hoffman W: The behavioral side effects of the antihypertensive agents. *Am Fam Physician* 1981;23(2);213–216.

Hutchins LN: Drug treatment of high blood pressure. *Nurs Clin North Am* 1981;16:365–377.

Jones LN: Hypertension: medical and nursing implications. *Nurs Clin North Am* 1976;11(2):283–295.

Kirschenbaum HL, Rosenberg JM: Clonidine and methyldopa. *RN* 1982;82(11):66–68.

Kirschenbaum HL, Rosenberg JM: Guanethidine and reserpine. *RN* 1984;84(2):31–33.

Kirschenbaum HL, Rosenberg JM: Hydralazine and minoxidil. *RN* 1982;82(12):42–43.

Lowther NB, Carter VD: How to increase compliance in hypertensives. *Am J Nurs* 1981;81(5):963.

Marcinek MB: Hypertension: What it does to the body. *Am J Nurs* 1980;80:928–932.

Marx JL: Hypertension: A complex disease with complex causes. *Science* 1980;194:821–825.

McKenney JM: Methods for modifying compliance behavior in hypertensive patients. *Drug Intell Clin Pharm* 1981;15:8–14.

Moser M: Hypertension: How therapy works. *Am J Nurs* 1980;80:937–941.

Pas DA, Lawlor MC: Beta-blocker agents: An update. *J Emerg Nurs* 1986;12(1);18–22.

Rangno RE, Nattel S, Lutterodt A: Prevention of propranolol withdrawal mechanism by prolonged small dose propranolol schedule. *Am J Cardiol* 1982;42:829–833.

Schoof CS: Hypertension — common questions patients ask. *Am J Nurs* 1980;65:894–899.

Taylor SH, Silke B, Lee PS: Intravenous beta-blockade in coronary heart disease. Is cardioselectivity or intrinsic sympathomimetic activity hemodynammically useful? *N Engl J. Med* 1982;306:631–635.

Ward GW, Bundy P, Fink JW: Treating and counseling the hypertensive patient. *Am J Nurs* 1978;78;824–828.

CHAPTER 40

Drugs Used for Ischemic Heart Disease and Other Vascular Disorders

Ischemia is a condition of insufficient blood flow to a tissue typically caused by pathological changes in small blood vessels. Ischemia can occur in the heart (ischemic heart disease) or in peripheral tissues as a result of peripheral vascular disorders. The primary cause of coronary ischemia is atherosclerosis of coronary vessels, and the two primary manifestations are angina pectoris and myocardial infarction. Peripheral ischemia has numerous causes and numerous effects. This chapter considers the drug therapies employed for these ischemic disorders.

Coronary Vessels and Coronary Atherosclerosis

The myocardium receives its entire blood supply through the right and left coronary arteries, distributive vessels that arise from the base of the aorta. The right coronary artery supplies the chambers on the right side of the heart. The left coronary artery divides soon after emerging from the aorta into two major branches — the anterior descending branch and the circumflex branch — that supply the left ventricle and atrium. The vessels themselves lie on the external surface of the heart and give rise to lesser arterial branches that penetrate into the myocardium.

Inflow of blood through coronary vessels occurs mainly during diastole. During systole, the coronary vessels are too compressed by the force of the myocardial contraction to permit much arterial flow. When heart rate is elevated, the myocardium spends less time in the relaxed diastolic condition, and the inflow of blood is consequently diminished. At the same time, the greater frequency of contractions increases the work of the heart and its requirement for oxygen. Since the extraction of oxygen from the coronary blood supply is close to optimal efficiency under normal circumstances, the principal means available for meeting increased oxygen demand is dilation of coronary arterioles. In addition, myocardial cells can, for short periods, switch over to principally anaerobic pathways of carbohydrate metabolism to meet energy demands. Under the best of circumstances, during times of physiological stress a delicate balance exists between the need of the body for increased cardiac output and the need of the heart itself for sufficient oxygen and nutrients to perform the added work.

This delicate balance is seriously disturbed by coronary artery disease. Coronary artery disease is usually related to progression of atherosclerosis in one or more of the three major coronary vessels. The initial atherosclerotic process consists of the lining of blood vessels with fatty streaks. Gradually these develop into white fibrous plaques, called atheromas. Plaques continue to expand and progressively clog the blood vessels. The center of a plaque may become necrotic, triggering hermorrhage, clotting, and calcification that further enlarge the occluding mass. Atherosclerotic plaques tend to occur where vessels bifurcate, turn, or rapidly diminish in diameter. The coronary vessels are prime sites for plaque formation.

Usually clinical symptoms appear only after 50–75% of the blood supply to a tissue area has been blocked after two to four decades of plaque formation. Subacute, intermittent ischemia, usually brought on by exercise and alleviated by rest, is manifested as angina pectoris. Abrupt reduction of blood supply to a region of the myocardium, almost always superimposed on coronary arteriosclerosis, results in myocardial infarction.

The causes of atherosclerosis are not well understood. It is a process that begins early in life and progresses gradually over the remaining decades. Nurses need to be aware of the risk factors that have been identified. (1) Men are more vulnerable to atherosclerosis than women during middle age, but after menopause the susceptibility is the same. Other risk factors include (2) race, (3) family history, (4) diabetes mellitus, (5) elevated serum lipids, (6) diets high in saturated fats, (7) hypertension, (8) obesity, (9) cigarette smoking, (10) overconsumption of alcohol, (11) lack of exercise, and (12) a stressful lifestyle. (13) Psychosocial factors have also been shown to contribute to atherosclerosis. People with so-called type A personalities appear to have an increased incidence of coronary heart disease. These individuals have an overly developed sense of urgency. They are easily provoked, impatient, have excessive drive, and are very competitive. The usual risk factors become more important to this population of people.

There is no single factor that causes atherosclerosis, but rather a combination of factors. For this reason, it is important to identify which factors one can control and, in cooperation with the client, determine means of reducing a number of such factors. While this approach works best when one begins teaching people early in life, it is also important for assisting older clients to regain health once they have developed early signs and symptoms of atherosclerosis.

Angina Pectoris

Angina pectoris (literally, a choking of the chest) is a clinical diagnosis very seldom possible to establish by objective proof, but sufficiently distinctive in its characteristics as to pose little problem in differential diagnosis. Angina pectoris is defined as episodes of substernal pain, described as a sensation of compression, tightness, or pressure, typically brought on by exertion and alleviated by rest. The pain is a manifestation of cardiac anoxia and occurs when metabolites formed in anaerobic metabolism, including lactic acid, accumulate and stimulate pain receptors surrounding the heart. The heart itself has no pain receptors; the pain signals originate from receptors in the substernal region. Anginal pain is typically referred pain, being felt in the left arm, neck, and jaws or less commonly the right arm. Anginal pain is usually described by clients as a tearing, ripping, or wrenching sensation that begins in the chest and radiates outward in all directions. Typically the pain lasts for a few minutes, subsiding when exercise is interrupted. In some people, it may be a barely perceptible ache felt beneath the sternum. In others, it may occur rapidly as a severe, crushing sensation. In contrast to supraventricular dysrhythmias, anginal sensations are seldom felt in the apical area of the heart. Atypically, anginal attacks may occur at night (nocturnal angina) during dreams, or while at rest (angina decubitus).

Myocardial anoxia occurs whenever oxygen demand exceeds the supply of oxygen from coronary perfusion. Myocardial anoxia is accompanied by electrophysiological changes that are reflected in the electrocardiogram (Figure 40–1). Relief occurs when myocardial oxygen demand is reduced or oxygen

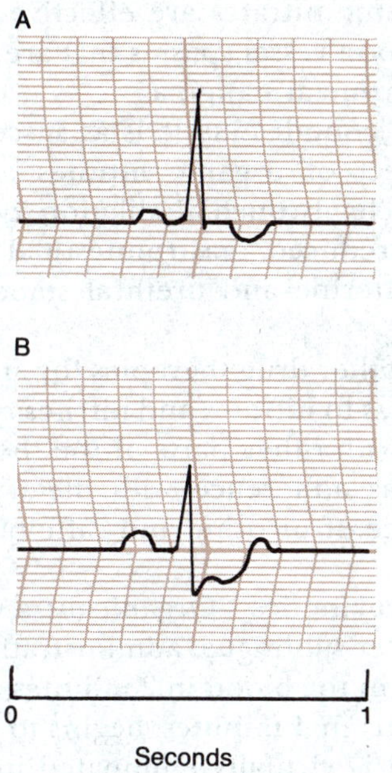

Figure 40–1
Typical ECG changes during an anginal attack. A. T-wave inversion. B. Depression of the S-T segment.

supply is increased. The determinants of cardiac oxygen consumption are heart rate, preload, contractility, and afterload. Any change in these factors will alleviate or intensify episodes of angina accordingly.

Angina pectoris is characteristically triggered by emotional crises, eating a large, heavy meal, especially in the evening, or physical exertion. The onset may be exacerbated by exposure to cold weather. Cigarette smoking, drinking caffeine-containing beverages, excessive alcohol consumption, or use of medications containing sympathomimetics, stimulants, or peripheral vasodilators can also trigger attacks.

The frequency of anginal attacks varies from rare, isolated attacks to several a day. In most clients, the characteristics of the condition are fairly stable or very gradually progressive. A sudden increase in frequency, duration, or intensity of attacks, or occurrence of attacks in less provocative situations (at rest, asleep, or with mild exercise) is indicative of **unstable angina,** a high-risk status that often indicates impending infarction.

Angina pectoris is almost invariably associated with extensive coronary arteriosclerosis and consequent occlusion of coronary blood flow. An exception is **variant angina** or **Prinzmetal's angina.** In this condition, attacks occur at rest and often with regularity at certain times of the day independent of the usual trigger factors. Cardiac ischemia in Prinzmetal's angina is caused by vasospasm of coronary vessels rather than atherosclerotic occlusion. This condition is often associated with peripheral vasospastic disorders: Raynaud's disease and migraine headaches.

The prognosis in angina pectoris is influenced by several factors. Mortality rates are greater when the client is old; when angiography indicates extensive occlusion; when there is concurrent hypertension, congestive heart failure, or history of myocardial infarction; or when more than one of the major coronary vessels is implicated.

Antianginal Drugs

Relief of typical angina depends on correcting the balance between oxygen utilization and oxygen delivery. Drug treatment of angina must either reduce myocardial oxygen requirements or increase oxygen availability. Oxygen requirements can be reduced by slowing the heart rate, reducing contractility, or reducing preload or afterload. The approach based on reducing cardiac output can be employed successfully but has the potential of diminishing coronary perfusion.

In theory, oxygen delivery can be improved by drugs that dilate coronary vessels, but sclerotic vessels dilate less readily than healthy vessels with the result that blood may actually be shunted away from the area of poor perfusion into the healthy vessels. In addition, so-called coronary vasodilators are never perfectly selective for coronary vessels; they produce some degree of systemic peripheral vasodilation that shunts additional blood away from the heart to other tissues. In the case of Prinzmetal's angina, drug efficacy is achieved by drugs that alleviate vasospasm, permitting normal flow through the vessel to the ischemic area.

Treatment of angina pectoris centers on four objectives: (1) reducing factors that promote continuing sclerotic process or that trigger anginal episodes; (2) alleviating painful attacks (with respect to both intensity and duration); (3) reducing the frequency of attacks; and (4) preventing the dangerous complications of angina pectoris: myocardial infarction and sudden death. The first objective is approached through client education and depends ultimately on the commitment of the client. The client should be urged to avoid smoking, overeating, overconsumption of caffeinated or alcoholic beverages, exercising immediately after meals, chronic stress, or use of sympathomimetic agents. In addition, clients must be taught to avoid those activities that tend to precipitate attacks, such as emotional and anxiety-producing situations.

The second objective, alleviating pain, is approached through acute medication in response to attacks. In general, this objective is the one most adequately realized in current practice. The third objective, reducing the frequency of attacks, requires chronic, prophylactic medication and is achieved to a variable degree. There is no evidence that the fourth objective is fully achieved by any current therapeutic approach. However, it is estimated that preventive measures and appropriate client teaching can give the individual who has angina about 5 years before the likelihood of having a myocardial infarction.

There are four classes of drugs currently in use for treatment of angina: (1) the nitrates, (2) dipyridamole, a coronary vasodilator, (3) the calcium channel blockers, and (4) the beta-blockers.

Organic Nitrates

Nitroglycerin was the original entry in this pharmacological family and remains the most important. First synthesized in 1846, nitroglycerin was quickly recognized to possess vasodilating properties. Today, five drugs are marketed in this family for administration by five routes. Nitroglycerin (Nitrostat) is marketed for sublingual and topical application and in a sustained release formulation for oral use. Isosorbide (Isordil and others) is available as the dinitrate salt in sublingual, chewable, and oral formulations. Amyl nitrite is available in the form of an inhalant. Pentaerythritol tetranitrate (Peritrate and others) is available in regular and sustained action oral forms, while erythrityl tetranitrate (Cardilate) is marketed in sublingual, chewable, and oral preparations. Only nitroglycerin and isosorbide are widely employed.

Mechanisms and Effects Organic nitrates act on specific receptors of vascular and visceral smooth muscle. Nitrates are universal dilators of vascular smooth muscle, acting on all regions of the vasculature, and on both the venous and arterial side of the circulation. At normal doses, organic nitrates dilate both venules and, to a lesser extent, the arterioles and thus reduce preload and afterload and reduce oxygen demand in the myocardium. The ability of nitrates to reduce oxygen utilization by the heart appears to be the major mechanism by which they alleviate pain in typical angina.

Two other factors may be relevant. Although organic nitrates do not increase total coronary blood flow in clients with typical angina, they do selectively increase the flow to the portion of the myocardium most vulnerable to ischemia — the subendocardium. Second, organic nitrates are effective spasmolytics, inhibiting blood vessel spasms that are the principal cause of Prinzmetal's angina.

Visceral smooth muscle is as susceptible to the relaxant effect of organic nitrates as is vascular smooth muscle. Bronchial dilation occurs, biliary pressure is reduced, gastrointestinal motility declines, and uterine and urethral smooth muscle is relaxed.

As with other drug therapies for angina, clinical responsiveness to nitrates and nitrites requires client compliance with other parts of the therapeutic regimen, such as adherence with dietary restrictions and avoidance of nicotine and caffeine.

Pharmacokinetics Organic nitrates are rapidly absorbed. After sublingual administration, nitroglycerin appears in the blood in 2 minutes, reaches peak concentrations in 4 minutes, begins to decline in 10 minutes, and is virtually eliminated in 30 minutes. When isosorbide is given sublingually in equivalent doses, it follows a similar time course. After topical administration of nitroglycerin ointment, absorption is more gradual, producing effects in 15 minutes with a duration of up to 3 hours. Oral administration is indicated only for chronic prophylaxis. Low oral doses of isosorbide, erythrityl tetranitrate, or pentaerythritol tetranitrate do not provide effective serum concentrations. Higher doses produce significant blood levels and effects in 15–30 minutes that last 2–6 hours. Nitroglycerin in oral, sustained release capsules or tablets produces effective serum concentrations for 8–12 hours.

Organic nitrates are inactivated in the liver virtually as rapidly as they reach it. This accounts for the short duration of action of organic nitrates. So-called long-acting organic nitrates are longer acting only to the extent that they are absorbed in a more sustained fashion after oral administration. The liver converts organic nitrates to more water soluble and substantially less active metabolites by removal of inorganic nitrite.

Clinical Indications Organic nitrates are indicated for acute relief of anginal episodes. Nitrates are useful both in typical and Prinzmetal's angina. Sublingual dosage forms are indicated in preference to oral formulations. Oral dosage forms are designated as possibly effective in long-term prophylaxis of angina, but the effectiveness of low doses has not been demonstrated and the use of high doses is associated with development of tolerance. *When nitrates are used for prophylaxis, clients should be instructed to keep careful records of the incidence of anginal attacks and the* *number of nitrate tablets used as an aid in adjusting prophylactic regimens.*

Adverse Effects and Contraindications Nitrates are remarkably selective for smooth muscle tissue. The principal adverse effects are related to **excessive vasodilation.** Vascular headache is common and often severe but becomes less prevalent with continued use of the nitrate. Other symptoms of hypotension include dizziness, faintness, and weakness. The skin may become flushed. Clients need to be warned that hypotensive effects are aggravated by concurrent use of alcohol and they should be advised not to drink alcoholic beverages. Body position is an important determinant of severity of symptoms related to nitrate-induced hypotension, severity being intensified when the client is erect and alleviated when the client reclines. *Nurses should instruct clients to sit down at the first sign of faintness or dizziness and to change position slowly, especially when arising from a recumbent position. Dangling and moving the feet for a few minutes before arising is helpful. Family members need to be informed of these precautions as well so that they can be supportive of the individual. Elderly people are especially prone to excess hypotension.*

Some clients develop **allergic reactions** to nitrates, exhibiting symptoms such as rash and exfoliative dermatitis. Amyl nitrite can cause **methemoglobinemia** (see Chapter 41).

Infrequent, sublingual use of organic nitrites is not associated with tolerance and clinical response occurs reliably. When high doses of nitrates are used orally, however, there is a significant decrease in the effect of nitrates on smooth muscle. **Withdrawal phenomena** have been noted, including myocardial infarction, increased blood pressure, anginal attacks, anxiety, and trepidation. *When prolonged therapy is scheduled for discontinuation, withdrawal should be conducted gradually.*

Preparations and Administration *Since nitroglycerin deteriorates rapidly, clients should be advised to keep their supply fresh, and not to use the drug when it is more than 3 months old. Nitroglycerin should be stored in a dark, airtight container and all but the portion in immediate use should be refrigerated. The drug should not be transferred to another container since some container materials (certain plastics) will absorb nitrites. The drug should be carried in a manner so as to protect it from bodily heat (not in a shirt pocket) or other heat sources to the extent possible. Nitroglycerin may be kept at bedside by hospitalized patients.*

If symptoms of angina pain are not relieved after taking the initial dose of drug, the individual may take additional doses every 5 minutes up to three tablets. If no relief occurs after three tablets, the family should seek medical help immediately. If the client is alone, he or she should call for emergency transportation.

Nitroglycerin may be used prophylactically as well. *Nurses can advise clients to take the drug before exercise, sexual intercourse, or events that are anticipated to be stressful. It is important to teach clients when not to use nitroglycerin as well. Clients with angina often become unduly anxious with the occurrence of slight pain or discomfort that has little or no relationship to the angina. Clients need to be taught how to make accurate judgments concerning the sources of pain.*

Transdermal nitroglycerin is a preparation that provides sustained release of drug over a 24-hour period. It is attached to an adhesive bandage, comes in different doses and strengths, and provides continual release of the drug into the systemic circulation. This results in active drug reaching the target organs (heart, extremities) before being metabolized by the liver. Steady-state plasma levels are attained within 2 hours after the patch is applied and continue as long as the client wears the patch, up to 24 hours. In the event that a client requires defibrillation or cardioversion, transdermal nitroglycerin systems should be removed because presence of the patch may alter electrical conductivity. *Transdermal nitroglycerin should be applied to the chest on areas without hair. Clients should be taught to rotate the transdermal pad to prevent irritation, but the extremities should not be used.*

In the event it is decided to terminate treatment with nitroglycerin, both the dosage and frequency of application must be reduced gradually over a period of 4–6 weeks to prevent sudden withdrawal reactions, common to all vasodilators in the nitroglycerin class.

Oral dosage forms of organic nitrates are generously designated by the Food and Drug Administration as "possibly effective" for angina prophylaxis. *Clients should be advised not to eat, drink, or smoke while sublingual tablets are under the tongue. Isosorbide dinitrate is best taken 1–2 hours before meals.*

Amyl nitrite
Inhalant
Recommended Doses: 0.18 or 0.3 ml by inhalation as required.

Erythrityl tetranitrate (Cardilate)
Tablets, sublingual tablets, chewable tablets
Recommended Doses: 5–10 mg sublingually or 10 mg orally prior to anticipated physical or emotional stress. Dosages may be titrated up to 100 mg/day.

Isosorbide dinitrate (Isordil, Sorbitrate, others)
Sublingual tablets, chewable tablets, tablets, sustained release tablets or capsules
Recommended Doses: 5–20 mg PO initially; for maintenance, 10–40 mg every 6 hours.

Nitroglycerin (Nitrostat)
Sublingual tablets, ointment in a lanolin-petrolatum base (Nitro-Bid, others), sustained release tablets and capsules, transdermal patches
Recommended Doses: Upon onset or anticipation of an attack of angina pectoris, one tablet is placed in the buccal pouch and allowed to dissolve. *As soon as anginal pain is alleviated, the remaining tablet may be expelled from the mouth, especially if any unpleasant side effects are noted. Clients should be advised not to eat, drink, or smoke while the sublingual tablet is under the tongue and not to swallow the pills.* The ointment is applied by squeezing a 1–2 inch column from the tube and applying it in a uniform thin layer to the skin of the chest. Some clients require as much as 4–5 inches of the ointment. The previous area of application should be thoroughly cleansed with each new application of the ointment. Capsules are taken every 8–12 hours on an empty stomach for prophylaxis against anginal attacks.

Pentaerythritol tetranitrate (Duotrate, Naptrate, Pentritol, Peritrate)
Tablets, sustained release capsules, sustained release tablets
Recommended Doses: 10–20 mg PO initially, titrated up to 40 mg, 3 or 4 times daily for quick-acting tablets; or one sustained release tablet every 12 hours.

Dipyridamole (Persantine)

Dipyridamole is a nonnitrate coronary vasodilator. It is fairly selective for coronary vessels at therapeutic doses. It decreases resistance to blood flow in small coronary vessels and increases coronary blood flow. Its mechanism appears to relate to the nucleotide adenosine. Adenosine is released by hypoxic myocardial cells and promotes vasodilation, a facet of normal autoregulation of coronary blood flow. Dipyridamole blocks uptake of adenosine by erythrocytes and other cells that would terminate its activity. The vasodilatory effect of adenosine on coronary capillaries is thus enhanced.

Despite its theoretical advantages, dipyridamole has not been convincingly shown to reduce frequency of anginal attacks. Dipyridamole does not improve exercise tolerance in standard treadmill tests. It has been designated as possibly effective for prophylaxis in angina pectoris but is not indicated for terminating attacks acutely.

Dipyridamole is relatively free of adverse effects. Gastrointestinal disturbances such as nausea, vomiting, and diarrhea occur occasionally. Excessive doses can produce peripheral vasodilation, hypotension, headaches, and vertigo. Dipyridamole is prescribed with surprising frequency considering its dubious value. *Blood pressure should be monitored during the period of dosage adjustment.*

Dipyridamole (Persantine and generic)
Tablets
Recommended Doses: 50 mg PO, tid, to be taken one hour before meals.

Calcium Channel Blockers

Calcium channel blockers have been available for clinical use in the United States since 1982 and have rapidly gained an important place in medical practice.

Mechanism and Effects Calcium channel blockers inhibit influx of calcium into muscle cells that ordinarily initiates contraction in response to excitation. Calcium channel blockers act directly on vascular smooth muscle (more so on the arterial than the venous side of the circulatory system) to reduce spasms and to promote vasodilation. They also act directly on the cells of the myocardium to decrease contractility, conductance in the A-V node, and automaticity. Thus the value of calcium channel blockers in angina is (1) to increase myocardial oxygen supply by increasing total coronary blood flow, redistributing blood to the subendocardial tissue, and relieving vasospasm; and (2) to decrease myocardial oxygen demand by reducing afterload, contractility, and heart rate.

Diltiazem (Cardiazem), nifedipine (Procardia), and verapamil (Calan, Isoptin), the three currently available calcium channel blockers, differ substantially in the preponderance of these various actions (Table 40–1). All three drugs are potent spasmolytics and all produce substantial coronary vasodilation. Nifedipine causes the most profound peripheral vasodilation, which in turn triggers reflexive activation of the sympathetic nervous system. The resultant sympathetic stimulation of the heart offsets direct depressant effects of nifedipine on cardiac muscle. Diltiazem produces only modest peripheral vasodilation and moderate cardiac suppression. Verapamil has the most profound effects on cardiac muscle, substantially decreasing contractility and suppressing A-V conduction rate. Verapamil is the only one of the three calcium channel blockers approved for use as an antidysrhythmic agent for supraventricular dysrhythmias (see Chapter 38). All three drugs are approved by the FDA for use in typical and Prinzmetal's angina. A fourth calcium channel blocker with distinctive characteristics, nitrendipine (Baypress), is currently undergoing clinical trials for use in hypertension (see Chapter 39).

Table 40–1
Comparisons Among the Calcium Channel Blockers

Activity	Diltiazem	Nifedipine	Verapamil
Spasmolytic action	+++	+++	+++
Coronary vasodilation	+++	+++	++
Peripheral vasodilation	+	+++	++
Contractility	0	↑↓	↓
Automaticity	↓	↑	↑↓
A-V nodal conduction	↓	0	↓↓
Sympathetic activity	↓	↑(reflexly)	↓

Key: +++ strong effect; ++ moderate effect; + small effect; 0 no change; ↑ increased; ↓ decreased; ↓↓ greatly decreased; ↓↑ decreased or increased.

Pharmacokinetics After oral administration, calcium channel blockers are well absorbed but subject to substantial first-pass elimination by the liver. The bioavailable fraction of an administered dose of nifedipine or diltiazem is only 45–65% and for verapamil about 10–22%. All three drugs are eliminated by liver metabolism, but both verapamil and diltiazem initially yield active metabolites. The half-lives range from 2 to 6 hours, so that administration 3 or 4 times daily is required. Protein binding in plasma is about 80% for diltiazem, 85% for verapamil, and 95% for nifedipine.

Clinical Indications Calcium channel blockers are indicated for oral prophylaxis in Prinzmetal's and typical angina pectoris. They decrease the frequency of anginal episodes, improve exercise tolerance, and therefore decrease requirements for nitroglycerin. Calcium channel blockers may be considered the treatment of choice for Prinzmetal's angina. Calcium channel blockers are an alternative to beta-blockers for typical angina. Calcium channel blockers offer some distinct advantages over beta-blockers: (1) they increase coronary blood flow while beta-blockers reduce it; (2) beta-blockers cause depression and fatigue; (3) beta-blockers are contraindicated in vasospastic (variant) angina; and (4) beta-blockers are contraindicated in clients with asthma, pulmonary disease, diabetes mellitus, and peripheral vascular diseases.

Adverse Effects and Contraindications The adverse effects of calcium channel blockers relate to three of their actions: (1) peripheral vasodilation, (2) negative inotropism, and (3) depression of S-A or A-V nodal conductance. Symptoms of **peripheral vasodilation** include dizziness, vertigo, nausea, fatigue, syncope, flushing, facial warmth, vascular headache, edema, and hypotension. This cluster of symptoms is far more common with nifedipine than with verapamil or diltiazem. *Patients should be advised to change positions gradually, especially when standing up from a recumbent position. If faintness occurs, the client should sit down immediately. The physician should be notified if the client exhibits swelling of the hands or feet, pronounced dizziness or nausea, or marked hypotension.*

Negative inotropism occurs mainly with verapamil (in about 1% of treated clients) and can lead to congestive heart failure or pulmonary edema. **Conduction blocks** and **bradycardia** occur with verapamil and diltiazem in 1–2% of clients. *The physician should be notified immediately if the client exhibits an irregular heart beat or shortness of breath.*

Drug Interactions Pharmacodynamic interactions of calcium channel blockers with other drugs relate to their adverse effects. Additive hypotension occurs with beta-blockers and other antihypertensive drugs, especially when nifedipine is selected. Additive depressant effects on contractility and A-V conduction are likely to occur if verapamil is used with beta-blockers or disopyramide. Both verapamil and nifedipine have been reported to increase plasma levels of digoxin, probably by reducing the rate of renal clearance. Use of calcium channel blockers may necessitate adjustment of digoxin dosing.

Preparations and Administration Nifedipine is the most widely prescribed of the three calcium channel blockers in current practice. *Monitoring of blood pressure is indicated during the period of dosage adjustment, and baseline hepatic and renal function should be* *evaluated before therapy with calcium channel blockers is begun.*

Diltiazem (Cardizem)
Tablets
Recommended Doses: For angina, 60–90 mg PO every 6–8 hours.

Nifedipine (Procardia)
Capsules
Recommended Doses: 10–30 mg PO every 6–8 hours.

Verapamil (Calan, Isoptin)
Tablets, injection solution (see Chapter 38)
Recommended Doses: 80–120 mg PO every 9 hours.

Beta-blockers

The general pharmacology of beta-blockers is discussed in Chapters 28 and 40 and the use of propranolol in dysrhythmias in Chapter 38. This section will address only the use of beta-blockers in angina pectoris.

Mechanism and Effects Beta-adrenergic drugs are effective in reducing the frequency and severity of anginal attacks of the typical variety, but they aggravate variant (Prinzmetal's or vasospastic) angina. Beta-blockers reduce requirements for nitroglycerin and improve exercise tolerance in typical angina. The value of beta-blockers in typical angina is their ability to reduce oxygen consumption by the heart by slowing heart rate, reducing the force of contraction, and decreasing afterload.

Pharmacokinetics Beta-blockers are well absorbed but subject to extensive and variable first-pass extraction by the liver. Bioavailability is consequently unpredictable and doses must be individualized. Propranolol (Inderal) has a half-life of about 4 hours and must be given three or four times daily. The other beta-blocker approved for angina, nadolol (Corgard), has the advantage of a long duration of action and can be taken once a day. Although tolerance does not develop to the therapeutic benefits of beta-blockers, abrupt withdrawal may precipitate significant withdrawal symptoms, including a rebound increase in anginal attacks and even myocardial infarction. Other withdrawal symptoms include tremulousness, sweating, severe headache, malaise, palpitation, and rebound hypertension. Long-term beta-blocker therapy should therefore be discontinued by gradually tapering size of dose (not frequency) over 1–2 weeks.

Clinical Indications Beta-blockers are indicated for oral prophylaxis of stable, exercise-induced angina pectoris. Because of the risk of serious adverse effects, beta-blockers should be reserved for those cases of angina characterized by intolerable pain not adequately controlled by nitroglycerin.

Exercise tolerance tests and an ECG evaluation should be conducted to determine baseline functioning before beta-blocker therapy for angina is instituted. If therapy does not result in increased exercise tolerance or reduced frequency of attacks after a reasonable trial priod, the drug should be discontinued.

Beta-blockers may be effective when combined with nitroglycerin in management of angina. Beta-blockers prevent reflex tachycardia and cardiac stimulation induced by nitroglycerin, while nitroglycerin counteracts the tendency of beta-blockers to increase preload. *As with other antianginal drugs, responsiveness to beta-blockers depends on client compliance with other facets of the therapeutic regimen. Typically, clients are told to stop smoking if they smoke and to lose weight if they are overweight. Client may be placed on bedrest during initial institution of drug therapy and stabilization of the condition.*

Adverse Effects and Contraindications Cardiotoxic effects of beta-blockers include severe bradycardia and precipitation of congestive heart failure. Beta-blockers are contraindicated in Prinzmetal's angina, peripheral vascular disorders, and diabetes mellitus. Propranolol has been known to exacerbate chest pains of clients with Prinzmetal's angina. Abrupt withdrawal of propranolol can produce a temporary exacerbation of angina, possibly culminating in myocardial infarction. *If it is decided to discontinue beta-blockers being employed for angina, drug withdrawal should be conducted gradually with constant monitoring. The client at home should be encouraged to record any sensations that occur as the drug level is reduced. In addition, nurses need to admonish clients against interrupting or ceasing use of the drug on their own, something which can sometimes occur when the client begins to feel better.* Beta-blockers are also contraindicated in individuals with bronchial asthma or pulmonary disease. *Any client receiving beta-blockers needs to be monitored for signs of respiratory distress. In particular, nurses should question these clients about incidents of nocturnal dyspnea.* Although not approved by the FDA for use in angina, selective β_1-antagonists such as metoprolol (Lopressor) minimize β_2-related adverse effects such as bronchial constriction.

Beta-blockers decrease heart rate and cardiac output and lower blood pressure. *Nurses need to ask clients whether they are experiencing nocturia and daytime oliguria, since often these are the first signs that there may be renal impairment resulting from a decrease in cardiac output.* The problem occurs because during the day

Nursing Observations for Drug Therapy in Angina

THERAPEUTIC GOAL Reduced incidence and severity of attacks; rapid relief from attacks when they occur.

PREADMINISTRATION ASSESSMENT

Baseline Data Complaints of chest pain especially upon exertion. Evaluate respiration, pulse, blood pressure, ECG, reflexes, affect, and orientation. Obtain laboratory tests including ECG and serum enzymes.

Contraindications/ Precautions History of cerebral hemorrhage, head trauma, orthostatic hypotension, or myocardial infarction; or current pregnancy or lactation. Determine if there is any history of allergic reactions to drugs.

EVALUATION OF DRUG RESPONSE

During Dosage Adjustment During hospitalization, carefully record the incidence and severity of anginal episodes and the identity and amounts of medication taken, including medications provided at bedside for self-administration.

For Therapeutic Benefit Improved understanding and control of precipitating factors should reduce the incidence of attacks. Proper use of antianginal medications for relief of acute attacks should provide relief of pain within 2–5 minutes without undue adverse reactions. At home, the client should keep a record of occurrence of attacks, their duration, alleviating factors, and response to drug therapy. In the hospital, take pulse and blood pressure before and during nitroglycerin therapy. Advise clients who are at home to take their pulses before and during therapy.

For Adverse Effects Monitor occurrence of headache, flushing, fainting or dizziness, hypotension, and other signs of excess peripheral vasodilation.

For Drug Interactions Monitor for additive hypotensive effect with alcohol or other drugs.

For Compliance Evaluate client's compliance with all facets of the therapeutic regimen by careful observation, interviewing, and review of progress. Report compliance problems to the physician and act as client-advocate when changes in the therapeutic regimen seem indicated.

the blood is shunted from the kidneys to parts of the body needing oxygen and nutrients. At night, when the body is at rest, blood flow returns to the kidneys at the previous level and urine production is increased. Clients may complain about loss of sleep because of needing to go to the bathroom frequently during the night.

Preparations and Administration

Nadolol (Corgard)
Tablets
Recommended Doses: 40 mg PO initially, once daily, gradually titrated in 40–80 mg increments at intervals of 3–7 days until optimal clinical response is obtained. The usual maintenance dose is 80–240 mg administered in one daily dose. Nadolol doses must be adjusted downward in renal failure in proportion to the extent of reduction in glomerular filtration rate (as determined by creatinine clearance).

Propranolol (Inderal)
Tablets
Recommended Doses: For prophylaxis of angina, 10 mg PO initially, 3 or 4 times daily, increased gradually (at 3- to 7-day intervals) to achieve optimal control to a maximum of 320 mg daily, in divided doses. The typical maintenance dosage range is 160–240 mg daily.

Important Nursing Implications for Antianginal Drugs

☐ Teach clients to place nitroglycerin tablets under the tongue or in the buccal pouch when using this drug for acute relief of anginal at-

Nursing Diagnoses and Interventions for Drug Therapy in Angina

Nursing Diagnoses	*Related Interventions*
TO ENHANCE DRUG BENEFITS OR REDUCE DRUG REQUIREMENTS	
Activity intolerance related to anginal attacks	Provide rest. Consider possible referral to a physical therapist.
Alterations in comfort: chest pain	Inform the physician if anginal attacks are not adequately controlled by the therapeutic regimen. With the physician's approval, clients with angina may be allowed to keep nitroglycerin at bedside for self-administration unless they exhibit signs of confusion.
Altered bowel function related to bed rest, life-style changes, or medications	Consider referral to a dietician.
Disturbances in self-concept, alterations in family processes, sexual dysfunction, or grieving related to required adjustments in life-style or role; fear related to present status and uncertain future	Provide support and encouragement; consider possible referral to a local heart association. Discuss life-style adjustments that can help provide the required changes in level of physical activity with minimal disruption of self-concept.
Impaired home maintenance management related to angina	Consider possible referral to a home health care agency.
TO MINIMIZE DRUG SIDE EFFECTS OR INTERACTIONS	
Increased risk of injury secondary to drug effects	Assure safety from falls and injury.
Sleep pattern disturbances related to medications and hospitalization	Initiate measures to minimize stress associated with hospitalization. Provide quiet atmosphere. Encourage use of nightly rituals preparatory to retirement.
Altered cardiac output related to the disorder or medications	Monitor for changes and report signs of edema, dyspnea, or fainting to the physician; provide life support measures if required.
TO ENSURE SAFE AND EFFICACIOUS DRUG USE	
Knowledge deficit related to the drug regimen	Teach the client and family members how to identify and alleviate factors that may precipitate attacks.
	Provide a list of prescription and over-the-counter drugs that may precipitate anginal attacks.
	Instruct the client concerning the nature of angina, the action of prescribed drugs, proper storage and administration procedures, and how to evaluate the adequacy of the regimen.
	Teach at least one responsible family member or friend how to administer an antianginal medication in the event that the client is unable to do it.
	Explain to the client the importance of losing excess weight, regular exercise, controlling elevated blood pressure, and avoiding tobacco, caffeine, and alcohol.
	Ensure that advice concerning risk factors is coordinated with that given by physician. Advise the client to avoid eating heavy meals, straining at stools, excessive exertion (especially in cold weather or early morning), and emotional outbursts. Advise the client to dress warmly in cold weather.

Ensure that the client is familiar with the potential adverse effects of any prescribed antianginal medication and methods of minimizing their occurrence and severity.

Remind the client that antianginal medications do not halt the progression of the disease.

Determine the adequacy of the client education steps by having the client repeat back each important point.

tacks. Clients should not eat, drink, or smoke while the tablet is in place and should not swallow it. When the attack is relieved, clients should expel the remaining part of the tablet from the mouth.

- ☐ Teach clients how to properly apply transdermal nitroglycerin to the chest, rotating the site and avoiding areas with hair. Encourage clients to report any changes in skin appearance (such as redness of blistering).
- ☐ Teach clients to store nitroglycerin properly, in light-resistant, airtight containers. All but the portion in immediate use should be refrigerated, preferably in a desiccator to protect the drug from moisture.
- ☐ Instruct hospitalized patients using nitrates or nitrites for acute relief of anginal attacks to keep a record of attacks and medication used.
- ☐ For clients in a hospital, monitor blood pressure and pulse when administering sublingual nitroglycerin.
- ☐ Teach clients to record the time when a tablet is taken in case it is necessary to repeat the dosage, to avoid intervals of less than 5 minutes.
- ☐ When drugs are used prophylactically for angina, teach clients to monitor blood pressure and radial pulse. Conduct an ECG assesment periodically.
- ☐ Instruct clients that medications used prophylactically for angina should not be discontinued abruptly. If this is done, the risk of anginal attacks will be elevated.
- ☐ Teach clients to recognize and report indications of excess vasodilation (fainting, lightheadedness, dizziness, headache), negative inotropism (edema, sudden weight gain), and gastrointestinal irritation (nausea, vomiting, diarrhea, or constipation).
- ☐ Advise clients that they should sit or lie down for 15–20 minutes at the first sign of faintness or dizziness to alleviate orthostatic hypotension caused by antianginal medications. Advise clients to avoid rapid changes in position. Dangling the feet before arising is also helpful.
- ☐ Advise clients that oral nitrates and calcium channel blockers should be taken with meals to reduce gastrointestinal irritation.
- ☐ Avoid getting nitroglycerin ointment on your skin when applying it to a client.

Myocardial Infarction

Myocardial infarction is the development of myocardial necrosis as a result of ischemia when blood flow to a portion of the myocardium is abruptly reduced. The major cause of myocardial infarction is atherosclerosis of the major coronary arteries. Occlusion of the coronary vessels may in some instances be acutely aggravated by thrombosis to initiate the attack. Less commonly, myocardial infarction can occur in the absence of atherosclerosis, due to vasospasm or the formation of a coronary embolism. The coagulation system may also contribute to the formation of the infarction.

The clinical presentation of myocardial infarction consists of severe precordial pain, heavy and crushing in character, similar to anginal pain but of greater intensity and duration. The pain does not respond to nitroglycerin or other antianginal medications. The pain is often experienced as radiating through the arms, back, and jaw. In severe infarctions, the patient may experience apprehensiveness, a sense of impending doom, nausea, vomiting, and profuse perspiration. The patient often appears pale and the skin is often cool.

Serum enzymology can be helpful in diagnosing myocardial infarction. When cardiac tissue becomes necrotic, myocardial cells rupture and spill their enzyme contents into the circulation. These enzymes can be detected in the plasma for several days after infarction (Figure 40–2). Creatinine phosphokinase activity rises most abruptly while glutamic oxaloacetic transaminase and lactic dehydrogenase produce longer lasting elevations. The electrocardiogram is very useful in identification and localization of myocardial infarcts (Figure 40–3). Other diagnostic techniques for confirming and assessing myocardial infarction include myocardial imaging and cardiac catheterization.

Foremost among the severe complications that accompany myocardial infarction are **dysrhythmias,** which occur in 90% of myocardial infarctions. Ventricular ectopic beats leading to ventricular tachycardia or fibrillation are the most common indications of dysrhythmia following myocardial infarction, but virtually all known dysrhythmias have been observed to occur. Fifty percent of patients die from the complication of dysrhythmia before receiving medical attention. Half of deaths from infarction occur within the first 2.5 hours following onset of pain. Ventricular dysrhythmias and sudden death occur with significant frequency during the 6 months following the acute phase of myocardial infarction.

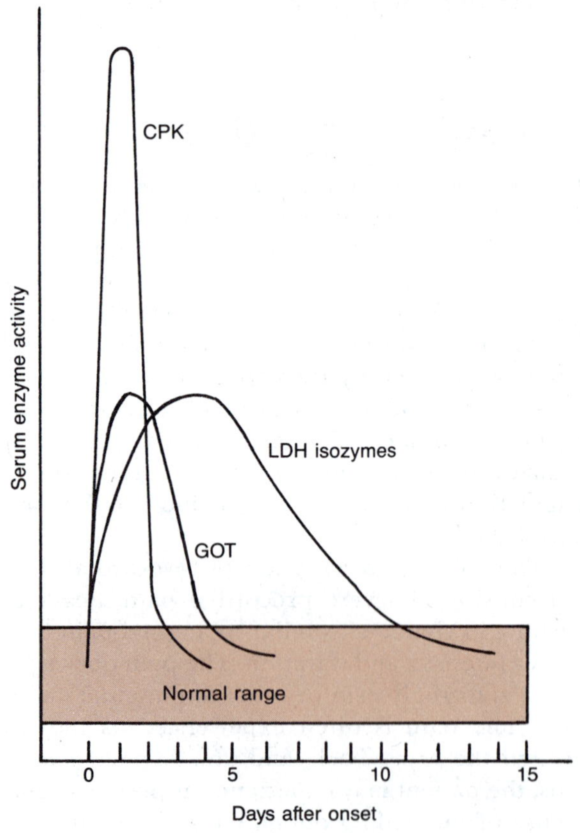

Figure 40–2
The typical pattern of changes in serum enzyme concentrations after a myocardial infarction: creatinine phosphokinase (CPK), glutamic oxaloacetic transaminase (GOT), lactic dehydrogenase (LDH).

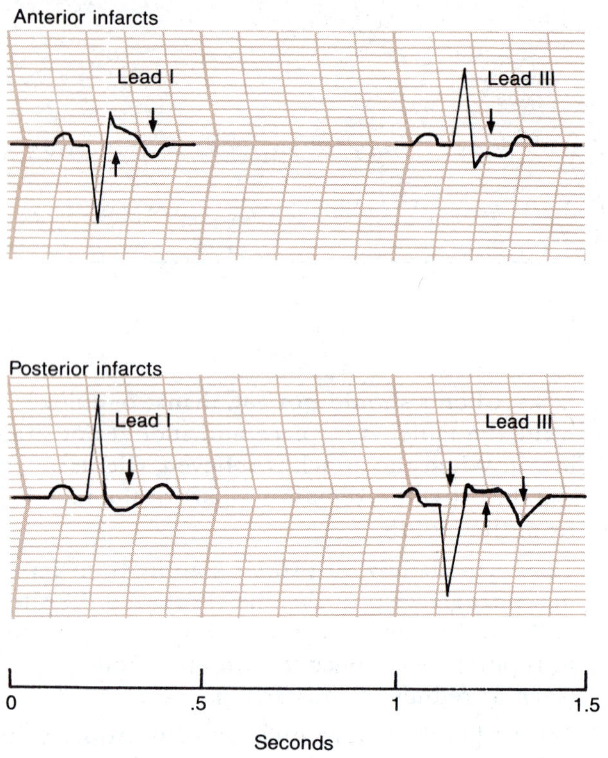

Figure 40–3
Typical lead I and lead III ECG tracings after an anterior or a posterior infarct.

A second major complication of acute myocardial infarction is **congestive heart failure** or **cardiogenic shock.** Severity of myocardial infarction is generally classified in relation to the extent of this complication: *class 1* exhibits no evidence of left ventricular failure; *class 2* exhibits mild to moderate left ventricular failure; *class 3* is associated with severe left ventricular failure and pulmonary edema; and *class 4* is accompanied by cardiogenic shock. Mortality is very high if cardiogenic shock occurs. Cardiogenic shock is defined as a drop in systolic blood pressure below 90 mm Hg or a fall of 30 mm Hg or more in a previously hypertensive individual, together with evidence of impaired perfusion of the skin, kidneys, and brain.

Other complications of myocardial infarction include subsequent thromboembolism, pericarditis, myocardial rupture, ventricular aneurysms, postmyocardial infarction syndrome, and emotional difficulties.

Management of Myocardial Infarction

The management of myocardial infarction is based on five objectives: (1) reducing the work of the heart, (2) reducing the peri-infarction zone, (3) preventing complications, (4) treating complications, and (5) providing support, comfort, and alleviation of distress for the patient. The drugs discussed in this section with respect to their use in myocardial infarction are given principal coverage in other chapters.

The early phase of management is critical to survival and often occurs outside of a clinical setting. Half of deaths from acute myocardial infarction occur before the patient reaches a medical facility. Patient denial is a major factor contributing to mortality in the early phase. Rapid recognition, alleviation of anxiety, and rapid transportation to a hospital are the important elements in early treatment. **Morphine** is useful for alleviating pain but causes significant hypotension. Elevating the legs will minimize hypotension induced by morphine. The main risks to survival in the early phase are ventricular dysrhythmias or, less commonly, heart block. Lidocaine (Xylocaine) is sometimes given routinely by intramuscular injection or intravenous infusion prior to transport of the patient. In the emergency room, monitoring of the ECG with a portable unit is initiated, an intravenous route is established, and the patient is transferred to a coronary care unit as quickly as possible. *The nurse should assure the patency of the intravenous site at all times.*

Emergency hospital treatment begins with management of dysrhythmias or shock. **Lidocaine** is given for ventricular premature beats, direct current shock for ventricular tachycardia or fibrillation, **atropine** for bradycardia, or **digitalis** to control ventricular response rate if an atrial dysrhythmia is present. The pharmacology of these drugs is discussed in the various chapters of this unit: the antidysrhythmic drugs in Chapter 38 and digitalis in Chapter 37. Vasopressors are employed to alleviate hypotension and to prevent shock (see Chapter 28). **Dopamine** (Intropin) or **dobutamine** (Dobutrex) may be given by intravenous infusion (5 to 30 mg/kg/min) to help maintain blood pressure. In-hospital mortality rates for acute myocardial infarction patients approximate 10%.

Once life-threatening complications are adequately controlled, attention next centers on reducing the peri-infarction zone. Myocardial infarction is not an absolute phenomenon. During the early phase, timely interventions may reduce ultimate tissue necrosis. The objective is to limit the extent of ischemia and ultimate tissue destruction by providing support to the cells adjacent to the region of infarction. Tactics employed are essentially the same as those used for alleviating angina pectoris: decreasing myocardial oxygen requirements or increasing oxygen availability. A carefully regulated, judicious reduction in blood pressure may be indicated in selected patients to reduce cardiac work. **Nitroprusside** (Nipride) or **nitroglycerin** (Nitrostat) (see Chapter 39) may be given by intravenous infusion for this purpose.

A special aim of the nurse in treatment of coronary patients should be to provide a quiet, calm, and restful environment and emotional reassurance. Visits from friends and families should be carefully regulated during the intensive phase immediately following a myocardial infarction. The nurse should take time to explain the equipment and procedures being employed to reassure the patient and significant family members concerning the quality of care being provided. The nurse should be especially attentive to the need to maintain a manner of optimism and competence. Rooms equipped with clocks and calendars help the patient maintain a sense of orientation and expectation of a brighter future.

General measures employed in myocardial infarction patients include prohibition of smoking, provision of a soft diet, and use of **laxatives** to maintain bowel function and minimize straining at stool. Milk of magnesia, 15–30 ml, twice per day, is a common laxative. Pain control is usually provided by **analgesics** such as morphine (4–15 mg per dose) or meperidine (Demerol) (50–100 mg per dose). **Diazepam** (Valium) may be given orally or intravenously if sedation is indicated.

After the acute phase of treatment has ended, long-term management is designed to minimize the risks of further episodes or postinfarction complications. **Propranolol** (Inderal) has recently been approved for use following myocardial infarction to reduce subsequent mortality. The mechanism by which propranolol confers protection is not established but may relate to prevention of postinfarction ventricular dysrhythmias. Postmyocardial infarction syndrome (Dressler's syndrome) is an autoimmune response to the presence of infarcted tissue. It occurs after several weeks and is characterized by fever, pericarditis, pleurisy, and joint pain. Aspirin or corticosteroids are employed in treatment.

Denial, depression, and anxiety are common during the recovery phase and should be addressed by factual, frank discussion of physical status, sound advice, and a positive program of rehabilitation. Nursing assessment should include evaluation of the client's level of anxiety and feelings concerning hospitalization, medication, being attached to tubes and monitoring equipment, and concerns for the future. Clients may be given antianxiety drugs during the

Nursing Observations for Use of Drugs in Myocardial Infarction

THERAPEUTIC GOAL	Reduce cardiac work, minimize the peri-infarction zone, prevent and treat complications, and provide support and comfort.
PREADMINISTRATION ASSESSMENT	
Baseline Data	Observe for fatigue, severe headaches, dyspnea, indigestion, edema, rales, anxiety, confusion, or pains in the chest, neck, shoulders, or back. Evaluate the ECG, myocardial imaging, cardiac catheterization. Obtain laboratory tests including serum enzymology, electrolytes, sedimentation rate.
EVALUATION OF DRUG RESPONSE	
For Therapeutic Benefit	Monitor ECG, blood pressure, pulse, and mental state.
For Adverse Effects	Monitor ECG, blood pressure, pulse, respiration, blood volume, bowel function, intake-output, mental status (confusion, disorientation, pain, agitation), weight, pulses, and edema.
For Compliance	Evaluate client's compliance with all facets of the therapeutic regimen by careful observation, interviewing, and review of progress. Report compliance problems to the physician and act as client-advocate when changes in the therapeutic regimen seem indicated.

postmyocardial infarction phase, but in the long run, nurses must help clients work on determining how best to reduce stress and render the environment less anxiety-provoking.

Peripheral Vascular Disorders

Peripheral vascular disorders are diseases involving the arteries, veins, and lymphatics of the extremities. These disorders can be caused by spasms, inflammation, occlusions, or other damage to the blood vessel endothelium. Symptoms include acrocyanosis (cyanosis of the extremities due to vascular dysfunctions), acroparesthesias (tingling sensations of like origin), and claudication (lameness or limping). Among the major examples of peripheral vascular disorders are arteriosclerosis obliterans (peripheral atherosclerotic disease), thromboangiitis obliterans (Buerger's disease), diabetic arteriosclerosis, gangrene, endarteritis, frostbite sequelae, thrombophlebitis, scleroderma, and Raynaud's disease and phenomenon (which are spastic conditions of peripheral vessels).

Four kinds of drugs have found use in peripheral vascular disorders but the efficacy of such drugs is not convincingly established: (1) alpha-adrenergic blockers, (2) β_2-adrenergic agonists, (3) direct-acting peripheral vasodilators, and (4) the hemorheological agent, pentoxifylline. The first three types of drugs share the therapeutic objective of dilating the vessels through which flow is impaired. Pentoxifylline (Trental) represents a different approach, affecting the blood itself rather than the vessels. The pharmacologies of the alpha-blocker tolazoline (Priscoline) and the β_2-agonists isoxsuprine (Vasodilan) and nylidrin employed for peripheral vascular disorders are discussed in Chapter 28. Tolazoline is designated as "possibly effective" for spastic peripheral vascular disorders, arteriosclerosis obliterans, thromboangiitis obliterans, causalgia (burning pain), diabetic arteriosclerosis, gangrene, endarteritis, frostbite sequelae, postthrombotic conditions, Raynaud's disease, and scleroderma. The beta-agonists are labeled as "possibly effective" for essentially the same set of conditions. Here we will consider the other two classes of agents employed for peripheral vascular disorders: peripheral vasodilators and hemorheological agents.

Peripheral Vasodilators

Cycladelate is a direct-acting vascular smooth muscle relaxant that does not affect adrenergic receptors. It has been designated by the FDA as "possibly effective" for therapy of intermittent claudication,

Nursing Diagnoses and Interventions for Use of Drugs in Myocardial Infarction

Nursing Diagnoses	*Related Interventions*
TO ENHANCE DRUG BENEFITS OR REDUCE DRUG REQUIREMENTS	
Activity intolerance related to diminished cardiac function and pain of ischemia	Provide bedrest until stabilization of acute attack. After recovery from a myocardial infarction, instruct clients to allow for sufficient periods of rest and to exercise regularly but to avoid overexertion.
Alterations in comfort: pain related to myocardial ischemia	Provide comfort measures; administer analgesics as provided by the physician's drug order.
Changes in self-concept and family processes related to limitations imposed by the disorder	Teach the client and family about the nature of the disorder and help them to accept and adjust to changes in roles necessitated by the disease.
Fear related to medical condition and uncertain future; Grieving related to actual or perceived limitations imposed by the disease	Provide emotional support and reassurance; maintain a positive attitude. Demonstrate efficiency and competence in caring for the client. Take time to discuss with clients their feelings and fears. Introduce the client to others who have successfully adjusted to a similar condition.
Sexual dysfunction related to fear or occurrence of anginal pain during sexual exertion	Provide emotional support and encourage understanding on the part of the sexual partner. Discuss taking nitroglycerin prior to sexual exertion.
Sleep pattern disturbances related to medical condition, unfamiliar environment, interventions	Provide a quiet, calm, restful environment during recovery. Limit the number and length of visits. Suggest to physician an order for diazepam. Encourage use of bedtime rituals.
TO MINIMIZE DRUG SIDE EFFECTS OR INTERACTIONS	
Alterations in bowel function: constipation related to medications or bed rest	Provide a soft diet, increase dietary bulk, or (with the physician's approval) administer a laxative such as milk of magnesia.
Alterations in cardiac output related to the infarction or medications	Confine to bed, elevate the legs, monitor the ECG, alleviate concomitant dysrhythmias, and prohibit smoking. Discourage use of caffeinated beverages.
TO ENSURE SAFE AND EFFICACIOUS DRUG USE	
Knowledge deficit related to drug regimen	Explain the equipment and procedures being used. Educate the client and family regarding the nature of the disorder and its management. Teach the client how to recognize quickly when his or her condition is changing in a direction that requires renewed medical attention. Help client understand and accept limitations dictated by the disorder. Explain the use of any prescribed medications, their rationale, effects, and proper administration. Provide a list of potential adverse effects and drug interactions involving medications prescribed and what to do if any occur.

Nursing Observations for Drug Therapy of Peripheral Vascular Disorders

THERAPEUTIC GOAL	Improve perfusion of affected tissues.
PREADMINISTRATION ASSESSMENT	
Baseline Data	Observe for claudication, cold extremities, local cyanosis, ulcerations, absence of hair on feet and toes, poor wound healing, persistent infections, changes in skin color, or fluctuating levels of consciousness. Evaluate peripheral pulses, touch sensitivity, tissue perfusion, and mental status.
EVALUATION OF DRUG RESPONSE	
For Therapeutic Benefit	Monitor perfusion of affected tissue and reversal or containment of complications related to ischemia.
For Adverse Effects	Monitor for orthostatic hypotension, reflex cardiac stimulation, gastrointestinal disturbances, or allergic reactions.
For Drug Interactions	Monitor for additive hypotension with other hypotensive drugs.
For Dietary Interactions	Monitor diet for excess fat, which aggravates peripheral vascular disorders.
For Compliance	Evaluate client's compliance with all facets of the therapeutic regimen by careful observation, interviewing, and review of progress. Report compliance problems to the physician and act as client-advocate when changes in the therapeutic regimen seem indicated.

arteriosclerosis obliterans, thrombophlebitis, nocturnal leg cramps, Raynaud's phenomenon, and selected cases of ischemic cerebral vascular disease. The principal adverse reactions to the drug are gastrointestinal disturbances (heartburn, pain) and mild reactions attributable to peripheral vasodilation (flushing, headache, tachycardia, or feelings of weakness). *If gastrointestinal irritation occurs, cycladelate should be taken with food or antacids.*

Nicotinyl alcohol is a precursor of niacin. Niacin relaxes blood vessels of the face, neck, and ears with little action on vessels of the lower extremities. Nicotinyl alcohol is designated as "possibly effective" for conditions of deficient circulation such as vascular spasm, varicose veins, decubital ulcers, chilblains, Menière's syndrome, and vertigo. Adverse reactions are limited to flushing and minor allergic symptoms such as rash.

Papaverine and **ethaverine** are related peripheral vasodilators that have possible value in peripheral vascular disorders associated with arterial spasm. The evidence for value of these agents is not substantial. Adverse reactions include gastrointestinal symptoms (including nausea, abdominal distress, anorexia, constipation, and diarrhea), hepatic allergic reactions, CNS symptoms (such as drowsiness, headache, and dizziness), increased heart rate or blood pressure, symptoms of peripheral vasodilation (flushing, sweating, hot face), and occasional rashes.

Preparations and Administration

Cycladelate (Cyclospasmol, Cyclan)
Tablets, capsules
Recommended Doses: 1,200–1,600 mg/day PO initially in 2–4 divided doses before meals and at bedtime. Cycladelate should be used cautiously if the client has a history of glaucoma, coronary artery disease, or cerebral vascular disease.

Ethaverine
Tablets (Ethaquin, Ethatab, Ethavex), capsules (Isovex), timed release capsules (Circubid)
Recommended Doses: 100 mg PO three times daily (or 150 mg timed release capsule twice daily) initially, may be increased up to 600 mg daily.

Nicotinyl alcohol (Roniacol, Rontinol)
Tablets, timed release tablets, elixir
Recommended Doses: 50–100 mg PO, 3 times daily, or 1 or 2 timed release tablets in the morning and the evening.

Papaverine (numerous trade names)
Tablets, timed release capsules, injection solution
Recommended Doses: 100–300 mg PO, 3–5 times daily, or 150 mg timed release capsule every 12 hours.

Nursing Diagnoses and Interventions For Drug Therapy of Peripheral Vascular Disorders

Nursing Diagnoses	*Related Interventions*
TO ENHANCE DRUG BENEFITS OR REDUCE DRUG REQUIREMENTS	
Activity intolerance related to tissue anoxia	Teach client to engage in light exercise to maintain blood flow and muscle tone but to avoid heavy exertion.
Alteration in comfort: pain related to tissue anoxia and spasm	Provide comfort measures; recommend an appropriate analgesic.
Alteration in tissue perfusion related to compromised peripheral circulation	Teach client to keep warm at all times since chilling causes vasoconstriction; apply local heat to the ischemic part; relax in positions that promote flow to affected tissues; avoid tight clothing such as round garters or girdles; and keep weight down. Teach clients not to sit with legs crossed.
Impaired home maintenance mangagement: inability to manage household routines	Assist clients to obtain community services. Help client identify methods of performing household routines while conserving energy.
Impaired skin integrity related to poor circulation	Avoid contact with caustic chemicals or other skin irritants; massage affected parts gently with an emollient; protect damaged skin with sterile dressings.
Increased risk of injury related to diminished somatosensory sensations	Provide safety measures; check temperature before applying local heat; discuss possible need to alter activities that would be dangerous with impaired dexterity.
Infection related to tissue ischemia and malnutrition	Advise client to wash the feet daily in warm, soapy water to minimize fungal infections. Recommend soaking of feet in potassium permanganate solution to control fungal infections.
TO ENSURE SAFE AND EFFICACIOUS DRUG USE	
Knowledge deficit related to drug regimen	Teach the client about the nature of the disorder and the rationale behind any prescribed drugs.
	Instruct the client about losing weight, not smoking, reducing dietary fats, avoiding cold exposure, care of the affected parts, and the prescribed exercise program.
	Provide clients with a list of adverse effects and drug interactions for prescribed vasodilators and what to do if any of these occur.

Hemorheological Agent

Pentoxifylline (Trental), introduced in 1984, represents a new approach to treatment of peripheral vascular disorders. Pentoxifylline is a xanthine derivative that improves peripheral blood flow and alleviates intermittent claudication by its effects on the viscosity of blood. Pentoxifylline increases the flexibility of erythrocytes, enhancing their ability to flow through the microcirculation. Pentoxifylline also decreases the concentration of fibrinogen in the blood and prevents aggregation of red blood cells and platelets. Pentoxifylline has been shown to be effective in alleviating claudication by such measures as increased walking distance after drug administration. After oral administration, pentoxifylline reaches peak plasma levels in 2–4 hours. The plasma half-life of pentoxifylline is 0.4–0.8 hours. Side effects of pentoxifylline are minimal, consisting mainly of some instances of nausea, dyspepsia, dizziness, and headache. Rarely, cardiovascular reactions, including angina, dysrhythmias, or hypotension, have been reported. If the patient is receiving antihypertensive medication, it may be necessary to adjust the dose of the antihypertensive agent.

Preparations and Administration

Pentoxifylline (Trental)
Controlled-release tablet
Recommended Doses: 400 mg PO, 3 times per day with meals. Clinical response can be expected in about 2–4 weeks. It is recommended that treatment be continued at least 8 weeks.

Case Study: Ischemic Heart Disease

R. B., a 53-year-old white man, was brought by ambulance to the emergency room at 8:00 PM on a blustery February night, accompanied by his wife. On the way from a restaurant to their parked car, R. B. had been overwhelmed by a crushing chest pain. R. B. is known to the hospital, having been under care for the past 6 years for angina pectoris. During this time, he has been on a medication regimen of dipyridamole (Persantine), 50 mg PO, 3 times a day 1 hour before meals, and sublingual nitroglycerin, as needed for acute relief of anginal attacks. Until 1 year ago, R. B. had experienced anginal attacks lasting a few seconds in response to physical exertion. In the last year, he experienced several attacks lasting several minutes occurring in the absence of unusual exertion.

R. B. was transferred immediately to the coronary care unit. His chest pain radiated down the inside of the left arm and to the neck. ECG analysis indicated an acute myocardial infarction with a normal rhythm.

The physician ordered cardiac monitoring, bedrest, diazepam (Valium), 5 mg, orally, 3 times daily, and a laxative. During the night, R. B. continued to experience transient episodes of chest pain. The physician ordered warfarin (Coumadin), 10 mg orally for 3 days; then 2.5 mg daily for 1 week. On the third night in the coronary care unit, R. B. had a severe episode of chest pain accompanied by frequent ventricular premature beats. The nurse administered lidocaine (Xylocaine) intravenously and reported the occurrence to the physician. The premature beats were eliminated by the lidocaine and the physician ordered the addition of procainamide, 50 mg/kg/day, orally, in divided doses at 3-hour intervals.

After 10 days of intensive care, R. B.'s condition stabilized and he was discharged on a regimen of propranolol (Inderal), 200 mg/day orally, in 4 divided doses, for 6 months, continuation of procainamide for 1 week, and dipyridamole and nitroglycerin as before.

1. Is R. B.'s angina pectoris better characterized as the typical or the vasospastic type? Is it stable or unstable?
2. Why does R. B. take both dipyridamole and nitroglycerin for angina? How effective are each of these for their respective purposes?
3. What factors may have contributed to the occurrence of the myocardial infarction at the time of admission?
4. Why was warfarin prescribed when R. B. continued to have frequent episodes of chest pain? How effective is it for this purpose?
5. Why were lidocaine and then procainamide administered? What side effects should R. B. watch for while he is receiving procainamide?
6. What are the potential side effects of procainamide?
7. Why was propranolol prescribed for R. B. after stabilization of the myocardial infarct?

Answers appear at the end of the book.

Recommended Readings

Antianginal Drugs

Abrams M: Nitroglycerine and long-acting nitrates. *N Engl J Med* 1980;302:1234–1236.

Braunwald E: Mechanisms of action of calcium-channel blocking agents. *N Engl J Med* 1982;307:1618–1627.

Butler JD, Harrison BL: Keeping pace with calcium channel blockers. *Nursing* 1983;13:38–43.

Fuller EO: The effect of antianginal drugs on myocardial oxygen consumption. *Am J Nurs* 1980;80:250–254.

Hanson MS, Woods SL: Nitroglycerin ointment. *Am J Nurs* 1980;80:1122–1124.

Klein DM, Cook D: Angina, physiology signs, and symptoms. *Nursing* 1984;14(2):44–46.

Leonard RG, Talbert RL: Calcium-channel blocking agents. *Clin Pharm* 1982;1:17–33.

Lute E: Calcium blockers: The important difference. *RN* 1984;84(6):36–39.

Moore K: Coronary artery spasm. *Nursing* 1983;13(8):49.

Rossi LP, Antman EM: Calcium channel blockers, new treatment for cardiovascular disease. *Am J Nurs* 1983;83(3):382–387.

Singh BN: Beta-adrenoreceptor blocking drugs and acute myocardial infarction. *Drugs* 1978;15:218–225.

Stowe HO: Review of calcium-channel blockers. *Nurs Pract* 1986;11(4):57–65.

Talma CL: Drugs used to treat angina pectoris. *Nurses' Drug Alert* 1981;5:28–30.

Walton C, Hammond B: Angina: Teaching your patient to prevent recurring attacks. *Nursing* 1978;8(2):32–38.

Drug Therapy for Myocardial Infarction

Chalmers CT et al: Evidence favoring the use of anticoagulants in the hospital phase of acute myocardial infarction. *N Engl J Med* 1977;297:1091–1096.

Chatterjee K, Parmley WW: Vasodilator treatment for acute and chronic heart failure. *Br Heart J* 1977;39:706–720.

Koch-Weser J: Vasodilator therapy of cardiac failure. *N Engl J Med* 1977;297:254–258.

Vedin JA, Wilhelmsson CE: Beta receptor blocking agents in the secondary prevention of coronary heart disease. *Annu Rev Pharmacol Toxicol* 1983;23:29–44.

Drug Therapy for Peripheral Vascular Disorders

Lamb C: Peripheral vascular disease — easing intermittent claudication. *Patient Care* 1983;17(4):123

Worthington de Toledo L: How vasodilators backfire (and when to expect it). *RN* 1982;45:41–45.

CHAPTER 41

Hematological Drugs

The hematological system consists of the constituents of the blood together with the supporting tissues, including the bone marrow, liver, spleen, and lymph nodes. The blood itself consists of formed elements (the red and white blood cells and platelets) and the plasma. In most respects, plasma is identical to and interchangeable with the interstitial fluid, but plasma contains a substantially higher concentration of protein than interstitial fluid, totaling about 7% of the overall plasma composition. These proteins consist 60% of albumins (which maintain intravascular osmotic pressure), 35% of globulins (including gamma-globulins of the immune system and alpha- and beta-globulins, which transport drugs, hormones, and proteins), and 5% of fibrinogen (the precursor of fibrin — the chief chemical constituent of clots).

The hematological system includes three subsystems, each with a specialized function: the erythropoietic, the hemostatic, and the leukopoietic. The last of these deals with the production and activities of the white blood cells in inflammatory and immune mechanisms, subjects taken up in Chapters 45 and 46. The erythropoietic subsystem consists of the red blood cells and carries out the transport of oxygen. The hemostatic subsystem is the clotting mechanism that serves to limit loss of blood when a break occurs in a blood vessel wall. This chapter addresses the erythropoietic and hemostatic functions of the hematological system, the disorders that can arise in these two subsystems, and the drugs used to treat or control such disorders.

The Erythropoietic System

The function of red blood cells (RBCs) is to transport oxygen from the lungs of the tissues. In addition, RBCs contain carbonic anhydrase, which catalyzes hydration of carbon dioxide, and hemoglobin, which helps buffer the blood and control acid-base balance. RBCs are produced in bone marrow. They are rich in hemoglobin, containing about 34 mg per 100 ml. About 40% of the blood consists of RBCs, with some 5 million RBCs per cubic millimeter of blood: the normal range for men is 4.6–6.2 million/mm^3; for women 4.2–5.4 million/mm^3.

Normally, RBC production is geared to the rate of loss of these cells so that total hemoglobin mass will be maintained. When production is inadequate or loss is excessive, anemia results. Normal production of RBCs requires sufficient dietary intake and gastrointestinal absorption of essential materials, including iron, protein, vitamins B_{12} and C, and folic acid. Also essential for RBC production is active bone marrow and liver storage of iron and vitamin B_{12}.

Nurses are often able to identify presence of anemia when assessing the client. Signs and symptoms of anemia include skin pallor and coldness, poor color in the nail beds, conjunctiva, lips, and mucous membranes of the mouth, purpuric lesions, easy bruising, bleeding gums, rapid heart beat or respiration, shortness of breath, headache, tinnitus, spots in the visual field, abnormal heart sounds, smooth, glossy tongue, glossitis, or stomatitis. Specific types of anemia may be suggested by evidence of occult bleeding (blood in stools or urine), increased menses, jaundice, renal impairment, or a family history of anemia.

Types of Anemia

Anemias are classified on the basis of etiology and the appearance and hemoglobin content of the red blood cells (Table 41–1). The three major categories are based on etiology: (1) anemias due to excessive blood loss, (2) anemias due to deficient red cell pro-

Table 41–1
Classification of Prevalent Anemias

I. Anemias Due to Excessive Blood Loss (Hemorrhage)

II. Anemias Due to Deficient Red Cell Production
- A. Hypochromic microcytic anemias
  - 1. Primary iron-deficiency anemia
  - 2. Secondary iron-deficiency anemias
    - a. Iron transport deficiency
    - b. Iron utilization deficiency (sideroblastic anemia)
    - c. Iron reutilization anemia (anemia of chronic disease)
- B. Normochromic normocytic anemias
  - 1. Hypoproliferative anemias
  - 2. Hypoplastic (aplastic) anemias
- C. Megaloblastic anemias
  - 1. Anemia due to vitamin B_{12} deficiency
  - 2. Anemia due to folic acid deficiency
  - 3. Anemia due to copper deficiency
  - 4. Anemia due to ascorbic acid deficiency

III. Anemias Due to Excessive RBC Destruction (Hemolytic Anemias)
- A. Defects extrinsic to the RBC
  - 1. Immunological anemias
  - 2. Anemia due to mechanical injury
- B. Defects intrinsic to the RBC
  - 1. Anemias due to defective RBC membrane
  - 2. Anemias due to abnormal RBC metabolism
  - 3. Anemias due to defective hemoglobin synthesis

duction, and (3) anemias due to excessive red cell destruction.

Anemias due to excessive blood loss are caused mainly by hemorrhage. The rate of blood loss as well as the total volume lost is critical. Sudden loss of one-third of the total blood volume could be fatal, while as much as two-thirds can be lost more slowly without fatality. Blood transfusion is the preferred method of restoring fluid volume and oxygen-carrying capacity. Administration of saline or plasma expanders can be a life-saving interim measure for restoring fluid volume but does not correct the deficient oxygen-carrying capacity. Whole blood transfusion is discussed in the final section of this chapter, treatment of fluid contraction in Chapter 42.

Anemias due to deficient RBC production include iron-deficiency anemias, hypoplastic anemias, and megaloblastic anemias. Primary and secondary **iron-deficiency anemias** are the most common type of anemias and often among the most treatable and preventable. **Hypoplastic anemias** are related to bone marrow failure, which can be due to diminished renal secretion of erythropoietin, hypometabolic states such as myxedema, or an actual loss of bone marrow mass due to infection or drugs. **Megaloblastic anemias** are deficiency conditions related to specific essential dietary requirements, including vitamin B_{12}, folic acid, ascorbic acid, and, rarely, copper.

Anemias due to excessive destruction of RBCs are called **hemolytic anemias** and can be due to extrinsic or intrinsic factors. Extrinsic factors that contribute to RBC hemolysis include mechanical injury (excessive shear or turbulence), presence of microorganisms (such as *Plasmodia, Clostridium perfringens,* or hemolytic streptococci), or immune disorders. In the last category are reactions to incompatible blood types and autoimmune hemolytic anemia. The mechanisms involved in immunological anemia are discussed in Chapter 46. The anemias due to intrinsic defects in RBCs are mainly hereditary and treatment is generally limited to periodic infusions of whole blood. **Hereditary RBC defects** include hereditary spherocytosis, glucose-6-phosphate dehydrogenase (G6PD) deficiency, sickle cell anemia, hemoglobin C disease, and thalassemias.

Oxygen-carrying capacity of RBCs can also be impaired in the absence of anemia when the iron in hemoglobin, normally in the ferrous form, is converted into the ferric form, which is much less efficient in transporting oxygen. Hemoglobin altered in this way is called **methemoglobin.** Methemoglobinemia is diagnosed if more than 1 percent of total hemoglobin has been converted to methemoglobin. Methemoglobinemia is produced by a variety of drugs (Table 43-3, page 745). The principal symptom is cyanosis.

Iron-Deficiency Anemia

Iron Requirements and Metabolism

Iron-deficiency anemias are the most common of all anemias. Sixty percent of bodily iron is found in hemoglobin, and the rest is stored in tissue or associated with myoglobin or iron-dependent enzymes. The body is remarkably efficent in conserving iron, which is a necessity because in spite of the abundance of iron in the earth's crust it is sparsely available in forms usable by most organisms. Over the course of a year, the total iron lost is only about 10% of the total bodily stores in males. Most of what is lost is contained in exfoliated mucosal cells, desquamated dermal cells, red cells eliminated in the feces, or iron in the bile or urine. Daily losses in men are about 1.0 mg; in women 1.4 mg. In the United States, a normal diet includes 8–20 mg. Iron-rich foods include liver, egg yolks, oysters, brewer's yeast, wheat germ, and dried beans and fruits. Moderate amounts of iron are also contained in lean meat, fish, fowl, cocoa, molasses, and green vegetables, especially spinach. It is common practice nowadays to add iron to flour. Milk and nongreen vegetables are low in iron.

While it might appear that a diet of 8–20 mg could easily replace the obligatory daily loss of 1.0–1.4 mg, absorption of iron is far from complete and is influenced by many factors. Digestion of food releases iron in two forms, inorganic and heme. Inorganic iron, the more abundant of the two, is only 5% absorbed. Heme iron is about 37% absorbed. Assuming an overall absorption of less than 10%, it is apparent that even under optimum conditions the diet can barely provide replacement for what is lost.

Dietary requirements in women are increased during pregnancy and menstruation. In pregnancy, daily requirements increase from 18 mg/day to 30–60 mg/day and cannot be met without use of supplements. Bleeding, even minor bleeding, increases requirements for iron. Each milliliter of blood contains about 0.5 mg of iron as hemoglobin; hence, even a few milliliters blood loss per day can be significant. Aspirin-like drugs increase gastrointestinal bleeding and it is recommended that iron supplements (20–50 mg/day) be provided to clients receiving long-term therapy with such drugs for arthritis or other inflammatory conditions.

Absorption of iron is a complex process (Figure 41-1). Iron sources bind to a carrier protein called **gastroferrin** and enter the intestinal mucosa, mostly

Figure 41–1

Iron metabolism. (1) Absorption of iron-gastroferrin (GF) complexes, (2) storage in ferritin (FR) complexes within tissue cells, (3) absorption into bloodstream and transport or iron-transferrin (TR) complexes, (4) incorporation into red blood cells, (5) reutilization of Fe^{++} from senescent cells, and (6) iron losses due to exfoliation of gastrointestinal (as well as epithelial and uterine) cells.

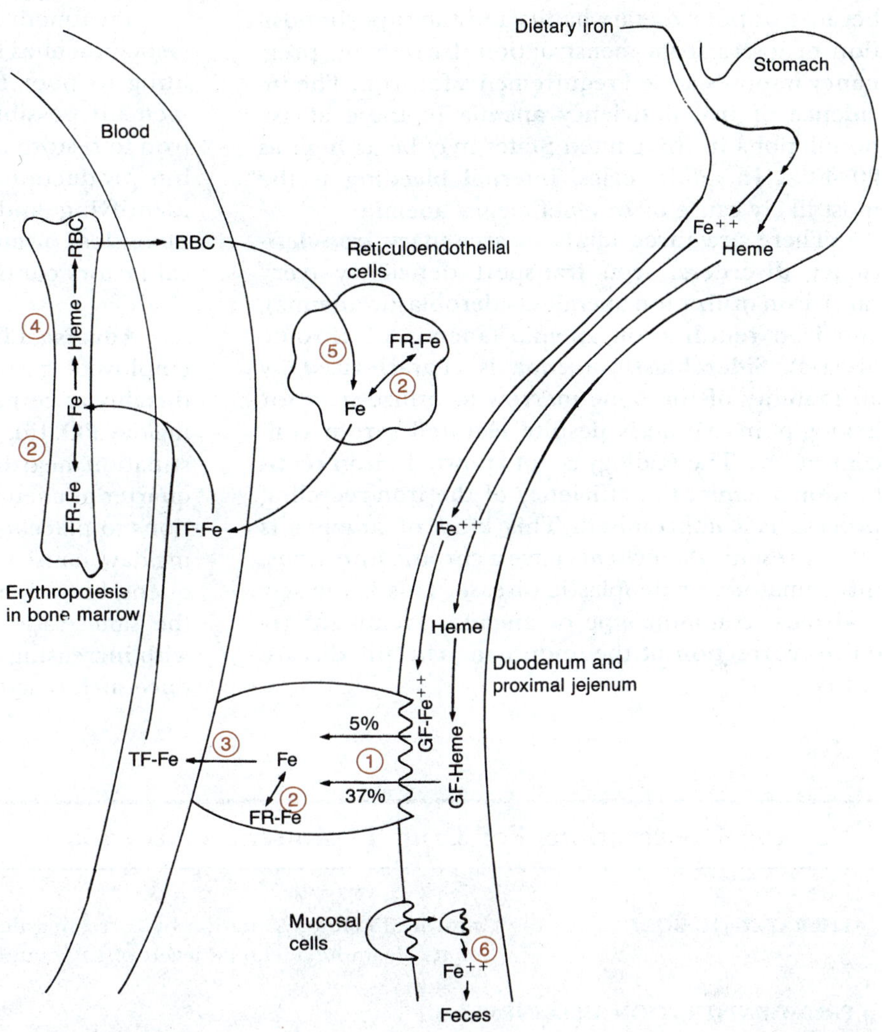

in the duodenum and proximal jejunum. Some of the absorbed iron is stored in the mucosal cells, attached to an iron binding protein called **ferritin,** and some is further absorbed into the plasma where it attaches to **transferrin,** a glycoprotein that shuttles iron throughout the vascular system, making it available to the bone marrow and storage tissues. About 25–40 mg of iron flows through the plasma attached to transferrin each day. Only 1–3 mg is obtained from the diet, the rest being **reutilization** of iron derived from catabolism of aging RBCs by reticuloendothelial cells. The average life span of a red blood cell is 120 days, so that each day 1/120 of the cells are destroyed and replaced by new cells.

Iron that is not immediately required by the bone marrow for production of new RBCs is stored in ferritin complexes in liver, spleen, bone marrow, and to some extent in every cell. In men, stored iron constitutes about 25% of the bodily total, but in women only about 10%, so males have a greater margin of safety before anemia develops. This is all the more true because of the greater iron losses in women. Normal menstruation increases iron losses by 0.5–1.0 mg/day but 10% of women lose more than 2 mg/day.

Types of Iron-Deficiency Anemia

Primary iron-deficiency anemia occurs when there is a decreased bioavailability of iron, an unmet increase in the iron requirement, or both. Decreased bioavailability can be related to dietary deficiency or absorption impaired by the influence of physiological abnormalities (such as achlorhydria or malabsorption syndromes), other dietary substances (starch, phytates, bicarbonate), or drugs. Iron deficiency is very common in toddlers, from ages 1 to 3, because of the requirements for rapid growth and the lack of iron in breast milk or most other infant foods. Adolescent girls may become iron-deficient because of poor dietary habits and the superimposition of losses from menstruation. In women, pregnancy imposes added requirements for iron. The incidence of iron-deficiency anemia in these at-risk populations in the United States may be as high as 20–40%. In adult males, internal bleeding is the most likely cause of iron-deficiency anemia.

There are three kinds of **secondary iron-deficiency disorders:** iron transport deficiency (very rare), iron utilization anemias (sideroblastic anemia), and iron reutilization anemia (anemia of chronic disease). **Sideroblastic anemia** is characterized by an inability of the bone marrow to utilize iron for hemoglobin synthesis despite elevated serum concentrations. The etiology is not known. In **iron reutilization anemia,** the efficiency of the iron-recycling process is compromised. This kind of anemia is often present when clients have a chronic infectious, inflammatory, or neoplastic disease. This is the second most common type of anemia. Treatment requires correction of the underlying chronic disease entity.

Iron Supplements for Iron-Deficiency Anemias

Treatment objectives for people with iron-deficiency anemias involve (1) correcting factors contributing to poor bioavailability or increased requirements if possible and (2) providing supplementary iron to restore normal iron availability for hemoglobin production. Top priority should be placed on identifying and correcting any sources of occult blood loss or any disease, dietary, or pharmacological factors contributing to impaired absorption.

Adverse Effects When iron supplements are employed, gastrointestinal intolerance occurs predictably at certain dosages. At a typical dose of 200 mg/day PO, tid, complaints of nausea, diarrhea, constipation, heartburn, and cramps occur in about one-quarter of clients (double the incidence of such reactions to placebos). When the dose is doubled to 400 mg/day, nausea and abdominal pain are more frequent, but other gastrointestinal symptoms occur at the same rate. A gradual phasing-in of treatment with increasing doses over the first few days may reduce such reactions. *Although iron absorption is reduced*

Nursing Observations For Drug Treatment of Anemia

THERAPEUTIC GOAL	Improve tissue oxygenation by correcting defect and/or reducing oxygen requirements. Promote adequate levels of RBCs and hemoglobin.
PREADMINISTRATION ASSESSMENT	
Baseline Data	Observe for tiredness, easy fatigability, skin pallor and coldness, lack of color in nail beds or mucous membranes, purpuric lesions, brittle or thin nails, altered menses, tarry stools, hematuria, bleeding gums, inflammation of the tongue or buccal mucosa, rapid heart beat or respiration. Evaluate for use of drugs that can cause hypoplastic anemia (Table 41–2), hemolysis (Tables 41–3 and 41–4), or methemoglobinemia. Evaluate diet for possible deficiencies in iron, folic acid, or vitamin B_{12}. Evaluate blood pressure, pulse rate, peripheral perfusion, respiration, skin color and lesions, liver function, bowel sounds, and neurological status. Obtain laboratory tests including red blood cell, reticulocyte, and platelet counts; serum iron and iron-binding capacity, blood smear, and hemoglobin level.
EVALUATION OF DRUG RESPONSE	
For Therapeutic Benefit	Evaluate changes in exercise tolerance, color, blood cell counts, hemoglobin, and reticulocytes.
For Adverse Effects and Drug Interactions	See discussions and Important Nursing Implications for individual drugs.
For Compliance	Evaluate client's compliance with all facets of the therapeutic regimen by careful observation, interviewing, and review of progress. Report compliance problems to the physician and act client-advocate when changes in the therapeutic regimen seem indicated.

when taken with meals, the decrease in gastrointestinal irritation and consequent improved compliance justify scheduling administration with meals. Patients should be advised that stools may acquire a black-green coloration when oral iron preparations are used.

Iron toxicity is a real risk, with fatalities occurring in toddlers who take 2–3 g or more. Iron intoxication is marked first by nausea, vomiting, and diarrhea, beginning 30 minutes after ingestion. Then pallor, lassitude, and drowsiness lead up to coma, cardiovascular collapse, and metabolic acidosis. Treatment consists of lavage, administration of an iron chelator, desferoxamine by nasogastric tube and slow intravenous infusion, and supportive measures for metabolic acidosis and shock.

Accidental poisoning in children is a common occurrence with a 50% fatality rate. *Therefore, nurses need to stress this danger to parents and grandparents. If parents suspect a child has taken ferrous tablets, emergency treatment can begin at home by inducing vomiting and by giving eggs or milk. The child should be taken to the emergency room, where specific iron-chelating agents are likely to be used.*

Preparations and Administration Iron supplements are usually provided by the oral route. Ferrous sulfate is the salt of choice. Ferric sulfate is much less well absorbed. Ferrous gluconate and ferrous fumarate are as effective as ferrous sulfate but more expensive and with no special advantages. Because iron absorption is inefficient, various special formulation techniques have been used to increase iron absorption. Sustained release formulations provide only about one-fifth the efficiency of absorption because iron is absorbed more rapidly in the proximal part of the intestine. So-called shotgun preparations, con-

Nursing Diagnoses and Interventions for Drug Treatment of Anemia

Nursing Diagnoses	*Related Interventions*
TO ENHANCE DRUG BENEFITS OR REDUCE DRUG REQUIREMENTS	
Activity intolerance related to hypoxia of anemia	Encourage client to obtain adequate rest to lower oxygen requirements. Counsel families to adjust life-style to promote rest for client. Oxygen therapy for acute breathlessness.
Alteration in oral mucous membranes related to hypoxia, atrophy, and inflammation of anemia	Teach the client proper mouth care, including use of soft toothbrush and a mouth wash. Refer client to a dental hygienist if necessary.
Infections related to increased tissue vulnerability secondary to anemia	Teach the client how to care for wounds and to avoid exposure to infection and injury.
TO MINIMIZE DRUG SIDE EFFECTS OR INTERACTIONS	
Alteration in bowel function related to atrophy of intestinal mucosa or iron therapy	Give oral iron preparations with meals to reduce gastrointestinal irritation; increase dietary bulk to avoid constipation.
TO ENSURE SAFE AND EFFICACIOUS DRUG USE	
Knowledge deficit related to drug regimen	Explain the nature of the type of anemia that is present, its prognosis, and the therapeutic measures recommended. Explain the need for adjustments in diet or activity if required. Provide the client with a list of potential adverse effects or drug interactions associated with each prescribed medication and explain what to do if any of these occur.

taining iron and multivitamins are no more effective than ferrous sulfate alone. The dose of ferrous sulfate should be based on the magnitude of the deficiency and weight of the client. Doses of 100–260 mg PO of elemental iron are typical, so the 65 mg tablet could be given 2–4 times per day. *If an oral solution is used, clients should be taught to dilute it in order to prevent staining of the teeth and to drink the solution through a straw.* Parenteral administration should be reserved for clients unable to take or tolerate oral iron. Responsiveness begins in 4–6 days and reaches maximum levels in 7–12 days. Oral therapy should be continued for several weeks after the client's hemoglobin levels have returned to normal.

About 1% of clients have gastrointestinal reactions of sufficient severity as to require discontinuation of oral iron medication. These clients may require parenteral administration, as will those for whom rapid replenishment of iron is essential (for instance, before surgery). *Sensitivity tests should be conducted before initiating parenteral administration.* Free iron, whether ferrous or ferric, cannot be used parenterally. The major parenteral preparation, iron dextran injection (Imferon), is a complex of iron with dextran. The product contains 50 mg/ml of iron in a colloidal solution and comes in 2 and 5 ml ampuls for intravenous or intramuscular use. Intravenous use of iron dextran should be limited to those situations in which the client has insufficient muscle mass for deep intramuscular injection, when stasis or edema are such that absorption is impaired, or when there is a possibility of uncontrolled intramuscular bleeding caused by the trauma of the injection.

When iron dextran is to be administered, nurses should use what is referred to as a Z-track technique, injecting the medication into the upper outer quadrant of the buttocks. The skin is pulled to one side as the needle is injected deep into the muscle so as to minimize staining or brown discoloration that might otherwise occur at the site of injection. Clients should be encouraged to walk around following the injection, since walking hastens absorption of the drug and reduces soreness and inflammation at the site of injection. However, the walking should not be overdone. After administration, nurses need to observe clients closely for evidence of allergic responses (including anaphylaxis), headache, dizziness, weakness, fever, and urticaria.

Megoblastic Anemias

Megaloblastic anemias are anemias characterized by presence of abnormally enlarged red blood cells. They are associated with deficiences of vitamin B_{12} (cyanocobalamin) and folic acid and rarely with copper or ascorbic acid deficiency.

Vitamin B_{12}-Deficiency Anemia

When the body is substantially depleted of vitamin B_{12}, a deficiency anemia and neurological symptoms develop. B_{12} deficiency may be due to dietary deficiency, poor absorption, or increased utilization of the vitamin, but the vast majority of cases are due to poor absorption. Vitamin B_{12}, like other B-complex vitamins, is a precursor of an essential coenzyme. It is found in foods of animal origin including meat, eggs, fish, milk, and cheese, especially organ meats and shellfish. Cooking reduces the amount of B_{12} available from such foods. Strict vegetarians could develop a dietary deficiency of vitamin B_{12} but seldom do in practice because of B_{12} in legumes. The recommended daily allowance of vitamin B_{12} is 2–3 μg in an adult, which is easily met by diets containing animal products.

Vitamin B_{12}-deficiency occurs with malabsorption diseases that affect the small intestine and especially the ileum, where B_{12} is normally absorbed. Bacterial and parasitic infections may also affect the absorption rate of this vitamin. Another cause of deficiency is surgical removal of large segments of the small intestines.

Pharmacokinetics of Vitamin B_{12} Vitamin B_{12} in food is typically attached to proteins. In the stomach, it is split off by the combined action of pepsin and the acid pH (Figure 41–2). The released B_{12} is bound to a glycoprotein secreted by gastric parietal cells, called **gastric intrinsic factor.** This complex is normally absorbed with great efficiency by mucosal cells of the intestine, but absorption is impaired in chronic pancreatitis, malabsorption syndrome, bacterial overgrowth, or by calcium chelators, aminosalicylic acid, anticonvulsants, biguanides, bile sequestrants, neomycin, alcohol, potassium chloride, and colchicine. Although only 1–2 μg of vitamin B_{12} is excreted daily, 3–8 μg undergo enterohepatic cycling. Therefore, if absorption is impaired, depletion of bodily stores occurs at a rate that is 2–5 times faster than would be predicted by normal daily loss of 1–2 μg.

Inside the ileal mucosal cells, vitamin B_{12} is separated from intrinsic factor and converted by the mitochondria to an active coenzyme form, 5′-deoxyadenosylcobalamin. At the basement membrane, this coenzyme is attached to a transport protein, transcobalamin II, and shuttled through the plasma to the liver and other tissues. Normal plasma levels of bound vitamin B_{12} are 0.2–0.9 μg/mL. In tissue cells, vitamin B_{12} is stored in attachment to cellular proteins: transcobalamins I and III. The liver, the main storage site for B_{12}, stores sufficient amounts of the

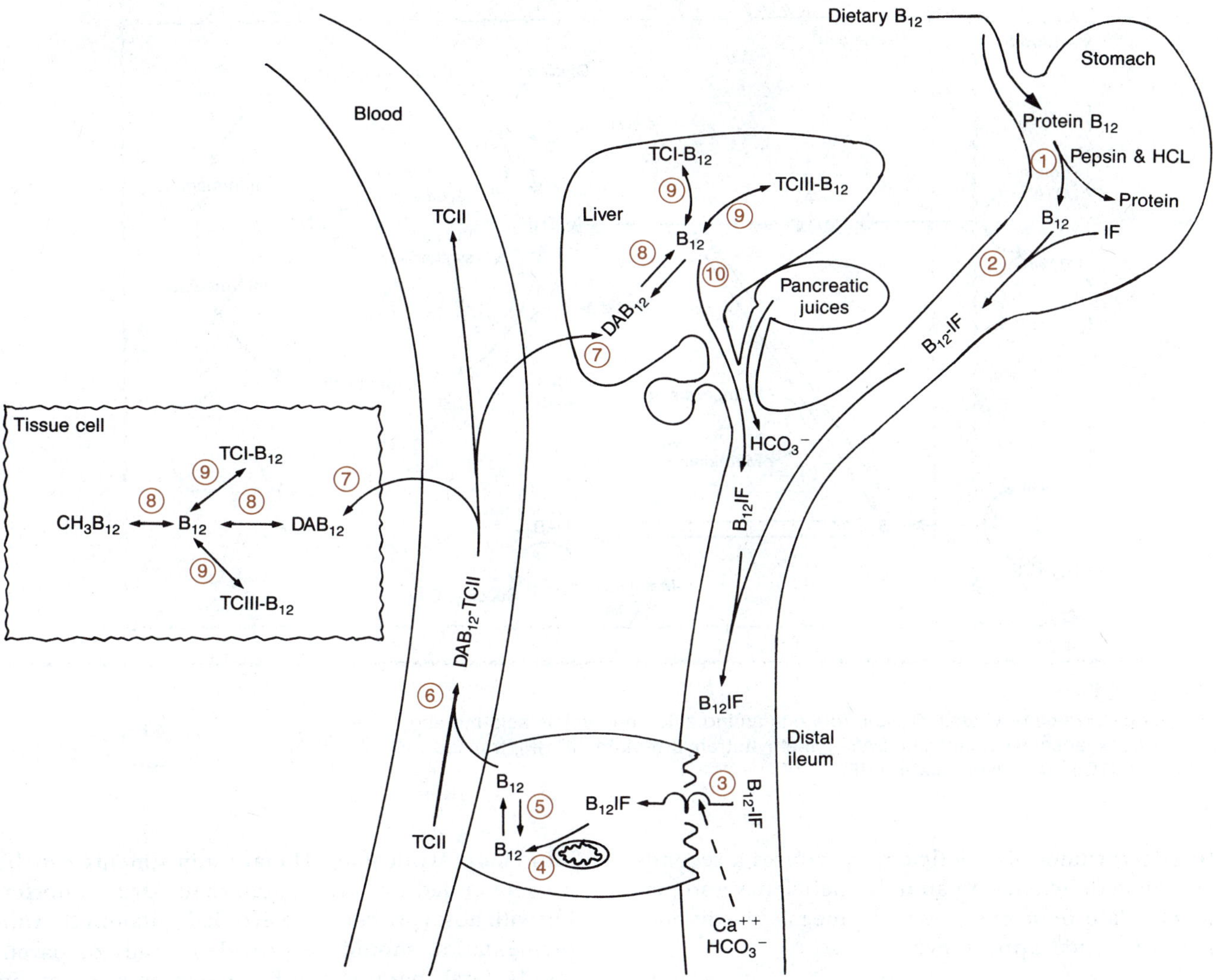

Figure 41–2
Vitamin B_{12} metabolism. (1) Liberation of B_{12} from dietary protein by digestion, (2) complexing of B_{12} with gastric intrinsic factor (IF), (3) absorption of the complex into mucosal cells, (4) cleavage of B_{12} from IF, (5) conversion to active coenzyme form, 5′-deoxyadenosylcobalamin (DAB_{12}), (6) transport of DAB_{12} through the blood in attachment to transcobalamin II (TCII), (7) uptake into tissue and liver cells, (8) interconversions between DAB_{12}, B_{12}, and methylcobalamin (CH_3B_{12}), (9) storage in tissue and liver cells in attachment to transcobalamin I (TCI) and transcobalamin III (TCIII), and (10) enterohepatic recycling of B_{12}.

vitamin to provide bodily needs for up to 3 years of complete dietary deficiency.

The most common cause of vitamin B_{12}-deficiency anemia is deficient production of gastric intrinsic factor. This form of B_{12}-deficiency anemia is what is commonly termed **pernicious anemia.** It is rarely hereditary, but more commonly acquired as a result of atrophy of the gastric mucosa.

Physiological Roles of Vitamin B_{12} Vitamin B_{12} occurs in three active forms (Figure 41–3). One form is a coenzyme for an important step in carbohydrate and lipid metabolism, another for the methylation of homocysteine to methionine, and the third participates in the activation of folic acid. This last role of vitamin B_{12} is of particular significance, providing a close association between vitamin B_{12} and folic acid.

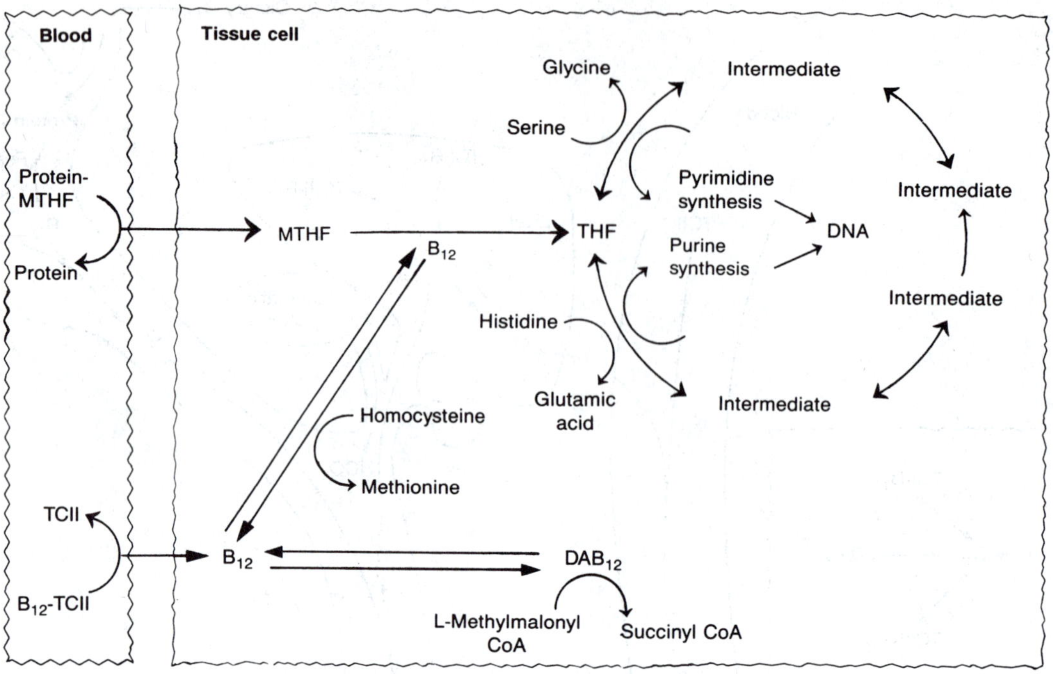

Figure 41–3
Physiological roles of vitamin B_{12} and folate in amino acid and nucleic acid metabolism: 5′-deoxyadenosylcobalamin (DAB_{12}), methyltetrahydrofolate (MTHF), transcobalamin II (TCII), tetrahydrofolate (THF).

In effect, vitamin B_{12} deficiency produces a secondary folate deficiency. Vitamin B_{12} deficiency and primary folate deficiency result in megaloblastic anemias of similar appearance.

Vitamin B_{12} Deficiency Severe vitamin B_{12} deficiency causes two main symptom clusters: megaloblastic anemia and neuropathy. A blood smear reveals the characteristic enlarged or megaloblastic cells. The neuropathy of B_{12} deficiency may occur before anemia. Peripheral nerves are affected first, spinal cord tracts next, and then the cerebral cortex. Myelinated neurons are the ones affected, swelling and undergoing demyelination and death. Clinical symptoms include parethesias, loss of vibratory sense in the extremities, ataxia, depression of deep-tendon reflexes, spasticity, and loss of position sense. Later, with cerebral involvement, symptoms include loss of memory, irritability, depression, paranoia, delusions, and hallucinations. Neurological damage is reversible only if it has been short term.

Treatment Treatment goals are elimination of the causes of deficiency if possible and replenishment of B_{12} stores. Bacterial overgrowth may be correctable with antibiotics or surgery (if due to blind-loop syndrome). Dietary adjustments can be recommended for strict vegetarians. Drugs interfering with absorption can be avoided. Vitamin B_{12} supplementation should be provided, orally or parenterally. Oral therapy with B_{12} is seldom adequate in pernicious anemia because absorption of B_{12} in the absence of intrinsic factor is only 1–2%. Oral therapy is useful to supplement deficient diets, however. Large doses have been given with some success to clients who refuse parenteral therapy. *Oral doses should be taken with meals to maximize the stimulation of intrinsic factor secretion.* Some oral preparations contain intrinsic factor from animal sources, but antibodies often develop to the animal intrinsic factor leaving the client refractory to further use of the preparation.

Parenteral treatment is conducted with either cyanocobalamin injection (Redisol, Rubramin) or hydroxycobalamin. The latter provides higher blood levels. There is also a depot, long-acting form of cyanocobalamin in sesame oil-aluminum monostearate gel. All are free of significant adverse effects. The object of parenteral B_{12} administration is repletion of bodily stores. A total dose of from 2,000 to 10,000 μg is required but must be given in frequent, divided doses since retention is poor when a few large doses are given. Doses of 100 μg are given daily at first (1–2 weeks), then 3 times per week until stores are replenished. Finally, maintenance injections of cyanocobalamin (100 μg, once per month) or hydroxycobalamin (1,000 μg, once every 2–4 months) are given for life. *The nurse should take an active role in educating the client about the need for compliance and lifelong treatment.*

With proper therapy, pernicious anemia responds in 2–3 days and is corrected in 6–8 weeks. Untreated vitamin B_{12} deficiency is fatal because of the progressive neuropathy.

Folic Acid-Deficiency Anemia

Folic acid deficiency anemia is of the megaloblastic variety and superficially indistinguishable from vitamin B_{12} deficiency. It is a common type of anemia, second in frequency only to anemias related to iron deficiency or iron reutilization.

Folic acid is a water-soluble vitamin. Like other water-soluble vitamins, it is a precursor of an essential coenzyme. The term *folacin* is used collectively for the vitamin precursor and the physiologically active metabolites to connote all substances with this characteristic nutritional value. The term *folic acid* is, strictly speaking, reserved for the dietary precursor form, which chemically is pteroylglutamic acid.

Folic acid is found in a variety of foods, including green leafy vegetables, liver, yeast, broccoli, asparagus, mushrooms, and fruits, especially oranges. Folate in food is somewhat unstable. It is broken down by light when foods are stored. Folate is heat labile and therefore its activity also decreases as much as 90% with cooking. Folate activity is also eluted into cooking fluids or canning fluids and potentially lost. Folate in citrus fruits is the most stable, perhaps due to protection by ascorbic acid.

The recommended daily allowance of dietary folate is 400 μg in adults. Normally, the minimum requirement to replace losses is net absorption of 50 μg. Marginal dietary intake is common, and folic acid deficiency is among the most frequent of dietary deficiencies. The normal American diet provides 50–500 μg of absorbable folate per day. People subsisting on low-quality diets and alcoholics are at risk populations. Requirements for folacin are elevated during pregnancy, lactation, infancy, malignancies (especially lymphomas), hypermetabolic disorders (such as hyperthyroidism), and during times of increased hematopoiesis.

Pharmacokinetics of Folate Dietary folates are freed by digestion in the intestines. Absorption of folate then occurs by active transport especially in the jejunum (Figure 41–4). Free folate is absorbed

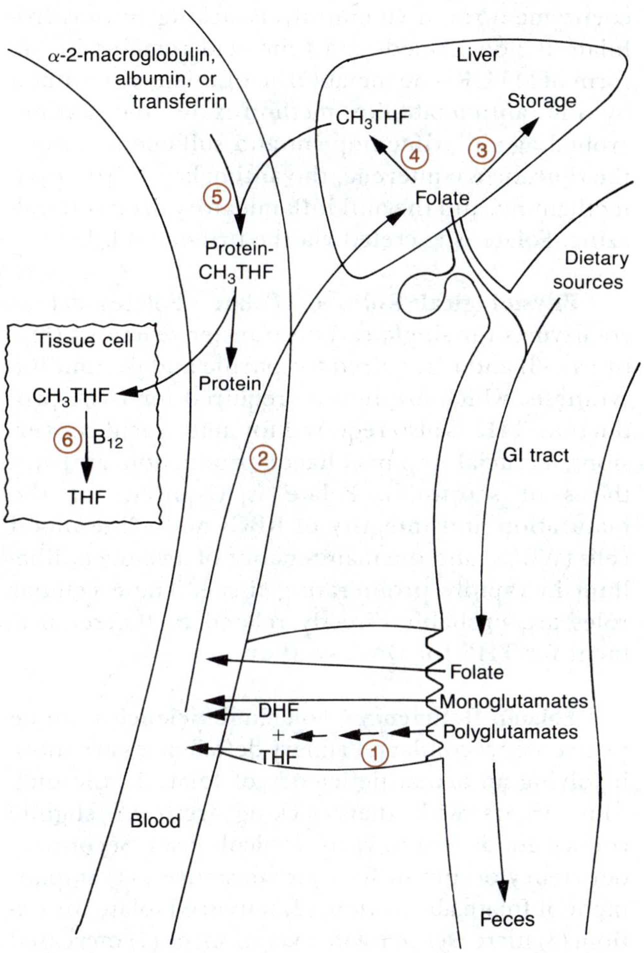

Figure 41–4
Metabolism of folate. (1) Active transport of dietary forms of folate, (2) transport to the liver, (3) liver storage, (4) conversion to transport form, methyltetrahydrofolate (CH_3THF), (5) attachment to transport proteins, (6) uptake into tissue cells, (7) vitamin B_{12}-dependent conversion to the active coenzyme form, tetrahydrofolate (THF).

as well as mono- and polyglutamates. Absorption is impaired in intestinal malabsorption conditions. Folate deficiency can itself further impair intestinal absorption (tropical sprue). Folate absorption is also impaired by anticonvulsants, bile sequestrants, biguanides, and alcohol. After absorption, folate derivatives enter the portal blood and reach the liver where folacin is stored (only a 2- to 4-month supply) or converted to its main transport form, 5-methyltetrahydrofolate (MTHF). This metabolite circulates in the blood attached to carrier proteins. Plasma levels vary from 3 to 21 ng/ml, rising shortly after meals. MTHF is taken up by cells and gives up its methyl group in a vitamin B_{12}-dependent step to form dihydrofolate and then tetrahydrofolate (THF), the active coenzyme form. If vitamin B_{12} is lacking, tetrahydrofolate is not formed, and folic acid remains in the form of MTHF. The metabolism of folate is inhibited by the antimetabolite methotrexate, the antimicrobial agents trimethoprim and sulfamethoxazole, the diuretic triamterene, the antimalarial drug pyrimethamine, and the anti-inflammatory drug sulfasalazine. Folate is excreted via the urine and bile.

Physiological Roles of Folate Folates act as coenzymes for single carbon transfer reactions (Figure 41–3) and is required for purine and pyrimidine synthesis, which are in turn required for DNA production. THF is also required for amino acid conversions, a crucial step in collagen production, and synthesis of serotonin. Folate is required for the maturation and integrity of RBCs and white blood cells (WBCs) and the maintenance of a viable epithelium in rapidly proliferating tissue. These cellular roles are probably directly related to the requirement for THF for DNA synthesis.

Folacin Deficiency Folacin deficiencies can be primary or secondary. Primary deficiencies are those involving an actual deficiency of folate in the diet. This occurs with diets lacking fresh or slightly cooked foods and in chronic alcoholism. Secondary deficiency occurs in four circumstances: (1) impairment of folate absorption, (2) impaired folate utilization, (3) increases in folate excretion, or (4) increased requirements for folate. Impaired absorption is usually related to malabsorption syndromes, blind-loop syndrome, or use of drugs such as oral contraceptives, alcohol, and antiepileptics. Utilization is impaired by folate antagonists (methotrexate, triamterene, trimethroprim, pyrimethamine, and sulfamethoxazole), vitamin B_{12} deficiency, and alcoholism. Excretion may be increased in liver disease or vitamin B_{12} dependency. Requirements are increased in pregnancy, lactation, infancy, lymphomas, hypermetabolic disorders, increased hematopoiesis (for example, in hemolytic anemias), and psoriasis.

Folacin deficiency is characterized by megaloblastic anemia, hypersegmented WBCs, and pancytopenia. Cellular morphology and blood cell counts are indistinguishable from B_{12}-deficiency anemia, but serum determination of the two vitamins provides differentiation. Normal serum folate is greater than 7 μg/ml. In folate deficiency, levels are below 3 μg/ml.

Neuropathy does not occur in folacin deficiency. Symptoms other than anemia include gastrointestinal problems (stomatitis, glossitis, and intestinal malabsorption), skin disturbances (exfoliative dermatitis, psoriasis, and eczema), and disorders of the reproductive system (abortion, toxemia of pregnancy, and infertility).

Treatment The goals of treatment are to (1) correct the underlying cause if possible, (2) restore folate levels, and (3) correct the hematological status. Therapy with folate consists of 1 mg/day given orally, for 2–3 weeks to replenish physiological stores followed by maintenance doses of 0.1–0.5 mg daily. Parenteral administration is required only in patients unable to take drugs orally. Response to folic acid therapy begins in 2–3 days and is normally complete in 6–8 weeks.

Folate preparations include folic acid, folic acid injection, and leucovorin calcium injection (folinic acid). Folic acid is also available in combinations with iron and other vitamins.

Prophylactic use of folate is appropriate in situations associated with elevated requirements such as pregnancy (0.3 mg/day), antiepileptic therapy (0.4–1.0 mg/day), chronic treatment with nonsteroidal antiinflammatory drugs (0.4–1.0 mg/day), use of bile sequestrants (0.4–1.0 mg/day), use of triamterene (Dyrenium) (0.4–1.0 mg/day), use of sulfasalazine (0.4–1.0 mg/day), use of oral contraceptives (0.4–1.0 mg/day), or use of antacids (0.4–0.8 mg/day).

Adverse effects do not occur with folic acid therapy, except that treatment of vitamin B_{12} anemia with folic acid alone is contraindicated because the anemia will improve but the neuropathy associated with B_{12} deficiency will continue to progress. Folic acid should not be taken by anyone undergoing therapy with methotrexate, since folic acid will antagonize its action.

Aplastic Anemia

Aplastic (or hypoplastic) anemias involve a reduced bone marrow mass with a consequent decline in hematopoiesis. The term *aplastic anemia* is used ambiguously for either pure RBC deficiencies or panhypoplasias (in which production of both RBCs and WBCs is deficient). Most often, there is at least some degree of WBC reduction as well as the anemia. Thus, the characteristic laboratory findings include a reduction in WBC count (usually $< 1{,}500$ per μl), in RBCs (usually < 1 million/ml), and in reticulocytes. This last is particularly illuminating since reticulocytes are newly formed RBCs and represent a direct indication of recent bone marrow activity. Serum iron is usually elevated in response to the anemia.

About one-half of cases of aplastic anemia are idiopathic, occurring mainly in adolescents or young adults. The other half are acquired in response to toxic effects of environmental chemicals (such as organic solvents, arsenic, organic phosphates), cancer therapy (either radiation or antineoplastic drugs), drugs (Table 41–2), or infections (viral infections, infectious hepatitis, and mycobacterial infections).

Onset usually occurs insidiously, over weeks or months, but it is occasionally rapid. The clinical symptoms depend on whether the hypoplasia is of the pure RBC type or a pancytopenia. In the former instance, the symptoms relate to anemia exclusively, with the usual triad of pallor, tachycardia, and fatigue. In panhypoplasia, there is usually thrombocytopenia with consequent purpura and bleeding around the nose, gums, and gastrointestinal tract. Lymphocytes are generally unaffected, but agranulocytosis may be profound, leading to complications of infection, potentially life-threatening.

The only long-term therapy for aplastic anemias is a bone marrow transplant. Siblings are evaluated for immunological compatibility. Otherwise treatment is symptomatic and supportive. Of immediate concern is control of infection and bleeding. Toxic causes are identified and eliminated. Blood or platelet transfusions can be employed but only if subsequent bone marrow transplantation is not anticipated. Androgens (1–2 mg/kg) have been used for their ability to stimulate hematopoiesis but are not effective in the majority of cases. Pure red blood cell aplasias often have an autoimmune origin and immunosuppressives such as corticosteroids or cyclophosphamide have been employed successfully.

Response to therapy is often limited. Partial or complete remissions do occur, but progression to death is more common. Death may occur in a few weeks or in a few years.

Hemolytic Anemias

Hemolytic anemias are caused by an excessively rapid rate of RBC destruction. Rapid rates of hemolysis can be caused by extrinsic factors such as immune attack or mechanical injury, or by intrinsic factors including defects in RBC hemoglobin synthesis, metabolism, or membrane structure. Hemolytic anemias related to intrinsic defects are almost always hereditary while those related to extrinsic factors are usually acquired.

A type of hemolytic anemia of particular relevance to pharmacotherapeutics is the group caused by drug **hypersensitivity reactions** (Table 41–3). These hypersensitivity reactions may be either type II or type III (see Chapter 46). Penicillin and methyldopa produce hemolytic anemia by type II hypersensitivity. Penicillin acts as a hapten, attaching to RBCs so that they are then treated as foreign cells by the humoral immune system. Methyldopa, on the other hand, triggers production of an antibody that is cross-reactive with a protein of RBCs. Methyldopa may also increase exposure of antigenic components within RBCs. Quinine and quinidine produce immune complexes (type III hypersensitivity) that attach to RBCs and platelets, leading to hemolytic anemia and thrombocytopenia respectively. Immunological hemolytic anemias are identified by a

Table 41–2
Drugs and Chemicals That May Cause Hypoplastic Anemia

Frequently	Occasionally
Antineoplastics	Acetazolamide
Chloramphenicol	Aspirin
Gold compounds	Benzene
Mephenytoin	Carbamazepine
Organophosphates	Cardiac glycosides
Phenylbutazone	Chlorthiazide
Quinacrine	Chlorinated insecticides
Trimethadione	Hair sprays
	Methyldopa
	Penicillin
	Phenytoin
	Quinidine
	Streptomycin
	Sulfonamides
	Sulfonylureas

Table 41–3
Drugs That Cause Immunological Hemolysis

Aspirin	Nitrofurazone
Cephalosporins	Penicillin
Chloramphenicol	Phenacetin
Chlorinated insecticides	Phenylbutazone
Chlorpromazine	Primaquine
Dimercaprol	Probenecid
Isoniazid	Quinacrine
Levodopa	Quinidine
Mefenamic acid	Quinine
Methyldopa	Stibophen
Methylene blue	Sulfonamides
Nitrofurantoin	Tetracycline

positive Coombs' test, which detects presence of antibodies on RBCs. Drug-induced hemolytic anemias are reversible when the causative drug is withdrawn. Hemolysis usually stops within 3 weeks. In severe cases, glucocorticoids can be used to suppress immunological activity.

Another type of hemolytic anemia relevant to clinical pharmacotherapeutics is **glucose-6-phosphate dehydrogenase (G6PD) deficiency.** This X-linked, inherited condition occurs commonly in black males (13%), less commonly in black females, Italians, Greeks, Arabs, and Sephardic Jews. The enzyme glucose-6-phosphate dehydrogenase participates in the hexose monophosphate shunt that provides hydrogen for reduction reactions. Patients with G6PD deficiency are generally asymptomatic except when exposed to oxidizing drugs (Table 41–4). The erythrocytes are unable to protect themselves from oxidation and hemolysis. Screening tests are available for testing G6PD sensitivity and should be employed routinely in high-risk populations, especially black males.

Hemolytic anemias related to impaired hemoglobin synthesis are usually hereditary. Full symptom expression occurs only in homozygotes. Heterozygotes are usually asymptomatic, less frequently mildly symptomatic. In **sickle-cell anemia,** an abnormal hemoglobin, HbS, is produced. The RBC has an abnormal sickle shape that causes it to lodge in small capillaries. About 10% of blacks have the sickle-cell trait (heterozygous). These individuals will produce 20–45% abnormal hemoglobin, but will usually not experience significant anemia or any reduction in life-span. About 0.3% of blacks are homozygous and have sickle-cell disease. These individuals will experience anemia, and severe, recurrent pains of the abdomen, back, and joints. The lodging of sickle-cells in small vessels causes progressive neurological, pulmonary, and renal dysfunction. Transfusions may be given during anemic crises. Otherwise treatment is symptomatic.

Table 41–4
Drugs and Nutrients Associated with Idiosyncratic Hemolysis in G6PD-Deficient Individuals

Aspirin	Phenacetin
Chloramphenicol	Primaquine
Dimercaprol	Probenecid
Fava beans	Quinacrine
Furazolidone	Quinidine
Isoniazid	Quinine
Nalidixic acid	Sulfonamides
Naphthalene (moth balls)	Sulfones
Nifurtimox	Sulfonylureas
Nitrofurantoin	Vitramin K analogs
Nitrofurazone	

The Hemostatic System

A remarkable characteristic of blood is its ability to flow freely through the blood vessels under normal circumstances and yet to form into tough clots to plug leaks as they occur. The hemostatic system of the blood is responsible for maintaining this delicate balance between the fluid and solid manifestations of blood, a balance so crucial that any substantial disturbance in it poses a threat to the life of the individual. The major blood constituents contributing to hemostasis are the platelets and the clotting factors.

Physiology of Coagulation

Clotting is initiated whenever damage occurs to blood vessel walls. The process culminates in formation of a fibrin-reinforced platelet plug. The clotting mechanism involves two principal components: platelet adhesion and the coagulation cascade (Figure 41–5). Both mechanisms are triggered by exposure of blood to collagen of connective tissue lying beneath the endothelial cells that line blood vessels, such as occurs when the vessel is damaged by injury or disease.

The platelet phase begins with adhesion of platelets to the exposed collagen strand. Under the influence of plasma thrombin, a phospholipid component of platelet cell membranes, arachidonic acid, is split off and is converted by prostaglandin synthetase into thromboxane A_2, a powerful stimulator of platelet degranulation and aggregation. Degranulation consists of the release of the rich stores of ADP contained within the platelet granules. The degranulated cells undergo viscous metamorphosis, spreading out along the collagen strand. The ADP released by degranulation as well as the thromboxane A_2 promote aggregation of additional platelets. These platelets lose their individual membranes, forming a sticky plug. The platelet mass by itself can quickly plug a capillary leak but will not be sufficiently stable for the long run unless it is further fortified by strands of fibrin, the end-product of the coagulation cascade. Normally the coagulation cascade proceeds simultaneously with the platelet phase.

The coagulation cascade can be initiated in either of two ways — by a mechanism intrinsic to the

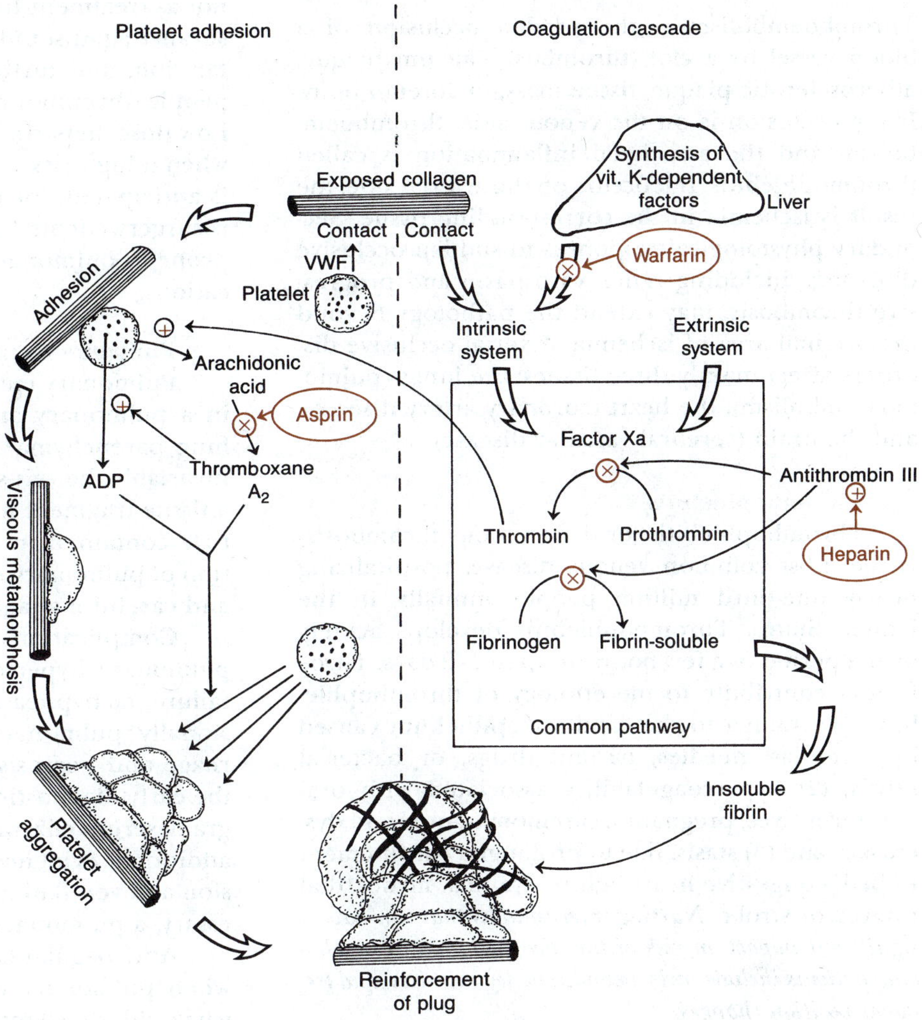

Figure 41–5
Platelet and coagulation phases of clotting, as described in the text. Aspirin inhibits platelet adhesion by inhibiting the enzyme (prostaglandin synthetase) that catalyzes formation of thromboxane A_2. Heparin activates a plasma protein antithrombin III, which inhibits factors Xa and thrombin. Oral anticoagulants, such as warfarin, inhibit the vitamin K-dependent hepatic synthesis of clotting factors.

blood or by another involving surrounding tissue. The intrinsic mechanism is initiated when blood comes into contact with exposed collagen of an injured blood vessel wall, which activates factor XII (Hageman factor). The action of this intrinsic mechanism will be augmented by an extrinsic mechanism if damage has also occurred to adjacent tissue cells, causing them to release tissue thromboplastin (factor III). In either event, the cascade of clotting factors culminates in activation of Stuart factor (factor X) and proceeds by a common pathway from this point on.

Activated Stuart factor catalyzes formation of thrombin from prothrombin. Thrombin catalyses conversion of the soluble plasma protein, fibrinogen, to soluble strands of fibrin. Thrombin also activates fibrin-stabilizing factor, which precipitates the fibrin strands onto the platelet plug. The fibrin strands effectively reinforce the plug and provide a scaffolding for later ingrowth of fibroblasts. Permanent repair of the rupture occurs gradually through the process of fibrosis.

Every clot consists of both platelets and fibrin, but the relative contribution of the two components depends upon the site of the vessel rupture. On the arterial side of the vascular system, where pressure is high and flow is rapid, the clot will consist of a large platelet head and a rather small fibrin tail. This is called a white or arterial thrombus. On the venous side, the relative contribution of fibrin is greater and the platelet mass is small. This is a red or venous thrombus. The drugs that affect the clotting factor cascade leading to fibrin formation are not the same as the drugs that inhibit platelet aggregation. Thus, the selection of drug therapy is based on the location of the clot.

Thromboembolic Disorders

Thromboembolism is the sudden occlusion of a blood vessel by a clot (thrombus), calcium plaque, atherosclerotic plaque, tissue mass, or foreign body. If the occlusion is on the venous side, thromboembolism and the associated inflammation is called thrombophlebitis. If it occurs on the arterial side, the result is ischemia in the corresponding tissue. Secondary physiological responses to sudden occlusive disorders, including reflex vasospasm and progressive thrombosis, may extend the pathology beyond the original area of ischemia. Arterial occlusive disorders affect mainly three tissues: the lungs (pulmonary embolism), the heart (coronary artery disease), and the brain (cerebral vascular disease).

Thrombophlebitis

Thrombophlebitis (or deep venous thrombosis) is the most common venous disease, hospitalizing nearly one-third million people annually in the United States. Thrombophlebitis develops acutely over a period of a few hours or up to 1–2 days. Three factors contribute to the etiology of thrombophlebitis: (1) trauma to the capillary epithelium caused by cannulas, needles, irritant drugs, or bacterial sepsis, (2) hypercoagulability associated with oral contraceptives, pregnancy, carcinomas, or blood dyscrasias, and (3) stasis, due to prolonged confinement to bed, congestive heart failure, trauma, myocardial infarct, or stroke. *Nursing interventions that can have a significant impact on risk of thrombophlebitis in convalescing patients include early ambulation, leg exercises, and frequent position changes.*

Presenting symptoms of thrombophlebitis are pain, swelling, and tenderness in the region of embolism. Deep venous thrombosis of the calf may be revealed by a positive Homans' sign: muscle pain is minimal on flexion of the ankle with the knee flexed, but severe with ankle flexion when the knee is extended. Increased restlessness and fever are also symptoms. Venography provides the strongest basis for diagnosis.

The foremost concern with thrombophlebitis is its association with pulmonary embolism as a secondary development. Emboli dislodged from deep peripheral veins usually pass quickly through the right side of the heart to become lodged in a pulmonary arteriole. *Some clients may want to rub or massage the calf because of the discomfort they feel. Nurses need to warn clients, relatives, and friends that this measure may split off a fragment of blood clot and cause an embolus to form. Elastic stockings may be advised during bedrest and once the individual begins to ambulate. For relief of pain in the legs, warm, moist compresses may be used unless there is also an arterial insufficiency.*

Anticoagulants are used in thrombophlebitis, not as treatment for the primary disorder, but as insurance against pulmonary embolism, myocardial infarction, and further venous thrombosis. For most people, thrombophlebitis subsides in a week or two. Low-dose heparin prophylaxis is also appropriate when a high risk of a primary deep-vein thrombosis is anticipated, for example, in orthopedic and neurosurgery clients. Surgery may be necessary for those prone to pulmonary emoblism or vena cava complications.

Pulmonary Embolism

Pulmonary embolism occurs when a clot lodges in a pulmonary artery, producing ischemia in the lung parenchyma. The origin of the clot is almost invariably the veins of the leg or pelvis. Occasionally a tissue fragment may be responsible, or even a particle contained in an intravenous infusate. Prevention of pulmonary embolism depends on prevention and careful management of thrombophlebitis.

Complications of pulmonary embolism include pulmonary hypertension with possible right heart failure, tachypnea and dyspnea, hypoxia, and occasionally pulmonary infarction leading to hemorrhage and necrosis. Symptoms and risk factors are the early diagnostic clues. Chest x-ray, electrocardiogram, serum enzymes, and blood cell counts provide additional evidence. Ultimately radioisotope perfusion and ventilation scans are conducted and, if necessary, a pulmonary angiogram.

Anticoagulants are employed as prophylaxis when pulmonary embolism is likely, for example, when elderly clients suffer leg or hip fracture. Anticoagulants are also used to prevent expansion of an existing embolism or formation of new ones. Thrombolytic drugs may help dissolve the existing clot.

Coronary Artery Disease

Coronary artery disease, usually initially manifested as angina pectoris, provides conditions in which the risk of clot formation in the blood vessels perfusing the myocardium is elevated. When a clot finally forms, myocardial infarction is the result. Angina is not appropriately treated with anticoagulants, but anticoagulants may be used electively in myocardial infarction in the hope of reducing the risks of secondary complications: pulmonary embolism, extension of the infarct, or thrombophlebitis. There is no clear evidence that anticoagulants or thrombolytic drugs accomplish this objective. Active bed exercises may be more important.

Cerebrovascular Disease

The lodging of a clot in a cerebral artery is commonly referred to as a stroke or a cerebrovascular accident. Cerebrovascular disease is the most widespread neurological disorder in developed countries. The stage is set for a stroke by the progression of atherosclerosis and hypertension. The immediate cause of the cerebral infarction is usually dislodgement of a thrombus from a prosthetic heart valve or fibrillating atrium. Neurological symptoms of cerebrovascular disease are variable and depend on the specific brain regions affected and the extent of the ischemia. The middle cerebral artery is the most commonly affected. Anticoagulants may be indicated for stabilization of stroke in evolution but are contraindicated in completed stroke because they may trigger hemorrhage and further brain damage.

Disseminated Intravascular Coagulation

Disseminated intravascular coagulation (DIC) is marked by diffuse fibrin deposits within the vasculature to an extent that depletes the clotting factors from the blood. It occurs in clients who are severely ill with conditions such as sepsis, heat stroke, cancer, liver failure, or septic abortion. Heparin is sometimes used in order to stop fibrin formation, allowing a repletion of clotting factors. At the same time, heparin may aggravate bleeding associated with DIC.

Anticoagulant, Antithrombotic, and Thrombolytic Drugs

Anticoagulants are drugs that inhibit the rate of formation of fibrin. In contrast, antithrombotic drugs inhibit the platelet phase of clotting, and thrombolytic drugs stimulate the fibrinolytic mechanism by which existing clots are dissolved. Anticoagulants work by inhibiting one or more steps in the clotting cascade. They do not dissolve existing clots but serve to prevent clot formation or the extension of existing clots. Formation of fibrin is the major contributor to formation of venous thrombi; somewhat less important in arterial thrombi. Low-dose anticoagulant therapy is used as primary prophylaxis for prevention of venous thromboembolism in patients undergoing surgery and secondary prophylaxis to prevent expansion of an existing embolism, progression of deep venous thrombi to pulmonary embolism, or formation of additional embolisms. The two types of anticoagulants are heparin and the oral anticoagulants. They differ from one another in many properties (Table 41–5).

Heparin

Heparin became available to medicine in 1938. It is obtained from animal sources and is a natural

Table 41–5
Comparisons between Heparin and Warfarin

Characteristic	Heparin	Warfarin
Source	Animal mast cells	Plant (clover)
Cost	Expensive	Inexpensive
Mechanism	Stimulation of antithrombin III	Inhibition of synthesis of vitamin K-dependent clotting factors
Effective in vivo	Yes	Yes
Effective in vitro	Yes	No
Route of administration	Parenteral, usually IV	Oral
Onset of action	Immediate	Delayed: 8–12 hours
Duration of action	4–6 hours	Days
Laboratory test for monitoring	Lee-White whole blood clotting	Prothrombin time
Toxic effect	Hemorrhage	Hemorrhage
Antidote	Protamine sulfate	Fresh plasma Vitamin K
Presence in breast milk	No	Yes
Safety during pregancy	Yes	No

constituent of the body, a so-called autacoid, presumably involved in regulating hemostasis. It is stored in mast cells in a macromolecular form. Its physiological role is not understood.

Mechanisms and Effects Heparin reduces blood coagulation by complexing with a plasma factor called antithrombin III. Antithrombin is an α_2-globulin that inhibits the activity of several clotting factors including thrombin. Heparin increases its anticoagulant influence. At low doses of heparin, the antithrombin-heparin complex is most effective in neutralizing factor Xa and thrombin (Figure 41–5). High doses of heparin over an extended period can cause a reduction in levels of antithrombin III, resulting in a compensatory increase in coagulability. Estrogens also lower antithrombin III, a fact that may contribute to the increased risk of thromboembolic disorders during pregnancy or use of oral contraceptives.

Pharmacokinetics Heparin is a large and polar molecule and is therefore poorly transported through physiological membranes. It is not effective orally. It is administered parenterally, usually intravenously or subcutaneously. Its effect is immediate in onset. A 10,000 unit intravenous bolus of heparin is effective for 4–6 hours, with a plasma half-life of 1.5 hours. Heparin is sometimes given by intravenous infusion or deep subcutaneous injection, which provides an 8–10 hour effect. Heparin is eliminated from the body by liver metabolism.

Heparin is effective as an anticoagulant *in vitro* (in a testtube) as well as *in vivo* (in a living organism) and is used in preventing formation of clots within cannulas employed for intravenous fluid administration or total parenteral nutrition. Heparin is used similarly in procedures requiring extracorporeal circulation including hemodialysis and vascular surgery. Coagulation is completely inhibited in vitro at a heparin concentration of 1 unit per milliliter of blood.

Adverse Effects and Contraindications The most important adverse effect of heparin is **hemorrhage.** Minor bleeding occurs in 4% of patients and major hemorrhage in 2%. Minor bleeding is usually occult, occurring from the genitourinary tract, nose, and gastrointestinal tract. Careful monitoring of doses is important. Hemorrhage within the brain or gastrointestinal tract is sometimes fatal. Heparin causes a mild and transient thrombocytopenia and rare hypersensitivity reactions. With long-term administration, osteoporosis, hypoaldosteronism, and alopecia occur in rare cases. Heparin may cause diuresis and loss of potassium. *Clients should be encouraged to eat potassium-rich foods.* Heparin is contraindicated in clients with active or suspected bleeding or inaccessible lesions, including those with gastrointestinal ulcers and closed-head injuries. It is contraindicated in people with hemophilia or blood dyscrasias, clients who have exhibited hypersensitivity reactions to heparin, severely hypertensive individuals, and those with visceral malignancies. Heparin is not used during regional or lumbar anesthesia.

If it becomes necessary to antagonize the action of heparin, either because an excessive dose has been given or because of hemorrhage, **protamine sulfate** can be employed effectively. Protamine sulfate forms a complex with heparin on a one-to-one basis. One milligram of protamine per 100 units of unmetabolized heparin provides complete antagonism. Protamine sulfate, in the absence of heparin, has a weak anticoagulant effect of its own. It is administered only by the intravenous route.

Preparations and Administration The dosage schedule for heparin is adjusted on the basis of coagulation monitoring with the aid of laboratory tests. Commonly employed tests are the **Lee-White whole blood clotting time** test (normal value 9–14 minutes) and activated partial thromboplastin time (APTT). The aim of heparin therapy is to increase clotting time twofold to threefold (20–30 minutes). *Long-term heparin therapy should be discontinued gradually, usually after a transition period of oral anticoagulant therapy, to avoid hypercoagulability.*

Heparin preparations are standardized on the basis of a comparison of in vitro activity. A unit of heparin activity is the quantity that prevents coagulation for 1 hour of 1.0 ml of citrated sheep plasma treated with $CaCl_2$ solution. Heparin preparations contain at least 120 units/mg. Heparin sodium injection (Hepathrom, Lipo-hepin, Liquaemin, Panheprin, and others) is provided in sterile water solutions. *Heparin should not be given by the intramuscular route. When heparin is given subcutaneously, it should be injected deep into the fat above the iliac crest or into abdominal fat layers. The site should be rotated. The nurse should use a fine-gauge needle, should* ***not*** *aspirate, and the area should* ***not*** *be massaged after administration since this could result in bleeding. When heparin is to be administered intravenously by continuous infusion or by intermittent infusion, a heparin lock is used.*

Oral Anticoagulants

In contrast to heparin, oral anticoagulants come from a plant source. In the early part of the twentieth century, cattle and sheep in the northern midwest sometimes died mysteriously. Examination of

Nursing Observations For Use of Anticoagulant Drugs in Thromboembolic Disorders

THERAPEUTIC GOAL	To minimize risk of further clot formation. The usual aim is to double prothrombin time from 11–12 seconds to 20–25 seconds.
PREADMINISTRATION ASSESSMENT	
Baseline Data	Observe for increases in local pressure, local edema, and tenderness along a vein, especially in the calf muscle; for pulmonary embolism: dyspnea, tachypnea, hypoxia, and pulmonary hypertension. Evaluate blood pressure, ECG, peripheral perfusion, respiratory rate and sound, liver function, skin integrity, and neurological status; for pulmonary embolisms: chest x-ray, radioisotope perfusion and ventilation scans, pulmonary angiogram. Obtain laboratory tests including urinalysis, prothrombin time, and partial thromboplastin time; for pulmonary embolism: serum enzymes and blood cell counts.
Contraindications/ Precautions	Hemorrhagic disorders, peptic ulcers, renal or hepatic disease, diabetes, tuberculosis, polyarteritis, subacute bacterial endocarditis, trauma, pregnancy, or lactation. Check for presence of an indwelling catheter. Check medication history for allergies to anticoagulants or tartrazine (used in some preparations).
Potential Interactions	Check medication chart for interacting drugs.
EVALUATION OF DRUG RESPONSE	
For Therapeutic Benefit	Monitor prothrombin time and partial thromboplastin time.
For Adverse Effects	Monitor for excess bleeding, bruising, tarry stools, gastrointestinal upset, bloody urine, nose bleeds, rash, or loss of hair.
For Drug Interactions	Monitor for increased anticoagulant action if client is using alcohol. Monitor the client's use of any prescription and nonprescription drugs for potential interacting substances (see drug discussions).
For Dietary Interactions	Monitor for excessive intake of vitamin K, an antagonist of oral anticoagulants. Vitamin K-rich foods include yellow and dark green vegetables.
For Compliance	Evaluate client's compliance with all facets of the therapeutic regimen by careful observation, interviewing, and review of progress. Report compliance problems to the physician and act as client-advocate when changes in the therapeutic regimen seem indicated.

the animals ultimately revealed that death was due to internal hemorrhage linked to ingestion of spoiled sweet clover and a resultant reduction in plasma prothrombin. This discovery led to the isolation of bishydroxycoumarin and development of a family of derivatives referred to collectively as the coumarins. The most widely used drug in this family is warfarin (Coumadin).

Mechanism and Effects The mechanism of coumarins is quite different from that of heparin. Coumarin drugs inhibit vitamin K-dependent hepatic synthesis of four clotting factors (II, VII, IX, and X) by competitive inhibition of vitamin K (Figure 41–6). The result is a gradual depletion of these factors. It takes about 8–12 hours of coumarin action for depletion to occur to an extent that begins to diminish the clotting ability of the blood. Moreover, coumarin-type anticoagulants are without effect in vitro. These drugs have no effect on platelet function nor any inhibiting effect on existing coagulation factors.

Disorders of hemostasis will modify the body's response to anticoagulants. Liver disease or hepatic congestion related to congestive heart failure will decrease formation of clotting factors in the liver and increase the impact of anticoagulants accordingly. In hypermetabolic states such as hyperthyroidism, response to oral anticoagulants is increased. In hypometabolic conditions such as myxedema, response is diminished. In pregnancy, the mother has decreased responsiveness to oral anticoagulants, but the re-

Nursing Diagnoses and Interventions for Use of Anticoagulant Drugs in Thromboembolic Disorders

Nursing Diagnoses	*Related Interventions*
TO ENHANCE DRUG BENEFITS OR REDUCE DRUG REQUIREMENTS	
Alteration in bowel function, respiratory function, or skin integrity related to immobility secondary to thromboembolism	Encourage leg exercise and early ambulation when appropriate; provide frequent position changes. Encourage adequate fluid intake and appropriate diet to counteract bowel problems.
Alteration in comfort: pain related to peripheral ischemia secondary to thromboembolism	Provide comfort measures such as elastic stocking during initial ambulation and warm, moist compresses over site of embolism.
Alteration in tissue perfusion related to thrombus	Provide rest to minimize oxygen requirements of the tissue; avoid massage of the calf as this can disrupt a clot fragment and lead to pulmonary embolism.
TO MINIMIZE DRUG SIDE EFFECTS OR INTERACTIONS	
Potential for injury related to uncontrolled bleeding after anticoagulant therapy	Teach the client the indications of occult bleeding and the necessity for avoiding risk of injury. Explain the importance of regular monitoring of therapy and avoidance of any interacting drug. For hospitalized clients, keep antidotes at hand for emergencies. Evaluate the home environment of outpatients to identify potential threats to their safety.
TO ENSURE SAFE AND EFFICACIOUS DRUG USE	
Knowledge deficit related to drug regimen	Teach the client about the nature of the disorder and the rationale for any prescribed medication.
	Teach clients how to measure dosages and keep track of how much medication has been taken.
	Provide the client with a list of potential adverse effects and drug interactions for each prescribed drug and explain what to do if any of these occur.
	Teach the client how to recognize indications of excessive bleeding tendency, such as tarry stools, blood in urine, nose bleeds, bleeding gums, or purpura.
	Explain the importance of blood tests in assessing the disorder and monitoring drug therapy. Tell the client not to use any other drug (prescription or nonprescription) without consulting with the physician who has prescribed the anticoagulant.
	Instruct the client concerning the importance of exact compliance with the regimen and frequent evaluation of therapy.
	Advise clients not to abruptly discontinue anticoagulant medication.
	Advise the client to wear an identification bracelet or tag indicating the medical condition and drug regimen.

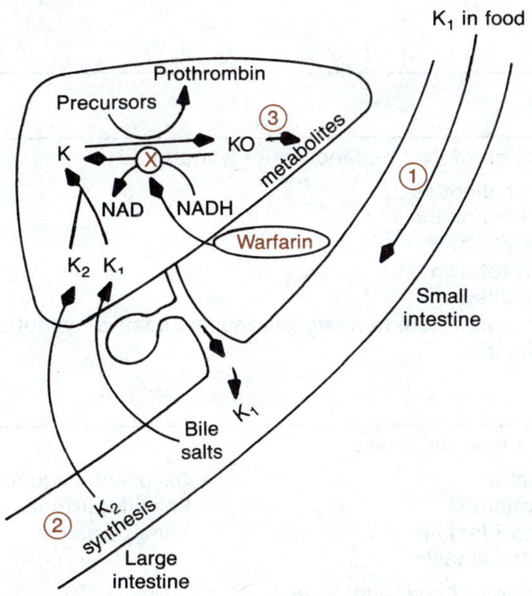

Figure 41–6
Vitamin K metabolism. (1) Dietary intake of vitamin K_1; (2) vitamin K_2 synthesis by intestinal bacteria; (3) interconversion between vitamin K and vitamin K epoxide (KO) linked to synthesis of vitamin K-dependent clotting factors such as prothrombin and inhibited by oral anticoagulants such as warfarin.

sponse of the fetus is unchanged. Since oral anticoagulants freely cross the placental barrier, elevated doses in pregnancy are ill-advised.

Pharmacokinetics Warfarin is rapidly and fully absorbed after oral administration. There is little difference in rate of onset when warfarin is given intravenously. In the plasma, warfarin is very highly bound (99%) to plasma albumin protein, a fact that creates a major potential for drug interactions by competition for protein binding sites. Warfarin is metabolized in the liver to inactive metabolites which are then excreted in the urine and bile. Warfarin has a half-life of 1.5–2.5 hours. Peak effect occurs after 1.5–3 days and the anticoagulant action persists for 2–5 days after a single dose. Other oral anticoagulants differ somewhat in time to peak effect and duration. Dicumarol (bishydroxycoumarin) produces its peak action 3–5 days after administration and the effect lasts 2–10 days. Phenprocoumon (Liquamar) produces its peak action in 2–3 days and has a relatively persistent effect, lasting 7–14 days. Anisindione (Miradon) produces its peak action in 2–3 days and the effect lasts 1–3 days.

Adverse Effects and Contraindications As with heparin, the principal adverse effect is **hemorrhage.** Monitoring of the magnitude of depression of coagulation is crucial, but bleeding may occur even when values from laboratory tests are within the normal range. The usual basis for adjusting doses of warfarin is measurement of **prothrombin time.** The object of therapy with oral anticoagulants is to double the normal prothrombin time value of 11–12 seconds to 20–25 seconds. When hemorrhage occurs, treatment consists of immediate withdrawal of the oral anticoagulant and administration of vitamin K orally or by injection. This should reduce bleeding significantly in a few hours and provide normal clotting values in 24 hours. *Outpatients should carry vitamin K with them in dosage units of 5–20 mg for use in the event of bleeding.* If more rapid reversal is required, fresh whole plasma can be administered. Oral anticoagulants occasionally cause **skin eruptions** as an allergic reaction. Contraindications for use of oral anticoagulants are bleeding disorders, ulcers, lumbar or regional anesthesia, and renal or hepatic insufficiency.

Drug and Diet Interactions Drug interactions involving oral anticoagulants are numerous and among the most important in clinical medicine. For one thing, relatively small changes in level of effect of oral anticoagulants can have dire consequences for the client, resulting in hemorrhage or conversely inadequate protection from thromboembolism. Only the cardiac glycosides have a comparably small margin of safety in the adjustment of the level of effect.

Interactions with oral anticoagulants occur in both directions and by several mechanisms. Drugs may alter the bioavailability of vitamin K, warfarin absorption, warfarin binding to plasma proteins, or warfarin catabolism in the liver (Table 41–6). **Antagonism of oral anticoagulants** may be produced by drugs that cause induction of liver enzymes (barbiturates, other hypnotics, antiepileptics, rifampin (Rifadin), griseofulvin (Fulvicin), and nafcillin (Nafcil)), since this hastens the metabolism of warfarin. Some drugs impair absorption of warfarin. This occurs with griseofulvin, aluminum hydroxide, colestipol (Colestid), and cholestyramine (Questran). Estrogens and estrogen-containing oral contraceptives increase the synthesis of procoagulant factors, necessitating an increase in the dose of an oral anticoagulant. Vitamin K is a competitive antagonist. Ingestion of a lot of foods rich in vitamin K can decrease the effect of cumarin therapy. *The client should be provided with a list of such foods and instructed to avoid sudden changes in dietary intake of these foods.*

Table 41–6
Drug Interactions of Oral Warfarin

Antagonism

Impaired absorption of warfarin	Induction of liver metabolism of warfarin
Cholestyramine	Antiepileptics
Colestipol	Antihistamines
Griseofulvin	Barbiturates
Increased coagulation factors	Griseofulvin
Estrogens	Nafcillin
Vitamin K	Nonbarbiturate nonbenzodiazepine sedative hypnotics
	Rifampin

Potentiation

Displacement of warfarin from albumin binding sites	Antithrombotic effect	
Aspirin	Aspirin	Oxyphenbutazone
Chloral derivatives	Clofibrate	Phenylbutazone
Clofibrate	Dipyridamole	Sulfinpyrazone
Diazepam	Indomethacin	
Diazoxide	Inhibition of coagulation factors	
Nonsteroidal anti-inflammatory drugs	Antimetabolites	
Phenytoin	Quinidine	
Sulfonamides	Quinine	
Sulfonylureas	Salicylates	
Decreased vitamin K availability	Possible drug-induced thrombocytopenia	
Broad-spectrum antibiotics such as neomycin	Acetazolamide	Lincomycin
Increased loss of vitamin K	Amitriptyline	Mefenamic acid
Hypolipemic drugs including:	Barbiturates	Methyldopa
Anabolic steroids	Benzodiazepines	Nalidixic acid
Clofibrate	Bromocriptine	Neuroleptics
Thyroid hormones	Carbamazepine	Nitrofurans
Inhibition of warfarin metabolism	Cardiac glycosides	Penicillins
Alcohol	Cephalosporins	Procainamide
Allopurinol	Chloramphenicol	Quinacrine
Chloramphenicol	Cimetidine	Quinidine
Cimetidine	Doxepin	Quinine
Disulfiram	Estrogens	Rifampin
Methylphenidate	Furosemide	Succinimides
Metronidazole	Gentamicin	Sulfonamides
Oxyphenbutazone	Gold compounds	Tetracycline
Phenylbutazone	Hydantoins	Thiazides
Sulfinpyrazone	Ibuprofen	Thiouracil
Sulfonamides	Levodopa	Valproate
	Lidocaine	

Potentiation of oral anticoagulants is more common than antagonism. Many drugs displace warfarin from plasma protein binding sites, increasing the pharmacologically active unbound fraction. Included in this category are aspirin, other nonsteroidal anti-inflammatory drugs, chloral hydrate, phenytoin, sulfonamides, sulfonylureas, and others. Since oral anticoagulants act competitively to inhibit the activity of vitamin K, a deficiency of this vitamin will increase the effect of a given dose of an oral anticoagulant. Broad-spectrum antibiotics destroy intestinal flora that ordinarily produce vitamin K for absorption. Hypolipemic drugs, thyroid hormone, anabolic steroids, and clofibrate increase losses of vitamin K. Thyroid hormone also increases the effect of oral anticoagulants due to hypermetabolism. Aspirin and aspirin-like drugs not only displace oral anticoagulants but also have an antiplatelet action of their own. In fact, aspirin-like drugs are being used experimentally as antithrombotic agents (see below). *Because aspirin is so widely used, the nurse needs to educate the client regarding this interaction in particular.* Other drugs that inhibit platelet aggregation include dipyridamole and sulfinpyrazone. Quinine, quinidine, salicylates, and antimetabolites potentiate the action of oral anticoagulants by inhibiting clotting factors. Phenylbutazone (Azolid), disulfiram (Antabuse), alcohol, allopurinol, (Zyloprim), cimetidine (Tagamet), chloramphenicol (Choromycetin), methylphenidate (Ritalin), sulfonamides, sulfinpyrazone (Anturane), and metronidazole (Flagyl) inhibit liver metabolism of oral anticoagulants. *Clients should be instructed not to begin or eliminate any medication without consultation. Other health care professionals involved in the client's care should be informed that the client is receiving anticoagulants.*

Preparations and Administration Prothrombin time should be determined daily when oral anticoagulants are first used. *The client should be instructed to take the medication at the same time each day. Doses may have to be adjusted during menstruation.*

Anisindione (Miradon)
Tablets
Recommended Doses: 300 mg PO on the first day, 200 mg on the second day, 100 mg on the third day, and 25–250 mg daily for maintenance.

Dicumarol (bishydroxycoumarin)
Tablets
Recommended Doses: 200–300 mg PO on the first day and 25–200 mg on subsequent days.

Phenprocoumon (Liquamar)
Tablets
Recommended Doses: For induction, 24 mg PO; for maintenance, from 0.75–6.0 mg daily. Phenprocoumon is the longest acting of the oral anticoagulants, with a duration of action of 7–14 days.

Warfarin (Coumadin, Panwarfarin)
Tablets, injection solution as warfarin sodium
Recommended Doses: 10–15 mg PO initially. Maintenance therapy requires 2–15 mg and continued weekly or monthly prothrombin determinations. Warfarin sodium for injection is seldom needed.

Important Nursing Implications for Anticoagulants

- ☐ Explain the rationale for treatment with anticoagulants, exact dosage ranges, and how to establish schedules so that doses are not missed.
- ☐ Whenever possible, include a responsible family member in the instructions.
- ☐ Explain to clients the need to take special precautions to avoid injury. Investigate or have someone from a community health agency investigate the home situation to identify obstacles that might prove to be a threat to the client's safety. Discuss with clients the cautionary measures essential when they use knives or other sharp tools. Advise clients to use an electric razor for shaving to avoid nicks and cuts, to use a thimble while sewing, to wear garden gloves to protect their hands and arms when working outdoors, and to avoid going barefoot, even indoors.
- ☐ Examine the mucosal membranes of clients for signs of bleeding when anticoagulants are used. Clients should be checked for bleeding gums, nose bleeds, petechiae, purpura, or blood in the urine or stools. Teach clients the signs and symptoms of adverse effects of anticoagulants and to report immediately any signs of hemorrhage. Also, warn women receiving heparin that menses may be increased and prolonged.
- ☐ Instruct clients about drugs that may interact with anticoagulants. For example, they need to be advised that salicylates can inhibit prothrombin and prolong bleeding.
- ☐ Advise women who use oral contraceptives of the potential risk of thromboembolism since oral contraceptives inhibit anticoagulant therapy. Others who use intrauterine devices as contraceptives need to be warned about possible hemorrhage.
- ☐ Advise clients to refrain from use of alcohol, since prolonged and heavy use of alcohol increases the effect of oral anticoagulants and the likelihood of bleeding.
- ☐ Teach clients about dietary influences on anticoagulant therapy. Yellow and dark green vegetables have high amounts of vitamin K, which counteracts the effects of anticoagulants. Therefore, the person on prolonged anticoagulant therapy should limit the amount of these foods. Nurses, in cooperation with dieticians and nutritionists, should work with the client to find appropriate substitutes.
- ☐ Remind clients of the importance of informing other health professionals (physicians, dentists, other nurses) that they are receiving anticoagulants so that interacting drugs can be avoided. Advise them to purchase all their medications from the same pharmacist, whenever possible, so that the pharmacy can maintain the client's medication profile and the pharmacist can identify potential drug interactions. Instruct clients to ask about over-the-counter drugs and to read labels on these drugs

to assure that ingredients they contain will not interact with the anticoagulant.

- ☐ Avoid administration of oral anticoagulants to pregnant or lactating women since these drugs freely pass the placental barrier and are secreted in breast milk.
- ☐ Advise all clients receiving oral anticoagulants to wear an identification bracelet stating what drugs they are taking so that appropriate action can be taken in an emergency.

Antithrombotic Drugs

Antithrombotic drugs, also called antiplatelet drugs, inhibit the platelet phase of clot formation. Clots formed on the arterial side of the circulatory system (white thrombi) have a large platelet component, so the use of antithrombotic drugs is most often directed toward arterial thromboembolic disorders. Antithrombotic drugs inhibit platelet function by a variety of mechanisms. Whether long-term administration of antithrombotic drugs actually decreases the incidence of thromboembolic disorders has yet to be definitely established. Antithrombotic drugs include aspirin, sulfinpyrazone (Anturane), dipyridamole (Pesantine) and the plasma expander, dextran (Macrodex).

Aspirin inhibits the enzyme prostaglandin synthetase (Figure 41–5). This in turn inhibits degranulation and aggregation. The effect of aspirin on platelets lasts several days while new platelets are being generated. Long-term studies of the effectiveness of aspirin in preventing cerebral or myocardial infarcts have not been conclusive.

Sulfinpyrazone is a uricosuric drug that has been used in gout. Sulfinpyrazone inhibits platelet adhesion and degranulation. This drug has been tested for use in preventing thromboembolism after myocardial infarction but has not been shown to be effective.

Dipyridamole is a vasodilator that has been effective when used in conjunction with warfarin (Coumadin) to prevent thromboembolism in clients with prosthetic heart valves. It is not effective alone. It is available in tablets.

Clofibrate (Atromid-S) is a hypolipidemic drug that inhibits platelet adhesiveness but without demonstrated value in secondary prophylaxis of thromboembolism. Dextran is under study as a means for reducing the risk of postoperative thromboembolic complications.

Thrombolytic Drugs

Thrombolytic drugs stimulate the fibrinolytic mechanism by which established clots are dissolved. They are indicated for treatment of acute thromboembolic disorders such as an established pulmonary embolism or iliofemoral thrombus. Thrombolytic drugs stimulate conversion of plasminogen to plasmin, an enzyme that digests fibrin strands. Thrombolytic drugs are thus able to dissolve an existing thromboembolism. On the negative side, these drugs profoundly alter hemostasis with the result that bleeding may occur and be difficult to control. There are currently two drugs available in this class: streptokinase (Streptase) and urokinase (Abbokinase).

Streptokinase is an enzyme obtained from a streptococcus bacterium. This enzyme catalyzes conversion of plasminogen to plasmin, promoting clot dissolution. Therapy is monitored through measurement of thrombin time. The aim is to increase thrombin time twofold to fivefold. There is a high risk of bleeding during treatment. Concurrent use of anticoagulants is contraindicated but after streptokinase treatment, heparin therapy is initiated, followed by oral anticoagulant treatment.

Urokinase has a similar mechanism of action, indications, and risks as streptokinase. It is an enzyme derived from human urine and its only known substrate is plasminogen. Urokinase is much more expensive than streptokinase. A course of therapy with streptokinase costs a few hundred dollars; with urokinase the cost is several thousand. Therefore, urokinase is reserved for clients allergic to streptokinase.

Streptokinase (Streptase and Kabikinase)
Powder for reconstitution and injection
Recommended Doses: 250,000 international units (IU) IV initially, followed by 100,000 IU/hour, IV, for 1–3 days.

Urokinase (Abbokinase)
Powder for reconstitution and injection
Recommended Doses: 4,100 IU/kg, IV, over 10 minutes. This is followed by continuous IV infusion at a rate of 4,400 IU/kg/hour for 12 hours.

Hemorrhagic Disorders

With the exception of the hemophilias, hemorrhagic disorders occur as symptoms and complications of other primary disease entities. **Purpura** is the most common hemorrhagic manifestation. It appears as an ease of bruising due to subcutaneous, or occasionally mucosal, bleeding. It occurs most commonly in postmenopausal women when the decline in estrogen causes thinning of the blood. It can also occur as an immune complex disorder following a streptococcal infection. Purpura has been noted with use of aspirin and in hypothyroidism.

Thrombocytopenia is a decrease in platelet count due to decreased production, increased destruction, increased utilization, or dilution. Typical signs include petechiae and ecchymoses (bleeding into the skin) and occult bleeding from the gastrointestinal, genitourinary, or vaginal mucosa. The bleeding may lead secondarily to anemia. Thrombocytopenia due to decreased platelet production is seen in panhypoplasia caused by infection, radiation or drug treatment for cancer, or certain other drugs. It also occurs as a result of marrow displacement in clients who have lymphoma or granuloma, or due to marrow diversion in clients with leukemia. Increased destruction of platelets can be caused by mechanical damage, hyperactivity of the spleen, or immune mechanisms. Quinine, quinidine, thiazides, and sulfonamides are known to trigger an immunological thrombocytopenia. Drugs most likely to induce thrombocytopenia are listed in Table 41-6. Increased utilization occurs in disseminated intravascular coagulation. Dilution occurs with use of plasma expanders.

Hemophilias are hereditary disorders of coagulation characterized by delayed clot formation. The client with hemophilia faces the risk of uncontrollable bleeding following minor injury. The most common forms are called hemophilia A, accounting for more than 80% of all cases, and B, accounting for about 10%. Hemophilia A involves a deficiency in factor VIII. Hemophilia B, or Christmas disease, is a deficiency in factor IX. Both of these conditions are inherited as recessive, sex-linked traits; therefore, clinical manifestations occur only in males. Women may be carriers of the abnormal gene to offspring. Treatment consists of administration of fresh plasma in acute situations and replacement therapy with purified preparations of the deficient factor.

Factor VIII (Factorate, Hemofil, Humafac, Koate, Profilate) is given intravenously in individualized doses based on weight and degree of deficiency. The typical maintenance dose is 250–500 units/day. Treatment is occasionally complicated by production of factor VIII inhibitors.

Factor IX is given in the form of a factor complex containing factors II, VII, IX, and X. These are the factors that are produced by vitamin K-dependent hepatic synthesis. Dosage is individualized.

Hemostatic Drugs

Hemostatic drugs are used to stimulate clotting as a means of terminating bleeding. Most such drugs are topical preparations used to control capillary bleeding. Vitamin K and the plasminogen inhibitors, on the other hand, are systemic hemostatic drugs, useful in alleviating certain bleeding conditions.

Vitamin K

Vitamin K may be administered to alleviate hemorrhage related to excessive doses of administered oral anticoagulant, or vitamin K deficiency. Vitamin K exists in two natural forms, vitamin K_1 (phytonadione) and vitamin K_2 (menaquinone), as well as a synthetic derivative called vitamin K_3 (menadione). In normal individuals, vitamin K is without significant pharmacological effects. In vitamin K deficiency, vitamin K drugs produce the same effects associated with dietary vitamin K: stimulation of synthesis of vitamin K-dependent clotting factors. Vitamin K is found in foods from both plant and animal sources. Vitamin K_1 is produced by photosynthetic plants and is found in green leafy vegetables, such as spinach, kale, cabbage, and collard greens. Vitamin K_2 is synthesized by bacteria, including those found in the human intestine. Liver is the main animal source of vitamin K. There is no established dietary requirement. When vitamin K is removed from the diet, apparently the intestinal flora synthesize enough to meet minimum requirements.

Vitamins K_1 and K_2 are fat-soluble vitamins. Like other fat-soluble vitamins, they are absorbed in the proximal part of the intestines after formation of micelles with bile salts (Figure 41-6). Vitamin K_3, by contrast, is water soluble and is absorbed along the entire length of the intestines, independent of bile salt availability.

Vitamin K Deficiency Vitamin K deficiency is seen only if dietary intake is inadequate and synthesis by intestinal flora is absent. Broad-spectrum antibiotics may produce a secondary vitamin K deficiency by destroying the intestinal flora. A more common occurrence is vitamin K deficiency in the first few days of life. At birth, the intestinal flora are not yet established and the infant's diet is slow in providing adequate amounts of vitamin K. Hypoprothrombinemia is common during this period. Oral administration of small doses of vitamin K at birth is recommended. Vitamin K_1 is nontoxic at any reasonable dose and is therefore preferred to vitamin K_3 which, though safe at low doses, may cause hemolytic anemia, hyperbilirubinemia, and kernicterus at moderate doses.

Secondary vitamin K deficiencies occur when absorption is inadequate, metabolism increased, or utilization impaired. Absorption may be diminished due to biliary obstruction, malabsorption syndromes, or use of mineral oil or bile sequestrants. Utilization is impaired in liver disease. Inducers of liver enzymes, including phenytoin (Dilantin), phenobarbital, and primidone (Mysoline), increase the rate of inactivation of vitamin K. It is wise to provide clients taking these medications with 1–5 mg daily supplements of vitamin K. Supplements of vitamin K and other fat-soluble vitamins are appropriate with use of bile sequestrants such as cholestyramine (Questran) and colestipol (Colestid), which reduce vitamin K absorption.

The most important cause of secondary vitamin K deficiency is the form that is intentionally induced by oral anticoagulants. When it is necessary to antagonize oral anticoagulants with vitamin K, vitamin K_1 is far more effective than vitamin K_3 and is preferred. The symptoms of vitamin K deficiency are entirely referable to the hemostatic system.

People who are deficient in vitamin K often give a history of frequent nose bleeds and bleeding gums or mucous membranes. Less frequently, presenting symptoms are cloudy urine.

Preparations and Administration Vitamin K preparations include vitamin K_1, or phytonadione, and vitamin K_3, or menadione.

Vitamin K_1 (Aquamephyton, Konakion, Mephyton)
Tablets, oral solutions, injection solutions dispersed in polysorbate and propylene glycol (Konakion) or polyethylated fatty acids and dextrose (Aquamephyton)
Recommended Doses: 5–20 mg PO; 10 mg IM.

Vitamin K_3 (Hykinone, Kappadione, Synkavite)
Tablets, injection solution in oil, as the sodium bisulfite salt, or as the sodium diphosphate salt
Recommended Doses: 5–10 mg PO; 25 mg/ml IM.

Plasminogen Inhibitors

The plasminogen inhibitors include aminocaproic acid (Amicar) and tranexamic acid (Cyklokapron).

Mechanisms and Effects Plasminogen inhibitors inhibit fibrinolysis (breakdown of clots) by inhibiting plasminogen activating substances. Tranexamic acid is about ten times more potent in this action than aminocaproic acid.

Clinical Indications Tranexamic acid is approved for short-term treatment (2–8 days) of clients with hemophilia to reduce requirements for transfusions after tooth extractions. Aminocaproic acid is approved for use in conditions of excessive bleeding associated with systemic or urinary hyperfibrinolysis. Although not FDA approved, additional uses of aminocaproic acid have included preventing recurrence of subarachnoid hemorrhage, management of certain types of thrombocytopenia, and prevention or treatment of attacks of hereditary angioneurotic edema.

Adverse Effects and Contraindications Plasminogen inhibitors promote the occurrence of **thrombosis,** as an extension and exaggeration of their therapeutic effect. *Nurses should be alert for indications of thrombosis, including leg pain or tenderness, chest pain, breathlessness or dyspnea, and unusual prominence of superficial veins.* Both of the available plasminogen inhibitors can cause nausea, cramps, diarrhea, and mild **hypotension.** *Because of the risk of orthostatic hypotension, inform clients receiving a plasminogen inhibitor to avoid rapid changes of position or prolonged standing in one place. Advise clients to sit or lie down if they begin to feel faint.* Aminocaproic acid, additionally, has been observed to cause muscle weakness or myalgia. *Nurses should instruct clients receiving aminocaproic acid to watch for occurrence of dark urine which might indicate myoglobinuria.* Aminocaproic acid can also cause neurologic symptoms (including dizziness, headache, tinnitus, delirium, hallucinations, and psychotic reactions), nasal stuffiness, conjuctival infusion, skin rash, and transient renal failure. Neither drug can be used if there is evidence of any active intravascular clotting process, such as disseminated intravascular coagulation. Use of tranexamic acid is also contraindicated in clients experiencing subarachnoid hemorrhage since it has been observed to cause cerebral edema and infarction in these individuals. Retinal damage has been reported in animal studies after high doses of tranexamic acid were administered chronically or subchronically. Such effects have not yet been reported in humans, although there have been instances of visual abnormalities, including loss of visual acuity or color vision, in patients using the drug in Europe. As a precaution, tranexamic acid should not be used in clients with acquired deficiencies of color vision since this condition would make difficult the assessment of potential visual toxicity.

Interactions with Drugs and Laboratory Tests Plasminogen inhibitors increase the risk of thromboembolic disorders developing in response to use of oral contraceptives or estrogen. Aminocaproic acid may elevate measurements of serum potassium levels because of its tendency to impair renal function.

Preparations and Administration

Aminocaproic acid (Amicar, generic)
Tablets, syrup, injection solution
Recommended Doses: Initially, 5 g orally or IV, followed by 1–1.25 g/hr thereafter to sustain a plasma level of 0.13 mg/ml

Tranexamic acid (Cyklokapron)
Tablets, injection solution
Recommended Doses: For dental extraction in clients with hemophilia, 10 mg/kg IV with substitution therapy immediately before surgery and 25 mg/kg orally (or 10 mg/kg IV) 3–4 times daily for 2–8 days. Or, 25 mg/kg orally, 3–4 times daily, beginning 1 day prior to surgery.

Topical Hemostatics

Topical hemostatics are designed to control surface capillary bleeding. They work by three mechanisms: (1) stimulation of natural hemostasis, (2) formation of artificial clots; or (3) presentation of a matrix that aids clot formation. Five such preparations are available.

Absorbable gelatin sponge (Gelfoam) is a sterile, water-soluble, gelatin-base foam of porous consistency that can be left in place over a surgical incision when suture is difficult or incomplete. The gel is completely absorbable, normally over a period of 4–6 weeks. It is moistened with saline or thrombin solution before application. *Care should be taken not to overpack a lesion cavity because gelatin sponge expands as it absorbs fluid. The nurse should be alert for signs of tenderness, redness, or swelling indicative of overexpansion.* Absorbable gelatin sponge acts as a mechanical barrier to bleeding and stimulates clot formation. There are no adverse effects. The cosmetic quality of the scar is not adversely affected.

Oxidized cellulose (Oxycel, Hemo-Pak, Surgicel) is a surgical gauze or cotton treated with cellulosic acid. This hemostatic substance stimulates clot formation through a reaction with hemoglobin. The hemostatic material is usually fully absorbed in 2–7 days, but occasionally several weeks is required. *Oxidized cellulose should not be premoistened with thrombin solution because the acid pH of cellulosic acid inactivates thrombin.* Oxidized cellulose is indicated for use in control of organ bleeding. It is contraindicated for application to epithelial surfaces because the cellulosic acid inhibits epithelial proliferation. It is also contraindicated for packing against fractures because the active ingredient inhibits bone regeneration. It is available in cotton pledgets, gauze pads, and gauze strips.

Three clotting factors, from human or animal sources, are used as topical hemostatics. **Thrombin,** isolated from bovine plasma, is available as a powder or as a sterile isotonic saline solution. It is applied topically, for example, to a vacant socket after tooth extraction. It stimulates the normal hemostatic mechanism by stimulating formation of fibrin. **Thromboplastin,** isolated from rabbits, is available as a powder for use as a topical hemostatic for surgical procedures and for determining prothrombin time in the laboratory. **Human fibrin foam** is sterile dried fibrin that can be applied to organs such as the liver, kidney, or brain during surgery to provide a matrix to control bleeding and to facilitate coagulation. It is fully absorbed.

Blood Transfusions

Blood transfusions entail the transfer of whole blood or a blood component from a donor to a recipient. Over 10 million such transfusions are conducted yearly in the United States. Transfusions can provide volume replacement, improved oxygen-carrying capacity, improved hemostasis, or increased immunological capability. These benefits are set against risks of immunological reactions, circulatory overload, metabolic complications, and infection. Transfusions should not be employed when safer alternatives exist. Because of the risks of infection and limited shelf life, procedures for collection and storage of blood are of critical importance and in many respects regulated by statutes.

Collection and Storage

Statutes governing blood collection, storage, and transportation include those established by the Food and Drug Administration, state and local health authorities, the American Red Cross, and the American Association of Blood Banks. Procedures have been greatly improved in recent years.

Prospective donors must meet certain criteria, some for their own protection, some for the protection of potential recipients. Donors are disqualified if they have had hepatitis, acquired immune deficiency syndrome, heart disease, cancer, severe asthma, bleeding disorders, or convulsions. A donor may also be temporarily refused by reason of exposure to malaria or hepatitis, pregnancy, major surgery, anemia, hypertension, hypotension, previous blood donation within the last 2 months, or if they are taking medications.

The usual donation of 450 mL of blood is collected into a special plastic bag with a nonwettable surface that minimizes clotting. The bag also contains an anticoagulant preservative, usually citrate phosphate dextrose (CPD) or adenine-supplemented citrate phosphate dextrose (CPDA-1). Blood can be stored with CPD for up to 21 days, or with CPDA-1 for up to 35 days. The dextrose in these preservatives provides an energy source for the RBCs. Even in the best of conditions, whole blood or packed red cells undergo deterioration during storage. The number of surviving RBCs declines, the pH falls, plasma hemoglobin rises, and plasma potassium increases.

In the blood bank, blood is examined and classified. The blood is screened for antibodies, the virus responsible for acquired immune deficiency syndrome (AIDS), and hepatitis B surface antigen. Classification is performed with respect to ABO and Rh typing.

Blood Typing

Red blood cells contain two specific surface antigens or agglutinogens, identified as A and B. The erythrocytes in group A blood possess only the A antigen; the plasma of group A blood will possess an antibody for the B antigen. Group B blood presents the opposite situation: RBCs with the B surface antigen and plasma with the A antibody. Group AB blood has erythrocytes with both surface antigens, but neither antibody in the plasma. Group O blood has RBCs without surface antigens but plasma containing both antibodies. Individuals with type A blood can be given type A or type O but not type B. Type B individuals can receive only types B or O. Type AB individuals can receive types A, B, AB, or O, but individuals with type O can be given only type O blood, since they have antibodies to both A and B antigens.

Transfusions conducted with blood that has not been properly matched with respect to the ABO system precipitates a severe immunological reaction that leads to hemolysis of the donor RBCs. In elective surgery, full compatibility can be assured by collecting blood from the client during the weeks prior to surgery.

Rh-factor is an additional element determining blood compatibility. It differs from the AB agglutinogens in that there is no natural antibody to Rh-factor. Patients who are Rh-negative are lacking in the factor but if exposed to Rh-positive blood will produce antibodies for the Rh-antigen. The consequence of Rh-antibody production, hemolysis of the donor RBCs, is not observed until the second exposure, during a second transfusion for example. A type of Rh-incompatibility reaction is erythroblastosis fetalis. If an Rh-negative mother gives birth to an Rh-positive child, exchange of blood during delivery may trigger formation of Rh-antibodies in the mother. If she then becomes pregnant with a second Rh-positive child, the Rh-antibodies will enter the fetal circulation via the placenta. This causes hemolysis of RBCs of the fetus, leading to anemia and possibly death. Erythroblastosis fetalis can be prevented by intramuscular administration of 300 μg of anti-Rh immune globulin (RhoGAM) to the mother at the time of delivery of the first Rh-positive baby. This drug destroys Rh-positive RBCs that might enter the maternal circulation in much the same manner as Rh-antibodies do, but the drug, unlike natural Rh-antibodies, is itself destroyed in a short time.

Individuals with O-negative blood have neither A- nor B-antigens on their RBCs nor Rh-factor. These individuals are known as universal donors since their blood is compatible for any recipient. Individuals with AB-positive blood have both A- and B-antigens and Rh-factor. These individuals are known as universal recipients since they can receive any type of blood without incompatibility reaction.

Blood Preparations

Blood obtained from donors is valuable not only for rapid replacement of blood lost during hemorrhage but also as a source of separate blood components. Blood components can be stored for longer periods of time than whole blood and provide a means of furnishing a single missing element in a deficiency condition without additional blood components that might trigger immunological reactions.

Whole Blood

Whole blood is less available than it once was because of the diversion of whole blood to the preparation of blood components. Whole blood is, nevertheless, still used for replacement in situations of rapid, massive blood loss due to hemorrhage or trauma. In situations of this sort, volume depletion is generally more critical than loss of specific blood components, so plasma expanders such as saline or dextran often suffice if whole blood is unavailable. Whole blood is also used in exchange transfusions in treatment of hemolysis in the newborn due to erythroblastosis fetalis. It is also used in management of hereditary defects of hemoglobin synthesis such as sickle-cell anemias. With whole blood transfusions, there is maximum risk of complications from incompatibility, immunological reactions, or hepatitis, because all blood components are present.

Packed Cells

When the major clinical goal is to increase oxygen-carrying capacity rather than to correct volume contraction, **packed red blood cells** can be utilized without the involvement of other blood components. Even when volume expansion is required, fluids such as saline can be given concurrently. RBC concentrates should not be administered with intravenous fluids other than saline. Ringer's solution causes clotting and 5% dextrose in water causes clumping and decreased RBC viability. Packed RBCs are useful in some types of anemia, such as certain hemolytic anemias, aplastic anemia, and sickle-cell anemia. They are also used for short-term prophylaxis against secondary complications of iron- or vitamin-deficiency anemias. **Frozen RBCs** are mixed with glycerol, frozen, and later thawed. This preparation is relatively expensive but is useful for clients who have unusual immunological or repeated febrile reactions. **Leukocyte-poor RBCs,** prepared by centrifugation, serve a similar purpose. **Washed RBCs** are used in patients who exhibit immunological reactions to donor plasma constituents.

Platelet packs or concentrates can be employed in thrombocytopenia, especially when severe or associated with bleeding. **Granulocyte transfusion** is new and experimental. It is used in sepsis associated with panhypoplasia caused by anticancer drugs.

Plasma and Plasma Components

Plasma is obtained from fresh blood after elimination of the formed elements. It can be concentrated, dehydrated, frozen, and reconstituted as required. The shelf life of frozen plasma is in excess of 2 years, but after thawing it must be used within 2 hours. It provides a source for all clotting factors except platelets and can be used effectively to control bleeding episodes. It is an ideal plasma expander.

As noted earlier in this chapter, specific **clotting factors** can be purified from plasma for use in clients with hemophilias. Factor VII, antihemophilic factor is employed in type A hemophilia. Prothrombin complex concentrates, containing factors II, VII, IX, and X, are available for type B hemophilia.

Normal human serum albumin is a hepatitis-free preparation of albumin, the major plasma protein fraction. It is excellent for use with fluids as a volume expander when the immediate concern is expansion of the intravascular compartment. It is also useful for treatment of hypoalbuminemia. It is available in 5 and 25 g/100 ml solutions. **Gamma-globulin preparations** find use in certain immune deficiency disorders and in prevention of viral hepatitis in exposed persons, such as health professionals.

Transfusion Procedures

An intravenous infusion, through an 18 gauge needle or larger, is begun usually with isotonic saline. Ringer's solution or 5% dextrose are not used because of incompatibility with whole blood or red blood cell concentrates. The blood unit is carefully checked (by two persons if specified by hospital regulations) to ensure that it is designated for the patient at hand, that the blood type is compatible, that it is the correct preparation, and that the expiration date is appropriate. The transfusion record is signed by the two specified persons. The unit of blood is mixed (and warmed if several units are to be given), attached to a "Y" blood-administration unit with filter set, and allowed to run into the isotonic saline. If the preparation for infusion is a RBC pack, 50–100 ml of saline are allowed to mix with the RBCs initially to reduce viscosity and facilitate flow. Flow rate is set so as to complete transfusion of a single unit in less than 2 hours. Packed cells are infused more slowly than whole blood. Dividing the transfusion of a given unit over 2 days should be avoided.

Observation during the first 15 minutes is especially important since this is the period during which most immunological and febrile reactions occur. If an adverse reaction is noted, the transfusion should be stopped and the blood bank should be notified. Upon completion of the transfusion, appropriate forms and the empty blood container are sent to the blood bank.

Complications of Blood Transfusion

One common type of complication of blood transfusion is **hemolytic transfusion reaction.** It occurs when the blood is incorrectly matched to the recipient with respect to ABO, Rh-factor, or plasma compatibility. ABO incompatibility reactions are more severe. The symptoms generally occur rapidly and consist of fever and chills, flushing, tachycardia, tachypnea, pain in the back and thighs, and burning sensations near the site of infusion. The transfusion should be stopped and vital signs monitored. Intake and output measures are begun, and the unused blood is returned to the blood bank. Possible complications of ABO incompatibilities include disseminated intravascular coagulation and renal failure. Mannitol (Osmitrol) (20 mg), an osmotic diuretic, is given by infusion to promote osmotic diuresis so as to ward off renal failure. Volume is maintained by continued saline infusion. Alkalinization of the urine (by administration of sodium bicarbonate) will reduce heme precipitation in the renal tubules. Rh-incompatibility reactions consist mainly of hemolysis and are usually mild, except in erythroblastosis fetalis.

Febrile reactions may develop after repeated transfusions. Symptoms include fever, chills, nausea, vomiting, headache, and back pain. These reactions are due to appearance of antigens to donor white blood cells. Specially prepared RBC packs, such as frozen-thawed or leukocyte-poor RBCs, can be used to eliminate febrile reactions in patients exhibiting this complication.

Allergic reactions sometimes occur to unknown antigenic components of donor blood. Symptoms are usually of the mild variety, including urticaria, edema, sore throat, eosinophilia, asthmatic reactions, dizziness, and headache. Rarely, violent anaphylactoid reactions occur.

Addition of too much fluid volume may result in **circulatory overload.** This is most likely to be problematic in patients with impaired cardiac function, possibly leading to congestive heart failure.

Complications of **massive transfusion** may include citrate or potassium accumulation. Citrate may cause hypocalcemia. With massive transfusions, 10 ml of 10% calcium gluconate should be given for every 2 units of blood. Potassium accumulation occurs in whole blood stored longer than a week. Most blood preparations do not contain concentrations of platelets comparable to those in the recipient's blood. Massive transfusion may dilute platelet concentration to the point that clotting is significantly impaired. Administration of platelet concentrations will correct this problem.

There is always a risk that transfusion will result in **transmission of infections.** Viral hepatitis may occur following infusions of whole blood or plasma. It is especially likely to occur from use of blood products that require pooling of blood from multiple donors, such as clotting factor concentrates and fibrinogen. Hepatitis risk is not eliminated by freezing plasma but is eliminated from plasma protein preparations by heating at 60° C for 10 hours. Blood banks routinely screen blood for evidence of hepatitis B surface antigens, but present methods identify only 30–60% of contaminated units. Current tests also fail to detect hepatitis A or other non-B viruses, and these now cause the majority of hepatitis infections from blood transfusion. The incidence with which the hepatitis antigen is found in donated blood varies by geographical region from 0.05% to as high as 2% of samples.

Other microorganisms that are occasionally transmitted by transfusion are bacteria and plasmodium (malaria). Although all donors are asked if they have had malaria, some are unaware that they have. Most bacteria do not proliferate in refrigerated blood, but a few gram-negative varieties do. Transfusion of heavily infested blood units may cause fatal sepsis. Blood should be warmed to room temperature only when multiple units are to be given, so that bacterial growth will be minimized. In recent years, there has been considerable concern about transmission of acquired immune deficiency syndrome (AIDS) as a result of blood transfusions. Screening procedures are now in place, but are less than 100% effective in identifying contaminated blood.

Case Study: Iron-Deficiency Anemia

Mrs. H. told the nurse that she bought all her foods at a nature health food store because they contained no additives or preservatives. In further discussion, however, the nurse uncovered the fact that in an effort to lose weight, Mrs. H. was following a fad diet that limited her intake to fresh fruits and a few vegetables. No grain foods were included, and she did not like many of the other foods that were allowed and might have provided sufficient iron and vitamin E. At the time of the nurse's assessment, Mrs. H. was complaining of constant fatigue and lack of energy and feeling faint much of the time.

After putting together a dietary profile, the nurse realized that Mrs. H. was following a diet almost designed to cause anemia because of its deficiency. The nurse was then able to discuss the changes that needed to be instituted to promote health. In time, Mrs. H. was able to report a lessening of fatigue, increased energy, and a loss of the desired weight. Her progress toward anemia was halted and she was able to achieve an improved state of health.

1. What foods might the nurse have suggested as dietary sources of iron?
2. If Mrs. H. had been unable to obtain sufficient iron even after correcting dietary deficiencies, the nurse would have referred her to a physician for medical help. What kind of preparation might have been prescribed?
3. Is it really very likely that a middle-class American would experience iron deficiency? What circumstances might contribute?

Answers appear at the end of the book.

Case Study: Pulmonary Embolism Secondary to Deep Vein Thrombosis

B. E., a 32-year-old woman, was admitted to the hospital suffering from sudden pleuritic chest pain. The admitting nurse noted that B. E. had a red, swollen area in her right calf. B. E. told her that she had just returned from a long trip by car and that the swelling had developed during the ride. The nurse took her vital signs, finding a blood pressure of 118/78, pulse of 105/minute, respirations at 27/minute, and a temperature of 100.5° F. There were no abnormal respiratory sounds. The medication history indicated that B. E. employed a combination birth control pill. The nurse reported her findings to the physician.

The physician ordered a chest x-ray, lung scan, measurement of blood gases, and a prothrombin time. Blood analysis indicated hypoxia and mild respiratory alkalosis. The x-ray and lung scans demonstrated a small mass in the right lung associated with a region of diminished perfusion but no ventilation defect. The condition was diagnosed as a pulmonary embolism secondary to deep vein thrombosis.

The physician ordered an initial intravenous injection of 10,000 units of heparin to be followed by 5,000 units every 6 hours; warfarin (Coumadin), 10 mg, PO, once daily (unless prothrombin time exceeds 25 seconds); diazepam (Valium) as needed for anxiety; oxygen as needed for hypoxia; daily determination of prothrombin time; and discontinuation of birth control pills. The nurse placed B. E. on bedrest, with the right leg elevated, with oxygen administered nasally, and a heating pad placed over the right calf. During the first day, the nurse monitored vital signs and examined the patient for signs of bleeding every 2 hours. She instructed B. E. to report immediately any occurrence of nose bleeds, purpura, ecchymosis, bloody stools, or blood in the urine. Respiratory rate and blood oxygen returned to normal after 24 hours and oxygen was discontinued. The patient showed no further signs of dyspnea or deep respirations. Prothrombin time measurements were taken each morning and increased daily, reaching 22 seconds on the fourth day. The physician changed the warfarin dosage to 5 mg/day, and subsequent prothrombin time measurements stabilized at 22 seconds.

The nursing staff began educating B. E. about her condition, the rationale for the drug treatments, potential adverse effects, dietary restrictions during warfarin therapy, the need to consult with the physician before using other drugs, and methods for decreasing likelihood of further thromboembolism in the future. When B. E. began menstruating on the sixth day, the nurse instructed her to monitor for unusual flow. The nurse scheduled a consultation with the hospital's gynecologist to provide B. E. with information concerning birth control alternatives to oral contraceptives.

On the eighth day after admission, a lung scan indicated that lung perfusion was improving. The physician ordered discontinuation of heparin. On the tenth day, the prothrombin measurement was 20 seconds. B. E. was discharged on a regimen of 5 mg warfarin daily, PO. She was scheduled for a follow-up evaluation in 5 days.

1. What was the relationship between the swelling in the calf and the pulmonary embolism?
2. Which of the initial vital signs were abnormal and consistent with a diagnosis of pulmonary embolism?
3. What was the reason for the hypoxia and respiratory alkalosis? Why was prothrombin time measured before any anticoagulant had been given?
4. Why was therapy initiated with both heparin and warfarin? Why was one given intravenously and the other orally?
5. What laboratory test might have been used to monitor heparin therapy? Why would prothrombin time not be appropriate?
6. Why was it necessary to discontinue the oral contraceptive?
7. Why was the nurse concerned about signs of bleeding?
8. What dietary restriction did the nurse likely indicate to B. E.?
9. Why was heparin discontinued before discharging the client?

Answers appear at the end of the book.

Recommended Readings

Drugs and Erythropoiesis

Callender ST: Treatment of iron deficiency, in Jacobs A, Worwood M (eds): *Biochemistry and Medicine.* New York, Academic Press Inc, 1974, pp 529–542.

Finck CA, Huebers H: Perspectives in iron metabolism. *N Engl J Med* 1982;306:1520–1528.

Drugs and Hemostasis

Brignoli ETB (ed): Using the antithrombotic agents. *Patient Care* 1980;14:62.

Chamberlain SL: Low-dose heparin therapy. *Am J Nurs* 1980;80:1115–1117.

Chatterjee K, Rouleau JL, Parmley WW: Medical management of patients with angina. *JAMA* 1984;252(9):1170–1176.

Griffin JP: Be prepared for the bleeding patient. *Nursing* 1986;16(6):34–42.

Hirsh J et al: Using the antithrombotic agents. *Patient Care* 1980;14:62.

Laffel GL, Braunwald E: Thrombolytic therapy — a new strategy for the treatment of acute myocardial infarction. *N Engl J Med* 1984;311(11):710–717, 311(12):770–776.

Lewis HD Jr et al: Protective effects of aspirin against acute myocardial infarction and death in men with unstable angina: Results of a Veterans' Administration study. *N Engl J Med* 1983;309:396–403.

Moore K, Maschak B: How patient education can reduce the risk of anticoagulation. *Nursing* 1977;7(9):24–29.

Rosenberg JM, Kirschenbaum JL: What to watch for with heparin. *RN* 1981;44(9):50–52.

Thompson DA: Teaching the client about anticoagulants. *Am J Nurs* 1982;82:278–281.

Weykei D: Current status of anticoagulant therapy. *Am J Med* 1982;72:659–664.

Blood Transfusions

Committee on Transfusion Practices, American Association of Blood Banks: The latest protocols for blood transfusions. *Nursing* 1986;16(10):34–42.

Querin JJ, Stahl LD: Twelve simple sensible steps for successful blood transfusions. *Nursing* 1983;13(11):34–44.

Smith L: Reactions to transfusions. *Am J Nurs* 1984;84(9):1096–1101.

UNIT VII

Drugs, Metabolism, and Nutrition

CHAPTER 42

Body Fluids and Electrolytes

Regulation of Body Fluids

The human body is composed largely of water — 50–70% of total body weight consists of this simple fluid. Since adipose (fat) tissue has a low water content, the water fraction is highest in persons who are thin. Water is an excellent solvent, facilitating dispersion of substances throughout the body and promoting ionization of many particles. The composition of body fluids, sometimes called the sea within us, must be carefully maintained by regulatory mechanisms of the body.

The fluid of the body is divided among various compartments, the two major ones being the intracellular and extracellular compartments. The intracellular comprises somewhat more than half the total body water. The extracellular includes the interstitial fluid and the plasma, and makes up about 35% of the total water of the body. The final 10% is found associated with the lungs, gastrointestinal tract, nephrourinary system, the eye, and other tissues.

The concentration of ions within the various fluid compartments controls fluid exchange between compartments. The total concentration of all solute particles within a fluid is usually expressed as *osmolarity*. The unit of measurement of osmolarity is the milliosmole (mosm). An osmole is 1 gram molecular weight of solute per liter of solvent, and a milliosmole is one-thousandth of an osmole. Membranes in the body are semipermeable, permitting passage of water but only certain solutes. If the fluids on the two sides of a membrane differ in osmolarity, water is drawn from the side of low osmolarity to the side of higher osmolarity. This tendency is called **osmotic pressure.** Only those solutes that cannot freely pass through the membrane contribute to osmotic pressure and hence water movement. Osmotic pressure between the intracellular and extracellular compartments is largely determined by sodium, the most abundant solute for which cell membranes provide an effective penetration barrier.

Disturbances of body fluid balance are common, occurring in many illnesses, including congestive heart failure, trauma, hypertension, diabetes, ulcerative colitis, and protracted diarrhea or vomiting. In each of these, nursing interventions designed to reestablish fluid balance often play a central role in restoring health. Three types of disturbances occur in the composition of body fluids: (1) disturbances of volume and osmolality, (2) disturbances of acid-base balance, and (3) disturbances of specific ion concentrations.

Disturbances of Volume and Osmolality

In the human body, intake and output of water are normally balanced. Water intake consists of drinking fluids (about 1,200 ml daily), water ingested in foods (approximately 1,000 ml daily), and water formed in metabolic processes (300–500 ml daily). Output of water occurs principally as urine and sweat, and to a lesser extent through expired water vapor, in the feces, as saliva, and as tears. Milk production contributes significantly to water loss in lactating females. Fluid homeostasis is maintained through the combined activities of the kidneys, lungs, pituitary gland, parathyroid glands, and adrenal glands, as well as other tissues less directly. When the balance between intake and output is upset, an abnormal state develops. Such fluid abnormalities are best characterized by considering two fundamental aspects of body fluid composition: volume and osmolality.

Disturbances of Fluid Volume

Dehydration (fluid contraction) is a reduction of water volume, while **overhydration** (fluid expansion) is an increase of water volume. Dehydration can be caused by excess losses, inadequate intake, or both. Vomiting, hemorrhage, bowel obstruction, diarrhea, and fever are common causes. Under clinical circumstances of dehydration, water is lost first from the extracellular compartment. Resulting changes in osmotic pressure then either increase or decrease intracellular water, altering the metabolic and functional capacity of the cells.

Symptoms of dehydration include sudden loss of weight; flushed, dry skin; loss of skin turgor; dry or cracked lips; and a reduction in urine output (urine flow rates less than 25 ml/hour suggest dehydration) or an unusually dark coloration or elevated specific gravity of the urine. Clients may complain of dry mouth and thirst. As dehydration worsens, clients may feel tired, weak, and ill. Orthostatic hypotension and rapid pulse and respiration may ensue. Nausea and vomiting may develop and further aggravate fluid and electrolyte imbalance.

Overhydration is most often associated with congestive heart failure, liver cirrhosis, renal disease, aldosteronism, excessive sodium ingestion, water intoxication, incorrect intravenous fluid therapy, or malnutrition. Water increases first in the extracellular compartment (usually the plasma compartment) but ultimately affects the intracellular milieu as well through changes in interstitial osmotic pressure. Acute weight gain, elevated venous blood pressure, edema, or ascites are signs that should alert the nurse to possible overhydration. Pulmonary edema should be suspected if basilar rales are present in spite of an adequate cough reflex, and can be confirmed by x-ray examination. Fear, pain, acute infection, and acute stress are frequent causes of water retention. Symptoms include poor attention, loss of coordination, sleeplessness, shouting and violent behavior, muscle weakness, and eventually delirium, convulsions, and coma. Hematological studies typically reveal a decrease in hemoglobin concentration or hematocrit.

Disturbances of Osmolality

Dehydration or overhydration may or may not be accompanied by changes in osmotic pressure. If osmotic pressure is disturbed, treatment must correct both the volume and osmolality imbalances. If osmotic pressure is not altered, treatment must correct the volume problem without disturbing osmotic balance. In either case, the clinicians involved must have an accurate profile of the fluid and electrolyte status of the individual under treatment. Disturbances of volume and sodium osmolality can be divided into six types, three involving volume contraction and three involving volume expansion (Table 42–1), since either contraction or expansion can be hypertonic, isotonic, or hypotonic.

Isotonic contraction is a proportionate loss of water and sodium and is often caused by intense diarrhea or vomiting. Water is not drawn out of the

Table 42–1
Characteristics of Volume/Osmolality Disorders

Type of volume/osmolality disorder	Clinical example	Volume: ECW	Volume: ICW	Plasma sodium concentration	Treatment
Hypertonic contraction	Excessive sweating	↓	↓	↑	Half-normal saline; 5% dextrose
Isotonic contraction	Severe diarrhea or vomiting	↓	0	0	Saline; plasma expander
Hypotonic contraction	Adrenal insufficiency	↓	↑	↓	Hypertonic saline and bicarbonate
Hypertonic expansion	Infusion of hypertonic saline	↑	↓	↑	Stop infusion
Isotonic expansion	Edema	↑	0	0	Diuretics
Hypotonic expansion	Water intoxication	↑	↑	↓	Fluid restriction or hypertonic saline and a diuretic

Key: ECW = extracellular water; ICW = intracellular water.

intracellular compartment in this kind of disturbance because osmotic pressure is unchanged. If the fluid loss occurs from a transcellular compartment, such as the gastrointestinal tract (due to vomiting or diarrhea), treatment is usually the administration of a fluid that resembles extracellular fluid, such as normal saline. This will replenish the two extracellular compartments, plasma and interstitial fluid, proportionately. If volume depletion is severe enough to compromise circulation, a plasma expander can be administered. Acid-base disturbances often accompany isotonic contraction — alkalosis from loss of acidic stomach fluid in prolonged vomiting, or acidosis from loss of alkaline diarrheal fluid in persistent diarrhea. When isotonic contraction is due to hemorrhage, the optimum therapeutic response is administration of properly matched whole blood. A plasma expander is the next most effective treatment, and in a crisis, normal saline may be given.

Hypertonic contraction occurs when water is lost in excess of sodium loss and is most often due to prolonged exposure to heat, such as sunlight, without an adequate source of water replacement. In the hospital, it may occur when a patient is unable to take water because of coma or delirium and too little water is provided parenterally. Other possible causes are osmotic diuresis, diabetes mellitus, and diabetes insipidus. Hypertonic contraction is alleviated by oral water or parenteral hypotonic saline.

Hypotonic contraction is sodium loss in excess of water loss, which occurs, for example, when the kidneys fail to reabsorb enough sodium, either because of inadequate aldosterone or chronic renal insufficiency. It also occurs when health care providers administer dextrose solutions lacking salt to treat isotonic contraction, or when individuals replenish water lost in exercise but not salt. In hypotonic contraction, reduced extracellular osmotic pressure causes water to be taken up into the intracellular compartment, further aggravating extracellular volume contraction. Hypotonic contraction is treated by administration of hypertonic saline and bicarbonate (to prevent acidosis due to bicarbonate dilution).

Isotonic expansion, also called **edema,** is a proportionate retention of water and sodium. It is a major factor in hypertension. Treatment centers on use of diuretics to increase sodium and water elimination. Edema can also occur when isotonic saline is administered in excess during intravenous fluid therapy. Nurses should be familiar with the signs of edema and its gradations.

Hypertonic expansion is seen when sodium retention occurs in excess of water retention. This disorder is usually iatrogenic, occurring when too much salt is given orally or too much hypertonic saline is given intravenously.

Hypotonic expansion occurs when water is retained in excess of sodium. The usual cause is water intoxication due to excessive intake of water. Clients in this situation complain of headache, nausea and vomiting, muscle pain and weakness, and abdominal cramps. If the condition is not corrected, the client will ultimately go into a stupor, coma, or convulsions. Less commonly, hypotonic expansion occurs with excess ADH secretion or excess intravenous administration of hypotonic fluids. Cardiac, liver, or renal failure are additional causes. When hypotonic expansion develops gradually, it is treated gradually by fluid restriction. When hypotonic expansion occurs rapidly, however, clients can become agitated, confused, or go into convulsions or coma. Treatment is therefore initiated quickly with intravenous administration of hypertonic saline (which corrects the hypotonic state immediately but temporarily aggravates the fluid expansion) and possibly a diuretic.

Preparations for Treating Disturbances of Volume and Osmolality

The preparations used for correcting disturbances of volume and osmolality include saline, dextrose, combinations of these two, balanced electrolyte solutions (Table 42–2), and plasma expanders. To these may be added single-salt solutions (discussed under Electrolytes, later in this chapter) as required by the individual patient.

Saline

Sodium chloride (NaCl) is available as **normal saline** (in isotonic solutions of 0.85 or 0.9%), as half-normal saline, or in hypertonic solutions of 3.0 or 5.0%. Normal saline contains 154 mEq of both sodium and chloride. It is used to replace body fluids in isotonic contraction, and in crises for any condition of volume contraction when osmolality has not been determined. Given adequate renal function, normal saline will provide the raw material for correcting volume depletion and restoring osmolar balance. Levels of sodium and chloride should be monitored when saline solutions are used to alleviate hyponatremia.

Normal saline is used for initiating and terminating red blood cell transfusions. It has the effect of minimizing clumping of cells. However, nurses should recognize that saline is contraindicated for those with renal dysfunction or congestive heart failure, those on sodium-free diets, and those with hypoproteinemia. **Hypertonic saline** is useful for clients experiencing hypotonic contraction while **half-normal saline with dextrose** is useful in hypertonic contraction.

Dextrose Solutions

Dextrose solutions in water or half-normal saline are valuable for providing water in excess of salt. They are virtually isotonic with blood so that water is not unduly drawn into the intracellular compartment. Appropriate rates of administration provide 1 L over a period of 3.5–5 hours, up to a maximum of 3 L/day. Fructose is available as an alternative in a 10% solution. Rapid intravenous injections of dextrose may cause glycosuria (producing "false-positives" in urine testing by diabetics). Dextrose and fructose are fully metabolized via normal pathways of carbohydrate metabolism.

Multiple-Salt Solutions

Multiple-salt solutions available commercially include **Ringer's solution** and others listed in Table 42–2. All are isotonic but they differ in the balance between electrolyte and nonelectrolyte components. High-electrolyte solutions contain mainly ionizable electrolytes; medium-electrolyte solutions contain dextrose and lesser amounts of electrolytes. Multiple-salt solutions are employed for maintenance or replacement, after normal hydration is established.

Plasma Expanders: Dextran

When vascular volume depletion must be corrected quickly, a plasma expander can be employed. **Plasma protein fraction** is a sterile solution of 5% human plasma proteins in normal saline. It is isotonic with plasma and contains not less than 83% albumin proteins. **Albumin human** is a sterile solution of purified human albumin protein in 5% or 25% concentrations in sodium chloride solutions that are close to normal.

Dextran is the major synthetic plasma expander. It is derived from a naturally occurring polysaccharide that consists of units of glucose linked together in large chains. These chains are partially hydrolyzed to yield strands of various lengths.

Mechanisms and Effects Dextran provides osmolar units that remain in the vascular compartment to hold water and maintain blood pressure. Dextran increases blood pressure, pulse pressure, central venous pressure, and cardiac output. It increases venous return to the heart, microcirculation, and urinary output. Dextran is slowly hydrolyzed in the body to glucose.

Clinical Indication Dextran is used in adjunctive treatment of shock or impending shock caused by hemorrhage, burns, surgery, or other trauma. It is

Table 42–2
Composition of Preparations for Treating Disturbances of Volume and Osmolality

Type	Glucose	Cations				Anions				
		Na^+	K^+	Ca^{++}	Mg^{++}	Cl^-	HCO_3^-	$PO_4^=$	Lactate	Acetate
I. Electrolyte solutions										
A. Saline (NaCl)										
1. 0.45% (half-normal)		73								
2. 0.85% (normal)		145								
3. 0.9%		154								
4. 3.0%		513								
5. 5.0%		856								
B. Dextrose in water										
1. 5%	50									
2. 10%	100									
3. 20%	200									
C. Dextrose in saline										
1. 5% in isotonic saline	50	145								
2. 5% half-normal saline	50	73								
3. 2.5% in half-normal saline	25	73								
D. Multiple electrolyte, high content										
1. Ringer's solution		147	4	5		156				
2. Hypotonic Ringer's		103	5	5	3	116				
3. Lactated Ringer's (Hartmann's solution)		130	4	3		109			28	
E. Multiple electrolytes, medium content										
1. Ionosol B		57	25		5	108	50		27	23
2. Normosol-M		140	5		3	98	50			
3. Plasma-Lyte		140	10	5	3	103	55		8	47
4. Polysal		140	10	5	3	103				55

Type	Content
II. Plasma Expanders	
A. Plasma protein fraction	5% in normal saline
B. Albumin human	5% in 130–160 mEq of NaCl 25% in 130–160 mEq of NaCl
C. Dextran	
1. 70 or 75 injection	6% dextran 70 or 75 in 0.9% NaCl, 5% dextrose, or 10% invert sugar-fructose/dextrose
2. 40 injection	10% dextran 40 in 0.9% NaCl or 5% dextrose

Key: Electrolyte concentrations in mEq/L; glucose in g/L.

also used prophylactically and therapeutically in the treatment of venous thrombosis and pulmonary embolism.

Adverse Effects and Contraindications The major drawback of dextran is a rather frequent incidence of allergic reactions, approaching 10%. Reactions include pruritus, urticaria, and joint pains.

If a client is poorly hydrated, dextran may actually attract water from the extravascular spaces, resulting in further dehydration. *Should this occur, nurses can expect the client to have dry skin and mucous membranes, an elevated temperature, decreased urinary output, and an elevated specific gravity.*

Preparations and Administration Dextran is provided in normal saline or 5% dextrose solutions. Dextran 70 (Macrodex) utilizes strands with molecular weights averaging 70,000; dextran 75 (Gentran 75) employs strands averaging 75,000; and dextran 40 (Rheomacrodex, Gentran 40) contains shorter strands of about 40,000 molecular weight. All of these molecular weights approximate those of albumin proteins.

Important Nursing Implications for Dextran

- ☐ Be certain to use the prescribed molecular weight — dextran 40, 70, or 75. If the order is not specific, it is a nursing responsibility to have the order clarified in writing before using the drug.
- ☐ Assess for signs of hypersensitivity such as generalized urticaria, pruritis, flushing, wheezing, and complaints of chill, fever, or tightness in the chest. Since these reactions are most apt to occur during the first few minutes of administration, nurses need to monitor vital signs closely for at least the first 20 minutes. At the first sign of a reaction, the infusion should be terminated and other means of sustaining circulation used. Nurses should *always* have on hand resuscitation equipment, epinephrine, ephedrine, steroids, and antihistamines in the event of a reaction. Unless treated immediately, allergic reactions could progress to anaphylactic shock and cardiac and respiratory arrest.
- ☐ When large doses of dextran are used, check for prolonged bleeding and clotting times, a decreased hematocrit, or decreased plasma protein levels, all of which are related to excessive dilution of blood constituents.
- ☐ Monitor pulse, blood pressure, and urine output at least every 5–15 minutes for the first hour after dextran is administered. At the first indication of renal dysfunction, dextran should be discontinued.
- ☐ Check urine specific gravity at regular intervals after giving dextran. Low specific gravity may be an indication that dextran is not being cleared by the kidneys and should be discontinued.
- ☐ Remember that dextran may alter certain tests for blood glucose, urinary protein, and bilirubin. The laboratory should be alerted to the fact that the client is receiving dextran before the various samples are sent for analysis.
- ☐ Determine the client's blood type before administering dextran since plasma expanders can interfere with blood typing and cross-matching.

Acid-Base Disturbances

Another type of disturbance of body fluids occurs when pH is altered. There are four fundamental types of acid-base imbalance: respiratory acidosis, respiratory alkalosis, metabolic acidosis, and metabolic alkalosis (Table 42–3). The usual means of assessing a suspected acid-base disturbance is by examination of blood pH, P_{CO_2}, and total CO_2. When the problem is caused by disturbed pulmonary function, adjustments in renal function may fully or partially compensate for the imbalance.

Respiratory Acidosis

In respiratory acidosis, poor ventilation brings about an increase in the partial pressure of carbon dioxide (P_{CO_2}) in the blood. This results in formation of carbonic acid, which ionizes to generate hydrogen ions and a drop in plasma pH. Clients most likely to develop respiratory acidosis include those who have bronchitis, pulmonary edema, chronic obstructive pulmonary disease (COPD), asthma, or pneumonia, or those who have been taking respiratory depressant drugs, such as morphine, sedatives, or alcohol. Others at risk include those receiving surgical anesthesia and those experiencing mechanical asphyxiation. The kidneys attempt to compensate for respiratory acidosis by increasing reabsorption of bicarbonate, which can be used to buffer the acidity. Chloride is excreted in place of bicarbonate in this process, so hypochloremia is a frequent concomitant of respiratory acidosis.

Unfortunately, the signs of acute respiratory acidosis are not very specific. A decreased rate and depth of respiration, a low blood pH, elevated P_{CO_2}, and slightly elevated serum sodium and potassium are usual indications. Some clients develop CO_2 narcosis, a serious complication in chronic respiratory acidosis.

Treatment for respiratory acidosis is based on improving respiration. Bronchodilators for asthma and COPD, antibiotics for bacterial pneumonias, elimination of respiratory depressants, or mechanical ventilation may be indicated. Oxygen must be used cautiously since this could suppress the respiratory drive. Bicarbonate administration is reserved for severe acidosis.

Respiratory Alkalosis

Respiratory alkalosis occurs when P_{CO_2} has dropped as a result of hyperventilation, usually related to an emotional disturbance, but sometimes drug-induced (as in salicylate toxicity). Often, the kidneys are able

Table 42–3
Acid-Base Disturbances

Type	Some common causes	Initial event	Compensation	Treatment
Respiratory acidosis	Poor respiration (hyperventilation)	↑P_{CO_2}	Kidney: ↑HCO_3^- reabsorption; ↓Cl^-	Improve respiration: artificial respiration, bronchodilators; if severe, administer bicarbonate.
Respiratory alkalosis	Hyperventilation (emotional); salicylates	↓P_{CO_2}	Kidney: ↓HCO_3^- reabsorption; ↓Cl	Rebreathing; administer 5% CO_2; sedation.
Metabolic acidosis	Diabetic ketoacidosis; renal insufficiency; lactic acidosis; severe diarrhea	↓HCO_3^- or ↑acid from metabolism	Lungs: ↓P_{CO_2} Kidneys: ↑HCO_3^- reabsorption	Alleviate metabolic disorder; IV sodium bicarbonate.
Metabolic alkalosis	Vomiting; potassium depletion; administration of HCO_3^-	↑HCO_3^-	Lungs: ↑P_{CO_2} (limited); Kidney: ↓HCO_3^- reabsorption (limited) Other: organic acid accumulation in plasma	Correct primary problem; administer sodium cloride; if severe, administer ammonium chloride.

to compensate adequately for the fall in P_{CO_2} by decreasing bicarbonate reabsorption. Rebreathing air from a paper bag can alleviate the condition by elevating the P_{CO_2}. *Nurses need to teach clients more appropriate breathing patterns when they suspect the problem is caused by hyperventilation or improper breathing methods.*

Metabolic Acidosis

Metabolic acidosis is a decrease in blood pH related to excessive production of acid products (as in lactic acidosis or ketoacidosis), impaired acid excretion (as in renal tubular disease or chronic pyelonephritis), depletion of bicarbonate (as in severe diarrhea), or administration of excess amounts of acid drugs (such as salicylates) or acid-forming salts (such as ammonium chloride). Symptoms of metabolic acidosis include headache and weakness. Such clients are likely to take frequent deep breaths and to exhibit a flushed face and elevated pulse rate and pressures.

To compensate for metabolic acidosis, the lungs increase the blowing off of CO_2, and the kidneys increase bicarbonate reabsorption and elimination of hydrogen in the form of titratable acids and ammonium. When metabolic acidosis is chronic, as in diabetic ketoacidosis, lactic acidosis, or renal insufficiency, treatment rests on alleviating or controlling the underlying pathological process. For acute metabolic acidosis, sodium bicarbonate is the treatment of choice. Typically, one or more ampuls of 7.5% sodium bicarbonate is added to a 5% dextrose infusion solution. Lactated Ringer's solution and tromethamine (Tram) are alternative treatments but offer no advantages and certain disadvantages.

Metabolic Alkalosis

Metabolic alkalosis is an increase in serum pH, usually due to excess excretion of hydrogen ion. The body is only poorly capable of compensating for this rather unnatural condition. A client's respiration may slow slightly, bringing about an elevated P_{CO_2}, but the ensuing hypoxia and hypercapnia (excess CO_2 in the blood) severely limit this mechanism.

Metabolic alkalosis is often secondary to hypokalemia. In severe potassium depletion, hydrogen is drawn into the intracellular compartment, causing intracellular acidosis but extracellular (or systemic) alkalosis. Also, one type of ion pump in the kidney secretes either potassium or hydrogen in exchange for sodium. In hypokalemia, more hydrogen is exchanged with sodium because of the lack of potassium. Thus, metabolic alkalosis is a frequent concomitant of diuretic therapy, vomiting, excess mineralocorticoid activity (hyperaldosteronism, steroid therapy, or Cushing's disease), or dietary deficiency in potassium. Clients who are placed on gastric suction or who have repeated episodes of diarrhea are also prone to metabolic alkalosis.

Symptoms of metabolic alkalosis include irritability, confusion, and muscle twitching. Treatment usually involves saline and correction of potassium and chloride deficits. Administration of sodium chloride in metabolic alkalosis is effective because it increases the availability of sodium for excretion with bicarbonate. In particularly severe cases, direct acidification of the plasma may be accomplished by administering 2.14% ammonium chloride (NH_4Cl) parenterally. Ammonium is converted to urea in the liver, furnishing hydrogen ions in the process. In mild or chronic cases, treatment is directed at relieving the cause.

Solutions Used for Acid-Base Disturbances

The solutions used for treatment of acute or severe pH imbalance are ammonium chloride, sodium bicarbonate, potassium chloride, sodium lactate, Shohl's solution, and tromethamine (Table 42–4).

Ammonium Chloride

Clinical Indications Ammonium chloride (NH_4Cl) is useful in metabolic alkalosis, providing hydrogen ions indirectly and replacing lost chloride directly. Sodium chloride and potassium chloride (KCl) should be given concurrently. Ammonium chloride is used to correct chloride depletion following diuretic therapy, especially when mercurial diuretics have been used, and to lower urinary pH in the treatment of urinary tract infections. It is also used to aid clients in excreting certain basic drugs.

Table 42–4
Drugs Used for Acid-Base Imbalances

Drug	Use
Intravenous fluid additives	
26.8% ammonium chloride	Metabolic alkalosis
7.5% potassium chloride	Hypokalemia (often accompanies metabolic alkalosis)
14.9% potassium chloride	Same as 7.5% KCl
7.5% sodium bicarbonate	Metabolic acidosis (reserve treatment for respiratory acidosis)
28.0% sodium lactate	Metabolic acidosis (if lactate is not elevated)
0.3 mol tromethamine (Tham)	Metabolic acidosis
Oral medications	
Shohl's solution (Bicitra) (citric acid and hydrated sodium citrate)	Metabolic acidosis

Ammonium chloride is also used occasionally as an expectorant to decrease viscosity of bronchial secretions.

Adverse Effects and Contraindications Adverse reactions to ammonium chloride include skin rash, headache, and symptoms of hypokalemia, hyperglycemia, and glycosuria.

Preparations and Administration Ammonium chloride is available as a 2.14% solution for injection (0.14 mEq/ml) or as an additive for intravenous infusion fluids (26.8% solution; 100 mEq in 20 ml). Ammonium chloride may be given orally to acidify urine (4–12 g/day at 4-hour to 6-hour intervals), as an expectorant (250–500 mg for adults every 2–4 hours or 75 mg/kg/day in equally divided doses for children), and intravenously for metabolic alkalosis. When employed intravenously, it must be infused slowly.

Clients given ammonium chloride may develop nausea, anorexia, vomiting, and diarrhea from gastric irritation. *Nurses can minimize this problem by suggesting that enteric coated tablets be used and by having clients take the drug immediately after meals.* However, when used as an expectorant, the drug must not be enteric coated. *Rather, the nurse should administer it in liquid or noncoated tablet form and clients should be encouraged to drink a full glass of water with the medication.* The combination of drug and water may help to decrease the viscosity of bronchial secretions.

Important Nursing Implications for Ammonium Chloride

- ☐ While the client is receiving ammonium chloride, periodically check serum pH, carbon dioxide combining power, and serum electrolytes to assure that serious acidosis does not occur. Urinary pH should also be checked (normal 4.8–7.8).
- ☐ When ammonium chloride is administered intravenously, monitor the client for indications of adverse reactions, including pallor, sweating, irregular breathing, dysrhythmia, asterixis (liver flap), and twitching. To counteract these reactions, the nurse should always have on hand intravenous sodium bicarbonate or sodium lactate.
- ☐ Nurses need to report changes in the client's behavior as well as signs of weakness or altered voiding pattern to the physician.

Sodium Bicarbonate

Sodium bicarbonate ($NaHCO_3$) is the preferred treatment for metabolic acidosis and a reserve treatment for respiratory acidosis. It is available in 7.5% solution (45 mEq in 50 ml) for addition to intravenous fluid therapy. Excessive amounts may cause metabolic alkalosis. Caution should be exercised in clients exhibiting cardiac or renal disease. Sodium bicarbonate is sometimes employed as a home remedy for alleviation of gastric acidity. It is a short-acting systemic antacid that rapidly neutralizes gastric acid to form sodium chloride and water. Use of sodium bicarbonate in this manner may result in metabolic alkalosis and retention of excess sodium.

Important Nursing Implications for Sodium Bicarbonate

- ☐ Assess clients for reversal of the symptoms of metabolic acidosis (dry skin and mucous membranes, polydipsia, polyuria, and air hunger).
- ☐ When clients receive sodium bicarbonate to counteract metabolic acidosis, monitor blood pH, Po_2, Pco_2, HCO_3^-, and other electrolytes to ensure that the client is not developing alkalosis. The nurse noticing symptoms of alkalosis can sometimes reverse the situation by having the client rebreathe expired air in a paper bag or rebreathing mask. The nurse should always have on hand a parenteral solution of calcium gluconate and 2.14% ammonium chloride solution in the event of severe alkalosis or tetany.
- ☐ Warn clients to avoid over-the-counter drugs that contain sodium bicarbonate (Alka-Seltzer, Bromo-Seltzer, Fizrin, and others), since these can result in electrolyte imbalance.
- ☐ Warn clients that oral preparations of bicarbonate taken with milk or calcium can produce a milk-alkali syndrome leading to symptoms of anorexia, nausea, and vomiting. Sometimes clients become mentally confused.
- ☐ At intervals during the day, use nitrazine paper to test the urine of clients who are receiving sodium bicarbonate for alkalinization in order to monitor the client's progress and adjust the doses of sodium bicarbonate.

Other Solutions Used for Acid-Base Disturbances

Potassium chloride (KCl) is available in 7.5 or 14.9% solutions for addition to intravenous fluid therapy in ampuls containing 20 or 40 mEq in 20 ml. *Potassium chloride must never be given as an undiluted bolus as doing so can cause fatal cardiac dysrhythmias.* During infusion, the electrocardiogram should be monitored and serum potassium levels should be periodically determined. Potassium chloride is used for hypokalemia, a common cause of metabolic alkalosis.

Sodium lactate is available in 28.0% solutions (100 mEq in 40 ml) as an additive for intravenous fluid therapy. It can be used to treat metabolic acidosis except for lactic acidosis. Sodium lactate offers no advantages over sodium bicarbonate and it is slower, since its benefit depends on its being metabolized to bicarbonate.

Shohl's solution provides an oral dosage form for metabolic acidosis. It consists of citric acid and hydrated sodium citrate. **Tromethamine** (Tham) is a synthetic buffer used for metabolic acidosis. It is contraindicated in uremia, chronic respiratory acidosis, and pregnancy. It provides no special advantage over sodium bicarbonate.

Electrolytes and Minerals

In the extracellular fluid, sodium is the principal cation (positively charged ion), while chloride is the principal anion (negatively charged ion). Bicarbonate is the third most plentiful ion in the extracellular compartment. Sodium concentrations approximately equal those of chloride and bicarbonate together. Other important cations are potassium, calcium, and magnesium. Additional anions are phosphate, sulfate, and various organic anions.

The intracellular compartment has a quite different ionic character. Within cells, the concentration of potassium is about 15 times that of sodium. The second most abundant intracellular cation is magnesium. Phosphate and sulfate occur in high concentrations intracellularly and constitute the major anions in this compartment. Negative charges associated with proteins are also prominent in the intracellular compartment.

The body must maintain levels of critical ions within acceptable limits. Serious clinical conditions and even death can occur when concentrations fall short of or surpass these limits. Disturbances of specific ion balance occur frequently and for many reasons. Often dietary factors or drugs contribute (Table 42–5). Preparations of several important ions are available for treatment of insufficiencies: they include salts of sodium, potassium, calcium, magnesium, and iodide. Calcium is discussed in Chapter 31 because of its close relationship to hormones of the thyroid and parathyroid glands. Ions that are used

Table 42–5
Effects of Drugs and Diet on Concentrations of Electrolytes and Minerals[a]

Mineral or electrolyte	Drug interactions	Dietary interactions
Sodium (Na)	↑Salt-containing drugs (see Table 42–6) ↓Diuretics	↑Salty foods ↓Salt-restricted diet
Potassium (K)	↑Triamterene, spironolactone, potassium salts ↓Diuretics (except potassium-sparing), laxatives, mineralocorticoids	↑Bananas, fruits, tomatoes, potatoes, lima beans, Coca Cola ↓Natural licorice
Calcium (Ca)	↑Calcium salts, vitamin D, thiazides ↓Glucocorticoids, anticonvulsants, hypnotics, methotrexate, antibiotics, gentamicin, phosphates, fatty acids, sodium etidronate, magnesium salts, high-ceiling diuretics	↑Dairy products, vitamin D, parathyroid extract ↓Vitamin D deficient diet, phytates
Magnesium (Mg)	↑Magnesium salts, antacids containing magnesium ↓Calcium salts, diuretics, mineralocorticoids, thyroid hormone, ADH, gentamicin, cisplatin	
Zinc (Zn)	↑Zinc salts ↓Alcohol, penicillamine, estrogen, glucocorticoids, diuretics	↑Animal proteins, especially shellfish; foods cooked in galvanized pots ↓Phytates
Copper (Cu)	↓Ethanol, penicillamine, glucocorticoids	↑Organ meat, shellfish, nuts, legumes, whole grain, chocolate ↓Phytates
Phosphate (PO_4)	↓Aluminum salts, calcium salts	↑Vitamin D
Chloride (Cl)	↑Carbonic anhydrase inhibitors ↓All other diuretics	↑Salty foods
Bromide (Br)	↑Bromides ↓Diuretics	
Iodine (I)	↓Diuretics	↑Seafoods, iodized salt
Fluorine (F)	↑Fluoride toothpastes	↑Fluoridated water

[a]Iron is not included (see Chapter 41).

therapeutically in other than deficiency states are lithium, ammonium, and fluoride.

Sodium (Na^+)

Hyponatremia (a less than normal sodium concentration) is observed in hypotonic fluid contraction and hypotonic fluid expansion (dilutional hyponatremia). **Hypernatremia** (excessive sodium concentration) occurs in hypertonic fluid contraction or expansion. Excess sodium retention and associated edema is a leading cause of hypertension, which, in turn, is a major factor in overall mortality rates, especially cardiac disorders. Hypertensive clients are typically placed on sodium-restricted diets along with other therapeutic measures (see Chapter 39). Many prescription and nonprescription drugs contain significant amounts of sodium (Table 42–6).

Table 42–6
Some Sodium-Containing Drugs

Prescription	OTC
Ampicillin	Alka Seltzer
Carbenicillin	AlternaGEL
Cefamandole	Amphogel
Cefazolin	Baking soda
Cefoxitin	Basaljel
Cephalothin	Bisodol
Cephapirin	Bromo Seltzer
Cephradine	Camalox
Chloramphenicol	Creamalin
Erythromycin	Delcid
Methicillin	Di-Gel
Nafcillin	Kolantyl
Oxacillin	Metamucil
Penicillin G sodium	Milk of Magnesia
Ticarcillin	Phosphaljel
	Rolaids
	Sal Hepatica
	Simeco
	Titralac

Nurses should advise clients on sodium-restricted diets to avoid self-administration of sodium-containing drugs and should provide clients with a list of such medications.

An important interaction of sodium occurs with lithium salts employed for manic-depressive disorder. Hypernatremia reduces lithium effectiveness. Hyponatremia increases lithium toxicity. *Nurses should advise patients receiving lithium to maintain stable intake of sodium and to avoid both sodium depletion and excessive sodium ingestion.*

Potassium (K^+)

Potassium is the cation in highest concentration in the intracellular fluid. Plasma concentrations are about 3.5–5.0 mEq/L, but intracellular concentrations are about 150 mEq/L. More than 95% of potassium is intracellular. Potassium is essential for intracellular osmolality, electrical excitability of nerve and muscle cells, secretory activity, and renal function. It is also a cofactor in several enzymatic reactions of carbohydrate metabolism.

A normal diet provides 40–100 mEq daily, but 10 mEq of this is lost in the feces without having been absorbed. The remainder is excreted in the urine since there is no net accumulation or loss of potassium under normal circumstances. Urinary excretion of potassium is generally a good measure of dietary potassium. Potassium-rich foods include fruits (especially bananas), fruit juices, vegetables (including potatoes, tomatoes, and lima beans), and colas (Table 42–7). Five to 10 mEq is the bare minimum daily requirement for dietary potassium to replace obligatory losses. In practice, dietary potassium never falls below this level or even approaches it, except in utter starvation or intravenous fluid therapy lacking adequate potassium. Apparently, then, hypokalemia is attributable to excess losses rather than inadequate intake in nearly all instances.

Hypokalemia

Hypokalemia is defined as serum concentrations of potassium of less than 3.5 mEq/L; severe hy-

Table 42–7
Potassium-Rich Foods

Food	Portion	Potassium content (mg)
Baked potato	1	844
Avocado	½	602
Raisins	½ cup	545
Sardines, drained[a]	3 oz	501
Flounder	3 oz	498
Orange juice	1 cup	496
Banana	1	451
Apricots, dried	¼ cup	448
Winter squash, cooked	½ cup	445
Cantaloupe	¼	413
Skim milk[a]	1 cup	406
Sweet potato	1	397
Salmon, fillet[a]	3 oz	378
Buttermilk[a]	1 cup	371
Whole milk[a]	1 cup	370
Cod	3 oz	345
Beef liver	3 oz	323
Apricots, fresh	3	313
Sirloin, trimmed	3 oz	307
Steak, round	3 oz	298
Haddock	3 oz	297
Pork	3 oz	283
Lamb leg	3 oz	274
Turkey	3 oz	255
Perch	3 oz	243
Tomato, raw	1	254
Tuna, dried	3 oz	225
Chicken	3 oz	198
Broccoli[a]	½ cup	127

[a]Also rich in calcium.

pokalemia occurs when concentrations drop below 3.0 mEq/L. Hypokalemia is most commonly due to loss of potassium-rich gastrointestinal secretions as a result of vomiting, suction, diarrhea, malabsorption, too frequent enemas, or use of laxatives. Also common is hypokalemia caused by excess potassium excretion in the urine (kaliuresis) caused by kidney disease, diuretics, ketoacidosis, excess mineralocorticoid activity, or ingestion of large amounts of natural licorice. Extracellular potassium depletion can also be the result of transfer of potassium into the intracellular compartment, as for example, in acute alkalosis. Potassium loss also occurs with extensive burns.

The symptoms of hypokalemia relate to impairment of potassium-mediated functions. Muscles become weak or even paralyzed. Respiratory hypoventilation or even paralysis may occur, as well as hypotension, tetany, and twitches. Smooth muscle dysfunction occurs in the form of paralytic ileus. Impaired neural functioning can result in acute organic brain syndrome. Cardiac manifestations include dysrhythmias and increased sensitivity to digitalis glycosides. Hypokalemia leads to a nephropathy in which the concentrating mechanism is impaired, resulting in polyuria and polydipsia. Secondary metabolic alkalosis and hypochloremia can develop. Indeed, the most common cause of metabolic alkalosis is hypokalemia.

Prevention or treatment of mild hypokalemia can often be achieved by dietary adjustments involving added servings of bananas, citrus fruits, and vegetables rich in potassium. Hypokalemia caused by potassium-depleting diuretics (thiazides, high-ceiling diuretics), can be reduced by addition of triamterene (Dyrenium), 100 mg/day, or spironolactone (Aldactone), 25 mg qid.

Treatment of hypokalemia not adequately alleviated by dietary adjustments is based on oral or intravenous administration of potassium salts. Several potassium salts have been used, including the chloride, acetate, bicarbonate, citrate, gluconate, and phosphate compounds. When alkalosis and hypochloremia are involved, which is the usual case, potassium chloride is the superior choice. For oral administration, a 10% potassium chloride solution can be employed. Oral potassium salts should be diluted in juice and given with or after meals to reduce gastric irritation, which is otherwise considerable. Other potassium salts in liquid form are more palatable but useful only in mild hypokalemia without alkalosis. These include potassium gluconate (Kaon elixir) and a combination of three potassium salts (acetate, bicarbonate, and citrate) called Potassium Triplex. Various potassium salts are available in tablets that must be dissolved prior to use. These include effervescent tablets of potassium bicarbonate, citrate, and chloride. The gluconate salt (Kaon) is available as a tablet. Time release tablets have been developed in which the potassium is gradually released from a wax matrix (Slow-K, Kaon-Cl). *Solutions should be used in preference to tablets since the latter have been known to cause intestinal lesions.* Enteric coated products are especially hazardous since they usually reach the intestines still intact.

Potassium chloride is available as an additive for intravenous fluid therapy in concentrations of 7.5% (20 mEq in 20 ml) and 14.9% (40 mEq in 20 ml). The daily dose should generally not exceed 100–200 mEq. The ECG should be monitored during intravenous infusion of potassium chloride and serum levels should be determined periodically. *Intravenous infusions of potassium should not be speeded up, since rapid administration can cause cardiac arrest.*

Hyperkalemia

Hyperkalemia is diagnosed when serum levels of potassium exceed 5 mEq/L. It occurs in renal failure (due to impaired potassium excretion), trauma injuries, and severe infections (which cause release of intracellular potassium), overly vigorous administration of potassium salts, or metabolic acidosis (which causes transfer of potassium from the intracelluar to the extracellular compartment). It may also be seen in clients who have had a rapid transfusion of stored blood, since potassium is released as red blood cells break down during storage.

Symptoms of hyperkalemia include muscle weakness, areflexia, paresthesias, and paralysis. Bradycardia and hypotension occur at serum levels of 7–8 mEq/L; ventricular fibrillation and cardiac arrest at higher concentrations. The ECG initially exhibits tall, peaked T waves, a short Q-T interval, and a widening of the QRS complex. *Nurses need to pay special attention to ECG tracings of clients following severe trauma to identify developing hyperkalemia.*

Treatment depends on the magnitude of the elevation in serum levels. Mild to moderate hyperkalemia (5–6 mEq/L) can often be managed by restricting dietary intake of potassium or discontinuing a potassium-sparing diuretic. Although slow and often ineffective, a cation exchange resin, sodium polystyrene sulfonate (Kayexalate), may be given orally or as an enema. Each gram of resin removes about 1 mEq of potassium.

When serum potassium levels exceed 6–7 mEq/L or whenever ECG abnormalities are observed, hyperkalemia is a medical emergency. Three treatment steps are initiated immediately:

1. Sodium bicarbonate is given intravenously (1–4 ampuls of 44.6 mEq over 3–5 minutes) and repeated every 10 minutes as required.
2. Calcium gluconate is given intravenously (5–10 ml of a 10% solution) to antagonize cardiac effects of potassium.
3. Glucose containing 1 unit of insulin per 3 g of glucose is given intravenously over 30 minutes to promote movement of potassium into the intracellular fluid.

These measures are followed by administration of sodium polystyrene sulfonate. As a last resort, hemodialysis is undertaken.

The risk of hyperkalemia is especially great for the elderly because their kidney function is often impaired and because they often take dietary supplements of potassium that are required when diuretics are taken for hypertension. Therefore, elderly clients should be assessed closely for changes indicative of hyperkalemia. Should these occur, clients need to eliminate potassium-containing foods and drugs. The event should be reported immediately to the physician since lethal levels of potassium can be reached in a few days.

Magnesium (Mg^{++})

Magnesium is the fourth most abundant cation in the body but the second most abundant intracellular cation. Normally, about 50% of magnesium is found in bone, 45% in the cells, and only 5% in the extracellular fluid. The normal concentration in plasma is between 1.5 and 2.2 mEq/L. The average American diet provides 20–40 mEq of magnesium per day, of which about one-third is absorbed. Absorption occurs from the initial segment of the small intestine. It involves an energy-dependent carrier process. Elevated calcium in the diet inhibits magnesium absorption, while a deficiency enhances absorption. Magnesium absorption is impaired in malabsorption syndromes. Magnesium is excreted in the urine. About 3–5% of what is filtered is not reabsorbed, but this value may be increased by diuretics, diabetic acidosis, hypercalcemia, or states of hypersecretion of aldosterone, antidiuretic hormone (ADH), or thyroid hormone. Magnesium is an essential cofactor for all phosphate reactions that utilize ATP or other nucleotide triphosphates. Magnesium also plays a role in the binding of macromolecules to cellular organelles (for example, binding messenger ribonucleic acid to ribosomes).

Hypomagnesia

Hypomagnesia is seldom due to dietary deficiency alone. Most commonly, marginal dietary intake is made worse by poor absorption (malabsorption syndromes, alcoholism), excessive excretion (diuretics, hypercalcemia, or alcoholism), or increased requirements (lactation) (Figure 42–1). It may also occur in clients who are on gastric suction. Hypomagnesia may occur with prolonged parenteral nutrition unless magnesium is provided in the fluid. Nasogastric suction may also cause acute depletion.

Symptoms of hypomagnesia relate to magnesium's neural and muscular functions. Psychiatric symptoms include irritability and psychotic symptoms. Skeletal muscles become hyperexcitable, leading to tetany, tremor, and fasciculations. Smooth muscle hyperexcitability causes hypertension and nausea. Treatment consists of oral, intramuscular, or intravenous administration of the sulfate or chloride salts of magnesium. Serum magnesium levels are monitored during therapy.

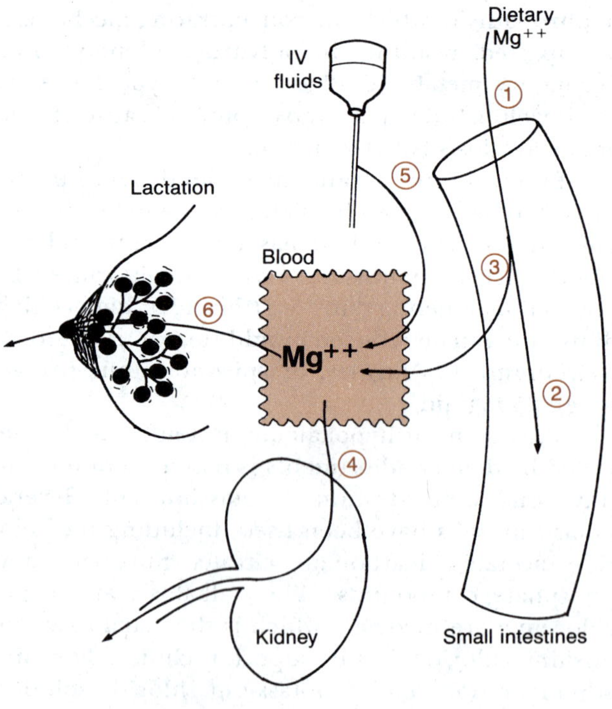

Figure 42–1
Causes of hypomagnesia: (1) too little dietary Mg^{++} (as in alcoholism); (2) excess loss of Mg^{++} due to formation of magnesium soaps in steatorrhea; (3) malabsorption syndrome; (4) urinary hyperexcretion caused by diabetic ketoacidosis, hyperaldosteronism, thyrotoxicosis, diuretics, cardiac glycoside, or alcoholism; (5) dilutional hypomagnesia from IV fluids lacking adequate magnesium or intermittent porphyria; and (6) increased requirement during lactation.

Hypermagnesia

Hypermagnesia occurs mainly in patients in renal failure who are given magnesium salts or antacids containing magnesium. Magnesium blocks calcium-induced release of neurotransmitters and hormones. Symptoms of hypermagnesia that are indicative of impaired release of acetylcholine and norepinephrine from peripheral nerve terminals include hyporeflexia, hypotension, cardiac dysrhythmias, and a curare-like neuromuscular blockade leading to weakness and even respiratory arrest. Central inhibition of transmitter turnover causes coma and hypothermia.

Hypermagnesia is diagnosed when serum concentrations exceed 2.2 mEq/L, and symptoms begin to appear at about 4.0 mEq/L. Acute treatment consists of administration of 10% calcium gluconate, which antagonizes virtually all of the magnesium-induced changes. High-ceiling diuretics and hemodialysis may be required in extreme cases. Treatment of chronic magnesium accumulation rests on determining and correcting the cause.

Phosphate ($PO_4^{=}$)

Phosphate pharmacokinetics are interrelated with calcium mechanisms. Phosphate, like calcium, is largely associated with bone, but both substances can be released into the serum by the action of parathyroid hormone. About 10% of phosphate is found in the serum; the normal range for serum phosphate is 1.45–2.76 mEq/L (2.5–4.8 mg/100 ml). Phosphate is absorbed from the intestines by an active carrier-mediated process that is stimulated by vitamin D, in much the same manner as calcium absorption. Large amounts of calcium or aluminum, such as from use of antacids, decrease phosphate absorption.

Hypophosphatemia is not common. Prolonged inadequate intake can occur in starvation, malabsorption syndromes, diarrhea, or regular use of antacids containing aluminum and calcium salts. These chronic deficiencies are best addressed by alleviating the cause. Oral supplements of phosphate are poorly tolerated due to a cathartic action. Low fat milk is a good source of phosphate. Acute hypophosphatemia is most likely to be seen in ketoacidosis of diabetes, alcoholism, or when prolonged intravenous fluid therapy is conducted without inclusion of phosphate. Symptoms include muscle weakness, lethargy, hemolytic anemia, impaired leukocyte and platelet function (due to depletion of adenosine 5′-triphosphate, ATP). Extreme hypophosphatemia can cause coma and death. Acute hypophosphatemia can be alleviated by intravenous infusion of monobasic potassium phosphate. For maintenance total parenteral nutrition, 15 mmol/day is usual. Larger doses are required in alcoholics or diabetics with ketoacidosis.

Zinc (Zn)

It is becoming increasingly apparent that some of the minerals found in the body in trace amounts are important to health (Table 42–8). Zinc is mostly associated with bones, teeth, hair, skin, liver, muscle, and the testes. It is an essential dietary requirement with a recommended daily allowance of 15 mg in adults. Zinc is obtained from ingestion of animal proteins such as meats, eggs, dairy products, fish, and especially shellfish. Lesser and variable amounts are obtained from vegetables and through contamination of foods cooked in galvanized tin pots.

Zinc is incompletely absorbed from the small intestines. Absorption can be critically impaired by dietary fiber and phytate from unleavened whole wheat bread. Most reports of zinc deficiency come from the Middle East, where whole wheat bread is a dietary staple. The inherited condition, acrodermatitis enteropathica, is related to deficient ability to absorb zinc.

In the plasma, zinc is bound to albumin, globulins, and amino acids. The portion bound to amino acids is excretable. When the concentration of serum albumin proteins is abnormally low (hypoalbuminemia) or the level of zinc-binding amino acids is unusually high, excretion of zinc is increased. Catabolic steroids elevate serum amino acids and lower zinc levels correspondingly. Decreased serum zinc levels have also been linked to use of estrogen in oral contraceptives.

Zinc is a component of certain metalloenzymes, notably carbonic anhydrase and alcohol dehydrogenase. Since alcohol dehydrogenase is required for activation of vitamin A, zinc deficiency can produce secondary vitamin A deficiency. Zinc is also required for protein and nucleic acid synthesis, in particular the incorporation of sulfur-containing amino acids into new proteins.

The symptoms of zinc deficiency include growth retardation, dwarfism, gonadal immaturity, anemia, delayed healing of wounds, and decreased acuity and abnormal sensations in the gustatory and olfactory senses. Treatment of zinc deficiency is achieved by oral supplements in the form of zinc sulfate ($ZnSO_4$) at doses of 30–150 mg/day.

Copper (Cu)

Most of the copper in the body is contained in muscle, bone, and the liver. Serum copper is largely

Table 42–8
Trace Minerals

Mineral	Physiological roles	Food sources	Recommended daily allowance
Chromium (Cr)	Glucose metabolism, regulation of insulin levels	Brewer's yeast, cheese, whole grains, meats	50–200 μg for adults
Copper (Cu)	Utilization of iron for producing red blood cells	Oysters, nuts, liver, kidney, whole grains, mushrooms	2–3 mg for adults; deficiency rare
Fluoride (F)	hardening of teeth and bone	Fluoridated drinking water	1.5–4 mg for adults; more for children
Iodine (I)	Production of thyroid hormones	Shellfish, iodized salt	150 μg after age 10; 175–200 μg during pregnancy or lactation
Iron (Fe)	Required for hemoglobin and myoglobin	Liver, red meats, dried beans and peas, enriched flour, prunes, raisins	10 mg after age 3; 30–60 mg during pregnancy or lactation
Manganese (Mg)	Coenzyme in protein and energy metabolism; bone structure and central nervous system function	Nuts, whole grains, tea, vegetables, fruits	2.5–5 mg for adults
Molybdenum (Mo)	Coenzyme in production of uric acid and metabolism of sulfites and aldehydes	Meats, grains, legumes	About 0.15–0.5 mg for adults
Selenium (Se)	Coenzyme	Fish, meat, grains	About 50–200 μg for adults
Zinc (Zn)	Constituent of several hormones and enzymes; needed for tissue repair and bone growth	Red meat, milk, liver, seafoods, eggs, grains	15 mg after age 10; 20–25 mg during pregnancy and lactation

(90%) bound to a globulin protein called ceruloplasmin. During pregnancy or use of oral contraceptives, blood copper levels increase because ceruloplasmin increases along with other plasma proteins.

The normal diet provides 2–5 mg/day. Copper in excess of the binding capacity of ceruloplasmin is free and quickly excreted in the bile and urine. Copper is actively removed from the plasma by the liver. Copper is a component of certain enzymes, notably cytochrome oxidase.

Copper deficiencies are rare. An inherited inability to absorb or transport copper is known. Copper deficiency is also sometimes associated with hypoproteinemia.

Copper excess occurs with acute excessive intake and in Wilson's disease. Symptoms of acute intoxication include nausea, vomiting, diarrhea, abdominal discomfiture, and muscle aches. Wilson's disease is a rare, inherited disease in which copper accumulates in red blood cells, the kidney, the liver, and the brain, ultimately damaging cells in these tissues. The reason for the positive copper balance is unclear, but it may be due to excessive absorption.

Treatment is based on preventing copper accumulation. Foods that contain high levels of copper (organ meat, shellfish, nuts, legumes, whole grain cereals, and chocolate) are eliminated from the diet. Penicillamine, a copper chelator, is used to improve elimination of copper. Penicillamine is begun at 250 mg/day and increased incrementally to 2–4 g/day. Penicillamine must be given on an empty stomach or absorption will be severely curtailed. Penicillamine induces vitamin B_6 and iron deficiencies, which, however, are correctable. Pyridoxine is given concurrent with penicillamine (25–50 mg/day) and serum iron is monitored.

Other Trace Metals

Cobalt (Co) is a component of vitamin B_{12}, but no deficiency condition has been identified for the metal itself. **Chromium** (Cr) is an essential trace element that participates in several enzymatic processes as well as in insulin-stimulated glucose utilization. Brewer's yeast is a good dietary source of chromium and has been observed to lower serum triglycerides and cholesterol and to reduce insulin requirements in some diabetics. Deficiency may occur in prolonged intravenous fluid therapy and undernutrition.

Selenium (Se) operates in concert with vitamin E in the selenium-glutathione peroxidase system. This antioxidant system protects the body from lipid peroxides by breaking them down. Selenium deficiencies have been reported in China to produce a childhood cardiomyopathy.

Manganese (Mn) is involved in several enzyme systems and is required for healthy bone structure. It is found in green leafy vegetables, unrefined grains, and tea. Deficiency has not been reported.

Halides

Chloride (Cl^-) is the major extracellular anion, accounting for more than 60% of extracellular anions. Very little chloride is found intracellularly. The normal serum concentration is 95–105 mEq/L. Chloride is filtered and reabsorbed in the renal tubule, but for the most part its rate of excretion varies passively in relation to primary changes in other anions. It is the companion ion for excretion with various cations (Na^+, K^+, and H^+) to the extent that other anions are unavailable.

Nearly all diuretics increase urinary chloride in proportion to elevations in sodium and potassium. The major exceptions are the carbonic anhydrase inhibitors that produce diuresis mainly by elevating bicarbonate excretion. Potassium chloride supplements are used to correct potassium deficiency induced by diuretics, but they also correct the chloride deficit.

Chloride levels are elevated in respiratory alkalosis and sometimes in metabolic acidosis. Chloride levels decline in respiratory acidosis and metabolic alkalosis. These changes are corrected automatically when the acid-base imbalance is adjusted.

Bromides were once used in medicine as hypnotics and anticonvulsants but are now obsolete. Bromides are excreted very slowly, causing an accumulation in the body. Symptoms of bromide intoxication include drowsiness, dizziness, impaired memory, and irritability. In severe cases, delirium, hallucinations, delusions, mania, lethargy, and ultimately coma ensue. Bromide, iodide, and chloride are all excreted by the kidney, so chloruretic drugs (most diuretics) can be used to hasten bromide elimination.

Iodine (I) is an essential dietary component. Recommended daily allowances for iodine are 150 μg for adults. Eighty percent of iodide is contained in the thyroid, where it is used in synthesis of the thyroid hormones. Seafoods are rich dietary sources, and iodized salt is commonly sold. Iodine deficiency results in endemic goiter. Iodine toxicity occurs when intake exceeds 2,000 μg because iodine in extremely high concentrations inhibits thyroid function, causing myxedema.

Fluoride (F^-) is found mainly in teeth and bones. Ideally, drinking water should contain 1 part per million. In many communities, fluoride is added to the water to that level, which significantly reduces incidence of dental cavities without promoting measurable toxicity. Stannous fluoride is used in many toothpastes. Incorporation of fluoride into the enamel of teeth makes them harder and resistant to decay. The action is most evident when fluoride is present during early development of the permanent teeth.

Case Study: Dehydration

L. T., a 55-year-old white male, appeared at a walk-in clinic complaining of feeling weak, tired, and ill. His wife said that L. T. had an elevated temperature and had lost his appetite. L. T. said he felt nauseated all the time and was afraid that eating or drinking might cause him to vomit. He already had diarrhea.

The nurse noted that L. T.'s skin was flushed and warm and that when she picked up the skin on his arm, it appeared inelastic — it did not resume the normal shape after having been grasped. She weighed L. T. and he told her he had lost 10 pounds in the last week. L. T.'s blood pressure was low (90/70). When the nurse asked L. T. for a urine sample, he replied that he would try but he had not been able to void much in the last few days. The sample of urine was a dark, amber color. L. T. also had a lack of moisture in the axillary region. The nurse defined his problem as dehydration. L. T. then saw the physician, who confirmed the nurse's findings. The physician diagnosed the cause of the dehydration as diarrhea resulting from ingestion of contaminated water. She had learned that L. T. had for 2 weeks prior to the onset of his current problems been swimming daily in a pond which, upon subsequent investigation, had been declared contaminated.

The physician prescribed a drug to treat the intestinal infection. L. T. refused to be hospitalized, so the nurse worked out a plan for the client to care for himself at home. She discussed the need for adequate fluid intake and worked with husband and wife to establish a schedule for food and fluid. Favorite fluids were discussed, as well as whether or not these might interact unfavorably with the medication L. T. was to take. L. T. was encouraged to include solid foods that are high in fluid content, such as cottage cheese, cantaloupe, and fresh fruit. Also, because of the diarrhea, it was felt there might be a need for foods high in potassium. Therefore, the couple were provided with a list of foods high in potassium as well as fluid. These included orange juice, skim milk, buttermilk (something L. T. said he particularly liked) and tomato.

Mr. and Mrs. T. were taught to maintain an accurate record of intake and output, including recordings of bowel function, consistency, and change. At the outset, it was determined that L. T. needed to take in at least 800–1,000 ml of fluid or more per day. Because of L. T.'s insistence on returning home, teaching of both the husband and wife was especially important if this goal was to be achieved.

1. Can you point out aspects of the nursing assessment that contributed to the nurse's finding of dehydration?
2. How did the nurse in this case use L. T.'s personal preferences to therapeutic advantage?

Answers appear at the end of the book.

Case Study: Hypokalemia

G. A., a 58-year-old alcoholic and diabetic, stated that he noticed an increased incidence of constipation, and his wife stated that his abdomen was becoming so distended that he could no longer fit into his clothes. The nursing assessment further revealed weakness, lethargy, and mental confusion. After evaluation of serum electrolytes, G. A. was given a diagnosis of hypokalemia.

In G. A.'s case, the physician, recognizing that oral administration is the safest way to replace potassium loss, suggested he be placed on a high potassium diet supplemented by potassium chloride, 10 g/day. The nursing plan included teaching G. A. about the foods high in potassium content and about side effects that could occur. The nurse made certain that Mr. and Mrs. A. understood the importance of reporting any adverse reactions, such as nausea, vomiting, or diarrhea. Because G. A. already had an enlarged abdomen, the nurse explained the importance of measuring G. A.'s girth to determine if it was increasing in size, since abdominal distention can indicate an adverse response. In addition, they were asked to report any abdominal pain or oliguria. The community health nurse was to follow G. A.'s progress.

The nurse explained to G. A. that potassium chloride tablets are large and may be difficult to swallow. He was told to take the pills always with a full glass of water, and while sitting or standing since, if he took them lying down, he might incur drug-induced esophagitis. He was also told not to allow the tablets to dissolve in the mouth. G. A. was admonished not to skip dosages and the nurse worked with Mr. and Mrs. A. to establish a schedule for taking the pills.

G. A. was also informed about foods and over-the-counter drugs that are sources of potassium (see Table 42–7). This was important because the selection and use of these are controlled solely by the client. The nurse also made an appointment for G. A. with a dietitian to discuss diet. Self-medication habits were discussed and the client was provided with a list of drugs to avoid, such as laxatives. The nurse also counseled G. A. to inform his dentist or any new physician that he was on potassium maintenance therapy. In addition, he was advised to wear a medic identification bracelet stating his drug regimen.

1. What was the connection between abdominal distention and potassium? What is the likely reason for G. A.'s abdomen being enlarged at the time of initial diagnosis of hypokalemia?
2. What other dosage form(s) of potassium chloride might have been selected in order to reduce risk of esophagitis or ulcerations?
3. What are some examples of foods and drugs that contain potassium?
4. Why should G. A. avoid use of laxatives?
5. Why was it important for G. A. to inform other health professionals that he was receiving potassium supplements?

Answers appear at the end of the book.

Recommended Readings

Boylan A, Marback B: Dehydration: subtle, sinister — preventable. *RN* 1979;42(8):37–41.

Cohen JJ, Kassirer JP: *Acid-Base.* Boston, Little Brown & Co, 1982.

Daly W, Papper S, Whang R (eds): *Clinical Fluid and Electrolyte Management.* Washington DC, US Veterans' Administration, 1976.

Elbaum M: Detecting and correcting magnesium imbalance. *Nursing* 1977; 7(8):34–35.

Felver L: Understanding the electrolyte maze. *Am J Nurs* 1980;80:1591–1596.

Gammon SS: Respiratory acidosis. *Nursing* 1982;12(8):65.

Gever LN: Administering sodium bicarbonate during a code. *Nursing* 1984;14(1):100.

Goldberger E: *A Primer of Water, Electrolyte, and Acid-base Syndromes,* ed 5. Philadelphia, Lea & Febiger, 1975.

Huey FL: What's on the market? A nurse's guide. *Am J Nurs* 1983;83(6):902–910.

Janusek LW: Metabolic acidosis: Physiology, signs, and symptoms. *Nursing* 14(7):44–45.

Janusek LW: Metabolic alkalosis: Physiology, signs, and symptoms. *Nursing* 14(8):60–61.

Koszuta LE: Choosing the right infusion control device for your patient. *Nursing* 1984;14(3):55–56.

Methany N, Snively W: *Nurses' Handbook of Fluid Balance,* ed 4. Philadelphia, J B Lippincott, 1983.

Michael A: Home IV therapy. *Am J Nurs* 1978;78(7):1223–1226.

Millam DA, Warren J: Using a local anesthetic for I.V. insertion: Boon or bain? *Nursing Life* 1985;5(1):52–53.

Morris ME: Intravenous drug incompatibilities. *Am J Nurs* 1979;79:1288–1296.

Newma KS, Diuhy RG: Hyperkalemia and hypokalemia. *JAMA* 1975;231:631–633.

Parent B: In line IV filters. *Nursing* 1981;11(8):58–60.

Snively W, Leitch G, Beshear D: Acid-base disturbances, a programmed text. *Am J Intravenous Ther* 1977–1978;4:22–40, 5:26–34, 5:36–56.

Taylor DL: Respiratory acidosis: Physiology, signs, and symptoms. *Nursing* 14(10):44–45.

Wittig P, Semmler-Bertanzi DJ: Pumps and contollers: A nurse's assessment guide. *Am J Nurs* 1983;83(7):1022–1025.

CHAPTER 43

Drugs and the Nephrourinary System

Physiology of the Kidney

The kidney is the single most important organ for maintaining body fluid composition, although the lungs and various other organs also participate in specialized ways. Not only is the kidney the chief means of excreting a large number of drugs and nonvolatile metabolic waste products, but it also plays a fundamental role in maintaining pH, controlling levels of electrolytes and water, and conserving their loss from the body. For nurses to make accurate clinical judgments concerning clients' responses to trauma or therapy, it is essential for them to understand kidney function.

The kidneys are a pair of organs located in the back of the peritoneal cavity, one on each side of the vertebral column. The parenchyma of each kidney consists of an outer region, the cortex, and a group of inner conical elements that together make up the medulla. The medullary cones are separated from one another by sections of cortex called the renal columns. The tips of the medullary cones, called the papillae, point toward the renal pelvis, the innermost section of the kidney.

The kidneys are highly vascularized and the renal blood vessels have unusually low resistance to blood flow. As a result, they normally receive about 25% of cardiac output, or 1,200 ml of blood per minute. The renal blood vessels are carefully regulated by sympathetic neurons, autacoids (bradykinin, angiotensin, and prostaglandins), and adrenal medullary hormones to ensure a constant rate of renal blood flow.

From a functional point of view, each kidney is composed of some 1–2 million similar structural units called **nephrons** (Figure 43–1). The nephron performs three fundamental physiological functions — filtration, reabsorption, and secretion — that ensure elimination of undesirable plasma constituents and retention of desirable substances. First, a portion of the water and smaller components of the plasma flowing through the blood vessels of the kidneys is filtered into tubules. The contents of this filtrate that are valuable are then reabsorbed into the blood vessels, while the remainder is ultimately excreted in the urine. Added to this filtrate are some molecules that are selectively secreted from the blood into the tubule, providing for elimination of these undesirable substances at a rate faster than could be achieved by filtration alone. Together the

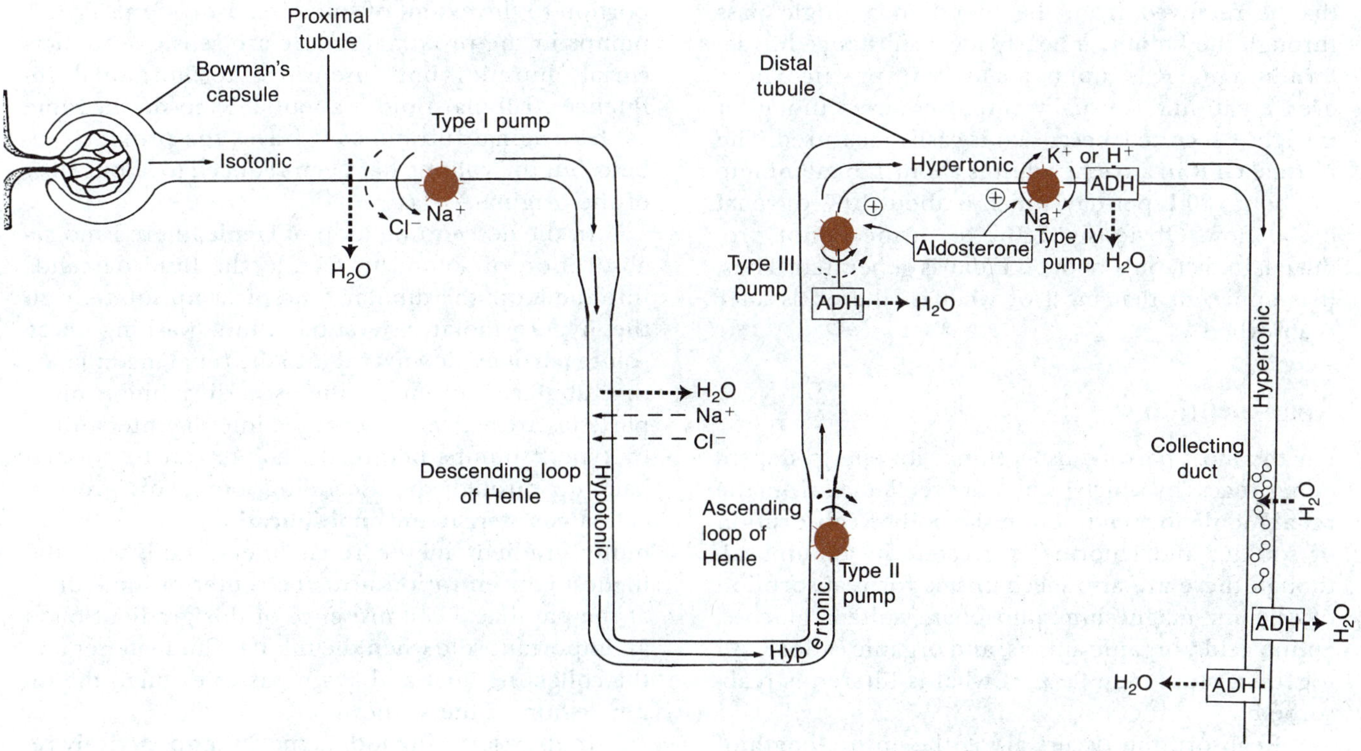

Figure 43–1
The nephron of the kidney showing ion pumps.

processes of filtration, reabsorption, and secretion allow the healthy kidney to control the composition of body fluids.

Filtration

Filtration occurs in the initial segment of the nephron called the renal corpuscle. This structure consists of a network of minute blood vessels, called the **glomerulus,** surrounded by the capsular ending of the renal tubule, called **Bowman's capsule.** As blood is forced into the glomerulus under pressure, part of it is filtered out of the blood vessels into Bowman's capsule. Generally blood components of less than about 30,000 molecular weight are at least partly filtered, and those less than 10,000 molecular weight are readily filtered. Substances readily filtered include water, electrolytes, glucose, urea, and other small solutes. Plasma proteins, lipids, cells, and substances bound to any of these do not pass through the glomerular membrane when it is healthy. Both the incoming and outgoing vessels of the glomerulus are arterioles, so filtration pressure is several times greater than that of other capillary beds.

Glomerular filtration rate (GFR) can be evaluated clinically by measurement of the rate of renal clearance of a substance that is neither secreted nor reabsorbed. Clearance is the fraction of a substance that is removed from the blood in a single pass through the kidney. A nearly ideal substance for determining GFR is inulin, a starch. In practice, however, creatinine is usually employed, even though it is slightly secreted, because it is easily measured. The normal GFR in a young adult is about 125 ml/minute or about 180 L per day, which is about 10% of renal blood flow. Obviously, 180 L of urine is not produced; in fact, only about 2 L/day is generated. Thus, it is apparent that most of what is filtered is later reabsorbed.

Reabsorption

For the most part, reabsorption is an energy-dependent process by which solutes are reclaimed from the renal tubule for retention in the body. Reabsorption of sodium and chloride is greatest in amount, although there are also mechanisms for reabsorption of calcium, magnesium, phosphate, sulfate, glucose, amino acids, organic anions, and organic cations. All together, more than 99% of what is filtered is reabsorbed.

Reabsorption occurs along the entire length of the nephron. From Bowman's capsule, tubular filtrate passes into the **proximal tubule.** This, in turn, leads into the **loop of Henle,** which first descends into the medullary portion of the kidney and then ascends back into the cortex. The ascending limb of the loop of Henle then opens into the **distal tubule.** The distal tubules from various nephrons join to form a common duct called the **collecting duct.**

The proximal tubule is especially well suited for reabsorptive function. The cells that line the proximal tubule have numerous microvilli that resemble the reabsorptive surface of the intestinal mucosa. About 70–80% of the filtrate of Bowman's capsule is reabsorbed in the proximal tubule. Organic anions and cations are primarily reabsorbed in the proximal tubule, by active carrier-mediated processes. Glucose is also reabsorbed in the proximal tubule — to the full extent that it is filtered, unless glucose levels exceed the maximum capacity of the reabsorptive mechanism. Many amino acids are similarly reabsorbed in the proximal tubule to a very high degree.

Electrolytes and water are reabsorbed throughout the tubule — to the largest extent in the proximal tubule. Sodium, the most abundant cation, is reabsorbed throughout the nephron, but the characteristics of sodium reabsorption vary by anatomical location. Reabsorption of major electrolytes involves the action of four kinds of transport mechanisms (Table 43–1). In the proximal tubule, type 1 pumps actively reabsorb sodium, carrying chloride in tandem, and water passively and isosmotically (in proportion to the extent of solute reabsorption). Type 1 pumps in the proximal tubule are sensitive to mercurial diuretics but insensitive to hormonal influences. Tubular fluid is about 285 mosm (the same as the original filtrate) as it leaves the proximal tubule, but the volume has been reduced to about 30% of the original.

In the descending loop of Henle, there is no reabsorption of solute. In fact, as the fluid descends into the loop, the tubular fluid picks up solute from the hyperosmolar interstitial fluid, washing these solute particles downward into the renal medulla. As the tubular fluid enters the ascending limb, solute particles are actively discharged into the interstitium by type 2 pumps before the solute can be washed back up through the ascending loop. This process, called **countercurrent multiplication,** creates an osmotic gradient in the renal interstitium, with the highest concentration near the center of the kidney at the papillae. (The presence of this gradient plays an important role when the tubular fluid later enters the collecting duct and again passes through the inner region of the kidney.)

In the ascending loop, type 2 pumps actively reabsorb chloride with sodium in tandem. Since the ascending limb is nearly impermeable to water, the tubular fluid becomes increasingly dilute (that is,

Table 43-1
Characteristics of the Reabsorption Mechanisms for Major Electrolytes

	Type 1	Type 2	Type 3	Type 4
Description	Sodium pump	Chloride pump	Sodium pump	Sodium-potassium or hydrogen exchange pump
Location	Proximal tubule	Ascending loop	Distal tubule	Distal tubule and collecting duct
Tandem ion movements	Chloride reabsorption	Sodium reabsorption	Chloride reabsorption	Potassium or hydrogen secretion
Passive water reabsorption	Yes, isosmotic	No	Yes or no — ADH dependent	Yes or no — ADH dependent
Hormonal sensitivity	No	No	Mineralocorticoid stimulation	Mineralocorticoid stimulation
Drug sensitivity	Inhibited by mercurial diuretics	Inhibited by high-ceiling diuretics	Inhibited by thiazide diuretics and mineralocorticoid antagonists	Inhibited by mineralocorticoid antagonists, triamterene, and amelioride

the water stays in and the sodium and chloride leave) and the interstitial fluid in the surrounding renal tissue becomes increasingly concentrated. The tubular fluid that reaches the end of the ascending loop of Henle is typically about 100 mosm and 20–25% of the original filtrate remains unabsorbed. Thus, much of the solute has been reabsorbed, but substantial water remains in the tubule. The type 2 pumps are sensitive to inhibition by high-ceiling diuretics.

The distal tubule provides the fine-tuning that is so important for electrolyte and water balance. Here, further solute and water reabsorption occurs under the control of aldosterone and antidiuretic hormone (ADH). First, in the initial portion of the distal tubule, the tubular fluid reaches the type 3 pumps, which reabsorb sodium, with chloride in tandem. The activity of the type 3 pumps is regulated by aldosterone and can be inhibited by thiazide diuretics.

Then, in the distal portion of the distal tubule and in the collecting ducts, the tubular fluid passes the type 4 pumps. These pumps, called **exchange pumps,** reabsorb sodium in exchange for potassium or hydrogen. The type 4 pumps are very important in potassium homeostasis and acid-base balance. When stimulated by presence of sodium in the tubules, the type 4 pumps secrete potassium and hydrogen and, if overly active, can produce hypokalemia and metabolic alkalosis. The type 4 pumps are stimulated by aldosterone and inhibited by potassium-sparing diuretics.

Electrolyte reabsorption by the type 3 and type 4 pumps may or may not be accompanied by water reabsorption. In the presence of ADH, water is reabsorbed and hypertonic urine is formed. At the end of the collecting duct, the concentration of tubular fluid might be approximately 1,200 mosm and equal in volume to about 1% of the original filtrate. In the absence of ADH, water is not reabsorbed and the urine formed is hypotonic, perhaps about 100 mosm with as much as 10% of the original filtrate being excreted.

Secretion

Secretion is the nephron's third fundamental function. Secretion provides for elimination of undesirable substances and waste products at a rate faster than could be achieved by filtration alone. During secretion, substances are transported from the blood in peritubular capillaries into the tubules — the opposite of reabsorption. Secretion occurs with many drugs. Some substances, mainly organic anions and cations, are secreted so effectively by the renal tubules that the blood is almost completely cleared of the substance in a single passage through the kidney. The most important aspect of tubular secretion is the mechanism by which hydrogen ion is secreted into the tubule. The human body is an acid-forming organism, so that net excretion of hydrogen ion is required if pH is not to be allowed to decline to values that would be toxic.

Hydrogen ion is made available for secretion from tubule cells into the tubule itself by the action of the enzyme carbonic anhydrase (CA), which occurs in high concentrations in cells lining the renal tubules (Figure 43–1). Carbonic anhydrase promotes hydration of carbon dioxide to form carbonic acid, which in turn breaks down into bicarbonate and hydrogen ions:

$$H_2O + CO_2 \xleftrightarrow{CA} H^+ + HCO_3^-$$

This reaction therefore furnishes a ready supply of hydrogen ions that can be secreted in exchange for sodium ions. Inhibitors of carbonic anhydrase are one of the classes of diuretic drugs.

Hormones Regulating Renal Function

The kidney is the target organ for the actions of ADH and aldosterone, but beyond that it is an important contributor to endocrine functions. It activates vitamin D (now recognized as a prohormone), degrades insulin, and synthesizes and releases renal hormones, including renin, erythropoietin (which promotes production of red blood cells), and kallikrein (a precursor of the plasma kinins, kallidin and bradykinin, which help regulate renal blood flow).

The kidney has a profound role in sodium homeostasis. Regulation of sodium reabsorption in the kidney is the single most important determinant of sodium levels in body fluids. There are three principal components in the capacity of the kidney to regulate levels of sodium. First, tubular reabsorption of sodium adjusts to changes in the glomerular filtration rate; if filtration decreases, so does reabsorption. This tends to ensure constant sodium excretion over a wide range of filtration rates — a process called glomerulotubular balance. Second, the kidney controls sodium reabsorption by means of the renin-angiotensin-aldosterone system. And third, sodium reabsorption is further regulated by the cardiac hormone, atrial natriuretic factor (ANF). The renin-angiotensin-aldosterone system has special importance to pharmacology and requires further consideration.

The Renin-Angiotensin-Aldosterone System

Renin is a renal hormone secreted by the cells of the macula densa. These specialized secretory cells are interposed between the distal renal tubule and the glomerulus. When the sodium load passing through the distal tubule decreases, renin secretion is stimulated. Renin secretion can also be triggered by decreased pressure in the afferent arterioles, by sympathetic nervous system stimulation (through β_2-receptors), by adrenal medullary hormones, or by vasopressin. It can be suppressed by ANF.

After release into the blood, renin acts as an enzyme, catalyzing conversion of an inactive plasma protein called **angiotensinogen** into **angiotensin I** (Figure 43–2). Angiotensin I is further converted into **angiotensin II** by the action of the enzyme **peptidyl dipeptidase** (PDP), also called **converting enzyme.** Angiotensin II is a highly active peptide, the most powerful vasoconstrictor known (about 40 times as potent as norepinephrine), and the main stimulator of **aldosterone** secretion by the adrenal cortex. Angiotensin II can be further converted into **angiotensin III** (which has significant angiotensin II-like activity of its own) and thence to smaller peptide fragments (which do not).

Aldosterone, secreted from the adrenal glands under the influence of angiotensin II and III, stimulates the type 3 and type 4 pumps of the distal convoluted tubule to promote reabsorption of sodium and water but increased excretion of potassium and hydrogen. The increased excretion of potassium and hydrogen is due to stimulation of the type 4 pumps. The results of aldosterone activity are expansion of body fluid volume and conservation of sodium. When aldosterone activity is excessive, hypernatremia, hypokalemia, and metabolic alkalosis may ensue. Aldosterone-sensitive sodium pumps are found in the serous membranes of distal tubule cells — that is, the side away from the tubular lumen (Figure 43–3).

Antidiuretic Hormone (Vasopressin)

The role of ADH evolved in conjunction with the emergence of life forms from sea to land, and the need to conserve water in a sometimes dry environment. ADH is a nonapeptide, having similar structure but different activity than its companion hormone in the posterior pituitary, oxytocin. ADH promotes water retention by allowing passive water reabsorption from the renal tubules as filtrate passes through the distal tubule and collecting duct. ADH also constricts vascular smooth muscle (a pressor effect), an action that has provided ADH with the alternative name *vasopressin.*

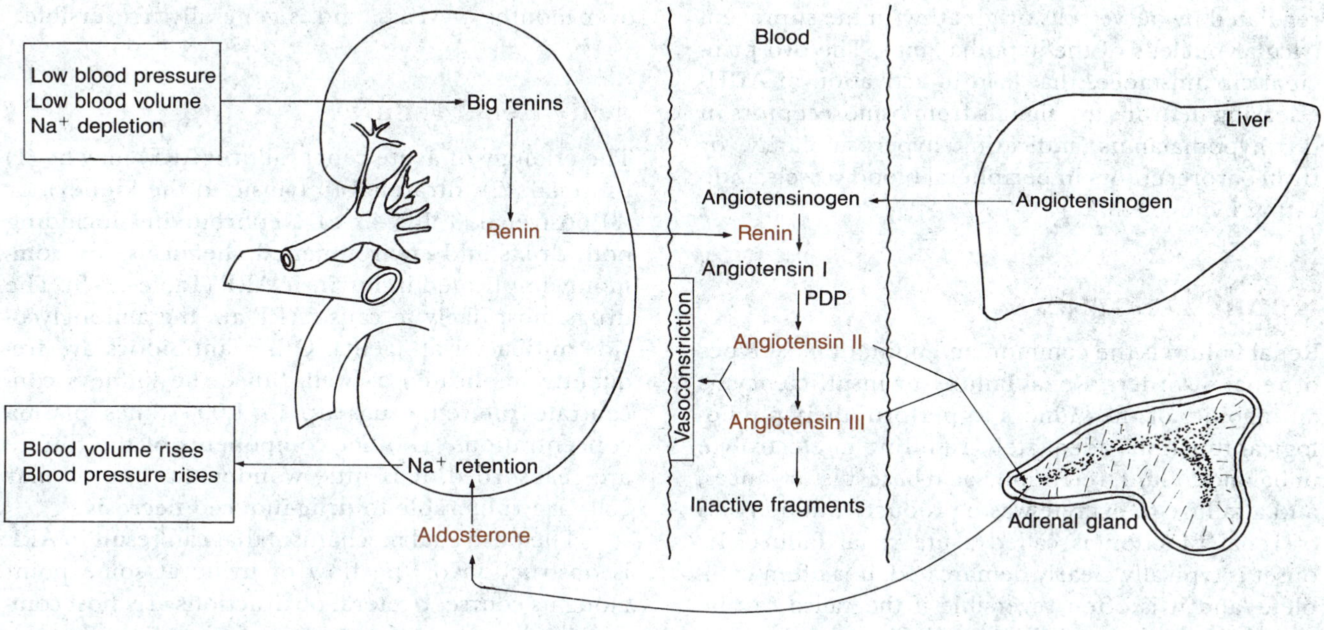

Figure 43–2

The renin-angiotensin-aldosterone system. Low blood pressure or volume or sodium depletion promotes release of renin, an enzyme that catalyzes conversion of the plasma protein angiotensinogen to angiotensin I. Angiotensin I is further converted by peptidyl dipeptidase (PDP) to angiotensin II and angiotensin III which stimulate release of aldosterone from the adrenal cortex. Aldosterone stimulates sodium pumps in the kidney to promote sodium and water retention and to correct the original deficiency.

Figure 43–3

Location and influence of aldosterone and ADH receptors. Aldosterone stimulates sodium pumps and exchange pumps in the serosal membranes of renal tubule cells, creating a gradient that draws sodium out of the renal tubule and pushes potassium and hydrogen into the tubule. ADH activates an adenylate cyclase-linked receptor on the serosal membrane of tubule cells that initiates formation of cyclic AMP, which promotes aggregation of proteins in the luminal membrane that serve as water channels.

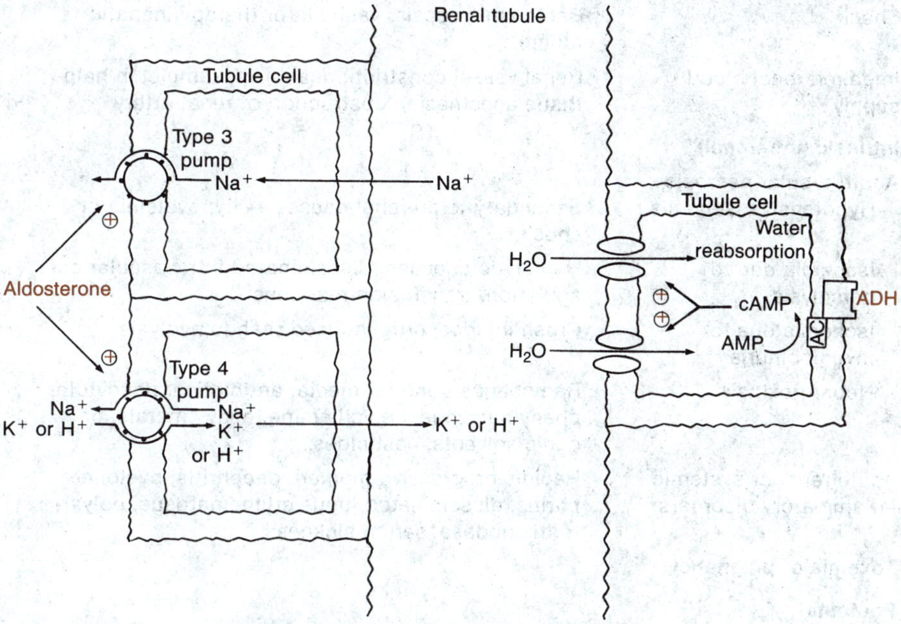

Release of ADH from the posterior pituitary is regulated by nerve cells originating in the supraventricular nucleus of the hypothalamus. The two principal circumstances that lead to activation of ADH-releasing neurons are signals from osmoreceptors in the hypothalamus, indicating hyperosmolarity, or from baroreceptors in peripheral blood vessels, indicating hypovolemia.

Renal Disorders

Renal failure is the common end-point of most types of renal disorders. Renal failure (or insufficiency) is an inability of the kidneys to perform their physiological functions adequately, resulting in electrolyte imbalance, fluid retention, acid-base disturbances, and a failure to excrete waste products. Sudden loss of renal function is called acute renal failure. Its onset is typically clearly demarcated, it is often complete, and it is often reversible if the cause can be rapidly identified and eliminated. Chronic renal failure, by contrast, is insidious in onset, developing over months or years, and is generally irreversible.

Acute Renal Failure

The etiology of acute renal failure (ARF) may be (1) prerenal, (2) intrarenal (intrinsic to the kidney), or (3) postrenal (Table 43–2). Nephrotoxins, including both drugs and environmental chemicals, are commonly implicated in intrinsic ARF (Table 43–3). The drugs most likely to cause ARF are the aminoglycoside antibacterial agents. Other antibiotics are frequently implicated as well. Since the kidneys concentrate filtered drugs up to 1,000 times plasma concentrations, as other components of the filtrate are reabsorbed, it is little wonder that the tubular cells are vulnerable to drug-induced necrosis.

The postrenal mechanism that can result in ARF is obstruction of the flow of urine at some point along its course. Ureteral obstructions are most common and can be due to trauma, infection, radiation,

Table 43–2
Causes of Acute Renal Failure

Type	Examples
Prerenal	
Hypovolemia	Hemorrhage, burns, excess diuresis, heatstroke
Cardiac failure	Congestive heart failure
Shock	Bacteremic sepsis, vasodilator therapy, hepatic failure
Impaired renal blood supply	Renal vessel constriction (as, for example, in halothane anesthesia), obstruction of renal artery
Intrinsic (Intrarenal)	
Acute tubular necrosis	
Hypotensive ischemia	Secondary to prerenal causes — hypovolemia or shock
Ischemia due to hemolysis	Hemolytic anemias, disseminated intravascular coagulation, transfusion reactions
Ischemia due to myoglobinuria	Crush injuries, drug-induced rhabdomyolysis
Nephrotoxins	Radiopaque contrast media, antibiotics, phenytoin, phenylbutazone, penicillamine, heavy metals, organic solvents, pesticides.
Acute renal or systemic inflammatory disorders	Rapidly progressive glomerulonephritis, pyelonephritis, disseminated lupus erythematosus, polyarteritis nodosa, serum sickness
Toxemia of pregnancy	
Postrenal	
Obstruction	Calculi (stones), cysts, prostate tumor, other neoplasms, clots, foreign objects

Table 43–3

Mechanisms of Nephrotoxicity Caused by Drugs and Chemicals

Mechanisms	Drugs
I. Ischemia	
A. Constriction of afferent arterioles	Amphotericin B, ergot alkaloids
B. Excess pigment	
1. Hemolysis in G6PD individuals	Aspirin, chloramphenicol, isoniazid, nalidixic acid, naphthalene, nitrofurantoin, phenacetin, primaquine, quinacrine, quinidine, quinine, sulfonamides, sulfonylureas
2. Immunological hemolysis	Chloramphenicol, insecticides, isoniazid, levodopa, mefenamic acid, methyldopa, penicillin, phenacetin, quinidine, quinine, stibophen, sulfonamides
3. Methemoglobin production	Acetanilid, aniline, benzocaine, coal tar, dapsone, dinitrophenol, ethoxazene, formaldehyde, lidocaine, mefenide, methylene blue, nitrates, nitrites, nitrofurantoin, nitroprusside, phenacetin, phenazopyridine, phenol, potassium salts, primaquine, resorcinol, silver nitrate, sulfonamides, sulfones, thiopental, triclocarban, various industrial chemicals
4. Rhabdomyolysis	Amphetamine, phencyclidine
II. Direct cytotoxic effect	
A. Tubulointerstitial necrosis	Amphotericins, antineoplastics, caffeine, heavy metals, nonsteroidal antiinflammatory drugs, oxalic acid (and ethylene glycol and methoxyflurane which form oxalic acid), paramethadione, penicillamine, phenytoin, pesticides, radiopaque contrast media, solvents, trimethadione
B. Nephrosis	Bismuth, captopril, gold, levamisole, mercury, penicillamine, probenecid
C. Proximal cell necrosis	Aminoglycosides, amphotericin B, bacitracin, cephaloridine, methicillin, polymyxin, rifampin, sulfonamides
III. Immunological	
A. Immune complex deposition	Captopril, gold, heroin, hydralazine, isoniazid, levamisole, penicillamine, phenytoin, procainamide
B. Allergic tubulointerstitial nephritis	Penicillins (especially methicillin), rifampin, sulfonamides, trimethoprim and sulfamethoxazole
IV. Growths	
A. Retroperitoneal fibrosis	Methysergide
B. Cysts and neoplasms	Diphenyl, pesticides
V. Obstructions	
A. Promotion of urate crystals	Antileukemic agents, mercaptopurine, phencyclidine, phenylbutazone, thiotepa, uricosurics
B. Drug crystals	Mercaptopurine, methotrexate, primidone, sulfonamides
VI. Nephrogenic diabetes insipidus	Demeclocycline, lithium
VII. Electrolyte disturbances	
A. Hypercalcemia	Calcium salts, milk-alkali, thiazides, vitamin D
B. Hypokalemia	Carbenicillin, diuretics, penicillins
C. Hyperkalemia	Potassium-sparing diuretics
D. Hypomagnesia	Alcoholism, diuretics

prostatic hyperplasia, or urinary **calculi** (kidney stones). About 0.1% of adults in the United States are hospitalized annually as a result of urinary stones. Calculi can be composed of calcium, oxalate, urate, cystine, xanthine, or phosphate. The likelihood of formation of kidney stones is increased by presence of elevated quantities of these substances in the urine and by factors that facilitate formation of crystals, including urinary stasis, changes in pH, or presence of foreign bodies. There are geographical regions, called "stone belts," where incidence of urinary calculi are high. The age group most at risk is 20–55 years of age. Most ureteral calculi originate in the kidney and move into the ureter, where they become lodged, causing excruciating, intermittent pain, called **colic.** Some calculi form in the bladder. Stones are usually eliminated by lithotripsy (mechanical crushing of the stone within the bladder or urethra) or surgical procedures.

The constellation of symptoms that occur clinically as a consequence of ARF is called **uremia** and results from the inability of the kidney to maintain its homeostatic and excretory functions. Widespread imbalances occur in the regulation of electrolytes, acid-base balance, sodium, potassium, phosphate, calcium, magnesium, and nitrogen. These imbalances lead to far-reaching clinical manifestations, including neurological, hematological, cardiovascular, visual, dermatological, gastrointestinal, and respiratory symptoms.

Dialysis is the mainstay of management of the patient with intrinsic ARF. If dialysis is not available, management of patients in ARF is considerably more complicated, requiring restriction of intake for all substances that are normally eliminated by the kidneys. *An important role of the nurse in management of patients with acute renal failure is regulation of fluid and electrolyte status. Water intake is restricted to equal measured urinary output, plus measured extrarenal output, plus 500 ml/day to balance insensible water losses. A weight chart is maintained as a basis for monitoring changes in body fluid retention. Small amounts of ice chips may be helpful in reducing the intense thirst that many patients experience from the water restriction.*

The role of the nurse in evaluation of renal function is most evident with respect to the recognition of signs and symptoms indicative of changing renal status. Nurses need to have a mental checklist of relevant observations and must educate clients to note and report such indicators of renal function.

Nurses need to recognize that many drugs exhibit an increased potential for toxicity when administered to clients who are in acute renal failure. Renal failure will prolong half-life and increase pharmacological effects and toxicity of drugs that are eliminated from the body mainly by renal clearance (Table 43–4), so doses will need to be reduced and plasma concentrations monitored. Renal failure also alters the elimination of liver metabolites of drugs, especially those formed by acetylation or hydrolysis, but this is seldom of consequence unless the metabolite is active. Drug administration should be more conservative for the client in renal failure. No drug should be given unless specifically indicated. Drugs that affect acid-base balance or electrolyte balance should be avoided (Table 43–5). If uremia is present, the protein binding of certain drugs (Table 43–4) will be significantly reduced by the high concentration of uric acid, necessitating dosage reduction.

Some drugs produce a harmless discoloration of urine as they are excreted (Table 43–6). Nurses need to forewarn clients of such effects so that the clients will not be unduly alarmed or suspect renal failure.

Table 43–4
Some Drugs Requiring Dosage Reduction in Renal Failure

I. Because of decreased excretion:

A. GFR < 50 ml/minute	B. GFR < 20 ml/minute
Antimicrobials	All drugs in list A, plus:
Aminoglycosides	Antimicrobials
Colistimethate	Ampicillin
Fluorocytosine	Amphotericin B
Tetracyclines	Carbenicillin
Vancomycin	Cephalosporins
Viomycin	Cycloserine
Others	Dapsone
Cyclophosphamide	Ethambutol
Digoxin	Lincomycin
Gold	Methicillin
Lithium	Neomycin
Mephobarbital	Penicillins
Methotrexate	Quinine
Phenobarbital	Sulfonamides
Probenecid	Others
Succinimides	Diazoxide
	Methyldopa
	Procainamide

II. Because of decreased binding in uremia

Barbiturates	Phenylbutazone
Benzylpenicillin	Phenytoin
Clofibrate	Salicylates
Diazepam	Sulfonamides
Diazoxide	Thyroxine
Furosemide	Triamterene
Morphine	Valproic acid
Pentobarbital	Warfarin
Phenobarbital	

Table 43–5
Drugs That Alter Acid-Base, Fluid, or Electrolyte Balance

Type of imbalance	Drugs
Acidosis	Ammonium chloride, nalidixic acid, nitrofurantoin, salicylates
Alkalosis	Calcium carbonate, carbenicillin
Hypervolemia	Carbamazepine, chlorpropamide, clofibrate, indomethacin
Hypermagnesia	Antacids
Hyperkalemia	Potassium penicillin G
Hypernatremia	Many (see Table 42–6)
Uremia	Anabolic steroids, glucocorticoids, tetracyclines

Chronic Renal Failure

Chronic renal failure (CRF) is a gradually developing state of renal dysfunction that typically passes through three stages of severity: (1) diminished renal reserve, in which there is measurable but asymptomatic loss of renal function, (2) renal insufficiency, and finally, (3) uremia. The causes of CRF are many and varied, and the progression of renal disease is not altered by any currently known treatment. During the phase of renal insufficiency, dietary management and careful avoidance of aggravating factors (such as hypovolemia, nephrotoxins, infections, hypercalcemia) can prolong the period of comfortable and productive life and delay the need for dialysis or kidney transplantation.

Antidiuretic Hormone as a Drug

Mechanisms and Effects The foremost effect of ADH is to promote reabsorption of water from the tubule of the nephron by increasing permeability of tubular cells to water in the distal tubule and collecting duct. Water reabsorption occurs by osmotic flow if the tubular wall is permeable to it in this region because the distal tubule and collecting

Table 43–6
Changes in the Appearance of Urine Caused by Drugs or Foods

Change in appearance	Possible causes
Milky urine	Phosphates
Pink, red, or red-brown	Anthraquinones, cinchophen, danthrone, doxorubicin, food pigments, metronidazole, nitrites, phenindione, phenolphthalein, phenothiazines, phensuximide, phenytoin, prochlorperazine
Yellow-pink (only if urine is alkaline)	Aloin, cascara, senna
Yellow-orange	Fluorescein, sulfasalazine
Orange, red-orange, or red-brown	Chlorzoxazone, ethoxazene, phenazopyridine, phenindione, rifampin
Yellow or green	Vitamin B_2, carotene-containing foods, methylene blue, quinacrine, yeast concentrate
Green	Anthraquinone, bile pigments, methylene blue, resorcinol, tetrahydronaphthalene, thymol
Blue or black	Methylene blue, aniline dyes, cascara, hydroxyquinone, melanin, naphthalene, naphthol, nitrites, nitrofurans, phenols, pyrogallol, quinine, resorcinol, rhubarb, senna, thymol
Purple or magenta	Fuchsin, phenolphthalein
Brown or tan	Bile (in jaundice), bismuth, chlorzoxazone, danthron, levodopa, metronidazole, methyldopa, mercury, naphthalene, nitrofurans, primaquine, quinine, sulfonamides

duct pass through the highly osmolar medullary region of the kidney on their way to the renal pelvis.

ADH receptors are located on the basement membrane of distal tubule cells in the luminal membrane, on the opposite side of the cell from the tubule (Figure 43–3). When activated by ADH, these receptors promote formation of adenosine 3′-5′-cyclic phosphate (cyclic AMP) in the tubule cells, which in turn promotes formation of water channels in the luminal membrane. These channels are very small, permitting passage of water but not even small solute particles. ADH also stimulates formation of prostaglandins that ultimately turn off the ADH action. Inhibitors of prostaglandin synthesis sensitize the kidney to ADH.

The other important effect of ADH is on smooth muscle. Stimulation of vascular smooth muscle results in a pressor action. The effect is direct, not mediated through sympathetic receptors nor antagonized by sympathetic blockers. The action is also nonspecific — all regions of the vasculature are affected, including coronary, gastrointestinal, and cutaneous blood vessels. At high doses, ADH can stimulate visceral as well as vascular smooth muscle, causing hypermotility of the gut and uterine contractions in women. ADH also increases factor VIII of the clotting cascade. During pregnancy, ADH can be destroyed by a peptidase that appears in the plasma (presumably for the purpose of metabolizing oxytocin to prevent premature uterine contractions).

Pharmacokinetics ADH of most mammals is identical to human ADH, but porcine ADH (called lypressin) differs slightly in structure and is less potent but more selective for antidiuresis (Table 43–7). The natural peptides with ADH activity are rapidly metabolized by peptidases and are thus short-acting drugs. A synthetic analogue of ADH, desmopressin, is more resistant to peptidases, and has a much longer duration of action, greater antidiuretic potency, and little pressor effect.

Table 43–7
Activity of ADH-like Peptides

	Activity[a]	
	Antidiuretic	Pressor
ADH	100	100
Lypressin	80	100
Oxytocin	1	1
Desmopressin	1,200	0.39

[a]Relative to ADH.

Clinical Indications ADH is used to treat diabetes insipidus, a deficiency of ADH resulting from dysfunction of hypothalamic/neurohypophyseal peptide-producing neurons. Diabetes insipidus can be either neurogenic (ADH-sensitive) or nephrogenic (ADH-insensitive), which occurs as a kidney defect. The main feature of diabetes insipidus is production of a large volume of dilute urine, typically with a specific gravity of less than 1.005 (osmolarity less than 200 mosm/L). The water loss is accompanied by thirst and polydipsia. Diabetes insipidus may be caused by lesions (such as cranial injuries, fractures, vascular accidents, tumors, or granulomas) or congenital defects that interrupt the hypothalamo-neurohypophyseal pathway, inhibiting delivery of ADH to the terminals in the neurohypophysis. Diagnosis of diabetes insipidus is established by measuring overnight urinary concentrating capacity. If diabetes insipidus is confirmed, ADH is administered to determine if it is ADH-sensitive or ADH-insensitive.

Nephrogenic diabetes insipidus occurs when the renal tubule is insensitive to ADH. It occurs in CRF involving the distal tubule and collecting ducts, including many cases caused by hypercalcemia, hypokalemia, metabolic diseases, hereditary tubulointerstitial diseases, and obstructions. Reversible ADH-insensitive diabetes insipidus can also be induced by drugs such as lithium, the antibiotic demeclocycline, and drugs that inhibit activity of microtubules, such as colchicine and vinca alkaloids. Irreversible nephrogenic diabetes insipidus has been caused by the anesthetic methoxyflurane. Since nephrogenic diabetes insipidus is ADH-insensitive, the principal means of therapy is with diuretics.

Adverse Effects and Contraindications Adverse effects of ADH are insignificant at low doses. The main concern is the proper adjustment of dose so as to avoid water intoxication. At high doses, adverse symptoms occur due to both pressor and water-retaining effects. The adverse effects due to the pressor action include facial pallor caused by constriction of surface blood vessels. Nausea, cramps, urge to defecate, and uterine cramps in women occur due to visceral smooth muscle stimulation. Coronary artery disease is a contraindication for use of any but the smallest doses of ADH because of the constrictor effects. All of these adverse effects are avoidable by selection of desmopressin (Stimate), since it lacks significant pressor activity. The only adverse effects associated with the renal action of vasopressin compounds are elevations in blood pressure and associated vascular headaches, and these occur only with doses of 40 μg or more.

Preparations and Administration ADH is available in a number of preparations that differ in specificity of action, duration, and routes of administration. Posterior pituitary is a desiccated powder of pituitary glands. It is available in capsules or as an inhalator. Posterior pituitary injection (Pituitrin) is a sterile aqueous extract for injection. These pituitary extract preparations have mixed oxytocic and vasopressin activity and are used mainly for their oxytocic effects.

Posterior pituitary injection (Pituitrin-S) is employed as a topical hemostatic for esophageal varices and abdominal surgery. There is a risk of serious cardiac and vascular complications due to the constrictor effects of vasopressin on coronary and other blood vessels. Vasopressin is never employed when sympathomimetics can be used effectively.

Vasopressin injection (Pitressin) is obtained from pituitary glands of cows and pigs or by synthesis. There is no oxytocin in this preparation, although vasopressin has a weak oxytocic effect. It is given intravenously for determining if urine-concentrating ability is affected by ADH in patients with diabetes insipidus. This test distinguishes ADH-sensitive from ADH-insensitive diabetes insipidus. It can also be used for transient polyuria. Vasopressin is of no value in chronic treatment of diabetes insipidus because of its short duration of action (about 3–4 hours).

Vasopressin tannate (Pitressin tannate) is an oil suspension of vasopressin for depot injection. Until recently, it was the treatment of choice for clients with diabetes insipidus. It is given intramuscularly every 1–3 days. Sterile abscesses and abdominal pain sometimes occur.

Lypressin (Diapid), synthetic lysine vasopressin, is provided as a nasal spray. It must be administered every 4–12 hours. Four times per day is typical, but the dosage regimen is individualized for each client.

Desmopressin acetate (Stimate) is the current drug of choice for diabetes insipidus, combining improved specificity of action (lack of pressor effect) and long duration (8–12 hours). It is used as a nasal spray. About 25% of patients can use the drug once a day with satisfactory results. The majority must use it twice a day, while a few patients require three doses daily. Dosage requirements vary from 5–40 μg and must therefore be individualized. The nighttime dose is first titrated to control nocturia, then the morning dose is adjusted to control daytime polyuria. A third dose may be required in the afternoon. The drug is stored at 4° C. and has a survival time of about 2 weeks at room temperature.

Diuretics

Diuretics are drugs that increase the volume of urine formed per unit of time. Usually they are ordered when clients have not been able to correct sodium and water retention through the use of diet and other drugs. Many classes of drugs have been used as diuretics, and they differ widely in their mechanisms of action. The most important indications for use of diuretics are the alleviation of essential hypertension and the mobilization of edema fluid. Diuretics are also used in acute renal failure to maintain an adequate urine volume. Most diuretics have pronounced effects on the reabsorption of ionic substances; the effects are important both to an understanding of the mechanism of action of these drugs and to an appreciation of clinical aspects of therapy that incorporates use of these agents.

Nine distinct classes of diuretics can be identified, but of these, two classes are obsolete (organic mercurials and acid-forming salts such as ammonium chloride) and will not be discussed here. One class, uricosuric diuretics, is under development but not yet available for clinical use. Two other classes, the carbonic anhydrase inhibitors and xanthines, are of minor importance. These groups will be discussed only briefly. That leaves four types of diuretics having significant clinical importance at the present time: (1) benzothiadiazides and related diuretics, (2) high-ceiling diuretics, (3) potassium-sparing diuretics, including two distinct types, and (4) osmotic diuretics, which have distinctive and limited applications. Five classes of diuretics are compared in Table 43–8. Various combination preparations are also marketed. Of the top 200 prescription drugs in 1983, 15 were diuretics. Ten of these 15 contained only a thiazide or a related sulfonamide diuretic; two contained a thiazide in combination with a potassium-sparing agent (including Dyazide, the most widely prescribed of all drugs); one a thiazide in combination with the antihypertensive drug, reserpine; one a high-ceiling diuretic alone; and one a potassium-sparing diuretic alone. Clearly, the thiazides and related drugs dominate the current market for diuretic prescriptions.

Benzothiadiazides and Related Diuretics

The benzothiadiazides, or thiazide-type diuretics, evolved out of research aimed at developing new carbonic anhydrase inhibitors. While many thiazides

Table 43–8
Characteristics of Major Diuretic Classes

	Thiazides	High-ceiling	Potassium-sparing	Osmotic	CA inhibitors
Site of action	Distal tubule sodium pumps	Ascending loop chloride pumps	Distal tubule Na^+-K^+(H^+) exchange mechanism	Osmotic gradient in proximal tubule and ascending loop	H^+ secretory mechanism
Route	Oral	Oral	Oral	IV	Oral
Maximum extent of diuresis[a]	+ + +	+ + + +	+	+ + + +	+ +
Time to peak (hours)	4–6[b]	1–2	2–6	Immediate	2–8
Effect on potassium	Hypokalemia sometimes	Hypokalemia	Hyperkalemia	Negligible hypokalemia	Hypokalemia
Acid-base effect	Negligible in net	Alkalosis	Acidosis	Negligible	Acidosis
Effect on GFR	Decrease	Little effect	Triamterene decreases. Spironolactone has no effect.	Increase	None
Effect on nitrogen compounds	Hyperuricemia Azotemia	Hyperuricemia	Azotemia	None	None
Other adverse effects	Allergic reactions GI disturbances	Hypovolemia Ototoxicity Allergic reactions		Dehydration	
Special indications	Primary choice for essential hypertension and mild to moderate edema	Severe edema Azotemia Disorders of electrolytes	Hyperaldosterism Hypokalemia	To increase renal elimination of poisons	Metabolic alkalosis Cor pulmonale

[a]+ + + +, strongest diuresis; + + +, substantial diuresis; + +, moderate diuresis; +, minimal diuresis.
[b]The peak for cyclothiazide occurs later (7–12 hours) and for metolazone and chlorthalidone earlier (2 hours).

are, in fact, inhibitors of carbonic anhydrase, this is not the main basis for their diuretic efficacy. Thiazides include the prototype chlorothiazide (Diuril), hydrochlorothiazide (HydroDiuril), hydroflumethiazide (Saluron), benzthiazide (Exna), cyclothiazide (Anhydron), methylclothiazide (Enduron, Aquatensen), trichlormethiazide (Naqua, Metahydrin, Diurese), and polythiazide (Renese). In addition, three sulfonamide diuretics are currently marketed that are structural analogues of the thiazides and are equivalent to them pharmacologically: chlorthalidone (Hygroton), metolazone (Zaroxolyn), and quinethazone (Hydromox). Another drug, indapamide (Lozol), is structurally distinctive, but pharmacologically equivalent. Indapamide is an indoline derivative first marketed in 1982.

Mechanisms and Effects The thiazide-type diuretics **inhibit the reabsorption of sodium** and its attendant chloride ion from the distal convoluted tubule by the type 3 pumps (Figure 43–4). The result is an elevated excretion of sodium, chloride, and water. Some of the thiazide diuretics have effects on carbonic anhydrase, but the extent of this action varies from agent to agent (Table 43–9). Inhibition of sodium reabsorption results in an increased intratubular sodium load in the distal tubule. With delivery of more sodium to the distal tubule, the sodium-potassium exchange mechanism is stimulated, generating an **increase in potassium secretion.** Potassium excretion frequently occurs to the point where hypokalemia results. On the other hand, thiazides usually exert their action without altering acid-base balance. Mild alkalosis may occur due to stimulation of sodium exchange for hydrogen ion, but those agents that significantly inhibit carbonic anhydrase may inhibit hydrogen ion secretion and raise urinary pH.

Other effects of thiazide diuretics include a **decrease in glomerular filtration rate** (which can be used to good effect in treatment of nephrogenic dia-

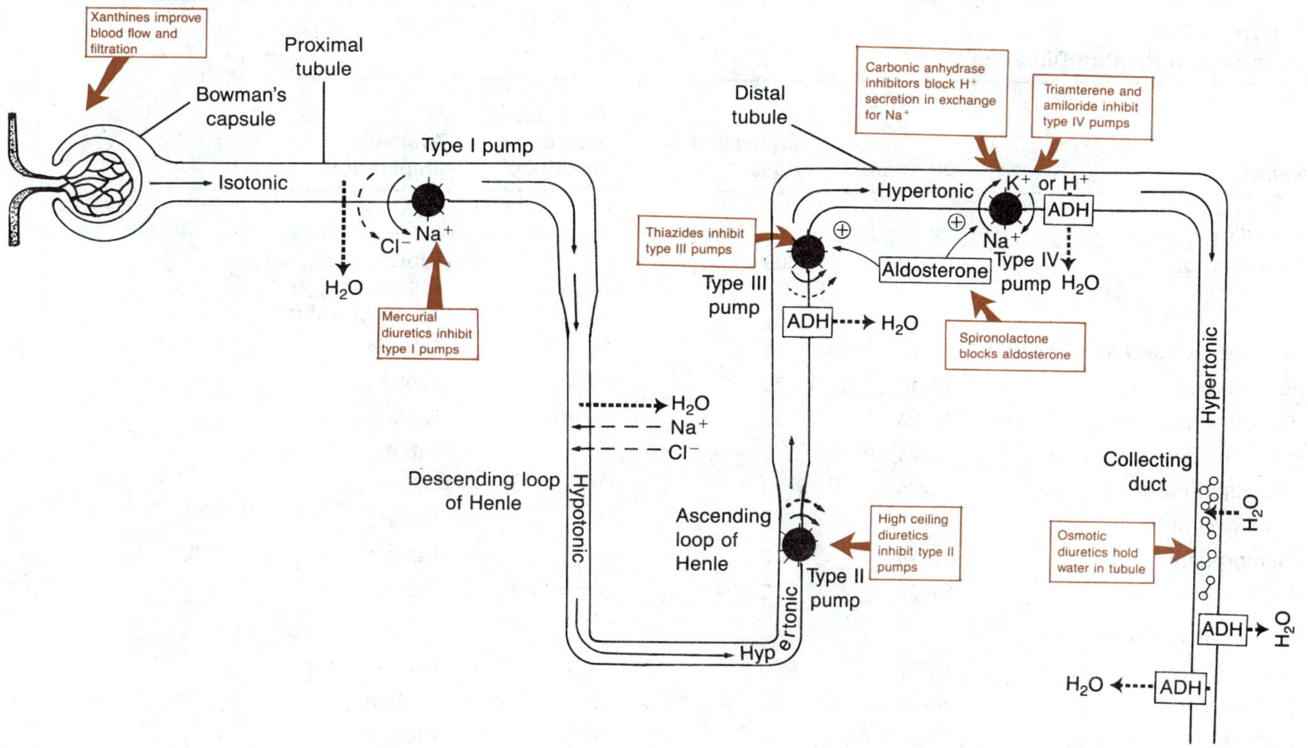

Figure 43–4
The mechanisms of diuretics.

betes insipidus), **a decrease in uric acid secretion** (leading to hyperuricemia and aggravation of gout), a **decrease in calcium excretion** (unlike most diuretics), **increased magnesium excretion** (leading to hypomagnesia), and **hyperglycemia** of unknown etiology. The decrease in GFR is not seen with use of metolazone, which otherwise shares the effects of this class.

Thiazides produce a hypotensive effect by **relaxing the vascular smooth muscle,** causing decreased peripheral resistance to blood flow. In hypertensive individuals in whom elevated blood pressure is attributable to edema, correction of hypervolemia also contributes to the antihypertensive efficacy. Some diuretic thiazide-like drugs (indapamide (Lozol), for example), and nondiuretic thiazide-like drugs (diazoxide (Hyperstat) and minoxidil (Loniten), discussed in Chapter 39) have a more powerful and direct action on vascular smooth muscle related to inhibition of calcium-induced vascular smooth muscle contractions.

Pharmacokinetics Thiazides are well absorbed from the intestines after oral administration. Anion exchange resins can interfere with thiazide absorption, and for that reason, thiazides should be given at least 1 hour before resin administration.

Thiazide-type diuretics are actively secreted into the urine unchanged by the organic anion transport system. Since elimination of thiazides is largely by renal excretion, their use in acute renal insufficiency is hazardous. Indapamide, however, is largely metabolized in the liver before excretion (in both the urine and the bile) and is safe for use in renal insufficiency. The renal mechanism by which thiazides are secreted is subject to competitive inhibition by other organic anions, such as probenecid. Inhibition of thiazide transport may or may not alter the diuretic effect. Thiazide diuretics readily cross the placental barrier and are excreted in breast milk.

Clinical Indications One major indication for use of thiazides is edema, especially that resulting from congestive heart failure, liver or kidney disease, or pregnancy. The most common use of thiazides is for essential hypertension. Thiazides exert an antihypertensive effect that is partly secondary to the diuretic action and partly a direct relaxant action on the vascular smooth muscle. The antihypertensive effect is achieved by a reduction in peripheral resist-

Table 43–9
Thiazide and Related Diuretics

Name	Duration	Equivalent dose	Carbonic anhydrase inhibition[a]	Available preparations
Thiazides				
Chlorthiazide	6–12	500	+ + + +	Tablets, oral suspension, injection powder
Hydrochlorothiazide	6–12	50	+ + +	Tablets
Benzthiazide	12–18	50	+ +	Tablets
Hydroflumethiazide	18–24	50	+ +	Tablets
Bendroflumethiazide	18–24	5	+	Tablets
Methyclothiazide	24	5	?	Tablets
Cyclothiazide	18–24	2	?	Tablets
Trichlormethiazide	18–24	2	+ +	Tablets
Polythiazide	24–36	2	?	Tablets
Related diuretics				
Chlorthalidone	48–72	50	+ + + +	Tablets
Quinethazone	18–24	50	?	Tablets
Metolazone	12–24	5	+ +	Tablets
Indapamide	18–24	2.5	?	Tablets

[a] + + + +, strongest CA inhibition; + + +, substantial inhibition; + +, moderate inhibition; +, minimal inhibition.

ance to blood flow as a result of dilation of small arterioles. The reduction in peripheral resistance is related to hyponatremia and correction of hypervolemia. Thiazides potentiate other antihypertensive agents. The thiazides are the first drugs normally employed in essential hypertension in the step approach (see Chapter 39).

A less frequent use of thiazides is in the treatment of diabetes insipidus, where they produce a paradoxical reduction in urine volume. Thiazides can also be used in management of hypercalciuria associated with recurrent calcium stones.

Adverse Effects and Contraindications The most important side effect of thiazides is **hypokalemia.** *Elderly patients and those on steroids or digitalis are most likely to suffer hypokalemic effects.* Clients experiencing hypokalemia require treatment with dietary adjustments, potassium supplements, or concurrent use of potassium-sparing diuretics. Blood measurements of electrolytes, uric acid, and blood urea nitrogen (BUN) should be conducted frequently for patients on prolonged thiazide therapy. Magnesium supplements may be required during diuretic therapy with thiazides to combat **hypomagnesia.**

Uric acid and BUN are measured in order to determine the extent of **hyperuricemia,** a frequent adverse effect of thiazides. Hyperuricemia occurs because thiazides, as organic anions, compete with uric acid for the proximal tubule organic anion transport mechanism, blocking uric acid secretion. Hyperuricemia is of consequence mainly in susceptible patients in whom attacks of gout may occur. Probenecid (Benemid) can be used to promote uric acid excretion, but may also alter the effects of the diuretic.

Thiazide-induced **hyperglycemia** may aggravate diabetes mellitus. *Nurses need to alert clients who take insulin that they may need to adjust the dosage. Nurses should assess clients for symptoms of diabetes, especially in those patients with preexisting active or latent diabetic conditions.*

Diuretic therapy is aimed at correcting body fluid retention. If the dosage is not optimized, **hypovolemia** or, conversely, continued edema may be evident. *Clients at home need to be taught self-monitoring and recording of blood pressure, fluid intake and output, and daily weight. Clients should be encouraged to report neurological symptoms indicative of fluid imbalances, such as headache, vertigo, and paresthesias. The nurse, client, and* *client's family should watch for signs of orthostatic hypotension, such as dizziness or fainting upon standing up abruptly. Xerostomia (dry mouth) may accompany fluid elimination and requires thorough oral hygiene to minimize risks of irritation to membranes and demineralization of teeth that can occur when salivary secretions are sharply diminished.*

Other adverse effects of thiazide include **gastrointestinal side effects:** upset stomach, heartburn, loss of appetite, constipation, or abdominal cramps. Nurses or clients may note changes in skin color indicating jaundice. Some clients develop a **rash** or **photosensitivity.** *The nurse should instruct clients concerning the possibility of unusual or delayed sunburn and the need to report such reactions to the physician.* Clients may also develop a **hemolytic anemia** in response to use of thiazides.

Drug Interactions Drug interactions are not uncommon with thiazides. To begin with, thiazides can enhance the antihypertensive action of other antihypertensives, and their own action may be potentiated by central nervous system depressants. Thiazides also inhibit blood pressure responses to catecholamines. Because of the hypokalemia associated with thiazides, digitalis action can be intensified to the point that maintenance doses may become toxic. Thiazides may intensify paralysis induced by curare because of hypokalemia. Concurrent use of steroids aggravates thiazide-induced hypokalemia. Clients with diabetes may require elevated doses of insulin because of the hyperglycemic action of thiazides. Lithium clearance by the kidney is decreased by thiazides, and its toxicity is correspondingly increased.

Preparations and Administration The preparations of thiazide diuretics are listed in Table 43–9. The drugs are equivalent in most pharmacological respects, differing only in the degree of inhibition of carbonic anhydrase, the lack of effect of metolazone on GFR, the additional direct effect of indapamide on vascular smooth muscle, and pharmacokinetic parameters (equivalent dose and duration of action). Doses and frequency of administration are dictated by the relative potencies and durations of action of the various drug selections (Table 43–9). Thiazide diuretics produce their effects within 1–2 hours after administration, and peak effect usually occurs in 3–6 hours. Duration is determined mainly by the extent of plasma protein binding. Drugs with durations of 18 hours or longer are given once a day; those with durations in the 6–18 hour range are usually given twice. Doses should be scheduled so as to avoid causing nocturia — no later than approximately 3:00 PM for the second dose for drugs given twice a day. Unit doses are given in the morning. *To encourage clients' compliance, it is best to work with them so they can adjust their activities to coincide with peak drug activity and so as not to interfere with work or leisure plans.*

For chlorthiazide (Diuril), the usual daily dose is 500 to 1,000 mg PO for hypertension or 1,000–2,000 mg for edema. Doses of other drugs are smaller in proportion to the differences in equivalent doses. The preparations vary tremendously (by a factor of 18) in cost per unit of effectiveness; high cost may adversely affect compliance.

High-Ceiling Diuretics

High-ceiling diuretics derive their name from the fact that their maximum efficacy is far greater than that of other contemporary diuretics. There are currently three high-ceiling diuretics available for clinical use: furosemide (Lasix), bumetanide (Bumex), and ethacrynic acid (Edecrin). The first two of these are structurally related to each other and the thiazides, though they differ from the thiazides in mechanism. Bumetanide was introduced in the United States in 1983 but has been available in Europe longer. Ethacrynic acid is structurally unrelated but similar in pharmacology. Furosemide (Lasix) is currently the second most widely prescribed diuretic preparation and among the top 10 prescription drugs.

Mechanisms and Effects High-ceiling diuretics are sometimes called **loop diuretics** because their principal effect occurs on the type 2 electrolyte pumps in the ascending loop of Henle. Like thiazides, high-ceiling diuretics **inhibit reabsorption of sodium and chloride.** However, high-ceiling diuretics are much more potent in achieving this effect. Thiazides may promote excretion of at most 10% of the sodium and chloride that is filtered, whereas the high-ceiling diuretics can generate excretion of 20–30% of the filtered sodium and chloride.

The high-ceiling diuretics do not alter carbonic anhydrase activity appreciably. Both hydrogen and potassium excretion are increased because of increased sodium load in the distal tubule resulting in stimulation of sodium exchange for these ions. **Metabolic alkalosis** and **hypokalemia** are therefore significant adverse effects of high-ceiling diuretics, and the nurse must be alert for indications of hypokalemia such as muscle cramps, weakness, dry mouth, anorexia, and mental confusion. The loop diuretics are not rendered ineffective by either alkalosis or acidosis.

Unlike thiazides, high-ceiling diuretics increase calcium as well as magnesium excretion, resulting in

hypocalcemia and **hypomagnesia.** Like thiazides, loop diuretics cause **hyperuricemia** by inhibition of uric acid secretion. High-ceiling diuretics seldom alter renal blood flow or GFR, except at very high doses. High-ceiling diuretics have no significant direct effects on tissues other than the kidney at normal doses.

Pharmacokinetics The high-ceiling diuretics are readily absorbed after oral administration. In the plasma, they are bound to plasma proteins in substantial quantities and compete with other drugs for protein-binding sites. Onset of diuresis occurs typically in 20–60 minutes. Excretion occurs principally via the kidney, both by filtration and by secretion. A lesser amount is excreted through the bile.

Clinical Indications The main indications for high-ceiling diuretics are congestive heart failure and renal or hepatic dysfunctions that lead to severe edema. They are also used in conjunction with intravenous infusions of normal saline to stimulate diuresis in clients who have electrolyte accumulation such as hypernatremia, hypercalcemia, and hypermagnesia. Furosemide, along with mannitol (Osmitrol), an osmotic duretic, is sometimes employed in incipient acute renal failure. With respect to essential hypertension, high-ceiling diuretics are reserved for clients requiring a potent diuretic or for those who are refractory to thiazides. The risks of hypokalemia and excessive diuresis leading to circulatory collapse are the limiting considerations in clinical application.

Adverse Effects and Contraindications Adverse effects of high-ceiling diuretics usually relate directly to the primary effects on electrolytes and fluid. **Excess diuresis** can lead to hypovolemic shock or neurological symptoms such as vertigo, headache, blurred vision, and, in the extreme, circulatory collapse. *The nurse should be attentive, especially in the elderly, to symptoms such as weakness, lightheadedness, and dizziness indicative of hypovolemia.* This is especially true among those who have chronic heart disease and have been on salt-restricted diets for a period of time. If not monitored closely, the resultant hypovolemia can lead to vascular thrombi, emboli, or circulatory collapse. *Hospitalized clients receiving high-ceiling diuretics intravenously need to be observed for changes in blood pressure or vital signs. The infusion rate is usually prescribed by the physician, and the nurse needs to check it frequently.* The usual flow rate does not exceed 4 mg/minute.

Hypokalemia is a common problem, again especially in the elderly. *Complaints of weakness, increased perspiration, feeling faint, lightheaded, or dizzy, may be early signs of electrolyte imbalance. Other indications of electrolyte disturbances are bladder spasm, muscle cramps, or unusual urinary frequency. The client and family members should be told to report such symptoms immediately. Nurses need to help clients adjust their diet to prevent or reduce the incidence of potassium depletion.* Most clients will likely require a fairly liberal salt intake to prevent **hyponatremia** and **hypochloremia.** However, those who have cirrhosis usually are on salt-restricted diets. *Clients receiving high-ceiling diuretics should have periodic serum and urine electrolyte determinations.*

Allergic reactions occur to high-ceiling diuretics, and in the case of furosemide and bumetanide, there is often cross-sensitivity with the structurally related thiazides. Skin rashes, exfoliative dermatitis, other eruptions, and jaundice are the allergic manifestations. *Nurses need to assess clients' sclera for evidence of jaundice. Nurses should advise clients receiving high-ceiling diuretics to avoid excessive exposure to direct sunlight.*

Leukopenia and **anemia,** as well as **thrombocytopenia** occur rarely. *Clients receiving high-ceiling diuretics should have periodic blood counts.* **Ototoxicity** is a special concern with high-ceiling diuretics, and they should not be used concurrently with antimicrobials. Hearing loss, tinnitus, or vertigo are early signs of toxicity.

High-ceiling diuretics are contraindicated in pregnancy and in nursing mothers. *High-ceiling diuretics may cause gastrointestinal disturbances and are best taken with meals.* Gastrointestinal side effects are much more common with ethacrynic acid than with furosemide. Precautions regarding clients who take digitalis and those who are prone to gout are the same as for thiazides. *When clients are taking digitalis, they need to be monitored carefully for digitalis intoxication and dysrhythmias.*

Clients who report redness and swelling and pain in joints may be experiencing uric acid accumulation. Clients receiving high-ceiling diuretics should have periodic uric acid determinations.

High-ceiling diuretics cause **hypoglycemia** rather than the hyperglycemia seen with thiazides. *Thus, a client complaining of feeling weak, tired, dizzy, or lacking energy should be suspected of having an adverse response to a high-ceiling diuretic. Those who have diabetes may need changes in insulin requirements. Clients receiving high-ceiling diuretics should have periodic blood sugar determinations.*

Drug Interactions High-ceiling diuretics are similar to thiazides in that they potentiate antihypertensive agents, intensify digitalis toxicity, and inhibit responsiveness to catecholamines. In addition, high-

Nursing Observations for Diuretic Therapy

THERAPEUTIC GOAL	Mobilization of retained fluid and reduction of blood pressure.
PREADMINISTRATION ASSESSMENT	
Baseline Data	Evaluate skin perfusion, swelling of hands, ankles, and feet, and abdominal protrusion. Measure blood pressure, pulses, and ECG. Evaluate respiratory rate, depth, and sounds. Assess renal output and neurological function. Obtain laboratory tests including baseline blood tests: electrolytes, BUN, creatinine, blood glucose, complete blood cell count, uric acid, and pH.
Contraindication/ Precautions	Pregnancy, lactation, renal or hepatic failure, gout, or electrolyte imbalances.
EVALUATION OF DRUG RESPONSE	
For Therapeutic Benefit	Monitor for increased fluid output, reductions in edema, weight, abdominal distention, improved skin tone, diminished pulmonary congestion, and diminished coughing.
For Adverse Effects	Monitor blood pressure regularly and look for symptoms of dehydration or orthostatic hypotension. Evaluate serum electrolytes or hypo- or hyperkalemia, hyponatremia, hypochloremia, hypo- or hypercalcemia, hypomagnesia, and metabolic alkalosis or acidosis. Watch for acute aggravations of hypokalemia related to prolonged diarrhea, vomiting, stress, or diet changes. Monitor serum uric acid levels for hyperuricemia and fasting blood glucose for hyperglycemia. Observe for evidence of thromboembolism since risk is increased by dehydration. Monitor blood cell counts for evidence of dyscrasias.
For Drug Interactions	Monitor potentiation of digitalis or neuromuscular preparations as a result of hypokalemia. Monitor for need to adjust doses of antidiabetic agents or antigout drugs. Monitor for interactions with lithium, alcohol, and steroids with mineralocorticoid activity.
For Dietary Interactions	Monitor dietary intake of potassium, sodium, and calcium to ensure that intake is appropriate to the requirements of the specific regimen.
For Compliance	Evaluate client's compliance with all facets of the therapeutic regimen by careful observation, interviewing, and review of progress. Report compliance problems to the physician and act as client-advocate when changes in the therapeutic regimen seem indicated.

ceiling diuretics inhibit renal excretion of salicylates and may therefore cause salicylate toxicity. Ethacrynic acid has a mutually antagonistic action with probenecid (Benemid). High-ceiling diuretics are bound to plasma proteins to a significant extent and will potentiate drugs such as warfarin (Coumadin) that are likewise highly bound. As with thiazides, clearance of lithium is reduced and its toxicity is thus increased. Absorption of high-ceiling diuretics is inhibited by phenytoin (Dilantin).

Preparations and Administration *Tablets of Lasix may change color, but their potency remains the same. However, solutions of Lasix should be discarded if they change in color. Both tablets and solutions should be stored at temperatures between 59° and 86° F and protected from light or freezing.*

Bumetanide is well absorbed. One milligram of bumetanide is equivalent in potency to 40 mg of furosemide.

High-ceiling diuretics should be scheduled so as to avoid nocturia that could disturb client sleep. A single daily dose should be given in the morning. If the client is to take the diuretic twice a day, taking it in the early morning (7:00 or 8:00 AM) and early afternoon (1:00 or 2:00 PM) should enable the client to complete the peak activity before it is necessary to go to bed.

Bumetanide (Bumex)
Tablets, injection solution
Recommended Doses: 0.5–2.0 mg PO in a single administration. Additional doses can be given at intervals no less than 4–5 hours up to a total of 10 mg/day.

Ethacrynic acid (Edecrin)
Tablets, powder for reconstitution and injection
Recommended Doses: 50 mg PO daily, increased as required.

Furosemide (Lasix)
Tablets, oral solution (orange flavored), injection solutions in vials and prefilled syringes
Recommended Doses: For edema, 20–80 mg/day PO initially in a single dose, titrated upward to as much as 600 mg/day. For hypertension, 80 mg/day PO initially in 2 divided doses, titrated to achieve a satisfactory blood pressure reduction. In children, 2 mg/kg initially. The usual IV or IM dose is 20–40 mg initially with increments of 20 mg at 2-hour intervals. High parenteral doses should be infused slowly at no more than 4 mg/-minute.

Potassium-Sparing Diuretics

Three agents, spironolactone (Aldactone), triamterene (Dyrenium), and amiloride (Midamor) are used alone as diuretics or in conjunction with thiazide or high-ceiling diuretics to reduce loss of potassium. Because of their ability to inhibit potassium secretion, they are known as potassium-sparing agents. The drugs in this group act by more than one mechanism.

Spironolactone (Aldactone)

Mechanisms and Effects Spironolactone is a synthetic steroid that acts as a competitive inhibitor of the mineralocorticoid, aldosterone (Figure 43–4). Aldosterone normally stimulates both the sodium pumps and the Na^+-K^+(H^+) exchange mechanism in the distal convoluted tubule in its role as the major regulator of electrolyte balance. Spironolactone inhibits both of these effects of aldosterone. Inhibition of aldosterone-stimulated sodium reabsorption promotes sodium excretion and diuresis. Inhibition of aldosterone-stimulated exchange of sodium for potassium and hydrogen promotes potassium retention and metabolic acidosis. The extent of response to spironolactone depends on the level of circulating aldosterone.

Pharmacokinetics Spironolactone is well absorbed after oral administration. Spironolactone is not active until it is converted in the liver to its primary metabolite, canrenone. This occurs rapidly. Both spironolactone and canrenone are more than 90% bound by proteins in the plasma. Canrenone has an elimination half-life of 13–24 hours. Ultimately, spironolactone metabolites are excreted in the urine.

Clinical Indications Spironolactone is indicated for treatment of hypertension or edema, alone or in combination with more potent diuretics, especially when hypokalemia needs to be corrected. In addition, spironolactone, but not triamterene, is indicated for treatment of hyperaldosteronism, and its effectiveness is diagnostic for the condition.

Adverse Effects Spironolactone may produce **hyponatremia** or **hyperkalemia.** *During early phases of therapy with spironolactone, nurses need to monitor serum electrolytes and report signs of imbalances to the physician. Nurses are responsible for teaching clients to report instances of dry mouth, thirst, lethargy, and drowsiness, or abdominal cramps, which are symptoms of hyponatremia. A client's complaints of weakness, heaviness of the legs, or paresthesias, or the client's family's complaints that the client is confused may be indicative of hyperkalemia. Nurses need to teach clients receiving spironolactone to avoid foods that are high in potassium and to avoid salt substitutes. Clients should be given a list of foods from which to choose as well as being taught how to calculate sodium and potassium levels that would be allowable.*

Clients may experience minor **gastrointestinal discomfort** (anorexia, nausea, vomiting, and diarrhea). **Neurological symptoms** may cause clients to complain of drowsiness, weakness, or headache, or they may develop ataxia. Relatives may notice that the client appears confused. Some male clients receiving spironolactone experience difficulty obtaining or maintaining erection, which may result in noncompliance.

Spironolactone has weak **androgenic properties,** promoting hirsutism, deepening of the voice, gynecomastia, and breast tenderness. *Women need to be told of the potential for menstrual irregularities. They may be inclined to discontinue drug therapy if they notice hirsutism or voice changes. Nurses will need to help female clients adjust to the problem or advocate a change in the regimen if such problems interfere with compliance.*

In animal studies, carcinogenicity has been demonstrated with spironolactone. Spironolactone crosses the placenta, and its active metabolite, canrenone, is excreted in breast milk. Spironolactone is therefore relatively contraindicated in pregnancy and in nursing mothers. Spironolactone is contraindicated in acute renal insufficiency and hyperkalemia. Serum potassium levels should be monitored when spironolactone is used. The risks of hyperkalemia are increased if potassium salts are employed concurrently or if the diet is unusually rich in potassium.

Drug Interactions Diuretic effects of spironolactone may be additive with those of other diuretic agents. The diuretic effect of spironolactone may cause an increase in the concentration of clotting factors in the blood, which may interfere with the action of oral anticoagulants. Hyperkalemia associated with use of spironolactone may be increased by concurrent use of captopril (Captoten), since captopril inhibits formation of aldosterone. Spironolactone may decrease vascular responsiveness to norepinephrine. Salicylates have been noted to reduce the action of spironolactone.

Preparations and Administration

Spironolactone (Aldactone)

Tablets, combinations with hydrochlorthiazide (Aldactazide, Spiractazide, and others)

Recommended Doses: For hypokalemia, 25–100 mg/day PO; for hypertension, 50–100 mg/day PO; for hyperaldosteronism, 100–400 mg/day PO. The daily amount is usually given in 2 administrations.

Triamterene (Dyrenium)

Mechanisms and Effects Triamterene is not an aldosterone antagonist and does not require presence of aldosterone to exert its diuretic and potassium-sparing action. It exerts a direct inhibitory action on the sodium-potassium exchange mechanism in the distal tubule (Figure 43-4). The drug has no significant action except on the kidney. The diuresis

Nursing Diagnoses and Interventions for Diuretic Therapy

Nursing Diagnoses	*Related Interventions*
TO MINIMIZE DRUG SIDE EFFECTS OR INTERACTIONS	
Alteration in nutrition related to need to adjust sodium and potassium intake appropriate to the medication	Teach clients to recognize signs of hypokalemia. Inform clients about potassium-rich foods. Instruct clients to adhere to the prescribed sodium restriction.
Alteration in urinary elimination related to diuretic-induced increase in urinary output	Provide easy access to bathroom. Encourage clients to take diuretics at times when bathroom attendance is most convenient.
Increased risk of injury related to potential orthostatic hypotension caused by diuresis	Warn clients to avoid standing quickly because faintness may occur; provide side rails and other safety measures as required.
Sexual dysfunction related to diuretic therapy	Provide encouragement and reassurance that impotence sometimes caused by diuretics is transient and reversible.
TO ENSURE SAFE AND EFFICACIOUS DRUG USE	
Knowledge deficit about the drug regimen	Explain the actions of each drug in the regimen, appropriate dosing, and when the drug is to be taken. Provide the client with a list of adverse effects and drug interactions for each prescribed medication and what steps to take if any of these occur. Teach clients how to monitor their blood pressure and weight and to keep a record of changes. Instruct clients about prescribed dietary adjustments and use of potassium supplements if required.

produced by triamterene is modest. It is accompanied by loss of sodium and chloride but retention of potassium and hydrogen ions. Triamterene does not inhibit carbonic anhydrase or interfere with uric acid secretion.

Pharmacokinetics Triamterene is well absorbed and has an onset of action within 2–4 hours. Maximum therapeutic benefit may not be seen until after several days of therapy. Triamterene is metabolized in the liver and excreted by the kidney.

Clinical Indications Triamterene is indicated for relief of edema and in hypertension, alone or in combination with other diuretics, for its added diuretic effect and potassium-sparing action. It is contraindicated in severe renal or hepatic diseases.

Adverse Effects Triamterene appears to produce few adverse effects and some that do occur can be managed successfully so that clients need not discontinue using the drug. **Gastrointestinal disturbances** occur only occasionally. *When they do occur, the nurse should advise the client to take the drug either with or after meals. If nausea and vomiting continue to occur, the nurse should recognize that these symptoms may be an indication of electrolyte imbalance or renal failure and should report them.*

The most important adverse effect of triamterene is **hyperkalemia.** *Nurses need to make certain that clients do not take potassium supplements, salt substitutes, or eat an excessively potassium-rich diet.* Triamterene-induced hyperkalemia may antagonize the effects of cardiac glycosides.

When working with clients who have renal insufficiency, who are elderly, or who have diabetes mellitus, it is important for nurses to be particularly cognizant of signs and symptoms of hyperkalemia. Since many of these clients are at home, nurses have an added responsibility of assuring that periodic evaluations of renal function (BUN, serum creatinine) are done if they are suspected of renal insufficiency. Any complaint of fatigue, inability to sleep, nausea and vomiting, or an unpleasant taste in the mouth should cause the nurse to investigate further. *Nurses need to encourage clients to report even seemingly minor complaints, since in the aggregate the complaints may be an early warning that more serious problems are imminent.*

Blood dyscrasias and **liver damage** have occurred rarely. Weakness, headache, dry mouth, rash, and photosensitivity are possibilities. Triamterene causes a functional **deficiency in folic acid** and supplements of this vitamin during triamterene use are appropriate.

There have been reports that triamterene increases blood glucose. *Blood glucose levels should be monitored periodically and clients with diabetes should be warned about possible hyperglycemia.*

Triamterene tends to cause a blue fluorescence to urine. Nurses need to alert clients to this fact and reassure them that it is a harmless response to the drug.

Drug Interactions Antihypertensive effects of triamterene are additive with those of other antihypertensive drugs. Hyperkalemia induced by triamterene is increased with concomitant use of potassium salts, other potassium-sparing diuretics, or captopril. Triamterene may increase toxicity of lithium by reducing its renal clearance.

Preparations and Administration The combination product containing triamterene and hydrochlorthiazide (Dyazide) is currently the most widely prescribed of all drugs.

Triamterene (Dyrenium)
Capsules, combination capsules with hydrochlorthiazide (Dyazide)
Recommended Doses: 100 mg PO initially, twice daily, taken after meals to minimize gastrointestinal irritation. The maximum daily dosage is 300 mg. For the combination product, 1 or 2 capsules, twice daily.

Amiloride (Midamor)

Amiloride became the third potassium-sparing diuretic with its introduction in 1981. Although chemically unrelated to spironolactone or triamterene, its pharmacological effects are similar.

Pharmacokinetics Amiloride is excreted unchanged by the kidneys. Although its duration of action is sufficient to allow once-a-day administration, it does not ordinarily accumulate. Accumulation may occur, however, in patients with renal insufficiency.

Adverse Effects and Contraindications Amiloride is not employed alone because of the risk that it will induce **hyperkalemia.** Hyperkalemia occurs in up to 10% of patients when the drug is used alone, but in only 1–2% of patients when amiloride is added to thiazide therapy. *Clients who have symptoms of hyperkalemia usually complain of weakness and fatigue. Nurses would note the presence of flaccid paralysis, paresthesias, and bradycardia. If the client is being monitored by ECG, the nurse would note abnormalities. Ultimately, left untreated, the client would go into shock.* Hyperkalemia is especially likely in the elderly and in patients with diabetes mellitus, renal impairment, or acidosis.

Those at risk of hyperkalemia or exhibiting the characteristic symptoms should be closely monitored for serum electrolytes, creatinine, and blood urea nitrogen. **Diabetic nephropathy** and **renal insufficiency** are contraindications for use of amiloride.

Drug Interactions Amiloride inhibits renal elimination of lithium and should not be used in patients on lithium therapy. Potassium supplements should usually not be employed with amiloride but may be required in very severe cases of hypokalemia. Amiloride-induced hyperkalemia can also be intensified by concurrent use of other potassium-sparing diuretics or captopril.

Preparations and Administration

Amiloride (Midamor)
Tablets, combination tablets with hydrochlorthiazide (Moduretic)
Recommended Doses: 5 mg PO, taken once daily with food. In severe cases of hypokalemia, the daily dose can be increased to 10 mg.

Osmotic Diuretics

Osmotic diuretics are substances that are filtered but not reabsorbed to any great extent. Since they are osmotically active, they cause water to remain in the tubular filtrate, to be excreted ultimately in the urine. They are active as diuretics only until they are themselves excreted. Mannitol, the most extensively used osmotic diuretic, has a very rapid diuretic action of short duration. These characteristics dictate both the limitations and the usefulness of the drug. Osmotic diuretics are of no value for long-term mobilization of edema fluid. Their most important use is in prophylactic treatment of acute renal failure (oliguria), because reduced glomerular filtration rate does not affect their action. Other uses are to hasten elimination of toxic substances, to reduce intraocular pressure, and to reduce elevated intracranial pressure. Potential adverse effects of mannitol include headache, nausea, chills, chest pain, electrolyte depletion, and hypovolemia. Use of the drug must be terminated if signs of heart failure develop.

Preparations and Administrations

Mannitol (Osmitrol)
Injection solutions
Recommended Doses: 50–200 g/day, IV.

Carbonic Anhydrase Inhibitors

The use of carbonic anhydrase inhibitors as diuretics was instrumental in defining the importance of carbonic anhydrase in renal physiology. The prototype drug of the class is acetazolamide (Diamox). Carbonic anhydrase inhibitors inhibit the availability of hydrogen ion for exchange with sodium and thus increase urine volume as water is drawn out with the sodium retained in the tubule. Hydrogen ion is retained in the body, causing metabolic acidosis, but potassium must be exchanged for sodium to a greater than normal extent, resulting in hypokalemia.

Carbonic anhydrase inhibitors are effective diuretics, but newer drug classes provide greater efficacy. Metabolic acidosis produced by carbonic anhydrase inhibitors is a limiting feature. The only remaining indications for these drugs are as adjunctive treatment of edema and in glaucoma, to reduce intraocular pressure as an interim measure when a delay in surgical intervention is anticipated. The effectiveness in glaucoma is due to the role of carbonic anhydrase in formation of aqueous humor. Acetazolamide is sometimes used during initiation of therapy for gout with probenecid in order to promote a dilute and alkaline urine so as to minimize the risk of formation of urate crystals in the nephrourinary tract.

Preparations and Administrations

Acetazolamid (Diamox)
Tablets, sustained release capsules, injection solution
Recommended Doses: For glaucoma, 250 mg to 1 g PO daily initially, in doses of 250 mg.

Dichlorphenamide (Daranide, Oratrol)
Tablets
Recommended Doses: For acute angle-closure glaucoma in adults, 100–200 mg PO initially, followed by 100 mg every 12 hours until intraocular pressure is reduced.

Methazolamide (Neptazane)
Tablets
Recommended Doses: For glaucoma, 50–100 mg PO 2–3 times daily.

Xanthines

Xanthines are seldom used as diuretics, although they exert a mild diuretic action. Theophylline has a greater diuretic potency than either caffeine or theobromine. Theophylline has been used with thiazides to enhance absorption of the thiazide. The action of xanthines is principally on the hemodynamics of the kidney, improving renal blood flow and increasing filtration. The xanthines, especially theophylline, also weakly inhibit tubular reabsorption of sodium and chloride. Xanthines are discussed in Chapters

14 and 52 in relation to their more important roles as CNS stimulants and bronchodilators.

Important Nursing Implications for Diuretic Therapy

- ☐ Note the extent of edema prior to the initiation of a diuretic regimen and monitor changes in edema as an indication of response to therapy. Question the client about the quantity of urine excreted, color of the urine (to determine concentration), amount of sweating, and intake of fluids and foods with high fluid content. If there appears to be evidence of fluid retention, place the client on intake-output monitoring. Have the client weigh himself or herself daily, using the same scale, type of clothing, and time of day to further monitor for fluid retention.
- ☐ Teach clients to monitor their weight, girth, and their intake and output both of fluids and those foods that have high moisture content such as fruits and vegetables to assure that they are excreting the necessary amounts of fluids.
- ☐ Teach clients and their families to take the client's pulse and blood pressure to monitor for possible hypovolemia that can result from diuretics.
- ☐ Caution clients against ingesting alcohol, since alcohol encourages diuresis and can produce severe hypotension when taken with diuretics.
- ☐ Encourage clients to report any gastrointestinal disturbances, rapid heart rate, or oliguria, since these may be indicative of electrolyte imbalance.
- ☐ If the client is on a low sodium diet, monitor the client for possible hyponatremia. This is particularly important when working with elderly clients. Client complaints of nausea, vomiting, and lethargy can be caused by the excessive excretion of sodium.
- ☐ Observe for indications of hypokalemia such as complaints of muscle weakness, cramps, fatigue, hypoactive reflexes, paresthesia, and mental confusion, or signs of cardiac dysrhythmia. Intensify client monitoring after reports of anorexia, vomiting, or diarrhea, since these events contribute to hypokalemia. Hypokalemia is especially dangerous when clients are also receiving digitalis, since digitalis toxicity is increased in hypokalemia.
- ☐ Potassium depletion may contribute to depleting chloride. When this happens, metabolic alkalosis may occur. Monitor clients with this problem to make sure they are taking sufficient potassium chloride to replace both potassium and chloride that is being lost in the urine.
- ☐ If hypokalemia occurs, assure that the individual eats foods especially high in potassium in order to maintain a serum potassium of at least 3.2 mEq/L. This will usually reverse symptoms of hypokalemia, often dramatically.
- ☐ Advise clients that increased dietary sodium will tend to aggravate hypokalemia by causing more sodium to be delivered to the distal tubule, where it is exchanged for potassium.
- ☐ Caution clients against eating licorice because of its potential to cause severe hypokalemia.
- ☐ Monitor clients employing a potassium-sparing diuretic for possible hyperkalemia and instruct them not to take potassium supplements or to increase dietary potassium.
- ☐ Monitor clients who have diabetes for hyperglycemia since diuretic compounds can cause hyperglycemia. Clients who have diabetes may need to increase the dosage of a hypoglycemic agent (insulin or oral hypoglycemic). Individuals who have undiagnosed latent diabetes may begin to exhibit more overt symptoms of diabetes under the influence of a diuretic.
- ☐ Monitor uric acid levels in the plasma. Thiazide and high-ceiling diuretics may increase plasma uric acid concentrations, producing or aggravating hyperuricemia. The result is complaint of acute arthritis, especially in clients who have a hereditary predisposition to gout or those who have chronic renal failure. Uricosuric drugs may be necessary to counteract the condition.
- ☐ Check clients for signs of hypersensitivity such as sore throat, rash, or jaundice.

Uricosurics and Other Drugs for Hyperuricemia and Gout

Hyperuricemia can occur, as we have seen, as a side effect of thiazide and high-ceiling diuretics. It also occurs as an independent disorder due to abnormalities of purine metabolism. Accumulation of uric acid leads to deposition of crystals of monosodium urate from supersaturated body tissue around the joints and tendons. The result is a recurrent acute inflammatory disease of the peripheral joints, called **gout.** The big toes are often the first sites of acute gouty inflammation. The crystalline deposits in the joints are called tophi. The patient experiences periodic attacks of pain, swelling, and tenderness of the joints. Women have, on the average, slightly lower levels of uric acid in the serum, and gout is nearly 20 times more common in men than women. Obesity is a predisposing factor and long-term management of gout often involves a program for gradual weight loss.

Uric acid has rather poor solubility, all the more so in acidic fluids. When high concentrations of urate appear in the urine, there is a risk that urate crystals will form into calculi, causing obstruction of the nephrourinary tract. Uncontrolled gout is associated with chronic arthritis, nephritis, and premature atherosclerosis.

Uric acid is freely filtered by the renal glomerulus and is both secreted and reabsorbed in the proximal tubule by an organic anion transport mechanism. Drugs (such as probenecid) that compete with uric acid for reabsorption by this pump can be used to enhance uric acid excretion, while those (such as thiazide diuretics) that compete mainly for secretion may cause uric acid retention and aggravation of gout.

Chronic gout can be prevented or ameliorated by prophylactic measures. Dietary intake of foods that are rich in purines, including organ meat, sardines, and sweetbreads, should be restricted and alcohol should be avoided. Clients should be advised to wear light clothing, to elevate the affected extremities whenever possible, and to maintain high fluid intake. Treatment of hyperuricemia includes the use of three distinctive kinds of drugs: uricosurics, an inhibitor of uric acid synthesis, and a drug that blocks uric acid binding sites.

Uricosurics

A uricosuric is a drug that enhances excretion of uric acid in the urine by inhibiting its reabsorption. Two uricosuric agents are currently available, probenecid (Benemid) and sulfinpyrazone (Anturane). In clients with gout, uricosuric agents increase the excretion of urates to nearly double at normal therapeutic doses, although much higher increases in excretion rates can be achieved with elevated doses. These drugs are used to alleviate chronic gout and prevent the formation of new tophi. There may even be reduction in size or even removal of existing tophi as uric acid deposits are mobilized. Uricosurics are not effective for alleviation of acute attacks of gouty pain and inflammation. In fact, uricosuric therapy for chronic gout should not be initiated during an acute attack because mobilization of urate from tophi may briefly increase severity and frequency of attacks.

Pharmacokinetics Probenecid and sulfinpyrazone are both completely absorbed after oral administration and reach peak plasma concentrations in 2–4 hours. They are transported in the blood mainly bound to plasma proteins (85–95%). The free fraction is filtered by the kidney and exerts its effect in the proximal tubule. The half-life is about 8–10 hours for both drugs. Liver metabolites of probenecid appear in the urine. If the urine is alkaline, probenecid reabsorption is markedly reduced, resulting in more rapid elimination. Sulfinpyrazone is excreted in the urine unchanged.

Adverse Effects and Contraindications Probenecid causes few adverse effects in most patients. Gastrointestinal irritation (nausea, constipation) occurs in about 2% of patients and is especially problematic in patients with gastric or peptic ulcers. *These side effects can be alleviated by taking the drug after meals.* Allergic reactions, such as mild rashes, occur in 2–4% of patients. Probenecid increases the risk of stones and may cause hemolytic anemia in individuals with glucose-6-phosphate dehydrogenase deficiency (see Chapter 41). Headache, sore gums, and skin flushing occasionally occur. Rare serious side effects include nephrotic syndrome, blood dyscrasias, and aplastic anemia.

Sulfinpyrazone (Anturane) is more potent as a uricosuric but causes more frequent adverse reactions. Gastrointestinal irritation occurs in 10–15% of patients; sulfinpyrazone should be taken with food, milk, or antacids. Sulfinpyrazone is contraindicated in patients with active peptic ulcer or gastrointestinal inflammatory diseases. Hypersensitivity reactions, such as rash and fever, have been observed. Severe blood dyscrasias are a risk with sulfinpyrazone, and the drug should therefore not be used in patients with preexisting dyscrasias.

Drug-Drug and Drug-Diet Interactions Uricosurics can potentially alter the excretion of all drugs normally handled by the organic anion-transport system. Similarly, such drugs can alter probenecid excretion. For example, probenecid or sulfinpyrazone will interfere with clinical tests utilizing organic acids, including the phenolsulfonphthalein test of kidney function, the sulfobromophthalein test of liver function, the para-aminohippurate test, and tests using iodopyracet (Diodrast) as a contrast agent. Probenecid also inhibits transport of the serotonin metabolite, 5-hydroxyindole acetic acid, out of the brain, an effect that is utilized in evaluating serotonin turnover by cerebral spinal fluid measurements. *Nurses should notify the laboratory that the client is receiving probenecid when tests are ordered.*

Aspirin and diuretics, including thiazide and high-ceiling drugs, interfere with the uricosuric effect of probenecid by competing for the carrier system. *Nurses should advise clients to use acetaminophen rather than aspirin if a nonnarcotic analgesic is required.* Sulfonamides, penicillins, and cephalosporins have prolonged presence in the body when given with probenecid or sulfinpyrazone. Oral hypoglycemics likewise have an increased half-life and pharmacological activity. *Clients with diabetes need to be taught to monitor their status carefully and to report any signs of change.*

Foods that have a high purine content may interfere with the action of probenecid. Organ meats, meat extracts, and meaty soups should be avoided. *Nurses, working with a dietitian, need to assist clients in devising a diet that restricts high purine foods.*

Preparations and Administration *Because increased excretion of uric acid tends to predispose clients to renal calculi (kidney stones), the nurse should encourage clients to maintain a high fluid intake (10–12 glasses of water daily) and a urinary output of at least 2,000 ml/day.* Alkalinization of urine (with oral sodium bicarbonate or potassium citrate) during the first phase of therapy is advisable. *If urinary alkalinizers are used, nurses need to assure that acid-base status is evaluated periodically. Nurses need also to alert clients to physical changes that would indicate a potential imbalance when urinary alkalinizers are being employed.*

Probenecid (Benemid)
Tablets
Recommended Doses: For gout, 500 mg/day PO in 2 divided doses initially, increased to 1,000 mg/day in 2 doses after 1 week, and finally 2,000 mg/day in 4 divided doses if required.

Sulfinpyrazone (Anturane)
Tablets, capsules
Recommended Doses: 200–400 mg PO daily initially in 2 divided doses, to be taken with milk or food. The maximum daily dose is 800 mg.

Colchicine

Colchicine is an effective drug for prevention and relief of acute attacks of gout. Colchicine is an alkaloid derived from the seeds and roots of *Colchicum autumnale,* the autumn crocus or meadow saffron. The effectiveness of *Colchicum* for acute gout was recognized by Von Stöorck in 1763 and may have been introduced into the United States by Benjamin Franklin. The active alkaloid was extracted in 1820.

Colchicine resembles the vinca alkaloids, drugs used in cancer chemotherapy, in its mechanism of action. It binds to cellular proteins associated with the microtubular system to disrupt spindle formation during metaphase and thereby interrupt mitotic division of cells. Rapidly proliferating tissues are most affected. Alopecia can result from the drug's action on hair follicles, and the intestinal mucosa may undergo exfoliation.

The mechanism by which colchicine produces relief in hyperuricemia is not fully established. Colchicine does not inhibit synthesis of uric acid nor increase its excretion. The mechanism appears to be related to the inflammatory response to urate in the joints. Colchicine depresses the central nervous system, producing hypothermia and hypoventilation. On the other hand, colchicine raises blood pressure by increasing sensitivity of blood vessels to sympathetic amines.

Pharmacokinetics Colchicine is rapidly absorbed after oral administration, reaching peak plasma concentrations in 0.5–2 hours. The drug and its metabolites exhibit enterohepatic cycling to a substantial extent, which, unfortunately, ensures that effects on the gastrointestinal mucosa will be intense and prolonged.

Colchicine has a very large volume of distribution and an extended presence in the body. Cumulative toxicity is a risk. In order to avoid cumulative toxicity, a given course of colchicine therapy for acute gout is not usually repeated within 3 days. *Clients need to be made aware of the potential toxic effect of too frequent use of colchicine.* The drug is excreted 80–90% in the feces, only 10–20% in the urine.

Clinical Indications Colchicine is indicated for prevention and relief of acute attacks of gout. *Nurses should advise clients to take colchicine at the first sign of an attack. Since early initiation of therapy at the first sign of an acute attack is crucial, patients should be instructed to carry colchicine with them at all times.* Relief is obtained in better than 95% of attacks. Colchicine is so effective in acute gout that it is often employed to confirm the diagnosis.

During the period between attacks (called the intercritical period) colchicine has proven to be very effective as a prophylactic agent, to reduce the frequency and duration of attacks. Colchicine can also be used in this way during instillation of allopurinol or uricosuric therapy, when the risk of acute attacks is elevated. Colchicine can also be used prophylactically in gout-prone patients prior to and following surgery when the risk of acute attacks is elevated. Tolerance does not occur to colchicine.

Adverse Effects and Contraindications **Gastrointestinal problems** are an almost universal aspect of use of colchicine, occuring in 80% of clients, and generally as the first indication of toxicity. The susceptibility of the alimentary tract is probably due to the rapid rate of proliferation of the intestinal mucosal cells and the recycling of the drug through the enterohepatic system. Nausea, vomiting, diarrhea, and abdominal pain are the most common complaints. To counteract diarrhea, clients may need to take an antidiarrheal agent. Hemorrhagic gastroenteritis can occur with high doses, causing bloody stools. Malabsorption of carbohydrates, vitamins (notably B_{12}), and other nutrients may occur.

The irritant effect of colchicine may extend to the esophagus, skin, and kidney. **Acute renal failure,** indicated by oliguria and hematuria, may occur. *Clients who will be taking colchicine for a long period of time need to be taught to monitor fluid intake and output.* Dialysis and lavage may be required to remove colchicine if renal failure occurs. In overdose situations, weakness and muscle paralysis set in. The pulse becomes rapid but pulse pressure is reduced.

Chronic use of colchicine may cause disturbances of the formed elements of the blood: agranulocytosis, aplastic anemia, megaloblastic anemia, or panhypoplasias (nonspecific bone marrow suppression). *Nurses need to be certain that baseline and periodic complete blood cell counts and hemoglobin determinations are conducted. Blood cell problems should be suspected when clients complain of sore throat, feeling fatigued, or if they report repeated incidents of fever. Clients need to be alerted to report any unusual bleeding or bruising, or incidents of sore mouth or bleeding gums since these signs are often indicative of agranulocytosis.* Myopathies and alopecia are other potential chronic adverse effects.

Drug Interactions Colchicine reduces absorption of vitamin B_{12}, possibly resulting in a B_{12} deficiency. Colchicine increases the response of the brain to depressant drugs and of the vasculature to sympathomimetic agents. The activity of colchicine is enhanced by alkalinizing agents and inhibited by acidifying agents.

Preparations and Administration If colchicine is administered intravenously, it is important that the drug not be diluted with fluids that can change the pH, since a precipitate may form. Sterile water may be used. *Care must be taken to avoid extravasation because of the local irritant effect of colchicine. Also, to avoid tissue irritation, a needle used to withdraw solution from a vial needs to be replaced by a fresh sterile needle for injecting the medication.* The injection should be slow, over 3–5 minutes.

Colchicine (generic)

Tablets, enteric coated tablets, sugar coated granules, injection solution, combination tablets with probenecid (ColBENEMID and others)

Recommended Doses: 1 mg PO initially, followed by additional 0.5 mg amounts every 2–3 hours, up to a total of 4–10 mg. More than 10 mg should not be repeated within 3 days because of drug accumulation. A single intravenous dose of 2 mg in 10–20 ml of normal saline is an alternative regimen. The prophylactic dose of colchicine is 0.5–2.0 mg PO every night or every other night. For treatment of chronic gouty arthritis complicated by frequent, recurrent acute attacks, 2 ColBENEMID tablets, which may be increased by 1 tablet every 4 weeks to a maximum of 4 per day.

Important Nursing Implications for Colchicine

- ☐ Instruct clients in advance to discontinue use of colchicine if any of the more serious side effects begin to develop.
- ☐ Instruct clients to begin a course of therapy with colchicine as quickly after onset of symptoms as possible.
- ☐ Nurses need to check for symptoms indicative of acid-base imbalance resulting from diarrhea.
- ☐ To reduce gastric upset in clients on colchicine, the nurse should advise them to take the medication with meals. If joint pain is still present and gastric upset persists, the client should not continue the medication.
- ☐ Advise clients to avoid drug accumulation by not repeating a course of therapy with colchicine until at least 3 days after the previous course.
- ☐ Conduct periodic blood tests for all clients receiving colchicine.
- ☐ Be especially cognizant of the problems faced by elderly clients with gout. Colchicine must be used with caution in elderly or debilitated patients because of the gastrointestinal, renal, cardiac, and bone marrow effects. Colchicine can be a particular problem if the individual has other disease states such as kidney disease, cardiovascular disorders, or liver impairment. Elderly clients, especially those who live alone, need to be assisted in keeping track of the amount of drug they take. They need to have particular attention given to side effects that

can cause rapid deterioration of their health. The family should be alerted to report immediately signs such as mental confusion, numbness, or tingling sensations of the feet or hands.

☐ Avoid extravasation when giving colchicine intravenously because of its vesicant properties.

Allopurinol (Zyloprim)

Mechanism and Effects Allopurinol provides an effective drug treatment for the primary hyperuricemia that causes gout, secondary hyperuricemias (which occur in association with proliferative hematopoietic diseases, thyroid disorders, hypertension, obesity, and certain hereditary diseases), drug-induced hyperuricemias, or for prophylaxis for recurrent urate stone formation. Its mechanism is distinct from that of both colchicine and the uricosurics. Both allopurinol and its active metabolite, alloxanthine, are inhibitors of the enzyme xanthine oxidase, which is required for the synthesis of uric acid. The half-life of the active metabolite alloxanthine (18–30 hours) is substantially greater than that of allopurinol (2–3 hours), so the active metabolite, though a weaker inhibitor, contributes more to the overall effect than the parent compound. Uric acid synthesis is not completely suppressed by allopurinol, but the urinary excretion of purines is divided among three substances — hypoxanthine, xanthine, and uric acid — improving solubility and preventing crystallization.

Unlike the uricosurics, allopurinol reduces excretion of uric acid because it reduces its synthesis. However, like the uricosurics, allopurinol is likely to cause an increase in acute gouty attacks during the first few months of therapy as uric acid from tophi is gradually mobilized. During the early period of therapy, clients may be prescribed colchicine concurrently with drugs that produce slight alkalinization of the urine to minimize risks of acute attacks and formation of urinary tract calculi respectively. Therapy is initiated at relatively low doses, and fluid intake is maintained at a high level to further alleviate the risks during the early phase.

Pharmacokinetics Allopurinol is absorbed fairly well, although about 20% is lost in the feces, unabsorbed. The peak plasma concentration occurs in about 30–60 minutes. Most of the drug is converted by xanthine oxidase as described above, with only 10–30% being excreted unchanged. However, any decrease in renal function can cause an accumulation of the drug in the kidneys. *Clients need to report immediately any change in the volume of urinary output, cloudy urine, or unusual color or odor in the urine.* Neither

Nursing Observations for Pharmacotherapy of Gout

THERAPEUTIC GOAL	Symptomatic relief from acute attacks, reduction in serum uric acid levels, and prevention of further episodes.
PREADMINISTRATION ASSESSMENT	
Baseline Data	Observe for pain in one or both large toes or other joints, redness or swelling of joints, or tophi. Evaluate vital signs. X-ray evaluation of joints. Obtain laboratory tests including serum uric acid levels.
EVALUATION OF DRUG RESPONSE	
For Therapeutic Benefit	Monitor subjective relief from pain when medications are used to alleviate acute attacks. Encourage the client to maintain a diary of the incidence and severity of attacks to assess prophylactic therapy. Monitor serum uric acid levels periodically.
For Adverse Effects and Drug Interactions	See the individual drug discussions.
For Compliance	Evaluate client's compliance with all facets of the therapeutic regimen by careful observation, interviewing, and review of progress. Report compliance problems to the physician and act as client-advocate when changes in the therapeutic regimen seem indicated.

allopurinol nor its active metabolite are bound to plasma proteins.

Clinical Indications Allopurinol is indicated for more serious cases of chronic hyperuricemia, with presence of tophi, kidney stones, nephropathy, or renal insufficiency. It is also used whenever milder cases are refractory to uricosurics. It is useful in primary, secondary, or iatrogenic types of hyperuricemia. It is not useful for alleviating acute attacks of gout, and in fact, may increase frequency or severity of such attacks during the first few months of use. Its use is never begun during an acute attack.

Adverse Effects and Contraindications Allopurinol is contraindicated in those who have exhibited a previous serious adverse reaction to the drug and in children and nursing mothers. Allopurinol is well tolerated by most patients. The most common adverse effects are **hypersensitivity reactions,** occurring in 3% of patients. Rashes and a variety of more worrisome skin eruptions (pruritus, purpura, exfoliative dermatitis) and febrile reactions occur. The risk of skin eruptions is increased when certain antibiotics, such as ampicillin, are taken at the same time as allopurinol. *Nurses should determine if the client is taking any antibiotics and the name of the drug used.*

Rare serious reactions include alterations in blood cells, hepatomegaly, peripheral neuritis, and cataracts. Mild responses include headache, vertigo, nausea, and vomiting. *Nurses should suggest that allopurinol be taken with or immediately after meals to minimize gastrointestinal symptoms.* Allopurinol can cause drowsiness.

Drug Interactions Allopurinol can be used to treat severe drug-induced hyperuricemia. It is seldom required for the low-level hyperuricemia produced by thiazides or high-ceiling diuretics but may be needed when 6-mercaptopurine or azathioprine is used in a vigorous antineoplastic regimen. 6-Mercaptopurine is a purine analogue and organic acid.

Nursing Diagnoses and Interventions for Pharmacotherapy of Gout

Nursing Diagnoses	*Related Interventions*
TO ENHANCE DRUG BENEFITS OR REDUCE DRUG REQUIREMENTS	
Alterations in comfort: pain related to gouty inflammation	Instruct the client to rest the inflamed joint, reduce dietary intake of purines, and eliminate extra weight.
Alteration in pattern of urinary output related to formation of urate crystals (stones)	Encourage the client to maintain a high level of fluid intake so that urine will be dilute. Monitor and teach clients to monitor intake-output. Alkalinize the urine if necessary by drug or dietary interventions.
Alterations in cardiac output related to hyperuricemia	Monitor blood pressure.
TO ENSURE SAFE AND EFFICACIOUS DRUG USE	
Knowledge deficit related to drug regimen	Teach the client about the nature of the disorder, the rationale for use of any prescribed medications, and appropriate administration, including when medications should be taken in relation to meals and occurrence of symptoms.
	Provide clients with a list of the adverse effects and drug interactions for each prescribed medication, and what to do if any of these should occur.
	Explain the importance of dietary restrictions in management of gout and how to design a meal plan to meet the restrictions.
	Advise clients to maintain a consistently high level of fluid intake to minimize risk of kidney stone formation.

It causes uric acid retention by competing for the secretory component of the organic anion transport mechanism in the proximal tubule of the nephron. The build-up of uric acid can be prevented with allopurinol. At the same time, allopurinol also blocks the inactivation of 6-mercaptopurine by xanthine oxidase, so doses of the antineoplastic drug must be reduced to one-quarter to one-third the normal amount.

Allopurinol prolongs the half-life and increases the activity of oral anticoagulants. The effect of oral hypoglycemics is likewise increased because allopurinol inhibits hepatic metabolism of these drugs.

Allopurinol may interfere with certain diagnostic tests. Clients taking allopurinol may have elevated serum triglycerides, total serum lipid levels, and serum enzymes used to evaluate liver function. There may be a decrease in serum glucose.

Preparations and Administration The immediate objective of allopurinol therapy is to lower serum uric acid concentrations to below 6 mg/100 ml. Doses must be adjusted downward for patients with renal impairment in proportion to the reduction in GFR. The precautions described above that are exercised during initiation of therapy should be recalled: concurrent prophylaxis with colchicine, initial low doses, slight alkalinization of the urine, and maintenance of ample fluid intake. Zyloprim is the most widely prescribed preparation for hyperuricemia and one of the top 50 prescription drugs.

Allopurinol (Zyloprim, Lopurin)
Tablets
Recommended Doses: 200–300 mg/day PO in a single dose. In severe cases, 400–600 mg/day PO in divided doses.

Drugs Affecting the Urinary Tract

Urinary Tract Infections and Anti-infectives

Bacteriuria is indicative of infection of the nephrourinary tract if urine is collected by strict aseptic technique. Clinical signs include chills and fever of sudden onset, increased frequency and urgency of micturition, urethral discharges, burning sensations or pain on urination, suprapubic, lower back, or flank pain, and nocturia. Infections can occur in the kidney and be accompanied by inflammation (pyelonephritis), but commonly they are confined to the lower urinary tract, the bladder, and urethra. Urinary tract obstruction predisposes to infection of the nephrourinary system because obstruction causes stasis. In the absence of obstruction or other complications, localization studies are not indicated, lower urinary tract infection is assumed, and treatment with an appropriate anti-infective agent is begun. If, however, infection is recurrent, nonresponsive to treatment, or complicated, localization studies are conducted in order to give appropriate direction to therapy.

Infective pyelonephritis can be acute or chronic. **Acute bacterial pyelonephritis** usually occurs by ascent of bacteria that have entered via the urethral meatus. Obstructions are frequently present in the urinary tract. Acute pyelonephritis is especially common in females during infancy and pregnancy, and after urethral catheterization or instrumentation. The condition is uncommon in males free of urinary tract disorders. In pyelonephritis, the kidneys are enlarged and neutrophils are abundantly present. Onset is typically rapid, with chills, fever, and flank, loin, or high back pain. The urine is frequently alkalinized due to presence of urea-splitting organisms. Urinary bacteria are typically 60% coated with antibodies. Antimicrobial therapy is instituted and continued for a minimum of 10–14 days.

Chronic bacterial pyelonephritis is most likely to occur in patients with obstructions or prior history of recurrent acute urinary tract infections. It leads to gradual renal failure and accounts for about 10–15% of end-stage chronic renal failure. Treatment depends on elimination of obstructions if possible and elimination of infecting organisms with antimicrobial drugs.

Lower urinary tract infection is a very common disorder, 10 times more frequent in females than males except during infancy, when there is no sex differential. In infancy, infections often occur by spread of infection through the blood system or lymphatics, but in children and adults, infection is almost always by the ascending route, often after sexual intercourse. Lower urinary tract infections include urethritis, cystitis (bladder infection), and, in males, prostatitis. In as many as 85% of uncomplicated cases, lower urinary tract infections are caused by the gram-negative bacterium, *Escherichia coli.* Men with urethral infections may have purulent white discharges, increased urgency and frequency of micturition, and burning sensations upon urinating. For women, symptoms of urethritis resemble those of cystitis: burning sensations and pain on urination, urinary urgency and frequency, nocturia, and suprapubic or lower back pain.

Nursing Observations for Anti-infective Therapy of Urinary Tract Infections

THERAPEUTIC GOAL	Elimination of the infection and maintenance of urinary output.
PREADMINISTRATION ASSESSMENT	
Baseline Data	Assess for dysuria, chills or fever of sudden onset, increased urinary frequency or urgency, urethral discharges, back pain, or nocturia. Monitor intake-output and appearance of urine. Conduct urethral catheterization and bladder washout tests as indicated to localize infection. Examine for evidence of obstructions. Obtain laboratory tests including urine culture, urinalysis, urine casts, and determination of infecting agent.
Contraindications/ Precautions	Check medication history for allergies to urinary tract antiinfectives.
EVALUATION OF DRUG RESPONSE	
For Therapeutic Benefit	Relief of pain and itching; urine cultures.
For Adverse Effects	Monitor for pulmonary hypersensitivity reactions and peripheral neuropathies when nitrofurantoin is used; CNS symptoms when nalidixic acid or cinoxacin is employed.
For Compliance	Evaluate client's compliance with all facets of the therapeutic regimen by careful observation, interviewing, and review of progress. Report compliance problems to the physician and act as client-advocate when changes in the therapeutic regimen seem indicated.

Nitrofurantoin (Furadantin, Macrodantin)

For urinary tract infections, antibiotics that are quickly excreted are valuable. Nitrofurantoin is a nitrofuran that is well absorbed from the intestine but rapidly excreted. The plasma half-life is only about 20 minutes in normal individuals and therapeutic concentrations are achieved only in the urinary tract. Its only use is in urinary tract infections. Nitrofurantoin interferes with carbohydrate metabolism in bacterial cells by inhibiting acetylcoenzyme A. It is bacteriostatic at low concentrations and bactericidal at higher concentrations.

Adverse Effects and Contraindications **Gastrointestinal disturbances** occur occasionally. *Clients who experience gastrointestinal irritation need to be advised to take the drug with milk or buttermilk to minimize the problem. They should not, however, use antacids, since these may interfere with absorption of the drug.*

Nitrofurantoin can stain the teeth. *Nurses should tell clients to avoid letting the drug come in contact with the teeth and to rinse the mouth thoroughly after taking the drug.*

Nitrofurantoin can cause the urine to be brown in color. *Nurses should reassure clients that this is not harmful. However, milky or foul smelling urine or perineal irritation or dysuria may indicate superinfection of the urinary tract.*

Hypersensitivity reactions occur occasionally to nitrofurantoin. People with a history of asthma, angioneurotic edema, anaphylaxis, or jaundice should likely not receive nitrofurantoin. Clients who are on prolonged therapy may develop subacute or chronic pulmonary sensitivity reactions. These pulmonary disorders are usually manifested as flu-like conditions: cough, malaise, chills, fever, and shortness of breath during normal exertion. The client may complain of chest pains, and the nurse listening to breath sounds may notice a decrease in sound and occurrence of rhonchi (a rattling in the throat resembling snoring). These problems are more pronounced among the elderly. *Nurses need to report occurrence of such symptoms immediately.* Usually the client recovers quickly once the medication is discontinued.

Another problem is not so easy to cure. Clients who report that they feel weak (muscle weakness) or dizzy, or who have tingling or numbness of the extremities or headaches may be developing **peripheral neuropathy,** which can be irreversible. Peripheral neuropathy is most likely to occur if the client has renal impairment, anemia, diabetes mellitus, electrolyte imbalance, or vitamin B deficiency. *Nurses should immediately report these symptoms and expect that the client will be taken off the drug.*

Interactions with Drugs or Food Presence of food in the stomach or simultaneous administration of anticholinergic drugs will increase absorption of nitrofurantoin by prolonging gastric emptying time. Antacids, on the other hand, decrease absorption of nitrofurantoin.

Preparations and Administration The macrocrystal preparation of nitrofurantoin (Macrodantin) is widely prescribed and offers the advantage of improved gastrointestinal tolerance with no reduction in efficacy. Clients placed on nitrofurantoin should receive the drug at equal intervals around the clock if they are to maintain therapeutic urinary levels.

Methenamine (Mandelamine, Hiprex, Urex)

Methenamine is a broad-spectrum antibiotic used to treat clients with urinary tract infections. Its mode of action is release of formaldehyde in an acidic environment, so it is effective only if the urine is acidic (as is normally the case). It is free of substantial toxicity. It must not be used with sulfonamides because an insoluble precipitate forms. The drug should be taken with food.

Quinolone Anti-infectives

Nalidixic acid (NegGram), cinoxacin (Cinobac), and norfloxacin (Noroxin) are related quinolone antimicrobials used for urinary tract infections. Nalidixic acid and cinoxacin are effective against most gram-negative bacilli (except *Pseudomonas*). Norfloxacin has a broader spectrum, inhibiting growth of most gram-positive and gram-negative aerobic bacteria. Nalidixic acid has a short half-life, necessitating administration 4 times daily; the longer duration of cinoxacin and norfloxacin permit less frequent administration (twice daily). Neurological problems, such as headache, dizziness, and nausea, are the most common side effects with these drugs. Gastrointesti-

Nursing Diagnoses and Interventions for Anti-infective Therapy of Urinary Tract Infections

Nursing Diagnoses	*Related Interventions*
TO ENHANCE DRUG BENEFITS OR REDUCE DRUG REQUIREMENTS	
Alteration in comfort: pain in abdomen, back, flank, or suprapubic area related to inflammatory reaction to infection or dysuria	Maintain adequate fluid intake and urine flow.
Alterations in patterns of urinary elimination: dysuria related to urinary tract infection or superinfection	Monitor intake-output and immediately report occurrence of oliguria. Monitor for indications of urinary tract superinfections.
Ineffective individual coping: depression related to chronicity of certain upper urinary tract infections	Provide emotional support and reassurance.
TO ENSURE SAFE AND EFFICACIOUS DRUG USE	
Knowledge deficit related to drug regimen	Educate the client about the nature of the disorder and the rationale for medications prescribed.
	Stress the importance of increased fluid intake.
	Stress the importance of round-the-clock administration of anti-infectives. Advise clients which medicatoins are to be taken with meals and which on an empty stomach.
	Advise clients if the drug administered is likely to cause coloration of the urine.
	Provide clients with a list of potential adverse effects and drug interactions for each medication prescribed and what to do if any of these should occur.

nal disturbances and allergic reactions occur occasionally. These drugs can cause erosions of cartilage in weight-bearing joints during maturation, so their use is contraindicated in children or pregnant women. Side effects occur more often with nalidixic acid than with the two newer agents in this group. Nalidixic acid potentiates coumarin anticoagulants, cinoxacin's effect is slowed by probenecid (Benemid), and norfloxacin's effect is inhibited by concurrent nitrofurantoin.

Other Antimicrobials

For clients with uncomplicated lower urinary tract infections, sulfonamides, tetracyclines, ampicillin, amoxicillin, trimethoprim, or the combination sulfamethoxazole and trimethoprim (Bactrim, Septra) are typical choices. If infections are recurrent, determination of the organism and sensitivity tests are important and tetracyclines, cephalosporins, nalidixic acid, nitrofurantoin, or sulfamethoxazole and trimethoprim are employed. The latter combination is the least likely to cause formation of resistant organisms, and the pair is favored for the same reason in chronic pyelonephritis. If acute or chronic pyelonephritis is complicated by renal insufficiency, the selection of an anti-infective is constrained by the effect of reduced renal function on the pharmacokinetics of various drugs. Drugs that depend on renal clearance for delivery to the urinary tract, such as nitrofurantoin and methenamine, should be used only if GFR (based on creatinine clearance) is greater than 50 ml/minute. No anti-infective should be used if creatinine clearance is less than 20 ml/minute.

When clients have abnormalities in the lower urinary tract that result in inevitable, chronic lower urinary tract infection, antimicrobial therapy should be reserved for short courses of therapy during periods of acute intensification. Aminoglycosides may be required when resistance has developed to other selections.

Some preparations for urinary tract infections consist of a combination of sulfonamides *or* methenamine with an antispasmodic (antimuscarinic drug) and a urinary tract analgesic, phenazopyridine. The additional ingredients are provided for relief of symptoms of urgency, frequency, and dysuria.

Preparations and Administration

Cinoxacin (Cinobac)
Capsules
Recommended Doses: 1 g PO daily, in 2–4 divided doses, for 7–14 days.

Methenamine (Mandelamine, Hiprex, Urex, others)
Tablets, tablets as methenamine hippurate, tablets as methenamine mandelate, enteric coated tablets, oral suspensions, granules
Recommended Doses: 1 g PO qid for methenamine or the mandelate salt, 1 g bid for the hippurate salt.

Nalidixic acid (NegGram)
Caplets, oral suspension
Recommended Doses: 1 g PO qid for 1–2 weeks. Long-term therapy is conducted at a total daily dose of 2g.

Nitrofurantoin (Furadantin, Macrodantin)
Tablets, capsules, capsules with macrocrystals, oral suspension, powder for injection
Recommended Doses: 100–150 mg PO, qid.

Norfloxacin (Noroxin)
Tablets
Recommended Doses: 400 mg PO twice daily for 7–10 days.

Urease Inhibitor

Some of the bacterial species that cause chronic urinary tract infections, such as *Proteus*, release an enzyme, urease, that liberates ammonia from urea. This action of urease results in alkalinization of the urine, a circumstance that in turn favors formation of kidney stones. Acetohydroxamic acid (Lithostat) was introduced in 1983 as an inhibitor of urinary urease. It is indicated as an adjunct to antibacterial therapy for prevention of alkalinization of urine caused by urease when urinary tract infection is produced by urea-splitting organisms. Acetohydroxamic acid does not directly acidify the urine but prevents alkalinization caused by urease activity.

Adverse effects of acetohydroxamic acid include neurological and psychiatric reactions such as headache, depression, anxiety, and nervousness (in 30% of patients during the first 48 hours); gastrointestinal disturbances (nausea, vomiting, and anorexia) in 20–25% of patients, and mild hemolytic anemia (in approximately 15% of patients). Allergic reactions consisting of rash occur in some patients, often triggered by consumption of alcohol. Acetohydroxamic acid reduces absorption of iron because it forms a chelate with iron and certain other heavy metals in the alimentary tract.

Acetohydroxamic acid (Lithostat)
Tablets
Recommended Doses: 10–15 mg/kg/day PO, 3 or 4 times daily.

Urinary Tract Alkalinizers and Acidifiers

Urinary tract **alkalinizers** are bases or salts of bases that are excreted as free base in the urine, with the result that urinary pH is elevated. Urinary tract alkalinizers can be used to correct acidosis (see Chapter 42), to minimize the risk of formation of crystals of uric acid or sulfonamides, to hasten excretion of drugs that are weak acids (such as aspirin), and to increase the antimicrobial effectiveness of aminoglycosides. The principal agents in this class are sodium bicarbonate and citrate (Citrolith, Polycitra, Bicitra).

Urinary **acidifiers** can be used to increase the solubility of calcium so as to prevent precipitation of calcium deposits in the urinary tract. They can also be used to increase the activity of certain urinary tract anti-infectives that require an acid pH, such as methenamine (Mandelamine), to enhance the excretion of drugs that are weak bases, or to aid in correction of systemic acidosis (see Chapter 42). The agents used as urinary acidifiers include ammonium chloride, ascorbic acid (which may or may not be effective in this regard), acid phosphates (K-Phos), and a combination product (pHos-pHaid) containing ammonium and sodium biphosphates and sodium acid pyrophosphate. Ammonium chloride was once employed as a diuretic and was particularly useful in combination with mercurials, which are now obsolete.

Preparations and Administration

Sodium bicarbonate
Tablets
Recommended Doses: For alkalinization of the urine, 325–2,000 mg PO, up to 4 times daily. The total daily dose should not exceed 16 g in those under 60 years of age or 8 g in those over 60.

Urinary Tract Stimulants

Neural regulation of bladder function involves efferent fibers of the parasympathetic, sympathetic, and somatic nervous systems. Neurogenic bladder occurs when efferent nerve innervation to the bladder is impaired for any reason — congenital abnormality, brain damage, spinal cord injury, or damage to local autonomic nerves that supply the bladder.

Direct- or indirect-acting cholinomimetics can be employed to help maintain urinary tract tone in neurogenic bladder and to alleviate nonobstructive urinary retention. Among the direct-acting cholinomimetics, bethanechol (Urecholine) is the agent of choice for this application. Among the indirect-acting agents, the cholinesterase inhibitor, neostigmine (Prostigmin), is commonly employed for clients with bladder atony and urinary retention. The pharmacology of both of these agents is addressed in Chapter 29.

Urinary Tract Spasmolytics

Painful spasms of the urinary tract can be relieved by use of antimuscarinic agents (discussed in Chapter 29). In addition, there are three agents available that act directly on the smooth muscle of the urinary tract to counteract spasm: flavoxate (Urispas), oxybutynin (Ditropan), and dimethyl sulfoxide (DMSO, Rimso-50). The former two drugs are indicated for relief of dysuria, urgency, nocturia, suprapubic pain, urinary frequency, and incontinence (involuntary urination during the day or night), but are not useful for relief of urinary tract infections. These agents are contraindicated in patients with obstructions or hemorrhage of the gastrointestinal tract or obstructive uropathies. **Flavoxate** should be used with caution in individuals with suspected glaucoma because it may increase intraocular pressure. Adverse effects of flavoxate include nausea and vomiting, dry mouth, hyperpyrexia, urticaria, dysuria, tachycardia and palpitations, eosinophilia, and leukopenia. Neurological deficits sometimes occur, especially in elderly individuals, including nervousness, vertigo, drowsiness, confusion, headache, and blurred vision.

Oxybutynin must be used cautiously in elderly patients or those with autonomic neuropathy, hepatic or renal disease, ulcerative colitis, or paralytic ileus. Symptoms of hyperthyroidism, coronary heart disease, congestive heart failure, cardiac dysrhythmias, hypertension, or prostatic hypertrophy may be aggravated. An excessive effect of oxybutynin leads to urinary retention and hesitancy. Other adverse effects include dry mouth, blurred vision, elevated intraocular pressure, drowsiness or insomnia, nausea and vomiting, constipation and intestinal bloating, impotence, suppression of lactation, dizziness, weakness, and allergic reactions such as urticaria or other skin eruptions. *Clients should be alerted to avoid driving when using this drug.*

Dimethyl sulfoxide (DMSO) is a liquid with diverse pharmacological activity, including anti-inflammatory, bacteriostatic, diuretic, vasodilating, local anesthetic, and spasmolytic properties. It is also an inhibitor of acetylcholinesterase. Currently, DMSO is approved only for symptomatic relief of interstitial cystitis. Its value in this condition is attributable mainly to its spasmolytic, anti-inflammatory, and local anesthetic properties. It has been investigated for a variety of other possible applications, including scleroderma, arthritis, tendonitis, retinitis pigmentosa, breast and prostate cancer, herpes virus infections, and stroke. For cystitis, DMSO is administered topically to the bladder by catheter or aseptic syringe and allowed to remain for 15 minutes, before the client is permitted to void. An analgesic lubricant gel is administered to the urethra prior to insertion of the catheter to prevent spasm. When administered topically to the skin, DMSO is substantially absorbed. It is eliminated in the urine and feces, in exhaled air, and through the skin. DMSO eliminated on the breath and through the skin gives a characteristic garlicky odor and taste. DMSO releases histamine and can produce anaphylactoid reactions. Other adverse effects when administered topically to the skin include local dermatitis, sedation, nausea, vomiting, headache, and stinging of the eyes. Transient chemical cystitis can occur when the drug is administered to the bladder. DMSO is available as an industrial, laboratory, and veterinary chemical as well as for clinical use. *The nurse should advise clients against the use of these preparations for medicinal purposes, since they often contain unidentified impurities that can be absorbed systemically after cutaneous administration.*

Preparations and Administration

Dimethyl sulfoxide (DMSO) (Rimso-50)
Solution
Recommended Doses: For bladder instillation, 50 ml.

Oxybutynin (Ditropan)
Tablets, syrup
Recommended Doses: For adults, 5 mg PO, 2 or 3 times daily; children over 5 may be given 5 mg twice daily.

Flavoxate (Urispas)
Tablets
Recommended Doses: For adults and children over 10 years, 100 or 200 mg, 3 to 4 times daily.

Urinary Tract Analgesics

Phenazopyridine is a urinary tract analgesic. After oral administration, it is absorbed systemically and rapidly excreted in the urine. The analgesic effect of phenazopyridine is a topical action on the mucosa of the urinary tract. This drug is indicated for symptomatic relief of pain associated with infections of the lower urinary tract. Phenazopyridine is compatible with concurrent antimicrobial therapy but does not substitute for diagnosis and treatment of the causative agent. Phenazopyridine can produce gastrointestinal disturbances, hemolytic anemia, methemoglobinemia, renal and hepatic toxicity, and a reddish-orange discoloration of the urine.

Preparations and Administration

Phenazopyridine (Azodine, Baridium, Pyridium, Pyridiate)
Tablets
Recommended Doses: For adults, 200 mg PO, 3 times per day, after meals.

Drugs for Enuresis

Enuresis is a mixed organic and functional disorder characterized by involuntary, frequent episodes of bed wetting by children over 5–6 years of age. It occurs much more commonly in boys than girls and is often familial. Imipramine (Tofranil), discussed in Chapter 20, is effective in reducing frequency of wets as long as it continues to be administered, but recidivism is high after drug withdrawal. Behavioral and other psychotherapeutic techniques produce better long-term results.

Case Study: Diabetes Insipidus

A married student nurse, M. T., revealed to one of her nursing instructors that she had diabetes insipidus and that it was a major deterrent to pursuing her master's degree. Upon learning that M. T. was not under the care of a physician, the instructor counseled M. T. to seek medical assistance and helped her to locate an appropriate clinic.

She was placed on vasopressin injection, 5–10 units, subcutaneously, 2 times daily. Because M. T. was a nurse, she did not need instructions regarding administering medication subcutaneously. However, the nurse at the clinic did review with her sites for injection. The nurse also worked with M. T. to monitor her response to therapy. M. T. was provided a chart on which to record her blood pressure and weight. M. T. was taught to assess her fluid balance so that she could determine when she needed medication and how much to take. Initially, M. T. measured fluid intake and output and specific gravity of urine. However, over time, the nurse was able to assist M. T. in assessing hydration status based on thirst, dryness of mucous membranes, and frequency of voiding. At times, M. T. found it necessary to restrict sodium and protein intake to decrease the volume of urine.

The nurse also worked with M. T.'s husband and sister to assure that M. T. was responding appropriately to the drug. For example, they were asked to report when M. T. showed evidence of headache, listlessness, drowsiness, or confusion — all of which are symptoms of water intoxication. If not reported quickly, this condition could lead to convulsions and coma.

M. T. was told to report any incidents of rash, urticaria, increased sweating, or facial pallor, since these are signs of hypersensitivity to the drug. Hypertension, abdominal cramping, and blanching of the skin are reactions to excessive doses of vasopressin. In addition, the nurse kept track of other possible problems such as uterine cramping, bradycardia, minor dysrhythmias, and premature atrial contractions.

1. Was M. T. experiencing nephrogenic or neurogenic diabetes insipidus?
2. Why would the hormone ADH, which acts primarily on the kidney, have any significant effect on blood pressure? On uterine contractions? Why might bradycardia occur in response to ADH?
3. Why might an excessive ADH action have led to water intoxication?

Answers appear at the end of the book.

Case Study: Diuretic Therapy

J. O., a 58-year-old male with a history of mild gout, had been asymptomatic without medication for the past 5 years. He had no history of other health problems. At a blood pressure clinic, J. O. was evaluated by a nurse and was found to have a blood pressure of 145/100. J. O.'s physician confirmed the nurse's finding and prescribed 50 mg PO hydrochlorthiazide, bid, a low-salt diet (2–3 g daily), and potassium chloride syrup, 20 mEq PO, 3 times daily. The physician instructed J. O. to take the potassium chloride syrup with a full glass of water immediately after meals. Before J. O. left his office, the physician took a blood sample in order to conduct baseline laboratory determinations of serum electrolytes, glucose, blood urea nitrogen (BUN), and creatinine. The values obtained were as follows (the normal ranges are given in parentheses): Ca^{++}: 5.0 mEq/100 ml (4.4–5.4 mEq/100 ml); Cl^-: 103 mEq/L (96–112 mEq/L); HCO_3^-: 25 mEq/L (22–26 mEq/L); K^+: 4.3 mEq/L (3.8–5.6 mEq/L); Mg^{++}: 1.8 mEq/L (1.5–2.5 mEq/L); Na^+: 142 mEq/L (135–150 mEq/L); PO_4: 2.2 mEq/L (1.45–2.76 mEq/L); pH: 7.35 (7.31–7.41); BUN: 13 mg/dl (8–20 mg/dl); creatinine: 0.9 mg/100 ml (0.7–1.4 mg/100 ml); and glucose: 100 mg/100 ml (70–110 mg/100 ml). J. O.'s weight was 190 lb (about 15 pounds in excess of the ideal weight for his height and build).

J. O. returned after 1 month for evaluation. His blood pressure was now 125/85. A blood sample drawn at that time indicated that all values remained well within normal limits. J. O. did not complain of any side effects.

J. O. did not return for further evaluation for 10 months. He had begun to experience swelling and pain in the big toe of his right foot. He had self-medicated for the pain, taking aspirin in amounts up to 5 g/day. J. O. was anxious, weak, and tired, and his reflexes were diminished. After assessment, the physician had J. O. hospitalized and ordered immediate blood tests.

The admitting nurse interviewed J. O. and learned that he had been taking the hydrochlorthiazide as prescribed by the physician but had stopped taking the potassium syrup because of its bad taste and because it irritated his stomach. The laboratory results were returned as follows: Ca^{++}: 5.1 mEq/100 ml; Cl^-: 88 mEq/L; HCO_3^-: 33 mEq/L; K^+: 2.9 mEq/L; Mg^{++}: 1.2 mEq/L; Na^+: 136 mEq/L; PO_4: 2.5 mEq/L; pH: 7.44; BUN: 23 mg/dl; creatinine: 1.0 mg/100 ml; and glucose: 103 mg/100 ml. Based on the nurse's assessment and the laboratory results, the physician ordered infusion of KCl for 4 hours at 10 mEq/hour; oral KCl, 20 mEq, tid, after completion of the KCl infusion; colchicine, 1 mg every 2 hours until relief of pain; and no aspirin or diuretic.

Colchicine was discontinued after 3 doses when the pain in the toe diminished. The nurse encouraged J. O. to remain in bed to rest the swollen joint. The nurse instructed J. O. concerning dietary sources of potassium in preparation for his return to diuretic therapy upon discharge. Blood tests were conducted daily and after 48 hours, all values had returned to normal. However, J. O.'s blood pressure was up to 145/100. J. O. was placed on Dyazide, a combination product consisting of 50 mg of triamterene and 25 mg of hydrochlorthiazide, twice daily. The nurse explained to J. O. that he would not now need to increase dietary intake of potassium.

1. What was the cause of the swelling and pain in the right big toe joint in this case?
2. Which of the laboratory values obtained when J. O.

was admitted to the hospital were abnormal? Explain the likely reason in each case.

3. What diagnosis would be appropriate for J. O.'s condition upon admission to the hospital? What is the likely basis for the neurological symptoms?
4. Which values would argue against a conclusion that the dose of hydrochlorthiazide being employed by J. O. was excessive?
5. Why did administration of K^+ correct the alkalosis as well as the hypokalemia?
6. Why did the physician prohibit administration of aspirin? How might aspirin have contributed adversely to J. O.'s condition?
7. What was the reason for administration of colchicine?
8. Why would J. O. likely fare better on Dyazide than on his original diuretic prescription? Since he will now be receiving only one-half as much hydrochlorthiazide daily, is it likely that his blood pressure will not be adequately controlled?
9. Why did the nurse indicate to J. O. that he should not substantially increase his dietary intake of potassium with his new regimen?

Answers appear at the end of the book.

Recommended Readings

General Sources

Brundage D: *Nursing Management of Renal Problems,* ed 2. St Louis, CV Mosby Co., 1980.

Diuretics

Brater DC: Pharmacodynamic considerations in the use of diuretics. *Annu Rev Pharmacol Toxicol* 1983;23:45–62.

Freis ED: Salt in hypertension and the effects of diuretics. *Annu Rev Pharmacol Toxicol* 1979;19:13–23.

Gever LN: Furosemide: A potent diuretic that requires careful patient monitoring. *Nursing* 1981;11(4):40–42.

Jacobsen JR, Kokko JP: Diuretics: Sites and mechanisms of action. *Annu Rev Pharmacol Toxicol* 1976;16:201–214.

Kemp G, Kemp D: Diuretics. *Am J Nurs* 1978;78:1006–1010.

Kirschenbaum HL, Rosenberg JM: What to watch out for with thiazides. *RN* 1983;83(7):28–30.

Perez-Stable EC, Materson BJ: Diuretic drug therapy of edema. *Med Clin North Am* 1971;55(2):359–372.

Phillips M: Diuretics. *Nurs Mirror* 1983;157(8):29–35.

Quinlan M: Edema: What really causes it. How to control it. *RN* 1984;84(4):55–57.

Todd B: Drugs and the elderly — when the patient is on diuretics. *Geriatr Nurs* 1981;2(2):149–150.

Drugs and Renal Disease

Bennett W et al: Drug therapy in renal failure: Dosing guidelines for adults. *Ann Intern Med* 1980;93:62–89.

Orr ML: Drugs and renal disease. *Am J Nurs* 1981;81(5): 969–971.

Drugs and the Urinary Tract

Keys TF, Edson RS: Antimicrobial agents in urinary tract infections. *Mayo Clin Proc* 1983;58(3):165–168.

Stamm WE: Guidelines for prevention of catheter associated urinary tract infections. *Ann Intern Med* 1975;82:386–390.

Drugs for Gout

Boss GR, Seegmiller JE: Hyperuricemia and gout: Classification, complications, and management. *N Engl J Med* 1979;300:1459–1468.

Kelley WN: Effects of drugs on uric acid in man. *Annu Rev Pharmacol Toxicol* 1975;15:327–350.

CHAPTER 44

Drugs and Nutrition

Drugs and foods, along with respiratory air, are the major kinds of chemical substances that are taken into the body, so it is inevitable that their interactions are many and varied. Diet not only affects drug therapy in many instances but has direct impact on the disease states often treated with drugs. An important part of nursing assessment is an evaluation of the client's dietary habits. The dietary pattern is probably best recorded on a dietary profile chart such as the one illustrated in Table 44–1.

The fraction of food that nourishes the body is **nutriment,** which includes some 40 individual **nu-**

Table 44–1
Dietary Assessment Form

			Frequency				
				Weekly			
Type of food	Likes	Dislikes	Daily 1×	4×	2×	Rarely	Never
Citrus fruits							
Oranges							
Grapefruit							
Orange juice							
Grapefruit juice							
Apples							
Pears							
Fresh vegetables							
Carrots							
Peas							
Beans							
Spinach							
Broccoli							
Collard greens							
Turnips							
Rutabagas							
Cabbage							
Brussel sprouts							
Frozen or canned vegetables							
Red meats							
Beef							
Lamb							
Pork							
Veal							
Poultry							
Chicken							
Turkey							
Duck							
Fish							
Organ meats							
Liver							
Breads							
White							
Whole wheat							
Dairy							
Milk							
Cheese							

trients. Nutrients are divisible into macronutrients and micronutrients. **Macronutrients** include the energy-yielding substrates of intermediary metabolism (carbohydrates, fats, and protein) and the amino acid building-blocks of proteins. **Micronutrients** include the vitamins and the minerals (discussed separately in Chapter 42). All of the micronutrients and some of the macronutrients are **essential,** meaning that they cannot be synthesized in the body but must be obtained from the diet. A balanced diet from four food groups (dairy, meat or protein-rich alternatives, vegetable-fruit, and bread-cereal) ensures adequate intake of each type of nutrient except when requirements are elevated by disease, stress, pregnancy, antinutritional effects of drugs, or other factors that elevate nutritional requirements.

Malnutrition is any type of disorder of nutrition. It may involve excessive or inadequate intake of one or more nutrients: vitamins, minerals, protein, or carbohydrates. It may be primary (related to intake) or secondary (related to absorption, utilization, loss, or unusual requirements). It may be acute, subacute, or chronic.

Macronutrient Imbalances and Related Drugs

The macronutrients include carbohydrates, fats, proteins, and amino acids. The major forms of malnutrition that relate to the macronutrients include obesity, undernutrition, and disorders of lipid, protein, amino acid, or carbohydrate metabolism.

Obesity

Obesity occurs when caloric intake chronically exceeds caloric expenditure. Body mass more than 20% in excess of the value taken from a table of standard heights and weights is the accepted criterion for obesity. Obesity involves organic, psychological, and interpersonal factors. The genetic influence in obesity is substantial, although the relative importance of genetic and environmental factors is not known. Other organic influences include endocrine imbalance (as in Cushing's disease) and brain injury (especially to the hypothalamus, which regulates energy balance). If obesity begins in childhood, it is likely to be **hyperplastic,** characterized by an increase in the number of fat cells, whereas obesity of adult onset is likely to be **hypertrophic,** characterized by increased size of fat cells rather than number. Hyperplastic obesity is more difficult to contend with; the excess weight is lost only with great difficulty and is regained easily.

Alcohol use contributes to both obesity and nutritional deficiencies. If the calories from alcohol are added onto an unchanged baseline of food intake, net caloric intake inevitably rises. But alcohol-derived calories are of little nutritional value. If baseline food intake is reduced in response to intake of calories from alcohol, deficiency of micronutrients and protein is likely.

Psychological factors contributing to obesity include psychogenic eating abnormalities such as **bulimia,** characterized by compulsive ingestion of large quantities of food, followed by intense feelings of guilt and in some cases frequent self-induced vomiting. Interpersonal factors, such as peer pressure, can either positively or negatively influence habits relating to eating, physical exercise, and appearance.

Obesity, regardless of the cause, is a serious health problem. It affects the individual's emotional integrity and increases the incidence of diseases such as adult-onset diabetes, hypertension, coronary artery disease, and liability to accidents. It is also a risk factor for premature death. Authorities believe obesity causes increased respiratory work, leading to alveolar hypoventilation, hypercapnia, and somnolence. Persons who are markedly overweight are at increased risk during any surgical procedure. Treatments for obesity include diets, increasing physical activity, behavior modification, self-help organizations such as Weight Watchers, surgery, and anorexic drugs. Controlled exercise such as walking, swimming, and bicycling performed for periods of 20–30 minutes burns approximately 300 calories per session.

Many cases of obesity can be managed by dietary restrictions and improved exercise habits alone. Most authorities recommend that clients should first be placed on a program of dietary restrictions, weight reduction, and exercise before drug therapy is instituted. However, drug therapy may be used to suppress a client's appetite as an adjunct to restricting caloric intake and instituting an exercise program.

Anorexics

Amphetamine and its derivatives are sometimes used to induce anorexia. Amphetamine itself is used less often now than it once was for appetite control, but more than a half-dozen less potent drugs of similar mechanism are currently marketed and increasingly used as diet aids. Some of these are benzphetamine (Didrex), chlorphentermine (Pre-sate), diethylpropion (Tenuate), fenfluramine (Pondimin),

Nursing Observations for Use of Anorexics for Obesity

THERAPEUTIC GOAL	Weight reduction.
PREADMINISTRATION ASSESSMENT	
Baseline Data	Measure weight and blood pressure. Evaluate cognitive and emotional status.
EVALUATION OF DRUG RESPONSE	
For Therapeutic Benefit	Weight reduction and maintenance of weight reduction.
For Adverse Effects	Monitor for overuse of anorexics and development of psychological dependence.
For Dietary Interactions	Monitor changes in caloric intake and the adequacy of the diet for supplying micronutrients.
For Compliance	Evaluate client compliance with all facets of the therapeutic regimen by careful observation, interviewing, and review of progress. Report problems of overcompliance to the physician and act as client-advocate when changes in the therapeutic regimen seem indicated.

mazindol (Sanorex), phendimetrazine (Plegine), phenmetrazine (Preludin), and phentermine (Ionamin, Wilpowr). Controlled studies consistently indicate that weight loss occurs with anorexics only if accompanied by stringent dietary controls and close professional supervision. Even then there is a high likelihood that the lost weight will be regained if supervision is relaxed. Amphetamine-like stimulants cannot be used in the evening or close to bedtime, when a lot of overeating occurs, since they frequently cause insomnia.

Another risk is that clients who suddenly reduce food intake with the aid of anorexics will experience deficiencies in one or another of the micronutrients. *Nurses must assist clients using anorexics in careful balancing of food groups or appropriate use of multivitamin supplements to ensure that deficiencies are avoided.*

Anorexics are effective for only 4–6 weeks if used on a daily basis, after which tolerance develops. There is a risk of psychological dependence with long-term use. Sudden withdrawal of anorexic therapy after use of high doses can result in fatigue and depression. This is usually accompanied by an increase in appetite, and if the client is not careful, any lost weight is quickly regained. There are also potential peripheral adverse effects, such as cardiac palpitations and increased blood pressure.

Anorexics should be taken 30–60 minutes before meals, and the last dose no later than 6 hours prior to bedtime. *Nurses need to stress the importance of adhering strictly to the dosage regimen.* The full pharmacology of the amphetamine-like stimulants and other anorexics is discussed in Chapter 14.

Undernutrition

Starvation is generalized inadequate intake of nutrients or impaired ability to utilize nutrients. It is accompanied by progressive structural and functional changes involving all physiological systems. The characteristic indications of starvation are weight loss or emaciation, muscle wasting, protrusion of bones, hair loss, and thin, elastic skin, often pale with patches of pigmentation. Cardiac output decreases and respiratory rate and volume decline. Gonadal atrophy occurs along with loss of libido and amenorrhea.

Primary inanition is starvation due to inadequate intake of nutrients in general as in famine, deprivation, or anorexia nervosa (weight phobia). Initial treatment consists of small feedings with bland foods or a formula consisting of skim milk, edible oil, sucrose, minerals, and vitamins. **Secondary inanition** may be due to (1) maldigestion (gastric or pancreatic diseases), (2) malabsorption syndromes, (3) impaired nutrient utilization (endocrine, metabolic, and other disorders), (4) increased nutrient requirements (hyperthyroidism, pregnancy, growth spurts, and periods of ill-health in general), and (5) increased nutrient losses (hemorrhage, burns, vomiting, diarrhea, or nephrosis).

One drug used to stimulate appetite is cypro-

Nursing Diagnoses and Interventions for Use of Anorexics for Obesity

Nursing Diagnoses	*Related Interventions*
TO ENHANCE DRUG BENEFITS OR REDUCE DRUG REQUIREMENTS	
Activity intolerance related to fatigue and dyspnea because of excess weight	Help the client develop an exercise program suitable to his or her condition, starting slowly and gradually increasing in level of exertion.
Alteration in nutrition: intake in excess of requirements	Help the client reduce and control caloric intake in keeping with requirements; teach client to keep a food diary.
Disturbance in self-concept related to self-perception and response of others to obesity	Provide moral support and encouragement; introduce client to appropriate self-help or therapy groups.
Ineffective individual coping: excess food consumptions in response to stress	Consider referring the client to a psychotherapist skilled in this area.
TO MINIMIZE DRUG SIDE EFFECTS OR INTERACTIONS	
Alterations in thought processes: excess stimulation	Urge client to reduce or eliminate use of anorexics.
Sleep pattern disturbance from use of stimulants	Instruct client not to take anorexics late in the day.
TO ENSURE SAFE AND EFFICACIOUS DRUG USE	
Knowledge deficit related to drug regimen	Teach the client about the nature of obesity, its relation to mortality statistics, and the importance of balancing caloric intake with requirements.
	Discourage the use of anorexics. If anorexics are part of the regimen, stress the importance of adjusting caloric balance for maintenance of any weight loss achieved while using anorexics.
	Warn clients about the potential adverse effects of anorexics and the risks associated with overuse.

heptadine hydrochloride (Periactin). It is an antihistaminic and antiserotonergic agent. It has been used for alleviation of anorexia nervosa and other anorexias. It is more effective in the anorexias other than anorexia nervosa. When used in anorexia nervosa, it is more effective in the subgroup of clients classified as restrainers, who restrict their food intake, than in the subgroup classified as bulimics, who engage in binge-purge cycles (periods of massive food intake followed by self-induced vomiting or diarrhea).

Disorders of Lipid Metabolism and Hypolipemic Drugs

The class of substances called lipids consists mainly of fatty acids; esters of fatty acids with glycerol including mono-, di-, and triglycerides; phospholipids; cholesterol and other steroids; and pigments such as hemoglobin and carotenes. In addition, lipids can affiliate with proteins to form lipoproteins. Dietary fat is composed mostly of triglycerides. The daily metabolism of triglycerides in humans is between 70 and 150 g as compared with 1–2 g of cholesterol or phospholipids. Lipids can be absorbed in a less fully digested state than proteins and carbohydrates, but they must be emulsified by the action of bile salts before absorption can take place.

Once absorbed, lipids are transported through the lymph ducts and blood vessels by association with proteins to form lipoprotein complexes. Some lipoproteins function as carriers for exogenous lipids from the intestines to fat cells, muscle cells, and the liver. Other lipoproteins are carriers for endogenous lipids, providing transport for lipids mobilized from the liver or promoting clearance and elimination. All of the lipids contained in the plasma are bound to proteins in the form of these lipoprotein complexes. Hyperlipemias, disorders in which the levels of triglycerides or cholesterol are elevated, are therefore always secondary to abnormally high quantities of lipoproteins — a condition called hyperlipoproteinemia.

Types of Lipoproteins

Five classes of lipoproteins have been identified based on size and density (Table 44–2). The largest are the chylomicrons, followed by very-low-density lipoproteins (VLDL, or prebeta), intermediate-density lipoproteins (IDL), low-density lipoproteins (LDL, or β-lipoproteins), and high-density lipoproteins (HDL, or α-lipoproteins).

Chylomicrons are composed 90% of triglycerides and only 5% cholesterol. Their chief role is the transport of absorbed fats from the intestines to target cells or storage sites. Chylomicrons typically appear in the blood over the period of 2–10 hours after a meal. Chylomicrons pass through the blood to fat, muscle, and liver cells where they are acted upon by lipase enzymes, producing fatty acids and glycerol for cellular energy requirements or storage.

VLDL, IDL, and LDL are probably metabolically interrelated, one giving rise to the next as first the triglycerides and finally the cholesterol is removed from the carrier protein. In the liver, triglycerides, and to a lesser extent cholesterol, mobilized from fat stores, are attached to VLDL for transport to peripheral tissues as needed. Here triglycerides are severed from the lipoprotein by action of tissue lipases. As more and more of the triglycerides are removed, the lipoprotein is transformed first to IDL and then to LDL. Cholesterol is not removed from the lipoprotein as readily as the triglycerides. The cholesterol content, only 12% in VLDL, increases to 30% for IDL, and 50% for LDL. Serum levels of LDL correlate strongly with atherosclerosis and the attendant risk of cardiovascular diseases.

HDL appears to function independently of the other lipoproteins. It originates in the liver and intestines, binds cholesterol preferentially and triglycerides secondarily, and facilitates the clearance and degradation of these lipids by the liver. In stark contrast to LDL, the levels of HDL correlate inversely with risk of atherosclerosis.

Cholesterol is currently more a focus of concern than the triglycerides because of its relationship to atherosclerosis, high blood pressure, dementia, angina, and xanthomas (yellow papules or plaques in the skin due to lipid deposits). Triglycerides are not clearly a risk factor in cardiovascular disorders, but elevated levels may lead to pancreatitis, eruptive xanthomas, hepatosplenomegaly, lipemia retinalis, hyperuricemia, and glucose intolerance. Normal levels of cholesterol are difficult to define since the correlation between levels and risk of coronary heart disease is continuous over a wide range of concentrations. As a practical matter, hypercholesterolemia is defined as a level above the 95th percentile for age-matched individuals. This value increases with age from 230 mg/100 ml in young adults to over 300 mg/100 ml in the elderly. As a general guideline, cholesterol levels about 220 mg/100 ml are considered a risk factor. For triglycerides, serum levels do not increase with age and values greater than about 200 mg/100 ml are abnormal.

If serum levels of triglycerides or cholesterol are significantly elevated, it is important to establish by laboratory testing which lipoproteins are involved, since this will determine both diagnosis and treat-

Table 44–2
Characteristics of Five Classes of Serum Lipoproteins

Type	Triglyceride (%)	Cholesterol (%)	Role	Correlation with hypertension
Chylomicra	90	5	Transport of exogenous fats from GI tract	No
Very-low-density lipoproteins	60	12	Transport of endogenous fats from liver	Weak
Intermediate-density lipoproteins	40	30	Transport of endogenous fats from liver	Weak
Low-density lipoproteins	10	50	Transport of endogenous fats from liver	Very strong
High-density lipoproteins	5	20	Clearance of serum fats	Inverse

ment. Usually inspection of plasma after overnight storage at 4° C and measurement of cholesterol and triglycerides is enough to characterize the type of hyperlipoproteinemia. Electrophoresis or ultracentrifugation are confirmatory procedures, but not usually required.

Hyperlipoproteinemia

Hyperlipoproteinemia is a major contributing factor in atherosclerosis, which in turn contributes to several life-threatening or incapacitating conditions, including coronary artery disease, myocardial infarction, chronic organic brain syndrome, cerebral vascular accidents, thrombosis and embolism, and other thromboembolic diseases. Hyperlipoproteinemia is not the only factor in atherosclerosis, since some individuals with the disease do not have elevated serum lipids while other individuals with hyperlipoproteinemia never develop atherosclerosis. Nevertheless, the correlation between atherosclerosis and hyperlipoproteinemia is sufficiently strong to have encouraged the introduction of drugs that lower circulating lipid levels into therapy for the disorder. Five types of hyperlipoproteinemias are recognized (Table 44–3).

Hyperlipoproteinemia is often unrecognized until significant clinical consequences have occurred. *The nurse who is knowledgeable about early indications and risk factors can help to initiate laboratory assessment and treatment that may prevent debilitating consequences. Nursing assessment should include family history, dietary patterns, and physical complaints. Because hyperlipoproteinemias are often genetically determined, nurses should suggest that relatives of clients with the condition be screened for abnormal lipid levels.* Some health care settings make use of random screening procedures for cholesterol and triglycerides.

Treatment of hyperlipoproteinemia is indicated both for the relief of presenting symptoms and as part of the effort to decrease the risk of cardiac disease. Treatment begins with dietary restrictions (Table 44–3). If triglycerides are elevated (types I, III, IV, and V), weight reduction and alcohol elimination are indicated and a low-fat diet is instituted. Other risk factors in cardiac disease, such as stress, smoking, or lack of exercise, may need to be addressed concurrently. Lowering of serum cholesterol has not yet been proved to decrease risk of cardiovascular mortality.

Clofibrate (Atromid-S) and Gemfibrozil (Lopid)

Mechanisms and Effects Clofibrate and gemfibrozil lower triglyceride and cholesterol concentrations by 25–80% by reducing levels of VLDL. The mechanism by which this change is brought about is not yet fully determined, but clofibrate has been noted to inhibit hepatic synthesis of cholesterol and to increase catabolism of VLDL, IDL, and LDL. Gemfibrozil is similar to clofibrate in both structure and pharmacology.

Pharmacokinetics Clofibrate and gemfibrozil are well absorbed after oral administration, with peak concentrations occurring 4 hours after administration. Effects begin about 2–5 days after therapy is begun. Clients will experience a rebound at about the second or third month of therapy, followed by further decreases in lipid levels. If improvement does not occur in 3 months, therapy with clofibrate or gemfibrozil should be discontinued.

Clinical Indications Clofibrate is the drug of choice for type III hyperlipoproteinemia, is variably effective in types II, IV, and V, but has no effect in type I. Gemfibrozil is approved for type IV hyperlipoproteinemia, for clients with very-high-serum triglycerides at risk of abdominal pain or pancreatitis and who cannot be successfully managed by dietary measures.

Adverse Effects and Contraindications Clofibrate is usually well-tolerated, but has a few serious side effects. Nausea, diarrhea, skin rash, alopecia, weakness, impotence, decreased libido, and breast tenderness have been reported. Rarely, muscle stiffness and malaise have occurred. The most common adverse effects of gemfibrozil are abdominal pain, nausea, vomiting, and flatulence.

Use of clofibrate and gemfibrozil has been associated with occurrence of **gall bladder disease,** so both clofibrate and gemfibrozil are contraindicated in clients with preexisting gall bladder disease. These drugs increase the risk of cholelithiasis (formation of stones in the gallbladder) and cholecystitis (inflammation of the gallbladder). *Nurses should pay particular attention to complaints of abdominal pain, especially pain that radiates toward the right shoulder. Also, any incidence of nausea and vomiting needs to be investigated since these signs may indicate cholecystitis or pancreatitis.* Both drugs are also contraindicated in patients with renal or hepatic dysfunction, biliary cirrhosis, hypothyroidism, or peptic ulcer.

Gemfibrozil and clofibrate may produce renal dysfunction. *Clients' complaints of blood in the urine (hematuria), decreased urinary output, or other symptoms of renal dysfunction need to be investigated.*

Antilipemic agents present a risk to the fetus if utilized by a woman during pregnancy. *Women of childbearing age who are sexually active need to be advised*

Table 44–3
Five Types of Hyperlipoproteinemia

Characteristic	Type I	Type II	Type III	Type IV	Type V
I. Diagnostic indications					
A. Plasma cholesterol	Normal or slightly increased	Greatly increased	Greatly increased	Normal or slightly increased	Normal or slightly increased
B. Plasma triglycerides	Greatly increased	Normal or slightly increased	Greatly increased	Greatly increased	Very greatly increased
C. Clinical presentation	Pancreatitis Eruptive xanthomas Hepatosplenomegaly Lipemia retinalis	Premature atherosclerosis Xanthelasma Tendon and tuberous xanthomas Juvenile corneal arcus	Premature atherosclerosis Planar xanthomas Tuberous and tendon xanthomas	Possibly premature atherosclerosis Glucose intolerance Hyperuricemia	Pancreatitis Eruptive xanthomas Hepatosplenomegaly Sensory neuropathy Lipemia retinalis Hyperuricemia Glucose intolerance
II. Etiological factors					
A. Secondary causes	Dysgammaglobulinemia SLE Diabetes mellitus (type I)	Excess dietary cholesterol Hypothyroidism Nephrosis Multiple myeloma Porphyria Obstructive liver disease	Dysgammaglobulinemia Hypothyroidism	Excess alcohol Oral contraceptives Diabetes mellitus Pregnancy Nephrotic syndrome Stress Glycogen storage disease	Alcoholism Diabetes mellitus (type I) Nephrosis Dysgammaglobulinemia
B. Extent of risk of atherosclerosis	Very great	Great	Great	Slight	Slight
III. Treatment					
A. Goals	Eliminate abdominal pain	Lower serum cholesterol	Lower serum cholesterol and triglycerides	Lower serum triglycerides	Lower serum triglycerides and eliminate abdominal pain
B. Diet					
1. Calories	Unrestricted	Unrestricted	Restricted	Restricted	Restricted
2. Fat	Restrict to 25–30 g/day	Unrestricted	40% of daily calories	40% of daily calories	30% of daily calories
3. Cholesterol	Unrestricted	300 mg/day	At least 300 mg/day	300 mg/day	Moderately restricted
4. Carbohydrates	Higher because of fat restriction	Unrestricted	35% of daily calories (eliminate concentrated sugars)	45% of daily calories (limit concentrated sugars)	50% of daily calories
C. Drugs	None	Cholestryamine	Clofibrate (primary choice) Nicotinic acid (secondary choice)	Clofibrate or gemfibriol (primary choices) Nicotinic acid (secondary choice)	Nicotinic acid (primary choice) Clofibrate (secondary choice)

about birth control measures and to continue to use birth control measures while they are taking the drug because of potential risks to the fetus. Males tend to have decreased libido in response to antilipemic agents.

Drug Interactions Gemfibrozil and clofibrate increase the effect of oral anticoagulants, necessitating dosage adjustment to prevent bleeding. Doses of oral hypoglycemics or insulin may have to be increased when gemfibrozil is administered. Smoking increases the likelihood of adverse responses to clofibrate and gemfibrozil, such as dysrhythmias and congestive heart failure. *Nurses need to advise clients not to use any over-the-counter medications while receiving an antilipemic drug without first consulting their physicians.*

Preparations and Administration *Nurses need to instruct clients not to alter the frequency or amount of dose of antilipemic drugs. The nurse should help the client establish a schedule that reminds the client to take the drug.*

When clients are taking one of these medications for xanthoma, therapy may continue for up to a year, as long as the client's lesions continue to be reduced in size. *Throughout the therapy, clients need to have frequent serum transaminase and other liver function tests. In addition, blood counts and renal function tests should be performed regularly to assure that adverse reactions such as leukopenia, anemia, eosinophilia, potentiation of anticoagulant effects, or renal dysfunction do not go undetected.*

Clofibrate (Atromid-S)
Capsules
Recommended Doses: 2,000 mg PO, in 2–4 divided doses.

Gemfibrozil (Lopid)
Capsules
Recommended Doses: 1,200 mg PO in 2 divided doses 30 minutes before the morning and the evening meals.

Anion-Exchange Resins

Mechanisms and Effects Cholestyramine resin (Questran) and colestipol hydrochloride (Colestid) are anion-exchange resins that act to sequester bile acid. Bile acids are required for formation of micelles, which are in turn required for absorption of dietary lipids. Thus, anion-exchange resins inhibit the absorption of dietary lipids. Anion-exchange resins consist of polymers with numerous ion-exchange sites that can complex with bile salts, causing them to be excreted in the feces. Chloride ions are released in the process. The resins themselves are not soluble and are neither digested nor absorbed.

Clinical Indications Bile sequestrants are indicated in type II disease, especially for clients whose triglyceride levels are not also elevated. When combined with a restriction in dietary cholesterol, resins are highly effective in limiting cholesterol absorption and enterohepatic reabsorption by preventing formation of micelles. A maximum fall in LDL of 25–35% is seen within 2 weeks, with initial benefit being noted in 4–7 days. *Nurses can expect to see a marked reduction in a client's serum cholesterol during the early weeks when the drug is administered. However, if the drug is discontinued or if the client does not adhere to the drug regimen, there will be a rapid rise in serum cholesterol.* Anion-exchange resins are also indicated for relief of pruritus in clients who have a partial biliary stasis.

Adverse Effects and Contraindications Adverse effects of bile sequestrants are usually related to the gastrointestinal tract. These include constipation, nausea, vomiting, cramps, and distention. Impaction can occur and may aggravate hemorrhoids if present.

Anion exchange resins may contribute to occurrence of peptic ulcer. *Nurses should be attentive to clients' complaints of abdominal discomfort or pain, heartburn, anorexia, nausea, or burning sensations in the stomach and should report occurrence of such symptoms to the clients' physicians.*

Anion-exchange resins have not been established as safe for use during pregnancy or breastfeeding.

Drug and Diet Interactions Bile sequestrants should not be taken with other drugs since these could bind to the exchange sites and be rendered ineffective. Other drugs should be administered at least 1 hour before or 4 hours after the resin. Absorption of fat-soluble vitamins is significantly impaired by bile sequestrants and vitamin deficiencies have occurred. *Clients should be taught to include foods high in vitamins A and D in their diets. Supplements may be required. Nurses need to ask clients from time to time whether they have noticed any abnormal bleeding of mucous membranes or presence of black, tarry stools (indicative of bleeding along the upper portion of the gastrointestinal tract) which may indicate need for a vitamin K supplement.*

Preparations and Administration The resins are mixed with water or juice. The resins have an unpleasant gritty texture but can be added to fruit juice or sauce to enhance palatability. *Constipation can be reduced by intake of ample fluids and bulk foods.*

Nurses should instruct clients to pour the contents of one packet of medication onto the surface of the preferred liquid and allow it to stand for 1–2 minutes without stir-

ring, only twirling occasionally. Then the mixture should be stirred until the suspension is uniform throughout and ingested. The vessel used should then be rinsed and the client should drink the rinse water to assure that all of the drug has been taken. It is important for the nurse to stress the need to mix the drug uniformly in the vehicle, since these agents are irritating to mucous membranes and can cause esophageal impaction if not thoroughly mixed.

Cholestyramine (Questran)
Powder
Recommended Doses: 16–32 g/day PO in 2–4 divided doses before or during meals and at bedtime.

Colestipol (Colestid)
Powder
Recommended Doses: 15–30 g/day PO.

Niacin

Niacin is a B-complex vitamin and a precursor of nicotinamide adenine dinucleotide (NAD) and other coenzymes that contribute to dehydrogenase reactions of intermediate metabolism, including the metabolism of lipids. Niacin in pharmacological doses lowers serum lipids by reducing VLDL and LDL, after 1–7 days of treatment, possibly by preventing VLDL production in the liver. It is effective in type III, IV, and V disorders, and in type II when combined with a bile sequestrant. The use of niacin is limited by adverse effects, notably flushing and pruritus. Tolerance often develops to these side effects after a few weeks, and gradual upward dosing at the beginning may minimize such problems. Niacin may also aggravate ulcers or cause vomiting, diarrhea, and dyspepsia. With prolonged therapy, dry skin and hyperpigmentation have been reported. Niacin can impair liver function, increasing serum transaminase activity and sometimes producing jaundice. Hyperglycemia, glucose intolerance, and hyperuricemia have occurred at pharmacological doses. The drug should be given at mealtime to minimize gastric irritation.

Preparations and Administration

Niacin
Tablets, timed release capsules
Recommended Doses: For lipid reduction, 3 g/day PO in 3 doses (as compared to 0.3–1.0 g/day as a vitamin supplement).

Other Drugs Lowering Lipid Proteins

It is well known that thyroid hormones lower serum lipid levels, but clinical use of these in hyperlipoproteinemia is constrained by the stimulatory effects of thyroid hormones on metabolism. **Dextrothyroxine,** the dextro isomer of natural T_4 (thyroxine), is relatively selective in lowering lipids with minimal effects on metabolism. Unfortunately, in a major clinical trial, it was found to increase mortality from coronary disease.

A secondary drug for hyperlipoproteinemia is **β-sitosterol,** a plant sterol resembling cholesterol in structure. It is not absorbed, but acts in the intestinal tract to decrease cholesterol absorption. Side effects include diarrhea, nausea, and bloating. Its efficacy has not been firmly established.

A new drug that lowers plasma cholesterol is **probucol** (Lorelco). If combined with dietary restrictions, probucol lowers plasma cholesterol by a modest 10–15% by lowering LDL. It is well tolerated. Experience with the drug has been limited. It is indicated only for type II disorders.

Vitamins

Micronutrients include minerals (discussed in Chapter 42) and the vitamins. Vitamins are micronutrients that are necessary for particular biochemical processes. All of them are essential. A healthy individual who enjoys a normal, balanced diet takes in sufficient vitamins to meet his or her normal nutritional needs. In industrialized countries vitamin inadequacies are seen principally in special populations such as the elderly, hospitalized patients, pregnant women, the economically disadvantaged, drug abusers, and persons on restrictive diets. However, a survey conducted in 1977 showed that overall intake of vitamins A, B_1, B_2, and C from the diet was lower for the average American than in 1955 or 1965. If this trend continues, vitamin deficiencies will become increasingly frequent. The mean caloric intake of women in the United States is lower today (down to 1,650 calories) than a decade or two ago, making it more difficult to derive sufficient vitamins from the diet. In many developing countries, malnutrition, and thus vitamin deficiency, is endemic.

Frank **vitamin deficiencies** lead to characteristic clinical syndromes that have been recognized and described for centuries, though only recently linked to specific micronutrients. **Hypovitaminemias** (marginal states of deficiency) may compromise health in less obvious ways.

Vitamin supplements may be required for both primary and secondary vitamin deficiencies. **Primary vitamin deficiencies** are those related to inadequate intake. Contributing factors include poverty, cultural or religious dietary restrictions, alcoholism, poor eating habits, fasting, anorexia, or food processing or preparation methods that destroy or eliminate vitamins. The causes of **secondary** (or functional) **vitamin deficiencies** fall into four general categories:

1. Poor absorption of vitamins due to maldigestion or malabsorption, as in infectious or inflammatory diseases of the gastrointestinal tract, prolonged diarrhea, or drug-induced malabsorption (Table 44–4)
2. Diminished ability to activate or utilize vitamins, as in liver cirrhosis, renal disease, or certain genetic deficiencies
3. Increased nutrient losses from renal failure, hemodialysis, or hypermetabolic states such as hyperthyroidism, pyrexial disease, or fever of infection
4. Increased nutrient requirements, as in childhood, pregnancy, numerous disease states, periods of unusual exertion, or during administration of antivitamins — drugs that interfere with particular vitamins (Table 44–5).

Recommended daily allowances for most vitamins and minerals have been established by the federal government (Table 44–6). These represent minimal daily requirements. Accepted special requirements in relation to life-cycle stages include the need for vitamin C and minerals in young boys, vitamin A and protein for both sexes during adolescence, and vitamins A, D, E, B_1, B_2, B_6, B_{12}, niacin, and folate, as well as protein and minerals in pregnant and lactating women. In primary avitaminosis, appropriate preparations are those that provide vitamins in quantities that do not exceed recommended daily requirements — larger quantities provide no added benefit. In secondary deficiencies, substantially larger amounts may be required. Vitamin supplements (Table 44–7) are also indicated during prolonged therapy with drugs that act as antivitamins. Some vitamin supplements must be specifically avoided during therapy with particular drugs because of the potential for interference with drug therapy or additive toxicity (Table 44–8).

Vitamin preparations designed for treatment of disease are designated drugs, while those that serve as dietary supplements are treated as foods under federal statutes. Many of the multivitamin products contain levels of vitamins that are many times in excess of the recommended allowances. Some also contain substances for which dietary necessity is not established and for which no deficiency conditions are known. At best, such preparations are expensive placebos, at worst potential sources of vitamin overdosage.

Vitamins are generally divided into a fat-soluble group (A, D, E, and K) and a water-soluble group (B and C). Water-soluble vitamins are less likely to cause toxicity when taken in large quantities, since any excess tends to be rapidly excreted, whereas fat-soluble vitamins readily accumulate in tissues. However, toxicity can occur even with water-soluble vitamins when doses are extreme. *In order to minimize risks of vitamin overdose, clients need to be counseled to keep vitamin preparations out of the reach of children.*

Table 44–4
Drugs That Induce Malabsorption

(1) By irritation of the mucosa	
Alcohol	
Aminoglycosides	
Antineoplastic drugs	
Broad-spectrum antibiotics	
Nonsteroidal anti-inflammatory drugs	
Tetracyclines	
(2) By creating a physical barrier	
Laxatives	
Liquid paraffin	
Mineral oil	
Phenolphthalein	
(3) By interference with bile or digestive enzymes	
Bile sequestrants	
Drugs causing allergic cholestasis (e.g., phenothiazines)	
Drugs causing pancreatitis (e.g., alcohol)	
(4) By inhibition of absorption of specific nutrients	
Folate:	Antiepileptics
	B_{12} deficiency
	Oral contraceptives
	Salicylazosulfapyridine
B_{12}:	Biguanides
	Para-aminosalicylic acid
	Potassium chloride
Vitamin K:	Phenindione

Fat-Soluble Vitamins

The existence of fat-soluble vitamins was first recognized just before World War I. We now recognize four vitamins in this group, vitamins A, D, E, and K. Vitamin K is discussed in Chapter 41 because of its close association with several clotting factors.

Vitamin A

Sources and Requirements Vitamin A enters the body as retinol itself (vitamin A_1), 3-dehydroretinol (vitamin A_2), and as provitamin A (carotene). Sources rich in retinol include dairy products, eggs, fish, kidney, and especially liver. Carotene is found especially in carrots, sweet potatoes, and yellow corn, and appreciably in green, leafy vegetables,

Table 44–5
Vitamins and Antivitamins

Vitamin	Antivitamins	Mechanism
A	Alcohol	Decreased absorption
	Antilipemic agents	Decreased absorption
	Emollients	Decreased absorption
D	Antilipemic agents	Decreased absorption
	Emollients	Decreased absorption
	Glucocorticoids	Decreased activation
	Phenytoin and other inducers	Increased elimination due to induction of liver enzymes
	Sodium etidronate	Decreased activation
E	Antilipemics	Decreased absorption
	Mineral oil	Decreased absorption
	Polyunsaturated fats	Increased requirement
B_1	Alcohol	Decreased intake, absorption, and utilization
	Antacids	Decreased absorption
	Digitalis	Increased requirement
	Raw fish	Increased metabolism
	Tea	Antagonism
B_2	Alcohol	Decreased intake, absorption, and utilization
	Boric acid	Decreased transport
	Oral contraceptives	Decreased levels
	Phenothiazines	Decreased activation
	Tetracyclines	Decreased absorption
	Tricyclic antidepressants	Decreased activation
B_3	Alcohol	Decreased intake, absorption, and utilization
	Antimetabolites (6-mercaptopurine and 5-fluorouracil)	Decreased activation
	Isoniazid	Secondary to B_6 deficiency
B_6	Alcohol	Decreased intake, absorption, and utilization
	Cycloserine	Forms complex with the vitamin
	Hydralazine	Forms complex with the vitamin
	Hydrazides	Forms complex with the vitamin
	Isoniazid	Forms complex with the vitamin
	Oral contraceptives	?
	Penicillamine	Forms complex with the vitamin
C	Alcohol	Decreased intake, absorption, and utilization
	Aspirin	Increased excretion
	Inducers such as phenytoin, barbiturates, tobacco, paraldehyde, aminopyrine	Increased metabolism
	Oral contraceptives	Decreased levels
	Tetracyclines	Decreased absorption

broccoli, winter squash, tomatoes, pumpkin, and yellow or green fruits such as apricots. Since meat, vegetables, and fruits all contain vitamin A, primary deficiencies occur mainly in people subsisting entirely on foods from the bread and cereal group.

Daily requirements for vitamin A (as well as D and E) are stated in International Units (IU) because preparations of fat-soluble vitamins are contained in oil (such as fish oil) and vary in purity. (Requirements for water-soluble vitamins are given in milli-

Table 44–6
Sources, Deficiency Symptoms, and Recommended Daily Allowances of Vitamins[a]

Vitamin	Typical food sources	Deficiency disease	Infants	Children				Males					Females						
			0–0.5 year	0.5–1.0	1–3	4–6	7–10	11–14	15–18	19–22	23–50	>50	11–14	15–18	19–22	23–50	>50	Pregnant	Lactating
Fat-soluble																			
Vitamin A (IU)	Dairy products, green vegetables, liver, eggs, carrots	Night blindness, keratinization of the skin, cornea, and conjunctiva	420	400	400	500	700	1,000	1,000	1,000	1,000	1,000	800	800	800	800	800	+200	+400
Vitamin D (μg)	Egg yolk, butter, milk, cod liver oil, salmon, shrimp	Rickets (children) and osteomalacia (adults)	10	10	10	10	10	10	10	7.5	5	5	10	10	7.5	5	5	+5	+5
Vitamin E (IU)	Egg yolk, liver, wheat germ, vegetable oils	Hemolytic anemia (controversial)	3	4	5	6	7	8	10	10	10	10	8	8	8	8	8	+2	+3
Water-soluble																			
Vitamin B_1 (thiamine) (mg)	Cereal, yeast, meat, beans, peas	Beriberi: fatigue, nervous system disturbances, Wernicke's encephalopathy.	0.3	0.5	0.7	0.9	1.2	1.4	1.4	1.5	1.4	1.2	1.1	1.1	1.1	1	1	+0.4	+0.5
Vitamin B_2 (riboflavin) (mg)	Yeast, liver, meat, green vegetables	Glossitis, dermatitis, corneal vascularization, anemia	0.4	0.6	0.8	1.0	1.4	1.6	1.7	1.7	1.6	1.4	1.3	1.3	1.3	1.2	1.2	+0.3	+0.5
Vitamin B_3 (niacin) (mg)	Yeast, liver, meat	Pellagra	6	8	9	11	16	18	18	19	18	16	15	14	14	13	13	+2	+5
Vitamin B_5[b] (pantothenic acid) (mg)	Liver, eggs, cheese	Not seen in humans; neurological disturbances, muscle disturbances	4–5	4–5	4–5	4–5	4–5	4–5	4–7	4–7	4–7	4–7	4–5	4–7	4–7	4–7	4–7	—	—
Vitamin B_6 (pyridoxine) (mg)	Yeast, liver, cereal, egg yolk, nuts, meat, fish, potatoes, peas	Neural hyperexcitability, convulsions, GABA depletion, edema	0.3	0.6	0.9	1.3	1.6	1.8	2.0	2.2	2.2	2.2	1.8	2.0	2.0	2	2	+0.6	+0.5
Vitamin C (ascorbate) (mg)	Fruits, green vegetables, and many foods	Scurvy	35	35	45	45	45	50	60	60	60	60	50	60	60	60	60	+20	+40

[a]Excluding vitamins K, B_{12}, and folic acid, which are discussed in Chapter 41.
[b]No official recommended daily allowances have been established.

grams.) Recommended daily allowances for vitamin A are 400–700 IU in children, 1,000 IU in adult males, and 800 in adult females. Recommended supplements for women are 200 IU during pregnancy and 400 IU during lactation.

Pharmacokinetics The pharmacokinetics of vitamin A are important because drugs may interact with vitamin A by altering pharmacokinetic parameters. Retinol esters are hydrolyzed by pancreatic lipase and β-carotene is cleaved by hydrolysis in the small intestine. Both reactions lead to formation of retinol (Figure 44–1). Retinol is then solubilized through formation of micelles with bile salts and acids. Thus, absorption of vitamin A is dependent on adequate exocrine activity of the pancreas and biliary system. Clients who have inadequate exocrine function of the pancreas, or liver or gallbladder disease can be anticipated to develop vitamin A deficiency even though they may be ingesting quantities of the vitamin that would otherwise be adequate. Optimal vitamin A absorption is also dependent on presence of dietary fat.

After absorption into mucosal epithelial cells of the intestines, retinol is reesterified with palmitic acid. Retinyl palmitate reaches the liver by way of

Table 44–7
Recommended Daily Vitamin/Mineral Supplements in Conjunction with Drug Therapy

Drugs	Recommended Daily Vitamin/ Mineral Supplements
Antiepileptics	
Phenytoin	Vitamin D: 400–800 IU Vitamin K: 1–5 mg Folic acid: 0.4–1.0 mg, but not more than 2.0 mg
Primidone	Vitamin K: 1–5 mg
Anti-inflammatory drugs	
Aspirin	Vitamin C: 50–100 mg Folic acid: 0.4–1.0 mg Iron: 20–50 mg
Indomethacin	Iron: 20–50 mg
Sulfasalazine	Folic acid: 0.4–1.0 mg
Antilipemics	
Cholestryramine or colestipol	Vitamin A: 2,000–5,000 IU Vitamin D: 200–800 IU Vitamin K: 2–25 mg Folic acid: 0.4–1.0 mg
Antimicrobials	
Neomycin	Vitamin A: 2,000–5,000 IU Vitamin D: 200–800 IU Vitamin K: 2–25 mg Folic acid: 0.4–1.0 mg
Tetracyclines	Vitamin B_2: 5 mg Vitamin C: 0.8–1.5 g Calcium: 0.8–1.5 g
Digitalis	Thiamine: 10–30 mg
Diuretics	
Thiazides and high-ceiling diuretics	Potassium-enriched diet or potassium supplements
Triamterene	Folic acid: 0.4–1.0 mg
Gastrointestinal drugs	
Antacids	Folic acid: 0.4–0.8 mg
Emollients	Vitamin A: 5,000–10,000 IU Vitamin D: 400–800 IU
Hydrazides	
Hydralazine, isoniazid, or penicillamine	Vitamin B_6: 25–100 mg Niacin: 15–25 mg Vitamin D: 400–800 IU
Oral contraceptives	
Estrogen/progestin combinations	Vitamin B_6: 1.5–5.0 mg Folic acid: 0.4–1.0 mg
Psychotropics	
Neuroleptics	Riboflavin: 2–5 mg
Tricyclic antidepressants	Riboflavin: 2–5 mg

the lymph and blood. Reserves of vitamin A in the liver and tissues of adults are adequate to preclude vitamin A deficiency unless dietary insufficiency is rather long term. Retinol is transported to target tissues (the retina, testes, skin, and mucosa) as required in attachment to retinol binding protein. In the target cells, retinol is reduced to retinal, the active form, by alcohol dehydrogenase.

Physiological Roles and Pharmacological Effects Retinal is the immediate precursor of rhodopsin, a visual pigment important in all types of vision, but especially night vision. Vitamin A is also required for spermatogenesis. Epithelial cells throughout the body, and especially those involved in mucous secretion and keratinization (formation of scales), are dependent on vitamin A for maintenance of structural and functional integrity. Vitamin A promotes epithelial cell differentiation.

Vitamin A Deficiency and Administration Night blindness was described as long ago as 1500 BC in Egypt; later, Hippocrates recommended eating beef liver (a source of vitamin A) to alleviate the condition. The connection between night blindness and vitamin A was made during World War I, shortly after the initial recognition of fat-soluble vitamins. Visual impairment related to vitamin A deficiency is the major cause of blindness in children in Third World countries.

In vitamin A deficiency, mucous-secreting epithelial cells of the skin, lungs, eye, and gastrointestinal and urinary tracts atrophy, leading to drying and increased keratinization. Susceptibility to infection is increased. Excess vitamin A leads to excess mucin production and inhibition of keratinization. *Nursing assessments if vitamin A deficiency is suspected would include observing the condition of the client's skin and mucous membranes. Clients who seem prone to infection or who tend to have skin lesions may have a deficiency in vitamin A.*

In the United States, primary vitamin A deficiency is seldom seen. When it does occur, it should

Table 44–8
Vitamin Restrictions in Relation to Drug Therapy

Drug	Vitamin Restriction
Isotretinoin	Avoid vitamin A supplements.
Levodopa	Avoid vitamin B_6 supplements.
Oral anticoagulants	Avoid vitamin K supplements.
Oral contraceptives	Avoid megadoses of vitamin C.

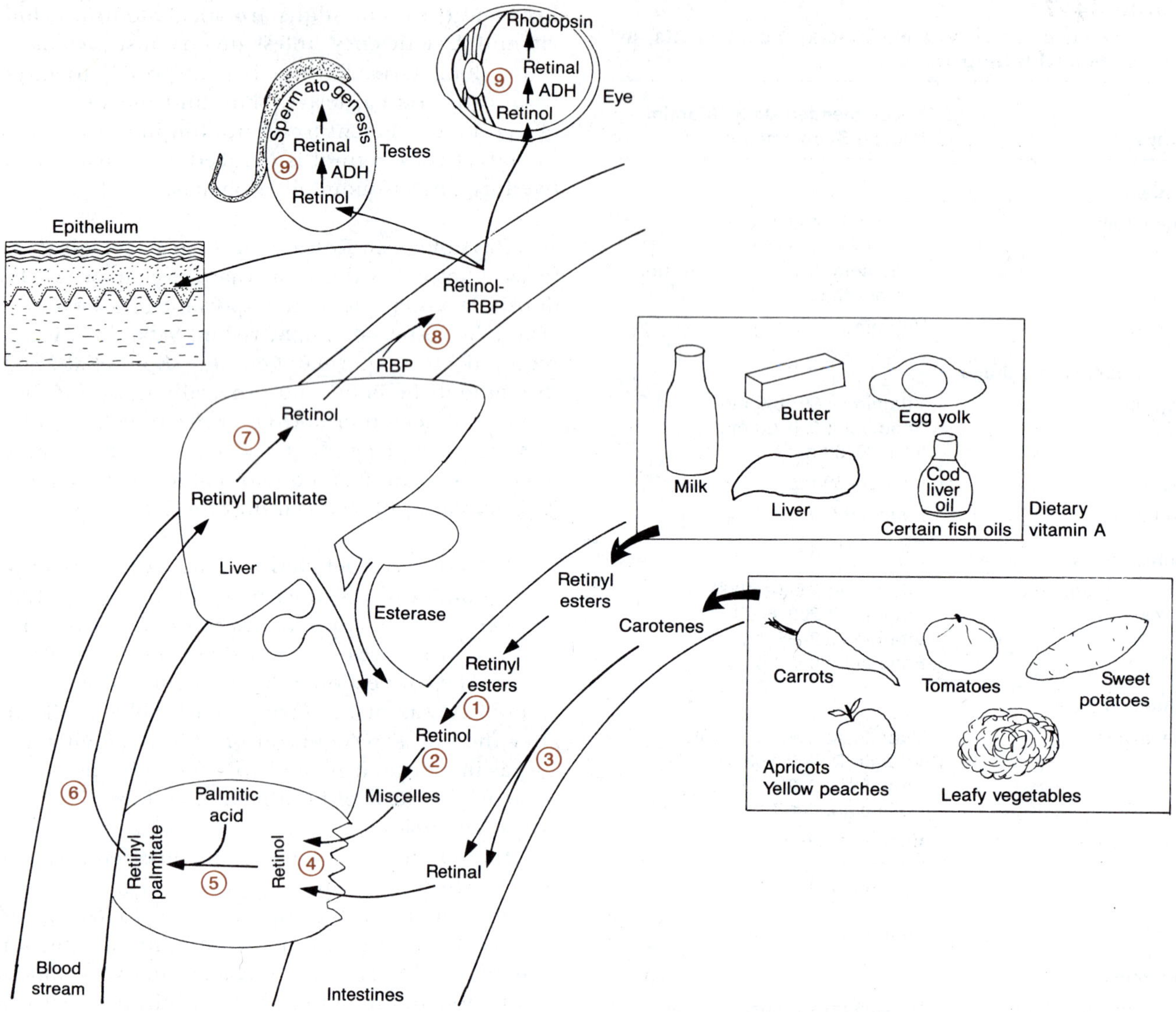

Figure 44–1
Vitamin A. (1) Hydrolysis of dietary retinyl esters; (2) incorporation into fat miscelles; (3) cleavage of dietary carotenes (provitamin A); (4) absorption of retinol; (5) reesterification with palmitic acid to form retinyl palmitate; (6) transport of retinyl palmitate to liver; (7) hydrolysis to retinol; (8) attachment to retinol binding protein for transport to target tissues; (9) activation by alcohol dehydrogenase (ADH) to retinal which can be converted to the visual pigment rhodopsin in the eye, stimulate spermatogenesis in the testes, and regulate sebaceous glands and keratinization in the skin.

be corrected by dietary adjustment. Secondary deficiency can be due to a variety of mechanisms. Absorption of vitamin A is impaired in obstructive jaundice, pancreatic diseases or operations, sprue, colitis, or with use of mineral oil or anion-exchange resins.

Vitamin A deficiency increases liability to carcinomas (cancers of epithelial tissues). Moreover, vitamin A administration can prevent progression of premalignant epithelial tumors to malignant ones. Although the role of vitamin A in occurrence of carcinomas is not fully known, vitamin A has been noted to exert a regulatory influence on transcription by interacting with ribonucleic acid (RNA). Liver accumulation of the natural vitamin A limits its usefulness in treatment of carcinomas. When large doses are given, very little reaches the target epithelial cells, and liver toxicity is apt to occur. Development of synthetic analogues may ultimately solve this pharmacokinetic problem.

Storage of vitamin A is impaired in liver cirrhosis and transport is diminished in hypoproteinemia. Alcohol can inhibit the conversion of vitamin A to retinal in the testes (and elsewhere), which may contribute to sterility in male alcoholics. Secondary vitamin A deficiency may require use of vitamin A concentrates, for example, during periods of increased need, such as pregnancy, lactation, infancy, and disease states involving impaired absorption.

Vitamin A doses should be based on the guidelines established by minimum daily requirements. During pregnancy and lactation, 1,000–1,200 IU is appropriate. Doses should not exceed 25,000 IU/day, as this may lead to hypervitaminosis after a few months. Vitamin A preparations consist of cod liver oil or halibut liver oil (either may be diluted with vegetable oil), or vitamin A concentrate in fish liver oil or vegetable oil. The fish liver oils contain vitamin D as well. The usual route of administration is oral. Ointments are available for topical administration and a water-miscible preparation (Aquasol A) can be given by intramuscular injection (slow and deep).

Vitamin D

Vitamin D is another fat-soluble vitamin that exists in multiple forms and derivatives. Its fundamental role is the regulation of calcium metabolism, together with calcitonin and parathyroid hormone (see Chapter 31 for a full discussion of calcium regulation). Vitamin D activity results in uptake of calcium from the intestines and normal mineralization of bone. Absence of vitamin D activity results in rickets in children or the analogous osteomalacia in adults. Substances with vitamin D potency are said to be **antirachitic.**

Sources and Requirements Vitamin D is available to the body from both endogenous and dietary sources. The endogenous source involves synthesis of the vitamin in the skin from a provitamin (Figure 44–2), when the skin is exposed to sunlight. Under normal circumstances, synthesis in the skin is the main source and a sufficient source of vitamin D. However, skin pigmentation, use of sun screens, duration and area of skin exposure, weather, and pollution are factors determining whether, in fact, endogenous production is sufficient.

Dietary sources rich in vitamin D include certain fish (shrimp, salmon, and especially fish liver), egg yolk, butter, and fortified products such as milk, cereal, and infant formulas. These foods contain vitamin D in two forms: vitamin D_2 and vitamin D_3, which have equivalent activity in man. There was once thought to be a third dietary form (D_1), but it was shown to be a mixture of antirachitic substances.

Recommended daily allowances of vitamin D are 10 μg in children and adolescents, 7.5 μg for young adults 19–22 years of age, and 5 μg thereafter, regardless of gender. Supplements of 5 μg daily are recommended in women during pregnancy or lactation.

Pharmacokinetics Vitamin D ingested in the diet is absorbed from the small intestines, mainly in the initial segments. Like other lipids, its absorption is promoted by bile salts and by the presence of dietary fat. Biliary obstruction or use of mineral oil or anion-exchange resins (which bind bile salts) will substantially impair vitamin D absorption.

Vitamin D is transported in plasma attached to a serum protein and is taken up by the liver or stored in lipid depots. Vitamin D is really a prohormone, requiring biotransformation in the liver and then the kidney before achieving biological activity. Competitive inhibition of the activating step in the liver by glucocorticoids contributes to osteoporosis that accompanies long-term treatment with such drugs. After both activating steps have occurred, the most potent of the resulting metabolites is **calcitriol;** it is formed preferentially in conditions of frank deficiency of vitamin D or calcium and phosphate. Formation of this very active form is stimulated by parathyroid hormone. Calcitriol enhances intestinal absorption of calcium and resorption of calcium from bone to overcome hypocalcemia. On the other hand, when serum calcium levels are normal, the hormone calcitonin shifts renal activation of vitamin D from formation of calcitriol to another metabolite, HCC (24,25-trihydroxycholecalciferol), which is able to stimulate intestinal absorption of calcium but not bone mobilization. Under these circumstances, calcium storage in bone takes place.

Physiological Role and Pharmacological Effects The two clearly established target tissues for vitamin D activity are the intestines and bone. In the intestines, vitamin D metabolites stimulate protein synthesis and thus modify the structure of the intestinal epithelium to enhance calcium and phosphate absorption. Some drugs, such as mineral oil, can inhibit calcitriol-stimulated calcium absorption from the intestines.

The effect of calcitriol on bone is to stimulate

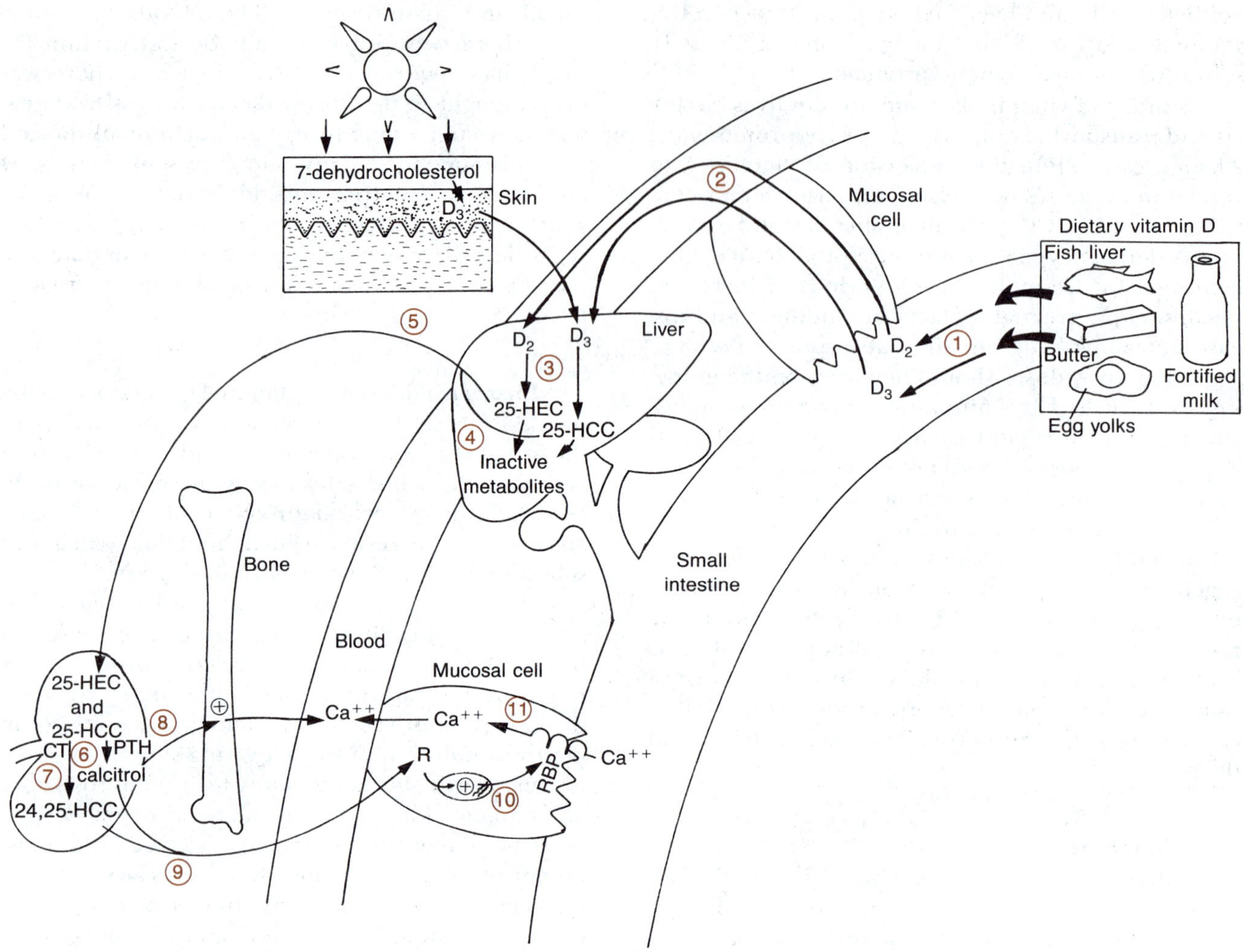

Figure 44–2

Vitamin D. (1) Dietary forms of vitamin D (D_2 and D_3) are absorbed in the small intestines and are transported through the blood (2) to the liver. Vitamin D_3 can also be synthesized in the skin (3) by exposure to sunlight. Vitamin D is activated in two steps, the first in the liver (4), yielding 25-hydroxyergocalciferol (25-HEC) or 25-hydroxycholecalciferol (25-HCC). If they escape destruction in the liver (5), these intermediaries are (6) transported to the kidney and further activated to either calcitriol (7) under the influence of parathyroid hormone, or 24,25-hydroxycholecalciferol (24,25-HCC) (8) under the influence of calcitonin (CT). Both of these active forms of vitamin D stimulate intestinal mucosal cells (9) to produce a binding protein (10) required for calcium absorption (11). Calcitriol also stimulates resorption of calcium from bone.

mobilization of calcium, an effect not shared by all vitamin D metabolites. The mechanism of this effect is not established, but might involve active transport of calcium across osteocytes by a mechanism analogous to intestinal absorption.

Other proposed target sites for vitamin D derivatives include muscle, the parathyroids, and kidneys. In the kidneys, vitamin D may have a direct effect of increasing calcium and phosphate reabsorption.

Vitamin D Deficiency and Administration The disorders associated with vitamin D deficiency are **rickets** in children and **osteomalacia** in adults. They are similar in etiology but differ in pathological expression because of the differing impacts of the deficiency on developing versus formed bones. In rickets, ossification of the skull will be slow if the defect is present in infancy. Bending of the ribs may occur in children who are old enough to sit up. Widening of the epiphyseal cartilage may occur at the ends of the long bones of the limbs. In osteomalacia, insufficient deposition of calcium causes the bones to become brittle and easy to break. Clients with osteomalacia may experience pain, deformity, and muscle weakness.

Usually, vitamin D deficiency is due to inadequate exposure to sunlight and poor diet, but diseases and drugs may be contributing factors. Malabsorption syndromes may impair vitamin D absorption. Liver disease or chronic glucocorticoids can impair liver hydroxylation of vitamin D, while inducers of liver enzymes increase liver catabolism of vitamin D and its metabolites. Renal failure or hereditary rickets may inhibit hydroxylation in the kidney. Thus, a complete history needs to include questions about liver disease, renal problems, or illness that could result in malabsorption. Diagnosis of vitamin D deficiency is based on a history of inadequate vitamin D intake or production, radiology, low serum levels of vitamin D metabolites, low serum phosphorus and calcium, and elevated serum alkaline phosphatase.

Nurses and dietitians need to collaborate with clients in establishing dietary habits and exposure to sunlight that will ensure appropriate quantities of vitamin D. Treatment of established deficiencies consists in most instances of ensuring adequate calcium, phosphorus, and vitamin D intake. The usual dose of vitamin D is 1,200 to 1,600 International Units per day. Vitamin D-resistant rickets, due to impaired formation of the active metabolites, is treated by administration of the metabolites themselves. For prevention of rickets, children may be given 200 IU/day initially, with doses increasing to 800 IU/day by 2 months of age. Premature babies and other high-risk infants may be given 800 to 1,200 IU daily. Vitamin D administration is also used to promote healing of bone fractures.

In addition to cod liver oil and oleovitamin combinations of vitamins A and D, there are three kinds of concentrated vitamin D preparations available. Vitamin D_2 and D_3 combinations are available in capsules of 50,000 IU and in solutions of 10,000 IU/g for oral administration. These dosage forms are intended for vitamin D-resistant rickets, which, however, is more rationally treated with preparations of vitamin D metabolites. Calcifediol (Calderol), the main circulating form of vitamin D, is available in 20 μg and 50 μg capsules. The usual dose is 50–100 μg PO daily. Calcitriol (Rocaltrol), the most potent renal metabolite of vitamin D, is available in 0.25 and 0.5 μg capsules. The usual maintenance dose is 0.5–1.0 μg PO daily. This preparation is especially appropriate for vitamin D-resistant rickets, osteodystrophy secondary to renal failure, and hypoparathyroidism. Doses of any vitamin D preparation should be titrated against serum calcium determinations, at first weekly and then monthly. Normal serum values are 8.5–10.5 mg/100 ml.

A client who has chronic renal failure is more prone than others to developing magnesium intoxication if he or she is also taking vitamin D. Therefore, nurses need to advise such clients to avoid taking antacids or laxatives that contain magnesium.

Hypervitaminosis D Hypervitaminosis D occurs when vitamin D ingestion is excessive (> 40,000 IU/day) or doses of vitamin D preparations have been inadequately adjusted (serum calcium above 12.0 mg/100 ml). The symptoms are essentially symptoms of hypercalcemia. Early symptoms of vitamin D toxicity include anorexia, nausea, and vomiting. Subsequent symptoms are weakness, nervousness, headache, somnolence, metallic taste, dry mouth, and pain in muscle and bone. Still later symptoms include polydipsia, polyuria, pruritus, conjunctivitis, pancreatitis, decreased libido, and cardiac dysrhythmias. *Special care is required in patients predisposed to dysrhythmias, such as those on digitalis preparations.* When symptoms of vitamin D toxicity are observed, use of vitamin D preparations should be curtailed, fluid intake should be increased, and a low-calcium diet instituted.

Clients receiving therapeutic doses of vitamin D need to be carefully supervised since the margin of safety between therapeutic and toxic doses is very narrow. *Nurses should warn clients of the hazards of overdoses.*

Progress of clients receiving vitamin D should be followed closely. *If the therapeutic dose is high, serum calcium phosphates and urea should be monitored. In addition, urine should be examined for calcium, casts, albumin, and the presence of erythrocytes. If a client develops hyperphosphatemia, the nurse needs to see that the dietary intake of phosphate is restricted.* The client may also be placed on aluminum gel to bind intestinal phosphate.

Once symptoms of vitamin D deficiency have been relieved, the dosage of vitamin D should be reduced to avoid hypercalcemia. *Nurses should stress the need to report any signs of toxicity to the physician immediately so that the client can be promptly taken off the vitamin. Should toxicity occur, nurses should be prepared to teach clients the need for a low-calcium diet and the foods necessary to increase acidification of the urine. In addition, such clients should be encouraged to increase their fluid intake.*

Vitamin E

Sources and Requirements Vitamin E refers to a group of fat soluble substances belonging to the family of **tocopherols.** The vitamin was isolated in 1936 from wheat germ oil. In addition, it is found in soybean oil, nuts, eggs, liver, and margarines. The role of vitamin E is less clear than for the other fat-soluble vitamins. What is known is that tocopherols are powerful antioxidants that help to maintain membrane stability by complexing with polyunsaturated phospholipids. For example, vitamin E helps to protect red blood cells against hemolysis. Recommended daily allowances for vitamin E are 8 IU for adult women and 10 IU for adult males. Vitamin E requirements increase if the diet is rich in polyunsaturated fats. Other antioxidants, such as the chemical element selenium, can substitute for vitamin E in most respects. Vitamin E is relatively lacking in both toxicity and pharmacological activity, except in treatment of deficiency states. However, clients who take excessive amounts of vitamin E may complain of unusual fatigue, muscle weakness, and gastrointestinal upset. Some have complained of blurred vision.

Pharmacokinetics Vitamin E absorption is similar to that of other fat-soluble vitamins and fats in general, being dependent on formation of micelles with bile salts and presence of adequate levels of dietary fats. In the blood, levels of vitamin E parallel levels of serum lipoproteins. It may be that vitamin E is normally bound to a carrier lipoprotein. Patients with hyperlipoproteinemia typically exhibit high levels of vitamin E. Anion-exchange resins that lower lipoprotein levels in serum produce similar declines in vitamin E.

Vitamin E Deficiency and Administration Symptoms of vitamin E deficiency are difficult to sort out from effects related to overall decreases in serum lipids because the two go hand in hand. At present, symptoms thought to be attributable to vitamin E deficiency include sterility and miscarriage, increased hemolysis of red blood cells, and a muscular dystrophy due to creatinuria and ceroid deposits in skeletal muscles. However, vitamin E administration appears to be effective in alleviating such symptoms only when they are caused specifically by vitamin E deficiency.

Vitamin E capsules (Aquasol E, E-Ferol) contain from 30 to 1,000 I.U.'s of alpha-tocopherol. It is also available for injection in dosage forms of 100–200 I.U.'s. The sole clinical indications are vitamin E deficiency and anemias not responsive to other treatments.

Water-Soluble Vitamins

The water-soluble vitamins have an early history that is tied to that of the fat-soluble vitamins. McCollum and Davis, in 1915, studied dietary factors in butter that contributed to growth. They separated butter into fat-soluble A and water-soluble B fractions, finding that each component contained substances necessary for growth. The term *vitamin* (originally *vitamine*) was applied to suggest a substance vital to life. The water-soluble B fraction ultimately proved to contain several distinct chemicals, and as these were identified, they were designated as B_1, B_2, and so forth. Currently, 10 substances are included as B-complex vitamins: thiamine (B_1), riboflavin (B_2), nicotinic acid (B_3), pantothenic acid (B_5), pyridoxine (B_6), biotin, folic acid, cyanocobalamin (B_{12}), choline, and inositol. Two of these, folic acid and cyanocobalamin, are discussed in Chapter 41 because of their involvement in hematopoiesis. The rationale for continuing to designate these disparate substances as a complex of vitamins is that they are often found together in food sources, especially yeast and liver, and consequently, deficiency states tend to involve more than one member of the group.

The other water-soluble vitamin, ascorbic acid, or vitamin C, was first isolated in 1932, although it had been known for some 200 years that citrus fruit could cure scurvy, a disease described since the Middle Ages.

Water-soluble vitamins function as precursors for coenzymes involved in the catabolism of macronutrients. Being water soluble, these vitamins do not accumulate, so that hypervitaminosis conditions are seldom a problem for this group.

Thiamine (Vitamin B_1)

Thiamine (thiamin, vitamin B_1) was the first B-complex vitamin to be discovered. The related deficiency disorder is a polyneuritis called *beriberi.* This disease was widespread in East Asia in the nineteenth century, after the introduction of rice processing mills that removed the thiamine-containing husks to produce polished white rice. The discovery that a water extract from the husks or the husks themselves could be used to treat beriberi led to the isolation of thiamine. Thiamine is a precursor of an important coenzyme, thiamine pyrophosphate (TPP). It is converted to the active coenzyme by reaction with ATP, which provides the pyrophosphate.

Sources and Requirements The best dietary sources of thiamine are whole wheat grains, nuts, eggs, yeast, and meat, especially pork. Secondary sources include milk, potatoes, and legumes (peas and beans). Some methods of food preparation — steaming of vegetables or baking of potatoes or grains for example — can reduce concentrations of thiamine. Cereals, flour, pasta, breads, and milk modifiers are often enriched with thiamine and other vitamins. Thiamine is involved mainly in metabolism of carbohydrates. Therefore, the human requirement for thiamine depends on the amount of carbohydrate in the diet, or approximately, caloric intake. The recommended daily intake of thiamine is 0.5 mg/1,000 kcal, or about 1.4 mg in adolescent and adult males, or 1.1 mg in adolescent and adult females (Table 44–6). Thiamine intake should be increased in lactating or pregnant females and in the elderly (who utilize it less efficiently).

Pharmacokinetics Absorption of thiamine occurs from the small intestine, especially the jejunum, by sodium-dependent active transport. Passive absorption is also significant when thiamine is present in high concentrations. Absorption is impaired in folic acid deficiency and alcoholism. After absorption, thiamine is phosphorylated in the liver, red blood cells, and cerebral cortex. About 1 mg of thiamine is completely degraded daily in tissues involved in carbohydrate metabolism. This approximates the minimum daily requirement.

Physiological Role and Pharmacological Effects Thiamine pyrophosphate is a coenzyme in the metabolism of carbohydrates. Pharmacological and toxic effects of thiamine are practically nonexistent except for relieving symptoms of deficiency. Body requirements for thiamine are directly proportional to carbohydrate intake and metabolic rate. Therefore, when the diet consists mostly of carbohydrates, the requirement for thiamine is increased.

Thiamine Deficiency and Administration Thiamine deficiency, or beriberi, is characterized by neurological disturbances, both central and peripheral, and cardiovascular problems. Central neurological manifestations include anorexia (which can further aggravate the deficiency) and Wernicke's-Korsakoff's syndrome (discussed more fully in Chapter 13 in relation to alcoholism). Peripheral neurological changes consist initially of tingling or burning sensations in the legs, leg pains, and calf muscle cramps. A nursing examination might reveal impaired reflexes, loss of vibratory and proprioceptive sensations, weakness and atrophy of leg muscles, tremors, and drooping of the feet and toes. Cardiovascular symptoms of beriberi appear as congestive heart failure. Heart disease and peripheral neuritis occur in fairly mild states of deprivation while Wernicke's encephalopathy usually appears only in severe deprivation.

Nurses need to take a complete dietary history to rule out potential causes of thiamine deficiency. The most common cause of thiamine deficiency is chronic alcoholism, which leads to a mixed primary and secondary deficiency. The primary component is diminished intake of thiamine and other nutrients because of anorexia and the high caloric content of alcohol. The secondary component may entail diminished absorption from mucosal cells into the blood supply or decreased conversion of thiamine to thiamine pyrophosphate in the liver (if hepatitis or cirrhosis has developed). *Since thiamine deficiency rarely occurs alone, nurses need to be aware of evidence of general vitamin deficiency. The presence of other disease states that contribute to vitamin deficiencies often precludes a neat diagnosis.*

Other conditions that may contribute to secondary thiamine deficiency due to impaired absorption include prolonged diarrhea or malabsorption syndromes, ulcerative colitis, regional ileitis, or surgical resection. Thiamine requirements may also be elevated by consumption of large amounts of raw fish (which contains thiaminase, an enzyme that destroys thiamine) or tea (which contains a thiamine antagonist). Digitalis has also been reported to increase requirements for thiamine.

Thiamine can be provided either through dietary adjustments or administration of concentrates. Dried yeast contains at least 0.12 mg of thiamine per gram. *Clients need to have a list of foods rich in thiamine, such as yeast, pork, beef, liver, whole grains, and fresh vegetables. The nurse must be fully knowledgeable about disease states that would preclude eating some of these foods. For example, clients who have cardiovascular disorders should not increase their intake of beef or pork but might instead increase their intake of whole grains and fresh vegetables. Refined flours and polished rice are poor sources of thiamine.*

With large doses, hypersensitivity reactions have been noted, though rarely. *Nurses should advise clients to preserve thiamine hydrochloride in tight, light-resistant, nonmetallic containers. Because thiamine is unstable in neutral or alkaline solutions, it should not be used with solutions such as acetates, barbiturates, bicarbonates, carbonates, or citrates.*

Thiamine Hydrochloride (Betalin S and others)
Tablets, injection solutions, elixir
Recommended Doses: For mild peripheral neuropathy, 10–20 mg/day PO typically in 3 or 4 divided doses. For more severe neuropathies, 20–30 mg/day PO. For Wernicke's encephalopathy or cardiovascular beriberi, 50–100 mg, subcutaneously or intravenously, twice per day.

Riboflavin (Vitamin B_2)

Sources and Requirements Water-soluble B vitamin was recognized to contain multiple active substances when it was separated into the heat-labile antiberberi factor (B_1) and another heat-stable factor, which was named B_2. The B_2 fraction was noted to have a yellowish appearance in direct proportion to its vitamin activity. The yellowish B_2 vitamin was given the name *riboflavin.* Riboflavin is a precursor of two coenzymes: flavin mononucleotide (FMN) and flavin adenine dinucleotide (FAD).

Riboflavin is an essential dietary substance, found in greatest concentration in milk, cheese, eggs, organ meats, whole grains, green leafy vegetables, legumes such as peas and lima beans, and especially dried yeast. Cereals, breads, flour, and milk modifiers are frequently enriched with riboflavin. The normal daily requirement is 0.6 mg/1,000 kcal or about 1.6 mg for young men or 1.2 mg for young women (Table 44–6). Higher intake is required in pregnant and lactating women.

Pharmacokinetics Most of the vitamin B_2 in foods is in the form of the two nucleotides, flavin adenine dinucleotide (FAD) and flavin mononucleotide (FMN), which are digested by the gastrointestinal fluids. The riboflavin so produced and any residual FMN are absorbed in the initial segment of the intestines. The presence of food with administered B_2 enhances its absorption, probably by slowing its transit time through the intestines. Conversely, hypermotility impairs absorption. *Nurses should expect that clients who have had prolonged episodes of diarrhea will also have signs of B_2 deficiency.* FMN is formed from riboflavin in the mucosal cells during absorption and is then bound to plasma albumin proteins during transport in the plasma. FMN can be displaced from these binding sites by boric acid leading to hyperexcretion. Riboflavin is stored mainly in the liver and kidneys and undergoes both biliary and renal excretion. *Clients should be reassured that the intense yellow color riboflavin imparts to urine is a harmless effect.*

Physiological Role The nucleotides (FMN and FAD) derived from riboflavin contribute to energy transfer reactions associated with lipid, amino acid, and carbohydrate catabolism as well as synthesis of certain sterols, purines, pyrimidines, and pteridines, and activation of vitamin B_6. Flavin coenzymes are also involved in the microsomal drug-metabolizing enzyme system.

Riboflavin Deficiency and Administration Riboflavin deficiency is associated with mucosal and cutaneous lesions. Nurses will often note that clients have lesions occurring in the angles of the mouth (angular stomatitis) and the lips. If these become infected by *Candida albicans,* they will take on a grayish appearance and are called perlèche. The client's tongue may have a magenta coloration and the lips and mouth may appear pale. They may have cutaneous lesions in the folds of the ears, eyelids, nose, and labia or scrotum. Glossitis and dermatitis may occur. On occasion, clients develop visual problems such as keratitis and vascularization of the cornea. Because glucocorticoid production is impaired in riboflavin deficiency, clients may develop an anemia. Primary deficiency is rare, but secondary marginal deficiencies can accompany chronic diarrhea, alcoholism, and liver disease. Riboflavin deficiency may be present in as many as 50% of chronic alcoholics. Thyroid hormone stimulates formation of flavonucleotides from riboflavin, so riboflavin utilization is impaired in hypothyroidism, and B_2 supplements or dietary adjustments are indicated. Riboflavin supplements are also indicated in conjunction with drug therapy involving phenothiazines and tricyclic antidepressants (since these inhibit formation of FMN) and tetracyclines (which impair absorption of riboflavin). No side effects or toxicities have been reported from riboflavin supplements, even at high doses.

Riboflavin (Lactoflavin)
Tablets, injection solutions
Recommended Doses: For symptoms of deficiency, 5–30 mg/day initially in divided oral doses until a response is seen; then 2–4 mg until recovery. For parenteral administration, 50 mg IM.

Niacin (Nicotinic Acid, Vitamin B_3)

The deficiency disease associated with niacin is called *pellagra* and has been described for centuries in Italy and North America where maize (Indian corn) is a dietary staple. Corn protein is low in the amino acid tryptophan, a precursor of niacin. The relation between niacin and pellagra was firmly established in 1937. Like B_1 and B_2, niacin is a precursor of coenzymes.

Sources and Requirements Niacin is obtained from dietary sources both directly and indirectly. The coenzyme forms are found in yeast, liver, and in lesser amounts in meats and legumes. The precursor, niacin, is used to fortify breads and cereals. The indirect source is endogenous production of niacin from tryptophan, at an efficiency of about 1 mg of niacin from 60 mg of ingested tryptophan. Tryptophan is itself an essential amino acid, derived entirely from dietary protein. The normal daily requirement is about 18 niacin equivalents for male adolescents and adults and 14 niacin equivalents for females. (A niacin equivalent is 1 mg of niacin or 60 mg of tryptophan.) Requirements for women are higher in pregnancy or lactation.

Pharmacokinetics Nicotinamide derived from digestion of niacin coenzymes, niacin itself, and tryptophan are all readily absorbed and reach the liver via the portal vein. In the liver, the vitamin precursors are used to produce the coenzyme forms called *pyridine nucleotides:* nicotinamide adenine dinucleotide (NAD) and nicotinamide adenine dinucleotide phosphate (NADP). These coenzymes are hydrogen receptors that participate in metabolism of glucose and certain drugs.

Tryptophan can be converted to niacin in a series of steps, the first of which is sensitive to stimulation by steroids (estrogen and glucocorticoids). Another of the reactions in the sequence is vitamin B_6 dependent, so deficiency of B_6 may lead to deficiency in niacin. Tryptophan is also the precursor of serotonin and, in malignant carcinoid tumor, tryptophan is diverted to the formation of serotonin, eliminating one source of niacin.

The conversion of niacin to NAD occurs in three steps. Excess niacin is excreted in the urine after metabolism in the liver.

Physiological Roles and Pharmacological Effects A good many of the dehydrogenase reactions of intermediary metabolism require one or the other of the pyridine nucleotides. The coenzymes combine with dehydrogenase enzymes and accept hydrogen removed in oxidation-reduction reactions. The reduced coenzymes (NADH and NADPH) can be reoxidized by flavoproteins. Dehydrogenase reactions involving NAD or NADP include many of the steps in carbohydrate, lipid, and protein metabolism, as well as steroid and triglyceride synthesis and the pentose shunt. Alcohol dehydrogenase, a liver enzyme involved in metabolism of ethanol and certain other drugs, and the drug metabolizing microsomal enzymes of the liver also utilize pyridine nucleotide coenzymes. Niacin in large amounts has a hypolipemic effect. It has been used to lower blood lipid levels in hyperlipemia.

Niacin can produce flushing from vasodilation, with itching or tingling sensations. *Nurses should stress to clients that they may feel a warm flushing in the face and ears within 2 hours after taking the medication.* Drinking alcohol while taking niacin will increase the flushing response. *Alcohol use should be curtailed when a client is receiving niacin therapy.*

Niacin has been reported to increase blood sugar levels as well as sugar and ketones in the urine. *Nurses need to warn clients with diabetes not to take niacin unless it is specifically ordered. If the drug is ordered for diabetic clients, nurses need to alert them to the possibility of hyperglycemia, glycosuria, and ketonuria and tell them that they may need to increase their insulin or oral hypoglycemic medication to combat the problem.*

Clients may develop hepatic dysfunction in response to niacin or nicotinamide administration. *Clients should be told to report dark colored urine, light colored stools, or itching. Clients should also observe the whites of the eyes for evidence of jaundice. Any change in skin color (suggesting possible jaundice) should of course be reported immediately.*

Some clients who are predisposed to gout may experience flank, joint, or stomach pain. They may also have a change in urine pattern. *These signs should all be reported immediately.* Some clients will experience photosensitivity reactions. Blurred vision may develop. Others may develop dermatitis. *Nurses need to alert clients that if such reactions occur, they should remain out of direct sunlight until the lesions have healed.*

Niacin Deficiency and Administration Niacin deficiency, or pellagra, is characterized by the symptom triad of dermatitis, diarrhea, and dementia. Mild deficiency is manifested in malaise. This is followed by cutaneous and mucous membrane lesions of several types, involving the skin, mouth, tongue, vagina, and urethra. Secondary infections may occur. Neurological disturbances occur in severe cases and culminate in psychosis, depression, mania, memory impairment, or delirium. Primary niacin deficiencies are seldom seen without involvement of other B-complex vitamins; therefore multivitamin preparations are often indicated. Secondary niacin deficiency may occur in prolonged diarrhea, liver cirrhosis, alcoholism, and with certain drugs. Alcohol can decrease niacin and tryptophan intake, absorption, and utilization for synthesis of pyridine nucleotides. Isonicotinic acid hydrazide (INH), a drug used in tuberculosis, inhibits conversion of tryptophan to niacin. Certain antimetabolites used in cancer chemotherapy (6-mercaptopurine and 5-fluorouracil) inhibit cellular production of pyridine nucleotides.

For some clients, dietary adjustments do not suffice and supplements are required. *Since niacin can cause clients to have nausea and hunger pangs, the drug should be taken with meals.* Nicotinamide is preferred to niacin for pellagra because it does not produce vasodilation or other side effects of niacin, but nicotinamide is less effective than niacin in reducing serum lipid levels. *Nurses can generally expect a therapeutic response to begin within 24 hours of the start of niacin or nicotinamide therapy. Usually small doses of niacin or nicotinamide given frequently during the day are more effective than a single daily dose because divided doses reduce urinary losses.*

Niacin
Tablets, injection solution
Nicotinamide
Tablets, capsules, injection solution
Recommended Doses: 300–1,000 mg daily in divided oral doses, or 100–250 mg subcutaneously, bid or tid.

Figure 44–3
Vitamin B_6. Formation of the active coenzyme, pyridoxal phosphate, from the dietary forms under the influence of flavomononucleotide (FMN), pyridoxal kinase (PK), and pyridoxine phosphate oxidase (PPO).

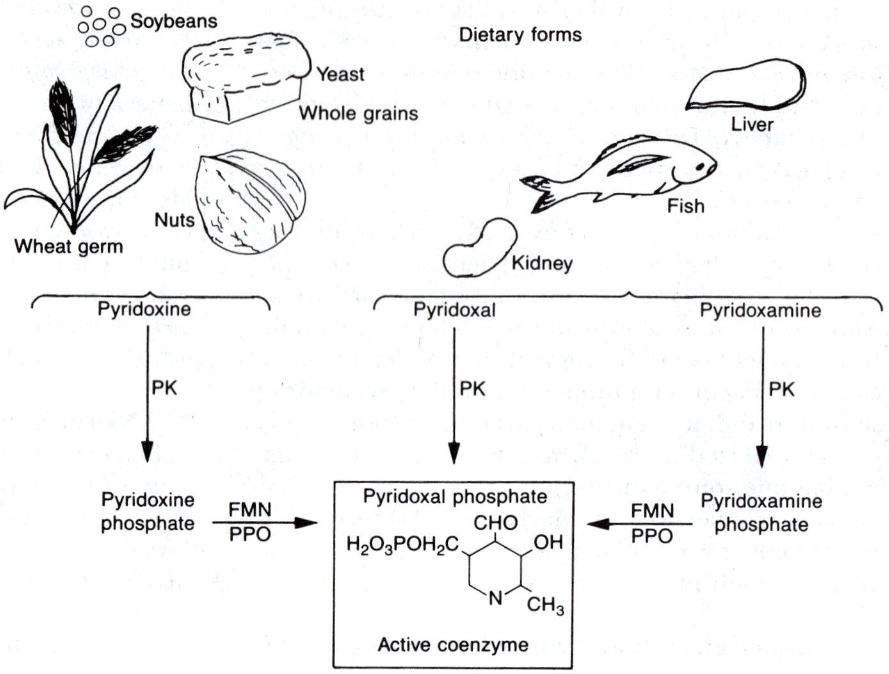

Pyridoxine (Vitamin B_6)

Sources and Requirements Vitamin B_6 consists of a group of three interconvertible precursor forms and an active coenzyme form (Figure 44–3). One precursor form, pyridoxine, is obtained from vegetable sources such as wheat germ, whole grains, nuts such as walnuts or peanuts, soybeans, and yeast. The other precursor forms are consumed in meats, especially liver and kidney, and fish such as herring and salmon. Vitamin B_6 is inactivated by high-temperature food processing.

Vitamin B_6 precursor forms are converted to pyridoxal phosphate, the active coenzyme form, which is necessary for certain metabolic steps involving amino acids. Therefore, human requirements for B_6 increase with protein intake. In adults, 1.5 mg of vitamin B_6 is required per day per 100 g of protein. The recommended daily allowance of protein is 44–56 g for adults, but actual intake may exceed 100 g in some individuals. The recommended daily intake of 2.2 mg of vitamin B_6 in adult males or 2.0 mg in females provides a cushion to provide for high protein intake.

Pharmacokinetics All dietary forms of B_6 are readily absorbed from the gastrointestinal tract, apparently by passive diffusion. In the liver, precursor forms of B_6 are converted to pyridoxal phosphate, the active coenzyme and the main circulating form. It is taken up by red blood cells and presumably other target cells. Excess vitamin B_6 is metabolized by the liver and then excreted in the urine.

Physiological Roles and Pharmacological Effects Vitamin B_6 is required for three main types of metabolic transformations, involving amino acid metabolism, synthesis of several neurotransmitters (gamma-aminobutyric acid, epinephrine, dopamine, and norepinephrine), and synthesis of heme.

Pyridoxine has no significant pharmacological actions other than in treatment of B_6 deficiency states. However, pyridoxine has been used adjunctively in treating nausea and vomiting associated with radiation therapy or "morning sickness" of pregnancy. Pyridoxine may suppress lactation in nursing mothers. Vitamin B_6 interferes with levodopa therapy of parkinsonism through a pharmacokinetic interaction. Vitamin B_6 increases peripheral decarboxylation of levodopa, decreasing its availability to the brain. *Therefore B_6 preparations or multivitamins containing B_6 should be avoided by clients receiving levodopa.*

B_6 Deficiency and Administration The symptoms of B_6 deficiency pertain to three systems: the nervous system, red blood cells, and skin. Early nervous system effects include depression and a peripheral sensory neuritis. More severe B_6 deficiency can cause convulsions. B_6 deficiency can cause anemia. Dermatological symptoms of B_6 deficiency take the form of seborrheic dermatitis around the eyes, nose, and mouth, accompanied by stomatitis and glossitis.

Primary B_6 deficiency is rarely seen in the United States, but secondary deficiencies occur. Absorption may be impaired in malabsorption syndromes and nutrient losses may be elevated in hemorrhage, burns, or other trauma injuries. In addition to the situations that generally affect all nutrients, there are specific genetic conditions and vitamin antagonists that relate to vitamin B_6. Some individuals have a genetic dependency on vitamin B_6 due to a defect in the ability to bind the coenzyme effectively. The defect can be overcome by elevated B_6 intake. Vitamin B_6 antagonists include isonicotinic acid hydrazide (INH), cycloserine, hydralazine, and penicillamine. *Vitamin B_6 supplements in the range of 25–100 mg/day are recommended when these drugs are employed.* In addition, there is inconclusive evidence that some women employing oral contraceptives may experience a functional vitamin B_6 deficiency, which may in certain cases contribute to premenstrual depression. Some clinicians believe that prophylactic use of B_6 supplements, from 1.5 mg to 5 mg daily, is justified in women using oral contraceptives.

Pyridoxine Hydrochloride
Tablets, injection solutions
Recommended Doses: 5 mg PO daily, up to 100 mg with B_6 antagonists such as isoniazid.

Pantothenic Acid

Pantothenic acid is a constituent of coenzyme A. It is widely distributed, so that specific deficiencies have not been reported. Organ meats and whole grain cereals are especially rich sources of pantothenic acid. Ordinary cooking does not diminish concentrations of this vitamin. Experimental deficiencies in human volunteers are associated with fatigue, headache, sleep disturbances, nausea, vomiting, abdominal cramps, paresthesias in the extremities, muscle cramps, and impaired coordination. The paresthesias that occur in starvation may be related to pantothenic acid deficiency. Precise daily requirements for pantothenic acid are not known but are provisionally estimated at 4–7 mg. The average American diet provides 8.7 mg daily. Calcium pantothenate is available in 10–250 mg tablets. It is also included in multivitamin preparation. There is no established therapeutic use.

Biotin

Biotin is a coenzyme for several carboxylation reactions, aiding in fixation of carbon dioxide. Biotin deficiencies are not seen in humans unless very large amounts of egg whites are consumed. Egg whites contain avidine, a protein that binds biotin in the intestines, making it unavailable for absorption. However, biotin is contained in egg yolks, so that whole eggs do not contribute to deficiency. Deficiency symptoms include loss of hair, dermatitis, incoordination, lassitude, inhibited lactation, anorexia, and electroencephalographic changes. Biotin dependency has been reported in which specific biotin-dependent carboxylase enzymes are unable to utilize biotin. Large doses of biotin (10 mg daily) are used to overcome this genetic abnormality. Symptoms occurring in children with biotin-dependent conditions include retarded mental and physical development, alopecia, and immune deficiencies. The average dietary intake is about 150–300 μg; the minimum requirement is not established. Some biotin is synthesized by bacterial flora. There is no official preparation of biotin, but it is frequently included in multivitamin preparations.

Choline and Inositol

Choline and inositol are not true vitamins since there is no clearly established dietary requirement. Choline needs can be met either through diet or endogenous biosynthesis by transmethylation of ethanolamine or by an extended pathway requiring B_{12} and folate. Dietary choline is provided in the form of choline itself or, more commonly, as lecithin, which is converted to choline. Free choline is not well absorbed, so lecithin is actually a better source of choline than choline itself. Inositol may or may not be synthesized endogenously, but no deficiency syndrome has been demonstrated in humans.

Choline is a precursor of the transmitter acetylcholine. Degeneration of cholinergic neurons is a facet of Alzheimer's disease and choline administration has been thought useful in reducing the associated cognitive impairment, although the evidence is not clear-cut at this time. Choline treatment has been advocated for tardive dyskinesias, Huntington's chorea, Gilles de la Tourette's syndrome, and Friedreich's ataxia.

Choline is also a constituent of several major phospholipids: lecithin, plasmalogens found in mitochondria, and sphingomyelin, a constituent of the myelin sheath of neural axons. Inositol is also found in the phospholipid, phosphatidylinositol, a constituent of cell membranes and serum lipoproteins. Both choline and inositol have a lipotropic action, reducing fat accumulation in the liver. They aid in mobilization and transport of fat molecules. Unofficial sources of choline currently available include choline bitartrate, choline dihydrogen citrate, choline chloride, and lecithin.

Vitamin C (Ascorbic Acid)

Sources and Requirements Vitamin C is found in large concentrations in citrus fruits and juices, other fresh fruits such as strawberries, black currants, and vegetables, including broccoli, cabbage, cauliflower, green beans, and peppers, peas, potatoes, and tomatoes. The related deficiency disease, scurvy, has been known for centuries; it was especially prevalent on long sea voyages and during the winter in Northern European countries where fresh fruits were not available. The connection between scurvy and citrus fruits was made in 1747 by James Lind, a physician in the British Royal Navy. The active constituent of citrus juices, ascorbic acid, was identified and named in the 1930s. Ascorbic acid is a six-carbon sugar similar to glucose, possessing antioxidant properties. The human requirement is about 60 mg, which provides for replacement of the amount lost daily (about 3–4% of body stores).

Pharmacokinetics Ascorbic acid is readily and almost completely absorbed. It is distributed in all tissue throughout the body and in plasma. Concentrations in white blood cells are often used to evaluate tissue concentrations since these vary less rapidly than plasma levels. A count of less than 0.1 mg/100 ml of white blood cells is diagnostic of scurvy. Excess ascorbic acid is excreted in the urine.

Physiological Roles and Pharmacological Effects Ascorbic acid is important for synthesis of collagen. Normal collagen synthesis is required for maintenance of connective tissue, the capillary endothelium, osteoid tissue of bone, and dentin of teeth. Collagen synthesis is also important in tissue repair following injury. Other metabolic activities dependent on ascorbic acid include synthesis of carnitine, hemoglobin, and adrenal steroids. Vitamin C is also important for activation of folic acid and drug metabolism by microsomal enzymes. Metabolism of many drugs is impaired in vitamin C deficiency.

Vitamin C in "megadoses" has been reputed to be effective in preventing or alleviating cold symptoms, but this claim has not been supported by several well-controlled studies.

Ascorbic Acid Deficiency and Administration Nurses will see ascorbic acid deficiency mainly among the elderly (especially those unable to get out and shop for fresh fruits and vegetables), among drug abusers, and in infants fed on formulas deficient in vitamin C. Vitamin C levels are reduced by alcohol, tobacco, anorexics, anticonvulsants, and tetracycline. Aspirin, which reduces vitamin C levels most significantly, does so by increasing ascorbic acid excretion. Atropine, ammonium chloride, and barbiturates also increase excretion of vitamin C. Women who are pregnant or lactating, and clients with elevated metabolism, as in hyperthyroid conditions, have increased requirements for vitamin C. Newborn infants, especially if premature, may require extra ascorbate for metabolism of the large amounts of dietary tyrosine. Individuals with diarrhea and achlorhydria have impaired ability to absorb vitamin C. Requirements for vitamin C are elevated during recovery from surgery, burns, or injuries, since vitamin C is necessary for wound-healing and in hemorrhagic states. Levels of vitamin C may be lowered during periods of stress because of its involvement in the formation of epinephrine, a compound released from the adrenal medulla during stress reactions.

The clinical symptoms of scurvy are preceded by tissue and plasma depletion of ascorbate. Clinical manifestations begin with perifollicular hyperkeratosis (accumulation of epithelial cells around the hair follicles) followed by skin and conjunctival hemorrhages and bleeding and swelling of the gums. In severe cases, loosening of teeth, gingivitis, and anemia are noted.

Elderly people, the indigent, those who go on fad diets, drug addicts, alcoholics, and people who are on restricted therapeutic diets may develop subclinical vitamin C deficiency. In addition, those who are subjected to prolonged IV therapy, parenteral hyperalimentation (providing nutrients through an indwelling central venous catheter placed into the superior vena cava), or chronic hemodialysis without receiving adequate supplementation are very likely to have marginal vitamin C deficiency. *Nurses providing care for such clients would notice that they become increasingly debilitated and have anorexia. Often such clients are sensitive to touch. They bruise easily, have sensitive, swollen, bleeding gums, and nosebleeds. If there are injuries, wounds are slow to heal. Clients may complain of joint pain; they may be irritable. When any client develops such symptoms, it is a nursing responsibility to investigate the possibility that the client is not receiving adequate amounts of vitamin C.* If the client can take foods orally, he or she should be given citrus fruits and fresh, leafy green vegetables. If they are unable to ingest the tablets in any form, they should be given vitamin C IM, 100–250 mg, twice a day. The vitamin may be added to IV fluids.

The established use for vitamin C is for prevention and treatment of marginal or frank deficiency. Prevention is most adequately achieved through inclusion of fresh fruits and vegetables in the diet. For infants, giving orange juice or adding vitamin C to formula is the usual method of ensuring adequate vitamin C. *Nurses should advise mothers not to heat orange juice or add vitamins to formula before heating, since vitamin C (and some of the other vitamins) are destroyed by heat.*

Vitamin C is frequently employed as a natural preservative for its antioxidant properties. High doses of vitamin C, such as those advocated for prevention or treatment of colds, can produce adverse effects. Vitamin C in megadoses impairs absorption of vitamin B_{12}. Kidney stones can result from excessive concentrations of oxalate derived from ascorbic acid. Rebound scurvy has been reported in individuals using large amounts for extended periods and in newborn children of mothers using large doses of vitamin C. Large doses of ascorbic acid also interfere with anticoagulant therapy. Women using oral contraceptives have lower concentrations of ascorbic acid in their white blood cells than control subjects. Small supplements may thus be appropriate, but use of vitamin C at levels in excess of 1,000 mg/day in conjunction with oral contraceptives is contraindicated.

Vitamin C
Tablets, oral concentrates, injection solutions, multivitamin preparations
Recommended Doses: For clients receiving aspirin for extended periods of time for inflammatory conditions, 50–100 mg PO daily.

Important Nursing Implications for Vitamins

- ☐ Teach people how to meet daily requirements for healthy living, including how to obtain appropriate quantities of vitamins and minerals through the diet.
- ☐ Explain the dangers of an inadequate diet.
- ☐ Teach clients about potential interactions of vitamins and minerals with drugs.
- ☐ Be aware of special demands of the body through the life span in assessing individual clients for potential vitamin deficiencies. Keep in mind that absorption of vitamins decreases with age.
- ☐ Recognize that people who consume large quantities of alcohol are at risk for vitamin deficiencies, including vitamins B_1, B_6, and folic acid.
- ☐ Keep in mind that people who live alone are prime candidates for vitamin deficiencies. They may become too depressed to have an interest in food, or they may see little reason to prepare a meal for "just one person."

Drug-Diet Interactions

Drug-diet interactions are increasingly recognized as important factors in drug therapy. The nurse can play a significant role educating the client in this area. Drug effects on specific micronutrients have been discussed for each specific micronutrient and are summarized in Tables 44–5, 44–7, and 44–8. Other drugs may have more global effects on nutrition by altering appetite, absorption in general, or one of the classes of macronutrients. In still other cases, drug-diet interactions may entail effects of foods and beverages on drug action.

Adverse Effects of Drugs on Nutrition

Drugs That Suppress Appetite

Anorexia may be caused when a drug suppresses the hypothalamic appetite control centers, elevates blood sugar levels, causes nausea or vomiting, alters taste sensitivity, produces a full feeling in the stomach, or provides calories (Table 44–9). If anorexia is brief, as in recovery following use of many general anesthetics, the impact on nutrition is not profound. On the other hand, chronic use of drugs eliciting anorexia, directly or indirectly, can have a significant role in lowering intake of nutrients.

Many of the nonsteroidal anti-inflammatory drugs, most notably indomethacin, cause untoward gastrointestinal effects leading to nausea or vomiting. Cardiac glycosides in high doses cause anorexia and can lead to emaciation. Wasting is also a common result of cancer chemotherapy. Antineoplastic agents, including those in antileukemia regimens, produce profound nausea, leading to loss of appetite. Compazine, corticosteroids, and tetrahydrocannabinol have been used to suppress nausea associated with cancer chemotherapy. *Nurses need to monitor the nutritional status of all such clients and to ensure appropriate use of oral or parenteral supplements.* Proper nutritional measures not only prevent wasting but improve tolerance for chemotherapy.

Glucagon suppresses appetite by elevating serum levels of glucose, but this is rarely of significance to nutrition since glucagon is chiefly employed acutely for alleviating insulin shock. Bulk-forming laxatives, such as methyl cellulose, plantago seed, polycarbophil, karaya gum, and guar gum reduce food intake in normal weight clients but have not been demonstrated to be effective in management of obesity.

Drugs that cause a decrease in taste sensitivity (hypogeusia) or that cause abnormal taste sensations (dysgeusia) often cause anorexia. Drugs producing

Table 44–9
Drugs Causing Anorexia

By direct suppression of appetite center	
	Amphetamine
	Benzphetamine
	Chlorphentermine
	Diethylpropion
	Fenfluramine
	Haloperidol
	Mazindol
	Phendimetrazine
	Phenmetrazine
	Phentermine
Secondary to nausea	
	Antimicrobials (many)
	Antineoplastics
	Cardiac glycosides
	Nonsteroidal anti-inflammatory drugs
Secondary to elevation of blood glucose	
	Glucagon
	Sympathomimetics
Secondary to "feeling full"	
	Bulk-forming laxatives
Secondary to altered taste sensitivity	
	Anorexics
	Captopril
	Carbonic anhydrase inhibitors
	Clofibrate
	Chloramphenicol
	Copper deficiency
	Disulfiram
	Griseofulvin
	Insulin
	Lithium
	Local anesthetics
	Metronidazole
	Penicillamine
	Phenindione
	Phenytoin
	Potassium iodide
	Tamoxifen
	Trazodone
	Tricyclic antidepressants
	Zinc deficiency
Secondary to intoxication, neuropathy, and empty calories	
	Alcohol

hypogeusia include penicillamine, clofibrate (Atromid-S) phenindione, phenytoin (Dilantin), and griseofulvin (Fulvicin). Disulfiram (Antabuse) and potassium iodide produce a metallic taste. Lithium produces a strange, unpleasant taste. Amphetamines decrease sweet and increase bitter sensitivity. Local anesthetics decrease sweet sensitivity and have variable effects on bitter and sour taste sensations. Insulin causes a decreased taste sensitivity to sweet and salt with long-term use.

Alcohol causes anorexia as well as specific antivitamin actions. Many factors contribute to alcohol-induced anorexia, including intoxication, withdrawal symptoms, encephalopathy, lactose intolerance, gastritis, and the high caloric concentration of alcohol. The nutrients most frequently affected by chronic alcohol consumption are folic acid, thiamine, riboflavin, niacin, ascorbic acid, pyridoxine, cyanocobalamin, protein, magnesium, and zinc.

Drugs That Stimulate Appetite

Obesity related to use of drugs is important since often clients will refuse to remain on a drug regimen that appears to cause them to gain weight. *Nursing support becomes very important, along with family support, to convince the client to remain on a given drug therapy under such circumstances.*

Drug-induced hyperphagia (stimulation of appetite) can be a factor in obesity (Table 44–10). Weight gain is often a complication of use of phenothiazines for psychoses or benzodiazepines, meprobamate (Equanil), and hydroxyzine (Vistaril) for anxiety. Tricyclic antidepressants, especially amitriptyline (Elavil), and monoamine oxidase (MAO) inhibitors, also can trigger weight gain, sometimes massive weight gain. Lithium, used for clients with manic-depressive disorder, has likewise been associated with weight gain. Marihuana use is known to stimulate appetite acutely, whereas nicotine (from tobacco smoking) is associated with weight gain during the withdrawal phase, when smokers quit.

Table 44–10
Drugs Associated with Hyperphagia

Anabolic steroids
Benzodiazepines
Cyproheptadine
Hydroxyzine
Insulin
Lithium
MAO inhibitors
Marihuana
Meprobamate
Oral hypoglycemics
Phenothiazines
Thyroid hormone
Tobacco withdrawal
Tricyclic antidepressants

Anabolic steroids trigger increase in muscle mass. Thyroid hormones on the other hand do not promote weight gain even though they increase metabolic rate, appetite, and food consumption. Insulin and oral antidiabetic drugs stimulate appetite by lowering blood glucose levels and may cause weight gain.

Drug Effects on Absorption

A fairly large number of drugs decrease absorption of nutrients (Table 44–4); a smaller number facilitate absorption of nutrients. Whether the diminished absorption of a given nutrient will result in clinical symptoms depends on the nutritional status of the client.

Drugs may induce malabsorption by a number of different mechanisms. One mechanism is mucosal irritation or damage. Alcohol irritates and inflames the intestinal epithelium producing a "structural" impairment that inhibits absorption. Neomycin, kanamycin, tetracyclines, and broad-spectrum antibiotics can cause diarrhea and malabsorption due to direct irritation and disturbance of the intestinal flora. Nonsteroidal anti-inflammatory drugs, especially indomethacin (Indocin), irritate the intestinal mucosa, causing ulcerative lesions, diarrhea, and impaired absorption. Colchicine, a drug used for clients with gout, causes histological abnormalities in the wall of the gut as well as inhibition of the intestinal enzyme, disaccharidase. The result is impaired absorption of fat, lactose, carotene, vitamin B_{12}, sodium, and potassium. Antineoplastic drugs, most notably methotrexate (Mexate), cause malabsorption due to desquamation of intestinal epithelial cells. Malabsorption caused by antineoplastic drugs may even continue in some individuals after therapy has been discontinued.

A second mechanism is the production of a physical barrier to absorption. Laxatives containing emollients such as mineral oil, phenolphthalein, and liquid paraffin dissolve fats and fat soluble vitamins, carrying the nutrients out in the feces. Laxatives and cathartics impair absorption of slowly absorbed nutrients by increasing motility.

A third mechanism is interference with activity of bile salts or digestive enzymes. Hypolipemic agents such as cholestyramine (Questran) and colestipol (Colestid) bind bile salts in the intestine, interfering with absorption of fats, fat-soluble vitamins, iron, and B_{12}. Drugs that induce cholestasis (such as the phenothiazines) or pancreatitis (such as alcohol) have a similar detrimental effect on absorption of fats and fat-soluble vitamins.

Fourth, drugs may selectively block transport of specific vitamins. Folate and vitamin B_{12} are the vitamins most vulnerable to malabsorption-related deficiency. The intestinal anti-inflammatory drug sulfasalazine (Azulfidine) decreases folate absorption. Oral contraceptives and antiepileptic drugs lower serum folate levels partly by impairing absorption. Vitamin B_{12} absorption is impaired by biguanides (metformin and phenformin, oral hypoglycemics formerly used in mild diabetes) and para-amino salicylic acid (an antituberculosis drug). Potassium chloride impairs vitamin B_{12} absorption by lowering the pH in the ileum. Phenindione (Hedulin), a rather toxic oral anticoagulant, interferes with vitamin K absorption.

Drugs That Affect Specific Macronutrients

Drugs may alter serum levels of glucose or lipids. Hypoglycemic drugs include aspirin and other nonsteroidal anti-inflammatory agents, barbiturates, MAO inhibitors, beta-adrenergic blockers, sulfonamides, and, of course, the antidiabetic drugs. Hyperglycemia is produced by glucocorticoids, catecholamines, narcotics, phenothiazines, phenytoin (Dilantin), coumarins, thiazide diuretics, and probenecid (Benemid). Serum lipid levels are increased by oral contraceptives, glucocorticoids, alcohol, growth hormone, and vitamin D. Serum lipid levels are reduced by antilipemic agents, salicylates, tetracyclines, glucagon, colchicine, dextrans, and L-asparaginase. Protein synthesis is inhibited by tetracyclines, neomycin, and anticancer drugs.

Effects of Foods and Beverages on Drug Therapy

The impacts of foods and beverages on drug activity include (1) the effects of the schedule of drug administration in relation to mealtime, (2) the effect of food and beverage pH on absorption, (3) foods and environmental chemicals that alter drug metabolism, and (4) specific drug-food interactions. The specific drug-food interactions have been addressed when relevant in other chapters and include the various interactions of alcoholic beverages (Chapter 13), the interaction of dietary tyramine with MAO inhibitors (Chapter 20), the interaction of dietary sodium with lithium (Chapter 21), the interaction of dietary pyridoxine with levodopa therapy (Chapter 22), the interaction of vitamin K with oral anticoagulants (Chapter 41), and the influence of goitrogenic foods on thyroid hormone therapy (Chapter 31). Here we discuss the remaining categories of influences of foods and beverages on drug therapy.

Drug Administration in Relation to Mealtime

Drug absorption may be decreased, delayed, or enhanced by presence of food in the gastrointestinal tract. *Nurses need to give clients precise instructions as to when to take medication in relation to mealtime so that absorption is not subject to undue variability.* Whether or not drug absorption will be altered by food depends on the characteristics of the drug, the formulation, and the type of food.

Many drugs should be taken on an empty stomach because of adverse effects of food on their absorption (Table 44–11). Meals slow gastric emptying time and delay passage of drugs ingested concurrently. Since most drugs are absorbed more rapidly in the intestines than in the stomach, meals tend to decrease or at least slow absorption. Most drugs are taken on an empty stomach with a sufficient volume of water to ensure rapid passage into the small intestines. Drugs in the penicillin family are particularly vulnerable to delayed and diminished absorption due to prolonged presence in the stomach. These drugs are unstable in the acid environment of the stomach and are also subject to digestion by gastric peptidases. Absorption of tetracyclines is severely hindered by meals, especially foods containing calcium, such as milk and other dairy products. Tetracyclines form nonabsorbable chelates with divalent ions in the intestines. Therefore, tetracyclines should not be taken within 2–3 hours of ingestion of dairy products or iron-rich foods. It is unwise, on the other hand, to curtail total daily intake of calcium in patients receiving tetracyclines, because tetracyclines deplete body calcium. In fact, calcium supplements at time intervals alternating with the tetracycline doses are appropriate.

Levodopa (an antiparkinsonian medication) and methyldopa (an antihypertensive drug) are absorbed from the stomach by transport mechanisms utilized by amino acids. Absorption of these drugs is inhibited by high-protein meals (meat, fish, eggs, beans). Therefore they should be taken at least 1 hour before or 3 hours after mealtime. Digitoxin absorption may be slowed, but not reduced, by food containing large amounts of fiber.

Drugs used for treatment of ulcers are most appropriately administered one-half hour before meals (Table 44–12). This includes the traditional antimuscarinic drugs (atropine, belladonna, methscopolamine, and propantheline), the new H_2-receptor blockers (cimetidine (Tagamet) and ranitidine (Zantac)), and chlordiazepoxide (Librium).

Nurses should anticipate that some drugs will be taken with meals even though their absorption is reduced because food will diminish irritation of the gastrointestinal mucosa (Table 44–13). Drugs in this category are aspirin, acetaminophen, and other

Table 44–11
Drugs to Be Taken on an Empty Stomach

Drug	Reason
Antimicrobials	
Cephalosporins Erythromycin Penicillins	Destruction in stomach is increased when gastric emptying time is prolonged.
Tetracyclines	Forms chelates with calcium in foods.
Isoniazid Lincomycin Rifampin Sulfonamides	Absorption is reduced by food.
Quinacrine	Improves contact with intestinal parasites.
Other	
Captopril Methylphenidate Phenmetrazine	Absorption is reduced by food.
Digoxin	Food delays absorption; high-fiber food reduces absorption.
Furosemide	Absorption is more rapid.
Lomustine	Reduces nausea and vomiting.
Penicillamine	Formation of chelates.
Unless gastrointestinal side effects occur	
Acetaminophen Aminophylline Barbiturates Ethambutol Furosemide	Food delays absorption but reduces gastrointestinal irritation.
Levodopa Methyldopa	Absorption is competitively inhibited by amino acids, but small amounts of food prevent nausea and vomiting.

Table 44–12
Drugs to Be Taken One-Half Hour Before Meals

Anticholinergics
Atropine
Belladonna
Chlordiazepozide (in Librax)
Dipyridamole
Homatropine
Methscopolamine
Methantheline
Propantheline
H_2-Blockers
Cimetidine
Famotidine
Ranitidine

Table 44–13
Drugs to Be Taken with Meals

To reduce irritant effect or diarrhea	
Allopurinol	Ammonium chloride
Antiadrenergic drugs	Antineoplastics (most)
Ascorbate (Vitamin C)	Aspirin
Bromocriptine	Chloral hydrate
Codeine	Colchicine
Corticosteroids	Cyproheptadine
Dihydroergotamine	Ethacrynic acid
Estrogens	Ethionamide
Iodine solution	Iron preparations
Isoxsuprine	Magnesium oxide
MAO inhibitors	Methysergide
Metronidazole	Nalidixic acid
Nonsteroidal anti-inflammatory drugs	Pepsin
Phenothiazines	Phentolamine
Potassium salts	Probenecid
Pyrantel pamoate	Pyrazinamide
Quinidine	Reserpine
Sulfasalazine	Sulfinpyrazone
Sulfonylureas	Theophylline
Thiazide diuretics	Valproate
Xanthines	
To improve absorption by presence of fat	
Adrenal steroids	
Spironolactone	
Vitamin A	
Vitamin D	
To improve absorption by slowing passage	
Carbamazepine	
Diazepam	
Griseofulvin	
Hydrochlorthiazide	
Nitrofurantoin	
Propoxyphene	
Riboflavin	
Sulfasalazine	
Triamterene	
To reduce first-pass extraction by liver	
Hydralazine	
Metaprolol	
Propoxyphene	
Propranolol	
To improve absorption by presence of intrinsic factor	
Cyanocobalamin (vitamin B_{12})	

prostaglandin synthetase inhibitors, as well as the MAO inhibitors, potassium salts, codeine, xanthines, and antiadrenergic drugs, such as reserpine (Serpasil). Metronidazole may be given with meals to reduce the likelihood of it causing epigastric distress and diarrhea.

Another group of drugs is taken with meals because their absorption is actually improved (Table 44–13). Nurses should suggest that vitamins A and D, adrenal steroids, and spironolactone should be taken with meals because they are better absorbed in the presence of dietary fat. Absorption of drugs that are slowly absorbed, such as riboflavin, propoxyphene, hydrochlorthiazide, griseofulvin (Fulvicin), and triamterene (Dyrenium), is more complete when the drug is taken with food because food slows passage through the gastrointestinal tract. Nurses should administer sulfasalazine (Azulfidine) with food because it must be metabolized by intestinal bacteria before it can exert its therapeutic benefit in inflammatory bowel disease. Nurses should also recognize that foods containing fiber and carbonated beverages are especially likely to delay gastric emptying, thus allowing drugs taken concurrently to be gradually passed on to the intestines. Tablets that have a slow rate of disintegration, like nitrofurantoin (Furadantin) and diazepam (Valium), may likewise benefit from a prolonged passage through the stomach.

Drugs that are normally subject to poor bioavailability because of extensive first-pass extraction by the liver may exhibit increased bioavailability if taken with meals because of competition between the food and drug for liver absorption and metabolism. This mechanism is postulated to operate for hydralazine (Apresoline), propranolol (Inderal), metaprolol, and propoxyphene (Darvon).

Effect of Food and Beverage pH on Absorption

The absorption of drugs that are weak acids or weak bases is affected by the pH of the gastric and intestinal fluids, and their urinary excretion is affected by the pH of the urine (see Chapter 4). Therefore, another potential influence of foods and beverages on drug action is their pH effects. The normal mixed diet results in a net metabolic production and urinary excretion of acid. Diets containing unusual portions of milk, cream, nuts, vegetables (except corn and lentils), and fruits (except cranberries, prunes, and plums) generate a higher (or alkaline) urinary pH (Table 44–14). Most beverages are acid, lowering gastrointestinal pH and ultimately urinary pH. Milk, beer, club soda, cream soda, root beer, and sarsaparilla are less acidic than cola, fruit juices, wine, or coffee. *Nurses need to inform clients that acidic beverages increase inactivation of acid-labile penicillin drugs in the stomach.* Coffee increases absorption of aspirin but decreases absorption of phenothiazines by its pH influence. Alcoholic beverages may cause premature disintegration of spansule capsules resulting in an exaggerated effect.

Table 44–14
Influences of Diet on pH

pH may be lowered by	
Acid-ash foods	
	Dairy: cheese and eggs
	Fruits: cranberries, plums, and prunes
	Meats: fish, fowl, and shellfish
	Nuts: brazil, filberts, peanut butter, peanuts, and walnuts
	Starches: bread, crackers, pasta, and pastries
	Vegetables: corn and lentils
Very acidic beverages (pH 2.2–3.6)	
	Juices: cherry, cider, cranberry, grapefruit, and lemon
	Sodas: cherry, cola, ginger ale, grape, lemon, and lemon-lime
	Wines
Moderately acidic beverages (pH 3.6–5.0)	
	Beer
	Juices: grape, pineapple, prune, and tomato
	Sodas: club, cream, root beer, and sarsaparilla
pH may be raised by	
Alkaline-ash foods	
	Fruits: all except cranberries, prunes, and plums
	Nuts: almonds, chestnuts, and coconuts
	Vegetables: all except corn and lentils
Alkaline beverages	
	Cream
	Milk

Foods and Environmental Chemicals That Alter Drug Metabolism

Both dietary and environmental chemical constituents have been identified that alter drug metabolism. Drug metabolism in the gastrointestinal tract, carried out mainly by the commensurate flora, is sharply decreased by certain antimicrobial drugs. More critically, liver drug-metabolizing enzymes can be induced by a variety of dietary and environmental substances. Ingestion of large amounts of cabbage or brussel sprouts, charcoal-broiled meats, or high-protein diets induces liver metabolism of theophylline. Alcohol, cigarette smoke, and marihuana smoke also induce liver enzymes. Environmental chemicals that induce liver enzymes include the insecticides, DDT, and lindane. On the other hand, energy or protein deficiencies reduce tissue enzyme levels and reduce drug metabolism. Deficiencies in water-soluble vitamins, which serve as essential coenzymes, can also reduce drug metabolism. This occurs especially with deficiencies in vitamin B_2, C, and niacin, which participate in the microsomal enzyme system.

Nutritional Aids

In this section, we consider uses and risks of nutritional aids. The nurse may be called upon to provide advice concerning nutritional aids or to supervise the utilization of nutritional aids in clients. The nutritional aids discussed in this section are special oral diets, parenteral nutrition, infant formulas, additives, preservatives, sweeteners, and health foods.

Special Oral Diets

Clients with impaired gastrointestinal function may require special oral diets, such as liquid diets, blenderized diets, low-residue diets, and elemental diets (Table 44–15). *When special oral diets are used, nurses must monitor the client's weight, assess the client for endocrine disorders that might alter nutritional requirements, and review factors that alter fluid requirements, such as fever, elevated environmental temperature, old age, or increased urine output. Nasal or oral tubes should be inserted carefully to avoid trauma. Care should be taken to ensure that the tube is in place, by aspiration or auscultation, before each feeding. If nutrients are to be inserted by tube for longer than one-half hour, the material should be warmed to about 105° F before administration. Nutrients should be gravity fed, not forced. Care should be taken to minimize air ingestion and tubes should be cleaned every 2 days.*

Liquid Diets

Simple liquid diets are the oldest technique for accommodating a diminished digestive capability. The client is restricted to bland liquids such as water, sugar water, light broths, or gelatin. Liquid diets have been employed successfully as household remedies for centuries to provide a brief respite for the gastrointestinal tract that is misbehaving because of acute intestinal flu. It is an inexpensive and simple approach, free of significant risk. Simple liquid diets provide too little nutrition to be useful in chronic disorders.

Blenderized Diets

A blenderized diet is a purée produced by a blender from a selection of foods that provide a nutritional balance. It is inherently variable, often unpalatable, and provides the gastrointestinal tract with only moderate rest. Digestion is required and there is substantial residue. Diarrhea is a frequent complication when blenderized diets contain lactose from dairy products.

Table 44–15
Therapeutic Diets

Type	Balanced?	Promoting of positive nitrogen balance	Level of digestion required	Level of residue	Ability to tube feed
Liquid diet	No	No	Minimal	Low	Good
Blenderized diet	Yes	No	Moderate	High	Moderate
Low-residue diet	No	No	Moderate	Low	Poor
Elemental diet	Yes	Yes	Minimal	Zero	Excellent

Low-Residue Diets

Low-residue diets are available as liquids and flavored powders. They are used to enhance caloric intake in clients with malabsorption syndrome or irritable bowel syndrome. The diet consists of a combination of proteins, fats, and carbohydrates. They do not provide all essential dietary requirements or promote positive nitrogen balance. Considerable digestion is required. Residue is reduced, but what remains is of a dense consistency.

Elemental Diets

Elemental or defined formula preparations represent a significant advance in enteral feeding. They are usually given by means of a polyethylene nasogastric catheter, less commonly by jejunostomy feeding. Elemental diets are appropriate when intestinal function is diminished but not absent, to replace or supplement oral nutrition. The diets consist of a combination of essential nutrients in a form that is readily absorbed, requiring little or no digestion. Residue is virtually zero. These preparations are not appropriate for oral use, being rather unpalatable. Enteric feeding is safer and less expensive than parenteral nutrition. A typical nasogastric infusion rate for a 1 kcal/ml solution is 125 ml/hour, but initial feedings are begun slowly and increased as tolerated. A typical elemental diet contains 150–230 g of carbohydrate per 1,000 kcal in the form of glucose, oligosaccharides, sucrose, or maltodextrin. The carbohydrate component typically provides 60–90% of the caloric value. Most of the rest of the caloric content is contributed by amino acids, 20–44 g per 1,000 kcal, in the form of egg albumin, hydrolyzed casein, whey, soy, or meat, or pure crystalline amino acids. Some preparations contain added amino acids to ensure positive nitrogen balance. One to 11 g of fat per 1,000 kcal is present in the form of safflower oil, soy oil, or medium chain triglycerides. Some preparations also contain essential fatty acids.

Parenteral Nutrition

Total parenteral nutrition (TPN) was introduced in 1969 and has become a fixture of medicine, not only in the hospital, but increasingly in the home. TPN is not without risks and complications and should be reserved for clients for whom oral or tube feeding is contraindicated or insufficient. TPN has been employed acutely or for as long as 10 years. The indications for TPN are mainly inadequacies of gastrointestinal capability, including intestinal obstruction, esophageal obstruction, enterocutaneous fistula, inflammatory bowel lesions, pancreatic or biliary fistula, necrotizing gastroenteritis, and short-bowel syndrome. TPN has also been used for nutritional support for patients undergoing chemotherapy or radiation treatments for cancer, for patients following major surgery, for victims of extensive burns or other trauma, for clients with severe anorexia nervosa, and for patients in coma. Acute renal failure and certain liver diseases are additional indications.

TPN is administered through a peripheral vein if the anticipated duration is less than 10 days or if TPN is supplemental to inadequate oral or enteral feeding. For longer periods of TPN, a central blood vessel must be used, generally the vena cava. Placement of the catheter in a central vein is a surgical procedure and significant risks are involved both in initial placement and subsequent complications. Strict aseptic technique must be followed during catheter placement. TPN solutions must be prepared under a laminar-flow, air-filtered hood by personnel free of upper respiratory tract infection or broken skin. Catheter tips must be sterilized daily to prevent sepsis and catheters must be flushed with saline and heparin before and after each feeding to prevent clotting. Tubing is changed every 24 hours. Central catheters must be changed every 2–3 months. Care must be taken to prevent air embolism or accidental dislodgement of the catheter.

The need for monitoring during TPN is extensive. Blood measurements should include sodium, potassium, chloride, calcium, phosphorus, magnesium, blood urea nitrogen, ammonia, glucose, plasma protein fractions, plasma transaminases, osmolarity, and pH. Urine measurements should include glucose, osmolarity, and electrolytes. General measurements include weight, volume infused, and urinary output. Signs of infection should be watched for closely.

Solutions employed for TPN contain two requisite components and up to three optional additives. The two invariant parts are a protein source and a calorie source. The protein source is provided by a solution of crystalline amino acids. The amino acids ensure a positive nitrogen balance, a necessary condition for the protein synthesis required during illness and convalescence. All of the commercially available amino acid solutions include each of the eight essential amino acids as well as six or seven of the nonessential ones.

The carbohydrate component is provided in the form of dextrose. Alternatives such as fructose, sorbitol, xylitol, and ethanol have not proved satisfactory, causing metabolic problems such as hyperuricemia, hyperbilirubinemia, lactic acidosis, and folate deficiency.

The three kinds of additives that can be employed are electrolytes, trace metals, and multivitamin infusion concentrate (MVI). The first two of these were discussed in the context of intravenous fluid therapy in Chapter 42. Multivitamin infusion concentrate contains all of the essential vitamins, except vitamins B_{12}, K, and folate, in amounts such that 2 ml of concentrate provide a reasonable approximation of parenteral requirements (Table 44–16). Vitamins B_{12}, K, and folate cannot be given in single-solution intravenous infusions because of instability in acidic aqueous media.

Another preparation designed for intravenous nutrition is an emulsion of 10% fat (Intralipid), produced from refined soybean oil, egg-yolk phospholipids, and glycerin. Use of this preparation ensures provision of the essential fatty acids. However, this preparation cannot be mixed with other solutions for parenteral alimentation. A full balance of vitamins, electrolytes, and macronutrients can be achieved with multisolution regimens.

Table 44–16
Vitamins for Total Parenteral Nutrition

Vitamin	Proposed parenteral requirements in adults	Amount in 2 ml or MVI concentrate
Fat-soluble		
A (IU)	3,300	4,000
D_2 (IU)	200	400
E (IU)	10	2
K_1 (μg)	—	—
Water-soluble		
Ascorbic acid (mg)	100	200
Niacin (mg)	40	40
Riboflavin (mg)	3.6	4
Thiamine (mg)	3.0	20
Pyridoxine (mg)	4.0	6
Vitamin B_{12}	5.0	—
Folic acid (μg)	400	—

Infant Formulas and Mother's Milk

It is reasonable to assume that the characteristics of mother's milk have evolved to provide a highly suitable, if imperfect, source of nutritional requirements for developing infants. Mother's milk is the standard of comparison for infant formulas. Although the current trend in American society is for more women to breast-feed their babies, about half who initially breast-feed continue no longer than 6 months. So the selection and proper use of formula preparations is an important matter, and nurses are often asked for advice by new mothers.

The nutrients provided by human milk, dairy milk, or formulas include protein, fat, carbohydrates, vitamins, minerals, and trace elements (Table 44–17). Newborn infants require protein as a source of amino acids for synthesis of protein that will support the rapid growth occurring in infancy. From birth to 6 months of age, the recommended daily allowance of protein is 2.2 g/kg; in the second half-year it is 2.0 g/kg. Most of the protein in human milk is highly soluble lactoalbumin, or whey. About one-third is casein proteins in the form of fine, soft curds. Breast milk protein is quickly digested and completely absorbed. Breast-fed babies feed frequently because breast milk is so rapidly digested. Colostrum, the special milk produced during the first few days after birth, is especially rich in amino acids, providing a solid nutritional support for initial growth and development.

Nearly half of the calories of milk is provided in the form of fat. Human milk contains fats composed of long-chain, unsaturated fatty acids which are readily digested and provide the essential fatty acids, linoleic, linolenic, and arachidonic acids. Breast milk

Table 44–17
Nutrients in Infant Foods

Type of food	Protein	Fat	Carbohydrate	Vitamins	Minerals
Breast milk	Only one-third casein; fully absorbed	Human milk fat; long-chain unsaturated fatty acids including essential ones	Lactose; requires disaccharidase for digestion	Optimum	Beneficially low in Na^+ and Ca^{++}; too low in Fe^{++}
Cow's milk	Mainly casein; twice as much as in breast milk; 50% absorbed	Butterfat; long and short-chain saturated fatty acids; less digestible or nutritious	Lactose but only one-fourth as much as breast milk	Low in fat-soluable vitamins; sterilization reduces heat-labile vitamins	Too much Na^+ and Ca^{++}; no Fe^{++}
Standard formulas	Cow's milk or nonfat cow's milk	Soy, coconut, and safflower oil; more digestible and nutritious than butterfat	Lactose similar to breast milk	Balanced	Fe^{++} added to some
Therapeutic formulas	Soy isolate, casein hydrolysate, beef-heart; better absorbed than cow's milk	Soy, coconut, corn, and safflower oils	Sucrose, corn syrup, tapioca starch; can be digested without disaccharidase	Balanced	Optimum
Special formulas					
Sodium-free	Casein	Coconut oil	Lactose	Balanced	No Na^+
Low-fat	Sodium caseinate or casein hydrolysate	Low plus medium chain triglycerides	Corn syrup solids, etc.	Balanced	Optimum
Phenylalanine-free	Casein hydrolysate	Corn oil	Corn syrup	Balanced	Optimum
Electrolyte replacement	None	None	Dextrose or glucose and corn syrup solids	None	Optimum
High-calorie	Casein and whey	Coconut and corn oils	Lactose; fortified	None	Optimum

fat content is variable, even for a given mother. Most of the fat content is secreted near the end of a feeding. Fore milk may have as little as 1.5 calories per ounce and hind milk as much as 30.

Lactose, the main carbohydrate in human milk, is readily digested (by most infants) in the intestines, and creates in the process an acid environment favorable to *Lactobacillus bifidus*, a beneficial bacterium, but unfavorable to other microorganisms. Human milk also contains a carbohydrate that promotes growth of *L. bifidus* but suppresses many other microorganisms.

The newborn infant has adequate stores of vitamins at birth, unless the mother was poorly nourished. Breast milk provides adequate amounts of all essential vitamins, with the possible exception of vitamin D. Being relatively low in electrolyte composition, it minimizes the work required of the immature kidneys. Both human milk and cow's milk contain little iron; in this one sense milk does not provide the infant complete nutrition. Iron stored in tissues at birth generally sustains the needs of the infant in its first year. But from age 1 to age 3, iron-deficiency anemia is prevalent, in fact, the most prevalent of all infant nutritional disturbances. The needs of the infant for iron can be furnished after 6 months of age through iron-rich solid foods (egg-yolks and certain grains, iron-enriched cereals) or with iron-fortified formulas or vitamin drops.

Breast milk enhances the infant's immunological and enzymatic resistance to infection. Breast milk contains the enzyme lysozyme, which destroys certain bacteria. Breast milk and especially colostrum are vehicles for transfer of immunoglobulin A, in effect transmitting some of the immunological history of the mother to the child. *Breast-feeding provides the firmest basis for ensuring sound nutrition in infancy. Mothers should be encouraged to elect this method of meeting infant nutritional needs. The father of the newborn and other family members and health care professionals should try to provide the emotional, physical, situational, and medical support needed by the mother who elects to breast-feed. Some mothers may benefit from participation in support groups such as La Leche League.*

Contaminants such as DDT, chlordane, dieldrin, polychlorinated biphenyls (PCBs), and strontium 90, a radioactive isotope, are found in breast milk and cow's milk alike, somewhat more in breast milk. Contaminants in breast milk are usually substances that have high lipid solubility, resistance to physiological or biological transformation, wide environmental distribution, and low excretion rates. In the United States, detectable levels of chlorinated insecticides are found in 60–80% of breast milk samples and PCBs in about 30%. The average level of contaminants in breast milk samples is about 0.1–0.2 ppm for chlorinated insecticides and 0.1 for PCBs. Samples with the highest levels of contamination provide levels of contamination approximately tenfold greater than the allowable daily intake levels for infants (however, these standards are established with a 100-fold to 1,000-fold margin of safety). *Nurses should advise women who are breast-feeding to minimize their exposure to such contaminants by careful selection of the foods they eat.*

Formulas

Three kinds of formulas are currently marketed: standard formulas, therapeutic formulas, and special formulas. **Standard formulas** are based on cow's milk without any special modifications. These are least expensive and most widely used. **Therapeutic formulas** provide closer approximation to mother's milk in certain respects and are prescribed for children who exhibit poor tolerance for cow's milk, whether by reason of allergy, poor digestion, gastrointestinal distress, or a need to restrict fat intake. **Special formulas** are employed for children with specific medical difficulties.

Cow's milk contains twice the protein content of human milk; formulas dilute this protein content by addition of water to enable the infant to tolerate it. The protein in cow's milk is mainly casein protein of low solubility that forms large, tough curds in contact with gastrointestinal fluids. The presence of these large curds in the stomach slows gastric emptying time and promotes gastrointestinal distress. Diluting the cow's milk is helpful, as is heating, which makes the curds softer and smaller. Even so, the curds typically remain in the stomach, only partly digested, for an average of 4 hours. Only about 50% of protein in cow's milk or formulas based on cow's milk is assimilated, the rest being excreted in the feces. The bottle-fed baby needs to ingest twice the volume of milk to obtain the same nutritional benefit as a breast-fed baby. The bottle-fed baby takes in extra calories in the process of obtaining adequate amino acids, contributing to obesity.

The total fat content in cow's milk and human milk is similar, but after dilution (which must be done to lower the protein concentration) the cow's milk in standard formulas contains only about 50% as much fat as human milk. The fat of cow's milk consists largely of butterfat, composed of long- and short-chain saturated fatty acids. Modern formulas supplement or replace milk fat with fat from vegetable oils, which are readily digestible and which provide medium-chain, unsaturated fatty acids. Corn, soy, and coconut oil are commonly used; the first two are more easily digested than coconut oil. The use of vegetable oils has been a significant advance in the quality of formulas.

After dilution, cow's milk has only about one-fourth the carbohydrate content of breast milk, but lactose is added to standard formulas to approximate breast milk. Cow's milk contains galactose and glucose in addition to lactose. Metabolism of galactose and glucose produces an alkaline environment, more favorable to pathogenic microorganisms.

The vitamin content of human milk and cow's milk differ, some vitamins being more concentrated in one, some in the other. Sterilization decreases concentrations of heat-labile vitamins. After dilution, cow's milk contains less of fat-soluble vitamins than human milk, and cow's milk is a particularly poor source for vitamin C. Bottle-fed babies require vitamin drops and an early start on supplementary feeding of semisolid foods. Vitamin drops must be added to formulas *after* sterilization of the bottles.

Cow's milk contains excessive sodium relative to its nutrient value, straining kidney function and contributing to water retention in infants. Calcium content is much higher in cow's milk and calcification of bones and skeletal growth is greater in bottle-fed infants. Breast-fed infants lag behind in skeletal growth as well as overall weight gain.

Therapeutic formulas utilize alternative sources of protein so as to improve assimilation and better mimic human milk. Soy isolate is frequently used and is better digested; it is contraindicated in children with cystic fibrosis. Other protein sources encountered in therapeutic formulas include beef heart and casein hydrolysates, which are partially "predigested" by enzymatic modification. Therapeutic formulas also utilize carbohydrate sources other than lactose, making them better tolerated by infants who are deficient (temporarily or permanently) in disaccharidase, the enzyme required for metabolism of lactose. Special formulas, used for babies with special requirements, include sodium-free, phenylalanine-free, electrolyte replacement, and high-calorie preparations.

Additives, Preservatives, and Artificial Sweeteners

Additives and preservatives are nutritional aids to the extent that they improve taste or retard spoilage of perishable foods. The use of preservatives reduces wastage and increases the range of foods that can be made available, but the use of these substances entails risks. For example, nitrites used in meats to prevent botulism can contribute to methemoglobinemia and are also metabolized to nitrosamines that are carcinogenic. Monosodium glutamate used as a preservative in many foods can cause angina-like symptoms called the "Chinese Restaurant Syndrome." Federal controls on use of additives and preservatives is becoming increasingly stringent.

Artificial sweeteners, used in foods, beverages, medicines, dentifrices, and cosmetics, play an important role in controlling caloric intake, especially for the 11 million individuals with diabetes and the 80 million self-determined dieters in the United States. Currently there are two artificial sweeteners approved by the Food and Drug Administration, two under FDA review, and others in various stages of development. Saccharin is 300 times sweeter than sucrose and has considerable versatility as to applications, but it has been reported to cause tumors in male rats. The FDA considered banning it in 1977, but a congressional moratorium kept it on the market. A second sweetener, aspartame, was approved in 1979. It is 180 times as sweet as sucrose and tastes more like the natural sweetener than does saccharin. Combinations of aspartame and saccharin work well together. Cyclamate, 30 times as sweet as sucrose, was banned in the United States in 1970 because of reports of carcinogenicity, but it continues to be used in more than 40 countries. It is currently being reviewed by the FDA in response to a petition. The FDA is also considering approval of acesulfame K, which is 200 times sweeter than sucrose. Two other sweeteners are already in use in Japan: thaumatin, which is 200 times sweeter than sucrose, and stevioside, 300 times sweeter than sucrose.

Health Foods

Some health foods provide a "healthy" alternative to modern diets of processed and synthetic foods, but some health foods and products are, in fact, hazardous, and many herbal remedies with implied health benefits are ineffective but harmless. Most herbal remedies consist of plant parts or an extract containing a large number of chemicals, just as coffee, tea, tobacco, marihuana, and opium each contain a plethora of active constituents. Herbal teas that contain harmful ingredients include comfrey, coltsfoot, life root, pokeroot, and sassafras. Certain other herbal teas (bayberry, betony, canaigre, Mormon, and raspberry), as well as ordinary tea, contain catechin tannin, which has been linked to esophageal cancer. Dolomite, a calcium and magnesium source, can also contain toxic concentrations of lead. Known effects and risks of herbs and health foods are summarized in Table 44–18.

Table 44–18
Risks and Reputed Benefits of Herbs and Health Foods

Herb or health food	Comment
Alfalfa	Claimed benefit in arthritis is not documented by scientific evaluation.
Angelica	A flavoring agent. No documented pharmacological activity but promoted variously as a bronchial tonic, diuretic, antirheumatic, or emmenagogue.
Apricot pits	Source of laetrile. Claimed to be effective in cancer, but there is no objective evidence of benefit. A potentially fatal source of cyanide.
Arnica	Employed topically as a counterirritant. Toxic if ingested.

(continued)

Table 44–18
Risks and Reputed Benefits of Herbs and Health Foods (*continued*)

Herb or health food	Comment
Bayberry tea	Contains catechin tannin, which has been linked to esophageal cancer.
Betony tea	Contains catechin tannin, which has been linked to esophageal cancer.
Black cohosh	Bitter taste. Claimed useful for indigestion, dysmenorrhea, and bronchitis, but there is no supporting evidence. Toxic reactions can occur, characterized by tachycardia, tremor, and vertigo.
Blessed thistle	Used in bitter tonics to alleviate flatulence and stimulate appetite. Claimed value in liver or gallbladder disease is not documented.
Blue vervain	Contains verbenalin, a weak parasympathomimetic. Claimed value as a diaphoretic, expectorant, or tranquilizer not supported by evidence.
Boneset	Diaphoretic and laxative activity. Lacks therapeutic value.
Borage	Claimed antidepressant, demulcent, diaphoretic, and diuretic activity.
Bran	Useful laxative effect.
Broom	Antidysrhythmic and oxytocic effects. Dangerous for self-administration.
Buchu	A weak diuretic and urinary tract antiseptic.
Burdock	Claimed value in gout, rheumatism, and syphilis and for use as a diuretic or diaphoretic, but without convincing evidence. Sometimes used as a tea.
Canaigre	Astringent properties. Often misrepresented as ginseng. Contains tannin, which is carcinogenic. No established therapeutic value.
Catnip	Used to make a tea. Sometimes smoked, but it is not clear whether or not it has a euphoriant effect.
Chamomile	Popular herbal tea. It has anti-inflammatory and spasmolytic activity when used as whole plant extract. The tea has much less activity. Some individuals experience allergic reactions such as contact dermatitis or anaphylaxis.
Chaparral	Has been employed in bronchitis and rheumatic pain for anti-inflammatory effect. Safety is not established.
Chicory	Often used as a coffee additive. Claimed value as a diuretic, laxative, or treatment for gallstones, hepatic disorders, and indigestion are undocumented.
Cocillana	Formerly used as an expectorant.
Collinsonia	Undocumented claims of value as an astringent, diuretic, or diaphoretic.
Coltsfoot (farfara)	Used to make a tea. Probably hepatotoxic.
Comfrey tea	Reputed treatment for ulcerations. Contains allantoin, which may have some value as an emollient but also contains hepatotoxic pyrrolizidine alkaloids.
Cucurbita seed	Somewhat effective for promoting expulsion of tapeworms. No known toxicity.
Damiana	Prepared as an alcoholic cordial. Claimed euphoriant and aphrodisiac. No reliable scientific data.
Devil's claw	Claimed value in rheumatism. Has anti-inflammatory and claimed oxytocic properties.

Table 44–18
Risks and Reputed Benefits of Herbs and Health Foods (*continued*)

Herb or health food	Comment
Dolomite	A calcium and magnesium source that sometimes also contains toxic concentrations of lead.
Echinacea	Bacteriostatic anti-infective properties. Used to promote wound healing. Active constituent is echinacoside. Reliable studies not yet conducted.
Eleuthero	Tranquilizing properties are due to a saponin glycoside in this plant. Related to ginseng.
Eyebright	Claimed value as ocular anti-inflammatory agent. Therapeutic value is doubtful.
Fenugreek	Useful as an emollient but no demonstrated pharmacological activity.
Garlic	Many claimed values. Antibacterial property is documented. Other claims not tested.
Gentian	Contains a bitter-tasting glucoside: gentiopicrin. Claimed to improved digestion and stimulate appetite.
Ginseng	Contains triterpenoid saponins. Widely used in the Orient for anemia, diabetes, gastritis, neurasthenia, impotence, and insomnia. Claimed aphrodisiac properties not supported by evidence. Long-term ingestion can lead to habituation and symptoms such as hypertension, nervousness, and sleepiness; or contrariwise, hypotension and sedation.
Goldenseal	Used to soothe eyes in ocular inflammations. Contains alkaloids, berberine, and hydrastine that possess weak antiseptic properties.
Gotu kola	Has sedative and anti-inflammatory effects and stimulates mitosis to hasten wound healing due to presence of several alkaloids. Relative safety and efficacy is unknown.
Hawthorne	Has coronary and peripheral vasodilating properties. Contains a flavonoid glycoside.
Hedge hyssop	Unsupported claims of value in liver and spleen ailments and as a diuretic and cathartic.
Hibiscus	An aromatic and mildly laxative tea.
Honey	A sucrose-rich nutrient. Demulcent properties may be useful in cough. Other claims not supported by evidence.
Hops	Mildly sedative properties when ingested. Mild euphoriant when smoked but can cause dizziness, intoxication, and jaundice.
Horehound	Herbal cough remedy with claimed expectorant properties.
Hydrangea	Diuretic and cathartic properties. Toxic effects occur when hydrangea is ingested.
Hyssop	Reputed value in removing lens opacities.
Kelp	A source of iodine. May stimulate production of thyroid hormone. May promote weight loss as a result; a risky approach.
Lecithin	A source of choline, the precursor of acetylcholine. Claimed value in gallstones, atherosclerosis, skin, and nervous disorders. Possibly useful in improving cognitive functioning somewhat in Alzheimer's disease.

(*continued*)

Table 44–18
Risks and Reputed Benefits of Herbs and Health Foods (*continued*)

Herb or health food	Comment
Life root	Has been used to promote menstrual flow. Contains hepatotoxic pyrrolizidine alkaloids.
Linden flowers	Provides a xanthine-free tea. Claimed values for headache, anxiety, and indigestion not supported by evidence.
Lovage	Weak diuretic properties.
Marigold	Aromatic plant extract applied topically to skin lesions. No proven value and potentially allergenic.
Mistletoe	Active substances, viscotoxins and phoratoxin, cause hypotension, bradycardia, decreased cardiac contractility, and vasoconstriction. Mistletoe tea is therefore potentially hazardous.
Mormon tea	A tannin-rich xanthine-free tea. Pleasant tasting, but tannin has been linked to esophageal cancer.
Muira puama	A Brazilian folk remedy containing a resin that stimulates the central nervous system. Claimed aphrodisiac properties unsubstantiated.
Onion	Claimed value in wound healing, lowering blood pressure, stimulation of bile, and treatment of common colds. Contains prostaglandin A_1. Real value not known.
Pangamic acid	So-called vitamin B_{15}. Claimed value in promoting glucose uptake by cardiac cells and related value in ischemic heart disease is not supported by data.
Parsley	Diuretic and uterine stimulant properties. No evidence of therapeutic value.
Passiflora	Used as a tea. Sedative properties but not well evaluated.
Pennyroyal	Claimed as a headache remedy but without supporting evidence. Has been used as a diaphoretic, stimulant, and to promote menstrual flow.
Poke root	A dangerously toxic tea that can cause gastroenteritis, hypotension, and respiratory depression. Claimed value for rheumatism, dysmenorrhea, and indigestion.
Pollen	Nutrient value but risk of allergies.
Propolis	Bee glue. No evidence for claimed antibiotic effect.
Raspberry	An herbal tea containing hazardous tannins.
Red bush tea	No xanthines and little tannin. A coffee substitute.
Rose hips	Variable quantities of ascorbic acid.
Sarsaparilla	A flavoring agent. Claimed effects in rheumatism and syphilis not founded.
Sassafras	A tea of pleasant taste but potentially carcinogenic and hepatotoxic.
Selenium	A trace metal that is toxic if daily intake exceeds 0.2 mg. No evidence for claimed prophylactic value against cancer.
Senega snakeroot	Has been used as an expectorant.
Senna	An herbal tea with laxative properties. Can cause diarrhea.
Tamarind	Claimed value for dysentery and fevers.
Tarragon	A flavoring agent with claimed but unsupported values as a sedative, diaphoretic, or promoter of menstrual flow.
L-Tryptophan	Precursor of serotonin. Possibly useful as an hypnotic.
Tumeric	Has broad-spectrum antimicrobial activity but no established therapeutic usefulness.

Table 44-18
Risks and Reputed Benefits of Herbs and Health Foods (*continued*)

Herb or health food	Comment
Uva ursi	An herbal tea with weak diuretic and antiseptic properties.
Valerian	A mild tranquilizer.
Wormwood	A flavoring agent and folk remedy used for flatulence and as a diaphoretic. Can cause severe toxic reactions, including tremors, stupor, dementia, and death.
Yarrow	Used as a tea. Similar to chamomile in activity and risks.
Yohimbe	Contains the α_2-adrenergic receptor blocker yohimbine. Claimed aphrodisiac properties. Stimulant and hallucinogenic properties. Hypotensive effects. Can aggravate diabetes and kidney or heart failure.

Case Study: Low-Cholesterol Diet

G. T., a 57-year-old male client, was placed on a low fat, low cholesterol diet after he had a heart attack. The nurse was given the responsibility for teaching G. T. his new dietary restrictions.

The teaching began during G. T.'s hospital stay. The nurse began by simply discussing with G. T. the role of diet in health care. Then, since the institution in which G. T. was hospitalized had films and tapes that were played over closed circuit television, the nurse suggested he watch certain segments, telling G. T. the time, and arranging to be with him to answer any questions he might have. As he progressed to the step-down unit, the nurse involved G. T. in classes held for clients with similar problems. Finally the nurse arranged classes for G. T. and his family, held at hours arranged for the convenience of the family and in advance of G. T.'s discharge.

Working with Mr. and Mrs. T, the nurse made a list of foods G. T. ate and the quantity of foods eaten. Together, they determined that G. T., while not eating a poor diet, was ingesting too much cholesterol. They then set a goal of decreasing cholesterol and saturated fats in the diet. In establishing a plan of action, the nurse worked with husband and wife to determine food likes and dislikes. G. T. was Polish by birth and especially liked Polish sausage. Instead of eliminating this food entirely from the diet, a system was established whereby G. T. could have a limited portion on identified special occasions. When Polish sausage was to be a part of the diet, the remainder of the foods for that day were specially low in saturated fats.

Later, another problem that confronted the nurse was potential effects of the dietary restrictions on the social interactions of Mr. and Mrs. T. While Mr. and Mrs. T. invited people to their home for dinners, friends and relatives did not reciprocate because, they said, they "didn't know what to fix." This was understandable to the nurse in the situation because most feel that "red meat" is essential every day and knew little about the preparation of fish and poultry. The nurse worked with Mr. and Mrs. T. and with other relatives to teach appropriate eating habits for health. G. T. learned about the role diet and nutrition could play in improving his overall health status. He learned to adjust his food intake according to his activities. He learned to adjust fluid intake as well. And in the process, G. T. became an active participant in health promotion and maintenance.

In evaluating the success of the plan, the nurse relied on comparing response with the original nursing assessment. When G. T.'s general appearance improved, his energy level improved, and his cholesterol level was lowered somewhat, it became apparent that the plan was working.

1. What is the relationship between cholesterol and occurrence of heart attacks that would justify placing G. T. on a low cholesterol diet?
2. Cite examples of how the nurse in this case worked with G. T.'s personal preferences to help achieve the therapeutic goal?
3. What might you have done differently or additionally if you had been the nurse working with G. T.?

Answers appear at the end of the book.

Case Study: Hypervitaminosis A

E. V., a 37-year-old woman, complained to her friend, a nurse, about constant abdominal discomfort. She said she had no pep or energy to do things, no appetite, and felt tired all the time. The nurse noted that E. V.'s skin was dry and scaling, something she had not noted before. When asked about other potential problems, E. V. stated she sweated all the time, her skin itched, and that her hair seemed to be falling out. The nurse, noting that many of E. V.'s fingernails seemed broken, was told that the nails had become brittle. Later, as the nurse was talking with E. V.'s son, the boy complained that his mother was no fun anymore; she was irritable and cranky much of the time. While in discussion with her friend, the nurse noted a bottle of vitamin A tablets. When asked about them, E. V. said she wanted to be sure her family did not suffer dietary deficiency. Upon recommendation of the nurse, E. V. made an appointment with her physician who ordered a plasma level of vitamin A. The results revealed a level of 1,200 IU/ml, a finding that confirmed the nurse's suspicions. Upon advice of the physician, the neighbor stopped taking vitamin A and her symptoms subsided within 1 week.

1. Which of the symptoms displayed by E. V. were consistent with a diagnosis of hypervitaminosis A?
2. Which other vitamins may produce clinical problems when taken in excess amounts? Why don't problems develop with others?

Answers appear at the end of the book.

Recommended Readings

Alfin-Slater R et al: Hyperlipidemia: What to do about the lipids to-do. *Patient Care* 1980;14:14.

Buchner LH: Special report: Vitamin C update. *Am J Nurs* 1983;83:440–441.

Fisher WR et al: The common hyperlipoproteinemias: An understanding of disease mechanisms and their control. *Ann Intern Med* 1976;85:497–508.

Giordane C, Conly D: Taking the worry out of hyperal. *RN* 1981;81(6):40–48, 81(7):50–53.

Grant JP: *Handbook of Total Parenteral Nutrition.* Philadelphia, WB Saunders, 1980.

Green ML, Harry J: *Nutrition in Contemporary Nursing Practice.* New York, John Wiley & Sons Inc, 1981.

Keithley JK, O'Donnell J: Look out for these drug-nutrient interactions. *Nursing* 1986;16(2):42–43.

Kolata G: Lowered cholesterol decreases heart disease. *Science* 1984;223:381–382.

Konstantinides NN, Shronts E: Tube feeding — managing the basics. *Am J Nurs* 1983;83(9):1312–1320.

Krause M, Mahon K: *Food, Nutrition and Diet Therapy,* ed 7. Philadelphia, WB Saunders, 1982.

Riordan J, Riordan M: Drugs in breast milk. *Amer J Nurs* 1984;84(3):329–332.

Roach ES, McLean WT: Neurologic disorders of vitamin B_{12} deficiency. *Am Fam Physician* 1982;25(1):111–115.

Roe DA: *Drug-induced Nutritional Deficiencies.* Westport, Conn, The AVI Publishing Co Inc, 1976.

Rolig EC: Vitamins: Physiology and deficiency states. *Nurse Pract* 1986;11(7):38–48.

Wilhelm L: Helping your patient "settle in" with TPN. *Nursing* 1985;15(4):60–64.

Williams SR: *Nutrition and Diet Therapy,* ed 5. St Louis, CV Mosby, 1985.

Wright T, Murray M: Potassium problems: Which patient's in danger? *RN* 1982;82(6):57–61.

UNIT VIII

Drugs and Inflammation

CHAPTER 45

Anti-inflammatory Drugs

The process of inflammation is critical to survival of the human organism and is a prelude to all tissue repair. Inflammation provides for isolation of the invading organisms and their ultimate destruction. At the same time, the swelling and pain of inflammation serve to restrict use of the injured tissue during the repair.

The body is periodically infiltrated by potentially dangerous microorganisms, such as viruses and bacteria. Inflammation limits infection and tissue damage by means of phagocytosis — the engulfment and digestion of microorganisms, foreign particles, or tissue debris. Specialized phagocytic cells form pseudopodia that protrude outward from the cell (Figure 45–1) to surround the foreign object. As the pseudopodia close, the cell membrane invaginates to form a vacuole, called a phagosome. Enzymes enter the phagosome as it forms to digest the engulfed material.

The Inflammatory Response

The inflammatory response is triggered by tissue damage caused by trauma or infection. Nearly 2,000 years ago, inflammation was characterized by the ancient Roman physician Celsus as *rubor et tumor cum calore et dolore;* these Latin words are translated as "redness and swelling with fever and pain." This statement remains a good description of inflammation. The inflammatory response has three phases: (1) redness, (2) edema, and (3) fever, pain, and phagocytosis.

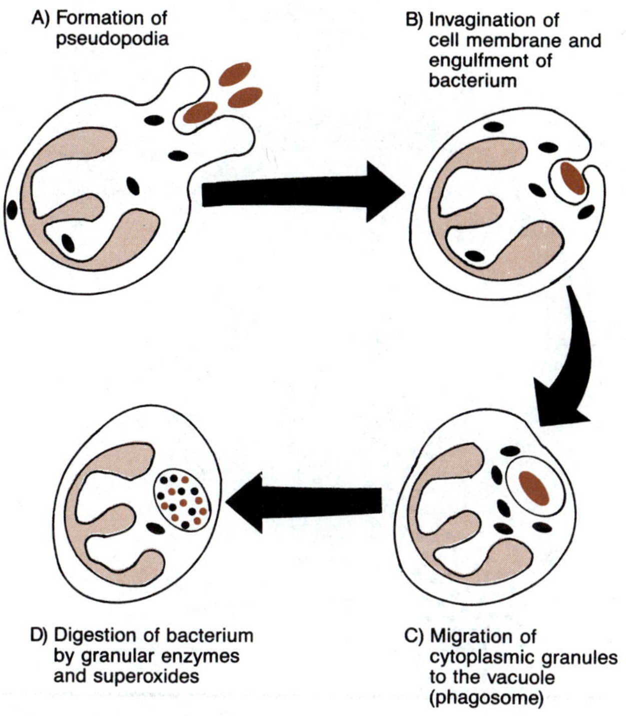

Figure 45–1
Steps in phagocytosis.

Redness, the first phase of inflammation is the congestion of blood in an area of tissue injury or infection. Congestion of blood is achieved by the combined action of various chemical mediators released from mast cells, including histamine, kinins, and prostaglandins. Histamine, for example, dilates arterioles but constricts venous capillaries, causing congestion of blood at the injured site and conferring a red coloration to the region. This accumulation of blood facilitates delivery of white blood cells that will be needed to combat infection and materials required for repairing injured tissue.

Histamine may also be the main mediator of **edema,** the second phase of inflammation. Histamine promotes contraction of endothelial cells that line small blood vessels, causing gaps to appear between adjacent cells. This permits serum constituents to leak outward into the interstitium in the area of tissue injury. Among the plasma components that leak into the interstitium in this manner are plasma kinins (most importantly bradykinin) and an enzyme called kallikrein that activates the kinins. Kinins dilate arterioles, further increase blood vessel permeability, trigger pain impulses, and promote accumulation of granulocytes. In this second phase of inflammation, the extracellular and lymphatic spaces surrounding the infection become clogged by fibrinogen clots, thus slowing the flow of fluids and invading agents away from the infected area. These events wall off the area of injury from surrounding healthy tissue.

The third phase of inflammation encompasses a wealth of physiological mechanisms: (1) release of chemical mediators, (2) chemotaxically directed migration, (3) opsonization, (4) phagocytic activity; and three mechanisms discussed elsewhere in this book: activation of pain receptors (Chapter 25), platelet aggregation (Chapter 41), and fever induction (Chapter 25). During the third phase, phagocytes migrate to the injured area, engulf tissue debris and microorganisms, and release chemical mediators that stimulate and attract other phagocytic cells and T lymphocytes. Production and delivery of phagocytic cells to the area of invasion is the function of the **reticuloendothelial system** (RES).

Components of the Reticuloendothelial System

The RES (a functional rather than an anatomical system) is composed of the reticulum cells that line the lymphatic and vascular channels, cells of the bone marrow and spleen, circulating leukocytes, and histiocytes (the fixed phagocytic cells found in tissues). Phagocytic activity is provided by four kinds of cells: (1) neutrophils, (2) eosinophils, (3) monocytes, and (4) macrophages. The first three of these cell types are circulating blood cells while the last is a fixed cell found in various tissues, especially tissues of the RES and the penetration barriers. Neutrophils and eosinophils belong to a class of white blood cells called granulocytes. The **neutrophils** are the most abundant and most active of the circulating phagocytic cells. The population of neutrophils is continuously replenished by production of new neutrophils in the bone marrow. Any significant reduction (to a level below 1,000/mm^3) in neutrophils (neutropenia) results in an increased risk of infection. **Eosinophils** are also phagocytic, though less active against bacteria than are the neutrophils. Eosinophils have a special role in parasitic infections caused by helminths and protozoa. They also play an important clean-up role in allergic reactions by degrading antigen-antibody complexes. A third class of granulocytes, the **basophils,** are only weakly phagocytic but contain large quantities of preformed chemical mediators such as histamine. Basophils resemble mast cells in both appearance and function (see Chapter 50).

Other than granulocytes, white blood cells include **monocytes** and **lymphocytes.** Lymphocytes, the functional unit of the immune system, are discussed in Chapter 46. Monocytes are precursors of tissue macrophages and the epitheloid cells that make up granulomas in diseases such as tuberculosis. **Macrophages** are the immediate source of phagocytic cells when a tissue is invaded. Like neutrophils, macrophages can engulf entire bacterial cells. Tissues of the RES, such as the spleen, are especially rich in macrophages. The spleen filters particles from the blood for phagocytosis by its macrophages.

At the onset of inflammation, the cells mediating the reaction are mainly the fixed tissue macrophages and mast cells at the site of injury. With the development of edema, additional phagocytic cells and platelets leak into the area of injury from the blood supply. Later, large numbers of phagocytic cells are drawn to the site of injury by specific chemotaxic influences.

Chemical Mediators of Inflammation

Three kinds of chemical mediators are released by activated phagocytic cells during the third stage of inflammation: (1) products of arachidonic acid metabolism, (2) lysosomal hydrolases, and (3) active oxygen species (Figure 45–2). Arachidonic acid, derived from phospholipid constituents of cell membranes, is the common precursor for the production of two groups of substances, one that includes several **prostaglandins** and **thromboxane A_2** and a smaller group including the **leukotrienes** and 12-hydroxyarachidonic acid (**HETE**). Prostaglandins are thought to be especially important in inflammation, contributing to vasodilation, chemotaxis, and sensitization of pain receptors. Thromboxane A_2 may be the major chemical mediator promoting increased platelet aggregation, while HETE is probably the major chemotaxic metabolite of arachidonic acid.

The second set of chemical mediators of inflammation are **lysosomal enzymes** released from phagocytic cells and platelets. Lysosomes are intracellular granules found in platelets and phagocytic cells that contain digestive enzymes. During the formation of phagocytic vacuoles, phagocytes introject enzymes from their lysosomal stores into the vacuole so that the enzymes can digest the engulfed particle. Some of the lysosomal enzymes spill out inadvertently into the extracellular fluid where they can attack proteins of both microbial and tissue cells. Tissue cells are less susceptible than microbial cells to the action of the proteolytic enzymes because they possess special proteins (α_1-antitrypsin and α_2-macroglobulin) that inhibit the proteolytic enzymes, but their protection is far from absolute, and excessive release of lysosomal contents causes the tissue damage often associated with inflammation. One of the major objectives of anti-inflammatory drug therapy is to limit release of the lysosomal enzymes responsible for tissue destruction.

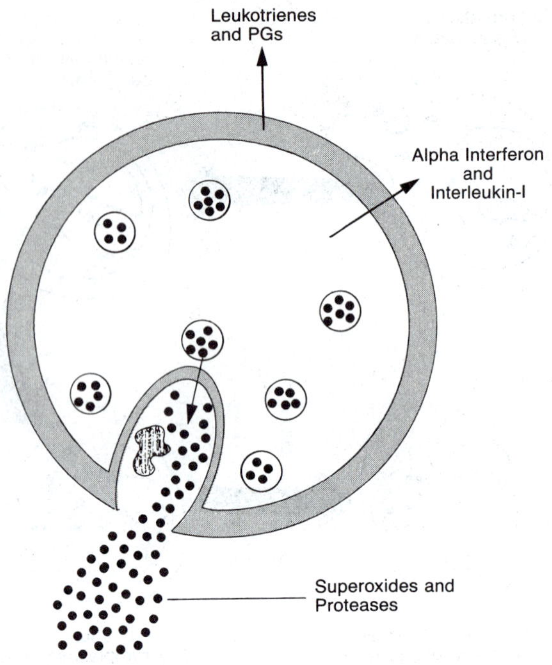

Figure 45–2
Mechanism of inflammation. Release of superoxides and proteases and formation of prostaglandins and leukotrienes during phagocytosis of foreign cells causes irritation and damage to host tissue cells. Release of interferon and interkukin-1 stimulates activity of T lymphocytes.

The third class of chemical mediators of inflammation are active oxygen species, known as **superoxides,** including hydrogen peroxide and free radicals derived from oxygen or hydroxyl groups. These particles are microbicidal but they can also injure tissue cells when they spill out of phagocytic vacuoles. Superoxides are formed within phagocytic cells by activity of the metabolic pathway called the hexosemonophosphate shunt. This pathway exhibits a burst of activity when phagocytic cells make contact with an opsonized particle.

During the inflammatory response, phagocytic cells also release an **endogenous pyrogen** that ultimately reaches the hypothalamus of the brain to initiate fever (see Chapter 25). The role of fever in the inflammatory response remains obscure, although there is evidence that the activity of phagocytic cells is enhanced by elevated body temperature. Macrophages also release **alpha-interferon,** which has antiviral activity and stimulates natural killer cells (a type of T lymphocyte), and **interleukin-1,** which stimulates formation and activity of T lymphocytes. The activities of T lymphocytes are discussed in Chapter 46.

Chemotaxis

Neutrophils, eosinophils, and monocytes all exhibit the ability to migrate to an area of inflammation under the direction of a variety of chemotactic substances. Chemotactic substances include HETE, some of the prostaglandins, some of the products of complement activation, and lymphokines released by sensitized T lymphocytes. Under the influence of these chemoattractants, a massing of leukocytes occurs in the area of injury.

Neutrophils within the central circulatory compartment are normally divided about evenly into two pools: a circulating pool that flows in the central stream of blood and a marginal pool that adheres to the postcapillary venules. **Margination** of neutrophils is promoted in the area of injury as a result of "sludging" caused by the slowed flow of blood and also due to the influence of activated kinins. Some of the white blood cells clinging to the capillary wall can pass through the vessel pores by a squeezing process called **diapedesis** (Figure 45–3): a little at a time the cells constrict to the size of the pores and pass through. Once outside the vessels, the white blood cells migrate to the site of injury by ameboid motion. The flow of the leukocytes is guided by the trail of chemotactic substances emanating from the area of injury.

Neutrophils are the first of the blood cells to arrive in the area of injury in large numbers to reinforce the tissue macrophages. Neutrophils begin to arrive at the injury site within a few minutes and reach maximum levels in 6–12 hours after injury. After 12 hours, macrophages, derived from circulating monocytes, take over primary responsibility for the inflammatory response. At the site of inflammation, monocytes are transformed into macrophages and begin to engulf microorganisms, cell fragments, and granulocytes destroyed during the earlier stages of the inflammatory process. Phagocytic activity of macrophages is stimulated by certain lymphokines, such as **gamma-interferon,** released by T lymphocytes (see Chapter 46). Any waste material that is not engulfed by the phagocytic cells accumulates in pockets within the area of inflammatory activity. This material, commonly known as **pus,** ultimately disintegrates or escapes to the body surface or through the extracellular spaces.

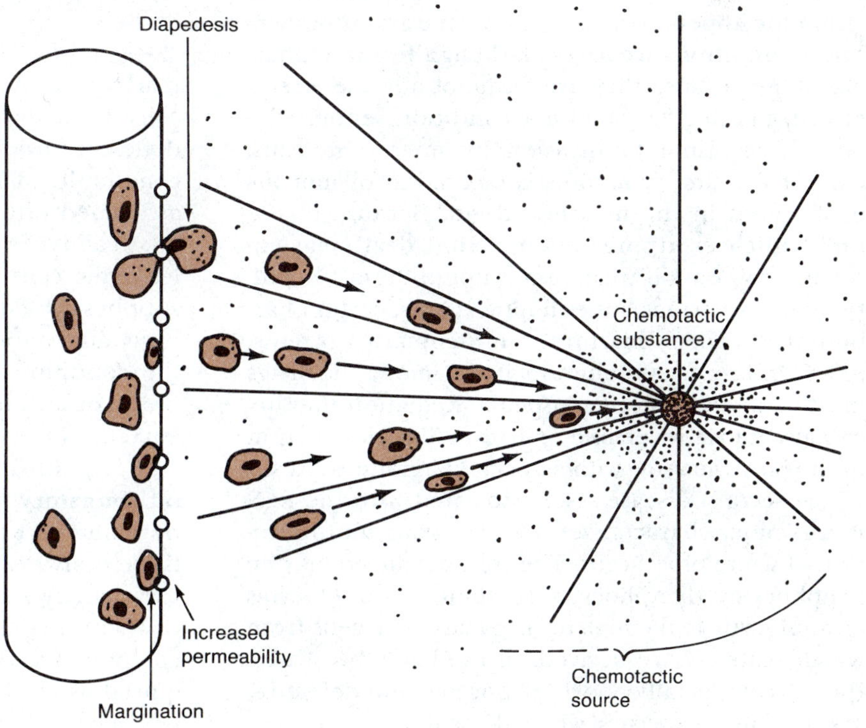

Figure 45–3
Movement of neutrophils by the process of chemotaxis toward an area of tissue damage. From A. C. Guyton, *Textbook of Medical Physiology*, 6th ed. Philadelphia: Saunders, 1981.

Opsonization

The ability of phagocytic cells to engulf particles can be greatly facilitated through a process called opsonization. An **opsonin** is a bodily substance that can attach to foreign particles or microbes to enhance their attractiveness to phagocytes. The term *opsonization* means "to prepare food for" and aptly describes the influence of opsonins. The opsonins include several humoral factors, such as lysozyme secreted by T lymphocytes, some of the components of complement, and immunoglobulins secreted by B lymphocytes (all discussed in Chapter 46). Immunoglobulins, the best understood of the opsonins, attach themselves to antigenic sites of microbes or particles (Figure 45–4). Phagocytic cells possess surface receptors that recognize and bind to the immunoglobulins, thereby capturing the attached particles. Opsonized particles and microbes are highly active stimuli for phagocytosis.

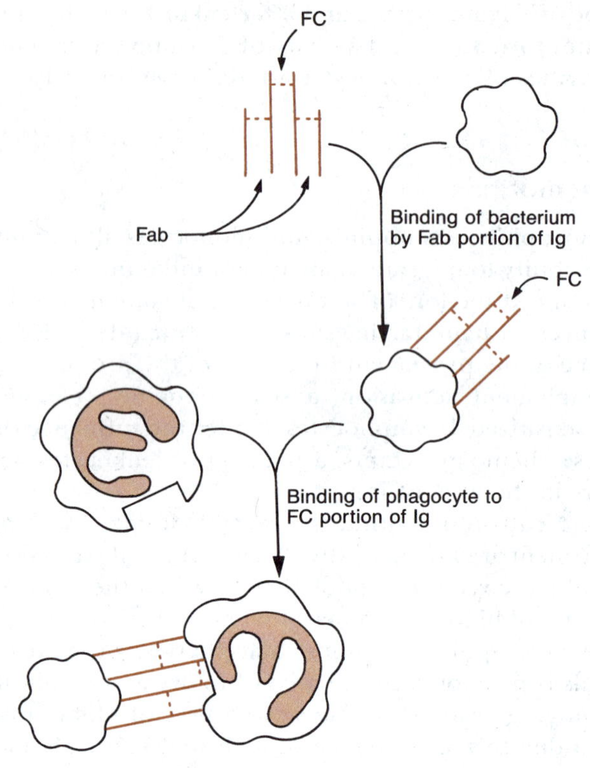

Figure 45–4
Opsonization. Attachment of an immunoglobulin to a bacterial cell facilitates its recognition and ultimate digestion by a phagocytic cell.

Diseases of the Reticuloendothelial System

There are three types of disease states related to inflammatory mechanisms: (1) a reduction in the number of any of the blood cells that mediate inflammation, (2) leukemia, and (3) inflammatory disorders. Abnormally low white blood cell counts include **leukopenia** (involving all WBCs) and **agranulocytosis** (granulocytopenia) (involving only the granulocytes). These conditions are particularly significant to pharmacology because they are frequent adverse effects of drugs (Table 45–1). Either condition renders the body susceptible to invasion by microorganisms. One of the first symptoms is ulceration of mucous membranes in the mouth and gut. Because of the rapid, unchecked spread of infection, death may ensue in a few days if treatment is not undertaken. Sulfonamides, various antiepileptic agents, certain barbiturates, phenothiazines, antineoplastic agents, phenylbutazone, and thiouracil are among the drugs most likely to induce leukopenia. Radiation therapy can also cause reversible or irreversible destruction of the bone marrow with associated agranulocytosis.

A second disease state associated with the RES is **leukemia,** characterized by cancerous multiplication of white blood cells. The cells produced may be lymphocytes (lymphocytic leukemia), granulocytes (granulocytic leukemia), or megakarocytic cells from which platelets are derived. In the latter two cases, the cells are usually poorly elaborated and defective. Tissue damage occurs when the colonizing cancer cells invade and attack lymph nodes, spleen, bone marrow, liver, or other regions rich in reticulum cells. When bone marrow destruction is substantial, deficient production of functional leukocytes or, commonly, of red blood cells, may follow. Anemia associated with a drop in red blood cells may be fatal. In all types of leukemia, the rapidly proliferating leukemic cells sap the body's nutrients and energy supplies, which, depending on severity, can cause the individual to become lethargic and weak. Untreated, the condition quickly worsens and the individual dies. The antineoplastic agents used for treatment of leukemias are discussed in Chapter 56.

The third type of disorder of the RES are the **inflammatory diseases.** Although inflammation is normally part of the reparative process of the body, there is always a risk that overly vigorous inflammatory activity will damage the host tissue by the action of lysosomal enzymes or phagocytic cells on tissue components. Anti-inflammatory drugs may be required when the inflammatory response is inappropriate or overly sustained. Inflammatory diseases are divided broadly into rheumatic and nonrheumatic

Table 45–1
Drugs That Most Frequently Cause Leukopenia

Drug class	Drugs
Anesthetics	Nitrous oxide
Antidysrhythmics	Procainamide, Quinidine
Antiepileptics	Mephenytoin, Trimethadione
Antihistamines	Tripelennamine
Antihypertensives	Captopril, Enalapril, Methyldopa
Antimicrobials	Aminoglycosides, Cephalosporins, Chloramphenicol, Griseofulvin, Nitrofurantoin, Penicillins, Sulfonamides, Tetracyclines
Antineoplastics	Alkylating agents, Antimetabolites, Cisplatin, Cytarabine, Procarbazine, Vinblastine
Antithyroid drugs	Propylthiouracil
Cardiac glycosides	
Diuretics	Acetazolamide, Thiazides
Hypolipemic agents	Clofibrate
Immunosuppressives	Azathioprine, Methotrexate
Neuroleptics	
NSAIDs	Aspirin, Cinchona Alkaloids, Gold Salts, Indomethacin, Pyrazolones, Sulindac
Oral anticoagulants	Warfarin
Oral hypoglycemics	Chlorpropamide, Tolbutamide
Sedative-hypnotics	Barbiturates, Meprobamate
Tricyclic antidepressants	

types (Table 45–2). Drugs used to treat inflammatory disorders include two major groups, the steroidal (glucocorticoid) and nonsteroidal (aspirin-like) agents. Other miscellaneous agents are used in specific situations. In general, rheumatic types of inflammation are best treated with nonsteroidal anti-inflammatory drugs (NSAIDs), while nonrheumatic disorders require steroid therapy.

In **rheumatoid arthritis,** the prototypical rheumatic disorder, the inflammatory response is initiated in response to accumulation of antigen-antibody complexes within the joints. Oddly, the antigen (called rheumatoid factor) and the antibody may both be immunoglobulins. Rheumatoid factor (RF) is synthesized by lymphocytes in the affected joints. The RF-antibody complexes stimulate phagocytic activity, releasing lysosomal enzymes that attack the tissues of the joints and cause pannus formation, cartilage destruction, osteoporosis, and finally ankylosis.

In the current therapeutic regimen for rheumatoid arthritis (see Table 45–3), the less toxic nonsteroidal anti-inflammatory drugs are employed first, along with such nondrug measures as rest, heat, and therapeutic exercise. The second level of intervention, if required, entails use of steroids by intraarticular injection, more potent NSAIDs such as phenylbutazone and indomethacin, antimalarials, analgesics, and additional nondrug measures such as orthopedic devices (splints, bars, a cane) and intensive physical and occupational therapy. The third level of intervention, for clients with still more difficult cases, involves use of gold salts, oral steroids, preventive surgery, and hospitalization. As the last resort, immunosuppressives, reconstructive surgery, placement in a rehabilitation center, and experimental methods may be required.

Other inflammatory disorders are summarized in Table 45–3 and discussed in the various chapters that deal with the organ system that is affected.

Table 45–2
Indications for Anti-inflammatory Drugs

Disease	Drugs employed
Rheumatic	
Rheumatoid arthritis	NSAIDs, gold salts, steroids, antimalarials, cytostatics
Rheumatoid variants	NSAIDs
Ankylosing spondylitis	
Reiter's syndrome	
Psoriatic arthritis	Methotrexate
Osteoarthritis	NSAIDs
Systemic lupus erythematosus	Salicylates, antimalarials, steroids, cytostatics
Gout	Colchicine, allopurinol, probenecid, NSAIDs
Nonrheumatic	
Psoriasis	Emollients, anthralin, tars, steroids, salicylates, PUVA, cytostatics
Contact dermatitis	Steroids (topical)
Polyarteritis	Steroids
Dermatomyositis	Steroids
Ulcerative colitis	Antidiarrheals, steroids, sulfasalazine, azathioprine
Multiple sclerosis	Steroids

Table 45–3
Drug Treatment of the Principal Inflammatory Disorders

Inflammatory disorder	Drug and nondrug treatments
Cardiovascular	
Cardiac	
Myocarditis	Steroids
Endocarditis	Antimicrobials, steroids
Pericarditis	Antimicrobials, NSAIDs, steroids, analgesics
Vascular	
Aortitis	Vasodilators, anticoagulants, steroids
Thromboangiitis obliterans (Buerger's obliterative arteritis)	Vasodilators
Thrombophlebitis	Oral anticoagulants
Vasculitis	
Polyarteritis nodosa	Steroids, immunosuppressives, antihypertensives
Polymyositis	Steroids
Granulomatous group (polymyalgia rheumatica, temporal arteritis, Wegener's granulomatosis)	Steroids
Pulmonary	
Bronchitis	Bronchodilators, antitrypsin, inhalation steroids, systemic steroids
Bronchiolitis	Usually none
Alimentary	
Stomatitis	Oral hygienic measures; nystatin as a lozenge
Gingivitis	Dental hygienic measures
Periodontitis	Dental hygienic measures
Esophagitis	Avoid drug or food causes; antacids, elevated head at night, cimetidine
Gastritis	Eliminate toxic causes; antacids
Appendicitis	Appendectomy
Pancreatitis	Gastric aspiration, analgesics, subtotal pancreatectomy, no alcohol
Peritonitis	Antimicrobials, surgery
Gastroenteritis	Supportive: rest, fluids, antiemetics, antidiarrheals, antimicrobials rarely
Regional enteritis	Antidiarrheals
Ulcerative colitis	Antidiarrheals, steroids, sulfasalazine, azathioprine
Diverticulitis	Supportive; surgery if severe
Proctitis	Antimicrobials
Hepatitis	
Acute	Supportive
Chronic	Steroids, azathioprine
Kidney and urinary tract	
Glomerulonephritis	Eliminate causative drugs; steroids
Tubulonephritis	Antimicrobials, diuretics, antihypertensives
Ureteritis	Antimicrobials
Interstitial cystitis	Bladder dilation; anticholinergics
Reproductive organs	
Female	
Salpingitis	Antimicrobials
Vulvitis	Compresses, hygiene, antihistamines, topical steroids
Vaginitis	Hygiene, antimicrobials
Male	
Balanoposthitis	Hygiene, antimicrobials
Prostatitis	Antimicrobials
Epididymo-orchitis	Antimicrobials; vasectomy
Thyroid	
Hashimoto's thyroiditis	T_3, T_4
Subacute thyroiditis	NSAIDs
Musculoskeletal and connective tissue	
Rheumatoid arthritis (RA)	Basic program: salicylates, rest, heat, therapeutic exercise, education
	Level 2: phenylbutazone, indomethacin, antimalarials, intraarticular steroids, physical and occupational therapy, orthopedic devices, analgesics, muscle relaxants
	Level 3: oral steroids, gold, preventive surgery, hospitalization
	Level 4: immunosuppressives, reconstructive therapy, rehabilitation center
	Level 5: experimental approaches

Table 45–3
Drug Treatment of the Principal Inflammatory Disorders (*continued*)

Inflammatory disorder	Drug and nondrug treatments
RA variants	
Ankylosing spondylitis	NSAIDs
Reiter's disease	NSAIDs
Psoriatic arthritis	NSAIDs
Osteoarthritis	NSAIDs
Lupus erythematosus	
Systemic	NSAIDs, antimalarials, steroids, immunosuppressives
Discoid	Topical steroids, antimalarials, systemic steroids,
Gout	Colchicine, probenecid, allopurinol, aspirin, phenylbutazone
Myositis	Steroids
Bursitis	NSAIDs, steroids
Tendonitis	Steroids
Osteomyelitis	Antimicrobials
Skin	
Dermatitis	
Contact	Eliminate cause; topical steroids
Atopic	Eliminate allergens; topical steroids, antihistamines, oral steroids as last resort
Seborrheic	Zinc pyrithione, selenium, sulfur and salicylic acid, tar shampoos; topical steroids
Nummular	Antimicrobials, topical steroids
Chronic — of hands and feet	Remove cause; topical steroids
Stasis	Topical steroids, zinc oxide
Perioral	Antimicrobials
Psoriatic	Anthralin, tars, emollients, steroids, salicylates, PUVA
Drug eruptions (dermatitis medicamentosa)	Stop offending drug; and:
Urticaria	Epinephrine, steroids, antihistamines
Morbilliform	Lubricant
Mucocutaneous	—
Acneiform	—
Fixed	—
Lichenoid	Antihistamines, intralesional steroids
Purpuric	—
Photosensitivity	Protect from sunlight
Erythema nodosum	Rest, antimicrobials, aspirin, steroids
Erythema multiforme	Compresses
Toxic epidermal necrolysis	Cloxacillin, methicillin
Exfoliative dermatitis	Petrolatum, oral steroids
Keloids, lichen planus	Intralesional steroids
Nervous system	
Meningitis	Antimicrobials
Encephalitis	Antimicrobials
Eyes	
Conjunctivitis	
Infectious	Topical antimicrobials
Allergic	Topical steroids
Keratitis	Topical antimicrobials
Blepharitis/hordeolum/chalazion	Topical antimicrobials
Uveitis	
Anterior (iritis, cyclitis)	Topical steroids
Posterior (choroiditis, chorioretinitis)	Systemic steroids
Ears and sinuses	
External otitis	Topical steroids, topical antibiotics
Otitis media	Oral antibiotics, decongestants
Sinusitis	Decongestants, antihistamines, oral antibiotics

Steroidal Anti-inflammatory Drugs

The general pharmacology of steroidal anti-inflammatory drugs is discussed in Chapter 33, since these drugs are related to one of the classes of steroids released by the adrenal gland. In this chapter, we consider only the mechanisms and indications of these drugs as they relate specifically to inflammation.

Mechanism of Action

Steroids inhibit inflammation whatever its cause. Whether the stimulus is thermal, mechanical, chemical, infectious, or immunological, corticosteroids suppress the intensity of the inflammatory response. Thus, the action of steroids is on the inflammatory mechanism itself rather than on the causative factor. Steroidal anti-inflammatory drugs alter many of the steps involved in inflammation (Figure 45–5). Thus far, four actions of steroids have been identified that appear to contribute to anti-inflammatory activity: (1) inhibition of phagocyte migration, (2) inhibition of recognition of opsonins by phagocytic cells, (3) inhibition of release of lysosomal enzymes, and (4) inhibition of formation of superoxides. All of these actions help to spare tissue cells in the region of inflammation from attack by lysosomal enzymes and superoxides released during inflammation.

Because steroids inhibit so many aspects of the inflammatory mechanism, extended use of steroidal anti-inflammatory drugs impairs resistance to infection. This is in marked contrast to the action of nonsteroidal anti-inflammatory drugs, which do not alter the ability of phagocytes to recognize, engulf, or kill opsonized microbes.

Clinical Use of Glucocorticoids in Inflammation

Steroidal anti-inflammatory drugs are employed in many nonrheumatic inflammatory disorders (Table 45–3). Steroids are employed in acute therapy for in-

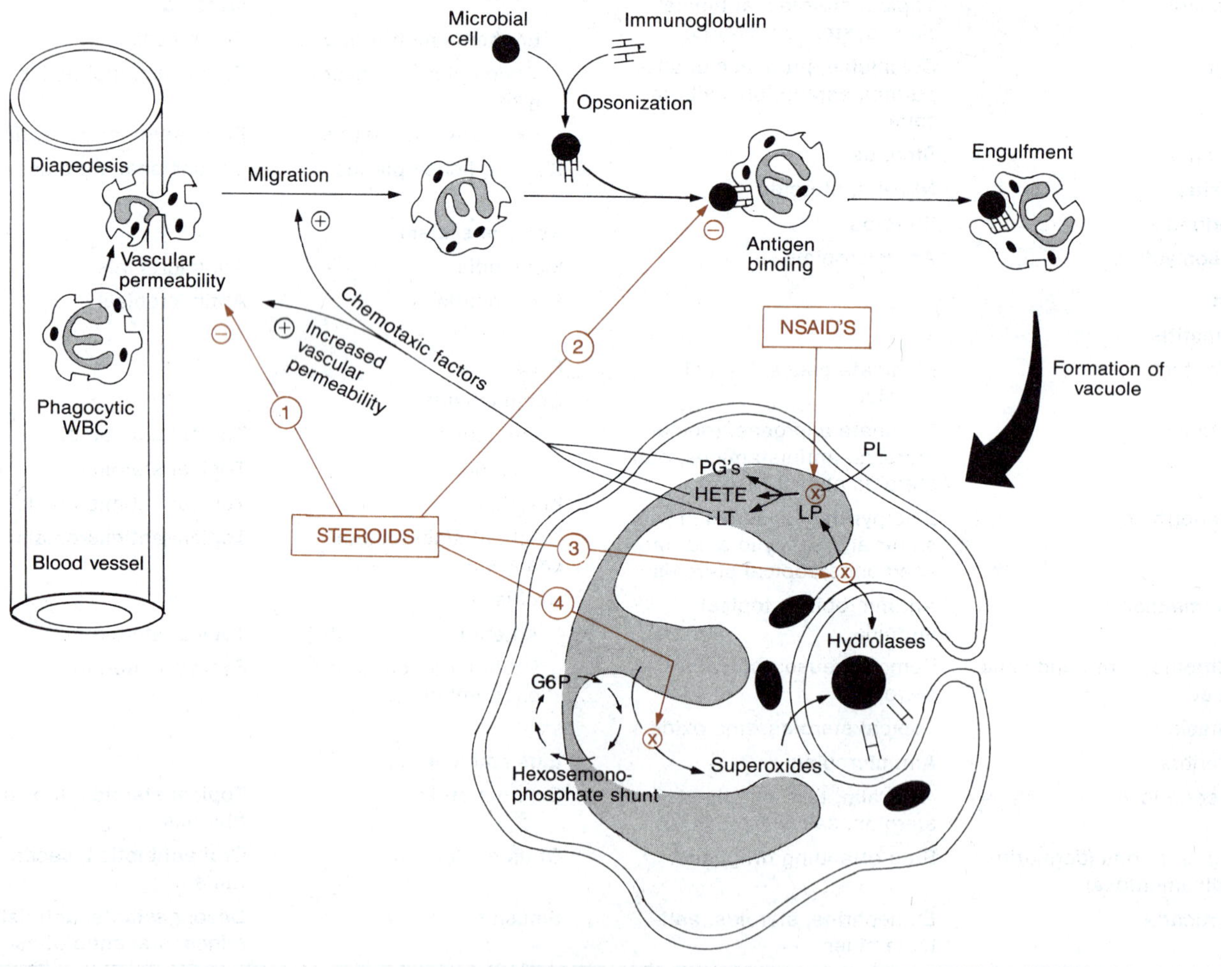

Figure 45–5
Anti-inflammatory mechanisms of steroids and nonsteroidal anti-inflammatory drugs (NSAIDs). Steroids inhibit vascular permeability to phagocytic white blood cells, impair antigen recognition by phagocytic cells, inhibit degranulation in phagocytic cells, and inhibit formation of superoxides. NSAIDs inhibit conversion of membrane phospholipids (PL) to various mediators of inflammation: prostaglandins (PGs), leukotrienes (LT), and HETE.

flammations of the myocardium, endocardium, or pericardium, along with antimicrobials when the cause of the inflammation is infectious. Steroids are often used in vasculitis and sometimes in arthritis. Steroids are useful for brief periods in myositis, tendonitis, and severe bursitis. They are employed systemically in severe ulcerative colitis, multiple sclerosis, chronic hepatitis, severe discoid or systemic lupus erythematosus, and posterior uveitis. Topical steroids find use in bronchitis (by inhalation), contact dermatitis, most other forms of dermatitis, urticaria, allergic conjunctivitis, allergic rhinitis, anterior uveitis, external otitis, and vulvitis.

Nonsteroidal Anti-inflammatory Drugs

The major group of nonsteroidal anti-inflammatory drugs (NSAIDs) are the aspirin-like drugs that share the ability to suppress the synthesis of prostaglandins. Drugs in this group are also antipyretic and analgesic, though only aspirin and acetaminophen are widely used for these purposes. The antipyretic and analgesic effects of aspirin-like drugs, as well as their general pharmacology, is discussed in Chapter 25. Here we will consider only the anti-inflammatory effects of aspirin-like drugs and the NSAIDs that are marketed expressly for anti-inflammatory applications.

Mechanisms and Effects The aspirin-like NSAIDs are inhibitors of the enzyme cyclooxygenase, the enzyme that initiates the synthetic sequence that leads from arachidonic acid to the family of prostaglandins (PGs). NSAIDs are said to inhibit *prostaglandin synthetase,* a term that is a shorthand for the group of enzymes that control the series of steps in the pathway from arachidonic acid to the PGs. Unlike steroids, aspirin-like drugs do not alter the ability of phagocytic cells to recognize, engulf, or kill microorganisms. Thus suppression of inflammation can be achieved with NSAIDs without diminished capacity to combat infection. NSAIDs do not prevent infiltration of leukocytes into an area of inflammation because the major chemotactic metabolite of arachidonic acid, HETE, is still formed in the presence of aspirin-like drugs. Formation of leukotrienes also continues in the presence of NSAIDs.

Clinical Indications NSAIDs are indicated primarily for inflammation and pain associated with rheumatic types of inflammatory disorders (Table 45–2). In **acute rheumatic fever,** NSAIDs suppress the acute inflammatory process but do not affect the progression of the disease. **Rheumatoid arthritis** is treated with NSAIDs, often in combination with gold compounds. Psoriatic arthritis, osteoarthritis, gouty arthritis, bursitis, and alkylosing spondilitis are other inflammatory conditions responsive to NSAIDs.

Shared Adverse Effects of NSAIDs Although some side effects of the NSAIDs are unique to a given drug, many are common problems for the class as a whole. The most commonly shared adverse effect is an **irritant effect on the gastrointestinal mucosa.** The invariable result is an increase in gastrointestinal bleeding; a frequent result is outright ulceration and consequent anemia. The consistent association of this side effect with the many NSAIDs suggests that it is related to prostaglandins.

Another side effect shared by most NSAIDs is an anticoagulant action due to inhibition of platelet agglutination. This effect is linked to inhibition of prostaglandin synthetase, which prevents formation of a substance that promotes platelet aggregation called thromboxane A_2. NSAIDs should be used with caution, if at all, in clients with abnormalities of blood coagulation or those receiving anticoagulants. NSAIDs should generally be discontinued for 1 week prior to surgery (including oral surgery) to minimize risks of postoperative bleeding. Many aspirin-like drugs are potentially nephrotoxic, especially when abused, an effect possibly related to prostaglandin.

Prostaglandins are involved in the uterine contractions of labor as well as those that accompany menstruation. A woman who takes aspirin-like drugs during the last trimester of pregnancy runs the risk of prolonging the pregnancy and labor as well as having an inordinate amount of bleeding during and after delivery. In addition there is a risk of hemorrhage in the neonate. *Nurses need to inform clients of these facts.*

Salicylates

History and Sources Though the NSAID class is now populated by a wealth of individual drugs (Table 45–4), the oldest representatives, the salicylate family, are still most widely used and most thoroughly researched. Salicylates are derived from salicylic acid, a substance originally found in willow bark, but now synthesized from phenol. Salicylic acid was first prepared from oil of wintergreen in 1844, but it proved too irritating for internal use. It is used topically as a keratolytic agent (Chapter 53). Salicylates are derivatives of salicylic acid by substitution at either the carboxyl group to make salicylic acid

Table 45–4
Comparisons of Nonsteroidal Anti-inflammatory Drugs

Drug	Daily maximum dosage (mg)	Anti-inflammatory effectiveness	Overall toxicity
Salicylates			
Aspirin	3,900	++	++
Diflunisal	1,500	++	+
Propionic acid derivatives			
Ibuprofen	3,200	++	+
Fenoprofen	3,200	++	+
Ketoprofen	300	++	+
Naproxen	1,100	++	+
Suprofen	800	+	+
Fenamates			
Meclofenamate	400	++	+++
Parachlorobenzoic acid derivatives			
Indomethacin	50	++++	++++
Sulindac	400	+++	+++
Tolmetin	1,800	+++	+
Pyrazolone derivatives			
Phenylbutazone	600	++++	++++
Oxyphenbutazone	600	++++	++++
Oxicams			
Piroxicam	20?	++	+

Key: +, lowest degree of effectiveness or toxicity; ++++, highest degree of effectiveness or toxicity.

esters or at the hydroxyl group, to make salicylate esters (Figure 45–6). Apart from salicylic acid and methylsalicylate, which are used topically, there are eight salicylates marketed for anti-inflammatory applications. **Aspirin** (acetylsalicylic acid) continues to be the most widely used anti-inflammatory/analgesic/antipyretic agent, and the standard of comparison for other salicylates and other NSAIDs.

Mechanisms and Effects Like other NSAIDs, salicylates are inhibitors of prostaglandin synthetase. Aspirin is an acetylated salicylate, whereas other salicylates available for clinical use are classified as nonacetylated salicylates. In comparison with aspirin, the nonacetylated salicylates are generally less potent inhibitors of prostaglandin synthesis and do not produce the inhibition of platelet aggregation that occurs with aspirin and most other NSAIDs. The pharmacokinetics and clinical indications of salicylates are discussed fully in Chapter 25.

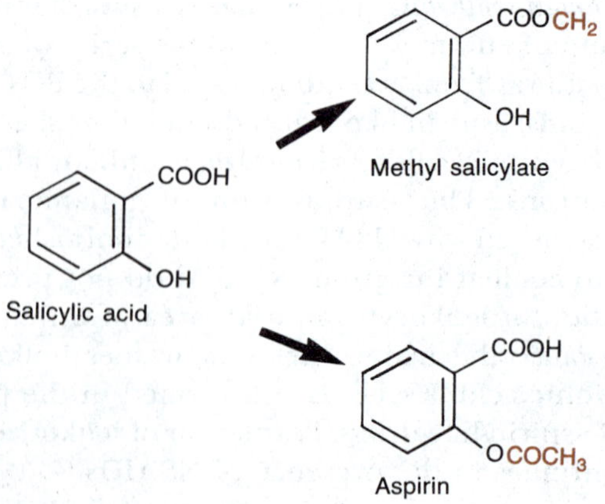

Figure 45–6
Salicylic acid derivatives involve substitution at either the carboxyl group (to form salicylic acid esters such as methyl salicylate) or the hydroxyl group (to form salicylate esters such as aspirin).

Adverse Effects and Contraindications The adverse effects of salicylates and toxic effects of salicylate overdose are discussed in detail in Chapter 25. It should be recalled that large doses of salicylates can cause **ototoxicity:** tinnitus and impaired hearing. In children, toxicity is characterized by agitation, **hyperpnea,** confusion, and lethargy. *Nurses need to assess children and other clients for presence of urticaria, wheezing, tightness in the chest, or shortness of breath. Clients who appear to be hyperventilating or who complain of feeling dizzy or suffering from severe headaches may be having adverse reactions to salicylates and should be further evaluated.* Children are also especially likely to develop **hypoglycemia,** sweating, and constipation. Clients with diabetes are also likely to experience hypoglycemia. Extended use of salicylates for inflammatory disorders can lead to **iron-deficiency anemia,** especially in women. *Clients who use high doses of salicylates over prolonged periods of time need to be assessed regularly for evidence of iron-deficiency anemia.*

Any history of hypersensitivity to a salicylate-containing drug preparation should suggest the need to consider an alternative drug selection. Clients with allergies to salicylates should be provided with a list of products that contain salicylates and taught how to identify from product labels whether or not the formulation contains a salicylate. Nurses need to be aware that clients with asthma, nasal polyps, perennial vasomotor rhinitis, or hay fever tend to have a high degree of hypersensitivity to salicylates.

When clients are receiving large doses or prolonged medication with salicylates, the nurse should educate the client to recognize and report symptoms of salicylism, such as petechiae, ecchymoses, bleeding gums, or tarry stools. Blood tests should be scheduled periodically to evaluate hematocrit and prothrombin time. The client should be reminded that self-administration of an aspirin-containing product in addition to the prescribed dose of aspirin could result in salicylism. Clients should be advised to maintain good hydration to minimize risks of formation of salicylate crystals in the urine.

Drug Interactions Aspirin is highly bound to plasma proteins and competes with other highly bound drugs (such as phenytoin (Dilantin) or penicillin) to produce mutual potentiation. Aspirin causes an acidification of the urine, which may alter the excretion of other drugs that are weak acids. The platelet and ulcergenic actions of aspirin may be additive with similar effects produced by other drugs.

Preparations and Administration Aspirin is often buffered, which hastens absorption, but may also increase gastric irritation and, with repeated use, speeds excretion and alkalinizes the urine. Some aspirin products are enteric coated; this minimizes the risks of gastric irritation. *Nurses need to educate clients concerning the differences between aspirin-containing products.* The anti-inflammatory doses of aspirin are greater than those used for antipyretic or analgesic applications and are often associated with significant adverse effects.

The great therapeutic value of aspirin together with its less-than-ideal spectrum of side effects has stimulated search for better salicylate drugs. Next to aspirin, the most widely used salicylate is sodium salicylate, which is less effective than aspirin. Sodium thiosalicylate is marketed for intramuscular use in inflammatory conditions, particularly in acute gout and rheumatic fever. Two salicylates with less severe gastrointestinal effects than aspirin are choline salicylate and magnesium salicylate. Salsalate is a molecule that hydrolyzes into two acetylsalicylic acid molecules, but only in the intestines. It is free of irritant effects on the stomach, but the intestine is still vulnerable. Another salicylate derivative, diflunisal, first marketed in 1982, appears to be lower in toxicity than aspirin. It has a long duration of action permitting twice-a-day regimens.

Aspirin
Numerous formulations
Recommended Doses: For antipyretic and analgesic applications, 650 mg PO, up to 4 times daily, at intervals of no less than 4 hours. For anti-inflammatory purposes, total daily doses of 3–5 g PO for adults, in individual 1 g doses. Maximum anti-inflammatory benefit from aspirin is achieved when plasma concentrations are maintained between 150 and 250 μg/ml. For anti-inflammatory uses in children, 100–125 mg/kg/day PO in divided doses at 4-hour to 6-hour intervals.

Choline salicylate (Arthropan)
Liquid
Recommended Doses: For adults and children over 12 years of age, 870 mg PO, repeated every 3–4 hours if necessary up to 6 times daily.

Diflunisal (Dolobid)
Tablets
Recommended Doses: For osteoarthritis, 500–1,000 mg PO daily in 2 divided doses.

Magnesium salicylate (Durasal, Mobidin, MSG-600, Triact, and Magan)
Tablets
Recommended Doses: 600 mg PO tid or qid initially, increased up to 3.6–4.8 g daily in divided doses at intervals of 3–6 hours. Not recommended for children under 12.

Salsalate (Arcylate and Disalcid)
Tablets, capsules
Recommended Doses: 325–1,000 mg PO 2–3 times daily. Take last dose at bedtime.

Sodium salicylate (Uracel, Parbocyl, and generic)
Tablets, enteric coated tablets, injection solution
Recommended Doses: 325–1,000 mg PO, 2–3 times daily.

Sodium thiosalicylate (Thiosol, Thiosul, others)
Injection solution
Recommended Doses: For gout, 100 mg IM every 3–4 hrs for 2 days, then 100 mg daily. For rheumatic fever, 100–150 mg IM every 4–6 hours for 3 days, then 100 mg twice daily.

Propionic Acid Derivatives

The propionic acid derivatives in the NSAID group available for clinical use in the United States are ibuprofen (Motrin), fenoprofen (Nalfon), suprofen (Suprol), ketoprofen (Orudis), and naproxen (Naprosyn, Anaprox, Syntex). One other drug in this group, flurbiprofen is marketed in Europe (Froben) and is undergoing clinical trials in the United States (Ansaid). Like the salicylates, propionic acid derivatives possess analgesic and antipyretic properties in addition to their anti-inflammatory value. Ibuprofen recently joined aspirin and acetaminophen as a third nonnarcotic analgesic available without prescription. Like other NSAIDs, propionic acid derivatives inhibit prostaglandin synthetase.

Pharmacokinetics Propionic acid derivatives are rapidly and completely absorbed after oral administration. Concurrent food ingestion delays absorption but does not reduce total absorption except in the case of fenoprofen. Absorption is not altered by concurrent use of antacids (aluminum or magnesium hydroxides). Propionic acid derivatives are metabolized in the liver and the metabolites are excreted in the urine. Binding of propionic acid derivatives to plasma proteins is very high (about 99%).

Clinical Indications Propionic acid derivatives are effective for suppressing inflammation associated with rheumatoid arthritis and osteoarthritis. Additional benefit is obtained from coadministration of gold salts in these conditions. There is no added benefit from combining propionic acid derivatives with salicylates. Suprofen is approved only for relief of mild to moderate pain or dysmenorrhea.

Adverse Effects and Contraindications Like all NSAIDs, propionic acid derivatives cause **gastrointestinal difficulties** (epigastric distress, nausea, vomiting, anorexia, bloating, flatulence, cramps, diarrhea, constipation, stomatitis, and ulcerations). Individuals prone to upper gastrointestinal tract disorders need to be closely supervised if given NSAIDs. *The nurse should consult with the physician before advising clients to take propionic acid derivatives with food or antacids if gastrointestinal upset occurs because concurrent food ingestion delays the bioavailability of drugs in this group.*

Skin eruptions occur in about 3–9% of individuals using propionic acid derivatives, including pruritus, rash, urticaria, ecchymoses, purpura, angioneurotic edema, and, rarely, erythema multiforme. Nondermatological **hypersensitivity reactions** to propionic acid derivatives have included allergic nephritis, serum sickness, anaphylactic reactions, and a systemic lupus erythematosus-like reaction. Known hypersensitivity to propionic acid derivatives is a specific contraindication for their use. Cross-sensitivity is often observed with other NSAIDs.

Minor **neurological reactions** (dizziness, headache, drowsiness, tinnitus) are among the most common side effects of propionic acid derivatives. Auditory examination should be performed prior to initiating drug therapy. More severe, but less common, neurological reactions include insomnia, depression, fatigue, confusion, inability to concentrate, tremor, hallucination, and dream disturbances. *Clients should be advised that propionic acid derivatives may interfere with performance of tasks requiring mental alertness or visual acuity.* **Visual problems** occur occasionally, including blurred vision, diminished acuity, scotomata, diplopia, disturbances in color vision, and conjunctivitis. *Nurses should recommend periodic opthalmic evaluation for individuals on long-term therapy.*

All types of **blood dyscrasias** have been reported, although not commonly. *Nurses should suggest that baseline hemoglobin and blood cell measurements be conducted before initiating drug therapy to provide a baseline for later comparisons. These measurements should be repeated every 3–6 months during long-term therapy.* Edema, fluid retention, congestive heart failure, hypertension, and dysrhythmias are occasional **cardiovascular reactions,** more common in elderly than in younger clients. *Clients receiving one of these drugs and having a history of cardiac decompensation should be monitored for signs of congestion or edema.* Jaundice, alopecia, gynecomastia, hyperglycemia, and hypoglycemia are other uncommon side effects. Ibuprofen and suprofen can cause elevations in several serum enzymes including SGOT, SGPT, and serum alkaline phosphate, suggesting **hepatic toxicity.** *It is best to conduct hepatic and renal function tests prior to instituting therapy with propionic acid derivatives to provide baseline data for comparison with tests taken during drug treatment.*

On the whole, propionic acid derivatives provide a somewhat more favorable balance of efficacy and side effects than do the salicylates (Table 45–4). Efficacy is comparable with the two classes of drugs but adverse reactions occur less commonly with the propionic acid derivatives.

Drug Interactions The most important kind of drug interaction with propionic acid derivatives is due to their high level of binding to plasma proteins. Propionic acid derivatives will produce mutual potentiation when used concurrently with other drugs that are similarly highly bound by plasma proteins, such as hydantoins, sulfonamides, and sulfonylureas. Inducers of liver enzymes increase the rate of metabolism of fenoprofen. Probenecid slows renal clearance of naproxen significantly. Naproxen interferes with some laboratory assays for 5-hydroxyindoleacetic acid (5-HIAA), the chief metabolite of serotonin.

Propionic acid derivatives prolong bleeding time in the same manner as the salicylates. They potentiate the effect of oral anticoagulants not only by a direct additive effect on the clotting mechanism but also by displacing them from plasma protein binding sites and inhibiting their metabolism. *The client should be advised to inform dentists or physicians who are to perform surgical procedures that he or she is taking the particular drug. Propionic acid derivatives are relatively contraindicated for use by oncology clients such as those with leukemia or those receiving chemotherapeutic agents because of the effect on bleeding time.*

Irritant effects of propionic acid derivatives on the gastrointestinal system are increased when other irritating drugs, such as alcohol or caffeine, are used concurrently. *Nurses should advise clients using NSAIDs of any type to avoid use of alcoholic beverages.*

Preparations and Administration Ibuprofen was approved for nonprescription use in 1984 and has recently appeared in new over-the-counter formulations. *Nurses should advise clients to take ibuprofen 1 hour before meals or 2 hours after meals. This is necessary because when administered with food the drug's absorption rate is slowed and drug plasma levels are reduced. However, if gastrointestinal problems occur, it may be determined that the client should take the drug with food or milk or that the dosage should be decreased.*

Fenoprofen (Nalfon)
Capsules, tablets
Recommended Doses: 300–600 mg PO tid or qid to a daily maximum of 3,200 mg.

Flurbiprofen (Ansaid)
Investigational

Ibuprofen (Motrin, Rufen, and generic formulations)
Tablets
Recommended Doses: For rheumatoid athritis or osteoarthritis, 300–600 mg PO tid or qid. The total daily dose should not exceed 3,200 mg.

Ketoprofen (Orudis)
Capsules
Recommended Doses: 75 mg PO initially, tid or 50 mg qid. The total daily dose should not exceed 300 mg.

Naproxen
Tablets (Naprosyn), tablets as the sodium salt (Anaprox)
Recommended Doses: 250–375 mg of the base (or the equivalent for the salt form) PO bid (morning and evening). The maximum daily dose should not exceed 1,100 mg.

Suprofen (Suprol)
Capsules
Recommended Doses: For mild to moderate pain or dysmenorrhea, 200 mg PO every 4–6 hours as needed up to 800 mg/day.

Fenamates

The fenamates include **meclofenamate** (Meclomen), **mefenamic acid** (Ponstel), and **flufenamic acid.** Mefenamic acid is approved only for use as an analgesic for periods not to exceed a week. Flufenamic is not available for use in the United States. Thus, only meclofenamate is used in the United States as an anti-inflammatory drug. Meclofenamate is well absorbed after oral administration, producing peak plasma levels in 0.5–1.0 hours. Absorption is unaffected by concomitant antacids, which can be used to good effect to diminish gastrointestinal toxicity of fenamates. Inactivation of meclofenamate involves both urinary and fecal excretion after hepatic metabolism. The half-life for elimination is about 2 hours. Meclofenamate is indicated for acute or chronic rheumatoid arthritis or osteoarthritis but is not recommended as an initial choice because of the severity of gastrointestinal side effects. Diarrhea occurs in 10–33% of individuals treated with the drug. Other less frequent GI symptoms include vomiting, abdominal cramps, flatulence, constipation, anorexia, stomatitis, and peptic ulcer. *Clients with a history of upper gastrointestinal disease will require close monitoring while using meclofenamate.* Nongastrointestinal symptoms are uncommon but some clients may develop edema, rash, urticaria, pruritus, dizziness, and tinnitus. Meclofenamate competes with other drugs such as warfarin (Coumadin) for plasma protein binding sites.

Preparations and Administration

Meclofenamate (Meclomen)
Capsules
Recommended Doses: For rheumatoid arthritis or osteoarthritis, 200–400 mg/day PO in 3 or 4 divided doses. The maximum daily dose is 400 mg/day.

Parachlorobenzoic Acid Derivatives

Three currently available anti-inflammatory drugs are derivatives of parachlorobenzoic acid: indomethacin (Indocin), sulindac (Clinoril), and tolmetin (Tolectin). The first two are methylated indoles and closely related to one another. Another methylated indole, etodolac (Ultradol), is undergoing clinical trials.

Indomethacin (Indocin)

Indomethacin is an especially potent inhibitor of the enzyme prostaglandin synthetase. In addition, it has a centrally mediated analgesic action along with the peripherally mediated analgesic effect typical of all NSAIDs. Indomethacin inhibits phosphodiesterase and the motility of polymorphonuclear leukocytes. Although indomethacin is an especially effective NSAID, it cannot be considered for routine use because of its high level of toxicity.

Pharmacokinetics Indomethacin is rapidly and completely absorbed after oral administration. When clients are fasting, peak concentrations are achieved within 3 hours after administration. Peak concentrations occur somewhat later if the drug is taken with food. Single oral doses of 25–50 mg produce serum concentrations of 1 or 2 μg/ml respectively, but chronic use, three times per day, produces concentrations 40% higher than the values for a single dose because of accumulation. In the plasma, indomethacin is 90% bound to plasma proteins. It is inactivated mainly by metabolism with a half-life of about 4.5 hours. About 60% of the drug and its metabolites are eliminated in the urine, and the remainder in the feces.

Clinical Indications Indomethacin is indicated for clients suffering from moderate to severe rheumatoid arthritis, osteoarthritis, ankylosing spondylitis, and acute gouty arthritis, if the condition is not sufficiently responsive to salicylate or propionic acid derivatives. For clients with severe rheumatoid arthritis, indomethacin is more effective than aspirin and equivalent in value to phenylbutazone. Indomethacin has also been used for promoting closure of a persistently patent ductus arteriosus in neonates — a cause of congenital cardiac failure.

Adverse Effects and Contraindications Indomethacin produces adverse effects in 35–50% of clients who are given the drug; in 20% of clients the severity necessitates discontinuation. **Gastrointestinal reactions** are common. Vomiting and diarrhea occur in more than 10% of clients. Nausea, anorexia, and abdominal pain are also frequent. Indomethacin promotes bleeding, ulceration, multiple ulcerative lesions, and even hemorrhage within the gastrointestinal tract; occult bleeding may be severe enough to lead to anemia. *The nurse should monitor clients on indomethacin for signs of occult bleeding, such as tarry stools, fatigability, pallor, or blood in the vomitus.*

Neurological side effects are also common with indomethacin. Headache, usually in the frontal region, is the most common of all adverse reactions to indomethacin, occurring in up to 25–50% of clients. Other neurological reactions include dizziness, lightheadedness, and vertigo, as well as tinnitus, auditory disturbances, deafness, corneal deposits, retinal disturbances, and blurred vision. *The nurse should encourage the patient to schedule periodic ophthalmic examinations while taking indomethacin.* Indomethacin can produce **psychiatric side effects** including confusion, severe depression, suicidal tendencies, hallucinations, and psychosis. Because of its effects on the central nervous system, indomethacin can aggravate preexisting psychiatric disorders, epilepsy, and parkinsonism and should be used cautiously in patients with any of these conditions. *Clients receiving indomethacin should be advised that driving an automobile or operation of machinery can be hazardous while on this drug.*

Other adverse reactions to indomethacin generally occur in less than 1% of clients. **Hematological reactions** include leukopenia, bone marrow depression, and anemia secondary to occult blood loss. **Hypersensitivity reactions** range from drug eruptions (pruritus, rash, urticaria, petechiae, exfoliative dermatitis, erythema nodosum, alopecia) to asthma-like and anaphylactic reactions. Cross-sensitivity is often observed between aspirin and indomethacin.

Cardiovascular side effects such as hypertension, tachycardia, chest pain, palpitation, and dysrhythmias have been reported. **Hyperglycemia** and **hyperkalemia** can occur as well. Indomethacin may promote **hepatic dysfunction.** *Periodic liver function tests should be scheduled. The nurse should advise the client that a green coloration to the urine may be indicative of indomethacin-induced hepatitis.*

Indomethacin should be avoided during pregnancy, especially during the last trimester, when it can cause prenatal closure of ductus arteriosus. In-

Nursing Observations for Nonsteroidal Anti-inflammatory Drug (NSAID) Therapy of Rheumatoid Arthritis

THERAPEUTIC GOAL	Reduce pain and inflammation and enhance mobility.
PREADMINISTRATION ASSESSMENT	
Baseline Data	Observe for difficulty and pain with movement, especially in the morning immediately after arising. Evaluate vital signs, weight, and swelling or deformities of the joints. Evaluate joint function including extention and ability to perform activities. Obtain laboratory tests including blood cell counts, erythrocyte sedimentation rate (ESR), hematocrit, hemoglobin, rheumatoid factor, and antinuclear antibodies.
Contraindications/ Precautions	Peptic ulcers, ulcerative colitis, renal or hepatic dysfunction, blood dyscrasias or clotting defects, pregnancy or lactation, or hearing impairment. Check medication history for allergies to salicylates or other NSAIDs.
Potential Interactions	Check current medication regimen for interacting drugs including oral anticoagulants, oral hypoglycemics, and other drugs highly bound by plasma proteins.
EVALUATION OF DRUG RESPONSE	
During Dosage Adjustment	Monitor serum levels of the NSAID.
For Therapeutic Benefit	Evaluate subjective relief of pain and tenderness, changes in swelling, mobility, and extension.
For Adverse Effects	Assess neurological function, blood pressure, pulse, peripheral perfusion, auscultation, bowel sounds, tarry stools, skin lesions, bleeding nose or gums, changes in liver function, complete blood cell counts, BUN, and creatinine. Compare findings with predrug status.
For Drug Interactions	Monitor for toxic interactions with anticoagulants, oral hypoglycemics (first generation), sulfonamides, phenytoin (Dilantin), diazepam (Valium), and probenecid (Benemid). Monitor for decreased efficacy of NSAIDs during diuretic therapy. Check for other interactions specific to the NSAID selected (see Drug Interaction sections for each drug).
For Dietary Interactions	Monitor for malabsorption or anorexia secondary to gastrointestinal irritation.
For Compliance	Evaluate compliance with all facets of the therapeutic regimen by careful observation, interviewing, periodic measurement of serum concentrations of the NSAID, and review of progress. Report compliance problems to the physician and act as client-advocate when changes in the therapeutic regimen seem indicated.

domethacin is readily excreted in breast milk. Since its safety in children has not been established, the drug should be avoided in nursing mothers and in children.

Drug Interactions Indomethacin does not directly alter the effect of **oral anticoagulants** but must nevertheless be used with caution in clients receiving such drugs because of the risk of indomethacin-induced occult bleeding and because indomethacin can inhibit platelet aggregation. **Probenecid** inhibits renal excretion of indomethacin, increasing its plasma concentrations. Indomethacin inhibits prostaglandin synthetase in the kidney (as well as elsewhere) and thus antagonizes the natriuretic and antihypertensive effects of potent diuretics such as **furosemide.** Indomethacin reduces renal clearance of **lithium,** causing a clinically significant elevation in lithium blood levels. Nurses should inform clients that concurrent administration of indomethacin with **aspirin** does not provide any added benefit over indomethacin alone, and there is even some laboratory evidence suggesting that these drugs can be antagonistic in some respects.

Preparations and Administration Since the adverse effects of indomethacin are for the most part dose dependent, every effort should be made to employ the lowest effective dose.

Indomethacin (Indocin and generic formulations)
Capsules
Recommended Doses: For moderate to severe inflammatory disorders (rheumatoid arthritis, osteoarthritis, ankylosing spondilitis), 25 mg PO, 2 or 3 times per day. If this dose is well tolerated, it can be increased if necessary in increments of 25 mg up to a maximum total daily dose of 150–200 mg.

Sulindac (Clinoril)

Sulindac is a prodrug. After oral administration, sulindac is 90% absorbed. In the central compartment, sulindac is metabolized by oxidation to a sulfone derivative, which is then reduced to a sulfide. The sulfide metabolite of sulindac is the active form. Sulindac is also conjugated in the liver to inactive metabolites.

Sulindac is about one-half as potent as indomethacin. Adverse reactions, though somewhat less frequent than with indomethacin, still occur in about 25% of patients. Adverse effects resemble those of indomethacin, including the high incidence of gastric bleeding and neurological problems. Sulindac is highly bound to plasma proteins and tends to displace aspirin and oral anticoagulants from these sites.

Preparations and Administration

Sulindac (Clinoril)
Tablets
Recommended Doses: 150 mg PO, twice a day. The maximum daily dose is 400 mg.

Tolmetin (Tolectin)

Based on a relatively brief period of clinical experience, tolmetin appears to present a favorable balance between efficacy and adverse reactions. Tolmetin is more effective than aspirin but less effective than indomethacin or phenylbutazone as an anti-inflammatory agent. The incidence of adverse effects appears to be less than for aspirin.

After oral administration, tolmetin is rapidly and completely absorbed, reaching peak plasma levels in 30–60 minutes. It is eliminated with a half-life of 1–3 hours.

Adverse effects are mainly those common to all NSAIDs: gastrointestinal irritation and an anticoagulant action. Tinnitus, skin rash, transient decreases in hemoglobin, infrequent agranulocytosis, dizziness, lightheadedness, and headaches have been reported. Of these, headache is the most common problem, occurring in about 10% of individuals. It is recommended that tolmetin not be used concurrently with salicylates since there is no evidence of increased benefit.

Preparations and Administration

Tolmetin (Tolectin)
Tablets, capsules
Recommended Doses: For rheumatoid arthritis or osteoarthritis, 400 mg PO tid. Total daily doses from 600 to 1,800 mg have been found effective in rheumatoid arthritis. Doses above 1,600 mg for osteoarthritis or 2,000 mg for rheumatoid arthritis are not recommended. For children over 2, 20 mg/kg/day initially in 3 or 4 divided doses. The maximum recommended dose in children is 30 mg/kg/day.

Pyrazolone Derivatives

The pyrazolone derivatives include one of current importance, phenylbutazone, as well as four agents that are now obsolete (aminopyrine, antipyrine, oxyphenbutazone, and dipyrone) because of unacceptable levels of toxicity. In addition, a new pyrazolone, apazone (azapropazone) is available in Europe though not in the United States. The mechanism of action by which pyrazolones produce their anti-inflammatory, analgesic, and antipyretic effects is the same as for aspirin and other NSAIDs, but pyrazolones exhibit distinctive toxicity.

Pharmacokinetics Pyrazolones are rapidly and completely absorbed after oral administration, reaching peak plasma concentrations in 2 hours. In the plasma, pyrazolones are highly bound (about 98%) to plasma proteins and therefore act as potent displacers of other drug and endogenous substances that share these binding sites. The pyrazolones are metabolized in the liver by conjugation — glucuronidation and hydroxylation. The half-life of phenylbutazone is long — about 50–100 hours — and it is metabolized initially to oxyphenbutazone, an active metabolite.

Clinical Indications In general, pyrazolones provide a higher level of anti-inflammatory efficacy together with a higher level of adverse effects and serious risks. Therefore, these drugs are reserved for severe cases of inflammatory disorders not adequately responsive to less toxic NSAIDs and for acute exacerbations of such conditions. Pyrazolones also find use for acute episodes of gouty inflammation.

Nursing Diagnoses and Interventions for Nonsteroidal Anti-inflammatory Drugs (NSAIDs) Therapy of Rheumatoid Arthritis

Nursing Diagnoses	*Related Interventions*
TO ENHANCE DRUG BENEFITS OR REDUCE DRUG REQUIREMENTS	
Activity intolerance related to fatigue and stiffness of arthritis	Encourage client to get adequate rest. After suppression of inflammation, passive and active exercises may enhance mobility, restore muscle mass, and prevent flexion contractures, but should not be fatiguing.
Disturbance in self-concept related to physical deformities and immobility	Provide support and encouragement. Assist client in enhancing positive features to distract from the deformities. Discuss methods of improving mobility and social function.
Self-care deficits or impaired home maintenance related to immobility and need for rest	Assess availability of community services or help from family or friends.
Social isolation and alterations in family processes related to inability to get around and to perform role functions	Provide support and encouragement; advise client to explain the limitation to family and friends. Introduce client to self-help groups.
TO MINIMIZE DRUG SIDE EFFECTS OR INTERACTIONS	
Alteration in comfort related to gastrointestinal irritation by NSAIDs	Instruct clients to take NSAIDs with meals or snacks. If gastric irritation persists, consult with physician about possible use of an enteric coated preparation or a drug that causes less gastrointestinal irritation.
Sensory-perceptual alteration related to decreased auditory acuity or tinnitus caused by NSAIDs	Provide safety measures related to any hearing deficits.
TO ENSURE SAFE AND EFFICACIOUS DRUG USE	
Knowledge deficit related to drug regimen	Teach the client about the nature of rheumatoid arthritis, the rationale for anti-inflammatory drug therapy, and safe and appropriate dosing with NSAIDs.
	Teach the client measures of rest and exercise appropriate to the condition.
	Instruct the client in the use of heat therapy for arthritic joints.
	Warn the client to avoid dietary quackery related to this disorder.
	Explain to clients that anti-inflammatory effects of NSAIDs may require 2–4 weeks of administration.

Adverse Effects and Contraindications The most dangerous adverse effects of pyrazolones are **blood dyscrasias:** aplastic anemia, leukopenia, agranulocytosis, and thrombocytopenia. The drop in white blood cells that leads to leukopenia or agranulocytosis can be precipitous, and several instances of fatal dyscrasias have been reported with pyrazolones. The obsolete pyrazolones, such as aminopyrine, were withdrawn because of their great propensity for producing dangerous agranulocytosis. *Clients receiving pyrazolones should be closely monitored with frequent blood tests to determine if blood cell abnormalities are evident. The nurse should stress the importance of the client attending all scheduled blood tests.*

Like other NSAIDs, pyrazolones cause **irritation of the gastrointestinal mucosa.** Mild irritation may result in nausea, vomiting, diarrhea, flatulence, or epigastric distress. More severe gastrointestinal reactions to pyrazolones include peptic ulcer, possibly with hemorrhage or perforation, and ulcerative stomatitis. *The nurse should be attentive for indications of occult bleeding, such as tarry stools, when pyrazolones are being administered. Administration of pyrazolones with meals will reduce the extent of GI irritation.*

The most common **hypersensitivity reactions** to pyrazolones are skin rashes, urticaria, and pruritus. Less common systemic reactions such as drug fever, arthralgia, anaphylactic shock, serum sickness, polyarteritis, vasculitis, and systemic lupus erythematosus sometimes occur. There can also be dangerous dermatological reactions such as erythema nodosum and erythema multiforme.

Phenylbutazone inhibits uptake of iodide and iodination of tyrosine by the thyroid gland. **Myxedema** and **goiter** are occasionally reported. Pyrazolones displace thyroid hormone from its plasma protein binding sites, which will lead to erroneous measurements if **thyroid functions tests** are conducted.

Pyrazolones promote retention of sodium, chloride, and fluids, which can be sufficiently severe as to precipitate cardiac decompensation and congestive heart failure. Hypertension, pericarditis, and myocarditis can result. Salt restriction may be required to control edema. *Clients receiving pyrazolones should be taught the signs of fluid retention and instructed to report such symptoms immediately.*

Pyrazolones are uricosuric, a useful effect in clients with gout, but an action that can also lead to formation of **urate crystals** in the kidney or ureters. **Neurological side effects** of pyrazolones include headache, drowsiness, lethargy, weakness, confusion, agitation, tremors, tinnitus, and hearing loss. **Visual disturbances,** such as blurred vision, optic neuritis, scotomata, retinal detachment or hemorrhage, or oculomotor palsy, can also occur.

Overall, the incidence of adverse effects with pyrazolones is a disturbing 20–45%, and 10–15% of clients must discontinue pyrazolone therapy. Since older clients experience adverse reactions to pyrazolones with great frequency, individuals over 60 should not receive pyrazolones for more than 1 week.

Drug Interactions Pyrazolones displace other drugs and endogenous ligands from plasma protein binding sites. Thus, pyrazolones increase the free fraction and pharmacological activity of oral anticoagulants, oral hypoglycemics, sulfonamides, and other NSAIDs. As an example, phenylbutazone increases bleeding time when coadministered with warfarin (Coumadin). Pyrazolones are potent inducers of hepatic microsomal enzymes, potentially speeding the metabolism of certain other drugs. Pyrazolones can, on the other hand, competitively inhibit hydroxylation of other drugs by the liver.

Preparations and Administration Pyrazolones are contraindicated for children under 15 years of age and in senile patients. *Pyrazolones should be stored between 59 and 86° F in light- and moisture-resistant containers.*

Phenylbutazone (Azolid, Butazolidin, Phenylzone, and generic formulations)
Tablets, capsules containing aluminum hydroxide gel and magnesium trisilicate to alleviate gastrointestinal irritation
Recommended Doses: For rheumatoid arthritis, ankylosing spondylitis, or osteoarthritis in adults, 300–600 mg PO daily initially in 3 or 4 divided equal doses. Maximum response is usually obtained at 400 mg daily. For acute attacks of gout, 400 mg initially, followed by 100 mg every 4 hours.

Oxicams

Piroxicam (Feldene) was marketed in 1982 — the first drug in a new chemical class called the oxicams. Its mechanism appears to be similar to that of other NSAIDs. It possesses anti-inflammatory, analgesic, and antipyretic activity and is approved for use in rheumatoid arthritis and osteoarthritis.

Piroxicam is well absorbed from the gastrointestinal tract regardless of presence of food or antacids. Piroxicam has a long half-life leading to accumulation for the first 7–12 days of use. Therefore clinical responsiveness develops progressively over the first few weeks of treatment.

Like other NSAIDs, piroxicam causes gastrointestinal irritation, such as nausea, epigastric distress, and peptic ulceration. The incidence of this appears to be less than for aspirin. Other adverse reactions include peripheral edema, reduction in levels of hemoglobin, dizziness, headache, rash, and rare cases of tinnitus.

Piroxicam is highly bound to plasma proteins and can be presumed to act as a displacer. It should not be employed concurrently with aspirin, since no added benefit is derived.

Preparations and Administration

Piroxicam (Feldene)
Capsules
Recommended Doses: 20 mg PO, once per day.

Important Nursing Implications for Nonsteroidal Anti-inflammatory Drugs

- ☐ Check client medical histories for evidence of allergies to NSAIDs before initiating drug therapy.
- ☐ Determine if clients taking aspirin-like drugs are experiencing epigastric distress, as well as nausea and vomiting, as a result of gastric irritation. Advise clients to take NSAIDs (except enteric coated preparations) with water, milk, or meals to minimize gastrointestinal irritation. Clients may also be advised to crush tablets into powder, chew tablets, dissolve them in water or juice before swallowing, or to take them with antacid.
- ☐ Advise clients using aspirin or other NSAIDs to avoid use of alcohol because of its potential for additive ulcergenic effects with NSAIDs.
- ☐ Observe for indications of occult bleeding such as tarry stools, bleeding gums, petechiae, or ecchymoses.
- ☐ Advise women taking aspirin for dysmenorrhea to take the drug 1–2 days prior to menstruation for best results. However, if menstrual flow is heavy, the nurse may need to encourage clients to avoid NSAIDs.
- ☐ Advise clients in the last trimester of pregnancy to avoid NSAIDs.
- ☐ Employ extreme caution when NSAIDs are utilized in individuals with impaired renal or hepatic function. Monitor such individuals for changes in renal and hepatic function by monitoring of creatinine clearance, serum enzymes, serum electrolytes, fluid retention, and hypertension.
- ☐ When pyrazolones are employed, monitor for changes in blood cell counts during therapy and teach clients to note and report any indications of possible agranulocytosis such as fever, malaise, or sore throat.

Other Anti-inflammatory Drugs

Gold

Gold therapy (chrysotherapy) is a useful alternative to NSAIDs and steroids for rheumatoid arthritis. The mechanism of action of gold in rheumatoid arthritis is not known with certainty. What is known is that gold accumulates both in synovial tissue and in macrophages and that it binds most readily to sulfur. It has been suggested that gold inhibits the phagocytic activity of macrophages and reduces escape of lysosomal enzymes that contribute to tissue inflammation. Gold may also inhibit cell-mediated immunity and inactivate the complement cascade (both discussed in Chapter 46). The action of gold in rheumatoid arthritis is palliative or preventive but not curative. The effective gold preparations are monovalent aurous salts.

Pharmacokinetics Two of the gold salts currently available, aurothioglucose and gold sodium thiomalate, are given by injection because absorption after oral administration is erratic. After intramuscular injection, peak concentrations are achieved in 4–6 hours. In the plasma, these gold compounds are 95% bound by plasma proteins. Gold distributes widely to the liver, kidneys, skin, eyes, bone, bone marrow, lymphatic tissue, and synovial tissue. Concentrations in synovial fluid reach about 50% of plasma concentrations. The half-life of gold is about 7 days after a single dose, but this value increases with successive doses to values as high as several weeks or even months. Elimination of gold is about 60–90% by renal excretion, the remainder appearing in the feces.

Auranofin is marketed in capsules for oral administration. It is approximately 25% absorbed, reaching peak serum concentrations in 1–2 hours. Auranofin is about 60% bound to plasma proteins in the blood. The plasma half-life for auranofin is 26 days; 60% of the absorbed drug is ultimately excreted in the urine.

Clinical Indications Gold is employed as an adjunctive in treatment of active rheumatoid arthritis, whether of juvenile or adult onset. Gold salts are indicated for rheumatoid arthritis of moderate severity; it is not required for mild cases and is ineffective in severe cases when damage to cartilage and bone is already established. Gold cannot repair existing damage to synovial tissue. Gold has also been used for treatment of psoriatic arthritis, Sjörgen's syndrome, nondisseminated lupus erythematosus, and pemphigus.

Clinical response to gold is often slow. With the parenteral dosage forms, response sometimes occurs in 6–8 weeks but may require months. With the oral dosage form, therapeutic response seldom occurs earlier than 3 or 4 months and may require 6 months.

Adverse Effects and Contraindications Adverse effects occur in 25–50% of patients receiving chrysotherapy. Toxicity is severe enough to require termination of therapy in about 10% of cases and results in death in about 0.4% of individuals. The most common adverse reactions relate to mucocutaneous tissue. *Nurses should alert clients to possible* **cutaneous reactions** such as puritus, erythema, exfoliative dermatitis, alopecia, and shedding of nails. *The nurse should advise clients who experience mild dermatitis in response to gold therapy to avoid sunlight since gold dermatitis may be aggravated by exposure to excessive sunlight.* Individuals with existing urticaria or eczema should not be given chrysotherapy. *At each session, the nurse should question the client concerning occurrence of itching or skin eruptions.*

Mucous lesions can occur throughout the alimentary tract or vagina resulting in oral lesions, stomatitis, glossitis, pharyngitis, tracheitis, gastritis, colitis, or vaginitis. Individuals with preexisting colitis should not be given gold therapy. *The nurse should regularly examine the skin, buccal mucosa, and urine (for hematuria) of patients receiving gold therapy.* Antihistamines and steroids (topical or systemic) may be useful in alleviating mucosal lesions.

Hematological reactions are another form of gold toxicity. Severe blood dyscrasias have been reported, including leukopenia, agranulocytosis, aplastic anemia, and thrombocytopenia. Aurotherapy is contraindicated in patients with hematological disorders. *Prior to initiating gold therapy, the nurse should arrange blood cell and platelet counts. After therapy is underway, these tests should be repeated frequently (weekly for 2–3 months; then every 2–3 weeks). Any rapid reduction in these counts suggests toxicity and the nurse should draw this to the attention of the physician. In addition, nurses need to instruct clients about symptoms that might suggest changes in blood cell levels.* Other drugs with the potential for promoting blood dyscrasias, including immunosuppressives, antimalarials, and pyrazolones should not be used in conjunction with gold.

Gold can produce adverse effects on kidney function. **Proteinuria** and **nephrosis** may occur in 1–3% of treated individuals. *At each treatment session, urine should be analyzed for evidence of proteinuria or hematuria before injecting the scheduled dose of gold. Clients should be advised to report immediately any changes in urine output or urine coloration.* Gold therapy should not be initiated in patients with renal disease.

Adverse effects of gold on liver function take the form of **hepatitis.** Individuals with preexisting liver disease or hepatitis should not receive gold treatment. **Interstitial pneumonitis** and **fibrosis** have occurred as a result of gold therapy. *Periodic chest x-ray and pulmonary function tests should be conducted during chrysotherapy.*

Other adverse effects of gold therapy include **nitroid** and **anaphylactic reactions.** Nitroid reactions are characterized by flushing, faintness, and dizziness. *Since allergic reactions to gold usually occur within 10 minutes of injection, the nurse should observe clients for at least 30 minutes after injection. Dimercaprol should be kept at hand as an antidote.*

Preparations and Administration The three gold salts marketed currently are auranofin (Ridaura), gold sodium thiomalate (Myochrysine), and aurothioglucose (Solganal). The latter two are parenteral dosage forms and contain approximately 50% gold; auranofin, an oral dosage form, contains about 29% gold. *Vials of gold salts should be agitated before withdrawal of the dose to assure uniformity. Gold preparations should be stored in light-resistant containers. Solutions of gold sodium thiomalate that are darker than pale yellow should not be used.* Oral administration of gold in the form of auranofin was approved in 1985.

It has been estimated that about 15% of clients given chrysotherapy experience complete remission, about two-thirds experience significant improvement, about 10% are nonresponsive, and about 10–20% must discontinue treatment because of toxicity.

Gold sodium thiomalate (Myochrysine)
Injection solution
Recommended Doses: For rheumatoid arthritis, 10 mg IM for the first injection, 25 mg for the second, and 25–50 mg in subsequent injections. The interval between injections is initially 1 week. Dosing is continued until there is significant clinical improvement up to a maximum of 1.0 g cumulative dose. The practice of employing smaller doses initially does not eliminate adverse reactions but does reduce their severity. If a favorable response is obtained, maintenance doses (25–50 mg) may or may not be employed, at intervals of every 2 weeks for 2–20 weeks and every third or fourth week indefinitely.

Aurothioglucose (Solganal)
Suspension
Recommended Doses: Same as for gold sodium thiomalate.

Auranofin (Ridaura)
Capsules
Recommended Doses: 6 mg PO daily, either in 1 or 2 administrations. Doses in excess of 6 mg daily are not recommended for initial therapy because of the incidence of diarrhea, but if response to auranofin is inadequate after 6 months, an increase up to 9 mg daily in 3 administrations of 3 mg each may be tried.

Antimalarials in Rheumatoid Arthritis

Several of the 4-aminoquinoline compounds with antimalarial activity have been found to be effective in the treatment of collagen diseases such as rheumatoid arthritis (RA) and systemic or discoid lupus erythematosus. Chloroquine, amodiaquine, and hydroxychloroquine have all been used effectively in RA, but hydroxychloroquine is most commonly employed because of its relatively low toxicity. Antimalarials are second-line drugs for RA because their potential for toxicity exceeds that of the best of the NSAIDs. The mechanism of action of antimalarials in RA is unknown, although it may involve a suppression of formation of RF, the antigenic factor of rheumatoid arthritis. Hydroxychloroquine is readily absorbed after oral administration, reaching peak plasma levels in 1–3 hours.

Adverse Effects and Contraindications Adverse effects of antimalarials are widespread, extending to the **CNS** (irritability, lassitude, emotional disturbances, psychosis, headache, vertigo, tinnitus, deafness, nystagmus, convulsions), neuromuscular function (extraocular palsies, weakness), **visual function** (impaired accommodation, opacities, photophobia, blurred vision, corneal deposits, abnormal retinal pigmentation, scotoma, field constriction, retinopathy), the **skin** (alopecia, bleaching of hair, pruritus, skin and mucosal hyperpigmentation, urticaria, psoriasis, lichenoid eruptions, maculopapular or morbilliform eruptions, purpura, and exfoliative dermatitis), the **gastrointestinal system** (anorexia, weight loss, nausea, vomiting, diarrhea, cramps), and the **hematopoietic system** (aplastic anemia, leukopenia, agranulocytosis, thrombocytopenia, and hemolytic anemia in glucose-6-phosphate dehydrogenase deficient individuals). *Visual examinations should be conducted at frequent intervals when antimalarial drugs are being used. Reflexes should be examined periodically to check for signs of muscle weakness. Blood cell counts should be conducted periodically.* Children are especially susceptible to toxic effects of 4-aminoquinolines; fatalities have occurred at low doses. Antimalarial drugs should be avoided in children and during pregnancy.

Preparations and Administration *The daily dose is taken in a single oral administration, with a meal or glass of milk to minimize gastrointestinal irritation. Hydroxychloroquine should be stored between 59 and 89° F.*

Hydroxychloroquine sulfate (Plaquenil)
Tablets
Recommended Doses: For RA in adults, 4–6 mg/kg PO daily. The dose may be adjusted downward after 5–10 days until the optimum maintenance dosage is determined (typically 200–400 mg daily).

Immunosuppressives in Rheumatoid Arthritis

Immunosuppressives represent a last resort in treatment of RA. Drugs such as azathioprine (Imuran) (see Chapter 50) and cyclophosphamide (Cytoxan) (see Chapter 56) are highly effective in suppressing the phagocytic cell activity that contributes to RA but are highly toxic. Immunosuppressives are thus reserved for individuals refractory to alternative treatments.

Case Study: Rheumatoid Arthritis

P. C. was a 72-year-old woman who came to the arthritis clinic because of increasing pain, tenderness, and immobility in her joints: her knees, hands, wrists, and right elbow. As best as she could recollect, the pain and stiffness had occurred off and on for about 5 years, gradually increasing in frequency and intensity. While assessing P. C., the clinic nurse learned that P. C.'s symptoms were most pronounced for a few hours after arising in the morning, that she often experienced fatigue in the late afternoon, and that she occasionally took aspirin to alleviate the pain. On physical examination, the nurse noticed minor deformities in the small joints of the fingers. Both knees exhibited swelling. The knees and the right elbow lacked full extension. Vital signs, including blood pressure, pulse, respirations, and temperature were normal. P. C. weighed 200 lb.

The physician reviewed the nurse's assessment and ordered x-rays of the joints, blood cell counts, hemoglobin determination, erythrocyte sedimentation rate, and rheumatoid factor (RF) determination. The x-rays revealed degenerative changes in the knees, hands, and right elbow; hip x-rays were normal. White blood cell count was normal but erythrocyte sedimentation rate was 26 mm/hour (normal: 0–10 mm/hour) and hemoglobin was 10.5 g/100 ml (normal: 12–16 g/100 ml in women). The determination of RF was positive. The diagnosis was rheumatoid arthritis with anemia.

The physician wrote a prescription for aspirin, 975 mg (3 tablets), qid, with meals or snack. The nurse worked with P. C. to establish a schedule of activity that would provide her with 12 hours of rest from ambulation each day. She explained the nature of rheumatoid arthritis to P. C. and the role of aspirin in suppressing inflammation. The nurse emphasized the importance of adhering to the prescribed regimen rather than taking the drug only when she felt she needed it for pain. P. C. was surprised to learn that aspirin was being used to suppress inflammation and not merely to alleviate pain. The nurse taught P. C. how to apply a heat pack to a tender joint. She also advised P. C. to reduce her weight and worked with her to devise a meal plan that would reduce caloric intake. Since P. C. had difficulty with ambulation, the nurse reviewed with P. C. her requirements for ambulation and together they were able to plan some adjustments in P. C.'s activities that would allow her to reduce the time she spent on her feet. The nurse spoke to P. C.'s adult son, who lived nearby, and he volunteered to help his mother once a week with her grocery shopping. The nurse also referred P. C. to a store that sold orthopedic shoes. She instructed P. C. to watch for symptoms of gastric distress (nausea, gastric pain), tarry stools, nosebleeds, or changes in hearing (such as diminished acuity or ringing in the ears).

After 3 weeks, P. C. returned for evaluation. The nurse obtained a blood sample and the serum salicylate concentration was found to be 225 μg/ml (therapeutic range: 150–300 μg/ml). After 6 months, evaluation of therapy revealed that there was diminished swelling and pain in the arthritic joints and ambulation was improved although still somewhat difficult. P. C. had purchased orthopedic shoes, which increased her foot comfort and improved ambulation. The minor deformities of the fingers were still evident, but joint swelling was diminished. P. C. had reduced her weight to 185 lb.

1. Are the symptoms reported by P. C. initially typical of rheumatoid arthritis?
2. What is the likely reason for the mild anemia present in this case?
3. Which laboratory finding was most crucial in distinguishing the cause of the arthritis?
4. Why was weight loss considered desirable in this case? Why was P. C. advised to increase her opportunities for rest?
5. Why did the nurse advise P. C. to watch for signs of gastrointestinal distress? Changes in hearing? Tarry stools and nosebleeds?
6. What is your evaluation of the extent to which P. C. was complying with the prescribed regimen? What evidence can you cite for your evaluation?
7. Was it alarming that there was no improvement in deformity of the finger joints after 6 months? How would you rate the client's progress?

Answers appear at the end of the book.

Recommended Readings

Brennan BE, Simon RR: Management of salicylate intoxication. *Drugs* 1982;24:335–340.

Clegg DO, Ward JR: Slow-acting anti-rheumatic drug therapy for rheumatoid arthritis. *Nurse Pract* 1987; 12(3):44–52.

Clive DM, Stoff JS: Renal syndromes associated with nonsteroidal antiinflammatory drugs. *N Engl J Med* 1984; 310:563–572.

Conner CS: Oral gold in arthritis. *Drug Intell Clin Pharm* 1984;18(10):804–805.

Ehrlich GE: Other NSAIDs of choice for rheumatoid arthritis. *Drug Intell Clin Pharm* 1984;18:39–41.

Gall EP: The use of drugs in rheumatic diseases. *Primary Care* 1984;11(2):369–380.

Garcia C: Gold therapy in arthritis treatment. *Nurse Pract* 1981;6(1):35, 38, 49.

Hadler NM: The argument for aspirin as the NSAID of choice in the management of rheumatoid arthritis. *Drug Intell Clin Pharm* 1984;18:34–38.

Hart FD, Huskisson EC: Non-steroidal anti-inflammatory drugs. Current status and rational therapeutic use. *Drugs* 1984;27:232–255.

Kantor TG, Kaplan H, Ward JR: NSAID therapy made a little simpler. *Patient Care* 1984;30(1):123.

Miller SB: NSAIDs: Examining therapeutic alternatives. *Geriatrics* 1982;37(3):70–78.

O'Duffy JD, Luthra HS: Current status of disease-modifying drugs in progressive rheumatoid arthritis. *Drugs* 1984;27:373–377.

Samuelsson B: Leukotrienes: Mediators of immediate hypersensitivity reactions and inflammation. *Science* 1983; 220:568–575.

Settipane GA: Adverse reactions to aspirin and related drugs. *Arch Intern Med* 1981;141:328–332.

Spruck M: Gold therapy. *Am J Nurs* 1979;79(7):1246–1248.

Strand CV, Clark SR: Adult arthritis: Drugs and remedies. *Am J Nurs* 1983;83(2):266–269.

UNIT IX

Drugs and the Immune System

CHAPTER 46

Host Versus Pathogens

Human beings share the environment with a multitude of tiny organisms of seemingly endless variety. With many of these microorganisms, our relationship is, fortunately, cooperative, or symbiotic. For example, the commensal flora (such as *Escherichia coli*) that thrive within the alimentary tract contribute crucial digestive and metabolic activities and help to inhibit colonization by potentially pathogenic microorganisms. With such commensal organisms, a tenuous balance has been established between the resistance of the host against pathogenic incursions of the foreign cells and the need of the microorganism for nourishment. Only a small minority of all microbes pose a threat to us. With such organisms, continued encroachment leads ultimately to tissue damage or dysfunction and clinical disease states.

Nonspecific Resistance

Resistance of the human host to pathogenic microorganisms derives from an array of defense mechanisms. Most of these defenses provide **nonspecific resistance,** operating against all organisms in general. Most important of these nonspecific mechanisms are the penetration barriers associated with the tissues that make up the portals of entry: the skin, alimentary tract, respiratory tract, genitourinary tract, external ear canals, and the epithelial surface of the eye. Special properties of the skin and mucosal membranes provide a degree of general protection against all microorganisms.

The outer, horny layer of the epidermis is composed of heavily keratinized, dead cells that form a tough, resistant barrier to penetration. The relative lack of moisture in this layer presents an unfavorable environment for most microorganisms. The continuous shedding and regeneration of skin helps to eliminate microorganisms that reside on the skin surface and also ensures repair of cutaneous lesions that might provide easy access for microorganisms to the interior of the body. Secretions of the sebaceous and sweat glands provide further protection by creating a hostile fluid environment. The low pH and high salt content of sweat inhibits growth of many microorganisms, and the fatty acids found in sebum inhibit growth of certain fungi.

Mucosal membranes of the nasal cavity and airways possess a special mucociliary lining designed to protect the underlying tissue from incursions and to remove microorganisms and debris. The cilia lining the airways lift phagocytized particles to the larynx where they can be harmlessly swallowed. Ciliated mucosal cells of the alimentary tract protect against attachment of microorganisms by their constant motion. Many microorganisms are destroyed by the acid environment or digestive enzymes of the stomach. Fluids that bathe mucosal surfaces — including mucus, tears, and saliva — contain **lysozyme,** an enzyme that breaks down (lyses) the cell walls of some bacteria. Mucosal secretions also contain phagocytic white blood cells to engulf microorganisms. The genitourinary tract is protected by its mucous coating and the external ear canal by the waxy secretion of associated glandular cells.

Inevitably, some microorganisms do reach the circulatory system. Certain tissues are protected from invasion of microorganisms from the blood by special **penetration barriers.** For example, the blood-brain barrier protects the central nervous system against invasion of microorganisms as well as entrance of many drug substances. The placental barrier protects the fetus from penetration of some microbes.

The reticuloendothelial system provides the active component of nonspecific resistance against microorganisms (see Chapter 45 for full discussion). The components of this system include the granulocytes (neutrophils, eosinophils, and basophils), the monocytes, and tissue macrophages. Macrophages, distributed diffusely through the various bodily tissues but most abundantly in tissues associated with portals of entry, provide a first line of defense. The monocytes and neutrophils, circulating in the plasma, provide rapid reinforcement of defenses at the site of an infection. Both of these classes of phagocytic blood cells are rapidly directed to an area of microbial invasion by chemotaxis. Microorganisms that have penetrated the body to reach the blood are gradually filtered and phagocytized as they pass through lymph nodes of the lymphatic system. Lymph nodes are strategically located near the major portals of entry to pick up microorganisms that manage to escape destruction and gain entrance at these portals.

Specific Resistance: The Immune System

In contrast to the mechanisms that confer nonspecific resistance, the immune system provides **specific resistance** — resistance against particular types of microorganisms, proteins, or other chemicals that the system has "learned" to recognize as foreign. Substances recognized as foreign by the immune system are called **antigens.** The immune system responds with increasing vigor when exposed repeatedly to a given antigen, exhibiting a degree of adaptability that the nonspecific mechanisms lack. The immune system is of major importance as a means of reestablishing the integrity of the host that has been compromised by excessive incursion of pathogens, enabling the body to recognize such foreign agents and destroy or neutralize them. The vast majority of invasions are adequately controlled by the combination of nonspecific defenses and the immune system. Of the remainder, many can be checked by antimicrobial drugs until the host defense mechanisms can regain the upper hand. The action of antimicrobial drugs is best understood in the context of this uneasy balance between host defense mechanisms and pathogenic invasions.

In some individuals, malfunction of the immune system is itself pathogenic, resulting in hypersensitivity reactions, leukemia, immune deficiencies, or autoimmunity. These situations will be discussed in Chapter 50. In this chapter, we will consider the physiology of the immune system.

Duality of the Immune System

Specific resistance, in the form of immune responses, is the function of the lymphoid system. The specialized mediators of immunity are a class of white blood cells called **lymphocytes.** Lymphocytes are derived from stem cells of the bone marrow that give rise to red blood cells, granulocytes, monocytes, and lymphocytes alike. During the later stages of fetal development and the first few months of life, stem cells destined to seed the lymphoid tissue migrate from the bone marrow. Stem cells reaching the thymus give rise to **T lymphocytes,** the "T" signifying the relationship of these lymphocytes to the *t*hymus. Other stem cells migrate to lymphoid tissue associated with the alimentary tract — the tonsils, appendix, and so forth. These stem cells give rise to **B lymphocytes,** so named because in birds, where they were first identified, the B cells are associated with a lymphoid tissue called the *b*ursa. Thus, stem cells ultimately give rise to the two distinct populations of lymphocytes that provide the basis for the duality of the immune response — cell-mediated immunity and humoral immunity.

The immunity conferred by T lymphocytes is called **cell-mediated** or *cellular immunity.* Cell-mediated immunity requires 1–3 days to develop after antigenic challenge and is thus also called *delayed immunity.* Early in life, T cells are entirely dependent on intact thymus function, but later many T cells originate in the lymph nodes, spleen, and bone marrow. About 75% of lymphocytes circulating in the blood are T lymphocytes. T lymphocytes are designed to kill virus-infected host cells but do not bind free antigen. T lymphocytes exert their toxic effect on infected cells by releasing lymphokines that promote lysis or phagocytosis (by monocytes or neutrophils).

Humoral immunity is provided by the activity of B lymphocytes. Most B lymphocytes remain within lymphoid tissue. A relatively small but functionally significant portion are free-floating in the bloodstream, comprising about 25% of all circulating lymphocytes. B cells in the plasma are short-lived, with a life-span of only about 15 days. B lymphocytes produce a large quantity of immunoglobulins that circulate in the plasma, ready to combine with free-floating antigens to promote phagocytosis, precipitation, neutralization, or lysis of antigen.

The two components of the immune system share a response sequence (Figure 46–1) consisting of (1) antigen recognition, (2) blast formation, (3) cloning, (4) differentiation of clones into various effector cells, and (5) release of effector substances to neutralize or destroy antigens or antigen-infected cells.

Antigen Recognition

An **antigen** is any substance capable of activating the immune response — culminating in formation of immune effector cells. Normally, antigens consist of foreign proteins or cells, but abnormally they may be endogenous tissue components. Only molecules of sufficient size, generally greater than 10,000 molecular weight, have antigenic potential. Most often, antigens are proteins or protein complexes with other organic chemicals as in the case of lipoproteins. Less frequently, they may be polysaccharides or other complex substances. The antigen may be a free-floating substance or a constituent of a foreign cell. Simple compounds, including most drugs, are not antigenic in themselves but some can act as **haptens** (incomplete antigens), attaching to protein to produce a complex that is antigenic. This kind of mechanism is involved in many types of drug allergies.

The receptors of B lymphocytes are immunoglobulins that extend from the cell surface. The receptors of T lymphocytes are believed to be gamma-globulin-like molecules on the cell surface. When the three-dimensional distribution of electrical charges on a complex molecule matches the receptors of a lymphocyte, the substance is antigenic and can initiate an immune response. Activation of T lymphocytes is a little more complicated than activation of B lymphocytes, requiring simultaneous binding of the T cell to an antigen and a host cell surface receptor. This additional requirement is the reason that activity of T lymphocytes is directed against infected host cells while the activity of B cells is directed mainly against circulating antigens. T lymphocytes are most sensitive to chronic infectious microorganisms such as fungi and Mycobacterium *tuberculosis,* antigenic components of tissue transplants, rhus antigen, and certain drugs applied topically to the skin.

Each lymphocyte possesses unique surface receptors; taken collectively, the population of lymphocytes present a vast, varied array of potential binding sites. If two antigens are sufficiently similar that the immune response triggered by one also operates against the other, the antigens are said to be **cross-reactive.** Microbial cells are sufficiently complex that they frequently contain several antigenic constituents or products. The antigenic component may be inside the cell (somatic or "O" antigens), on the cell surface (surface antigens), in the capsule of mycobacteria (capsular antigens), in the cilia of motile species (flagellar or "H" antigens), or secreted by the cell as an exotoxin. A microbial cell may activate more than one type of lymphocyte, producing a sequential response involving, for example, IgM-releasing B lymphocytes, then IgG-releasing lymphocytes, and finally T lymphocytes.

Blast Formation, Cloning, and Differentiation

Binding of an antigen to a lymphocyte receptor initiates an immune response involving blast formation, cloning, and differentiation into the various effector

Figure 46–1
Steps in the immune response.

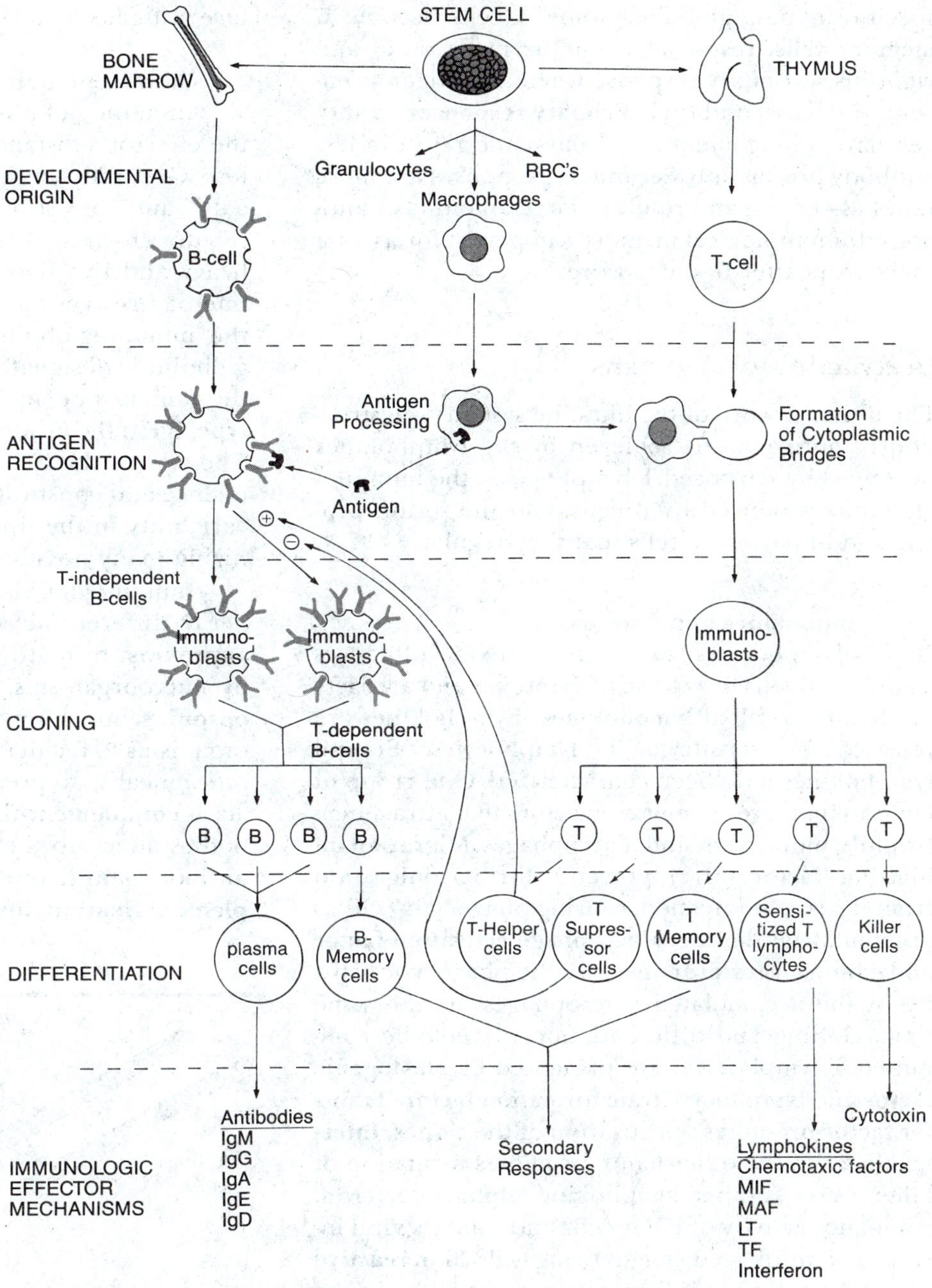

cells that perform the functions of immunity. Clonal proliferation can also be stimulated, in the case of T lymphocytes, by a substance released from active macrophages called **interleukin-1.** The activated lymphocyte is first converted into a blast cell capable of rapid mitosis to produce numerous clones of itself. If the reaction is a cell-mediated response involving T lymphocytes, some of the clones differentiate into **sensitized lymphocytes,** also called **committed T cells.** Most of these are activated to release lymphokines targeted against the antigenic cells. Some become **T memory cells** capable of mediating subsequent responses to the particular antigen. Still others become **helper** or **suppressor cells** that modify responses of B lymphocytes to the antigen.

A similar pattern of clonal proliferation occurs if the response is a humoral immune reaction. B cells with surface receptors that match the antigen are transformed into blast cells, producing numerous clones. Most of the clones differentiate into **plasma**

cells, specialized secretory factories that produce the specific immunoglobulin. Some B cells become **B memory cells,** responsible for the more rapid and vigorous secondary response when an antigen is encountered a second time. **Primary responses** to antigen have a long latency (4–5 days) and result in less antibody production. **Secondary responses** are more rapid (2–3 days) and result in large amounts of antibody. Immunological memory can persist for as long as 20 years after first exposure.

Destruction of Antigens

The ultimate work of the immune system — destruction of antigens — is achieved by the lymphokines produced by sensitized T lymphocytes, the immunoglobulins produced by B cells, and the serum proteins and phagocytic cells that they regulate.

Lymphokines and Cytotoxin

T lymphocytes exert their toxic influences against antigens by release of **cytotoxin** and a variety of chemicals called **lymphokines.** Lymphokines are released by sensitized T lymphocytes. Several lymphokines have been characterized. One group of lymphokines are **chemotaxic factors** that attract neutrophils, monocytes, and macrophages. **Migration inhibition factor** (MIF) prevents further migration from the site of infection, causing phagocytic cells to accumulate at the site. **Macrophage activation factor** and **gamma interferon** increase the phagocytic activity of the accumulated macrophages. At the same time, cloning and differentiation of yet-to-be committed T lymphocytes are promoted by **blastogenic factor** and **lymphocyte transformation factor. Transfer factor** promotes sensitization of the clones. **Interleukin-2,** on the other hand, promotes formation of killer cells. Another lymphokine, **alpha interferon,** stimulates activity of killer cells and inhibits viral invasion of uninfected, neighboring cells. **Skin reactive factor** activates the inflammatory mechanism in the skin.

Killer cells, a separate class of T lymphocytes, release **cytotoxin,** also called lymphotoxin. There are two groups of killer cells. **Natural killer cells** are always present among the circulating lymphocytes and can be activated by alpha-interferon released by macrophages. **Lymphokine-activated killer cells** are produced and activated by interleukin-2 released from sensitized lymphocytes. Administration of the combination of lymphokine-activated killer cells and interleukin-2 has been introduced as an experimental treatment for certain cancer conditions not responsive to conventional therapies (see Chapter 56). Cytotoxin destroys any microbial cell with surface antigens by a cytolytic action.

Immunoglobulins

Immunoglobulins, also called **antibodies,** are the effector substances of the humoral immune system. Generally, immunoglobulins have the shape of a "Y" and consist of two heavy and two light chains (Figure 46–2) (IgM is larger, being composed of five heavy and five light chains). The heavy chains are one of five types and determine the class to which the immunoglobulin belongs. Thus, the immunoglobulin is designated as IgG if the large chain is of the gamma type, IgM if the mu type, IgA if the alpha type, IgE if the epsilon type, and IgD if the delta type. The tips of the "Y" have a variable amino acid sequence and constitute the antigen-binding sites. The variability in the tips provides the ability for recognizing many possible antigens.

Immunoglobulins inactivate antigens in a number of different ways. Some immunoglobulins act as **antitoxins,** to neutralize soluble exotoxins released by microorganisms. Some immunoglobulins act as **opsonins,** attaching to cell surface antigens of microorganisms to facilitate phagocytosis. The term *opsonization* means "to prepare food for." IgM and IgG can act as **complement-fixing sites.** The tips of these antibodies attach to the antigen while the stems of the antibodies initiate a reaction sequence called **complement fixation,** involving serum proteins, that ulti-

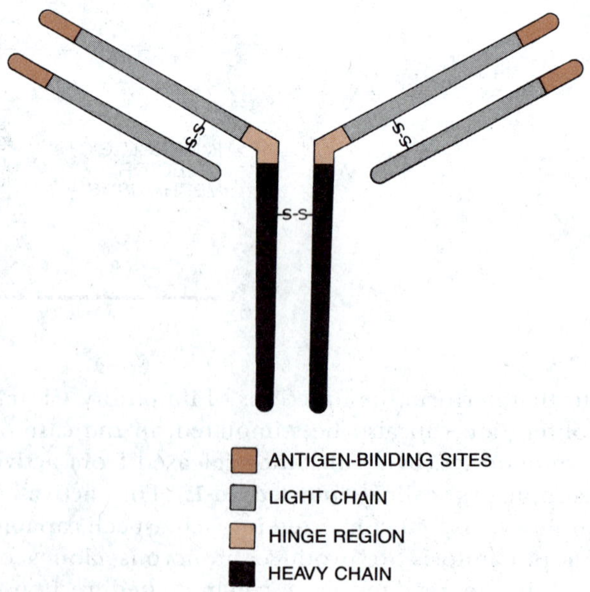

Figure 46–2
Structure of an immunoglobulin.

mately destroys the antigen. Sometimes immunoglobulins act as **precipitins** to precipitate antigens or **agglutins** to agglutinize antigens.

The five classes of immunoglobulins exhibit differing characteristics (Table 46–1). **IgM** constitutes about 7% of the total immunoglobulins in the body. Because it is a larger molecule than the other immunoglobulins, it has greater antigen-binding capacity but also has limited capacity to cross bodily membranes. IgM is largely confined to the plasma. Its size makes it an excellent site for fixation of complement and a good antitoxin. The large tail of IgM promotes phagocytosis by macrophages, the so-called opsonic effect. IgM is the first immunoglobulin to appear when infection occurs. When a given antigen is encountered for the first time (a primary immune response), IgM carries the main responsibility for immunological protection. The large number of binding sites make it ideal for initial interaction with novel antigens. Large quantities of IgM in the blood indicate continuing or recent infectious processes, since the half-life of IgM is only 1 day. IgM is responsible for immunological reactions to natural blood group antigens (ABO). It is the major antibody for polysaccharides and has special affinity for gram-negative bacteria.

IgG is the most abundant of the immunoglobulins, comprising 70–80% of the total. IgG is not an important part of primary immune responses, but after a **sensitizing dose** of an antigen, a subsequent **eliciting dose** provokes a rapid and vigorous humoral immune response that is mediated mainly by

Table 46–1
Characteristics of Immunoglobulins

Characteristic	IgM	IgG	IgA	IgE	IgD
Heavy chain	Mu	Gamma	Alpha	Epsilon	Delta
Binding capacity	High	Average	Average	Average	Average
Size	Large	Moderate	Moderate	Moderate	Moderate
Complement-fixing capacity	Great	Moderate	None	None	Unknown
Subclasses	2	4	2	Unknown	Unknown
Distribution					
Plasma	90%	40%	Low	Low	Low
Lymph and other extracellular fluids	10%	60%	0%	0%	Unknown
Mucosal secretions	0%	0%	100%	Most	Unknown
Approximate prevalence	7%	75%	18%	0.02%	0.2%
Half-life (days)	1	23	6	2	3
Transfer to offspring	None; occurs in fetus in 5th or 6th week	Via placenta	Via colostrum and milk	None	None
Antigens	Microbes, ABO antigens	Microbes	Microbes	Reagenic antigens	Unknown
Functions	Primary immune response Good opsonins Good antitoxins Presence indicates active or recent infection	Secondary immune response Good antitoxins	Protection of mucosal surfaces	Immediate (atopic) allergic reactions Attaches to mast cells and basophils to trigger release of autacoids and formation of prostaglandins and leukotrienes	Unknown Located mainly on B-cell surfaces; may be antigen receptor site

IgG. IgG is the major antibody active against viruses, most bacteria, and bacterial exotoxins. Three of the four IgG subclasses (IgG_1, IgG_2, and IgG_3) are effective in triggering complement fixation. The smaller size of IgG in relation to IgM allows it to freely enter extracellular fluids including the lymph, cerebrospinal fluid, and synovial and peritoneal fluids. IgG freely crosses the placental barrier and provides passive immunological protection for the fetus until it is able to produce its own IgM and later IgG antibodies.

IgA is barely present in the serum, but is abundant in seromucosal secretions and in the colostrum. Presence in the colostrum provides transfer to the newborn child who is breast-fed, which is a strong argument for breast-feeding infants. Presence of IgA in mucosal secretions protects the surface tissues of the body from infection. Large amounts of IgA are produced in the gastrointestinal and respiratory tract mucosa. It is also found in tears and saliva. IgA interacts with microorganisms.

IgE is also found mainly in seromucosal secretions but is found in measurable concentrations in the serum. Interaction of IgE with mast cells and basophils produces the distinctive symptoms of IgE-mediated allergic reactions. These symptoms include anaphylaxis, drug eruptions, hay fever, asthma, urticaria (hives), allergic rhinitis, and allergic conjunctivitis. These reactions are characterized by rapid onset and are therefore called **immediate-type** hypersensitivity reactions. The antigens that interact with IgE are often called **allergens.** IgE is sometimes called **reaginic antibody** or **atopic antibody.**

Little is known about **IgD** except that most of it is attached to the surfaces of B lymphocytes. It is speculated that IgD may serve as the antigen receptor for T-independent B lymphocytes.

Complement Fixation

Complement consists of a group of nine serum proteins (C_1–C_9) that contribute to the destruction of antigenic cells. They interact in a cascade of reactions in a manner analogous to the more familiar cascade of clotting factors. The first protein in the sequence, C_1, is activated by antigen-antibody complexes if the antibody is IgG, or especially IgM. C_1 attaches to the tail end of these immunoglobulins. The remaining proteins of complement attach sequentially, forming a ring that punctures the membrane of the antigenic cell. In addition, C_4 can neutralize viruses; C_3 promotes phagocytosis, production of antibodies, and release of histamine and other substances of anaphylaxis; and C_5, C_6, and C_7 promote chemotaxis of neutrophils (polymorphonuclear cells). The toxic effects of complement are sometimes directed against host cells in autoimmunity.

Host Defense Mechanisms in Relation to Antimicrobial Therapy

The actions of antimicrobial drugs occur in the context of the ongoing opposition between host defense mechanisms and infectious activities of pathogenic microorganisms. In most situations, antimicrobial drugs serve to shift the balance in favor of host defense mechanisms by stopping the spread of the infectious microbe. Antimicrobial agents seldom effect a cure if host defense mechanisms are substantially impaired. In the normal host, levels of both immunoglobulins and phagocytic white blood cells rise in direct proportion to the severity of an infection. Antimicrobial drugs do not improve host defense mechanisms but act directly on the pathogenic microorganisms. Nonspecific, supportive measures, such as oxygenation, correction of fluid, electrolyte, or nutritional imbalances, and bedrest may, on the other hand, improve the vigor of host defense processes. When host defense mechanisms are fully intact, many infections do not require antimicrobial drug therapy.

The extent of impairment of host defense mechanisms and the severity of infection may alter parameters of drug therapy. Parenteral therapy or large doses of potent antimicrobial drugs may be used for severe infections. Combinations of agents may be required in the compromised host where single drug therapy would be adequate in the host with normal immune function. The aim of therapy may have to be redefined: a drug with bacteriostatic (proliferation-suppressing) action might be perfectly adequate in a host with vigorous defense mechanisms but one with a bactericidal (killing) effect may be required when defenses are severely compromised. Thus, drug therapy for infections begins with assessment of host defense mechanisms and organ function.

Local conditions at the site of infection may also be relevant. Presence of large quantities of pus may necessitate a more vigorous approach since pus reduces activity of many antimicrobial drugs. Accumulation of hemoglobin at the site of infection leads to binding and inactivation of certain antimicrobial agents. If the infection is in the stomach, urinary tract, or areas bathed by the cerebrospinal fluid, the local pH is usually low, necessitating selection of drugs that are active in an acidic environment. Some antimicrobial drugs (such as aminoglycosides, macrolides, and lincosamides) lose activity at low pH, but others (such as nitrofurantoin and chlortetracycline) are more active.

Human Pathogens

The pathogens responsible for infectious disorders in humans are diverse — in size, complexity, and type. Six types of pathogens are recognized at present: (1) prions, (2) viruses, (3) bacteria, (4) protozoa, (5) fungi, and (6) parasitic worms. Only three of these types are true microorganisms — namely, bacteria, protozoa, and fungi. Prions and viruses are not truly living organisms, being mere particles of fragmentary cellular material. Parasitic worms, on the other hand, are far too complex to qualify as microorganisms.

Prions are recently discovered infectious agents responsible for Creutzfeldt-Jakob disease (a dementia) and scrapie, a veterinary disease in sheep. Formerly called slow viruses, prions are probably responsible for two other types of dementia — kuru, which occurs among cannibalistic tribes in New Guinea, and Gerstmann-Straussler syndrome. Prions may even be involved in Alzheimer's disease. Prions appear to be composed mainly if not entirely of a protein that forms rod shaped aggregates. They are capable of reproducing only by infecting certain mammalian cells. The mechanisms of their reproduction are not yet established, and there are no specific drug therapies for infectious diseases related to prions.

Viruses are similarly dependent on occupation of host cells for replication. Viruses consist of an inner core of nucleic acid strands (DNA or RNA, but not both) encapsulated in a symmetrical protein coat called a capsid, and sometimes in an additional outer layer called an envelope. Viruses shed their coats upon entering host cells and redirect the genetic machinery of the host cell to synthesize new viral components: nucleic acids and capsid proteins. The nature of viruses is discussed more completely in Chapter 48.

The true microorganisms belong to the kingdom of **protists,** the group of single-celled or simple multicellular organisms that have evolved from the common ancestors of plants and animals. These prototypes of higher organisms share many of the properties of both plants and animals. Protists consist of two groups: lower and higher protists. The **lower protists** are always single cells and **procaryotic,** meaning that their nuclear material is not contained within a nuclear membrane. Other internal cellular structures are similarly rudimentary in appearance. The lower protists include **bacteria** and the **cyanobacteria** (or blue-green algae). The simplest of all bacteria are **rickettsiae** and **chlamydiae,** two very small and simple microorganisms barely more complicated than viruses. Like viruses, these nonmotile bacteria are obligate (surviving only within host cells), but they possess cell walls similar to other bacteria, contain both DNA and RNA, possess ribosomes, and multiply by binary fission. The nature of bacteria and their varieties are discussed more fully in Chapter 47. A wealth of antibacterial drugs are available for clinical use.

The **higher protists** include algae, slime molds, fungi, and protozoa. Higher protists are **eucaryotic,** possessing well-developed membranous boundaries for their nuclear material as well as other internal organelles. Eukaryotic cells possess mitochondria. Algae and slime molds are not pathogenic nor parasitic since they contain chlorophyll and are autotrophic (self-nourishing). **Fungi,** on the other hand, contain no chlorophyll and are heterotrophic, obtaining nourishment from organic material derived from living or recently dead organisms. Most fungi that cause infections in humans, such as the *Tinea* group, belong to one subdivision of fungi called *Fungi imperfecti* (*Deuteromycotina*). Unicellular varieties of fungi are called **yeasts** and multicellular varieties are **molds.** The yeasts belong to the subdivision of fungi called *Ascomycotina,* and include the important pathogen *Candida.*

Protozoa, the simple, single-celled ancestors of the animal kingdom, are also heterotrophic and frequently pathogenic to humans. Fungi and protozoa, and the drugs used to combat parasitic infections by these microorganisms, are discussed in Chapter 48.

Parasitic worms, or **helminths,** differ from other infectious pathogens in being somewhat developed, multicellular organisms with differentiated tissues and organs. Helminths include round worms (Nemathelminths) and flat worms (Platyhelminths), and both groups include pathogenic varieties. Infectious round worms include the hookworm and filarial worm; flatworms include tapeworms (Cestodes) and flukes (Trematodes). Helminths and antihelmintic drugs are discussed further in Chapter 48.

Nursing Measures to Control Spread of Infectious Disorders

Infections result from the introduction of a pathogen into a susceptible host. To be successful, the pathogen must have an environment conducive to its growth, a method of exit, and a means of transportation to a new site. Altering any of those factors helps to control spread of infection. Knowledge about the requirements of particular organisms helps to define strategies that may be successful in combating their presence. For example, some microbes are aerobic and some anaerobic and will thus colonize different parts of the body.

Pathogens enter the body through breaks in the skin or mucous membranes, through kissing, contact of the mouth with the hands, consumption of contaminated foods, inhalation through the respiratory system, and via the genitourinary system during sexual intercourse. It is often the nurse who must teach clients about modes of transmission and the preventive measures that must be taken at the entry site to prevent further infection or transmission. Nurses may need to teach clients proper hand washing. Nurses may need to advise clients about safe and unsafe sexual practices and use of condoms. If there is an infection on the skin, the nurse might need to teach clients appropriate sterile techniques for applying dressings and disposing of old dressings. Dressings that are contaminated should be incinerated. Sometimes it may be advisable to use no dressing since dressings may provide the optimum conditions of warmth and moisture to support proliferation of microbes.

Microorganisms may be transmitted by fomites (such as glasses, dishes, silverware) or by vectors (insects, flies, and mosquitoes). A susceptible host may be infected by bacteria transported in food, water, or on air currents. Appropriate hand washing and maintaining clean premises help to break the chain of infection.

Many airborne microorganisms exit from a host through coughs and sneezes. Others are transmitted in vomitus and saliva, and some via infected urine or vaginal secretions. Bacteria and viruses may be present in the bloodstream and exit through instruments used to withdraw blood. Sometimes microbes from a local infection drain onto the skin surface. To prevent transmission at the point of exit requires appropriate procedures for applying and discarding dressings, hand washing, use of gloves, decontamination of instruments or vessels used in caring for clients, and teaching clients important points to remember in handling potentially contaminated materials in the home.

The spread of microorganisms requires the availability of susceptible hosts. Nurses, especially those who work with clients in community settings, have a special responsibility to identify those most at risk of infection: (1) those with exogenously impaired defense mechanisms (including people being treated with corticosteroids, antineoplastic agents, immunosuppressive drugs, or systemic antimicrobial drugs), (2) clients undergoing instrumentation and diagnostic examination of the gastrointestinal, respiratory, or urinary tracts, and (3) clients with certain medical conditions and chronic diseases such as malignancies, diabetes, or collagen diseases. More generally, the person who is fatigued, has poor nutrition, and poor health habits is at increased risk. In assessing susceptibility of clients to the chain of infection, nurses must often consider social, cultural, and educational factors that may contribute to the client's health care problem. For example, people who live in unsanitary conditions and those subjected to overcrowding and malnutrition have reduced resistance to infection. Crowding also facilitates spread of infections by social contacts.

Recommended Readings

Bullock B: Immunity, in Bullock B, Rosendahl P: *Pathophysiology: Adaptations and Alterations in Function.* Boston, Little Brown & Co, 1984, pp 109–136.

Rose RR, Barron AL: *Microbiology: Basic Principles and Clinical Applications.* New York, Macmillan, 1983.

CHAPTER 47

Antibacterial Drugs

The Nature of Bacteria

Bacteria belong to the kingdom of protists, simple organisms derived from the common ancestors of plants and animals. Bacteria are unicellular microorganisms classified as **lower protists** because their cell structure is primitive (Figure 47–1). Bacterial cells are procaryotic — that is, they lack a true nucleus. The nuclear material of bacterial cells, consisting of both deoxyribonucleic acid (DNA) and ribonucleic acid (RNA), is loosely organized within the cell without any surrounding membrane. The ribosomes are small and lack clear demarcation. Mitochondria are lacking, and the analogous processes of respiration occur within sac-like invaginations of the cytoplasmic membrane called mesosomes.

The external structures of bacterial cells largely determine the relative sensitivities of various bacterial strains to antibacterial drugs (Figure 47–2). Every bacterial cell has a cytoplasmic membrane, but most bacteria possess one or two additional protective layers. Most bacteria have a **cell wall** surrounding the cytoplasmic membrane. The cell wall is a rigid but permeable structure composed of carbohydrate-protein (peptidoglycan) subunits. The transpeptidase enzymes required for synthesis and maintenance of the cell wall are attached to the outer surface of the cytoplasmic membrane or sometimes contained in the periplasmic space between the cytoplasmic membrane and cell wall. Antibacterial drugs of the penicillin and cephalosporin families interact with these enzymes to inhibit cell wall synthesis. If the bacterial cell is unable to maintain its cell wall, the denuded cell becomes shapeless and vulnerable. One unusual group of bacteria, the *Mycoplasma,* are unable to produce a cell wall, and have an amorphous appearance resembling that of other bacteria that have been acted on by antibiotics.

Some bacterial strains form an additional layer external to the cell wall. Some bacteria possess an **outer membrane** that hinders access of antibacterial drugs to the transpeptidase enzymes that synthesize the cell wall. Others produce a viscous **capsule** or **slime layer** that surrounds the cell wall, composed of polysaccharide or protein units. The presence of a capsule or slime layer increases resistance of a bacterium to both antibacterial drugs and host defense mechanisms. Some encapsulated bacteria, such as *Clostridium perfringens,* can even survive within a phagocytic white blood cell without disintegration.

Many bacteria possess **flagella** that provide motility. Some bacteria possess a single flagellum extending from one end, some possess two flagella extending from opposite poles, and some have numerous flagella extending around the entire exterior surface. Some bacteria possess fine filaments called **pili** that serve to provide adherence to surfaces or attachment to other bacterial cells for exchange of nuclear material (conjugation).

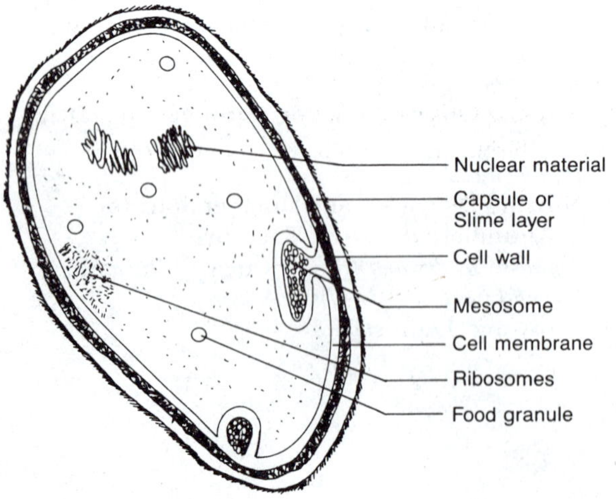

Figure 47–1
A bacterial cell. Note the lack of a nuclear membrane, the mesosome, the lack of a mitochondrion, the cell wall in addition to the cell membrane, the capsule or slime layer, and the primitive ribosomes.

Classification of Bacteria

In addition to morphological considerations, bacteria can be classified on the basis of (1) their relation to host cells, (2) their shape, (3) their requirement for oxygen, and (4) their reaction to various stains. In relation to the host cells, most bacteria exist as **extracellular pathogens.** Mycobacteria are unique among bacteria in their ability to survive either intracellularly or extracellularly. They are described as **facultative pathogens.** *Rickettsiae* and *Chlamydiae,* the two simplest bacterial forms, are **obligate pathogens,** surviving only within host cells.

Bacteria occur in four basic shapes (Figure 47–3). **Cocci** are round bacteria. Cocci often clump together, in twos to form diplococci, in long chains to form streptococci, or in irregular clumps to form staphylococci. **Bacilli** are straight and rod shaped whereas **vibriones** are curved and rod shaped. Both bacilli and vibriones have rigid structure. Some bacilli are encapsulated (Figure 47–3). **Spirochetes** are long, flexible, spiral shaped bacteria that propel themselves by undulation.

Bacteria that require oxygen for survival are classified as **aerobic.** Those that can survive in the absence of oxygen are **anaerobic.** This characteristic

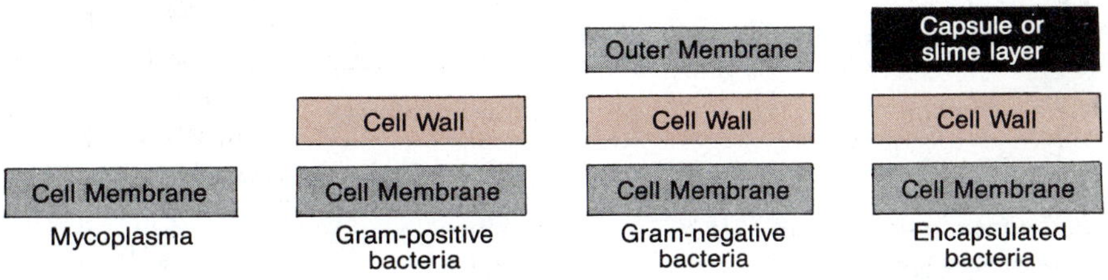

Figure 47–2
Surface structures of four kinds of bacteria.

of bacteria influences the selection of tissue sites that each type can colonize.

The most commonly employed method for characterizing and visualizing bacteria is **Gram's stain.** Bacteria are stained with aniline dyes, treated with a solution of iodine and potassium iodide (Lugol's solution), and then washed with alcohol. How the bacterium reacts to the stain depends on whether it has an additional membrane outside of the cell wall. If the bacterium does not have an outer membrane, the dye becomes fixed to the cell wall and is not removed by the subsequent alcohol wash. These bacteria are called gram-positive. Those bacteria having an outer membrane, in which the coloration is eluted by alcohol, are called gram-negative. Because Gram staining is determined by the outer structure of the bacterium, it is often predictive of whether a bacterium will be sensitive to various antibacterial agents, notably penicillin G. Bacterial responses to Gram's stain are indicated in Table 47–1.

General Principles of Antibacterial Drug Therapy

History and Sources The introduction of antimicrobial agents is arguably the most important development in clinical therapeutics of this century or any other. Judicious use of antimicrobial agents can effect true cures, something seldom achieved by other pharmacological treatments. Millions of people have been relieved of infections that would otherwise have been fatal, and many millions more have experienced more rapid recovery and reduced pathology from less serious infections. The seeds of this great medical advance lie in the folk medicine

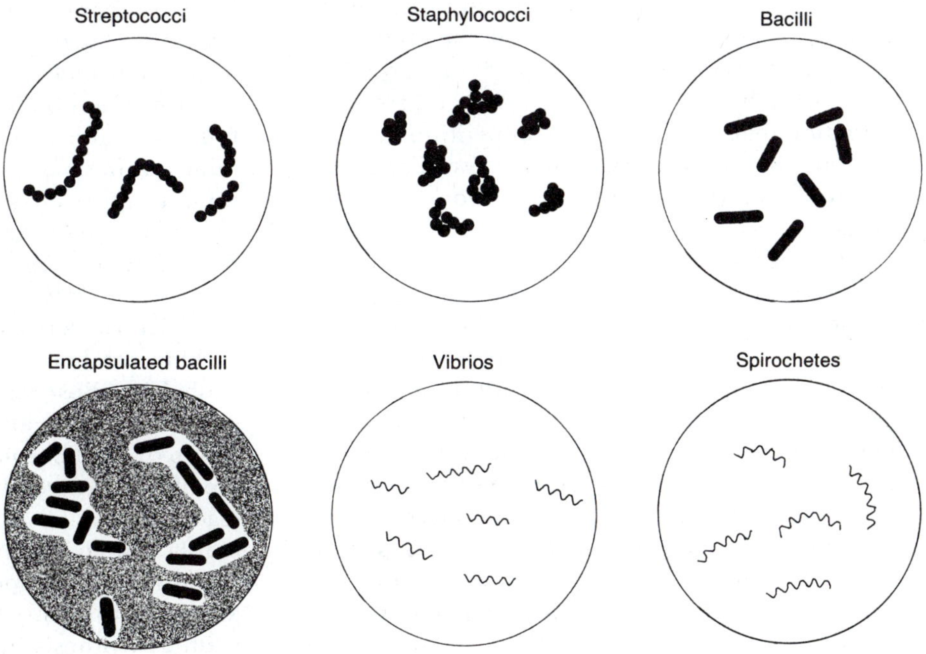

Figure 47–3
Classification of bacteria by shape and appearance.

Table 47-1
Gram Response of Bacteria

Microorganism	Gram response
Cocci	
Diplococcus pneumoniae	Positive
Staphylococcus	Positive
Streptococcus	Positive
Neisseria gonorrhoeae	Negative
Neisseria meningitidis	Negative
Bacilli and vibriones	
Bacillus anthracis	Positive
Clostridium	Positive
Corynebacterium diphtheriae	Positive
Bacteroides	Negative
Escherichia coli	Negative
Haemophilus	Negative
Pasteurella	Negative
Proteus	Negative
Pseudomonas	Negative
Shigella	Negative
Vibrio cholerae	Negative
Spirochetes	Require special stains

of the early history of civilization. Records as old as 2,500 years report the application of moldy soybean curd to dermatological infections such as carbuncles and boils. Application of plant parts or soil to infections was practiced for centuries prior to modern medicine. Louis Pasteur ushered in the era of microbiology during the second half of the nineteenth century and along with it microbial chemotherapy, noting that certain bacteria could inhibit proliferation of other bacteria. Pasteur recognized from his observation that the concept of competition between life forms disclosed by Darwin for the higher life forms applied with equal force to the world of microorganisms.

The modern era of antimicrobial chemotherapy began in 1936 with the introduction of the first sulfonamide. The purification of penicillin in the 1940s opened up what is now called the "golden age of miracle-drugs." From the early, serendipitous beginnings, the business of developing antibiotics has become a large-scale, methodical, and very lucrative enterprise. Dozens of useful agents are now available to clinical practice. Yet, in spite of the successes, the range of opportunities for further progress is enormous. Many infectious processes remain untreatable, especially infections involving viruses and prions. Mycobacteria continue to present special problems for therapy as well. Adverse effects occur frequently with use of antimicrobial drugs and the development of resistant organisms necessitates a continuing search for new and increasingly effective agents. Undoubtedly, the field of antimicrobial chemotherapy will continue to exhibit rapid development.

Early antimicrobial drugs, with the exception of the sulfonamides, were obtained from natural sources such as fungi and bacteria. The term **antibiotic** refers to such naturally occurring antimicrobial drugs — chemicals produced by microorganisms that act upon other microorganisms. Most antibiotics have been derived from actinomycetes, an order exhibiting features of both fungi and bacteria. Streptomycin is an example of a drug obtained from a member of this order. Some antibiotics, including penicillin and the cephalosporins, have been derived from true fungi and a smaller fraction from bacteria. Many of the antimicrobial drugs used today are still derived from such natural sources, but many others are synthetic or semisynthetic. In 1983, 43 of the 200 most widely prescribed drugs were antimicrobial agents; all but 5 of these were antibacterial drugs. An even dozen were penicillins, 3 were cephalosporins, 7 were tetracyclines, 8 were macrolides, 5 sulfonamides with or without trimethoprim, and 4 were urinary tract antibacterial agents.

Mechanisms and Effects Antimicrobial drugs that destroy bacteria are said to be **bactericidal;** those that merely inhibit growth of the microbes are **bacteriostatic.** Most agents serve to limit proliferation of the bacterial colony until the body's own defense mechanisms can cope with the intruder. Some agents are bacteriostatic at a moderate dose and bactericidal at higher doses.

Antimicrobials act against bacteria by one of four mechanisms (Table 47-2). (1) Some agents inhibit synthesis of the cell wall of bacteria, either by inhibiting the enzymes involved in synthesis of cell wall components or by activating enzymes that break the wall down. The denuded bacteria become vulnerable, are unable to replicate, and ultimately burst. Antibacterial agents that operate by this mechanism include the beta-lactam antibiotics (penicillins and cephalosporins), vancomycin (Vancocin), bacitracin, cycloserine (Seromycin), and ristocetin. (2) Another group of antimicrobial drugs acts directly on the cell membrane, increasing membrane permeability and leading ultimately to cell lysis. This category includes amphotericin B (Fungizone), nystatin (Mycostatin), polymyxin (Aerosporin), and colistin (Coly-Mycin M). (3) A third mechanism is the interference with protein synthesis in susceptible bacterial cells. This category subsumes at least three distinct mechanisms

Table 47–2
Mechanisms of Antibacterial Drugs

Mechanism	Principally bacteriostatic		Principally bactericidal
Inhibit cell wall synthesis			Penicillins
			Cephalosporins
			Vancomycin
			Isoniazid (?)
			Bacitracin
	Cycloserine	— or —	Cycloserine
Alter membrane permeability			Polymyxins Nystatin Amphotericin B
Inhibit protein synthesis			
Inhibition of transcription	Novobiocin		Rifampin
	Nalidixic acid		
	Cinoxacin		
Binding to 30S ribosomal subunit	Tetracyclines		
	Spectinomycin		
	Aminoglycosides (low concentrations)	— or —	Aminoglycosides (high concentrations)
	Viomycin		
	Capreomycin		
Binding to 50S ribosomal subunit	Chloramphenicol		
	Macrolides		
	Lincosamides		
Antimetabolites	Sulfonamides		
	Sulfones		
	Trimethoprim		
	Ethambutol		
	PAS		
Unknown	Ethionamide		Pyrazinamide

at the molecular level (Table 47–2). (4) The fourth group of drugs act as antimetabolites, inhibiting one or another metabolic step within the bacterial cell. Drugs acting in this way include the sulfonamides, trimethoprim (Proloprim), para-aminosalicylate (Teebacin), and ethambutol (Myambutol).

Pharmacokinetics The usual aim in antimicrobial therapy is to achieve a drug concentration at the site of infection that is several times the minimum inhibitory concentration (MIC) for the microorganism in question. Achieving this goal depends upon pharmacokinetic factors, including absorption, penetration of distribution barriers, protein binding, renal excretion, and liver metabolism. Oral administration is usually the preferred route if the patient is able to receive oral therapy, if an effective serum concentration can be achieved, and if gastrointestinal irritation from the drug is not excessive. Some antimicrobial agents — including the aminoglycosides, polymyxins, polyenes (amphotericin B and nystatin), and acid-labile penicillins (methicillin and carbenicillin) — are ineffective when taken orally. Even when a drug is orally effective, intravenous therapy may be preferred when an infection is sufficiently serious that adequate plasma concentrations must be achieved with certainty and promptly. *Care must be taken when administering antimicrobial drugs intravenously to ensure that the agents are properly reconstituted, administered in an appropriate intravenous fluid vehicle, used only while fresh, and not mixed with incompatible electrolytes, vitamins, or other drugs.* Sulfonamides, penicillins, tetracyclines, methicillin, kanamycin, and vancomycin are incompatible with multivitamin solutions or with heparin. Tetracyclines are incompatible with alkaline solution or divalent cations. Methicillin and carbenicillin are acid-labile and therefore incompatible with acid media. Penicillin is hydrolyzed in alkaline carbohydrate solutions. Kanamycin and vancomycin are inactivated by sodium bicarbonate. Methicillin should not be mixed with kanamycin or tetracyclines. Cephalothin is incompatible with polymyxins, tetracyclines, kanamycin, calcium, or heparin; it is also ineffective when pH deviates significantly from neutrality in either direction.

Many of the antibacterial drugs are polar and do not readily cross the blood-brain barrier under normal circumstances, achieving concentrations in the brain that are only 1–5% of plasma values. This includes penicillins, cephalosporins, and ampicillin. However, in meningitis, the integrity of the blood-brain barrier is generally compromised, allowing greater than normal penetration of these and other drugs. Chloramphenicol (Chloromycetin) crosses the blood-brain barrier readily in any case.

Many of the antibacterial drugs reach effective (and for some, potentially toxic) concentrations in the fetus when administered to a woman during pregnancy. Penicillins, cephalosporins, sulfonamides, tetracyclines, lincomycin (Lincocin), chloramphenicol (Chloromycetin), streptomycin, and isoniazid (Laniazid, Nydrazid) readily pass the placental barrier. Of these, tetracyclines, chloramphenicol, and streptomycin are established teratogens and are contraindicated during pregnancy. Many antibiotics are contraindicated in nursing mothers because they appear in breast milk in substantial amounts and have been reported to result in adverse effects in nursing infants. Included in this category are chloramphenicol, sulfonamides, streptomycin, and tetracyclines. Another group of antibiotics may be used, but they necessitate close observation of the infant for possible adverse effects. In this group are erythromycin, isoniazid, kanamycin (Klebcil, Kantrex), third-generation cephalosporins, and penicillin G and V. Antibiotics that either are not excreted in the milk or that appear in small amounts without apparent clinical significance are first- and second-generation cephalosporins, oxacillin (Bactocill, Prostaphlin), and ampicillin (Omniphen).

Most antimicrobial drugs are eliminated primarily by renal excretion. Renal insufficiency requires caution in using such agents, especially since toxicity of antimicrobial agents is often directed toward the kidney. Special care is required with use of aminoglycosides, polymyxins, vancomycin (Vancocin), and flucytosine (Ancobon) since these are eliminated exclusively by the kidneys. Cephalosporins, penicillins, trimethoprim (Proloprim), sulfonamides, nitrofurantoin (Furatantin), most tetracyclines, and chloroquine (Aralen) are other drugs eliminated mainly by renal excretion. Tetracyclines may aggravate uremia associated with renal insufficiency because they are catabolic. Neonates, the elderly, and clients with impaired renal function should receive lower doses of those antibiotics that are excreted by the kidneys and should be monitored with extra care for signs of toxicity.

The minority of antibacterial drugs that are eliminated mainly by liver metabolism must be used with caution in patients with impaired hepatic function. Dosage adjustments are typically required for chloramphenicol, clindamycin (Cleocin), lincomycin (Lincocin), rifampin (Rifadin), isoniazid (Nydrazid), and erythromycin (Ilotycin) in patients with liver diseases, and in the elderly, or in neonates.

Many of the antibacterial preparations have a limited shelf-life and lose potency as they age. *Expiration dates should be checked on all medications to be used, especially those in reconstituted solutions. Nurses should counsel clients to dispose of any unused antimicrobial medications and to avoid the temptation to economize by hoarding such medications.*

Resistance and Antibacterial Therapy

Resistance

Antibacterial therapy is complicated by the fact that many strains of bacteria are resistant to various antibacterial drugs. The resistance of a bacterial strain to a drug may be inherent or acquired. Most gram-negative bacteria, for example, are inherently resistant to penicillin G. Their external membranes provide a barrier to drug penetration and a periplasmic space for storage of an enzyme called **penicillinase** that metabolizes penicillin G. Bacteria often possess enzymes capable of metabolizing other antimicrobial drugs. The production of these enzymes may be increased by prolonged contact of the bacteria with the drug substrate. Presence of a capsule or slime layer or alterations in cell membrane structure may prevent penetration of the drug in some bacteria. Or the binding sites to which the drug attaches may decrease in number.

The rapid rate of reproduction of bacterial cells permits relatively rapid evolutionary shifts in genetic composition. If in a population of bacterial cells, a few cells possess genetic characteristics that make them resistant to a given antimicrobial drug, these hardy cells will survive in the presence of the drug and their descendants will form a relatively resistant strain. The development of resistant strains as a result of this process has occurred repeatedly in the less than 50 years of antimicrobial drug therapy. When a bacterial strain develops resistance to a particular antimicrobial drug, it is likely that **cross-resistance** will occur to other closely related anti-infective agents. Resistance can be transferred between bacterial cells during bacterial conjugation or by the intercession of bacteriophages that transfer bacterial DNA from one bacterial cell to another.

Choosing the Antibacterial Agent

Since no one drug is effective against all strains of bacteria, an important part of rational antimicrobial chemotherapy is determination of the infecting microorganism. Ideally, the organism is identified by routine laboratory tests, including microscopic examination and Gram staining. Identification of the organism allows the clinician to select a drug to which the particular bacterium is not inherently resistant. Whether or not the organism can be clearly identified, its sensitivity to various antibacterial drugs will need to be determined by culturing it in media in petri dishes. Filter disks impregnated with commonly used antimicrobial drugs in standardized concentrations are placed in the culture media and the relative abilities of the various agents to inhibit growth of the microorganism are noted. The results provide a rational basis for drug selection.

Often a physician will initiate treatment before obtaining results from a culture. The physician makes assumptions about the most likely cause of the infection. Such assumptions are often guided by awareness of local epidemiological events. A broad-spectrum drug, one effective against a wide variety of strains, is usually selected. Even when therapy is initiated in this way, cultures are required to confirm or correct the preliminary judgment. Prescription of antibiotics without determination of the causative agent, either before or following initiation of drug treatment, is unsound medical practice. Once drug therapy is initiated, the appropriateness of the drug selection needs to be verified by careful monitoring of the client's response. *The nurse, the client, and in many cases family members need to assess the individual for evidence of beneficial results.*

Although there are many exceptions, a general guideline to the susceptibility of organisms to various antimicrobial drugs can be described in relation to Gram staining. Penicillin G and other narrow-spectrum penicillins, erythromycin, lincomycin, clindamycin, vancomycin, and bacitracin are effective mainly against gram-positive cocci and bacilli. Aminoglycosides and polymyxins act mainly on aerobic gram-negative bacilli. Broad-spectrum penicillins, cephalosporins, sulfonamides, trimethoprim, tetracyclines, and chloramphenicol are widely effective against gram-negative and gram-positive species alike. The agents most effective against the various pathogenic bacteria are summarized in Table 47–3.

Use of Antimicrobial Drug Combinations

Combinations of antimicrobial agents are frequently employed, especially when there is more than one microorganism involved and the organisms exhibit different drug susceptibilities. The requirement for determining drug sensitivities should not be relaxed when multidrug regimens are anticipated. Use of multidrug regimens against a single infecting organism has the advantage of retarding the development of resistance. There is little likelihood that a given cell will simultaneously possess characteristics affording it resistance against two drugs of differing mechanisms. Multidrug therapy may also be indicated when undertaking rapid and vigorous treatment of life-threatening infections of unknown etiology.

One advantage of combination drug therapy may be a reduction in side effects. When more than one drug is used, each drug may be given at a dose that is low enough to minimize severity of adverse effects. In some cases, however, combination treatment can increase the risk of adverse reactions — especially allergic reactions, which occur with an intensity that is not very closely related to dose — simply because it increases the number of drugs the client is exposed to. The risk of superinfections is greater when two or more drugs are given.

For purposes of matching drugs for simultaneous use, antibacterial agents can be grouped into two sets. Penicillins, aminoglycosides, bacitracin, and polymyxins can be used effectively together to provide increased antibacterial activity. Sulfonamides, trimethoprim, tetracyclines, chloramphenicol, erythromycin, and novobiocin (Albamycin) can also be used in pairs to good effect. Simultaneous use of one drug from each of these groupings is usually not of value and may actually inhibit therapeutic benefit.

Common Misuses

Antibacterial drugs are among the most commonly misused clinical agents. This misuse has implications for both individual therapy and for society collectively. The frequent offenses include (1) failure to match the drug to the specific invading agent, (2) use of drugs for infections that do not respond to any available drugs, (3) treatment of symptoms of indeterminate origin, such as fever, (4) improper dosage

Table 47–3
Primary and Secondary Drug Selections for Principal Bacterial Infections

Pathogenic organisms	Disease(s) produced	Primary choices	Alternative choices
Gram-positive cocci			
Staphylococcus aureus	Abscesses, bacteremia, cellulitis, endocarditis, food poisoning, furunculosis, impetigo, meningitis, osteomyelitis, pneumonia, septicemia		
Not penicillinase producing		Penicillin G	Cephalosporins Vancomycin Clindamycin
Pencillinase producing		A penicillinase-resistant penicillin	Cephalsoporins Vancomycin
Staphylococcus epidermidis	Carbuncles, furuncles, toxic epidermal necrolysis, septicemia		
Not penicillinase producing		Penicillin	
Penicillinase producing		A penicillinase-resistant penicillin	
Streptococcus agalactiae (beta-type, group B)	Bacteremia, septicemia (especially in neonates)	Ampicillin Penicillin G	Aminoglycosides Cephalosporins Chloramphenicol Erythromycin
Streptococcus faecalis	Endocarditis, bacteremia, urinary tract infection	Ampicillin Penicillin G with an aminoglycoside	Vancomycin
Streptococcus penumoniae	Pneumonia, meningitis, otitis, sinusitis, arthritis, bacteremia	Penicillin G	Cephalosporins Erythromycin Chloramphenicol Clindamycin
Streptococcus pyogenes (beta-type, group A)	Scarlet fever, rheumatic fever, erysipelas, pharyngitis, impetigo, otitis, sinusitis, pneumonia, bacteremia, cellulitis	Penicillin G Penicillin V	Cephalosporins Erythromycin Vancomycin
Streptococcus viridans	Bacterial endocarditis	Penicillin	Erythromycin Clindamycin
Peptostreptococcus	Bacteremia, endocarditis, abscesses, sinusitis	Penicillin G	Cephalosporins Clindamycin Chloramphenicol Erythromycin
Gram-positive bacilli			
Bacillus anthracis	Anthrax	Penicillin G	Erythromycin Tetracyclines Cephalosporins Choloramphenicol
Clostridium botulinum	Botulism	Penicillin G	Chloramphenicol Cephalosporins Clindamycin
Clostridium perfringens	Gas gangrene	Penicillin G	Chloramphenicol Cephalosporins Clindamycin
Clostridium tetani	Tetanus	Penicillin G	Tetracyclines Erythromycin
Corynebacterium diphtheriae	Diphtheria	Penicillin G	Erythromycin Cephalosporins Rifampin
Listeria monocytogenes	Meningitis, bacteremia, endocarditis	Ampicillin	Aminoglycosides Chloramphenicol Erythromycin Tetracycline

Table 47–3
Primary and Secondary Drug Selections for Principal Bacterial Infections (*continued*)

Pathogenic organisms	Disease(s) produced	Primary choices	Alternative choices
Gram-negative cocci			
Neisseria gonorrhoeae	Gonorrhea	Ampicillin Amoxicillin Penicillin G Tetracycline Streptomycin	Erythromcyin Spectinomycin Cefoxitin Trimethoprim-sulfamethoxazole
Neisseria meningitidis	Meningitis, pneumonia	Penicillin G	Chloramphenicol
Streptococcus moniliformis	Rat-bite fever	Penicillin	
Gram-negative bacilli and vibriones			
Acinetobacter	Bacteremia, nosocomial infections	Gentamicin	Amikacin Cefoxitin
Bacteroides fragilis	Abscesses of brain, lung, or abdomen	Chloramphenicol Clindamycin	Carbenicillin Ticarcillin Metronidazole Penicillin G Cefoxitin
Bordetella pertussis	Whooping cough	Erythromycin	
Burcella	Brucellosis	Tetracyclines Streptomycin	Chloramphenicol Trimethoprim-sulfamethoxazole
Calymmatobacterium granulomatis	Granuloma inguinale	Tetracycline	Streptomycin
Enterobacter aerogenes	Pneumonia, urinary tract infection, wound infections	Second-generation cephalosporins Gentamicin Tobramycin	Carbenicillin Ticarcillin
Escherichia coli	Urinary tract infections, septicemia, respiratory infections, peritonitis	Ampicillin Sulfonamides Trimethoprim-sulfamethoxazole	Cephalosporins Tetracyclines Nitrofurantoin
Haemophilus ducreyi	Chancroid	Tetracyclines	Sulfonamides Streptomycin
Haemophilus influenzae	Respiratory infections, meningitis, otitis, sinusitis	Amoxicillin Ampicillin Chloramphenicol	Trimethoprim-sulfamethoxazole Second generation cephalosporins
Klebsiella penumoniae	Pneumonia, urinary tract infections, septicemia	Cephalosporins	Gentamicin Tobramycin Chloramphenicol
Legionella pneumophila	Legionnaires' disease	Erythromycin	Rifampin
Pasteurella multocida	Animal bite wound infections, abscesses, bacteremia, meningitis	Penicillin G	Tetracyclines
Proteus mirabilis	Urinary tract infections, other infections	Ampicillin Gentamicin Tobramycin	Cephalosporins
Proteus-indole sensitive Morganella marganii, Proteus vulgaris, Providencia rettgeri	Urinary tract infection	Gentamicin Tobramycin	Carbenicillin Ticarcillin Cefoxitin
Pseudomonas aeruginosa	Urinary tract infections, pneumonia, burn-wound infection, septicemia	Carbenicillin Ticarcillin	Gentamicin Tobramycin

(continued)

Table 47–3
Primary and Secondary Drug Selections for Principal Bacterial Infections (*continued*)

Pathogenic organisms	Disease(s) produced	Primary choices	Alternative choices
Pseudomonas mallei	Glanders	Streptomycin and tetracycline	Chloramphenicol
Pseudomonas pseudomallei	Melioidosis	Tetracycline and chloramphenicol	Trimethoprim-sulfamethoxazole
Salmonella	Typhoid	Ampicillin Chloramphenicol	Trimethoprim-sulfamethoxazole
	Food poisoning	None	
Serratia	Nosocomial infections	Gentamicin	Amikacin Cefoxitin
Shigella dysenteriae	Bacillary dysentery	Ampicillin Trimethoprim-sulfamethoxazole	Chloramphenicol
Vibrio cholerae	Cholera	Tetracycline	Trimethoprim-sulfamentoxazole Chloramphenicol
Yersinia pestis	Bubonic plague	Streptomycin	Tetracyclines Chloramphenicol
Mycobacteria			
Mycobacterium leprae	Leprosy	Sulfones Rifampin	Clofazimine Amithiozone
Mycobacterium tuberculosis	Tuberculosis	Isoniazid with rifampin	Isoniazid with rifampin and ethambutol or streptomycin
Spirochetes			
Borrelia burgdorferi	Lyme disease	Penicillins Tetracycline	Erythromycin
Leptospira	Meningitis	Penicillin G	Tetracycline
Treponema pallidum	Syphilis	Penicillin G	Tetracyclines
Treponema pertenue	Yaws	Penicillin G	Tetracyclines
Actinomycetes			
Actinomyces israelii	Lesions	Penicillin G	Tetracycline Cephalosporins Chloramphenicol
Nocardia	Lesions	Sulfonamides Ampicillin	Minocycline Tetracycline Cycloserine Trimethoprim-sulfamethoxazole
Primitive bacteria			
Chlamydia psittaci	Psittacosis (parrot fever)	Tetracyclines	Chloramphenicol
Chlamydia trachomatis	Trachoma	Tetracyclines Sulfonamides	Erythromycin Chloramphenicol
Mycoplasma pneumoniae	Atypical pneumonia	Erythromycin Tetracyclines	
Rickettsia prowazeckii	Epidemic typhus	Chloramphenicol Tetracyclines	
Rickettsia rickettsii	Rocky Mountain spotted fever	Chloramphenicol Tetracyclines	
Rickettsia typhi	Endemic typhus	Chloramphenicol Tetracyclines	

or duration of treatment, and (5) general, or broad-spectrum, prophylaxis. The result for the individual is prolonged illness or unnecessary risk of adverse effects. The risk for society is to encourage the development of resistant strains of bacteria.

An exceptional feature of antimicrobial drug therapy is that errors of dose and duration are usually in the direction of too little for too short a time period. When antimicrobial drugs are used at doses that fail to achieve adequately inhibitory concentrations at the site of infection or when treatment is prematurely discontinued, there is a substantial risk that there will be too many surviving organisms for the host's defenses to handle successfully. This is especially likely to occur if the drug is merely bacteriostatic. Infection that has been arrested may reestablish itself, and the surviving cells will be those most resistant to the improperly employed drug as well as to the host defenses. If these survivors are allowed to reestablish themselves and proliferate, the resurgent infection is likely to be more resistant to treatment than the original one.

The nurse can play an important role in assuring that antimicrobial chemotherapy is appropriately vigorous and not terminated prematurely. *The nurse should assure that the client understands that antimicrobial chemotherapy is conducted (with rare exceptions) around the clock, day and night. The nurse should carefully explain to each client receiving antibiotics the importance of completing the full course of therapy regardless of how quickly annoying manifestations subside, unless significant side effects occur.* Antimicrobial drug therapy is usually continued for 10–14 days. Symptoms should be absent for at least 2–3 days before withdrawing the drugs.

Use of residual antimicrobial drugs from old prescriptions provides no benefit and entails definite risks. *Clients should be instructed to discard leftover medications and not to give any medications to friends or relatives with similar or different symptoms. Nurses are responsible for teaching clients the danger of self-medication with systemic antimicrobial drugs.*

Most lay people do not understand that the familiar antibiotic drugs are mainly effective against bacterial infections and have no value in viral infections. *Nurses may need to instruct clients concerning why an antibiotic drug has not been prescribed when the physician makes such a decision.*

Prophylactic use of antimicrobial drugs is seldom justified. An exception is protection of individuals who are at identifiable risk of infection because of immune deficiency, such as those with acquired immune deficiency syndrome (AIDS), and those receiving antineoplastic agents. Broad-spectrum prophylaxis following surgical procedures is generally no longer accepted as good practice, but prophylaxis against predictable infectious complications of certain procedures is generally accepted. For example, people with valvular heart disease are frequently given penicillin during dental procedures as a precaution against endocarditis induced by *Streptococcus viridans*. Penicillin is used for the same purpose in healthy individuals following oral surgery and as prophylaxis against *Pneumococcus* in clients undergoing splenectomy. Individuals with chronic bronchitis may require prophylactic tetracycline or ampicillin during epidemics of bacterial influenza or pneumonia to guard against exacerbation of airway distress. Antibiotics are sometimes employed prophylactically to guard against sepsis in clients who have suffered penetrating wounds. Prophylactic use of antimicrobial drugs affords little protection but entails the usual adversities of antimicrobial drug therapy. Disturbance of the commensal flora is likely to result in superinfection. Allergic reactions and other toxic effects may occur.

Side Effects Common to Many Antibacterial Drugs

Although some side effects are unique to specific antibacterial drugs, others occur commonly and still others are shared by all antimicrobial agents. (Unique side effects will be considered later for each drug group.) Two types of side effects are nearly universal risks when anti-infective agents are employed: hypersensitivity reactions and superinfection.

Hypersensitivity Reactions

Hypersensitivity reactions occur frequently, especially with parenteral administration. Reactions vary in manifestations from rash, urticaria, and pruritus to anaphylactic shock, hemolytic anemia, nephropathy, and pseudomembranous enterocolitis. The last of these, enterocolitis, is an inflammatory reaction of the bowel in which membrane-like plaques of exudate replace interstitial mucosa that has necrotized. Allergic reactions to antibiotics occur invariably upon secondary exposure to the allergy-inducing medication, but the initial exposure (sensitizing dose) may have been incidental, for example, from ingestion of cow's milk, beer, Roquefort cheese, poultry, or other foods or beverages containing an antibiotic. Many allergic reactions are predictable based on the client's previous history of drug reactions. *The nurse should question clients thoroughly regarding previous allergic reactions to drugs. Also, nurses should check if the client has a medical identification bracelet or card. The nurse should note identified drug sensitivities in each client's records and hospital chart, and a special notation must be posted on the physician's order sheet, Kardex, medication records, or other areas according to the policy of the particular institution.*

Anyone receiving a particular antimicrobial drug for the first or second time should be observed for one-half hour for signs of allergic reaction. Reddening or edema at the site of an injection is an early indication. Clients need to be taught the variety of symptoms that may indicate allergy and urged to report these promptly. Redness of the skin, itching, and skin eruptions may seem mild and may not be reported unless clients are asked to watch for these signs of allergy. Allergic symptoms normally disappear once the drug has been discontinued, although for some clients the adverse response may last for 5 or more days. *If hypersensitivity to an antimicrobial drug occurs, the nurse should be certain that the client is aware of the allergic nature of the reaction so that the drug can be avoided in the future.*

The nurse and the client should also watch for signs of anaphylaxis. Sweating, fainting, shortness of breath, irritability, cyanosis, unconsciousness, convulsions, and feelings of constriction in the chest should all be mentioned as signs of anaphylaxis to assist clients in reporting an accurate history. *When administering antimicrobial drugs, the nurse should have on hand the standard aids for treating anaphylaxis: epinephrine, diphenhydramine or another potent antihistamine, hydrocortisone, a hand tourniquet, and equipment for emergency endotracheal intubation.* Some outpatient clinics or other facilities may elect to send clients home with epinephrine or hydrocortisone and instructions on the circumstances under which these should be used. In this event, it is safest to provide the client with the telephone number of the nurse practitioner or clinical specialist and instructions to call before proceeding to use these agents, so as to assure appropriate responses to the problem.

Clients should be warned to avoid excessive exposure to sunlight, since some antimicrobials are photosensitizing. The nurse should avoid contact of antibiotics with the skin since many are known to cause contact dermatitis.

Superinfection

Superinfection, the other type of side effect that can occur with any antibacterial drug, is a significant risk. Superinfection occurs when the normal microbial flora of the body are disturbed by antimicrobial drug administration to the extent that microbes normally held in check are able to penetrate and produce tissue damage. Superinfection can occur in the intestines, mouth, sinuses, respiratory tract, genitourinary tract, or on the skin. The microflora of these orifices and surfaces are finely balanced ecosystems. In the gastrointestinal tract alone, an estimated 10^{15} cells of 400 different microbial varieties are normally found. Antimicrobial drugs disrupt the delicate balance of endogenous microbes. The result is frequently a superinfection — a new infection superimposed on the existing one under treatment. The microorganisms most likely to be responsible for superinfection are *Proteus, Staphylococci, Pseudomonas, Candida, Tinea,* and *Clostridium.* The new organism is frequently relatively drug resistant, as evidenced by its ability to flourish during antimicrobial drug therapy. The risk of superinfection is greatest when the drug employed is broad-spectrum, since these have the greatest disruptive effect on the natural flora. Extended periods of use also contribute to occurrence of superinfection. When superinfection occurs, the drug in use should be discontinued and chemotherapy initiated for the new infection.

When antibacterial drugs are being administered, the nurse should periodically examine the individual's tongue for signs of bacterial or fungal growth that would indicate superinfection. Large stools, diarrhea, or nausea may be indicative of superinfection in the lower digestive tract. Other indications include anogenital itching, vaginal discharge, glossitis, or stomatitis. *Since many clients who receive antimicrobial drugs are at home, it is important to help them learn to keep accurate records of drug responses.*

Other Side Effects Common to Many Antibacterial Drugs

Other side effects that occur commonly though not universally with antibacterial drugs include nephrotoxicity, ototoxicity, hepatotoxicity, neuromuscular blockade, gastrointestinal irritation, and hematological disorders. **Nephrotoxicity** and **ototoxicity** appear to be etiologically related phenomena since the drugs that cause one generally cause the other. This relationship is discussed in Chapter 55 and presumably occurs because the cochlear and kidney are both engaged in redistributing ions by active processes. Aminoglycosides are the antibacterial drugs most likely to cause adverse effects on the kidney and auditory apparatus. Polymyxin B, bacitracin, amphotericin, colistin, cephalosporins, rifampin, and sulfonamides are also directly nephrotoxic. Penicillins, sulfonamides, and nitrofurantoin can produce nephrotoxicity by allergic mechanisms. When nephrotoxicity does develop, there is likely to be a sharp decrease in renal excretion of the antibacterial agent as well as other drugs, possibly resulting in drug accumulation and further toxicity. *The nurse should monitor intake and output in clients receiving antibiotics that are potentially nephrotoxic, and clients who are at home should be taught the importance of observing intake* *and output ratios. Clients should be taught to report signs of hematuria such as cloudy or pink urine. If the drug is known to be potentially nephrotoxic, pretreatment evaluation should include measurement of blood urea nitrogen (BUN) and creatinine. Nursing assessment should also include evaluating the client's hearing and determining whether the client has any ringing in the ears (tinnitus) or problems with balance. If the drug to be employed is known to be ototoxic, it is wise to obtain baseline audiometry before beginning therapy and to repeat the procedure periodically thereafter.*

Hepatotoxicity is a less common toxic response to antibacterial drugs. Isoniazid (Nydrazid) can cause hepatitis. Erythromycin can cause obstructive jaundice in clients who have an allergic reaction to the drug. Tetracycline has been observed to cause fatty liver. *Observable indications of possible liver toxicity include fatigue, loss of appetite, malaise, nausea, vomiting, dark urine, yellowish skin, or scleral discoloration.*

Gastrointestinal side effects occur frequently to antibacterial drugs that are given orally for two reasons. First, many of the drugs produce a direct irritant effect on the gastrointestinal mucosa. Second, antimicrobial agents may promote gastrointestinal upset by disturbing the normal intestinal flora. *Usually, the nurse should remind clients to take oral antibiotics with a liquid or light snack to reduce the problem of gastrointestinal irritation. However, the absorption of some antibiotics is adversely affected by particular foods; tetracyclines, for example, are affected by dairy products. Clients should be instructed to avoid foods or beverages that are highly acidic if the antibiotic is acid-labile. Therefore, nurses need to review the characteristics of the drug and teach clients when it is to be given in relation to meals. The common symptoms of gastrointestinal irritation are diarrhea, nausea, vomiting, and anorexia.*

Aminoglycosides, polymyxin, and bacitracin can cause **neuromuscular blockade** that is additive to that produced by curare, hypokalemia, and drugs with local anesthetic properties. **Hematological toxicity** is not common with antibacterial drugs except in individuals with glucose-6-phosphate dehydrogenase (G6PD) deficiencies. In these individuals, penicillins, sulfonamides, chloramphenicol, nalidixic acid, and nitrofurantoin can cause hemolytic anemia. Chloramphenicol can rarely cause aplasic or iron-deficiency anemias. Whenever possible, complete blood cell counts should be conducted before therapy begins to provide a baseline against which to measure changes resulting from antibacterial agents. Sometimes antibacterial drugs contribute to a vitamin K deficiency by destroying intestinal bacteria that normally synthesize this vitamin. *Nurses should alert clients to watch for signs of increased bleeding such as an exaggerated tendency to bleed when there is a small cut.*

General Antibacterial Agents

Antibacterial drugs are grouped into families on the basis of structure and pharmacological activity. There are four major groups and several lesser groups and individual agents. The major groups are (1) the beta-lactam antibacterial drugs (including penicillins and cephalosporins), (2) the aminoglycosides, (3) tetracyclines and chloramphenicol, and (4) sulfonamides and trimethoprim. Lesser groups include the macrolides, lincosamides, and peptide antibiotics. Vancomycin and spectinomycin are miscellaneous agents not belonging to any group.

Beta-Lactam Antibacterial Drugs

Both penicillins and cephalosporins contain in their structures a four-sided carbon ring called a beta-lactam ring. For the penicillins, a second five-membered ring with one sulfur atom, called a thiazolidine ring, is fused to the beta-lactam ring. The cephalosporins also have a second ring, but it is a six-sided ring, also containing a sulfur.

The penicillins and cephalosporins are among the most important antibiotics. In 1928, Alexander Fleming, a British bacteriologist, noted that a mold that was contaminating one of his bacterial cultures inhibited the growth of bacteria in its vicinity and caused the bacterial cells to lyse. He identified the mold as *Penicillium notatum* and named the antibacterial substance **penicillin,** but after a few inconclusive experiments he dropped his work with the mold. It was not until 1939 that Howard Florey and his colleagues at Oxford University recognized the significance of Fleming's observation and began work to purify penicillin. World War II gave impetus to a joint effort by the United States and Great Britain to discover the structure of penicillin and undertake its large-scale manufacture. By the end of the war in 1945, its structure was firmly established and penicillin was being manufactured in quantities large enough to be helpful in treating battlefield wounds.

In 1941 other investigators observed that certain bacteria possessed an enzyme capable of destroying penicillin, an enzyme that they named **penicillinase.** Bacteria capable of producing this enzyme were resistant to the effects of penicillin. The researchers also noted that penicillin was much more effective against some bacteria than against others. These observations led to a concerted effort to develop new antibiotics that would be resistant to penicillinase and effective against a broader spectrum of microbes. The group of penicillin-related antibacterial drugs now includes a wide selection of semisynthetic and synthetic agents that differ in the extent to which they are absorbed, the extent to which they are protein-bound in plasma, the breadth of their antibacterial action, and their resistance to breakdown by bacterial enzymes (Table 47–4).

The beta-lactam antibiotics inhibit the synthesis of bacterial cell walls by attaching to enzymes that normally produce the peptidoglycan chains that compose the wall. The structural components of the cell walls are unable to assemble properly, and the cells become susceptible to disruption. Beta-lactam antibiotics are bacteriocidal for susceptible organisms. Some bacteria produce beta-lactamases (penicillinases or cephalosporinases) that destroy the beta-lactam ring of drugs in this class. The various drugs differ widely in their susceptibility to this enzymatic attack; moreover, the various bacterial species and strains vary widely in their ability to produce beta-lactamase enzymes.

As a class, the beta-lactam antibacterial agents are the most broadly effective and least toxic of antimicrobial drugs. The penicillins have developed in a series of steps leading to five generations of drugs differing in oral effectiveness, resistance to beta-lactamase inactivation, and breadth of antibacterial activity: (1) the original agents, penicillin G and penicillin V, (2) the penicillinase-resistant penicillins, (3)

Table 47–4
Characteristics of Penicillins

Drug	Oral effectiveness	Protein bound (%)	Beta-lactamase resistant	Broad-spectrum
First-generation penicillins				
Penicillin G (benzylpenicillin)	Some	60	No	No
Penicillin V (phenoxymethyl penicillin)	Yes	80	No	No
Penicillinase-resistant				
Isoxazolyl penicillins				
Cloxacillin	Yes	95	Yes	No
Dicloxacillin	Yes	96	Yes	No
Floxacillin	Yes	?	Yes	No
Oxacillin	Yes	90	Yes	No
6-Aminopenicillanic acid derivatives				
Methicillin	No	40	Yes	No
Nafcillin	Yes	90	Yes	No
Broad-spectrum penicillins				
Ampicillin-like				
Amoxicillin	Yes	20	No	Yes
Ampicillin	Yes	20	No	Yes
Bacampicillin	Yes	20	No	Yes
Cyclacillin	Yes	20	No	Yes
Hetacillin	Yes	20	No	Yes
Antipseudomonal				
Azlocillin	No	?	No	Yes
Carbenicillin	Yes	50	No	Yes
Mezlocillin	No	?	No	Yes
Piperacillin	No	?	No	Yes
Ticarcillin	No	45	No	Yes
Amidinopenicillin				
Amdinocillin	No	10	Yes	Yes

the ampicillin-like broad-spectrum penicillins, (4) the antipseudomonal broad-spectrum penicillins, and (5) amidinopenicillins. The cephalosporins can likewise be placed into three generations of agents.

Penicillin G and Penicillin V

Pharmacokinetics Penicillin G provides poor and variable absorption after oral administration. Under the best of circumstances, only about one-third of the administered dose is absorbed. Penicillin G is acid-labile and therefore destroyed by stomach acid. Penicillin V is absorbed more completely and more readily than penicillin G after oral administration, and is preferred for that reason for oral administration.

After parenteral administration, penicillin G produces a reliable blood level that is, however, short-lasting. Only about one-fifth the oral dose of penicillin G is required when it is given intramuscularly. Blood levels reach their peak in less than 1 hour after parenteral injection and 1–2 hours after oral administration. The aqueous suspension of penicillin G procaine provides extended absorption after intramuscular injection. A plateau plasma concentration is maintained for about 4 hours and gradually declines over the next 15–20 hours. Benzathine penicillin has an even longer effect, though peak levels of antibiotic are reduced. Absorption occurs over several weeks. After absorption, benzathine penicillin is converted by hydrolysis to penicillin G.

In the blood, penicillin G is bound 60% to plasma proteins; penicillin V is bound to a somewhat greater extent. Penicillin G distributes unevenly, having a volume of distribution equal to about 50% of the body water. It is taken up by the liver, kidney, intestines, lymph, and synovial fluid but does not penetrate into the brain or cerebral spinal fluid when the meninges are healthy. When penicillin does enter the brain, neurotoxic effects may occur, including lethargy, neuromuscular impairments, hallucinations, or seizures. Psychiatric symptoms may include anxiety, depression, or combativeness.

Penicillin is eliminated by the kidneys, by filtration (10%) and active secretion (90%). The renal secretory mechanism is the organic anion carrier. Probenecid and other organic acids can slow excretion of penicillin by competing for this pump. The rate of clearance is much less in neonates due to the immaturity of renal function.

Clinical Indications Penicillin G (also called benzylpenicillin) is still considered the drug of choice for a wide range of bacterial infections (Table 47–3). Penicillin G and penicillin V (the phenoxymethyl derivative) have similar effectiveness against gram-positive bacteria, but penicillin V is less potent against gram-negative organisms. Penicillin G is more widely effective against gram-negative species (Table 47–5). Penicillin G and V are highly effective against *Staphylococcus* that do not produce penicillinase, but many strains of both *Staphylococcus aureus* and *Staphylococcus epidermidis* have developed resistance by producing the beta-lactamase enzyme that inactivates penicillin. Penicillin G is the drug of choice for most infections of *Streptococci,* including the α-type (*Streptococcus viridans*), the β-type, group A (*Streptococcus pyrogenes*), the β-type, group B (*Streptococcus agalactiae*), enterococci (*Streptococcus faecalis*), *Streptococcus moniliformis,* and *Streptococcus pneumoniae.* Penicillin G and V lack effectiveness against the anaerobic cocci — *Peptostreptococcus.*

Most strains of gram-positive bacilli are likewise susceptible to penicillin G and V, including *Bacillus anthracis, Clostridium, Corynebacterium,* and *Listeria monocytogenes.* Among the gram-negative bacteria, penicillin G is active against *Salmonella, Shigella, dysenteriae, Pasteurella multocida;* effective against some *Escherichia coli, Enterobacter aerogenes,* and *Proteus mirabilis;* effective only at high doses against *Bacteroides fragilis;* and ineffective against *Acinetobacter, Haemophilus influenzae,* indole-sensitive *Proteus* species, *Pseudomonas aeruginosa,* and *Serratia.* Penicillin inhibits *Actinomyces israelii* and is the initial drug of choice for most spirochete infections. Penicillins have no effectiveness against fungi, viruses, protozoa, or rickettsiae.

Adverse Effects and Contraindications The adverse effects of penicillin G and penicillin V include those that are common to all antibacterial drugs: **superinfection** and **hypersensitivity reactions.** Hypersensitivity reactions occur in as many as 5–10% of individuals given penicillin. *Before initiating therapy with a penicillin drug, every effort should be made to obtain as precise a history as possible of previous exposure and reactions to antimicrobial agents. A scratch test or intradermal test can be used to assess risk, using benzylpenicilloyl-polylysine (Pre-Pen).* Allergic reactions may occur immediately or after weeks of therapy. Cross-sensitivity between penicillins and cephalosporins occur in about 10% of sensitive individuals.

There is no evidence of teratogenicity with any of the penicillins. However, penicillin may be excreted in breast milk and can result in sensitization of nursing infants.

Sodium penicillin G and potassium penicillin G provide significant **electrolyte loads** that can be problematic in individuals with impaired renal func-

Table 47–5
Antibacterial Spectra of Penicillins and Cephalosporins

Bacterial species	Penicillin V	Penicillin G	Penicillinase resistant	Ampicillin group broad spectrum	Antipseudomonal group broad spectrum	Cephalosporins: First-generation	Cephalosporins: Second-generation	Cephalosporins: Third-generation
Gram-positive Cocci								
Staphylococcus aureus								
Not penicillinase producing	Yes	Yes*	Yes	Yes	Few	Yes	Yes	Yes
Penicillinase–producing	No	No	Yes*	No	No	Weak	Yes	Yes
Methicillan–resistant	No	No	No	No	No	No	Yes	Yes
Staphylococcus epidermidis								
Not penicillinase producing	Yes	Yes*	Yes	Yes	Yes	Yes	Yes	Yes
Penicillinase producing	No	No	Yes*	No	No	Yes	Yes	Yes
Methicillin resistant	No	No	No	No	No	Yes*	Yes	Yes
Streptococcus agalactiae (beta-type, group B)	Yes	Yes*	Yes	Yes*	Yes	Yes	Yes	Yes
Streptococcus faeclis (enterococci)	Yes	Yes*	Yes	Yes*	Yes	No	No	No
Streptococcus pneumoniae	Yes	Yes*	Yes	Yes	Weak	Yes	Yes	Yes
Streptococcus pyrogen (beta-type, group A)	Yes	Yes*	Yes	Yes	Weak	Yes	Yes	Yes
Streptococcus viridans (alpha-type)	Yes	Yes*	Yes	Yes	Yes	Yes	Yes	Yes
Peptostreptococcus (anaerobic)	No	No	No	No	Yes*	Yes	Yes	Yes
Gram-positive Bacilli								
Bacillus anthracis	Most	Most*	Most	Yes	Yes	Yes	Yes	Yes
Clostridium	Most	Most*	Most	Yes	Yes	Yes	Yes	Yes

Corynebacterium	Most	Most*	Most	Yes	Yes	Yes	Yes	Yes
Listeria monocytogenes	Yes	Yes	Yes	Yes*	Yes	Yes	Yes	Yes
Gram-negative Cocci								
Neisseria gonorrhoeae	No	Yes	Yes	Yes*	Yes	Yes	Yes	Yes
Neisseria meningitidis	No	Yes*	Yes	Yes	Yes	Yes	Yes	Yes
Streptococcus moniliformis	Yes	Yes*	Yes	Yes	Yes	Yes	Yes	Yes
Gram-negative Bacilli								
Acinetobacter	No	No	No	Few^R	Yes	No	No	No
Bacteroides fragilis	No	Weak	Weak	Very weak	Yes*	No	Yes*	Weak
Enterobacter aerogenes	No	Some	Some	Few^R	Most	No	Yes*	Yes
Escherichia coli	No	Some	Some	Yes*	Yes	Most	Yes	Yes
Haemophilus influenzae	No	No	No	Yes*	Yes	50%	Yes*	Yes
Klebsiella pneumoniae	No	No	No	Few^R	Yes*	Yes*	Yes	Yes
Pasteurella multocida	No	Yes	Yes	Yes	Yes*	No	No	No
Proteus mirabilis	No	Most	Most	Most^R	Yes*	Yes	Yes	Yes
Proteus (indole-positive)	No	No	No	Few^R	Yes*	Yes	Yes	Yes
Pseudomonas aeruginosa	No	No	No	Few^R	Yes*	No	No	Yes*
Salmonella	No	Yes	Yes	Most^{R*}	Yes	Most	Most	Most
Serratia	No	No	No	Few	Yes*	No	Yes	Yes*
Shigella dysenteriae	No	Yes	Yes	Yes*	Yes	Most	Most	Most
Actinomycetes								
Actinomyces israelii	No	Yes*	Yes	Yes	Yes	Yes	Yes	Yes
Nocardia	No	No	No	Yes*	Yes	No	No	No
Spirochetes								
Treponema	No	Yes*	Yes	Yes	Yes	?	?	?
Leptospira	No	Yes*	Yes	Yes	Yes	?	?	?

Key:
- Yes: Some or all drugs in the group are effective.
- No: Not effective.
- *: A primary drug choice for the indicated organism.
- R: Resistance has developed in some strains.
- Most: Effective against most strains.
- Weak: Weakly effective.
- Some: Effective against some strains.
- Few: Effective against a few strains.

Nursing Observations for Antibacterial Drug Therapy

THERAPEUTIC GOAL	Eliminate infection or keep infection in check until host defense mechanisms gain control.
PREADMINISTRATION ASSESSMENT	
Baseline Data	Assess infected area; assess temperature, blood pressure, pulse, respiratory rate and sounds, bowel sounds, urinary output, skin lesions, and neurological function. Review laboratory tests: cultures and sensitivity pattern of organism; urinalysis and liver function tests.
Contraindications/ Precautions	Check medical history for contraindications specific for each class of antimicrobial drugs, such as renal or hepatic failure, pregnancy or lactation, allergies, urinary or gastrointestinal obstructions, porphyria, myasthenia gravis, or hearing defects.
Potential Interactions	Check current medication regimen for oral contraceptives, other antimicrobials, and other interacting medications (specific for each class of antibacterial agents).
EVALUATION OF DRUG RESPONSE	
For Therapeutic Benefit	Watch for resolution of symptoms of infection.
For Adverse Effects	Assess for allergic reactions, gastrointestinal irritation, superinfection, liver dysfunction, and other drug-specific side effects (see Adverse Effects for each group of drugs).
For Drug Interactions	Discuss with female clients who are using oral contraceptives the possibility that antibacterial medications may diminish the effectiveness of oral contraception. Monitor for decreased effectiveness of other antimicrobial drugs, and other drug-specific interactions (see Drug Interactions for each group of drugs).
For Dietary Interactions	Assess for interaction of acidic foods with acid-labile penicillins; dairy products and antacids with tetracyclines.
For Compliance	Evaluate the client's compliance with all facets of the therapeutic regimen by careful observation, interviewing, and review of progress. Report compliance problems to the physician and act as client-advocate when changes in the therapeutic regimen seem indicated.

tion or hypertension or who are receiving cardiac glycoside treatment. *Potassium penicillin G and sodium penicillin G should not be considered interchangeable. The physician may have ordered penicillin G potassium because the client is on a sodium-restricted diet. When high doses are being used, injection of penicillin salts should be conducted slowly to reduce the risk of electrolyte imbalance.* Sodium penicillin G contains 20 mEq of sodium per million units of penicillin; potassium penicillin G contains 1.7 mEq of potassium and 0.33 mEq of sodium per million units.

Other adverse effects of penicillins include **gastrointestinal symptoms** (diarrhea, flatulence, epigastric distress, vomiting, stomatitis, enterocolitis), **liver reactions** (cholestatic or nonspecific hepatitis), **hematological reactions** (anemia, granulocytopenia), and **renal damage** (interstitial nephritis). *Clients receiving high parenteral doses should have intake and output monitored. Any evidence of renal problems, such as oliguria, hematuria, or changes in the intake-output ratio are important. Dehydration increases the concentration of drug in the kidney and can contribute to renal irritation and damage. Neonates, young infants, elderly, debilitated clients, those with impaired renal function, and those receiving high doses of penicillin should be observed especially closely for signs of toxicity. These clients should be given renal, hepatic, and hematological examinations at regular intervals.*

Neuromuscular irritability occurs in some individuals, most often in those receiving in excess of 20 million units per day or those with renal impairment, hyponatremia, or underlying disease of the central nervous system (such as myasthenia gravis or epilepsy). *It is important that these clients know the precautions to take to prevent seizure.* Usually penicillin-induced seizures begin with twitching of the face and extremities.

Drug Interactions Antacids tend to delay absorption of oral penicillins, but they may also protect penicillin from being destroyed by gastric acids increasing the overall bioavailability of the drug.

Preparations and Administration *Oral penicillin G should be taken on an empty stomach.* When injected, penicillin G benzathine is a repository form providing extended action, but the blood levels obtained are low. Penicillin G procaine is another repository form for injection. It provides a 12-hour duration of action. Penicillin V has the advantage of greater stability in the presence of acid, providing more reliable oral absorption. Its disadvantage is its weaker activity against gram-negative organisms.

Penicillin tablets and dry powders for reconstitution are stored in tightly closed containers at room temperature and should be protected from excessive heat. Oral suspensions or syrups and injection solutions are stable for 2 weeks under refrigeration or for 24 hours at room temperature.

Penicillin G benzathine (Bicillin)
Tablets, dosage units for IM injection (Bicillin L-A, Permapen)

Penicillin G potassium
Tablets, powder for oral solutions
Recommended Doses: From 300,000 to 1,200,000 units PO daily in adults, depending on the identity of the microorganism being treated. Seven to 14 days of treatment is common.

Penicillin G procaine
Injection units, combination with penicillin G benzathine
Recommended Doses: 300,000 units IM once or twice daily.

Penicillin G (aqueous)
Powder for injection
Recommended Doses: Up to 100,000 units/ml can be given IM; up to 20 million units (total) can be given by continuous IV infusion.

Penicillin V (phenoxymethyl penicillin)
Tablets, powder for oral suspensions

Penicillin V potassium
Tablets, powder for oral suspensions

Penicillinase-Resistant Penicillins

The penicillinase-resistant penicillins include six drugs. Two of these, methicillin and nafcillin, are derivatives of 6-aminopenicillanic acid. The other four are isoxazolyl penicillins: cloxacillin (Tegopen, Cloxapen), dicloxacillin (Dynapen and others), oxacillin (Prostaphlin, Bactocill), and floxacillin.

Pharmacokinetics The isoxazolyl drugs resist acid and thus are well absorbed after oral administration. Methicillin is completely inactivated by gastric acid and nafcillin is inactivated to a variable extent. Methicillin (Azapen, Celbenin, Staphcillin) is marketed therefore only for parenteral use; nafcillin (Unipen, Nafcil) is available for both parenteral and oral applications, but the oral route is not recommended.

Clinical Indications The most important use of drugs in this group is for treatment of penicillinase-producing strains of *Staphylococcus aureus* and *Staphylococcus epidermidis.* In recent years, some strains have begun to develop resistance to drugs in this group as well; such strains are designated as **methicillin-resistant,** but the term implies resistance to any drug in the methicillin group. Moreover, in the case of *Staphylococcus aureus,* methicillin-resistant strains are often resistant to first-generation cephalosporins, aminoglycosides, erythromycin, clindamycin, and tetracyclines. Vancomycin and the second- and third-generation cephalosporins are the drugs of choice for strains resistant to methicillin. Cephalosporins are often effective against methicillin-resistant strains of *Staphylococcus epidermidis.*

Preparations and Administration Methicillin contains 3 mEq of sodium per gram. High doses of methicillin cause interstitial nephritis more frequently than do other penicillins. *Methicillin solutions are stable for 24 hours at room temperature or 4 days under refrigeration.* It is always administered intramuscularly or intravenously. Nafcillin provides a sodium load of 3 mEq/g. The sodium of oxacillin sodium is about 3 mEq/g. Floxacillin is not marketed in the United States.

Cloxacillin sodium (Tegopen, Cloxapen, and generic)
Capsules, powder for oral solutions
Recommended Doses: For mild infections in adults or children over 20 kg, 250 mg PO every 6 hours. For severe infections, the dose is doubled. For children under 20 kg, 50–100 mg/kg/day PO in 4 equal doses.

Dicloxacillin sodium (Dynapen, Dycill, Veracillin, Pathocil)
Tablets, powder for oral solutions
Recommended Doses: For adults and children over 40 kg, 250 mg PO every 6 hours. For smaller children, 25 mg/kg/day PO in 4 divided doses at 6-hour intervals.

Nursing Diagnoses and Interventions for Antibacterial Drug Therapy

Nursing Diagnoses	*Related Interventions*
TO MINIMIZE DRUG SIDE EFFECTS OR INTERACTIONS	
Alteration in bowel elimination with penicillins: diarrhea	Advise clients to notify the physician if diarrhea occurs.
Alteration in comfort related to gastrointestinal irritation when macrolides, tetracyclines, or chloramphenicol are used	Instruct the client about foods that can and cannot be taken with the medication to reduce irritation.
Alteration in urinary elimination patterns with sulfonamides	Force fluids to maintain dilute urine to minimize risk of crystals.
Alteration in respiratory function related to allergic reaction to antibacterial drugs	Evaluate drug history for indication of allergies; observe client after first dose; advise client to immediately report rash or difficulty breathing.
TO ENSURE SAFE AND EFFICACIOUS DRUG USE	
Knowledge deficit related to regimen	Explain the nature of the infectious condition, the rationale for use of the antibacterial agent, and expected therapeutic response.
	Teach the client how to determine the proper dose, when to administer the drug, and when to take the drug in relation to food intake.
	Advise the client to complete the full course of therapy even though symptoms of infection will usually resolve before the last dose is scheduled to be taken.
	Provide the client with a list of adverse effects, drug-drug interactions and drug-food interactions for each drug in the regimen and advise the client what to do if any of these occur.
	Explain any storage requirements such as protection from light (sulfonamides and tetracyclines). Warn clients to discard any unused antimicrobials and not to employ leftover medications.

Methicillin sodium (Azapen, Celbenin, Staphcillin)
Powder for injections, piggyback units, bulk package

Nafcillin sodium (Unipen and Nafcil)
Capsules, tablets, powder for oral solutions, powder for injection

Oxacillin sodium (Prostaphlin, Bactocill)
Capsules, powder for oral solutions, powder for injection solutions
Recommended Doses: For adults, 500 mg PO, qid.

Ampicillin-like Broad-Spectrum Penicillins
Prototypical of the broad-spectrum penicillins is ampicillin. Other members of this group include amoxicillin (many brands), bacampicillin (Spectrobid), cyclacillin (Cyclapen-W), and hetacillin (Versapen).

Clinical Indications The agents of this group are broad-spectrum but not penicillinase-resistant, and resistance to their action is a commonplace phenomenon. Their spectrum of activity is less broad today than when they were first introduced. Drugs in this group are generally less effective than penicillin against penicillin-sensitive organisms and should thus not be employed as routine substitutes for penicillin. The most important gains in activity with this class relate to certain gram-negative species of bacteria. Ampicillin or other members of this group are often the first choices for infections due to *Escher-*

ichia coli, Haemophilus influenzae, Salmonella, Neisseria gonorrhoeae, and *Shigella dysenteriae.* Ampicillin was once widely effective against *Acinetobacter, Enterobacter aerogenes, Klebsiella pneumoniae,* indole-sensitive *Proteus* varieties, and *Pseudomonas aeruginosa,* but most strains of these organisms are now resistant.

Preparations and Administration All drugs in this group are available in oral formulations; only ampicillin is used parenterally. *After reconstitution, ampicillin oral solutions are stable for 14 days if refrigerated.* Ampicillin can be given intravenously by slow direct injection, by drip, or piggyback. *The nurse should be careful when administering ampicillin by IV infusion that the infusion solution is one that is compatible with the drug.* The sodium load of this preparation is approximately 3 mEq/g. Ampicillin may be administered with probenecid (Benemid) to extend its duration of action, or with sulbactam, a β-lactamase inhibitor, to increase its activity against penicillinase-producing bacteria. The latter combination was marketed in 1987 as Unasyn. Ampicillin undergoes enterohepatic recycling and is excreted in the bile as well as by the kidney. Ampicillin has been noted to cause false-positive glucose urine tests if Benedict's, Clinitest, or Fehling's solutions are used. *Nurses should advise clients with diabetes receiving ampicillin to use clinistix or Tes-Tape to test for glucosuria.*

Amoxicillin is better absorbed than is ampicillin and food does not impair its absorption. Ampicillin and amoxicillin (Amoxil) were the most widely prescribed penicillin preparations in 1983. Amoxil was among the top 10 prescription drugs. In 1984 amoxicillin was marketed in a combination with potassium clavulanate (Augmentin). Clavulanic acid is a weak beta-lactam agent structurally related to the penicillins. Its chief value is that it binds irreversibly to beta-lactamase enzymes to protect amoxicillin from breakdown. Augmentin has been approved for use in lower respiratory tract infections caused by beta-lactamase producing strains of *Haemophilus influenzae;* for otitis media or sinusitis caused by beta-lactamase producing strains of *Branhamella catarrhalis* and *Haemophilus influenzae;* for cutaneous infections caused by beta-lactamase-producing *Staphylococcus aureus, E. coli,* or *Klebsiella* species; and urinary tract infections caused by beta-lactamase-producing strains of *E. coli, Klebsiella* species, or *Enterobacter* species.

Hetacillin (Versapen) and bacampacillin (Spectrobid) are prodrugs, being hydrolyzed to ampicillin in the body. Absorption of hetacillin is altered by concurrent food administration; hetacillin should generally be taken 1–2 hours before meals. An advantage of bacampicillin is that it can be given twice daily as compared to the 3 times required for amoxicillin or 4 times for ampicillin.

Amoxicillin (Amoxil, Larotid, Trimox, Utimox, Wymox, and others)
Capsules, chewable tablets, powder for oral suspensions, combination tablets with potassium clavulanate (Augmentin), combination oral suspension with clavulanic acid.
Recommended Doses: For infections in adults, 250–500 mg PO of amoxicillin every 8 hours.

Ampicillin (Omnipen, Amcill, Amcap, Penbritin, Polycillin, Totacillin, Pfizerpen-A, and others)
Capsules, powder for injection (as the sodium salt), powder for oral suspensions, combination with probenecid (Principen with Probenecid, Probencilin, Probampacin, Polycillin-PRB), combination with sulbactam (Unasyn).
Recommended Doses: Vary according to the agent of infection being treated.

Bacampicillin (Spectrobid)
Tablets
Recommended Doses: 400 or 800 mg PO every 12 hours.

Cyclacillin (Cyclapen-W)
Tablets, powder for oral suspensions
Recommended Doses: 250–500 mg PO every 6 hours.

Hetacillin (Versapen)
Capsules, powder for oral suspensions

Antipseudomonal Broad-Spectrum Penicillins

This second and newer group of broad-spectrum antibacterial agents now includes five drugs: **azlocillin** (Azlin), **carbenicillin** (Geopen, Pyopen), **mezlocillin** (Mezlin), **piperacillin** (Pipracil), and **ticarcillin** (Ticar).

Clinical Indications The most important extensions of spectrum afforded by this group of agents are increased activity against *Pseudomonas aeruginosa,* indole-sensitive *Proteus, Serratia, Proteus mirabilis, Pasteurella multocida, Klebsiella pneumoniae, Bacteroides fragilis,* and *Peptostreptococcus.* Carbenicillin, ticarcillin, mezlocillin, and azlocillin are indicated primarily for *Pseudomonas aeruginosa* and *Proteus* species. Piperacillin sodium is useful against *Bacteroides fragilis* and *Clostridium difficile.* Piperacillin and azlocillin have the greatest in vitro activity against *Pseudomonas aeruginosa.* Piperacillin has a tendency to deplete potassium stores. *Nurses should observe for indications of hypokalemia when piperacillin is employed.*

Preparations and Administration *Solutions of carbenicillin are stable for 24 hours at room temperature and 72 hours under refrigeration.* Azlocillin is administered only intravenously by slow injection or infusion. The sodium load of piperacillin is 1.98 mEq/g.

Azlocillin (Azlin)
Powder for injection

Carbenicillin
Powder for injection as the disodium salt (Geopen, Pyopen), film coated tablets as carbenicillin indanyl sodium (Geocillin)

Mezlocillin (Mezlin)
Powder for injection
Recommended Doses: 3 g every 4 hours or 4 g every 6 hours, IM or IV. Intramuscular injection is often painful. The concentration should not exceed 10%.

Piperacillin sodium (Pipracil)
Powder for injection
Recommended Doses: 24 g/day, IM or IV.

Ticarcillin (Ticar)
Powder for injection solutions

Amidinopenicillins

Amdinocillin (Coactin) was introduced in 1985, the first of a new group of amidinopenicillins of distinctive activity.

Mechanisms and Effects Amdinocillin binds to a different site (penicillin-binding protein 2) in bacterial cells than other penicillins (which bind to penicillin-binding proteins $1B_s$ and 3). The action of amdinocillin is synergistic with that of other beta-lactam antibiotics, making it a useful drug for combination therapies against severe infections. Amdinocillin causes formation of abnormal spherical forms of bacterial cells by preventing cell elongation.

Clinical Indications Amdinocillin has an antibacterial spectrum that is distinctive from that of other penicillins. It is active alone against *E. coli, Klebsiella* species, *Salmonella* species, *Enterobacter* species, *Citrobacter* species, and *Serratia* species, and in combination with other beta-lactam antibiotics against *Proteus mirabilis, Morganella morganii,* and *Providencia* species. Amdinocillin is indicated for urinary tract infections caused by susceptible strains of *E. coli, Klebsiella* species, and *Enterobacter* species.

Preparations and Administration

Amdinocillin (Coactin)
Powder for injection
Recommended Doses: When used alone, 60 mg/kg/day, IM or IV, in divided doses at 4-hour intervals. In combination with other beta-lactam antibiotics, 40 mg/kg/day, IV or IM, in divided doses at 6-hour intervals. Treatment should be continued at least 2 days after the signs of infection have abated.

Cephalosporins — First Generation

The early cephalosporins were derived from the fungus *Cephalosporium acremonium,* which was gathered in 1948 from a sewer outlet to the sea off the coast of Sardinia. The first cephalosporin was introduced into medicine in 1960. The first-generation cephalosporins now include seven agents — four with oral effectiveness and three without (Table 47–6). Two others, cephaloglycin (Kafocin) and cephaloridine (Loridine) were marketed but have been discontinued.

Mechanisms and Effects The cephalosporins resemble the penicillins in both structure and pharmacology. The spectrum of cephalosporins is broad. Even the first-generation drugs are active against many gram-negative as well as gram-positive organisms. First-generation cephalosporins are effective against *Klebsiella* species, *Proteus mirabilis,* most *Escherichia coli,* most *Salmonella* and *Shigella,* and 50% of *Haemophilus influenzae* strains, in addition to the gram-positive *Staphylococci* and *Streptococci.* The individual drugs vary widely in their resistance to bacterial beta-lactamase. Two of these cephalosporins, cephalothin (Keflin) and cephapirin (Cefadyl), produce active metabolites, though the diacetylated products are somewhat less active than the parent compounds.

Pharmacokinetics The half-lives of the injectable first-generation cephalosporins vary from 30 minutes for cephapirin to 2 hours for cefazolin. Peak serum levels occur in about 1 hour, except for cefazolin, which reaches its peak level in 3 hours. Renal excretion accounts for 70–90% of the elimination of cefazolin; both metabolism and renal elimination contribute significantly to inactivation of cephapirin and cephalothin.

Clinical Indications One indication for first-generation cephalosporins is for *Klebsiella pneumoniae,* but these drugs are also useful alternatives to penicillins in individuals allergic to the older group of drugs. Cross-sensitivity occurs in only 10% of individuals allergic to penicillins. *Care must still be taken when using cephalosporins in clients with known allergies to penicillins.*

Preparations and Administration Cephalothin, cephapirin, and cefazolin are not employed orally. Cephalothin sodium is used almost exclu-

Table 47–6
Characteristics of Cephalosporins, Oxa-Beta-Lactams, and Carbapenems

Drug	Orally effective	Protein bound (%)	Beta-lactamase resistant	Bacterial spectrum
First-generation cephalosporins — orally effective				
Cefaclor	Yes	25	No	Broad
Cefadroxil	Yes	20	Somewhat	Broad
Cephalexin	Yes	10	Somewhat	Broad
Cephradine	Yes	24	Considerable	Broad
First-generation cephalosporins — not orally effective				
Cefazolin	No	80	Little	Broad
Cephalothin	No	65	Considerable	Broad
Cephapirin	No	47	Somewhat	Broad
Second-generation cephalosporins				
Cefamandole	No	56–78	Yes	Broader
Cefoxitin	No	72	Yes	Broader
Cefuroxime	No	33–50	Yes	Broader
Cefonicid	No	98	Yes	Broader
Ceforanide	No	80	Yes	Broader
Third-generation cephalosporins				
Cefoperazone	No	82–93	Yes	Broadest
Cefotaxime	No	51	Yes	Broadest
Ceftazidime	No	10–17	Yes	Broadest
Ceftizoxime	No	30	Yes	Broadest
Cetriaxone	No	85–95	Yes	Broadest
Cefotetan	No	78–91	Yes	Broadest
Oxa-beta-lactam				
Moxalactam	No	?	Yes	Broadest
Carbapenems				
Imipenem/ cilastatin	No	20	Yes	Broadest

sively by intravenous injection or infusion because it causes considerable pain when injected intramuscularly. *Deep gluteal injection minimizes but does not eliminate painful reactions. When IM injections are to be used, the powder should be diluted with 4 ml of sterile water or, alternatively, lidocaine (Xylocaine) (without epinephrine) to minimize pain. The water should be slightly warmed to increase solubility. Unused solutions should be discarded after 96 hours if refrigerated or after 12 hours at room temperature. When cephalothin is to be given by intravenous infusion, phlebitis occurs commonly. It is best to discontinue other intravenous solutions because of possible incompatibilities.* As with penicillins, probenecid (Benemid) can be used with cephalosporins to slow their renal elimination.

The orally effective first-generation cephalosporins are cephalexin, cefaclor, cefadroxil, and cephradine. Cephalexin is the most widely employed cephalosporin, the second most widely used antimicrobial drug, and the eleventh most widely prescribed of all drugs (as of 1983). *The oral suspension and pediatric drugs are stable for no more than 14 days under refrigeration. They should be kept in a tightly covered container and shaken well before use.* Administration of cephalexin with food slows but does not alter total absorption.

Cefaclor is currently the next most widely used cephalosporin and among the top 50 prescription drugs. It is less well absorbed by a factor of 2 than cephalexin but is more active against gram-negative bacilli. *Absorption of cefaclor is not affected by food.* The distinctive feature of cefadroxil is its longer half-life (70–80 min) than cephalexin (30–70 min) or cefaclor (36–54 min).

PARENTERAL DRUGS

Cefazolin (Ancef, Kefzol)
Powder for injection solutions

Cephalothin sodium (Keflin)
Powder for injection

Cephapirin (Cefadyl)
Injection solution

ORAL DRUGS

Cefaclor (Ceclor)
Capsules, oral suspensions
Recommended Doses: For adults, 250 mg to 1 g PO daily in 3 doses. For children, 20 mg/kg/day PO in divided doses at 8-hour intervals.

Cefadroxil (Duricef, Ultracef)
Capsules, tablets, oral suspensions
Recommended Doses: For adults, 1 or 2 g PO daily in 2 divided doses. For children, 30 mg/kg/day PO in divided doses every 12 hours.

Cephalexin (Keflex)
Capsules, tablets, pediatric drops, oral suspensions
Recommended Doses: For adults, 1–4 g/day PO in 2 or 4 divided doses. For children, 25–50 mg/kg/day in 4 doses.

Cephradine (Velosef, Anspor)
Capsules, tablets, oral suspensions, powder for injection
Recommended Doses: For adults, 250 mg PO every 6 hours or 500 mg every 12 hours. For children, 25–50 mg/day PO in 2–4 divided doses.

Cephalosporins — Second Generation

In recent years, new cephalosporins have been developed that have a broader spectra than the first-generation drugs. The *second-generation* drugs include cefamandole (Mandol), cefonicid (Monocid), ceforanide (Precef), cefoxitin (Mefoxin), and cefuroxime (Zinacef).

Mechanisms and Effects One significant feature of these drugs is their resistance to inactivation by bacterial beta-lactamase enzymes. In addition, second-generation cephalosporins provide improved activity against *Bacteroides fragilis, Enterobacter aerogenes, Haemophilus influenzae,* indole-positive *Proteus* species, and *Serratia.* Cefoxitin is superior to the other members of this group against *Bacteroides fragilis, Serratia,* and indole-positive *Proteus* but less effective against *Enterobacter aerogenes* and *Haemophilus influenzae.* Cefuroxime (Zinacef) has the special feature of penetration into the cerebral spinal fluid, a property shared with third-generation cephalosporins but not with first-generation or other second-generation drugs. Accordingly, it is useful for treating meningitis caused by susceptible organisms. None of the second-generation cephalosporins are orally effective. Cefonicid (Monocid) and ceforanide (Precef), the newest of the second-generation cephalosporins, offer no advantages in spectrum over other second-generation cephalosporins, but are longer acting, allowing less frequent administration.

Preparations and Administration Both cefoxitin and cefamandole have half-lives approximating 1 hour. Cefamandole has been reported to cause reactions like those of disulfiram (Antabuse) (see Chapter 13) to alcohol consumption. The sodium load of cefuroxime is 24 mEq (54.2 mg)/g.

Cefamandole nafate (Mandol)
Injection solutions
Recommended Doses: For severe infections in adults, 1–2 g IM or IV every 4–6 hours. Twelve grams daily is recommended for life-threatening infections. For children, 50–150 mg/kg/day IM or IV in 4–6 divided doses.

Cefonicid (Monocid)
Powder for injection solutions in vials, piggyback vials, or bulk vials
Recommended Doses: 1 g daily in a single dose, IM or IV.

Ceforanide (Precef)
Powder for injection solutions in vials or piggyback containers
Recommended Doses: 0.5–1.0 g, IM, IV, or IV infusion, every 12 hours.

Cefoxitin (Mefoxin)
Powder for injection
Recommended Doses: For intermittent intravenous injections, 1 or 2 g in 10 ml of sterile water over 3–5 minutes. For continuous IV infusion, add to dextrose or saline solutions or combinations.

Cefuroxime sodium (Zinacef)
Infusion solution
Recommended Doses: For adults, 750–1,500 mg, tid or 1,500 mg every 6 hours for life-threatening or less sensitive infections.

Cephalosporins — Third Generation — and Oxa-Beta-Lactams and Carbapenems

The **third-generation** cephalosporins include cefotaxime (Claforan), cefoperazone (Cefobid), ceftizoxime (Cefizox), ceftriaxone (Rocephin), ceftazidime (Fortaz), and cefotetan (Cefotan), all introduced in the 1980s. In addition, two new beta-lactam drugs, moxalactam (Moxam), an oxa-beta-lactam, and imipenem (Primaxin), a carbapenem, though structurally distinctive from the penicillins, cephalosporins, and each other, have the extended spectrum of antibacterial activity typical of the third-generation cephalosporins.

Mechanisms and Effects Like the second-generation drugs, all of these agents are stable against bacterial beta-lactamase. Like cefuroxime (Zinacef), the third-generation cephalosporins effectively penetrate the cerebral spinal fluid. Moxalactam is especially capable of penetrating the CNS, but imipenem does not effectively penetrate the CNS.

The third-generation cephalosporins, moxalactam, and imipenem are notable for their extended spectra against gram-negative bacilli, especially *Serratia marcescens, Pseudomonas aeruginosa,* and *Bacteroides fragilis.* Cefoperazone is the most active of the six third-generation cephalosporins against *Pseudomonas aeruginosa* but the least active against most other gram-negative organisms. Moxalactam and imipenem are the most effective against *Bacteroides fragilis,* being comparable to the second-generation drug cefoxitin. Imipenem has the broadest spectrum of any currently available antibacterial drug, being active against all gram-positive and gram-negative bacteria except chlamydiae and resistant strains of staphylococci, *Streptococcus faesium, Pseudomonas maltophilia, Pseudomonas cepacia, Flavobacterium,* and anaerobic corynebacteria.

Adverse Effects Cefoperazone and moxalactam have been reported to cause **disulfiram-like reactions** to alcohol consumption within 72 hours after administration of the antibacterial drug. Other adverse effects of drugs in this group are those typical of antibacterial agents: hypersensitivity reactions, gastrointestinal disturbances, bleeding disorders, and pain at the injection site. None of these are common. Imipenem is less likely to cause superinfection than are the third-generation cephalosporins.

Preparations and Administration Cefotaxime sodium (Claforan) is administered intramuscularly or intravenously. It contains 2.2 mEq of sodium per gram of drug. The sodium content of cefoperazone sodium is 1.5 mEq/g, while that of ceftizoxime (Cefizox) is 2.6 mEq (20 mg)/g. Moxalactam provides 3.8 mEq (88 mg) of sodium per gram of drug.

When imipenem is administered alone, it is metabolized rapidly by the renal enzyme dehydropeptidase-I (DHP-I) and is ineffective. It therefore must be administered in combination with an inhibitor of DHP-I, cilastatin.

Cefoperazone sodium (Cefobid)
Powder for injection solutions
Recommended Doses: For adults, 2–4 g/day, IM or IV in 2 divided doses at 12-hour intervals.

Cefotaxime sodium (Claforan)
Powder for injection solutions
Recommended Doses: For adults, 1 g every 6–8 hours. The maximum daily dose is 12 g for serious infection.

Cefotetan (Cefotan)
Powder for injection in vials
Recommended Doses: 1 or 2 g IV or IM every 12 hours for 5–10 days.

Ceftazidime (Fortaz)
Powder for injection in vials, infusion packs, and bulk packages
Recommended Doses: For adults, 1 g every 8–12 hours, IV or IM, varying with the site of infection and causative agent.

Ceftizoxime sodium (Cefizox)
Frozen injection solutions or powder for injection in conventional or piggyback vials
Recommended Doses: For adults, 1–2 g every 8–12 hours; for severe infections, 3–4 g may be given at 8-hour intervals.

Ceftriaxone (Rocephin)
Powder for injection in vials, piggyback units, and bulk containers
Recommended Doses: For adults, 1 or 2 g in 1 or 2 doses, IM or IV. For meningitis in children, 50–75 mg/kg/day (to a maximum of 2 g) in divided doses every 12 hours.

Imipenem/Cilastatin (Primaxin)
Powder for infusion
Recommended Doses: For adults with normal renal function, 250–1,000 mg every 6–8 hours to a maximum of 4 g/day or 50 mg/kg/day, whichever is less. Doses of 250–500 mg are infused over 20–30 minutes; doses of 1,000 mg over 40–60 minutes. If nausea occurs, the rate of infusion should be reduced.

Moxalactam disodium (Moxam)
Powder for injection
Recommended Doses: 2–4 g/day, IM, IV, or IV infusion, in divided doses at 8-hour intervals.

Important Nursing Implications for Beta-Lactam Antibacterial Agents

☐ Before administering a beta-lactam antibiotic, conduct a careful review of the client's medication history for evidence of allergies to any of these drugs. Clients should be clearly informed when they are about to be given a penicillin drug.

- ☐ Observe clients for 30 minutes after administering the first or second dose of an antibiotic drug for indications of anaphylaxis or other allergic reactions. Reddening or edema at the site of injection may be an early indication of an allergic response.
- ☐ Advise clients who do experience allergic responses to inform all health care practitioners in the future about their drug allergy.
- ☐ Carefully monitor renal and hepatic function and blood tests in the elderly, infants, and clients receiving high-ceiling diuretics or other potentially nephrotoxic drugs, since these clients are especially liable to renal, hepatic, and hematopoietic side effects of beta-lactam antibiotics.
- ☐ Advise clients to avoid excessive exposure to sunlight while using beta-lactam antibiotics because of the potential for photosensitivity reactions.
- ☐ Periodically examine clients receiving antibiotics for indications of superinfection such as bacterial growth on the tongue, unusually large stools, diarrhea, nausea, anogenital itching, vaginal discharge, glossitis, or stomatitis.
- ☐ If the client has any dietary restrictions involving sodium or potassium, check the drug selection for its sodium or potassium load.
- ☐ Oral doses of most beta-lactam antibiotics are taken on an empty stomach — at least 1 hour before meals or 2 hours after meals, with a full glass of water.
- ☐ The expiration date should always be checked before administration of an antibiotic.
- ☐ If the client is to take the drug in a liquid oral form, it is important that the individual measure the dose with a specifically marked device since household teaspoons vary in measure.
- ☐ Carefully follow the instructions for reconstituting injection solutions provided with each drug. The powder should be loosened by tapping the vial against the palm of the hand. The amount of diluent should be drawn up into a syringe and, holding the vial horizontally, the nurse should rotate the vial while directing the stream of fluid against the wall of the vial. Afterward the vial should be shaken vigorously until all the powder is dissolved.
- ☐ Select the IM site carefully so as to ensure that the solution is not injected into or near a nerve. It is wise to ask the client about prior injections. The client may know of an anomaly that will suggest a different site should be chosen. Large muscle masses should be chosen and, as usual, the nurse should check for the back-flow of blood before injecting the drug. Injection sites should be rotated and a chart marked to indicate areas used. If the client experiences pain at a site where such sensitivity is unusual, the nurse should mark the client's chart to indicate that the area should be avoided in the future.
- ☐ Be aware that some physicians may prescribe use of procaine or lidocaine, 1% or 2%, without epinephrine, to be used as the diluent for penicillin injections in order to prevent pain at the site of administration. Penicillin preparations containing procaine are for intramuscular injection only — never intravenous administration.
- ☐ Reinforce the need to complete courses of therapy with antibiotics even after overt symptoms have disappeared.
- ☐ Teach clients to discard unused antibiotics since they lose their potency during storage.

Aminoglycosides

The aminoglycoside antibiotics are a group of eight antimicrobial drugs, seven of which are used for treatment of infections caused by gram-negative bacteria not responsive to less toxic agents. The eighth aminoglycoside, paromomycin, is used only for intestinal amebiasis and is discussed in Chapter 48. The original aminoglycoside, streptomycin, was discovered in 1944 as a result of a concerted effort by Waksman and colleagues to isolate effective antibacterial agents from fungi of the actinomycetes group. Four years of work culminated in the isolation of a potent and broad-spectrum antibacterial drug from *Streptomyces griseus.* The drug was named **streptomycin.** Other aminoglycosides are derived directly from other species of actinomyces, except amikacin, which is a semisynthetic derivative of kanamycin. The aminoglycoside family now includes streptomycin, neomycin (Mycifradin, Neobiotic), gentamicin (various brands), tobramycin (Nebcin), kanamycin (Kantrex, Klebcil), amikacin (Amikin), and netilmicin (Netromycin). On the whole, this class of drugs exhibits a great deal of homogeneity with respect to antibacterial spectra, adverse effects, pharmacokinetics, and cross-sensitivity.

Mechanisms and Effects Aminoglycosides inhibit proliferation of bacteria by interfering with protein synthesis in bacterial cells. They cause the ribosomes to misread the genetic code of the messenger RNA and may also inhibit subsequent phases of protein synthesis. Aminoglycosides are bacteriostatic at low concentrations, but bactericidal at doses 3 or 4 times higher.

Aminoglycosides can exert their action only to the extent that they are able to penetrate the outer bacterial structures — the outer membrane, the cell wall, and the cytoplasmic membrane. Aminoglycosides do not cross cell membranes passively because they are polar molecules. However, many bacteria actively transport the aminoglycosides into the cell interior. This energy-dependent transport process does not occur in anaerobic bacteria or facultative bacteria grown under anaerobic conditions. These organisms have a **natural resistance** to aminoglycosides, as do most mammalian cells. Coadministration of drugs of the penicillin family greatly enhances the effectiveness of aminoglycosides by improving the ability of the aminoglycosides to penetrate bacterial cell walls. *However, aminoglycosides and penicillins should not be physically mixed for simultaneous administration because they are chemically incompatible.* Some strains of bacteria exhibit natural or acquired resistance to aminoglycosides because their ribosomes have less affinity for binding aminoglycosides. Other bacteria contain enzymes that destroy aminoglycosides. The major cause of acquired resistance to aminoglycosides is an increase in activity of bacterial enzymes that inactivate the drugs. Amikacin is the most resistant to the enzymes, being susceptible only to acetylation.

Pharmacokinetics All of the aminoglycosides are highly polar compounds. This accounts for several aspects of their pharmacokinetics. Aminoglycosides are not absorbed to an appreciable extent after oral administration. The only oral uses of aminoglycosides are for surgical prophylaxis or treatment of intestinal infections. After parenteral administration, aminoglycosides are rapidly absorbed, reaching peak levels in 0.5–1.5 hours.

The polarity of aminoglycosides prevents their penetration into most cells and into the eye, the cerebral spinal fluid, and the brain. Some penetration into the CNS does occur when the integrity of the meninges is compromised by meningitis. The volume of distribution of aminoglycosides approximates the volume of extracellular fluid. Aminoglycosides are not substantially bound to plasma proteins. Streptomycin is about 30% bound, but the other aminoglycosides are less than 10% bound by plasma proteins.

The half-lives of all of the available aminoglycosides approximate 2–3 hours, and slightly more than half of a parenterally administered dose is excreted within 24 hours. Aminoglycosides are secreted into the bile by an active hepatic process, but this contributes little to overall elimination. Renal extraction accounts for nearly 100% of the elimination of these compounds. Urine concentration can reach 50–200 μg/ml. The tendency of these drugs to concentrate in the renal tubule contributes to the considerable risk of renal toxicity of aminoglycosides.

Clinical Indications Because of the severity of toxicity caused by aminoglycosides, they are employed only for infections resistant to other drug selections. They are most commonly used for aerobic, gram-negative organisms not responsive to penicillins, but with the advent of newer penicillins and cephalosporins with extended spectra, the clinical requirement for aminoglycosides has narrowed. Aminoglycosides can also be used for gram-positive organisms either in combination with penicillins, or as an alternative to penicillins or cephalosporins for strains that are resistant to the primary drug choices. The spectra of the available aminoglycosides are listed in Table 47–7.

Streptomycin has important though infrequent use against a number of infections that are rare in the United States, including *Yersinia pestis* (bubonic plague), *Haemophilus ducreyi* (chancroid), *Francisella tularensis* (tularemia), *Calymmatobacterium granulomatis* (granuloma inguinale), and *Brucella* (brucellosis). Streptomycin and gentamicin are sometimes employed in combination with a penicillin for bacterial endocarditis caused by *Streptococcus faecalis.* Aminoglycosides are, however, totally ineffective against streptococcal pneumonias. Kanamycin is generally less effective than other aminoglycosides.

Neomycin is used almost exclusively for topical application: to the skin or by oral administration for intestinal infections. It is frequently used as an intestinal antiseptic agent preceding bowel surgery. However, the drug is contraindicated among those who have intestinal obstruction or ulcerative colitis. When the drug is used to prepare clients for bowel surgery, the individual should be placed on a low-residue diet. Usually a saline laxative is given prior to instituting neomycin therapy and daily enemas may also be ordered. The parenteral dosage form is seldom used and is absolutely contraindicated among those with renal disease, impaired hearing, or myasthenia gravis.

Gentamicin, tobramycin, and amikacin have similar spectra and usefulness, although amikacin has the additional advantage of resistance to bacterial degratory enzymes. These three are primary or secondary choices for *Enterobacter aerogenes, Escher-*

Table 47–7
Antimicrobial Spectra of Aminoglycosides

Microorganism	Streptomycin	Neomycin	Gentamicin	Tobramycin	Kanamycin	Amikacin	Netilmicin
Gram-positive cocci							
Staphylococcus	Yes		Yes	Yes	Yes	Yes	Yes
Streptococcus	Yes	Some	Yes	Some		Yes	
Streptococcus faecalis	Yes*	Yes	Yes*	No			
Streptococcus pneumoniae	No	No	No	No	No	No	
Gram-positive bacilli							
Listeria monocytogenes		Yes					
Gram-negative cocci							
Neisseria gonorrhoeae	Yes				Yes		
Neisseria meningitidis		Yes					
Gram-negative bacilli							
Acinetobacter (Mima-Herellea)					Yes	Yes*	
Bordetella pertussis		Yes					
Brucella	Yes*						
Calymmatobacterium granulomatus	Yes*						
Citrobacter freudii			Yes	Yes		Yes	
Enterobacter aerogenes	Yes	Yes	Yes*	Yes*	Weak	Yes*	Yes
Escherichia coli	Yes	Yes	Yes*	Yes	Yes	Yes*	Yes
Francisella tularensis	Yes*						
Haemophilus ducreyi	Yes*						
Haemophilus influenzae	Yes	Yes			Yes		
Klebsiella pneumoniae	Yes	Yes	Yes*	Yes*	Weak	Yes*	Yes
Pasteurella multocida		Yes					
Proteus mirabilis	Yes		Yes*	Yes*	Yes	Yes*	Yes
Proteus (indole-positive)	Yes	Yes	Yes*	Yes*	Yes	Yes*	Yes
Pseudomonas aeruginosa		Some	Yes*	Yes*	No	Yes*	No
Salmonella		Yes	Yes*				
Serratia			Yes*	Yes	Weak	Yes*	Yes
Shigella dysenteriae		Yes	Yes		Yes		
Vibrio cholerae		Yes					
Yersinia pestis	Yes*						
Mycobacteria							
Mycobacterium tuberculosis	Yes*			No		Yes*	

Key:
Yes: Effective against indicated bacterial species.
No: Not effective.
Weak: Weakly effective.
Some: Effective against some strains.
*: Important therapeutic applications.
Blank: Effectiveness not established.

ichia coli, Klebsiella pneumonias, Proteus, and *Serratia.* Gentamicin is additionally effective against *Salmonella.* Streptomycin and amikacin can be used for clients who have tuberculosis that is not adequately controlled with the combination of isoniazid and rifampin (Rifamate) or isoniazid and ethambutol. Tobramycin (Nebcin) is usually reserved for organisms resistant to gentamicin.

Kanamycin has value in hepatic coma because of its ability to decrease production of ammonia by intestinal bacteria. The intraperitoneal route has been used in administration for hepatic coma, but this is hazardous because of systemic absorption. Administration by this route is especially likely to contribute to neuromuscular blockade of respiratory muscles.

Adverse Effects and Contraindications Aminoglycosides exhibit a common set of adverse effects, though differences in incidence occur between drugs. The adverse effects of aminoglycosides include renal toxicity, ototoxicity, neuromuscular blockade, hypersensitivity reactions, and superinfection. Renal insufficiency is a major factor contributing to accumulation of aminoglycosides and toxicity. Doses of aminoglycosides should be reduced in proportion to a decrease in the kidney's glomerular filtration rate (GFR) from normal, as determined by creatinine clearance. *The nurse can aid in minimizing the risk of aminoglycoside toxicity by ensuring that the client is well hydrated. Hydration serves to reduce the extent to which aminoglycosides will be concentrated in the renal tubules.*

Renal toxicity of aminoglycosides is due in part to the concentrating effect of the kidney on these drugs. Aminoglycosides accumulate to high levels in the renal cortex and urine. The nature of the toxicity is an acute tubular necrosis. The urine exhibits elevated protein and tubular cell casts when tubular necrosis occurs. The condition is reversible if the drug is withdrawn promptly. The renal toxicity of aminoglycosides can be self-enhancing because toxicity decreases the GFR and thus promotes still higher concentrations of the drug within the kidney. *Urinalysis and tests of renal function should be conducted periodically when aminoglycosides are used for extended periods of time. The nurse should watch for evidence of decreased renal function such as oliguria, increased specific gravity of urine, an elevated BUN or creatinine level, or signs of uremia.* The likelihood of toxicity with aminoglycosides is higher in elderly clients and neonates, especially premature infants, because renal function is often diminished in the elderly and incompletely developed in infants. Neomycin is the most nephrotoxic of the currently available aminoglycosides and has therefore been withdrawn from systemic use. The incidence of nephrotoxicity is higher for gentamicin, kanamycin, and netilmicin (about 3–8%) than for tobramycin or streptomycin (about 1%).

Ototoxicity occurs with all aminoglycosides, and entails both auditory and vestibular deficits. Interestingly, the drugs differ in their propensity for auditory versus vestibular toxicity (Table 47–8). Vestibular toxicity is often preceded by a moderate headache for a day or two, followed by nausea, vomiting, loss of balance, vertigo, and increased incidence of coordination errors involving continuation of ocular or bodily movements past an intended point. Auditory toxicity is caused by accumulation of aminoglycosides in the perilymph of the inner ear. An early symptom is a high-pitched tinnitus. This is followed by a gradual loss of auditory acuity. Hearing loss rapidly becomes irreversible if the drug is not discontinued within a few days. When treatment with aminoglycosides is contemplated for more than a few days, an audiogram should be taken initially and then periodically during treatment to guard against changes in auditory acuity. The elderly are especially susceptible to ototoxicity, because auditory acuity declines as a natural course of events with aging.

An unusual adverse effect of aminoglycosides is **neuromuscular blockade.** Although the extent of neuromuscular blockade is seldom enough to cause respiratory paralysis, nurses may occasionally notice a client developing apnea or even prolonged paralysis when doses are excessive or the drugs are instilled into the intrapleural or intraperitoneal spaces from whence they have rapid access to neuromuscular receptors of the respiratory muscles. The neuromuscu-

Table 47–8
Ototoxic Potential of Aminoglycosides and Vancomycin

Drug	Auditory	Vestibular
Amikacin	+ + +	–
Gentamicin	+	+ +
Kanamycin	+ + +	+
Neomycin	+ + + +	+
Netilmicin	+	–
Streptomycin	+	+ + +
Tobramycin	+ +	+ +
Vancomycin	+ + +	–

Key: –, does not occur; +, seldom occurs; + +, sometimes occurs; + + +, often occurs; + + + +, most likely to occur.

lar blocking action is additive with that of curare and drugs with local anesthetic properties. Even a modest degree of neuromuscular blockade may be problematic for clients with myasthenia gravis or parkinsonism. Neomycin has the strongest neuromuscular blocking effect of the aminoglycosides, followed by streptomycin, kanamycin, amikacin, gentamicin, and tobramycin. The neuromuscular blocking action can be antagonized by administration of a cholinesterase inhibitor (such as neostigmine) or a calcium salt.

Hypersensitivity reactions are less common with aminoglycosides than with penicillins, but a full gamut of reactions can occur. Skin eruptions occur in about 5% of individuals and include morbilliform, maculopapular, urticarial, and erythematous reactions. Exfoliative dermatitis can also occur. More severe allergic reactions include blood dyscrasias (agranulocytosis, neutropenia, thrombocytopenia, aplastic, or hemolytic anemias) in about 0.7% of individuals, and drug fever or anaphylaxis.

Prolonged therapy with aminoglycosides may result in **superinfection** by nonsusceptible organisms. When such overgrowth occurs, aminoglycoside therapy should be terminated and the new infection treated.

Drug Interactions The drug interactions of aminoglycosides relate to both toxicity and efficacy. With respect to toxicity, the ototoxic, nephrotoxic, and neuromuscular blocking actions described above are all increased when an aminoglycoside is used concurrently with another drug having one of these actions. Nephrotoxicity is additive with that of cephaloridine, polymyxin B (Neosporin), colistin (Coly-Mycin S), vancomycin (Vancocin), or high-ceiling diuretics. High-ceiling diuretics also increase the ototoxicity of aminoglycosides. Neuromuscular blockade is additive with that produced by curariform agents, drugs with local anesthetic properties (including quinidine (Cin-Quin, Quinidex) and propranolol (Inderal)), and drugs causing hypokalemia.

The efficacy of aminoglycosides against many organisms, especially gram-positive cocci, is enhanced by concurrent administration of penicillin-like drugs. As noted earlier, aminoglycosides should not be mixed with such drugs in a single administration vehicle, because the drugs are physically incompatible.

Preparations and Administration Streptomycin sulfate is given only intramuscularly. *Solutions of streptomycin should be used immediately after reconstitution.* Neomycin, though available in an injectable form, is used only orally for amebiasis or to suppress intestinal bacteria preoperatively.

Amikacin (Amikin)
Injection solutions
Recommended Doses: For severe infections, 15 mg/kg/day, IM or IV, in 3 divided doses.

Gentamicin (Apogen, Bristagen, Garamycin, U-Gencin)
Injection solutions as the sulfate salt in ampuls or piggyback units
Recommended Doses: A loading dose of 1–2 mg/kg is infused initially over 30–60 minutes, followed by maintenance doses. For maintenance, 2 or 3 mg/kg/day, IM or IV, in divided doses (usually every 8 hours) for 7–10 days. Dosage adjustment is required if renal impairment is present.

Kanamycin sulfate (Kantrex, Klebcil)
Injection solutions, capsules as the sulfate salt
Recommended Doses: For adults, up to 1.5 g/day IM or IV. For suppression of intestinal bacteria, 1.0 g every hour for 4 hours, followed by 1.0 g every 6 hours for 36–72 hours. For treatment of hepatic coma, 8–12 g are given per day in divided doses.

Neomycin (Mycifradin, Neobiotic, and generic)
Tablets, oral solution
Recommended Doses: For suppression of intestinal flora, 40 mg/lb PO for 1 day. Treatment should not exceed 3 days. For infectious diarrhea due to enteropathic *E. coli,* 50 mg/kg/day for 2–3 days.

Netilmicin sulfate (Netromycin)
Injection solutions
Recommended Doses: 4–6.5 mg/kg/day, IM or IV, in 2 or 3 divided doses.

Streptomycin sulfate
Powder for injection
Recommended Doses: Depends on the nature of the infection; 1–4 g daily for 7–10 days is typical.

Tobramycin (Nebcin)
Injection solutions
Recommended Doses: Up to 5 mg/kg/day, IM or IV.

Important Nursing Implications for Aminoglycosides

- ☐ During prolonged therapy, monitor plasma concentrations of aminoglycoside antibiotics to ensure that levels are appropriate.
- ☐ Assess clients for indications of toxicity, including vertigo, loss of acuity of hearing, tinnitus, and ataxia. Clients should be given periodic audiograms if treatment with aminoglycosides is prolonged.

- ☐ Watch for indications of nephrotoxicity such as changes in urinary output. Renal function tests should be conducted when aminoglycoside administration is prolonged. Advise clients to maintain good hydration to minimize risks of nephrotoxicity.
- ☐ Observe for indications of neuromuscular blockade, especially if aminoglycosides are used in conjunction with curariform agents, local anesthetics, or skeletal muscle relaxants or in clients with myasthenia gravis or hypokalemia.
- ☐ Observe clients for signs of superinfection or allergic reactions. Teach clients to recognize indications of superinfection or allergic reactions to aminoglycosides.

Tetracyclines

The first of the tetracyclines, chlortetracycline, was introduced in 1948. It has been followed by eight additional agents in this family. Chlortetracycline and demeclocycline (Declomycin) are derived from *Streptomyces aureofaciens;* oxytetracycline (Terramycin) from *Streptomyces rimosus.* Tetracycline (Achromycin, Tetracyn), methacycline (Rondomycin), doxycycline (Vibramycin), and minocycline (Minocin) are semisynthetic derivatives. Meclocycline, a tetracycline introduced in 1980, is marketed in a cream formulation for topical use in acne vulgaris (see Chapter 53), but oral tetracyclines are probably more effective. The seven members of the class exhibit very similar spectra of effectiveness, toxicities, and other features.

Mechanisms and Effects Tetracyclines inhibit bacterial protein synthesis by combining with the ribosomes, thereby inhibiting access of transfer RNA to the messenger RNA acceptor site. The action of tetracyclines is primarily **bacteriostatic,** being exerted selectively on bacterial cells that are actively replicating. Activity requires that the drug enter the bacterial cell. In gram-negative bacteria, most of the tetracyclines diffuse across the outer cell membrane passively through hydrophilic pores; the more lipid-soluble members of the family, minocycline and doxycycline, are able to pass through the lipid phase of the membrane. Penetration of the inner membrane is by an energy-dependent, carrier-mediated process. Host cells are less affected than bacterial cells because they do not actively transport tetracyclines. Tetracyclines are broadly effective against many gram-negative and gram-positive organisms, but resistance has developed in some bacterial species.

Pharmacokinetics Tetracyclines are well absorbed after oral administration, although the extent of absorption varies from agent to agent (Table 47–9). Chlortetracycline, oxytetracycline, and tetracycline are least well absorbed, most rapidly excreted, and least bound to plasma proteins.

Demeclocycline and methacycline also exhibit incomplete absorption, but their longer half-lives permit them to be given just twice daily for most purposes. Absorption of demeclocycline, methacycline, oxytetracycline, chlortetracycline, and tetracycline is significantly impaired by antacids, iron, or dairy products such as milk because they form chelates with calcium. *The nurse should advise clients using tetracyclines not to ingest milk products, antacids, or iron within 1 hour of administration of these tetracyclines.*

Doxycycline and minocycline are realiably and completely absorbed allowing use of smaller doses. Absorption of these two tetracyclines is not affected by food, a distinct advantage. Since residual concentrations of these drugs in the intestines are less, gas-

Table 47–9
Pharmacokinetic Parameters of Tetracyclines

Drug	Absorption	Time to peak effect (hours)	Half-life (hours)	Usual number of daily doses
Tetracycline Chlortetracycline Oxytetracycline	Incomplete; variable	2–4	6–9	4
Demeclocycline Methacycline	Incomplete; variable	2–4	10–16	2
Doxycycline Minocycline	Complete; reliable	2	17–20	1

trointestinal irritation and floral imbalance is correspondingly reduced.

Absorption of tetracyclines occurs from the stomach and initial segment of the intestines where the low pH favors their absorption. *Nurses should warn clients that absorption of tetracyclines is greatly impaired by concurrent administration of antacids, especially those containing divalent ions, including aluminum, calcium, or magnesium salts.* Presence of food also reduces absorption of most tetracyclines. *It is usually best to advise clients to take the drugs on an empty stomach unless gastrointestinal irritation occurs.* Tetracyclines penetrate into all extracellular fluid compartments, although concentrations in the cerebral spinal fluid are usually too low to provide therapeutic benefit except by intravenous injection.

Tetracyclines are excreted by renal and biliary mechanisms. Renal extraction is quantitatively greater, but biliary excretion is apparently also important, because biliary obstruction will increase plasma levels and retention of tetracyclines. Chlortetracycline, and especially doxycycline, are more dependent on biliary excretion than are other tetracyclines. Doxycycline is thus the favored agent for individuals with reduced renal function. Renal excretion of tetracyclines is entirely as a result of filtration, and declines in proportion to the glomerular filtration rate. Tetracycline should be used cautiously, in reduced doses if at all, in individuals with impaired renal function. Included in this group are some elderly individuals and especially neonates, who will have much greater plasma levels of tetracyclines if dosage adjustments are not made in relation to the lesser renal function.

Clinical Indications Tetracyclines are effective against a wide range of bacteria (Table 47–10). Tetracyclines are often a first choice for infections caused by *Vibrio cholerae* (cholera), *Pseudomonas pseudomallei* (melioidosis), *Calymmatobacterium granulomatis* (granuloma inguinale), *Rickettsia, Chlamydia, Neisseria gonorrhoeae* (gonorrhea), *Brucella* (brucellosis), *Haemophilus ducreyi* (chancroid), *Borrelia recurrentis* (relapsing fever), and *Mycoplasma pneumoniae* (atypical pneumonia). Tetracyclines are also used as secondary choices in infections due to *Proteus mirabilis, Escherichia coli, Staphylococci, Pasteurella multocida* (abscesses), *Francisella tularensis* (tularemia), *Yersinia pestis* (bubonic plague), *Streptobacillus moniliformis, Treponema pallidum* (syphilis), and *Treponema pertenue* (yaws).

Table 47–10
Antibacterial Spectra of Tetracyclines, Chloramphenicol, sulfonamides, and Trimethoprim-Sulfamethoxazole

Bacterial species	Tetracyclines	Chloramphenicol	Sulfonamides	Trimethoprim-Sulfamethoxazole
Gram-positive cocci				
Peptostreptococcus	Some*	Yes*		
Staphylococcus aureus	Some	Yes		Yes
Streptococcus				
agalactiae	Some^R	Yes*		
faecalis				Yes
group D	No			Yes
pneumoniae	Most^R	Yes*	Yes	Yes
pyrogenes	Most^R	Yes	Yes	Yes
viridans				Yes
Gram-positive bacilli		Yes*		
Bacillus anthrax	Yes*	Yes*	Yes	Yes
Clostridium perfringens	Some			
Other Clostridium	Some*			
Corynebacterium diptheriae			Yes	Yes
Erysipelothrix rhusiopathiae		Yes*		
Listeria monocytogenes		Yes*		

Table 47–10
Antibacterial Spectra of Tetracyclines, Chloramphenicol, sulfonamides, and Trimethoprim-Sulfamethoxazole (*continued*)

Bacterial species	Tetracyclines	Chloramphenicol	Sulfonamides	Trimethoprim-Sulfamethoxazole
Gram-negative cocci				
Neisseria gonorrhoeae	Most	Yes	Yes[R]	
Neisseria meningitidis	Yes	Yes*	Few[R]	Yes
Gram-negative bacilli				
Bacteroides fragilis	Some	Yes*		
Bordetella pertussis		Yes	No	
Brucella	Yes*	Yes	Yes	Yes*
Calymmatobacterium granulomatis	Yes*		Yes	
Campylobacter fetus		Yes*		
Enterobacter aerogenes	Some[R]	Some	No	Yes
Escherichia coli	Few[R]*	Yes*	Yes*	Yes*
Francisella tularensis	Yes*		No	
Fusobacterium nucleatum		Yes*		
Haemophilus ducreyi	Yes*		Yes*	Yes
Haemophilus influenzae	Some[R]	Yes*	Yes*	Yes*
Klebsiella pneumoniae	Few[R]	Some*		Yes
Pasteurella multocida	Yes*			
Proteus mirabilis		Yes	No	Yes
Proteus (indole-positive)	Few[R]		No	Yes
Pseudomonas aeruginosa		No	Yes	No
Pseudomonas mallei	Yes*	Yes*		
Salmonella		Yes	Yes	Yes*
Serratia		Some		Yes
Shigella	Some	Yes*	Some[R]	Yes*
Vibrio cholerae	Yes*	Yes*	Yes	Yes*
Yersinia enterocolitica	Yes*		Yes	
Yersinia pestis	Yes*		Yes	Yes
Actinomycetes	Yes*	Yes*	Yes	Yes
Spirochetes				
Borrelia recurrentis	Yes*		No	
Leptospira	Yes*		No	
Treponema	Yes*		No	
Primative bacteria				
Chlamydia	Yes*	Yes*	Yes	Yes
Mycoplasma pneumoniae	Yes*	Yes		
Pneumocystis carninii			Yes	Yes*
Rickettsii	Yes*	Yes*	No	

Key:
Yes: Effective against indicated bacterial species.
No: Not effective.
Some: Effective against some strains.
Most: Effective against most strains.
R: Resistance has been observed in some strains.
*: A clinical use as a primary or secondary choice.
Blank: Effectiveness not established.

Adverse Effects and Contraindications The toxic effects of tetracyclines include gastrointestinal irritation; hypersensitivity reactions and photosensitivity; renal toxicity; hepatic toxicity; damage or coloration of teeth, nails, or bones; a catabolic effect; blood cell dyscrasias; and superinfections.

Gastrointestinal irritation occurs in some individuals when they take tetracyclines orally. Symptoms include nausea, vomiting, epigastric distress, and abdominal discomfiture. *When symptoms of gastrointestinal distress occur, the nurse should advise clients to take the drug with food, but not with dairy products or antacids. In the absence of gastrointestinal irritation, it is better to take tetracyclines 1–2 hours before meals to maximize absorption.* Clients may develop diarrhea in response to tetracyclines due either to gastrointestinal irritation or superinfection. The latter cause requires termination of drug therapy, the former does not. Nurses will note that when diarrhea is due to irritation, the client usually describes the stools as fluid and frequent. Examination of the stools reveals no elevation in white blood cells in the feces.

Hypersensitivity reactions to tetracyclines include various kinds of drug eruptions: rashes, urticaria, fixed drug eruptions, photosensitivity to sunlight, exfoliative dermatitis, and pruritic reactions involving the eyes, vulva, anus, or vagina. *Patients should be instructed to avoid prolonged exposure to sunlight or sunlamps and to report any skin eruptions.* Anaphylaxis and febrile reactions also occur. Cross-sensitivity occurs between all drugs in this group.

Renal toxicity to tetracyclines occurs most commonly in individuals with preexisting renal insufficiency or existing renal infections. Tetracyclines should generally not be used when such conditions exist, but doxycycline is considerably safer than other tetracyclines for individuals with impaired renal function because it is excreted entirely by the biliary system. Nephrogenic diabetes insipidus has been reported in response to demeclocycline.

Ototoxicity, which often accompanies renal toxicity, occurs with minocycline but has not been reported with other tetracyclines. Only the vestibular function is affected.

Hepatic toxicity occurs in response to tetracyclines most frequently in pregnant women. The first sign, jaundice, may be followed by damage to hepatic cells, azotemia, and hepatic shock. Oxytetracycline and tetracycline produce less hepatic toxicity than other tetracyclines.

A unique adverse effect of tetracyclines occurs because of their ability to chelate with divalent cations. Tetracyclines become deposited in the teeth, bones, and nails. The nails and teeth may become pigmented, at first a fluorescent yellow hue, later a rusty brown color. Discoloration of the first set of teeth is most likely to occur when tetracyclines are used in the mother in the second half of pregnancy or in a neonate during the first 6 months. Discoloration of the permanent teeth frequently follows use of tetracyclines in children from age 6 months to 7 years, the period during which these teeth are being formed. Tetracyclines depress bone growth acutely, but the effect is reversible when drug treatment is completed.

Tetracyclines have a **catabolic effect** that can aggravate uremia by increasing production of nitrogen-containing metabolites. The negative nitrogen balance can lead to weight loss if dietary intake of proteins is marginal. **Blood cell dyscrasias** may occur when tetracyclines are given for extended periods of time. Characteristic toxicities are leukocytosis, thrombocytopenic purpura, and abnormalities of lymphocytes and granulocytes. Tetracyclines sometimes cause **elevation of intracranial pressure** in infants and in the elderly.

Tetracyclines are contraindicated for use in pregnancy, children under 12 years of age, and in individuals with renal insufficiency or renal infection. A syndrome of severe gastrointestinal and renal distress has occurred in individuals taking out-of-date tetracyclines. *The nurse should instruct clients to discard any unused portion of a tetracycline prescription.*

Drug Interactions The major interactions of tetracyclines are pharmacokinetic and were addressed above: namely, the absorption of tetracyclines is impaired by concurrent ingestion of dairy products or antacids containing magnesium, calcium, or aluminum salts, or sodium bicarbonate. Four other important drug interactions occur. Tetracyclines impair the effectiveness of antibiotics in the penicillin family. Agents from the two groups should not be employed concurrently. The thrombopenic effect of tetracyclines can increase the anticoagulant effect of anticoagulant drugs. Nephrotoxic effects of tetracyclines and the ototoxic effect of minocycline are additive with drugs having similar toxicity. Doxycycline, the tetracycline most dependent on the liver for its elimination, has a reduced half-life when liver enzymes have been induced by phenytoin (Dilantin), barbiturates, or other enzyme-inducing agents.

Preparations and Administration Tetracycline is available in both parenteral and oral dosage forms. Achromycin V, a brand of tetracycline, was the most widely prescribed tetracycline preparation as of 1983. *Tetracyclines decompose with age and exposure to light. Solutions should be considered stable at room tem-*

perature for no more than 12 hours. Powdered drug should be refrigerated.

Demeclocycline (Declomycin)
Capsules, tablets
Recommended Doses: For adults, 150 mg PO qid or 300 mg bid. For children over 8, 3–6 mg/lb/day PO in 2 or 4 divided doses.

Doxycycline (Vibramycin)
Capsules, tablets, oral suspension, syrup
Recommended Doses: For adults, 200 mg orally the first day in 2 doses at a 12-hour interval followed by 100 mg/day thereafter in 1 or 2 doses. For children over 8, 2 mg/lb PO on the first day in 2 doses; 1 mg/lb in 1 or 2 doses on subsequent days.

Methacycline (Rondomycin)
Capsules
Recommended Doses: The same as for demeclocycline.

Minocycline (Minocin)
Capsules, syrup
Recommended Doses: For adults, 200 mg PO initially followed by 100 mg every 12 hours. In children over 8, 4 mg/kg PO initially and 2 mg/kg every 12 hours thereafter.

Oxytetracycline (Terramycin)
Injection solutions, powder for injection solutions, capsules, tablets, syrup
Recommended Doses: For adults, 250 mg IM once daily or 300 mg in divided doses; or 250–500 mg IV every 12 hours. For children over 8, 15–25 mg/kg up to 250 mg per injection; or 10–20 mg/kg/day IV in 2 divided doses, with 12 mg/kg/day being usual. Oral doses are the same as for tetracycline.

Tetracycline (Achromycin, Tetracyn)
Powder for injection solutions, syrup, capsules, tablets, combinations with amphotericin (Mysteclin-F) or nystatin (Achrostatin V, Tetrastatin, Terrastatin, Declostatin) for candidal infections
Recommended Doses: For adults, 1–2 g daily in 2 or 4 divided doses. It is recommended that treatment continue at least 1–3 days after symptoms of infection subside.

Important Nursing Implications for Tetracyclines

- ☐ Tetracyclines should not be administered to pregnant women (especially during the second and third trimesters) or children under 7 because of potential adverse effects on bone and teeth.
- ☐ Observe clients receiving tetracyclines for indications of superinfection such as black, furry, bacterial or fungal overgrowths on the tongue, diarrhea, and vaginal or anorectal itchiness.
- ☐ Instruct clients to avoid excessive exposure to sunlight while receiving tetracyclines because of the possibility of photosensitivity.
- ☐ Monitor renal, hepatic, and hematopoietic function during prolonged therapy with tetracyclines for indications of toxicity.
- ☐ Observe clients receiving tetracyclines concurrently with anticoagulants for indications of excess bleeding. This indicates a need to reduce the dose of the anticoagulant.
- ☐ Advise clients not to take tetracyclines with milk or other dairy products, antacids, or iron preparations.
- ☐ Store tetracyclines in light- and moisture-resistant containers and protect from extremes of heat. Observe listed expiration dates. Decomposition products of tetracyclines can be toxic.

Chloramphenicol

Mechanisms and Effects Chloramphenicol was isolated from *Streptomyces venezuelae* in 1947. Its mechanism resembles that of tetracyclines as well as clindamycin (Cleocin) and erythromycin. It binds to bacterial ribosomes to inhibit protein synthesis, resulting in a bacteriostatic action. Chloramphenicol also inhibits ribosomes within mitochondria of host cells, perhaps because of the resemblance of these to bacterial ribosomes. This action is exerted especially on red blood cells.

Pharmacokinetics Chloramphenicol is rapidly absorbed after oral administration reaching peak plasma concentrations in 1–2 hours. The drug distributes to all body fluids including the cerebral spinal fluid and, in fact, reaches higher levels in the brain than in the plasma. It crosses the placental barrier and appears in breast milk. Chloramphenicol is excreted in the urine, partly unchanged, and partly as metabolites. The elimination half-life is 1.6–3.3 hours.

Clinical Indications The antibacterial spectrum of chloramphenicol is broad (Table 47–10), but its toxicity limits its use to organisms not susceptible or poorly susceptible to other antibacterial drugs. Chloramphenicol is a primary selection for infections due to *Rickettsia, Salmonella, Haemophilus influenzae, Pseudomonas pseudomallei, Campylobacter fetus,* and *Bacteroides fragilis.* It is a secondary choice for anaerobic *Streptococci, Streptococci pneumoniae, Neisseria meningitidis, Bacillus anthracis, Listeria monocytogenes, Erysipelothrix rhusiopathiae, Clostridium perfringens, Escherichia coli, Klebsiella pneumoniae, Shigella, Brucella, Yersinia pestis, Francisella tularensis, Fusubacterium nucleatum, Actinomyces israelii,* and *Chlamydia.* Chloramphenicol is particularly useful in treating clients with bacterial meningitis because of its ability to penetrate into the cerebral spinal fluid (Table 47–11).

Adverse Effects and Contraindications Adverse reactions to chloramphenicol include blood dyscrasias, gastrointestinal irritation, neurotoxicity, hypersensitivity reactions, and the gray syndrome in infants. The occurrence of **blood dyscrasias** is the limiting feature of chloramphenicol. Chloramphenicol has a suppressant effect on the bone marrow that can result in pancytopenia or reduced levels of a single class of blood cells: leukopenia, thrombocytopenia, or aplastic anemia. The hematological toxicity of chloramphenicol is sometimes fatal, although only one in 30,000 individuals experiences bone marrow suppression. Aplastic anemia is the most common hematological reaction. Bone marrow suppression may occur weeks or even months after therapy with chloramphenicol is discontinued. *Baseline blood studies should be conducted before initiating therapy with chloramphenicol and repeated throughout therapy. Clients should be advised to report immediately symptoms of sore throat, fever, easy fatigability, or abnormal bleeding tendencies.*

Gastrointestinal irritation is similar to that caused by many other antibacterial drugs: nausea, vomiting, and diarrhea. Peritoneal irritation and altered taste sensations also occur. **Nephrotoxicity** is uncommon, but blurred vision, paresthesias, optic and peripheral neuritis, and depression have been reported. *The nurse should monitor the intake-output ratio for indications of nephrotoxicity.* **Hypersensitivity reactions** include skin eruptions (rashes, urticaria), anaphylaxis, and drug fever.

Neonates have limited ability to metabolize chloramphenicol, which requires glucuronidation by the liver. In addition, renal excretion of the unchanged drug is slow in neonates. As a result, infants are highly prone to chloramphenicol toxicity unless doses are very sharply reduced. Because of drug accumulation, chloramphenicol produces a characteristic, sometimes fatal, reaction called the **gray syndrome** in infants. It typically occurs from 3–9 days after treatment is initiated with chloramphenicol. Symptoms include abdominal distention, emesis, pallid cyanosis, vasomotor collapse, dyspnea, and death. *Mothers taking chloramphenicol should be advised against breast-feeding.*

Drug Interactions Chloramphenicol is an inhibitor of liver microsomal enzymes, thus prolonging the action of phenytoin (Dilantin), alcohol, barbiturates, oral anticoagulants, and oral hypoglycemics. This interaction has resulted in fatalities. *Nurses should advise clients to avoid use of alcohol during therapy with chloramphenicol. Clients with diabetes who usually employ oral hypoglycemic agents may be required to use insulin instead during chloramphenicol treatment.* Drugs that induce liver enzymes decrease the half-life of chloramphenicol.

Preparations and Administration *Chloramphenicol should be taken on an empty stomach with a full glass of water.*

Chloramphenicol (Chloromycetin, Mychel-S, and generic)

Table 47–11
Penetration of Antibacterial Drugs into the CSF

Good penetration with meninges intact	Penetration when meninges inflamed	Little or no penetration into CSF
Chloramphenicol	Penicillins	Aminoglycosides
Flucytosine	Second- and third-generation cephalosporins	Amphotericin B
Isoniazid	Moxalactam	First-generation cephalosporins
Metronidazole	Rifampin	Clindamycin
Sulfonamides	Trimethoprim	Lincomycin
		Polymyxin B
		Vancomycin

Capsules, oral suspension, powder for injection solutions, injection solution
Recommended Doses: For adults and children, excepting neonates, 50 or 100 mg/kg/day orally in 4 divided doses at 6-hour intervals. The recommended dose in neonates is 25 mg/kg/day in 4 doses at 6-hour intervals.

Important Nursing Implications for Chloramphenicol

- ☐ Assess clients receiving chloramphenicol for indications of hypersensitivity reactions such as rash.
- ☐ Conduct periodic blood cell counts and monitor clients for indications of possible agranulocytosis such as fever or sore throat.
- ☐ Assess clients given chloramphenicol for evidences of superinfection, such as black, furry overgrowths on the tongue, rectal or vaginal itching, or diarrhea.
- ☐ Instruct clients not to use alcohol during therapy with chloramphenicol.

Sulfonamides and Trimethoprim

Sulfonamides, the oldest of the effective antimicrobials, dominated chemotherapy for bacterial infections until the introduction of penicillins. Domagk received the Nobel prize in 1938 for his discovery of sulfonamides in 1932. Though sulfonamides were out of vogue for three decades after the penicillins became available, the last decade has seen a resurgence of their use, especially the combination of sulfamethoxazole and trimethoprim. Sulfonamides are not antibiotics, since they are not derived from a biological source. Instead, they are synthetic derivatives of sulfanilamide, which is a subunit of certain azo dyes. Twelve sulfonamides are currently marketed in preparations for oral, parenteral, dermatological, ophthalmic, and vaginal administration.

Mechanisms and Effects Sulfonamides have a **bacteriostatic** action on a broad spectrum of gram-negative as well as gram-positive bacteria (Table 47–10). Since sulfonamides serve only to hold bacterial proliferation in check, ultimate eradication of the infection depends upon adequate functioning of the immune system and phagocytic cells. Sulfonamides are not effective against viruses, fungi, or protozoa.

Sulfonamides inhibit expansion of bacterial infections by blocking an important step in bacterial metabolism (Figure 47–4). Sulfonamides are competitive inhibitors of the bacterial enzyme that initiates the metabolic sequence using para-aminobenzoic acid (PABA) as a substrate. As an inhibitor of the final step in the sequence, trimethoprim has a synergistic effect with sulfonamides, and the combination of these drugs has become a mainstay of chemotherapy. Sulfonamides can also be used effectively in combination with tetracyclines, but the effect obtained when sulfonamides are used in conjunction with penicillins is unpredictable.

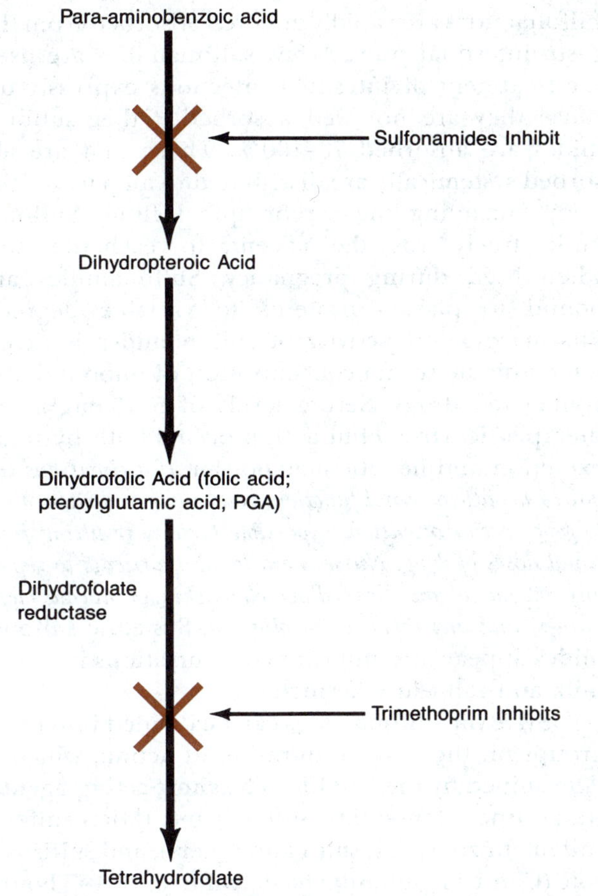

Figure 47–4
Sites of action of sulfonamides and trimethoprim in metabolism of tetrahydrofolate.

Resistance to sulfonamides has been acquired by some strains of bacterial species usually susceptible to sulfonamides. Cross-resistance occurs within the sulfonamide family but not with other antibacterial drug groups. Many strains of *Neisseria gonorrhoeae, Neisseria meningitidis,* and *Shigella* have acquired resistance. Some bacterial species have natural resistance to sulfonamides, including *Pseudomonas aeruginosa, Enterobacter aerogenes, Francisella tularensis, Bordetella pertussis, Mycobacteria, Leptospira borrelia, Treponema,* and *Rickettsiae.*

Pharmacokinetics Trimethoprim and most sulfonamides are rapidly and well absorbed from the gastrointestinal tract. A few sulfonamides are used for treatment of intestinal infections expressly because they are not well absorbed. Other sulfonamides are absorbed 70–100%. Those that are absorbed systemically are distributed to all parts of the body, including the cerebrospinal fluid. Sulfonamides freely cross the placenta to reach the fetus when used during pregnancy. Sulfonamides are bound to plasma proteins to variable degrees. Pharmacological activity of sulfonamides is determined by the serum concentration of unbound, unconjugated drugs. Serum levels of 5–15 mg% are therapeutic. Drug elimination occurs both by renal excretion and hepatic metabolism. *If a client has impaired hepatic or renal function, both nurse and client need to give special attention to possible toxicity resulting from usual doses of drug. Nurses need to advise clients to report any evidence of jaundice (yellow sclera, skin, or mucous membranes) and any incidents of oliguria.* Systemic sulfonamides appear in significant concentrations in breast milk and can cause kernicterus.

Systemic sulfonamides can be divided into three groups on the basis of duration of action, which is determined by the half-life. The **short-acting agents,** sulfacytine (Renoquid), sulfadiazine (Microsulfon), sulfamethizole (Thiosulfil and others), and sulfisoxazole (Gantisin, Sulfasox) have half-lives of 4–7 hours. The **intermediate-acting drugs,** trimethoprim and sulfamethoxazole (Bactrim, Septra), have half-lives of 10–12 hours. Sulfamethoxazole and trimethoprim have well-matched pharmacokinetic properties that help to ensure a nearly constant ratio (20:1) when the two are used together. The **long-acting sulfonamides,** sulfamethoxypyridazine and sulfadimethoxine, are no longer available because their use was associated with a high incidence of erythema multiforme.

Clinical Indications Although sulfonamides have been replaced for many purposes, they are often primary drug choices for urinary tract infections caused by *E. coli* and for diseases caused by *Yersinia enterocolitica* (yersiniosis), *Nocardia,* and *Chlamydia trachomatis* (trachoma). In addition, sulfonamides are useful secondary choices for infections caused by *Brucella, Haemophilus ducreyi, Haemophilus influenzae, Vibrio cholerae, Salmonella, Serratia,* and susceptible strains of *Shigella.* The widespread use of sulfonamides in Third World nations can be attributed to the inexpensiveness of sulfonamides and the prevalence of sensitive pathogens. Sulfonamides are also appropriate for meningitis caused by susceptible organisms because of their ability to penetrate the cerebral spinal fluid (Table 47–11). Sulfonamides that are highly soluble in urine are particularly effective for clients with kidney infections (pyelonephritis), which are usually caused by organisms susceptible to sulfonamides — *E. coli, Klebsiella, Enterobacter, Proteus,* or *Staphylococcus aureus.* The combination of trimethoprim and sulfamethoxazole is frequently used in preference to a sulfonamide alone for infections caused by *E. coli, Haemophilus influenzae, Serratia, Yersinia enterocolitica, Vibrio cholerae,* and *Pneumocystis carinii.*

Some of the sulfonamides have specialized uses. Sulfadiazine is approved for use as an alternative to penicillin for prophylaxis against recurrent rheumatic fever. Sulfasalazine, a sulfonamide that is not absorbed appreciably, is useful for treating clients with ulcerative colitis. Sulfapyridine, an older sulfonamide, is employed topically for an autoimmune inflammatory disorder of the skin called dermatitis herpetiformis, although dapsone is usually a preferred treatment. Mafenide and silver sulfadiazine are sulfonamides used topically on burns to protect against infection. These agents are discussed in Chapter 53. Sulfacetamide and sulfisoxazole are available in ophthalmic solutions or ointments for treatment of conjunctivitis, corneal ulcers, and other superficial infections of the eye caused by susceptible organisms. Sulfisoxazole, sulfathiazole, sulfabenzamide, and sulfacetamide are available for treatment of vaginitis caused by *Haemophilus vaginalis,* in the form of vaginal creams and vaginal tablets. Intravenous infusions of the combination of trimethoprim and sulfamethoxazole (Bactrim, Septra) are currently being employed in critically ill patients with acquired immune deficiency syndrome (AIDS).

Adverse Effects and Contraindications The adverse effects of sulfonamides include hypersensitivity reactions, hematological reactions, gastrointestinal irritation, neuropathies and psychiatric problems, crystalluria and renal toxicity, goiter, hypoglycemia, reduced sperm count, and alopecia. There are a large variety of serious side effects with sulfonamides, but the total incidence of these is only about 0.1%.

Hypersensitivity reactions are frequent with sulfonamides and account for the majority of side effects of these drugs. Allergic reactions are especially likely with long-term use. Mild dermatological hypersensitivity reactions include urticaria, pruritus, skin eruptions, purpura, and photosensitivity reactions. Very serious reactions include erythema multiforme, erythema nodosum, epidermal necrolysis, and exfoliative dermatitis. Dermatological reactions are three times more common with the trimethoprim-sulfisoxazole combination than when sulfisoxazole is used alone. Systemic allergic reactions are similarly varied: anaphylactoid reactions, serum sickness, periorbital edema, conjunctival or scleral injection, arthralgia, allergic myocarditis, eosinophilia, polyarteritis nodosum, lupus erythematosus-like reactions, and drug fever. Cross-sensitivity is frequent but not universal between sulfonamide drugs.

Hematological reactions include aplastic anemia, hemolytic anemia, agranulocytosis, leukopenia, thrombocytopenia, hypoprothrombinemia, and methemoglobinemia. Some cases of anemia are due to allergic reactions, some to bone marrow suppression, and some occur in patients with deficiency of glucose-6-phosphate dehydrogenase. *The nurse should watch for symptoms indicative of hematological reactions: sore throat, fever, pallor, hematuria, cloudy urine, and fatigability.*

Gastrointestinal irritation occurs in only 1–2% of individuals given sulfonamides. Typical manifestations are nausea, vomiting, cramps, diarrhea, or anorexia. Sulfasalazine (Azulfidine) is most likely to cause such reactions, because it remains in the intestines. *The nurse should instruct patients to take sulfasalazine with food if gastrointestinal irritation occurs. Other sulfonamides are taken at least 1–2 hours before meals with a full glass of water.* Sulfonamides infrequently cause hepatitis, jaundice, pancreatitis, stomatitis, or toxic nephrosis.

A troublesome problem with sulfonamides is the risk of **crystalluria,** the formation of sulfonamide crystals in the urine due to poor solubility at low pH. The result can be renal or urinary tract lesions. Sulfadiazine and sulfamethoxazole are especially likely to cause formation of crystals, sulfisoxazole less so. The risk of crystals can be reduced by three interventions: (1) alkalinization of the urine by administration of sodium bicarbonate, (2) maintenance of good hydration, or (3) use of combinations of sulfonamides. Combinations of sulfonamides reduce risk of crystals for the simple reason that although pharmacological activity is comparable and additive, the drugs have independent solubilities. With the newer, more soluble sulfonamides, there is less reason to use combinations, although some are still marketed. Urinary tract obstructions increase the risk of crystal formation because of urinary stasis. *The nurse should monitor renal output in patients receiving sulfonamides. Fluid intake should be at least 2,500 ml/day (unless the client is fluid-restricted) to ensure a urine output of at least 1,200 ml/day. Urine pH should be measured daily and alkalinization with sodium bicarbonate undertaken if the urine becomes too acidic or if visual inspection reveals presence of crystals or blood.* Sulfasalazine may cause a yellow discoloration of the urine.

Central nervous system effects of sulfonamides include both neurologic and psychiatric reactions. The **neurological side effects** range from headache, vertigo, dizziness, tinnitus, insomnia, fatigue, lassitude, and drowsiness to ataxia, hearing loss, peripheral neuritis and neuropathies, and convulsions. **Psychiatric reactions** include depression, psychosis, and hallucinations.

The sulfonamides are chemically related to the thiazide diuretics, sulfonylurea hypoglycemics, and the antithyroid drugs, and can produce lesser degrees of the actions associated with each of these drug classes: diuresis, hypoglycemia, hypothyroidism, and goiter. Other side effects include suppression of sperm production and alopecia.

Contraindications for use of systemic sulfonamides are (1) hypersensitivity to sulfonamides or drugs of related structure, (2) pregnancy, lactation, or infancy, (3) urinary tract obstruction, and (4) porphyria (because sulfonamides can precipitate acute attacks).

Drug Interactions Sulfonamides are highly bound to plasma proteins and will displace other drugs that are similarly highly bound. This is most significant when the competing drug is an oral anticoagulant or cardiac glycoside.

In the kidney, sulfonamides are transported by the organic anion carrier system in the proximal tubule and will alter transport of other drugs using this system such as methotrexate and tolbutamide. Drugs or foods that acidify the urine increase the risk that sulfonamide crystals will form, whereas urinary alkalinizers decrease the risk. Sulfonamides should not be used with methenamine, since the latter drug forms formaldehyde in the urine, a substance that can precipitate sulfonamide crystals. Sulfonamides produce false positives in urinary glucose measurements.

Sulfonamides can retard the metabolism of other drugs that are acted upon by the same liver enzymes that degrade the sulfonamide. For example, certain sulfonamides produce a disulfiram-like potentiation of the effects of alcohol. *Nurses should advise clients to refrain from use of alcohol while receiving sulfonamides.* The half-lives of phenytoin (Dilantin) and first-generation oral hypoglycemics are also prolonged in this manner when coadministered with sulfonamides.

Preparations and Administration The combination of trimethoprim and sulfamethoxazole (Bactrim, Septra) is far and away the most widely prescribed sulfonamide-containing preparation. Sulfamethizole and sulfacytine are seldom used. Oral sulfonamide combinations, so-called "triple sulfas," consisting of equal parts (162 or 167 mg) of sulfadiazine, sulfamerazine, and sulfamethazine, as tablets or suspensions, are also seldom employed. Triple sulfa combinations in vaginal creams and tablets, containing sulfathiazole, sulfacetamide, and sulfabenzamide, are more commonly employed (for topical treatment of vaginitis due to *Haemophilus vaginalis*). Local irritant effects can occur, including pruritus, urticaria, and vulvitis. *The client should be advised to stop treatment if local irritation occurs.* Ophthalmic preparations are discussed in Chapter 54 and burn preparations in Chapter 53.

The infusion solution combination of trimethoprim and sulfamethoxazole is diluted within 2 hours prior to use in 125 ml of 5% dextrose in water. *It should not be mixed with other drugs because of the potential for incompatibilities. The solution should be discarded if cloudy or if a precipitate forms.*

Sulfacytine (Renoquid)
Tablets
Recommended Doses: For adults and children over 14, 500 mg PO initially, followed by 250 mg qid for 10 days. The drug is not indicated for children under 14.

Sulfadiazine (Microsulfon and generic)
Tablets
Recommended Doses: For prophylaxis against recurrent attacks of rheumatic fever, 1 g PO daily for clients weighing more than 30 kg or 0.5 g daily for clients weighing less than 30 kg. For susceptible infections, 2–4 g PO as a loading dose for adults, followed by 2–4 g/day in 3–6 divided doses. For children, the loading dose is 75 mg/kg PO, followed by maintenance doses of 150 mg/kg/day in 4–6 divided doses.

Sulfamethizole (Thiosulfil, Microsul, Proklar, Urifon, Urobak)
Tablets
Recommended Doses: For adults, 0.5–1.0 g PO, 2 or 4 times daily. For children over 2 months, 30–45 mg/kg/day PO in 4 divided doses.

Sulfamethoxazole (Gantanol, Methoxal)
Tablets, oral suspension
Recommended Doses: For adults, 2 g PO initially followed by a maintenance dose of 1 g tid in the morning and evening. For children over 2 months, 50–60 mg/kg PO initially, followed by a maintenance schedule of 25-30 mg/kg, morning and evening.

Sulfapyridine
Tablets
Recommended Doses: For treatment of dermatitis herpetiformis, 500 mg PO qid.

Sulfasalazine (Azulfidine and generic)
Tablets, enteric coated tablets
Recommended Doses: For adults, 3–4 g/day PO in divided doses initially, reduced to 2 g daily in 4 divided doses for maintenance after the condition is controlled. For children, 40–60 mg/kg/day PO in 3–6 divided doses until the condition is under control; followed by 30 mg/kg/day in 4 doses for maintenance.

Sulfisoxazole (Gantrisin, Sulfasox, and generic)
Tablets, syrup (chocolate flavored), pediatric suspension (raspberry flavored), long-acting emulsion (vanilla-mint flavored) (Lipo Gantrisin), injection solution
Recommended Doses: For adults, 2–4 g PO loading dose followed by 4–8 g/day in 4–6 divided doses. For children over 2 months, 75 mg/kg PO loading dose and 150 mg/kg/day maintenance dose in 4–6 divided doses to a maximum of 6 g/day. Sulfisoxazole for injection (SC, IM, or IV), is used only in clients unable to take oral medication.

Trimethoprim-sulfamethoxazole (Bactrim, Septra)
Tablets, double-strength tablets, oral suspensions (fruit-licorice or cherry flavor), infusion solution
Recommended Doses: For urinary tract infections in adults, 160 mg trimethoprim and 800 mg sulfamethoxazole PO every 12 hours for 10–14 days. For urinary tract infections or otitis media in children over 2 months, 8 mg/kg trimethoprim and 40 mg/kg sulfamethoxazole PO each day in 2 divided doses at 12-hour intervals for 10 days. For IV infusion, the contents of a 5 ml ampul (80 mg trimethoprim and 400 mg of sulfamethoxazole) are added to 125 ml of 5% dextrose in water for infusion over 60–90 minutes.

Oral sulfanomide combinations, containing sulfadiazine, sulfamerazine, and sulfamethazine
Tablets, suspension
Recommended Doses: For adults, 2–4 g PO initially, then 2–4 g daily in 3–6 divided doses. For children over 2 months, 175 mg/kg PO initially, then 150 mg/kg/day in 4–6 divided doses, to a maximum of 6 g daily.

Vaginal creams and tablets, containing sulfathiazole, sulfacetamide, and sulfabenzamide
Recommended Doses: Twice daily for 4 days to 2 weeks. *Instruct the client to insert the cream or tablet high into the vagnia.*

Important Nursing Implications for Sulfonamides

☐ Monitor the urinary output of clients receiving sulfonamides for changes that might indicate nephrotoxicity. Advise clients to drink at least 2,500 ml of water daily while receiving sulfonamide medications to ensure a urine output of at least 1,200 ml/day. Visually examine the urine for evidence of crystals. Report any evidence of possible crystalluria to the physician. Alkalinization of the urine with sodium bicarbonate may be required.

- ☐ Observe clients and teach them to watch for indications of allergic reactions to sulfonamides such as rash or eruptions.
- ☐ Conduct periodic blood cell counts to check for occurrence of blood dyscrasias. Teach clients to recognize and report indications of anemia (fatigue and pallor), thrombocytopenia (purpura and occult bleeding), and agranulocytosis (fever and sore throat).
- ☐ Observe clients for indications of diuresis or hypoglycemia.
- ☐ Provide clients with a list of drugs that may interact with the sulfonamide that is being administered.
- ☐ Monitor clients for interactions of sulfonamides with other drugs that are highly bound to plasma proteins, such as nonsteroidal anti-inflammatory drugs, antiepileptics, oral anticoagulants, oral hypoglycemics, and digoxin.
- ☐ Do not administer sulfonamides to women during the final trimester of pregnancy.
- ☐ Instruct clients not to administer sulfonamides with antacids or emollient laxatives, since these inhibit absorption of the antibiotic.

Other General Antibacterial Drugs

The Macrolides

The macrolide antibacterial drugs include erythromycin, its various salts, and troleandomycin. Erythromycin was discovered in 1952, as a substance produced by *Streptomyces erythreus.* The name *macrolide* refers to the multiple lactone rings that compose the nucleus of these antibiotics.

Mechanisms and Effects Erythromycin and troleandomycin (Tao) inhibit protein synthesis by binding to the same site of bacterial ribosomes that is bound by chloramphenicol. The macrolides are usually bacteriostatic but can be bactericidal depending on dose and the microorganism upon which they are acting. The macrolides are most active against gram-positive cocci (Table 47–12). Acquired resistance has not developed commonly to erythromycin in most species but does occur in many strains of *Staphylococcus aureus.* Cross-resistance occurs between macrolides and lincosamides.

Pharmacokinetics Erythromycin base (E-Mycin, Ilotycin, and others) is absorbed from the initial segment of the intestines but is inactivated by gastric acid. It must be administered in an enteric coated formulation to be effective. Various esters of erythromycin have been developed in an attempt to increase acid stability. These include stearate, estolate, and ethylsuccinate esters. The stearate ester does not produce significantly more absorption than erythromycin base, but the esolate and ethylsuccinate esters do provide improved stability and absorption. Erythromycin lactobionate and erythromycin gluceptate (Ilotycin) are available as powders for reconstitution and IV injection, but this route is reserved for patients unable to tolerate oral medication.

After absorption, macrolide antibiotics distribute into all body fluids. Penetration into the cerebral spinal fluid is limited unless the meninges are inflamed. Erythromycin crosses the placental barrier, but in reduced concentrations, and is excreted in breast milk. Plasma binding is about 72% for erythromycin. Erythromycin is concentrated in the liver and excreted in the bile and urine. Only 10–15% is excreted unchanged in the urine. Erythromycin has a half-life of 1.1–3.5 hours.

Clinical Indications Erythromycin and troleandomycin have similar spectra. The latter drug has no special advantages over the older agent and is seldom used in practice. Erythromycin is employed most often for infections caused by gram-positive organisms and is used as an alternative to penicillin in patients sensitive to that class of drugs. Erythromycin is especially useful against *Staphylococcus aureus, Streptococcus pneumoniae,* and *Streptococcus pyrogenes.* It is also highly effective against gram-positive bacilli, including *Clostridium tetani, Bacillus anthrax, Listeria monocytogenes, Erysipelothrix rhusiopathiae,* and *Corynebacterium diphtheriae.* Erythromycin is an excellent alternative treatment for *Neisseria gonorrhoeae.* A few species of gram-negative bacilli are also inhibited by erythromycin, including some strains of *Bacteroides fragilis, Bordetella pertussis, Flavobacterium meningosepticum, Fusobacterium nucleatum,* and *Legionella pneumophilia* (erythromycin is the drug of choice for Legionnaire's disease). Erythromycin is highly active against *Mycoplasma pneumoniae,* the causative agent of atypical pneumonia. *Chlamydia trachomatis* and *Treponema pallidum* are also inhibited by erythromycin.

Adverse Effects and Contraindications The adverse effects of macrolides include mild and serious hypersensitivity reactions, superinfection, hepatoxicity, gastrointestinal irritation, and rarely,

Table 47–12
Antibacterial Spectra of Miscellaneous Antibacterial Drugs

Bacterial species	Macrolides	Lincosamides	Vancomycin	Spectinomycin	Polymyxins	Bacitracin
Gram-positive cocci						
Peptostreptococcus	Yes*	Yes*				
Staphylococcus						
aureus	Some[R]*	Yes*	Yes*			
epidermidis	Yes		Yes			
Streptococcus						
faecalis	Yes*	No	Yes*			
pneumoniae	Yes*	Yes	Yes			
pyrogenes			Yes*			
viridans		Yes	Yes			
Gram-positive bacilli						
Bacillus anthrax	Yes*					
Clostridium perfringens	Yes	Yes*	Yes			
Other Clostridium	Yes*	Yes	Yes			
Corynebacterium diphtheriae	Yes*	Yes	Yes			
Erysipelothrix rhusiopathiae	Yes*					
Listeria monocytogenes	Yes*					
Gram-negative cocci						
Neisseria gonorrhoeae	Yes*	No		Yes*		Yes
Neisseria meningitidis	Weak	No			No	Yes
Gram-negative bacilli						
Bacteroides fragilis	Few*	Yes*				
Bordetella pertussis	Yes*					
Enterobacter aerogenes					Yes	Yes
Escherichia coli					Yes	
Flavobacterium meningosepticum	Yes*					
Fusobacterium nucleatum	Yes*	Yes*				Yes
Haemophilus influenzae	Weak	No				Yes
Legionella pneumophilia	Yes*				Yes	
Pasteurella multocida	Yes				Yes	
Proteus mirabilis					No	
Proteus (indole-positive)					No	
Pseudomonas aeruginosa					Yes*	Yes
Pseudomonas mallei						Yes
Salmonella					Yes	
Actinomycetes						
Actinomyces israelii		Yes	Yes			Yes
Nocardia						Yes
Spirochetes						
Borrelia	Yes				Yes	
Treponema pallidum	Yes*					

Table 47–12
Antibacterial Spectra of Miscellaneous Antibacterial Drugs (*continued*)

Bacterial species	Macrolides	Lincosa-mides	Vancomycin	Spectino-mycin	Polymyxins	Bacitracin
Mycobacteria						
Mycobacterium fortuitum	Yes					
Mycobacterium scrofulaceum	Yes					
Primative bacteria						
Chlamydia trachomatis	Yes*					
Mycoplasma pneumoniae	Yes*					

Key: Yes: Active against the indicated bacterial species.
No: Not effective.
Weak: Weakly effective.
Some: Effective against some strains.
Few: Effective against a few strains.
R: Some instances of acquired resistance have been noted.
*: Clinical use as a primary or alternative choice.
Blank: Effectiveness not established.

transient auditory impairment. **Hypersensitivity reactions** vary from rashes and urticaria to anaphylaxis, jaundice, fever, leukocytosis, and eosinophilia. Superinfection occurs with erythromycin to a similar extent as with penicillin drugs.

Hepatic toxicity is due to infiltration of leukocytes and may result in cholestasis. Liver toxicity usually occurs only with high doses or prolonged treatment. Under these circumstances, periodic liver function tests should be conducted. Erythromycin estolate (Ilosone) is more likely to cause hepatotoxicity than other preparations of macrolides and should not be used in patients with a prior history of hepatic disease. **Irritant effects** of macrolides on the alimentary tract are manifested as nausea, vomiting, and abdominal cramps. *Although food decreases absorption of erythromycin, the drug may be taken with meals if gastrointestinal irritation occurs when the drug is taken on an empty stomach.* Intravenous administration of macrolides also results in irritation at the site of administration — that is, phlebitis and pain. **Ototoxicity** with erythromycin is considerably less severe than that produced by aminoglycosides, occurring only at high doses. It is reversible with drug elimination. The only contraindication for macrolides is a history of sensitivity to drugs in this group or the lincosamides.

Drug Interactions Macrolides have a synergistic effectiveness when used with sulfonamides against *Haemophilus influenzae.* The product Pediazole is a combination preparation of erythromycin ethylsuccinate and sulfisoxazole that is marketed (as a powder for making oral suspensions) for use in treating acute otitis media caused by *H. influenzae.* Erythromycin and lincosamides have a mutually antagonistic effect and should not be used concurrently. Macrolides (and lincosamides) decrease renal clearance of theophylline, thus elevating serum concentrations of the xanthine. Appropriate dosage adjustment for theophylline is required when treatment with any of these antibacterial drugs is instituted.

Preparations and Administration The parenteral forms of erythromycin must be prepared in sterile water without preservatives to avoid precipitation.

Erythromycin base (E-Mycin, Ilotycin, and others)
Enteric or film coated tablets
Recommended Doses: Vary according to the organism, but 250 mg PO every 6 hours is typical for adults and 30–50 mg/kg/day in 3 or 4 divided doses is usual for children.

Erythromycin estolate (Ilosone)
Capsules, tablets, chewable tablets, drops, oral suspension, powder for oral suspension
Recommended Doses: Same as for erythromycin base.

Erythromycin ethylsuccinate
Chewable tablets, film coated tablets, suspensions, powder for oral suspensions, powder for preparation of oral drops
Recommended Doses: For adults, 400 mg PO qid.

Erythromycin lactobionate (generic)
Erythromycin gluceptate (Ilotycin gluceptate)
Powders for injection
Recommended Doses: 1–4 g IV daily in divided doses.

Erythromycin stearate
Film coated tablets
Recommended Doses: Same as for erythromycin base.

Troleandomycin (Tao)
Capsules, oral suspension
Recommended Doses: For adults, 250–500 mg PO qid. For children, one-half the adult dose.

Important Nursing Implications for Macrolides

- ☐ Monitor clients receiving erythromycin or troleandomycin for indications of superinfection such as furry overgrowths on the tongue, vaginal or rectal itching, or diarrhea.
- ☐ Observe clients receiving either of these drugs for allergic reactions such as rash or anaphylaxis.
- ☐ Assess for indications of hepatotoxicity (such as jaundice), especially when the esolate form of erythromycin is employed.
- ☐ Avoid letting these drugs touch the skin since they can produce contact dermatitis.
- ☐ Administer macrolide antimicrobial drugs on an empty stomach, or with food if gastrointestinal irritation occurs.

Lincosamides

Mechanisms and Effects The lincosamides include lincomycin (Lincocin), an antibiotic produced by *Streptomyces lincolnensis,* and clindamycin (Cleocin), a synthetic congener of lincomycin. Lincomycin was discovered in 1962. These agents are bacteriostatic, acting to inhibit protein synthesis by binding to the ribosomes in a manner similar to macrolides and chloramphenicol. Lincosamides and these antibiotics of related mechanism can inhibit each other and should not be employed concurrently. Lincomycin produces more untoward reactions than clindamycin with no advantage in activity, so it is seldom employed.

Pharmacokinetics Clindamycin is more completely and reliably absorbed than lincomycin. Concurrent administration of kaolin inhibits oral absorption of both lincosamides. Clindamycin achieves peak plasma levels in 1 hour and is eliminated 90% by hepatic metabolism, 10% by renal elimination of unchanged drug. Clindamycin distributes to all body fluids except the cerebral spinal fluid.

Clinical Indications The lincosamides are active mainly against *Staphylococcus aureus, Peptostreptococcus, Clostridium perfringens, Bacteroides fragilis,* and *Fusobacterium nucleatum.* Clindamycin is used mainly in individuals allergic to penicillins or for microbes resistant to penicillins or cephalosporins.

Adverse Effects and Contraindications Adverse effects of lincosamides include hypersensitivity reactions, hematopoietic reactions, gastrointestinal irritation, hypotension, and ototoxicity. The reported **hypersensitivity reactions** include rash, urticaria, vaginitis, anaphylaxis, serum sickness, and rare instances of erythema multiforme and exfoliative dermatitis. Skin reactions occur in about 10% of individuals treated with clindamycin. Rare **blood cell dyscrasias** produced by lincosamides include neutropenia, agranulocytosis, thrombocytopenic purpura, aplastic anemia, and pancytopenia.

Gastrointestinal irritation ranges from nausea, vomiting, glossitis, stomatitis, persistent diarrhea, and pruritus ani to potentially fatal pseudomembranous colitis. *The nurse should instruct clients to take oral medications with a full glass of water to prevent esophageal irritation. To minimize diarrhea, food should be avoided 1–2 hours before and after ingestion of lincosamides. If diarrhea occurs in spite of this precaution, kaolin may be administered, but no sooner than 2 hours after and at least 3–4 hours before taking the antibiotic again. In rare instances, lincomycin-induced diarrhea has been fatal. Nurses need therefore to stress the importance of observing stools for blood and mucus and reporting appearance and quantity of fecal material expelled. This is especially important for elderly or debilitated clients, who can easily become dehydrated and develop electrolyte imbalance.*

Ototoxic effects of lincosamides include both tinnitus and vertigo. Like the macrolides, lincosamides interfere with renal excretion of theophylline. Also, like aminoglycosides, lincosamides can produce a degree of neuromuscular blockade that can be additive to that produced by curare or anesthetics.

Preparations and Administration Lincosamides are best taken one to two hours after meals with a full glass of water. Absorption of clindamycin is less influenced by concurrent food ingestion than is absorption of lincomycin. Lincomycin (Lincocin) is seldom used.

Clindamycin (Cleocin)
Capsules, flavored granules, injection solution
Recommended Doses: In adults, 150–450 mg PO every 6 hours. For children, 8–20 mg/kg/day in 3 or 4 divided doses.

Lincomycin (Lincocin)
Capsules, pediatric capsules, syrup (raspberry flavor syrup), injection solution
Recommended Doses: For adults, 500 mg PO every 6 or 8 hours. For children over 1 month old, 30–60 mg/kg/day PO in 3 or 4 doses.

Vancomycin (Vancocin)

Mechanisms and Effects Vancomycin is an antibiotic produced by *Streptomyces orientalis,* another actinomycete. It is structurally unrelated to aminoglycosides. Its mechanism is similar to that of the penicillins: it binds to the subunits that are used to make bacterial cell walls, causing deterioration of the cell wall in bacteria that are proliferating. It is bactericidal for most gram-positive bacteria, although only bacteriostatic against *Streptococcus faecalis.*

Pharmacokinetics Absorption of vancomycin is poor after oral administration, but after intravenous administration, effective plasma concentrations persist for about 6 hours, which is also the half-life of the drug. Vancomycin is 10% bound by plasma proteins and distributes into most body fluids. Vancomycin appears in the cerebral spinal fluid if meningitis is present. Elimination is almost exclusively by renal extraction.

Clinical Indications The special value of vancomycin is its effectiveness against not only penicillin-resistant *Staphylococcus aureus* but even the methicillin-resistant strains. Although a very few strains of *Staphylococcus aureus* have natural resistance to vancomycin, there is no evidence that acquired resistance has developed since vancomycin was discovered in 1956. Vancomycin can be used effectively in combinations with aminoglycosides to achieve a synergistic effect against *Streptococcus faecalis.* It is reserved for infections caused by susceptible organisms for which penicillins or cephalosporins are inappropriate due to resistance or hypersensitivity.

Adverse Effects and Contraindications Adverse reactions include **hypersensitivity reactions** (rash, urticaria, drug fever, eosinophilia, and anaphylactoid reactions), **neutropenia, nephrotoxicity,** and **ototoxicity.** Vancomycin can produce nephrotoxic and ototoxic effects but is less likely to do so than are the aminoglycosides. Ototoxicity is usually caused by excessive plasma levels of the drug. *Nurses need to assure that renal function tests and audiograms are performed before initiation of therapy with vancomycin.* Elderly recipients of the drug are especially vulnerable to both renal and ototoxicity. If there is preexisting renal or hearing impairment, vancomycin should be avoided. Concomitant use of other nephrotoxic or ototoxic antibiotics (including aminoglycosides, cephaloridine, and peptide antibiotics) should also be avoided.

Phlebitis and pain at the site of IV injections can occur, and thrombophlebitis can result from prolonged intravenous administration. Vancomycin is contraindicated for persons known to be allergic to the drug.

Preparations and Administration

Vancomycin (Vancocin)
Powder for injection solution, powder for oral solutions
Recommended Doses: For adults, 2 g PO in 2 or 4 divided doses. For children, 20 mg/lb/day PO in divided doses. The intravenous dose is 500 mg in a large volume of fluid, every 6 hours or 1 g every 12 hours for adults; and 44 mg/kg/day by continuous infusion in children.

Spectinomycin (Trobicin)

Mechanisms and Effects Spectinomycin, an antibiotic derived from *Streptomyces spectabilis,* is pharmacologically but not structurally similar to the aminoglycosides. It binds to the ribosomes to inhibit bacterial protein synthesis.

Pharmacokinetics Spectinomycin is administered intramuscularly. Absorption occurs rapidly from the site of injection, producing peak plasma levels in 1 hour. Spectinomycin is not significantly bound by plasma proteins and is excreted unchanged in the urine.

Clinical Indications The activity of spectinomycin is exerted on a number of gram-negative bacteria but is generally less effective than other drugs that inhibit the same organisms, and resistance frequently develops. *Neisseria gonorrhoeae,* however, is notably sensitive to spectinomycin and the drug has thus found a place in clinical practice for treatment of proctitis, urethritis, or cervicitis caused by this gram-negative cocci when the infecting strain has been established to be sensitive to the drug and the individual is unable to tolerate tetracyclines or penicillins. Spectinomycin is not effective in treating syphilis.

Adverse Effects and Contraindications The adverse effects of spectinomycin include allergic reactions (urticaria, drug fever), nonspecific effects (such as dizziness, nausea, and insomnia), and soreness at the site of injection. Since spectinomycin is normally given just once, adverse effects are minimal.

Preparations and Administration

Spectinomycin (Trobicin)
Powder for injection
Recommended Doses: 2 g (in 5 ml), injected deeply into the upper outer quadrant of the gluteus muscle.

Peptide Antibiotics

Mechanisms and Effects The polymyxins are the major group of peptide antibiotics. Polymyxin B (Aerosporin) is derived from *Bacillus colistinus.* The polymyxins are surface-active drugs or detergents that disrupt the structure of bacterial cell membranes by interaction with the phospholipid component. The result is an increase in permeability of the bacteria cell membrane that is **bactericidal.** Differences in sensitivity of microorganisms are determined by access of the drug to the membrane. Polymyxins act only on gram-negative bacilli (Table 47–12). The activity of polymyxins is usefully additive to that of sulfonamides.

Pharmacokinetics Neither polymyxin B nor colistin (Coly-Mycin S) is absorbed from mucosal surfaces, the skin, or even large burn injuries. Oral administration does not provide any systemic activity. Peptide antibiotics are most useful for topical applications. Occasionally, they are injected intramuscularly for systemic effects. Intramuscular injections of polymyxins often result in sharp pain at the site of injection, sometimes radiating along the peripheral nerve. To diminish this problem, a sulfamethylated form of colistin, colistimethate (Coly-Mycin M), is often used. Colistimethate is not itself biologically active, but after absorption, it is slowly hydrolyzed to colistin.

Clinical Indications The topical use of polymyxins for dermatological infections is discussed in Chapter 53. These drugs are also useful topically for infections of the eyes (corneal ulcers) and the ears (external otitis) because these infections are commonly due to *Pseudomonas aeruginosa,* which is highly sensitive to polymyxins. Systemic use is limited to severe urinary tract infections caused by *P. aeruginosa,* but even this application has virtually disappeared with the advent of new penicillins and aminoglycosides that inhibit this microbe. Polymyxins are typically used in combination with synergistic antibacterial drugs against highly resistant strains. Rarely, polymyxins are used intrathecally for meningitis. Polymyxins cannot otherwise penetrate the central nervous system. Intrathecal injection is sometimes associated with meningeal irritation.

Adverse Effects and Contraindications Systemic use of polymyxins is constrained by significant risk of **nephrotoxicity.** The nature of the toxicity is a renal tubular necrosis, resulting in proteinuria, hematuria, and azotemia. Nephrotoxicity is most likely when doses are high or treatment is prolonged or when other nephrotoxic drugs are used concurrently.

Neurotoxicity also occurs. Neurological symptoms include diplopia, ptosis, dizziness, paresthesias, areflexia, slurred speech, and general weakness. *Complaints of dizziness or general weakness or nursing observations of slurred speech, dyspnea, or facial flushing should be reported immediately.* Polymyxins produce a neuromuscular blockade similar to aminoglycosides. *Nurses should observe clients for apnea or restlessness. They should have on hand calcium gluconate, oxygen, and equipment for respiratory support.* Polymyxins should not be used in individuals with parkinsonism or myasthenia gravis. Clients also receiving magnesium, quinidine, or neuromuscular blockers are at particular risk of neuromuscular blockade.

Hypersensitivity reactions seldom occur with polymyxins, but rashes, fever, and urticaria are occasionally reported. Large oral doses cause gastrointestinal irritation.

Preparations and Administration Bacitracin, a peptide antibiotic, though available in an injection solution, is no longer used systemically because of the frequency with which it causes nephrotoxicity. Topical use of bacitracin is discussed in Chapter 53. The antibacterial spectrum of bacitracin is indicated in Table 47–12.

Colistimethate sodium (Coly-Mycin M)
Powder for injection
Recommended Doses: 2.5–5 mg/kg/day IM in 2–4 divided doses. Parenteral doses of any of the polymyxins must be sharply reduced if there is indication of renal impairment.

Colistin sulfate (Coly-Mycin S)
Oral solution
Recommended Doses: 5–15 mg/kg/day PO in 3 divided doses.

Polymyxin B (Aerosporin)
Numerous topical ointments, injection solution
Recommended Doses: 25,000–30,000 units/kg/day IM, IV, or intrathecal, in divided doses at intervals of 4 or 6 hours.

Chemotherapy of Mycobacterial Diseases

Mycobacteria are a group of nonmotile bacilli that present distinct problems for chemotherapy. They are facultative pathogens, able to survive either intracellularly or extracellularly within the host. The most important mycobacteria are two species that have plagued humankind for millions of years: *M. tuberculosis* and *M. leprae*. *M. tuberculosis* causes tuberculosis and *M. leprae* leprosy. Worldwide, both conditions remain major health problems. Leprosy has never been a significant health problem in the United States. The incidence of tuberculosis in the United States has declined dramatically during the last quarter-century but remains a significant health problem involving some 25,000 new cases each year. Historically, treatment of both tuberculosis and leprosy presented such grave difficulties that afflicted individuals were treated in specialized sanitariums. In the case of leprosy, a great deal of social stigma was attached to the disease, and afflicted individuals were isolated into leper colonies.

Tuberculosis and Antitubercular Drugs

Tuberculosis is caused by *M. tuberculosis* or, uncommonly, by *M. bovis*, which infects cows and may contaminate cows' milk. Four characteristics of these bacilli have important implications for the disease and its treatment: (1) their facultative nature complicates therapy in that both intracellular and extracellular varities must be eradicated; (2) they are obligate aerobic bacteria, and thus exhibit preference for highly oxygenated tissue such as the lungs; (3) they are on the whole slow-growing organisms, making them resistant to bactericidal drugs that act mainly on rapidly proliferating cells; and (4) they exhibit a great potential for mutation and readily develop resistance to drug treatments. In the absence of complete eradication of the mycobacteria through vigorous and extended drug therapy, tuberculosis is a chronic, lifelong conflict between the microorganism and the host defenses, characterized by acute exacerbations, extended periods of latency, and reactivation by gradual extension of pathology. The characteristic pathological development of tuberculosis is the occurrence of tubercles, fibrosis, and necrosis in the lungs. The tubercles are composed of giant and epitheloid cells derived from macrophages.

Infection occurs by inhalation of infectious droplets produced by the coughing of already infected individuals. Such droplets can persist in stagnant air for extended periods, so there is no requirement of direct physical proximity to a person with the disease. Prevalence of new cases of tuberculosis is greatest in older persons, especially non-Caucasian males. Active disease may follow initial exposure to the pathogen by as much as 1–2 years. Diagnosis is established by means of the tuberculin skin test and chest x-rays.

Treatment of tuberculosis is successful only if the organism is completely eradicated. Otherwise relapse inevitably occurs. Because the mycobacteria replicate at such a slow rate, chemotherapy must be continued for extended periods, 6–9 months or 18–24 months depending on the selection of drugs. The drugs employed for tuberculosis can be divided into first-line and second-line agents. **First-line drugs** for tuberculosis include isoniazid (Laniazid, Nydrazid, Teebaconin), rifampin (Rifadin, Rimactane), ethambutol (Myambutol), and streptomycin. These drugs provide a favorable ratio of efficacy versus adverse effects. The **second-line drugs** include amikacin, kanamycin (Kantrex, Klebcil), cycloserine (Seromycin), pyrazinamide, ethionamide (Trecator), aminosalicylic acid (Parasal, Teebacin), capreomycin (Capastat), viomycin, and amithiozone. The vast majority of cases of tuberculosis can be treated with a combination of first-line drugs. Second-line drugs are reserved for unusually resistant strains.

Treatment of clients with tuberculosis is usually conducted with combinations of drugs in order to reduce the risk that resistance will develop. Resistance to single-drug regimens is commonplace because of the high rate of mutation in *M. tuberculosis* and because of the extended period of treatment that is required. Cross-resistance does not occur between isoniazid, the primary drug choice for the disease, and other antitubercular drugs. Although resistance does occasionally develop to even the two-drug regimens, the likelihood of this happening is much less.

Isoniazid

Isoniazid, also known as INH (short for isonicotinylhydrazide), is considered to be the primary drug choice for tuberculosis. Isoniazid has advantages of oral effectiveness, inexpensiveness (a factor to be considered because of the extended period of therapy), good efficacy, and a generally acceptable level of toxicity.

Mechanisms and Effects The mechanism of INH has not been clearly determined. Isoniazid is bactericidal against *M. tuberculosis* cells during their replicative stage but bacteriostatic for latent cells. Isoniazid is initially highly effective against *M. tuberculosis* and *M. bovis,* but when the drug is used alone, resistance develops rapidly as less vulnerable mutant cells of the organism selectively replicate to produce resistant strains. Resistance appears to involve a diminished uptake of the drug into the bacterial cells. Isoniazid readily penetrates nonresistant mycobacterial cells. *Appropriate microbiological studies should be conducted periodically during therapy with isoniazid to detect any bacterial resistance.*

The current best hypothesis regarding the molecular basis for the action of isoniazid relates to the unique character of the cell wall of mycobacteria. Its composition includes large quantities of mycolic acids. Isoniazid may inhibit the synthesis of the precursor molecules that make up mycolic acid. Since mycolic acid is a unique constituent of the cell walls of mycobacteria, such a mechanism would explain the selective nature of the antimicrobial action of INH for mycobacteria.

Pharmacokinetics Isoniazid is rapidly absorbed after oral administration, reaching peak levels in the serum in 1–2 hours. The drug diffuses readily into all bodily tissues and fluids and is about 20% bound in the plasma to plasma proteins. Isoniazid is inactivated entirely by hepatic metabolism, which is followed by renal excretion of the inactive metabolites and conjugates. Acetylation is the major pathway providing inactivation. This has important implications for therapy because rate of acetylation exhibits genetic variability. Approximately 50–60% of North Americans are classified as **slow acetylators,** as are most Scandinavians, Jews, and Arabs. Blacks, Eskimos, and Orientals are much more likely to be **rapid acetylators.** The half-life of isoniazid when given to rapid acetylators averages a little over 1 hour; in slow acetylators the average is 3 hours. The average blood level in slow-acetylators tends to be two or three times that of rapid acetylators. Rapid-acetylators are more prone to liver toxicity of INH while slow acetylators are more prone to extrahepatic toxicities. Hepatic toxicity is believed to be due to an acetylated metabolite of INH, which accounts for the greater incidence of this reaction in rapid acetylators. In spite of the differences in serum levels in the two populations, there is no evidence of differential clinical responsiveness. Dosage recommendations do not routinely take into account differences in rate of acetylation.

Clinical Indications Isoniazid is used only for tuberculosis. In current practice, it is almost always used together with rifampin or ethambutol for treatment of established tuberculosis infection. *Nurses should advise clients that the therapeutic effects of isoniazid will usually become evident in about 2–3 weeks, at which time clients should notice a decrease in fever and night sweats, less coughing, less sputum, less fatigue, an increase in appetite, and a gain in weight. However, clients should be advised that these improvements should not be taken as reason to decrease scheduled rest periods.*

Isoniazid is also used alone for prophylaxis in household members or other close associates of individuals with recently diagnosed tuberculosis. Prophylaxis is also indicated for individuals who test positively as tuberculin skin test reactors and who have circumstances (leukemia, hematological diseases, silicosis, or use of immunosuppressives) that predispose them to activation of latent disease or who show x-ray evidence of nonprogressive tuberculous disease.

Adverse Effects and Contraindications Most significant of the adverse effects of INH is the risk of severe or even fatal **hepatitis.** Individuals under 35 have only a 0.3% risk of hepatitis; those over 50 have a 2.3% risk. Rapid acetylators are more likely to experience hepatotoxicity. Risk is also increased in individuals receiving additional hepatotoxic drugs, including rifampin, and in individuals with alcohol-induced liver disease. Liver status can be monitored through serum enzymology, but there are differing opinions as to how routine this should be. Monthly monitoring is considered appropriate by some. Acetylhydrazine, an acetylated metabolite of INH is known to cause hepatotoxicity and is a likely factor in the hepatitis associated with isoniazid. Jaundice occurs in about 0.6% of individuals receiving isoniazid. *The nurse should periodically interview clients receiving isoniazid to determine if indications of hepatotoxicity are present, such as fatigue, loss of appetite, malaise, nausea, dark urine, or scleral icterus (discoloration due to jaundice).*

Hypersensitivity reactions to isoniazid represent the most frequent though not the most significant form of adverse reaction. The most prevalent manifestations are rash, occurring in 2% of individuals, and drug fever, occurring in 1.2%. Other reported skin eruptions include maculopapular, morbilliform, urticarial, and pruritic varieties.

Hematological reactions to INH have included agranulocytosis, eosinophilia, thrombocytopenia, and anemia. Anemia is most likely to occur in individuals with marginal vitamin B_6 deficiency, which is aggravated by isoniazid.

Vitamin B_6 (pyridoxine) is also directly involved in the **neurological side effects** of isoniazid. Those most susceptible to neurological difficulties from isoniazid administration are adolescents, slow acetylators, and clients who are malnourished or diabetic. These side effects are avoidable by concurrent administration of adequate pyridoxine supplements. From 50 to 100 mg of pyridoxine per day is recommended for adults; children receiving INH seldom require any B_6 supplementation because of the adequacy of dietary intake even for the expanded need during isoniazid therapy. In the absence of adequate vitamin B_6, isoniazid frequently causes peripheral neuritis, in up to 20% of individuals. *Complaints of numbness, tingling, and burning sensations should alert the nurse to impending peripheral neuritis.* Central neurological dysfunction can also develop, such as optic neuritis and atrophy, slurred speech, dizziness, tinnitus, ataxia, muscle twitches, paresthesias, mood changes, hallucinations, and stupor. *Nurses should observe clients for behavioral changes and instruct the clients' families to note these as well. Because of the risk of optic neuritis, clients should have a vision test and ophthalmoscopic examination before initiation of isoniazid therapy and periodically during treatment if they complain of visual symptoms.* Overdoses or normal doses in epileptic individuals can trigger convulsive seizures, possibly intractable and fatal. Vitamin B_6 is a coenzyme for production of gamma-aminobutyric acid (GABA), the major inhibitory transmitter of the brain. All of the neurological symptoms are circumvented by vitamin B_6 supplementation.

Some clients receiving isoniazid may experience **orthostatic hypotension.** Other side effects of isoniazid include metabolic acidosis, dry mouth, epigastric distress, urinary retention, and hyperglycemia. *Diabetic clients should be observed closely for any change in status.*

Interactions with Other Drugs, Nutrients, and Tests The relationship between INH and the micronutrient, vitamin B_6, has just been mentioned. INH also interacts with alcohol in beverages, the two agents causing additive hepatotoxicity. *Nurses should instruct clients to avoid alcohol ingestion.* Among other antituberculosis drugs, rifampin increases the hepatotoxicity of isoniazid, and cycloserine the CNS toxicities.

Isoniazid interacts with certain drugs with respect to hepatic metabolism. Para-hydroxylation of phenytoin is inhibited by INH, and previously appropriate doses of phenytoin may cause severe ataxia and sedation when INH therapy is initiated. Para-aminosalicylic acid (PAS) inhibits acetylation of INH, increasing plasma levels and toxicity of the latter drug. Disulfiram also inhibits metabolism of isoniazid, increasing its CNS toxicity.

Absorption of isoniazid is reduced by both laxatives and aluminum hydroxide- or magnesium-containing antacids. *Clients should be warned not to use these laxatives within 1 hour of taking isoniazid because of their interference with isoniazid absorption.*

Isoniazid may produce false-positive results for diabetic clients who use Benedict's solution. *Nurses should advise them to use Clinitest since the drug appears not to affect this test.*

Preparations and Administration The usual treatment period is 6–9 months when INH is used in combination with rifampin for active tuberculosis. When combined with ethambutol, which is only bacteriostatic, the conventional treatment period is 18–24 months. It is imperative that treatment be continued for the full designated period and that compliance be maintained reliably because of the ability of *M. tuberculosis* cells to assume a dormant status for long periods. *The nurse should explain to clients and their families the need for extended therapy and reliable compliance and reinforce the education at each visit. Clients should understand that absence of symptomatology is not equivalent to a cure, and that reinfection invariably follows premature discontinuation of therapy. Isoniazid is administered on an empty stomach, at least 1 hour before or 2 hours after meals.*

Isoniazid (Niconyl, Teebaconin, Laniazid, Panazid, and generic)
Tablets, injection solution, powder for injection solution
Recommended Doses: For active tuberculosis, 5 mg/kg/day (up to 300 mg/day) PO for adults, in a single dose; or 10–20 mg/kg/day PO (up to 300–500 mg/day) in children, in a single dose. For prophylaxis, the adult dose is 300 mg PO once per day and for infants or children 10 mg/kg/day PO (300 mg/day maximum) in a single dose.

Rifampin

Rifampin is an antibiotic obtained from *Streptomyces mediterranei.* Introduced in 1967, rifampin has a broad spectrum of activity against many gram-positive and gram-negative bacteria including *E. coli, Klebsiella, Proteus, Pseudomonas, Staphylococcus aureus, N. meningitidis, M. tuberculosis,* and most of the atypical strains of mycobacteria except *M. fortuitum.*

Mechanisms and Effects Rifampin is an inhibitor of transcription and thus of protein synthesis. It is bactericidal and tuberculocidal. Mycobacteria can develop resistance to rifampin in a single generation because 1 in every 10–100 million tubercle bacilli is inherently resistant. Therefore, rifampin is never used as the sole drug in a regimen for tuberculosis.

Pharmacokinetics Rifampin is rapidly and completely absorbed after oral administration, producing peak plasma levels in 2–4 hours. *Absorption is altered by food: rifampin is thus administered on an empty stomach.* Absorption is also inhibited by concurrent administration of PAS. Rifampin is cleared from the blood mainly (70–95%) by the liver, where it is deacetylated. The elimination half-life averages 3 hours. Rifampin induces its own metabolism with chronic administration, reducing its half-life by 40% after 2 weeks. The induction produced by rifampin affects other drugs as well, including glucocorticoids, oral contraceptives, oral anticoagulants, digitoxin, and dapsone.

Clinical Indications Rifampin is approved for two clinical indications. It is used in conjunction with isoniazid (or occasionally ethambutol), but never alone, in chemotherapy for tuberculosis. The combination of INH and rifampin can usually provide complete eradication of *M. tuberculosis* — a clinical cure — in about 6–9 months. Rifampin is also the drug of choice for prophylaxis against meningitis infections caused by *Neisseria meningitidis.* It is used prophylactically for individuals exposed to persons within a household who are infected with the meningococcal organism or in asymptomatic carriers to eliminate the microorganism from the nasopharyngeal mucosa.

Adverse Effects and Contraindications Adverse effects of rifampin are not common, occurring

Nursing Observations for Antitubercular Drug Therapy

THERAPEUTIC GOAL	Complete eradication of the infection.
PREADMINISTRATION ASSESSMENT	
Baseline Data	Asymptomatic at first; later observe for cough, fever, night sweats, malaise, and weight loss. Sputum may be bloody, green and purulent, or yellow and mucoid. Chest x-ray, vital signs, and respiratory rate and sounds. Conduct liver, neurological, and visual evaluation prior to initiating usual three-drug regimen. Obtain laboratory tests including tuberculin skin tests and sputum culture for acid-fast bacilli.
EVALUATION OF DRUG RESPONSE	
For Therapeutic Benefit	Resolution of symptoms, chest x-rays, and tuberculin skin tests.
For Adverse Effects	Assess for allergic reactions, gastrointestinal disturbances, hepatic dysfunction, hematological reactions, neurological and visual impairments, and orthostatic hypotension.
For Drug Interactions	With isoniazid, discuss potential changes in requirements for hypoglycemic drugs in diabetic clients, reduced absorption when laxatives are employed, potentiation of phenytoin (Dilantin) toxicity, and increased toxicity with disulfiram (Antabuse); with rifampin monitor for induction of liver enzymes. Watch for para-aminosalicylic acid (PAS) to potentiate isoniazid but to antagonize rifampin.
For Dietary Interactions	Monitor clients for adequate vitamin B_6 when isoniazid is used; observe for additive hepatotoxicity if alcohol is employed with isoniazid; observe for inhibition of rifampin absorption by concurrent food ingestion.
For Compliance	Evaluate the client's compliance with all facets of the therapeutic regimen by careful observation, interviewing, and review of progress. Report compliance problems to the physician and act as client-advocate when changes in the therapeutic regimen seem indicated.

in less than 4% of individuals treated with the drug. Hypersensitivity reactions and gastrointestinal distress are the most likely symptoms. **Hypersensitivity reactions** include rash, drug fever, flu-like symptoms, urticaria, acneiform eruptions, eosinophilia, mucosal sores on the tongue or oral surfaces, and exudative conjunctivitis. **Gastrointestinal disturbances** reported are nausea, vomiting, anorexia, gas, diarrhea, cramps, and epigastric distress. Some individuals experience **mild neurological symptoms** such as visual disturbances, mental confusion, muscle weakness, impaired concentration, or numbness of the extremities.

Hepatic injury is the most important though an infrequent problem. Jaundice or even renal-shock syndrome may result. Old age, use of alcohol, and concurrent use of other hepatotoxic agents, including INH, are predisposing factors. **Hematological reactions** sometimes occur, such as hemolytic anemia, leukopenia, or thrombocytopenia. Rifampin crosses the placental barrier and has possible teratogenic potential (evidence is based on limited animal studies). It should be avoided during pregnancy. *Nurses should encourage clients to take rifampin consistently since there is a higher incidence of adverse reactions if therapy is intermittent. Clients receiving rifampin should be advised that this drug may produce a harmless orange coloration of bodily fluids such as the urine, saliva, sweat, and tears and may stain some contact lenses.*

Drug Interactions The interactions of rifampin include the effect of PAS on rifampin absorption and the influence of rifampin-induced induction of liver enzymes on a variety of drugs as described above with respect to the pharmacokinetics of rifampin. The major pharmacodynamic interaction is the additive nature of the hepatotoxic potential exhibited by rifampin and other drugs, such as alcohol and INH.

Preparations and Administration Rifampin is administered once daily, at least 1 hour before or 2 hours after meals.

Rifampin (Rifadin, Rimactane)
Capsules
Recommended Doses: For tuberculosis in adults, 600 mg/day PO; for children, 10–20 mg/kg PO to a maximum of 600 mg/day. The same doses are employed for prophylaxis against meningococcal infection (*Neisseria meningitidis*).

Ethambutol

Ethambutol is bacteriostatic, not bactericidal. It is never used alone in tuberculosis, but has traditionally been used in conjunction with INH. When tuberculosis is treated with INH and ethambutol, treatment must be continued for 18–24 months, a duration that often taxes the individual's commitment to comply reliably with the treatment program. For that reason, the alternative combination of rifampin and INH is gaining favor. Ethambutol inhibits growth of *M. kansasii* as well as *M. tuberculosis*. It acts as an antimetabolite. Resistance can develop to ethambutol, but only very slowly and infrequently. There is no cross-resistance with other antituberculosis drugs.

Pharmacokinetics Ethambutol is about 75–80% absorbed, reaching peak plasma levels in 2–4 hours after oral administration. Ethambutol is accumulated in red blood cells to twice the plasma concentration. Plasma protein binding is only 20%. The elimination half-life is about 3 hours; thus, daily doses do not result in accumulation. Ethambutol is inactivated 80% by renal excretion, 20% by metabolism.

Clinical Indications Ethambutol is used with INH or in triple drug therapy (INH, rifampin, and ethambutol) for tuberculosis.

Adverse Effects and Contraindications Ethambutol is well tolerated. Adverse effects occur in less than 2% of individuals attributable to ethambutol. The most common effect is a **reduction in visual acuity,** occurring in 0.8% of individuals. This effect appears to be due to optic neuritis and depends on dose and duration. *Clients should be advised to report any change in visual acuity to the physician immediately. The usual first indication is a change in color vision affecting perception of green wavelengths. Baseline evaluation of visual acuity should be undertaken before initiating therapy and periodically (monthly is recommended) thereafter.* Snellen eye charts are a useful test of visual acuity. Blurred vision is a less frequent feature of the visual effects of ethambutol.

Hypersensitivity reactions to ethambutol include pruritus, dermatitis, fever, malaise, joint pain, leukopenia, and anaphylactoid reactions. **Neurological symptoms** that have occurred include headache, dizziness, mental confusion, disorientation, hallucinations, and numbness and tingling of the digits. **Gastrointestinal irritation** is uncommon and results in nausea, vomiting, abdominal pain, and anorexia.

Preparations and Administration

Ethambutol (Myambutol)
Tablets
Recommended Doses: For treatment of initial tuberculosis infections, 15 mg/kg PO, once daily. For retreatment, 25 mg/kg.

Nursing Diagnoses and Inverventions for Antitubercular Drug Therapy

Nursing Diagnoses	*Related Interventions*
TO ENHANCE DRUG BENEFITS OR REDUCE DRUG REQUIREMENTS	
Noncompliance related to requirement for long-term therapy	Stress the importance of completing the full course of therapy for permanent resolution.
Social isolation related to need to protect others from infection	Explain the need, provide emotional support, and allay unreasonable fears of family members regarding transmissibility.
TO MINIMIZE DRUG SIDE EFFECTS OR INTERACTIONS	
Alterations in thought processes related to drug regimen	Ask client and family members to observe for changes in mood or mental function such as hallucinations, confusion, or stupor.
Sensory-perceptual alterations: visual disturbances, paresthesias, or numbness related to the drug regimen	Schedule client for initial and periodic visual assessment. Assess client for evidence of paresthesias or numbness.
TO ENSURE SAFE AND EFFICACIOUS DRUG USE	
Knowledge deficit related to drug regimen	Isolate the client in accordance with hospital procedures. Explain to the client appropriate measures to minimize exposure of others to the disease.
	Explain the nature of tuberculosis infections and the rationale for the regimen selected.
	Explain to clients the importance of complete eradication of the infecting agent, why therapy must be continued for such a long period of time, and the importance of completing therapy even if there is no remaining overt symptomatology.
	Instruct clients to take rifampin on an empty stomach and warn clients that it may impart a harmless orange color to bodily fluids.
	Provide clients with a list of adverse effects and drug interactions for each drug and what to do if any of these occur.

Aminoglycosides and Related Drugs for Tuberculosis

Once the mainstay of chemotherapy for tuberculosis, **streptomycin** is now limited to the role of a third drug added to isoniazid and ethambutol or isoniazid and rifampin. Other aminoglycosides employed in a similar role are **kanamycin** (Kantrex, Klebcil) and **amikacin** (Amikin). Strains resistant to any one of these drugs are resistant to all. Two related drugs employed as second-line drugs in tuberculosis are **viomycin** and **capreomycin.** Viomycin is an antibiotic produced by actinomycete; capreomycin derives from *Streptomyces capreolus.* The two drugs are closely related, and although not strictly aminoglycosides, have pharmacological mechanisms, antibacterial spectra, and adverse effects closely similar to that class of drugs. Like the aminoglycosides, neither agent is absorbed adequately from the gastrointestinal system and both cause ototoxicity, nephrotoxicity, hepatotoxicity, hematological reactions, and hypersensitivity reactions equivalent to the aminoglycosides. Microorganisms resistant to these drugs exhibit cross-resistance to aminoglycosides. Viomycin is not marketed in the

United States. Capreomycin sulfate (Capastat) is available as a powder, 1 g in a 5 ml vial, for reconstitution and deep intramuscular injection. The recommended dose is 1 g daily for 60–120 days followed by 1 g, 2 or 3 times weekly for the remainder of the 18–24 month treatment period.

Second-Line Drugs for Tuberculosis

Para-aminosalicylic acid, or PAS (Parasal, Teebacin) was once an important agent in chemotherapy for tuberculosis and continues to have an ancillary role. PAS is bacteriostatic against *M. tuberculosis* but has an additional benefit based on its pharmacokinetic interactions when used in combinations for tuberculosis. PAS competes for the hepatic acetylation pathway with INH, thus enhancing blood levels of the latter drug. On the other hand, when used with rifampin, PAS competes for the absorption mechanism, reducing bioavailability of rifampin. When both drugs are being employed, they should be administered at least 1 hour apart. PAS presents a less favorable set of adverse reactions than ethambutol and has generally been supplanted by that agent for arresting tuberculosis. PAS competes for the organic anion transport mechanism with probenecid (Benemid) and other drugs. Thus probenecid elevates levels of PAS. Doses of oral anticoagulants often have to be reduced when PAS is employed because of thrombocytopenia produced by PAS. PAS causes gastrointestinal irritation, hypersensitivity reactions, hematological reactions (leukopenia, agranulocytosis, hemolytic anemia, and thrombocytopenia), goiter and myxedema, hypokalemia, and acidosis. *Gastrointestinal irritation caused by PAS can be reduced by administering it with food or antacids.*

Ethionamide (Trecator) and **pyrazinamide** are analogues of nicotinamide. Both are bacteriostatic and used only when standard drug regimens for tuberculosis have failed. The principal adverse effect of pyrazinamide is hepatic toxicity. Pyrazinamide is available in 500 mg tablets and is given in a dose of 20–35 mg/kg/day in 3 or 4 doses after meals. Ethionamide is limited by the severity of CNS toxicity (depression, optic neuritis, blurred vision, diplopia, drowsiness, convulsions, olfactory disturbances), peripheral neuropathies (impotence, paresthesias), gastrointestinal disturbances (stomatitis), allergic reactions (rashes, acneiform eruptions, allergic jaundice, thrombocytopenia), postural hypotension, hepatitis, alopecia, and endocrine disturbances (gynecomastia and increased difficulty with management of diabetes mellitus).

Cycloserine (Seromycin) is a fairly effective but rather toxic antituberculosis drug. This antibiotic, produced by *Streptomyces orchidaceus,* produces serious nervous system symptoms including drowsiness, somnolence, confusion, disorientation, headache, vertigo, tremor, convulsions, memory loss, aggressiveness, irritability, and psychosis. It is reserved for instances of tuberculosis not responsive to conventional approaches.

Preparations and Administration

Cycloserine (Seromycin)
Capsules
Recommended Doses: 500–1,000 mg PO daily in divided doses.

Ethionamide (Trecator)
Tablets
Recommended Doses: For adults, 0.5–1.0 g/day PO in divided doses.

Para-aminosalicylic acid (Parasal, Teebacin, and generic)
Tablets
Recommended Doses: For adults, 12–15 g/day PO in 2 or 3 divided doses. For children, 200–300 mg/kg/day PO in 3 or 4 divided doses.

Important Nursing Implications for Antitubercular Drugs

- ☐ Provide clients the support necessary to enable them to complete the long courses of administration required for treatment of tuberculosis.
- ☐ Explain the importance of adhering to prescribed regimens without interruption, even though overt symptoms may have diminished or disappeared.
- ☐ When the person with tuberculosis is being treated as an outpatient, educate family members to take an active role in monitoring the individual for signs of adverse drug reactions.
- ☐ Encourage periodic microbiological evaluations to determine the continued sensitivity of the mycobacteria to the prescribed regimen and to ensure that levels of mycobacteria are continuing to decline.
- ☐ Ensure that clients receiving antitubercular drugs receive periodic evaluations of their progress.
- ☐ Teach clients to recognize and report allergic reactions to antitubercular drugs.
- ☐ Encourage clients to undertake periodic visual examinations as a guard against isoniazid-induced optic neuritis.

- ☐ Advise clients to avoid use of alcohol during isoniazid therapy.
- ☐ Ensure that adult clients receive vitamin B_6 supplements during isoniazid therapy.
- ☐ Make sure that clients understand when each drug is to be taken in relation to food intake and antacid regimens (if applicable).

Leprosy and Leprostatics

The other major disease caused by mycobacteria is leprosy. Although a rare disease in the United States, the World Health Organization estimates that over 10 million individuals are afflicted with leprosy worldwide. Although a few of the agents effective in tuberculosis also find use in treatment of leprosy, most of the drugs for the two major mycobacterial diseases are uniquely active against one or the other of the two mycobacterial species.

The most important class of drugs for treatment of leprosy are the **sulfones.** The two members of this class marketed in the United States are **dapsone** (Avlosulfon) and **sulfoxone** (Diasone). These bacteriostatic agents are antimetabolites, interfering with bacterial nutrition in a manner similar, but not identical, to sulfonamides. Though effective against a wide spectrum of gram-positive and gram-negative bacteria, their use is limited by toxicity to treatment of all forms of leprosy and dermatitis herpetiformis. Sulfoxone is a prodrug, inactive until it is metabolized to dapsone. The pharmacology of the two drugs is thus identical. Sulfones are well absorbed and widely distributed, ultimately accumulating in the skin, muscle, kidney, and liver. Infected skin accumulates sulfones in higher concentrations than normal skin. Adverse effects of sulfones include hemolysis and methemoglobinemia, gastrointestinal disturbances, central and peripheral neurological problems, hepatotoxicity, and especially severe dermatological hypersensitivity reactions. The relatively high levels of the sulfones in the skin probably account for the severity of cutaneous reactions. Exfoliative dermatitis can occur and is frequently fatal. Erythema multiforme and toxic epidermal necrolysis are additional risks.

Some experts recommend use of drug combinations in treating leprosy to decrease the risk that a resistant strain will develop. **Rifampin** (Rifadin, Rimactane) is often the second drug added. This drug is also an antituberculosis agent and is discussed in the preceding section. Two other leprostatics are **clofazimine** (Lamprene) and **amithiozone** (Panrone, Tibione). Clofazimine is used as a second drug in combinations with dapsone or for individuals infected by strains resistant to sulfones. Clofazimine appears to interfere with transcription by binding to DNA. Its bactericidal action occurs only after 50 days of drug treatment. Clofazimine remains in the body for several days after a single administration, and thus administration twice a week is adequate. Clofazimine is well absorbed after oral administration. Clofazimine can cause a temporary red discoloration of the skin in light-skinned individuals. Amithiozone is effective against both *M. leprae* and *M. tuberculosis.* It is used in leprosy only when the condition is resistant to sulfones because it is generally a less effective drug and may cause bone marrow suppression.

Preparations and Administration

Amithiozone (Panrone, Tibione)
Recommended Doses: 50 g/day PO initially, gradually increased to 200 mg/day.

Clofazimine (Lamprene)
Tablets
Recommended Doses: 100–300 mg PO.

Dapsone (Avlosulfon)
Tablets
Recommended Doses: 25 mg twice per week initially, gradually building up to 100 mg 4 times per week by week 21 of treatment. Treatment usually lasts for 24 weeks.

Sulfoxone (Diasone)
Enteric coated tablets

Case Study: Pneumonitis—Bacterial vs. Viral

T. M. came to the clinic with symptoms of chills, shakes, fever of 103° F, unrelenting nonproductive cough, rapid pulse, and rapid, shallow respirations. The nurse measured T. M.'s blood pressure (120/80) and examined his eyes, nose, and throat. There were no ocular symptoms, but the nose and throat were both inflamed. Respiratory sounds were noted in the left lung.

The physician ordered a chest x-ray, which revealed opacity in the lower lobe of the left lung. A complete blood cell count indicated leukocytosis. A sputum sample was cultured for determination of the infecting organism, which was identified as a penicillinase-producing *Staphylococcus aureus*. The physician ordered cloxacillin, 250 mg every 6 hours for 10 days.

Before administering the cloxacillin, the nurse reviewed T. M.'s medication history for any indications of allergic reactions to penicillin or any other antimicrobial drug, and she asked T. M. if he recalled any such reaction. There was no evidence of allergy. After administering the first dose of cloxacillin, the nurse instructed T. M. to remain at the clinic for 30 minutes. She used the first 10 minutes of this time to explain to T. M. about pneumonia and the treatment regimen. She instructed T. M. that he should expect his fever to subside in 2–3 days but that he should nevertheless complete the full 10-day regimen of cloxacillin. She explained the importance of taking the medication every 6 hours around the clock even though it meant being awakened once during the night. He was told that he should call the clinic immediately if he developed a rash or difficulty breathing. She advised T. M. to stay at home in bed until resolution of symptoms. Two weeks later T. M. was reexamined; all symptoms had disappeared and all parameters had returned to normal.

Two years later T. M. experienced a similar bout of symptoms, including chills, fever, nonproductive cough, malaise, and headache. He went to the clinic, where he was again assessed by the nurse. Temperature was elevated (103° F), respiration rapid and shallow, and pulse rapid. Laboratory tests were conducted, revealing presence of influenza, type A in the sputum sample. The physician recommended that T. M. be admitted to the hospital. In the hospital, T. M. was put on bedrest, increased oral fluids, and aspirin for fever and pain. T. M. asked the nurse why he was not being given a "penicillin drug" like he had received the last time. The nurse explained the differences between viral and bacteria pneumonia and the reason for not using a penicillin drug in this case. T. M.'s temperature returned to normal after 4 days and other symptoms resolved as well. T. M. was discharged on the sixth day. A follow-up chest x-ray after 2 weeks showed that the pneumonitis had resolved completely.

1. Which symptoms and laboratory findings during T. M.'s first episode were likely due to pneumonia?
2. What was the basis for selecting cloxacillin? Could methacillin have been employed just as well?
3. Why did the nurse ask T. M. to remain at the clinic for 30 minutes after administration of the antibiotic?
4. Why should T. M. take the medication for the full 10 days even if symptoms resolve sooner?
5. Why should T. M. take the medication round the clock?
6. How would you have explained to T. M. why an antibiotic was not given for his second episode of pneumonia?

Answers appear at the end of the book.

Recommended Readings

General Sources

Arking L, Saravolatz, L: Antimicrobial treatment: A coordination challenge for nursing. *Nurs Clin North Am* 1980;15:689–701.

Cunha BA, Parkey GA: Antimicrobial selection: Criteria beyond efficacy. *Current Prescribing* 1980;6(1):65–66.

Mandell GL, Douglas RG, Bennett JE: *Antiinfective Therapy.* New York, John Wiley & Sons, 1985.

May C: Antibiotic therapy at home. *Amer J Nurs* 1984; 84(3):348–349.

Tobey L, Covington T: Antimicrobial drug interactions. *Am J Nurs* 1975;75(9):1470–1473.

Treloar D: Cephalosporins — the third generation. *RN* 1986;49(1):28–29.

Van Scoy RE, Wilkowske CJ: Prophylactic use of antimicrobial agents. *Mayo Clin Proc* 1983;58(4):241–245.

Welch HG: Antibiotic resistance: A new kind of epidemic. *Postgrad Med* 1984;76(6):63–66.

Beta-Lactam Antibacterial Agents

Gever LN: Cefotaxime and monolactam. *Nursing* 1982; 12(10):79–80.

Smith BR: Cefsulodin and ceftazidine: Two antipseudomonal cephalosporins. *Clin Pharm* 1984;3(4):373–385.

Thompson RL, Wright AJ: Cephalosporin antibiotics. *Mayo Clin Proc* 1983;58(2):79–87.

Wright AJ, Wilkowske CJ: The penicillins. *Mayo Clin Proc* 1983;58(1):21–32.

Tetracyclines and Chloramphenicol

Kucer A: Good antimicrobial prescribing: Chloramphenicol, erythromycin, vancomycin, tetracyclines. *Lancet* 1982;2:425–429.

Marks MI, Laferriere C: Chloramphenicol: recent developments and clinical indications. *Clin Pharm* 1982; 1:315–320.

Wilson WR, Cockerill FR III: Tetracyclines, chloramphenicol, erythromycin, and clindamycin. *Mayo Clin Proc* 1983;58(2):92–98.

Aminoglycosides

Edson RS, Key TF: The aminoglycosides. *Mayo Clin Proc* 1983;58(2):99–102.

Langslet J, Habel ML: The aminoglycoside antibiotics. *Am J Nurs* 1981;81:1144–1146.

Yoshikawa TT: Proper use of aminoglycosides. *Am Fam Physician* 1980;21(5):125–130.

Sulfonamides and Trimethoprim

Cockerill FR III, Edson RS: Trimethoprim-sulfamethoxazole. *Mayo Clin Proc* 1983;58(3):147–153.

Schiffman DO: Evaluation of an anti-infective combination: trimethoprim-sulfamethoxazole. *JAMA* 1975;231: 635–637.

Wormser GP, Keusch GT, Rennie CH: Cotrimoxazole (trimethoprim-sulfamethoxazole): An updated review of its antibacterial activity and clinical efficacy. *Drugs* 1982;24: 459–518.

Other Antibacterial Drugs

Geraci JE, Hermans PE: Vancomycin. *Mayo Clin Proc* 1983;58(2):88–91.

Schwartz J, Swanson L, Bartle B: Anti-infective therapy — clinical perspective of erythromycin. *Continuing Practice* 1982;9:26–31.

Drugs for Mycobacterial Infections

Glassroth J, Robins AG, Snider DE: Tuberculosis in the 1980's. *N Engl J Med* 1980;302(26):1441–1448.

Mangione RA, Sause RB: Antimicrobial management of pulmonary tuberculosis. *Pharm Times* 1984;50:74–83.

Modderman ES: Dapsone, still the first choice in leprosy. *Pharm Int* 1980;1(10):198–202.

VanScoy RE, Wilkowske CJ: Antituberculous agents: Isoniazid, rifampin, streptomycin, ethambutol, and pyrazinamide. *Mayo Clin Proc* 1983;58(4):233–240.

CHAPTER 48

Systemic Antiviral, Antifungal, Anthelmintic, and Antiprotozoal Drugs

Chapter 47 discussed drugs employed for systemic bacterial infections. This chapter considers drugs used for alleviating infections caused by any of the nonbacterial pathogens: viruses, fungi, worms, and protozoa. There are no broad-spectrum antiviral, antifungal, anthelmintic, or antiprotozoal drugs; rather, each drug is effective against only a limited number of organisms. As a result, these drug classes include many different agents, no one of which will be encountered by the nurse with frequency, although each is important for its own limited applications.

Chemotherapy for Systemic Viral Infections

The Nature of Viruses

Viruses challenge our thinking as to what is and what is not living substance. The smallest of viruses is barely larger than a good sized macromolecule. Viruses are not complete or independent microorganisms but merely genetic fragments capable of replication only within host cells. Even the largest of viruses lack the organelles and membranous structures found in all cellular organisms.

An individual viral particle, called a **virion,** contains a central core of genetic material and viral proteins (Figure 48–1). This material is surrounded by a protein coat called a **capsid.** The capsid is often a symmetrical, icosahedral (20-sided) structure, but in some viruses it is either helical or complex. Many viruses that infect bacteria, for example, have a globular head and a tailpiece that give the appearance of a miniature tadpole. The capsid is sometimes surrounded by an additional outer amorphous layer called an **envelope.**

Viruses can survive and replicate only within host cells. They are designated as obligate parasites because of this exclusively intracellular existence. In effect, viral particles make use of the host's own biochemical facilities, subverting them to the business of viral replication. The very simplicity of viruses

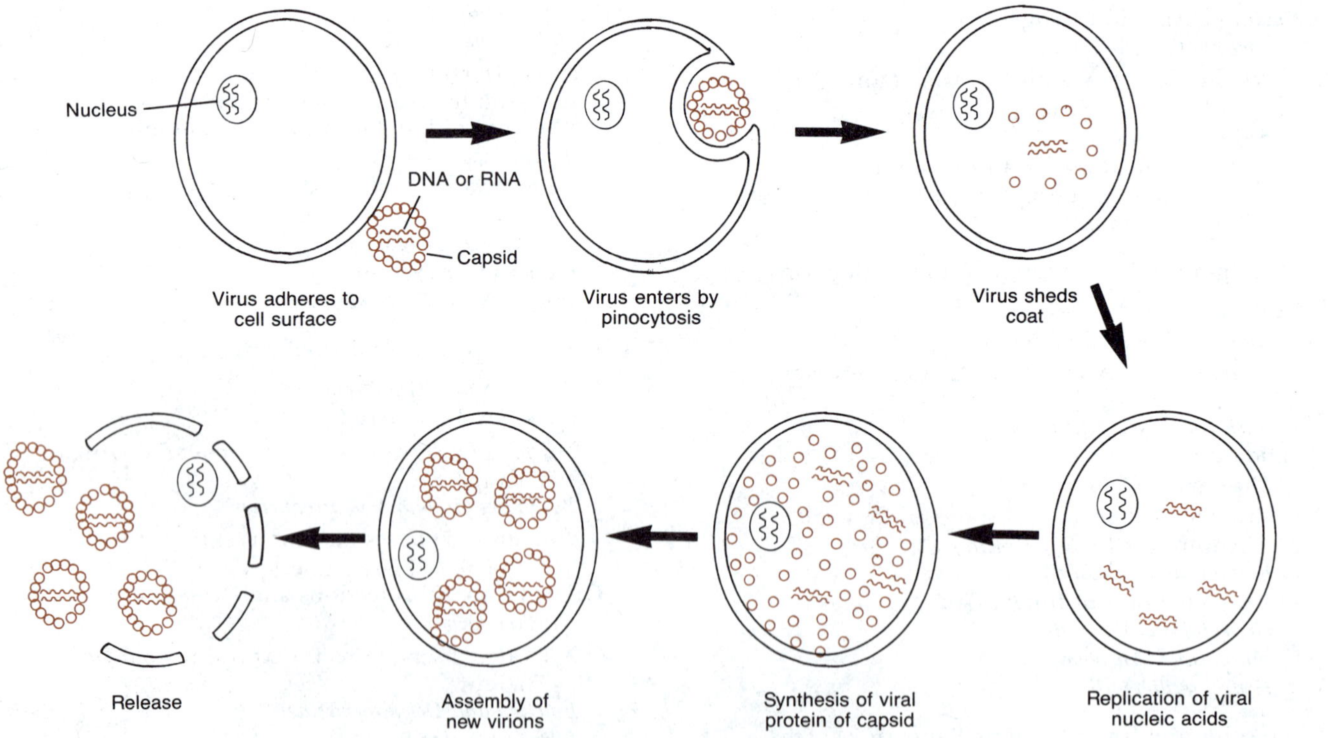

Figure 48–1
Viral replication. The virus is adsorbed to the cell surface (A), then penetrates the cell by pinocytosis (B). Inside the cell, the virus sheds its capsid (C), leaving denuded viral ribonucleic acids, which subvert the synthetic machinery of the cell to the production, first, of new viral nucleic acids (D) and, subsequently, protein (E) for viral capsids. The new viral particles are assembled (F) and escape from the cell when it bursts (G).

and their interrelationship with host cells has severely hampered progress in developing effective antiviral agents that do not also produce an unacceptable attack on host cells. Major strides have been made in the development of viral vaccines, but relatively little has been accomplished to date with respect to development of drugs to curtail viral infection that is underway. Nevertheless, some progress is evident and the rate of advance appears to be accelerating. Viral replication is now more clearly understood and this understanding suggests several target points for drug control.

Viral Replication

Viral replication is conceptualized as involving seven steps (Figure 48–1). After gaining entrance into the body, a virion adheres to the cell surface of a host cell. This adherence, or adsorption, of the virion to the host cell is believed to be based on electrostatic attraction to the cell membrane, without involvement of specific receptors. Adsorption of the virus to a host cell surface initiates invagination of the host cell membrane and pinocytosis; the virion is swallowed into the host cell's interior. After incorporation of the virion, its capsid (and envelope, if it has one) is stripped away by digestive enzymes of the host cell, freeing the nucleic acid core (either DNA or RNA, but not both). After a latency period, the viral nucleic acids begin to serve as templates for replication of viral components, using the DNA or RNA polymerase enzymes of the host cells or, in some cases, a unique polymerase enzyme of the virus itself. Replication of viral nucleic acids occurs first, followed by production of viral proteins (which form the capsid or which direct synthetic activity). Then, the viral nucleic acids and proteins are assembled into new virions. These are ultimately released from the host cell into the extracellular fluids, often by bursting of the host cell. The progeny virions can then spread to infect other cells.

The steps in viral replication provide the potential sites for action of antiviral drugs. Adsorption can be inhibited by polyionic chemicals, such as the anticoagulant heparin, but there are as yet no clinically useful antiviral drugs that operate by this mechanism. Pinocytosis of virions is inhibited by amantadine (Symmetrel), one of the most important antiviral drugs. However, amantadine prevents cellular penetration for only a few viral types. The antimalarial drug, chloroquine (Aralen), also has an inhibitory effect on this step, but not to a clinically useful extent.

The most fruitful approach to interfering with viral replication has employed drugs that interfere with the polymerase enzymes that build the new strands of viral DNA stepwise, utilizing purine and pyrimidine bases as building blocks. The use of the natural nucleotide bases by the polymerase enzymes can be inhibited by administration of analogues of the natural bases. Such analogues act as antimetabolites and are incorporated into newly synthesized viral genomes in place of the analogous normal bases to produce defective nucleic acid strands. Most of the currently available antiviral drugs are nucleic acid analogues.

There are as yet no drugs available for general clinical use that affect any of the late stages of viral replication, although some possibilities are under study. For example, there is evidence that the late viral synthetic stage involving messenger RNA and protein production is inhibited by rifampin (Rifadin). Viral assembly can be inhibited by rifampin and guanidine. And the spread of virions may be altered by endogenous interferon or drugs promoting interferon production.

Host Viral Defenses

Both components of the immune system (B cells and T cells) play a role in combating viruses. Many viruses are pathogenic only during the first exposure. Immunological memory in the form of memory cells provides a rapid and vigorous secondary immune response to subsequent exposure, preventing development of clinical symptoms. The T cells contribute to defense against viruses by releasing interferon. This substance is also produced by cells of many other tissues during viral infections.

Classification of Pathogenic Human Viruses

Most human viruses are pathogenic only in humans and are spread from human to human by social contact. Viruses are classified on the basis of (1) their nucleic acid content, (2) the symmetry of their capsids, and (3) the presence or absence of an envelope (Table 48–1).

The DNA viruses include adenoviruses, papovaviruses, hepatitis viruses, herpes viruses, and poxviruses. **Adenoviruses** possess a 20-sided (icosahedral) capsid but lack an exterior envelope. More than 30 serotypes of adenoviruses are known. Some types occur mainly in children, some mainly in adults. Adenoviruses account for about 5% of acute febrile respiratory illnesses requiring clinical attention. Other adenoviral infections include keratoconjunctivitis, pharyngoconjunctival fever, pneumonia, and enteritis. Vaccines exist for two of the serotypes that have the potential of causing local epidemics, particularly in military encampments. There is no effective drug treatment.

Interferon

Interferon was first recognized in 1957 and is now known to encompass a family of glycoproteins that vary not only from species to species, but even from tissue to tissue. Interferon is active against all types of viruses. Tissue cells produce interferon in response to intracellular presence of foreign nucleic acids such as occurs after viral penetration and uncoating (Figure 48–2). Macrophages and lymphocytes also release interferon. Interferon does not appear to protect cells that produce it, but after release into the extracellular fluid, it protects surrounding cells from the action of the virus. Interferon protects cells that are not yet infected by stimulating them to synthesize an antiviral protein. Interferon also inhibits rapidly proliferating cells such as occur in tumors and may help prevent formation of neoplasms under normal circumstances. Interferon also stimulates the type of T lymphocytes known as killer cells.

There is considerable interest in the potential for interferon as a drug, but only in recent years has sufficient interferon become available to permit its study, and clinical trials as well as basic research are underway. Early results suggest possible value in rabies virus, hepatitis B virus, herpes zoster, and lymphomas. Two interferon products were introduced at the end of 1986 for treatment of hairy cell leukemia (see Chapter 56). The final place of interferon in medicine will probably not be known for many years.

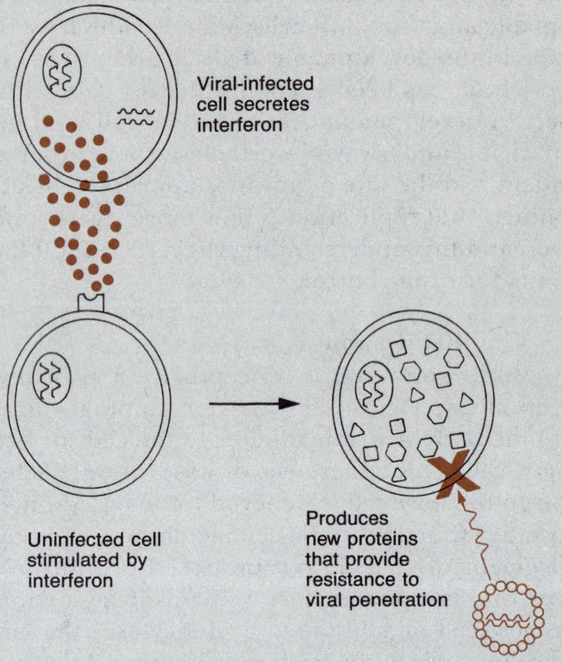

Figure 48–2
Mechanism of interferon. Interferon produced by a virus-infected cell (A) is released and stimulates adjacent cells (B) to produce proteins (C) that increase resistance to viral penetration.

Papovavirus is the agent responsible for warts, small benign tumors of the skin. This virus has universal distribution, and warts are often recurrent. There is no vaccine or drug regimen for this condition, but caustics are used effectively to remove individual warts (see Chapter 53).

Viral hepatitis may be caused by hepatitis A virus, hepatitis B virus, or non-A, non-B hepatitis virus. Hepatitis viruses, though not yet officially classified, are DNA-type viruses with icosahedral capsid symmetry and no envelope. Hepatitis viral vaccines were introduced in 1986.

The **herpes viruses** include some of the most prevalent viruses and the ones for which development of drug therapy is most advanced. **Herpes simplex type 1** causes frequently concurrent skin and eye infections — keratoconjunctivitis. Herpes labialis and cold sores are other forms of infection caused by herpes simplex type 1. This virus can also cause an encephalitis that is frequently fatal. There are several agents (such as idoxuridine (Dendrid, Herplex, Stoxil)) that are effective by topical administration (to the skin or eye) for treating keratoconjunctivitis (see Chapter 53). The newest agent, acyclovir, is also useful parenterally for severe mucosal and cutaneous infections by herpes simplex virus. **Herpes simplex type 2** is responsible mainly for genital infections (herpes vulvovaginitis), less commonly for cutaneous infections. Acyclovir is uniquely effective against the type 2 herpes virus. There is no effective herpes vaccine. Also in the herpes family of viruses is (1) the **beta encephalitis virus,** (2) **herpes zoster** (varicella), which is responsible for chickenpox in children and the recurrent segmental infections of herpes zoster in adults, (3) **cytomegalovirus** (an agent causing hepatitis, mononucleosis, congenital defects, or disseminated infections), and (4) **Epstein-Barr virus,** the causative agent of infectious mononucleosis and Burkitt's lymphoma.

The poxviruses include **variola major,** the cause of smallpox, and **vaccinia virus,** a cause of eczema and encephalitis. Development of smallpox vaccine, a major event in medicine, obliterated this formerly epidemic disease.

Table 48–1
Viruses That Are Infectious to Humans

Viral classification	Infectious disease
I. DNA type	
A. Icosahedral capsid symmetry	
1. No envelope	
a. Adenovirus	Respiratory and ophthalmic infections
b. Papovavirus	Warts
c. Hepadnavirus	
i. Hepatitis A virus	Hepatitis
ii. Hepatitis B virus	Hepatitis
iii. Non-A, Non-B Hepatitis virus	Hepatitis
2. Envelope present	
a. Herpes simplex type 1	Encephalitis, keratoconjunctivitis, epithelial keratitis
b. Herpes simplex type 2	Genital infections, skin eruptions
c. Herpes zoster	Skin infections
d. Varicella zoster	Chickenpox
e. Herpes simiae (beta virus)	Encephalitis
f. Cytomegalovirus	Mononucleosis, hepatitis, disseminated infections
g. Epstein-Barr virus	Infectious mononucleosis, Burkitt's lymphoma
B. Complex capsid	
1. Envelope present	
a. Pox virus	
i. Variola major	Smallpox
ii. Vaccinia virus	Dermatitis, encephalitis
II. RNA type	
A. Icosahedral capsid symmetry	
1. No envelope	
a. Reovirus	Mild respiratory and intestinal infections
b. Picornavirus	
i. Enteroviruses	
(a) Poliovirus	Poliomyelitis
(b) Coxsackievirus	Aseptic meningitis, respiratory infections, myocarditis
(c) Echovirus	Aseptic meningitis, respiratory infections, myocarditis, gastroenteritis
ii. Rhinovirus	Respiratory infections
2. Envelope present	
a. Togavirus	
i. Alpha virus	
(a) Equine encephalitis	Encephalitis
ii. Flavivirus	
(a) Yellow fever virus	Yellow fever
(b) Dengue virus	Fever, rash, headache, arthritis
iii. Rubivirus (rubella)	German measles
B. Helical capsid	
1. Envelope present	
a. Orthomyxovirus (influenza)	Influenza

(continued)

Table 48–1
Viruses That Are Infectious to Humans (*continued*)

Viral classification	Infectious disease
b. Paramyxovirus	
i. Parainfluenza	Bronchitis, pneumonia
ii. Morbillivirus	Measles, subacute sclerosing panencephalitis
iii. Pneumovirus (respiratory syncytial virus)	Pneumonia
iv. Mumps virus	Mumps
c. Rhabdovirus	Rabies
C. Capsid symmetry unknown	Leukemia
1. Envelope present	
a. Retrovirus	
i. Oncovirus	
(a) Human T-cell Lymphotropic Virus-I (HTLV-I)	Leukemia
(b) HTLV-II	Leukemia
(c) HTLV-III (Human immunodeficiency virus, HIV)	Acquired immune deficiency syndrome (AIDS)

The RNA viruses include reoviruses, picornaviruses, togaviruses, orthomyxoviruses (influenza), paramyxoviruses, rhabdoviruses, and retroviruses. The **common cold** (acute coryza) is caused by several of these: rhinoviruses, echoviruses, coxsackieviruses (all examples of picornaviruses); influenza virus; parainfluenza and pneumovirus (both paramyxoviruses); and corona virus (another RNA virus). Spring, summer, and fall colds are usually caused by one of the picornaviruses; winter colds are typically due to paramyxoviruses or influenza. **Reoviruses** are common inhabitants of the respiratory tract but are usually not infectious, causing only mild respiratory tract infections mainly in children.

Among the enteroviral subgroup of picornaviruses are poliovirus, coxsackieviruses, and echoviruses. **Poliovirus,** widely epidemic in the 1950s, has been largely controlled by an effective vaccination program. **Coxsackieviruses** can cause aseptic meningitis or myocarditis in addition to common colds. They affect children more than adults and are more prevalent during the warm months. There are some 30 serotypes of coxsackievirus. **Echoviruses** cause colds, aseptic meningitis, diarrhea, paralytic disease, myocarditis, or pericarditis. Like coxsackieviruses, echoviruses affect children more than adults and are prevalent in the warm months.

The togaviruses include most of the varieties that are transmittable to humans from nonprimate species. Viruses with this characteristic are designated as **arboviruses.** The togaviruses include various **equine encephalitis viruses, yellow fever virus, dengue virus,** and probably **rubella** (German measles). The togaviruses are characterized by an icosahedral capsid and an envelope. Vaccines exist for German measles and can be made for the equine encephalitis viruses. Equine encephalitis is frequently fatal.

Infection caused by RNA viruses having a helical capsid include influenza, parainfluenza, **measles, mumps,** pneumonia (pneumovirus), and **rabies.** Vaccines exist for influenza, measles, mumps, and rabies. In addition, immunoglobulins and antirabies serum are available for treatment of rabies. Amantadine is an effective drug for treatment of influenza. Rabies and pneumovirus infections are high-mortality conditions. Pneumovirus, also called respiratory syncytial virus, often contributes to sudden death in children or the elderly.

Human immunodeficiency virus (HIV), a **retrovirus,** is the virus responsible for acquired immune deficiency syndrome (**AIDS**), a condition that has become an epidemic during the mid-1980s, and has affected an estimated 2 million Americans as of early 1987. This virus, also called T-cell lymphotrophic virus Type III (HTLV-III), AIDS-associated retrovirus (ARV), or lymphadenopathy-associated virus (LAV), is spread almost exclusively by sexual contact (especially anal intercourse), sharing of syringes and needles used for intravenous injections, or blood transfusions. Populations currently at special risk include homosexuals, intravenous drug abusers, prostitutes, and hemophiliacs, but the virus is rapidly penetrating into the general population through heterosexual activity. *The risk of transmission to health care workers appears to be small, but two nurses have been infected as a result of accidentally pricking the skin with a contaminated needle. Another health care worker who had acne contracted AIDS, presumably through hand contact with breaks in the skin. Health care personnel working in operating rooms are advised to wear protective goggles and gloves to ensure that bodily fluids do not contact mucosal membranes or broken skin.* HIV preferentially infects the class of lymphocytes known as T_4 cells — cells that direct much of the immune response to infectious microorganisms. After infecting T_4 lymphocytes, HIV may remain latent for as much as 10 years, but when activated, often by an infection, it replicates rapidly causing death of the infected T_4 lymphocytes. This results in an immune deficiency which predisposes the patient to opportunistic infections by commensal flora, especially *Pneumocystis carinii* and cytomegaloviruses, which are ultimately fatal.

Systemic Antiviral Drugs

Amantadine (Symmetrel)

Mechanisms and Effects Amantadine is a synthetic antiviral drug. It inhibits the uncoating of susceptible viruses following their penetration into host cells, a mechanism that is distinct from other antiviral drugs.

Pharmacokinetics Amantadine is well absorbed (about 90%) after oral administration. Peak serum levels (0.2 mg/ml) are achieved in 1–8 hours after a single dose of 100 mg. The half-life of amantadine is fairly long (15 hours); as a result, accumulation occurs when the drug is employed in the usual schedule of 100 mg every 12 hours, reaching the maximum tissue concentration after 48 hours. Amantadine is widely distributed, freely crossing the blood-brain barrier and reaching all body fluids, including saliva and breast milk. Elimination is achieved largely (90%) by the kidney; liver metabolism eliminates the remaining 10%. The dose of amantadine should be reduced in the elderly or in any clients with impaired renal function in proportion to any decline in the kidney's glomerular filtration rate (GFR).

Clinical Indications Amantadine is approved for prophylaxis against influenza type A during epidemics, especially for high-risk clients such as the elderly and persons with severe cardiovascular, pulmonary, metabolic, neuromuscular, or immune deficiency disorders. Prevention by early immunization is preferred, but when this is not feasible, amantadine is indicated for prophylaxis. Clients should take amantadine if they anticipate contact or as soon as possible after coming in contact with someone infected with the virus. It is usually recommended that the drug be continued for 5–6 weeks during the periods of high infection. Amantadine has also been found to produce a palliative effect when given within 48 hours after onset of influenza symptoms due to the type A virus. Though not approved for use against other viral infections, there is evidence that the antiviral action of amantadine extends to parainfluenza, pseudorabies, and Russian influenza, though not to type B influenza. Amantadine is also employed in parkinsonism (see Chapter 22).

Adverse Effects and Contraindications Amantadine produces relatively little toxicity. The most frequent serious reactions include depression, psychosis, orthostatic hypotension, and congestive heart failure. *Clients should be advised to report occurrence of shortness of breath, edema, or orthostatic hypotension; all are possible indications of congestive heart failure. The nurse should carefully observe clients given amantadine who have any degree of diminished cardiac function.*

Psychiatric effects include hallucinations, confusion, anxiety, and irritability. *Nurses should advise clients receiving amantadine to report any unusual changes in mood or mental functions.* Neurological difficulties such as ataxia, dizziness, fatigue, weakness, slurred speech, and visual disturbances have been reported. *Nurses should advise clients that this drug may impair their driving ability.* Seizures have occurred rarely in individuals given amantadine. *When giving amantadine, the nurse should carefully observe clients with a history of seizures for signs of impending seizure activity.*

Some clients complain of gastrointestinal symptoms such as nausea, vomiting, anorexia, diarrhea, or constipation. Atropine-like anticholinergic effects such as dry mouth, urinary retention, and visual disturbances occur especially when other anticholinergic drugs are used concomitantly. *The nurse should advise clients to report signs of urinary retention such as swelling of the extremities or difficulty in urinating.* Hypersensitivity reactions, such as rash, dermatitis, leukopenia, and neutropenia, occur only rarely with amantadine. Rare instances of oculogyric episodes (eyes fixed in a lateral gaze) similar to those produced by neuroleptics have been observed.

Drug Interactions Amantadine exhibits two kinds of interactions. The anticholinergic effects of amantadine are additive with those caused by other

Nursing Observations for Amantadine Therapy of Influenza Type A

THERAPEUTIC GOAL	Prevention or rapid resolution of type A influenza in high-risk populations, such as the elderly or those with cardiovascular, pulmonary, metabolic, neuromuscular, or immune deficiency disorders.
PREADMINISTRATION ASSESSMENT	
Baseline Data	Observe for chills, fever, malaise (especially in the legs and back), headache, photophobia, sore throat, nonproductive cough, flushing, weakness, and fatigue. Evaluate blood pressure (sitting, standing, and prone), pulse, perfusion, heart sounds, edema, respiratory rate and sounds, renal output, and neurological status before giving amantadine. Obtain laboratory tests including BUN and serum creatinine before giving amantadine.
Contraindications/ Precautions	Renal or liver disease, pregnancy or lactation, congestive heart failure, psychosis, or seizures. Check medication history for allergic reactions to amantadine.
Potential Interactions	Check current medications for use of anticholinergics.
EVALUATION OF DRUG RESPONSE	
For Therapeutic Benefit	Resolution of symptoms or prevention of infection with influenza type A.
For Adverse Effects	Assess for orthostatic hypotension, congestive heart failure, anticholinergic symptoms, gastrointestinal irritation, mood changes or psychotic symptoms, neurologic symptoms, urinary retention, and allergic reactions.
For Drug Interactions	Monitor for additive anticholinergic effects with other anticholinergic drugs and additive stimulation with CNS stimulants.
For Compliance	Evaluate the client's compliance with all facets of the therapeutic regimen by careful observation, interviewing, and review of progress. Report compliance problems to the physician and act as client-advocate when changes in the therapeutic regimen seem indicated.

anticholinergic drugs. Psychiatric effects of amantadine are additive with those of CNS stimulants.

Preparations and Administration Prophylactic dosing for influenza A virus should begin as soon as possible when exposure is likely and continued for at least 10 days following a known exposure or up to 90 days during periods of possible exposure. If influenza A vaccine is used concurrently, amantadine is continued for 2–3 weeks after vaccination. The divided dose should be used if side effects occur with the single daily dose.

Preparations and Administration

Amantadine (Symmetrel)
Capsules, syrup
Recommended Doses: For adults, 200 mg/day PO in 1 or 2 doses. For children over 9 years of age, 100 mg, twice per day. For children from age 1–9, 2–4 mg/lb daily in 2 or 3 equal portions of syrup.

Antimetabolites

Mechanisms and Effects All systemic antiviral drugs except amantadine and ribaviran are analogues of (and therefore antimetabolites for) the pyrimidine or purine bases that are constituents of the nucleotide building blocks of nucleic acids. Six such drugs are currently available. Four, **zidovudine, idoxuridine, cytarabine,** and **trifluridine,** are analogues of the pyrimidine base thymidine. Idoxuridine (Dendrid, Herplex, Stoxil) and trifluridine (Viroptic) are available only in topical preparations (see Chapters 53 and 54). Cytarabine (Cytosar-U) is classified as an antimetabolite for use in cancer chemotherapy, primarily for acute myelocytic leukemia (Chapter 56). It is marketed only for that application, but like the related antimetabolites has antiviral activity. It has been used experimentally in eye infections caused by herpes zoster virus. Zidovudine (AZT, Retrovir) is a thymidine analogue currently available as an investigational new drug for adminis-

Nursing Diagnoses and Interventions for Amantadine Therapy of Influenza Type A

Nursing Diagnoses	*Related Interventions*
TO MINIMIZE DRUG SIDE EFFECTS OR INTERACTIONS	
Alteration in cardiac output related to orthostatic hypotension or congestive heart failure caused by amantadine	Report any signs of diminished cardiac function to the physician. Advise client to report episodes of dizziness or fainting and to avoid standing up too quickly. Make sure the client and family know the symptoms of congestive heart failure and to report such symptoms immediately.
Alteration in urinary elimination related to amantadine	Advise clients to report signs of urinary retention such as swelling of the extremities or difficulty urinating.
Disturbance in self-concept related to neurological and psychological effects of amantadine	Provide emotional support and encouragement to aid coping with neurological problems and mood changes.
Increased risk of injury related to neurological effects and seizure liability caused by amantadine	Provide safety measures as required; watch for signs of impending seizures. Warn clients that driving may be hazardous due to drowsiness caused by amantadine.
Sensory-perceptual alterations related to visual disturbances caused by amantadine	Instruct client to report any visual disturbances that occur during amantadine therapy. Warn clients that visual impairments may make driving hazardous.
TO ENSURE SAFE AND EFFICACIOUS DRUG USE	
Knowledge deficit related to drug regimen	Explain the nature of the infection and the rationale for using amantadine. Provide clients with a list of adverse effects and drug interactions of amantadine and what to do if any of these occur. Instruct clients how to safely administer the drug.

tration under a compassionate use protocol for patients with acquired immune deficiency syndrome (AIDS) or AIDS-related complex (ARC).

Two of the antiviral antimetabolites are analogues of the purine base adenosine: **vidarabine** (Vira-A) and **acyclovir** (Zovirax). Both are available in parenteral as well as topical dosage forms and acyclovir in an oral dosage form. The topical forms of these drugs are discussed in Chapters 53 and 54. Here we consider only the use of the parenteral and oral forms.

Pharmacokinetics Slow intravenous infusion is the only acceptable method of administration of vidarabine. After intravenous administration, vidarabine is rapidly converted to an active hypoxanthine metabolite. The parent compound and the metabolite may actually have a synergistic action. The half-life of vidarabine of about 3.3 hours precludes accumulation. Serum levels reflect the rate of infusion. Vidarabine readily penetrates into the cerebrospinal fluid (CSF). It is excreted in the urine, 50% as the hypoxanthine metabolite, 1–3% as the parent compound, the rest as other metabolites.

Acyclovir is slowly and incompletely absorbed (15–30%) after oral administration, but absorption is unaffected by food. Peak plasma concentrations are achieved in 1.5–2 hours. In the blood, acyclovir is 9–33% bound by plasma proteins. Acyclovir distributes widely into all tissues; concentrations in the

CSF reach approximately 50% of serum levels. Elimination is 60–90% by renal excretion of the unchanged drug, so the rate of clearance is dependent on renal function.

Based on preliminary studies, zidovudine appears to be about 60% absorbed after oral administration. It is cleared from the blood mainly by hepatic metabolism, with a half-life of approximately 1 hour. Concurrent administration of probenecid (Benemid) slows both its metabolism and renal excretion.

Clinical Indications Vidarabine is active against herpes simplex type 1 virus, herpes zoster, and cytomegalovirus but not against herpes simplex type 2 or other viruses. Mortality from herpes simplex viral encephalitis is reduced two-thirds by parenteral use of vidarabine.

Acyclovir is active against herpes simplex virus type 2, as well as herpes simplex type 1, herpes zoster, cytomegalovirus, and Epstein-Barr virus. Acyclovir is the first drug with significant activity against herpes simplex virus type 2, the usual cause of herpes genitalis. The parenteral dosage form of acyclovir is indicated for treatment of severe initial clinical episodes of herpes genitalis or recurrences of the infection. Milder genital infections by herpes simplex type 2 are adequately and more safely treated with topical or oral dosage forms of acyclovir. *Nurses need to advise clients that the drug does not prevent the transmission of the infection to others. Clients should be cautioned to avoid sexual intercourse when lesions are visibly present.* Acyclovir has not yet been approved for use in infections caused by susceptible viruses other than herpes simplex type 2.

Zidovudine is indicated for use in patients with AIDS or AIDS-related complex who have had at least one documented bout of pneumonia caused by *Pneumocystis carinii* and who are not currently receiving chemotherapeutic, nephrotoxic, or immunosuppressant drugs. Zidovudine therapy initially increases the number of T_4 lymphocytes (the helper-inducer cells infected by the AIDS virus), although ultimately the levels of T_4 lymphocytes fall back to and below the pretreatment levels as the disease progresses. Thus, zidovudine therapy prolongs the life of the AIDS victim, but does not halt the progression of the disease toward death. During the period of time that T_4 lymphocytes are elevated by administration of zidovudine, patients often exhibit such signs of clinical improvement as fever reduction, increased energy, weight gain, and a reduced incidence of opportunistic infections.

Adverse Effects and Contraindications Toxic effects of vidarabine are relatively few and fall into the categories of gastrointestinal, central nervous system, hematological, and hypersensitivity reactions. **Gastrointestinal side effects** are transient and usually mild. Clients may complain of anorexia, nausea, vomiting, and diarrhea. **CNS side effects** include neurological reactions (tremor, dizziness, ataxia) and psychiatric reactions (hallucinations, confusion, psychosis). **Hematological reactions** include mild and uncommon instances of reduced hemoglobin or hematocrit or white blood cell counts. **Allergic reactions** are limited to rash and pruritus. The only contraindication for vidarabine is known allergy to the drug.

After intravenous administration of acyclovir, nurses may notice **phlebitis** at the site of injection (14% of clients). A few clients have **hypersensitivity reactions** (rash or urticaria in 5% of clients) or **CNS symptoms** (tremors, agitation, lethargy, and confusion). There is a risk that acyclovir will form **crystals** in the nephrourinary tract if serum levels or renal concentration is excessive. Since bolus administration is likely to produce conditions conducive to formation of crystals, intravenous administration of acyclovir is always by infusion. Nevertheless, 5% of clients exhibit an increase in creatinine levels, indicative of renal injury. Renal excretion of acyclovir is slowed by probenecid (Benemid).

The most important side effect of zidovudine in AIDS patients is **depression of the bone marrow.** In preliminary clinical trials, significant bone marrow depression occurred in 25% of patients, necessitating frequent blood transfusions. Another frequent side effect is **headache.** Less frequent side effects include restlessness, agitation, and insomnia.

Preparations and Administration Vidarabine has only limited solubility. *When preparing the injection solution, shake the vial well before withdrawing a dose of drug and transferring it to IV fluid.* Vidarabine should be dissolved in a large volume of IV infusion fluid (at least 1 liter of IV fluid per 450 mg of vidarabine or 1 mg of drug per 2.2 ml of IV fluid). *The IV solution should be agitated thoroughly, but the nurse should avoid any unnecessary shaking. The solution should be run through an in-line filter (0.45 micron or smaller) to ensure removal of undissolved particles. Nurses need to monitor the infusion so as to maintain a constant flow rate over 12–24 hours.*

Acyclovir solutions for injection are prepared in sterile or bacteriostatic water for injection containing benzyl alcohol, but bacteriostatic water containing parabens as preservatives must not be used since this will result in drug precipitation. *When high concentrations are infused, extravasation at the infusion site may result in phlebitis or inflammation. After administration of either acyclovir or vidarabine, the nurse should make certain that blood products, protein, or other colloidal fluids are not used.*

Preparations and Administration

Acyclovir (Zovirax)
Capsules, powder for injection solutions
Recommended Doses: 5 mg/kg infused in dextrose or an electrolyte solution over 1 hour, repeated every 8 hours for 7 days for mucosal or cutaneous herpes simplex or for 5 days for herpes genitalis. For oral treatment, 200 mg, tid, continued indefinitely as prophylaxis against recurrent herpes virus infections; or 200 mg every 4 hours while awake, for 5 days, to halt active infection and hasten the healing of existing lesions. *Nurses need to advise clients not to exceed the recommended dose, frequency of application, or length of treatment.*

Vidarabine (Vira-A)
Injection solution
Recommended Doses: 15 mg/kg/day for 10 days infused slowly after dilution in an appropriate intravenous solution over 12–24 hours each day.

Zidovudine (AZT, Retrovir)
Capsules (investigational new drug, compassionate use protocol)
Recommended Doses: For AIDS or ARC, as of April, 1987, 200 mg every 4 hours.

Ribavirin (Virazole)

Ribavirin, an antiviral drug introduced in 1986, is active against respiratory syncytial virus, influenza virus, and herpes simplex virus, but its mechanism is unknown. Ribavirin is administered by aerosol and is indicated for use in selected hospitalized infants or young children with severe lower respiratory tract infections due to herpes simplex virus. After administration by aerosol, ribavirin is absorbed systemically. The plasma half-life approximates 9.5 hours. Since ribavirin has been employed only in infants with life-threatening diseases involving impaired respiratory function, the role of ribavirin in deterioration during treatment, such as worsening of respiratory status and cardiac arrest, has not been determined. Rash and conjunctivitis have occurred and have been linked to use of ribavirin aerosol.

Preparations and Administration

Ribavirin (Virazole)
Powder for injection solution
Recommended Doses: Administered by aerosol mask for 12–18 hours per day for 3–7 days.

Chemotherapy for Systemic Fungal Infections

The Nature of Fungi

Fungi are a varied group of eukaryotic protists, distributed throughout the world, and characterized by the absence of chlorophyll and the presence of a rigid cell wall. The group includes yeasts, molds, and mushrooms. Yeasts are simple one-celled organisms; molds and mushrooms are more complex and multicellular.

Most of the fungi that are pathogenic to humans belong to one of the five classes of fungi — the class Deuteromycetes (or *Fungi Imperfecti*). This class includes fungi that cause histoplasmosis, coccidiodomycosis, blastomycosis, and the tinea dermatophytoses. Candida, by contrast, belongs to the Ascomycotes class. The fungus causing cryptococcosis belongs to the Basidiomycotes class. The other two classes, Zygomycotes and Mastigomycotes are seldom pathogenic to humans. The major systemic fungal infections and their drug treatments are summarized in Table 48–2. Many fungal infections have limited geographical distributions; for example, coccidioidomycosis is limited to the southwestern United States, blastomycosis to Africa and North America, and paracoccidioidomycosis to South America.

Some fungal infections occur only as opportunistic infections. *Candida* and *aspergillis,* for example, are always part of the **commensal flora** but become pathogenic in clients with extensive burns or impaired immune resistance due to disease or immunosuppressive drugs. Systemic fungal infections are often chronic, with slowly developing pulmonary lesions. From the lungs, fungal infections disseminate to tissues that are characteristic for each type of organism. Diagnosis of a systemic fungal infection is usually confirmed by identification of the organism in an appropriate body fluid: blood, urine, cerebrospinal fluid, or sputum, for example. This method is less reliable when the fungus is prevalent and commensal. Histopathology is also usually distinctive when infections have a fungal origin.

Polyenes

Amphotericin B (Fungizone)

Amphotericin B is a polyene antibiotic derived from a soil actinomycete, *Streptomyces nodosus.* After a quarter century of clinical use, this drug remains the most important one for systemic mycotic (fungal) in-

Table 48–2
Drug Therapy for Systemic Fungal Infections

		Drug selections	
Disease	**Site and locale**	**Primary choices**	**Alternate choices**
Cryptococcosis	Opportunistic infections of the lungs with possible dissemination to the skin, bones and kidneys. Worldwide, southeastern United States	Amphotericin B and flucytosine	None
Candidiasis	Opportunistic dermatophytoses, septicemia, endocarditis, meningitis, osteomyelitis Universal distribution	Amphotericin B Ketoconazole	Amphotericin B and flucytosine
Histoplasmosis	Lungs with possible dissemination to oropharynx, alimentary tract, and lymphatics Ohio and Mississippi River valleys	Amphotericin B	
Coccidioidomycosis	Lungs with possible dissemination to the skin, lymphatics, spleen, liver, bones, kidneys, meninges, and brain Southwestern United States	Amphotericin B	Miconazole
Blastomycosis	Lungs with possible dissemination to the skin North America and Africa	Amphotericin B	Hydroxystilbamidine
Paracoccidioidomycosis	Skin, mucous membranes, lymphatics, and other organs South and Central America	Amphotericin B	Sulfonamides
Sporotrichosis	Skin, superficial lymph nodes, occasionally disseminating to the lungs or other tissues Worldwide, especially hot, arid climates	Amphotericin B	None
Aspergillis	Opportunistic infections of the lungs with possible general dissemination Worldwide	Amphotericin B	Flucytosine

fections. Amphotericin B can be either fungistatic or fungicidal depending on its concentration at the site of action. Polyene antifungal drugs bind to sterol molecules in membranes of sensitive yeasts and fungi. Bacteria do not contain sterol in their membranes and are thus insensitive. The interaction of polyene antifungal drugs with sterol constituents of mycotic membranes leads to an increase in permeability of the membrane and leakage of potassium ions outward and sodium ions inward and cell viability is lost.

Amphotericin is active against a wide variety of fungi (Table 48–3), notably *Cryptococcus neoformans, Candida albicans, Histoplasma capsulatum, Coccidioides immitis, Blastomyces dermatitidis* and *braziliensis, Torulopsis glabrata,* and the dermatophytes. Some strains of *Sporotrichum schenckii,* the dermatophytes, and *Aspergillus* are sensitive, but some of these as well as mutant strains of *Candida albicans* are resistant. The antifungal activity of amphotericin B is synergistic with that of flucytosine, and certain antibiotics (rifampin (Rifadin) or tetracycline) with little or no antifungal activity of their own augment the effect of amphotericin B.

Pharmacokinetics Amphotericin B is not well absorbed from the gastrointestinal tract and is therefore given by intravenous injection. After injection, the drug circulates in the plasma bound to serum lipoproteins and in tissues is largely bound to cholesterol constituents of membranes. Amphotericin B does not effectively penetrate into the cerebrospinal fluid, vitreous humor, or amniotic fluid. It is largely metabolized before excretion, with an elimination half-life of about 15 days.

Clinical Indications Clinical indications for amphotericin B include cryptococcosis, systemic forms of candidiasis, histoplasmosis, coccidiodomycosis, blastomycosis, and infections caused by

Table 48–3
Antifungal Spectra of Systemic Antifungal Drugs

	Polyenes		Imidazoles				
Fungal infections	**Amphotericin B**	**Nystatin**	**Miconazole**	**Ketoconazole**	**Flucytosine**	**Griseofulvin**	**Hydroxystilbamidine**
Systemic							
Cryptococcosis	S	A	S	S	S	N	
Candidiasis	S	S	S	S	S	N	
Histoplasmosis	S	A	A	S	N	N	
Coccidioidomycosis	S		S	S	N	N	
Blastomycosis	S	A	P	P		N	A
Paracoccidioidomycosis			S	S			
Sporotrichosis	S		P	P	N	N	
Aspergillosis	S						
Chromomycosis	A				A	N	
Rhodoturuliosis	A						
Superficial							
Candidiasis	A		S	S	A	N	
Tinea versicolor						N	
Dermatophytoses							
Trichophyta	A	T		A		S	
Epidermophyton	A	T		A		S	
Microsporum	A	T		A		S	

Key:
S: Systemic use of the drug is indicated.
A: Active systemically, but not a primary drug choice.
P: Poor level of activity.
N: Not active.
T: Topical use of the drug is indicated.
Blank: No information.

sensitive strains of *Mucor, Rhizopus, Absidia, Entomophthora, Basidiobolus, Sporotrichum schenckii,* and *Aspergillus fumigatus.* Prior to introduction of amphotericin B, infections caused by many of these fungi were fatal.

Adverse Effects and Contraindications Adverse reactions to amphotericin B are frequent, varied, and often pronounced. **Fever** occurs in half of patients upon initial administration, often accompanied by headache, chills, nausea, vomiting, and anorexia. These symptoms typically subside within the first 4 hours. Other common reactions include malaise, generalized joint and muscle pain, epigastric distress, phlebitis at the site of injection, and anemia (normochromic, normocytic). Indications of **renal impairment** are evident in 80% of patients receiving amphotericin B. These signs include azotemia, hypokalemia, renal tubular acidosis, hypomagnesia, fibrosis and hyalinization of the glomeruli, and nephrocalcinosis. Anuria or oliguria may rarely occur. *Careful monitoring of patients' input and output is important. The nurse can help to reduce the occurrence of nephrotoxicity by ensuring that patients maintain adequate hydration. Nurses should also report immediately appearance of blood or sediment in the urine, since this can be an early indication of renal damage that is reversible if the drug is discontinued at this early stage.*

Cardiovascular disturbances occur only rarely, but include cardiac arrest, dysrhythmias, and both hypertension and hypotension. **Hematological side effects** such as anemia, leukopenia, agranulocytosis, eosinophilia, leukocytosis, or thrombocytopenia are also rare. **Hypersensitivity reactions** include maculopapular rash, pruritus, and anaphylactoid reactions. *Patients who are hypersensitive to amphotericin B should not be given it.*

Neurological disturbances, including tinnitus, loss of auditory acuity, blurred vision, diplopia, convulsions, and peripheral neuropathies are uncom-

Nursing Observations for Antifungal Drug Therapy

THERAPEUTIC GOAL	Eradication of the infecting fungal agent.
PREADMINISTRATION ASSESSMENT	
Baseline Data	Observe for respiratory symptoms, neurological problems, and symptoms specific to each disease. Evaluate ECG, pulse, respiratory rate and sound, bowel sounds, neurological status. Obtain laboratory tests including microscopic identification of the organism in an appropriate body fluid; complete blood cell counts, BUN, creatinine, urinalysis, liver function.
Contraindications/ Precautions	Renal or hepatic dysfunction, pregnancy or lactation, or bone marrow depression. Check medication history for allergic reactions to antifungal drugs.
Potential Interactions	Check current drug regimen for interacting drugs.
EVALUATION OF DRUG RESPONSE	
For Therapeutic Benefit	Monitor resolution of symptoms of infection and elimination of organism from body fluid specimen cultures.
For Adverse Effects	Assess renal and hepatic function, complete blood cell counts, fever, pain, skin rash, gastrointestinal reactions, and changes in cardiac function. During initial dosage adjustment for amphotericin B, monitor serum electrolytes and conduct hemograms, urinalysis, and renal function tests.
For Compliance	Evaluate the client's compliance with all facets of the therapeutic regimen by careful observation, interviewing, and review of progress. Report compliance problems to the physician and act as client-advocate when changes in the therapeutic regimen seem indicated.

mon. Ototoxic, nephrotoxic, and neurotoxic effects of other drugs can be additive with similar adverse effects of amphotericin B. *Any patient's complaints of ringing in the ears or vertigo should be reported. Hearing loss is not always evident to patients, so nurses should be attentive to indirect clues and check with friends and family about any change in hearing.*

Corticosteroids should be avoided when amphotericin B is being employed. The combination increases risk of superinfection.

Preparations and Administration Amphotericin B is administered only to hospitalized patients. *Patients need to know that 6–10 weeks of therapy is usually necessary to assure an adequate response and that relapse will not usually occur. Some infections may take 9–11 months to be cured.* No optimum dosage schedule has been established for amphotericin B.

When the drug is reconstituted for intravenous infusion, it may be added to solutions of 5% dextrose in water, with a pH above 4.2. If the pH is less than this, it is necessary to add a sterile buffer. The infusion solution must not contain preservatives since these will precipitate amphotericin B; strict aseptic technique must therefore be observed in preparation of solutions. Use of an in-line filter during IV infusion is not usually recommended, but there may be occasions when this is unavoidable. In those instances, the mean pore diameter should be no less than 1 micron; otherwise the concentration of amphotericin B received by the patient will be reduced. Amphotericin B is light sensitive, but no significant deterioration occurs within the 6–8 hours required for infusion of a single dose. If precipitate or particles appear in a solution of amphotericin, it should be discarded.

Local inflammation or thrombosis may occur at the site of amphotericin B injection, especially if extravasation occurs. Among children the risk of thrombophlebitis may be reduced by using a pediatric scalp vein needle, inserting it into the most distal vein possible, alternating veins, and using heparin. *It is important for the nurse to check the IV frequently for leakage. This is especially critical among the elderly, who have lost tissue elasticity as a consequence of the normal aging process.*

During the initial therapy, the nurse should monitor vital signs every 30 minutes for at least 4 hours, observing the individual closely for adverse effects. During the period when drug dosage is being established, hemograms, serum measurements of potassium, magnesium, and calcium, and renal function tests (including urinalysis) should be performed on alternate days and then weekly. Liver function tests should also be done periodically throughout therapy. These tests will help identify hematological changes such as leukopenia, coagulation defects, anemia, or thrombocytopenia, or signs of acute liver failure. If blood urea nitrogen exceeds 40 mg/dl, if nonprotein nitrogen exceeds 100 mg/dl, or if serum creatinine exceeds 3 mg/dl, the nurse should withhold the drug and report the findings to the physician, who may either reduce the dosage or discontinue the drug.

Preparations and Administration

Amphotericin B (Fungizone)
Powder for reconstitution in sterile water and addition to a 5% dextrose infusion solution
Recommended Doses: Up to 1 mg/kg if given daily or up to 1.5 mg/kg if given on alternate days. The recommended rate of infusion is to give the daily dose over 6 hours.

Nystatin (Mycostatin, Nilstat, generic)

Another polyene antibiotic used as an antifungal agent is nystatin. The drug is derived from *Streptomyces noursei* and its name is a contraction of New York State, where it was discovered. Nystatin is used for treatment of infections caused by Candida species. After oral administration, nystatin is poorly absorbed and does not generate significant plasma concentrations if renal function is normal. Thus, oral administration of nystatin approximates topical application to the alimentary tract. Oral tablets are seldom used but are officially indicated for **intestinal candidiasis.** The principal use of nystatin is in creams, powders, ointments, suspensions, drops, and vaginal tablets for topical use in candidal infections of mucosal membranes or cutaneous surfaces.

Nursing management of clients requiring nystatin is extremely important — some say as important as the drug treatment in preventing reinfection and eliminating deep-seated infections. *For oral candidiasis (thrush), the oral suspension should be swished around so that it contacts each side of the mouth. Before administering the drug, the client's mouth should be cleared of food and the client instructed to keep the medication in contact with the oral mucosa for a few minutes before swallowing it. Nurses should advise clients to brush their teeth or rinse their mouths thoroughly after each meal. Either the nurse or a dental hygienist should teach the client proper flossing methods. Dentures should be removed and cleaned thoroughly after each meal.*

The nurse needs to instruct clients who require vaginal tablets to insert the medication high in the vagina. If the woman is sexually active, she should be told to advise her sexual partner to use a condom to prevent reinfection. Nurses should advise clients to continue therapy even during menstruation. If the client is not pregnant, she may take cleansing douches for aesthetic reasons before insertion of the tablet. Vaginal tablets can be employed as oral lozenges for treatment of candidiasis of the mouth or esophagus.

The mechanism of nystatin is the same as that of amphotericin B. Nystatin produces little toxicity and has not been reported to result in allergic reactions. *Nevertheless, nurses should instruct clients to report occurrence of redness, swelling, or irritation.* Gastrointestinal reactions are mild, including nausea, vomiting, or diarrhea.

Preparations and Administration

Nystatin (Mycostatin, Nilstat, and generic)
Tablets
Recommended Doses: For intestinal candidiasis, 500,000–1,000,000 units PO, 3 times per day, to be continued at least 48 hours after alleviation of clinical symptoms.

Imidazoles

Of the five imidazoles currently available for treatment of fungal infections, three — clotrimazole (Lotrimin, Mycelex), butoconazole (Femstat), and econazole (Spectazole) — are available in topical preparations only and are discussed in Chapter 53; one, miconazole, is available in topical (Monistat-Derm) and intravenous (Monistat I.V.) dosage forms; and the fifth, ketoconazole, is available only in an oral dosage form (Nizoral tablets). Systemic uses of miconazole and ketoconazole will be discussed here. These two imidazoles have similar antifungal spectra (Table 48–3), and are indicated for treatment of cryptococcosis, systemic candidiasis, histoplasmosis, coccidioidomycosis, paracoccidioidomycosis, and chronic mucocutaneous candidiasis. Imidazoles cause destruction of fungal cell membranes by inhibition of synthesis of ergosterol by fungi. These drugs also inhibit mitochondrial function in fungal cells.

Miconazole (Monistat)

Miconazole is given by intravenous infusion or topically as a cream. The topical use of this drug is discussed in Chapter 53. This drug penetrates effectively into joints, the eyes, peritoneal fluid, sputum,

Nursing Diagnoses and Interventions for Antifungal Drug Therapy

Nursing Diagnoses	*Related Interventions*
TO ENHANCE DRUG BENEFITS OR REDUCE DRUG REQUIREMENTS	
Alteration in bowel elimination pattern: diarrhea related to fungal infection	Give small frequent meals; intensify hygienic measures.
Alteration in comfort: headache or gastrointestinal pain related to fungal infection	Give analgesics or antiemetics as required; provide emotional support.
TO MINIMIZE DRUG SIDE EFFECTS OR INTERACTIONS	
Alteration in urinary elimination related to use of amphotericin B	Monitor fluid intake-output; tell client to report difficulty voiding, blood or sediment in urine, or cloudy or pink urine; monitor for granular or hyaline casts in the urine.
Alteration in tissue perfusion related to renal or liver dysfunction, bone marrow depression, or thrombus caused by drug therapy	Monitor for edema or signs of jaundice; tell client to report fever, chills, yellowing of eyes or skin, dark urine, or pale stools; observe for thrombus formation or thrombophlebitis at the site of injection with amphotericin B.
Sensory-perceptual alteration related to ototoxicity, diplopia, or peripheral neuropathies with amphotericin B	Instruct clients to report any decrease in auditory acuity or ringing in the ears, blurring of vision, or diminished touch sensitivity.
Increased risk of injury related to neurological impairments related to use of amphotericin B	Provide safety measures as required.
TO ENSURE SAFE AND EFFICACIOUS DRUG USE	
Knowledge deficit related to drug regimen	Teach the client about the nature of the disorder and the rationale for drug selection.
	Instruct the client about safe storage of medication and proper dosage, and administration of each drug in the regimen.
	Teach the client the potential interactions for each drug in the regimen and what to do if any of these occur.
	Teach clients to watch especially for signs of allergy, dyscrasias, or hepatic dysfunction.

saliva, but only sparingly into the cerebrospinal fluid. Intrathecal administration is required for treatment of meningitis caused by susceptible organisms. In the plasma, miconazole is 90% bound to plasma proteins and can potentiate oral anticoagulants by displacement. Miconazole is inactivated mainly by metabolism. Adverse effects relating to intravenous administration of miconazole include phlebitis at the site of infusion (in 29% of clients), allergic reactions (pruritus or rash), gastrointestinal side effects (nausea, vomiting, diarrhea, anorexia), febrile reactions, flushing, and drowsiness. *Gastrointestinal effects can be reduced by prior administration of an antihistaminic or antiemetic drug, or administration of miconazole more slowly and at a time further removed from mealtime.* Miconazole and amphotericin B are mutually antagonistic and should not be coadministered.

Preparations and Administration

Miconazole (Monistat)
Injection solution
Recommended Doses: For adults, 1,000–3,600 mg/day IV for coccidioidomycosis, 1,200–2,400 mg/day for cryptococcosis, 600–1,800 mg/day for candidi-

asis, and 200–1,200 mg/day for paracoccidioidomycosis. Treatment durations range from 1 week to more than 20 weeks.

Ketoconazole (Nizoral)

Ketoconazole was introduced in 1981 and is an important new drug. It has a broad antifungal spectrum (Table 48–3), is effective orally, and produces fewer adverse effects than amphotericin B. Ketoconazole is approved for treatment of candidiasis, oral thrush, coccidioidomycosis, histoplasmosis, chromomycosis, and paracoccidioidomycosis. It is the drug of choice for chronic mucocutaneous candidiasis. Several clinical trials have indicated effectiveness against dermatophytes as well. Adverse effects of ketoconazole are mild: nausea or vomiting in 3% of clients, abdominal discomfort and pruritus in 1–2% each.

Although normally well absorbed, ketoconazole is mildly basic and requires adequate stomach acid for dissolution and absorption. *Nurses should instruct clients who are receiving antacids, H_2-receptor blockers, or anticholinergics to take ketoconazole at least 2 hours after their antiulcer medication(s).* Individuals with pronounced achlorhydria should dissolve tablets of ketoconazole in 0.2 N HCl and ingest the mixture, using a straw to avoid contact of the solution with the teeth.

Preparations and Administration

Ketoconazole (Nizoral)
Tablets
Recommended Doses: 200 mg/day PO in a single dose, preferably with a meal in order to minimize occurrence of nausea and vomiting. The duration of therapy usually exceeds 6 months for systemic fungal infection, but candidiasis may respond more quickly (in a minimum of 1–2 weeks).

Other Systemic Antifungal Drugs

Griseofulvin (Fulvicin, Grifulvin V, Grisactin, Gris-PEG)

Griseofulvin is an antibiotic obtained from *Penicillium griseofulvin.* As an antifungal drug, griseofulvin has a limited spectrum of effectiveness. It is fungistatic against the three species of dermatophytes, *Trichophyton, Epidermophyton,* and *Microsporum,* but it is ineffective against other fungi or bacteria. Griseofulvin interferes with mitotic division of dermatophyte cells by disrupting the microtubules that direct mitosis.

Pharmacokinetics After oral administration, griseofulvin is absorbed to a variable extent. Absorption is improved when the drug is taken with food, especially foods with a high fat content. Griseofulvin is available in an ultramicrocrystalline formulation that improves absorption by a factor of 2. Peak plasma levels of griseofulvin occur after about 4 hours. Griseofulvin has great affinity for the skin, being deposited in keratin precursor cells and ultimately appearing in the horny layer bound to keratin. Dermatophytes are prevented from growing in the new skin, hair, and nails. Gradually, infected skin and skin appendages are shed and replaced by healthy, fungus-free tissue. Griseofulvin has a serum half-life of about 24 hours and is inactivated mainly by metabolism followed by renal excretion of metabolites.

Clinical Indications Griseofulvin is indicated exclusively for infections of the skin, nails, and hair caused by dermatophytes. It is useful for treatment of tinea corporis, tinea pedis, tinea cruris, tinea capitis, tinea barbae, and tinea unguium. Determination of the infecting organism should be conducted prior to instituting griseofulvin therapy to ensure that the infection is due to a sensitive organism.

Adverse Effects and Contraindications Adverse reactions to griseofulvin are not common. Most are **allergic reactions,** such as rash, urticaria, photosensitivity, erythema multiforme, serum sickness, and rare instances of angioneurotic edema. *Clients should be warned to avoid intense natural or artificial sunlight because of the potential of photosensitivity reactions.* **Neurological difficulties** occur uncommonly, such as headache, paresthesias, lethargy, fatigue, mental confusion, vertigo, syncope, blurred vision, and peripheral neuritis. Griseofulvin may alter taste sensitivity, which can lead to anorexia. Griseofulvin infrequently causes **hematological reactions** such as leukopenia, neutropenia, and punctate basophilia. *Blood tests should be conducted before initiating drug therapy and at least weekly thereafter.* **Gastrointestinal symptoms** include nausea, vomiting, diarrhea, gastritis, stomatitis, and flatulence. **Hepatotoxicity** and **renal toxicity** occur rarely. *Clients should have periodic renal and hepatic function tests performed to identify any evidence of nephrotoxicity or hepatotoxicity.*

Drug Interactions Griseofulvin reduces the activity of oral anticoagulants such as warfarin (Coumadin), requiring dosage adjustment for the latter drug. Barbiturates impair the absorption of griseofulvin, necessitating an increase in the dose of griseofulvin. Central nervous system depression produced by alcohol and other sedative-hypnotics is additive with neurological effects of griseofulvin.

Nurses should caution clients that use of alcohol with griseofulvin may cause excessive flushing and tachycardia.

Preparations and Administration Griseofulvin is marketed in microsize and ultramicrosize formulations. *Perhaps the most important nursing function with respect to griseofulvin therapy is to encourage clients to continue taking the medication until the infection is completely eradicated. This may take as long as a year.*

Griseofulvin (Fulvicin, Grifulvin V, Grisactin, Gris-PEG)
Microsize capsules, microsize tablets, microsize oral suspension, ultramicrosize tablets
Recommended Doses: For adults, 500 mg PO daily of the microsize preparation or 250 mg daily of the ultramicrosize preparation in single or divided doses. Difficult infections such as tinea unguium and tinea pedis may require doses as high as 1 g daily of the microsize preparation. For children, the dose is 5 mg/lb/day of the microsize drug. For children weighing 30–50 lb, the dose is 125–250 mg daily of the microsize drug; for those weighing over 50 lb, it is 250–500 mg/day of the microsize drug. The duration of therapy is typically 2–4 weeks for tinea corporis, 4–6 weeks for tinea capitis, 4–8 weeks for tinea pedis, and at least 4 months for tinea unguium.

Flucytosine (Ancobon)

Flucytosine is an orally effective antifungal drug of limited usefulness. This antimetabolite agent is fungistatic against *Cryptococcus neoformans* and some strains of *Candida albicans.* Organisms develop resistance to the drug rather quickly, and flucytosine is therefore rarely used alone. Its chief use is as an add-on to therapy with amphotericin B for cryptococcosis and candidiasis. After oral administration, flucytosine is well absorbed and widely distributed. It is not significantly bound by plasma proteins and is eliminated mainly (80%) by renal excretion with a half-life of 3–6 hours. Adverse effects of flucytosine include bone marrow suppression (anemia, leukopenia, thrombocytopenia), gastrointestinal symptoms (nausea, vomiting, diarrhea), hypersensitivity reactions (rash), and neurological effects (headache, vertigo, confusion, hallucinations, and sedation). *Gastrointestinal effects can be minimized by taking capsules a few at a time over a 15-minute period.*

Preparations and Administration

Flucytosine (Ancobon)
Capsules
Recommended Doses: 50–150 mg/kg/day PO in divided doses at 6-hour intervals. Dosage adjustment is necessary for renally impaired clients.

Hydroxystilbamidine

This drug has limited usefulness because of the severity of its adverse effects. It has a fungistatic action against *Blastomycosis dermatitidis* and is used only in conjunction with amphotericin B for that condition.

Preparations and Administration

Hydroxystilbamidine
Powder for injection solution
Recommended Doses: 225 mg every 24 hours.

Important Nursing Implications for Systemic Antifungal Drugs

- ☐ Continue treatment with systemic antifungal drugs at least 48 hours after indications of infection are eliminated. Premature discontinuation of therapy invites relapse.
- ☐ Stress to clients the importance of precise compliance with the drug regimen.
- ☐ Monitor clients for evidence of superinfections such as growths on the tongue, vaginal or rectal itching, or diarrhea.

Chemotherapy for Infectious Parasitic Worms

Helminths

Helminths are the group of invertebrates known commonly as worms. Some of these are parasitic, causing infections in humans. Worms are the parasites most common in human beings; they infect approximately one billion people worldwide. The helminths are soft-bodied animals, easily visible in their mature state, containing differentiated muscle tissue and specialized nervous, digestive, excretory, and reproductive structures. The two major groups of helminths are the roundworms (nematodes) and flatworms (platyhelminths). The flatworms are further divided into two subgroups: the cestodes (or tapeworms) and trematodes (or flukes). All three groups — nematodes, cestodes, and trematodes — have representatives that are pathogenic to humans (Table 48–4).

Nematodes are cylindrical and bilaterally symmetrical. They have a tough outer cuticle. Important nematodes include hookworms, pinworms, whipworms, and threadworms. Hookworms have special cutting plates, or hooks, at their mouths that provide attachment to host tissue. Nematodes are pointed at

Table 48–4
Drug Selections for Infections Caused by Parasitic Worms

Parasitic worm	Disease	Distribution	Source of infection	Symptoms of infection	Drug selections
Intestinal nematodes					
Ascaris lumbricoides	Ascariasis (giant roundworms)	Worldwide, especially warm, moist climates	Contaminated vegetables or soil	Bronchial symptoms, abdominal pain, or eosinophilia	Pyrantel pamoate Mebendazole Piperazine Thiabendazole Diethylcarbamazine
Enterobius	Enterobiasis (pinworm)	Worldwide, mainly in children	Eggs from contaminated fomites	Perianal or perineal itching	Pyrantel pamoate Mebendazole Piperazine Pyrvinium pamoate Thiabendazole
Strongyloides stercoralis	Strongyloidiasis (threadworm)	Southern United States and moist tropics	Fecal contamination of soil	Gastric pain, diarrhea	Thiabendazole Pyrvinium pamoate
Trichuris tichiura	Trichuriasis (whipworm)	Warm, moist climates; seldom in the United States	Fecal contamination of soil	Diarrhea, abdominal cramps, anemia	Thiabendazole Mebendazole
Ancylostoma duodenale	Uncinariasis (common hookworm)	Moist climates	Fecal contamination of soil	Abdominal pain, anemia, cardiac failure, weight loss	Thiabendazole Mebendazole
Necator americanus	Uncinariasis	Warm, moist climates	Fecal contamination of soil	Abdominal pain anemia, cardiac failure, weight loss	Bephenium hydroxynaphthoate Pyrantel pamoate
Tissue nematodes					
Brugia malayi	Filiariasis	Tropics and subtropics	Mosquito bites	Lymphangitis, orchitis, and chyluria	Diethylcarbamazine
Drancunculus medinensis	Draconiasis	India, Near East, Africa, West Indies	Water infested with crustacea	Skin ulcers	Niridazole Thiabendazole Metronidazole
Loa loa	Loiasis	Africa	Fly bites	Subcutaneous swellings	Diethylcarbamazine
Mansonella ozzardi	Monsonelliasis	Central and South America		Usually asymptomatic	Diethylcarbamazine
Onchocerca volvulus	Onchocerciasis (river blindness)	South and Central America; Central Africa	Black fly bites	Fibrous nodules of the skin and subcutaneous tissue	Diethylcarbamazine
Dipetalonema streptocerca	No name	Africa		Usually asymptomatic	Diethylcarbamazine
Trichinella spiralis	Trichinosis	Worldwide; rare in tropics	Pork sausage	Intestinal distress and fever	Thiabendazole
Cestodes					
Hymenolepis nana	Cysticercosis (dwarf tapeworm)	Worldwide; Southern United States	Eggs on objects	Diarrhea or abdominal pain	Quinacrine Niclosamide Paromomycin

(continued)

Table 48–4
Drug Selections for Infections Caused by Parasitic Worms

Parasitic worm	Disease	Distribution	Source of infection	Symptoms of infection	Drug selections
Diphyllobothrium	Diphyllobothriasis (fish tapeworm)	Worldwide; Northern Minnesota and Michigan; Canada	Freshwater fish	Intestinal symptoms or pernicious anemia	Quinacrine Niclosamide Paromomycin
Taenia saginata	Taeniasis saginata (beef tapeworm)	Worldwide	Poorly cooked beef	Abdominal distress or asymptomatic	Quinacrine Niclosamide Paromomycin
Taenia solium	Cysticercosis (pork tapeworm)	South America; Asia, Eastern Europe	Poorly cooked pork	Abdominal distress	Quinacrine Niclosamide Paromomycin
Trematodes					
Schistosoma	Schistosomiasis (blood flukes)		Snail infested waters		
S. hematobium		Africa; Near East		Dysentery, fibrosis of intestinal or bladder wall, hematuria	Niridazole Metrifonate Praziquantel Hycanthone Antimonials Stibophen
S. japonicum		Orient		Dysentery, fibrosis of intestinal, hepatic, or bladder wall	Niridazole Antimonials Praziquantel Metrifonate
S. mansoni		Africa; Latin America		Dysentery, fibrosis of intestinal, hepatic, or bladder wall	Oxamniquine Antimonials Praziquantel Hycanthone Stibophen
Paragonimus westermani and *Kellicotti*	Lung flukes	Africa; Orient; Latin America	Crabs or crayfish	Brochiolar distress	Bithional Chloroquine
Clonorchis sinensis	Chinese liver flukes	Orient	Freshwater fish	Hepatic colic, cholecystiasis	Chloroquine Antimonials Bithional
Fasciola hepatica	Large liver fluke	Sheep-raising countries	Watercress	Hepatic colic, cholecystiasis	Emetine Bithional
Fasciola buski	Giant intestinal fluke				Tetrachloroethylene Hexylresorcinol

both ends but lack segments. Most nematodes exist as separate male and female sexes.

Cestodes are flat and elongated, consisting of many segments. The tapeworms are hermaphroditic, with each worm containing both male and female sex organs. Tapeworms produce eggs that must develop through multiple stages to reach adulthood. Often, development occurs in intermediate hosts. In most cases, it is the adult cestode that infests the intestinal tract of humans. Humans are thus the final or definitive host.

Trematodes are the group of worms known as flukes. They can infect the blood, intestines, liver, or lungs of humans. Blood flukes, called **schistosomes,** are elongated, round, and bisexual. Flukes infecting all other tissues are flat, leaf-shaped, and hermaphroditic. Human infection by flukes results from swimming in infested water or from ingesting pork, beef, fish, crustaceans, or water plants infected by flukes.

Identification of worm infections is a critical step in rational therapy, since anthelmintic drugs have quite specific spectra of activity. Identification is usually made on the basis of ova or larvae found in the human host's feces, urine, or sputum. The pathological effects of worms are often quite indirect: they may block the intestines or lymph passages, secrete toxic chemicals, or compete with the host for nourishment. It is often advisable to treat all family members simultaneously when undertaking treatment for intestinal nematodes. *Clients should be instructed to launder underwear, sheets, towels, and nightclothes daily and to disinfect toilets daily during therapy.*

Nursing assessment and management requires a review of the client's personal hygiene habits. Nurses need to teach clients and their families effective measures to prevent reinfestation, emphasizing washing hands thoroughly after using the toilet, keeping hands away from the mouth, and, in some sections of the country, avoiding hookworm by not walking barefoot outdoors. Because pinworms can be transmitted easily from person to person, all members of a family need to be treated simultaneously.

Anthelmintics Employed for Nematode Infections

Mebendazole (Vermox) and Thiabendazole (Mintezol)

Mebendazole and thiabendazole are benzimidazole compounds, possessing potent vermicidal activity against all of the major intestinal nematodes as well as *Trichinella spiralis* and *Dracunculus medinensis* (Table 48–5). These drugs appear to block glucose uptake by susceptible helminths, ultimately depleting the stores of glycogen in the organisms. After oral administration, mebendazole is poorly absorbed, with only 5–10% reaching the serum for ultimate excretion in the urine. Most remains in the intestines and is excreted in the feces. Thiabendazole, on the other hand, is absorbed rapidly, producing peak plasma levels in 1–2 hours. Inactivation is by liver conjugation. The two drugs are employed for pinworm, treadworm, roundworm, hookworm, and whipworm infections and cutaneous larva migrans (creeping eruption). The adverse effects of these drugs usually relate to the gastrointestinal tract: nausea, vomiting, anorexia, diarrhea, and epigastric distress. Thiabendazole produces additional adverse effects because of systemic absorption. These include CNS reactions (fatigue, drowsiness, giddiness, headache, tinnitus, blurring of vision) and hypersensitivity reactions (rash urticaria, cholestasis, fever, chills, angioderma, erythema multiforme, and anaphylaxis).

Preparations and Administration

Mebendazole (Vermox)
Chewable tablets
Recommended Doses: One tablet in the morning and in the evening for 3 consecutive days. This treatment course can be repeated after 3 weeks if a cure is not evident.

Thiabendazole (Mintezol)
Chewable tablets, oral suspension
Recommended Doses: For treatment of strongyloidiasis, ascariasis, uncinariasis, trichuriasis, or cutaneous larva migrans, 10 mg/lb per dose PO for clients less than 150 lb and 1.5 g for clients over 150 lb; 2 doses daily for 2 successive days. Treatment for enterobiasis is continued only 1 day and for trichinosis for 4 successive days. Thiabendazole is best given after meals.

Piperazine (Antepar, Vermizine)

The salts of piperazine are effective in treatment of pinworms and roundworms. They paralyze these worms, enabling the host to expel them in the feces. The action is similar to that of curare but is exerted more powerfully against parasites than against the mammalian host. Piperazine is absorbed to a variable but significant extent. The absorbed portion is excreted in the urine. Piperazine is indicated for treatment of infections due to pinworms (enterobiasis) and roundworms (ascariasis). Adverse effects are usually mild. Gastrointestinal reactions (nausea, vomiting, cramps, and diarrhea) can be reduced if clients take the medication with food. CNS effects (headache, ataxia, tremors, vertigo, weakness, hyporeflexia, blurred vision, nystagmus, convulsions, impaired memory), hypersensitivity reactions (urticaria, rash, erythema multiforme, purpura, fever, arthralgia, rhinorrhea, lacrimation, and bronchospasm), and cataracts have been reported. The drug is contraindicated for clients who have convulsive disorders, since these conditions can be aggravated by the drug. Piperazine can cause extrapyramidal movement disorders (choreiform movements) or aggravate those caused by neuroleptics.

Preparations and Administration

Piperazine (Antepar, Vermizine)
Tablets or syrup as the citrate salt
Recommended Doses: For adults, 3.5 g/day PO in a single daily dose, for 2 consecutive days. For children, 75 mg/kg/day for 2 consecutive days, 1 dose per day.

Table 48–5
Spectrum of Activity of Anthelmintics

Type of worm	Antimonials	Bephenium hydroxynaphthoate	Dichlorophen	Diethylcarbamazole	Hycanthone	Levamisole and Tetramisole	Mebendazole and Thiabendazole	Metrifonate	Metronidazole	Niclosamide	Niridazole	Oxamniquine	Paramomycin	Piperazine	Praziquantel	Pyrantel pamoate	Pyrvinium pamoate	Quinacrine	Stibocaptate
Intestinal Nematodes																			
Ascariasis		+		*		*	*							*		*			
Enterobiasis							*							*		*	*		
Strongyloidiasis							*										+		
Trichuriasis		+					*												
Uncinariasis		*					*									+			
Tissue nematodes																			
Filiariasis				*															
Draconiasis							+		+		+								
Loiasis				*															
Mansonelliasis				*															
Onchocerciasis				*															
Trichinosis				*			*												
Cestodes																			
Cysticercosis			+							*					+			*	
Diphyllobothriasis										*					+			*	
Taeniasis saginata			+							*					+			*	
Trematodes																			
Schistosomiasis																			
hematobium	+				*			*			*		*		*				*
japonicum	*										*		*		*				*
mansoni	+				*							*	*		*				*

Key: * A primary drug choice.
+ A secondary drug choice.

Pyrantel Pamoate (Antiminth)

Pyrantel pamoate is the drug of choice for pinworm and roundworm infections. It is partly absorbed, but the absorbed portion is excreted rapidly. Adverse effects are usually limited to gastrointestinal symptoms such as anorexia, nausea, vomiting, diarrhea, or cramps. Occasionally, skin rash or CNS effects, such as dizziness, headache, drowsiness, or insomnia, occur.

Preparations and Administration

Pyrantel pamoate (Antiminth)
Oral suspension
Recommended Doses: 11 mg/kg (maximum 1 g) PO per dose, the entire dose taken at once, with milk or fruit juice if desired.

Pyrvinium Pamoate

Pyrvinium pamoate is a cyanide dye that is active primarily against pinworms. This drug is not significantly absorbed. Adverse effects occur mostly in the alimentary tract: nausea, vomiting, cramps, and diarrhea. Allergic reactions such as photosensitivity occur occasionally. *Nurses should advise clients that pyrvinium pamoate will stain if spilled and will produce a red coloration to the stools and vomitus. The teeth will be stained if the tablet is not swallowed whole.*

Preparation and Administration

Pyrvinium pamoate
Film coated tablet, oral suspension
Recommended Doses: 5 mg/kg PO in a single dose. The treatment may be repeated after 2 or 3 weeks.

Other Drugs Active Against Intestinal Nematodes

Tetramisole and **levamisole** are closely related drugs active against many nematodes, but employed in humans only for ascariasis. Levamisole (Ketrax) is given in a single oral dose of 120–150 mg. These drugs are more often used in veterinary practice than in medical practice.

Bephenium hydroxynaphthoate is effective against many nematodes but has been replaced by newer drugs for most purposes. It is occasionally employed against hookworms. A single dose is usually effective. It is administered on an empty stomach.

Diethylcarbamazine

Diethylcarbamazine is the most broadly effective drug against tissue infections due to nematodes. It is considered the drug of choice for filariasis, loiasis, mansonelliasis, onchocerciasis, and trichinosis. Diethylcarbamazine works on tissue nematodes by increasing their vulnerability to phagocytosis. This piperazine derivative produces no severe adverse effects. Diethylcarbamazine is freely absorbed, producing peak plasma levels in about 3 hours. The drug is mainly metabolized before renal excretion. Diethylcarbamazine distributes well into all body compartments except for fat tissue. Mild adverse reactions are common, including gastrointestinal irritation and allergic reactions to protein fragments released by dying parasites. Swelling of lymph nodes is typical. Eosinophilia, often already present due to the infection, may be briefly intensified by the drug.

Anthelmintics Employed for Cestode Infections

Niclosamide (Yomesan)

Niclosamide is active against all major cestodes that infect humans. The drug is not significantly absorbed and is free of systemic toxicity. Mild gastrointestinal upset occasionally occurs. *The drug should be given after or with food to prevent gastrointestinal upset.*

Preparations and Administration

Niclosamide (Yomesan)
Chewable tablets available from the Parasitic Diseases Division of the Centers for Disease Control

Nursing Observations for Anthelmintic Drug Therapy

THERAPEUTIC GOAL	Eradication of infecting worm.
PREADMINISTRATION ASSESSMENT	
Baseline Data	Assess client for abdominal pain and diarrhea (indicative of trichuriasis), fever, wheezing, and abdominal cramps (indicative of ascariasis), abdominal pain and iron-deficiency anemia (evidence of hookworm disease), epigastric pain (indicating strongyloidiasis), fever and abdominal, preorbital, and muscle pain (suggesting trichinosis), chest pain, cough, and bloody sputum (indicating heartworm), dermatitis, liver dysfunction, and fever (for possible schistosomiasis), or epigastric pain, diarrhea, and weight loss (if tapeworm is suspected). Evaluate gastrointestinal output and sounds, neurological status, visual function, and skin color and lesions. Obtain laboratory tests including liver and renal function tests and cultures for parasites and ova.
Contraindications/ Precautions	Renal or hepatic failure, cardiac impairment, pregnancy or lactation, or convulsive disorders. Check medical history for drug allergies.
EVALUATION OF DRUG RESPONSE	
For Therapeutic Benefit	Evaluate eradication of the worm by periodic cultures.
For Adverse Effects	Monitor for allergic reactions, gastrointestinal irritation, liver dysfunction, and neurological symptoms.
For Drug Interactions	Monitor for interactions specific for each drug (see drug discussions).
For Compliance	Evaluate the client's compliance with all facets of the therapeutic regimen by careful observation, interviewing, and review of progress. Report compliance problems to the physician and act as client-advocate when changes in the therapeutic regimen seem indicated.

Recommended Doses: For adults, 2 g PO taken in a single dose and washed down with water. The alimentary tract may be purged 2 hours before administration of niclosamide. For children weighing 11–34 kg, 1 g PO. For children under 2, 0.5 g PO. *Nurses should tell clients to follow the tablets with a small amount of water.*

Quinacrine (Atabrine)

Quinacrine is effective against intestinal cestodes, as well as certain protozoa. (This drug is given primary coverage later in the chapter as an antimalarial agent.) *Nurses need to advise clients that the urine and skin may become yellow while they are taking quinacrine. They should also remind clients to keep the drug out of the reach of children and not to drink alcohol.*

Preparations and Administration

Quinacrine (Atabrine)
Tablets
Recommended Doses: For tapeworm in adults, 3 or 4 doses of 200 mg PO at 10-minute intervals, each dose with sodium bicarbonate to minimize nausea and vomiting. The day before treatment is begun, the client is required to take only semisolid or liquid food, no food after the evening meal, and an enema or laxative. On the day of treatment, breakfast is omitted, the first dose of 400 mg is taken at 8 AM and a second dose at 8:30 AM. Sodium bicarbonate may be taken before each dose to decrease vomiting. If there is no laxative effect in 90–120 minutes, a laxative is taken.

Nursing Diagnoses and Interventions for Anthelmintic Drug Therapy

Nursing Diagnoses	*Related Interventions*
TO ENHANCE DRUG BENEFITS OR REDUCE DRUG REQUIREMENTS	
Alteration in comfort: gastrointestinal pain or pain from other infected tissue	Provide frequent, small meals; analgesics and antipruritics as required.
Alteration in self-concept related to diagnosis	Provide emotional support and encouragement in coping with diagnosis.
TO MINIMIZE DRUG SIDE EFFECTS OR INTERACTIONS	
Alteration in comfort: gastrointestinal irritation from the drug regimen	Give the medication with food unless absorption is overly impaired by this tactic.
TO ENSURE SAFE AND EFFICACIOUS DRUG USE	
Knowledge deficit related to drug regimen	Teach the client about the disease, hygienic measures to prevent reinfection, and the rationale for each drug used in treatment. Clients may require instruction in such hygienic measures as handwashing after using the toilet, daily showers, frequent washing of underwear and bedclothes, keeping nails trimmed.
	Instruct the client about drug storage, dosage, and administration.
	Provide the client with a list of adverse effects and drug interactions for each drug in the regimen and instructions as to what to do if any of these occur.
	If the worm is transferred between family members, advise these individuals to undergo medical examination.
	Stress the importance of compliance for success in eradicating the infection and preventing spread to others.

Anthelmintics Employed for Schistosomiasis

Antimonials

Trivalent antimonial compounds inhibit utilization of glucose by species of Schistosoma, a genus of trematodes that infect the smaller blood vessels of the host. Unfortunately, antimonials produce considerable toxicity. Intravenous injection tends to cause a severe cough and frequently pneumonia. Pain occurs in the muscle and joints, mainly the knees, wrists, and ankles. Bradycardia, headache, fainting, edema, and hypersensitivity reactions (rash and anaphylactoid reactions) also occur. Antimony potassium tartrate is still the drug of choice for *Schistosoma japonicum.* Stibocaptate (Astiban), available from the Center for Infectious Diseases, is effective against all three varieties of Schistosomes.

Hycanthone (Etrenol)

Hycanthone is active against *Schistosoma hematobium* and *Schistosoma mansoni.* Hycanthone is less toxic than an earlier drug, lucanthone, from which it is derived. Nevertheless, transient side effects are frequent, including gastrointestinal disturbances, headache, and weakness. The drug is contraindicated in pregnancy and infancy and in clients with liver impairment. Hycanthone should not be used concurrently with drugs known to impair liver function.

Preparations and Administration

Hycanthone mesylate (Etrenol)
Powder for injection
Recommended Doses: 2.5–3.0 mg/kg in a single deep intramuscular injection. Treatment can be repeated after 1–3 months.

Metrifonate (Bilarcil)

Metrifonate is an organophosphate cholinesterase inhibitor. It is active against *Schistosoma hematobium* but also inhibits pseudocholinesterase in the host.

Preparations and Administration

Metrifonate (Bilarcil)
Scored tablets: 100 mg supplied by the Centers for Disease Control
Recommended Doses: 5–15 mg/kg given orally three times at 2-week intervals.

Niridazole (Ambilhar)

Niridazole (Ambilhar) is effective against *S. hematobium* and *S. japonicum.* Niridazole is slowly but almost completely absorbed. It is eliminated in equal portions in the urine and feces. Adverse effects of niridazole include electrocardiographic changes, neurological effects (agitation, confusional states, hallucinations, insomnia, paresthesias, headache, and convulsions), gastrointestinal irritation (nausea, vomiting, diarrhea, anorexia, and cramps), skin rashes, hepatic toxicity, and inhibition of spermatogenesis. The drug is contraindicated in clients with epilepsy, psychotic disorders, anemia, or poor nutritional status.

Preparations and Administration

Niridazole
Tablets available from the Centers for Disease Control
Recommended Doses: 25 mg/kg/day PO in 2 doses per day for 5–10 days.

Oxamniquine (Vansil)

Oxamniquine is indicated for *Schistosoma mansoni* infections. It is well absorbed, reaching peak plasma levels in 1–1.5 hours. The plasma half-life is 2.5 hours. The drug is eliminated by the kidney after hepatic metabolism. Adverse effects include transient dizziness and drowsiness, gastrointestinal irritation, urticaria, and convulsions.

Preparations and Administration

Oxamniquine (Vansil)
Capsules
Recommended Doses: 12–15 mg/kg in a single oral dose to be taken with food.

Praziquantel (Biltricide, Droncit)

Praziquantel is active against all three of the species of schistosomes that infect human beings, *S. hematobium, S. japonicum,* and *S. mansoni,* and is currently considered to be the drug of choice. It is readily absorbed after oral dosing and eliminated changed and unchanged in the urine with a half-life of 1 hour. Side effects appear to be mild but frequent. Malaise, headache, dizziness, and abdominal disturbances have been reported, one or another of these occurring in 90% of clients. Hypersensitivity reactions (fever or urticaria) occur rarely.

Preparations and Administration

Praziquantel (Biltricide)
Tablets
Recommended Doses: Three doses of 20 mg/kg PO at 4–6 hour intervals, administered with meals but not chewed since the drug has a very bitter taste.

Chemotherapy for Protozoal Infections

The protozoa are a large family of microorganisms, occupying an entire phylum in the animal kingdom. There are four subphyla of protozoa, and each includes examples that are pathological to humans. The **Sarcodina** are the **amebae,** simple protozoa that move by changing their shapes, bulging and retracting their protoplasm. Sarcodina reproduce asexually by simple binary fission. One type of ameba, *Entamoeba histolytica* causes amebic dysentery.

The subphylum of protozoa called the **Ciliophora** (or **ciliates**) include the harmless paramecia often observed by high school biology students under the microscope. Most ciliates are nonparasitic, but **Balantidium coli** causes a recurrent dysentery when it infects the human intestines.

A third subphylum of protozoa, the **Mastigophora** (or **flagellates**) are characterized by the presence of elongated thread-like projections called **flagella** that are employed for propulsion. Pathogenic flagellates can infect the intestines or the blood of humans. The **intestinal flagellates** include **Trichomonas** and **Giardia.** The **hemoflagellates** include **Trypanosoma** and **Leishmania.**

The fourth subphylum of protozoa is the sporozoa. These complex protozoa exhibit alternating sexual and asexual phases of reproduction, the asexual stage occurring in human or other vertebrate hosts. **Malaria** is the preeminent example of a disease caused by a sporozoa, the plasmodium.

Malaria and Antimalarials

It is estimated that 15–20 million people worldwide suffer from malaria. Malaria is caused by protozoa of the genus **Plasmodium.** There are four species of Plasmodium that can infect man — *Plasmodium falciparum, Plasmodium vivax, Plasmodium malariae,* and *Plasmodium ovale.* The first of these produces a severe infection, which, if untreated, is commonly fatal. When treated adequately, however, remission is complete, and relapses do not occur. The other three varieties are all milder but can entail relapses up to 2 years after the initial infection.

Control of malaria is dictated by the life cycle of the Plasmodium species and its relation to the intermediate host — the female *Anopheles* mosquito. Plasmodium exhibits two phases in its overall cycle — the asexual cycle, which occurs in humans, and the sexual cycle, which occurs in the mosquito (Figure 48–3). The mosquito ingests both forms of Plasmodium, but only the sexual form survives. Fertilization of the female gametocytes leads to production of zygotes that develop into sporozoites. When an infected mosquito bites a human, the sporozoites carried by the mosquito enter the human's bloodstream. Initially, the sporozoites accumulate mostly in liver parenchyma cells, where they multiply asexually and

Figure 48–3
The Plasmodium life cycle in malaria.

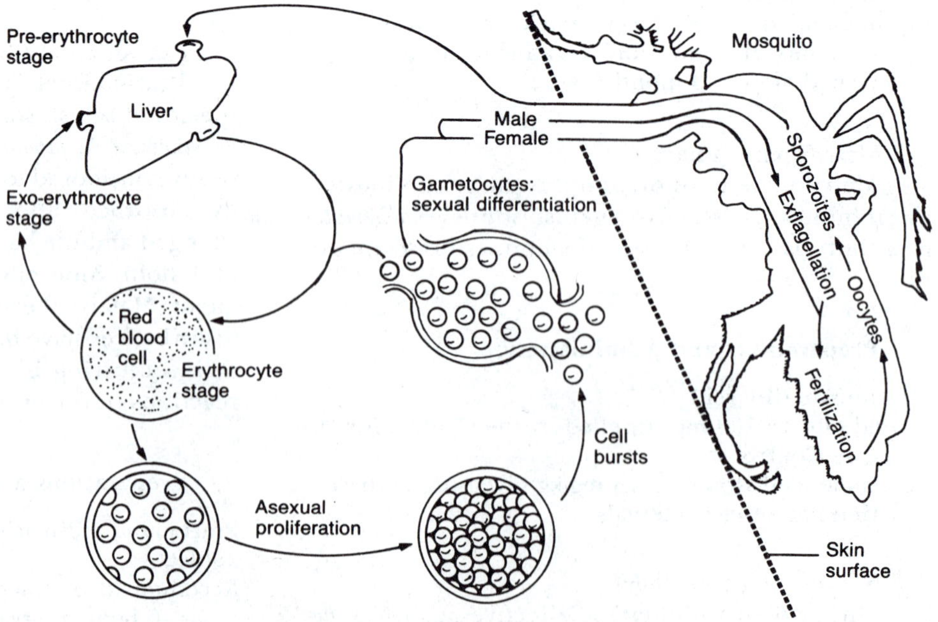

mature into merozoites. During this phase, known as the **tissue phase,** the human host is free of clinical symptoms. The mature merozoites then enter the bloodstream and invade red blood cells (erythrocytes) to commence the **erythrocytic phase.** In all types of malaria except that caused by *P. falciparum,* some merozoites invade other tissues and form secondary tissue colonies capable of triggering relapses. Merozoites multiply within the erythrocytes and cause these cells to burst, liberating cellular debris, protein, and young parasites. The disruption of erythrocytes produces the prominent clinical manifestations, including recurring chills and fever. Some merozoites develop into sexual forms, which can then be transferred by the mosquito to other human hosts.

The various drugs used in treatment of malaria differ in their point of attack in the life cycle of the parasite (Table 48–6). Efforts to eradicate the mosquito are helpful but have not been completely successful. Antimalarial drugs are frequently classified by the stage of the cycle that is altered by the drug. **Primary tissue schizonticides,** also called causal prophylactic agents, destroy the liver colonies of sporozoites shortly after infection. Primaquine, chloroguanide, and pyrimethamine have this effect. **Blood schizonticides** destroy merozoites released into the blood, producing a clinical cure or suppression of symptoms. Blood schizonticides include quinine, chloroquine (Aralen), amodiaquine (Camoquin), chloroguanide (Paludrine), and pyrimethamine (Daraprim). **Clinical prophylaxis** for the traveler can be provided by these agents. **Secondary tissue schizonticides** are used in the relapsing types of malaria to destroy the secondary tissue colonies. **Primaquine** is effective in this regard. **Gametocides** are drugs that destroy the sexual forms of the Plasmodium and thereby prevent spread of the disease to other human hosts. The antimalarial drugs are divisible broadly into two groups: the quinoline derivatives and the inhibitors of folinic acid synthesis.

Table 48–6
Activity of Antimalarial Drugs

Type of antimalarial action	Drugs
Primary tissue schizonticides	
(Causal prophylactic agents)	Primaquine (especially against *P. falciparum*)
	Chloroguanide (poor against *P. vivax*)
	Pyrimethamine (poor against *P. vivax*)
Blood schizonticides	**Quinolines**
(Clinical prophylactic agents)	Chloroquine
	Amodiaquine
	Hydroxychloroquine
	Quinine
	Folacin inhibitors
	Chloroguanide
	Pyrimethamine
	Tetracycline
	Sulfonamides
Secondary tissue schizonticides	
(Radical curative agents)	Primaquine
Gametocides	Primaquine

Quinoline Antimalarials

History and Sources The quinoline group includes primaquine, quinine (Quine), quinacrine (Atabrine), chloroquine (Aralen), amodiaquine, hydroxychloroquine (Plaquenil), and mefloquine. Until 1930 **quinine** was the only effective antimalarial drug. This alkaloid is the major active constituent of cinchona, a powder made from the bark of the cinchona tree of South America. Quinine and quinidine, the important antidysrhythmic drug (see Chapter 38), are optical isomers. Quinine, a blood schizonticide, has an effective suppressant action in acute malarial attacks, but it is not well tolerated, causing marked irritation of the gastrointestinal system, with nausea, vomiting, and gastric pain, when taken orally.

During World War I, the Germans, finding their supply of quinine interrupted, initiated development of synthetic antimalarial agents. This led to the preparation of **quinacrine,** but not until 1930. Ironically, it was the Allies who ultimately benefited from this effort. By the time World War II was underway, quinine refinement had shifted into the hands of German drug companies, and the Allies, finding themselves without adequate supplies of quinine, initiated production of quinacrine. Field trials demonstrated that it was more effective than quinine in suppressing symptoms of malaria, but its toxicity was considerable. Investigation of structurally related drugs began. Quinacrine, though available as Atabrine in 100 mg tablets, is no longer employed for malaria. Its sole remaining indication is for treatment of giardiasis. Hundreds of quinoline derivatives were tested during World War II for potential use in malaria, including 4-aminoquinolines, 8-aminoquinolines, and 4-quinoline-methanol derivatives. From the series of 4-aminoquinolines, **chloroquine, amodiaquine,** and **hydroxychloroquine** have entered clinical practice. Although chloroquine (Aralen) was available as early as 1934, it was initially believed to be too toxic. Later tests showed it to have a better therapeutic index than the drugs available at the time as well as most of the other agents in the 4-aminoquinoline series. Chloroquine has gradually superseded quinine and quinacrine, although the older drugs remain available to treat strains of plasmodium that have developed resistance to chloroquine.

Mechanisms and Effects Drugs in the quinoline group are potent and resistance to their action develops only slowly, although after several decades of use of these drugs, resistant strains of Plasmodium species have emerged. The mechanism of the quinolines remains obscure. Some of the quinolines bind to DNA molecules of schistosomes, impairing replication. However, some of the quinolines do not produce this effect. It is possible that more than one mechanism contributes to the schizonticidal activity of these drugs.

Chloroquine-resistant strains have been reported in South America and elsewhere, though infrequently. Some such strains exhibit cross-resistance to other 4-aminoquinolines, but others respond to quinine, mefloquine, or folinic acid inhibitors. Amodiaquine (Camoquin) and hydroxychloroquine (Plaquenil) are congeners of chloroquine. They are comparable to chloroquine in both efficacy and adverse responses. **Primaquine** is also an aminoquinoline derivative, but with a substitution in the 8-carbon position.

Pharmacokinetics Chloroquine is readily absorbed from the gastrointestinal tract. In the plasma, more than half the drug is bound to plasma protein. It is metabolized into a large number of products, but about 70% of the parent compound is excreted slowly in the urine unchanged. Primaquine is rapidly absorbed after oral administration and is quickly metabolized and excreted.

Clinical Indications Chloroquine acts on the erythrocytic phase of the Plasmodium cycle and thus suppresses clinical symptoms. A complete (or radical) cure is achieved only in clients infected with *Plasmodium falciparum;* relapses associated with other malarial organisms are not prevented. Chloroquine, hydroxychloroquine, and other antimalarials are also used as anti-inflammatory drugs in rheumatoid arthritis. Chloroquine is effective in treatment of extraintestinal amebiasis such as hepatic amebiasis caused by *Entamoeba histolytica.*

Primaquine has the distinction of acting on the sexual and secondary tissue forms of the protozoa. It is therefore effective in preventing spread of malaria and in preventing relapses in types of malaria other than that caused by *P. falciparum.* If administered during the initial tissue phase of the cycle, primaquine can effect radical cure of the malaria caused by *P. vivax.* It is ineffective in the erythrocyte phase, so acute attacks require concurrent administration of chloroquine or another agent.

Mefloquine is a 4-quinoline-methanol derivative that has demonstrated effectiveness against strains of *P. falciparum* that are resistant to most other antimalarial drugs, so-called multidrug-resistant strains. It appears to be a well-tolerated drug based on limited experience. It is currently indicated only for treatment of resistant strains of plasmodia.

Adverse Effects and Contraindications At low or moderate doses, the toxicity of chloroquine is quite low. At higher doses, severe toxic effects may occur, including psychoses, neuropathies leading to deafness, retinopathy, corneal damage causing blindness, and gastrointestinal disturbances. The drug can cause congenital defects if used during pregnancy. *Adverse reactions (such as neuropathies and visual problems) are reversible if quickly detected. Therefore nurses need to carefully observe and test the visual function of clients. Blurred vision, double vision, seeing halos, corneal insensitivity, light sensitivity, and impaired color perception are indicators of visual toxicity. Renal excretion of chloroquine can be hastened by acidification of the urine with ammonium chloride. Periodic blood tests should be conducted during prolonged treatment.*

Primaquine produces few side effects in most Caucasians. The range of reactions is usually limited to mild gastrointestinal irritation (cramps and epigastric distress), mild anemia, cyanosis due to methemoglobinemia, and leukocytosis. Higher doses can cause leukopenia. *Periodic blood tests should be conducted to check for leukopenia.* A special problem exists when primaquine is used in blacks and in ethnic groups of Caucasians having darker skin colorations (Sephardic Jews, Iranians, Greeks). These are the genetic groups having a high frequency of glucose-6-phosphate dehydrogenase (G6PD) deficiency. This trait, while it imparts some protection from malaria, results in a vulnerability of erythrocytes to oxidant drugs. Primaquine yields several metabolites with oxidant properties, and these produce a severe hemolytic action in individuals with the G6PD deficiency. *The nurse should be alert to signs indicative of red blood cell hemolysis, such as darkening or redness of the*

Nursing Observations for Antimalarial Drug Therapy

THERAPEUTIC GOAL	Alleviation or prevention of symptoms of malaria; eradication of blood and tissue forms of plasmodia.
PREADMINISTRATION ASSESSMENT	
Baseline Data	Observe for chills, fever, sweats, malaise, headache, and possibly delirium. Evaluate blood pressure, pulse, ECG, respiratory rate and sounds, neurological status, vestibular and auditory function, ophthalmological function, skin color and lesions, and bowel sounds. Obtain laboratory tests including blood smear for identification of plasmodium; urinalysis, BUN, serum creatinine, complete blood cell counts.
Contraindications/ Precautions	Renal or hepatic failure, pregnancy or lactation, or bone marrow depression. Check medication history for allergies to antimalarial agents.
Potential Interactions	Check current medications for interacting drugs, including nephrotoxic agents or hemolytic agents.
EVALUATION OF DRUG RESPONSE	
For Therapeutic Benefit	Blood smears to determine if plasmodia have been eradicated; monitor improvement in clinical symptoms of malaria.
For Adverse Effects	Monitor for liver or renal dysfunction, blood dyscrasias, defects of vision, hearing, or balance, and gastrointestinal disturbances.
For Drug Interactions	Monitor for increased ototoxicity, renal dysfunction, or hemolytic problems with other drugs having similar adverse effects.
For Compliance	Evaluate the client's compliance with all facets of the therapeutic regimen by careful observation, interviewing, and review of progress. Report compliance problems to the physician and act as client-advocate when changes in the therapeutic regimen seem indicated.

urine. A progressive decrease in urine production may also indicate developing anemia.

Preparations and Administration

Amodiaquine
Tablets
Recommended Doses: For prophylaxis, a single weekly dose of 520 mg PO. For an acute attack in adults, amodiaquine is given in a dose of 780 mg on the first day followed by 520 mg on days 2 and 3.

Chloroquine (Aralen)
Tablets, injection solution
Recommended Doses: For prophylaxis, 5 mg/kg PO (maximum 300 mg), once per week beginning 2 weeks prior to possible exposure and continuing 6–8 weeks after leaving the endemic area. For alleviation of acute attacks, 600 mg for an adult or 10 mg/kg for a child initially, followed in 6 hours by a second dose that is one-half the initial dose. This smaller dose is then repeated, 1 per day, on the second and third days of treatment.

Hydroxychloroquine (Plaquenil)
Tablets
Recommended Doses: For prophylaxis, 5 mg/kg up to 310 mg PO. For an acute attack of malaria, 620 mg in adults or 10 mg/kg in children initially, followed by half that amount 6 hours later, and once per day on days 2 and 3.

Mefloquine
Tablets available for investigational purposes from the Walter Reed Army Institute of Research

Primaquine phosphate
Tablets
Recommended Doses: For radical cure in adults, 26.3 mg PO, once per day for 14 days or 79 mg once per week for 8 weeks. The latter regimen results in lower incidence of hemolytic reaction. For children, 0.3 mg (base)/kg/day for 14 days or 0.9 mg (base)/kg/day, once per week for 8 weeks. Treatment with primaquine is begun at the end of a course of suppression with chloroquine or a chloroquine congener.

Inhibitors of Folic Acid Production

Mechanisms and Effects The second group of drugs that are active against plasmodia are inhibitors of folic acid synthesis. Plasmodia normally produce folic acid and tetrahydrofolate (THF) from para-aminobenzoic acid (PABA). THF is needed as a coenzyme in carbohydrate metabolism, amino acid conversions, and purine and pyrimidine metabolism. Antimalarial drugs that inhibit formation of THF include chloroguanide, chloroguanide triazine pamoate, pyrimethamine, trimethoprim, sulfonamides, dapsone, and sulfones.

Agents in this class are slow to bring about clinical improvement and are particularly likely to induce acquired resistance in the parasites, especially if inadequate doses are used or result from poor absorption. All drugs in this group act only as blood schizonticides, promoting clinical prophylaxis or cure but not destroying tissue forms of plasmodium. Effective therapy with agents in this group requires use of combinations. Most commonly, one or more agents in this group are added to a regimen that already includes a quinoline derivative such as chloroquine. A combination of pyrimethamine and a long-acting sulfonamide or dapsone may be effective without a quinoline derivative, but improvement occurs slowly. The most frequent use of inhibitors of THF synthesis is to suppress clinical symptoms caused by chloroquine-resistant strains of *P. falciparum.* If suppression is continued for 10 weeks or more, a suppressive or clinical cure may be effected. *Since resistance frequently develops during prolonged therapy, the nurse should watch for signs of relapse.*

Chloroguanide (Paludrine) was the first drug of this group employed for malaria. Initially an effective agent, its utility has diminished because of the great frequency with which strains of plasmodia have developed resistance to the drug. **Chloroguanide triazine pamoate** (cycloguanil pamoate) is a long-acting version of chloroguanide that can afford protection for several months after an intramuscular injection. Unfortunately, the drug does not circumvent the problem of resistance that occurs with chloroguanide.

Two diaminopyrimidines, **pyrimethamine** and **trimethoprim,** are inhibitors of the enzyme dihydrofolate reductase. Trimethoprim is employed primarily with sulfonamides for bacterial infections. Pyrimethamine has relatively greater activity against dihydrofolate reductase in protozoa than in bacterial or mammalian cells. Trimethoprim, on the other hand, has greater effect on bacteria and protozoa and almost no effect on mammals. Pyrimethamine is usefully combined (in Fansidar) with a sulfonamide to produce a synergistic inhibition of THF synthesis following the same rationale as the combination of trimethoprim with sulfonamides for improved antibacterial efficacy (see Chapter 47).

A long-acting sulfonamide used alone or in combinations for malaria is **sulfalene** (Kelfizina). It is used almost exclusively in partially immune clients for *P. falciparum* strains known to be sensitive to the drug. **Dapsone,** a sulfone used primarily in leprosy, has effectiveness in malaria comparable to that of sulfonamides. **Tetracyclines** are used in malaria only in desperate situations for multidrug-resistant strains. The problems with long-term use of tetracyclines (see Chapter 47) greatly limit their value in malaria.

Clinical Indications Pyrimethamine is used for chemoprophylaxis against susceptible plasmodial strains, but the more rapid-acting quinolines are preferred. Pyrimethamine is usually reserved for conjoint treatment with chloroquine or a chloroquine analogue. These combinations produce a synergistic effect in suppressing clinical symptoms of malaria. Pyrimethamine is also employed with triple sulfonamides for treatment of toxoplasmosis.

A combination of pyrimethamine with the long-acting sulfonamide, sulfadoxine, was first marketed in the United States (as Fansidar) in 1982. It is indicated for treatment and prophylaxis of malaria due to susceptible strains of plasmodia, though chloroquine continues to be the drug of choice. The sulfadoxine-pyrimethamine combination is useful for chloroquine-resistant strains.

Adverse Effects and Contraindications The clinically effective dose of pyrimethamine is close to toxic levels. The typical adverse effects include gastrointestinal irritation, such as anorexia and vomiting. *Pyrimethamine should be given with meals to reduce the likelihood of emesis.* More serious adverse effects are mainly hematological: leukopenia, megaloblastic anemia, thrombocytopenia, or pancytopenia. Excessive doses may cause acute intoxication and CNS toxicity including convulsions.

Adverse effects of pyrimethamine-sulfonamide combinations include gastrointestinal, neurological, allergic, and hematological reactions — the combined set of side effects of the two agents. The use of these preparations is contraindicated during pregnancy and lactation because of the risk of kernicterus with sulfonamides and teratogenicity with pyrimethamine.

Chloroguanide is very well tolerated, producing only mild and infrequent side effects such as vomiting, abdominal cramps, and diarrhea.

Nursing Diagnoses and Interventions for Antimalarial Drug Therapy

Nursing Diagnoses	*Related Interventions*
TO MINIMIZE DRUG SIDE EFFECTS OR INTERACTIONS	
Activity intolerance related to anemia caused by primaquine	Advise clients to watch for darkening of the urine due to hemolysis.
Alteration in bowel elimination: diarrhea with antimalarials	Provide and teach hygienic measures.
Alteration in comfort: gastrointestinal irritation from drugs	Provide frequent, small meals; advise clients to take irritating drugs with or after meals to reduce upset.
Alteration in tissue perfusion related to renal or liver failure or bone marrow suppression by antimalarial drugs	Instruct clients to report sore throat, pallor, jaundice, and purpura; monitor fluid intake-output and report significant changes to the physician.
Sensory-perceptual alterations: visual disturbances or defects of the eighth cranial nerve (hearing and balance) in response to antimalarial drugs	Teach client to report changes in vision, hearing, or balance. Provide safety measures necessitated by defects of vision, hearing, or balance.
TO ENSURE SAFE AND EFFICACIOUS DRUG USE	
Knowledge deficit related to drug regimen	Teach the client about the nature of malaria, the need to completely destroy all forms of the parasite. Give the rationale for each drug in the regimen.
	Instruct the client on proper storage, dosage, and administration of each drug in the regimen. These drugs must be kept out of reach of children.
	Provide the client with a list of adverse effects and drug interactions for each drug in the regimen and what to do if any of these should occur.
	Advise clients who will be traveling in regions where malaria is prevalent to obtain drug prophylaxis and to take these drugs reliably.
	Warn clients that chloroquine can cause a brown coloration of the urine.

Preparations and Administration

Pyrimethamine (Daraprim)
Tablets
Recommended Doses: For chemoprophylaxis in adults and children over 10 years of age, 25 mg PO once per week. For children 4–10 years of age, 12.5 mg PO once weekly. For infants and children up to 4 years of age, give 6.25 mg PO weekly. For treatment of acute attacks, pyrimethamine alone is recommended only in areas where all strains of plasmodia are sensitive. The recommended adult dosage is 50 mg PO daily for 2 days.

Sulfadoxine-Pyrimethamine (Fansidar)
Tablets
Recommended Doses: For prophylaxis, a single dose (2–3 tablets) 2 or 3 days before entering an area where malaria is endemic, and continued once per week while in the area and 4–6 weeks thereafter. For treatment of malaria, a single dose (2 or 3 tablets), alone or (usually) in combination with a quinoline derivative.

Important Nursing Implications for Antimalarial Drugs

- ☐ Conduct periodic blood cell counts during prolonged therapy for evidence of leukopenia.
- ☐ If the client experiences gastrointestinal disturbances, suggest that oral antimalarials be taken with meals or snacks.

☐ Monitor clients receiving chloroquine for evidence of neuropathies or alterations in visual function (such as blurred vision, halos, light-sensitivity, or impaired color vision).

☐ Monitor the urine of clients receiving primaquine for redness that could indicate drug-induced hemolysis.

☐ Monitor clients for signs of relapse since resistance develops frequently during prolonged therapy.

Other Protozoal Infections and Drugs

Most protozoa, unlike the Plasmodium species responsible for malaria, have simple life cycles and an extracellular existence. The three groups excluding sporozoa are distinguished from each other on the basis of their method of locomotion. The amebae move by displacing their protoplasm into bulges called pseudopodia. Flagellates possess whiplike appendages called flagella, while ciliates have numerous short hairlike surface elements called cilia. With respect to life cycle, these three groups of protozoa pass through two stages: the **trophozoite** and the **cyst.** The active, pathogenic, feeding form is the trophozoite. The cyst form, which exists for many but not all protozoa, is important in transmission of infection from host to host. In the cyst stage, the protozoal cell is small and covered by a tough, protective wall or membrane. The cyst form can survive in hostile environments that would be lethal to the trophozoite form. Transmission of protozoal infections often involves asymptomatic cyst carriers who contaminate food or water supplies.

Amebae

Since there is no drug effective against all types of protozoa, determination of the identity of the infecting organism is important for effective treatment of protozoal infection (Table 48–7).

By far the most prevalent parasitic protozoan of the ameba group is **Entamoeba histolytica.** This ameba causes the disease commonly known as **dysentery,** characterized by diarrhea, gastrointestinal irritation, and ulcerations extending from the descending colon to the rectum. Some individuals are asymptomatic carriers; others experience severe clinical manifestations. *E. histolytica* may spread by infiltration into the blood to the liver, kidney, lungs, or brain to cause abscesses. This form of infection by *E. histolytica* is called **extraintestinal dysentery.** The most common type involves the right lobe of the liver. In the United States, *E. histolytica* is found mainly in the South and Southwest, among socially disadvantaged populations. Homosexuals are also susceptible to acquisition of the infection from anal-oral contact.

Several varieties of nonpathogenic entamoebae are found in the human intestinal tract. They are clinically important only in that they complicate diagnosis of dysentery since some of these nonpathogenic varieties are difficult to distinguish from *E. histolytica.* A few amebae other than *E. histolytica* are occasionally pathogenic in humans. *Acanthamoeba* and *Naegleria* can cause a primary amebic meningoencephalitis (PAM). *Acanthamoeba* is a free-living soil ameba that has been linked to a few cases of subacute PAM. Naegleria grow in warm, stagnant water and has caused acute, usually fatal, PAM. Over 100 cases have been reported in the United States, occurring in individuals who had recently swum or water-skied in warm, polluted bodies of water.

Flagellates

The major pathogenic flagellates for humans are *Giardia lamblia, Trichomonas vaginalis, Trypanosoma,* and *Leishmania.* **Giardia lamblia** usually infects the duodenum, less frequently the gallbladder. Clinical indications of giardiasis are epigastric distress, nausea, diarrhea, flatulence, and steatorrhea (fatty stools). **Trichomonas vaginalis** is a widespread protozoan, infecting approximately 25% of women in the United States. The organism is transmitted through sexual contact and is thus a venereal disease. Females may experience vulvovaginitis, cervicitis, and leukorrhea, a frothy white discharge from the vagina. The vaginitis may be intensely itchy. Males are usually asymptomatic carriers. Urethritis and prostatitis occur occasionally.

Trypanosomes and Leishmaniae are hemoflagellates, infecting the blood and thereby reaching various internal organs. **Trypanosoma gambiense** and **Trypanosoma rhodesiense** produce the West and East African varieties of sleeping sickness, respectively. Early stages of these diseases are characterized by swelling of lymph nodes, endothelial proliferation, perivascular infiltration, pruritus, and fever. Later, the CNS is involved as meningomyelitis develops. In the later stage, headaches, neuralgia, impaired concentration, somnolence, and finally terminal coma ensue. **Trypanosoma cruzi** is the causative agent of the South American disease called Chagas' disease. It occurs rarely in the United States. *T. cruzi* is considerably more resistant to currently available drugs than other species of trypanosomes. *T. cruzi* infects the lymph nodes, spleen, liver, lung, brain, and especially the heart.

Leishmania donovani causes a disease called kala azar, black disease, or Dumdum fever. It is prevalent in Mediterranean countries, Africa, South

Table 48–7
Drug Treatments for Protozoal Infections Exclusive of Malaria

Protozoan	Disease	Drug Selections: Primary choices	Drug Selections: Alternate choices
Amebae			
Entamoeba histolytica			
Intestinal	Dysentery	Metronidazole	Iodoquinol Paromomycin
Extraintestinal	Liver, kidney, lung, or brain abscesses	Metronidazole Emetine Chloroquine	
Asymptomatic cyst passers		Diloxanide furoate	
Flagellates			
Giardia lamblia	Mild to severe GI upset: nausea, diarrhea, epigastric pain, flatulence	Metronidazole Quinacrine	Tinidazole Furazolidone
Trichomonas vaginalis	Opportunistic and venereal infections of vagina which can cause cervicitis or vulvovaginitis	Metronidazole	Tinidazole
Trypanosoma			
T. gambiense and *T. cruzi*	Chagas' disease: infection of spleen, heart, liver, lymphatics, and bone marrow	Nifurtimox	
T. rhodesiense (sleeping sickness)			
Early	Swelling of lymph nodes, fever, perivascular infiltration	Suramin Diamidines	
Late	CNS involvement: meningoencephalitis, somnolence, coma	Arsenicals	
Leishmania			
L. donovani (kala azar)	Visceral infections: spleen, liver, lymph nodes, and bone marrow	Antimonials Diamidines	
L. tropica (oriental sore)	Skin lesions	Stibogluconate Diamidines	Antimonials
L. mexicana	Cutaneous ulcerations, especially around ear	Cycloguanil pamoate Metronidazole	
Ciliates			
Balantidium coli	Ulcerative lesions of intestines, diarrhea, and dysentery	Oxytetracycline Iodoquinol	
Sporozoa			
Toxoplasma gondii	Lymphadenopathy, malaise, fever, muscle pain, congenital defects	Sulfonamides and pyrimethamine	Sulfonamide alone (first trimester of pregnancy)
Pneumocystis	Pneumocystitis in immunodeficient individuals	Trimethoprim-sulfamethoxazole	Pentamidine

America, central Asia, India, and China. This protozoan infects white blood cells of the spleen, liver, lymph nodes, and bone marrow. The resulting impairment of host defenses increases susceptibility to other infections. **Leishmania tropica** causes so-called oriental sore. It is found in the Mediterranean countries and Africa. **Leishmania mexicana** produces cutaneous ulcerations of somewhat similar appearance. This disease is found in Mexico and tropical South America.

Ciliates and Nonplasmodium Sporozoa

The only pathogenic protozoan in the ciliate group is **Balantidium coli.** Infections caused by this organism are intestinal, resembling the dysentery of amebiasis. The other major disease caused by a sporozoan besides malaria is toxoplasmosis, which is caused by **Toxoplasma gondii.** This protozoan is frequently carried by cats. Like plasmodia, *T. gondii* has both sexual and asexual reproductive stages. The sexual stage occurs only in cats. Toxoplasmosis can be acquired by human adults by ingesting contaminated food. Typical symptoms are malaise, fever, muscle pain, and lymphadenopathy. Occasionally, toxoplasmosis disseminates, producing severe disease that can result in hepatitis, pneumonitis, myocarditis, or meningoencephalitis. Of particular concern is **congenital toxoplasmosis,** acquired by the fetus through placental transfer of *T. gondii.* In the first trimester, the fetus is extremely vulnerable to congenital defects from toxoplasmosis. Pyrimethamine, the most useful agent against *T. gondii,* cannot be employed during pregnancy because it is teratogenic. Treatment of congenital toxoplasmosis is conducted with sulfonamides, which also present risks to the fetus.

Nitroimidazoles

The nitroimidazoles include **metronidazole** (Flagyl) and two related drugs, **tinidazole** (Fasigyn) and **nimorazole** (Naxogin, Nulogyl), that are available in some parts of the world but not in the United States. Metronidazole was the first orally effective agent for *Trichomonas vaginalis.* Until the introduction of this drug, the only available therapeutic approach was topical treatment with vaginal suppositories — adequate for mild cases but not for severe infections. Topical treatment of male partners was not feasible so that reinfection of the female was common. Topical treatment also met with compliance difficulties. Metronidazole is amebicidal and trichomonacidal, and also kills *Giardia lamblia* and obligate gram-negative anaerobic bacilli. Metronidazole is believed to inhibit DNA synthesis in sensitive organisms.

Pharmacokinetics Metronidazole is usually well absorbed, but some clients do not achieve satisfactory plasma concentrations of the drug at normal doses and fail to respond. Absorption does not appear to be influenced by food. Peak serum concentrations are usually achieved in 1–2 hours. Metronidazole distributes widely through the body and penetrates into the brain. Binding to plasma proteins is insignificant. Hepatic metabolism is the major route of elimination. The elimination half-life of metronidazole is about 8 hours.

Clinical Indications Metronidazole is the drug of choice for amebic dysentery (intestinal amebiasis) as well as extraintestinal forms of infection by *E. histolytica.* In the latter condition, metronidazole may be used alone or in combinations with emetine and chloroquine. Metronidazole is an alternative to quinacrine for treatment of *Giardia lamblia,* although quinacrine remains the first choice. Metronidazole has replaced older topical treatments for *T. vaginalis* and is highly effective both in women and their asymptomatic male sexual partners. Diagnosis of trichomoniasis should be confirmed by a wet smear or by cultures. Males who are asymptomatic are frequently the source of reinfection for women. *Therefore nurses should recommend that couples being treated with metronidazole refrain from sexual intercourse during the treatment period and that males receive therapy even when they have a negative culture to avoid reinfection of the female partner. Women should also be advised not to wear pantyhose or other tight clothing since occlusive clothing encourages growth of trichomona.*

Adverse Effects and Contraindications The most frequent adverse reactions are due to **gastrointestinal hyperexcitability** and include vomiting, epigastric distress, abdominal cramps, diarrhea, or conversely, constipation. *The nurse should advise clients to take metronidazole with food to minimize gastrointestinal upset.*

More severe but uncommon side effects include hematological reactions (mainly leukopenia), **neurological reactions** (vertigo, dizziness, incoordination, ataxia, confusion, weakness, decreased libido, depression, irritability, insomnia, convulsions), and **peripheral neuropathy** (mainly paresthesias). *Nurses should warn clients that any symptoms such as tremors, lack of coordination, paresthesias, numbness, or impairment of pain or touch sensations should be reported immediately and the drug discontinued.* Metronidazole rarely causes **allergic reactions** such as serum sickness, arthralgia, fever, urticaria, and erythematous eruptions.

An unpleasant metallic taste may be imparted by this drug. A metabolite of metronidazole imparts a dark pigmentation to the urine. *To allay clients' concern, nurses should inform them that this may occur.* Rarely, polyuria or incontinence occurs. Metronidazole may cause an overgrowth of *Candida albicans,* resulting in vaginal candidiasis, furry tongue, glossitis, or stomatitis. *Nurses need to advise clients to report any symptoms of candidal overgrowth. The client might notice color changes of the tongue, glossitis, stomatitis, and possibly a furry tongue. Women may note a milky or curd-like vaginal discharge. The client may require treatment with an anticandidal agent.*

Metronidazole is contraindicated in individuals with a history of dyscrasias, active organic brain syndrome, or known hypersensitivity to the drug. *Blood*

Nursing Observations for Antiprotozoal Drug Therapy

THERAPEUTIC GOAL	Eradication of the infection.
PREADMINISTRATION ASSESSMENT	
Baseline Data	Observe for diarrhea or dysentery (if amebiasis is suspected), flatulence and malabsorption (indicative of giardiasis), sharply demarcated ulcerations of the skin (indicating oriental sore), fever, edema, skin eruptions, tremors, headache, and coma (for possible trypanosomiasis), or posterior uveitis, muscle weakness, headache, and diarrhea (suggesting toxoplasmosis). Evaluate gastrointestinal function and sounds, respiratory rate and sounds, and neurological function. Obtain laboratory tests including cultures to identify infecting organism, BUN, and urinalysis before antiprotozoal drugs are given.
Contraindications/ Precautions	Renal or hepatic failure, pregnancy, or lactation. Check medication history for allergies to the drug being considered.
Potential Interactions	Check current medications for sympathomimetics, MAO inhibitors, or nephrotoxic drugs.
EVALUATION OF DRUG RESPONSE	
For Therapeutic Benefit	Conduct cultures periodically to monitor eradication of the protozoan.
For Adverse Effects	Monitor for changes in liver, gastrointestinal, or neurological function. Observe for indications of superinfection.
For Drug Interactions	Monitor for additive ototoxic and nephrotoxic effects when paromomycin is used with other drugs having similar toxicity, hypertensive crisis with furazolidone and pressor drugs, and alcohol intolerance (with furazolidone and metronidazole).
For Dietary Interactions	Monitor for nutritional deficits due to diarrhea and malabsorption.
For Compliance	Evaluate client's compliance with all facets of the therapeutic regimen by careful observation, interviewing, and review of progress. Report compliance problems to the physician and act as client-advocate when changes in the therapeutic regimen seem indicated.

studies should be ordered to determine the presence of dyscrasias prior to initiating metronidazole administration.

Metronidazole should not be used during the first trimester of pregnancy and should be used only with caution in the second trimester. For women who are in the second or third trimester of pregnancy, the therapy should extend over a 7-day period. A 1-day course of therapy produces high serum levels that may reach the fetal circulation.

Drug Interactions Metronidazole can cause a disulfiram-like reaction when alcohol is consumed while the drug is in the system. *Clients should be advised to refrain from use of alcohol during metronidazole therapy.* If used concurrently with disulfiram, the metronidazole-disulfiram combination can produce confusion even in the absence of alcohol consumption. Metronidazole can potentiate the anticoagulant effect of warfarin (Coumadin), necessitating dosage adjustment of the anticoagulant.

Preparations and Administration *As with all antimicrobial regimens, clients should be advised to complete the full course of therapy and not to discontinue the drug merely because overt symptoms have been relieved.*

Metronidazole (Flagyl)
Tablets
Recommended Doses: For acute amebic dysentery in adults, 750 mg PO tid for 5–10 days. For extraintestinal infection by *E. histolytica* in adults, 500–750 mg PO tid for 5–10 days. For all forms of amebiasis in children, 35–50 mg/kg/day PO in 3 divided doses for 10 days. For *T. vaginalis*, optional 1-day or 7-day courses of therapy with metro-

nidazole are listed. The 1-day course entails administration of 2 g PO in 1 or 2 doses on the same day. The 7-day course calls for 250 mg PO tid for 7 days. Cure rates are a little higher for the 7-day regimen. The selection of the length of treatment is based in part on whether the individual is liable to comply with the prescribed schedule.

Emetine and Dehydroemetine

Emetine is the active ingredient of the age-old Brazilian folk preparation ipecac. In 1912 the effectiveness of emetine against amebae was demonstrated in vitro. It is useful in both extraintestinal and intestinal forms but does not readily destroy cysts. The clinical efficacy of emetine is monitored by laboratory examination of stool specimens. *Stool specimens should be sent to the laboratory while they are still warm to facilitate identification of ameba that may be present.*

Adverse Effects and Contraindications **Electrocardiographic changes** occur in 90% of patients and may appear after several days of emetine administration. *An ECG should be taken at least after every fifth dose, on completion of therapy, and 1 week later.* There may be an inversion of the T wave, prolonged Q-T interval, and other changes resembling those that occur after a myocardial infarction. These abnormalities may persist in some patients as much as 2 months after the drug has been discontinued. *Nurses should assess clients for indications of serious cardiovascular reactions, such as shortness of breath, the presence of precordial pain, and tachycardia.* Clients who are permitted to ambulate are especially likely to develop tachycardia. Pulse rate and quality and blood pressure should be taken and recorded at least 3 times each day.

Emetine is also liable to produce **neuromuscular toxicity.** *Nurses should monitor neuromuscular function and report signs of weakness, fatigue, listlessness, muscular stiffness, tenderness, or pain. These symptoms usually occur before more serious symptoms and serve as guides to avoiding overdose.*

Fluid intake and output should be monitored to determine if renal toxicity is developing. Nurses should report oliguria or changes in intake-output ratio. Nurses should also record and report the number of client stools, unusual odor or consistency of stools, and presence of mucus or blood in the stools.

Preparations and Administration Dehydroemetine and emetine have similar efficacy and adverse effects. Local irritation (aching and tenderness) may occur after injection. Since emetine is a general protoplasmic toxin, adverse effects can occur in the liver, heart, kidneys, or other tissues. It should be used only in hospitalized patients placed on bedrest during therapy and for several days afterward. *Nurses need to advise patients to remain sedentary for several weeks after the drug has been discontinued.*

Emetine is very irritating to tissues and nurses must therefore avoid splashing or otherwise allowing the drug to come into contact with mucous membranes. In addition, the nurse should make a record of the injection sites used and check them daily for signs of irritation.

Nurses should assure that clients remain under medical supervision and nursing guidance once discharged. Clients should be instructed to have repeated fecal examinations for at least 3 months to assure ameba have been eliminated. In addition, nurses need to have health teaching sessions for clients and their families that include personal hygiene, handwashing after using toilet facilities and before preparing or eating foods, and the risks of eating raw foods.

Preparations and Administration

Dehydroemetine
Injection solution available from the Parasitic Diseases Division of the Centers for Disease Control
Recommended Doses: 1–1.5 mg/kg/day in a single deep SC or IM injection for 5 days. Doses must usually be halved and monitoring intensified when the drug is employed in elderly, debilitated, or underweight clients because of the potential severity of adverse effects in these groups.

Emetine
Injection solution
Recommended Doses: 1 mg/kg/day, up to 65 mg/daily by IM or deep SC injection, preferably the latter, in 1 or 2 doses daily, for a maximum of 10 days. For acute fulminating amebic dysentery, treatment continues only long enough to control the symptoms (3–5 days). For extraintestinal amebiasis such as amebic hepatitis, the drug is given for 10 days. Another amebecide should then be given as an immediate follow-up to guarantee eradication. The course of treatment should not be repeated in less than 6 weeks.

8-Hydroxyquinolines

A number of halogenated quinolines have demonstrated value in amebiasis. **Diiodohydroxyquin** (iodoquinol, Yodoxin) and iodochlorhydroxyquin (clioquinol, Vioform) are available in the United States; others, such as chlorquinaldol and chiniofon are available elsewhere. These agents act only against intestinal *E. histolytica.* Absorption after oral administration is variable, and most of the drug is excreted in the feces. Toxicity is low, consisting of gastrointestinal reactions (nausea, vomiting, cramps, diarrhea,

Nursing Diagnoses and Interventions for Antiprotozoal Drug Therapy

Nursing Diagnoses	*Related Interventions*
TO ENHANCE DRUG BENEFITS OR REDUCE DRUG REQUIREMENTS	
Alteration in comfort: pain and irritation related to disease, drugs, and superinfections	Provide frequent, small meals; intensify oral hygiene to prevent superinfection; provide appropriate treatment for superinfections; drugs that contribute to gastrointestinal irritation may be taken with meals.
Alteration in nutrition related to gastrointestinal infection	Provide nutritional supplements as required.
TO MINIMIZE DRUG SIDE EFFECTS OR INTERACTIONS	
Sensory-perceptual alterations related to visual, vestibular, and auditory side effects of antiprotozoal drugs	Instruct clients to immediately report such side effects and advocate adjustments in the regimen.
TO ENSURE SAFE AND EFFICACIOUS DRUG USE	
Knowledge deficit related to drug regimen	Teach the client about the nature of the infection, hygienic measures to prevent reinfection, and the rationale for the treatment approach. Clients may require instruction in hygienic measures such as handwashing after using the bathroom, avoidance of tight-fitting clothing over infected areas, and daily showers. Instruct the client about storage, dosage, and administration of each antiprotozoal drug employed. Provide the client with a list of adverse effects and drug interactions for each drug in the regimen and instructions as to what to do if any of these occur. Emphasize the importance of compliance for complete eradication of the infection. Shorter, higher dose regimens can be considered for clients assessed as poor compliance risks.

and pruritus ani), occasional skin eruptions, and mild systemic allergic responses such as chills and fever. *Clients should be instructed to take 8-hydroxyquinolines after food to reduce gastrointestinal upset.* Prolonged therapy with high doses has caused optic neuritis and atrophy. Iodoquinolines liberate iodide and thus may distort certain tests of thyroid function. *The nurse should instruct clients about the importance of completing the entire course of treatment.*

Preparations and Administration

Iodoquinol (Yodoxin and generic)
Tablets
Recommended Doses: For adults, 650 mg PO tid taken after meals for 20 days. For children, 40 mg/kg/day (maximum 1.95 gm) in 3 divided doses for 20 days.

Substituted Acetanilides

Diloxanide furoate is a substituted acetanilide with unique clinical value. It is relatively ineffective against intestinal or extraintestinal ameboid trophozoites but is highly active against cyst forms of *E. histolytica.* It is the drug of choice for treatment of asymptomatic passers of cysts. The drug is absorbed 60–90%. The ester is hydrolyzed in the process. Diloxanide is excreted mainly in the urine as a glucuronide metabolite. Diloxanide appears on the basis of limited experience to be low in toxicity.

Preparations and Administration

Diloxanide furoate
Recommended Doses: For adults, 500 mg PO tid for 10 days. A second course may be given immedi-

ately after the first if cysts continued to appear in the feces. In children, 20 mg/kg/day in 3 divided doses for 10 days.

Amebicidal Antibiotics

Paromomycin (Humatin) is the only directly amebicidal antibiotic and thus has replaced erythromycin and tetracycline for treatment of amebic dysentery. Paromomycin is an aminoglycoside with properties similar to other members of that class (see Chapter 47). After oral administration, very little paromomycin is absorbed, limiting its efficacy and toxicity to intestinal effects for the most part. GI upset and diarrhea are typical. Paromomycin is effective against intestinal *E. histolytica,* but less so than metronidazole. It is also active against most cestodes (Table 48–4).

Preparations and Administration

Paromomycin (Humatin)
Capsules, syrup (root beer flavored)
Recommended Doses: For intestinal amebiasis in both adults and children, 25–35 mg/kg/day PO, in 3 doses with meals, for 5–10 days.

Metallic Antiprotozoal Drugs: Arsenicals and Antimonials

Both arsenicals and antimonials have demonstrated activity against flagellate protozoa. As early as 1940, **arsenicals** were observed to exhibit trypanocidal activity. Although nonmetallic trypanocides are more satisfactory for treating clients who have an early diagnosis, before the CNS has become involved, arsenicals remain the drugs of choice when trypanosomiasis has progressed to produce meningoencephalitis. The three arsenicals in use currently are **melarsoprol** (Arsobal), **carbarsone,** and **tryparsamide.** Tryparsamide and carbarsone are pentavalent arsenicals and present a less favorable balance of efficacy to toxicity than the trivalent arsenical melarsoprol. The various strains of Trypansomae do not exhibit cross-resistance between these two kinds of arsenicals. Melarsoprol is usually given by slow intravenous infusion under hospital supervision. Penetration of melarsoprol into the CSF is adequate to allow it to suppress protozoa that have invaded the brain and meninges. Excretion is rapid. Adverse effects, especially reactive encephalopathy, are common. Hemolytic reactions often occur in patients with G6PD deficiencies.

Preparations and Administration

Melarsoprol (Arsobal)
Recommended Doses: 3.6 mg/kg/day IV for 3–9 days. This protocol can be repeated if required after 7–10 days.

Sodium stibogluconate is an **antimonial** with efficacy against *Leishmania donovani,* the cause of kala azar, and *Leishmania tropica,* the cause of oriental sore. It is more effective against *L. donovani* and is the drug of choice for infections by that organism. Adverse effects are less severe than with trivalent antimonial compounds. Typical side effects include joint pain (especially in the wrists, knees, and ankles), bradycardia, headache, fainting, dyspnea, hemolytic anemia, hepatic dysfunction, and anaphylactoid reactions.

Preparations and Administration

Sodium stibogluconate
Injection solution
Recommended Doses: 6 ml, once a day, for 6–10 days.

Diamidines

Two diamidine drugs are effective against trypanosomes: stilbamidine and pentamidine (Pentam 300). These nonmetallic trypanocides are highly effective in early cases of sleeping sickness but have little value in late cases and lack activity against *T. cruzi* (the cause of Chagas' disease). Pentamidine is also effective against *Pneumocystis carinii,* an increasingly frequent cause of pneumonia in compromised patients. Trimethoprim-sulfamethoxazole, the usual choice for *P. carinii,* causes a high incidence of adverse effects in patients with acquired immune deficiency syndrome (AIDS), one of the populations at greatest risk of pneumonia due to this protozoan. Diamidines are given parenterally (preferably intramuscularly). Adverse reactions can be quite severe, but usually not life-threatening. Typical responses to injection are dizziness, fainting, tachycardia, headache, and dyspnea. Changes in blood sugar (in either direction) and transient renal impairment have been reported. Pentamidine isethionate (Lomidine) has been available from the Parasitic Diseases Division of the Centers for Disease Control in Atlanta for several years, as 200 mg of powder in an ampul for reconstitution and injection. In 1984 pentamidine began being marketed commercially.

Preparations and Administration

Pentamidine (Pentam 300)
Injection solution
Recommended Doses: For trypanosomiasis, 4 mg/kg given IM or IV, once daily on alternate days, for about 20 days. For treatment of pneumocystitis, 4 mg/kg once daily for 14 days.

Suramin (Germanin)

Another drug that is effective in sleeping sickness is a nonmetallic dye, suramin (Germanin). It is not effective against *T. cruzi.* In clients with infections caused by *T. rhodesiense* and *T. gambiense,* suramin can be used alone if the disease is in the early stage, or combined with an arsenical if there is CNS involvement. The combination is quite effective. Side effects of suramin include hypersensitivity reactions, which vary in intensity in relation to nutritional status of the patient. Rapid adverse reactions may include nausea, vomiting, urticaria, and shock. Other allergic manifestations may occur later, after 24 hours or more, such as photophobia, papular eruptions, hyperesthesia of the palms and feet, and lacrimation. Hematological reactions occur occasionally.

Preparations and Administration

Suramin (Germanin)
Powder for injection
Recommended Doses: For sleeping sickness, 1 g given once daily on days 1, 3, 7, 14, and 21, and weekly thereafter for 5 more weeks. An initial dose of 200 mg tests for hypersensitivity.

Nitrofurans

The nitrofurans include four currently available antimicrobial drugs, each with distinct clinical uses. Nitrofurantoin is a urinary tract anti-infective discussed in Chapter 43. Nitrofurazone is a topical burn preparation discussed in Chapter 53. Two nitrofurans have antiprotozoal spectra. **Furazolidone** (Furoxone) is an oral drug active against *Giardia lamblia* (no less so than metronidazole or quinacrine). **Nifurtimox** (Lampit) is the most effective known treatment for *T. cruzi,* the protozoan that infects millions of South Americans to produce Chagas' disease. Side effects of nitrofurans include gastrointestinal irritation, allergic reactions, hematological reactions, colitis, proctitis, pruritus ani, and disulfiram-like reactions.

Preparations and Administration

Furazolidone (Furoxone)
Tablets or oral liquid available from the Center for Disease Control
Recommended Doses: For protozoal enteritis due to *G. lamblia* in adults, 100 mg PO qid; for children 1–4 years of age, 17–25 mg of the liquid 4 times daily; for children 1 month to 1 year, 8–17 mg of liquid PO, 4 times daily. For adults with Chagas' disease, 5–7 mg/kg PO daily for 2 weeks, gradually increased at 2-week intervals until a dose of 15–17 mg/kg/day is given by week 10. For children under 15 with Chagas' disease, 25 mg/kg/day PO in 4 divided doses for 15 days, followed by 15 mg/kg/day in 4 doses for 75 days.

Case Study: Candidiasis

L. R., a 21-year-old female college student, returned to the University Health Services Clinic for a follow-up appointment after completing a 10-day course of therapy with ampicillin for pneumonia. She told the nurse that she had felt better a few days after her last visit to the clinic but that during the last 4 days she has been experiencing abdominal pain, sore throat, and vaginal itching. Examination of L. R.'s mouth revealed perlèche and thrush. The tongue was inflamed with creamy white patches. A vaginal examination revealed presence of a white discharge and white patches on the vaginal wall and vulva. The nurse scraped off a portion of a patch for a culture, which was determined to be *Candida albicans.* Based on the culture and the characteristic lesions, the nurse concluded that L. R. had mucocutaneous candidiasis.

The nurse observed that L. R. was somewhat pale and thin. L. R. indicated that she was having a very busy semester and would sometimes skip meals. The nurse took a blood sample for blood cell and electrolyte evaluation, which later verified that L. R. was anemic. The nurse discussed with L. R. the importance of maintaining adequate nutrition, especially during periods of intensified activity and infection. She gave L. R. a pamphlet discussing nutritional issues oriented to concerns of college students. The nurse also explained to L. R. the relationship between the course of therapy with the antibiotic and the present symptoms.

The nurse reviewed her assessment and findings with the physician, who prescribed ketoconazole (Nizoral), one 200 mg tablet taken daily, for 2 weeks, at which time a follow-up appointment was scheduled. The nurse asked L. R. if she used any nonprescription medications and learned that once or twice a week, L. R. took Maalox "for heartburn." The nurse instructed L. R. not to take the ketoconazole tablets within 2 hours of the antacid and to take the ketoconazole with meals unless this caused vomiting. The nurse advised L. R. to inform her in the unlikely event that vomiting did occur so that an appropriate drug remedy could be prescribed. She told L. R. to be sure to swallow the tablet intact and not to chew it. She advised L. R. that if she was having sexual relations, her partner might be a source of reinfection for her, even if he exhibited no apparent symptoms himself. The nurse also discussed oral hygiene with L. R., emphasizing regular flossing and brushing of the teeth. The nurse wrote down a list of possible adverse reactions that could occur with ketoconazole and told L. R. to notify the physician if she experienced abdominal pain, pronounced fever or diarrhea, fatigue, anorexia, yellow skin or sclera, dark urine, or pale stools. She warned L. R. that driving might be dangerous because ketoconazole may cause drowsiness or dizziness.

1. What is perlèche? Thrush?
2. Would a positive culture for *Candida albicans* be a sufficient basis for diagnosing candidiasis without the characteristic lesions?
3. What factors have most likely predisposed L. R. to candidiasis? What is the likely connection with the antibiotic therapy? Would another antibiotic have been less likely to contribute to occurrence of candidiasis?
4. Name at least three other drugs that are active against *Candida albicans.* Can these be employed orally?
5. Why did the nurse tell L. R. not to take ketoconazole with Maalox? Why is it best to take it with a meal?
6. If nausea or vomiting does occur (the incidence is 3–10%), what kind of a drug might be given with the ketoconazole?
7. Why is it advisable for L. R. not to chew the tablet?
8. If L. R. notices yellow skin or sclera, pale stools, dark urine, or pruritus, what is the likely cause?

Answers appear at the end of the book.

Recommended Readings

Antiviral Agents

Buchanan RA: Advances in antiviral chemotherapy. *Can Med Assoc J* 1979;120:7–10.

Dolan R: Amantadine and influenzae. *Am Fam Physician* 1979;19:127–130.

Douglas RG: Antiviral drugs. *Med Clin North Am* 1983;67(5):1163–1172.

Hermans PE, Cockerill FR III: Antiviral agents. *Mayo Clin Proc* 1983;58(4):217–222.

Hirsch MS, Swartz MN: Antiviral agents. *N Engl J Med* 1980;302:903–907.

Lefrock JL, Smith BR: Antiviral agents. *Am Fam Physician* 1983;27(1):237–240.

Mannering GJ, Deloria LB: The pharmacology and toxicology of the interferons: An overview. *Annu Rev Pharmacol Toxicol* 1986;26:455–516.

Mindal A et al: Intravenous acyclovir treatment for primary genital herpes. *Lancet* 1982;1:697–700.

Schoeneck CLE: Acyclovir: A recently developed antiherpes agent. *Crit Care Nurse* 1985;5(4):8–10.

Serota FT et al: Acyclovir treatment of herpes zoster infections. *JAMA* 1982;247:2132–2135.

Smith RA, Sidwell RW, Robins RK: Antiviral mechanisms of action. *Annu Rev Pharmacol Toxicol* 1980;20:259–284.

Whitley RJ et al: Vidarabine: Preliminary review of its pharmacological properties and therapeutic use. *Drugs* 1980;20:267–282.

Antifungal Agents

Cohen J: Antifungal chemotherapy. *Lancet* 1982;2:532–537.

Comer JB: Amphotericin B: Ten common questions. *Am J Nurs* 1981;81:1166–1167.

Gever LN: Giving amphotericin B for systemic fungal infections. *Nursing* 1984;14(7):8.

Goldman P: Metronidazole. *N Engl J Med* 1982;75:190–197.

Hermans PE, Keys TF: Antifungal agents used for deep-seated mycotic infections. *Mayo Clin Proc* 1983;58(4):223–231.

Medoff G et al: Antifungal agents useful in therapy of systemic fungal infections. *Annu Rev Pharmacol Toxicol* 1983;23:303–330.

Sohn CA: Evaluation of ketoconazole. *Clin Pharm* 1982;1:217–224.

Antiparasitic Agents

Archer S: The chemotherapy of schistosomiasis. *Annu Rev Pharmacol Toxicol* 1985;25:485–508.

Harries J: Amoebiasis: A review. *J Roy Soc Med* 1982;75:190–197.

Loken S: Giardiasis: Diagnosis and treatment. *Nurse Pract* 1986;11(12):20–32.

Miller MJ: Protozoan and helminth parasites — a review of current treatment. *Prog Drug Res* 1976;20:433–464.

Rosenblatt JE, Edson RS: Metronidazole. *Mayo Clin Proc* 1983;58(3):154–157.

Yoshikawa TT: Antiparasitic drugs. *Am Fam Physician* 1980;21(3):132–138.

Rozman RS: Chemotherapy of malaria. *Annu Rev Pharmacol Toxicol* 1973;13:127–152.

Wang CC: Current problems in antiparasitic chemotherapy. *Trends Biochem Sci* 1982;7:354–356.

Wyler DJ: Malaria — resurgence, resistance, and research. *N Engl J Med* 1983;308: part 1, 875–878; part 2, 934–940.

CHAPTER 49

Serums and Vaccines

Immunity and Immunization

Immunity is a characteristic of vertebrates that helps to ensure their survival. It protects them against invasion of foreign substances and enables the organisms to build up resistance, thereby protecting them from repeated infections by the same pathogen.

The susceptibility of a given organism to infection by microorganisms reflects both innate and acquired characteristics of the organism. Each species is inherently resistant to infection by many microorganisms — a phenomenon referred to as **innate resistance.** Over the course of a lifetime, each member of a species develops resistance to some microorganisms that were originally infectious — a resistance known as **acquired immunity.** Acquired immunity is unique for each individual, reflecting the history of the individual's exposure to pathogenic microorganisms and the capabilities of his or her immune system for developing and maintaining specific immunity. The typical form of acquired immunity is that which occurs after an attack of an infectious disease. The immune system develops the capacity to eradicate the infectious microorganism, and this capability becomes part of the stored weapons of the individual's immune system, for later use as required. The response capacity is stored in the form of T or B lymphocytic memory cells.

Acquired immunity can be either natural or artificial: **natural immunity** results from exposure to infectious microorganisms, while **artificial immunity** results from exposure to vaccines. Both natural and artificial immunity can be either active or passive. **Active immunity** is resistance to microorganisms achieved by activation of the individual's own immune system (Table 49–1). Natural active immunity is acquired by exposure to microorganisms in the environment. **Passive immunity** is the direct transfer of antibodies to an individual who has not developed an immune response. Natural passive immunity is acquired either by the transfer of immunoglobulins across the placenta to the fetus during pregnancy, by the ingestion of immunoglobulins contained in breast milk by breast-feeding infants, or by administration of immunoglobulins. Active immunity provides immunity that is longer in duration, slower in onset (5–14 days after exposure to antigen), and highly effective in combating subsequent antigen contacts. Passive immunity, by comparison, is immediate in onset but lasts only as long as a few days or weeks and affords only moderate protection.

In this chapter, we are concerned primarily with artificial immunity, immunity that is conferred by therapeutic interventions. Active artificial immunity is produced by administration of vaccines: suspensions of live attenuated or dead microorganisms, cell extracts of microorganisms, or soluble toxins released by microorganisms. Vaccines act as antigens to activate immune responses that resemble those triggered by the living, active pathogen or exotoxin. Passive artificial immunity is achieved by administration of serums that contain antibodies against a microorganism or toxin. The serums are usually obtained from animals that have been inoculated with the pathogenic microbe or toxin. There is a high risk of allergic reactions to immune serums because of presence of animal protein in these products.

Table 49–1
Types of Acquired Immunity

Type	How acquired
Natural immunity	
Actively acquired	Occurs as a result of previous infections
Passively acquired	Transfer of immunoglobulins from mother to offspring via the placenta or breast milk
Artificial immunity	
Actively acquired	Vaccination with live attenuated or dead organisms, or exotoxins
Passively acquired	Injection of serum containing antibodies

Immunization: Pros and Cons

What Has Been the Impact of Immunization Programs?

The answer to this question is less clear than one might imagine or wish. No doubt, there has been a remarkable decline in the frequency and severity of infections caused by the agents for which vaccines exist during the time period since introduction of the vaccines. However, it is not established whether the decline can in fact be attributed to the use of vaccines. In the case of whooping cough, diphtheria, tetanus, cholera, and typhoid, the occurrence of these diseases was already declining precipitously before introduction of vaccination, and it is not evident that the rate of decline has accelerated appreciably as a result of vaccination. The declines preceding the vaccination era have been generally attributed to improvements in hygiene and, to a lesser extent, improvements in nutrition. These factors may be more important than vaccination in accounting for the further decline in incidence of related diseases that has occurred since the introduction of vaccination. The strongest evidence for effectiveness of vaccination concerns smallpox, poliomyelitis, measles, mumps, and rubella. Smallpox was eradicated worldwide by a vigorous vaccination program during the 1970s. The diminished incidence of the other diseases in this list since the introduction of vaccination clearly exceeds what could be attributed to factors other than vaccination. For example, the overall incidence of measles in the United States dropped from about 400,000 cases annually in the early 1960s to about 30,000 cases annually in the mid-1970s.

How Long Does Immunity Last?

There is considerable evidence developing that immunity conferred by vaccination is not lifelong, but rather that it wears off after a number of years — perhaps a decade. For example, when outbreaks of whooping cough or measles occur, those who were immunized more than ten years earlier are as likely to experience infection as those that are not, illustrating that immunity has worn off. Natural immunity to infectious diseases of childhood such as measles was traditionally considered to be a lifetime proposition, but it is no longer clear that natural immunity was ever as long-lasting as once thought. Prior to the widespread control of measles by vaccination, an individual who had experienced the disease as a child would be reexposed to the virus periodically as a result of social contacts over the course of a lifetime. Because of immunological resistance to the virus, such exposures would not have resulted in clinical symptoms but could have provided regular "booster" exposures to reinforce the immunological memory. One consequence of near eradication of a pathogenic microbe is that it deprives immune individuals (whether immune from previous exposure or vaccination) of the opportunity for the natural booster effect of periodic contact with the infectious agent. Some opponents of immunization contend that artificial immunity is less durable than natural immunity, but it is more likely that modern immunity for the near obsolete infectious diseases, whether artificial or natural, is less durable than it used to be because of near absence of contact with the pathogenic antigen that would be necessary in order to reinforce immunity periodically.

The Problem of Delaying Occurrence of Infectious Diseases

In the United States there has been a clear shift in the age groups susceptible to epidemic attacks of measles and mumps as a result of immunization programs. Outbreaks now occur predominantly in teenagers and young adults (when the immunity provided by innoculations during childhood is wearing off), with only sporadic cases in young children. Unfortunately, measles, mumps, and rubella are all diseases that are considerably less well tolerated after puberty than before (historical accounts of exposure of primitive peoples to measles virus for the first time give evidence of a much higher death rate among adolescents and young adults than in prepubertal children). Moreover, adults immunized with the original (now discontinued) killed measles vaccine are susceptible to an intensified form of measles called atypical measles syndrome (AMS), characterized by abrupt onset, high fever, headache, abdominal pain, and cough, followed in 1–2 days by the familiar skin eruption. AMS can last for 12 weeks or longer.

In the case of mumps, complications occur particularly after puberty. Postpubertal males have a 20% likelihood of experiencing orchitis, and in some of these cases, testicular atrophy and sterility can occur. Other complications of mumps that are more common in clients after puberty include meningoencephalitis, pancreatitis, prostatitis, myocarditis, nephritis, and polyarteritis. Rubella is also more severe postpuberty than in childhood. Arthritis, purpura, encephalitis, and testicular pain are complications occasionally seen in young adults but seldom in children. The congenital rubella syndrome (discussed below) presents unique risks for women of childbearing years and their offspring.

Unnatural Aspects of Artificial Immunity

One of the criticisms voiced against achieving immunity by vaccination has related to the method of antigen presentation. The bodily defenses, like those of a medieval fortress, are organized in concentric rings — the outermost line of defense being the barriers to penetration, the innermost being the lymphocytes and phagocytic cells of the blood. In the course of daily living, the average human encounters many different microorganisms in small numbers. The body protects itself effectively from most of these potential pathogens at the level of the outermost defenses. The mucosal membranes comprise the major penetration barriers through which most substances and pathogens gain penetration into the body if at all, except in the circumstances of severe burns or penetrating wounds. Associated with the mucosal membranes are tissue monocytes and immunoglobulins, especially of the IgA class. Natural acquired immunity most frequently involves enhanced immunological or nonspecific resistance at the level of the mucosal membranes (mucosal immunity) because pathogenic antigens are typically presented first to these resistance barriers. By contrast, with the exception of the oral polio vaccine, the antigenic substances of vaccines are presented in an artificial manner directly to the most central defense component. Injected intramuscularly, such antigens diffuse freely into the blood without the need to pass through normal external barriers to penetration. Relative to natural immunity, active artificial immunity places all of the burden for resistance to infection on the central defense mechanisms of the blood compartment and provides no impetus for enhancing resistance at the level of the penetration barriers.

In addition, one might raise other questions concerning artificial immunity. Is the presentation of large amounts of attenuated antigen comparable to natural exposure that would typically occur in small amounts, gradually? How does immunization impact on developmental aspects of immune functioning? Is there a risk of traumatizing the immune system or, conversely, depriving it of sufficient "exercise" against natural antigens so that we undermine its normal progression to a vigorous and experienced defense system? Is there a limitation in the total immunological memory capacity that might be taxed by presentation of large amounts of antigen directly to the central compartment? Unfortunately, our current level of understanding of the immune system does not permit conclusive answers to these kinds of questions. Neither the advocates nor the opponents of immunization can present an irrefutable case.

Current Recommendations of Official Agencies

Recommended schedules of immunization are generated by two agencies. The Immunization Practices Advisory Committee makes its recommendations to the Public Health Service; the Committee on Infectious Diseases provides its recommendations to the American Academy of Pediatrics. Currently, the schedules recommended by the two agencies for immunization of normal infants and children are identical (Table 49–2).

Responsibility for immunization programs is frequently the domain of the nurse. *Nurses should review with the parents of juvenile clients the recommended health maintenance schedule to determine which inoculations have been given. This will provide a history of the child's immunization and indicate where the parents or guardians might not be in compliance with health maintenance requirements.* A record showing sparse attention to the immunization schedule may suggest that the parents or guardians cannot be relied upon to comply with the established requirements, or there may be other valid reasons why the requirements have not been met. Cultural factors, beliefs about health care, or presence of other health problems may have precluded compliance. *The nurse should investigate further to determine the reason for noncompliance.*

A documented history of having had the clinical diseases for which a vaccine exists renders vaccination for that disease unnecessary. Many states and locales have immunization requirements for retention in the public school systems. *The nurse should provide an immunization schedule to parents and should encourage them to maintain their own complete written record of immunizations for their children. Blank forms are available for this purpose.* For children who were not immunized during infancy for one reason or another, an alternative schedule for immunization has been developed (Table 49–3).

Occurrence of puncture wounds is always reason to reassess the status of the individual's tetanus vaccination. *If a person suffering a puncture wound has not received a tetanus immunization within the past 10 years, the nurse should recommend or arrange for a booster shot of tetanus toxoids.* Special immunizations are often required for foreign travel, with requirements that are specific for each region of the world (Table 49–4).

Table 49–2
Recommended Schedule of Immunizations for Normal Infants and Children

Age	Vaccine
2 months	DPT[a], TOPV[b]
4 months	DPT, TOPV
6 months	DPT
15 months	MMR[c]
18 months	DPT, TOPV
4-6 years	DPT, TOPV
14-16 years	Td[d]

[a]DPT is diphtheria and tetanus toxoids and pertussis vaccine.
[b]TOPV is trivalent oral poliovirus vaccine.
[c]Measles-mumps-rubella (MMR) immunization can be conducted using combined or individual vaccines.
[d]Td is the adult type of combined tetanus and diphtheria toxoids; repeat every 10 years.

Agents for Active Immunization

Viral Vaccines

Measles (Rubeola) Virus Live Attenuated Vaccine

Effectiveness Measles, though usually less serious in young children than after puberty, is not always benign in young children because of the risk of complications such as pneumonia, otitis media, and

Table 49–3
Recommended Schedule of Immunizations for Children or Adolescents Not Immunized During Infancy

Visit	Vaccine
Under 6 years of age	
First visit	DPT[a], TOPV[b]
One month later	MMR[c]
Two months after first visit	DPT, TOPV
Four months after first visit	DPT
Ten–18 months after first visit or preschool	DPT, TOPV
Age 14–16 years	Td[d]
Six years and over	
First visit	Td, TOPV
One month later	MMR
Two months after first visit	Td, TOPV
Eight–14 months after first visit	Td, TOPV
Age 14–16 years	Td

[a]DPT is diphtheria and tetanus toxoids and pertussis vaccine.
[b]TOPV is trivalent oral poliovirus vaccine.
[c]Measles-mumps-rubella (MMR) immunization can be conducted using combined or individual vaccines.
[d]Td is the adult type of combined tetanus and diphtheria toxoids; repeat every 10 years.

secondary bacterial infections. Most severe of the complications of measles is encephalitis (in about 1 per 600–1000 cases) and subacute sclerosing panencephalitis (in about 1 per 100,000 cases), a particularly dreadful occurrence since it is a slowly progressing, chronic brain disease that can affect children months or years after a measles infection.

During the period 1963–1967, measles vaccination was conducted with a killed measles vaccine. Unfortunately, the killed measles vaccine proved to have very limited value in providing immunization against the wild virus. Moreover, some individuals receiving the killed measles vaccine actually became sensitized to measles virus, so that upon contracting the disease they experienced an exaggerated form of the condition which became known as atypical measles. *The nurse should examine the immunization records of clients to identify individuals who received measles vaccination between 1963 and 1967, and should urge them to be immunized anew with the modern measles vaccine.*

The measles virus live attenuated vaccine is very effective, inducing immunity to measles in 97% of susceptible individuals. The protection lasts at least 8 years but appears to be less than lifelong. Epidemics of measles in the United States now tend to occur mainly in adolescents and young adults with only sporadic cases in children. The measles vaccine produces a modified measles infection, and symptoms such as fever and rash often occur.

Indications The current recommendation is that children receive measles vaccination at 15 months of age. Children not immunized in infancy may receive measles vaccine later. Infants who live in regions where measles infection is likely to be contracted earlier than 15 months may be immunized at an earlier age, but response failures are greater and the child should be reimmunized after age 15 months. Children living in institutional settings are especially liable to measles and should therefore be immunized. Other high-risk children include those who are malnourished or who have diseases such as tuberculosis, cystic fibrosis, heart disease, chronic pulmonary diseases, or asthma. Immunization conducted after exposure to measles provides only slight protection; given 2 or more days before exposure, protection is substantial. Adolescents and young adults vaccinated in infancy may require reimmunization due to waning immunity, especially if a measles epidemic in the area makes exposure likely.

Adverse Effects and Contraindications The measles vaccine is contraindicated for use in individuals who have known hypersensitivity to eggs, chicken, chicken feathers, or neomycin (the vaccine includes 25 μg of neomycin). Nurses should take the client's temperature before vaccination and should postpone immunization in individuals with fever. The measles vaccine should not be employed in clients who are immunodeficient as a result of ongoing therapy with adrenocorticotropic hormone (ACTH), corticosteroids, antimetabolites, alkylating agents, or radiation therapy. Measles vaccine also should not be given to clients who have blood cell dyscrasias, leukemia, lymphomas, malignant neoplasms involving the bone marrow or lymphatics, or primary immune deficiency disorders such as hypogammaglobulinemia. In such individuals, short-term passive immunity can be achieved by administration of human measles immune globulin.

Use of the measles vaccine is contraindicated during pregnancy because natural measles is known to increase fetal risk. Vaccination of postpubertal females should entail a preliminary evaluation of the risk of pregnancy and women should be advised of the need to avoid pregnancy during the three months following vaccination.

The most common adverse reactions to measles vaccination are moderate fever (101–103° F) and

Table 49–4
Immunizations for Foreign Travel

Vaccine or drug prophylaxis	World regions
Required	
Cholera vaccine	Asia, Middle East, Africa
Smallpox vaccine	Virtually eradicated
Yellow fever vaccine	Tropical regions of South America and Africa
Recommended	
Hepatitis A virus vaccine	Africa, Asia, South America, Central America, rural Mexico, Philippines, South Pacific Islands
Malaria prophylaxis	Endemic areas (especially central Africa and southeast Asia)
Plague vaccine	Cambodia, Laos, and Vietnam
Rabies vaccine	Areas where rabies are endemic in wild or domestic animals
TB vaccine	For children who test tuberculin-negative who will be traveling to areas where tuberculosis is prevalent
Typhoid	Areas where sanitation is poor or typhoid is endemic
Typhus	Rural areas of Africa, Asia, and South America

rash. Less frequently, high fever (>103° F) occurs with the possibility of febrile convulsions. In about one per million vaccinations, the nurse may observe serious neurological reactions — encephalitis or encephalopathy — but the risk of these same reactions to natural measles is about one per thousand. Subacute sclerosing panencephalitis, which occurs in about 5–10 per million cases of wild measles, has been reported in about 1 per million vaccinated individuals.

Local reactions at the site of injection, such as swelling, redness, and vesiculation, occur occasionally, most frequently in individuals vaccinated with the killed measles virus, discontinued since 1967. Anaphylaxis occurs only rarely in response to measles vaccine, but epinephrine should be kept on hand just in case.

Administration and Storage Measles vaccine is given only subcutaneously. This vaccine should not be given within 1 month of other live virus vaccines, except for the live oral poliovirus vaccine, or when used in the measles-mumps-rubella combination preparations. Vaccination with measles virus should not be conducted less than 3 months after transfusions involving blood, plasma, or human immune serum globulin. Tuberculin tests may be temporarily suppressed (falsely) following vaccination.

Measles vaccine should be stored at 10° C or below until reconstitution and between 2° and 8° C afterward. The vaccine should be used within 8 hours after reconstitution and should be protected from light at all times. The usual dose is 0.5 ml of the reconstituted vaccine. Measles live attenuated vaccine (Attenuvax) is provided in single dose vials with a diluent-containing disposable syringe and needle.

Rubella Virus Live Vaccine

Effectiveness The rubella vaccine is highly effective, producing immunity against natural rubella virus in about 99% of those immunized. The immunization persists for at least 6 years but probably not for a lifetime.

Indications The current recommendation is that rubella vaccination be conducted at 15 months of age. It may be given as early as 12 months but should not be given in children less than 12 months of age since they may still have maternal rubella-neutralizing antibodies that will interfere with vaccination. As with measles, the prime age of susceptibility to infection by wild rubella virus is rapidly shifting toward late adolescence and early adulthood.

Vaccination of postpubertal females must be undertaken only with utmost caution. It is well established that maternal rubella infection during pregnancy poses substantial risks to the fetus. It would be ideal to reestablish immunity in women prior to childbearing years, but this objective must be weighed against the extreme risk that vaccination might occur concurrent with inadvertent pregnancy. If vaccination is contemplated in a postpubertal female, and testing reveals susceptibility to rubella, the woman must agree not to become pregnant for at least 3 months after vaccination. She should also be informed that arthralgia and arthritic symptoms often occur when young adult women are vaccinated for rubella, 2 and 4 weeks after immunization.

Adverse Effects and Contraindications Adverse reactions are uncommon, but symptoms resembling natural rubella may occur. Typical in this category are moderate fever (101–103° F), lymphadenopathy, rash, urticaria, sore throat, headache, and general malaise. Fever over 103° F is less common. Irritation at the site of injection includes such reactions as inflammation, erythema, induration, and pain. Joint pain seldom occurs in children immunized with rubella vaccine, but incidence increases in female patients with age. Anaphylaxis occurs only rarely in response to rubella vaccination. *The nurse should have epinephrine on hand in case of an anaphylactoid reaction.* Encephalitis is a rare but serious complication that has reportedly occurred in reaction to rubella vaccination. Hematological reactions such as thrombocytopenic purpura can also occur.

Rubella vaccine contains neomycin and is contraindicated in clients hypersensitive to that drug. Vaccination with rubella vaccine should be postponed in clients with fever due to infections. Immunization is contraindicated in immunosuppressed individuals such as those receiving ACTH, corticosteroids, anticancer drugs, or radiation therapy, or those with blood dyscrasias, leukemia, lymphomas, neoplasms involving the bone marrow or lymphatics, or immunodeficiency states. Rubella vaccine is contraindicated during pregnancy or when there is any risk of inadvertent pregnancy.

Administration and Storage Rubella vaccine is given only subcutaneously. Rubella vaccine should not be given within 1 month, before or after, of other live virus vaccines except measles or mumps. Vaccination should not be conducted within 3 months of transfusions with whole blood, plasma, or human immune serum globulins. Prior to reconstitution, rubella vaccine is stored at 2–8°C. The vaccine must be used within 8 hours after reconstitution. The vaccine is reconstituted by injecting the diluent from the syringe supplied into the vial. The reconstituted vaccine should be stored protected from light to 2–8°C. Rubella live virus vaccine (Meruvox II) is supplied in single-dose vials with diluent-containing disposable syringes. Rubella vaccine is available in combinations with mumps vaccine (Biavax II), measles vaccine (M-R-Vax II) and both measles and mumps (M-M-R II). Adverse effects and contraindications for these preparations are the combined ones for each of the vaccines in the combination.

Mumps Virus Live Vaccine

Effectiveness A single vaccination with the live mumps virus vaccine provides immunity in 97% of children and 93% of adults. The duration of immunological protection persists up to 10 years but is not lifelong. The incidence of mumps in adolescents and young adults is increasing as immunity that is initiated in infancy begins to wane.

Indications The current recommendation is that infants be vaccinated for mumps at 15 months, along with their vaccinations for measles and rubella. The vaccine is not recommended for infants less than 12 months of age.

Adverse Effects and Contraindications Mild fever occurs occasionally, but fever seldom exceeds 103°F. Parotitis and orchitis have occurred rarely following mumps vaccination, but prior exposure to wild mumps virus is a factor in some of these cases. *Nurses should be alert for signs of either of these reactions.* The vaccine is propagated in chick embryo cultures, but the incidence of allergic reactions is very low. The most common allergic manifestation has been urticaria. Purpura and encephalitis have occurred very rarely. Clients may complain of tenderness at the site of injection.

Mumps vaccine is contraindicated in clients with impaired immunity, active infectious conditions, or hypersensitivity to neomycin. Mumps vaccination should not be conducted during pregnancy, although adverse consequences have not been definitely established.

Administration and Storage Mumps vaccine is given subcutaneously, preferably in the outer aspect of the upper arm. The mumps vaccine (Mumpsvax) is furnished in single-dose vials with a diluent-containing disposable syringe. Prior to reconstitution, the vaccine should be stored at 2–8°C. After reconstitution, the vaccine should be stored at 2–8°C and protected from light. It should be used within 8 hours of reconstitution. The total volume of reconstituted vaccine constitutes a single dose. The dose is the same for all patients regardless of age or weight.

Poliovirus Live Oral Trivalent Vaccine

Effectiveness and Indications The trivalent oral poliovirus vaccine (TOPV, or Sabin vaccine) produces active immunity by simulating the natural infectious disease. The recommended series for primary immunization entails three oral administrations. The TOPV is recommended in preference to the inactivated poliomyelitis vaccine (IPV, or Salk vaccine) for several reasons. The oral route is easier and better tolerated by patients. The oral vaccine also promotes development of immunity at the level of the mucosal barriers as well as in the blood. Booster shots are not required after vaccination using TOPV. TOPV does not alter preexisting active poliomyelitis. The immunity produced by TOPV is comparable to that acquired by having the disease. TOPV is indicated for prevention of poliomyelitis due to types 1, 2, or 3 polioviruses.

Adverse Effects and Contraindications Adverse reactions are infrequent but potentially severe. Paralytic poliomyelitis has occurred rarely not only in patients themselves but even in nonvaccinated individuals in close contact with the patient. When TOPV is to be administered to an infant, it should first be determined if adults or older children in the same household have been previously vaccinated. If not, consideration should be given to vaccinating these individuals first, with at least two doses of IPV.

Immunization of a child should be postponed if the child is experiencing diarrhea or vomiting or has an acute fever due to active infection. If the patient is immunodeficient for any reason, IPV is used in preference to TOPV because the mild poliovirus infection produced when TOPV is used could be greatly intensified in the absence of normal immunological resistance. Viral vaccines other than measles, mumps, or rubella, or combinations of these should not be used concurrently, since many of these interfere with the immunological response to TOPV. TOPV should not be given before age 6 weeks.

Administration and Storage TOPV (Orimune, Trivalent) is furnished as a mixture of types 1, 2, and 3 polioviruses in 0.5 ml single-dose pipettes or in 10-dose vials with a dropper. The drug should be stored in the freezer compartment of a refrigerator and thawed before use. The vaccine should not be refrozen if at any time its temperature exceeds 8°C. Once thawed, the vaccine may be used for up to 30 days if stored below 8°C. Once opened, the contents of a vial should be used within 7 days.

The primary immunization series consists of three doses. For infants, the first should be given at 6–12 weeks of age, usually with the first dose of diphtheria-pertussis-tetanus (DPT) vaccine. The second dose is given 8 weeks later; the third is given 8–12 months after the second. For children or adolescents not immunized in infancy, the same interval between doses is used. Immunization is not indicated for adults unless they are at increased risk. The dose for TOPV is 2 drops (0.5 ml), which is the entire content of the single-dose pipette.

Influenza Virus Vaccine

Effectiveness and Indications Influenza virus vaccine consists each year of a mixture of influenza viral strains that are expected to be prevalent that year. The vaccine affords protection only against the strains included in the vaccine, typically three strains. Influenza virus vaccine is strongly recommended by the U.S. Public Health Service for individuals at special risk, including those with acquired or congenital heart disease, chronic obstructive pulmonary diseases, chronic renal failure with azotemia, or immunodeficiencies. Vaccination is also recommended for persons over age 65 because of the increased mortality from influenza in that age group. Some sources recommend vaccination for school personnel due to their increased exposure.

Adverse Effects and Contraindications Adverse reactions seldom occur in adults. Younger persons commonly experience adverse reactions, such as fever, malaise, myalgia, and local irritation at the site of infection (tenderness, redness, induration). High fever in children under 3 years may occasionally cause febrile convulsions. Hypersensitivity reactions are extremely rare. The vaccine used in 1976 was associated with an incidence of Guillain-Barré syndrome (GBS) of about 10 cases per million vaccinated individuals, but no elevated risk of GBS has been observed in the years since then. GBS is a paralytic condition, reversible in most cases, but fatal in about 5% of individuals. In addition, about a dozen people developed encephalopathies other than GBS associated with the influenza vaccine in 30 years of use. Most had brief neurological disorders followed by full recovery. Influenza virus vaccine is contraindicated in clients with a history of allergic reactions to chicken eggs, since the vaccines are grown in chicken embryo cells. If there is doubt as to whether the person is hypersensitive to egg protein, a skin test can be conducted using the vaccine. Vaccination should usually be postponed in individuals with active febrile respiratory infections. Although there is no clear evidence indicating risk to the fetus when the vaccine is used during pregnancy, vaccination during the first trimester should be avoided. Increased frequency of fetal abnormalities has not usually been linked to influenza virus, whether the wild virus or the vaccine, being reported only in the pandemics of 1918–1919 and 1957–1958.

Administration and Storage Influenza virus vaccine (Fluogen, Fluaz, Fluzone-Connaught) is provided in 5 ml vials containing 10 adult doses. Influenza virus vaccine is given intramuscularly, or less commonly subcutaneously, but never intravenously. Intramuscular administration produces fewer local reactions than when the vaccine is given subcutaneously. The deltoid or the lateral aspect of the thigh is the usual site for IM injection. Influenza viruses are provided as whole-virus or split-virus preparations. For children under 13, only the split-virus preparations are recommended because the incidence of adverse reactions is lower. The usual vaccination procedure for influenza virus vaccine is a single 0.5 ml dose. Children under 35 months are given half doses: 0.25 ml. Influenza virus vaccine must be stored at 2–8°C.

Hepatitis B Vaccine

Effectiveness and Indications Hepatitis B vaccine stimulates the formation of antibodies against the hepatitis B virus. The vaccine is 80–95% effective in preventing acute hepatitis B infections. The percentage of clients who develop immunity is higher when three innoculations are conducted than when only two innoculations are performed (about 95% versus 85%). Injection of the vaccine into the buttocks results in a lower rate of response (about 80%) than when the deltoid muscle is utilized. Revaccination of those who do not respond to an initial series of injections results in immunity in only one-third of cases. The hepatitis B vaccine is effective against all known subtypes of hepatitis B virus. Vaccination with the hepatitis B vaccine may not prevent development of hepatitis B infections when administered to individuals already infected with virulent hepatitis B virus. Immunosuppressed clients may require higher doses of the vaccine because of the diminished responsivity of their immune system. Vaccination against hepatitis B is recommended for persons of all ages, especially those at special risk of hepatitis infections, including health care personnel, patients undergoing hemodialysis, patients requiring frequent transfusions or administration of preparations derived from blood, cancer patients, infants born to mothers who test positive for hepatitis B surface antigen, Alaskan Eskimos, Indochinese and Haitian refugees, sexually-active male homosexuals, prostitutes, morticians, prisoners, intravenous drug users, and military personnel in certain parts of the world.

Adverse Effects and Contraindications Serious adverse reactions seldom occur in response to the hepatitis B vaccine. Mild tenderness, swelling, erythema, or pruritus may occur at the site of injection. Mild gastrointestinal symptoms (nausea, diarrhea, cramps, or vomiting) and neurological symptoms (headache, dizziness, paresthesia, or insomnia) have been reported occasionally. Some clients experience a degree of fatigue or a febrile reaction with sweating, chills, malaise, and achiness. As a precaution, nurses administering the vaccine should have epinephrine immediately available in the event of a systemic hypersensitivity reaction. The vaccine should be administered cautiously to individuals with compromised cardiopulmonary function or those who may respond adversely to a mild febrile reaction. The safety of this product for use during pregnancy or in mothers who are nursing infants has not been established.

Administration and Storage Hepatitis B vaccine is intended for intramuscular injection. The preferred site of injection is the deltoid muscle in adults or the anterolateral thigh in infants and young children. Injection into the buttocks results in unreliable absorption. Subcutaneous injections may be employed in persons at special risk of hemorrhage, but the incidence of reactions at the site of administration is higher when this route is employed. The available preparations of hepatitis B vaccine include plasma-derived inactivated human hepatitis B surface antigen (Heptavax-B) and recombinant vaccine produced by yeast cells (Recombivax). Both types of hepatitis antigen are available in pediatric and adult injection solutions. The usual immunization sequence involves three innoculations, the second and third administrations following 1 and 6 months respectively after the initial dose. The recommended doses for prophylaxis are 0.5 ml each administration in children from birth to age 10, 1.0 ml in older children and adults, and 2.0 ml (1.0 ml at each of two sites) for dialysis or immunocompromised patients. The hepatitis B vaccine should be stored at 2°–8° C. Freezing impairs the potency of the vaccine. The vaccine requires no dilution or reconstitution.

Smallpox Vaccine

The risk of smallpox in the United States and worldwide is so small that routine vaccination is no longer indicated. Adverse reactions to smallpox vaccination include encephalitis, encephalopathy, myelitis, acute infectious polyneuritis, eczema, eye infections with possible blindness, and generalized vaccinia. Complications have resulted in disability or death. The incidence of adverse reactions with revaccination is very low. Vaccination and revaccination is contraindicated during pregnancy, in immunodeficient patients, in clients with disorders of gamma globulin synthesis, for individuals with skin wounds, burns, or diseases and for their families' members, and for infants exhibiting failure to thrive. Smallpox vaccination is performed by needle puncture through a drop of vaccine placed on the skin. The site is first cleansed using a suitable cleansing agent and allowed to dry. The vaccination site should be protected from direct exposure to sunlight for several days, but an occlusive shield or pad should not be applied. Patients should be instructed not to touch the site. Inadvertent spread of the vaccine to the eyes has led to serious ocular infections and even blindness. Successful vaccination should produce a vesicle after 6–8 days. Smallpox vaccine (Dryvax) is furnished in packages of dried vaccine for 25 or 100 vaccinations, with a container of diluent and sterile bifurcated (forked) needles.

Yellow Fever Vaccine

Yellow fever vaccine is indicated for travelers over 6 months of age planning to visit countries requiring a certificate of vaccination against yellow fever. Immunity develops in about 7 days after vaccination and is long-lasting — at least 10 years. About 10% of patients vaccinated with this preparation experience fever or malaise, but otherwise adverse reactions are rare. *Nurses should warn clients that they may develop low-grade fever, malaise, or myalgia.* Reversible and mild encephalitis has developed rarely in very young infants given this vaccine. The vaccine should not be used during pregnancy, before age 6 months, in patients who are immunodeficient, or in those who are hypersensitive to chicken protein. Yellow Fever Vaccine-Connaught is furnished in 5 and 20 dose ampuls for needle injection and 100 and 200 dose ampuls for jet injector use. This vaccine must be maintained continuously at below 5°C and should be frozen until reconstitution and use. When use is anticipated, the vaccine should be removed from the freezer, the diluent added, and the injections given promptly (within 60 minutes after reconstitution). The vaccine should be shaken thoroughly before withdrawing each dose. A single dose is given, 0.5 ml subcutaneously. Reimmunization is required after 10 years if there is continuing need for protection.

Rabies Vaccines

Two types of rabies vaccines are available: rabies vaccine, duck embryo vaccine (DEV) and rabies vaccine, human diploid cell cultures (HDCV). These products are indicated for preexposure immunization of high-risk individuals or postexposure immunization. Both products are effective, but HDCV eliminates the risk of hypersensitivity reactions in individuals who may be sensitive to chicken protein. Adverse reactions are infrequent. Nurses should inform clients that they might anticipate local reactions such as swelling, induration, erythema, and slight pain. Slight headache, fever, or nausea occur occasionally. Rabies vaccine is given by IM injection into the deltoid region. The recommended schedule for preexposure immunization with HDCV in the United States is a three-injection sequence on days 0, 7, and 21 or 28. The dose at each scheduled injection is 1.0 ml. The recommended postexposure schedule with HDCV in the United States calls for 5 doses of 1.0 ml given IM on days 0, 3, 7, 14, and 28. The vaccine is stored at 2–8°C until reconstituted for use.

Bacterial Vaccines

Bacillus Calmette-Guerin (BCG) Vaccine

BCG vaccine is a live attenuated bacterial vaccine composed of a strain of *Mycobacterium bovis.* It is indicated for individuals who test negative to a tuberculosis skin test and who are repeatedly exposed to persons with untreated or persistent sputum-positive pulmonary tuberculosis. The BCG vaccine has also been used in circumscribed communities where there is a high rate of new tuberculosis infections, when traditional surveillance and treatment programs are inadequate or inapplicable. The overall incidence of side effects is low, although adverse reactions can occur up to 1 year after immunization. However, nurses should inform clients that they should report any reactions such as local ulceration and swelling of the lymph nodes. Health care professionals should follow the client's progress so as to identify other potential problems such as osteomyelitis and disseminated BCG infections. BCG vaccine should not be given to patients with significant burns, skin infections, or recent smallpox vaccination. Clients receiving isoniazid (Rifamate) therapy may experience interference with BCG vaccine. The vaccine is contraindicated in immunodeficient individuals and those who are tuberculin-positive. Use during pregnancy should be avoided. BCG vaccine is provided in 1 ml ampuls for reconstitution. The immunizing dose is 0.1 ml injected intradermally, except in newborn infants who receive one-half that dose: 0.05 ml. If vaccination has been effective, a small red papule appears at the site of injection in 7–10 days, expands to a maximum diameter of 8 mm in 5 weeks, scales, ulcerates, and dries, shrinking to a small pink or bluish scar in 6 months. In the absence of an overt reaction of this type, success of vaccination can be ascertained by means of a tuberculin test 2–3 months after immunization. If negative, vaccination may be repeated. After vaccination with BCG, a person can no longer be accurately tested for tuberculosis infection, since the tests do not differentiate between virulent infection and continuing immunity.

Meningococcal Vaccines

Meningococcal vaccines provide immunity only against *Neisseria meningitidis,* Group A or Group C. It does not afford protection against other bacterial or viral pathogens that cause meningitis. The meningococcal vaccine is indicated for individuals at risk because of presence in an area of an epidemic or in household contact with individuals infected with *N. meningitidis,* Group A or C. The type A vaccine is usually restricted to use in individuals over 3 months of age; the type C vaccine is indicated for individuals over 2 years of age. Adverse reactions include headache, fever, chills, malaise, cramps, and local tenderness, soreness, or induration at the site of injection. The vaccine should not be used during an acute illness or during pregnancy. The vaccine is provided in formulations of the A type, the C type, or mixed A and C meningococci. Each type is furnished in 10-dose vials or 50-dose vials for use with a jet injector. The standard dose is 0.5 ml, which contains 50 μg of the meningococcal isolate. Diluent is supplied for reconstitution. Epinephrine should be at hand in the event of anaphylactoid reactions.

Cholera Vaccine

Cholera vaccine is indicated for immunization of individuals who are to be exposed to *Vibrio cholerae.* The vaccine consists of a mixture of two serotypes and provides immunity that is short-lasting (3–6 months) and incomplete. Exposure to massive amounts of the microorganism will still cause infection. Systemic reactions to this vaccine are usually short-lived, subsiding in at most 48 hours. They include aches and pains, fever, malaise, headache, tachycardia, hypotension, and flushing. Local reactions include erythema, tenderness, swelling, induration, and, uncommonly, necrosis or ulceration. Cholera vaccine is given subcutaneously, intramuscularly, or intradermally in individuals over 5 years of age. Cholera vaccine is supplied in 1.5 ml vials. The usual dose is 0.5 ml. Booster doses are required at 6-month intervals if extended protection is required.

Typhoid Vaccine

Typhoid vaccine is indicated for individuals who must travel to a region in which typhoid fever is endemic or who are in intimate household contact with an infected individual. Nurses should advise clients of possible systemic reactions to typhoid vaccination, such as headache, fever, malaise, and myalgia. There may also be local reactions such as tenderness, erythema, and induration. Prior to giving the vaccine, the nurse should note any evidence of respiratory or other infections; if they are present the immunization should be postponed. The nurse should have epinephrine at hand in the event the client goes into an anaphylactic reaction. The vaccine is provided in 5, 10, and 20 ml vials. Primary immunization is accomplished with two doses given at an interval of 4 weeks or more. The dose in individuals 10 years of age or over is 0.5 ml on each occasion; children under 10 are given half-doses of 0.25 ml on each occasion. Booster shots must be given at least every 3 years if exposure continues.

Plague Vaccine

Plague vaccine consists of inactivated *Yersinia pestis.* It is recommended for individuals who live in known plague areas. This includes portions of central Asia, southern India, Pakistan, Nepal, Java, Vietnam, South Africa, South America, Saudi Arabia, and the southwestern United States. The vaccine is especially valuable in protecting people who work with rodents and rabbits in plague areas, since these species are a major reservoir for *Y. pestis.* The plague vaccine provides a degree of protection against the insect-borne form of plague, called bubonic plague, improving chances of recovery in those who are infected. Protection is of limited duration, and unfortunately, each booster shot is associated with increasing local reactions. Primary immunization after age 10 consists of two SQ doses of 0.5 ml at an interval of 4 or more weeks followed by a third 0.2 ml dose 4–12 weeks after the second dose. Children are immunized on the same schedule, but doses are reduced to one-fifth of the adult dose for children under 1 year, two-fifths for children 1–4, and three-fifths for children 5–10 years of age. Booster injections are required at 6-month intervals.

Pneumococcal Vaccine, Polyvalent

This vaccine consists of capsular antigens from 14 types of pneumococci, which together account for at least 80% of bacterial pneumonias. Pneumococcal vaccine is indicated for clients at special risk of morbidity or mortality from pneumococcal pneumonia: clients with chronic heart disease, chronic pulmonary disorders, chronic metabolic disorders, individuals in chronic care facilities or convalescing from severe diseases, clients who have had splenectomy, and high-risk individuals over 50. Nurses can expect the drug to cause systemic and local reactions typical of vaccines: fever, local soreness, erythema, and induration. Anaphylactoid reactions are rare. Pneumococcal vaccine should not be used in clients who are pregnant, who have febrile respiratory illness or other active infections, who have Hodgkin's disease, who are receiving chemotherapy or nodal radiation, or who have known hypersensitivity to the vaccine. The vaccination should not be repeated in less than 3 years. The usual vaccination regimen is 0.5 ml in a single SQ or IM dose, preferably in the deltoid muscle or lateral midthigh. Pneumococcal vaccine (Pneumovax, Pnu-Immune) is provided in single-dose and 5-dose vials and prefilled syringes.

Mixed Respiratory Vaccine (MRV)

MRV contains many strains of bacteria that produce respiratory infections. Its proposed use is for individuals who have bacterial hypersensitivities that are manifested as asthma, severe rhinitis, or urticaria. The Food and Drug Administration has not endorsed this product because effectiveness has not been conclusively demonstrated and the product lacks uniformity of content and potency. Adverse reactions consist primarily of allergic manifestations, ranging from mild exaggeration of the patient's usual allergic symptoms to severe anaphylactoid reactions. Epinephrine should be at hand when MRV is employed. The recommended initial dose for prophylaxis is 0.05 ml given subcutaneously. Doses may be increased at 4-day to 7-day intervals to a maximum of 0.5–1.0 ml. The recommended maintenance dose is 0.5 ml once every week or once every 2 weeks.

Toxoid Vaccines

Diphtheria-Pertussis-Tetanus (DPT) Vaccine

Diphtheria, tetanus, and pertussis vaccines are usually given together as a 3-in-1 preparation.

Effectiveness Tetanus and diphtheria toxoids consist of the toxin produced by tetanus and diphtheria bacilli respectively, modified by treatment with formaldehyde to eliminate toxicity but not anti-

Nursing Observations for Immunizations

THERAPEUTIC GOAL	Routine protection from diphtheria, pertussis, tetanus, polio, measles, mumps, and rubella. Protection from certain other infectious agents when the person is at special risk.
PREADMINISTRATION ASSESSMENT	
Baseline Data	Observe for signs of infection as a contraindication. Evaluate blood pressure, pulse, peripheral pulses, and respiratory rate and sounds before administering vaccines.
Contraindications/ Precautions	Acute infection, immunodeficiency, or pregnancy.
Potential Interactions	Check current medications for glucocorticoids, immunosuppressives, antineoplastics, or gamma globulin therapy.
EVALUATION OF DRUG RESPONSE	
For Therapeutic Benefit	Monitor long-term prophylaxis against the corresponding infectious disorder. If successful vaccination is crucial, monitor serum titers.
For Adverse Effects	Monitor pain, fever, discomfort, and allergic reactions.

genic potential. The toxins are adsorbed onto aluminum hydroxide to improve antigenic potency. Immunization with absorbed toxoid preparations affords a high level protection for a period of 5–10 years. Pertussis vaccine is effective but the most risky of the routinely employed vaccines.

Clinical Indications The recommended schedule for primary DPT immunization calls for four administrations between 2 months and 6 years of age. The recommended schedule in normal infants provides initial injections at 2, 4, and 6 months; and the fourth or reinforcing injection at 18 months. A booster shot is given between 4 and 6 years of age. Immunization is maintained by additional booster shots at 10-year intervals, but DPT is not recommended for this purpose. After age 6, the combined tetanus and diphtheria toxoids (adult type, Td) is recommended.

Adverse Effects and Contraindications Adverse reactions occur to all three components and since individual products are available, we will consider the adverse reactions of each independently. Tetanus toxoid commonly produces local irritation at the site of injection, including redness, induration, and occasionally formation of nodules or abscesses. Severe systemic reactions are rare, but mild to moderate reactions are fairly common, especially when booster doses are given to individuals over 25. Edema, itching, and hives may occur. Fever, chills, malaise, aches and pain, hypotension, flushing, and tachycardia are typical reactions in adults. Neurological complications such as paralysis have occurred rarely.

Diphtheria toxoid produces both local and systemic reactions, more so in individuals who have received large numbers of booster injections. Systemic reactions include fever, malaise, hives, pruritus, hypotension, flushing, aches and pains, and tachycardia. Local reactions are the usual redness, tenderness, and induration.

Pertussis vaccine has been associated with severe and even fatal reactions. Most of the dangerously severe reactions occur within 48 hours, but some have occurred after as long as a week. Severe reactions are characterized by extreme fever (>105° F), shock, screaming, convulsions, encephalopathy, and thrombocytopenic purpura.

There is an elevated risk of sudden infant death syndrome (SIDS) following DPT injection. The recommended age for DPT administration is also the peak age for SIDS. It is not clear to what extent DPT contributes to SIDS or which component (if any) is involved.

DPT is not recommended for use in children over 6 years of age. Immunization should be postponed if the child is febrile or experiencing an acute infectious disorder. *When a second or subsequent DPT injection is being contemplated, the nurse should ask the parents about the child's reactions to previous injections.* Pertussis vaccination should be discontinued if any of the following reactions occurred in response to DPT: fever in excess of 103°F, convulsions, syncope, neurological symptoms, screaming, collapse, purpura, somnolence, shock, or encephalopathy. DPT should not be used in immunodeficient individuals.

Administration and Dosages Although both tetanus toxoid and diphtheria toxoid are available singly, the two are almost always administered in combination, usually with pertussis vaccine as well. The triple vaccine is marketed as Tri-Immunol, Triogen, Triple Antigen, and as a generic in single dose 0.5 ml vials and in 7.5 ml vials. The dose for all individuals at each scheduled injection is 0.5 ml. The injection is given IM, preferably in the midlateral muscle of the thigh or in the deltoid.

Diphtheria and tetanus toxoids are available without pertussis vaccine in pediatric and adult formulations. The pediatric formulation is recommended for patients under 6 in whom pertussis vaccine is contraindicated. The adult formulation (Td) contains a full dose of tetanus toxoid but a reduced dose of diphtheria toxoid in order to reduce the severity of hypersensitivity reactions. It is recommended for anyone over 6 years of age. The dose for either formulation is 0.5 ml.

Important Nursing Implications for Vaccines

- ☐ Keep current with the immunization requirements of various health agencies.
- ☐ Routinely assess the immunological status of adolescents, immigrants, new parents, and other high-risk groups.
- ☐ Provide clients who inquire with factual information to aid them in weighing the pros and cons of immunization.
- ☐ Before administering any vaccine, check for possible contraindications, including pregnancy, current use of glucocorticoids or immune serums, recent blood transfusion, a significant fever, leukemias, lymphomas, and history of allergy to the vaccine or any component of the vaccine.

Nursing Diagnoses and Interventions for Immunizations

Nursing Diagnoses	*Related Interventions*
TO MINIMIZE DRUG SIDE EFFECTS OR INTERACTIONS	
Alteration in comfort: pain at the site of injection	Apply heat to the area of swelling or give a nonnarcotic analgesic if required; provide adequate rest and relaxed environment; warn parents that infants may be fussy or irritable for up to 24 hours after vaccination and instruct them to intensify comfort measures. Teach clients to move the arm (not to hold it stiff) after the injection to promote absorption and reduce pain.
Alteration in tissue perfusion related to anaphylactic reaction to immunization	Provide emergency measures such as epinephrine or tourniquets as required.
TO ENSURE SAFE AND EFFICACIOUS DRUG USE	
Knowledge deficit related to drug regimen	Discuss the reasons for immunization or for withholding immunization as appropriate. Provide client with a record of immunization and explain how to keep it current. Explain the possible adverse reactions indicating clearly which are to be considered routine and which should be reported immediately. If the vaccination poses a hazard for a fetus, warn sexually active female clients to maintain reliable birth control for the requisite period of time.

- ☐ Encourage elderly clients and those with respiratory ailments to obtain annual influenza virus vaccinations.
- ☐ Do not give two or more vaccines concurrently unless compatibility has been specifically established.
- ☐ After injecting the agent, record the date, name of the agent or product, the manufacturer, lot number, amount of agent used, the site of injection, and the client's response in the client's medical record.
- ☐ Observe each client for a period of one-half hour after immunization for indications of allergic reactions, such as rash, hives, serum sickness, or anaphylaxis. Keep epinephrine, oxygen, antihistamines, corticosteroids, respiratory apparatus, and a tourniquet (if the vaccine or serum is injected into an arm) available for emergency management of anaphylaxis.
- ☐ Help parents keep a permanent, accurate record of immunizations for each of their children. Such records are often required by schools, camps, day care centers, and other programs for children.
- ☐ Teach clients about adverse reactions to immunization and which are normal and which, by contrast, need to be reported. Explain that transient fever may occur and that aspirin or acetaminophen may be used to reduce elevated temperature.
- ☐ Store vaccines in accordance with the instructions for each preparation. Most vaccines must be refrigerated until immediately before use and must be frozen during longer periods of storage.

Agents for Passive Immunization

Immune Serums

Immune serums contain gamma globulins in a concentration of about 16.5%. These gamma globulins are obtained from humans or horses, depending on the product. Immune serum globulin (ISG, or gamma globulin) is obtained from donors from the general population. Immune globulins for pertussis, hepatitis B, tetanus, varicella zoster, and Rh_0 (D) are obtained from hyperimmune individuals. Rabies immune globulin is obtained from either hyperimmune human beings or from horses. These products provide rapid but short-lived protection against the corresponding specific antibodies, or, in the case of the nonspecific immune globulin, against a variety of infectious microorganisms.

Immune serums are contraindicated in individuals who have allergies to gamma globulins or the preservative thimerosal, or who are known to possess antibodies for IgA. Individuals with isolated IgA immunodeficiency are likely candidates to develop antibodies to administered IgA, with anaphylaxis as a possible consequence. Immune serums should thus be used only if absolutely required in such individuals. Immune serums must be given intramuscularly. Individuals with severe clotting defects may be at risk when any kind of intramuscular injection is performed. Immune serums should never be given intravenously. Immune serums may interfere with development of immunity from vaccinations. If it is necessary to administer an immune serum within 3 months after vaccination, revaccination should be conducted 6 months or more after the final administration of immune serums. Although allergic reactions to immune serums are not common, they may be severe. Epinephrine should be on hand for relief of anaphylactoid reactions. Local tenderness and stiffness at the site of administration is commonplace but subsides after several hours.

Immune Serum Globulin (ISG)

ISG provides passive immunization against hepatitis A, hepatitis B, rubeola (measles), varicella, rubella, and various bacteria including Proteus species and *Pseudomonas aeruginosa.* The value of ISG against hepatitis A is greatest if given before or soon after exposure. ISG is not indicated for use more than 2 weeks after exposure to hepatitis A. ISG is less effective than the specific hepatitis B immune globulin for hepatitis B and should be used only if the specific immune serum globulin is not available. ISG is useful during early pregnancy for protection of mother and fetus against rubella when vaccination would entail unacceptable risks. Use of ISG for this purpose should be limited to women known to have been exposed to rubella; routine prophylaxis is not justifiable. ISG has been found effective as an adjunct to antibiotic therapy for various severe bacterial infections. ISG is useful in alleviating immune deficiency conditions such as agammaglobulinemia.

ISG (Gamastan, Gammagee, Gammar, Immu-G, Immuglobin, Immune Globulin) is available in 2–10 ml vials. It should be stored at 2–8° C and used before the expiration date. Typical doses are 0.02 ml/kg for hepatitis A, 0.06 ml/kg for hepatitis B, 0.2 ml/kg for measles, 0.6 to 1.2 ml/kg for varicella, 20 ml during pregnancy for women exposed to rubella, and

0.55–3.3 ml/kg as an adjunct in treating bacterial infections. For replacement therapy in immunoglobulin deficiency conditions, 1.2 ml/kg is given initially, followed by 0.66 ml/kg at 3-week to 4-week intervals thereafter indefinitely.

Specific Immune Globulins

Pertussis immune globulin (Hypertussis) is indicated for prophylaxis and treatment of pertussis. It is given only by IM injection. For prophylaxis, the usual dose is 1.25 ml in infants or 2.5 ml in older children. For treatment, the usual dose is 1.25 ml repeated once between 24 and 48 hours later.

Hepatitis B immune globulin (H-BIG, Hep-B-Gammagee, HyperHep) is indicated for prophylaxis after exposure to hepatitis B. The recommended dose is 0.06 ml/kg given by IM injection. Treatment is repeated once after 28–30 days.

Tetanus immune globulin (Homo-Tet, Hu-Tet, Hyper-Tet, Immu-Tetanus, Tet-CONN-G-Connaught, T-I-Gammagee, generic) is indicated for those exposed to tetanus who have not been immunized or who are of uncertain immunological status. The usual prophylactic dose is 250 units given by IM injection. Doses for treatment have not been definitely established, but use of 3,000–6,000 units has been reported.

Varicella-zoster immune globulin (VZIG) is indicated for passive immunization of immune deficient children after exposure to varicella-zoster. Supplies of the drug are limited, necessitating restriction of treatment to children who meet established criteria of immunodeficiency and likelihood of exposure. Dosage is adjusted in accordance with the weight of the child. VZIG is given only by IM injection.

Rabies immune globulin, human (RIG) and antirabies serum, equine origin (ARS) are indicated for passive protection of individuals exposed or possibly exposed to rabies. RIG or ARS is given in conjunction with rabies vaccine, as promptly after exposure as possible. Rabies serums should not be repeated and are contraindicated in individuals known to be allergic to gamma globulin or other constituents of the respective products. The incidence of allergic reaction is lower with RIG than ARS. RIG (Hyperab) is provided in 2 ml and 10 ml vials containing 150 IU per ml. The recommended dose is 20 IU/kg to be given with the first vaccination dose. Up to half the dose can be used to infiltrate the wound. The remainder is given IM. ARS is available in 1,000 unit vials. The recommended dose is 1,000 units/40 lb. Part of the dose can be infiltrated into the wound if feasible. The rest is given IM.

Rh_0 (D) immune globulin suppresses the immune response in Rh_0 (D) negative individuals to Rh_0 (D) positive blood. The immune response might occur during birth or abortion when the child or fetus is Rh_0 (D) positive and the mother is Rh_0 (D) negative. Use of this product is indicated whenever a Rh_0 (D) negative mother has not been previously sensitized and the baby is Rh_0 (D) positive. If pregnancy is incomplete and typing of the fetus's blood is not feasible, the fetus should be assumed to be Rh_0 (D) positive unless the father is definitely known to be Rh_0 (D) negative. Rh_0 (D) immune globulin (Gamulin Rh, HypRho-D, RhoGAM) is provided in vials along with a cross-match 1 : 1,000 dilution solution. Before administration of Rh_0 (D) immune globulin to the mother, a minor cross-match test is conducted using one drop of a 5% suspension of the mother's red blood cells and the cross-match solution furnished with the immune globulin.

Antitoxins and Antivenins

Another means of providing passive immunization is the administration of antitoxins and antivenins. These products are obtained from the blood of horses immunized against specific toxins. Available preparations include antitoxins for diphtheria and tetanus and antivenin for rattlesnake, North American coral snake, and black widow spider venoms. The antivenin products are indicated for treatment of bites by the corresponding snakes or spider. The antitoxins are employed for postexposure treatment of individuals not protected from tetanus or diphtheria by vaccination.

Antitoxin and antivenin products can cause both local and systemic reactions. Local reactions usually consist of pain and inflammation within 7–12 days, which typically subside in 2 days. Repeated injections produce more severe reactions including necrosis and sloughing. Systemic reactions are hypersensitivity reactions and may include serum sickness (in 5–10% of treated individuals) or anaphylaxis. *Preliminary sensitivity tests should be conducted before administration of the treatment dose, including a scratch test and a conjunctival test.* Negative results with both of these tests do not preclude an allergic reaction, but the likelihood is greatly diminished. If preliminary sensitivity tests are positive or ambiguous, desensitization can be conducted by serial injection of diluted antitoxin or antivenin at 15-minute intervals. Epinephrine should be at hand in the event of anaphylaxis.

Diphtheria antitoxin is available in vials containing 10,000 or 20,000 units. This product neutralizes the toxins produced by *Corynebacterium diphtheriae.* The antitoxin is warmed to 90–95°F before IM injection or slow IV infusion. The usual dose (if sensitivity tests are negative) is 10,000 units.

Tetanus antitoxin is available in vials of 1,500 or 20,000 units. This preparation is used only when tetanus immune globulin is unavailable. Active immunization can be initiated concurrently. The usual dose for prophylaxis is 1,500 to 5,000 units IM or SQ. For treatment, 50,000 to 100,000 units is given, at least partly IV, the rest IM.

Antivenin crotalidae polyvalent is an antivenin produced by immunizing horses with venoms from four types of snakes of the pit viper family. This antivenin is capable of neutralizing venoms of rattlesnakes, copperheads and cottonmouth moccasins, Cantils, and bushmasters of North, Central, and South America, Japan, and Korea. The antivenin is supplied in packages containing the vials of antivenin, vials with vehicle (10 ml of bacteriostatic water), and vials of 1 : 10 dilute horse serum for sensitivity testing. The usual dosage (if sensitivity testing is negative) is 20–40 ml (2–4 vials) if the bite resulted in minimal envenomation; 50–90 ml (5–9 vials) for moderate envenomation; and 100–150 ml (10–15 vials) if envenomation is severe. This antivenin is given by slow IV infusion.

Antivenin micrurus fulvius is used to treat bites of two of the three kinds of poisonous coral snakes found in Texas, Arizona, and New Mexico. It is ineffective against the third kind of coral snake *(Micrurus euryxanthus)*. The product is provided in packages containing one vial of antivenin and one vial of diluent (bacteriostatic water). Sensitivity testing to horse serum should be conducted initially if practical. If the patient is not dangerously allergic to horse serum, the content of 3–5 vials (30–50 ml) are given by slow IV injection into tubing or by addition to an IV drip. The first 1–2 ml should be given in 3–5 minutes. If allergic symptoms are not evident, infusion should be continued at the maximum safe rate at which the IV fluid can be given until the full 30–50 ml has been given.

Antivenin latrodectus mactans is used for bites of the black widow spider. After testing for sensitivity to horse serum, the antivenin is reconstituted in 2.5 ml of sterile water and given by IV infusion in 10–50 ml of saline over 15 minutes.

Case Study: Immunizations

Mrs. D. A. was notified by the grade school that her 6-year-old son Joseph attends that a measles epidemic was occurring. D. A. called the nurse at the pediatric clinic to ask if she should bring Joseph and her other children in for shots. In addition to Joseph, D. A.'s children are Christine, 17 years old and attending high school, and Matthew, 1 year old, at home with his mother. Since both the younger children had been brought to this pediatric clinic since birth, the nurse was able to determine from the clinic records that Joseph's immunization schedule was entirely up to date and that he was fully protected. Matthew, on the other hand, had received only the three DPT and trivalent polio shots according to the standard schedule, at 2 months, 4 months, and 6 months. The nurse explained that infants do not normally receive measles-mumps-rubella (MMR) vaccination until 15 months of age, since younger children were at higher risk of adverse reactions such as fever. The nurse recommended that under the circumstances of the local epidemic, Matthew should receive a measles vaccination earlier than usual. The full MMR vaccination would be given at a later date.

The clinic had no records of vaccination for Christine. D. A. had several immunization forms that indicated that Christine had received vaccination for measles in 1967 at 2 years of age. The nurse asked D. A. if the record specified the type of vaccine and learned that Christine had received the killed virus type of immunization for measles. The nurse also determined that to the best of D. A.'s recollection, Christine had never had measles. The nurse explained to D. A. that this type of vaccine had not proved reliable and that Christine was probably not protected. D. A. stated that she had never heard of anyone as old as Christine having measles and that it would probably not be necessary for her to have the vaccination. The nurse informed D. A. that in recent years, measle epidemics have occurred with increasing frequency in late adolescence and the young adult years and that the disease is less well tolerated in this age group than in children. In addition, should Christine develop measles during pregnancy, there would be a risk of adverse effects to the fetus. Based on this information, D. A. agreed to bring Matthew and Christine in for vaccination.

Before administering the vaccine, the nurse asked if either of the children had allergies to eggs and if they were receiving any drugs (she asked about cortisone or other steroids in particular). She examined both Matthew and Christine for evidence of active infection. Speaking alone with Christine, the nurse told her that vaccination for measles should not be given during pregnancy and asked if there were any possibility that she was pregnant. Christine indicated that although she had been sexually active at times in the last year, she had not missed a period and had just had her period 1 week earlier. The nurse advised her that the vaccination could be harmful to the fetus if conception were to occur up to 2 months after inoculation. Christine indicated that she was not currently "going with" any particular boy and agreed that she would not have intercourse during the next 2 months without first establishing reliable contraception.

Christine and D. A. were told that mild soreness at the site of injection might be expected and possibly low-grade fever. Matthew might be irritable or fussy during the next 24 hours. If fever were to occur, Matthew could be given baby aspirin or baby acetaminophen. D. A. was warned not to exceed the recommended frequency or doses and told how to observe for symptoms of salicylate intoxication. D. A. was instructed to contact the pediatric clinic if the reaction to immunization were anything more severe. The nurse had one of the clinic's secretaries transpose the several partial records that D. A. had concerning Christine's immunization history onto one form and gave one copy to D. A. and filed another at the clinic. These activities took about 10 minutes following the immunizations, so the nurse asked D. A. to remain in the clinic waiting room for another 20 minutes for observation before leaving.

1. What is DPT vaccine? MMR vaccine?
2. If D. A. had indicated that Christine had definitely had measles as a child, would vaccination still be required?
3. Why is measles becoming more prevalent now in adolescence and young adult years? In what sense is it less well tolerated after puberty?
4. Why did the nurse inquire about allergies to eggs? Use of steroids?
5. What are the risks to the fetus if Christine becomes pregnant soon?
6. The request of D. A. that she stay a total of 30 minutes after the shots so the children could be observed is a precaution against occurrence of what kind of reaction?

Answers appear at the end of the book.

Recommended Readings

Conner CS: Literature analysis of influenza vaccine for 1981–1982. *Drug Intell Clin Pharm* 1981;15:913.

Feng CS: An immunization program for the geriatric patient. *Geriatrics* 1982;37(10):76–84.

Gurevich I: Viral hepatitis. *Am J Nurs* 1983;83(4):571–586.

Hayman LL: Varicella. *Nursing* 1983;13(4):41.

Hook EW: Typhoid fever today. *N Engl J Med* 1984;310(2):116–118.

Krugman S, Katz SL: Childhood immunization procedures. *JAMA* 1977;237:2228–2230.

Nichols AO: Taking the fear out of rabies treatment. *Nursing* 1983;13(6):42–43.

Selekman J: Immunization: What's it all about? *Am J Nurs* 1980;80:1440–1445.

CHAPTER 50

Drugs Used for Disorders of the Immune System

The body's ability to establish immunological resistance to foreign substances is a vital part of homeostasis and critical to the ability to stay healthy. There is a wide range of immunological competence, with resistance generally declining with age. Knowledge of the characteristics of altered immune responses, including the contribution of genetic and drug factors, is increasingly important to modern nursing.

Drugs bear a relationship to disorders of the immune system in two respects. On the positive side, drugs may be useful in the treatment or diagnosis of certain pathological conditions of the immune system. On the negative side, drugs are among the most frequent causes of hypersensitivity (allergic) reactions of all types. In this chapter we will examine the major disorders of the immune system with special reference to drug issues. Disorders of the immune system are divisible into two major groups: immunodeficiencies and hypersensitivities.

Immune Deficiency

Immune deficiency states are characterized by an increased vulnerability to infection, the immune system being one of the major mechanisms by which the body ordinarily protects itself from pathogenic microorganisms. There is a physiologically normal immunodeficiency in the fetus and in young infants because of incomplete development of immune capacity. Infants are dependent on maternally derived immunoglobulins, obtained by placental transfer and later breast-feeding, for immunological defense. In other circumstances, severe immunodeficiency is life-threatening or fatal. Immune deficiency states can be either nonspecific or specific. In the latter, there is a failure or reduced efficiency of one or both branches of the immune system: the B cells that mediate humoral immunity or the T cells that provide cell-mediated immunity. Nonspecific deficiencies occur when there are disturbances in immune-associated mechanisms such as the complement cascade, phagocytosis, or chemotaxis. Immunodeficiency may occur as a primary disorder or it may be secondary to a variety of medical disorders. In nephrotic syndrome, for example, gamma globulins may be lost in the urine to an extent that undermines humoral immunity. Immunosuppression may be caused by malignancy, malnutrition, aging, immunosuppressive drugs, and drugs that suppress the bone marrow. Cell-mediated immunity may exhibit diminished responsivity in Hodgkin's disease, leprosy, sarcoidosis, or miliary tuberculosis.

Cell-mediated immunity may be severely impaired (culminating in death from infection) when T cells are infected by a virus, leading to an **acquired immune deficiency syndrome** (AIDS). The occurrence of this condition has reached epidemic proportions in the United States in recent years. Ninety-four percent of victims are male. Promiscuous male homosexuals and bisexuals are at greatest risk, followed by Haitian refugees, individuals with hemophilia A, intravenous drug users, and users of volatile nitrites. Of the women who have acquired the condition, more than half are intravenous drug users and an additional 18% have male sexual partners who are intravenous drug users.

Most primary specific immunodeficiency states are hereditary, but intrauterine conditions that occur during fetal development are also important. Thus, the fetus exposed to rubella during the early months of development may exhibit selective deficiency of IgA at birth. Defects that affect only humoral immunity are **hypogammaglobulinemias.** Occasionally the condition is selective for one class of immunoglobulins. A program of replacement therapy with immune serum gamma globulins can be beneficial for patients with hypogammaglobulinemias. This preparation is discussed in Chapter 49. Complete deficiency of cell-mediated immunity due to congenital absence or hypoplasia of the thymus is called **DiGeorge syndrome.** This condition is almost always fatal in infancy; survival is possible only by complete isolation of the individual in a special aseptic chamber. Partial deficiencies of cell-mediated immunity are associated with recurrent infections. Combined deficiency of both the B cell and T cell components of the immune system generally reflect an absence of bone marrow precursor cells and is rapidly fatal if the deficiency is substantial or associated with frequent infections. Treatment of immune deficiency conditions is at best difficult. In addition to gamma globulin therapy (which provides only IgG), fresh frozen plasma transfusions can be employed to provide IgG, IgA, and IgM; lymphocytes from HLA-identical donors can be infused; bone marrow transplantation can be attempted in severe combined immunodeficiency; thymus implantation can be attempted in DiGeorge syndrome; or extracts of lymphocytes can be given subcutaneously for chronic mucocutaneous manifestations of T cell deficiency (chronic candidiasis, for example).

Hypersensitivity Reactions: Type I

The current classification of hypersensitivity reactions identifies four types. Types I, II, and III are produced by the humoral immune system; type IV by the T cells of cell-mediated immunity. Type I reactions are distinctive from the other types in that they are mediated by IgE and occur with great rapidity. Type I hypersensitivity reactions provide the greatest range of opportunity for chemotherapeutic intervention. Type I hypersensitivity reactions (Table 50–1) come closest to what the lay person thinks of when the term *allergy* is employed. The term **allergen** is reserved for antigens that evoke this type of hypersensitivity reaction. Many of the steps that are involved in type I reactions have been elucidated.

Table 50–1
Type I Hypersensitivity Reactions

Characteristics

IgE-mediated

Explosive onset

Antigen equals allergen (such as pollens, dust, food, animal dander, feathers, drugs)

Diagnostic tests: Skin scratch tests, elimination diets

Treatments: Avoidance, symptomatic relief, desensitization

Includes

Atopic allergies: Hay fever, asthma, hives, allergic rhinitis, conjunctivitis, rashes, drug eruptions

Anaphylaxis: Rapidly developing hypotension and shock from massive activation of mast cells, with itching, hives, asthmatic constriction of bronchioles, and GI distress. May be termed anaphylactic reaction when drug-induced.

The Type I Allergic Reaction

One unusual feature of type I reactions is that they develop almost explosively, in seconds or minutes after contact with an appropriate allergen. The body is in a sense primed for this rapid response. Preparation occurs during an initial exposure to an allergen and the allergic reaction occurs upon subsequent exposures.

Type I allergic reactions are closely related to one of the five classes of immunoglobulins — IgE. B lymphocytes capable of synthesizing a particular IgE antibody are coated with receptors that are a sample of the specific antibody that the cell is prepared to manufacture in quantity if activated. When an antigen is encountered that has binding sites that can attach to these surface receptors, the lymphocyte is stimulated to produce millions of molecules of its specific IgE (Figure 50–1). This does not, however, constitute the allergic reaction. The production and release of a specific IgE initiates the preparatory step that sets the stage for an allergic reaction when the specific antigen is next encountered. The IgE that is released during this preparatory stage attaches to two kinds of cells that are instrumental in type I allergic reactions: **mast cells** and **basophils.** These two kinds of cells are similar, except that mast cells are tissue cells while basophils are free-floating white blood cells. Mast cells are widely distributed throughout the body, in the skin, lymphoid organs, and in mucosal membranes of the eye, nose, mouth, respiratory tract, and intestines. Each mast cell possesses from 100,000 to 500,000 receptors for IgE molecules. The stems of the Y-shaped IgE molecules attach to the receptors of the mast cells and basophils and the two arms of the Y extend outward and the individual is primed for an allergic reaction when the allergenic substance is next encountered.

The allergic reaction is activated when an antigen forms a bridge between two adjacent IgE mole-

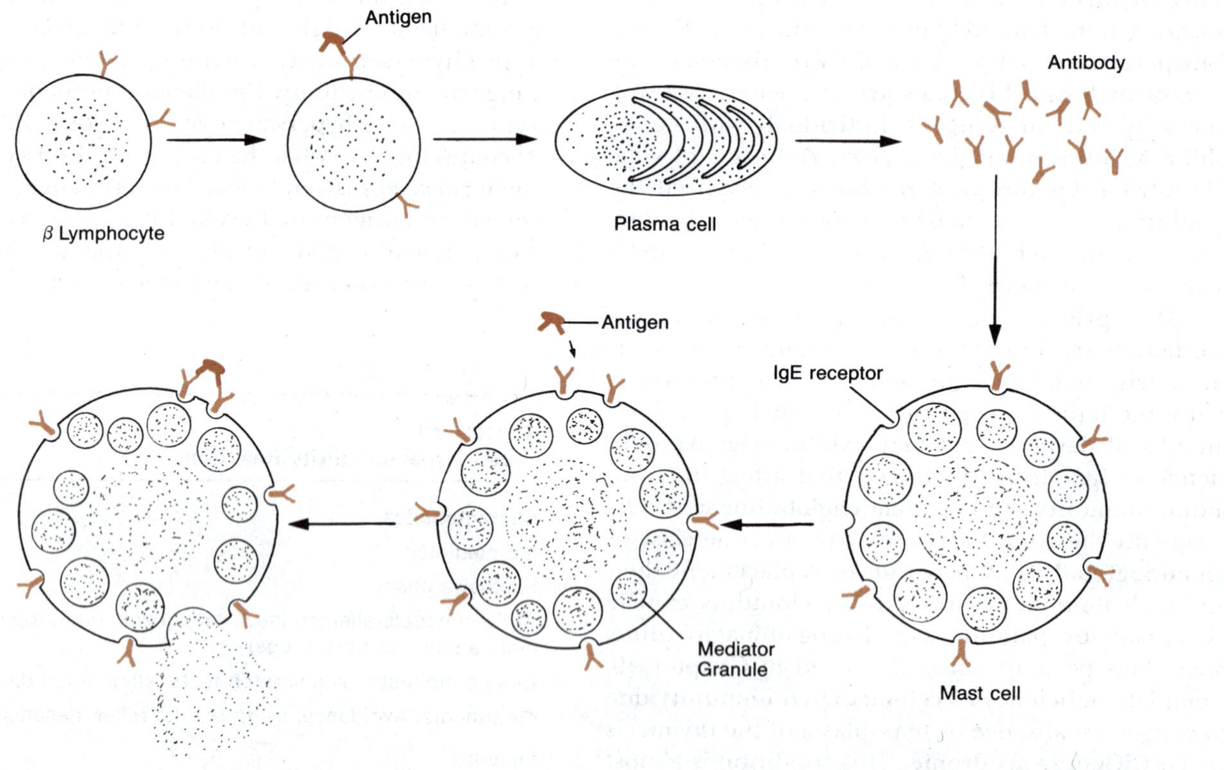

Figure 50–1
Events of a type I allergic reaction. When an IgE-producing B lymphocyte encounters an antigen that matches its specific immunoglobulin, it is transformed into a plasma cell that manufactures and releases its unique antibody. The IgE molecules travel through the blood to attach to mast cells. When next the same antigen is encountered, attachment of antigen to the IgE units on the mast cells triggers release of histamine and other mediators of inflammation.

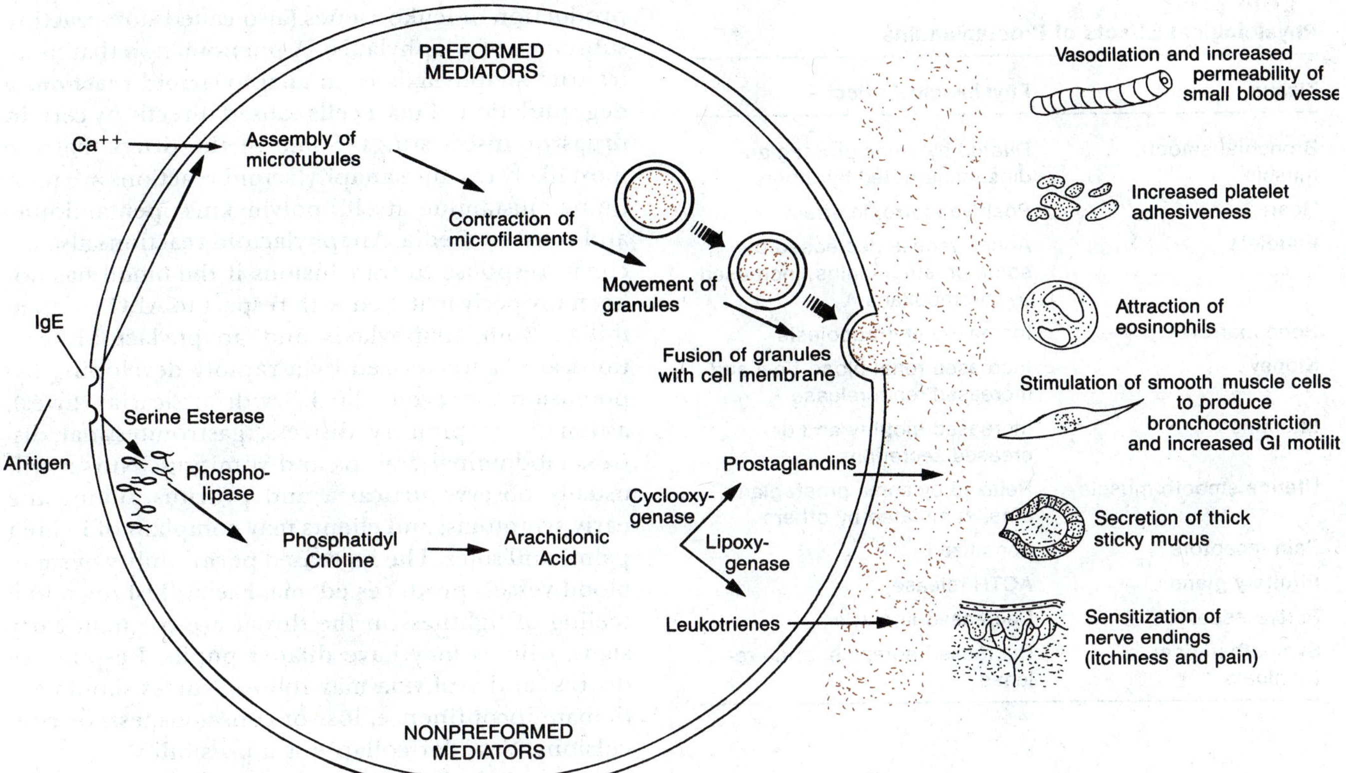

Figure 50–2
Mediators of type I allergic reactions.

cules protruding from the surface of a mast cell or basophil (Figure 50–2). Formation of this bridge activates an enzyme, called serine esterase, within the membrane of the mast cell or basophil. Serine esterase initiates a chain reaction that modifies the structure of the basophil or mast cell membrane, setting into motion events within these cells that ultimately lead to release of a variety of chemicals that are the mediators of the allergic response. The mediators of the allergic responses are of two types. One type consists of **preformed chemical mediators** that are stored within granules in the mast cells and basophils; the other type, **nonpreformed chemical mediators,** are produced only after the allergic reaction has begun.

The preformed mediators of immediate hypersensitivity reactions include histamine, serotonin, heparin, chemotaxic factors, and chemicals that activate phagocytic white blood cells. These substances are contained in about 1,000 granules within each mast cell and basophil. When one of these cells is activated by antigen, the preformed chemical mediators are released by exocytosis into the surrounding extracellular fluid. The exocytosis event (also called degranulation) is directed by a network of microtubules and microfilaments within the cell that control the movement of granules toward the outer cell membrane, ultimately promoting a fusion of the granule with the cytoplasmic membrane, leading to extrusion of the granular contents.

The nonpreformed chemical mediators are two classes of chemical substances called **prostaglandins** and **leukotrienes.** When the allergic reaction is triggered, enzymes are activated that break down the cell membrane, ultimately producing arachidonic acid. Arachidonic acid is converted (by the enzyme cyclooxygenase) to prostaglandins and (by the enzyme lipoxygenase) to leukotrienes. Prostaglandins are a large family of substances that produce a bewildering variety of effects on various bodily tissues (Table 50–2).

Taken together, the preformed chemical mediators, the prostaglandins, and the leukotrienes produce the manifestations of type I allergy. The principal targets of their activity are smooth muscle cells, small blood vessels, mucous glands, eosinophils,

Table 50–2
Physiological Effects of Prostaglandins

Tissue	Physiological effect
Bronchial smooth muscle	Dilated by some prostaglandins, constricted by others
Heart	Positive inotropic effect
Platelets	Adhesiveness decreased by some prostaglandins, increased by thromboxane A_2
Bone marrow	Increased erythropoiesis
Kidneys	Increased renal blood flow and increased renin release
Intestines	Increased motility and decreased secretions
Uterine smooth muscle	Relaxed by some prostaglandins, stimulated by others
Pain receptors	Sensitized
Pituitary gland	ACTH release
Fatty tissue	Decreased lipolysis
Sympathetic nerve terminals	Decreased norepinephrine release

platelets, and pain receptors of the skin. The overall effects of these mediators of allergy are constriction of the airways, stimulation of gastrointestinal motility, dilation and increased permeability of small blood vessels, stimulation of mucous glands to produce a thicker and stickier mucus, activation of phagocytic white blood cells, attraction of eosinophils, increased platelet adhesiveness, and sensitization of pain receptors resulting in itchiness or pain.

A variety of drugs can either modify degranulation or modify the action of one or another of the chemical mediators of immediate-type allergic reactions. **Sodium cromoglycate** inhibits calcium influx that is required for initiation of the activity of the microtubules that leads to degranulation. **Corticosteroids** and **beta-adrenergic agonists** (which elevate adenosine 3′ : 5′ cyclic phosphate, cyclic AMP, in mast cells) inhibit the contraction of the microfilaments necessary to direct movement of granules to the outer membrane. **Antihistamines** block the effects of released histamine, whereas **aspirin-like drugs** inhibit the formation of prostaglandins.

Anaphylaxis and Atopic Reactions

Type I allergic reactions can be localized (atopic), or they can be systemic. The systemic type I hypersensitivity reaction is called **anaphylaxis.** The reaction is attributable largely to release of histamine and production of leukotrienes (also called slow-reacting substance of anaphylaxis). A phenomenon that mimics true anaphylaxis is an **anaphylactoid reaction,** a degranulation of mast cells caused directly by certain drugs or insect stings. Some of the drugs that are most likely to cause anaphylactoid reactions are morphine, histamine itself, polymyxins, pentamidine, and contrast media. Anaphylactoid reactions also occur in response to transfusions if the blood has not been properly matched with respect to ABO compatibility. Both anaphylaxis and anaphylactoid reactions are characterized by a rapidly developing hypotension or even shock, with urticaria (hives), asthmatic respiratory distress, gastrointestinal distress (abdominal cramps and vomiting). Nurses will usually observe urticaria and pruritus among the early symptoms, and clients may complain of itching palms and soles. The increased permeability of small blood vessels produces edema. Facial flushing and a feeling of tightness in the throat are frequent early signs. Clients may have dilated pupils. Respiratory distress and asphyxia may follow. Nurses should anticipate incontinence, loss of consciousness, or convulsions. Vascular collapse is a possibility.

Anaphylaxis requires rapid treatment. If the client is receiving drug therapy, the medication should be stopped immediately. Epinephrine solution should be injected to counter the action of histamine on the blood vessels and bronchioles. Corticosteroids may be required to aid in the client's recovery following the attack. A patent airway must be maintained and oxygen may be used to counteract asphyxia.

Atopic allergic reactions are limited to a particular body tissue that has been exposed to the allergen: the skin, mucosal membranes, gastrointestinal tract, or the airways. The common atopic allergic reactions that nurses can expect to encounter include hay fever, asthma, allergic rhinitis, allergic conjunctivitis, hives, rashes, drug eruptions, and gastrointestinal irritation from food allergy.

Allergens

The substances that can act as allergens to precipitate type I allergic reactions include pollens, dust, certain foods, animal danders, feathers, and drugs. Although different individuals will have distinctive sensitivities to particular allergens, certain substances tend to be allergenic for a large number of people while other substances are seldom or never allergenic. Pollens produced by plants of the ragweed family are allergenic to millions of Americans, yet some equally abundant pollens, such as that produced by the nettle plant, do not produce allergic reactions. Dust is potentially allergenic because it provides a haven for the dust mite, *Dermatophagoides farinae,* a tiny organism that subsists on cutaneous scales shed by humans. Some individuals are allergic to the animal proteins found in the dander of household pets, or in feathers, wool, or other material of animal origin. The foods most likely to be allergenic include cow's milk, eggs, wheat, cirtrus fruits (especially grapefruit and oranges), melons, strawberries, corn, tomatoes, nuts, peanuts, fish, shellfish, chocolate, spices (such as cloves, mustard, or black pepper), and additives. Food allergies are less common, however, than allergies to airborne substances. Allergies to airborne substances occur in more than 10% of the population of the United States. Most drugs are not allergenic in most individuals for the simple reason that drugs are usually rather small molecules of only modest chemical activity. Drug preparations, such as serums and vaccines, that contain animal protein are most frequently allergenic. Serums cause allergic reactions in about 10% of treated individuals. Most other drugs are allergenic only by their ability to act as haptens. A **hapten** is a small molecule that can attach to a bodily protein (the **carrier**), thereby producing an allergenic complex. In effect, the immunological reaction is directed against a hapten-modified host protein. Most drug eruptions are atopic skin allergies produced in this way.

It is not entirely understood why some individuals are allergic to a large number of substances, some to only a few, and others not at all. It is clear that a hereditary factor influences allergenicity, but it has been estimated that 18% of the population carries the gene or genes for allergy yet allergy is manifested in only about 40% of these carriers. Children with two allergenic parents have a nearly 60% chance of being allergenic; those with one allergenic parent have a nearly 40% chance; but even those with no allergenic parents have a greater than 10% chance of being allergenic.

A second factor that contributes to allergenicity is the type of feeding received by infants. Individuals who were bottle-fed as infants have nearly double the likelihood of developing allergies as individuals who were fed only on mother's milk during earliest infancy. The increased incidence of allergies in bottle-fed infants applies not only to gastrointestinal allergies but to other kinds of type 1 allergies as well. The connecting link between bottle-feeding and allergies is probably the incidence of gastrointestinal infections. Breast-fed infants have a lower incidence of gastrointestinal infections because mother's milk provides antibodies that confer protection against potentially pathogenic viruses and bacteria. Other studies have established that occurrence of gastrointestinal infections during infancy predisposes to allergies, perhaps by allowing undue exposure to foreign proteins that are able to transverse an intestinal mucosa that has been compromised by infection.

Allergy Testing

A convenient method for identifying the allergen responsible for allergenic reactions of an individual is the **direct skin test.** Skin tests are performed using extracts prepared from common allergens such as windborne pollens, animal dander, house dust, allergenic foods, molds, insect venums, horse serum, or drugs. The test solutions can be applied to scratches in the skin, injected intradermally, or applied by pricking the skin with a needle through a drop of extract. Control tests are conducted with diluent and histamine or morphine. The latter two drugs provide positive controls to test the reactivity of the site selected. Allergenic substances typically produce wheal and flare reactions within 15–20 minutes after application. Less commonly, sensitivity testing is conducted at other tissue sites, including nasal challenge, opthalmic testing, or bronchial inhalation. Numerous commercial diagnostic allergenic extracts are available from Barry, Hollister-Stier, Berkeley Biologics, Greer Laboratories, and Dome.

Treatment of Type I Hypersensitivity Reactions

There are three approaches to treatment of type I allergies: avoidance of the allergen, symptomatic relief, or desensitization therapy. **Avoidance,** which consists of eliminating contact with the allergen, is the best approach when it is feasible. If the allergenic substance is a specific food, a drug, or a dander from a household pet, avoidance is often a viable approach. Frequent damp dusting and damp mopping may provide some relief if the allergen is the dust mite. Vacuuming may be more effective in removing dusts and pollens than sweeping or dusting in some cases. Pollens are more difficult to avoid, but some locales have lower pollen counts than others.

Symptomatic relief entails the use of mainly two classes of drugs, antihistamines, and sympathomimetics (see Chapter 28). Corticosteroids have limited value, being excluded from use in conditions that are either mild or long-lasting. They are reserved for antiallergic purposes for the treatment of severe, self-limited reactions such as seasonal asthma, reactions to bee stings, severe contact dermatitis, serum sickness, or infiltrative lung disease.

Desensitization Therapy

Desensitization (immunotherapy) entails the subcutaneous administration (in the lateral aspect of the arm) of gradually escalating doses of an allergenic extract. Injections are never given intramuscularly or intravenously. The principle behind this form of therapy is the stimulation of production of IgG antibodies for the antigenic substance, which act as blocking antibodies, competing with the IgE receptors for the antigen. Effective immunotherapy depends on generating at least a twofold increase in neutralizing IgG antibodies. Levels of IgE, on the other hand, may rise initially during therapy, but ultimately fall if therapy is successful. Antigen-triggered release of histamine from basophils falls by 50% or more in successful treatment.

Desensitization therapy is indicated only for bee stings and airborne allergens that cannot be avoided and only when the severity of the allergy is great. The allergens employed in desensitization protocols include pollens, house dust, molds, and venoms. Animal dander desensitization is employed only for individuals unable to avoid exposure due to occupational requirements (such as veterinarians or researchers handling laboratory animals).

Desensitization therapy is initiated with dilute concentrations such as 1 part in 10^8 up to 1 part in 10^5. The once weekly injections are gradually increased in concentration until the maximum tolerated dose is reached. Desensitization is maintained thereafter by a maintenance schedule of injections, typically once per month. Injections given year round provide optimum benefit even if contact with the allergen is seasonal. Dosage adjustments may have to be made if local reactions are severe, if systemic reactions occur, if a new extract product is employed, or during contact if environmental sources of the allergen is temporarily elevated (as during the pollen season if the allergen is a pollen).

After administration of an allergenic extract, the client should be observed for at least 1 hour, since the most severe reactions occur within this time period. Adverse reactions may indicate that the dose was incorrectly calculated, that the dose was incremented too rapidly, or, during initial therapy, that the individual's sensitivity is unusually great. Adverse reactions range from mild to life-threatening. When clients complain of mild soreness, swelling, and redness at the site of injection, nurses should reassure them that such reactions are to be expected. However, nurses must also warn clients that excessively large, painful, or persistent reactions sometimes occur. An **Arthus reaction** may occur in which tissue at the site of injection undergoes a sequence of inflammation, edema, abscess, gangrene, necrosis, and sloughing. Nurses can expect systemic symptoms to include swelling of the entire extremity into which the allergen has been injected. Clients may also develop urticaria, pruritus, edema, joint or muscle pain, wheezing, dyspnea, sneezing, cough, hoarseness, fever, chills, dizziness, headache, nausea, throat tightness, tachycardia, flushing, cyanosis, lacrimation, and perspiration. Life-threatening allergic manifestations include anaphylactic shock, serum sickness, neurological reactions, and renal disease.

Mild reactions such as slowly developing urticaria can be treated with an antihistamine. Rapidly developing reactions of moderate severity such as sneezing, asthma-like reactions, flushing, and pruritus are treated with epinephrine given subcutaneously (0.1–1.0 mg, SQ or IM, in the arm opposite from the one in which the allergen was injected) and a double dose of an oral antihistamine. A tourniquet may be applied to the arm above the injection site but should be released briefly every 10–15 minutes. Reactions of anaphylaxis are treated first by volume expansion with intravenous fluids followed by epinephrine (1–2.5 ml of a 1 : 10,000 solution IV over 10 minutes). Oxygen and artificial respiration may be required and should be available whenever desensitization therapy is undertaken. Antihistamine or corticosteroids may be utilized after blood pressure has been stabilized sufficiently. A bronchodilator may be required to alleviate respiratory distress. Desensitization therapy should be considered as a last resort and should be undertaken only by physicians experienced in administering allergens.

When desensitization therapy is conducted for clients allergic to hymenoptera venom (from stings of bees, wasps, or yellow jackets), nurses should warn the clients that they can have severe reactions to stings in spite of desensitization therapy. *The nurse should advise such individuals to carry an emergency supply of epinephrine for subcutaneous self-administration and should make certain that the client and a responsible member of the client's family know how to use it. The nurse should alert the client to the need to carry a card stating that he or she is allergic to insect stings and indicating what should be done immediately in the event of stinging.* The older method of desensitization using whole body hymenoptera insect preparations has been supplanted by hymenoptera venom extract (Albay, Pharmalgen Treatment Kit). Treatment can be conducted using individual venoms (from honeybee, yellow jacket, yellow hornet, white-faced hornet, or wasp) or a mixed vespid venom preparation (from the yellow jacket, yellow hornet, and white-faced hornet).

When clients have known hypersensitivity to insect stings or bites, the best therapy is prevention.

Nurses should instruct susceptible clients to avoid wearing perfumes and bright colors, since these attract insects. Clients should be instructed to avoid excessive exposure of the skin, especially the neck. The client may have to wear high-necked clothing, scarves, or other clothing accessories. Clients should be warned to avoid sitting or lying on the grass or in areas where there are bushes, flowers, shrubs, or trees and they should not go barefoot.

Histamine and Antihistamines

The hypersensitivity reactions of the immediate type (type I) occur with considerable frequency, and their management by chemical interventions is a major medical concern. Until the 1940s, the only drugs available for treatment of allergies, anaphylaxis, asthma, and related conditions were those that were effective in alleviating such symptoms of allergy as blood vessel dilation and bronchial constriction. For example, epinephrine was used both to constrict blood vessels and to dilate the bronchioles.

During the 1920s and 1930s, it became apparent that an important mediator of allergic reactions was the widely distributed endogenous autacoid called **histamine.** We now know that histamine is but one of several mediators of immediate-type allergic reactions. Research in the 1920s and 1930s culminated in 1937 in the development of a specific antihistaminic drug. The first clinically useful antihistamines appeared in Europe in 1942 and in the United States in 1945–1946. The first two antihistamines introduced in the United States, diphenhydramine (Benadryl) and tripelennamine (PBZ), continue to be used today, along with some 20 other drugs in this group.

The pharmacology and clinical applications of antihistamines are entirely attributable to their ability to antagonize the actions of histamine. Antihistamines occupy, and thereby block, the receptors for histamine, preventing access to the autacoid to its receptors. Thus, the effects of antihistaminic drugs are indirect, reflecting only a decreased activity of histamine in bodily tissues.

Histamine

Distribution and Release of Histamine

Histamine is widely distributed throughout the body, being found in highest concentrations in the lungs, skin, intestines, and stomach — four areas that are exposed to environmental chemicals and pathogens. A large percentage of histamine is associated with mast cells and with basophils, the cells involved in generating type I allergic reactions. Within these cells, histamine is stored in granules, together with heparin, hydrolytic enzymes, and the other preformed chemical mediators of type I hypersensitivity reactions. An additional pool of histamine is found in the brain, contained within nerve cells, where histamine may be acting as a neurotransmitter.

Release of histamine from mast cells and basophils can be triggered by allergens acting on IgE surface receptors of the histamine-containing cells, by agents causing tissue damage, or by drugs that promote degranulation directly without cell damage (Table 50–3). Horse serum is an example of an agent that produces histamine release by an IgE-mediated hypersensitivity reaction.

Table 50–3
Releasers of Histamine

Type I Hypersensitivity Reactions (Anaphylactic or Atopic)	
Allergens acting on IgE receptors	Horse serum, pollens, dander, house dust, certain foods
Anaphylactoid Reactions	
Cytotoxic agents	Mechanical, thermal, chemical, or radiant insult; venoms
Enzymes	Phospholipase A_2, chymotrypsin, eosinophil peroxidase
Polysaccharides	Dextran, dextrin, mannan
Lectins	Canavalin A, others
Anaphylatoxins	Polypeptide cleavage fragments from complement proteins
Basic drugs	
Alpha-blockers	Phentolamine, tolazoline
Anticholinergics	Atropine
Antimicrobials	
Diamidines	Pentamidine, propamidine, stilbamidine
Other	Quinine
Antineoplastics	Bleomycin
Ganglionic blockers	Trimethaphan
Narcotics	Codeine, meperidine, morphine, nalorphine
Neuromuscular blockers	Atracurium, decamethonium, metocurine, pancuronium, succinylcholine, *d*-tubocurarine
Spasmolytic	Dimethyl sulfoxide (DMSO)
Stimulants	Amphetamine, strychnine
Monoamines	Phenylalanine, tyramine
Basic polypeptides	Polymyxin B, bradykinin, substance P, neurotensin, somatostatin, protamine, ACTH, PTH
Basic amino acids	Arginine, lysine, carnosine, ornithine
Electrolytes	Calcium

Drugs that produce degranulation directly (not as a result of an allergic reaction) include several that are widely employed. The polysaccharide dextran, often used as a plasma expander, can cause histamine release. Frequently drugs, polypeptides, or amino acids that are bases release histamine. Three of the neuromuscular blocking drugs, *d*-tubocurarine, succinylcholine, and decamethonium, are basic drugs and histamine releasers. Among the narcotics, morphine, codeine, nalorphine, and meperidine (Demerol) release histamine. Antimicrobials that cause histamine release include polymyxin B (Neosporin), quinine, and the diamidine group of antiprotozoal drugs (stilbamidine, pentamidine (Pentam 300), and propamidine). Other drugs causing histamine release include amphetamine, atropine, papaverine, strychnine, and the alpha-blockers, tolazoline (Priscoline) and phentolamine (Regitine). Severe reactions caused by massive histamine release by nonallergic mechanisms are called **anaphylactoid reactions.**

Histamine Receptors

The actions of histamine in the body are mediated by two distinct classes of receptors, called H_1- and H_2-receptors. The major effects of histamine — bronchoconstriction, increased permeability of venules, and sensitization of sensory nerve endings (causing itchiness) — are brought about by H_1-receptors (Table 50–4). Gastric acid secretion and cardiac stimulation are H_2-receptor effects. Both H_1- and H_2-receptors contribute to capillary dilation. H_2-receptors predominate in the central nervous system (although these receptors can be blocked by large doses of H_1-blocking antihistamines) and are linked with adenylate cyclase and promote formation of cyclic AMP.

Table 50–4
Histamine Receptors Mediating the Various Effects of Histamine

Histamine effect	Type of receptor
Vascular Effects	
Capillary dilation	H_1 and H_2
Increased permeability of venules	H_1
Cardiac Effects	
Increased force of contraction	H_1 and H_2
Increased heart rate effect	H_2
Slowed AV conduction	H_1
Visceral Smooth Muscle	
Bronchoconstriction	H_1
Intestinal stimulation	H_1
Exocrine Glands	
Gastric acid secretion	H_2
Minor stimulatory effect on salivary, lacrimal, pancreatic, intestinal, and bronchial exocrine glands	H_1 and H_2
Nervous System	
Stimulation or sensitization of peripheral nerve endings	H_1
Cyclic AMP accumulation in brain	H_2

Effects of Histamine

Histamine is mainly important for its role as an endogenous substance (although the effects of administered histamine provide an indication of the roles performed by endogenous histamine). The influences of histamine can be grouped into several categories, including effects on the vascular system, the heart, the smooth muscle, the exocrine glands, and the nervous system.

In the vascular system, histamine **dilates blood vessels,** resulting in a decrease in peripheral resistance and flushing, and **increases the permeability of venules**. The dilatory effect involves principally the finer blood vessels and is most obvious in the region of the face and upper body involved in the blush response. Dilation of cranial blood vessels can result in vascular headache. Vasodilation caused by histamine is mediated by both H_1- and H_2-receptors. It can be fully blocked by simultaneous administration of both an H_1-blocker and an H_2-blocker but not by either type alone. In large part, the increase in permeability is due to a shrinkage of the endothelial cells that line the vessels. This creates gaps between the cells where plasma can seep through the basement membranes of the vessels and accumulate in the surrounding tissues to create edema and increased lymph flow. Increased permeability of venules in response to histamine is mainly if not entirely an action mediated by the H_1-receptor. The vascular effects of histamine contribute to the process of inflammation.

Histamine causes **cardiac stimulation.** Histamine increases the force of contraction (an H_1- and H_2-receptor effect) and the heart rate (an H_2-receptor effect) and slows atrioventricular conduction (an H_1-receptor effect).

The most important effect of histamine on the smooth muscle is **bronchoconstriction.** Clients with asthma or chronic obstructive pulmonary disease are especially susceptible to this action. Histamine-induced constriction of bronchial smooth muscle can have fatal consequences. Bronchoconstriction caused by histamine is mediated by H_1-receptors. Smooth muscle in other tissues is much less affected by histamine. For example, histamine increases contractile activity of the intestines to a modest extent.

Exocrine glands are stimulated by histamine acting on H_2-receptors. The most important influence in this category is the powerful effect of histamine on **secretion of gastric acid,** an effect interdependent with the influence of acetylcholine on these cells. It appears that acetylcholine sensitizes gastric secretory cells to the influence of histamine.

Within the brain, histamine acts as a **neurotransmitter.** It is concentrated in and around the hypothalamus and in afferent pathways to the cerebral cortex and hippocampus. Most of the histamine receptors in the brain are of the H_2-type. However, large doses of H_1-receptor blockers can inhibit effects of histamine at these H_2-receptors in the brain. Histamine also has an influence on peripheral nerve endings. Histamine-induced **sensitization of peripheral nerve endings** produces itching sensations when the autocoid is injected intradermally or released in atopic allergies.

The roles of endogenous histamine, to the extent that they are understood, relate most especially to inflammation and type I (immediate) hypersensitivity reactions. With respect to inflammation, histamine is important for promoting accumulation of blood at a site of injury or microbial invasion and for promoting capillary permeability that allows phagocytic blood cells to mass in the area of inflammation. The nature of the inflammatory mechanism is described more fully in Chapter 45. With respect to type I allergic reactions, histamine stored in mast cells and basophils shares with the other chemical mediators of allergy the responsibility for producing the tissue responses such as bronchoconstriction and sensitization of nerve endings that comprise type I hypersensitivity reactions.

H_1-Histamine Blockers

Histamine itself acts as an agonist on both H_1- and H_2-receptors, but the two classes respond differently to many other drugs. All histamine antagonists developed between 1937 and 1972 were active exclusively at H_1-receptors. The first H_2-receptor blockers were produced in 1972 and cimetidine was the first approved for clinical practice in 1977. Because for 40 years the term *antihistamine* meant a drug that could block effects of histamine at H_1-receptors, it remains force of habit to refer to the classical H_1-antagonists simply as antihistamines, while the newer H_2-antagonists are known by their more precise designation as H_2-blockers. H_2-blockers are discussed in Chapter 51 as antiulcer drugs. This chapter deals only with the H_1-blockers.

Pharmacological Effects The classical antihistamines block all of the H_1-mediated effects of histamine, without altering its release or preventing its H_2-mediated actions. H_1-blockers do not produce direct effects of their own except to the extent that a given antihistamine may possess other properties in addition to the antihistaminic action. The nature and extent of the clinical response to antihistamines depends in large measure on the level of histamine activity preexisting at the time of administration of the drug.

H_1-blockers antagonize the smooth muscle stimulatory effects of histamine. Antihistamines produce **bronchodilation** only when the bronchioles are constricted in response to histamine. Bronchodilation is accomplished less rapidly with antihistamines than with β_2-sympathomimetics. **Relaxation of the gut** occurs in response to H_1-antihistamines, but there is no significant change in secretion of gastric acid since this is a H_2-mediated effect.

H_1-blockers substantially but incompletely **reverse vasodilation caused by histamine.** The reason that the antagonism is incomplete is that capillary dilation caused by histamine is mediated through both H_1- and H_2-receptors. Concurrent administration of an H_2-blocker with the H_1-blocker will completely reverse histamine-induced vasodilation. The **reversal of capillary permeability** achieved by H_1-blockers is more complete, since this is largely an H_1-mediated effect of histamine. The edema associated with histamine effects on capillary permeability is likewise reversed.

Histamine sensitization of peripheral nerve endings is prevented by H_1-blockers. Antihistamines are **antipruritic** to the extent that they alleviate histamine-induced itch. As a result, antihistamines inhibit the flare stage of the triple response of inflammation, which depends upon stimulation of sensory nerve endings by histamine.

In type I hypersensitivity reactions, H_1-blockers alleviate only that part of the response that is caused by histamine release from mast cells and basophils. Effects attributable by the other chemical mediators of allergy are not attenuated by antihistamines. Thus, edema and itch are substantially eliminated by antihistamines, but allergic bronchoconstriction (largely produced by a leukotriene) and hypotension (mainly produced by prostaglandins and leukotrienes) are little altered. Anaphylactoid reactions produced by histamine-releasing drugs respond very well to treatment with antihistamines, but anaphylaxis produced through activation of IgE receptors does not respond satisfactorily to antihistamines alone.

In the central nervous system, the usual response to antihistamines is CNS depression that varies in accordance with drug selection and dose from a mild sedation to intense depression and somnolence. There is also individual variability. With continued use, the extent of CNS depression tends to diminish. CNS depression produced by antihistamines is additive to that produced by other CNS depressants, such as alcohol, sedative-hypnotics, neuroleptics, anxiolytics, and narcotics.

Less commonly, antihistamines elicit indications of increased CNS excitability, such as restlessness, nervousness, or insomnia. Antihistamines lower the seizure threshold and may initiate seizure activity in seizure-prone individuals. Dizziness and tremors are occasional CNS reactions. CNS excitability is most likely to occur when toxic doses are employed.

Many, but not all, of the H_1-blockers possess substantial anticholinergic as well as antihistaminic activity. For example, the ethanolamine group of antihistamines have anticholinergic properties equivalent to those of atropine, but the ethylenediamine group is essentially devoid of anticholinergic activity. Antihistamines with anticholinergic properties are useful in parkinsonism. They produce additional adverse reactions attributable to the blockade of cholinergic receptors, including dryness of mouth, blurred vision, urinary retention, and the other symptoms of the anticholinergic syndrome. Anticholinergic effects of these drugs are potentially additive with those of other anticholinergic substances and are increased by concurrent use of MAO inhibitors.

Pharmacokinetics After oral administration, H_1-blockers are well absorbed. Onset of action occurs in 15–30 minutes, peak effect develops in 1–2 hours, and the action subsides in 3–6 hours for most of the agents. Inactivation of antihistamines is mainly by hepatic metabolism.

Clinical Indications H_1-blockers are used orally and parenterally for a wide variety of purposes. Antihistamines are used orally for alleviation of symptoms associated with type I hypersensitivity reactions. H_1-blockers provide dramatic relief of the symptoms of perennial or seasonal **allergic rhinitis** or **allergic conjunctivitis** such as reactions caused by hay fever or ragweed allergies. They are especially effective in this application if taken prophylactically — before substantial contact with the allergen. H_1-blockers are highly effective in acute **urticaria** (hives) and **angiodermatitis** and less effective but helpful in chronic urticaria.

Antihistamines are employed orally or parenterally as adjuncts in the treatment of **anaphylaxis** and **anaphylactoid** reactions. Epinephrine and supportive measures take precedence over administration of antihistamines. Antihistamines provide more benefit in anaphylactoid reactions than in anaphylaxis, since most symptoms of anaphylactoid reactions are attributable to histamine release whereas symptoms of anaphylaxis involve numerous chemical mediators in addition to histamine.

Many of the antihistamines are effective for nausea associated with **motion sickness.** Though less effective than scopolamine in motion sickness, the antihistamines such as promethazine (Phenergan) and cyclizine (Marazine) offer a longer duration of action and fewer side effects than scopolamine. *The first dose is given 30 minutes before departure for travel.* Caution must be exercised in using antihistamines for the nausea of early pregnancy, since some of those used as antinausea agents are teratogenic.

Diphenhydramine (Benadryl) is often the antihistamine selected for parenteral applications requiring a potent agent. Diphenhydramine is a useful alternative to benztropine (Cogentin) or trihexyphenidyl (Artane) as an **antiparkinsonian** agent. However, current evidence suggests that the value of diphenhydramine in parkinsonism can be attributed to its anticholinergic rather than its antihistaminic properties. Antihistamines have been employed in **migraine,** but their value is limited to the nonspecific benefit provided by mild sedation.

Antihistamines are used as **sleep-aids** in nonprescription preparations. Generally the antihistamines that are most likely to cause sedation are selected for this application. Sleep-aids are discussed in Chapter 13.

The most frequent use of antihistamines is as a component of many nonprescription **cold formulations.** Histamine is released during common colds in response to cellular injury caused by viral invasion as part of the inflammatory response to infection and tissue damage. Use of antihistamines in coryza does not hasten the elimination of the infection, but it may suppress symptoms attributable to activity of histamine.

Adverse Effects and Contraindications Adverse effects of antihistamines are commonplace but usually not severe. **Allergic reactions** occur rarely to all of the antihistamines, more commonly when they are applied topically to the skin or administered parenterally than when they are taken orally. Allergic manifestations include rash, urticaria, photosensitiv-

Nursing Observations for Treatment of Type I Allergic Reactions with Antihistamines

THERAPEUTIC GOAL	Alleviate allergic manifestations such as hypotension, skin eruption, itching, or respiratory distress.
PREADMINISTRATION ASSESSMENT	
Baseline Data	Observe presence of wheezing, rhinitis, conjunctivitis, hives, angioderma, rash, fainting, or dizziness. Evaluate blood pressure, pulse, perfusion, respiratory rate and sounds, constriction of nares, bowel sounds, abdominal swelling, urinary output, skin lesions, and neurological function.
Contraindications/ Precautions	Check medical history for contraindications for specific antihistamines, including gastrointestinal or bladder obstructions, glaucoma, prostatic hypertrophy, pregnancy, or lactation. Check medication history for allergies to antihistamines or tartrazine (contained in some antihistamine products).
Potential Interactions	Check current medications for use of CNS depressants, anticholinergic agents, sympathomimetics, or MAO inhibitors.
EVALUATION OF DRUG RESPONSE	
For Therapeutic Benefit	Monitor for alleviation and prevention of allergic manifestations.
For Adverse Effects	Assess for gastrointestinal irritation, sedation, anticholinergic side effects (thickening of respiratory mucus, urinary retention, dry mouth, or aggravation of glaucoma).
For Drug Interactions	Monitor additive CNS depression, additive gastrointestinal irritation, and additive anticholinergic properties.
For Dietary Interactions	Monitor for additive CNS depression with alcohol.
For Compliance	Evaluate the client's compliance with all facets of the therapeutic regimen by careful observation, interviewing, and review of progress. Report compliance problems to the physician and act as client-advocate when changes in the therapeutic regimen seem indicated.

ity, diaphoresis, chills, and anaphylactic shock. Known hypersensitivity to antihistamines is a specific contraindication for their use.

The most common adverse effect of antihistamines is **CNS depression.** All antihistamines produce a degree of sedation; some produce outright somnolence. The ethanolamines produce the greatest degree of CNS depression; ethylenediamines somewhat less; alkylamines and piperazine produce very little. *Clients taking antihistamines should be warned that operation of a motor vehicle or machinery may be hazardous and that the depressant effects are additive with those of alcohol and other CNS depressants.*

Antihistamines may cause **gastrointestinal disturbances,** including nausea, vomiting, diarrhea, constipation, and epigastric distress. The incidence of gastrointestinal symptoms is greatest for the ethylenediamines, less for the alkylamines, and least with the ethanolamines. *Administration of antihistamines with meals reduces gastrointestinal disturbances.* Some clients on chronic regimens experience anorexia or conversely increased appetite and weight gain. Antihistamines are contraindicated for clients with pyloric obstruction.

Other side effects are relatively uncommon. Antihistamines can cause blurred vision and diplopia and should be avoided in individuals with narrow angle glaucoma. The drying effect of antihistamines may result in thickening and drying of the sputum in the bronchioles. For this reason, antihistamines should be avoided in asthmatic clients. *Dry mouth may occur but can be alleviated by rinsing the mouth, chewing gum, or sucking lemon drops.* Antihistamines can cause urinary frequency, urinary retention, or difficult urination and should be avoided by individuals with obstruction of the bladder neck or prostatic hypertrophy. Adverse cardiac effects can include hypotension, palpitations, tachycardia, and extrasystoles. Hemolytic reactions can occur, most commonly in clients with glucose-6-phosphate dehydrogenase deficiency. *Patients on long-term therapy with antihistamines should be given periodic blood tests with complete blood cell counts.*

Neurological side effects other than sedation include dizziness, vertigo, tinnitus, acute labyrinthitis, paresthesias, tremor, and convulsions. *Neurological side effects associated with overdose, including convulsions and possibly culminating in death, are especially likely in infants and children. Warn clients to keep antihistamines out of the reach of children.* CNS stimulatory effects are most pronounced with the alkylamine group and phenindamine. Possible psychiatric side effects are confusion, restlessness, excitation, nervousness, irritability, insomnia, euphoria, and hysteria.

Antihistamines are contraindicated for use by nursing mothers and should be avoided during pregnancy. Teratogenicity has been attributed to some of the antihistamines, especially the piperazine group. Others have not been linked specifically to teratogenic effects but on the other hand have not been established as safe for use in pregnancy. Antihistamines present risks to the neonate as well as the fetus.

Because antihistamines suppress the emetic response, toxicity of poisons that normally induce vomiting may be increased. *Nurses need to warn clients who use antihistamines that these drugs may mask the usual signs of toxicity from poisons, such as nausea, vomiting, and ototoxicity.*

The phenothiazine antihistamines may cause adverse reactions not shared by other antihistamines: allergic jaundice, extrapyramidal reactions, and orthostatic hypotension. Phenothiazine antihistamines should be avoided in clients with a history of cardiovascular disease, liver dysfunction, or ulcers.

Elderly individuals are especially liable to certain side effects of antihistamines. These include sedation, confusion, dizziness, extrapyramidal reactions, and hypotension. Dosage may need to be lowered in older clients.

Classes and Preparations of Antihistamines

The classes of antihistamines differ somewhat in their clinical applications (Table 50–5) and in the incidence of adverse effects, including CNS depression, gastrointestinal disturbances, anticholinergic effects, and teratogenicity (Table 50–6). Almost all of the antihistamines are marketed for treatment of atopic allergies (marked by urticaria, allergic rhinitis, and so on) and many have additional uses. Doses and dosing intervals are given in Table 50–5.

Ethanolamines

Diphenhydramine (Benadryl), one of the oldest of the antihistamines, is the prototype of the ethanolamine group. The ethanolamine drugs produce the highest degree of drowsiness of any of the antihistamines and have the most severe anticholinergic side effects. Nearly 50% of individuals given normal doses experience somnolence. This action is put to beneficial effect when doxylamine or diphenhydramine are used in sleep-aid preparations. Carbinoxamine is less depressant than other drugs in this group. On the positive side, ethanolamines seldom produce gastrointestinal disturbances. Although it is recommended that all antihistamines be avoided during pregnancy, dimenhydrinate (Dramamine), a member of the ethanolamine group, is considered an acceptable risk for use in treating nausea and vomiting of pregnancy for women unwilling to tolerate the inconvenience. The anticholinergic properties of diphenhydramine make it a useful drug for treatment of parkinsonism. This drug has also been noted to have substantial antitussive efficacy.

Preparations and Administration

Bromodiphenhydramine (Ambodryl)
Tablets

Carbinoxamine (Clistin)
Tablets, repeat action tablets, elixir

Clemastine (Tavist)
Tablets

Dimenhydrinate (Dramamine, others)
Tablets, oral liquid, suppositories, injection solution

Diphenhydramine (Benadryl and others)
Capsules, tablets, syrups, elixir, injection solutions

Doxylamine
Tablets (Decapryn) for allergies, tablets (Unisom) as a sleep-aid, syrup

Ethylenediamines

The ethylenediamines provide the greatest specificity of action at H_1-receptors. For example, pyrilamine (Allertoc) is 40,000 times more potent at H_1-receptors than at muscarinic receptors for acetylcholine. The extent of CNS depression is less than that produced by ethanolamines but is still substantial. In fact, pyrilamine, a member of this group, is used as a sleep-aid. Drugs in this group find use in topical preparations for the skin (pyrilamine or tripelennamine (PBZ) for relief of itching) and for the eye (antazoline or pyrilamine for allergic conjunctivitis). Gastrointestinal reactions are more common with ethylenediamines than with any other group of antihistamines.

Table 50–5

Antihistamine Uses and Regimens

	Applications											Regimens	
Drug	**Atopic Allergies**	**Anaphylaxis and Serum Sickness**	**Colds**	**Antinausea**	**Motion Sickness**	**Antitussive and Antiparkinsonian**	**Topical for Allergic Conjunctivitis**	**Topical Antipruritic**	**Oral Antipruritic**	**Sedation**	**Sleep aid**	**Dose (mg)**	**Dosing Interval (hour)**
Ethanolamines													
Bromodiphenhydramine	+											25	4–6
Carbinoxamine	+		+									4–8	6–8
Clemastine	+											1.34	12
Dimenhydrinate				+	+							50	4
Diphenhydramine	+	+			+	+		+		+	+	25–50	6–8
Doxylamine	+										+	12.5–25	4–6
Phenyltoloxamine	+		+					+				50	4–6
Ethylenediamines													
Antazoline							+					0.5% solution	3–4
Pyrilamine	+		+				+	+			+	25–50	6
Thonzylamine	+											50–100	4–6
Tripelennamine	+		+					+				25–50	4–6
Alkylamines													
Brompheniramine	+	+	+									4–8	6–8
Chlorpheniramine	+	+	+									4	4–6
Dexchlorpheniramine	+		+									2	4–6
Dimethindene	+											2.5	12
Pheniramine	+		+				+					20	4–6
Triprolidine	+		+									2.5	6–8
Piperazines													
Buclizine				+	+							50	4–6
Chlorcyclizine			+					+				25	8
Cyclizine				+	+							50	4–6
Meclizine				+	+							25–50	12–24
Phenothiazines													
Methdilazine	+											8	6–12
Promethazine	+		+	+	+					+		25	12–24
Trimeprazine	+								+			2.5	6–8
Antiserotonergic/antihistamines													
Azatadine	+											1–2	12
Cyproheptadine[a]	+											4	8
Other													
Diphenylpyraline	+											2	4
Phenindamine			+									25	4–6
Pyrrobutamine			+									7.5	8–12
Terfenadine	+											60	12
Thenyldiamine			+									7.5	8

[a]Also useful in cold urticaria, postgastrectomy dumping syndrome, intestinal hypermotility of carcinoid syndrome, anorexia nervosa, and migraine.

Table 50–6
Comparisons Among Classes of Antihistamines

Class	CNS depression	GI disturbance	Anticholinergic effects	Teratogenicity	Risk of CNS stimulation	Extrapyramidal disorders
Ethanolamines	+++	+	+++	?	+	0
Ethylenediamines	++	+++	0	?	+	0
Alkylamines	+	++	0	?	+++	0
Piperazines	+	+	+	Yes	+	0
Phenothiazines	++	+	+++	?	+	+

Key: +++, substantial; ++, moderate; +, mild; 0, does not occur.

Preparations and Administration

Pyrilamine maleate (Allertoc, generic, and others)
Tablets and capsules for antiallergy purposes, tablets and capsules as sleep-aids (Compoz, Nervine, Nytol, Sleep-Eze, Sominex, Nytol)

Tripelennamine (PBZ and generic)
Tablets, long-acting tablets, sustained release tablets, elixir

Alkylamines

The alkylamines are the least sedative of the antihistamines. They are therefore useful drugs for daytime applications; chlorpheniramine (Chlor-Trimeton), the prototype of this group is the most widely used antihistamine in combination formulations for colds and coughs. Alkylamines are relatively devoid of anticholinergic activity. The incidence of gastrointestinal disturbances is intermediate between that of ethylenediamines and ethanolamines. Neurological problems attributable to CNS stimulation occur more commonly with alkylamines than with other antihistamines. Restlessness, excitation, and even convulsions can occur if excessive doses are ingested, especially by children.

Preparations and Administration

Brompheniramine (Dimetane, Bromamine, and others)
Tablets, timed release tablets, elixir

Chlorpheniramine (Chlor-Trimeton and others)
Tablets, chewable tablets, timed release capsules or tablets, syrup

Dexchlorpheniramine (Polaramine)
Tablets, repeat action tablets, syrup

Dimethindene (Forhistal, Triten)
Timed release tablets

Pheniramine (Inhiston)
Tablets

Triprolidine (Actidil)
Tablets, syrup

Piperazines

Piperazines are used mainly for alleviating motion sickness. Evidence from animal studies has suggested that drugs in this group may be teratogenic. Although clear evidence of teratogenicity in humans is lacking, piperazines are contraindicated for use in pregnancy. The incidence of drowsiness, depression, and gastrointestinal disturbances is low with the piperazine antihistamines.

Preparations and Administration

Bucladin-S (Bucladin-S)
Tablets

Chlorcyclizine
Combination cold pills and dermatological creams

Cyclizine (Marezine)
Tablets, injection solution

Meclizine (Antivert, Bonine, generic)
Tablets, chewable tablets, capsules

Phenothiazine Antihistamines

Promethazine (Phenergan), the prototype of this group, is used as an antinausea drug and to produce sedation, especially in preoperative or postoperative applications. Other phenothiazine antihistamines are employed in atopic allergies. The phenothiazine antihistamines have side effects that are additional to those that they share with other antihistamines. Phenothiazines can cause extrapyramidal reactions (parkinsonism, akathisias, dyskinesias) and hypotension. The phenothiazine antihista-

Nursing Diagnoses and Interventions for Treatment of Type I Allergic Reactions with Antihistamines

Nursing Diagnoses	*Related Interventions*
TO ENHANCE DRUG BENEFITS OR REDUCE DRUG REQUIREMENTS	
Ineffective airway clearance related to asthmatic bronchial constriction or thickening of secretion from drug therapy	Give antihistamines and other medications for allergic reactions as soon after onset of the attack as possible. Teach clients measures to avoid exposure to the allergen. Employ a vaporizer or humidifier to help loosen viscous respiratory secretions.
TO MINIMIZE DRUG SIDE EFFECTS OR INTERACTIONS	
Alteration in comfort related to dry mouth or gastrointestinal irritation caused by antihistamines	Provide oral hygiene and sugarless lozenges to alleviate dry mouth; take drug with food to reduce GI irritation.
Alteration in urinary elimination due to drug-induced urinary retention	Recommend that the client void before each dose of the drug.
Risk of injury related to dizziness and sedation from drug therapy	Provide appropriate safety measures. Advise clients that driving or operating dangerous equipment may be hazardous when taking these drugs.
Sensory-perceptual alterations related to aggravation of glaucoma by anticholinergic antihistamines	Check for history of glaucoma. Schedule tonometric evaluation if visual symptoms or headaches arise.
TO ENSURE SAFE AND EFFICACIOUS DRUG USE	
Knowledge deficit related to drug regimen	Teach clients about the nature of the allergy, measures for avoiding the antigen, and rapid administration of appropriate drug doses.
	Provide clients with a list of adverse effects and drug interactions for each drug in the regimen and explain what the client should do if any of these occur.

mines should be avoided in individuals with cardiovascular disorders, liver impairment, or ulcers.

Preparations and Administration

Methdilazine (Tacaryl)
Tablets, chewable tablets, syrup

Promethazine (Phenergan, others)
Tablets, syrups, suppositories

Trimeprazine (Temaril)
Tablets, syrup, spansule capsules

Other Antihistamines

Cyproheptadine (Periactin) and **azatadine** (Optimine) are potent blockers of serotonin as well as histamine receptors. Sedation occurs to a moderate degree. Cyproheptadine's antiserotonergic properties are useful in treatment of clients with postgastrectomy dumping syndrome or intestinal hypermotility of carcinoid syndrome. Cyproheptadine tends to stimulate appetite and weight gain, an effect put to good benefit when cyproheptadine is used in adolescents with anorexia nervosa. Cyproheptadine is useful in prophylaxis against migraine, though less so than methysergide or propranolol.

Phenindamine is found in combination preparations for colds. Like the alkylamines, it has a higher than typical liability of causing paradoxical excitatory effects, especially in children when doses are excessive. **Diphenylpyraline** (Diafen, Hispril) is used in atopic allergies. **Terfenadine** (Seldane) is a new antihistamine introduced in 1985. It is potent but nonsedating and lacks anticholinergic properties. However, it occasionally causes unique adverse responses such as alopecia, galactorrhea, bronchospasm, dysmenorrhea, and nightmares. It is relatively long-acting, allowing an interval of 12 hours between doses.

Astemizole (Hismanal) is a nonsedating H_1-blocker that is structurally unrelated to other antihistamines. Its long action (the elimination half-life is approximately 100 hours) allows it to be administered once per day and makes it a good choice for clients requiring long-term therapy. However, it is slow to act, requiring 1–4 hours to achieve peak plasma concentrations, making it a poor choice for quick relief of acute symptoms. Astemizole is available in Europe and has investigational status in the United States.

Preparations and Administration

Astemizole (Hismanal)
Tablets
Recommended Dosage: For type I allergic reactions, 10 mg/day.

Azatadine (Optimine)
Tablets

Cyproheptadine (Periactin, others)
Tablets, syrup

Diphenylpyraline (Diafen, Hispril)
Tablets, timed release capsules

Phenindamine
Combination preparations for colds.

Terfenadine (Seldane)
Tablets

Important Nursing Implications for Antihistamines

- ☐ Review the client's medical history for contraindications for antihistamines such as urinary retention, bronchial asthma, lactation, hyperthyroidism, peptic ulcer, pyloric or nephrourinary obstructions, cardiovascular disease, or increased intraocular pressure.
- ☐ Remember that the first priority in treating anaphylaxis is administration of epinephrine. An antihistamine provides little immediate benefit and can be given later.
- ☐ Warn clients not to drive an automobile or engage in other kinds of potentially hazardous activities while using an antihistamine, especially those with the greatest sedative effects.
- ☐ Caution clients about the potential for additive CNS depression if antihistamines are used in conjunction with alcohol or other depressant drugs.
- ☐ If the antihistamine being used has anticholinergic properties, advise clients that dryness of mouth can be alleviated by chewing gum, sucking on hard candy, or frequent mouth rinses.
- ☐ Avoid use of antihistamines that have anticholinergic properties in clients with asthma because of potential thickening of respiratory mucus.
- ☐ Monitor for potential additive anticholinergic effects with other anticholinergic drugs.
- ☐ When antihistamine therapy is prolonged, periodic blood cell counts should be conducted.
- ☐ Avoid use of antihistamines for nausea associated with pregnancy or for colds during pregnancy.
- ☐ Oral doses of antihistamines are taken with food or water to reduce incidence of gastrointestinal irritation.
- ☐ Administer antihistamines for motion sickness about 30 minutes before anticipated travel.
- ☐ Instruct clients to store antihistamines in airtight, light-resistant containers.

Hypersensitivity Reactions: Types II, III, and IV

Type II and type III hypersensitivity reactions are produced by the humoral immune system, like the type I reactions, but are mediated by IgG, IgM, and complement, rather than IgE (which mediates type I reactions). Type IV reactions are produced by the T cells of cell-mediated immunity. All of these types of immune reactions can be suppressed for medical purposes by use of immunosuppressive drugs.

Type II Hypersensitivity: Cytotoxic Reactions

Type II hypersensitivity reactions are humoral immune responses directed against tissue cells with antigenic components (Table 50–7). The antigenic component may be an exposed or abnormal cell constituent, antigenic components of a heterograft, or an antigen or hapten of endogenous origin that has attached to the cell membrane. Cytotoxic immune reactions have been identified that affect blood cells, somatic nerve endings, cutaneous cells, liver cells, thyroid cells, and basement membrane cells of the renal glomeruli and alveoli. Cytotoxic reactions culminate in cell lysis brought about mainly by complement fixation. Type II hypersensitivity reactions are identified by the presence of unusual amounts of

Table 50–7
Type II Hypersensitivity Reactions

Characteristics

Phagocytosis or lysing of tissue cells triggered by:
- Attachment of a hapten or allergen to the cell surface
- Exposure of a normally sequestered antigenic cell component
- Cross-reactivity between a drug-induced antibody and a cell protein

Mediated by IgG, IgM, and complement

Includes

Hyperacute rejection reactions due to HLA or ABO incompatibility

Disorders triggered by extrinsic allergens — usually after 2–4 weeks of exposure to allergen
- Quinidine-induced thrombocytopenia
- Penicillin- or methyldopa-induced hemolytic anemia
- Phenothiazine-induced cholestasis

Autoimmunity — chronic
- Involving blood cells
  - Coombs positive hemolytic anemia
  - Antibody-induced thrombocytopenia
  - Leukopenia
- Involving the stomach
  - Pernicious anemia
- Involving the kidneys and lungs
  - Goodpasture's syndrome
- Involving the skin
  - Pemphigus
  - Bullous pemphigoid
- Involving the pancreas
  - Insulin-dependent diabetes mellitus (also involves type IV hypersensitivity)
- Cytotoxic receptor reactions
  - Myasthenia gravis
  - Insulin resistance
  - Graves' disease
  - Adrenergic insensitivity

antibody for the diseased tissue in the serum or on the cells of the tissue itself.

The most rapid kinds of cytotoxic hypersensitivity reactions are those caused by **HLA or ABO incompatibility.** Cytotoxic reactions are directed against heterografts when there has been a failure to achieve adequate HLA (tissue antigen) compatibility, resulting in early graft rejection. Similarly, rapidly developing hemolytic reactions can occur when blood infusion is conducted with that has not been properly matched with respect to ABO compatibility.

Drug-induced cytotoxic reactions occur when a drug acts as a **hapten,** attaching to a body cell or protein, modifying it to an extent that the cell or protein is no longer recognized as self and acquires antigenicity. The cell or protein to which the hapten attaches is called the **carrier.** Most examples in this category involve attachment of drugs to blood cells with subsequent cytotoxic destruction of the cells. For example, quinidine can attach to platelets, triggering immunological attack on the platelets that culminates in thrombocytopenia. Penicillin can bind to red blood cells, leading to hemolytic anemia. Quinine, quinidine, and stibophen do not themselves act as haptens, but form antigen-antibody complexes that can then act as haptens, binding to RBCs to cause hemolytic anemia.

Some autoimmune disorders are chronic cytotoxic hypersensitivity reactions directed against one's own tissue cells, such as Coombs positive hemolytic anemia, antibody-induced thrombocytopenic purpura, leukopenia, pernicious anemia (antibody neutralization of gastric intrinsic factor), pemphigus and bullous pemphigoid (bullous skin disorders occurring in middle age or old age), and Goodpasture's syndrome (in which the cytotoxic reaction is directed against the basement membrane of the renal glomeruli and pulmonary alveoli).

Other disorders that may possibly have an autoimmune basis involving cytotoxic hypersensitivity include progressive systemic sclerosis, mixed connective tissue disease, and some cases of infertility (involving antispermatozoal antibodies). In clients with insulin-dependent diabetes mellitus, immunity may be directed against beta-cells of the pancreas, involving both cytotoxic humoral immunity and cell-mediated immunity (type IV).

In some disorders, it is believed that type II immune reactions may be directed against specific receptor populations. It appears likely that immunity directed against TSH receptors contributes to Graves' disease; that immunity against neuromuscular cholinergic receptors is involved in myasthenia gravis; and that cytotoxic reactions against insulin receptors contributes to insulin resistance. It is also probable that adrenergic drug resistance in some asthmatics is due to cytotoxic attack on adrenergic receptors.

Type III Hypersensitivity: Immune-Complex Disorders

Type III hypersensitivity reactions (Table 50–8) occur when antigen-antibody complexes become

Table 50–8
Type III Hypersensitivity Reactions

Characteristics

- Caused by deposition of soluble immune complexes
- Mediated by IgG, IgM, and complement

Includes

- Disorders triggered by drug administration
  - Vasculitis
    - SLE-like reactions caused by hydralazine, procainamide, penicillamine, phenytoin, captopril, isoniazid
    - Drug-induced polyarteritis caused by sulfonamides, iodides, penicillin, arsenicals, gold salts, hydantoins, mercurials, phenothiazines, and thiouracils
    - Arthus reactions caused by repeat injections of allergenic extracts, immune serums
    - Serum sickness caused by horse serum, penicillins, sulfonamides, cephalosporins, phenylbutazone, sulfonylureas, thiazides, viral hepatitis
  - Tissue deposition
    - Kidney
      - Drug-induced nephrotic syndrome caused by trimethadione, probenecid, penicillamine, pollens, venums, poison ivy
      - Drug-induced nephropathy caused by aminoglycosides, other antibiotics
    - Lungs
      - Drug-induced infiltrative lung disease caused by gold salts, penicillin, sulfonamides, nitrofurantoin, imipramine, mephenesin, para-aminosalicylic acid
- Autoimmunity
  - Vasculitis
    - SLE
    - Polyarteritis
  - Tissue deposition
    - Joints
      - Rheumatoid arthritis
    - Kidney
      - Glomerulonephritis
    - Lungs
      - Hypersensitivity pneumonitis (also involves type IV reaction)
      - Bronchopulmonary aspergillosis (also involves type I reaction)
      - Infiltrative lung disease

lodged in blood vessels or other tissues. Type III reactions are mediated by IgG, IgM, and complement and are identified by occurrence of vasculitis or presence of soluble immune-complexes. Antibody-antigen (immune) complexes that become deposited in tissue or walls of blood vessels attract and activate complement, thereby promoting tissue cell lysis, attraction of phagocytic neutrophils, and ultimately, release of proteolytic enzymes and superoxides from the lysosomes of the phagocytic cells. The result is tissue damage and dysfunction. The most common site of immune complex deposition is in the walls of blood vessels. The result is **vasculitis,** which is inflammation of blood vessels. Some of the types of vasculitis thought to involve immune-complex deposition in blood vessels include systemic lupus erythematosus (SLE) and polyarteritis (vasculitis of the medium-sized muscular arteries).

Immune-complex vasculitis can also occur as an autoimmune disorder or as a reaction to drug administration. One example of a drug-induced immune-complex disorder is the **Arthus reaction,** a local reaction at the site of administration of an antigenic drug, caused by severe, localized vasculitis, leading to gangrene, necrosis, and sloughing of dermal tissue. Another drug-induced immune-complex vasculitis is **serum sickness,** so named because it was originally identified as a reaction to horse serums employed in passive immunization (see Chapter 49). However, it is now recognized as a potential response to penicillin, certain other antibiotics, sulfonylureas, thiazides, phenylbutazone, and viral hepatitis. Serum sickness is characterized by diffuse vasculitis, with edema, swelling, pain, and fever. **Drug-induced SLE reactions** can be caused by hydralazine, procainamide, penicillamine, phenytoin, captopril, or isoniazid, and **drug-induced polyarteritis** by sulfonamides, iodides, penicillin, arsenicals, gold salts, hydantoins, iodides, mercurials, phenothiazines, sulfonamides, and thiouracils.

Other than the vasculature, the tissues most likely to be sites of immune-complex deposition are the kidneys, lungs, and joints. The kidneys are vulnerable in immune complex deposition because of their filtering function. **Glomerulonephritis** is believed to be a type III autoimmune disorder. Drug-induced immune-complex disorders affecting the kidney include **nephrotic syndrome** caused by trimethadione, probenecid, penicillamine, pollens, venums, and poison ivy; and **nephropathy** caused by aminoglycosides and other antibiotics.

The lungs are also especially susceptible to type III allergic reactions. **Infiltrative lung disease** occurs as a type III autoimmune disorder or as a reaction to administration of such drugs as gold salts, penicillin, sulfonamides, nitrofurantoin (Furadantin), imipramine (Tofranil), mephenesin, or para-aminosalicylic acid. **Hypersensitivity pneumonitis,** which occurs in people with occupations that expose them to airborne animal or vegetable proteins (farmers and workers who process hens, mushrooms, malt, cheese, fishmeal, or coffee) involves both type III and type IV hypersensitivity. **Bronchopulmonary aspergillosis,** on the other hand, involves both type I and type III reactions.

Rheumatoid arthritis (RA) is probably an immune-complex autoimmune disorder in which immune-complex deposition in the joints activates immune attack against synovial tissue. The antigen in RA is rheumatoid factor (RF), itself an immunoglobulin. RF-IgG complexes accumulate in joints and attract complement.

Type IV Hypersensitivity: Cell-Mediated Reactions

Type IV hypersensitivity reactions (Table 50–9) are mediated by T lymphocytes transformed by contact with appropriate antigens into sensitized lymphocytes or killer cells. Type IV reactions develop gradually, in a minimum of 24 hours after contact with antigen, and reach peak intensity in 2–3 days when the reaction is acute. Recovery occurs in 3–14 days if the source of antigen is removed. Delayed-hypersensitivity skin tests and patch tests can be used to identify allergens causing contact dermatitis — the atopic form of type IV hypersensitivity.

The major examples of type IV hypersensitivity are **contact dermatitis** (including photoallergic contact dermatitis) late **allograft rejections, granulomas** due to intracellular pathogens, **Hashimoto's thyroiditis, encephalomyelitis** associated with rabies vaccination, **insulin-dependent diabetes mellitus** (also involves type II mechanisms), and **hypersensitivity pneumonitis** (also involves type III mechanisms).

Table 50–9
Type IV Hypersensitivity Reactions

Characteristics
Involves cell-mediated immune response
Produced by sensitized T lymphocytes and killer cells
Delayed onset (typically 24 hours to onset; 48–72 hours to peak)
Includes
Late allograft rejection
Drug-induced or plant-induced reactions
Contact dermatitis to plants (e.g., poison ivy) or drugs such as penicillins, sulfonamides, neomycin, antihistamines, phenothiazines, benzocaine, hexachlorophene
Photoallergic contact dermatitis from after-shave lotions, sulfonamides, sunscreens
Encephalomyelitis from rabies vaccine
Autoimmunity
Granulomas due to intracellular pathogens
Thyroiditis
Hypersensitivity pneumonitis (also involves type III reaction)
Insulin-dependent diabetes mellitus (also involves type II reaction)

Immunosuppressives

In recent years, a frontier of medicine has been opened up in the area of tissue grafts and organ transplants. The potential for prolonging life by transplantation of healthy organs to replace diseased ones is immense, but the problems involved may be equally immense. Tissue cells contain a wide variety of antigens, and the uniqueness of each individual's antigen profile substantially limits the compatibility of tissue transplanted from donor to recipient. There are at least 30 antigens that contribute to transplantation compatibility: consequently, typing such tissues is highly complicated. The most influential antigenic influences are the human leukocyte A **(HLA)** and major blood group **(ABO)** antigens. HLA antigenicity is governed genetically by at least four closely linked loci on closely associated genes. There is some evidence suggesting that individual susceptibilities to atopic allergies and certain autoimmune disorders may be controlled by the HLA genotype of the individual. With respect to transplantation, the likelihood and severity of rejection reactions is directly related to the extent of antigenic differences between the donor and the recipient.

The most rapid rejection reactions occur when an individual has been presensitized to the HLA antigens of the transplant by previous blood transfusion, transplantation, or pregnancy. In this event, rejection is hyperacute and is a type II hypersensitivity reaction mediated by the humoral immune system. The more common type of rejection reaction is a cell-mediated (type IV) hypersensitivity reaction. Suppression of acute allograft rejection reactions can sometimes be achieved with immunosuppressive therapy. After successful suppression of an acute rejection reaction, it is often possible to maintain the graft with a modest degree of immunosuppression. It is rarely possible to eliminate immunosuppressives completely after a transplantation except for isografts (between identical twins) or autografts (from one location to another in the same individual). The drugs used as immunosuppressives include antimetabolite and alkylating drugs employed in cancer (discussed in Chapter 56) and corticosteroids (discussed in Chapter 45). Three drugs used mainly as immunosuppressives are azathioprine (Imuran), cyclosporine (Sandimmune), and muromonab-CD3 (Orthoclone).

Azathioprine (Imuran)

Azathioprine is an antimetabolite related to 6-mercaptopurine. Both are purine analogues and are incorporated into DNA of proliferating cells in place of the natural purine bases to produce abnormal DNA. Rapidly proliferating cells are affected more by this action than are cell populations with slow turnover rates. The immunosuppressive effect of azathioprine is due to the fact that lymphocytes proliferate rapidly, especially in response to antigenic challenge.

Pharmacokinetics Azathioprine is given intravenously or orally. In the blood, azathioprine is about 30% bound to plasma proteins. It is quickly removed by the liver and metabolized, in part to mercaptopurine, an active metabolite. Inactivation of azathioprine and mercaptopurine is mainly by liver metabolism, but sufficient amounts are excreted by the kidney so that pharmacological activity and toxicity are doubled in anuric clients. This is especially relevant when the transplanted organ is a kidney, since renal function in the transplanted kidney is initially depressed. *The nurse should monitor the fluid intake-output ratio for any evidence of an abrupt drop in urinary output that would alter the activity of azathioprine. Kidney function tests should be performed at least weekly.* Blood levels of azathioprine and mercaptopurine bear little relation to efficacy since the drugs are removed from the blood rapidly but are present in tissue for longer periods.

Clinical Indications Azathioprine is indicated for use in suppressing rejection of renal homotransplants. It has also been approved for use in clients with rheumatoid arthritis refractory to conventional treatments. There are no other approved applications, but the drug is being studied for use in autoimmune disorders, including systemic lupus erythematosus, autoimmune hemolytic anemias, and idiopathic thrombocytopenic purpura.

Adverse Effects and Contraindications Azathioprine produces serious side effects similar to those associated with antineoplastic agents. Reversible or irreversible **bone marrow suppression** may occur. *Complete blood cell counts should be performed at least once a week. The nurse should monitor the client for signs of leukopenia (occurrence and persistence of infections) and thrombocytopenia (purpura, oral lesions, or bleeding). Poor color, dark urine, clay-colored stools, or shortness of breath may indicate that anemia is developing.* If leukocyte counts are observed to decline sharply, azathioprine should be discontinued or the dosage reduced. Hematological reactions are the most common adverse reactions to azathioprine.

An inevitable hazard of immunosuppression is the elevated **risk of infection** by all classes of pathogenic microorganisms. Fatalities from uncontrollable infections sometimes occur. *The nurse should advise clients receiving azathioprine to avoid contact with individuals with infections (such as colds), to report immediately indications of infection (sore throat, fever, chills, malaise, nasal or sinus congestion, common colds), and to maintain scrupulous hygiene.*

Azathioprine can produce a negative nitrogen balance which may be persistent in some clients. If used during pregnancy, azathioprine, like all antimetabolite agents, is potentially teratogenic. As with other antineoplastic/immunosuppressive agents, rapidly proliferating cells of the gastrointestinal mucosa are adversely affected, leading to nausea, vomiting, diarrhea, steatorrhea, and possible pancreatitis. *Bland foods and antiemetic drugs may help to relieve nausea and vomiting.* Cholestasis and jaundice may occur. *The nurse should monitor the client for signs of jaundice (clay-colored stools, yellow or orange skin, scleral discoloration, dark urine).* As with antineoplastic agents, alopecia occurs. Hypersensitivity reactions occur occasionally in the form of skin rashes or drug fever; their presence represents a specific contraindication for use of this drug. *Nurses should advise women of childbearing years to practice birth control during therapy and for 4 months after therapy has been discontinued.*

Drug Interactions Allopurinol is a potent inhibitor of the metabolism of both azathioprine and mercaptopurine. It is sometimes employed concurrent with azathioprine. When allopurinol is employed with azathioprine, the dose of the immunosuppressive drug should be reduced to one-third the usual dose.

Clients should be warned that vaccinations or other immunity-conferring agents may cause unusually severe reactions because of the immunosuppressant effect of azathioprine. Therefore clients must inform health care professionals that they are taking azathioprine. In addition, they should wear or carry a card or other item that identifies them as receiving immunosuppressant therapy.

Preparations and Administration *After reconstitution in sterile water, the sodium salt of azathioprine is stable for 24 hours at room temperature.* Intravenous injection may be employed during the first 1–4 days after renal homotransplantation if the patient is unable to accept oral therapy. *IV infusion is conducted by addition of azathioprine to a sodium chloride or 5% dextrose infusate.* Oral doses are to be preferred whenever possible. Azathioprine therapy is usually instituted 1–5 days prior to kidney transplantation and is restarted within 24 hours after transplantation. Most clients require maintenance doses for life. *The nurse should advise clients not to discontinue the drug unless directed to do so by the physician.*

Azathioprine (Imuran)
Tablets, injection solution as the sodium salt
Recommended Doses: 3–5 mg/kg/day, PO or IV, initially. After stabilization, doses are adjusted downward if control over immunological rejection can be satisfactorily maintained. The usual maintenance dose is 1–2 mg/kg/day.

Cyclosporine (Sandimmune)

Cyclosporine is a major new agent introduced in 1983 as an immunosuppressive. This drug is a cyclic polypeptide of 11 amino acid residues. It is used in conjunction with glucocorticoids in prophylaxis against organ rejections involving kidney, liver, or heart transplants. In combination with a glucocorticoid, it appears to be more effective than azathioprine alone or azathioprine and a glucocorticoid. It has important advantages with respect to adverse effects, causing less of an increase in susceptibility to infections and no suppression of the bone marrow. The doses of glucocorticoids used with cyclosporine are often less than those employed with azathioprine.

Pharmacokinetics Cyclosporine is available for oral and intravenous use. After oral administration, absorption is erratic and incomplete (typically about 30%). Blood levels should be monitored periodically when the drug is given orally and employed in making dosage adjustments.

Clinical Indications Cyclosporine is indicated for prophylaxis against organ transplant rejection and lifelong maintenance of immunosuppression in clients who have received kidney, liver, or heart transplants. Investigative applications include rheumatoid arthritis, systemic lupus erythematosus, multiple sclerosis, and psoriasis.

Adverse Effects and Contraindications The most important adverse effect with cyclosporine is a dose-dependent **nephrotoxicity.** The reported incidence has been 20% in clients receiving kidney transplants, 33% in those receiving heart transplants, and 41% in those given liver transplants. Nephrotoxic reactions can often be diminished by reducing dosage. Although increased susceptibility to infections is less than occurs with azathioprine, the client should be advised to exercise caution against contact with individuals with infections and to report signs of infection. Other adverse effects of cyclosporine include hypertension, tremor, nausea and vomiting, hirsutism, and hyperplasia of the gums.

Drug Interactions Cyclosporine should be used cautiously with other immunosuppressives (glucocorticoids, azathioprine, or muromonab-CD3) as this could produce dangerous susceptibility to infection. Concurrent use of other nephrotoxic drugs, such as aminoglycosides should be avoided. Ketoconazole and amphotericin B have been noted to increase blood levels of cyclosporine.

Preparations and Administration Oral administration is recommended in all clients able to tolerate oral dosing. Maintenance therapy is often a lifetime proposition for transplant recipients.

Cyclosporine is not soluble in water. The oral solution utilizes a vehicle consisting of olive oil, alcohol, and polyoxyethylated oleic glycerides. *The nurse should instruct the client to dissolve this solution in milk, chocolate milk, or orange juice immediately before ingestion. The nurse should also advise the client to take the drug at the same time each day. The contents of a bottle of the oral solution should be utilized within 2 months of being opened.*

The injection solution utilizes a vehicle of polyoxyethylated castor oil and alcohol. One milliliter of the commercial formulation is diluted in 20–100 ml of normal saline or 5% dextrose for infusion over 2–6 hours.

Cyclosporine (Sandimmune)
Oral solution, injection solution
Recommended Doses: 15 mg/kg/day PO initially, given in a single daily dose. The first dose is given 4–12 hours before the transplantation procedure, then continued daily for 1–2 weeks, and then gradually tapered at 5% per day to the maintenance level of 5–10 mg/kg/day. Prednisone is usually given concurrently. The initial dose of prednisone is 2 mg/kg/day, which is gradually tapered downward until the maintenance dose of 0.15 mg/kg/day is reached within 2 months.

Muromonab-CD3 (Orthoclone)

Muromonab-CD3, introduced in 1986, represents a novel approach to achieving immunosuppression. This drug is an antibody, produced in mice, to an antigenic component (called CD3) of human T cells. Muromonab-CD3 binds to and blocks the activity of T cell, thereby suppressing their role in acute allograft rejection.

Pharmacokinetics Muromonab-CD3 is given by intravenous injection. With daily administration of 5 mg, accumulation occurs for the first 3 days, after which serum trough levels stabilize at approximately 0.9 μg/ml.

Clinical Indications Muromonab-CD3 is used to alleviate acute allograft rejection of kidney transplants. It is used in a 10–14 day course of therapy.

Adverse Effects and Contraindications The incidence of side effects occurring during the first 2 days of therapy with muromonab-CD3 is higher than that occurring with conventional immunosuppressives. *Nurses should monitor clients receiving this drug especially closely during the first 48 hours of therapy.* Adverse reactions most often observed during this period include fever (73% of clients), chills (57%), dyspnea (21%) and wheezing (11%), chest pain (14%), nausea (11%) and vomiting (13%), diarrhea (10%), and tremor (10%). Febrile reactions can be extreme (>104° F) in about 2% of patients. *An antipyretic should be administered if fever exceeds 100° F).* Methylprednisolone sodium succinate, 1 mg/kg IV, is sometimes given prior to the first dose and hydrocortisone sodium succinate, 100 mg IV, 30 minutes after administration of muromonab-CD3 to reduce adverse reactions to the initial dose. Acetaminophen and antihistamines have also been given with the first dose for this purpose.

The most serious early reaction to muromonab-CD3 is severe, potentially fatal, **pulmonary edema,** and for this reason the first dose of the drug should be given only in a facility with cardiopulmonary resuscitation equipment and fluid overload should be ruled out (by chest x-ray and analysis of changes in weight) before administering the drug.

After the first few days of treatment, the major adverse effect of muromonab-CD3 is increased risk of infection. Infections most commonly observed are cytomegalovirus, herpes simplex, *Staphylococcus epidermidis,* and *Pneumocystis carinii.* Use of muromonab-CD3 is contraindicated for clients allergic to any component of the preparation.

Drug Interactions Other immunosuppressive drugs should be reduced or eliminated during therapy with muromonab-CD3. Maximum daily doses of other immunosuppressives being given concomitantly with muromonab-CD3 are 0.5 mg/kg for prednisone and 25 mg for azathioprine. Cyclosporine doses should be reduced or discontinued. Preestablished maintenance immunosuppressive doses should be recommenced 3 days before completing the course of therapy with muromonab-CD3.

Preparations and Administration The product should be refrigerated (at 2–8° C) but not frozen. The solution should not be shaken. When preparing for injection, the solution should be drawn into the syringe through a low protein-binding 0.20–0.22 μm filter.

Muromonab-CD3 (Orthoclone)
Injection solution
Recommended Doses: 5 mg by IV bolus (not infusion), once daily, for 10–14 days.

Case Study: Pollen Allergy

L. C., a 44-year-old male, had a history of allergic rhinitis during pollen season. Over the years he had learned to manage the condition adequately by a combination of strategies: minimizing yard work during periods of high pollen count, air-conditioning the two rooms in his house where he spent the most time, and taking an allergy preparation when the familiar symptoms of puffy, itchy nose and eyes, congestion of nasal passages, runny nose, and irritability began. When L. C. first began self-medicating for his allergic condition, he used a product (Novated A capsules) containing a combination of pseudoephedrine and chlorpheniramine. Although the preparation was effective in lessening the symptoms of allergy, he did not like the "buzz" that he experienced, finding that the drug seemed to interfere with his intellectual processes. As a result, L. C. had been using diphenhydramine (Benadryl) in recent years. He found that this drug relieved the itchiness, puffiness, runny nose, and irritability without the "buzz," but did not alleviate the nasal congestion as well as the previous regimen.

In the last year, L. C. had begun to experience a degree of sleepiness when he took diphenhydramine that he found unacceptable. A friend of L. C.'s was a nurse and he decided to call her to ask her advice on a suitable alternative to the diphenhydramine that might be less sedating but would not produce the "buzz" he had experienced with the pseudoephedrine and chlorpheniramine combination. The nurse agreed to research the question and call him back with a suggestion.

1. What type of drug is pseudoephedrine? Chlorpheniramine? What is the contribution of each in relieving symptoms of allergic rhinitis?
2. What was the likely cause of the "buzz" experienced with the combination of pseudoephedrine and chlorpheniramine?
3. Is sedation a likely side effect of diphenhydramine?
4. What alternative might the nurse suggest for L. C.?

Answers appear at the end of the book.

Case Study: Systemic Lupus Erythematosus (SLE)-Like Reaction to Medication

B. B., a 66-year-old black man, came to his physician complaining of pleuritic pain, photophobia, and generalized body aches, especially pronounced in the knees and elbows. Physical examination revealed further the presence of a facial rash and oral lesions. B. B. had been treated by this physician over a period of 12 years for hypertension. He had been treated initially with a thiazide diuretic alone, with satisfactory blood pressure control. Later, when diastolic pressure could no longer be contained below 95 with the diuretic alone, propranolol (Inderal) was added to the regimen. Then, 8 months ago a vasodilator, hydralazine (Apresoline), was added as the condition was no longer adequately controlled by the two-drug regimen. B. B. had no history of medical problems other than hypertension.

The physician had B. B. admitted to the hospital for evaluation. He ordered a blood test: hemoglobin was 11.5 g/100 ml (normal range in males: 14–18 g/100ml), erythrocyte sedimentation rate was 84 mm/hour (normal range in males: 0–10 mm/hour), and a lupus erythematosus (LE) cell test was positive. The physician ordered discontinuation of hydralazine and administration of prednisone, 10 mg, bid. After 5 days of this regimen, the body aches had been alleviated and B. B. was discharged, with prednisone continued for 2 months and then gradually tapered off. Prazosin (Minipress) was added to the hypertension regimen of hydrochlorthiazide and propranolol as a substitute for hydralazine. B. B. had no recurrence of the body aches, but follow-up blood tests at 4-month intervals exhibited a positive LE cell test after 4 and 8 months, but a negative result after 12 and 16 months.

1. The criteria for SLE proposed by the American Rheumatism Association are (1) facial erythema, (2) discoid lupus erythematosus, (3) Raynaud's phenomenon, (4) alopecia, (5) photosensitivity, (6) oral or nasopharyngeal ulceration, (7) arthritis without deformity, (8) LE cells, (9) chronic false-positive serological test for syphilis, (10) proteinuria, (11) cellular casts, (12) pleuritis or pericarditis, (13) psychosis or convulsions, or (14) leukopenia, thrombocytopenia, or hemolytic anemia. At least four of these must be present to diagnose SLE. Which of these were evidenced by B. B. based on the information provided?
2. What was the likely cause of the SLE?
3. What is the prognosis for B. B.?
4. What other drugs are associated with a risk of drug-induced SLE-like reactions? What signs and symptoms should the nurse watch for when drug-induced SLE-like reactions are a possibility?

Answers appear at the end of the book.

Recommended Readings

Anderson D: AIDS: An update on what we know now. *RN* 1986;49(3):49–56.

Barrows JJ: Dealing with anaphylaxis — stat. *Nursing Life* 1985;5(3):33–39.

Bennett J: AIDS beyond the hospital: What we know about AIDS. *Am J Nurs* 1986;86(9):1015–1021.

Brodoff AS: Keeping current on allergy treatment. *Patient Care* 1984;18(3):137–147.

Buissert PD: Allergy. *Sci Am* 1982;247(2):86–95.

Crutcher JE, Kantner TR: The effectiveness of antihistamines in the common cold. *J Clin Pharmacol* 1981;21:9–15.

Griffin JP: Acquired immune deficiency syndrome: A new epidemic. *Crit Care Nurse* 1983;3(2):21–28.

Harmon AL, Harmon DC: Anaphylaxis, sudden death anytime. *Nursing* 1980;10(10):40–43.

Lagunoff D, Martin TW, Read G: Agents that release histamine from mast cells. *Annu Rev Pharmacol Toxicol* 1983;23:331–351.

Montefusco C, Goldsmith J: Cyclosporine immunosuppression in organ graft receipts: Nursing implications. *Crit Care Nurse* 1984;4(2):117–119.

Norman PS: Allergic rhinitis. *J Allergy Clin Immunol* 1985;75(5):531–548.

Randall BJ: Reacting to anaphylaxis. *Nursing* 1986;16(3):34–40.

Reinhardt D, Borchard U: H1-receptor antagonists: Comparative pharmacology and clinical use. *Klinische Wochenschrift* 1982;60:983–990.

Rosenberg JM, Kirschenbaum HL: What to watch for with antihistamines. *RN* 1981;44(5):70–72.

Steele SM: AIDS: Clarifying values. *Nursing Health and Care* 1986;7(5)f:247–248.

UNIT X

Drugs and the Systems That Interface with the External Environment

CHAPTER **51**

Drugs Used for Disorders of the Alimentary Tract and Liver

The alimentary tract, consisting of the mouth, esophagus, stomach, intestines, bowel, and anus, has three major functions: the movement, digestion, and absorption of food. From the food ingested every day, these processes provide the body with the nutrients, electrolytes, and water necessary for survival.

Physiology of the Alimentary Tract

The smooth muscle walls of the gastrointestinal tract are organized for two kinds of movements: mixing movements, which constantly stir up the contents, and propulsive movements, which force the contents from one segment of the tract to the next. Mixing is caused by local rhythmic contractions of the muscle walls, while propulsion is the result of progressive waves of contractions along the gut (peristalsis). The propulsion of food through the alimentary tract is also partly regulated by the tone of the pyloric, ileocecal, and anal sphincters — ringlike bands of muscle fiber that control the natural orifices. The entire alimentary tract is controlled by the enteric nervous system, which is under autonomic control. The parasympathetic nervous system promotes motor and secretory activities of the tract. Conversely, the sympathetic nervous system inhibits passage of material through the intestine by relaxing the smooth muscle of the gut wall and constricting the ileocecal and anal sphincters. At the same time, invagination of the gut wall is increased, promoting absorption.

There are numerous secretory glands throughout the alimentary tract as well as highly specialized secretory tissues, the exocrine pancreas, and the liver. Together, the secretory glands and tissues serve the two principal functions of digestive-enzyme secretion and lubrication. Important glandular cells include the goblet cells, which secrete a lubricating mucus (composed of mucin, leukocytes, inorganic salts, and epithelial cells) and Paneth's cells, which secrete a watery fluid resembling extracellular fluid to facilitate absorption of various substances. The digestive enzymes are secreted in the saliva, gastric juices, and pancreatic secretions and are also found in the epithelial cells of the intestinal mucosa. In all areas of the alimentary tract, there is a balance between digestive secretions and mucous secretions that protects the tissue from autodigestion.

Most nutrients as well as some water and electrolytes are absorbed by the small intestine through the villi that line the folds of the intestinal mucosa. The outer layer, or brush border (it looks like the bristles on a thick brush), greatly increases the absorptive surface. The basement membrane, a rich network of capillaries, absorbs nutrients into the portal vein of the circulatory system, while the central lacteal takes substances into the lymphatic system. Absorption occurs either by active transport, diffusion, or facilitated diffusion. The blood of the portal vein, containing newly absorbed substances, flows directly to the liver, which stores the nutrients, metabolizes potential toxins, and phagocytizes pathogens.

Drugs That Affect the Mouth

Drugs used expressly for effects on the mouth, including mouthwashes, gargles, and dentrifrices, have little pharmacological activity. Some drugs used for other purposes, however, have significant oral side effects; for example, anticholinergic drugs cause dryness of mouth, thrombocytopenic drugs may cause oral bleeding, and other drugs may alter taste sensitivity (see Chapter 44).

Many preparations marketed as **mouthwashes** simply provide a pleasant, aromatic ingredient that masks unpleasant breath odor. Even mouthwashes that contain an antiseptic are usually not in contact with oral surfaces long enough to affect bacteria. Clients' use of mouthwashes sometimes complicates nursing assessment since breath odors are often indicators of health problems. Cepacol mouthwash is used in some hospitals and is available commercially as a solution or lozenge. As a gargle for sore throat, dilute sodium chloride solution (0.9%, which is normal saline) is as effective as any commercial gargle.

The numerous **dentifrices** usually consist of a mild abrasive, a foaming agent, and substances added to produce an appealing taste. For children, toothpastes containing fluoride are superior in preventing cavities. In adults, the value of brushing and flossing teeth is the mechanical cleansing action, which removes food debris and plaque. The toothpaste contributes only by providing a mild abrasive and a pleasant taste.

Stomach and Duodenum Disorders and Drugs

Drugs that affect the stomach or duodenum are used to induce or suppress emesis, to treat hyperacidity and peptic ulcers, to aid digestion in hypochlorhydria, and to reduce gas and flatulence.

Nausea, Vomiting, and Drugs

Vomiting is a physiologic response to noxious stimuli, characterized by forceful oral expulsion of the contents of the upper alimentary tract. Nausea, the feeling that vomiting is imminent, is experienced as an epigastric sensation. Nausea often is a component of a diverse set of autonomic symptoms, called the vasovagal reaction, which results from enhanced activity of the parasympathetic branch of the autonomic nervous system. The symptoms of the vasovagal reaction, in addition to nausea, include perspiration, salivation, pallor, bradycardia, and hypotension.

The stimulus for nausea or vomiting may have a peripheral or central origin. Drugs or harsh foods as well as excessive distention can irritate the gastric mucosa. At other times, stimuli from the central nervous system (elevated intracranial pressure, emotional disorders, stress, pain, or vascular headaches) may act directly on the medullary control centers to activate nausea or vomiting responses. Nausea or vomiting may also be initiated by the direct action of drugs, toxins, or metabolic products on a sensitive region of the medulla called the **chemical trigger zone** (CTZ), which relays impulses to the vomiting center. The vomiting center then simulates skeletal muscles of the diaphragm and abdomen as well as to visceral muscles of the stomach and esophagus to produce the emetic response.

It is important to determine the type of vomiting (Table 51-1), since this helps in identifying disease states associated with it. Nausea and vomiting are sometimes caused by drugs such as apomorphine, narcotics, and cardiac glycosides that stimulate the CTZ directly. Other drugs, such as alco-

Table 51-1
Types of Oral Expulsions

Type	Description	Possible causes
Regurgitation	Passive ejection of fluid from the stomach immediately after it is swallowed Small amount of material brought up without nausea or muscle contractions May smell sour because of contact with HCl	Seen in infants with immature cardiac sphincter; reduced by upright position when feeding infant Heartburn, esophagitis
Rumination	Ejection of vomitus by manipulation such as finger on the base of the tongue	Psychopathologic condition Seen frequently in people who fear weight gain
Vomiting	Ejection of undigested food or poorly digested food. Forceful	Associated with disease states Also caused by certain medications
Cyclical vomiting	Occurs repeatedly Difficult to establish physical base as cause	May be associated with psychological stress Could be interpreted as convulsive disorder
Pernicious vomiting	Severe, long-term repeated vomiting	Occurs in pregnancy when normal morning sickness lasts beyond 3 months
Projectile vomiting	Forceful Projected some distance from the mouth	Associated with increased intracranial pressure Also pyloric stenosis in infants
Retching	Stomach contracts to eject food No vomitus present Stomach empty	Associated with acute gastrointestinal disorders where stomach is extremely irritated

Adapted from Brenda Bigelow-Kemp and Adele Pillitteri, *Fundamentals of Nursing: A Framework for Practice*, Table 35-5. Copyright © 1984 by Brenda Bigelow-Kemp and Adele Pillitteri. By permission of Little, Brown and Company.

hol, aspirin, other nonsteroidal anti-inflammatory agents, nitrofurantoin (Furadantin), and anticancer drugs, promote nausea and vomiting by irritating the gastrointestinal mucosa. Radiation therapy for cancer has a similar effect on the gastrointestinal mucosa. Although vomiting is essentially a protective mechanism designed to enable the body to eject harmful substances from the stomach before they are fully absorbed, it can endanger life if excessive amounts of fluid and electrolytes are lost.

The color, odor, consistency, and contents of vomitus are important clues to its origin. Vomitus that is bright red or very dark brown (due to conversion of hemoglobin to hematin by the action of stomach acid) indicates gastrointestinal bleeding. Black or dark brown granular vomitus is indicative of an old episode of bleeding. Green-colored vomitus contains bile and originates in the duodenum. Vomitus that is brown, odorous, and fecal stained comes from the intestinal tract, and is commonly seen in clients who have intestinal obstruction.

Emetic Drugs

To rid the stomach of toxic substances, it may be desirable to induce vomiting by administering an emetic drug, although gastric lavage is an alternative more commonly used in hospital settings. **Ipecac syrup** is a useful nonprescription emetic. Nurses are sometimes asked about the advisability of using ipecac following accidental or intentional poisonings. *Explain that ipecac should not be used if the individual has ingested strong alkalis, acids, other corrosive materials, strychnine, petroleum distillates, volatile oils, or rapidly acting CNS depressants.* When ipecac is used, the victim is given 3 teaspoonsful of ipecac, followed by 1–2 glasses of tepid water for adults or $\frac{1}{2}$–1 glass of water for children. Vomiting should occur in 15–30 minutes and will likely continue for 20–25 minutes. If vomiting does not occur within 30 minutes, the dose may be repeated one more time. If vomiting still does not occur, the individual should be brought to an emergency room for gastric lavage and administration of activated charcoal to recover both the poison and the ipecac. When ipecac is absorbed rather than vomited, clients may develop bloody diarrhea, shock, cardiac dysrhythmias, or go into convulsions or coma.

Apomorphine is often the emetic employed in clinical settings. Administered subcutaneously or intravenously, apomorphine produces emesis by an action on the chemical trigger zone of the medulla. Apomorphine produces its emetic effect within 15 minutes in adults and within 1–2 minutes in children. In adults, 200–300 ml of water or evaporated milk immediately before injecting the drug may produce a more effective emesis. Just prior to vomiting, the client will usually complain of nausea and excessive salivation. Once vomiting ceases, the client usually falls asleep for about 2 hours. If the individual has ingested an absorbable poison, activated charcoal may be administered before or after apomorphine. *After administration of apomorphine, the client should be monitored closely for at least 2 hours. Vital signs should be taken and the client observed for adverse effects such as salivation and nausea, lacrimation, prespiration, restlessness, tremors, euphoria, and tachycardia.* Use of apomorphine is contraindicated in clients hypersensitive to morphine derivatives, clients who have ingested a corrosive substance, or clients who are inebriated from a CNS depressant.

Antiemetic and Antinausea Drugs

Clinical Indications When vomiting occurs, it is generally acute, and drug suppression is neither feasible nor necessary; eliminating its cause and general support measures are usually sufficient. When vomiting is prolonged or recurrent, medical intervention is directed at identifying and alleviating the underlying disorder. Antiemetic drugs should not be used to suppress vomiting of unknown etiology. In current medical practice, antiemetic drugs are employed for motion sickness, with cancer chemotherapy, and for postoperative nausea and vomiting. Over-the-counter drugs and home remedies (such as hot tea) are widely used for alleviating the "upset stomach" associated with overeating, but there is no firm evidence that these treatments are effective. Antiemetic drugs are sometimes self-administered and nurses are often asked about the advisability of requesting prescribed antiemetic agents for the nausea or vomiting of pregnancy ("morning sickness"). Since the use of antiemetics poses a potential hazard for the fetus, nurses should recommend nondrug alternatives.

Antiemetic drugs currently in use fall into four categories: (1) phenothiazines, (2) antihistamines, (3) anticholinergics, and (4) other. There is not a clear distinction among the first three groups, however, because both the phenothiazines and the antihistamines used as antiemetics have profound anticholinergic properties. Antiemetic drugs are most effective in preventing vomiting or alleviating nausea that is related to activation of the CTZ — for example, nausea or vomiting caused by motion, nauseating odors, or centrally acting emetic drugs. Antiemetic agents are substantially less effective when nausea or vomiting is caused by gastrointestinal irritation or distention.

Phenothiazines indicated for suppression of nausea and vomiting include chlorpromazine (Thorazine), prochlorperazine (Compazine), perphenazine (Trilafon), promethazine (Phenergan), triflupromazine (Vesprin), and thiethylperazine (Torecan). In practice, prochlorperazine is the most widely used. Many of the phenothiazines are extensively employed in psychotic disorders (see Chapter 18). The doses required for antiemetic applications are smaller than those used for clients with psychosis, and the severity and variety of adverse reactions are correspondingly diminished. At antiemetic doses, adverse reactions are generally limited to anticholinergic side effects and orthostatic hypotension. Phenothiazine antiemetics are contraindicated in pregnancy.

Nonprescription antihistamines used to suppress nausea and vomiting (mainly for motion sickness) include meclizine (Bonine, Vertrol), cyclizine (Marezine), buclizine (Bucladin), diphenhydramine (Benadryl), and dimenhydrinate (Dramamine, others). The first three should be avoided during pregnancy, teratogenicity having been observed in animal studies. Adverse effects of these antihistamines include sedation and anticholinergic effects such as dry mouth, blurred vision, and urinary retention. Hydroxyzine (Atarax, Vistaril), a prescription antihistamine used frequently as an antianxiety drug (see Chapter 19), is also effective in suppressing nausea and vomiting. When used as a preanesthetic sedative, it has the added benefit of suppressing the nausea and vomiting that often occur with anesthetics. The complete pharmacology of the antihistamines, including preparations and recommended doses, is discussed in Chapter 50. *Nurses should warn clients that antihistamines that are used as antiemetics cause drowsiness, which can be additive with that produced by alcohol or other CNS depressants.*

Scopolamine, a classic antimuscarinic drug that produces a full array of anticholinergic side effects, can be employed to alleviate motion sickness. Other drugs marketed for control of nausea and vomiting include trimethobenzamide (Tigan), benzquinamide (Emete-Con), dronabinol (Marinol), diphenidol (Vontrol), and phosphorated carbohydrate solution. Trimethobenzamide is widely prescribed, although its value has not been clearly established. It is sometimes used as an antiemetic during surgical procedures. Adverse reactions to trimethobenzamide are similar to those caused by phenothiazines: anticholinergic effects, hypotension, blood dyscrasias, allergic reactions, and parkinsonian-like symptoms.

Benzquinamide is a drug used in hospital settings for postoperative nausea and vomiting because it is less likely to produce hypotensive responses. However, both hypertension and hypotension are possible reactions. Nurses should also observe clients for other adverse responses such as skin reactions (hives and rash), drowsiness, anticholinergic symptoms, cardiac dysrhythmias, and CNS stimulation (restlessness, excitement, nervousness, and insomnia). Benzquinamide is not advised for clients with cardiovascular disease or those receiving preanesthetic or cardiovascular drugs. Also, because of drug interaction, clients receiving pressor agents such as epinephrine-like drugs should only be given a fraction of the usual dose of benzquinamide.

Dronabinol (Marinol) was introduced in 1985 for use in treating nausea and vomiting associated with cancer chemotherapy that does not respond to conventional treatment. Dronabinol is delta-9-tetrahydrocannabinol, the principal active ingredient of marihuana.

Diphenidol is used for the vertigo, nausea, and vomiting associated with labyrinthine disturbances that occur in Ménière's disease or after surgery on the middle or inner ear. It is also employed postoperatively and in conjunction with cancer chemotherapy. Diphenidol has a suppressant effect on both the chemical trigger zone and the vestibular apparatus. Adverse reactions include auditory and visual hallucinations and disorientation. Complaints of drowsiness, depression, sleep disturbances, gastrointestinal irritation, and dry mouth may indicate the presence of other adverse responses. The usual oral dose is 25 mg, which can be repeated every 4 hours as required. It is also available for parenteral use.

Phosphorated carbohydrate solution (Emetrol) is a nonprescription preparation consisting of a mixture of invert sugars and phosphoric acid used to adjust gastric pH to 1.5–1.6. However, its efficacy has not been adequately demonstrated. Although it is claimed that this hyperosmolar carbohydrate solution delays gastric emptying time by a direct action on the wall of the stomach, there is no evidence that nausea or vomiting is influenced by gastric emptying time. The preparation is devoid of significant adverse effects except in diabetic clients, in whom the high sugar content of the medication could cause hyperglycemia. If large doses are used, osmotic diarrhea can occur.

Preparations and Administration

Benzquinamide (Emete-Con)
Injection solution
Recommended Doses: 50 mg, IM; or 25 mg, intravenously.

Chlorpromazine (Thorazine)
Formulations: See Chapter 18
Recommended Doses: As antiemetic, 10–25 mg PO, up to 4 times per day.

Dimenhydrinate (Dramamine)

Nursing Observations for Use of Antiemetic Drugs for Nausea and Vomiting

THERAPEUTIC GOAL	Provide comfort measures, if nausea or vomiting are acute. For chronic nausea or vomiting, identify the underlying cause. Discuss with physician use of antiemetic drugs when nausea or vomiting is caused by motion sickness or cancer chemotherapy or when the exertion of vomiting threatens to disrupt the wound in the postoperative patient.
PREADMINISTRATION ASSESSMENT	
Baseline Data	Observe for anorexia, vomiting, weight loss, or behavior indicating presence of nausea. Distinguish between episodes of vomiting, retching, regurgitation, or coughing. Determine frequency and duration of episodes. Determine the time of day and relationship to meals. Evaluate vital signs, fluid intake and output, weight changes, and skin turgor. Check for constipation. Examine vomitus for color, odor, consistency, or presence of mucus, bile, or blood. Evaluate contributing factors such as recent general anesthesia, influenza, motion, nauseating odors, elevated intracranial pressure, organic disorders of the upper alimentary tract, metabolic disorders (uremia, ketoacidosis, or viral hepatitis), or use of drugs that cause nausea and vomiting. Obtain laboratory tests including serum electrolytes, blood cell counts, and platelet counts if vomiting is prolonged. If ingestion of a poison is suspected, a sample of vomitus may be analyzed for presence of particular chemicals.
EVALUATION OF DRUG RESPONSE	
For Therapeutic Benefit	Monitor for relief of nausea and vomiting and ability to resume nutrition.
For Adverse Effects	Monitor for anticholinergic symptoms (dryness of mouth, blurred vision, and urinary retention), orthostatic hypotension, sedation, allergic reactions, parkinsonian-like symptoms, and other drug-specific adverse effects (see individual drug discussions).
For Drug Interactions	Monitor for increased toxicity of poisons that would normally elicit emesis before complete absorption.

Tablets, liquid, injection solution
Recommended Doses: As antiemetic in adults, 50–100 mg orally, up to 4 times per day. For children 2–5 years of age who experience motion sickness, 12.5–25 mg PO up to 3 times daily, with the initial dose given 30–60 minutes before travel.

Diphenidol (Vontrol)
Tablets
Recommended Doses: For adults, 25 mg PO every 4 hours. For children, 0.4 mg/lb, up to 25 mg, every 4 hours.

Dronabinol (Marinol)
Liquid capsules
Recommended Doses: 5 mg/m^2 orally, 1–3 hours prior to chemotherapy, repeated every 2–4 hours up to 6 doses daily. The initial amount can be increased in increments of 2.5 mg/m^2 up to a maximum of 15 mg/m^2 per dose.

Perphenazine (Trilafon)
Tablets, repetabs, concentrate, injection solution
Recommended Doses: For suppression of vomiting, 8–16 mg daily in divided oral doses. For rapid control of vomiting, 5–10 mg intramuscularly or 1 mg per injection intravenously up to 5 mg.

Phosphorated Carbohydrate Solution (Eazol, Emetrol, Especol, Nausetrol)
Oral solution
Recommended Doses: For adults, 15–30 ml PO at 15 minute intervals. For children, 5–10 ml at 15 minute intervals.

Prochlorperazine (Compazine)
Tablets and sustained release capsules as the maleate salt; syrup and injection solution as the edisylate salt; suppositories
Recommended Doses: As antiemetic, 5–10 mg, up to 4 times per day, orally, IM, or rectal suppository.

Nursing Diagnoses and Interventions for Use of Antiemetic Drugs for Nausea and Vomiting

Nursing Diagnoses	*Related Interventions*
TO ENHANCE DRUG BENEFITS OR REDUCE DRUG REQUIREMENTS	
Alteration in comfort related to nausea and vomiting	Provide comfort measures. Minimize noxious odors. Apply cool cloth to the forehead. Remove food from the client's sight and reduce other contributing factors when possible.
Alteration in nutrition: intake less than requirements related to vomiting or anorexia due to nausea	Provide the client with a liquid diet. Provide foods the client enjoys and can tolerate. Encourage client to drink small amounts of fruit juices. Avoid hot or cold liquids.
Alterations in oral mucous membranes related to irritation by vomitus	Intensify oral hygienic measures. Encourage flossing and use of a soft toothbrush. Encourage use of a mouthwash to alleviate distaste associated with vomiting.
TO ENSURE SAFE AND EFFICACIOUS DRUG USE	
Knowledge deficit related to drug regimen	Teach clients about foods and drugs that may contribute to occurrence of nausea and vomiting. Carefully explain the dosage and administration of antiemetic drugs. Advise women who have nausea or vomiting related to pregnancy (morning sickness) to refrain from use of antiemetic drugs. If the severity of the problem is intolerable, encourage the client to discuss the problem with the obstetrician to obtain appropriate medication. Provide the client with a list of adverse effects and drug interactions for each drug in the regimen and explain what to do if any of these occur.

Promethazine (Phernergan and others)
Tablets, syrup, suppositories, injection solution
Recommended Doses: For nausea and vomiting, 25 mg orally at 4–6 hour intervals. For children, 0.25–0.5 mg/kg intramuscularly every 4–6 hours.

Scopolamine
Capsules (Triptone), transdermal therapeutic system (patches) that delivers 0.5 mg scopolamine for 3 days after administration.
Recommended Doses: 0.25 mg PO, 1 hour before anticipated travel, repeated in 4 hours if necessary. Maximum daily dose: 1mg. The patch is applied to the postauricular skin at least 4 hours before the antiemetic effect is required.

Triflupromazine (Vesprin)
Injection solutions
Recommended Doses: For adults, 5–15 mg intramuscularly every 4 hours up to 60 mg daily or 1 mg intravenously up to 3 mg daily. For children over 2.5 years of age, 0.2–0.25 mg/kg intramuscularly up to 10 mg/day.

Trimethobenzamide (Tigan)
Capsules, suppositories, injection solution
Recommended Doses: 250 mg PO, up to 4 times daily.

Important Nursing Implications for Antiemetic Drugs

- ☐ Instruct clients not to use antiemetic drugs for vomiting of unknown origin.
- ☐ Advise women who are pregnant to avoid use

of antiemetic drugs. Suggest other methods for minimizing nausea and vomiting such as eating frequent small meals or snacks. If the client persists in wanting an antiemetic drug for morning sickness, provide her with a list of drugs to avoid (those with the highest risk of teratogenicity) and warn her to limit the use of any drug to very brief periods.

- ☐ Warn clients that drowsiness is often a side effect of antiemetic medications and urge them to avoid driving or other hazardous activities while using a drug in this group.
- ☐ Advise clients that depressant effects of antiemetic drugs may be additive with those of other CNS depressants, including alcohol.
- ☐ Teach clients to recognize the symptoms of allergic reaction to any antiemetic drug that is prescribed or self-administered.
- ☐ Antiemetics taken to suppress motion sickness should be taken about 30 minutes before anticipated travel time.
- ☐ Employ nursing measures to promote the antiemetic activity of administered antiemetic drugs. Comfort measures, ice chips, a warm drink, and a quiet environment help.

Peptic Ulcer and Antiulcer Drugs

Pathophysiology of Peptic Ulcers

Peptic ulcer is a localized lesion of the mucous membrane of the upper gastrointestinal tract (Figure 51–1). The lesions may be single or multiple. The crater formed by the ulcer extends through the mucosal lining or, in severe cases, all the way through the smooth muscle, producing a perforation of the entire gastric or intestinal wall. Peptic ulcers occur most commonly in the duodenal bulb (**duodenal ulcers**) and in the lesser curvature of the stomach (**gastric ulcers**). Less commonly, ulcers can form in the pyloric channel or in the lower end of the esophagus. Peptic ulcers occur in approximately 10% of the population in the United States and are responsible for about 4 million hospital days per year.

Ulcers can occur acutely as a complication of surgery, trauma, toxicity, or other diseases. The hemorrhaging that results from the penetration of blood vessels in the stomach wall can be life-threatening. If recognized quickly and dealt with adequately, acute ulcerations heal with minimal scar tissue formation and are unlikely to recur. Recurrent ulcers are far more common and are a major public health problem. The healing process usually requires 4–8 weeks, although pain often subsides within about 1 week. During healing, granular connective tissue forms at

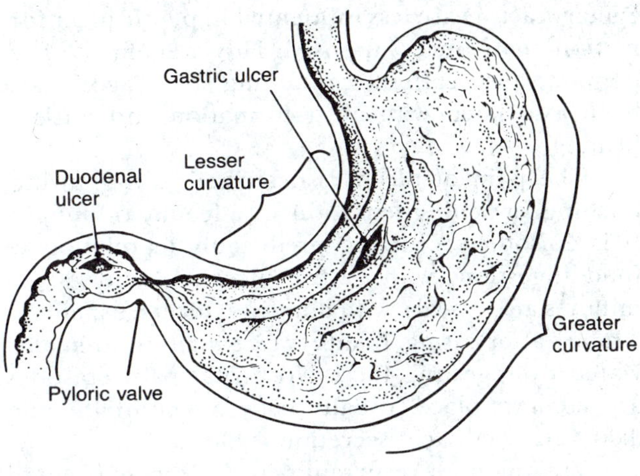

Figure 51–1
Common sites of peptic ulcers. From Barbara L. Bullock and Pearl Philbrook Rosendahl, *Pathophysiology: Adaptations and Alterations in Function*, Fig. 35-5. Copyright © 1984 by Barbara L. Bullock and Pearl Philbrook Rosendahl. Reprinted by permission of Little, Brown and Company.

the base of the ulcerous crater and spreads outward toward the circumference; it may adhere to adjacent structures, causing later complications. In more than one-half of clients, peptic ulcers recur within 2 years after healing.

The pathogenesis of peptic ulcers is not known, but they appear to be caused by disruption of the normal balance between digestive secretions and protective secretions. Hydrochloric acid secreted by the stomach as part of the digestive process is the major ulcer-promoting factor; the digestive enzyme pepsin may contribute as well. However, many individuals with elevated levels of secretion are free of ulceration. It may be that individuals who are susceptible to peptic ulcers have weaker protective factors, collectively called the **gastric mucosal barrier.** These include the integrity of the surface columnar epithelial cells, the viability of the tight junctions between the cells, the degree of permeability of the lipid layer of the cells, and the quantity and quality of the mucous coating.

The etiology of peptic ulcer is even less well understood at this time. Peptic ulcers may be neurogenic in part, occurring in response to chronic stress, but ulcers sometimes occur in individuals who experience very little tension or anxiety. There appears to be a genetic influence, but ulcer is not a hereditary disease determined by a single chromosome. Of the variety of drugs that are ulcergenic, the most important (since they are the most common) are alcohol, aspirin, caffeine, and probably nicotine. But while use of these drugs increases the risk of ulcer, the drugs are not implicated clearly in all cases. Dietary factors are less influential in peptic ulcer formation than once supposed. However, fatty diets, pepper, and caffeine-containing beverages have been associated with ulcer formation and impede healing.

The pain of ulcers is described as a gnawing, burning, or aching sensation, or a feeling of hunger. It is episodic, occurring predictably in relation to food ingestion: with gastric ulcers, usually 30–90 minutes after meals; with duodenal ulcers, usually 2–3 hours after eating. In either case, pain is often alleviated by ingesting food. Nocturnal pain episodes are commonplace, usually between midnight and 3:00 A.M., when acid secretion is elevated.

Treatment of recurrent peptic ulcers may entail (1) nondrug measures, including dietary adjustments and stress-reduction, (2) primary drug treatments, and (3) supplemental drugs, if required. The American Dietetic Association recommends a well-balanced diet for people with ulcers. Usually, only pepper, caffeine, alcohol, and sometimes nicotine are eliminated or sharply curtailed, as are any foods specifically identified by the individual as aggravating factors. Late-night snacks are eliminated if nocturnal episodes of pain are a factor. Frequent small meals reduce total daily acid secretion and make better use of the buffering capacity of food. The primary drug selections for peptic ulcers are (1) antacids and (2) blockers of H_2-histamine receptors. Prostaglandins, such as misoprostol (Cytotec), are under investigation for use in treatment.

Antacids

Mechanisms and Effects Antacids increase the pH of the gastric contents, which promotes healing of peptic ulcers and alleviates other forms of hyperacidity. The agents currently in use are all weak bases, capable of combining with hydrochloric acid to form salts and water. It is not necessary for an antacid actually to neutralize stomach pH (raising it to a neutral 7.0); if the drug raises pH three units (from a typical value of 1.3 up to a value of 4.3), it effects a thousandfold reduction in hydrogen ion concentration. Elevation of stomach pH also reduces activity of pepsin.

Antacids are classified as absorbable (or systemic) and nonabsorbable (or nonsystemic). In reality, the distinction is less absolute than the terms imply, since many so-called nonabsorbable antacids are absorbed to some extent and may yield systemic toxicity. Sodium bicarbonate, the major systemic antacid, can produce acid-rebound, risk of systemic alkalosis, and sodium overload. It is no longer used for neutralizing gastric contents in peptic ulcers. Its use in alleviating systemic acidosis is discussed in Chapter 42.

The nonabsorbable antacids currently in use are bases or salts of three metals: magnesium, aluminum, and calcium. Selection of an antacid is based on three primary considerations: acid-neutralizing capacity (Table 51–2), the risk of adverse effects, and palatability. Factors that influence compliance, such as cost, are additional factors in choosing a drug. In general, calcium carbonate has the greatest capacity for neutralizing acid, but it also has the greatest risk of producing systemic toxicity. Aluminum compounds often do not provide sufficient acid-neutralizing capacity to be useful alone; moreover, aluminum is more readily absorbed than magnesium. Magnesium compounds provide the greatest margin of safety and have nearly the acid-neutralizing capacity of calcium carbonate. Aluminum and magnesium compounds can be advantageously combined, for reasons that will be discussed below. The majority of products available consist of such a combination with or without additional ingredients (see Table 51–2).

Antacids increase the secretion of gastric juices, in particular hydrochloric acid. Hypersecretion of HCl may persist when antacid therapy is discontinued. It occurs especially with calcium carbonate but may also occur after use of magnesium hydroxide.

Pharmacokinetics Antacids are available as liquid suspensions, chewable tablets, tablets for ingestion, capsules, and powders. Liquid suspensions provide superior activity because of their large surface area for interaction with acid. Calcium carbonate, magnesium hydroxide, and sodium bicarbonate provide rapid neutralization of stomach acid and consequently their effects are little affected by gastric emptying time. Magnesium carbonate and magnesium oxide provide slower neutralization, and aluminum hydroxide and salts have the slowest rate of activity.

Although both aluminum hydroxide and magnesium hydroxide are absorbed to a small extent, systemic accumulation occurs only in clients with renal insufficiency or after excessive self-dosing. When systemic accumulation does occur, adverse effects are due mainly to the metal ion rather than systemic alkalosis. Calcium carbonate absorption can be more problematic. If use is excessive, dangerous hypercalcemia may occur, especially if renal function is impaired, milk or cream is ingested concurrently, or gastrointestinal hemorrhage is present. The duration of action of antacids is determined by gastric emptying time (as much as 2–4 hours after eating or less than 1 hour when fasting).

Table 51–2

Forms, Contents, and Neutralizing Capacity of Representative Antacid Drugs

		Content (mg/tablet or 5 ml liquid)							
Antacid	Forms	$AL(OH)_3$	$Mg(OH)_2$	$Mg_2Si_3O_8$	$CaCO_3$	Other antacid	Simethicone	Sodium	Neutralizing capacity[a]
AlternaGel	Liquid	600						<2.5	16.0
Aludrox	Tablets	233	83					1.4	10.0
	Liquid	307	103					2.3	12.0
Amphojel	Tablets	300						1.8	8.0
	Liquid	320						<2.3	10.0
Basaljel	Capsules					400[b]		2.8	12.0
	Tablets					400[b]		2.1	13.0
	Liquid					400[b]		2.4	12.0
Basaljel Extra Strength	Liquid					1,000[b]		23	22.0
Camalox	Tablets	225	200		250			1.0	18.0
	Liquid	225	200		250			2.5	22.3
Delcid	Liquid	600	665					<15	42.0
Di-Gel	Tablets	282[c]	85				25	<5	9.0
	Liquid	200	200				20	<5	10.5
Gelusil	Tablets	200	200					0.8	11.0
	Liquid	200	200				25	0.7	12.0
Gelusil-II	Tablets	400	400				30	2.1	21.0
	Liquid	400	400				30	1.3	24.0
Gelusil-M	Tablets	300	200				25	1.3	12.6
	Liquid	300	200				25	1.2	15.0
Kolantyl Gel	Liquid	150	150					<4.6	10.5
Maalox	Tablet #1	200	200					0.7	9.7
	Liquid	225	200					1.4	13.3
Maalox Plus	Tablets	200	200				25	0.8	11.4
	Liquid	225	200				25	1.2	13.3
Maalox TC	Tablets	600	300					0.5	28
Mylanta	Tablets	200	200				20	0.77	11.5
	Liquid	200	200				20	0.68	12.7
Mylanta-II	Tablets	400	400				40	1.3	23.0
	Liquid	400	400				40	1.14	25.4
Phosphaljel	Liquid					233[d]		7.0	2.2
Riopan	Tablets					480[e]		<0.1	13.5
	Liquid					540[e]		<0.1	15.0
Riopan Plus	Tablets					480[e]	20	<0.1	13.5
	Liquid					540[e]	20	<0.1	15.0
Silain-Gel	Liquid	282	285				25	4.8	15.0
Titralac	Tablets				420	150[f]		<0.3	7.5
	Liquid				1,000	300[f]		11	19.0
Triconsil	Tablets	80		80		200[g]		50.6	?
Win Gel	Tablets	180	160					<2.5	12.3
	Liquid	180	160					2.5	11.6

[a]Acid neutralizing capacity (mEg/L) per tablet or 5 ml
[b]Aluminum carbonate
[c]Aluminum hydroxide and magensium carbonate
[d]Aluminum phosphate
[e]Magaldrate
[f]Glycine
[g]Sodium bicarbonate

Clinical Indications Antacids are prescribed by physicians mainly for treatment of active peptic ulcers and esophagitis due to reflux. They also relieve symptoms of gastritis, hyperacidity, heartburn, or hiatal hernia. Since antacids are readily available as nonprescription drugs, they are self-administered for a variety of appropriate situations but are also widely abused.

For active peptic ulcers, antacids are generally used in intensive regimens of 15–30 ml administered hourly for several weeks to maintain a pH of 5 or more. In less severe cases, the antacid may be taken 4–7 times daily, once or twice after each meal and at bedtime. Antacid regimens of this sort have been demonstrated to promote healing of peptic ulcers, provided that compliance is adequate. Ironically, antacids are all too often overused for inappropriate conditions and underutilized when intensive therapy is required.

Adverse Effects and Contraindications The adverse effects of antacids are summarized in Table 51–3. The shared adverse effects of antacids are those that relate to alterations in pH. Within the stomach itself, elevation of pH may increase susceptibility to infection by pathogens that are ordinarily inhibited by the acid environment. Systemic alkalosis is not uncommon when calcium carbonate is

Nursing Observations for Use of Antiulcer Medications for Peptic Ulcer

THERAPEUTIC GOAL	(1) Promote healing of the ulcer by decreasing ulcer-promoting and increasing protective mechanisms, and (2) prevent complications such as penetration, perforation, hemorrhage, and obstruction.
PREADMINISTRATION ASSESSMENT	
Baseline Data	Question client about presence of (1) localized epigastric pain which has a gnawing, burning, or aching quality; (2) episodic pain 30–90 minutes (gastric) or 2–3 (duodenal) hours after meals; (3) nocturnal epigastric pain, especially between midnight and 3:00 A.M. Evaluate location and quality of pain and relationship to meals; check for occult blood in the stools; conduct gastrointestinal x-rays and gastroscopy. Before initiating drug therapy, palpate the abdomen and take blood pressure, pulse, and ECG. Assess client's gastrointestinal output, skin integrity, and neurologic status. Obtain laboratory tests including complete blood cell counts, hematocrit, hemoglobin, and liver and renal function tests.
Contraindications/ Precautions	Hepatic or renal failure, pregnancy, or lactation. Check medication history for drug allergies.
Potential Interactions	Check current regimen for interacting drugs.
EVALUATION OF DRUG RESPONSE	
For Therapeutic Benefit	Monitor pain relief and healing of the ulcer.
For Adverse Effects	Monitor for diarrhea, constipation, dizziness, drowsiness, headache, urinary retention, symptoms of pyloric obstruction, acid-rebound, and other drug-specific adverse effects.
For Drug Interactions	Monitor for additive effects on gastrointestinal motility. Watch for use of ulcergenic drugs. Observe for other drug-specific interactions including decreased effect of anticoagulants, beta-blockers, theophylline, benzodiazepines, phenytoin, and digoxin when cimetidine is employed.
For Dietary Interactions	Assess for ulcergenic effects of irritant foods and the influence of frequency, size, and timing of meals on episodes of pain.
For Compliance	Evaluate the client's compliance with all facets of the therapeutic regimen by careful observation, interviewing, and review of progress. Report compliance problems to the physician and act as client-advocate when changes in the therapeutic regimen seem indicated.

Table 51–3
Adverse Effects of Antacids

Antacid	Gastrointestinal infection	Metabolic alkalosis	Acid rebound	Diarrhea	Constipation	Milk-alkali syndrome	Hypermagnesia	Aluminum encephalopathy	Hypophosphatemia
Sodium bicarbonate	+	++	++	—	—	+	—	—	—
Calcium carbonate	+	+	++	—	++	++	—	—	—
Aluminum hydroxide	+	+/−*	—	—	++	—	—	+/−*	+
Magnesium hydroxide	+	+/−*	+	++	—	—	++	—	—
Aluminum and magnesium hydroxide combinations	+	+/−*	—	+	+	—	+	—	+

Key: *, only if renal insufficiency is present; —, does not occur; +/−, occurs rarely; +, occurs occasionally; ++, occurs often.

employed but occurs with aluminum and magnesium hydroxides only in clients with impaired renal function. Calcium carbonate use may cause the **milk-alkali syndrome** (especially if milk or cream is ingested as well), which can be recognized by the characteristic symptoms of hypercalcemia and hyperphosphatemia. Clients with these symptoms should be observed closely because severe milk-alkali syndrome may lead to impairment of kidney function, which will in turn aggravate the hypercalcemia. Acute renal failure and azotemia may result.

Acid rebound occurs most severely when calcium carbonate is the antacid employed. It is occasionally noted with magnesium hydroxide but seldom with aluminum hydroxide or salts. Acid rebound is likely to occur during sleep, causing episodes of nocturnal pain.

Antacids frequently alter gastrointestinal motility. Aluminum-containing antacids cause **constipation,** probably from the mild astringent effect caused by formation of complexes with membrane proteins of intestinal mucosal cells. Magnesium compounds, on the other hand, have a **cathartic** effect. Thus, aluminum and magnesium antacids are often combined to offset the opposing effects on intestinal motility. Calcium carbonate usually has a mild constipating action.

Prolonged use of aluminum hydroxide together with low dietary intake of phosphate may cause **hypophosphatemia** from the formation of insoluble aluminum phosphate salts. Long-term hypophosphatemia leads to osteomalacia and myopathies (see Chapter 42). Aluminum accumulation in the brain can result in encephalopathy, but accumulation occurs only in clients who also have renal insufficiency. Aluminum salts slow gastric emptying time and are therefore contraindicated if pyloric obstruction is present.

Magnesium accumulation when magnesium compounds are employed is likewise limited to persons with renal insufficiency. **Hypermagnesia** is associated with neurologic, neuromuscular, and cardiovascular dysfunctions. Magnesium trisilicate, a salt found in some combination antacids, may cause formation of silicate renal stones. Less commonly, fecal stones composed of $Mg(OH)_2$ or $MgCO_3$ occur when magnesium hydroxide is employed.

Interactions of Antacids with Drugs and Nutrients Antacids can alter the absorption of various drugs and nutrients. The important role of pH in the absorption of weak acids and bases is discussed in Chapter 4. Antacids tend to decrease absorption of weak acids such as salicylates, naproxen, indomethacin, and sulfadiazine. On the other hand, antacids can increase absorption of weak bases. Some drugs such as quinidine and quinine are poorly soluble in alkaline fluid and may precipitate when given with antacids.

Aluminum compounds retard gastric emptying time, while calcium and magnesium antacids hasten gastric emptying. Aluminum has been observed to retard absorption of barbiturates, digoxin (Lanoxin), isoniazid (Nydrazid), naproxen (Naprosyn), pheny-

Nursing Diagnoses and Interventions for Use of Antiulcer Medications for Peptic Ulcer

Nursing Diagnoses	*Related Interventions*
TO ENHANCE DRUG BENEFITS OR REDUCE DRUG REQUIREMENTS	
Ineffective individual coping: excessive anger, anxiety, or resentment contributing to occurrence of peptic ulcers	Provide physical and mental rest. Consider referral for humor therapy if available. Provide relaxed environment, understanding, and patience.
TO MINIMIZE DRUG SIDE EFFECTS OR INTERACTIONS	
Alteration in bowel elimination: constipation related to dietary restrictions, antacids, or anticholinergics	Adjust diet. Eliminate anticholinergics, or balance a constipating antacid with one that increases intestinal motility.
Alteration in bowel elimination: diarrhea related to H_2-blockers or antacids	Employ an antacid that reduces intestinal motility.
Alteration in comfort: pain related to the ulceration or headache caused by H_2-blockers	Eliminate ulcergenic foods and drugs; instruct clients to take late-night snacks for nocturnal episodes; suggest client eat more frequent smaller meals; provide nonnarcotic analgesics for relief of headache as required.
Sensory-perceptual alterations: dizziness caused by H_2-blockers	Provide safety measures as required.
TO ENSURE SAFE AND EFFICACIOUS DRUG USE	
Knowledge deficit related to drug regimen	Educate the client about the nature of peptic ulcers, the role of stress, diet, and drugs, and the rationale for the prescribed regimen.
	Teach the client to keep a diary to determine activities that provoke stress and ulcer attacks. Help client to identify effective methods of countering social or vocational stress.
	Teach the client to take H_2-blockers immediately before meals to decrease food-induced acid secretion.
	Teach the client to relieve nocturnal episodes of ulcer pain by setting an alarm for 1 hour before the usual time of attacks to take an antacid.
	Stress the importance of compliance with the therapeutic regimen 4–6 weeks after overt symptoms of peptic ulcers have subsided.
	Advise the client to refrain from use of ulcergenic drugs, such as caffeine, nicotine, alcohol, and aspirin, and from ulcergenic foods, including fats and pepper.
	Provide client with a list of adverse effects and drug interactions for each drug in the regimen and explain what to do if any of these occur.
	Teach clients how to recognize indications that a complication is developing.

toin (Dilantin), propranolol (Inderal), quinidine (Cin-Quin), benzodiazepines, and warfarin (Coumadin). Antacids other than aluminum speed delivery of drugs to the intestines, where most absorption occurs. Enteric coated formulations are more rapidly disintegrated because of more rapid delivery to the intestines and the elevated pH. Antacids also frequently alter motility. The cathartic effect of magnesium, when it occurs, impairs absorption of poorly absorbed drugs when bioavailability depends on the transit time through the alimentary tract.

Antacids may also interact chemically with substances in the alimentary tract. Aluminum will form complexes with many drugs, including propranolol, antimuscarinics, phenothiazines, digoxin, tetracyclines, and sulfadiazine, impairing their absorption rates. Magnesium compounds bind with digoxin and tetracyclines, decreasing the bioavailability in each case. Most antacids inhibit absorption of oral iron. If an antacid is absorbed sufficiently to cause alkalinization of the urine, elimination rates of weak bases, such as quinidine and amphetamines, are decreased; elimination of weak acids such as aspirin is increased. *To avoid alterations in absorption kinetics, oral medications should not be taken within 2 hours after using an antacid.*

Preparations and Administration Aluminum compounds employed in antacid preparations include aluminum hydroxide, aluminum phosphate, dihydroxyaluminum aminoacetate, dihydroxyaluminum sodium carbonate, and aluminum carbonate. Aluminum hydroxide is the usual form found in antacid combinations. Aluminum phosphate, found only in Phosphajel, is especially ineffective. Dihydroxyaluminum sodium carbonate (found only in Rolaids) is partially a systemic antacid because it incorporates a sodium bicarbonate moiety. Aluminum carbonate (Basaljel) has better neutralizing capacity than aluminum hydroxide and causes less hypophosphatemia.

Magnesium compounds employed as antacids are magnesium hydroxide, magnesium oxide, magnesium trisilicate, magnesium carbonate, and magaldrate. Magnesium hydroxide is the most widely utilized. Magnesium carbonate is slower acting and releases carbon dioxide, which may cause belching. Magnesium oxide is slower acting than the hydroxide but is otherwise comparable. Magaldrate, a complex of magnesium and aluminum hydroxides, has the advantage of reacting with acid in successive stages and presents aluminum hydroxide in a usable form for acid neutralization.

Other antacids include calcium carbonate and sodium bicarbonate. Calcium carbonate is seldom used alone because of its untoward effects but is incorporated into several combination products. Sodium bicarbonate is utilized in effervescent tablets such as Alka-Seltzer, Bromo Seltzer, and Bisodol. It is well absorbed and will produce systemic alkalosis if used on a regular basis. Many antacid formulations contain simethicone, a defoaming agent that reduces gastroesophageal reflux.

Important Nursing Implications for Antacids

- ☐ Make certain that clients know how to recognize the potential adverse effects that occur with the kind of antacid prescribed.
- ☐ Advise clients who frequently self-medicate with antacids to seek medical evaluation. Advise the client if there are potential interactions between the antacid and other drugs the client is taking.
- ☐ Check the sodium content of prescribed and self-administered antacids to determine if the preparation provides a level of sodium that will interfere with maintenance of any dietary restrictions the client may have.
- ☐ Advise clients that antacid liquids or chewable tablets provide better neutralizing capacity than tablets that are swallowed.
- ☐ Advise clients who use liquid antacids to substitute the chewable tablets should they experience loss of appetite.
- ☐ Antacids taken immediately after meals tend to slow gastric emptying, prolonging digestive activity in the stomach. Therefore, instruct clients to take their scheduled antacids 1–3 hours after meals.
- ☐ Instruct clients that antacid suspensions must be vigorously shaken before a dose is taken.
- ☐ If a client uses chewable tablets, discuss the need to pulverize the tablet thoroughly before swallowing it.
- ☐ Stress the importance of maintaining the prescribed schedule of antacid administration even after overt symptoms of the ulcer have subsided.

Pepsin Inhibitor

Sucralfate (Carafate), a drug marketed in 1981 as an antiulcer agent, is a complex of aluminum hydroxide with sulfonated sucrose, which has an antipepsin activity. Sucralfate is a nonabsorbable tenacious substance that is thought to combine with proteins secreted from ulcer sites in the duodenum.

It covers the ulcer and protects it from further attack by inhibiting pepsin activity.

Although the sucralfate complex includes aluminum hydroxide, it does not neutralize acid to the extent that antacids do. Sucralfate may be used in conjunction with antacid therapy, but the antacid should not be administered within 30 minutes before or after sucralfate. Sucralfate has some ability to sequester bile acids and may possibly cause deficiencies of fat-soluble vitamins if used for an extended period of time. Constipation is the most common side effect, occurring in 2% of patients. There are no systemic adverse effects since the drug is not absorbed.

Preparations and Administration

Sucralfate (Carafate)
Tablets
Recommended Doses: For adults, 1 g PO qid taken on an empty stomach, 1 hour before meals and at bedtime.

Histamine (H_2) Blocking Drugs

Secretion of hydrochloric acid in the stomach is partly regulated by H_2-histamine receptors. Conventional antihistamines block only H_1-histamine receptors and thus have no effect on acid secretion. A major advance in recent years has been the development and introduction of drugs that block H_2-histamine receptors. The first such drug to be marketed was cimetidine (Tagamet). Ranitidine (Zantac) was added in 1983 and famotidine (Pepcid) in 1986. H_2-blockers have revolutionized treatment of peptic ulcers in a few short years of use.

Mechanisms and Effects H_2-receptor blockers inhibit both basal and induced secretion of gastric acid. Gastric acid secretion that follows meals, distention of the gastric fundus, or administration of gastrin, histamine, cholinomimetics, insulin, or caffeine are all reduced by pretreatment with H_2-receptor blockers. Pepsin and hydrochloric acid secretory rates are reduced proportionately. H_2-blockers do not suppress secretion of proteins, gastrin, or pancreatic juices, and do not significantly alter gastric emptying time. The H_2-blockers currently in use (cimetidine, famotidine, and ranitidine) are relatively specific for H_2-histamine receptors.

Pharmacokinetics H_2-blockers are incompletely absorbed after oral administration (cimetidine, about 60%; ranitidine, about 50%; famotidine, about 45%). The rate of absorption is altered by factors that change gastric emptying time. Food ingestion, anticholinergics, and antacid preparations consisting mainly of aluminum hydroxide retard gastric emptying time, slowing absorption and prolonging the duration of action of H_2-receptor blockers. Cimetidine reaches peak concentrations in 1–1.5 hours and is 85% bound by plasma proteins. Famotidine reaches peak plasma concentrations in 1–3 hours and is only 15–20% bound to plasma proteins. Cimetidine is excreted unchanged in the urine, ranitidine is metabolized in the liver, and famotidine is eliminated two-thirds by renal excretion, one-third by liver metabolism. All three drugs appear in breast milk. Cimetidine crosses the placental barrier; placental transfer is not determined for the other two drugs.

Clinical Indications All three H_2-blockers are approved for short-term treatment of active peptic ulcers, prophylaxis against recurrence, and alleviation of hypersecretory states, such as Zollinger-Ellison syndrome. Ranitidine may be more effective than cimetidine in the latter condition, in which rates of acid production are extremely high. Some clients with peptic ulcer refractory to cimetidine respond to ranitidine. The H_2-blockers are as effective as antacids in promoting healing of ulcers. As with antacid therapy, there is a high risk of recurrence after therapy is discontinued. H_2-blockers can be successfully employed in combination with antacids or anticholinergics. The antisecretory effect of H_2-blockers is enhanced by concurrent use of anticholinergics, but the use of anticholinergics is justifiable only in severe cases not adequately manageable with H_2-blockers and antacids.

Adverse Effects and Contraindications H_2-blockers are well tolerated by most clients. Adverse effects are infrequent and seldom significant. However, some clients may complain of headache, malaise, dizziness, constipation, diarrhea, nausea, cramps, and skin rash. Rarely, H_2-blockers adversely affect CNS function, leading to symptoms such as confusion, delirium, slurred speech, or hallucinations. At the first indication of such reaction, drug therapy should be discontinued. Cimetidine has a weak antiandrogenic effect not shared by the other two drugs. Cimetidine can cause gynecomastia and reduction in sperm count in males, or galactorrhea in females as a result of its antiandrogenic properties. *Clients should be educated about these symptoms and told to report gynecomastia or galactorrhea to the physician if they occur.*

Some clients receiving cimetidine have developed increased prothrombin time. Occasionally, clients receiving H_2-blockers develop leukopenia, agranulocytosis, thrombocytopenia, or anemia. *Cli-*

ents should have periodic evaluations of blood count and renal and hepatic functions during therapy with one of these drugs.

If the client is elderly, severely ill, or has impaired renal function, fluid intake and output should be monitored during therapy with H_2-blockers. Some clients have developed paralytic ileus. *An absence of bowel sounds, bowel movements, or flatus should be reported to the physician immediately.*

Drug Interactions Cimetidine is a weak inhibitor of the cytochrome oxidase system of the liver that is responsible for oxidation of warfarin (Coumadin), propranolol (Inderal), diazepam (Valium) and several other benzodiazepines, and theophylline. Cimetidine can therefore potentiate activity of these drugs. Ranitidine does not significantly alter metabolism via this system.

Preparations and Administration *Clients should take H_2-blockers with meals so that the peak effect will coincide with the period of peak gastric acid secretion.* Antacids are often employed concurrently to control ulcer pain and should be taken 1 hour before or 1 hour after an H_2-blocker. Although pain often subsides within 1 week, it is important that the drug regimen be continued until healing of the ulcer is complete (4–8 weeks). Relapse is common when therapy is discontinued, and especially if discontinued prematurely. *Clients should be instructed to report immediately any recurrence of abdominal pain, bloody stools, or other indications of ulcer reactivation.* Prophylaxis for recurrent ulcer is provided by 400 mg of cimetidine taken at bedtime.

Cimetidine (Tagamet)
Tablets, oral solution, injection solution
Recommended Doses: For active peptic ulcers, 300 mg PO, 4 times a day, at mealtime and at bedtime. For maintenance, 400 mg PO at bedtime.

Famotidine (Pepcid)
Tablets, injection solution
Recommended Doses: For acute therapy, 40 mg PO once a day at bedtime. For maintenance, 20 mg PO at bedtime.

Ranitidine Hydrochloride (Zantac)
Tablets, injection solution
Recommended Doses: For acute therapy, 150 mg PO twice daily. For maintenance, 20 mg PO at bedtime.

Antimuscarinics in Peptic Ulcer

Antimuscarinics have been used in peptic ulcers for decades with variable results. Gastric secretions are stimulated by acetylcholine released by the vagus nerve. The effect is mediated by muscarinic receptors. The efficacy of antimuscarinics, however, is not very great and they produce a wide range of anticholinergic side effects. In addition, antimuscarinics are specifically contraindicated when peptic ulcer is accompanied by pyloric obstruction, since these drugs slow gastric emptying by inhibiting opening of the pylorus. Anticholinergics are most appropriately used in clients with duodenal ulcer where the delay in gastric emptying time is not a problem. Anticholinergics have been classified as effective for adjunctive therapy of peptic ulcers (that is, they should not be used alone).

Gastrointestinal Stimulants

Mechanisms and Effects Metoclopramide (Reglan) stimulates motility in the upper gastrointestinal tract without altering gastric, biliary, or pancreatic secretory activity. It accelerates gastric emptying because it relaxes the pyloric sphincter and increases gastric contractions. It also speeds transit in the upper intestine but has little effect on motility of the colon.

Metoclopramide is a dopamine antagonist, blocking both intestinal and CNS dopamine receptors. Because of the effect on central dopamine receptors, metoclopramide causes neuroleptic-like sedation and extrapyramidal reactions (in about 1 of 500 clients). The inhibition of dopamine receptors in the gut has the effect of sensitizing the gastrointestinal tissues to the actions of acetylcholine. The pharmacological actions of metoclopramide are diminished by anticholinergic drugs and increased by cholinomimetics.

Pharmacokinetics Metoclopramide has an onset of action in 1–3 minutes after intravenous administration or 10–15 minutes after intramuscular injection. When used orally, metoclopramide is well absorbed, acting in 30–60 minutes but is subject to considerable first-pass extraction. Its half-life is about 4 hours and effectiveness persists for 1–2 hours after onset of action. The drug is both metabolized in the liver and excreted unchanged in the urine.

Clinical Indications Metoclopramide is useful orally in stimulating gastric emptying in clients with recurrent diabetic gastroparesis, in whom delayed gastric emptying causes symptoms such as nausea, vomiting, anorexia, or persistent fullness. Metoclopramide has been found useful in hastening the healing of gastric ulcers and preventing relapse but is ineffective for duodenal ulcers. Metoclopramide may be used parenterally to facilitate small bowel intubation when the tube does not freely pass the pylourus using conventional procedures. It is also employed to hasten transit of barium given for purposes of radiologic examination of the stomach or small intestines.

Adverse Effects and Contraindications Metoclorpramide causes drowsiness, fatigue, lassitude, or restlessness in about 10% of patients receiving the drug. *Nurses should warn clients that drowsiness caused by the drug may impair the ability to drive or to perform other hazardous tasks.* Metoclopramide is contraindicated in clients with gastrointestinal obstruction, hemorrhage, or perforation, which would be aggravated by increased motility. It is also contraindicated in patients with pheochromacytoma, epilepsy, extrapyramidal disorders, or previous allergic reactions to the drug.

Drug Interactions The depressant effects of metoclopramide are additive to depressant influences of other CNS drugs.

Preparations and Administration

Metoclopramide (Reglan)
Tablets, injection solution
Recommended Doses: For relief of delayed gastric emptying, 10 mg initially, PO, 30 minutes before meals and bedtime. For facilitation of small bowel intubation or barium transit, a single 10 mg dose IV.

Antiflatulents

Simethicone and activated charcoal are sometimes employed to reduce intestinal gas and to alleviate flatulence. Simethicone acts on fluids in the stomach and intestines, altering the surface tension of gas bubbles and causing them to coalesce and release their contents of gas. Simethicone can be employed to alleviate pain from excessive gas in the intestines or stomach, which often occurs in diverticulitis, peptic ulcer, functional dyspepsia, or irritable bowel syndrome and after surgery.

Charcoal is occasionally employed to absorb gas in the digestive tract. It can also be used to absorb ingested toxins (see Chapter 57). Charcoal absorbs not only toxic substances but also nutrients and digestive enzymes and therefore should not be used on a routine basis. Charcoal should also be avoided when prescription drugs are being employed orally, since charcoal will alter absorption of many drugs.

Preparations and Administration

Charcoal
Tablets, capsules (Charcocaps)
Recommended Doses: 650–2,600 mg, up to 3 or 4 times daily. Tablets of charcoal are chewed or dissolved in the mouth.

Simethicone (Mylicon, Silain)
Tablets, chewable tablets, drops, combinations with antacids
Recommended Doses: 40–80 mg after meals or at bedtime, as needed.

Digestants

Digestants are drugs that supposedly promote the digestion of foods in the alimentary tract. The three categories of digestants currently on the market are (1) gastric acidifiers, (2) digestive enzymes, and (3) bile extracts. These agents are formulated into various combinations, often with additional constituents such as antacids, antiflatulents (simethicone), anticholinergics, and sedatives (phenobarbital or phenyltoloxamine citrate, an antihistamine). These products are used for symptomatic relief of indigestion, without evidence of benefit. The range of conditions for which digestants have demonstrable value is limited.

Gastric Acidifiers

Gastric acidifiers include diluted hydrochloric acid and glutamic acid hydrochloride (Acidulin). Theoretically, acidifiers should be of value in gastric achlorhydria. However, conventional doses of acidifiers do not significantly lower stomach pH. Also, because acid may damage teeth, acidifiers must be sipped through a straw or administered in capsules. Hydrochloric acid is administered at mealtimes as 5–10 ml of 10% hydrochloric acid further diluted into 125–250 ml of water.

Preparations and Administration

Glutamic Acid Hydrochloride
Tablets, capsules
Recommended Dose: One to three tablets or capsules before meals.

Digestive Enzymes

Digestive enzymes include the gastric enzyme, pepsin, and pancreatic enzymes. Pepsin can be used when secretion of gastric juices is insufficient (as in clients with pernicious anemia or gastric carcinoma) and aids in digesting proteins. It is not generally necessary to treat conditions of gastric insufficiency aggressively since the intestinal contribution to digestion is much more important that the gastric contribution and usually sufficient to provide adequate nutrition. Among the disorders likely to lead to deficient secretion of pancreatic enzymes are cystic fibrosis, chronic pancreatitis, pancreatectomy, pancreatic cancers that cause ductal obstructions, and pancreatic insufficiency. Pancreatic enzymes are effective in treating these deficiency conditions, aiding in digestion of fats, triglycerides, and carbohydrates.

Pancreatic enzymes preparations include pancreatin and pancrelipase. Both preparations are derived from bovine or porcine pancreatic tissue. They differ only in the level of activity of the three principal component enzymes: amylase, protease, and lipase. Adverse effects are uncommon. High doses may cause nausea and vomiting. Occasionally, hypersensitivity to these animal proteins occurs, in which event administration must be discontinued. Enteric coated formulations are advantageous since pancreatic enzymes can be destroyed by pepsin in the stomach. Cimetidine is sometimes employed with pancreatic enzyme preparations to suppress pepsin activity in the stomach so that the pancreatic enzymes can reach the duodenum intact. *Nurses should advise clients to take pancreatic enzyme preparations before or with meals. The dose should be adjusted in parallel with food intake. Related nursing management includes teaching the client to maintain a proper balance of nutrient groups (fats, protein, and starches) to enhance digestion and absorption.*

Preparations and Administration

Pancreatin (Elzyme, Viokase)
Tablets, enteric coated tablets, powder
Recommended Doses: 1–3 capsules or tablets PO after meals.

Pancrelipase (Cotazym, Ilozyme, Ku-Zyme HP, Pancrease)
Tablets, capsules, capsules containing enteric coated microspheres, powder packets
Recommended Doses: 1–3 capsules or tablets PO before or with meals or snacks.

Bile Extracts

Bile extracts are useful for conditions involving the biliary tract. Bile is the thick, viscid, yellow-brown or green-brown secretion of the liver and gallbladder that enters the duodenum by way of the bile duct. Bile is composed of pigments (bilirubin and biliverdin) from red blood cell decomposition, cholesterol, lecithin, mucin, bile salts, and other components. The bile salts are salt forms of the bile acids cholic acid and chenodeoxycholic acid. They contribute to digestion by promoting formation of micelles by emulsifying ingested lipids. Bile salts are themselves absorbed as components of the micelles and partake in enterohepatic cycling. The main therapeutic value of administered bile extracts is to stimulate bile flow, which occurs in proportion to the amount of administered drug. In fact, exogenously administered bile acids may slightly decrease excretion of bile pigments and are therefore ineffective in alleviating jaundice.

Chenodeoxycholic acid (also known as chenodiol) reduces the cholesterol content of bile by decreasing absorption of cholesterol from the small intestines and inhibiting synthesis of cholesterol within the liver. The decreased cholesterol content of the bile halts formation of cholesterolic gallstones and promotes dissolution of existing stones. Long-term use of chenodeoxycholic acid causes the loss of microvilli in patches along the biliary epithelium and may also cause hepatotoxicity. **Dehydrocholic acid** and **ketocholanic acids** decrease viscosity of bile and can be useful in flushing the biliary ducts; for example, they are used after surgery on the biliary tract. All bile acid preparations are useful as laxatives to alleviate uncomplicated constipation. The principal adverse effect of dehydrocholic acid and ketocholanic acid is diarrhea.

Preparations and Administration

Chenodeoxycholic Acid (Chenix)
Tablets
Recommended Doses: Initially, 250 mg PO, bid, for 2 weeks, increased by 250 mg/day each week until reaching the recommended final dose of 13–16 mg/kg/day in 2 divided oral doses, morning and evening. Therapy for gallstones typically requires 24 months of treatment.

Dehydrocholic Acid (Decholin, Hepahydrin, Neocholan, and others)
Tablets
Recommended Doses: 250–500 mg PO, after meals.

Ketocholanic Acids (Ketochol)
Tablet
Recommended Doses: 250–500 mg PO, after meals.

Ox Bile Extract
Enteric coated tablets
Recommended Doses: 150–600 mg PO with or after meals.

Intestinal Disorders and Drugs

Most of the absorption of nutrients occurs along the 12-ft length of the small intestine. To achieve this remarkable result, the small intestine performs three physiologic functions: digestion, movement of its contents, and selective absorption. In the duodenum, digestion is promoted by secretions from the pancreas, gallbladder, and liver. In the more distal portions of the small intestine, large quantities of enzymes contribute further to digestion. As digestion proceeds, the intestinal contents are propelled through the bowel by peristaltic contractions of the intestinal smooth muscle. At the same time, segmental contractions produce a kneading action on intestinal chyme. The propulsive peristaltic movements are regulated neurally to ensure adequate time for the small intestine to absorb nutrients and, later, the large intestines to absorb water. Unduly increased motility results in diarrhea; excessively low motility produces constipation.

If digestion is sufficiently complete and motility is adequately regulated, nutrient absorption will depend mainly on the integrity of the absorptive surface and absorptive mechanisms. Malabsorption may occur if (1) the endothelial cells of the intestinal villi are compromised by inflammation (enteritis), (2) the absorptive surface is reduced by surgical resection, (3) absorptive mechanisms are biochemically or genetically deficient, or (4) flow through mesenteric vascular or lymphatic vessels is insufficient. Vitamin supplements are often useful in alleviating secondary symptoms caused by malabsorption of micronutrients (see Chapter 44).

The most specific clinical indications of intestinal dysfunction are thus diarrhea, constipation, and malabsorption. In addition to these are the less specific symptoms of abdominal pain, nausea, vomiting, and anorexia, any of which may be indicative of intestinal problems or other kinds of disorders. For the most part, the use of drugs for intestinal effects is limited to the symptomatic relief of diarrhea and constipation. Primary treatment for underlying intestinal disorders seldom depends mainly on drugs that act specifically on the intestines. The four principal classes of agents that have important pharmacological actions on the intestines are (1) laxatives and cathartics, (2) antidiarrheal agents, (3) intestinal stimulants, and (4) intestinal antimicrobial drugs.

Constipation, Laxatives, and Cathartics

Constipation is difficult or infrequent passage of stools. It is a symptom of imprecise definition, subject to individual interpretation based on expectations of frequency and consistency of stools. The normal frequency of defecation varies from once in 3 days to three times per day. Acute constipation is a sudden change in the pattern of defecation for a given individual. The feces may be hard and dry, defecation may be infrequent or absent, or there may be a feeling of incomplete or difficult evacuation. Constipation of sudden onset is often related to psychological factors that interfere with the normal defecatory reflex. Acute constipation is also frequently observed as an adverse reaction to opiates, anticholinergics, ganglionic blockers, tricyclic antidepressants, calcium and aluminum antacids, iron or bismuth salts, or lead poisoning. Other causes of acute constipation include pregnancy, bowel obstruction, adynamic ileus, and general anesthesia.

Chronic constipation is often caused by dysfunction of the large intestine, which may be secondary to conditions such as major infections, hypothyroidism, hypercalcemia, porphyria, or uremia. Most commonly, however, it is due to defective neurologic regulation of the colon, as in irritable bowel syndrome or colon atony. Constipation may contribute to distention of the colon and hemorrhoids, complications which may in turn aggravate constipation. The patient with chronic constipation may be drawn into abuse of laxatives, which may further compromise bowel function.

When constipation is assessed to be clinically significant, management centers on five objectives: (1) prevention or elimination of impaction, (2) alleviation of psychogenic factors, (3) treatment of organic factors, (4) restoration of a normal frequency of defecation, and (5) promotion of a normal consistency of stools. Impaction in the lower bowel is corrected by means of flushing of feces by enema or breaking up of feces by digital maneuvers. Otherwise, impaction or constipation is managed acutely by use of laxatives.

Constipation can often be controlled by appropriate intake of fibrous foods, fluids, raw fruits and vegetables, stewed prunes, and whole grain cereals. Routine exercise, decreased emotional tension, and a regular schedule for defecation are also methods of managing bowel habits. If these adjustments prove inadequate for establishing appropriate bowel habits, it may be necessary to resort to laxatives.

A **laxative** effect occurs when a substance promotes elimination of a soft, formed stool. A **cathartic** (or **purgative**) effect is more vigorous, providing more complete and fluid evacuation of the bowel. The two kinds of actions are generally achieved by the same selection of drugs: a higher dose for the cathartic response and a lower dose for the laxative action. Thus the drugs in this class are appropriately referred to as laxative-cathartics, or for convenience, by either name alone.

Laxative-cathartics have rather limited medical application but are widely abused by the public. Adverse reactions to cathartics probably occur more frequently than do conditions necessitating their use; however, there are some legitimate uses for them, such as promoting excretion because of poisons or parasites; promoting soft stools after hemorrhoid removal, myocardial infarction, or cerebral vascular accident; or preparing for intestinal surgery. Proper treatment of constipation should involve adjustment of dietary and defecatory habits. When constipation is caused by organic disease, such as obstruction, anal or rectal problems, infection, drugs, or hypothyroidism, the treatment of the underlying cause is the therapeutic objective. Laxative-cathartics can be divided on the basis of mechanism of action into four categories: (1) bulk-forming drugs, (2) osmotic/saline agents, (3) contact agents (formerly called stimulant or irritant laxatives), and (4) emollient agents.

Bulk-Forming Laxative-Cathartics

Dietary fiber is the most natural means of promoting formation of soft stools that can be easily passed. Bulk-forming laxative-cathartics are related preparations, consisting of polysaccharides from natural sources. The diet in industrialized countries is often lacking in adequate fiber content, which contributes to constipation. Nurses should encourage clients therefore to augment their diets with bran cereals and whole meal bread, which provide excellent sources of fiber. Coarse bran is more effective than processed fine bran because of its large particle size. Other rich fiber sources are carrots, apples, oranges, and brussels sprouts. Ingestion of reasonable amounts of bran should be considered the treatment of choice for symptoms of constipation.

Mechanisms and Effects Dietary fiber and the related bulk-forming preparations increase the water content of the feces due to the hydrophilic properties of the constituent polysaccharides. The mass of the stool is increased as well, offering a physical stimulus to peristalsis, and transit time through the colon is hastened.

Clinical Indications Bran and other bulk-forming polysaccharides are effective in alleviating constipation, and to a lesser extent, the diarrhea of irritable bowel syndrome.

Nursing Observations for Use of Laxative/Cathartics for Constipation

THERAPEUTIC GOAL	(1) Prevent or eliminate impaction, (2) alleviate psychogenic factors, (3) treat organic factors if possible, (4) restore normal frequency of defecation, and (5) promote normal consistency of stools.
PREADMINISTRATION ASSESSMENT	
Baseline Data	Observe clients for evidence of a sharp reduction in frequency or quantity of stools, feelings of incomplete evacuation, unusually dry and hard stools, or straining at stools. Evaluate fluid intake-output, bowel sounds, quantity and quality of stools, presence of blood in the stools, and vital signs. Presence of impacted stools can be assessed by digital rectal examination.
EVALUATION OF DRUG RESPONSE	
For Therapeutic Benefit	Monitor occurrence of bowel movement within 12–24 hours after use of a laxative; observe for promotion of soft stools when used subacutely during recovery from removal of hemorrhoids, myocardial infarction, or a cerebral vascular accident.
For Adverse Effects	Monitor for diarrhea, intestinal cramps, and allergic reactions in adults. Observe for diarrhea in infants being breast-fed by mothers receiving laxatives. If mineral oil is administered, monitor for lipid pneumonitis and pruritus ani.
For Dietary Interactions	Monitor for additive effects with dietary fiber or elevated fluid intake.
For Compliance	Evaluate the client's compliance with all facets of the therapeutic regimen by careful observation, interviewing, and review of progress. Report compliance problems or excessive use of laxative-cathartics to the physician and act as client-advocate when changes in the therapeutic regimen seem indicated.

Adverse Effects and Contraindications Adverse effects of bulk-forming laxative-cathartics are minimal. Ingestion of these agents should be accompanied by ample quantities of water or other fluids, especially if the patient has any difficulty with swallowing. On rare occasions, impaction of the dry preparations can occur in the esophagus or intestines. *The nurse should instruct clients to stir powdered bulk-laxatives briskly into an 8-oz glass of cool water, milk, or juice immediately before drinking it.* Flatulence sometimes occurs when dietary fiber content is initially increased. However, it can usually be controlled by increasing fluid intake, altering the selection of fiber sources, or adjusting intake.

Preparations and Administration The bulk-forming laxative preparations currently available include psyllium (plantago) preparations, methylcellulose, carboxymethylcellulose, nondiastatic barley malt extract, polycarbophil, guar gum, and gum karaya. Occasionally, dried ripe seeds of the plantago plant are employed as whole seeds (Siblin), but such preparations have been generally displaced by powdered preparations of the seeds, which provide less irritation. Powdered and granulated preparations include 100% psyllium (Konsyl), 95% psyllium and sodium bicarbonate (Hydrocil Instant), 50% psyllium hydrophilic mucilloid and 50% dextrose (Hydrocil, Laxamead, Metamucil, and others), psyllium hydrophobic mucilloid, citric acid, and sodium bicarbonate (Metamucil Instant Mix), psyllium hydrocolloid and sodium bicarbonate (Effersyllium Instant Mix), and hemicellulose with 50% dextrose (Mucilose). Hemicellulose is also available as flakes (Mucilose Flakes).The effervescent preparations are to be avoided in clients on low-sodium diets because of the sodium content. Preparations with high dextrose content must be avoided by clients with diabetes. The powdered preparations are stirred into water, milk, or another suitable beverage, drunk as a suspension, and washed down with additional fluid.

As noted earlier, bulk-laxatives can also be somewhat effective in alleviating diarrhea, restoring normal stool consistency by absorbing free fecal water. Polycarbophil (Mitrolan) exhibits this dual activity, alleviating both constipation and diarrhea, regulating water and bulk content of stools. It is especially useful in irritable bowel syndrome and diverticulosis, conditions in which diarrhea and constipation may occur alternately.

Nursing Diagnoses and Interventions for Use of Laxative/Cathartics for Constipation

Nursing Diagnoses	*Related Interventions*
TO ENHANCE DRUG BENEFITS OR REDUCE DRUG REQUIREMENTS	
Alterations in bowel elimination: constipation	Increase dietary fiber or fruit juices. Encourage regular exercise, avoidance of stress, and greater attention to the defecatory reflex. Use an enema or digital manipulation to alleviate impaction. Increase fluid intake.
TO ENSURE SAFE AND EFFICACIOUS DRUG USE	
Knowledge deficit related to drug regimen	Educate clients so as to correct any misconceptions about normal defecatory function. Teach the client about the importance of adequate fluid intake and inclusion of foods containing bulk and juices in the diet for promoting soft stools. Discuss with clients overuse of laxatives and unrealistic conceptions concerning defecatory function. Provide client with a list of adverse effects and drug interactions for each drug in the regimen and explain what to do if any of these occur.

Methylcellulose
Oral liquid, syrup (orange flavored) (Hydrolose), combinations with carboxymethylcellulose (for example, Evactol)
Recommended Doses: For adults, 5–20 ml of liquid or 15 ml of syrup PO, or 1–6 g daily of the combination preparation. Ample water should be taken concurrently.

Polycarbophil (Mitrolan)
Chewable tablets
Recommended Doses: For adults, 1–4 g PO as needed.

Osmotic Laxative-Cathartics

The osmotic laxative-cathartics include magnesium salts, sodium phosphates, and lactulose.

Mechanisms and Effects Osmotic cathartics are soluble sugars or salts that are poorly absorbed from the alimentary tract. They promote retention of water in the fecal material by an osmotic effect. The added fluid volume promotes peristalsis and soft fluid stools.

Lactulose, a synthetic disaccharide, acts as a colon-specific osmotic laxative-cathartic. Related to lactose, it is not hydrolyzed by intestinal enzymes but reaches the colon unchanged. In the colon, it is metabolized by the commensal bacteria to organic acids, mainly lactic acid. The colon pH is reduced, causing formation of ammonium ion, and ammonia that is normally absorbed from the colon is trapped in its ionic form and ultimately excreted. The retention of osmotically active particles promotes water retention and softening of the stools. The reduction in colonic pH may also contribute by stimulating motility in the large intestine.

Clinical Indications Osmotic agents are highly effective for short-term alleviation of constipation, evacuation before diagnostic or surgical procedures, or for treatment of certain poisonings. Most osmotic agents are inappropriate for long-term use.

Lactulose is indicated for treatment of constipation and is useful for chronic applications, unlike many of the laxative-cathartics. Lactulose increases the frequency of bowel movements. It is also effective in preventing or alleviating portal-systemic encephalopathy because of its ability to reduce blood concentrations of ammonium.

Adverse Effects and Contraindications Although the extent of absorption of salts employed as osmotic laxatives is small, long-term use may result in electrolyte imbalances, pH imbalances, or toxic effects due to accumulation of the constituent cations. The salts employed as laxatives are salts of magnesium (magnesium sulfate, magnesium hydroxide, magnesium citrate) or sodium (monosodium phosphate, sodium phosphate, or sodium biphosphate). Magnesium tends to accumulate in body fluids if renal function is impaired and thus should not be used in patients with renal insufficiency. Sodium salts are contraindicated in clients with congestive heart failure or hypertension, and the phosphate component can result in hypocalcemia if use is prolonged.

Lactulose, upon initial administration, may cause intestinal cramps and flatulence; excessive doses may cause diarrhea. Lactulose contains small amounts of galactose and therefore should not be used for patients on galactose-restricted diets.

Preparations and Administration Magnesium sulfate (epsom salt) is a traditional laxative-cathartic. *Magnesium sulfate has a bitter taste and is best taken with lemon juice. Nurses need to advise clients using magnesium salts to watch for early signs of hypermagnesia: profound thirst, sedation, confusion, muscle weakness, and feelings of warmth.* Sodium phosphates are on the whole more palatable than magnesium salts. Lactulose is a prescription drug.

Lactulose (Cephulac, Chronulac)
Syrup
Recommended Dose: 15–30 ml PO daily.

Magnesium Citrate (citrate of magnesia, Citroma, Citro-Nesia)
Flavored oral solution.
Recommended Doses: 240 ml PO (a glassful).

Magnesium Hydroxide (Milk of Magnesia)
Flavored liquid suspension
Recommended Doses: For adults, 15–30 ml PO.

Magnesium Sulfate (Epsom Salt)
Recommended Doses: 15 g PO.

Monosodium Phosphate
Effervescent granules for dissolution in water (Sal Hepatica)
Recommended Doses: 1–2 teaspoons PO.

Sodium Phosphate
Powder for oral solution combination powder with sodium biphosphate for oral solutions.

Contact Laxative-Cathartics

The contact laxative-cathartics include (1) anthraquinones, (2) diphenylmethane agents, (3) docusates, (4) castor oil, and (5) bile acids. The anthraquinones occur widely in nature — in *Cascara sagrada,* senna (the dried leaves of *Cassia senna*), rhubarb, and aloe. The diphenylmethane laxative-cathartics include phenolphthalein and biscodyl. Docusates include the sodium, calcium, and potassium salts of docusate. Castor oil is derived from the seeds of *Ricinus communis,* the castor bean (the cathartic effects of seeds from this plant were known by the ancient Egyptians). Dehydrocholic acid, a synthetic bile acid, is also used for laxative purposes.

Mechanisms and Effects Contact laxative-cathartics act primarily by decreasing net absorption of electrolytes and water across the intestinal mucosa. The resulting increase in fluid volume then stimulates peristalsis and speeds transit. Apparently, the decrease in net absorption is due more to an increase in back diffusion than a decrease in forward absorption. The drugs within the group of contact laxative-cathartics differ somewhat in their sites of action: some acting primarily on the intestines and others acting primarily on the colon.

The anthraquinone contact agents act only on the large intestine. As a result, onset of action generally requires 6 hours after administration. With the diphenylmethane group, there is a high degree of individual variability in response. At standard doses, some patients fail to respond, while others experience severe griping. The action of diphenylmethane agents is mainly on the colon, thus requiring about 6 hours to act. Phenolphthalein is absorbed to about 15%. Since phenolphthalein turns pink at high pH, if urine is alkaline, phenolphthalein will impart a pinkish hue.

The docusates are **stool-softeners.** They act as detergents, allowing mixing of organic and aqueous media and increase the water content of fecal matter, softening the stool. Their maximal laxative action is less than for other contact agents. Recent studies, however, suggest that the mechanism of docusates is similar to that of other contact agents. Docusates are indicated for clients with hemorrhoids, chronic constipation, or painful conditions of the anus or rectum.

Castor oil acts on the small intestine, and therefore produces a prompt and complete evacuation. It is generally reserved for achieving purgative effects. It is not metabolized in the stomach and tends to slow gastric emptying time. The main use of castor oil in modern medicine is to prepare patients for x-ray examination of the viscera.

Adverse Effects and Contraindications The most important adverse effect of anthraquinones is excessive catharsis. Melanosis coli, a hyperpigmentation of the mucosa of the colon, has been reported in some patients. Controversy exists as to whether anthraquinones are excreted in breast milk. Senna probably is not, but the other drugs in this class should be avoided by nursing mothers.

Diphenylmethane derivatives have been associated with allergic reactions, from drug eruption to severe, even fatal, reactions, resembling lupus erythematosus. *Clients should discontinue the drug immediately if skin eruptions occur.* Excessive catharsis may cause fluid and electrolyte imbalance.

Docusates are well tolerated. Adverse effects include intestinal cramps and nausea. When castor oil is employed, abdominal contractions may be severe and painful in some patients, while others experience little distress.

Drug Interactions Any drug that increases intestinal motility has the potential for impairing absorption of drugs that are slowly absorbed because of the reduced transit time. Contact laxative-cathartics may possibly decrease absorption of oral anticoagulants, vitamins A and K, estrogens, isoniazid, and sulfonamides. Docusates, on the other hand, may increase intestinal absorption of certain drugs, including mineral oil and danthron.

Preparations and Administration The tablet preparation is less reliable than the fluid. The aromatic fluid extract is preferred to the plain fluid extract because of the extreme bitter taste of the former. Senna dates back to before 900 A.D. as an Arabian remedy. It is capable of producing a complete evacuation, but usually the effect is accompanied by powerful and painful contractions of the bowels.

Biscodyl (Cenalax, Codylax, Deficol, Dulcolax, Fleet Biscodyl, Laxadan, Nuvac, Sk-Biscodyl, Theralax)
Enteric coated tablets, suppositories
Recommended Doses: For adults, 10–15 mg PO or 10 mg suppository; for children over 6, 5–10 mg PO or 10 mg suppository; for children under 2, 5 mg suppository.

Cascara Sagrada
Tablets, fluid extract, aromatic fluid extract
Recommended Doses: 0.5–1.5 ml PO for the fluid extract or 5 ml for the aromatic fluid extract.

Castor Oil (Emulsoil, Alphamul, Neoloid)
Liquid, emulsion
Recommended Doses: Dose depends on concentration. *Castor oil is given on an empty stomach because it tends to slow gastric emptying time.*

Danthrone (Dorbane)
Tablets, oral liquid
Recommended Doses: 37.5–150 mg PO with the evening meal or 1 hour after. *Danthrone is most effective if taken with a full glass of water.*

Docusate Calcium (Surfak)
Capsules
Recommended Doses: 240 mg PO daily.

Docusate Potassium (Dialose, Kasof)
Capsules
Recommended Doses: For adults, 240–300 mg PO daily.

Docusate Sodium (Colace, Doxinate, others)
Tablets, capsules, oral solutions, syrups, suppositories
Recommended Doses: For adults, 50–240 mg PO daily.

Phenolphthalein (Ex-Lax, Feen-a-Mint, others)
Tablets, chewable tablets, gum tablets, mints, wafers, tablets, powder
Recommended Doses: 30–194 mg PO, preferably at bedtime for evacuation the next morning.

Senna (Senexon, Senokot, Senolax, S-Prep, Black-Draught, and Dasafru)
Tablets, granules, powder, syrup, liquid, and suppository formulations

Emollient Laxative-Cathartics

Mechanisms and Effects Oils have an emollient effect on the alimentary tract, penetrating and softening the stool and interfering with absorption of water. Mineral oil (or liquid paraffin) is an indigestable oil and thus is very potent as an emollient. Digestible oils such as olive oil, corn oil, or cottonseed oil produce a similar effect when large quantities are ingested.

Adverse Effects and Contraindications Mineral oil is absorbed to some extent into mucosal cells, the more so when used in combination with docusate agents. Absorption of mineral oil is associated with an inflammatory response in tissues in which it accumulates. If significant amounts of mineral oil reach the lungs, a condition called **lipid pneumonitis** occurs. An annoying aspect of the use of mineral oil is seepage of the oil from the anus, which may cause pruritus ani and embarrassing staining.

Drug and Nutrient Interactions Mineral oil is an organic solvent. When administered at meal time, it interferes with absorption of fats and fat-soluble vitamins. Vitamins A and K are particularly affected and corresponding deficiency states may result with chronic use of mineral oil.

Preparations and Administration *Mineral oil is usually given at bedtime, on an empty stomach, with a glass of fruit juice to increase palatability.*

Mineral Oil (Nujol, Agoral Plain, Zymenol, others)
Liquid, jelly, emulsion, suspension, or combination enema preparations, such as Fleet mineral oil enema
Recommended Doses: 15–30 ml PO for adults, 10–15 ml for children.

Important Nursing Implications for Laxative-Cathartics

- ☐ Teach clients that it is usually best to refrain from use of laxatives and to allow adequate time for formation of a normal stool and initiation of the defecatory reflex.
- ☐ Review the medical records of clients for contraindications for use of laxatives such as inflammatory, hemorrhagic, or obstructive diseases of the alimentary tract, undiagnosed abdominal pains, pregnancy, breast-feeding, chronic constipation, or anemia.
- ☐ Advise clients that bulk-forming laxatives are the only safe ones for repeated use.
- ☐ Warn clients who use contact laxative-cathartics that they may experience irritation of the rectal skin and mucosa, fluid and electrolyte loss, cramping, belching, and diarrhea.
- ☐ Instruct clients (especially pregnant women) that the use of emollient laxatives may result in deficiencies of fat-soluble vitamins. The resultant deficiency in vitamin K is especially hazardous to the fetus.
- ☐ Warn clients that emollient laxatives may cause anal leakage and lipid pneumonia. Instruct clients not to use mineral oil since this drug is especially likely to cause lipid pneumonia.
- ☐ Teach clients who use magnesium sulfate the symptoms of hypermagnesia.
- ☐ Advise clients who use bulk-forming laxatives to maintain a high fluid intake. Clients with stenosis, adhesions, or dysphagia should not use these drugs.

Diarrhea and Antidiarrheals

Diarrhea may be defined as an increased frequency or fluidity of bowel movements; feces are typically liquid or semiformed. Since there is considerable variation from individual to individual, the standard of comparison is the client's own normal pattern. Diarrhea is a symptom that can result from a variety of mechanisms. **Osmotic diarrhea** occurs when nonabsorbable solutes cause water to be retained in the bowel. Examples include osmotic laxative-cathartics and sugar substitutes such as hexitols, sorbitol, and mannitol, often found in dietetic candy and chewing gum. **Secretory diarrhea** occurs when net absorption of electrolytes and water from the intestines is reversed, so that fluid is secreted into the bowel. This occurs in certain infections of viral (echo), bacterial (*Escherichia coli,* salmonella, shigellosis), or parasitic (*Entamoeba histolytica, Giardia lamblia*) origin. It also can be caused by contact laxative-cathartics, excess dietary fat, bile acids, and hormones such as calcitonin and vasoactive intestinal peptide (VIP).

Malabsorptive diarrhea occurs in malabsorption syndrome due to retention of unabsorbed nutrients in the bowel. **Exudative diarrhea** occurs when the intestinal mucosa is seriously compromised by ulceration, tumor formation, or inflammation, allowing outflow of mucus or blood. Diarrhea can also occur when intestinal transport time is substantially decreased due to **resectioning** or **hypermotility.** A large number of drugs cause hypermotility, directly or indirectly, including many antimicrobials, antacids, colchicine, laxatives, antineoplastics, digitalis, quinidine, cholinomimetics, and antiadrenergic agents. Diarrhea is often attributed to **gastroenteritis,** a nonspecific term employed when the identity of the infectious pathogen or toxic substance is undetermined. Diarrhea is clinically significant not only as an indicator of underlying pathology but also as a potential cause of fluid and electrolyte imbalance, or, if prolonged, nutritional deficiency.

The therapeutic objectives in management of diarrhea include (1) preventing or correcting fluid or electrolyte imbalances, (2) treatment of causative factors, (3) restoration of normal frequency and consistency of stool formation, (4) alleviation of associated symptoms, and (5) prevention of perianal irritation. Pharmacological intervention with antidiarrheals is helpful with respect to the first and third of these objectives. Intestinal anti-infectives may be helpful with respect to the second objective, if the cause is an intestinal infection. Nonpharmacological measures are also important. Dietary or drug factors promoting diarrhea should be eliminated. Diarrhea may cause temporary depletion of disaccharidase, leading to acute lactose intolerance. It is therefore wise to eliminate milk and milk products for a few days after the diarrhea is corrected. Rest is recommended since exercise increases bowel activity.

Provision of oral fruit juices or glucose and electrolyte solutions is usually sufficient to treat fluid and electrolyte difficulties. Unless the diarrhea is mild, oral fluids (such as hot broths or tea) should be avoided. Hot and cold fluids tend to increase peristalsis; therefore these substances should be avoided. Tepid fluids are all right for clients with mild diarrhea. Parenteral fluids may be required in severe cases. If the client's kidneys are functioning, potassium is usually added to the intravenous fluid to replace the large amounts commonly lost in severe diarrhea. If the kidneys are not functioning adequately, potassium should not be added because of the risk of producing potassium overload and cardiac dysrhythmias.

Four kinds of drugs find use in management of diarrhea: (1) opiates and their congeners, (2) anticholinergics, (3) absorbents, and (4) intestinal flora modifiers.

Opiates and Congeners

Mechanisms and Effects The antidiarrheal properties of opiates have been known for thousands of years. The value of these drugs is partly due to a slowing of gastric emptying time but is largely related to their effect on gut motility. Opiates increase nonpropulsive, segmental contractions, but inhibit propulsive, peristaltic movements. They mainly depress the slow cholinergic phase of peristaltic contractions, although loperamide, a synthetic congener, depresses the rapid, prostaglandin-mediated phase as well. Opiates produce a wide range of other pharmacological effects through actions on the central nervous system (see Chapter 25).

The classical opiates employed for diarrhea include opium tincture, paregoric (camphorated opium tincture), and codeine. All three lack specificity for the intestinal tract, causing marked CNS depression. With codeine, a low dose will have minimal effect on the CNS, but the duration of the antidiarrheal action will persist only for about 2 hours. Higher doses produce longer antidiarrheal effects but substantial CNS depression. Codeine is an ingredient in the combination preparation, Kaodene β1. Paregoric is included in Corrective Mixture with Paregoric. Opium tincture or powder is contained in some 20 combination preparations for diarrhea, including Donnagel-PG and Diabismul. There is no adequate justification for use of these agents given the improved selectivity found in newer congeners.

Diphenoxylate (Lomotil) and loperamide (Imodium) are two **opiate congeners,** related to the narcotic meperidine and developed expressly for their selectivity of action on the bowel. Diphenoxylate produces measurable CNS narcotic action only at doses about 3–4 times the maximum daily dose for diarrhea. With loperamide, selectivity is even greater. Analgesia occurs with loperamide only at serum concentrations 1,000 times those associated with normal antidiarrheal doses. Twenty-seven 2 mg capsules of loperamide were found in one study to produce a serum concentration of only about one one-hundredth that required for analgesia. Loperamide has been shown to be devoid of abuse liability in both animal studies and in humans. Thus, while these drugs are opiate congeners, diphenoxylate and especially loperamide are for all practical purposes free of significant systemic opiate effects. A subtherapeutic dose of atropine sulfate is added to diphenoxylate preparations to discourage abuse even more.

Pharmacokinetics Diphenoxylate is rapidly metabolized to difenoxine, an active metabolite. The parent compound has a half-life of 2.5 hours, but the active metabolite has a long half-life of 12–14 hours. Difenoxine and subsequent metabolites are excreted more in the feces than in the urine. Loperamide has a half-life of 10.8 hours, which contributes substantially to its selectivity. It is poorly absorbed and most of what is absorbed is recycled by the enterohepatic shunt. Less than 1% of an administered dose reaches the systemic circulation.

Adverse Effects and Contraindications Adverse effects of diphenoxylate and loperamide are uncommon. Constipation, abdominal discomfiture, paralytic ileus, and skin rash may occur occasionally. CNS depression has been noted with diphenoxylate and anticholinergic side effects from the atropine included in diphenoxylate products. Overdoses with diphenoxylate or loperamide can be treated with naloxone, lavage, and supportive therapy. *Neither opiates nor opiate congeners should be used when diarrhea is caused by organisms that penetrate the intestinal mucosa, such as* Salmonella, E. coli, *or* Shigella, *because the antiperistaltic action of these drugs may promote penetration of*

Nursing Observations for Use of Antidiarrheal Drugs

THERAPEUTIC GOAL	(1) Relieve symptoms by decreasing propulsive movements of the gut, (2) prevent electrolyte imbalance, (3) treat causative factors, (4) restore normal frequency and consistency of stools, and (5) prevent perianal irritation.
PREADMINISTRATION ASSESSMENT	
Baseline Data	Assesse for increased frequency or fluidity of bowel movements. Question the client about recent exposure to unusual food or water sources, medications, use of laxative-cathartic drugs, or individuals with intestinal infections. Determine precise meaning of "diarrhea" to the client, since clients' expectations regarding defecatory function vary sharply. Determine if the client has concurrent symptoms such as fever, chills, nausea, vomiting, malaise, or weakness. Assess abdominal pains or cramps and where they are located. Evaluate bowel sounds; palpate for areas of tenderness, monitor intake-output of solids and liquids, vital signs, and quality and quantity of stools; observe for presence of blood, mucus, or unusual odor in stools and dehydration. Obtain laboratory tests including culturing of stool specimens and assessment of fluid and electrolyte balance.
EVALUATION OF DRUG RESPONSE	
For Therapeutic Benefit	Monitor for decreased frequency of passage of stools and passage of well formed stools.
For Adverse Effects	Monitor for constipation, abdominal discomfiture, paralytic ileus, and skin rash with narcotic congeners. Monitor for CNS depression when opiates are employed. Monitor for dry mouth, diplopia, aggravation of glaucoma, tachycardia, urinary retention, and paralytic ileus if anticholinergic drugs are employed.
For Dietary Interactions	Monitor for diminished efficacy of antidiarrheal medications if diet is rich in fiber or fluid.
For Compliance	Evaluate the client's compliance with all facets of the therapeutic regimen by observing, interviewing, and reviewing progress. Report compliance problems to the physician and act as client-advocate when changes in the therapeutic regimen seem indicated.

the pathogen. Abdominal distention may indicate toxic megacolon or ulcerative colitis due to excessive delay of intestinal motility when antidiarrheals are employed.

Diphenoxylate should be used cautiously for clients with cirrhosis of the liver or severe liver disease because hepatic coma may occur. Children with Down's syndrome may develop signs of atropinism even when using recommended doses.

Drug Interactions Used in conjunction with monoamine oxidase inhibitors, diphenoxylate has been reported to precipitate a hypertensive crisis.

Preparations and Administration Lomotil is currently the most widely prescribed antidiarrheal and among the top 100 of all prescription drugs. Imodium is the second most widely prescribed antidiarrheal and in the top 200 of all prescription medications. Its high degree of specificity makes it the drug of choice for diarrhea in adults and in children old enough to ingest capsules.

Diphenoxylate (Lomotil, others)
Tablets with atropine, liquid with atropine
Recommended Doses: For adults, 5 mg PO initially, 4 times daily. In children over 2 years of age, 0.3–0.4 mg/kg PO initially, daily in 3–5 divided doses. The drug is not recommended for children under age 2.

Loperamide (Imodium)
Capsules
Recommended Doses: 4 mg PO initially, followed by 2 mg after each bout of diarrhea, up to 16 mg daily.

Important Nursing Implications for Narcotic-Congener Antidiarrheal Agents

- ☐ Instruct clients to seek full medical evaluation about the cause of the diarrhea.
- ☐ Teach clients the dangers of using antidiarrheal drugs for acute infectious diarrhea caused by penetrating bacteria such as *Escher-*

Nursing Diagnoses and Interventions for Use of Antidiarrheal Drugs

Nursing Diagnoses	*Related Interventions*
TO ENHANCE DRUG BENEFITS OR REDUCE DRUG REQUIREMENTS	
Alteration in bowel elimination: diarrhea	Advise clients who plan to visit places where they are likely to encounter unfamiliar intestinal pathogens to avoid uncooked foods, dairy products, and tap water. Intensify perianal hygienic measures to minimize irritation. Teach use of emollients; eliminate milk and milk products temporarily; provide juices or glucose and electrolyte solutions. Increase rest. Provide immediate access to a bedpan or restroom as required.
TO ENSURE SAFE AND EFFICACIOUS DRUG USE	
Knowledge deficit related to drug regimen	Advise clients to see a physician if persistent diarrhea occurs.
	Instruct clients having a problem of diarrhea to keep track of passage of stools, noting frequency, consistency, and unusual contents if the client is not already under direct medical care.
	Teach clients having diarrhea how to observe for early indications of hypokalemia, such as muscle weakness, twitches, or tetany, hypotension, mental fatigue, polyuria, and polydipsia.
	Provide client with a list of adverse effects and drug interactions for antidiarrheal drugs that are prescribed and explain what to do if any of these occur.

ichia coli, Salmonella, Shigella, or *Campylobacter jejuni,* since penetration is increased if elimination during diarrhea is diminished.

- ☐ Do not use loperimide or diphenoxylate for clients with pseudomembranous colitis.
- ☐ Teach clients to recognize symptoms indicative of an allergic reaction to an antidiarrheal medication.
- ☐ Instruct clients to discontinue use of antidiarrheal drugs for acute diarrhea after no more than 48–72 hours.

Anticholinergics

Anticholinergics are effective in alleviating diarrhea but lack adequate selectivity. Doses of atropine and other belladonna alkaloids required to relieve diarrhea produce profound anticholinergic influences on other systems. Potential effects are dry mouth, diplopia, pupillary dilation, aggravation of glaucoma, tachycardia, dizziness, urinary retention, and paralytic ileus. Many of the combination preparations, prescription and nonprescription alike, contain atropine, from 0.025 mg to as much as 0.5 mg per tablet, capsule, or 5 ml of liquid. The small doses are ineffective and the larger doses are likely to produce unwanted effects.

Absorbents

Absorbents, including kaolin, pectin, activated attapulgite, and bismuth salts, are contained in many antidiarrheal formulations to absorb bacteria and fluid and to improve the consistency of the stool. These effects, however, have not been demonstrated. Kaolin is hydrated aluminum silicate, and pectin is a carbohydrate obtained from rinds or pomace of fruits. Though generally safe when used at recommended doses, absorbents may occasionally cause constipation from impaction of the absorbent substance. In addition, absorbents may diminish the effect of medications taken concurrently. For example, kaolin with pectin can interfere with absorption of digoxin (Lanoxin) and lincomycin (Lincocin).

Intestinal Flora Modifiers

Lactobacillus organisms exist normally in the intestines, helping to digest food and suppress pathogenic microorganisms. In diarrhea, the normal flora may be disrupted, which is most obviously the case when diarrhea is caused by use of broad-spectrum antimicrobial drugs. Preparations containing *Lactobacillus* organisms have been marketed for use in suppressing diarrhea, canker sores, and fever blisters caused by a disturbance of the flora. However, there is no convincing evidence from clinical trials supporting efficacy of these preparations. In any case, a diet of milk, buttermilk, or yogurt, and lactose or dextrose, nutrients utilized by *Lactobacillus,* is just as effective in promoting recolonization.

Preparations and Administration

Lactobacillus Acidophilus/Lactobacillus Bulgaricus (Bacid, DoFUS, Lactines)
Capsules, packets of granules, chewable tablets
Recommended Doses: 2–4 Bacid capsules are taken with water or milk before meals. One DoFus capsule is taken daily. Lactinex packets are added to cereal, milk, juice, or water 3 or 4 times daily; lactinex tablets are taken 4 at a time, 3 or 4 times daily.

Sulfasalazine in Ulcerative Colitis

Ulcerative colitis is a chronic diffuse disease of the colon, involving inflammation and ulceration. Onset usually occurs between ages 15 and 40. The etiology is not known, although there is a familial pattern in its occurrence. The disease may begin focally and spread throughout the colon or it may be diffuse from the beginning. In the majority of cases, the disease exhibits a remitting course, with alternating periods of remission and exacerbation. In one-third of cases, the condition is chronic, characterized by mild, persistent symptoms. In the remaining 10% of cases, the condition is fulminant, progressing rapidly to death.

The classic sign of ulcerative colitis is bloody diarrhea from the inflammation and bleeding that occur throughout the mucosal lining of the colon. In addition, as the bowel fills with bloody, mucoid material, the client experiences a characteristic cramping pain, rectal urgency, and diarrhea. There is usually an electrolyte imbalance. Over time, the colon becomes thickened. Clients develop malabsorption and, because of the repeated blood loss, an iron-deficiency anemia. Dehydration is common and clients may also develop intestinal obstruction.

Certain drugs can produce syndromes resembling ulcerative colitis or aggravate existing ulcerative colitis. Such syndromes have been reported by clients who have taken oral contraceptives, antimetabolites (5-fluorouracil or 6-mercaptopurine), lithium carbonate, toxic levels of ^{131}gold, and many antimicrobials, including sulfonamides, penicillins, aminoglycosides, tetracyclines, macrolides, and chloramphenicol. The antibiotic-associated condition is called **pseudomembranous enterocolitis,** so named because characteristic membrane-like plaques of exudate gradually form in place of necrotizing mucosal cells.

Medical interventions in ulcerative colitis vary in relation to severity of the condition. In mild cases, nonspecific measures may suffice, including rest and antidiarrheal medications, and the avoidance of irritants such as raw fruit and vegetables and drugs known to aggravate the condition. In moderate to severe cases, sulfasalazine (Azulfidine) and steroids are employed. Blood or intravenous fluid replacement is sometimes required if hemorrhage is significant. Colectomy is sometimes required when hemorrhage is massive.

Mechanisms and Effects The mechanism by which sulfasalazine produces its beneficial influence in inflammatory disease of the intestines is not known, but it apparently is not due to its antimicrobial activity.

Pharmacokinetics Sulfasalazine is metabolized in the intestines. *Nurses should question clients about use of this drug because other antibiotics may alter the intestinal flora and hence the metabolism of sulfasalazine.* One major metabolite, sulfapyridine, is absorbed and later excreted in the urine. Therefore, sulfasalazine can cause systemic toxicity.

Clinical Indications Many physicians prefer to use sulfasalazine instead of corticosteroids in patients with moderately severe ulcerative colitis, reserving the steroids for severe cases. Sulfasalazine is also employed in regional enteritis and granulomatous colitis. For clients with the remitting type of ulcerative colitis, relapses are frequent when sulfasalazine is discontinued. Long-term sulfasalazine treatment often reduces the frequency of relapses.

Adverse Effects and Contraindications Adverse reactions of sulfasalazine include Heinz-body anemia, hemolytic anemia in glucose-6-phosphate dehydrogenase deficient individuals, and agranulocytosis. Allergic reactions, including rashes, fever, and arthralgias, occur in as many as 20% of patients receiving sulfasalazine. Nausea occurs frequently, but can be minimized by having the drug taken with meals. *If the client develops nausea, vomiting, or bloody diarrhea, it may be necessary to discontinue the drug. Nurses should also warn clients that sulfasalazine may impart an orange color to the urine if it is alkaline, and the skin may become yellow.*

Drug Interactions Phenobarbital decreases urinary excretion of sulfapyridine, thereby increasing its toxicity potential. Sulfasalazine can inhibit the absorption of folic acid, resulting in a folic acid deficiency anemia.

Preparations and Administration

Sulfasalazine (Azulfidine and generic)
Tablets, enteric coated tablets
Recommended Doses: For treatment of active ulcerative colitis in adults, 3–4 g PO daily in divided doses. Therapy can be initiated at 1–2 g daily to reduce initial reactions of nausea. Daily doses as high as 8 g are employed, but risks of toxicity increase with dose. For children, 40–60 mg/kg PO daily in 3–6 doses. For maintenance, 500 mg qid in adults; 7.5 mg/kg qid in children.

Hemorrhoids and Hemorrhoidal Preparations

Hemorrhoids are anorectal swellings caused by varicosities of the veins of one or more of the hemorrhoidal plexuses. They commonly occur in pregnant women and may be **internal** (lying beneath the mucosa of the rectum just above the anorectal juncture) or **external** (lying beneath the ectodermal wall of the anal canal). Hemorrhoids may become prolapses. Therapeutic management of hemorrhoids may be conservative, such as eliminating aggravating factors and focusing on symptomatic relief, or aggressive, such as surgical excision of hemorrhoidal tissue or cryosurgery. Some authorities consider diarrhea, constipation, and straining at stools to be additional predisposing or aggravating influences, but others question the role of these factors. Hygiene of the anal area should be sufficient to maintain cleanliness but not overmeticulous to the point of excessive abrasive influence.

There are several dozen nonprescription preparations marketed for symptomatic relief of hemorrhoids, consisting of various combinations of components from five drug categories: local anesthetics (benzocaine, pramoxine, diperodon, cyclomethycaine, piperocaine); vasoconstrictors (epinephrine, ephedrine, or phenylephrine); astringents (zinc oxide, bismuth subgallate or subcarbonate, tannic acid, or witch hazel); antiseptics used as preservatives, and emollient bases. In addition to the over-the-counter preparations, there are steroid-containing prescription creams, ointments, suppositories, and aerosol foams for use by patients with hemorrhoids. There is no clear evidence that any of these preparations is effective even for symptomatic relief. The pharmacology of each of the constituent drugs may be found elsewhere in this book.

Liver Disorders and Drugs

Because of its importance in metabolism, the liver plays a major role in determining the pharmacokinetics of drug elimination. Impairments in liver function prolong the half-life of many drugs (Table 51–4), increasing their duration of action, peak effect, and potential for toxicity. The liver itself is often one of the tissues negatively affected by drug toxicity. Toxic influences of drugs on the liver include drug-induced hepatitis, cirrhosis, cholestasis, and liver failure. Liver toxicity has wide-ranging consequences because the liver is involved in such a diversity of bodily activities.

Physiology of the Liver

The hepatic lobule is the functional unit of organization within the liver. Each lobule consists of an array of cells that is organized like the spokes of a wheel around a central vein. Each spoke consists of a layer of hepatocytes that surround channels called the bile *canaliculi.* The canaliculi receive the bile produced by the hepatocytes and converge into the network of bile ducts. The spokes are separated from one another by sinusoids, lateral extensions of the central vein that bring blood into close contact with the hepatocytes. Kupffer cells line the sinusoids and ingest foreign materials.

The liver receives both arterial and venous blood. The arterial blood provides oxygen to meet the needs of liver cells. The venous blood supply is provided by the portal vein. Before reaching the liver, the portal vein receives the blood from the intestinal mucosa, picking up in the process the newly absorbed materials from the alimentary tract. This unique pattern of blood flow ensures that the liver will absorb nutrients, destroy microbes, and detoxify chemicals before the blood containing the materials reaches the circulation at large. Under normal circumstances, the Kupffer cells are able to destroy 99% of invading microbes in the first pass of blood through the liver.

The liver has five major functions: (1) elaboration and secretion of bile ingredients, including bile salts and cholesterol, (2) recycling of red blood cell components following hemolysis, (3) detoxification of blood by phagocytosis of foreign cells and particles and biotransformation of chemicals, (4) synthesis of important blood proteins required for clotting, transport, and other functions, and (5) lipid, carbohydrate, and vitamin metabolism. Many of the metabolic functions of the liver are regulated by hormones of the endocrine system, including glucagon, insulin, growth hormone, anabolic and catabolic steroids, epinephrine, and thyroid hormones (the influences of these hormones were discussed in earlier chapters).

The plasma proteins that circulate in the bloodstream are synthesized by and large in the liver. Albumin, the most abundant of the plasma proteins, is produced exclusively in the liver. The plasma proteins provide the colloidal oncotic pressure that contributes to pressure within blood vessels as well as the binding sites for drugs and nutrients being transported through the circulatory network.

Table 51–4
Some Drugs with a Prolonged Half-life in Liver Disease

Acetaminophen	Meprobamate
Barbiturates	Morphine
Carbenicillin	Nortriptyline
Chloramphenicol	Pentazocine
Chlordiazepoxide	Phenylbutazone
Chlorpromazine	Phenytoin
Desipramine	Prednisone
Diazepam	Quinidine
Digoxin	Rifampin
Isoniazid	Theophylline
Lidocaine	Tolbutamide
Meperidine	

Hepatic Disorders

The major disorders associated with the liver include jaundice, fatty liver, hepatitis, and cirrhosis.

Jaundice

Jaundice is the yellowish discoloration of the skin and other tissues due to accumulation of excess bilirubin in the circulation. It occurs when bile spills out of the liver into the systemic circulation. Serum bilirubin is normally less than 1 mg/100 ml. Jaundice is usually apparent when levels of bilirubin exceed 2–2.5 mg/100 ml in serum. The principal source of bilirubin is breakdown of heme from red blood cells. Normally, 250–350 mg of bilirubin is formed daily (mainly from destruction of senescent red blood cells) and is destroyed by the liver. Jaundice can result from either excess formation or insufficient elimination of bilirubin. The terms *cholestasis* or *obstructive jaundice* are used to denote jaundice caused by impaired bile flow, which results in regurgitation of bile into the bloodstream. The bile ducts may be obstructed by gallstones, neoplasms, excess turbidity of biliary secretions, or constriction of the ducts.

A variety of drugs induce jaundice. Anabolic steroids (androgens and estrogens) can cause bile to leak out of hepatic cells or canals. Other drugs can induce cholestasis by provoking a hypersensitivity reaction, resulting in jaundice and eosinophilia. Drugs causing this type of reaction include the phenothiazines, tricyclic antidepressants, sulfonylureas, oral hypoglycemic agents, and sulfonamides. Thiouracil and tetracyclines can cause jaundice with variable amounts of necrosis as well.

Choleretics are drugs used to stimulate liver production of bile salts. Bile salts or acids can themselves be administered and act as choleretics, since they are absorbed into the portal circulation and are ultimately resecreted by the liver. **Hydrocholeretics** are drugs that lower the concentration of bile and increase its volume, which can be an aid in flushing minor obstructions out of the bile ducts. Dehydrocholic acid (Decholin) is used for this purpose.

Cholestyramine is an ion-exchange resin that binds bile acids. Being a resin, cholestyramine is not absorbed from the gastrointestinal tract. It has been used as an antidiarrheal when poor absorption of bile acids is a contributing factor and for relief of biliary tract obstructions by promoting more rapid flow of bile. The complete pharmacology of cholestyramine is discussed in Chapter 44.

Hepatitis

Hepatitis consists of an inflammation of the liver marked by jaundice, fever, and enlargement and necrosis of the liver. The two main causes of hepatitis are viruses and drugs. The hepatitis A virus causes epidemic, infectious hepatitis, which is relatively mild and generally terminates in 4–6 weeks, with complete restoration of function. The hepatitis B virus causes sporadic, infectious hepatitis of the

Table 51–5
Drug-Induced Hepatotoxicity

Type of hepatotoxicity	Drugs	
Acute hepatitis Toxic mechanism	Acetaminophen L-Asparaginase Carbon tetrachloride Cytarabine Cytotoxic antibiotics Dactinomycin Mithramycin Mitomycin Ethanol Ferrous salts 5-Fluorodeoxyuridine	Griseofulvin Heavy metals Indomethacin Insecticides Isoniazid[a] 6-Mercaptopurine[a] Methyldopa[a] Niacin Salicylates Tetracyclines Valproic acid[a]
Allergic mechanism	Allopurinol Halothane[a] MAO inhibitors Methimazole Nitrofurantoin Para-aminosalicylic acid[a]	Penicillins Phenylbutazone[a] Phenytoin Propylthiouracil Rifampin Sulfonamides (long-acting)
Cholestasis Toxic mechanism	Azathioprine Carbamazepine	Estrogens 17-Alpha-methyltestosterone
Allergic mechanism	Acetohexamide Butyrophenones Chlorpropamide Erythromycin estolate Gold Ibuprofen	Methylthiouracil Organic arsenicals Phenothiazines Thiouracil Thioxanthenes Tricyclic antidepressants
Cirrhosis	Alcohol Arsenic	Methotrexate
Neoplasm	Chlorambucil DDT	Oral contraceptives

[a]May progress to hepatic failure.

serum which can be fatal. Non-A, non-B virus or viruses also exist but are poorly characterized. Viral hepatitis, especially type B, may result in chronic hepatitis, which may in turn progress to cirrhosis. A vaccine for hepatitis B is available (see Chapter 49).

Alcohol is the most prominent among the drug causes of hepatitis, with hepatitis being an early manifestation of alcohol-induced liver disease. Other drugs that induce hepatitis are listed in Table 51–5. Carbon tetrachloride, miscellaneous insecticides and industrial solvents, heavy metal poisons, and phosphorus are direct hepatotoxins that can cause hepatitis. The hepatic allergens that cause hypersensitivity jaundice may induce necrosis as well. Severe fulminating hepatic necrosis is observed at times when isoniazid (Laniazid, Panazid, Teebaconin), iproniazid, phenylbutazone (Azolid, Butazolidin), urethane, 6-mercaptopurine (Purinethol), aminosalicylic acid (PAS, Parasal, Teebacin), or halothane (Fluothane) are used. With halothane, usually only transient jaundice occurs, but severe necrotic damage has been reported. This extreme reaction to halothane is believed to be a hypersensitivity reaction.

Most people with hepatitis are treated by nonspecific measures. Removal of hepatotoxins is a preliminary measure when hepatitis is drug-induced. Corticosteroids are rarely employed, but there is no definite evidence of value; some data even suggest that steroids increase mortality rates.

Fatty Liver and Cirrhosis

Fatty liver is the accumulation and infiltration of fat among the hepatocytes. It is a common response to hepatic damage, excess dietary fat, inadequate dietary protein (as in starvation), and excess alcohol consumption. The liver becomes enlarged, soft, and greasy. Fatty deposits do not themselves impair function of hepatocytes, but typically, chronic fatty liver ultimately gives way to fibrosis and cirrhosis.

Cirrhosis of the liver is a chronic disease, in which the anatomy of the liver is distorted by fibrotic nodular formations. It can lead to ascites (intraperitoneal accumulation of plasma-like fluid), hepatic coma, hepatic failure, blood-clotting deficiencies, and jaundice. The most common causes are alcoholism, severe hepatitis, intrahepatic or biliary obstructive jaundice, and hemochromatosis (iron toxicity). Alcoholism alone accounts for nearly one-half of these instances of cirrhosis. Treatment of clients with cirrhosis involves removal of contributing hepatotoxins and management of the complications brought on by the cirrhotic process. Initially reversible, cirrhosis is later irreversible, and finally fatally progressive. Cirrhosis ranks eighth among leading causes of mortality in the United States. Management of cirrhosis may involve diuretics for ascites, vitamins and iron for anemia and other signs of vitamin deficiency, and drugs such as neomycin and lactulose for hepatic coma.

Case Study: Peptic Ulcer

T. C., a 53-year-old man, was admitted to the hospital after 36 hours of vomiting that began shortly after food ingestion. The admitting nurse conducted the initial patient assessment. T. C. complained of episodes of gnawing epigastric pain, which began about 8 weeks earlier, increasing in frequency and intensity during the previous week. Abdominal palpation revealed epigastric tenderness. Auscultation of the bowel revealed normal sounds. The nurse learned that during the last 2 days, T. C. had passed stools sparingly and that blood was present in the stools. The nurse noted a pale appearance and T. C. indicated that during the last few days he had felt increasingly tired. Vital signs were blood pressure 145/95, temperature 98.6° F, pulse 80, and respirations 24.

The nurse reviewed T. C.'s medical history from the records on hand and by interview with the client. T. C. had a 10-year history of essential hypertension for which he was prescribed hydrochlorthiazide and methyldopa. He insisted that he took these medications regularly. He had a 1-year history of congestive heart failure secondary to essential hypertension, for which he was prescribed digitoxin and a low-sodium diet. T. C. occasionally employed an antacid (containing aluminum and magnesium hydroxides) and aspirin for his epigastric pains. T. C. smoked approximately one pack of cigarettes, consumed two to four alcoholic drinks (usually Scotch), and drank 4–5 cups of coffee per day. T. C. revealed that he was under a lot of pressure because of significant changes that the institution where he was an administrator had been undergoing during the past year.

The nurse reviewed her findings with the physician and laboratory tests were ordered. The results were subnormal hematocrit, subnormal hemoglobin, subnormal serum iron level, increased iron-binding capacity, and stool guaiac test of 1+. The medical team suspected that T. C. had a peptic ulcer, with pyloric obstruction, gastrointestinal bleeding, and secondary iron-deficiency anemia. Presence of the ulcer was confirmed by endoscopy, which revealed a 2.5 cm lesion in the upper portion of the duodenum.

The physician ordered cimetidine, 300 mg PO, 4 times daily, an iron/vitamin supplement, and regular use of the magnesium-aluminum antacid to which T. C. was accustomed (since he found this palatable), 1 hour after each meal and at bedtime. The nurse on this medical team who was responsible for providing client education asked T. C. to demonstrate his technique for measuring and taking the antacid. T. C. was accurate in measuring the antacid, but he did not shake the suspension adequately before pouring it and he washed the antacid down with a full cup of water. The nurse explained to him the importance of shaking the suspension and washing the measured amount down with only a small amount of liquid so that gastric emptying would not be hastened and the antacid would remain active in the stomach for as long as possible. Since antacid can interfere with absorption of many drugs, including both cimetidine and digoxin, the nurse worked with T. C. to schedule his drug dosages to be sure none of the other medications would be taken within 2 hours of the antacid. The schedule was also designed to allow digoxin and methyldopa to be taken with food to minimize gastrointestinal irritation sometimes associated with these drugs. The nurse reviewed with T. C. dietary adjustments that might be helpful, suggesting that he avoid substances that irritate the gastric mucosa (including alcohol, coffee, tea, and pepper) and substances that are especially potent stimulators of gastric secretions (such as the nicotine in tobacco smoke as well as meat gravies and meat-based soups). It was suggested that T. C. use acetaminophen rather than aspirin when he felt the need for an analgesic, and since T. C.'s ulcer was in the duodenum, to lie down after meals when possible to delay gastric emptying. The nurse discussed with T. C. the role of stress in peptic ulcers and adjustments that might be made in his schedule to allow him opportunities to unwind. The nurse also reviewed the potential adverse effects of cimetidine and antacids with T. C., provided him with a list of these, and discussed what he should do if any of these arose. The overall therapeutic plan was reviewed with T. C., emphasizing the need to continue the regimen for at least 4–6 weeks after elimination of overt symptoms. A plan for regular follow-up visits to the clinic was then established.

1. Which of the presenting symptoms and laboratory findings suggest peptic ulcer? Pyloric obstruction? Anemia?
2. How many factors can you identify in this case that may be contributing to the occurrence of peptic ulcer?
3. Why might anemia occur as a secondary complication in peptic ulcer?
4. What is the basis for the effectiveness of each of the antiulcer medications — cimetidine and antacids — prescribed for T. C.?
5. Why would an anticholinergic drug not be indicated for treatment of T. C.'s condition?
6. Why is acetaminophen preferable to aspirin when T. C. requires an analgesic?
7. Would there be any difference in the therapeutic regimen or the nursing measures in this case if the peptic ulcer had been gastric rather than duodenal?
8. Why does T. C. need to continue the medication after his symptoms are relieved?

Answers appear at the end of the book.

Recommended Readings

General Sources

Gitnick MD (ed): *Current Gastroenterology.* New York, John Wiley & Sons Inc, 1984.

Sleisenger MH, Fordtran JS: *Gastrointestinal disease: Pathophysiology, diagnosis, management.* Philadelphia, WB Saunders Co, 1983.

Emetics and Antiemetics

DiGregorio GJ, Froncillo RJ: Antiemetics. *Am Fam Physician* 1982;26(1):200–202.

DiPalma JR: Drugs for nausea and vomiting of pregnancy. *Am Fam Physician* 1983;28(4):272–274.

Harrington RA et al: Metoclopramide: An updated review of its pharmacological properties and clinical use. *Drugs* 1983;25(5):451–494.

Lovan WD: Motion sickness. *Am Fam Physician* 1984;28(6):117–120.

Manoguerra AS, Krenzelok EP: Rapid emesis from high-dose ipecac syrup in adults and children intoxicated with antiemetics or other drugs. *Am Hosp Pharm* 1978;35:1360–1362.

Wood CD: Antimotion sickness and antiemetic drugs. *Drugs* 1979;17:471–479.

Antiulcer Drugs

Banarer M, Ritschel WA: Antacid suspensions: A dilemma between acid neutralizing capacity and palatability. *Cont Pharm Practice* 1982;5:246–249.

Brogden RN et al: Ranitidine: A review of its pharmacology and therapeutic use in peptic ulcer disease and other allied diseases. *Drugs* 1982;24:267–303.

Feinberg LE: Treating duodenal ulcer: antacids or cimetidine? *Am Fam Physician* 1980;21(6):83–86.

Feldman M: Inhibition of gastric acid secretion by selective and nonselective anticholinergics. *Gastroenterology* 1984;86(2):361–366.

Ippoliti AF et al: Cimetidine versus intensive antacid therapy for duodenal ulcer. A multicenter trial. *Gastroenterology* 1978;74:393–395.

Isenberg JI: H2 receptor antagonists in the treatment of peptic ulcer. *Ann Intern Med* 1976;84:212–214.

Mar DD: Antacid therapy. *Am J Nurs* 1981;81(4):788–789.

Martin F et al: Comparison of healing capacities of sulcralfate and cimetidine in short-term treatment of duodenal ulcer: Double-blind randomized trial. *Gastroenterology* 1982;82:401–405.

Rosenberg J: Antacids. *RN* 1982;82(9):54–65.

Antidiarrheals

Awouters F, Niemegeers CJE, Janssen PAJ: Pharmacology of antidiarrheal drugs. *Annu Rev Pharmacol Toxicol* 1983;23:279–307.

Galambos JT et al: Loperamide: A new antidiarrheal agent in the treatment of chronic diarrhea. *Gastroenterology* 1976;70:1026–1029.

Heel RC et al: Loperamide: a review of its pharmacological properties and therapeutic efficacy in diarrhea. *Drugs* 1978;15:33–52.

Maresca JG, Stringari S: Assessment and management of acute diarrheal illness in adults. *Nurse Pract* 1986;11(11):15–28.

Netchvolodoff CV, Hargrove MD: Recent advances in the treatment of diarrhea. *Arch Intern Med* 1979;139:813–816.

Schiller LR et al: Mechanisms of antidiarrheal effects of loperamide. *Gastroenterology* 1984;86(6):1475–1480.

Laxatives

Aman RA: Treating the patient, not the constipation. *Am J Nurs* 1980;80:1634–1635.

Binder HJ: Pharmacology of laxatives. *Annu Rev Pharmacol Toxicol* 1977;17:355–367.

Thompson WG: Laxatives: Clinical pharmacology and rational use. *Drugs* 1980;19(1):49–58.

Drugs and the Liver

Bossone CM: The liver: A pharmacological perspective. *Nurs Clin North Am* 1977;12:291–303.

Gannon RB, Pickett K: Jaundice. *Am J Nurs* 1983;83:404–407.

Mar D: Drug induced hepatotoxicity. *Am J Nurs* 1982;82:124–126.

CHAPTER 52

Drugs Used for Respiratory Disorders

Respiration is the most immediately vital of the functions required for maintenance of life; disruption of the steady flow of oxygen is one of the most rapid causes of death. Respiration involves three distinct sequential processes: (1) pulmonary ventilation, (2) gas transport, and (3) cellular respiration. Pulmonary ventilation is the function of the respiratory system (Figure 52–1), which includes the airways (the mouth, nasal passages, pharynx, larynx, trachea, bronchi, and bronchioles), the lungs, the pleural sac, the muscles of respiration, and the diverse regulatory components (chemoreceptors and neural elements). Drugs are used to treat a variety of effects on the respiratory system: to alleviate asthma, to improve ventilation in clients with chronic obstructive pulmonary disease, to increase blood concentrations of particular gases, to stimulate or depress respiration, to reduce symptoms of upper respiratory tract infections, to treat pneumonia, and to alleviate allergic rhinitis. At other times, drugs used in medicine for a variety of disorders may have adverse effects on pulmonary function.

Asthma and Antiasthmatic Drugs

Bronchial asthma is characterized by a hypersensitive tracheobronchial tree that overreacts to a variety of stimuli with severe reflex bronchodilation (bronchospasm). Bronchospasms are paroxysmal contractions of the bronchial smooth muscles, which wrap in spirals around the bronchioles. When they contract, they constrict the bronchioles. Although bronchospasm is the major factor in asthmatic attacks, two other factors during an attack contribute to obstruction of airflow: secretion of large amounts of thick, white mucus and inflammation of the bronchial mucosa resulting in mucosal swelling.

In adults, about 10–20% of cases are extrinsic asthma, also known as allergic asthma because it is an IgE-mediated reaction to allergens such as pollens, molds, dust, and dander. Extrinsic asthma tends to run in families. Often, individuals in this category experience or later develop other kinds of allergies as well, such as hives and dermatoses. About 30–50% of cases appear to be purely intrinsic, occurring by nonallergic mechanisms, triggered by stress, emotion, or chemical irritants, or, most commonly, infection. In clients with mixed asthma conditions, both intrinsic and extrinsic factors play a role. Systemic drugs have also been noted to trigger asthmatic attacks (Table 52–1), with aspirin the most commonly implicated. In children, the proportion of cases that

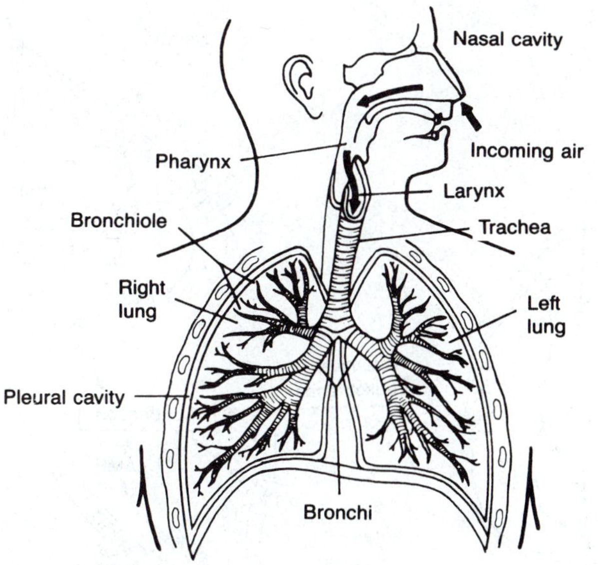

Figure 52–1
The respiratory system. From H. A. Braun, F. W. Cheney, Jr., and C. Paul Loehman, *Introduction to Respiratory Physiology*, 2d ed. Boston: Little, Brown, 1980.

Table 52–1
Systemic Drugs That May Precipitate Asthmatic Attacks

Acetylcysteine	Immunologicals
Antimicrobials	Allergenic extracts
Cephalosporins	Antisera
Chloramphenicol	Vaccines
Erythromycin	Lidocaine
Ethionamide	Mercurials
Griseofulvin	Monoamine oxidase inhibitors
Isoniazid	Neuromuscular blockers
Neomycin	Curare
Nitrofurantoin	Gallamine
Penicillamine	Succinylcholine
Penicillins	Nonsteroidal anti-inflammatory drugs
Polymyxins	Aspirin
Streptomycin	Ibuprofen
Sulfonamides	Indomethacin
Tetracyclines	Mefenamic acid
Beta-blockers	Phenylbutazone
Cannabis	Phenothiazines
Carbamazepine	Psillium
Cholinesterase inhibitors	Sodium dehydrocholate
Cholinomimetics	Verapamil
Estrogens	Vitamin K
Formaldehyde	
Histamine	

are of the extrinsic type is much higher; early onset is an indication that allergic mechanisms are probably involved. The incidence of attacks in children often declines with maturation.

Asthma occurs as attacks separated by extended symptom-free periods. An attack may come on with explosive suddenness or develop slowly. During an attack, the airways narrow, which triggers paroxysms of wheezing as the client tries to force air through them. The extent of wheezing during an attack is *not* a reliable indicator of the severity of the episode. Fatigue and hypercapnia occurring late in a severe attack may reduce ventilation so that wheezing is less prominent but hypoxia progressively severe. Clients may exhibit dyspnea, tachypnea, shortness of breath, unproductive cough, use of accessory muscles of respiration, sweating, dehydration, tachycardia, elevated blood pressure, difficulty talking, and dilated pupils.

Chemical Mediators

The tone of bronchial smooth muscles is determined by a variety of chemical mediators (Figure 52–2). One important factor is the balance between parasympathetic and sympathetic influences. Acetylcholine released from postganglionic parasympathetic fibers acts on muscarinic receptors to stimulate bronchoconstriction. Asthmatic patients exhibit an exaggerated sensitivity to cholinomimetic drugs, a response that can be blocked by antimuscarinic agents such as atropine. Normally, the cholinergic influence is balanced by an adrenergic influence involving β_2-receptors and a smaller population of β_1-receptors. The beta-receptor influences are mediated by cyclic 3′,5′-adenosine monophosphate. Cyclic AMP has a dual effect in promoting bronchodilation: not only does it act directly on bronchial smooth muscle to bring about relaxation, but it also acts on IgE-sensitized mast cells to inhibit degranulation (the release of chemical mediators).

Mast cells are directly implicated in those cases of asthma that are either entirely or partly extrinsic. Contact between an antigenic substance and IgE attached to the cell surface of mast cells can trigger release of preformed chemical mediators including histamine, serotonin, heparin, and eosinophil chemotaxic factor of anaphylaxis (ECF-A). IgE-mediated allergic reactions also stimulate synthesis of nonpreformed chemical mediators: prostaglandins and slow-reacting substance of anaphylaxis (SRS-A). This last substance is composed of three closely related substances in the leukotriene family. Histamine acts quickly to produce bronchoconstriction; SRS-A produces a more powerful bronchoconstriction that is slower in onset but longer in duration. Taken together, the mechanisms controlling tone of bronchial smooth muscles provide a basis for understanding the beneficial effects of drugs used in therapy for asthma. Useful drugs are those that ultimately in-

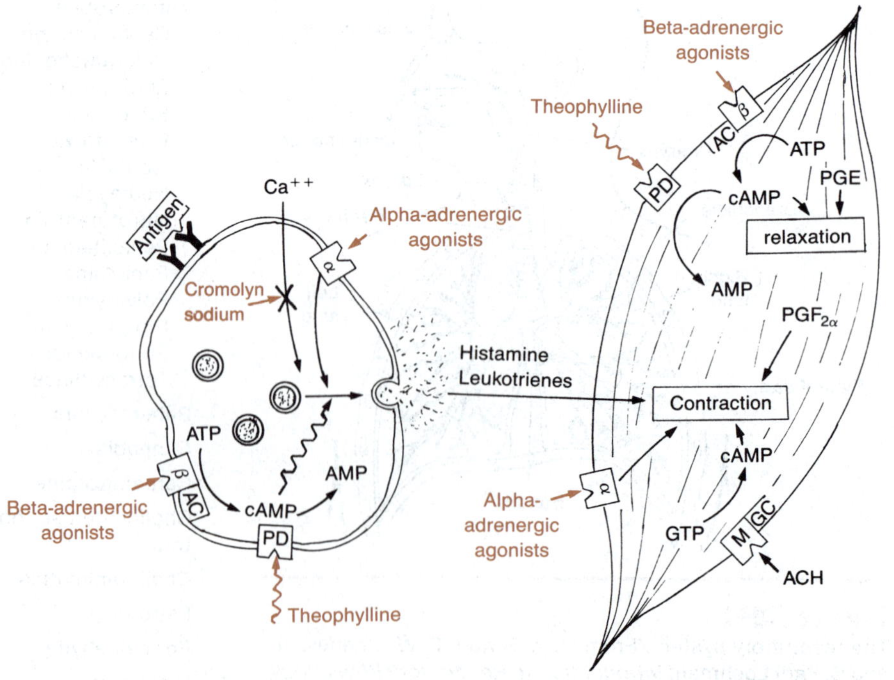

Figure 52–2
Mechanisms of asthma. Calcium-regulated release of chemical mediators of type I allergic reactions, following interaction of antigens with immunoglobulin receptors or stimulation of alpha-adrenergic receptors of mast cells, can be suppressed by drugs that inhibit calcium influx (cromolyn sodium) or that increase adenosine 3′:5′-cyclic phosphate (cAMP), either by stimulating its production (beta-adrenergic agonists) or by inhibiting its breakdown by phosphodiesterase (PD) (theophylline). The chemical mediators, as well as alpha-adrenergic agonists, acetylcholine, and prostaglandin F2α, contract bronchial smooth muscle causing bronchoconstriction, but drugs that increase cyclic AMP and prostaglandin E relax bronchial smooth muscle.

crease cyclic AMP levels in the bronchial smooth muscle cells.

Treatment of Asthma

Drug therapy is the mainstay of treatment of asthma, for both managing and preventing attacks, but nondrug measures are also important. Most important among the nondrug components of treatment is identification and elimination, or control, of causative agents in the environment. Skin tests can be conducted to test the allergenic potency of suspected allergens. It may be possible to eliminate contact with allergens, such as animal dander, chemical irritants such as cigarette smoke, fumes, or environmental factors such as humidity, temperature changes, or changes in air pressure. If the allergen is a pollen, hyposensitization therapy may be possible.

For acute management of attacks that have progressed to advanced stages, oxygen therapy and intravenous fluid and electrolytes are usually required in addition to specific antiasthmatic drugs. The antiasthmatic drugs belong to five classes: (1) beta-adrenergic agonists, (2) methylxanthines, (3) anticholinergics, (4) cromolyn sodium, and (5) steroids. Important considerations in drug selection include accurate assessment of the stage of the asthmatic attack, a recognition of primary drug choices versus those reserved for clients with recalcitrant or severe asthma, and the selection of an optimum route of administration.

Beta-Adrenergic Agonists

Sympathomimetics that act on β_2-receptors are effective for symptomatic relief of the bronchospasm of acute asthmatic attacks. These agents can also be useful for bronchospasm associated with chronic obstructive lung disease. Aerosol preparations incorporating long-acting, selective β_2-agonists also have a place in long-term prophylaxis in clients with severe asthma in conjunction with theophylline. The efficacy of a sympathomimetic depends on its ability to activate β_2-receptors. The ability to activate other receptors does not increase the drug's efficacy but will add side effects (Table 52–2). Therefore, a selective β_2-agonist (Table 52–3) is generally preferred, provided that one is available that has an appropriate duration of action and effectiveness when given by the desired route of administration.

Adverse Effects and Contraindications The adverse effects of a given preparation are determined mainly by the selectivity of the drug for adrenergic receptors and the route of administration.

Table 52–2
Adverse Effects of Sympathomimetics

Mediated by	Adverse effects
α_1-Receptors	CNS excitation: restlessness, anxiety, insomnia, anorexia
	Vasoconstriction: hypertension, pallor, possible hemorrhage
	Urinary retention
	Nasal edema
	Pupillary dilation
α_2-Receptors	CNS depression
β_1-Receptors	Cardiac stimulation: tachycardia, palpitations, dysrhythmias, angina (due to increased cardiac work)
β_2-Receptors	Vasodilation: hypotension, angina (due to decreased coronary blood flow), vascular headaches, flushing, cardiovascular collapse
	Tremor

The ideal situation for minimizing adverse effects is topical application (inhalation) of a β_2-selective drug. However, many asthmatics are unable to inhale an aerosol preparation effectively during an acute attack. Therefore, inhalation preparations are most useful in maintenance applications.

The most important adverse effects of β_2-receptor activation are tremor, vascular headaches, flushing, and vasodilation. In the extreme, clients may have severe hypotension and cardiovascular collapse, but this happens only when unreasonable quantities of drug are used. The agents that also activate β_1-receptors stimulate the heart and may cause tachycardia, palpitations, dysrhythmias, and anginal pain.

Beta-2-agonists also elevate blood glucose levels. *Clients with diabetes should be warned to intensify urine testing and to watch for symptoms of recurring hyperglycemia (increased thirst, increased voiding, or a rise in blood glucose).*

The least selective drugs, the ones that also stimulate alpha-receptors, can cause restlessness, anxiety, insomnia, anorexia, urinary retention, and hypertension. *Insomnia is common but can be minimized if the client takes the last dose of drug for the day several hours before bedtime. Clients should be encouraged to record intake and output to detect evidence of urinary retention.* A sharp rise in blood pressure can lead to hemorrhage.

Since beta-agonists reduce bronchial secretions, mucus plugs may become difficult to dislodge. *Nurses are responsible for teaching clients postural drainage and*

Table 52–3
Comparisons Among Bronchodilators

	Adrenergic agonist spectrum					
Drug	**Alpha**	**Beta-1**	**Beta-2**	**Acceptable routes**	**Onset (minutes)**	**Duration (hours)**
Albuterol			+++	Inhalation	5	4
Bitolterol		+	+++	Inhalation	3–4	5–8
Ephedrine	+++	++	++	Oral	15–60	3–5
Epinephrine	+	+	+++	Inhalation	2–3	0.25–0.5
	+++	+++	+++	Intramuscular	Variable	6–24
	+++	+++	+++	Subcutaneous	5–15	1–8
Ethylnorepinephrine	+	+++	+++	Intramuscular	5–10	1–2
	+	+++	+++	Subcutaneous	5–10	1–2
Isoetharine		+	+++	Inhalation	5	1–3
Isoproterenol		+	+++	Inhalation	2–3	1–2
		+++	+++	Intravenous	0	<1
		+++	+++	Sublingual	15–30	1–2
Metaproterenol		+	+++	Inhalation	5	1.5–3
		++	+++	Oral	15–30	4
Salbutamol			+++	European name for albuterol		
Terbutaline		+	+++	Oral	30	4–8
		+	+++	Subcutaneous	5–15	1.5–4

Key: + + +, highly potent; + +, moderately potent; +, weakly active; blank, no activity

breathing exercises to overcome this problem. Hypersensitivity reactions are rare with sympathomimetics, but when they occur they represent a specific contraindication for use. Beta-1-stimulants are contraindicated in clients with cardiac dysrhythmias or coronary artery disease.

Drug Interactions The action of sympathomimetics is intensified by monoamine oxidase inhibitors and thyroid hormones. Beta-1-agonists are contraindicated for use with anesthetics or in clients who have developed digitalis toxicity. Two or more adrenergic agonists are seldom used concurrently because of additive adverse effects.

Preparations and Administration The beta-agonists available for parenteral administration are epinephrine (Sus-phrine, Asmolin, and others), ethylnorepinephrine (Bronkephrine), isoproterenol (Isuprel), and terbutaline (Brethine, Bricanyl). **Epinephrine** is the most frequently used. For acute relief of an asthmatic attack in the early stages, epinephrine is typically given at a dose of 0.2–1.0 mg, subcutaneously or, less commonly, intramuscularly. Onset of action occurs in 3–5 minutes. *Since epinephrine is nonspecific in its action on adrenergic receptors, nurses should observe clients for signs of increased nervousness, restlessness, and sleeplessness.*

Epinephrine solutions should be stored in light-resistant containers. Oxidation causes epinephrine to change color to pink or brown. Solutions that become colored should be discarded. Clients and their families should be taught how to administer epinephrine subcutaneously. Clients should be taught not to withdraw solution from the vial before it is needed. Prior to withdrawing the solution, the vial or ampul should be thoroughly shaken to assure dispersion of particles. After inserting the needle, the client should draw the plunger back to assure the needle has not been inadvertently introduced into a vein, since intravenous injection of epinephrine can cause sudden hypertension and possibly cerebral hemorrhage. Once the client is assured the needle is correctly placed, the material should be injected, the needle withdrawn, and the area massaged to hasten absorption.

Since epinephrine induces vasoconstriction and reduces tissue oxygenation, which favors the growth of anaerobic bac-

Nursing Observations for Use of Antiasthmatic Drugs in Asthma

THERAPEUTIC GOAL	Relief of respiratory distress, dyspnea, and hypoxia associated with acute attacks and reduced incidence and severity of attacks over time.
PREADMINISTRATION ASSESSMENT	
Baseline Data	Observe for episodic respiratory distress, wheezing, rales, nonproductive cough, dyspnea, shortness of breath, use of accessory respiratory musles, sweating, dehydration, and anxiety. Evaluate blood pressure, pulse rate, respiratory rate, depth and sounds, vital capacity, neurologic and psychologic status. Note presence of infection. Evaluate pulse pressure for pulsus paradoxus of greater than 20–30 mm Hg. Obtain baseline pulmonary function tests before initiating new drug regimens. Obtain laboratory tests including arterial gas levels (↑ PCO_2; ↓ PO_2)
Contraindications/ Precautions	Check medical history for contraindications for particular antiasthmatic agents, such as hepatic or renal impairments, peptic ulcer or gastritis, coronary disease, or pregnancy or lactation. Check the medication history for a history of allergic reactions.
Potential Interactions	Check current medications for potential interactions with specific antiasthmatic agents.
EVALUATION OF DRUG RESPONSE	
During Dosage Adjustment	Monitor serum levels and blood glucose when a xanthine is initially employed.
For Therapeutic Benefit	Monitor vital signs, respiratory function, and arterial blood gases, alleviation of symptoms of respiratory distress, intake-output, level of consciousness, and occurrence of respiratory infection.
For Adverse Effects and Drug Interactions	Monitor for adverse effects and drug interactions specific for each drug in the regimen (see individual drug discussions).
For Compliance	Evaluate the client's compliance with all facets of the therapeutic regimen by careful observation, interviewing, and review of progress. Report compliance problems to the physician and act as client-advocate when changes in the therapeutic regimen seem indicated.

teria, particularly Clostridium welchii, *it is best to avoid intramuscular administration. When it is administered IM, it is best to avoid the buttock area.*

Isoproterenol does not act on alpha-adrenergic receptors but is nonspecific for β_1- and β_2-receptor sites. Thus, isoproterenol will produce cardiac stimulation along with its beneficial effects in asthma. The oral preparations are used primarily in maintenance therapy but are less useful than oral methylxanthines. Ephedrine was once the treatment of choice. Its effect on bronchial smooth muscle is weaker but more prolonged than that with epinephrine; hence it is useful only for mild to moderate bronchitis, seasonal or chronic. *Clients using the sublingual glossets should be given specific instructions not to swallow the tablets.*

The nurse should advise clients that excessive use of aerosol preparations can lead to tachyphylaxis (loss of drug effectiveness) or even a paradoxical constriction of airways after the primary drug action has subsided. Clients who are expected to self-administer the drug by nebulizer should be given specific instructions on use of the nebulizer. The client should clear the nose, exhale, place the nebulizer in the mouth with the lips tightly sealed around it, and inhale deeply, holding the breath for several seconds. After inhalations, clients should rinse the mouth and throat with water to avoid inadvertently swallowing residual drug and to prevent the oropharynx from becoming dry. Nurses should stress the importance of starting therapy with the first symptoms of bronchospasm and of using the least number of inhalations possible to provide relief. At least 1–2 minutes should elapse before further inhalations to prevent excessive dosage. The mouthpiece of the nebulizer unit should be rinsed with warm water at least once daily to prevent clogging with mucus. After washing, the mouthpiece should be immersed in 70% alcohol to sanitize it.

Nursing Diagnoses and Interventions for Use of Antiasthmatic Drugs in Asthma

Nursing Diagnoses	*Related Interventions*
TO ENHANCE DRUG BENEFITS OR REDUCE DRUG REQUIREMENTS	
Alteration in respiratory function and impaired airway clearance related to bronchospasm and increased respiratory secretions	Teach the client appropriate respiratory technique for acute attacks: upright sitting position and pursed-lip exhalation, with postural drainage if necessary. Between attacks, teach the client breathing exercises to follow and provide coaching during attacks. Administer oxygen. Employ an intermittent positive pressure breathing machine.
Anxiety related to respiratory distress and anticipation of recurrence	Provide support and reassurance. Teach relaxation techniques; consider referral to a psychotherapist for training in relaxation techniques.
TO MINIMIZE DRUG SIDE EFFECTS OR INTERACTIONS	
Alteration in cardiac output related to cardiac stimulation by antiasthmatic drugs	Monitor for cardiac dysrhythmias. Teach client to avoid over-the-counter preparations containing xanthines and to limit dietary intake of caffeine. Use aerosols in preference to oral sympathomimetics and selective β_2-agonists in preference to nonselective sympathomimetics.
Alteration in comfort related to irritant effect on gastric mucosa produced by xanthines	Assess for signs of gastric irritation; take xanthines with meals. Teach client self-monitoring.
Altered tissue perfusion related to diuretic effects of xanthines	Assess for dehydration and ensure adequate fluid intake; measure urine output.
Sleep pattern disturbance related to stimulatory effects of antiasthmatic drugs	Minimize evening and nighttime doses; assess for behavioral changes related to sleep deprivation.
TO ENSURE SAFE AND EFFICACIOUS DRUG USE	
Knowledge deficit related to asthma or antiasthmatic drugs	Teach client about the nature of asthma, environmental factors that tend to trigger attacks (smoking, allergens, irritants, weather, and infections), and the rationale for the medical regimen. Instruct client in the practice of breathing exercises and relaxation techniques. Explain the value of regular, moderate exercise. Teach client to recognize the signs and symptoms of exacerbation of respiratory problems or complications of asthma. Show client the proper technique for administration of aerosol preparations if required. If the client is a child, assure that family members have appropriate information for preventing attacks and for countering attacks when they occur. Teach client the proper use of positive pressure breathing devices or proper administration of oxygen if home administration of these is expected. Provide client with a list of adverse effects and drug interactions for each drug in the regimen and explain what to do if any of these occur.

PARENTERAL FORMULATIONS

Epinephrine (Sus-Phrine, Asmolin, others)
Injection solutions, solutions for nebulization (AsthmaNefrin, Vaponefrin, microNEFRIN), aerosols (AsthmaHaler, Bronitin Mist, Medihaler-Epi, Primatene Mist, and Bronkaid Mist).

Ethylnorepinephrine (Bronkephrine)
Injection solutions
Recommended Doses: 0.5–1.0 ml SC or IM.

Isoproterenol (Isuprel)
Injection solutions
Recommended Doses: For advanced stages of status asthmaticus in children, 0.01–0.02 mg IV repeated as required.

Terbutaline (Brethine, Bricanyl)
Injection solution
Recommended Doses: 1 mg/ml SC.

ORAL FORMULATIONS

Ephedrine
Capsules, syrup
Recommended Doses: For adults, 25–50 mg PO, every 3–4 hours. For children, 3 mg/kg/day PO in 4–6 divided doses.

Fenoterol (Berotec) — Investigational
Oral dosage forms

Isoproterenol (Isuprel)
Sublingual tablets
Recommended Doses: For adults, 10–20 mg PO per administration up to 60 mg daily. For children, 5–10 mg PO per administration up to 30 mg daily.

Metaproterenol (Alupent, Metaprel)
Tablets, syrup
Recommended Doses: For adults, 20 mg PO 3–4 times daily. For children over 9 or over 60 lbs., 20 mg PO 3–4 times daily. For children 6–9 or less than 60 lbs., 10 mg PO 3–4 times daily.

Phenylpropanolamine (generic and others)
Tablets, capsules, timed release capsules, elixir
Recommended Doses: For adults, 25 mg PO every 4 hours or 50 mg every 6–8 hours to a maximum of 150 mg/day. For children 6–12 years of age, 12.5 mg PO every 4 hours or 25 mg every 8 hours. For children 2–6 years of age, 6.25 mg PO every 4 hours or 12.5 mg every 8 hours.

Pirbuterol (Exirel)
Experimental
Recommended Doses: For adults, 10–15 mg PO, 3–4 times daily up to 60 mg/day.

Pseudoephedrine (Sudafed, First Sign, Cenafed, Neo-Fed, others)
Tablets, timed release capsules (D-Feda, Gyrocaps, Novafed, Sinufed, others), timed release capsules as the sulfate salt (Afrinol Repetabs), liquid (Cenafed, D-Feda, Novafed, Sudafed, Sympton 2, and generics)
Recommended Doses: For adults, 60 mg PO every 6 hours or 120 mg of the timed release formulation every 12 hours. For children, 6–12 years of age, 30 mg PO every 6 hours. For children 2–5 years of age, 15 mg PO every 6 hours.

INHALATION

Albuterol (Proventil, Ventolin)
Aerosol
Recommended Doses: For adults or children 12 or older, 2 inhalations every 4–6 hours.

Bitolterol (Tornalate)
Aerosol
Recommended Doses: For adults and children over 12 years of age, 2 inhalations separated by at least 3 minutes followed by a third if required.

Fenoterol (Berotec) — Investigational
Aerosol, nebulizer solution, powder for inhalation

Isoetharine
Solution for nebulization (Dispos-a-Med, Bronkosol, and generic), aerosol (Bronkometer)
Recommended Doses: With the hand nebulizer, 3–7 inhalations, with the aerosol nebulizer, 1–2 inhalations.

Isoproterenol (Isuprel)
Aerosols (Isuprel, Norisodrine Aerotrol, Medihaler-Iso), solutions for nebulization (Aerolone, Dispos-a-Med, Vapo-Iso, and Isuprel), powder for aerohalor inhalation (Norisodrine)
Recommended Doses: For acute relief of dyspnea, one inhalation initially followed after 2–5 minutes by a second if required. For maintenance, 1–2 inhalations, 4–6 times daily.

Metaproterenol (Alupent, Metaprel)
Aerosol, solution for nebulization
Recommended Doses: Two to three inhalations per administration to a maximum of 12 daily.

Pirbuterol (Exirel)
Aerosol
Recommended Doses: 1–2 inhalations every 4 hours to a maximum of 12 inhalations daily.

Methylxanthines

The methylxanthines include caffeine, theobromine, theophylline, and salts and derivatives of the latter. These drugs share several pharmacological actions: (1) CNS and respiratory stimulation, (2) cardiac stimulation, (3) dilation of coronary, pulmonary, and general systemic blood vessels by a direct relaxant effect on vascular smooth muscle, (4) constriction of cerebral blood vessels, (5) relaxation of visceral smooth muscle, (6) stimulation of skeletal muscles, and (7) diuresis. The methylxanthines are employed clinically or socially for at least four of these effects: CNS stimulation (see Chapter 14), constriction of cerebral blood vessels (see Chapter 26), diuresis (see Chapter 43), and relaxation of visceral smooth muscle (the relevant action in asthma). The available methylxanthines differ in their relative potencies in eliciting each of these effects (see Table 14–3). Caffeine is the most potent in producing skeletal muscle, respiratory, and CNS stimulation (see Chapter 14). Theophylline has the most potent effect on visceral smooth muscle, and is thus the methylxanthine most often used for asthma.

Mechanisms and Effects The methylxanthines competitively inhibit phosphodiesterase, the enzyme that degrades cyclic AMP, thus elevating cyclic AMP levels. In bronchial smooth muscle cells, cyclic AMP produces relaxation of muscle fibers. Elevation of cyclic AMP in mast cells also contributes to the antiasthmatic effect of theophylline. The current understanding is that cyclic AMP in mast cells inhibits release of both histamine and slow-reacting substance of anaphylaxis.

Pharmacokinetics The methylxanthines employed in asthma are theophylline and its salts and derivatives. These various agents produce equivalent pharmacological effects but are not equivalent on a weight basis because of differing amounts of theophylline in the various compounds (Table 52–4). After oral administration, theophylline is well absorbed. Concurrent food ingestion has little effect on theophylline absorption. **Antacids** (magnesium or aluminum hydroxides) decrease the rate of absorption of theophylline but not the extent.

The therapeutic window for theophylline plasma concentrations is 10–20 μg/ml. When long-term maintenance therapy is anticipated, the dosage regimen should be individualized initially by monitoring serum levels. After initial titration and stabilization, subsequent monitoring can be reduced in frequency. Monitoring of serum drug levels is especially important when higher than typical doses are required to achieve a response. Serum levels above 20 μg/ml are associated with toxicity.

Methylxanthines are eliminated mainly by metabolic transformation in the liver and subsequent excretion by the kidneys. Only a small amount of theophylline (<10%) is excreted unchanged. Differences in elimination kinetics from one person to another account for most of the variability in plasma concentrations. **Tobacco** smoking induces liver enzymes and metabolism of theophylline. The half-life of theophylline in adult nonsmokers averages 7–9 hours but is 4–5 hours in adult smokers. Charcoal broiled foods have also been reported to induce liver enzymes and hasten theophylline elimination. Theophylline elimination is also more rapid in children; the half-life averages 3.5 hours in children. On the other hand, the rate of clearance for theophylline can be reduced with the concurrent use of **cimetidine** (Tagamet), **oral contraceptives,** and certain **antibiotics**, including clindamycin (Cleocin), erythromycin, lincomycin (Lincocin), and troleandomycin (Tao). The half-life of theophylline can also be increased in liver disease, kidney dysfunction, congestive heart failure, or febrile conditions.

In theory, enteric coated tablets and sustained release capsules offer an advantage in maintaining stable serum concentrations of theophylline, but in

Table 52–4
Comparison of the Salts and Derivatives of Theophylline

Drug	Percentage theophylline	Equivalent dosage (mg)
Theophylline anhydrous	100	200
Theophylline monohydrate	91	220
Theophylline ethylenediamine (aminophylline) anhydrous	86	232
Theophylline ethylenediamine (aminophylline) dihydrate	79	254
Oxtriphylline	64	312
Theophylline sodium glycinate	49	400
Theophylline calcium salicylate	48	416

practice, these preparations often provide unreliable absorption.

Clinical Indications Methylxanthines are indicated both for acute relief of asthmatic attacks and for prophylaxis of asthma. Intravenous infusion of aminophylline, the theophylline salt, is a preliminary step in treatment of severe asthmatic eipsodes. For maintenance applications, oral preparations are generally employed. Rectal administration does not provide reliable absorption and may be irritating. Methylxanthines also find use in brochospasms associated with chronic bronchitis or emphysema.

Adverse Effects and Contraindications Adverse effects of methylxanthines fall most heavily on the gastrointestinal system, CNS, cardiovascular system, and the kidneys. Nausea and vomiting are the most common early signs of theophylline toxicity, but they do not occur reliably enough to provide a dependable warning of more severe reactions. Methylxanthines are ulcergenic and may aggravate or reactivate preexisting ulcers. Other **gastrointestinal symptoms** are epigastric pain, diarrhea, and intestinal bleeding. *If gastrointestinal symptoms occur, the nurse should advise the client to take theophylline preparations with meals or snacks.*

Central nervous system symptoms of xanthine intoxication begin with irritability, restlessness, anxiety, dizziness, and insomnia. With increasing levels of theophylline, clients begin to develop hyperreflexia, muscle twitching, and major convulsions. Convulsions have been reported to occur without previous obvious indications of developing toxicity. *The client should be advised to report occurrence of indications of restlessness or anxiety.*

Clients who have adverse reactions involving the **cardiovascular system** may exhibit palpitation, sinus or ventricular tachycardia, premature beats, ventricular fibrillation, reduced peripheral resistance, marked hypotension, or circulatory collapse. These effects derive from the positive inotropic and chronotropic actions of methylxanthines on the heart and the relaxation of peripheral blood vessels. *Prior to administering methylxanthines, nurses need to determine if the client has any history of cardiovascular disease such as myocardial injury or hypertension since these clients will require close monitoring.* Adverse renal effects include diuresis that may cause dehydration, which is especially critical among elderly clients. Evidence of renal damage may also occur, including proteinuria and increased excretion of red blood cells and renal tubular cells.

Other untoward effects of methylxanthines include **hyperglycemia** (due to liver glycogenolysis), **decreased clotting time**, **leukocytosis**, and persistence of benign breast tumors. **Allergic reactions** rarely occur to theophylline itself but sometimes occur to diphylline and the ethylenediamine component of aminophylline. *Prior to administering methylxanthines, nurses need to assess clients for evidence of hypersensitivity to xanthine compounds.* The use of methylxanthines is contraindicated in clients with peptic ulcer, liver or kidney impairment, hypotension, preexisting dysrhythmias, coronary artery disease, or hypersensitivity to any xanthine.

When theophylline overdose occurs, treatment is based on how far the symptoms have advanced. If the patient is conscious and not in seizure, vomiting should be induced by administration of ipecac syrup; gastric lavage, cathartics, and activated charcoal may also be employed. Intravenous diazepam (Valium) is employed as an anticonvulsant in clients with a methylxanthine-induced seizure. Otherwise, during a seizure or the subsequent postseizure coma, treatment is supportive. Attention focuses on maintaining an airway, oxygenation, and adequate blood pressure.

Drug Interactions Drugs that alter elimination of theophylline were discussed above in the pharmacokinetic section. The CNS stimulation of methylxanthines is potentially additive to that of other drugs, such as alpha-sympathomimetics, amphetamine, and cocaine, which can lead to excess stimulation. Nurses need to warn clients to avoid drinking beverages that contain caffeine such as coffee, cocoa, tea, and cola drinks as well as to avoid over-the-counter medications that contain xanthines. Methylxanthines and propranolol have mutually antagonistic effects. The diuretic effect of methylxanthines is additive with that of other diuretics. Aminophylline increases the rate of excretion of lithium; therefore lithium doses may require adjustment.

Preparations and Administration Only aminophylline (theophylline ethylenediamine) and dyphylline (dihydroxypropyl theophylline) are available for parenteral administration. The methylxanthines are available in innumerable formulations for oral administration. These include capsules, tablets, liquid, elixirs, syrups, suspensions, and timed release capsules and tablets. Suppositories are also available for rectal administration in the case of aminophylline, but they provide no particular advantage. Methylxanthines are available as individual agents and in various combinations with expectorants, sedatives, beta-sympathomimetics, and other ingredients.

PARENTERAL FORMULATIONS

Aminophylline
Injection solutions (*Dyphilline solutions must be protected from light.*)
Recommended Doses: For clients not currently receiving a methylxanthine, a loading dose of 6 mg/kg IV, infused in a concentration of 25 mg/ml or less at a rate of 25 mg/minute or less. This loading dose should be reduced if an oral methylxanthine has been administered recently. For maintenance infusions, monitoring of serum levels is imperative. An overly rapid rate of infusion will result in CNS and cardiovascular toxicity. The usual intramuscular dose is 500 mg for aminophylline or 250–500 mg of dyphylline. *Intramuscular injections should be done slowly. Clients should be warned that there may be some pain.*

Dyphylline
Injection solutions (Dilin, Dilor, Lufyllin, Neothylline, generic)
Recommended Doses: Same as for aminophylline.

ORAL FORMULATIONS

Aminophylline
Tablets, elixir (Mini-Lix or Lixaminol), oral liquid (Somophyllin), timed release tablets (Phyllocontin, Aminodur); combinations with expectorants (e.g., Mudrane-2), dextromethorphan (Lixaminol AT), ephedrine and amobarbital (Amesec), or ephedrine, phenobarbital, and an expectorant (Mudrane).
Recommended Doses: For adults, 500 mg PO for an acute attack, 200–315 mg every 6–8 hours for maintenance. In children, for acute asthmatic episodes, 7.5 mg/kg; for maintenance 5 mg/kg every 6 hours.

Dyphylline (Airet, Dilor, Dyflex, Lufyllin, Neothylline)
Tablets, long-acting tablets, liquids and elixirs; combinations with guaifenesin
Recommended Doses: For adults, 15 mg/kg PO every 6 hours.

Oxtriphylline (Choledyl)
Tablets, elixir, pediatric syrup
Recommended Doses: For adults, 200 mg, 4 times daily.

Theophylline (Bronkodyl, Elixophyllin, Slo-phyllin, Theoclear, and others)
Capsules, tablets, chewable tablets, elixirs, syrups, liquids, suspensions, and timed release formulations; combinations with the expectorant guaifenesin (e.g., Cerylin, Quibron), the expectorant potassium iodide (e.g., Theokin Elixir), ephedrine and phenobarbital (e.g., Tedral), pseudoephedrine and butabarital (Theo-Sed), ephedrine and hydroxyzine (e.g., Marax, Theophozine), ephedrine, guaifenesin, and an antihistamine (Bronitin), or ephedrine, guaifenesin, and a barbiturate (e.g., Duovent).
Recommended Doses: 200–250 mg PO every 6 hours in adults, 100 mg every 6 hours in children.

Theophylline Sodium Glycinate
Tablets (Synophylate), elixirs (Theofort, Synophylate)
Recommended Doses: For adults, 330–660 mg PO, 2 or 3 times daily, after meals.

Anticholinergics

Mechanisms and Effects Anticholinergic drugs were at one time widely used in treatment of asthma, but with systemic administration, the classical anticholinergic drugs such as atropine produced widespread side effects in the central nervous system, eye, cardiovascular system, and in the respiratory system itself (drying and thickening of the sputum). As a result, anticholinergic drugs were gradually displaced by newer drugs such as the beta-agonists and the methylxanthines. Recently, anticholinergic drug therapy for asthma has reemerged in the form of ipratropium bromide (Atrovent), a drug which can be administered topically as an aerosol to the respiratory system with little systemic absorption (less than 5% of the administered dose). Also, ipratropium is unable to cross the blood-brain barrier, so even the small fraction that does reach the systemic circulation is unable to enter the brain. Thus ipratropium selectively dilates the bronchioles with few systemic side effects. Ipratropium also has little effect on ciliary activity, mucus formation, or viscosity of sputum within the respiratory system itself.

Pharmacokinetics Bronchodilation occurs within a few minutes when ipratropium is given in an aerosol and lasts 1–2 hours with normal doses. The small amount of ipratropium that is absorbed systemically after administration in an aerosol reaches peak plasma levels in about 3 hours and is eliminated mainly by metabolism with a half-life of about 3–4 hours.

Clinical Indications Ipratropium is indicated for use as a bronchodilator in asthma or chronic bronchitis. Ipratropium appears to be approximately equal in effectiveness with beta-agonists or methylxanthines in alleviating these conditions.

Adverse Effects and Contraindications Systemic adverse effects are rare and mild when they do occur. Such reactions have included visual disturbances, dizziness, drowsiness, and a slight bradycardia. Mild local side effects that are common include dryness of mouth, a bad taste in the mouth, and throat irritation. Infrequently, local adverse effects have included an increase in sputum viscosity with a consequent decrease in its clearance by the mucociliary system.

Drug Interactions Ipratropium has been used successfully in combinations with theophylline and beta-agonists for treatment of both asthma and chronic bronchitis, but the response was not statistically greater than when ipratropium was used alone.

Preparations and Administration

Ipratropium Bromide (Atrovent)
Aerosol
Recommended Doses: For adults, 40 μg by inhalation 4 times daily

Cromolyn Sodium

Mechanisms and Effects Cromolyn sodium is employed only for prophylaxis against antigen-induced bronchospasms in extrinsic asthma. Cromolyn inhibits the degranulation of sensitized mast cells that occurs in contact with an antigen. Release of both histamine and slow-reacting substance of anaphylaxis is suppressed. The drug does not block histamine receptors, relax bronchial smooth muscle, or suppress inflammation.

Clinical Indications Cromolyn is used adjunctively in severe bronchial asthma when adequate prophylaxis with either methylxanthines alone or methylxanthine-sympathomimetic combinations cannot be achieved without intolerable side effects. It frequently allows a reduction in dosage requirements for the primary antiasthmatic drugs.

Adverse Effects and Contraindications Some clients who respond well to cromolyn will experience rebound asthmatic attacks when the drug is eliminated. *Thus, nurses need to warn clients not to discontinue medication abruptly without consulting the physician.* Hypersensitivity reactions occasionally occur, in the form of rash or urticaria. Other adverse effects include nausea, headache, dizziness, lacrimation, increased urinary frequency and dysuria, swollen glands, and angioderma. Some clients will experience bronchospasm, cough, nasal congestion, or pharyngeal irritation in response to cromolyn inhalation. *Gargling with water after the treatment may help to minimize throat irritation. Nurses should advise clients to notify the physician immediately if respiratory symptoms such as wheezing occur.*

Preparations and Administration Cromolyn is poorly absorbed after oral administration and is currently available only in capsules for use in a spinhaler apparatus for administration by inhalation. *Clients will need to be taught how to use the spinhaler device and instructed not to swallow cromolyn capsules. Before using the turboinhaler, the client should clear as much mucus as possible. The inhaler mouthpiece is then placed between the lips with the head tilted backward, and the client should inhale deeply and evenly and hold the breath for a few seconds before exhaling. The client should repeat this procedure until the entire dose is inhaled.* Cromolyn should be protected from heat and light. *Nurses need to stress that the effectiveness of cromolyn depends upon administration at regular intervals.*

Cromolyn (Intal)
Capsules for use in an inhalator device
Recommended Doses: For adults and children over 5, 20 mg inhaled 4 times daily.

Corticosteroids for Asthma

Mechanisms and Effects Since inflammation of the tracheobronchial mucosa contributes to the airway obstruction of asthma, intravenous corticosteroids can be used to good effect for acute management of severe asthma attacks. *Clients with a history of severe attacks should be advised to wear a medic alert bracelet to indicate the need for systemic steroids during severe asthmatic episodes.*

Clinical Indications There are inherent risks with the chronic use of glucocorticoids for prophylaxis (see Chapter 32), including suppression of the immune response and consequent increased susceptibility to infection. For this reason, glucocorticoids are used only when adequate prophylaxis cannot be achieved by other measures such as methylxanthines, beta-sympathomimetics, and cromolyn sulfate. The recent introduction of steroid aerosols has provided a means of delivering glucocorticoids directly to their sites of action in bronchial asthma, while minimizing adverse systemic effects. However, the glucocorticoids employed in respiratory inhalant preparations are rapidly absorbed from the respiratory tract so that use of these agents should still be reserved for clients who cannot be managed adequately otherwise. Glucocorticoids do not produce bronchodilation nor inhibit bronchospasms and should not be used as the primary measure for relief of bronchospasms. *Clients should be advised not to employ inhalation steroids in the attempt to abort acute attacks.*

Adverse Effects and Contraindications Local adverse effects of glucocorticoids include the occurrence of superinfections. Infections by *Candida albicans* or *Aspergillus* are frequently found in the mouth and pharynx, and less frequently in the larynx of clients using inhalation corticosteroids. As many as 75% of clients reportedly exhibit positive cultures for oral *Candidus,* although only a fraction of these have clinically significant infections. *Clients should be advised to notify the physician if sore throat occurs.* Concomitant antifungal medication is sometimes required. *Rinsing the mouth and gargling after each administration with warm water or mouth wash will reduce occurrence of candidiasis.* Systemic effects are modest if the normal dosage range is not exceeded. For example, little or no suppression of endogenous glucocorticoid production is observed at prescribed doses. There is no evidence that exceeding the normal dosage increases the chances of a favorable response.

Sometimes steroid inhalation therapy is begun while in the process of discontinuing a systemic corticosteroid regimen. Corticosteroids given by inhalation will not suppress the withdrawal syndrome associated with discontinuation of long-term systemic glucocorticoid administration. Thus, withdrawal of the systemic medication should be gradual even if inhalation therapy is begun. Adrenal insufficiency is common and deaths have occurred as a result of overly rapid withdrawal from systemic steroids. Withdrawal from systemic steroids is also associated with unmasking of suppressed allergic conditions and pulmonary infiltrative eosinophilia.

Preparations and Administration The glucocorticoids available for application by inhalation are beclomethasone, dexamethasone, triamcinolone (Azmacort), and flunisolide (AeroBid). *Clients who are using a bronchodilator concurrently should administer the steroid after the bronchodilator to maximize access and penetration of the steroid. Clients prescribed more than one inhalation per treatment should be instructed to allow at least 1 minute between inhalations.*

Beclomethasone (Beclovent, Vanceril)
Recommended Doses: For adults, 2 inhalations, 3 or 4 times per day. The total daily dose should not exceed 20 inhalations per day. For children 6–12 years of age, the typical dose is 1 or 2 inhalations, 3 or 4 times daily as required.

Dexamethasone (Decadron Phosphate Respihaler)
Recommended Doses: For adults, 3 inhalations, 3 or 4 times per day, initially. For children, 2 inhalations, 3 or 4 times per day.

Important Nursing Implications for Antiasthmatic Drugs

- ☐ Take the client's medication history for indications of hypersensitivity to a particular drug. Check the medical history for contraindications for use of specific drugs.
- ☐ Teach clients that many nonprescription preparations contain sympathomimetic amines or xanthines that can interact with regimens for asthma.
- ☐ Instruct clients in the proper use of nebulizers and aerosols.
- ☐ Teach clients to rinse the mouth carefully after use of inhalation preparations to prevent dryness and irritation and systemic absorption of the drug.
- ☐ Warn clients who use inhalation preparations that overuse will lead to tolerance and even rebound increases in airway resistance.
- ☐ Advise clients who have a history of severe asthmatic attacks to wear a medical identification tag or bracelet.
- ☐ Instruct clients who have hypertension, hyperthyroidism, heart disease, or diabetes mellitus to use sympathomimetics only with extreme caution and as little as possible.
- ☐ Teach clients that sympathomimetic amines often require special storage procedures. They should be protected from air, light, and extremes of temperature. Solutions that have changed color should be discarded. Dyphylline solutions must also be protected from light.
- ☐ Teach clients and members of their families who are responsible for them how to administer epinephrine subcutaneously for emergency situations.
- ☐ Observe clients, especially children, using sympathomimetic amines or xanthines for indications of excess stimulation, such as nervousness or insomnia.
- ☐ Advise against the use of methylxanthines by clients who have peptic ulcer, liver or kidney impairment, hypotension, preexisting dysrhythmias, coronary artery disease, or hypersensitivity to any xanthine.
- ☐ Warn female clients who are pregnant that theophylline crosses the placental barrier and may harm the fetus. Warn women who are breast-feeding that theophylline is excreted in breast milk.

- ☐ Recognize that dosage requirements for oral theophylline may be higher in cigarette smokers, since tobacco smoke induces liver enzymes and the metabolism of theophylline specifically.
- ☐ Advise clients to take oral xanthine preparations with food to reduce the incidence of gastrointestinal irritation or without food to hasten response.
- ☐ Do not mix theophylline in a syringe with any other drug. Theophylline is incompatible especially with alkali-labile drugs including epinephrine and other sympathomimetic amines and penicillin G.
- ☐ Monitor clients using glucocorticoid preparations by inhalation for indications of superinfection, such as sore throat. Advise clients to gargle after each administration to reduce this risk.

Chronic Obstructive Pulmonary Disease

Chronic obstructive pulmonary disease (COPD) encompasses two overlapping conditions: chronic bronchitis and emphysema. Although these two diseases occur as independent conditions in some clients, the majority of patients with chronic obstructive pulmonary disease exhibit indications of both. COPD is one of the leading causes of death in the United States.

Etiology

Chronic bronchitis occurs as a complex interaction of individual susceptibility and exposure to bronchial irritants. The irritant most often implicated is cigarette smoke. Individual susceptibility may be related to pulmonary disorders during childhood, an inherited partial inability to inhibit proteolytic enzymes from acting on lung tissue protein, or other factors. Pulmonary obstruction in chronic bronchitis involves mainly the small, near-terminal airways. Tobacco smoke is known also to induce hypersecretion of mucus by bronchial glands, which causes the familiar "smoker's cough," but it is probably not important in the pathogenesis of chronic bronchitis.

The etiologic basis of chronic emphysema is better understood. The principal cause of emphysema is destruction of lung protein by nonspecific proteolytic enzymes, or **proteases**, released by macrophages, granulocytes, and bacterial cells as a by-product of mechanisms that protect the lungs from infection. Elastin, the most abundant protein in pulmonary connective tissue is a potential substrate. The proteases can therefore also be referred to as elastases. In the normal lung, tissue proteins such as elastin are protected from the degratory activity of proteases by protease inhibitors of serum and tissue origin. The most important is a serum antiprotease called *α_1-antitrypsin.* It forms tight complexes with free proteases which are subsequently phagocytized and eliminated by the reticuloendothelial system.

Emphysema occurs when the lungs are inadequately protected from free proteases (Figure 52–3). One mechanism by which this occurs is a genetically determined deficiency in α_1-antitrypsin that is observed in about 9% of clients with COPD, especially cases of juvenile onset. Cigarette smoking also impairs antielastase activity of the lung tissue. Antielastase activity in lung tissue declines with aging, but the rate of decline is markedly accelerated in cigarette smokers. Tobacco smoke contains oxidizing agents that inactivate α_1-antitrypsin. In addition, hydrogen cyanide in cigarette smoke activates certain proteases that can destroy elastin. The result is a dangerous shift in the balance between elastase and antielastase activity, and the activated and uninhibited elastases gradually damage lung connective tissue. Infection is a third factor that can contribute to an imbalance. Purulent sputum, with its elevated count of bacteria and phagocytic cells, contains large concentrations of free proteases that can disturb the delicate balance.

COPD is characterized by a progressive exertional dyspnea and cough without definite cause. Other common symptoms are wheezing, recurrent infections, weight loss, weakness, or decreased libido. Sputum production is variable. Evaluation of pulmonary function consistently reveals obstructed airflow, but other physical signs are variable. Pulmonary hyperinflation, sitting in the "tripod position," pursed-lip breathing, depressed diaphragm, and a prolonged expiratory phase of respiration are typical. Clinical presentation and measurements of pulmonary function and blood gases may provide a basis for differentiating chronic bronchitis from emphysema (Table 52–5); but, as noted earlier, most cases of COPD are a composite of both conditions.

Treatment

Treatment of COPD is usually limited to relief of symptoms, reversal of airway obstruction, alleviation of complications, and minimization of exacerbating circumstances. Broad-spectrum antibiotics are used

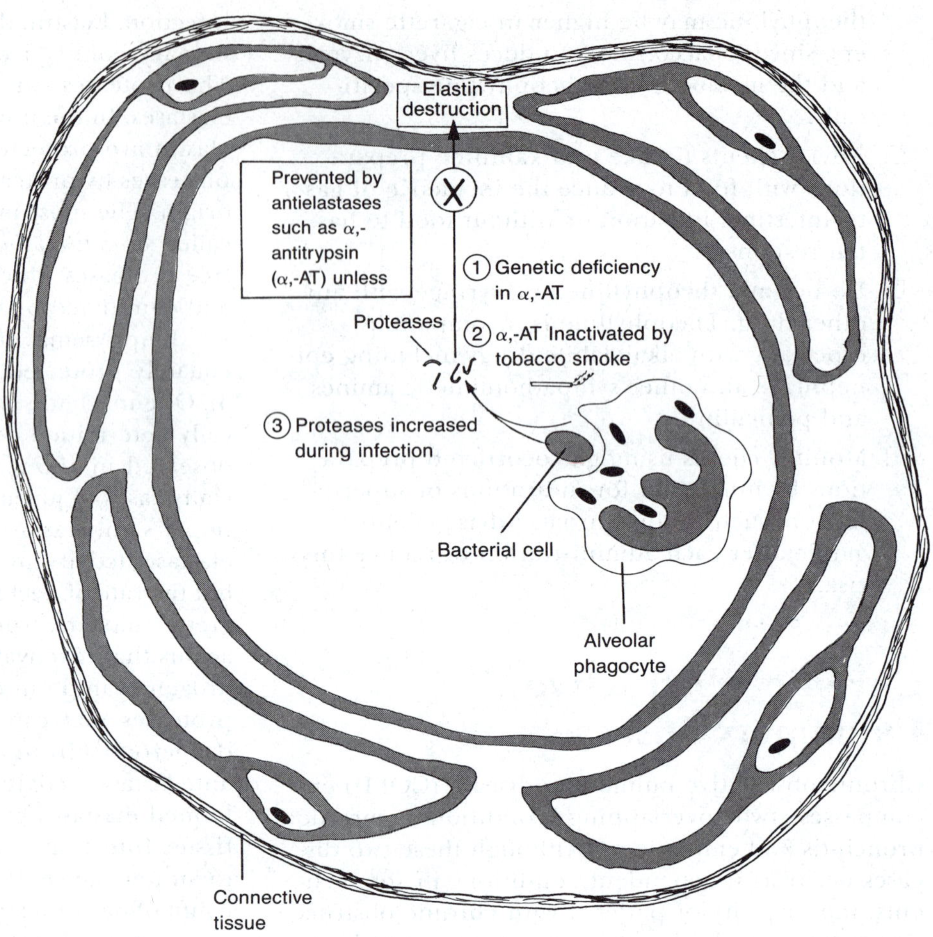

Figure 52–3
Mechanism of chronic bronchitis. Elastin in lung tissue is normally protected by antielastases from destruction by proteases released incidentally by phagocytic cells during engulfment of bacteria. This protection may not be adequate (1) if the person has a genetic deficiency in ability to produce the antielastase α_1-antitrypsin (α_1-AT); (2) if α_1-AT is inactivated by an oxidant in tobacco smoke; or (3) when protease release is elevated during pulmonary infection.

at the first sign of bronchial infection as a precaution against accumulation of purulent sputum. Inhalation of water or saline mist or acetylcysteine (see the next section) by nebulization helps to liquefy respiratory secretions, promoting upward movement of sputum and mucus. Maintaining adequate systemic hydration also helps prevent accumulation of hyperviscous secretions. Bronchodilators are used to alleviate airway obstruction to the extent possible. Improvement usually occurs at first, but the gradual progression of exertional dyspnea and airway obstruction is not abated. A regular exercise program geared to the level of respiratory difficulty of the patient will slow the rate of progression. When COPD has progressed to the extent of severe hypoxemia, hyperbaric oxygen is helpful in forestalling pulmonary hypertension and cor pulmonale. Diuretic therapy, dietary sodium restriction, and ultimately digitalis may be required for controlling heart failure. Although not yet available for clinical use, a number of synthetic protease inhibitors are under development that will ultimately revolutionize the treatment of emphysema.

Mucokinetic Agents

Mucokinetic agents are substances that produce a decrease in viscosity of thick mucus and sputum, thereby facilitating the removal of the secretions by the mucociliary escalator system. A variety of drugs have been used for this purpose over the years, including iodides, ammonium chloride, and tyloxapol (Alevaire), but none of these have demonstrated any advantage over humidification with normal or hypotonic saline. **Acetylcysteine** (Mucomyst), on the other hand, is an effective mucolytic agent. Acetylcysteine is a derivative of the endogenous amino acid cysteine. It possesses a free sulfhydryl group that helps to break disulfide linkages in mucoproteins. It also liquifies DNA found in sputum. The protein and DNA of respiratory secretions increase during infection and inflammation due to cell breakdown. These

Table 52–5
Differential Features of Asthma, Chronic Bronchitis, and Emphysema

Features	Asthma	Chronic bronchitis	Emphysema
Clinical presentation			
Age of diagnosis	Any	55–75	45–65
Cough	Yes	Yes	Only after dyspnea
Sputum	Scanty except in acute attack	Copious	Scanty
Recurrent infections	No	Frequently	Occasionally
Chest x-ray	Normal	Normal or fibrotic, enlarged heart, flattened diaphragm	Normal or prominent vessels
Pulmonary Function			
Compliance	Normal or decreased during an attack	Normal or decreased	Increased
Airway resistance	Elevated	Elevated	Near normal
Diffusing capacity	Normal	Variable	Low
Pulmonary artery pressure	Chronically normal	Elevated	Normal or slightly elevated
Blood gases			
Pa_{O_2}	Chronically normal; low during attack	Decreased	Normal
Pa_{CO_2}	Chronically normal; elevated in severe attack	Increased	Normal

constituents of phlegm are mainly responsible for its viscosity. Acetylcysteine loosens and liquifies respiratory secretions within a few minutes after inhalation of 1–10 ml of a nebulized 10% or 20% solution. The maximum effect occurs in 5–10 minutes. The treatment can be repeated 3 or 4 times daily. *Acetylcysteine should not be mixed with other drugs. Acetylcysteine will react with rubber and certain metals, so care should be taken to select a nebulizer constructed of plastic or nonreactive metals such as stainless steel or aluminum.*

Side effects are uncommon. Stomatitis, nausea, vomiting, and rhinorrhea have been reported. Nausea is in part related to the unpleasant odor produced by hydrogen sulfide released by the action of the drug. *Clients should be encouraged to continue use since this effect subsides with successful treatment.* Bronchospasm may occur if acetylcysteine is used in asthmatics. Acetylcysteine is sometimes used with isoproterenol in such patients. Acetylcysteine may occasionally increase the volume of liquified phlegm to the extent that suction is required to aid removal.

Therapeutic Gases

Oxygen and Hypoxia

Oxygen comprises approximately 20.9% of air at sea level. It is essential to aerobic metabolism and for maintaining life in most organisms. *Hypoxia* is a deficiency of oxygen at the tissue level, regardless of mechanism. *Hypoxemia* is a condition of reduced concentration of oxygen in the blood. Often the two occur in concert, but hypoxia can occur without hypoxemia and vice versa. Hypoxemia is important only in so far as it contributes to hypoxia. There are six types of hypoxia; the first three of which are associated with hypoxemia: (1) reduced oxygen content in inspired air that occurs at high altitudes and in poorly ventilated, enclosed spaces, (2) inadequate delivery of inspired air to the alveoli, which is seen in asthma, chronic bronchitis, emphysema, myasthenia gravis, sleep apneas, and overdoses of CNS depressants or neuromuscular blockers, (3) inadequate exchange of gases between the lung and blood in conditions where there is impairment of alveolar function, (4) inadequate transport capacity for oxygen in the blood due to inadequate hemoglobin (anemic hypoxia), (5) inadequate blood flow to a given tissue (ischemic hypoxia); or (6) abnormal requirement for or deficient utilization of oxygen by a tissue (histotoxic hypoxia) such as occurs in cyanide poisoning.

The tissues most vulnerable to the effects of hypoxia are the brain, heart, and kidney. The cerebral cortex of the brain is perhaps the most susceptible, exhibiting histologic changes in as little as 3–4 minutes of total circulatory occlusion. Cardiac output and heart rate initially increase as a compensatory response in acute hypoxia, but when hypoxia is prolonged, cardiac failure ultimately occurs. Oxygen is administered whenever hypoxia cannot be alleviated by direct treatment of causes.

Pharmacokinetics When administered by inhalation, oxygen normally diffuses readily across the walls of the alveoli into the blood. In the blood, oxygen is transported in two forms: in association with hemoglobin of red blood cells and in solution in the plasma. Normally most of the blood oxygen is attached to hemoglobin, but when oxygen is administered in high concentration or in a hyperbaric chamber, the amount of oxygen in simple solution may be enough to supply tissue requirements. If this occurs, oxygen attached to hemoglobin does not dissociate when it reaches the systemic capillaries. The result is that hemoglobin is unavailable for transport of carbon dioxide. Normally, 25% of the carbon dioxide in venous blood is carried in attachment to hemoglobin. Thus, excessive oxygenation of blood may reduce the ability of the body to eliminate carbon dioxide. The consequence may be carbon dioxide narcosis.

Nitrogen levels in the body may also be altered when oxygen is administered in concentrations above 21%. Any increase in oxygen above 21% is at the expense of nitrogen, which ordinarily constitutes 79% of inspired air. Bodily nitrogen is in equilibrium with atmospheric nitrogen. Since nitrogen is neither utilized nor generated in cellular metabolic activities, there is usually no net exchange. Inhalation of air containing less than 79% nitrogen, however, will lead to nitrogen elimination by the lungs. This effect of high concentrations of oxygen on nitrogen can be put to good effect in alleviating abdominal distention or headache resulting from pneumoencephalography, conditions usually caused by excessive retention of nitrogen. On the other hand, nitrogen depletion can result in collapse of body spaces ordinarily partly filled with nitrogen, such as the alveoli, the Eustachian tubes, the paranasal sinuses, and the gut, with painful or debilitating consequences.

Clinical Indications When hypoxia is due to airway obstruction, first thought is given to alleviating the obstruction, by administration of theophylline, beta-sympathomimetics, or glucocorticoids, for example. If bronchoconstriction is unresponsive to bronchodilators, oxygen is administered. Dyspnea is an indication for oxygen only if it is related to hypoxia. Oxygen-helium mixtures are sometimes used in obstructive dyspneas because the low density of helium facilitates air flow. Oxygen is most frequently used for conditions in which exchange of gases across the alveolar membranes is impaired (for example, in pulmonary fibrosis, pulmonary edema, excessive shunting of deoxygenated pulmonary arterial blood to the systemic circulation, and pneumonia). Oxygen inhalation can be helpful in maintaining tissue oxygenation in anemia or congestive heart failure. For clients who have had a myocardial infarction or cerebrovascular accidents, early administration of oxygen can minimize the ultimate extent of necrosis by alleviating hypoxia in cells at the margin of ischemia. Oxygen is employed in carbon monoxide poisoning to hasten the conversion of carboxyhemoglobin to oxyhemoglobin. Even in histotoxic hypoxia caused by cyanide, oxygen administration has some marginal benefit. During anesthesia, oxygen is used as a diluent for volatile liquid and gaseous anesthetics and enhances the safety of general anesthesia. Oxygen has been used successfully to alleviate vascular headaches due to hypoxia, alcohol "hangover," or postictal states.

Hyperbaric oxygen (oxygen administered at more than one atmospheric pressure) is often employed for oxygen therapy of carbon monoxide poisoning or localized circulatory disturbances such as stroke or peripheral vascular spasms. It has also been used successfully in treatment of people with infections caused by anaerobic bacilli such as *Clostridium perfringens,* the pathogen responsible for gas gangrene.

Adverse Effects Oxygen in low concentrations can be given safely for long periods of time, but in high concentrations oxygen is potentially toxic.

Administration of oxygen can cause respiratory arrest by suppressing the hypoxic drive of respiration, which can occur when the other drives, especially the hypercapnic drive, are compromised by disease or drugs. If an elevated concentration of oxygen is administered to a person with chronic hypercapnia or labored respiration from narcotic overdose, **apnea** may result from inhibition of the hypoxic drive by oxygen.

Oxygen concentrations above 80% for more than 12 hours can have an **irritant effect** on the respiratory tract. Oxygen also suppresses the mucociliary escalator system. The result of these effects can be cough, nasal congestion, and sore throat of progressive severity.

Oxygen administration to premature infants must be carried out within specific guidelines in order to avoid **retrolental fibroplasia.** Oxygen should be administered only to infants who clearly require it and only for as long as necessary. A concentration of between 35% and 40% is usually appropriate.

Severe **CNS toxicity** can occur when hyperbaric oxygen of high concentration is administered. The typical symptoms are paresthesias, vertigo, nausea, mood changes, and ultimately coma or convulsions.

Preparations and Administration Oxygen is provided in pressurized steel cylinders fitted with valves for easy administration. Gas tanks are color coded for quick identification and avoidance of errors (oxygen tanks in the United States are colored green). Oxygen can be administered by a variety of techniques.

Nasal cannulas and catheters are a simple means of delivering oxygen in concentrations up to 50%. The soft rubber or plastic tube is lubricated with a water-soluble jelly and inserted into a nostril through the external nares and nasopharynx to the epiglottis. The appropriate distance can be easily gauged by measuring the distance from the tip of the nose to the tragus of the ear, less 1 cm. The tip must not enter the esophagus because it will cause the client to swallow air, leading to gastric distention and discomfort. The catheter is attached to the forehead or nose with tape. Humidified oxygen is passed through the tube, typically at a flow rate of 3–4 L of oxygen per minute. Humidification prevents drying of the respiratory mucosa. Nasal tubes tend to become obstructed with respiratory secretion and must therefore be removed and cleaned several times daily. Advantages of nasal tubes include freedom of movement for the patient and easy access for medical personnel.

When concentrations higher than 50% are required, an **oxygen mask** is effective. A well-fitted mask can deliver 100% oxygen if required and is well tolerated by the client. Masks that are not disposable must be carefully sterilized to prevent transmission of infections.

Oxygen tents, face tents, and hoods allow regulation of temperature and humidity, and patient comfort. On the other hand, they restrict access for medical personnel, allow loss of oxygen, and may cause feelings of claustrophobia. A tent can deliver oxygen in concentrations only up to 50%; a face tent can provide concentrations up to 70%, while hoods can deliver 90–100% oxygen. Care must be taken to minimize loss of oxygen by carefully securing the tent sides and covering the mattress with a plastic or rubber sheet. These devices are less often used than nasal tubes or oxygen masks, being reserved for use in pediatric care. Hyperbaric oxygen is administered in special pressure chambers.

Carbon Dioxide

Carbon dioxide has profound importance in regulating both the pH of body fluids and respiration, but it has considerably less value than oxygen as a therapeutic gas. Normally, the hundreds of milliliters of carbon dioxide produced each minute at rest are transported to the lungs and discharged into the atmosphere. The usual partial pressure of carbon dioxide in inspired air is very low, less than 1 mm of Hg. When carbon dioxide is added to inspired air, the partial pressure of carbon dioxide in the blood increases until a new equilibrium is established where the gradient at the alveoli permits outward diffusion and elimination at a rate equal to the rate of production. The new equilibrium is characterized by elevated blood levels of carbon dioxide and a lower than normal pH (respiratory acidosis).

Pharmacological Effects Carbon dioxide has four principal pharmacological actions. The effect that generally occurs at lowest concentrations of carbon dioxide is stimulation of respiration. Specialized chemoreceptors located in both the medulla and peripheral arteries are specifically attuned to monitoring carbon dioxide levels. Inhalation of even small concentrations of carbon dioxide activates these receptors in seconds. The signals generated by these receptors quickly reach the medullary respiratory center, stimulating an increase in both rate and depth of respiration.

Carbon dioxide can also exert diffuse, nonspecific influence on neural functioning in the brain. Low doses depress the cerebral cortex but have little effect on subcortical centers. Inhalation of concentrations of approximately 25–30% cause substantial activation and possible convulsions. Concentrations above 50% produce widespread depression of both cortical and subcortical areas.

The remaining two effects of carbon dioxide are opposing direct and indirect influences on cardiovascular function. The direct effect is a depression of smooth muscle of the myocardium and peripheral blood vessels. The indirect effect is due to widespread activation of the sympathetic nervous system. At the level of the blood vessels, the direct relaxant effect predominates to a small degree so that there is a slight reduction in peripheral resistance overall. At the level of the heart, the indirect, sympathetically mediated effect predominates, resulting in increased heart rate and cardiac output. The overall effect on blood pressure is an elevation of systolic and diastolic pressures and pulse pressure.

Clinical Indications There are few unequivocal indications for administration of carbon dioxide. It can be useful for alleviating respiratory alkalosis, such as that caused by aspirin-induced hyperventilation. Carbon dioxide also can be used to stimulate respiration, but if continued more than a few minutes, significant respiratory alkalosis will occur. However, when used in 5–7% concentrations with general anesthetics, it stimulates respiration, speeds induction, decreases sensations of asphyxiation, and reduces struggling. Carbon dioxide can be used in an analogous manner during recovery from anesthesia to increase the rate of elimination of anesthetic gases and to suppress postoperative hiccups or atelectasis (complete or partial collapse of the lungs). Other methods provide better results. Carbon dioxide is sometimes employed in conjunction with oxygen in carbon monoxide poisoning to accelerate dissociation of carboxyhemoglobin. A drawback is that carbon dioxide inhalation superimposes respiratory acidosis on the metabolic acidosis typically present in carbon monoxide poisonings.

Adverse Effects At concentrations of 5–7%, the principal side effects of carbon dioxide inhalation are increased respiration, an acidic taste, tachycardia, increased blood pressure, and slight respiratory acidosis. Concentrations of about 10% cause early signs of CNS intoxication and symptomatic activation such as paresthesias, restlessness, dizziness, headache, and sweating. Still higher concentrations may result in carbon dioxide narcosis. Abrupt withdrawal of concentrations above 5% may result in headache or dizziness, but this can be avoided by a more gradual termination of inhalation therapy.

Preparations and Administration Carbon dioxide is provided in pressurized cylinders, often in combination with oxygen. It is usually administered in 5–10% concentrations by means of a close-fitting mask for no more than 3 minutes at a time and is discontinued as soon as the desired effect on respiration is achieved. A less sophisticated technique for administering carbon dioxide is to have clients rebreathe their own exhaled air by breathing into a paper bag. This technique should not be used for more than a few minutes because it depletes the oxygen in the inspired air.

Respiratory Stimulants and Depressants

Respiration is controlled by three drives: the neurogenic, hypoxic, and hypercapnic drives. The neurogenic drive arises in the respiratory center of the medulla oblongata, which includes a region controlling inspiration and a region controlling expiration. The two regions are mutually inhibitory and alternate in their firing patterns, thereby generating the rhythmicity of respiration. The hypoxic drive is related to arterial oxygen concentration, and the hypercapnic drive to carbon dioxide concentration and pH of the blood. The hypercapnic drive is stronger than the hypoxic drive.

Analeptics were once widely used to combat respiratory depression from sedative-hypnotic overdose, but are seldom employed in modern medicine. Treatment of sedative-hypnotic overdose is now based on supportive therapy without the use of analeptics, called the **Scandinavian method.** One drug remains available for the rare circumstances under which an analeptic might be employed: doxapram.

Ammonia, a reflex respiratory stimulant, is available in the form of an inhalant ("smelling salts") to stimulate respiration reflexly in treating or preventing loss of consciousness from fainting or mild concussion. Inhalation of ammonia vapors has an irritant effect on the mucosal membranes of the airways stimulating sensory receptors in the pharynx and esophagus. Respiratory rate and depth and blood pressure are all increased. Aromatic ammonia is provided as an inhalant and in alcohol solution (aromatic ammonia spirits), which is taken orally, 2 ml diluted in ample water.

Most CNS drugs cause respiratory depression if taken in a high enough dose. Two classes of psychotropic drugs, the narcotics and the sedative-hypnotics, are notoriously effective in suppressing respiration. These two classes of drugs generally rank first and second each year as causes of fatal drug overdoses. The cause of death is almost always respiratory arrest. All told, sedative-hypnotics and narcotics account for more than one-half of drug overdoses in most years. Occasionally, there is therapeutic benefit derived from the ability of sedatives to suppress respiration, when they are employed to correct respiratory alkalosis due to drug-induced or psychogenic hyperventilation.

Upper Respiratory Infections and Cold Remedies

Pulmonary Defense Mechanisms

The respiratory system, along with the skin and alimentary tract, is one of the major interfaces between the internal physiologic milieu and the external environment. Each breath of inspired air brings with it an abundance of particulate matter. Even after the filtering of the air by the nares and the trapping of large particles on the mucosal surfaces of the upper respiratory tract, inanimate particles and microorganisms remain in the air that reaches the bronchioles and lungs. The respiratory system must therefore continuously remove inspired debris and defend itself and the body at large from pathogenic influences. Two kinds of specialized defense mechanisms operate in the airways: the mucociliary escalator system and the airway reflex mechanisms.

The **mucociliary escalator system** consists of a protective blanket of mucous secretions along the tracheobronchial tree that is kept in constant upwardly directed motion by the cilea of the surface epithelial cells (Figure 52–4). The mucous blanket is comprised of two layers: the gel layer, produced by goblet cells, and the sol layer, produced by bronchial glands. Inspired particles and microbes adhere to the gel layer and are transported out of the respiratory tract. During times of respiratory infection, the goblet cells increase in number and secretory activity, which causes the respiratory mucus to become overly viscous and resistant to movement. The result is respiratory congestion. Cileated epithelial cells found over most of the airway surface slowly move the mucus layer upward to the trachea, a process called **mucokinesis.** The sol layer is a watery secretion and reaches the surface of the lumen through ducts. Drugs that stimulate secretory activity of the bronchial glands reduce viscosity of the respiratory mucus.

The **airway reflexes** provide a second defense system for the respiratory tract. Included in this category are the sneeze and cough reflexes and reflex bronchoconstriction. The **sneeze** reflex provides a defense against irritants. The **cough** reflex acts as an aid to the mucociliary escalator system in promoting clearance of the trachea and bronchi of foreign matter. **Reflex bronchoconstriction,** a reflexive narrowing of the airways triggered by dust, pollens, fumes, or gases, also helps to protect the alveoli from damage.

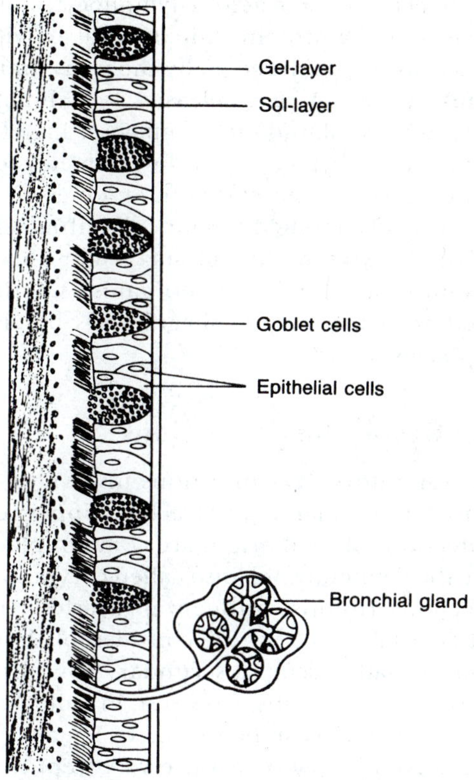

Figure 52–4
Structures of the mucociliary escalator system.

The lungs provide additional defense mechanisms. **Alveolar macrophages** efficiently destroy lung bacteria, although some more effectively than others, especially when their activity is impaired by hypoxia, acidosis, alcohol consumption, or smoking of tobacco. Viral infections not only produce their own set of primary symptoms but also reduce the ability of the alveolar macrophages to combat bacterial growth. Thus, bacterial infections are sometimes secondary, occurring about 6–10 days after an acute viral infection.

Immunologic defense of the lungs is conducted by both T lymphocytes and B lymphocytes. When a **T lymphocyte** recognizes a microbial antigen for which it is sensitized, it releases lymphokines that attract macrophages to the site of infection and stimulate their activity. Activated T-lymphocytes also release interferon, a protein with antiviral activity that protects cells not yet infected by the virus. Immunoglobulins of the IgA class released by pulmonary **B lymphocytes** are abundant on mucosal membranes that line the respiratory tract. IgA attaches to antigens in the airways, increasing their adhesion to the sol-gel layer. IgG and IgM immunoglobulins released by B lymphocytes of the plasma enter the lungs to opsonize antigenic microorganisms, stimulating their recognition and phagocytosis by alveolar macrophages.

Upper Respiratory Infections

Upper respiratory tract infections involve the nasopharynx, pharynx, larynx, or trachea. Upper respiratory infections of viral origin are commonplace and include the common cold (also called coryza, catarrh, or infectious rhinitis), influenza, measles, and rubella. Bacterial infections are considerably less common and usually occur as secondary complications of severe viral infections. However, in children, sore throat (pharyngitis) can be caused by bacteria of the beta-hemolytic *Streptococcus* variety ("Strept throat"). Since untreated **bacterial pharyngitis** can lead to serious complications, including rheumatic fever and glomerulonephritis, it is a wise precaution to have any child with a pronounced sore throat evaluated by a physician. *The nurse should recognize the characteristics that distinguish bacterial pharyngitis, influenza, and the common cold (Table 52–6).*

Bacterial pharyngitis is characterized by rapid onset, marked soreness in the throat, and is frequently accompanied by such symptoms as fever, headache, swollen glands, malaise, nausea, vomiting, or tachycardia. Presence of streptococci can be established by overnight culture. Although antibiotics have little effect on the primary symptoms associated with bacterial pharyngitis, they do prevent such local complications as middle ear infections (otitis media), sinusitis, and mastoiditis, and the serious systemic complications such as rheumatic fever and glomerulonephritis.

Somatic concomitants such as fever, swollen glands, malaise, and joint or muscle aches occur to only a modest extent with common colds but may be pronounced in **influenza.** Influenza occurs in epidemics, often in two waves, striking socially active family members in the first wave and institutionalized or homebound individuals in the second wave. Influenza is caused by myxoviruses that are classified as types A, B, and C. Each of these types exists in multiple strains. After contact with a given viral strain, an individual develops resistance to that specific strain for a number of years. A given strain can recycle after several years of absence. Vaccination produces a similar relative immunity for 1–2 years but is specific for a given strain. Vaccination is indicated mainly for aged and debilitated individuals who are at special risk of complications. Pregnant women due to deliver during the winter months should also receive vaccination with the prevalent strain if an epidemic is in progress. Amantadine is an effective antiviral agent against influenzas of the A type.

The **common cold** is the least severe of the upper respiratory infections. In healthy individuals, it is self-limited. After an incubation period of 1–4 days, symptoms progress rapidly for a few days, then subside and resolve in 5–10 days, although some symptoms may remain well into the second week. Significant fever is seldom seen in adults with common colds but a fever as high as 101–102°F is common in children. In spite of its relative mildness, the common cold is probably the most costly disease in the United States, accounting for more lost time from school and work than any other condition. There is a clear seasonal pattern to the occurrence of colds: one peak in September when school opens, one in midwinter, and one in spring. The winter peak is caused by paramyxo- and myxoviruses, whereas colds during other seasons are usually caused by picornavirus infections. Nearly 50% of the population will have one or more colds each winter, whereas only about 20% have a cold during the summer. Incidence of colds declines with age. Children typically experience 6–12 colds per year, young adults 3–6, and elderly people 2–3.

Cold-producing viruses spread directly from person to person and cannot be transmitted via food, water, or animals. Viral shedding (exhalation of exfoliated infected mucosal cells) often begins before onset of cold symptoms; thus transmission of the virus can occur before an infected person is aware of the infection. Whether contact with a given virus results in infection or not depends on both the virulence of the particular pathogen and individual susceptibility. Predisposing factors include fatigue, emotional distress, a history of nasopharyngeal allergies, irritation of the airways by chemicals, vocal straining, cold exposure, or midcycle hormonal patterns in women.

All levels of the upper respiratory tract are potential sites for common cold infections. Involvement of the nasopharynx results in **rhinitis** (inflammation of the nasal cavities) with an initial watery nasal discharge (rhinorrhea) that later becomes a tenacious, viscous, mucoid secretion consisting of

Table 52–6
Comparisons of the Major Kinds of Pharyngitis (Sore Throat)

	Bacterial	Viral upper respiratory tract infections	
Characteristic	**Pharyngitis**	**Coryza**	**Influenza**
Common language synonyms	Strep throat	Common cold	Flu, grippe
Occurrence	Limited epidemics; more common in children	Seasonal fluctuation but always common; more common in children	Epidemic in winter
Onset	Sudden	Less rapid	Sudden
Extent of nonrespiratory symptoms (e.g., fever, malaise, aches, vomiting)	Extensive	Mild	Extensive
Cough	Not usually	Mild to severe, nonproductive	Severe, productive
Lymph nodes	Enlarged and tender	Slight enlargement, not tender	Slight enlargement, not tender
Complications	Otitis media Sinusitis Rheumatic fever Glomerulonephritis	Usually none	Secondary bacterial infections (e.g., pneumonia) Encephalitis Myocarditis Myoglobinuria Death
Leukocyte count	Elevated	Normal	Normal if uncomplicated
Drug treatments	Antibiotics Symptom relief with analgesics, antitussives, decongestants, etc.	Self-limited Symptom relief with analgesics, antitussives, decongestants, etc.	Self-limited Symptom relief with analgesics, antitussives, decongestants, etc.

sloughed epithelial cells and leukocytes. Infectious rhinitis can be distinguished from allergic rhinitis only by careful consideration of differential features (Table 52–7). If viral penetration extends to the pharynx, the result is **pharyngitis,** an inflammatory condition characterized by a sore and raspy dry throat. The common cold is the most common cause of pharyngitis, but tobacco smoking, alcohol consumption, inhalation of gaseous irritants, streptococcal infection, influenza, scarlet fever, measles, smallpox, and tonsillitis are other possible causes. Involvement of the larynx results in **laryngitis.** The characteristic symptom of laryngitis is hoarseness or loss of vocalization. Laryngitis can also be caused by straining the voice.

Certain strains of viruses cause considerably more damage to the airway epithelium than others. If swelling is great and exudation prolific, obstruction may occur in one or more passages. Obstruction is especially likely in children because the passages are smaller and the child is unlikely to make a conscious effort to clear clogged passages. These circumstances provide ideal conditions for secondary bacterial infections. The most frequent secondary bacterial infections are sinusitis, otitis media, bronchitis, bacterial pneumonia, and tonsillitis. Secondary bacterial infections are indicated by a general worsening of symptoms such as cough and congestion, or addition of symptoms such as earache, headache, or fever.

There is as of yet no reliable chemical intervention that reduces the frequency of colds or

Table 52–7
Comparisons of Allergic and Infectious Rhinitis

Characteristic	Allergic	Infectious
Etiology	IgE-mediated allergic reaction	Virus
Occurrence	Often worst in spring, fall	Often worst in winter
Personal or familial history of allergy	Common	Occasional
Nonrespiratory symptoms	Rare	Occasional
Pruritus/sneezing	Common	Rare
Conjunctivitis	Yes	No
Discharge	Watery	Mucopurulent

shortens recovery time. The only reliable prophylaxis is avoiding contact with infected individuals. Minimization of the predisposing factors cited above may also be modestly helpful. There is no evidence that vitamin C, multivitamins, or antibiotics have any prophylactic value. When a cold is accompanied by fever, bedrest is advisable, especially for preadolescent children with all but the mildest colds. Use of a vaporizer may help to relieve congestion of airways. The cold remedies that are widely used consist of one or more drugs from four pharmacological categories: (1) nasal decongestants, (2) expectorants, (3) cough suppressants, and (4) antihistamines.

Nasal Decongestants

The factors that contribute to nasal congestion or stuffiness are swelling of the nasal mucosa and hyperactivity of nasal secretory glands. Both of these parameters are subject to influences of autonomic nervous system impulses. Sympathetic activity suppresses secretory activity of mucous glands and constricts mucosal blood vessels resulting in shrinkage of mucous membranes. Parasympathetic activity, on the other hand, increases secretory activity and dilates nasal blood vessels, contributing to engorgement and swelling of the mucosal lining. Thus a widening of the nasal passages can be achieved by administration of either a sympathomimetic or an anticholinergic drug, and both classes of drugs have been used as nasal decongestants. However, relatively few cold preparations now contain an anticholinergic. Sympathomimetics offer a good deal more selectivity because of the breakdown of sympathetic receptors into α_1, α_2, β_1, and β_2 classes.

Mechanisms and Effects Nasal decongestion is mediated through alpha-receptors. The optimum nasal decongestant is thus a sympathomimetic that is selective for alpha-receptors. Sympathetic agonists that act on alpha-receptors and also activate beta-receptors (such as ephedrine) can be effective, but they produce a wider range of side effects.

Preparations and Administration Nasal decongestants are available as sprays, drops, inhalants, and gels for topical installation; and tablets, capsules, and timed release capsules for systemic use. Topical application provides a more prompt and dramatic nasal decongestion but is also associated with more frequent adverse effects. Decongestants can cause mucosal irritation and ischemia due to vasoconstriction. If used for more than 3 or 4 days, topical decongestants cause a rebound congestion (rhinitis medicamentosa) that may promote continued use of the decongestant, which only aggravates the problem. *Nurses need to assure that clients are so informed.* Of the topical application forms, sprays offer the most reliable delivery to the deep recesses of the nasal cavities. *Nasal sprays should be administered with the head upright, by squeezing the flexible plastic container the prescribed number of times, with the tip inserted in one nostril. This procedure is then repeated in the other nostril. If stuffiness is extreme, the nose should be blown after a few minutes and the application repeated.*

Nasal drops do not provide for uniform distribution and usually deliver part of the dose into the pharynx. However, for children under 6, drops are usually the most convenient means of administration. *When applying drops, the head should be tilted back and the drops placed in each nostril without touching the dropper to the nasal mucosa. After application, the patient should recline, breathing through the mouth, for 5 minutes to allow the drug to seep into the nasal passages.*

Nasal inhalants utilize volatile sympathomimetics along with aromatics such as thymol, menthol, camphor, and eucalyptol. Irritation of mucosal membranes is greater, delivery is less reliable, and there can be loss of potency due to evaporation if the cap is poorly placed. The gel preparation is seldom employed and unreliable.

Oral preparations have a longer duration of action without risk of rebound congestion but less dramatic effectiveness. In addition, oral nasal decongestants produce systemic side effects that are mild and only of concern in vulnerable populations. Alpha-sympathomimetics taken orally can elevate blood pressure, but the magnitude of the effect is trivial except in hypertensive individuals. Cardiac stimulation occurs to a small extent, but is important only in clients predisposed to dysrhythmias. Ephedrine, which is not selective for alpha-receptors, causes hyperglycemia and should not be used by persons who have diabetes. Oral nasal decongestants should not be used in conjunction with MAO inhibitors or guanethidine (Ismelin).

The individual sympathomimetics also differ in duration of action (and hence frequency of administration), doses, appropriateness for use in young children, and dosage forms (Table 52–8). For ephedrine, only the 0.5% concentration is recommended by the Food and Drug Administration, and that only for adults and children over 6. Ephedrine is not FDA approved for oral use as a nasal decongestant, although it is approved by this route for prophylaxis of bronchial asthma. It is nevertheless found in some combination cold remedies. *Ephedrine is light-sensitive and should be stored in a dark container.* It is not selective for alpha-receptors.

Table 52–8
Nasal Decongestants

	Dosage[a] and (minimum interdose interval)		
Drug	**Adults**	**Children 6-12**	**Children 2-6**
Topical			
L-Desoxyephedrine	2 inhalations of 50 mg inhaler (2 hours)	1 inhalation of 50 mg inhaler (2 hours)	NR
Ephedrine	2-3 drops or sprays of 0.5% (4 hours)	1-2 drops or sprays of 0.5% (4 hours)	NR
Naphazoline	1-2 drops or sprays of 0.05% (6 hours)	1-2 drops or sprays of 0.25% (6 hours)	NR
Oxymetazoline	2-3 drops or sprays of 0.05% (8-10 hours)	2-3 drops or sprays of 0.05% (8-10 hours)	2-3 drops of 0.025% (8-10 hours)
Phenylephrine	2-3 drops or sprays of 0.5% (4 hours)	2-3 drops or sprays of 0.25% (4 hours)	2-3 drops of 0.125% (4 hours)
Propylhexedrine	2 inhalations of 250 mg inhaler (2 hours)	2 inhalations of 250 mg inhaler (2 hours)	NR
Tetrahydrozoline	2-4 drops or sprays of 0.1% (3 hours)	2-4 drops or sprays of 0.1% (3 hours)	2-3 drops of 0.05% (3 hours)
Xylometazoline	2-3 drops or sprays of 0.1% (8-10 hours)	2-3 drops or sprays of 0.05% (8-10 hours)	2-3 drops of 0.05% (8-10 hours)
Oral			
Ephedrine	12.5-25 mg (4 hours)	3 mg/kg/day (4 hours)	3 mg/kg/day (4 hours)
Phenylpropanolamine	25 mg (4 hours)	12.5 mg (4 hours)	6.25 (4 hours)
Phenylephrine	10 mg (4 hours)	5 mg (4 hours)	2.5 mg (4 hours)
Pseudoephrine	60 mg (6 hours)	30 mg (6 hours)	15 mg (6 hours)

Key: NR = Not recommended.
[a]Dosage is for each nostril for topical decongestants.

Phenylephrine has very good selectivity for alpha-receptors. Like all nasal decongestants, it can cause mucosal irritation when applied topically but it is one of the most effective drugs in this family. Pseudoephedrine is not selective for alpha-receptors and is only used orally. Phenylpropanolamine has good selectivity for alpha-receptors and minimal CNS stimulant properties. Peak action occurs about 3 hours after ingestion.

Six other selective alpha-sympathomimetics are available for topical application only. If systemic absorption occurs, naphazoline and tetrahydrozoline act as CNS depressants, due to their ability to act on α_2-receptors in the brain. They are not recommended for children under 6 years of age. Oxymetazoline and xylometazoline are long-acting. They are typically taken just twice a day, in the morning and evening. Both oxymetazoline and xylometazoline are active at α-$_2$-receptors as well as α_1-receptors, producing CNS depression rather than excitation. Propylhexedrine and levodesoxyephedrine are used in nasal inhalers because of their aromatic properties and are not marketed in other forms.

Ephedrine (Vatronol, Ephedsol, Nasdro No. 3, and generic)
Drops

Levodesoxyephedrine (Vicks Inhaler)
Nasal inhaler

Naphazoline (Privine)
Drops or spray

Oxymetazoline (Afrin, Duration, St. Joseph Decongestant for Children)
Spray, drops, or mentholated vapor spray

Phenylephrine (Neo-Synephrine, Alconefrin, Rhinall, Sinex)
Drops, sprays, jelly; combinations with antihistamines (pyrilamine or pheniramine) in sprays or drops (e.g., Dristan Nasal Mist); combination oral cold remedies (countless)

Phenylpropanolamine (Propadrine and generic)
Tablets, capsules, timed release capsules, elixir; combination cold remedies (countless)

Propylhexedrine (Benzedrex)
Nasal inhaler

Pseudoephedrine (Sudafed, Novafed, Cenafed, and D-Feda)
Tablets, timed release capsules, oral liquid

Tetrahydrozoline (Tyzine)
Drops or spray

Xylometazoline (Otrivin, Neo-Synephrine II Long Acting, others)
Drops or spray

Expectorants

Expectorants are drugs claimed to reduce the viscosity of bronchial secretions by stimulating production of the more liquid constituents by the bronchial glands. Some expectorants (guaifenesin, sodium iodide, potassium iodide, hydrogen iodide, calcium iodide, iodinated glycerol, ammonium chloride, ammonium carbonate, and ipecac syrup) are said to do this reflexively by causing gastric irritation. Terpin, by contrast, is said to act directly on the secretory glands of the lower respiratory tract. Despite widespread use, there is no evidence that any of these agents decrease the viscosity of sputum. The FDA advisory review panel on nonprescription respiratory system preparations did not classify any expectorant as "generally recognized as safe and effective." Adverse effects of **guaifenesin** are limited to vomiting, nausea, gastric irritation, drowsiness, and hypersensitivity reactions. Side effects with **iodide preparations** include metallic taste, skin eruptions, nausea, vomiting, gastrointestinal irritation, swelling of salivary glands, and fever. **Ammonium chloride** can cause metabolic acidosis and alter excretion of drugs due to acidification of the urine but not at the doses recommended when it is used as an expectorant (300 mg every 2–4 hours in adults). **Terpin** is marketed in combination with alcohol and codeine. Adverse effects of the combination are related to alcohol and codeine.

Preparations and Administrations

Guaifenesin
Recommended Doses: For adults, 200–400 mg PO every 4 hours

Antitussives

The cough reflex helps remove phlegm by forcefully expelling secretions from the larger airways. The cough reflex is initiated by the action of irritants on sensory nerves in the lungs and respiratory tract. Cough can be either productive or nonproductive. **Productive cough** provides the valuable function of removing phlegm from the lungs and should usually not be treated with suppressant medications. A cough can be nonproductive either because the phlegm is too viscous to be expelled (**nonproductive congested cough**), or because no significant amount of phlegm is present or remains present in the lungs (**nonproductive dry cough**). In the former case, one might wish, in theory, to treat the condition with a drug capable of decreasing the viscosity of phlegm — an expectorant. However, there are no unequivocally effective expectorants at this time. When a cough is nonproductive, dry, and without congestion, an opportunity exists for effective, safe, and satisfying drug intervention. This kind of cough tends to be self-perpetuating because the rapid flow of air that occurs during the cough reflex can itself be irritating to the mucosal wall of the airways. Suppression of the cough provides relief and may facilitate needed rest and sleep. *Nurses should teach clients when it is and is not advisable to suppress a cough with a medication.*

The effective antitussive drugs now in use act directly on the cough center of the medulla to suppress the cough reflex. The best of the agents available are remarkably effective in alleviating cough and have minimal adverse effects. Historically, the narcotic analgesics, and codeine in particular, have been the agents of choice for cough suppression. In recent decades equally effective but safer nonnarcotic drugs have emerged. Several of the nonnarcotic agents are derivatives (or congeners) of narcotics that share only the action on the cough center. Other nonnarcotic antitussives are totally unrelated to the narcotics and belong to diverse chemical groups.

Narcotic Antitussives

Although nearly all of the natural opiates and synthetic narcotics can suppress cough, codeine is preferred because it has a better relative potency against cough in relation to other narcotic actions. For example, on a weight basis, codeine is one-half as potent as morphine in suppressing cough but, only about one-tenth as potent in eliciting other narcotic responses. Under usual conditions of use and provided that recommended doses are not exceeded, codeine can be employed for cough suppression with little risk of dependence. Codeine is a controlled substance, however, because of the risk of misuse. Individuals with a history of narcotic dependency should be prescribed other cough remedies.

Adverse Effects and Contraindications Antitussive doses of codeine are well tolerated. The CNS depressant effects of codeine are noticeable in children and some adults, with symptoms of drowsiness and lightheadedness. The depressant effect of codeine is additive to that of other CNS depressants. Like other opiates, codeine has antimotility properties on the intestines and may cause constipation and nausea. Atopic allergic reactions characterized by pruritus occur rarely, mainly in histamine-sensitive patients. Respiratory system effects may include a drying effect on the respiratory mucosa, which precludes use of codeine in clients with asthma or chronic obstructive lung disorders with high-viscosity sputum and congestion. The respiratory depressant effect of codeine is usually not measurable at antitussive doses, but as a precaution, use of codeine should be avoided in clients with respiratory insufficiency of any kind. Hydrocodone is another narcotic available for use in adults only as an antitussive.

Preparations and Administration

Codeine
Tablets and soluble tablets, combination remedies for coughs and colds (numerous)
Recommended Doses: For antitussive effects in adults, 10–20 mg PO every 4–6 hours to a maximum of 120 mg per day. For children 6–12 years of age, 5–10 mg PO every 4–6 hours, not to exceed 60 mg per day. For children from 2–6 years of age, 2.5–5.0 mg PO every 4–6 hours up to 30 mg in a day.

Hydrocodone Bitartrate (Codone, Dicodid)
Tablets
Recommended Doses: For adults, 5–10 mg PO, 3 or 4 times per day.

Narcotic Congener Antitussives

Three nonnarcotic opiate derivatives are available for use as antitussives: dextromethorphan, levopropoxyphene, and noscapine. **Dextromethorphan** is currently the most widely used antitussive.

Mechanisms and Effects Dextromethorphan is the dextro-isomer of levorphanol, a potent narcotic analgesic. Apparently, narcotic receptors in most brain areas are stereospecific to a considerable extent, exhibiting affinity for only the levorotatory isomer of this pair. Narcotic receptors in the cough center, on the other hand, are not stereospecific and respond equally well to the dextro- and levo-isomers. Thus dextromethorphan produces the cough suppression characteristic of narcotics without other narcotic actions. The potency of dextromethorphan is comparable to 15 mg of codeine. Codeine may have a slight advantage in particularly recalcitrant cough because its antitussive potency can be increased if the dose is elevated to 30 mg, while the effect of dextromethorphan is already maximal at the normal dose of 15 mg.

Levopropoxyphene is the levo-isomer of dextropropoxyphene, a weak narcotic marketed as Darvon. At doses of 50–100 mg, its antitussive potency is comparable to 30 mg of dextromethorphan. It exhibits no analgesic properties.

Noscapine is a naturally occurring nonnarcotic opiate alkaloid related to papaverine. Although not widely encountered, on the basis of limited data it appears to be safe and effective. It is equipotent to codeine.

Adverse Effects and Contraindications Adverse effects of dextromethorphan are insignificant. Slight drowsiness or constipation is occasionally reported, but these effects are considerably less than with codeine. Frank overdoses in children have caused ataxia and stupor, but if emesis occurs there is quick recovery. There is no contraindication for use of dextromethorphan except for known hypersensitivity to the drug. Dextromethorphan should not be used with MAO inhibitors.

Adverse reactions to levopropoxyphene include nausea, vomiting, epigastric distress, skin rash, urticaria, dry mouth, drowsiness, dizziness, and nervousness. The only reported side effects of noscapine are uncommon incidents of nausea or drowsiness.

Preparations and Administration

Dextromethorphan
Chewable capsules, lozenges, syrups, liquid; combination cold and cough remedies (countless)
Recommended Doses: For adults, 10–20 mg PO every 4 hours or 30 mg every 6–8 hours. For children age 6–12 years, 5–10 mg PO every 4 hours or 15 mg every 6–8 hours. For children age 2–6 years, 2.5–5 mg PO every 4 hours or 7.5 mg every 6–8 hours.

Levopropoxyphene (Novrad)
Capsules, oral suspension
Recommended Doses: For adults, 100 mg PO every 4 hours; for children, 0.5 mg/lb every 4 hours.

Noscapine (Tusscapine)
Syrup, chewable tablets, combination with the nasal decongestant phenylephrine (Conar Suspension)

Other Centrally Acting Nonnarcotic Antitussives

Three other centrally acting antitussives are available that are chemically unrelated to the narcotics: diphenhydramine, carbetapentane, and chlorphedianol.

Mechanisms and Effects Diphenhydramine is a familiar and potent antihistaminic and anticholinergic agent with antitussive properties. Carbetapentane is a centrally acting antitussive that structurally resembles atropine and the local anesthetics. Its antitussive potency is comparable to codeine. Chlorphedianol is a slow but long-acting antitussive, comparable in potency to codeine. It possesses anticholinergic and local anesthetic properties.

Adverse Effects and Contraindications The principal side effects of diphenhydramine are drowsiness and anticholinergic symptoms such as dry mouth, aggravation of glaucoma, pupillary dilation, and urinary retention. Adverse reactions to carbetapentane are infrequent and mild. Clients given chlorphedianol occasionally experience CNS excitation, including hyperirritability, hallucinations, and nightmares. Anticholinergic symptoms such as dryness of mouth, vertigo, and visual disturbances may occur. Nausea and vomiting and hypersensitivity reactions (such as urticaria) are occasionally noted.

Drug Interactions Diphenhydramine has additive CNS depressant effects with other CNS depressants as well as additive anticholinergic effects with other anticholinergic agents (such as antidepressants).

Preparations and Administration For many years, diphenhydramine was available only by prescription, but in 1981 the FDA approved the first nonprescription cough remedy containing this drug (Benylin). Diphenhydramine preparations also contain ammonium chloride and sodium citrate, traditional but ineffective expectorants.

Carbetapentane
Combination cough and cold remedies (e.g., Cophene-X and -XP and Rynatuss Pediatric Suspension)
Recommended Doses: 15–30 mg PO, 3 or 4 times daily.

Chlorphedianol (Ulo)
Syrup
Recommended Doses: For adults, 25 mg PO, 3 or 4 times daily. For children ages 6–12 years of age, 12.5–25 mg PO, 3 or 4 times daily. For children ages 2–6 years of age, 12.5 mg PO, 3 or 4 times daily.

Diphenhydramine (Benylin, Benachlor, Tusstat, Nordryl, Eldadryl, Diphenadril, Diphenallin, Diphen-Ex, Valdrene) Syrup
Recommended Doses: 10 ml PO every 4 hours up to 40 ml per day in adults. For children ages 6–12 years, 5 ml PO every 4 hours up to 20 ml/day; for children ages 2–6 years, 2.5 ml PO every 4 hours up to 10 ml/day.

Peripherally Acting Antitussive

Benzonatate is chemically related to tetracaine and procaine and is unique among the antitussives in having a peripheral mechanism of action. Its antitussive action is based on its ability to anesthetize stretch receptors in the respiratory passages, lungs, and pleura, which reduces afferent impulses to the cough center and interrupts the cough reflex. Adverse reactions include sedation, headache, mild dizziness, nasal congestion, eye irritation, pruritus, skin eruptions, constipation, nausea, chills, and hypersensitivity reactions.

Preparations and Administration

Benzonatate (Tessalon)
Perles (a soft, spherical, gelatin capsule)
Recommended Doses: For adults and children over 10 years of age, 100 mg tid. The perles are swallowed whole.

Antihistamines

Although antihistamines are widely incorporated into cold preparations, there is no evidence that these drugs reduce liability to colds or shorten their duration. Histamine is released along with other chemical mediators during the inflammatory process that follows viral penetration of the respiratory mucosa. It is possible that antihistamines may reduce this component of the bodily response to the common cold infections. Antihistamines often relieve the sensations of itching or tickling in the nose that contributes to sneezing. The complete pharmacology of antihistamines is addressed in Chapter 50. The most important adverse effect of antihistamines is drowsiness.

Pneumonia

Pneumonia, the generic name for acute infections of the alveoli of the lungs, can be caused by any of a large number of microorganisms. The selection of an appropriate antibiotic for treatment is based on identification of the specific pathogen. The gram-positive bacteria that cause pneumonia are *Diplococcus pneumoniae, Staphylococcus* organisms, *Streptococcus* organisms, *Bacillus anthracis,* and *Corynebacterium diphtheriae.* Penicillin G is the drug of choice except for certain staphylococci, which may require a penicillinase-resistant penicillin. Among gram-negative bacilli, *Klebsiella* organisms, *Haemophilus influenzae, Pasteurella* organisms, and occasionally gram-negative bacilli of the normal body flora can cause pneumonia. Ampicillin is the most prescribed agent, although streptomycin is used for *Franciscella,* and a cephalosporin is used for *Klebsiella.* For clients with viral pneumonias, relief is symptomatic. *Actinomyces* organisms can produce pneumonia and are treated with penicillin G. *Nocardial* pneumonia is treated with a sulfonamide and streptomycin. Streptomycin, because of its curare-like action, may depress respiration. Sulfonamides may cause necrosis and inflammation of small and medium-sized arteries, possibly including the pulmonary artery.

Mycoplasmal pneumonia is treated with erythromycin and tetracycline. When pneumonia is caused by a fungus, amphotericin B may be administered in spite of its toxicity. Rickettsial organisms can also produce pneumonia and are treated with tetracycline. The complete pharmacology of antibacterial drugs is found in Chapter 47 and of antifungal drugs in Chapter 48.

Glucocorticoids in Allergic Rhinitis

Flunisolide (Nasalide) was introduced in 1981 in the form of a topical nasal spray for relief of symptoms of seasonal or perennial rhinitis. Because of the range of adverse effects of glucocorticoids, flunisolide should be reserved for patients who are unable to tolerate antihistamines or decongestants. Flunisolide alleviates sneezing, runny nose, and stuffiness when they are due to allergic mechanisms. It should not be used when infection of the nasal mucosa is present; it may actually help to spread the infection by suppressing the inflammatory and immune defense mechanisms (see Table 52–7 for a comparison of allergic versus infectious rhinitis). Although adverse systemic effects were not reported in clinical trials, flunisolide is absorbed systemically after topical administration to the nasal mucosa and might cause adverse systemic effects if used too frequently or in excessive amounts.

Preparations and Administration

Flunisolide (Nasalide)
Nasal spray: 6.25 mg in 25 ml
Recommended Doses: two sprays (50 μg) in each nostril twice daily. The maximum total daily dose should not exceed 8 sprays per nostril. The nasal passages should be cleared before application. If the nasal passages are congested, a topical decongestant should be administered just prior to flunisolide. Therapy may be continued up to 3 weeks, but relief often occurs in a few days.

Adverse Pulmonary Effects of Drugs

Systemic drugs and environmental allergens may trigger a variety of allergic reactions related to the lungs. Drugs capable of inducing asthmatic attacks are listed in Table 52–1. Other allergic drug reactions involving the lungs include anaphylaxis, eosinophilic pulmonary infiltration, systemic lupus erythematosus, and polyarteritis nodosa. **Infiltrative reactions with eosinophilia** occur in response to gold salts, penicillins, sulfonamides, nitrofurantoin, imipramine, mephenesin, and para-aminosalicylic acid. **Systemic lupus erythematosus-like syndromes** are caused by several d ugs, most commonly hydralazine (Apresoline, Unipres), penicillamine, procainamide, phenytoin (Dilar tin), captopril (Capoten), and isoniazid. Drugs implicated as causes of **polyarteritis nodosa** are arsenicals, gold salts, hydantoins, iodides, mercurials, penicillin, phenothiazines, sulfonamides, and thiouracils. **Anaphylactoid reactions,** which cause respiratory symptoms of wheezing, coughing, sneezing, and dyspnea, occur with histamine, morphine, polymyxin, and contrast media, among other drugs.

Adverse pulmonary reactions to drugs can occur by nonallergic mechanisms as well. Tobacco smoke, the most abundantly encountered respiratory irritant, contains some 15 carcinogens, toxic gases such as hydrogen cyanide and carbon monoxide, and oxidants that inhibit α_1-antitrypsin. Drugs that produce excessive hypotension, such as potent ganglionic blockers, can also produce interstitial pulmonary **edema** and **fibrosis.** Lung edema has also been reported with aspirin, iodide, naloxone, phenoxybenzamine, phenylbutazone, protamine sulfate, and thiazides. Lung fibrosis has been produced by aluminum salts, bleomycin (Blenoxane), nitrofurantoin (Furadantin), pindolol (Visken), practolol, and salazosulfapyramine. Another group of drugs capable of causing **interstitial pneumonitis** includes bleomycin, furazolidone (Furoxone), gold salts, hydralazine, naproxen (Anaprox), nitrofurantoin, penicillamine, phenytoin, sulindac (Clinoril), and thiazides.

Case Study: Asthma

R. D., a 26-year-old graduate student had a 15-year history of asthmatic attacks, averaging about 10 per year. He had observed that the attacks were often triggered when he visited friends who owned dogs or cats, and the attacks seemed seasonal. Skin tests conducted by his physician confirmed that he was allergic to pollens or dander. Sometimes stress or upper respiratory tract infections contributed to occurrence of attacks as well. A typical attack for R. D. was characterized by wheezing, mild dyspnea, and shortness of breath. R. D. was able to employ aerosol therapy (albuterol) for his attacks and he had been instructed in proper use of the aerosol by the nurse at the clinic that he visited. He seldom experienced asthmatic attacks in the evening and thus had no problem with insomnia from the medication. During the pollen season, R. D. used theophylline tablets prophylactically. He did not usually use them at other times because he had noted episodes of epigastric pain when he used theophylline for extended periods of time.

One day, an asthma attack began with deep cough, cold sweats, and dyspnea, about 4 hours before R. D. was scheduled to conduct a seminar. R. D. had also had a cold for about 3 days. He attempted to relieve the attack with albuterol aerosol but was so congested that he was unable to inhale the spray effectively. One hour after his attack began, R. D.'s respiratory rate was noticeably increased and he was brought to a nearby hospital by a fellow graduate student.

Upon initial examination, he had a pulse rate of 115, respiratory rate of 30, body temperature of 102°F, and bilateral wheezing and rales. The attending physician ordered an arterial blood sample for measurement of blood gases and a venous blood sample for complete blood cell counts and serum bicarbonate. While awaiting the laboratory results, emergency therapy was initiated with epinephrine, SC; oxygen by face mask; and an intravenous line with slow infusion of 5% dextrose. Laboratory results were returned after 30 minutes as follows: P_{CO_2} 53 mm Hg (normal: 35–45 mm Hg); P_{O_2} 65 mm Hg (normal: 80–100 mm Hg); HCO_3^- 24 mEq/L (normal: 22–26 mEq/L); and pH 7.33 (normal: 7.31–7.41). One hour after admission, R. D. continued to exhibit respirations at 28/minute. The physician ordered aminophylline, 250 mg by IV push. Before administering this order, the nurse checked the chart to see if any aminophylline had been given previously to this patient. The aminophylline administration resulted in noticeable improvement within 15 minutes. Respiratory distress diminished, respiratory rate declined, use of accessory muscles for respiration diminished, and the client was noticeably relieved.

One hour later arterial gases were reevaluated and indicted a P_{CO_2} of 47, P_{O_2} of 80, HCO_3^- of 25 mEq/L, and pH of 7.34. The next day R. D. was discharged in stable condition with instructions to take theophylline tablets as needed until his cold symptoms resolved and to employ aerosol as required for acute symptoms.

1. Is R. D.'s case of asthma best characterized as intrinsic, extrinsic, or mixed?
2. Why would albuterol aerosol be expected to cause fewer adverse effects than oral ephedrine?
3. Do you concur with R. D.'s suspicion that his episodes of epigastric pain were due to prolonged use of theophylline?
4. What factors were likely responsible for the severity of R. D.'s attack that led to hospitalization?
5. Why was the nurse careful to determine if aminophylline had been given recently (within the last 6 hours) before administering the ordered dose?
6. Explain the laboratory values at the height of the attack and after its resolution?

Answers appear at the end of the book.

Recommended Readings

Antiasthmatic Drugs

Clark TJ: Choice of drug treatment in asthma. *Pharmacol Ther* 1982;17:221–228.

Fernandez E: Update on the pharmacologic approach to asthma: Xanthine and adrenergic bronchodilators. *Resp Ther* 1984;14(4):42–44.

Fernandez E: Update on the pharmacologic approach to asthma: anticholinergics, corticosteroids, and cromolyn sodium. *Resp Ther* 1984;14(5):29–30.

Flenley DC: New drugs in respiratory disorders. *Br Med J* 1983;286:871–875, 955–959.

Kirilloff LH, Tibbals SC: Drugs for asthma: A complete guide. *Am J Nurs* 1983;83(1):55–61.

Melethil S, Carlson JD, Haug MT: Predictability of theophylline levels. *Drug Intell Clin Pharm* 1982;16:695–697.

Newman SP: Factors influencing the efficacy of inhaled bronchodilators. *Resp Ther* 1983;13(4):37–45.

Rifas EM: Teaching patients to manage acute asthma: The future is now. *Nursing* 1983;13(4):77–82.

Webber-Jones JE, Bryant MK: Over-the-counter bronchodilators. *Nursing* 1980;10(1):34–39.

Antitussives and Mucolytics

Barbieri EJ: Mucolytics. *Am Fam Physician* 1981;24(3):181–185.

Chasnoff IJ, Diggs G, Schnoll SH: Fetal alcohol effects and maternal cough syrup abuse. *Am J Dis Child* 1981;135:968.

Kuhn JJ et al: Antitussive effect of guaifenesin in young adults with natural colds. Objective and subjective assessment. *Chest* 1982;82:713–718.

Pepper GA: OTC vs. Rx for coughs and colds. *Nurse Pract* 1986:11(10):66–77.

Richardson PS: The principles of drug action on cough and on sputum characteristics. *Europ J Resp Dis* 1980 [Suppl] 61(110):67–79.

Zanjanian MH: Expectorants and antitussive agents: are they helpful? *Ann Allergy* 1980;44:290–295.

Chronic Obstructive Pulmonary Disease

Blair GP et al: Treatment of COPD with corticosteroids: Comparison of daily versus alternate-day therapy. *Chest* 1984;86(4):534–528.

Dunlap CI, Marchionno P: Help your COPD patient take a better breath — with inhalers. *Nursing* 1983;13(5):42–43.

Gross NJ, Skorodin MS: Role of the parasympathetic system in airway obstruction due to emphysema. *N Engl J Med* 1984;311(7):421–425.

Hudson LH: Management of COPD: State of the art. *Chest* 1984 [Suppl] 85(6):765–815.

Therapeutic Gases

D'Agostino JS: Set your mind at ease on oxygen toxicity. *Nursing* 1983;13(7):55–56.

Ellmyer P, Thomas NJ: A guide to your patient's safe home use of oxygen. *Nursing* 1982;12(1):56–57.

CHAPTER 53

Drugs Used for Skin Disorders

Physiology of the Skin

The skin, which is the largest organ of the body, has five major functions: (1) protection of the body from the external environment, (2) maintenance of the internal fluid environment, (3) temperature regulation, (4) somatosensory sensitivity, and (5) synthesis of vitamin D. An examination of the layers of the skin — epidermis, the dermis, and the subcutaneous tissue — demonstrates how the skin performs these functions.

The Epidermis

The epidermis, the outermost layer of skin, has four sublayers and continuously regenerates itself. The deepest layer of epidermis, called the **basal layer** or stratum germinativum (Figure 53–1), is only one cell thick. It lies immediately over the dermis and is held to it by interlocking processes. Formation of new cells by mitosis occurs mainly in the basal layer. Also found in the basal layer are the melanocytes that synthesize melanin, which colors the skin and provides a protective sunscreen for the deep layers of the epidermis and dermis.

As cells migrate upward, they take on a polygonal shape in the **spinous layer,** or **stratum spinosum.** The process of keratinization (the gradual transformation of cells into tough scales) begins in this layer as the cell synthesizes keratin, keratohyalin, and fibrillar and amorphous proteins. Cells reaching the top of the spinous layer flatten and become diamond-shaped as they proceed into the **granular layer,** or stratum granulosum. As they proceed through the granular layers, epidermal cells form a cytoplasmic grid, consisting of fibrils, amorphous proteins, and keratin. The basal, spinous, and granular layers together comprise the **prickle cell layer,** or **stratum malpighii.**

The outermost layer of epidermis is the **cornified** or **horny layer,** or **stratum corneum,** which provides a tough barrier of low permeability that shields the body from temperature fluctuations, pathogens, and toxic chemicals and minimizes water loss. As granular cells approach the cornified layer, the internal matrix is fully formed. The cell membranes thicken, and the cell finally expels its nucleus, organelles, and keratohyalin-containing granules, leaving only the cell membrane and keratin-fibril matrix. Released keratohyalin cements these cell fragments together, producing the tough layer of cornified cells. The total transit time for the average epidermal cell

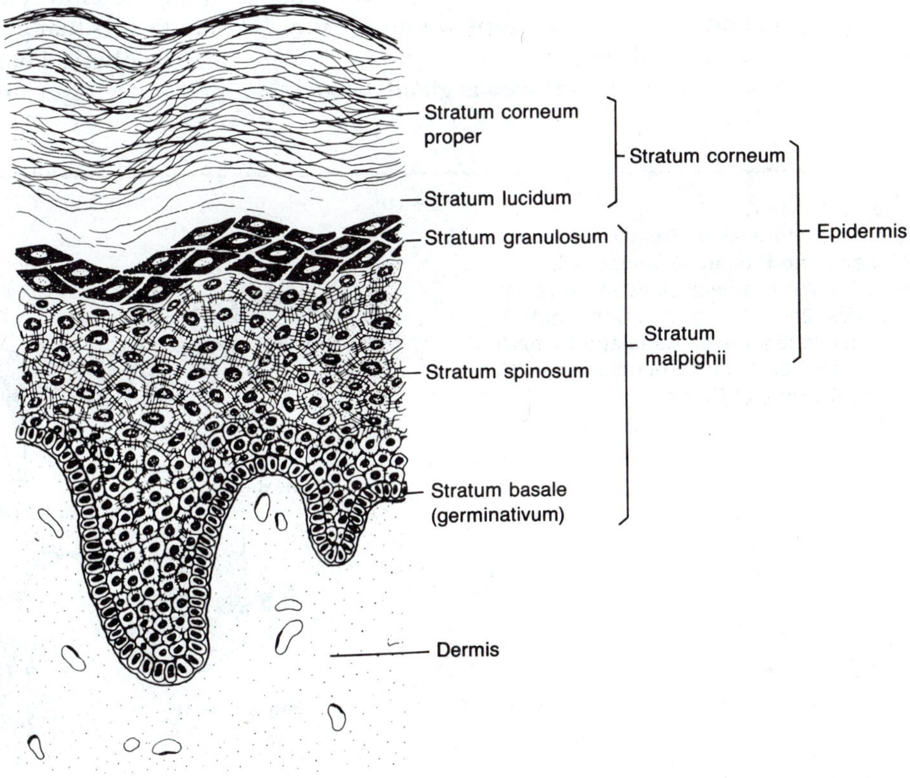

Figure 53–1
The epidemis in a region of "thick skin," showing the various layers. From M. Borysenko and T. Beringer, *Functional Histology,* 2d ed. Boston: Little, Brown, 1984.

from basal layer to surface is about 12–25 days. The outermost layer of cornified cells are gradually shed in a process called **exfoliation.**

The Dermis

The dermis lies between the epidermis and subcutaneous tissue (Figure 53–2) and consists of two layers: the papillary and the reticular. The papillary layer, next to the epidermis, consists of fibroblasts, collagen strands, elastic fibers, and ground substance. The deeper reticular layer has more collagen but fewer fibrocytes and less ground substance. Fibroblasts secrete fiber precursors (procollagen, proelastin, and microfibrillar proteins) and other components of the ground substance (which is composed of water, electrolytes, glucose, mucopolysaccharides, hyaluronic acid, and proteins). Intertwining collagen and elastic fibers provide the strength and elasticity characteristic of the dermis.

The dermal layer contains sensory nerve terminals, hair follicles, sweat and sebaceous glands, blood vessels, mast cells, and macrophages. The **hair follicles** extend from the dermal reticular layer to the skin surface (Figure 53–3) and are surrounded by epithelial root sheaths. Bodily hair protects the scalp from excessive sunlight and the eyes from sweat, filters inspired air as it flows through the nasal passages, and contributes to sexual attractiveness. The piloerector muscles cause the hair to stand up straight ("on-end"), producing "goose bumps," and promoting secretion of sebum.

Sebum is produced by **sebaceous glands** associated with the root sheath of the hair follicle (Figure 53–3). Sebaceous glands are widely distributed in the skin, being absent only in the palms, soles, and dorsa of the feet. Cells of the sebaceous glands accumulate lipids and waxes; in the process they become bloated and burst. The oil content is then secreted into the hair follicle and excreted onto the skin surface to lubricate the skin.

Two types of sweat glands are found in the dermal layer. **Eccrine sweat glands,** which secrete an odorless sweat, are distributed over the entire skin, especially in the soles, palms, and axilla. They are second in importance only to the kidney in regulating fluid and electrolyte balance. Sweat produced by **apocrine sweat glands** emits an odor when acted upon by skin surface bacteria. The sweat of apocrine glands has a milky appearance because it contains species-specific chemicals, called **pheromones,** that serve to attract the opposite sex. Apocrine glands are located in the axilla, nipples, breasts, anogenital region, external ear canal, and eyelids.

The blood vessels that supply the skin, found mainly in the reticular layer of the dermis, participate in temperature regulation of the body. **Mast cells,** which are found in the dermis surrounding the blood vessels, secrete autacoids, including histamine and heparin, that participate in inflammatory mechanisms. **Macrophages** in the dermal layer devour foreign particles, microbes, and cell debris during immune reactions and inflammatory processes. Other skin factors that provide protection against infection are the physical barrier provided by the tough cornified outer layer and the chemical barrier provided

Figure 53–2
Structure of the skin. From Josephine M. Sana and Richard D. Judge, eds., *Physical Assessment Skills for Nursing Practice,* 2nd ed., Fig. 6-3. Copyright © 1982 by Josephine M. Sana and Richard D. Judge. Reprinted by permission of Little, Brown and Company.

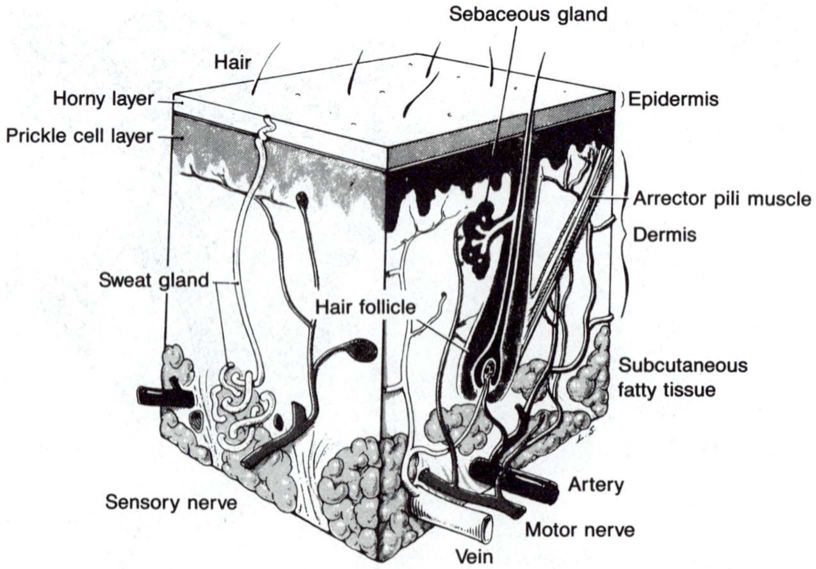

Figure 53–3
Some cutaneous appendages. From M. Borysenko and T. Beringer, *Functional Histology,* 2d ed. Boston: Little, Brown, 1984

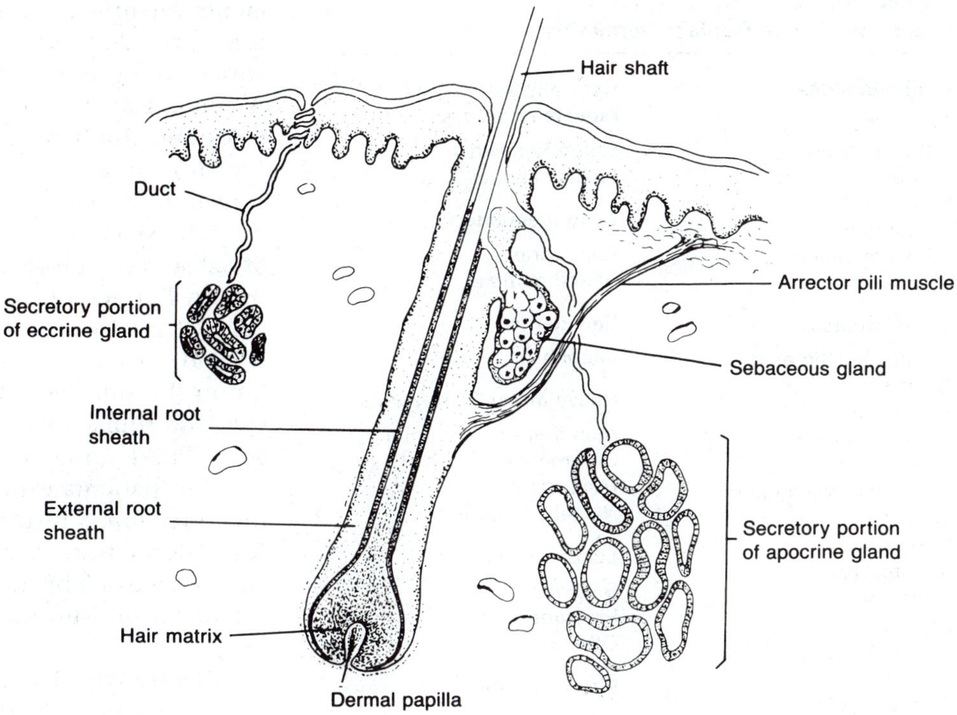

by presence of hyaluronic acid in the dermal ground substance.

Subcutaneous Tissue

The subcutaneous tissue lies beneath the dermis and consists mainly of fat with interdigitating elastic fibers, blood vessels, nerves, lymphatic vessels, and muscle fibers. The subcutaneous tissue is a pliable support base for the dermis that insulates heat and absorbs shock; it also provides a depot for fat that provides a caloric reserve. In some areas (the eyelids, areola, and genitalia), it is either thin or absent.

The characteristics and treatments of the numerous disorders that afflict the skin are summarized in Appendix 53A at the end of the chapter.

Inflammations of the Skin and Drug Treatments

Dermatitis

Contact Dermatitis

Superficial inflammation of the skin is referred to as **dermatitis** or **eczema.** It may have an endogenous or exogenous etiology. Exogenous dermatitis, called **contact dermatitis,** may be caused by chemicals (Table 53–1) or mechanical irritation. The inflammation is often limited to the area of contact, although it sometimes spreads. Soaps or detergents, acids, alkalis, or phenol cause chemical irritation; contact with wool or fiberglass causes mechanical irritation. Other major causes of contact dermatitis include plants (poison ivy, oak, or sumac) ingredients in topical medications, compounds of nickel, mercury, or chromate, chemicals used in clothing, cosmetics, dyes, and industrial chemicals. Most chemicals cause contact dermatitis by a delayed (type IV) hypersensitivity reaction. Some chemicals produce allergic contact dermatitis only after exposure to sunlight. Such phototoxic reactions are most common with sunscreening agents, topical sulfonamides, aftershave lotions, perfumes, coal tar, and oils.

Treatment of contact dermatitis hinges on removing the causative agent, but acute measures include wet wrappings, antipruritics, topical steroids, and systemic steroids. In areas of low humidity, use of humidifiers may be helpful. Bathing may need to be restricted. The client should be advised to avoid extreme temperatures. Application of emollients after bathing may help to retain skin moisture. Clients should be advised to keep rooms well ventilated and to wear loose, soft clothing to prevent mechanical irritation of the skin.

Table 53–1
Drugs that Cause Contact Dermatitis

Antihistamines	**Centrally acting skeletal muscle relaxants**
Antizoline	Chlorphenesin
Chlorcyclizine	Meprobamate
Diphenhydramine	**Decongestants**
Promethazine	Ephedrine
Pyrilamine	Phenindamine
Tripelennamine	**Emollients**
Others	Lanolin
Antimicrobials	**Heavy Metal Compounds**
Aminosalicylic acid	Aluminum compounds
Bacitracin	Chromates
Bleomycin	Mercurials
Chloramphenicol	Nickel compounds
Gentamicin	**Local anesthetics**
Iodochlorhydroxyquin	Benzocaine
Isoniazid	Procaine
Neomycin	Others
Nitrofurazone	**Phenothiazines**
Novobiocin	Chlorpromazine
Penicillins	Others
Propamidine	**Sunscreens**
Quinine	*p*-Aminobenzoic acid
Streptomycin	Cinnamates
Sulfonamides	Glyceryl PABA
Tetracyclines	Padimate A
Antiseptics and disinfectants	
Balsam Peru	
Benzoyl peroxide	
Carbanilides	
Formaldehyde	
Hexachlorophene	
Iodine	
Mercurials	
Parabens	
Phenol	
Quaternary ammonium compounds	
Resorcinol	
Salicylanilides	
Sulfur	

Rhus Dermatoses

Contact dermatitis caused by poison ivy, poison oak, or poison sumac is called a **Rhus dermatitis.** Three kinds of products are marketed for treatment of Rhus dermatoses: (1) nonprescription topical agents for acute relief of the itch, pain, and discomfort, (2) prescription, systemic preparations for prophylaxis, and (3) a prescription, systemic preparation for acute relief. The topical preparations contain odd combinations of antiseptics (phenol, benzalkonium chloride, phenylcarbinol), local anesthetics (benzocaine), protectants (zinc oxide, zirconium oxide, calamine, colloidal oatmeal), and rubefacients (menthol, camphor, methyl salicylate). They are provided as creams, lotions, ointments, sprays, and gels with product names such as Albitox, Aveeno, Calamatum, Calamine, Calamycin, Calamox, and Rhulicream. Two preparations (Ivy-Chex, Ivy-Rid) contain a specific antitoxin that inactivates urushiol, the active toxin of poison ivy.

The systemic prophylactic preparations consist of extracts of poison ivy for injection (Aqua Ivy, Poison Ivy Extract) or in oral solution (Ivy-Safe); poison oak extract in oral solution (ImunOak); combined ivy and oak extracts in oral capsules or injectable solution (Poison Ivy/Oak Extract); or a combined ivy, oak, and sumac extract for injection (Rhus-All Antigen). These antigenic preparations are contraindicated in patients with febrile respiratory illness, active infection, a history of kidney damage, or active Rhus dermatitis. A preparation named Rhus Tox Antigen is available in an injection solution for acute treatment of Rhus dermatitis.

Dermatitis of Endogenous Origin

Endogenous varieties of dermatitis include atopic, seborrheic, or exfoliative dermatitis and localized forms such as dermatitis of hands and feet, pruritus ani, pruritus vulvae, and neurodermatitis. **Atopic dermatitis** has a strong hereditary component. Persons with this disorder have a low threshold for itching and are especially sensitive to irritants such as wool, furs, chemicals, stress, temperature and humidity changes, and bacterial infections. The itching triggers scratching and rubbing reflexes that cause the characteristic skin lesions: erythema (redness and swelling of the skin) and lichenification. The areas of the body most often affected are the front of elbow, back of knee, neck, wrists, and eyelids. Atopic dermatitis is an IgE-mediated (type I) hypersensitivity reaction.

Seborrheic dermatitis is an inflammatory skin disease characterized by redness and scaling of the scalp, and sometimes the face or other areas of the body. **Dandruff** and **cradle cap** in young infants are mild, noninflammatory forms of this disorder. Seborrheic dermatitis has a familial trend but is also affected by climate and generally becomes worse in the winter. Treatment involves the application of antiseborrheic shampoos.

Localized neurodermatitis often has a strong psychogenic component and is most common in females between 20 and 50. Itching occurs in a circumscribed area, such as the back of the head, arms, anus, or vulva. Excessive scratching then causes the lesions, which usually appear as dry, scaly plaques. Antipruritics and topical corticosteroids are often useful. **Pityriasis rosea** is a mild, self-limited, acute inflammatory condition characterized by scaly patches, usually on the trunk.

Exfoliative dermatitis is a severe inflammatory disease of the skin with erythema and scaling. The skin becomes red, scaly, thickened, and crusty, and the condition may be life-threatening. Treatment involves removing possible causes (infections, topical or systemic medications, or primary dermatitides). **Lichen planus,** by contrast, is a chronic, recurrent inflammatory condition characterized by scaly, papular patches typically distributed on the flexor surfaces of the limbs, the trunk, the penis, the vaginal mucosa, and the mouth. An indistinguishable condition (lichenoid eruptions) can occur as a drug reaction. Antipruritics (oral antihistamines) and topical steroids are useful treatments, but steroid therapy is seldom effective unless applied intralesionally or with occlusive wrapping.

Topical Anti-Inflammatory Drugs

The availability of glucocorticoids in topical dosage forms has greatly improved clinical management of inflammatory dermatitides. The general pharmacology of glucocorticoids is discussed in Chapter 32 and topical preparations are listed in Table 32–7.

Glucocorticoids not only provide an anti-inflammatory action when applied to the skin but also are antipruritic and decrease edema by constricting blood vessels. The topical route is ideal for skin inflammations because it places the drug in direct contact with the area of lesion and minimizes occurrence of adverse systemic effects. To be effective, glucocorticoids must be absorbed from the skin surface into the underlying skin layers. The objective with topical application of glucocorticoids is to ensure adequate absorption so as to provide therapeutic benefit but not so much absorption as to cause an unacceptable level of systemic toxicity.

Pharmacokinetics The factors that influence the absorption of topical glucocorticoids fall into three categories: formulation characteristics of the topical preparation, application factors, and characteristics of the skin at the site of application. **Formulation characteristics** are concerned with the active ingredient(s) and the nature of the vehicle. The potency (high, intermediate, or low) of the active glucocorticoid is a crucial factor in efficacy (Table 53–2). The vehicle can have a variety of influences on efficacy as well. Client compliance is adversely affected if the vehicle has an unpleasant odor, stains clothing, or stings when applied. The vehicle also influences absorption of the active ingredient. Specially formulated vehicles that are hydrophilic or emollient provide stability and solubility of the therapeutic agent while permitting its release into the skin. Ointment bases generally provide the greatest absorption, followed by creams and then lotions. Unfortunately, market surveys of consumer preferences in cosmetics indicate that consumers prefer lotions, then creams, and ointments last. The potent glucocorticoids are provided mainly as creams and ointments, further enhancing their relative efficacy. For the intermediate and low potency agents, there is a large selection of vehicles with the result that efficacy varies considerably. Thus, hydrocortisone, usually a low-potency glucocorticoid when applied topically in a water miscible base, approaches intermediate potency when applied in the form of a cream in a hydrophilic base. The site of application and the nature of the lesion also influences vehicle selection. Hirsute areas such as the scalp are best treated with lotions or aerosols. Most lesions are treated with creams or lotions; dry, scaly lesions are best soothed and hydrated by use of an ointment.

Table 53–2
Potency of Topical Corticosteroids

High potency
Amcinonide (Cyclocort)
Clobetasol (Temovate)
Desoximetasone (Topicort)
Diflurasone (Florone, Maxiflor)
Fluocinonide (Lidex, Topsyn)
Halcinonide (Halog)
Intermediate potency
Betamethasone (Benisone, Diprosone, Uticort, Valisone)
Clocortolone (Cloderm)
Fluocinolone (Fluonid, Synalar)
Flurandrenolide (Cordran)
Triamcinolone (Aristocort, Flutex, Kenalog, Spencort, Tri-acet)
Low potency
Alclometasone (Aclovate)
Desonide (Tridesilon)
Dexamethasone (Hexadrol, Decaderm)
Flumethasone (Locorten)
Hydrocortisone (various)
Methylprednisolone (Medrol)
Prednisolone (Meti-Derm)

Application factors also influence absorption. Absorption is enhanced by increasing the amount applied, increasing contact time, or increasing frequency of application. Unfortunately, topical preparations are often prescribed or self-administered without the degree of concern for dosage (per unit of surface area) that is routinely considered when prescribing systemic medications. *The nurse should provide specific instructions about application to guide the client in judging how much of the topical medication to apply at each dosing interval. Clients should be taught to apply a thin film to the affected area since excess increases the danger of systemic toxicity and is uneconomical.* Typically, topical steroids are applied 3–4 times per day.

When topical steroids are employed for inflammatory conditions characterized by scaling (such as psoriasis or lichen planus), the outer scales should be removed. Scales can be softened for removal by soaking in a bath (which may contain oatmeal soap or other products designed to facilitate softening), and then rubbed, brushed, or picked off. When cosmetic considerations permit, the area of inflammation should be shaved as well. The topical preparation is then rubbed into the affected area thoroughly.

A special technique for applying topical glucocorticoids is an **occlusive dressing.** This method increases absorption by a factor of 10 (for example, from 1% to 10% for hydrocortisone). After the topical medication has been applied, the area is covered with a soft, plastic wrap such as polyethylene or plastic film, and the edges are sealed to the adjacent, unaffected skin with tape or another suitable closure. For treatment of the scalp, a shower cap can be useful; for the hands, surgical gloves are convenient. Whole body plastic suits are available when glucocorticoids must be applied extensively. The occlusive dressing remains in place for at least 7–8 hours but not more than 12 hours daily. Most clients find application of the dressing at bedtime most convenient, but it can be applied at the end of a workday and removed at bedtime if it interferes with sleeping comfort. Occlusive dressings should be continued for a few days after lesions have cleared to minimize the risk of recurrence of the inflammation. Occlusive dressing may cause folliculitis from bacterial or candidal infection, hyperthermia from heat retention, or systemic glucocorticoid side effects from increased absorption.

Absorption of topically applied glucocorticoids is influenced by **skin characteristics** at the site of application, such as perspiration, hydration, pH, temperature, and, especially, the thickness of the stratum corneum (which acts as a barrier to penetration). Mucous membranes lack a stratum corneum, therefore permitting much greater absorption of steroids. The scrotum, vulva, and eyelids have only a thin stratum corneum, while the soles of the feet have an unusually thick outer layer. The portion of a topically applied dose of hydrocortisone that is absorbed from the arch of the foot is only about 0.1%; 1% is absorbed from the forearm, 2% on the back, 4% from the scalp, 6% from the forehead, and about 40% from the scrotum. Systemic absorption is enhanced when skin is inflamed and especially if abrasions or exudative lesions are present, indicating breaks in the outer skin layers. The skin of the elderly and the very young offers less resistance to drug penetration.

Clinical Indications Topical corticosteroids are indicated for most inflammatory dermatoses, but there is a wide range of responses. Seborrheic dermatitis, atopic dermatitis, localized neurodermatitis, pruritus ani, psoriasis, and the later phase of both allergic and irritant contact dermatitis generally respond well to topical corticoids even without use of occlusive dressings or unusually potent formulations. High concentrations of potent corticoids, occlusive dressings, or intralesional therapy are used to treat other conditions, such as discoid lupus erythematosus, lichen planus, keloids, pemphigus, granuloma annulare, infiltrative dermopathy of hyperthyroidism, acne cysts, and psoriasis in areas having a thick stratum corneum (the soles, palms, knees, and elbows). The early phase of contact dermatitis and the inflammatory response to superficial fungal (dermatophyte) infections generally do not respond to corticosteroids regardless of dose or method of application.

Adverse Effects and Contraindications The adverse effects of topical corticosteroids include some related to systemic absorption and others relating to the skin itself. The likelihood of excess systemic absorption is directly related to the presence of factors that enhance absorption, such as use of potent agents or high doses, application to a large surface area, application too frequently or for too long a duration, use of occlusive dressings, or application to skin that is abraded, intensely inflamed, very old, very young, or lacking in stratum corneum. *If several of these risk factors are present, the client may develop the systemic adverse effects of Cushing's syndrome such as hypopigmentation, purpura, and striae. In practice, nurses will seldom see these symptoms resulting from topical use of corticosteroids. Adrenal suppression is the systemic adverse effect that most often occurs, especially in children, but the extent of suppression from topical applications is seldom of clinical importance.*

Adverse effects related to local effects on the skin are more frequent with high-potency preparations and occlusive dressings. Clients complain of **skin reactions** that include allergic contact dermatitis, dryness, itching, atrophy, hypopigmentation, and purpura. When high-potency products are ap-

Nursing Observations for Use of Dermatologics for Dermatitis or Psoriasis

THERAPEUTIC GOAL	Resolution of the condition if acute; control of the condition and management of discomfort if chronic.
PREADMINISTRATION ASSESSMENT	
Baseline Data	Note presence of rash, papules, macules, redness, scaling, swelling, stinging, or pruritus; observe for flaking and scaling of the skin, papules, and plaques, especially on elbows, knees, and scalp as indications of psoriasis. Evaluate skin integrity, color, texture, turgor, temperature, moisture, presence of lesion, rashes, or edema.
EVALUATION OF DRUG RESPONSE	
For Therapeutic Benefit	Monitor improvement in appearance of lesions and related itchiness
For Adverse Effects and Drug Interactions	Monitor for adverse effects and drug interactions specific for each drug (see individual drug discussions). Note that some dermatologics, such as corticosteroids, may be absorbed systemically to a great enough extent as to warrant monitoring for potential systemic toxicity.
For Compliance	Evaluate the client's compliance with all facets of the therapeutic regimen by careful observation, interviewing, and review of progress. Report compliance problems to the physician and act as client-advocate when changes in the therapeutic regimen seem indicated.

plied to the face (as for example in rosacea or acne) for extended periods of time, drug eruptions may emerge that resemble the disorders for which the drugs are being used. *There is a temptation on the part of clients to treat an eruption with higher doses or still more potent agents. On the other hand, withdrawal of the medication leads to temporary worsening but eventual clearing. Thus, nurses need to caution clients to use the designated medication in the prescribed amount so as to avoid worsening the condition.*

Clients may develop **ocular problems** such as glaucoma and cataracts when topical corticosteroids are used in the vicinity of the eyes. There is also the risk of secondary infections when occlusive dressings are employed. Topical corticosteroids are contraindicated in clients with infections and known allergies to corticosteroids, in pregnant women (because of possible risks to the fetus), or if adverse systemic or topical responses have occurred previously.

Psoriasis and Antipsoriatic Agents

Psoriasis is a common disorder affecting 1–2% of people in the United States, excluding mild cases. Caucasians are affected more than blacks. Usually there is a family history of the disorder. Psoriasis begins most commonly between 10 and 30 years of age. The condition typically fluctuates in severity, with exacerbations often triggered by injury, irritation, sunburn, topical medications, steroid withdrawal, or respiratory infections. The characteristic appearance of psoriasis is one of well-demarcated regions of erythematous plaques that yield thick gray flakes (Figure 53–4). In intertriginous zones, such as between the toes, under the breasts, or in the perianal

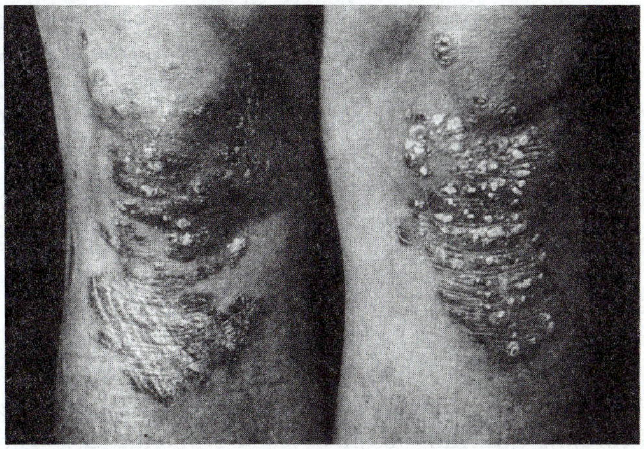

Figure 53–4
Psoriasis. From K. Arndt, *Manual of Dermatologic Therapeutics,* 3d ed. Boston: Little, Brown, 1983.

region, the psoriatic scales may soften, allowing formation of painful fissures. Certain drugs, such as lithium, can dry the skin and aggravate psoriasis.

The lesions are usually distributed on the scalp, the extensor surface of the limbs (elbows, knees), and the trunk, especially the back and buttocks; they may extend in some instances to the external genitalia, perianal region, ears, neck, and even to the palms and soles. Fingernail and toenail involvement is common, consisting of pitting, discoloration, separation at the margins, or accumulation of debris under the nail plate. This psoriatic nail dystrophy is often correlated with **psoriatic arthritis,** which comprises about 6% of cases of psoriasis. The treatment of psoriasis varies, depending on severity.

Topical Corticosteroids

Topical corticosteroids are widely employed in psoriasis and have an antimitotic and anti-inflammatory effect. Evidence suggests that corticosteroids induce cellular production of a substance that inhibits release of arachidonic acid from cell membranes; this limits formation of prostaglandins that are involved in directing inflammatory activity. Topical corticosteroids are generally effective in psoriasis, except in skin areas where a thick stratum corneum precludes adequate absorption (the soles and palms).

Emollients and Keratolytics

Emollients such as petroleum jelly or mineral oil are widely used in psoriasis to provide a protective coating for healthy skin adjacent to psoriatic plaques that may limit spread of the disease. In addition, an emollient lubricates the plaque, easing the removal of scales and reducing formation of fissures in intertriginous areas. Other methods used to soften psoriatic scales include occlusive dressings and **keratolytics.** A commonly employed keratolytic is salicylic acid, usually applied as an ointment. Propylene glycol is also used for this purpose. Ammoniated mercury (Mercuronate, Emersal) has been used as a keratolytic in psoriasis, but hypersensitivity reactions and damage to renal tubules has reportedly occurred, limiting the usefulness of this drug. Keratolytics are discussed later in the chapter as nonspecific dermatologics.

Tars

Preparations that contain **coal tar** are often employed topically for psoriasis; a few preparations contain pine tar or oil of cade from juniper. Tar products have an irritant effect on the skin and suppress DNA synthesis and mitosis. The antimitotic action is potentiated by exposure of the treated skin surface to ultraviolet (UV) light. Tars are indicated for use in seborrheic dermatitis and psoriasis. Adverse reactions to tars include allergic reactions, photosensitivity, and folliculitis. The preparations will stain clothing and bedding and have an unpleasant odor.

Although tar products contain a number of identified carcinogens, a study of clients using coal tar for 25 years did not provide evidence for increased tumors, cutaneous or otherwise. Tar-containing preparations include ointments, creams, gels, lotions, pastes, solutions, soaps, and shampoos.

Preparations and Administration

Coal tar
Cream (Cotasol), gel (Estar, psoriGel), solution in alcohol (Wright's), aqueous solution (various), lotion (Tar Doak), paste (Tarpaste), soap (Mazon), shampoo (Neutrogena T/Gel, Tersa-Tar, or Pentrax Tar. Combination creams, ointments, or lotions with allantoin (Alphosyl, Pso-Rite), which stimulates normal mitotic activity; menthol (Tarbonis), an antipruritic; zinc oxide (Supertah, Medotar), an antiseptic and protectant; precipitated sulfur and salicylic acid (Sulpik T, Pragmatar), which are keratolytics; salicylic acid and antiseptics (Tarlene, Mazon, Oxipor); or a mixture of antiseptics (Unguentum Bossi).

Pine tar (Packer's Pine Tar)
Shampoo

Polytar
Shampoo (juniper, pine, and coal tar), soap (vegetable and mineral tars)

Anthralin

Anthralin (dithranol) suppresses the mitotic activity of epidermal cells by inhibiting synthesis of deoxyribonucleic acid (DNA) and ribonucleic acid (RNA). It is a potent drug that works in some cases of psoriasis not responsive to tars or other treatments. Anthralin may cause kidney irritation if not used properly. Proper use entails application of concentrations up to 0.4% on stable, chronic plaque patches. *Prior to using anthralin, the client should have a skin patch test for hypersensitivity to the drug. Anthralin should not be applied to intensely inflamed areas, acute eruptions, or fissures. It should not be applied near the eyes because it can produce corneal opacity, keratitis, and conjunctivitis. Application to the face, genitalia, or intertriginous areas should likewise be avoided.* Anthralin can stain clothing, linen, and even the skin.

Anthralin ointment should be applied at bedtime and left in place for 8–12 hours. Warm mineral oil can be used in the morning to aid in removing the ointment. If erythema occurs in normal skin adjacent to the site of application, the concentration or frequency of use of anthralin should be

Nursing Diagnoses and Interventions for Use of Dermatologics for Dermatitis or Psoriasis

Nursing Diagnoses	*Related Interventions*
TO ENHANCE DRUG BENEFITS OR REDUCE DRUG REQUIREMENTS	
Alteration in comfort: pruritus from the disorder	Wrap lesions in wet dressings, calamine lotion, creams, or ointments; systemic antipruritics if required.
Disturbance in self-concept related to appearance and response of others; impaired social interactions due to fear of embarrassment or negative reactions	Provide emotional support, encouragement, and positive regard; when appropriate, teach client nondrug measures such as use of nonprescription skin cleansers or improved skin hygiene. Consider referral of client and family for psychological counseling.
Impairment of skin integrity due to lesions and inflammation	Treat secondary infections as required with antimicrobial drugs. Provide care and protection of lesions.
TO ENSURE SAFE AND EFFICACIOUS DRUG USE	
Knowledge deficit related to drug regimen	Teach client with allergic dermatitis to avoid contact with the allergenic substance.
	Teach client to avoid any cosmetics or topical drugs that are even mildly irritating and to apply such substances sparingly unless required for medical purposes.
	Provide the client with a list of adverse effects and drug interactions for each drug in the regimen and explain what to do if any of these occur.
	Teach client appropriate methods for application of topical dermatologics.

reduced. Nonocclusive bandages can be employed to prevent contact of the drug with normal skin. When the drug is applied to the scalp, a thin film of petroleum jelly should be applied to protect uninvolved skin adjacent to the area of lesion, especially the ears or margin of the scalp. Pillows should be covered with plastic to prevent staining, and the client should be advised to shampoo the hair in the morning. After shampooing, the scales can be removed by using a fine-tooth comb. Blond, white, or gray hair may be discolored.

The lowest effective concentration should be employed. Higher concentrations can be used effectively and safely for short intervals (1–2 hours) with minimal staining or adverse effects. *Anthralin preparations should be stored in tight containers between 50° and 86° F, protected from light.*

Preparations and Administration

Anthralin
Ointment (Anthra-Derm), unguent (Lasan)

Ultraviolet Light and Psoralens

Another treatment for psoriasis is to expose the skin to **ultraviolet light.** Ultraviolet light suppresses mitotic activity of basal cells in the epidermis. Treatment spas for psoriatic individuals have existed for centuries in various parts of the world that are blessed with plentiful sunshine, although the beneficial effects of brief periods of exposure are short-lived. On the other hand, most cases of psoriasis will clear with 20–40 sessions of phototherapy in combination with topical steroids, tars, or anthralin, and recalcitrant cases may respond to the further addition of drugs from the psoralen family. The combination of a psoralen drug and ultraviolet light is called **psoralen photochemotherapy.** Psoralen compounds include **trioxsalen** (Trisoralen) and **methoxsalen** (Oxsoralen). These drugs are also discussed later in the chapter as melanizing agents. Although trioxsalen is the safer choice as a melanizing agent, methoxsalen is more effective for photochemotherapy.

Methoxsalen is a photosensitizer that increases epidermal penetration of ultraviolet light. When methoxsalen is given systemically (0.6 ml/kg) twice per week in conjunction with phototherapy, 90% of cases of psoriasis clear within 20 sessions and 97% within 30 sessions. This is all the more remarkable because only people with the most severe psoriasis receive this treatment.

Unfortunately, photochemotherapy must be reserved for severe refractory cases because of significant adverse effects. Acutely adverse effects, such as erythema, pruritus, nausea, headache, and dizziness are mild and rarely occur. With chronic therapy, the skin often ages, thins, and exhibits characteristic freckles. Cutaneous carcinoma and neuritis have also been associated with photochemotherapy, and nail dystrophy and toxic hepatitis occur rarely. When photochemotherapy is employed, care must be taken to protect the skin and eyes from sunlight until the drug is substantially metabolized after 12–24 hours. To prevent risk of cataracts, ultraviolet-blocking sunglasses must be worn throughout the day after administration of methoxsalen. Photochemotherapy is contraindicated during pregnancy and in clients with bullous disorders, skin cancer, photosensitivity disorders, carcinomas, or cataracts. Photochemotherapy is contraindicated in clients with a history of exposure to arsenic or x-rays, since such individuals are at increased risk of carcinomas. Methoxsalen is administered 2 hours prior to exposure ultraviolet light.

Preparations and Administration

Methoxsalen (Oxsoralen)
Capsules

Antimetabolites

Systemic antimetabolites, like psoralen photochemotherapy, are a last resort for treatment of severe, recalcitrant cases of psoriasis. The usual antimetabolite employed for psoriasis is **methotrexate,** although hydroxyurea and aminopterin have been used. Methotrexate inhibits cell proliferation. Inhibition of proliferation of epidermal cells provides the therapeutic value in psoriasis. However, at the same time, inhibition of cell proliferation occurs in the bone marrow, intestinal and buccal mucosa, hair follicles, testes, and urinary bladder, resulting in serious adverse effects such as anemia, leukopenia, thrombocytopenia, bleeding, ulcerative stomatitis, diarrhea, hemorrhagic enteritis, oral bleeding, alopecia, oligospermia, and cystitis. In addition, methotrexate, especially in high doses, cause a cumulative hepatotoxicity (liver atrophy, fatty liver, fibrosis, cirrhosis, and necrosis). Other hepatotoxic drugs, including alcohol, must be avoided during methotrexate therapy. *Before being placed on methotrexate therapy, clients must be warned that the drug can cause serious and even fatal adverse reactions.* Because the rapid proliferation of cells necessary for fetal development is adversely affected, methotrexate is contraindicated in pregnancy. *Women should be advised to use contraceptive measures both during treatment and for at least 8 weeks after methotrexate treatment is terminated.* Preexisting disorders of blood cells, the kidney, or liver are additional contraindications.

Methotrexate is readily absorbed after oral administration, reaching peak serum concentrations in 1–2 hours. It is 50% bound by plasma proteins and may be potentiated by other highly bound drugs such as phenytoin, salicylates, sulfonamides, sulfonylureas, and tetracyclines. The drug is excreted largely unchanged by the kidney with an elimination half-life of 24–48 hours.

Preparations and Administration

Methotrexate
Tablets, powder or solution for injection
Recommended Doses: For psoriasis, 10–35 mg PO 1 day each week in 1–3 doses or 25–50 mg IM once weekly. Psoriasis typically clears in 3–6 weeks, after which minimal maintenance doses can be instituted to maintain control.

Retinoids

Etretinate (Tegison), a synthetic retinoid related to vitamin A, was introduced in 1986 for treatment of recalcitrant psoriasis. It is reserved for cases not responsive to corticosteroids, tars, psoralens and ultraviolet light, or methotrexate. Approximately 13% of clients with severe psoriasis respond to the recommended 4–9 month course of therapy. Etretinate does not provide a cure for psoriasis and relapse typically occurs within 2 months after treatment is discontinued. The adverse effects associated with etretinate resemble the symptoms of hypervitaminosis A. The most serious problems include intracranial hypertension, hepatitis, skeletal hyperostosis, and opacities or abrasions of the cornea. Less serious but more common adverse reactions are peeling of skin from the palms, soles, face, or fingertips, loss of hair, chapped lips, drying of the nasal mucosa, dry skin, itching, rash, bone or joint pain, and fatigue. Side effects occurring less often have included photosensitivity, nosebleeds, eyelid or eyeball abnormalities, and gastrointestinal complaints. *Etrinate should be administered with food to minimize gastrointestinal upset.* Etretinate is contraindicated for use during pregnancy because of a serious risk of birth defects.

Preparations and Administration

Etretinate (Tegison)
Capsules
Recommended Doses: For initial treatment, 0.75–1.0 mg/kg/day PO in divided doses. For maintenance, 0.5–0.75 mg/kg/day.

Drug Eruptions

Drug eruptions are the most common of all adverse reactions to drug therapy. Most chemicals that are administered systemically elicit drug eruptions in a fraction of clients (see Appendix 53B at the end of the chapter). The frequency, severity, and latency of eruptions varies tremendously. Dermatologic reactions vary from a mild rash or fixed drug eruption to life-threatening lupus-like reactions, toxic epidermal necrolysis, exfoliative dermatitis, or Stevens-Johnson syndrome. Most skin eruptions are hypersensitivity reactions caused by sensitized lymphocytes that ordinarily occur after a sensitizing dose has stimulated formation of the sensitized lymphocytes. A later exposure to an eliciting dose of the same drug triggers the reaction. Less commonly, skin eruptions may be due to accumulation of the drug in the skin, pharmacological actions of the drug on the skin, or actions on cutaneous appendages or blood vessels. With multiple drug regimens, the last drug added is most likely to be the cause of skin eruptions, although some eruptions appear only after years of using an offending agent. Rash most often appears hours or days after drug administration, whereas urticaria (hives) occurs usually in minutes.

Benign Skin Eruptions

Skin rash is a nonspecific designation: the rash may be measles-like **(morbilliform);** it may consist of small, solid, and flat spots **(maculopapular);** or it may consist of diffuse, reddish, inflammatory swelling **(erythema).** Most drugs produce a rash of generalized distribution, but a few produce recurrent eruptions in a particular circumscribed patch of skin or mucous membrane **(fixed drug eruption)** each time the drug is employed.

Other kinds of relatively benign skin eruptions occur less commonly than rash. **Acneiform eruptions,** resembling acne but without comedones (blackheads or whiteheads), are most common with steroids. **Lichenoid eruptions** resemble lichen planus, appearing initially as angular papules (solid elevations) that merge to become a patch of scaly plaques. Clients with **erythema nodosum** have painful red nodules usually on the leg above the shin bone or on the arms. Sulfonamides, oral contraceptives, and halides are the most common drug causes, but this condition is more often associated with upper respiratory tract infections.

Next to rashes, **urticaria** is the most often encountered eruption; it appears as characteristic fluid-filled wheals or pockets of edema. Urticaria, also called *hives,* is an anaphylactoid reaction limited to the skin. Clients may have the same reaction from certain foods, vaccines, insect bites or stings, viral infections, and food additives (preservatives, colorings, and other agents). The characteristic fluid-filled wheals of urticaria are caused by local release of histamine from mast cells in the dermis. Acute urticaria responds well to oral antihistamines, although systemic corticosteroids are sometimes required. Even without medication, the hives disappear in a few days if the causative factor is eliminated. In the majority of cases, chronic hives resolve without specific treatment after 1–2 years. Clients should avoid stress, caffeine, alcohol, nicotine, and aspirin. Oral antihistamines can be useful but are less effective than in acute urticaria.

Purpura is a dermatologic manifestation of internal bleeding from cutaneous blood vessels that usually indicates impaired coagulation. Often purpura is related to drug-induced thrombocytopenia, but in other cases it is due to nonplatelet factors. Purpura appears as flat, purple, nonblanching skin spots.

Photosensitivity reactions are induced by a wide variety of topical or systemic drugs. Photosensitivity eruptions appear as erythematous rash or areas of gray-blue patches. They can be of immunologic origin **(photoallergic reactions)** if the drug acts as a hapten, stimulating formation of cutaneous antibodies. Alternatively, they can be of nonimmunologic origin **(phototoxic reaction)** if the drug itself is toxic to the skin after photoactivation (producing a form of contact dermatitis) or if the drug increases the penetration and toxic actions of ultraviolet light on the epidermis.

Life-Threatening Skin Eruptions

Erythema multiforme is a skin eruption that ranges in severity from mild to fatal. Vivid red blisters appear symmetrically over the distal extremities, face, lips, and oral mucosa that may be accompanied by malaise and fever. The term **Stevens-Johnson syndrome** is often applied to the life-threatening form in which the large blisters extend to the oral mucosa, pharynx, eyes, and anogenital area. Clients taking penicillin, sulfonamides, and barbiturates are most likely to develop this syndrome. Herpes simplex, echovirus, coxsackievirus, mycoplasma pneumoniae, vaccines, and exposure to x-rays can also cause erythema multiforme, but often the causative factor is never identified.

Three other types of drug eruptions are life-threatening. **Discoid lupus erythematosus (DLE)** is related to systemic lupus erythematosus, an inflammatory disease of connective tissue. In DLE, symptoms are largely confined to the skin, although more severe cases are likely to be associated with internal symptoms typical of systemic lupus. DLE is a chronic autoimmune disorder in which antibodies are formed against the nuclear protein of connective tissue cells in the dermis. Although it often occurs without apparent drug involvement, certain drugs have been noted to cause DLE in the absence of other factors or prior history. *Clients who have systemic lupus should be cautioned that exposure to sunlight can also be an initiating or aggravating factor; thus protection from overexposure to the sun is a principal objective of treatment.*

Discoid lupus erythematosus is characterized by formation of erythematous circumscribed macules and scaling plaques, keratotic plugging of hair follicles, telangiectasia (vascular lesions or angiomas formed from distended small cutaneous vessels), and ultimately skin atrophy. The drugs most often implicated are procainamide (Pronestyl), hydralazine (Apresoline), penicillamine (Cuprimine), isoniazid, antiepileptics, and phenothiazines. Monitoring of antinuclear antibodies and lupus erythematosus tests provide a means of guarding against development of DLE in clients using these drugs. Management of established DLE entails topical steroids, systemic antimalarial drugs (chloroquine, hydroxychloroquine, or quinacrine), or, in recalcitrant cases, systemic corticosteroids.

Exfoliative dermatitis may occur as a drug eruption or a secondary development in atopic, psoriatic, or contact dermatitis, or fungal infections. Common drug causes are antimicrobials (sulfonamides, penicillin, isoniazid) or antiepileptics (phenytoin (Dilantin), barbiturates). The condition consists of a rapidly developing, widespread erythema of the skin that develops into crusting and scaling.

Toxic epidermal necrolysis, also called *scalded skin syndrome* or *Ritter-Lyell syndrome,* is a condition in which large sections of skin peel off in sheets. In infants, this disease usually occurs in response to a penicillin-resistant staphylococci, but in adults, it is usually a drug toxicity. Antimicrobials and antiepileptics are the most commonly implicated agents. This condition is often fatal because of electrolyte and fluid imbalance. Management is similar to that employed for burn victims.

Skin Infections and Topical Anti-Infectives

Although the skin routinely comes into contact with a variety of pathogenic organisms, the stratum corneum ordinarily provides an adequate barrier to penetration. Pathogens that do penetrate are for the most part destroyed by chemical and immunologic mechanisms in the lower skin strata. Some microorganisms are inherently pathogenic, causing systemic infection whenever they gain entry into the body or superficial infections when confined to the outer epidermis. Other microorganisms that are normally nonpathogenic may result in opportunistic infections if host defense mechanisms are impoverished by drugs, burns, anemia, cancer, metabolic disorders, wounds, or insertion of foreign bodies or therapeutic instruments. Often, hospitalized patients have compromised defense mechanisms for one or more of these reasons and are thus susceptible to nosocomial (hospital-acquired) infections. The pathogens most often implicated in these infections include *Staphylococcus aureus, Escherichia coli, Enterobacter, Klebsiella, Providencia, Serratia, Pseudomonas, Proteus, Candida,* and *Flavobacterium.*

Medical asepsis, the sanitizing of instruments and surfaces, is used to minimize hospital-acquired infections. The chemicals employed in sanitization are called **disinfectants,** and destroy organisms on equipment or other inanimate objects but would be toxic to living tissue. An ideal disinfectant is germicidal, rapidly effective, penetrating, active in the presence of organic matter such as blood, sputum, or fecal matter, stable in the presence of detergents, noncorrosive, and inexpensive.

Surgical asepsis by contrast aims at destroying all microorganisms in the area of a wound or incision. Surgical asepsis is achieved primarily through **sterilization** of instruments, utensils, and fluids. The accepted methods of sterilization include autoclaving (steaming under pressure) of most utensils; treatment with ethylene oxide, a gaseous sterilant, for heat-labile substances and heat-sensitive instruments; and hot air ovens for glassware.

Drugs employed on skin or mucous membranes to prevent growth of microorganisms are called **antiseptics.** Although some antiseptics are dilute versions of disinfectants, most are distinct agents because of the special requirements for effectiveness in antiseptic applications.

Antiseptics

The therapeutic index is a crucial consideration for antiseptics, since the agent must be considerably more toxic to the surface pathogens than to the adjacent living tissue. The relative effectiveness of the various topical antiseptics has not been well studied, but most antiseptic agents exhibit a broad antimicrobial spectrum. Vegetative forms of bacteria are the most sensitive to antiseptics, followed by fungi, lipophilic viruses, tubercle bacilli, and hydrophilic viruses, in that order. Bacterial and fungal spores, however, are resistant to most antiseptics.

Topical antiseptics and antimicrobials are less effective than commonly thought by most lay people and even medical personnel. Although topical therapy seldom provides a benefit comparable to systemic antimicrobial treatment, topical agents are indicated in certain instances: (1) in preoperative preparation, (2) as an adjunct to systemic antimicrobials for recalcitrant infections, and (3) as an alternative to systemic anti-infectives for resistant superficial infections or when the patient is hypersensitive or otherwise adversely affected by systemic drugs.

Antiseptics act by a variety of mechanisms. Some, such as phenol and alcohol, denature microbial proteins. Others, such as the quaternary ammonium compounds, disrupt the cell membranes of microorganisms by lowering the surface tension of the aqueous medium, resulting in cell lysis. Still others, such as the heavy metal compounds, inhibit essential metabolic steps of microbial cells: mercury and silver compounds, for example, inhibit sulfhydryl enzymes.

Before applying antiseptics, the nurse should ensure that dirt, soil, organic matter, or other contaminants are removed from the area since such materials not only harbor microorganisms but also provide a physical barrier restricting access of the antiseptic and may chemically inactivate particular antiseptics. The nurse should understand that various antiseptic drugs differ in spectrum and effectiveness and are not interchangeable. The wide variety of drugs used as antiseptics are summarized in Table 53–3. Here we will discuss only two of the more useful ones.

Hexachlorophene

Hexachlorophene (pHisoHex, Germa-Medica, Septisol) is widely used in hospitals, although with increasing caution in the last decade. It is found in various soaps, shampoos, creams, lotions, and ointments and is effective mainly against gram-positive bacteria. It is an excellent choice for preoperative scrubs or for hand cleaning by dentists or persons involved in food preparation, because most potentially pathogenic bacteria found on the hands are gram-positive. If used daily, hexachlorophene accumulates in the skin, creating a film that provides a 95–99% reduction in gram-positive bacteria.

The lack of effectiveness of hexachlorophene against gram-negative bacteria and nonbacterial microbes is a distinct disadvantage when hexachlorophene is used repeatedly without other anti-infectives. After a week or more of daily use, an excess of gram-negative bacteria, candida, and other nonsusceptible organisms appear on the skin, often resulting in infection.

The use of hexachlorophene for bathing young infants in hospital nurseries is controversial. Hexachlorophene has been effective in controlling epidemic staphylococcal infections that sometimes occur in hospital nurseries and which can culminate in fatal toxic epidermal necrolysis. Conversely, daily bathing of infants increases the number of gram-negative infections and can result in significant systemic absorption, especially if the infant is underweight, premature, or has excoriated skin. Neurologic problems, including lethargy, twitching, diplopia, convulsions, brain damage, and death can result. *The AMA recommends that hexachlorophene not be used routinely to bathe infants.*

Systemic toxicity can also occur in adults when hexachlorophene is applied excessively to the skin, or especially when applied to mucosal membranes (such as the vagina) or burned, abraded, or denuded skin. The risk of systemic toxicity can be reduced by immediately rinsing hexachlorophene from the skin with ethanol. This procedure eliminates the extended bacteriostatic action of hexachlorophene that occurs when it is allowed to remain as a film on the epidermis, however, making it no more effective than nonmedicated soap. An occasional individual will experience hypersensitivity reactions to hexachlorophene even in the absence of systemic absorption. *Hexachlorophene should be stored in tight, opaque containers.*

Preparations and Administration

Hexachlorophene

Liquid soap (Germa-Medica MG, Septi-Soft, pHiso-Hex, Soy-Dome Cleanser, WescoHEX), solution (Septisol), foam (Septisol), sponge (pHiso Scrub)

Recommended Doses: For surgical scrubbing, a preliminary wash (30 seconds) with hexachlorophene is followed by a 2- to 4-minute sudsy scrub with or without a hard brush. The hexachlorophene is then thoroughly rinsed off.

Table 53–3
Properties of Antiseptic Agents

Antiseptic	Characteristics
Phenol-type	
Phenol	Denatures protein of pathogens. Effective against bacteria, fungi, and lipophilic viruses. Ineffective against hydrophilic viruses and spores of bacteria and fungi. Frequently toxic to host cells. Found in Chloraseptic and Cepastat mouthwashes, mouth sprays, and lozenges.
Cresol	More potent and toxic than phenol. Used as a saponated cresol solution (Lysol) to disinfect inanimate objects and surfaces.
Metacresol	An isomer of cresol found in Obtundia cream and spray.
Thymol	A relative of cresol found in many gargles, mouthwashes, and vaginal deodorants. Probably ineffective in concentrations used.
Chlorothymol	Similar to thymol.
Hexachlorophene	Most widely used phenol-type antiseptic. Found in pHisoHex, Germa-Medica, Septisol, and in various soaps, shampoos, creams, lotions, and ointments. Effective only against gram-positive bacteria. When hexachlorophene is used routinely, gram-negative bacteria proliferate on the skin.
Resorcinol	Germicidal spectrum similar to phenol but less potent. Used in topical lotions and ointments. Dubious value in dermatitis.
Hexylresorcinol	Odorless, nonstaining relative of resorcinol. Used for minor cuts, scrapes, burns, and scalds. Found in Listerine and Sucrets throat lozenges.
Parabens	Widely employed as preservatives in various dermatologic preparations. Frequently implicated as a cause of contact dermatitis.
Tricosan	Active against gram-positive bacteria. Found in Rhulicaine and Solarcaine, products marketed for relief of minor burns, scrapes, or cuts.
Alcohols/aldehydes/acids	
Ethanol	Effective against most pathogenic bacteria at concentrations of 50–70%. Poorly effective against viruses, fungi, or spores. Cannot be applied to open wounds because of irritant effect.
Isopropanol	More germicidal than ethanol.
Formaldehyde	Used to disinfect inanimate objects, to preserve cadavers, or to fix histologic specimens. Kills all organisms at concentrations between 2% and 8%. Can be used to harden the palms or soles in treating hyperhidrosis.
Glutaraldehyde	Used as a sterilizing agent (Cidex). Less volatile then formaldehyde, but corrosive, explosive, unstable, and irritating to tissue.
Acetic acid	Used in some vaginal douches. Suppresses trichomonas, candida, and other organisms and is spermatocidal.
Lactic acid	Used similarly to acetic acid. Less volatile, so contact time is increased.
Boric acid	A mild, nonirritating antiseptic of modest value used in ophthalmic and otic preparations. Potential systemic toxicity. Should be applied only to intact tissues and never extensively.
Benzoic acid	Employed mainly as a preservative. Inhibits bacteria and fungi and is nontoxic unless ingested in large amounts.
Halogens	
Iodine	Effective against all pathogens and spores. Efficacy unaffected by body fluids, exudates, or tissue debris. Stains tissue and clothing. Corrodes the gastrointestinal tract if taken orally. Often dissolved in alcohol (iodine tincture).
Povidone-iodine	A loose complex that releases iodine after application. Povidone is also weakly antibacterial. Used as a surgical scrub. Relative to hexachlorophene, provides greater initial suppression of bacteria but shorter period of effectiveness. Found in Betadine, Pharmadine, and Frepp.
Chlorine	Effective as a sanitizing agent. Kills most bacteria, but acid-fast bacteria (such as *Mycobacterium tuberculosis*) are resistant.
Chlorophors	Sodium hypochlorite, oxychlorosene, chlorinated lime, and halazone are chlorophors, used as indirect sources of chlorine. Sodium hypochlorite is used in root canal therapy and to disinfect swimming pools.

Table 53–3
Properties of Antiseptic Agents (*continued*)

Antiseptic	Characteristics
Oxidizing agents	
Hydrogen peroxide	Sometimes used to cleanse wounds. Has weak antiseptic action, creates an effervescence of liberated oxygen that can help free tissue debris.
Benzoyl peroxide	Releases oxygen more gradually. Especially effective against anaerobic bacteria. Found in acne products such as Clearasil and Dry and Clear.
Potassium permanganate	Antiseptic and antifungal activity but its value is impaired by tissue debris.
Dyes	
Gentian dye	Active against gram-negative bacteria and fungi but causes permanent pigmentation of tissue.
Amanacrine	Active against many bacteria and fungi. Used in some topical vaginal preparations.
Heavy metals	
Mercurials	Only bacteriostatic, have poor therapeutic index, and do not penetrate tissues well. Mercurials include nitromersol (Metaphen), hydroxyphenylmercuric chloride (with cresols as Mercresin), phenylmercuric nitrate (Phe-Mer-Nite tincture), hydroxyphenylacetate, and thimerosal (Mersol, Merthiolate).
Silver nitrate	Highly germicidal but also caustic to tissue. Forms staining bluish black precipitates with chloride ions, so poor tissue penetration. Used as an ophthalmic solution in neonates to prevent gonococcal infections of the eye but frequently causes conjunctivitis.
Silver sulfadiazine	An organic silver compound used to prevent sepsis in severe burns. The silver is released slowly so precipitation is minimal. The sulfadiazine component provides broad antibacterial activity typical of sulfonamides, but resistance may develop. This drug may cause a burning sensation when applied. Requires monitoring of serum sulfa concentrations and sulfonamide side effects.
Zinc salts	Used as antiseptics as well as astringents, corrosives, and antiperspirants in ointments, lotions, powders, pastes, and shampoos for poison ivy, chafing, acne, pruritus, dermatitis, psoriasis, tinea, and seborrheic dermatitis of the scalp.
Surface-active quaternary ammonium compounds	
Benzalkonium	Acts as a detergent. Broadly bactericidal, but some gram-negative bacteria are resistant. Activity reduced by organic material, elevated pH, or soaps. Products include solutions (Germicin, Spensomide), tinctures (Zephiran), and aerosols (Bactine).
Cetylpyridinium	Used in various mouthwashes (Cepacol, Scope).
Methylbenzethonium	Found in topical diaper rash products (e.g., Diaparene).
Benzethonium	Found in topical diaper rash products (e.g., Methakote).
Biguanides	
Chlorhexidine	More effective against gram-negative than gram-positive bacteria. Marketed as a tincture (Hibitane) or emulsion (Hibiclens). Safer than hexachlorophene for washing neonates. Hypersensitivity can occur.
Sulfur	
Sulfur	Broadly germicidal. Dries oily skin. Chronic use can cause dermatitis. Used in acne preparations, such as Transact, Xerac, Liquimat, Fortex, Acne-Aid, Epi-Clear, and Postacne.
Salicylanilides and carbanilides	
Dibromsalan	Suppresses gram-negative bacteria but can cause contact dermatitis. Used in deodorant soaps.
Tribromsalan	Similar to dibromsalen.
Cloflucarban	Suppresses gram-negative and gram-positive bacteria. Used in deodorant soaps.
Triclocarban	Similar to cloflucarban. Used in Dial soap.

Benzalkonium

Benzalkonium is a detergent (surface-acting agent) that interferes with the stability of microbial cell membranes. It is broadly bactericidal, but some gram-negative bacteria are resistant and its germicidal efficacy is reduced by the presence of organic material, elevated pH, or soaps. Benzalkonium is used for general antisepsis and preoperative preparation. *The skin should be rinsed thoroughly before applying benzalkonium.* Some people experience contact dermatitis with chronic use. *Occlusive dressings should not be used with benzalkonium or other surface-active antiseptics since this procedure will increase skin irritation. Surface-acting agents should not be used concomitantly with iodine, kaolin, lanolin, silver nitrate, potassium permanganate, zinc oxide, or other heavy metal salts. Antiseptics in the surface-acting group should be kept in airtight containers away from light. Benzalkonium is not an adequate disinfectant for sterilizing surgical instruments. It may be corrosive to metal instruments.*

Preparations and Administration

Benzalkonium
Aqueous solutions (Germicin, Spensomide, Zephiran), tincture (Zephiran), aerosol (Bactine)

Superficial Bacterial Infections and Topical Antibacterials

Bacterial Infections of the Skin

The most common bacterial infections involving the skin are impetigo, folliculitis, furuncles and carbuncles, and erysipelas. **Impetigo** is an acute, superficial infection caused by a group A beta-hemolytic streptococcus or less commonly by *Staphylococcus aureus.* It occurs most commonly in children, but it may occur in adults in poor health. In severe impetigo infections, ulcerations may occur, in which case the condition is called **ecthyma. Folliculitis** is usually caused by *Staphylococcus aureus.* It appears as an inflammation of the hair follicles in which a pustule or nodule is located at the follicular opening. The infection may be superficial or may extend deep into the follicle, necessitating systemic antibiotics.

Furuncles or *boils* are acute perifollicular nodules caused by staphylococci that often develop following folliculitis. Furuncles appear most commonly on the face, neck, breasts, and buttocks. Maceration, irritation of the skin, or poor hygiene are predisposing factors. **Carbuncles** are clusters of large, deep furuncles that drain through the deeper skin layers, often causing extensive sloughing that leaves large scars. Topical antibacterials may be useful with mild furuncles, but severe furuncles and all cases of carbuncles require systemic antibacterial therapy. **Erythrasma,** mainly a disease of the tropics, is a superficial cellulitis caused by *Corynebacterium minutissimum.* Erythrasma responds well to systemic antibacterials such as erythromycin or tetracycline.

Topical Antibacterial Drugs

The main value of topical antibacterials is for prophylaxis against bacterial infection of minor skin abrasions, since these drugs have only a modest value in treating established superficial skin infections. For example, impetigo, folliculitis, and erysipelas clearly respond better to systemic antibacterial therapy. Mild cases of furuncles may be advantageously treated with topical agents, but severe cases require systemic medication. Carbuncles always require systemic treatment.

Neomycin (Myciguent) is an aminoglycoside antibiotic. Like other agents in this family, neomycin causes a misreading of the genetic code by bacterial ribosomes. It has a broad spectrum of activity, being effective against both gram-positive and gram-negative bacteria. *Staphylococcus aureus* is sensitive as are some varieties of *streptococci,* but *Streptococcus pyrogenes, Streptococcus viridans,* fungi, and viruses are resistant. Neomycin is highly toxic when used systemically, causing hepatotoxicity and neurotoxicity and is, in any case, poorly absorbed from the gastrointestinal tract after oral administration. As a topical agent, it is relatively devoid of adverse effects, although skin rash (an allergic dermatitis) occasionally develops. *Nurses need to caution clients to cease treatment if irritation occurs and to report the problem immediately to the physician. Once a client develops a reaction to neomycin, he or she should be warned about possible sensitivity to other aminoglycoside antibiotics. The client should wear an identification bracelet warning of sensitivity. The client and family need to be given the names of drugs in this group to which the client may be sensitive.*

Bacitracin (Baciguent) is bactericidal only against gram-positive spirochetes, cocci, and bacilli. It is a surface-acting agent that impairs microbial membrane function. Because of nephrotoxic effects that accompany systemic use, bacitracin is now used only in topical applications, principally for prophylaxis against infection of minor wounds. Hypersensitivity reactions to topical application occur rarely.

Polymyxin B (Aerosporin) is effective only against gram-negative bacteria, and thus has a complementary spectrum to that of bacitracin. It disrupts the cell membrane of susceptible organisms by a detergent action. Polymyxin B is not significantly absorbed from the intestine if given orally; therefore, its major uses are in skin infections that involve gram-negative bacteria (especially *Pseudomonas).* It is

Nursing Observations for Use of Topical Anti-Infectives for Skin Infections

THERAPEUTIC GOAL	Eradication of the infection, control of the infection and associated symptoms of pruritus and discomfort, prevention of damage to healthy skin, and prevention of secondary infection.
PREADMINISTRATION ASSESSMENT	
Baseline Data	Note skin characteristics: color, texture, turgor, vascularity, moisture, and temperature. Observe for inflammation, lesions, blisters, drainage, or erythema. Look for predisposing factors such as recent hospitalization (a nosocomial infection), trauma injuries, emotional stress, or sexual contact with a carrier. Obtain laboratory tests including culture of exudate or tissue to determine identity of the pathogen.
EVALUATION OF DRUG RESPONSE	
For Therapeutic Benefit	Monitor evidences of skin infection for eradication or control of the pathogen.
For Adverse Effects or Drug Interactions	Monitor for adverse effects and drug interactions specific for each kind of medication (see individual drug discussions).
For Compliance	Evaluate the client's compliance with all facets of the therapeutic regimen by careful observation, interviewing, and review of progress. Report compliance problems to the physician and act as client-advocate when changes in the therapeutic regimen seem indicated.

occasionally employed by parenteral routes for severe systemic infections of the meninges or urinary tract. Hypersensitivity reactions are not common, and systemic effects do not occur after topical application because of poor absorption, even when the medication is applied to open lesions. Polymyxin B is an ingredient of numerous topical powders, tablets, and ophthalmic solutions.

Three topical antibacterials marketed in formulations designed to prevent bacterial colonization of extensive burn injuries, mafenide (Sulfamylon), nitrofurazone (Furacin), and gentamycin (Garamycin), are discussed later in the chapter in the section on treatment of burns. Other topical antibiotics are seldom used. **Tetracyclines,** including tetracycline (Achromycin), chlortetracycline (Aureomycin), and oxytetracycline (Terramycin), are available singly or in combinations as ointments or powders for topical application. However, topical administration of tetracyclines should be avoided because of the high frequency of sensitization reactions.

Preparations and Administration

Bacitracin
Ointment, combination ointments and powders, generally with neomycin and polymyxin B.

Chloramphenicol (Chlormycetin)
Cream

Erythromycin (Ilotycin)
Ointment

Neomycin
Ointment or cream (Myciguent); nonprescription combinations, usually with bacitracin and polymyxin B (e.g., Neosporin, Mycitracin, Triple Antibiotic, Tri-Salve, Mity-Mycin).

Superficial Viral Infections and Drug Treatments

Herpes Viral Infections

The common viral infections of the skin are herpes virus infections, warts, and molluscum contagiosum. The herpes viruses responsible for infections include herpes simplex type I, herpes simplex type II, and herpes zoster. Herpes simplex type I produces cold sores, erosive lesions of the lips, perioral region, and mucous membranes of the mouth (Figure 53–5). Primary infections typically clear up spontaneously after 1–2 weeks, but sensory nerve cells supplying the region of infection are frequently invaded and remain infected for the rest of the patient's life, periodically precipitating herpes eruptions. The dormant virus can be activated by febrile infections, emotional stress, excessive exposure to sunlight, certain foods, or drugs. Herpes simplex type II, or herpes progenitalis, causes vesicular le-

Nursing Diagnoses and Interventions for Use of Topical Anti-Infectives for Skin Infections

Nursing Diagnoses	*Related Interventions*
TO ENHANCE DRUG BENEFITS OR REDUCE DRUG REQUIREMENTS	
Alteration in comfort related to pain and pruritus from skin infections	Employ antipruritics and analgesics as required; apply emollients, humectants, or drying agents as appropriate. Teach clients to avoid excessive warmth and rough fabrics.
Impairment of skin integrity related to lesions	Protect lesions from environment as appropriate. Protect surrounding uninfected areas with emollients as appropriate. Avoid secondary infections.
Impaired self-esteem related to appearance and need to prevent infection of others	Teach client how to avoid exposing others to the infection. Teach methods of asepsis and sterilization if required, and isolation during most contagious phase (with herpes zoster). Teach client to avoid picking lesions. Teach client to sterilize clothes and bedding for parasitic infections. Discuss ethical considerations of preventive health behavior.
TO ENSURE SAFE AND EFFICACIOUS DRUG USE	
Knowledge deficit related to drug regimen	Teach client about the nature of the infection, likely sources of infection, likely course of the disease, and the rationale for the medical regimen. Teach client not to use topical anti-infectives when infections are serious or persistent but to seek medical help. Topical anti-infectives are as specific in their spectra of antimicrobial activity as systemic drugs. Inform client of the importance of determining the identity of the pathogen when the infection is on the skin surface. Advise client not to treat unidentified infections with medications purchased over the counter. Educate client about prevention of skin infections and the need to protect others from infection if the condition is contagious. Teach client nondrug measures of skin care: good hygiene, avoidance of chemical irritants, and avoidance of excessive exposure to sunlight or wind. Provide the client with a list of adverse effects and drug interactions for each drug in the regimen and explain what to do if any of these occur. Teach client proper application of topical anti-infective drugs. Before application, the skin should be cleansed and rinsed of dirt, organic matter, or other contaminants. Carefully instruct client if the antiseptic or anti-infective is one that is harmful when applied to healthy skin adjacent to an infection, to sensitive skin or mucous membranes, or with occlusive dressings.

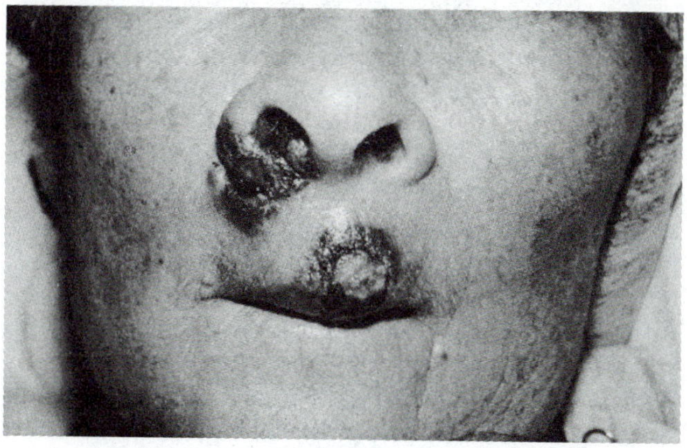

Figure 53–5
Lesions caused by the herpes simplex virus. From Theodore Rosen, Marilyn B. Lanning, and Marcia J. Hill, *The Nurse's Atlas of Dermatology.* Copyright © 1983 by Theodore Rosen and Marilyn B. Lanning. Reprinted by permission of Little, Brown and Company.

sions primarily in the mucosal membranes of the genitalia. It is usually transmitted by direct sexual contact and has become increasingly common in recent years. Various complications can occur from herpes infections, including a recurrent stomatitis, vulvo vaginitis, a severe encephalitis, and keratitis (an ophthalmic condition characterized by inflammation, vascularization, and scarring of the lens). Herpes zoster causes chickenpox and "shingles" and requires systemic medication (see Chapter 46).

Drugs for Treating Herpes Simplex Virus

Herpes simplex virus is one of the few viruses for which specific antiviral drugs exist. Four principal antiviral preparations are available for topical use in herpes simplex; three of these are used mainly for treating herpes simplex keratitis and have limited value in alleviating the epithelial lesions. **Idoxuridine** is an antimetabolite for herpes viruses, substituting for thymidine, a natural component of herpes DNA. Some strains of herpes are resistant, however. Idoxuridine occasionally causes irritation, inflammation, pruritus, or edema when applied to the eyes, and photosensitivity and other allergic reactions sometimes occur. Although idoxuridine is mutagenic in laboratory animals, it has not yet been shown to be carcinogenic in humans but should be used cautiously by pregnant women.

Vidarabine is available in topical preparations for herpes keratoconjunctivitis or epithelial keratitism and for systemic administration in herpes encephalitis. Systemic absorption does not occur after topical administration, and vidarabine causes less irritation to the cornea. Like idoxuridine, vidarabine has mutagenic potential. When clients apply this medication to the eye, adverse reactions include lacrimation, foreign body sensation, irritation, photophobia, and sensitivity; when using the medication systemically, clients may have gastrointestinal reactions (nausea, vomiting, diarrhea, anorexia). Psychiatric reactions (hallucinations, psychosis, confusion, ataxia) and blood cell dyscrasias may occur as well.

Trifluridine is used topically in herpes and alleviates keratoconjunctivitis and epithelial keratitis. When the drug is applied to the eyes, clients complain of transient stinging. Other adverse effects on the eye include superficial punctate keratopathy, epithelial keratopathy, and hypersensitivity reactions.

Acyclovir (Zolvirox), first marketed in 1982, represents an important advance in treatment of epithelial and mucosal lesions associated with Herpes simplex. Acyclovir is active against both type I and type II herpes simplex virus and is the first agent that usefully treats genital lesions associated with type II herpes simplex. Acyclovir ointment is indicated for treatment of initial herpes genitalis. Intravenous infusion or oral administration of acyclovir is indicated for severe cases in clients with no immune system disorders. Acyclovir is very effective in reducing the healing time of initial infections; unfortunately, it does not decrease spontaneous recurrence of infection from herpes viruses that have invaded sensory nerve cells nor does it prevent transmission of the infection. Acyclovir is well tolerated when administered topically. With intravenous administration, phlebitis may occur at the site of injection. After oral or intravenous administration, the principal adverse effects are rash or hives, and occasional instances of lethargy, agitation, confusion, or tremors. Acyclovir is excreted by the kidney; if the maximum dose is exceeded, there is a risk of crystal formation in the renal tubules. Probenecid (Benemid) and acyclovir compete for the same renal tubular secretory mechanism and therefore retard each other's elimination. Oral and injectable forms of acyclovir are discussed more fully in Chapter 48.

Oral lesions caused by herpes simplex virus are frequently painful, requiring symptomatic relief. Mouthwashes containing local anesthetics such as lidocaine (Xylocaine), tetracaine (Protocaine), hexylcaine (Cyclaine), dyclonine (Dyclone), cyclomethycaine (Surfacaine), or benzocaine (Hurricaine) are useful. Diphenhydramine oral elixir is also helpful.

Preparations and Administration

Acyclovir (Zolvirox)
Ointment, powder for injection, oral capsules

Idoxuridine (Dendrid, Herplex Liquifilm, Stoxil)
Ophthalmic solution or ointment

Trifluridine (Viroptic)
Ophthalmic solution

Vidarabine (Vira-A)
Injection solution, ophthalmic ointment

Warts and Caustics

Warts are benign epithelial tumors caused by a papovavirus, a small DNA-type virus. Common warts are firm, round, well-demarcated protuberances that are known as plantar warts when they occur on the palms of the hands and the soles of the feet; facial warts sometimes appear as flat warts. No treatment for warts is ideal. Cryosurgery (with liquid nitrogen or solid CO_2) is generally effective for common warts; surgery is useful for solitary warts. Chemical caustics have been used for removal of warts as well as moles and hyperplasias. Some agents in this category include glacial acetic acid, phenol, trichloroacetic acid (Tri-Chlor), dichloroacetic acid (Bichloracetate), podophyllum (Podoben, Podofin), salicylic acid (Freezone, Salacid, Wart-off, and others), lactic acid, cantharidin (Verrex, Verusol, and others), formaldehyde, glutaraldehyde, tretinoin, and silver nitrate. Caustics destroy tissue to which they are applied and must be applied judiciously.

Superficial Fungal Infections and Topical Antifungal Drugs

Superficial fungal infections are probably the most common type of infectious disorders, occurring in perhaps 10% of the population in the United States and a much higher percentage worldwide. Of the thousands of types of fungi, fewer than 100 varieties are pathogenic to humans. Many of the pathogenic fungi, which occur as yeasts or molds, are obligate parasites that can survive only on living protoplasm. Some are dimorphic, growing as yeasts at one temperature and molds at another.

Diagnosis of superficial fungal infections entails inspection, sometimes under special lighting, microscopic examination, or culturing of specimens. For systemic infections, serologic laboratory tests further aid in establishing the diagnosis. Most mycotic infections are superficial and chronic. Systemic mycotic infections are increasingly common and fatal in about 5% of instances (see Chapter 48).

A given variety of fungus can produce differing symptoms at various anatomic sites. For example, *Trichophyton mentagrophytes* can cause tinea pedis (athlete's foot), tinea cruris ("jock itch"), or tinea capitis (ringworm). The anatomic site of infection can influence selection of a drug for treatment. A relatively strong drug that might be acceptable for use on the scalp or hands might be too irritating for use on the lips, eyelids, or genitalia. An ointment would be inappropriate for use on the scalp but could be the formulation selected for less hairy areas. Keratolytic agents can be useful for chronic, scaly, thickened lesions, while wet compresses may have value for oozing lesions. Generally, localized fungal infections are more intensely inflamed, since the intensity of the inflammation is primarily responsible for limiting spread of the infection. Widespread distribution of fungal infection indicates a weak immunologic response and will not respond well to treatment. Each dermatophyte responds differently to the various antifungal drugs available. Sensitivity testing is not necessarily required for acute, localized infections but can be advantageous for treatment of recalcitrant, chronic, and widespread infections. The common superficial fungal infections are dermatophytosis, tinea versicolor, and candidiasis.

Dermatophytosis

Dermatophytosis is a superficial infection caused by fungi of the *Microsporum, Trichophyton,* and *Epidermophyton* genera. These fungi invade only dead tissue such as the stratum corneum, nails, and hair. There are numerous infective dermatophytes, but only 10 of these account for 95% of infections. It is often difficult to differentiate the exact organism involved in a given case. For this reason, traditional classification of dermatophyte infections has been based on the anatomic site involved. **Tinea pedis** (athlete's foot), which is especially common, is usually found in the webspace of the toes, especially the third and fourth interdigital spaces. When it occurs as vesicular lesions on the plantar skin of the sole, it can be very painful and can impede ambulation. Some cases are characterized by scaly lesions over the entire plantar surface of the feet and sometimes one or more hands as well.

Many drugs are effective against dermatophytes (Table 53–4), but some have broader spectra or greater potency than others. Topical imidazoles are potent and have a broad effectiveness. Lotrimin and Monistat are both widely prescribed and are two of only three antifungal drugs that appear in the top 200 prescription drugs. Econazole was introduced in 1983 and butoconazole in 1986. Another imidazole, **tioconazole,** was approved by the Food and Drug Administration in 1983 but has yet to be marketed. Adverse effects are uncommon with the imidazoles, but occasionally erythema or general urticaria is observed.

Fatty acids, such as **propionic acid, glyceryl tri-**

Table 53–4
Uses of Antifungal Drugs

Drug	Food preservative	Tinea versicolor	Dermatophytes	Candida
Food additives				
Benzoic acid	+			
Parabens	+			
Propionic acid	+			
Sorbic acid	+			
Topical agents — moderate potency				
Castellani paint[a]			+	+
Gentian violet			+	+
Glyceryl triacetate			+	
8-hydroxyquinolone			+	+
Propionic acid			+	
Salicylanilide			+	
Selenium sulfide		+		
Sodium thiosulfate		+		
Thymol in chloroform			+	+
Undecylenic acid			+	
Whitfield's ointment[b]			+	
Topical agents — higher potency				
Candicidin				+
Chlordantoin				+
Ciclopirox		+	+	+
Haloprogin			+	
Imidazoles				
Butoconazole				+
Clotrimazole		+	+	+
Econazole		+	+	+
Miconazole		+	+	+
Nystatin				+
Tolnaftate			+	
Systemic agents — oral				
5-Fluorocytosine				+
Griseofulvin			+	
Imidazole				
Ketoconazole		+	+	+
Systemic agents — IV				
Amphotericin B				+
Imidazole				
Miconazole			+	+

[a]Fuchsin, phenol, resorcinol, acetone, and alcohol.
[b]Benzoic acid and salicylic acid.

acetate, and **undecylenic acid** are effective only for tinea pedis. Undecylenic acid is the most potent of the group. Propionic acid is found in antifungal combinations such as Sopronol, Prophyllin, and Verdefam. **Salicylanilide** is used mainly for tinea capitis. **Tolnaftate** and **haloprogin** are more broadly effective against dermatophytes. Haloprogin can be irritating however. Occasionally, combinations of nonspecific antiseptics are employed for dermatophyte infections. Examples are **Castellani paint,** which contains phenol, resorcinol, acetone, and alcohol, and **Whitfield's ointment,** which contains benzoic acid and salicylic acid.

Clients with tinea pedis should be advised not to wear occlusive footwear such as rubber boots. Nurses should advise them to wash their feet daily, to wear cotton socks, and to change socks at least daily. Similarly, people with other types of dermatophyte infections should wear freshly laundered clothing each day. A lotion should be used in preference to a cream in intertriginous zones to avoid maceration. Clients should be instructed to complete the full course of therapy to minimize the likelihood of recurrence of infection.

IMIDAZOLES

Butoconazole (Femstat)
Vaginal cream

Clotrimazole (Lotrimin or Mycelex)
Cream or solution

Econazole (Spectazole)
Cream

Miconazole
Cream or lotion (Monistat-Derm)

OTHER DRUGS FOR DERMATOPHYTES

Glyceryl Triacetate (Triacetin)
Cream (Enzactin), ointment (Fungacetin)

Haloprogin (Halotex)
Cream

Tolnaftate (Tinactin and Aftate)
Creams, powders, solutions, gels, aerosols, and liquids

Undecylenic Acid (Desenex, Cruex, Caldesene, etc.)
Liquid, foam, ointment, cream, powder, aerosol, or soap, combinations (numerous)

Tinea Versicolor

Tinea versicolor is caused by a yeast, *Pityrosporon orbiculare* (formerly called *Malassezia furfur).* It is the most superficial of fungal infections. The lesions consist of white or brown patches, usually asymptomatic but occasionally pruritic (Figure 53–6). The lesions become apparent mainly in the summer when infected areas fail to tan.

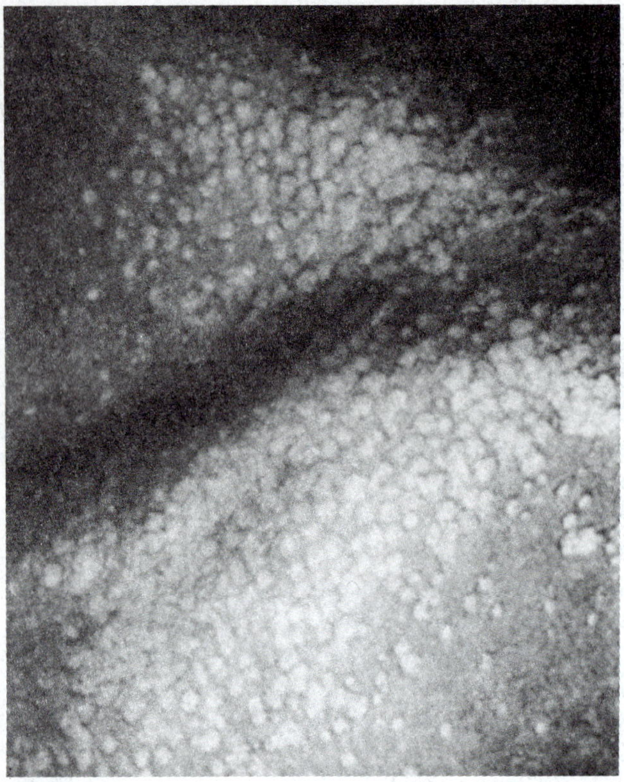

Figure 53–6
Tinea versicolor on the anterior trunk. From J. Noble, *Textbook of General Medicine and Primary Care.* Boston: Little, Brown, 1987.

There are fewer agents that are effective against *Pityrosporon orbiculare* than against dermatophytes, yet an adequate array of selections exists (see Table 53–4). The selection of an agent depends in part on the extensiveness of the infection. **Selenium sulfide** and **sodium thiosulfate** are preferred for widespread infections on the basis of cost if for no other reason. The topical imidazoles are useful for infections of limited distribution but are too expensive for long-term use over large areas of the body. The topical antifungal agent, **ciclopirox** (Loprox) is broadly effective and active against tinea versicolor. For severe, refractory cases of tinea versicolor, the imidazole agent, **ketoconazole,** can be given orally and toxicity appears to be remarkably low. Ninety-five percent of cases respond to 3 weeks of ketoconazole in a once-a-day regimen of 200 mg.

Preparations and Administration

Selenium sulfide
Lotion (Selsun Blue, Sul-Blue, Exsel)

Sodium thiosulfate
Lotion together with 1% salicylic acid, and isopropyl alcohol (Tinver)

Candidiasis

Candidiasis is a superficial infection of the skin and mucous membranes caused by *Candida albicans,* a normally commensal yeast. Overgrowth of *Candida albicans* occurs in favorable conditions, for example, in areas of moisture, when the normal flora is disturbed by a broad-spectrum antibiotic, or when the immunologic system is suppressed by glucocorticoids. There are six principal candidal syndromes, each requiring distinctive treatment.

The most common form is **oral thrush,** in which a creamy exudate appears on the tongue and buccal mucosa. Oral thrush is usually precipitated by use of antibiotics or corticosteroids but clears spontaneously when the precipitating factor is eliminated. Recovery can be hastened with local application of appropriate antifungal agents. Oral nystatin suspension (Mycostatin or Nilstat oral suspension) can be held in the mouth for 5 minutes, 3 times per day for 10 days. Alternatively, miconazole or clotrimazole cream can be applied gently to the buccal mucosa. Ketoconazole can be employed systemically at 200 mg/day for 10 days to 2 weeks.

Perlèche is a candidal infection in the cracks at the side of the mouth. Drooling, licking the sides of the mouth, or otherwise keeping the corners of the mouth moist precipitates the infection. The use of irritating cosmetics and inappropriate dental occlusion may predispose individuals to perlèche. Vitamin B_2 deficiency often causes maceration to occur in the mucosa in the angles of the mouth (angular stomatitis); if these become infected with *Candida albicans,* perlèche results. Therapy is directed at correcting the cause. Active lesions should be treated with an antifungal cream.

Candida intertrigo occurs when candida flourishes in moist intertriginous zones. The infection appears as a well-demarcated patch of erythema, often pruritic, sometimes exudative. Usually there are satellite papules or pustules. Patches may occur in the crural area, perianal area, webspaces of the toes or (rarely) the fingers, or as a diaper rash in the groin and gluteal folds. Intertrigo is most likely to occur among obese people or those who have a debilitating disease requiring bedrest. The condition is often associated with illnesses that cause high fever and perspiration. Treatment involves drying out the skin area with heat, air, or powder. Dusting powders are useful **absorbents** (Table 53–5). The most widely employed absorbent powders are talc, zinc oxide, magnesium or zinc stearate, boric acid, starch, and bismuth subcarbonate or subnitrate. Most powders become ineffective if moisture is great enough to cause caking. Stearates of magnesium and zinc are noncaking. Bismuth subnitrate, boric acid, tannic acid, and sulfur are *not* safe and effective for use as protectants, according to the FDA advisory review panel on nonprescription protectants.

High-potency creams or lotions, such as nystatin or the imidazoles, are helpful for treatment of difficult-to-dry creases and folds. Topical steroids can be used concomitantly to suppress inflammatory erythema. Oral ketoconazole has also proved successful. *Nurses should advise clients to rub the preparation well into the affected areas. There may be some skin discoloration with amphotericin B ointment. If it is embarrassing to the client, the physician may order a lotion instead. Both ointment and lotion will discolor fabrics. Clients should be warned of this possibility and advised to wash the fabric with soap and warm water immediately after use to prevent staining.*

Topical medications should be kept from the eyes. Topical administration may also cause sensitive clients to develop pruritus, irritation, and allergic dermatitis. Amphotericin B should not be used concurrently with glucocorticoids unless it is required to control a drug reaction.

Candidal **vulvovaginitis** has become rather common and is seen usually in women taking antibiotics, especially of the tetracycline group. Other predisposing factors are pregnancy or diabetes mellitus. Topical imidazoles, candicidin (Candeptin, Vanobid), chlordantoin (Sporostacin), oral ketoconazole, or the traditional colored paints (Genetian violet or Castellani paint) are alternative treatments. Infection of the glans penis by candida is not common but may occur in diabetic males or those whose partners have vulvovaginitis. Asymptomatic males may provide a source of recurrent candidiasis for females, and therefore both partners should be treated.

Candida paronychia is a candidal infection of the nails, seen in children who suck their fingers or thumbs, or adults whose occupation, chores, or hobbies keep their hands moist for long periods of time. This form of candidal infection resists therapy because of the difficulty in delivering an antifungal agent to the yeast cells under the nail. Thymol in chloroform is used because of its penetrating properties.

The most problematic form of candidal infection is **chronic mucocutaneous candidiasis** *(Candida granuloma).* Crusty red pustules appear at various sites, especially the nose and forehead. Until recently, the only effective treatment for chronic mucocutaneous candidiasis was intravenous therapy with miconazole or amphotericin B, a procedure re-

Table 53–5
Properties of Skin Protectants

Drug	Absorbent (drying agent)	Humectant (moisturizing agent)	Lubricating (emollient or demulcent)	Mechanical barrier	FDA classification
Allantoin		+			I
Aluminum hydroxide gel	+				I
Bismuth subnitrate	+				II
Boric acid	+				II
Calamine	+		+		I
Cocoa butter		+	+		I
Collodion				+	III
Dimethicone	+	+	+	+	I
Glycerin		+	+		I
Gum arabic			+		III
Kaolin	+				I
Lanolin			+		I
Petrolatum		+	+		I
Shark liver oil		+	+		I
Starch	+				I
Sulfur	+				II
Talcum powder	+				III
Tannic acid	+				II
Urea			+		III
Vegetable oils			+		III
Zinc carbonate	+		+		I
Zinc oxide	+		+		I

Key: I = recognized as safe and effective; II = not recognized as safe and effective, has unacceptable indications; III = insufficient data.

quiring repeated hospitalizations. Oral ketoconazole has revolutionized treatment of this condition.

Ectoparasitic Infestations and Drug Treatments

The two major ectoparasitic infections of the skin are scabies and lice. **Scabies** is caused by a mite that lays eggs in burrows tunneled into the stratum corneum. Mites frequently infest all members of a household, complicating therapy. Scabies is characterized by intense nocturnal pruritus and a gradual onset of rash. *Treatment can be effected by application of a miticide over the entire body surface from the neck to the soles of the feet and on normal and inflamed skin alike.* One application, if correctly applied, provides complete elimination of the mite. A second application 24 hours later provides insurance. *Nurses may need to advise all members of the family to be treated concurrently, and to wash sheets, towels, and clothing in hot water at the same time.*

The standard drug selection for eliminating mites is **lindane** (gamma benzene hexachloride). If ingested orally, lindane can cause convulsions in humans, but absorption after topical application is trivial, although skin eruptions occur occasionally. Another agent used as a miticide is **crotamiton** (Eurax). It is reputed to be less effective than lindane but has the advantage of being antipruritic. For treatment of scabies in young children or infants, **benzyl benzoate** lotion is less toxic though less effective.

Lice usually infect the hairy areas of the body. *Pediculus capitis* is the head louse; *Phthirus pubis*, the crab louse, infects the genital area. Body lice *(Pediculus corporis)* live in the undergarments, while head and genital lice live directly on the body. Lindane or permethrin shampoos are used to rid the head of lice. Lindane ointment can be applied to the pubic area to eliminate crab lice. *When applying lindane, a fine brush is used to ensure thorough application to hairy portions. A second application after 7–10 days is occasionally required, but repeated administration should be avoided because of risk of skin irritation. Clients should be instructed not to apply lindane to the face and to avoid contact of the drug with the eyes.* Genital dermatitis in males is especially likely with repeated application. *Bedding, clothing, and combs must be simultaneously decontaminated by boiling.* Reinfestation occurs commonly unless the effort to rid all lice is meticulous.

Pyrethrins, which are extracted from chrysanthemum flowers, are only moderately effective against lice. Pyrethrins are often combined with piperonyl butoxide, which inhibits metabolism of the pyrethrins by lice. **Permethrin,** on the other hand, is a newly introduced synthetic pyrethroid that is highly effective, comparing favorably in efficacy with lindane. A single administration of permethrin completely eliminates lice in 97–99% of individuals. Adverse reactions to permethrin are usually limited to mild itching, numbness of the scalp, mild erythema, or rash. Neither pyrethrins nor permethrin should be administered to individuals with a history of allergies to either drug or to chrysanthemums. *Before application of permethrin or pyrethrins, the hair should be shampooed, rinsed, and towel-dried. The hair is then saturated with the medication. Treatment can be repeated if necessary after 7 days.*

Isobornyl thiocyanoacetate (Barc) is a potentially toxic pediculicide. Applied as a cream, isobornyl thiocyanoacetate destroys lice in 10 minutes but is potentially irritating to the eyes, mucous membranes, and even the skin. It must be applied twice to be effective. Another agent that controls lice or mites is **Pedi-Bath,** a bath additive that contains colloidal sulfur and balsam Peru, both of which have scabicidal properties.

Preparations and Administration

Isobornyl thiocyanoacetate
Cream

Lindane (Kwell or GBH)
Cream

Permethrin (Nix)
Cream rinse

Pyrethrins
Gel (A–200 Pyrinate, Blue, TISIT), liquid (RID, Triple X, Pyrin-Aid, Pyrinyl, Barc, A–200 Pyrinate, or TISIT), shampoo (Vonce)

Pruritus and Antipruritics

Pruritus is a sensation of itching and represents a dermatologic symptom rather than a disease. It occurs most commonly in conjunction with skin disorders but can be caused by systemic disease, drugs, or psychogenic factors. Pruritus often occurs in connection with ectoparasitic infestations, insect bites, contact dermatitis, atopic dermatitis, urticaria, lichen planus, herpes infections, miliaria, neurodermatitis, and ichthyosis (dry skin). Systemic causes of pruritus include uremia, jaundice, lymphomas, and leukemias. Pruritus often accompanies drug eruptions but can also be a drug reaction in its own right without accompanying rash or other skin lesions. Drug-induced pruritus is most commonly observed with salicylanilides and barbiturates.

Treatment of pruritus centers on identification and elimination of the cause. The use of topical antihistamines should be limited to the temporary relief of contact dermatitis from poison ivy or oak, insect bites or stings, sunburns, or hives. Topical antihistamines cause irritation and inflammation in some individuals, and a prior history of allergic reactions to these agents is a specific contraindication to use. **Diphenhydramine** is less likely to cause sensitivity reactions than other antihistamines. *Topical antihistamines should not be applied to raw, blistery, pustulent, or open skin, or near the eyes or genitalia.*

Severe pruritic conditions may require oral antipruritic therapy with a phenothiazine. Promethazine (Phenergan), a phenothiazine with antihistaminic properties is widely used for this purpose. Prochlorperazine (Compazine) and chlorpromazine (Thorazine) are also used as oral antipruritics.

Preparations and Administration

Diphenhydramine
Cream (Benadryl), cream with calamine (Caladryl), cream or lotion with cyclomethycaine sulfate (Surfadil), lotion with calamine and camphor (Caladryl), spray or gel with tripelennamine, benzalkonium chloride, and menthol (Didelamine), lotion with zinc oxide (Ziradryl)

Phenyltoloxamine
Lotion with benzocaine and calamine (Histacalma)

Pyrilamine
Cream with neocalamine, benzocaine, camphor, menthol, and benzalkonium chloride (Tyrohist), ointment with neocalamine and zinc oxide (Caleate), lotion combination with two other antihistamines, pheniramine and chlorpheniramine (Derma-Pax)

Tripelennamine
Combinations with diphenhydramine; lotion with zirconium oxide, benzocaine, calamine, camphor, and menthol (Rhulihist); cream (PBZ)

Cornification, Emollients, and Keratolytics

Cornification refers to the formation of the horny layer by the process of keratinization. Excessive keratinization is responsible for several clinical conditions: dry skin (ichthyosis), keratoses, and calluses. Dry skin or xeroderma can occur as a mild, acquired disorder with aging. It can also be caused by prolonged exposure to low humidity and air movement or overly frequent degreasing. Other cases can occur as inherited conditions, some of which can be severe. Dry skin is controlled by administration of emollients, usually twice a day.

Keratoses are conditions of excess keratinization. Keratosis can result from chronic exposure to sunlight, menopause, or internal cancer. Emollients and keratolytics are used for cosmetic purposes in keratoses. Calluses are areas of hyperkeratinization appearing at a site of trauma; corns are cone-shaped calluses of the toes. Keratolytic agents are employed in their treatment along with properly fitted shoes.

Emollients and Demulcents

Emollients are fats and oils used to lubricate and soothe irritated skin; some of these also promote hydration of dry skin (see Table 53–5). Demulcents are water-soluble substances that have a similar application. Both types of agents are frequently used as vehicles for various topical preparations. Glycerin and acacia (gum arabic) are examples of demulcents often used as suspending or emulsifying agents.

Vegetable oils and hydrocarbons are among the most valuable emollients. Olive oil, cottonseed oil, and peanut oil are used to produce oily suspensions. Cocoa butter (theobroma oil) is a yellowish white, solid oil extract from the seeds of *Theobroma cacao,* which melts at body temperature and is often used as a base for suppositories or as a lubricant in massage linaments. Lanolin (hydrous wool fat) is derived from sheep wool with 25–30% water and is used in many ointments. Petrolatum, known as petroleum jelly (Vaseline), is a commonly used hydrocarbon emollient base.

Vitamins A and D, sometimes in the form of cod liver oil, can be added to lanolin-petrolatum base for application to the skin (Moruguent, Desitin). Petrolatum can be combined with white wax (bleached beeswax) to make white ointment, with yellow wax (unmodified beeswax) to make yellow ointment, or with spermaceti, a wax obtained from whales. White wax, yellow wax, and spermaceti are all used to harden ointments. Rosewater ointment consists of rosewater, rose oil, white wax, spermaceti, and almond oil. Cold cream is similar except mineral oil replaces the almond oil. Urea (carbamide) is a useful agent for alleviating dry skin and hyperkeratotic conditions, combining emollient and keratolytic properties. It is available as a lotion or cream (Aquacare, Nutraplus, Carmol, Rea-Lo).

Keratolytics

Keratolytics are drugs that dissolve keratin and thus remove the outer scaly layer and soften the skin. Keratolytics are useful in removing corns and warts, in softening scales for removal in seborrheic dermatitis and psoriasis, for reducing keratinization in the hyperkeratinization disorders (ichthyosis and keratoses), and in treatment of acne. Salicylic acid, resorcinol, allantoin, urea, lactic acid, and benzoic acid are the favored keratolytic agents, with salicylic acid perhaps the most important. **Salicylic acid** is provided as a cream (Calicylic), ointment, or gel (Saligel, Keralyt, Hydrisalic). Many of the keratolytic preparations are provided in a base of collodion or flexible collodion. After evaporation of the vehicle, nitrocellulose derivatives in the collodion bases form a rigid or flexible film, which prevents escape of fluid, promotes absorption of the active constituent, and protects the lesion from irritation. Salicylic acid is available in a flexible collodion base (Wart-Off Liquid). Salicylic acid and lactic acid are marketed in combination in a flexible collodion base (Duofilm, Salactic Film). Salicylic acid is also marketed in collodion bases with zinc chloride (Freezone, Gets-It) and with acetic acid (Compound W).

Drugs for Disorders of Skin Appendages

The Sebaceous Glands

The sebaceous glands produce the sebum that lubricates and protects the skin. **Acne vulgaris** is a disease of the sebaceous gland, the associated duct, and ultimately the skin. Acne vulgaris typically emerges in puberty from the rising levels of circulating androgens: testosterone in males and adrenal 17-ketosteroids in males and females alike. These androgens promote hypertrophy of sebaceous glands and an increase in sebum production. Sebum secreted by the sebaceous glands into the sebaceous duct consists of lipids and waxes, but these are partly hydrolyzed to free fatty acids by lipase enzymes contained in anaerobic bacteria — *Propionibacterium acnes (P. acnes)* and *Propionibacterium granulosum (P. granulosum).* The free fatty acids have an irritating effect on the portion of the follicular sheath lying above the entrance of the sebaceous duct (Figure 53–3), and the epithelial cells of the root sheath begin to keratinize excessively. These abnormal cells adhere tightly and are not readily flushed out by the flow of sebum. The follicular opening narrows and is ultimately occluded, preventing excretion of sebum. The follicle swells, forming a comedo (plural, *comedones)* or superficial cyst. Ultimately, the follicle may rupture, spilling its content of free fatty acids, bacteria, and sebum over the surface of the skin and inducing inflammation.

The lesions of superficial acne include closed and open comedones, superficial cysts, inflamed papules, and pustules (Figure 53–7). Closed comedones (whiteheads) occur in small follicles with openings narrowed by hyperkeratinization. Open comedones (blackheads) occur in larger follicles when keratinous plugs clog the orifice. The lesions of deep acne include inflamed nodules and pus-filled cysts; deep pits and scarring can occur when these lesions open.

Acne tends to grow worse in the winter and improve in the summer due to the salutary effect of sunlight, which dries the skin. Acne also fluctuates

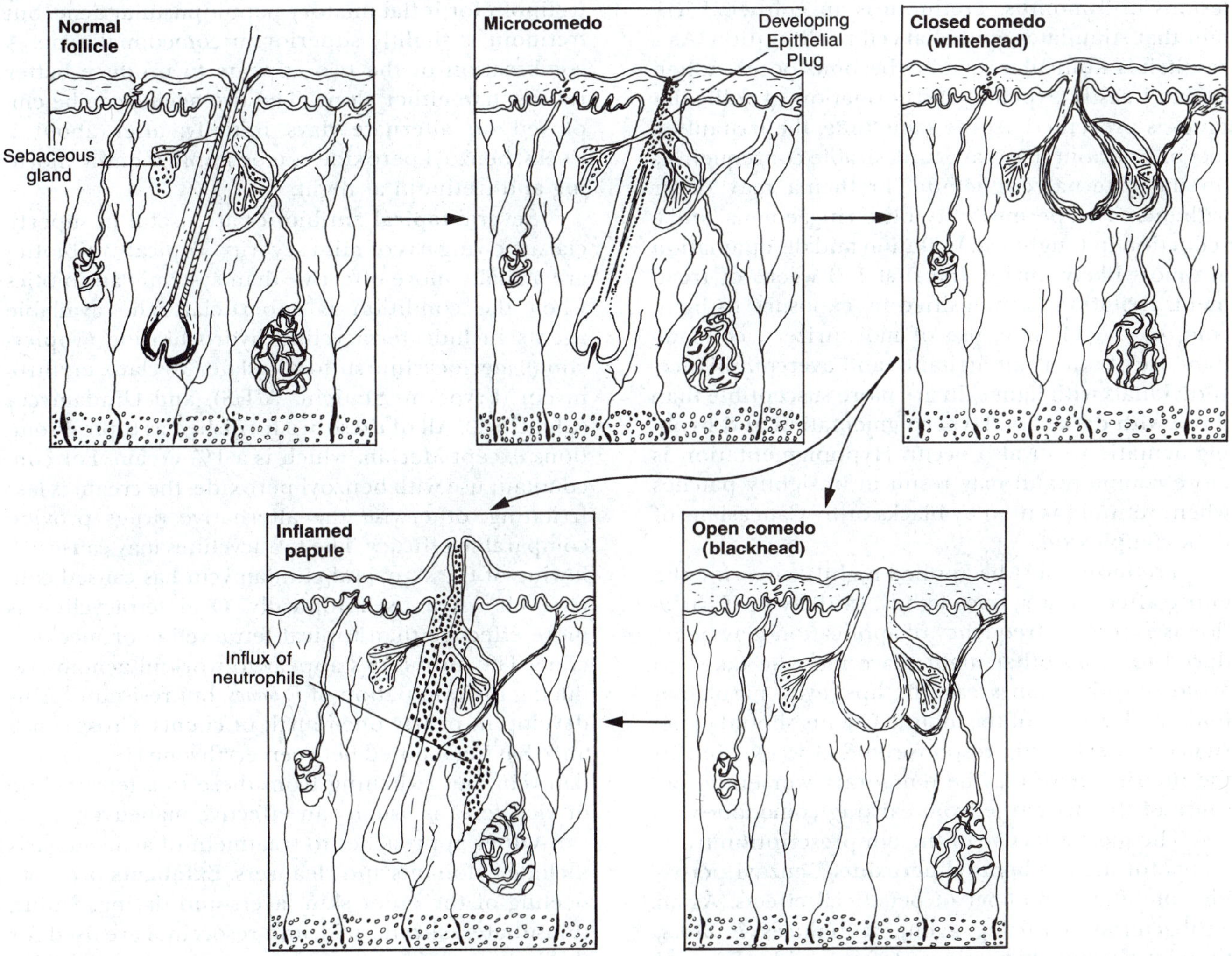

Figure 53–7
Typical sequence of events during formation of a comedo.

with the menstrual cycle in women, being worst during menses when estrogen levels drop. Although most cases begin at puberty and spontaneously remit in the early twenties, a few cases arise de novo in the twenties or thirties, usually in women using glucocorticoids, moisturizers, or other acnegenic drugs (see Appendix 53B). Therapy must be individualized for therapeutic requirements, skin sensitivity, and the client's compliance. Baseline physical examination with laboratory testing is required when systemic medication is anticipated.

Topical Medications for Superficial Acne Vulgaris

Topical medications are preferred for superficial acne but are not useful in deep acne. The most effective therapy for superficial acne is **tretinoin** (retinoic acid or vitamin A acid). Seventy-five percent of patients experience at least a 50% reduction in lesions in 3 months. Tretinoin is an epithelial irritant that stimulates epithelial cell proliferation. As a result, intrafollicular squames become loosely adherent and easily expelled and formation of follicular plugs is prevented. At the same time, the irritant effect of tretinoin may have undesirable consequences on the external epithelium. Erythema may occur with increased permeability, blistering, edema, and a reduction in toughness. Irritation and desquamation are most likely during the first 1–3 weeks of treatment. Irritation is intensified by exposure to light, cold, or dry climate, use of moisturizers, concomitant use of other skin irritants, and overcompliance. Individuals with light skin are more susceptible than those with dark skin. Hyperpigmentation and hypopigmentation can also occur. Hypopigmentation is more common and may result in unsightly patches when tretinoin is used by blacks or by Caucasians of dark complexion.

Tretinoin must be applied nightly, covering the entire affected area once lightly. Initially or if irritation is excessive, frequency of application may be reduced to every other night. Care must be taken to avoid sensitive skin areas: the lips, eyes, nasolabial folds, and creases of the mouth. Clients should experience a therapeutic response in 2–3 weeks, but in the interim there may be temporary worsening because of the discharge from existing comedones.

The most effective of the nonprescription treatments for acne is **benzoyl peroxide.** Benzoyl peroxide combines a number of beneficial effects. As an antibacterial oxidizing agent, it reduces *P. acnes,* thereby slowing formation of fatty acids. Benzoyl peroxide also possesses weak keratolytic properties, softening existing plugs to permit evacuation of comedones; it also reduces the rate of sebum production by the sebaceous glands. Benzoyl peroxide is also an exfoliant, promoting shedding of outer scales and hastening resolution of inflammatory papulopustular lesions.

Gel formulations of benzoyl peroxide are the most effective, followed by lotions, then washes. Three months of treatment with 10% benzoyl peroxide will reduce lesions by 75% in most patients. Skin irritation may occur, especially in fair-skinned individuals. *Nurses should warn clients to avoid letting the medicine come into contact with the eyes, eyelids, nostrils, or lips. Mild peeling may also occur during the first few days of use. Initiating treatment at the 5% concentration for a few weeks may be helpful in individuals prone to skin irritation. Since contact dermatitis occurs in about 3% of individuals, an initial patch test with a 2-day observation period is a useful precaution. Benzoyl peroxide may be worn under make up.*

Benzoyl peroxide is slightly more effective than tretinoin for inflammatory papulopustular acne, but tretinoin is slightly superior in comedonal acne. A combination of the two appears to produce better results than either alone. The two agents can be employed on alternate days initially; after about 2 weeks, benzoyl peroxide can be applied in the morning and tretinoin at night.

Several **topical antibiotics** are useful in superficial acne vulgaris of mild severity. Topical antibiotics are actually more effective than systemic antibiotics when the condition is superficial. The available agents include tetracycline hydrochloride (Topicycline), meclocycline sulfosalicylate (Meclan), erythromycin (Eryderm, Staticin, A/T/S), and clindamycin (Cleocin T). All of these are furnished as topical solutions except Meclan, which is a 1% cream. For concomitant use with benzoyl peroxide, the cream is less irritating; otherwise the alternative drugs provide comparable efficacy. The tetracyclines may cause yellowing of the skin, and clindamycin has caused colitis even when used topically. Oral tetracycline is more effective than topical tetracycline or meclocycline. The antibiotics appear to work in acne by reducing the population of *P. acnes,* but resistant forms develop in nearly one-fourth of clients. Cross-resistance has been noted between erythromycin and clindamycin, but switching from these to a tetracycline or vice versa is usually an effective maneuver.

Other approaches to treatment of acne vulgaris include exfoliants and cleansers. **Exfoliants** promote peeling of the outer skin layers and drying. Sulfur, thiosulfate, salicylic acid, and resorcinol are used for this purpose. These preparations are less effective than benzoyl peroxide in severe cases but are adequate for mild conditions.

Salicylic acid, in concentrations of 5–10%

(higher than those found in combination products) has a tretinoin-like action of inhibiting formation of keratinous plugs. Salicylic acid is available as a 5% cream (various), a 10% cream (Calicylic), a 5% gel (Saligel), or a 6% gel (Keralyt, Hydrisalic).

In addition to the above products, various **cleansers** are aggressively promoted for use in acne vulgaris, including medicated soaps, liquid cleansers, and abrasive cleansers. There is no evidence, however, that any of these products are beneficial. Ordinary soap is as effective as the special products marketed as cleansers for acne.

Preparations and Administration

Benzoyl Peroxide
Liquid cleanser (Desquam-X Wash), lotion (Oxy, Teen, Topex, Zeroxin, Persadox, Dry and Clear, others), gel (PanOxyl, benzac, Xerac, Desquam, Fostex, Dermodex, etc.), cream (Persadox); combination lotions with chlorhydroxyquinoline (Vanoxide, Loroxide) or sulfur (Sulfoxyl), combination ointments with chlorhydroxyquinoline (Quinolor), combination cream with bentonite (Clearasil)

Sulfur
Gels (Transact, Xerac), lotions (Postacne, Liquimat, Acne Aid, Epi-Clear), creams (Fortex), powder (Bensulfoid); combination preparations with resorcinol (Sulvesor, Acne Aid, Acne-Dome, Exzit, Sulforcin, Acnomel, Rezamid, Clearasil, Cenac) or with salicylic acid (Sebasorb, Therac, Acno, Akne Drying, Acnotex)

Thiosulfate
Combination preparations with salicylic acid (Komed), with resorcinol, and salicylic acid (Microsyn), and others.

Tretinoin (Retin-A)
Cream, gel, liquid, saturated swabs

Systemic Medications for Deep Acne Vulgaris

The deep forms of acne vulgaris are treated with systemic medications. The main therapy consists of oral antibiotics. Oral retinoids are a new approach that may revolutionize therapy for deep acne. Estrogens and antiandrogens can be employed usefully in teenage girls and women, and sulfones and steroids provide useful adjuncts for refractory cases.

The usual oral **antibiotics** used for clients with acne vulgaris are the tetracyclines and erythromycin. When high-dose therapy is conducted for 6–12 weeks, most clients experience a 50–70% reduction in lesions in 6–8 weeks. If clearing occurs, maintenance doses may be continued indefinitely. Ultimately, oral therapy is discontinued in preference for topical management. Oral antibiotics appear to work partly by reducing levels of *P. acnes* and partly by an anti-inflammatory action. The risks of oral antibiotic therapy should not be overlooked. Most prominent among these is vaginal candidiasis due to superinfection. Tetracyclines are also likely to cause dyspepsia, photosensitization, yellowish skin pigmentation, vertigo, and headache and must be discontinued during pregnancy. They must not be taken with milk or other calcium-rich foods since calcium impairs absorption of these drugs. Treatment failure after 12 weeks is frequently due to lack of compliance or inadequate administration.

Estrogens suppress androgen-stimulated activity of the sebaceous glands. The same effect has been produced in clinical trials in Europe with the **antiandrogen,** cyproterone acetate. Estrogen therapy is limited to female clients because of feminizing effects. The most convenient means of utilizing estrogen therapy is to place the client on oral contraceptives, employing an estrogen and progesterone combination for 21 days with an interruption of about 10 days to permit menses. Estrogen therapy, like treatment with tretinoin, often results in a brief worsening of acne as existing comedones are expressed. The adverse effects of oral contraceptives (such as nausea, weight gain, spotting, breast tenderness, depression, hypertension, thromboembolism, and vaginal moniliasis) should be considered by the client in risk/benefit assessment (see Chapter 34).

Synthetic **retinoids,** derivatives of vitamin A, represent a new approach to treatment of acne conglobata and severe inflammatory acne. Isotretinoin (Accutane) was approved by the FDA in 1982. Both comedones and papulopustular inflammations respond well; facial acne responds best, and female clients better than males. Isotretinoin appears to work by inhibiting production of sebum. Remarkably, when therapy is terminated after 4 months, most clients remain clear for prolonged periods. The main adverse effects are dry skin, facial dermatitis, conjunctivitis, arthralgias, and drying of the nasal mucosa with consequent nosebleeds. All adverse effects noted are dose dependent and reversible when medication is terminated.

Systemic **sulfones** are used only in severe cases of deep acne where scarring is likely without vigorous therapy. Sulfones such as dapsone (Avlosulfon) are employed as add-ons to a regimen of antibiotics, retinoids, topical tretinoin, and benzoyl peroxide. A daily dose of 100–200 mg of dapsone is given in divided doses. Adverse effects of sulfones include hemolytic anemia, methemoglobinemia, agranulocytosis, cholestasis, and nephrotic syndrome (see Chapter 47 for a full discussion of sulfones).

Oral **glucocorticoid** therapy for severe acne is likewise reserved for the most recalcitrant cases of acne conglobata and acne fulminans. Steroids themselves can produce an acneiform eruption as well as the many complications associated with long-term glucocorticoid medication. Fluorinated steroids tend to worsen acne.

The Sweat Glands

Disorders of the sweat glands usually involve the apocrine glands, although eccrine glands may be involved less commonly. **Hyperhidrosis** is excess sweating, caused by overactivity of the sweat glands, that usually involves the axillae, palms, soles, groin, or regions of inflamed skin. The sweat is often odorous because of the activity of surface bacteria and yeasts on apocrine excretions. Hyperhidrosis can be organic, drug-induced, or psychogenic. Organic causes include hypermetabolic endocrine disorders such as hyperthyroidism and any fever-provoking infectious condition. Drug causes of excess sweating include cholinomimetics and sympathomimetics. Cocaine intoxication, amphetamine intoxication, and hallucinogen hallucinosis all entail an increase in perspiration. Profuse sweating is also observed in the withdrawal syndromes for both narcotics and sedative-hypnotics. Psychogenic causes of sweating include generalized anxiety and panic attacks. Hyperhidrosis is itself a major factor in occurrence of contact dermatitis and fungal infections. Since the sweat glands are mainly regulated by acetylcholine-releasing sympathetic efferents, systemic anticholinergics suppress sweating, but the range of side effects that occur with use of cholinolytics is too great to justify this approach.

Antiperspirants and Deodorants

Antiperspirants are drugs that decrease the rate of perspiration, while deodorants are agents that reduce the bacterial flora, thereby reducing odor caused by degradation of perspiration by the microorganisms. Perspiration is odorless until acted upon by microorganisms, and periodic washing will remove a sizable fraction of the epithelial flora. Nevertheless, antiperspirants and deodorants are vigorously promoted and widely used in modern American society. Aluminum hydroxychloride (or aluminum chlorohydrate) is the most widely marketed antiperspirant. Other aluminum salts such as aluminum chloride and aluminum sulfate are less desirable because they hydrolyze to form acids that are damaging to clothing. The phenolsulfonate salts of both aluminum and zinc are low-acidity compounds that can be usefully employed in aerosol formulations, since they are soluble in alcohol.

Antiperspirants diffuse into the sweat ducts where they form a hydroxide gel that obstructs the duct. Acidic aluminum salts are also astringent, producing a necrotizing effect on the sweat ducts, and allergic reactions occur occasionally. Antiperspirants are available in a wide variety of application forms, from aerosols and sprays to pads, sticks, liquids, and roll-on creams.

Widely used deodorants are benzalkonium, methylbenzethonium chloride, neomycin, and vitamin E. The first two are topical antiseptics. Vitamin E is not antiseptic but has antioxidant properties that retard degradation of perspiration; neomycin is a topical antibacterial agent. All of these agents can produce allergic and irritant reactions.

Hair Follicles

The hair shaft is constantly being generated at its base by mitotic activity of matrix cells that surround the dermal papilla. Each hair shaft has a limited life-span: for example, the life-span of scalp hair ranges from 3 to 10 years. When a hair shaft reaches the end of its active life of generation (anagen), the inferior portion of the root shaft disintegrates, melanin synthesis ceases, and the hair turns white. This phase of involution (catagen) is followed by a period of inactivity (telogen). Finally the defunct hair shaft is pushed out of the root sheath by emergence of a newly developing hair shaft. Abnormalities related to generative activity of the hair follicles include alopecia (baldness), hirsutism (hypertrichosis), and ingrown hairs.

Alopecia is partial or complete loss of hair. It is often genetic and tends to occur with aging. Male-pattern baldness is common with a strong familial component. Toxic alopecia can occur in response to systemic, febrile illnesses, myxedema, syphilis, pregnancy, or cancer chemotherapy. Drugs known to cause alopecia are listed in Table 53–6. Minoxidil has recently been introduced as a topical treatment for baldness, but any hair grown under its influence is quickly lost when the drug is discontinued.

Hirsutism (hypertrichosis) is hair growth in areas ordinarily devoid of hair. Familial factors are common. In women, hirsutism may suggest virilism caused by an endocrine disturbance or a drug that has led to elevation of circulating 17-ketosteroids. Hirsutism occurs commonly during menopause or with administration of androgenic or glucocorticoid steroids. In neonates, hirsutism may be present as a result of drug teratogenicity, as for example, in the fetal alcohol syndrome. Excess hair growth can occur

Table 53–6
Drugs Causing Alopecia and Hirsutism

Alopecia	Hirsutism
Aminoglycosides	Androgens
Anorexics	Corticosteroids
Anticoagulents	Minoxidil
Antiepileptics	Oral contraceptives
Carbamazepine	Phenytoin
Hydantoins	
Oxazolidones	
Valproic acid	
Antineoplastic Drugs	
Colchicine	
Dactinomycin	
Ethionamide	
Gold salts	
Hydroxychloroquin	
^{131}Iodine	
Indomethacin	
Lithium	
Methimazole	
Oral contraceptives	
Propionic acid derivatives	
Quinacrine	
Sulfonamides	
Thallium salts	
Tricyclic antidepressants	
Vitamin A (hypervitaminosis)	

as a side effect of minoxidil (Loniten) or phenytoin (Dilantin). Treatment of hirsutism depends on eliminating the cause. Electrolysis of hair follicles provides the only permanent treatment, but cosmetic benefit can be achieved by periodic plucking, shaving, bleaching, or application of chemical depilatories.

Chemical depilatories are of two types. Most preparations consist of a substituted mercaptan (usually calcium thioglycolate) and an alkaline-reacting substance (calcium hydroxide or strontium hydroxide). These agents cause hair shafts to swell and deteriorate to a soft mass that is easily wiped off the skin. At concentrations of 2.5–4%, thioglycolates produce depilation in 5–15 minutes with minimal irritation to the skin. Higher concentrations do produce skin irritation and do not significantly hasten depilation. Alkaline sulfides are also useful chemical depilatories. They are two to three times more rapid than thioglycolate but are more irritating, have a strong odor of hydrogen sulfide, and are poisonous if ingested. Alkaline sulfides are now used only for removal of coarse hair of the axillae, which is very slow to respond to calcium thioglycolate.

Melanocytes

Melanin synthesis by melanocytes provides normal pigmentation as well as seasonal adjustments in pigmentation from sunlight and alterations in pigmentation at puberty. Abnormalities of melanocyte activity result in hypo- or hyperpigmentation. Chronic hypopigmentation, called **albinism,** is a rare autosomal recessive disorder in which melanin is not produced. Such individuals have white hair, pink eyes, and pale skin and must protect themselves from sunlight. **Vitiligo,** which is more common, is characterized by hypopigmented patches from a lack of melanocytes in a particular skin area. Vitiligo is common in Addison's disease and is also seen in clients who have diabetes mellitus, thyroid disorders, or pernicious anemia. Vitiliginous lesions usually burn when exposed to the sun. Hypopigmentation is often a characteristic of newly healed skin following inflammatory lesions, infections, or burns.

Melanizing agents can be used to promote repigmentation of the skin in vitiligo. The two closely related drugs of the psoralen family, trioxsalen and methoxsalen, are the major melanizing drugs. The psoralens stimulate existing melanocytes and melanocyte proliferation. Exposure to ultraviolet light is an integral part of the treatment protocol since the psoralens are effective in stimulating melanocytes only after photoactivation. The melanizing agent is taken daily, in the form of an oral tablet or capsule, 2 hours before a carefully titrated exposure to sunlight or ultraviolet radiation from a sunlamp. Methoxsalen topical solution is applied directly to the vitiliginous area in conjunction with oral therapy. Repigmentation begins to occur in a few weeks, but several months may be required to bring about a substantial darkening and increased tolerance to sunlight. Adverse effects of this regimen are minimal, but some clients experience nausea, gastrointestinal irritation, acute lupus erythematosus, or photoporphyria. Other photosensitizing drugs must not be used concurrently.

Preparations and Administration

Trioxsalen (Trisoralen)
Tablets
Recommended Dose: 10 mg PO daily.

Methoxsalen (Oxsoralen)
Capsules, topical solution
Recommended Dose: 20 mg daily.

Hyperpigmentation is usually caused by excess melanin production. This occurs in Addison's disease, pregnancy, and with use of oral contraceptives. Silver deposition, as when silver nitrate is employed in burn therapy, can also cause darkening of the skin. During pregnancy or use of oral contraceptives, hyperpigmentation may appear in the form of melasma, sharply demarcated, dark brown spots on the face. Treatment is effected by topical administration of monobenzone or hydroquinone, **demelanizing agents** that inhibit synthesis of melanin. Hydroquinone is the safer of the two and is indicated for bleaching of melasmatic blemishes such as freckles, old age spots, and melasma of pregnancy or oral contraception. The drug is contraindicated in miliaria, sunburn, skin irritation, or when depilatory agents are being used. Occasional skin rash is the only adverse effect. Clinical response is slow, often requiring 4 months of application. Protecting the treated area from ultraviolet light hastens the response significantly. For this reason, some preparations provide hydroquinone in an opaque base that shields UV light (Eldopaque). At night, nonopaque creams, lotions, ointments (Eldoquin), or solutions (Melanex) serve equally well. Hydroquinone is applied twice daily. Monobenzone, which may cause dermatitis, is recommended only for final depigmentation in disseminated vitiligo. It is available as an ointment (Benoquin) which is applied to pigmented areas 2–3 times daily.

Trauma

Special drug preparations are available for burn, excessive exposure to sunlight, and decubitus ulcers, the three kinds of trauma that frequently affect the skin more than other tissues.

Burn and Burn Preparations

Each year in the United States, there are over 2 million burn injuries of which approximately 250,000 require hospitalization and about 25,000 result in fatalities. All age groups are affected, men and boys marginally more frequently than women and girls. Burns can be caused by thermal or electrical agents or by chemicals that are acids or alkalis. Drug products that are available to aid in management or prevention of burns include protectants, local anesthetics, topical antibacterial drugs, and sunscreens.

Protectants

For treating minor burns, a protectant should be selected that provides lubricating and moisturizing capabilities (Table 53–5). Petrolatum is probably more effective than most alternatives. Protectants do not accelerate the healing process but protect the burn from further irritation, lubricate the outer layer, and permit normal healing to proceed.

Local Anesthetics

Local anesthetics provide a safe and effective means of achieving analgesia when burn injuries are painful. However, a local anesthetic should be employed only within the approved concentration range (Table 53–7). The selection of an agent to be applied should be adjusted on the basis of the skin integrity. Both efficacy and systemic toxicity require penetration of the drug into the skin. *Higher concentrations are safe when they are applied to intact skin, especially to body areas where the stratum corneum is thick. The lower end of the approved range is appropriate for application to skin that is mildly damaged.* The selection of an agent is also influenced by skin integrity in the area of anticipated application. For example, benzocaine produces little systemic toxicity and is safer for application to damaged skin. Lidocaine can be safely applied to intact or mildly irritated skin and is much less likely to cause allergic reactions than benzocaine.

Some of the available formulations should be avoided because they contain concentrations below the lower limit for effectiveness. Thus, Rhulicaine, Benzocol, Morusan, Solarcaine, Clo-Vi-Nol, and Unguentine have less than 5% benzocaine and Pontocaine ointment has less than 1% tetracaine. A few preparations exceed the upper recommended concentration for lidocaine (various 5% ointments). Still other preparations contain irritant antiseptics such as phenol (Anbesol), parabens (Xylocaine 4% solution, Xylocaine jelly, Cyclaine), or benzalkonium chloride (Anestacon, Americaine Anesthetic Lubricant, Americaine

Table 53–7
Effective and Safe Concentrations of Local Anesthetics

Drug	Effective and safe concentrations (%)
Benzocaine	5–20
Benzyl alcohol	10–33
Butamben	1
Dibucaine	0.25–1
Dimethisoquin	0.3–0.5
Diperodon	0.25–1
Dyclonine	0.5–1
Lidocaine	0.5–4
Pramoxine	1
Tetracaine	1–2

First Aid, Aerocaine, Dulzit, and Cetacaine). Still others contain irritating astringents such as menthol (Derma, Dermoplast, Medicone, Medicone Dressing, Pontocaine ointment), sulfur (Foille), or camphor. The safest formulations are those that contain only the active local anesthetic and an inert base. Preparations in this category include benzocaine, lidocaine (Xylocaine, Lida-Mantle), dibucaine (Nupercainal, Anesta-Caine, D-Caine, others), pramoxine (Tronothane), dimethisoquin (Quotane), diperodon (Diothane), butamben (Butesin Picrate), tetracaine (Pontocaine), and dyclonine (Dyclone). Aerotherm combines two local anesthetics: benzocaine and benzyl alcohol.

Local anesthetics should not be applied more than 4 times per day and should never be used in large amounts or over a large surface area. Clients should be given specific instructions regarding duration of treatment. The burn should be cleansed and neutralized before applying the local anesthetic.

Topical Antibacterials for Burns

The use of nonprescription antibiotics for home treatment of minor burns is of questionable value. For one thing, efficacy is not clearly established. Beyond that, use of such drugs could favor development of resistant organisms and allergic reactions can occur with bacitracin or neomycin. Polymyxin B alone is not effective against gram-positive organisms. If use of a nonprescription antibiotic is desired, a combination of polymyxin B and bacitracin without neomycin (Bacimycin, for example) probably offers the best balance between broad-spectrum efficacy with least risk of allergic reaction.

Second- and third-degree burns often require treatment with potent antimicrobials to minimize the risk of sepsis. The drug selected must be one that is minimally irritating to the wound, effective across a broad spectrum, and not likely to produce untenable systemic toxicity. In practice, a half dozen drugs have been singled out for use in preventing burn sepsis.

One of the best choices is **mafenide** (Sulfamylon). Mafenide, a sulfonamide drug, has a broad antibacterial activity, destroying most gram-positive and gram-negative organisms. It is an inhibitor of carbonic anhydrase and thus has the potential for inducing metabolic acidosis. However, the burn patient is typically in metabolic alkalosis due to CO_2 loss from the wound, and therefore the ability of mafenide to inhibit carbonic anhydrase is often a positive feature. Disadvantages of mafenide are risk of fungal colonization of the wound and pain that occurs when it is applied. *Wounds should be cleansed and debrided before application of mafenide. Mafenide can be continued up to 60 days until healing is well underway.* Sulfamylon is provided as an 85 mg/g cream.

Silver nitrate is the classic drug choice for preventing burn sepsis, but it is employed only in closed dressings. Gauze dressings are saturated with silver nitrate in a warm solution and applied to the wound. The gauze is covered with a warm blanket or other appropriate wrap to prevent water evaporation and undue heat loss. Silver nitrate is effective against the major pathogens that tend to colonize the burn eschar. Disadvantages include skin discoloration by silver nitrate, risk of methemoglobinemia from systemic absorption of the nitrate moiety, absorption into the body of large amounts of fluid from the dressing, and absorption into the dressing of electrolytes from the body.

Silver sulfadiazine, which combines the antimicrobial activities of silver and sulfadiazine, is applied as a cream for use in open dressings. Significant absorption can occur and can lead to systemic adverse reactions typical of sulfonamide drugs, including allergic reactions. The antibacterial spectrum is very broad, but fungi may flourish in or below the eschar. Silver sulfadiazine (Silvadene) is available as a 10 mg/g cream.

The other agents less commonly used in burn therapy are gentamicin (Garamycin) and nitrofurazone (Furacin, Furazyme, others). **Nitrofurazone** is a synthetic agent that is bactericidal for all types of bacteria that are present in surface infections, including many that are resistant to antibiotics. It inhibits enzymes involved in both anaerobic and aerobic carbohydrate metabolism in bacteria. When applied topically, nitrofurazone produces little toxicity, although contact dermatitis occurs occasionally. *Nitrofurazone should be applied only to the affected part. Adjacent healthy skin can be protected by application of zinc oxide. Nitrofurazone should be stored in an airtight, opaque container away from heat.* **Gentamicin** is absorbed only slowly when applied topically as an ointment, but when applied as a cream, absorption is more rapid and plasma concentrations can be substantial. Gentamicin produces systemic adverse effects similar to streptomycin: nausea, vomiting, headache, transient skin rash, and most important, nephrotoxicity and ototoxicity. Because of these toxic potentials, gentamicin is not used systemically except for life-threatening infections.

Sunburn

Sunburn is caused by excessive exposure to sunlight or ultraviolet light. The severity of sunburn depends on three factors: (1) the extent of exposure (time and intensity), (2) the susceptibility of the skin (fair or dark, tanned or pale), and (3) the adequacy of protective measures undertaken (clothing, chemical sunshields). In addition to the immediate painful inflammation of sunburn, chronic adverse effects on the skin are now recognized. A strong correlation exists between incidence of skin cancer and exposure to sunlight. Excessive exposure to sunlight also promotes signs of premature aging: drying, thinning, wrinkling, inelasticity, cracking, growths, and subcutaneous hemorrhagic lesions.

Midrange ultraviolet light (UV-B, 290–320 nm) is the most potent in eliciting erythema and burns. Long-wave radiation (UV-A, 320–400 nm) is less likely to cause erythema or burn but can augment the adverse effect of UV-B. UV-A is the wavelength that is most often involved in photosensitizing chemicals that cause photosensitivity disorders. Germicidal ultraviolet radiation (UC-V, 200–290 nm) is not found in sunlight but in artificial sources and is only mildly erythemagenic.

Sunscreens are agents that block the penetration of sunlight into the skin, whether by providing a physical barrier or a chemical one. Physical sunscreens such as titanium dioxide scatter and reflect UV radiation, while chemical sunscreens absorb it. **Suntan lotions** are not very efficient at blocking the sun's rays from the skin; they are qualitatively similar to sunscreens but less effective in preventing ultraviolet penetration. Sunscreens are useful prophylaxes against sunburn and some prevent photosensitivity reactions when drugs known to be photosensitizers are in use. Each sunscreen agent absorbs UV light efficiently only within a certain spectrum of wavelengths. A drug selected for prophylaxis against sunburn should be an efficient absorber in the UVB range, while a drug selected for preventing photosensitivity reactions should be efficient in the UV-A range. Since all of the effective drugs on the market absorb at least in the UV-B range, drugs that also absorb in the UV-A range are broad-spectrum. *The nurse should make sure that patients understand the need for a sunscreen when photosensitizing medications are employed and should aid in the selection of an appropriate agent.*

Another factor that must be considered in selecting an appropriate agent is the screening potential of the product. The various products differ substantially in the maximum protection against sunlight that each affords. The FDA has assigned a skin protection factor (SPF) for each agent, which is listed on the preparations container (15 is the maximum). Light-skinned Caucasian people who burn easily require an agent having an SPF of 8 or more. Those of medium skin color who burn moderately and tan gradually require a product with an SPF of 4–5. Those who burn minimally or rarely and tan well require a product with an SPF of 2–3. Dark skinned individuals who never burn have no need for a sunscreen preparation.

PABA (*p*-aminobenzoic acid) should be administered 2 hours before exposure to allow absorption into the skin. Photoallergic contact dermatitis sometimes occurs with PABA, padimate A, glyceryl PABA, and cinnamates. Titanium dioxide may provide such an occlusive barrier on the skin that excess sweat retention (miliaria) may be noted.

Decubitus Ulcers

The decubitus ulcer, or **bedsore,** is an ulceration of the skin and subcutaneous tissue that overlies a bony prominence due to sustained pressure or friction of a body part resting against an external object. Decubitus ulcers occur when beds, wheelchairs, casts, splints, or other objects persistently impinge on bodily tissue. Decubitus ulcers result from an interplay of external and internal factors. The external factors are pressure, shearing force, friction, and moisture. Pressure, the most important factor, is greatest over the bony prominences when an individual is lying down. The internal factors that contribute to decubitus ulcers include loss of skin sensibility, obesity, malnutrition, motor paralysis, muscle atrophy, muscle spasticity, trauma, incontinence, infection, heat and moisture, local capillary defects, or edema. When a combination of these extrinsic and intrinsic factors impairs local circulation excessively, the result is the ischemic necrosis that characterizes these ulcers.

The prevention and alleviation of bedsores is an important function of the nurse, whether dealing with hospital patients or serving bedridden clients in the community. Frequent inspection for bedsores is prerequisite to adequate care. Existing bedsores often require debridement by surgical techniques or application of debriding agents (see below). Prevention of bedsores is achieved by (1) measures that minimize external factors that contribute to pressure, shearing force, moisture, or friction, (2) measures that stimulate local blood flow to prevent ischemia, (3) measures for achieving proper hygiene and healthy skin, and (4) measures to achieve good nutrition.

Care must be taken to promote adequate blood circulation in the ulcer-prone areas. The recumbent position of bedridden patients should be changed every 2 hours, day and night. For patients with spinal injuries, a turning frame facilitates this maneuver. When appropriate, the patient should be given passive or active exercises to help maintain muscle tone and vascularity. Hydrotherapy in a whirlpool bath is also helpful. Massage of the patient's back and bony prominences with an appropriate lotion or nonalcoholic linament is an effective precaution (see below).

Good hygiene is an important aspect of preventing bedsores. Soap and water baths are the usual means of maintaining cleanliness. If water cannot be tolerated due to skin disease, an inert oil can be substituted. Care should be taken to maintain adequate but not excessive skin moisture. Excessive moisture that promotes infection can be prevented with absorbent powders or protectants. Dry skin that lacks strength and pliancy can be prevented by addition of a small amount of bath oil to bath water or using a lubricating emollient or lotion after washing.

Soap and Bath Oils

Ordinary soap consists of sodium salts of three fatty acids: palmitic, oleic, and stearic acids. Alkaline substances are used to make soap from fat by breaking down the fatty acid esters into fatty acids and glycerin, a process called *saponification.* Soaps are usually made from olive or coconut oils. All soaps are alkaline, and excess alkalinity may cause skin irritation. Antiseptics such as cresol, thymol, or sulfur may be added to produce medicated soaps, but these substances also may be irritating. Too frequent use of soap can result in dry skin for which bath oils or emollients may be helpful.

Bath oils fall into two categories: floating oils or dispersible oils. The difference between the two is the presence of an emulsifying (surfactant) agent in the dispersible formulations. The floating oils do not mix with water, leave an oily scum on the sides and bottom of the tub, lack cleansing or water softening properties, and form oily patches on the skin rather than spreading evenly. For these reasons, dispersible oils are more popular. All of the dispersible oils contain a surfactant. The emollient oils found in bath oils include mineral oil, lanolin, vegetable oils, and fatty acid esters.

Rubefacients, Linaments, and Counterirritants

Reflex vasodilation is the first phase of skin inflammation. Drugs known as rubefacients or counterirritants are mild irritants that induce vasodilation without causing subsequent phases of inflammation. The local vasodilation produced by rubefacients produces a sensation of warmth and feeling of comfort. Used in linaments, rubefacients can produce a useful counterirritant effect in alleviating muscle aches, arthritis, sprains, or neuralgia. *Rubefacients can be used to prevent bedsores but should not be applied to skin that is irritated or sensitive, nor should they contact muscous membranes or the eyes.* The principal counterirritants are methyl salicylate, camphor, menthol, thymol, eugenol, and eucalyptol. A variety of counterirritant preparations are available in the form of gels, creams, ointments, lotions, and linaments. *Methyl salicylate should be kept out of reach of children.*

Debriding Agents

Enzymes that digest tissue can be applied topically to necrotic debris to achieve chemical debridement, which clears the wound and promotes healing. The topical debriding enzymes include sutilains, collagenase, fibrinolysin, desoxyribonuclease, trypsin, and papain. Sutilains (Travase) and trypsin (Granulex) are proteolytic. Collagenase (Biozyme-C, Santyl) metabolizes collagen, the major protein of connective tissue. Fibrinolysin digests fibrin, while desoxyribonuclease breaks down DNA. The last two of these enzymes are provided in combination (Elase or Elase-Chloromycetin). Papain (Panafil, Panafil White) digests collagen in the presence of urea. Chymopapain (Chymodiactin), a proteolytic enzyme introduced in 1982, can be applied intrathecally to digest tissue that has been forced from a herniated lumbar disc that is exerting pressure against a nerve.

Before application of a topical debriding enzyme, the wound should be thoroughly cleaned with water or saline. Antiseptics such as iodide, hexachlorophene, heavy metal compounds, nitrofurazone, or benzalkonium chloride should not be employed prior to or during use of debriding enzymes, since these antiseptics have the potential of inactivating the debriding agents. Excess necrotic tissue is removed surgically with scissors and forceps. Any ointment previously applied must be removed before application of fresh enzyme. Crosshatching of thick eschar can be performed to hasten digestion. After thorough moistening of the eschar, ointment is applied directly to the wound tissue with a sterile tongue depressor or gauze. The treated wound is then covered with a thin layer of moist gauze or other nonadhering dressing. Dressings are changed 1–3 times daily and kept moist at all times, since enzyme activity depends on adequate moisture. Care must be taken not to allow the ointment to contact healthy skin. A protectant such as zinc oxide can be used on normal skin adjacent to the wound, and patients are instructed not to move the part so as to avoid displacing the medication and dressing. Treatment is discontinued when the wound is cleared of debris or if hypersensitivity reactions occur. The normal time required for debridement ranges from 2 to 4 days with the fibrinolysin-desoxyribonuclease combination to 11 days with collagenase.

To cleanse exudative ulcers and wounds, a nonenzymatic debriding agent called **dextranomer** is available that consists of a hydrophilic dextran polymer in the form of beads. Each hydrophilic bead absorbs about 4 ml of water, thereby removing exudates that may retard healing. Only low molecular weight particles are taken up into the beads, so that plasma proteins are left behind.

When saturated, the beads become grayish yellow and should be removed. *When used in decubitus ulcers, the cavity should not be tightly packed to allow for expansion of the beads as they absorb fluid. To minimize the possibility of cross contamination, the contents of a container should be limited to the use of one patient. Before application of dextranomer beads, the wound should be cleansed with sterile water or saline and left moist. The wound area is covered with beads to a thickness of about 3 mm. A light bandage can be applied to hold the beads in place. Removal of beads can be accomplished by irrigating 1–4 times per day. Dextranomer beads are dangerously slippery if spilled on the floor.*

Preparations and Administration

Dextranomer (Debrisan)
Beads

Case Study: Burn Injury

R. N., a nurse, was visiting at the summer home of friends when a cup of very hot coffee was spilled on the 2-year-old child, Alice. The child began crying immediately, and in a few seconds the skin turned red and appeared scalded. As the mother picked up the child, R. N. noted that the coffee had spilled on an area encompassing the left arm and left side of the chest and abdomen. The nurse instructed the mother to quickly remove the child's shirt and went into the kitchen, returning with washclothes and a pan of cold water. R. N. gently applied cold compresses to the area of redness while the mother comforted the child. While R. N. was applying the compresses, she mentally noted that the burn appeared to be superficial and, using the "rule of 9," she estimated that about 4% of the body surface area was involved. The burn on the arm extended from about the middle of the forearm to the middle of the upper arm. After 45 minutes of application of cold compresses, Alice had calmed down but continued to weep. The mother asked R. N. about application of a local anesthetic spray, a topical antibacterial preparation, or a powder; the nurse suggested application of petrolatum, which was also on hand in the medicine cabinet. R. N. ensured that the burn area was free of dirt or debris before applying the petrolatum. She suggested leaving the area open initially; later Alice was given a light, loose clean shirt to put on. R. N. then suggested that the mother check the status of the child's tetanus immunizations, since tetanus is a frequent complication of even minor burns.

1. Would Alice's burn injury qualify as "minor"? Why?
2. What properties of petrolatum make it a useful protectant for use in burn injuries? Why would a powder be less useful?
3. If R. N. had thought it necessary to apply a local anesthetic after first aid, what properties would be desirable in the product utilized? What instructions would the nurse likely have given the mother about using a local anesthetic?
4. Did the nurse err in advising against use of an antibacterial agent and suggesting that the burn area be left exposed initially?

Answers appear at the end of the book.

Recommended Readings

General Sources

Arndt KA: *Manual of Dermatologic Therapeutics with Essentials of Diagnosis,* ed 3. Boston, Little Brown & Co, 1983.

Acne Medications

Eady EA et al: Use of antibiotics in acne therapy: Oral or topical administration? *Antimicrob Chemother* 1982;10:89–115.

Melski JW, Arndt KA: Topical therapy for acne. *N Engl J Med* 1980;302:1419.

Olsen TG: Therapy for acne. *Med Clin North Am* 1982;66(4):851–871.

Peck GL: Retinoids: Therapeutic use in dermatology. *Drugs* 1982;24:341–351.

Antipruritics

Winkelmann RK: Pharmacologic control of pruritus. *Med Clin North Am* 1982;66(5):1119–1133.

Antipsoriatics

Amann L: Psoriasis — looking for a cure. *Nurs Times* 1979;75:407–410.

Anderson T: Psoriasis. *Med Clin North Am* 1982;66(4):769–794.

Anderson TF, Voorhess JJ: Psoralen photochemotherapy of cutaneous disorders. *Annu Rev Pharmacol Toxicol* 1980;20:235–257.

Arnold V, Rose S: Photochemotherapy for psoriasis. *Am J Nurs* 1979;79(3):466–468.

Kaidbey KH, Kligman AM: Clinical and histologic study of coal tar phototoxicity in humans. *Arch Dermatol* 1977;113:592–595.

Antiseptics

Block SS: *Disinfection, sterilization, and preservation,* ed 3. Philadelphia, Lea & Febiger, 1983.

Hargiss CO, Larson E: Guidelines for prevention of hospital acquired infections. *Am J Nurs* 1981;81(12):2175–2183.

Hnatko SI: Alternatives to hexachlorophene bathing of new born infants. *Can Med Assoc J* 1977;117:223–226.

Burn Preparations and Sunscreens

Kaidbey KH, Kligman AM: Appraisal of efficacy and substantivity of new high-potency sunscreens. *J Am Acad Dermatol* 1981;4:566–570.

Moleski RJ: Burn wound: Topical therapy for infection control. *Drug Intell Clin Pharm* 1978;12:28–35.

Pegg SP: Role of drugs in management of burns. *Drugs* 1982;24:256–260.

Warshauer DM, Steinbaugh JR: Sunlight and protection of the skin. *Am Fam Physician* 1983;27(6):109–114.

Drug Eruptions

Bickers DR: Treatment of selected photosensitivity diseases. *Med Clin North Am* 1982;66(5):927–939.

Fisher AA: *Contact Dermatitis,* ed 2. Philadelphia, Lea & Febiger, 1975.

Drugs and Decubitus Ulcers

Ahmed MC: Choosing the best method to manage pressure ulcers. *Nurses' Drug Alert* 1980;4(15):113–120.

Arnell I: Treating decubitus ulcers. *Nursing* 1983;13:50–55.

Nierman MM: Treatment of dermal and decubitus ulcers. *Drugs* 1978;15:226–230.

Emollients

Berliner H: Aging skin (parts 1&2). *Am J Nurs* 1986;86(10):1138–1141, 86(11):1259–1262.

Steinbaugh JR: Dry skin. *Am Fam Physician* 1983;27(3):171–174.

Topical Anti-Infectives

Allen HB et al: Selenium sulfide: Adjunctive therapy for tinea capitis. *Pediatrics* 1982;69:81–83.

Borgers M: Mechanism of action of antifungal drugs, with special reference to the imidazole derivatives. *Rev Infect Dis* 1980;2:520–534.

Estes S: Diagnosis and management of scabies. *Med Clin North Am* 1982;66(4):955–963.

Gossel T, Wuest R: Treatment of lice, mite, and tick infestations. *Calif Pharm* 1977, pp. 20–23.

Jones H: Therapy of superficial fungal infection. *Med Clin North Am* 1982;66(4):873–893.

Lewis MR: Tinea versicolor. *Nurse Pract* 1986;11(2):30–35.

McLaury P: Head lice: A pediatric social disease. *Am J Nurs* 1983;83:1300–1303.

Orkin M, Maibach HI: Current concepts in parasitology: This scabies pandemic. *N Engl J Med* 1978;298:496–498.

Rosen T, Rudolph AH: Identifying and treating bacterial and fungal infections of skin. *Geriatrics* 1978;33:71–82.

Smith E, Raimer S: Common viral infections of the skin and their treatment. *Med Clin North Am* 1982;66(4):807–817.

Topical Steroids

Miller JA, Munro DD: Topical corticosteroids: clinical pharmacology and therapeutic use. *Drugs* 1980;19:119–134.

O'Malley B: Mechanisms of steroid hormone actions. *J Invest Dermatol* 1977;68:1–4.

Robertson DB, Maibach HI: Topical corticosteroids. *Int J Dermatol* 1982;21:59–67.

Appendix 53A
Characteristics and Treatments of Skin Diseases

Skin disease	Typical population	Usual distribution	Type of lesion	Typical treatments
General inflammatory dermatitides				
Atopic dermatitis	Older children or adults	Feet, hands, face	Erythema, vesicles, papules, plaques, pruritus	Avoid irritants; topical steroids
Contact dermatitis	Any	Face, arms, anogenital area, axillae, eyelids, feet, hands, legs, lips	Bullae, scaly papules, pruritus	Remove causative agents; topical steroids; antipruritics
Exfoliative dermatitis	Any	Widespread	Erythema, scaling	Remove causative agents; topical steroids; oral steroids
Localized neurodermatitis	Females more than males; usually age 20–50	Occipital region, arms, legs, ankles	Erythema, scaly plaques, hyperpigmentation, pruritus	Topical steroids
Nummular dermatitis	Middle-aged	Usually on legs	Erythema, coin-shaped scaly vesicles	Topical steroids
Seborrheic dermatitis	Adults, infants	Scalp, face, occasionally on back, chest, ears, anogenital area	Plaques	Antiseborrheics; topical steroids
Granuloma annulare	Children or adults	Feet, legs, hands, fingers	Papules or nodules	Intralesional steroids; topical steroids with occlusive dressing
Papular inflammatory dermatitides				
Psoriasis	Mainly whites, onset 10–40 years of age	Abdomen, chest, back, legs, arms, scalp, feet, anogenital region	Scaly papules	Antipsoriatics (lubricants, keratolytics); topical steroids; antimetabolites; PUVA
Pityriasis rosea	Young adults	Chest, back, and proximal extremities	Scaly macules	Self-limited
Lichen planus	Adults	Arms, legs, trunk, mouth, anogenital region	Scaly papules, pruritus	Antipruritics; topical steroids and occlusive wrap
Drug eruptions				
Rash	Users of various drugs	Anywhere	Erythema, maculopapullar, morbilliform	Eliminate offending drug; lubricants; topical steroids
Acneiform	Especially clients on steroids	Areas rich in sebaceous glands	Pustules, papules	Eliminate offending drug
Urticaria	Any	Anywhere	Wheals, pruritus	Eliminate offending drug; oral antihistamines
Fixed Drug	Any	Reappear at same site	Rash	Eliminate offending drug; topical steroids
Purpura	Any	Lower extremities, elsewhere	Hyperpigmentation due to bleeding	Eliminate offending drug
Photosensitivity	Users of various drugs	Where skin is exposed to sunlight; where drug is applied if topical	Erythema, macules, gray-blue patches	Eliminate offending drug; sunscreen
Erythema nodosum	Young adults, especially those receiving sulfonamides, halides, or oral contraceptives	Forearms especially	Nodules	Eliminate offending drug; systemic steroids

Appendix 53A
Characteristics and Treatments of Skin Diseases (*continued*)

Skin disease	Typical population	Usual distribution	Type of lesion	Typical treatments
Erythema multiforme	Any	Palms, soles, mucus membranes or widespread	Bullae, erythema	Eliminate offending drug; systemic steroids
Exfoliative dermatitis	Any	Widespread	Erythema, profuse scaling	Eliminate offending drug; petrolatum; oral steroids
Discoid lupus erythematosus	Females more than males; late 30s	Face, ears, and scalp or whole body	Macules, plaques, erythema	Avoid sunlight exposure; use sunscreen; topical steroids; systemic antimalarials
Toxic epidermal necrolysis	Infants, adults	Widespread	Peeling sheets of skin with scalded appearance	Oral antibiotics for infant form; systemic steroids for adult form
Autoimmune disorders of the skin				
Pemphigus	Middle or old age	Mouth, pharynx, esophagus	Bullae	High-dose systemic steroids
Bullous pemphigoid	Adults	Widespread on skin	Bullae	High-dose systemic steroids
Dermatitis herpetiformis	15–60 years of age	Elbows, knees, sacrum, buttocks, face	Bullae, vesicles, papules	Dapsone; sulfapyridine
Bacterial infections				
Impetigo	Children	Arms, legs, and face	Vesicles, pustules	Systemic antibacterials
Erysipelas	Any	Face, arms, and legs	Vesicles, bullae, erythema	Systemic antibacterials
Folliculitis	Any	Hairy areas	Pustules, nodules	Systemic antibacterials
Furuncles/carbuncles	Young adults; males more than females	Neck, face, breasts, buttocks	Boils	Moist heat; systemic antibacterials
Fungal infections				
Dermatophytes	Any	Feet, nails, head, crural fold, trunk	Erythema, vesicles, bullae	Griseofulvin (systemic) or topical antifungals
Candidiasis	Any but especially diabetics, pregnant females, females using oral contraceptives	Intertriginous zones, vulvovaginal area, mouth, nails, perianal area	Erythema, pruritus	Topical nystatin; clotrimazole; miconazole
Tinea versicolor	Young adults	Abdomen, back	Colored patches	Selenium sulfide, imidazoles
Viral infections				
Herpes simplex	Children, young adults	Oral mucosa, genitals, pruritus	Vesicles, pustules	Idoxuridine, vidarabine, trifluridine
Herpes zoster	Before age 50	Band across the trunk or face, pruritus	Vesicles, pustules	Corticosteroids, wet compresses, aspirin
Warts				
Common	Older children, young adults	Fingers, elbows, knees, face, scalp	Nodules	Freezing, surgery, caustics
Plantar	Older children, young adults	Soles, palms	Nodules	Keratolytics

(*continued*)

Appendix 53A
Characteristics and Treatments of Skin Diseases (*continued*)

Skin disease	Typical population	Usual distribution	Type of lesion	Typical treatments
Parasitic infestations				
Pediculosis	Any, especially children	Hair of scalp or pubis	Pruritus, erythema	Pediculicides
Scabies	Any	Whole body	Pruritus, burrows, vesicles	Miticides
Pruritus	Any	Anyplace	Itching	Antipruritics
Disorders of cornification				
Corns/calluses	Heavy use of hands or feet	Feet, hands, bony prominences	Hyperkeratotic growths	Better fitting footwear; keratolytics
Xeroderma (dry skin)	Elderly; family history of dry skin; overly meticulous bathers	Lower legs especially	Scaling, pruritus	Emollients; reduce use of soaps
Keratosis pilaris (horny plugs)	Any	Arms, thighs, buttocks	Keratotic papules	Petrolatum or cold cream
Disorders of skin appendages				
Sebaceous glands				
Acne				
Superficial	Adolescents, especially males	Face, back, chest	Erythema, comedones, cysts, papules, pustules	Frequent washing, sunlight, benzoyl peroxidase, retinoic acid, topical antibiotics
Deep	White, adolescent males	Trunk, buttocks	Nodules, pits, cysts	Oral antibiotics, steroids, sulfones, oral retinoids
Acne rosacea	Middle age	Center of face	Papules, pustules	Avoid flush reactions; tetracyclines
Perioral dermatitis	Females, 20–60 years old	Circle around mouth	Papules	Tetracyclines
Sweat glands				
Hidrademitis suppurativa	Any	Axillae, groin, nipples, anus	Erythema	Eliminate antiperspirants; systemic antibacterials
Miliaria rubra	Any	Axillae	Erythema, pruritis	Avoid sweat-provoking conditions; topical steroids
Hyperhidrosis	Any	Palms, soles, axillae, groin	Wetness	Antiperspirants
Hair follicles				
Alopecia				
Male pattern	Older men	Scalp	Loss of hair in frontal and parietal areas	Hair transplants; hair piece; minoxidil
Female pattern	Postmenopausal females	Scalp	Thinning of hair in frontal and parietal areas	Usually none required
Alopecia areata	Any	Scalp; rarely whole body	Sudden hair loss	Topical steroids
Hirsutism	Adrenal virilism in females and children	Face, limbs, trunk	Excess hair	Electrolysis of follicles; shaving; plucking; waxing; chemical depilatories
Ingrown hairs	Black males	Beard area	Pustules	Let beard grow

Appendix 53A
Characteristics and Treatments of Skin Diseases (*continued*)

Skin disease	Typical population	Usual distribution	Type of lesion	Typical treatments
Melanocytes				
Hyperpigmentation	Females in pregnancy, on oral contraceptives, or aging	Face, arms	Melasma	Demelanizing agents
Hypopigmentation	Albinos, Addison's disease, diabetes mellitus, pernicious anemia	Trunk, limbs	Blanched areas	Cosmetics; melanizing agents
Nails				
Paronychial infections	Individuals experiencing prolonged exposure of hands to water	Nails	Inflammation, purulent pockets	Warm soaks; antibacterials or antifungals
Trauma				
Burns	Any	Any part	Superficial erythema; partial-thickness; full-thickness	Protectants; local anesthetics; anti-infectants
Sunburn	Sunbathers; people with outdoor occupations	Face, back, arms, neck, legs, breasts	Erythema, blistering	Sunscreens; local anesthetics
Decubitus ulcer	Bedridden patients with loss of sensibility or immobility	Over bony prominences	Ulcer	High-protein diet; exercises; rubs; debriding agents
Intertrigo	Obese people	Intertriginous areas	Chafing	Protectants; absorbents
Tumors				
Malignant carcinomas	Adults	Any part of epithelium	Nodules, ulcerations, plaques	Electrodesiccation and curettage; surgical incision; x-ray; topical fluorouracil
Melanomas	Pregnant females more than nonpregnant; males	Pigmented skin	Pigmented tumor	Surgical incision
Benign				
Moles	First appear in childhood, adolescence, or pregnancy	Anywhere	Pigmented macules, papules, or nodules	Surgical removal
Keloid	More common in blacks than whites	Upper back, chest, deltoid area	Fibroblastic growth	Intralesional steroids

Appendix 53B
Skin Eruptions Produced by Representative Drugs

	Not life-threatening								Life-threatening			
Drug	**Rash (erythematous or morbilliform)**	**Acneiform eruptions**	**Urticaria**	**Lichenoid reactions**	**Purpura**	**Fixed drug eruptions**	**Photosensitivity**	**Erythema nodosum**	**Erythema multiforme**	**Toxic epidermal necrolysis**	**Discoid lupus erythematosus**	**Exfoliative dermatitis**
Analgesics												
Migraine												
Ergots					X	X						
Methysergide	X										X	
Narcotics	X		X		X	X			X	X		
Nonnarcotics												
Acetaminophen	X		X			X						
Phenacetin	X		X			X						
Antialcoholic												
Disulfiram						X						
Antihistamines	X					X	X			X		
Anti-inflammatory drugs												
Nonsteroidal												
Allopurinol	X				X							X
Indomethacin	X		X					X				X
Pyrazolones	X				X	X	X		X	X	X	X
Salicylates	X		X		X	X	X		X			
Steroidal-direct		X			X							
-withdrawal											X	
Antimicrobials												
Amebicides												
Chloroquine				X		X	X					
Antibacterials												
Cephalosporins	X		X									X
Chloramphenicol	X		X			X			X			
Clindamycin	X		X						X			
Dactinomycin	X	X										
Erythromycin	X		X									
Gentamicin	X						X					
Lincomycin	X						X		X			
Neomycin	X									X		
Novobiocin	X		X						X			
Penicillin	X		X		X	X			X	X	X	X
Streptomycin	X		X		X	X					X	X
Sulfonamides	X		X		X	X	X	X	X	X	X	X
Tetracyclines	X		X		X	X	X		X	X	X	X

Appendix 53B
Skin Eruptions Produced by Representative Drugs (*continued*)

	Not life-threatening								Life-threatening			
Drug	**Rash (erythematous or morbilliform)**	**Acneiform eruptions**	**Urticaria**	**Lichenoid reactions**	**Purpura**	**Fixed drug eruptions**	**Photosensitivity**	**Erythema nodosum**	**Erythema multiforme**	**Toxic epidermal necrolysis**	**Discoid lupus erythematosus**	**Exfoliative dermatitis**
Antifungals												
Clotrimazole	X											
Griseofulvin	X		X		X	X	X				X	X
Miconazole	X											
Antihelmintics												
Bithional							X					
Piperazine	X		X		X				X			
Antimalarials												
Chloroguanide				X		X	X					
Quinacrine						X						
Quinine	X					X	X					
Antiprotozoals												
Arsenicals				X		X	X		X			X
Antitubercular												
Aminosalicylic acid	X			X		X					X	X
Ethionamide	X	X										
Isoniazid	X				X						X	X
Rifampin	X	X	X		X				X		X	
Leprostatic												
Amithiozone									X			
Sulfones	X								X	X		X
Urinary tract anti-infectives												
Methenamine	X					X						
Nalidixic acid	X						X					
Nitrofurans	X		X							X		X
Antineoplastics												
5-Fluorouracil	X						X					
6-Mercaptopurine	X						X					
Methotrexate	X		X				X					
Nitrogen mustards	X						X					
Autonomic drugs												
Belladonna alkaloids	X					X			X			
Beta-blockers	X				X							

(*continued*)

Appendix 53B

Skin Eruptions Produced by Representative Drugs (*continued*)

	Not life-threatening								Life-threatening			
Drug	**Rash (erythematous or morbilliform)**	**Acneiform eruptions**	**Urticaria**	**Lichenoid reactions**	**Purpura**	**Fixed drug eruptions**	**Photosensitivity**	**Erythema nodosum**	**Erythema multiforme**	**Toxic epidermal necrolysis**	**Discoid lupus erythematosus**	**Exfoliative dermatitis**
Decongestants												
Ephedrine					X	X						
Epinephrine						X						
Cardiovascular drugs												
Antidysrhythmics												
Procainamide			X								X	
Quinidine				X	X	X					X	
Antihypertensives												
Clonidine	X		X									
Hydralazine	X					X	X				X	
Methyldopa	X			X							X	
Reserpine	X					X					X	
Digitalis					X	X					X	
Nitrates	X											X
CNS drugs												
Analeptic												
Strychnine						X						
Antidepressants	X		X		X		X					
Antiepileptics												
Carbamazepine	X		X				X	X	X			X
Hydantoins	X	X	X			X	X		X	X	X	X
Oxazolidones	X						X		X		X	
Primidone	X										X	
Succinimides	X		X						X		X	
Valproic acid	X											
Antimanic												
Lithium		X										X
Antiparkinsonian												
L-dopa	X										X	
Antipsychotics												
Phenothiazines	X			X	X	X	X				X	X
Anxiolytics												
Benzodiazepines	X		X			X						

Appendix 53B
Skin Eruptions Produced by Representative Drugs (*continued*)

	Not life-threatening								Life-threatening			
Drug	Rash (erythematous or morbilliform)	Acneiform eruptions	Urticaria	Lichenoid reactions	Purpura	Fixed drug eruptions	Photosensitivity	Erythema nodosum	Erythema multiforme	Toxic epidermal necrolysis	Discoid lupus erythematosus	Exfoliative dermatitis
Sedative-hypnotics												
Barbiturates	X		X		X	X	X		X	X		X
Benzodiazepines	X											
Bromides		X	X			X		X				
Chloral hydrate	X				X	X						
Ethchlorvynol	X		X			X						
Meprobamate	X		X		X	X			X			X
Methaqualone	X		X									
Piperidinediones	X											
Stimulants												
Amphetamine						X						
Methylphenidate	X		X		X				X			X
Pemoline	X											
Dermatologics												
Antipsoriatics												
Anthralin						X	X					
Methoxsalen							X					
Tars							X					
Antiseptics/disinfectants												
Hexachlorophene							X					
Iodine						X						
Salicylanilides							X					
Counterirritant												
Methyl salicylate										X		
Sunscreens												
p-aminobenzoic acid							X					
Cinnamates							X					
Digalloyl trioleate							X					
p-dimethylaminobenzene							X					
Glyceryl *p*-aminobenzoate							X					

(*continued*)

Appendix 53B
Skin Eruptions Produced by Representative Drugs (*continued*)

	Not life-threatening								Life-threatening			
Drug	Rash (erythematous or morbilliform)	Acneiform eruptions	Urticaria	Lichenoid reactions	Purpura	Fixed drug eruptions	Photosensitivity	Erythema nodosum	Erythema multiforme	Toxic epidermal necrolysis	Discoid lupus erythematosus	Exfoliative dermatitis
Diuretics												
Acetazolamide	X									X		
Furosemide	X		X		X		X		X			X
Mercurials	X		X			X						X
Spironolactone	X		X									
Thiazides	X			X	X		X		X		X	X
Triamterene	X						X					
Endocrine drugs												
ACTH		X	X		X							
Androgens		X										
Antithyroid												
Iodides		X	X		X			X				
Thiouracils	X		X				X		X		X	
Estrogens												
Diethylstilbestrol					X	X	X	X	X			
Others							X	X	X			
Hypoglycemics												
Insulin	X		X	X								
Sulfonylureas	X		X		X		X		X			X
Oral contraceptives	X	X					X	X			X	
Endogenous pigments												
Porphyrins							X					
Foods[a]	X		X				X					
Gastrointestinal drugs												
Antacids												
Magnesium hydroxide							X					
Antidiarrheal												
Loperamide	X											
Anti-infective												
Sulfasalazine	X								X	X	X	X
Laxative-cathartics												
Karaya gum						X						
Phenolphthalein						X			X	X		
Emetic												
Ipecac						X				X		

Appendix 53B

Skin Eruptions Produced by Representative Drugs (*continued*)

	Not life-threatening								Life-threatening			
Drug	**Rash (erythematous or morbilliform)**	**Acneiform eruptions**	**Urticaria**	**Lichenoid reactions**	**Purpura**	**Fixed drug eruptions**	**Photosensitivity**	**Erythema nodosum**	**Erythema multiforme**	**Toxic epidermal necrolysis**	**Discoid lupus erythematosus**	**Exfoliative dermatitis**
Heavy metal antagonist												
Penicillamine	X										X	
Heavy metal compounds												
Antimony salts						X						
Bismuth salts						X						
Gold salts	X	X		X	X	X	X			X	X	X
Silver salts							X					
Hematopoietic												
Anticoagulants												
Phenindione	X				X							X
Warfarin	X		X		X							
Hematologics												
Dextran			X									
Serums	X		X									
Industrial chemicals[b]							X					
Local anesthetics							X			X		
Nutrients/electrolytes/additives												
Additive												
Saccharin						X	X					
Electrolyte												
Potassium						X						
Vitamin												
Cyanocobalamin		X										
Perfumes[c]							X					
Vaccines												
Measles virus									X			X
Smallpox							X		X			
Various						X						

[a]Foods most likely to produce rashes (atopic dermatitis) or urticaria include eggs, milk, wheat, citrus fruits (especially grapefruit and oranges), melons, strawberries, corn, tomatoes, nuts, peanuts, fish, shellfish, chocolate, spices (cloves, mustard, black pepper), and additives. Foods that cause photosensitivity include celery, citrus fruits, lady's thumb tea, parsley, parsnips, smartweed tea, and wild carrots.

[b]Industrial chemicals that cause photosensitivity include acridine, anthracene, benzene, eosin dye, methylene blue, naphthalene, phenanthrene, phenazine dyes, phenolic compounds, pyridine, toluene, and xylene.

[c]Perfumes that cause photosensitivity include bergamot, 6-methyl-coumarin, musk ambrette, psoralens, rose bengal, and sandalwood.

UNIT XI

Drugs and the Special Sensory Organs

CHAPTER 54

Drugs Used for Disorders of the Eye

Anatomy of the Eye

The eyeballs, deeply recessed in the orbits in the skull, are held in place and moved by the six **extraocular muscles:** the medial, lateral, superior, and inferior recti and the superior and inferior oblique muscles. These muscles are controlled by the third, fourth, and sixth cranial nerves, which arise from the oculomotor, trochlear, and abducens nuclei of the brainstem.

The outer sheath of the eyeball is the white, nontransparent **sclera** that covers the entire eyeball except where the cornea covers the iris and pupil and where the optic nerve gathers on the posterior surface before entering the brain. Inside the sclera, the eye is divided into two chambers, the large **posterior chamber** and the smaller **anterior chamber.** The inner wall of the posterior chamber is the light-sensitive retinal layer. The **retina** itself is a screen of neural elements extending about 100 degrees and backed by the **choroid,** which absorbs light so as to reduce reflection and scattering. The retina contains the receptor cells called *rods* and *cones.* Between the scleral and retinal layers is a small space, the **suprachoroidal space,** that contains the numerous small blood vessels of the eye.

In the back of the posterior chamber is the **blind spot** at the point where the optic nerve forms. One million fibers project from the eye along each of the two optic nerves. At the optic chiasm, half of the fibers cross over to join the opposite optic tract, so that the right visual field is represented in the occipital lobe of the left hemisphere and the left visual field is represented in the right hemisphere. Slightly lateral to the blind spot is the fovea centralis where visual acuity is greatest. Filling the posterior chamber is the **vitreous humor,** a viscous fluid.

Separating the posterior and anterior chambers is the lens and the system of suspensory ligaments that hold the **lens** in place. The lens, which focuses the light on the retina, is a gelatinous mass of proteinous fibers within a thin elastic sheath. The lens is normally transparent, but the transparency may gradually decline with aging, from exposure to x-rays or heat, or as a result of trauma, diabetes, inflammation, or use of glucocorticoids, resulting in an opaque area in the lens called a **cataract.**

The lens focuses light by changing its shape in a process called **accommodation,** which is controlled by the suspensory ligaments called *zonular fibers.* The zonular fibers are attached to the lens at one end and the **ciliary muscle** at the other. When the ciliary muscle is relaxed, the zonular fibers are taut and the lens is stretched outward in accommodation for far vision. For near vision, the ciliary muscle contracts, releasing the tension on the zonular fibers, and the lens rebounds to its more biconvex shape. This process occurs more readily in young people; with aging, the lens becomes more rigid and rebounds less fully, resulting in a gradual recession of the closest point that can be focused. The ciliary muscles that regulate accommodation are controlled by parasympathetic nervous system efferent fibers.

In front of the lens lies the anterior chamber, which is filled with the **aqueous humor.** Secreted by the ciliary bodies, the aqueous humor undergoes continuous turnover (Figure 54–1). The fluid flows into the anterior chamber through the space between the iris and lens, and the excess normally drains out of the anterior chamber through the trabeculae and spaces of Fontana into the canal of Schlemm. From there, discharged aqueous humor drains into the venous capillaries of the blood supply of the eye. If the rate of formation of new aqueous humor exceeds the drainage rate, intraocular pressure rises in the anterior chamber, resulting in glaucoma.

The doughnut-shaped **iris** protrudes medially

Figure 54–1
The flow of aqueous humor.

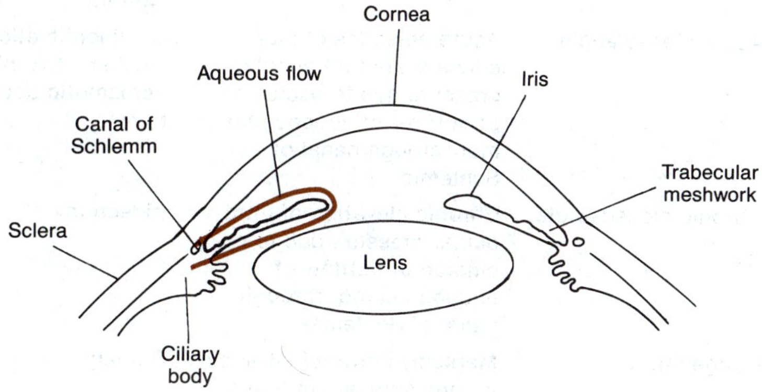

from the ciliary body, just anterior to the lens. The iris surrounds the pupil and controls the quantity of light that reaches the lens by dilating or constricting. The sphincter muscle within the iris forms a circle around the pupil and it contracts under parasympathetic influence to constrict the pupil. The dilator muscle extends radially in the iris from the pupil outward. It contracts under sympathetic influence to dilate the pupil. Thus pupillary constriction (miosis) is produced by drugs (miotics) that are either parasympathomimetic (cholinergic) or sympatholytic (antiadrenergic). Dilation (mydriasis) is produced by drugs (mydriatics) that are either sympathomimetic (adrenergic) or parasympatholytic (anticholinergic). The iris is variably pigmented, the specific hue (brown, blue, gray, green, or hazel) being genetically determined.

At the front of the eye, overlying the iris and anterior chamber is the **cornea,** which replaces the sclera as the outer membrane in this portion of the eyeball. The cornea is normally transparent and provides passage and rough focusing of light. It contains no blood vessels, obtaining oxygen by direct diffusion from surface air and nutrition from the aqueous humor of the anterior chamber. The outer layer of the cornea is epithelial and fairly resistant to infection, although injury increases susceptibility to infection and may promote scarring that interferes with vision.

The eyelids, eyelashes, eyebrows, and tears protect the eyeballs as do the blinking and corneal and conjunctival reflexes. The eyebrows prevent the flow of sweat from the forehead into the eye. The eyelashes are sensitive to foreign objects close to the eyes and trigger the blink reflex, which also occurs every few seconds as a means of spreading lacrimal fluid evenly over the surface of the eyeball. Tears provide lubrication and help to wash away debris. They are formed in the lacrimal glands located above and behind the outer canthus (corner of the eye), and drain via excretory ducts into the inner canthus, where they accumulate as the lacrimal lake. Tears drain from the lacrimal lake through two openings at the inner canthus into the lacrimal ducts, the lacrimal sac, and finally via the nasolacrimal duct into the nose. Tears contain lysozyme, a bactericidal protein. In spite of the protective mechanisms, the eye is subject to a variety of disorders. Drugs play a major role in two kinds of ocular disorders: glaucoma and inflammatory-infectious diseases (Table 54–1).

Glaucoma and Antiglaucoma Agents

Glaucoma is an eye disorder in which increased intraocular pressure occurs. If sufficiently severe and prolonged, the increased pressure leads to impaired vision that can range from a slight reduction in acu-

Table 54–1
Drug Treatments for Ocular Disorders

Disorder	Description	Treatments
Glaucoma		
Open-angle	Chronic elevation of intraocular pressure due to collapse of trabecular network	Cholinomimetics, sympathomimetics, beta-blockers, cholinesterase inhibitors, carbonic anhydrase (CA) inhibitors
Acute closed-angle	Acute episodes of markedly elevated intraocular pressure due to occlusion of outflow of aqueous humor through canal of Schlemm	Cholinomimetics, beta-blockers, CA inhibitors, hyperosmotic agents; iridectomy
Chronic closed-angle	Chronic elevation of intraocular pressure due to occlusion of outflow of aqueous humor through canal of Schlemm	Iridectomy
Congenital	Markedly elevated intraocular pressure within first 6 months of life	Surgery

Table 54–1
Drug Treatments for Ocular Disorders (*continued*)

Disorder	Description	Treatments
Glaucoma		
Secondary	Elevated intraocular pressure due to posterior synechia, iritis, cataracts, intraocular tumors, hemorrhage, trauma, or retinal vein occulsion	Topical or systemic steroids, surgery, CA inhibitors, etc.
Corticosteroid-induced	Adverse response to prolonged use of steroids	Eliminate steroid; employ cholinomimetics, beta-blockers, cholinesterase inhibitors, CA inhibitors
Inflammation/infections		
Conjunctivitis		
Acute	"Pink-eye." Inflammatory response to viral or bacterial infection or allergy	Topical antimicrobials; steroids if allergic origin
Chronic	Chronic conjunctival inflammation caused by viruses, bacteria, allergies, or chronic exposure to irritants	Eliminate irritant factors; short courses of antimicrobials
Eyelids		
Blepharitis	Inflammation of lid margins with scaling and crusting caused by bacterial infection	Topical antibacterial drugs
Hordeolum	Inflammation of meibomian glands usually caused by staphylococci	Topical antibacterial drugs
Chalazion	Chronic enlargement of meibomian gland with inflammation due to occlusion of its ducts	Hot compresses, topical antibacterials, curettage
Keratitis	Inflammation of superficial keratin layer of cornea, caused by:	
Superficial punctate	Viral infection or irritation	Topical antibiotics or eliminate irritant
Herpes simplex	Herpes simplex virus	Idoxuridine, vidarabine, trifluradine
Herpes zoster	Herpes zoster virus	Acyclovir
Uveitis		
Iritis	Inflammation of the iris caused by bacterial or viral infections or hypersensitivity reactions	Cycloplegic mydriatics; steroids
Cyclitis	Inflammations of the ciliary body; causes similar to iritis	Cycloplegic mydriatics; steroids
Choroiditis/chorioretinitis	Inflammation of the choroid or choroid and retina often associated with granulomatous diseases	Systemic steroids; topical mydriatics

ity to complete blindness. An imbalance between the rate of formation of aqueous humor and the rate of drainage causes a build-up of fluid and a rise in the intraocular pressure. Glaucoma can be primary, secondary, or congenital. Antiglaucoma drugs have an important role in treatment of primary glaucoma and in some types of secondary glaucoma but are not useful in congenital glaucoma, which is treated by surgical intervention. Secondary glaucoma can be due to iritis, intraocular tumors, large cataracts, or prolonged use of glucocorticoids.

Primary glaucoma manifests itself in two distinct types: open-angle (chronic, wide-angle) and closed-angle (also called narrow-angle, congestive, angle-closure) glaucoma (Figure 54–2). **Open-angle glaucoma,** the more common form, is a chronic disorder of gradual onset, with the slow loss of peripheral vision progressing to loss of central vision. It is usually familial, rarely unilateral, and rarely occurs before age 30. Open-angle glaucoma is caused by a gradual loss of patency in the trabeculae and spaces of Fontana. Collapse of these pores obstructs outflow of the aqueous humor, causing a buildup of fluid and pressure in the anterior chamber.

Closed-angle glaucoma occurs as an episodic condition with acute attacks of greater or lesser severity. It is caused by acute occlusion of the canal of Schlemm by the dilated iris. Attacks are typically unilateral and accompanied by pain, increased intraocular pressure, and reduced visual acuity. During an acute attack, the eye is widely dilated, the cornea has a steamy appearance, and the ciliary injections show clearly as red streaks across the sclera (Figure 54–3). A client with closed-angle glaucoma might complain of severe ocular pain, blurred vision, and seeing halos around lights. Primary closed-angle glaucoma constitutes about 10% of all glaucomas and is more common in females. Drug therapy is useful in alleviating acute attacks, but surgical procedures (iridectomy) are generally required for correction of the condition.

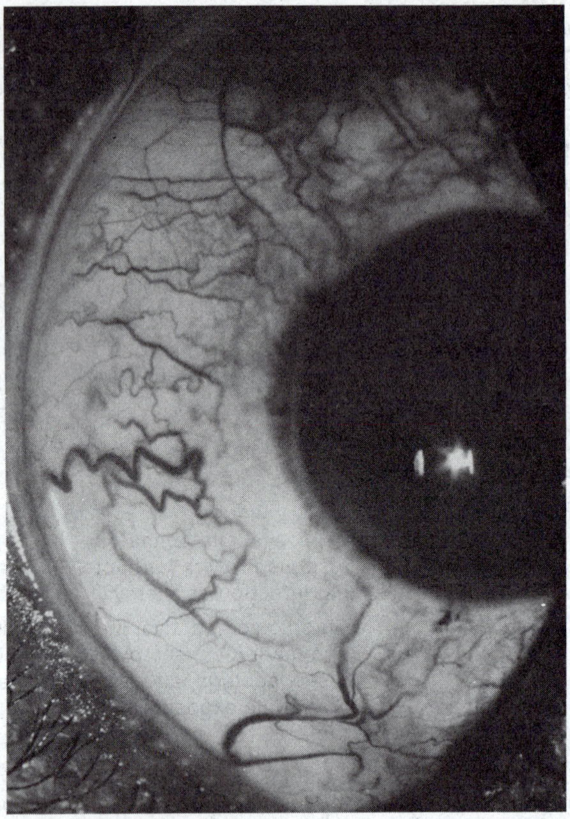

Figure 54–3
Pupillary dilation, ciliary injection, and steamy cornea of acute glaucoma. From D. L. Epstein, *Chandler and Grant's Glaucoma.* Philadelphia: Lea & Febiger, 1986.

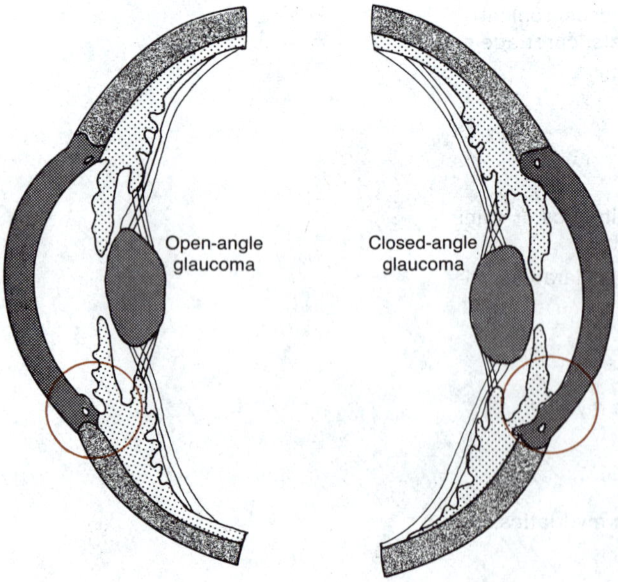

Figure 54–2
Comparison between open (wide) angle and closed (narrow) angle glaucoma.

Treatment

Parasympathomimetic drugs are useful in open-angle glaucoma because contraction of the sphincter and ciliary muscles enhances the tone of the trabecular meshwork, facilitating outflow. Other classes of drugs useful in open-angle glaucoma include sympathomimetics, the beta-blockers, carbonic anhy-

Table 54–2
Mechanism of Antiglaucoma Drugs

Drug	Decreased production of aqueous humor	Increased drainage of aqueous humor	Pupillary diameter	Lens
Cholinomimetics	+	+++	Constricted	Accommodation
Cholinesterase inhibitors	0	+++	Constricted	Accommodation
Sympathomimetics	+++	++	Dilated	No change
Beta-blockers	+++	+	No change	No change
Carbonic anhydrase inhibitors	+++	0	No change	No change
Osmotic agents	+++	0	No change	No change

drase inhibitors, and osmotic agents. Sympathomimetics are specifically contraindicated in closed-angle glaucoma, but otherwise drug management entails use of the same agents employed in open-angle glaucoma.

Reduction of intraocular pressure can be achieved either by decreasing production of aqueous humor or by increasing its outflow (Table 54–2). The direct and indirect cholinomimetics act primarily to increase drainage while the sympathomimetics, beta-blockers, and carbonic anhydrase inhibitors act primarily to decrease the rate of formation of aqueous humor. Drug therapy for glaucoma is begun with the weakest available topical preparation. Pilocarpine hydrochloride, 0.5% is the usual starting point. Timolol (Timoptic) is a good alternative and can be used alone or in combination with other agents. Carbachol (Carbacel, Isopto Carbachol) is more potent than pilocarpine and can be substituted when clients do not respond to the weaker drug. Sympathomimetic drugs are usually added to a regimen including a cholinomimetic, but occasionally they are used alone, primarily in clients who experience visual disturbances in response to the cholinergic agents. Carbonic anhydrase inhibitors are used as adjunctive therapy in those who are refractory to other drugs or drug combinations because of the systemic adverse effects. Long-acting cholinesterase inhibitors are likewise reserved for refractory cases. Osmotic diuretics are used only for controlling acute episodes of angle-closure glaucoma.

Cholinomimetics

Direct-acting cholinomimetic drugs are choline esters, chemically related to the natural transmitter, acetylcholine. Applied topically to the eye, cholinomimetic agents produce all of the ocular responses associated with parasympathetic nerve stimulation: (1) contraction of the sphincter muscle of the iris resulting in pupillary constriction; (2) contraction of the ciliary muscle, promoting accommodation; and (3) dilation of intraocular blood vessels. These drugs promote drainage of aqueous outflow by improving the patency of the trabecular meshwork and may also dilate collector channels and veins peripheral to the canal of Schlemm that receive the discharged aqueous humor. Cholinergic agonists may also have a modest ability to decrease the rate of production of aqueous humor. In closed-angle glaucoma, miosis produced by cholinomimetics opens the angle of the anterior chamber to facilitate drainage.

Acetylcholine itself is available as the chloride salt (Miochol) for intraocular administration. It is not employed in glaucoma, however, because of its very short duration of action, typically just a few minutes. From 0.5 to 2 ml of a 1:100 solution of acetylcholine is sometimes instilled in the eye to obtain rapid and complete miosis after removal of a cataract, peripheral iridectomy, penetrating keratoplasty, or in other ocular therapies. Transient lenticular opacities may occur.

Pilocarpine

Pilocarpine is the mainstay of drug treatment of glaucoma, especially open-angle glaucoma. Pilocarpine therapy can be continued indefinitely with this chronic form of glaucoma as long as it is effective in reducing intraocular pressure and causes no deterioration in visual function. In closed-angle glaucoma, pilocarpine is useful for control of acute attacks (frequently in conjunction with carbonic anhydrase inhibitors or osmotic diuretics) and in preparing a client for surgery. Pilocarpine also is used to antagonize the effect of mydriatics after surgery or ophthalmoscopic examination.

Adverse Effects and Contraindications Adverse effects of pilocarpine are usually confined to visual disturbances when applied topically to the eye. Systemic absorption is uncommon at usual doses. Pilocarpine should be used cautiously in clients with conditions that may be exacerbated by cholinergic activity. *It is important, therefore, that nurses acquire data concerning clients' cardiovascular condition prior to therapy so as to establish a predrug baseline assessment for those with bradycardia or congestive heart failure. Nurses should also closely observe clients who have a history of bronchial asthma, peptic ulcer, gastrointestinal spasm, urinary obstruction, hyperthyroidism, or parkinsonism.*

Adverse visual effects sometimes occur. During early phases of treatment with pilocarpine, hourly tonometric tests may be done because the drug may cause an initial transitory increase in intraocular pressure. Pilocarpine may produce spasm of the ciliary muscle with myopia and loss of visual acuity. These effects are most likely in younger clients at the initiation of therapy. *Nurses should warn clients of possible impairment of distance vision and if fluctuating myopia persists, the situation should be reported and alternative drugs, such as timolol (Timoptic) or epinephrine, should be considered.*

Older clients and those with lens opacity may complain that pilocarpine impairs visual acuity, especially in poor lighting. This complaint should be reported and may be a reason to change the prescription. *Nurses should also warn clients of possible worsening of night vision.* Other ocular effects include conjunctival vascular congestion and temporal or superorbital headaches. *Clients should be advised that headaches and browaches may occur so that they will understand that these are drug-induced events.*

Hypersensitivity reactions to pilocarpine are uncommon but are a contraindication to use when they occur. Contact dermatitis or folliculitis of the conjunctiva may occur with prolonged use. Rare but severe adverse reactions include retinal detachment and vitreous hemrrohages. Pilocarpine is contraindicated in certain kinds of secondary glaucoma when pupillary dilation would have adverse consequences.

Preparations and Administration The effect of pilocarpine begins in about 10–15 minutes and peaks after 30–60 minutes. Effects on the pupil may last as long as 20 hours, but accommodation of the lens lasts 2–3 hours. Intraocular pressure may rise transiently upon instillation of drops but then falls for up to 8 hours. Individuals with darkly pigmented irises tend to require higher doses, but adverse reactions also increase with concentrations above 4%. The choice of a concentration depends on the severity of the glaucoma and the client's response. The drug may sting for a few seconds after instillation, especially at higher concentrations and when first used. Pressing a finger lightly against the lacrimal sac for about 1 minute prevents drainage into the nasal chamber. Excess solution should be wiped away.

Fixed combinations of pilocarpine and epinephrine (E-Carpine, E-Pilo, PE) restrict the flexibility required to achieve optimal dosing. There is no evidence that combinations of pilocarpine with physostigmine achieve better results than either agent alone.

The **pilocarpine ocular therapeutic system** (Ocusert) provides a unique mode of application of pilocarpine for glaucoma. An elliptically shaped polymeric membrane (Figure 54–4) containing pilocarpine is placed in contact with the conjunctival surface. Pilocarpine gradually passes through the

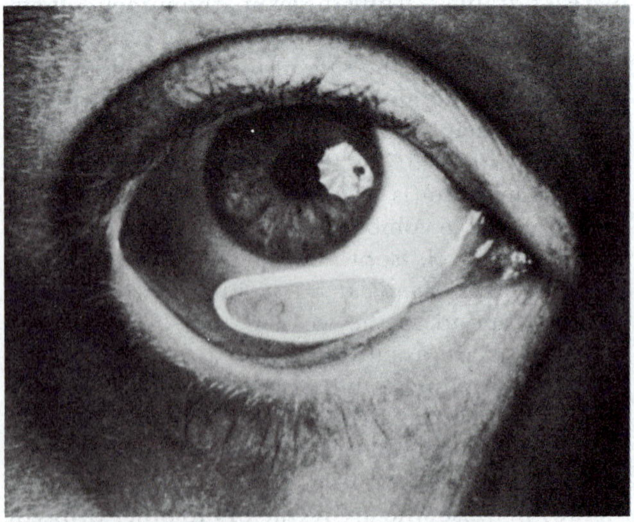

Figure 54–4
The Ocusert therapeutic system in place on the lower lid. From G. Gorin, *Clinical Glaucoma.* New York: Marcel Dekker, Inc., 1977.

membrane from the central reservoir at a steady rate of release for about 7 days. Drug is flushed from around the module by normal tear secretion so that a uniform concentration gradient is maintained. During the first 6 hours after insertion, pilocarpine is released from the preparation at three times the rated value, but from 6 hours to 1 week after insertion, there is a steady flow of drug at 20 μg/hr (Ocusert Pilo-20) or 40 μg/hr (Ocusert Pilo-40), plus or minus 20%. The Ocusert Pilo-20 preparation is generally appropriate for clients who have been previously managed with pilocarpine solutions from 0.5% to 1%, while the Ocusert Pilo-40 preparation substitutes for solutions from 2% to 4%.

The use of the membrane system offers several advantages. Slow, steady release (zero-order delivery) of pilocarpine allows for control of intraocular pressure that is continuous and achieved at a much lower total dose. Risks of systemic toxicity are eliminated. Ocular side effects of miosis and ciliary spasm are substantially reduced as well. Compliance of clients with the treatment regimen, frequently a problem in glaucoma due to the mildness of the symptoms, is greatly improved since the frequency of drug administration is reduced. There are some drawbacks, however. The unit is difficult to insert and remove, especially for clients with poor dexterity, and occasionally it slips out. *Clients should be advised to check the placement of the unit at bedtime and upon arising.* The unit occasionally ruptures, leading to a sudden increase in pilocarpine effects. Some clients experience conjunctival irritation or even inflammation with initial use. *Nurses should advise clients to contact the nurse or physician if irritation or sensitization occurs and to stop using the medication until examined by the physician.*

Ocusert is placed in the lower or upper cul-de-sac. Since pilocarpine induced myopia and the effect of the unit are somewhat greater during the first 6 hours of use, it is usually best to insert a new one at bedtime. The lower cul-de-sac is the usual placement site, but if the unit tends to slip out onto the cheek, placement in the upper cul-de-sac provides better retention. It may be helpful to gently maneuver the unit from the lower lid to the upper lid at night to improve retention: this can be easily accomplished by gentle manual manipulation through the closed lid. If the unit is lost, the pilocarpine effect continues for a few hours. New units should be refrigerated until use.

Pilocarpine Hydrochloride (Adsorbocarpine, Akarpine, Almocarpine, Isopto Carpine, Pilocar, Pilocel, Pilomiotin, and Piloptic)
Ophthalmic solutions, combination solutions with epinephrine (E-Carpine, E-Pilo, PE) and physostigmine (Isopto P-ES, Miocel)
Recommended Doses: One to two drops is instilled in the eye every 4–8 hours. The usual concentration range is 0.5%–4.0%.

Pilocarpine Nitrate (P.V. Carpine Liquifilm)
Solutions in alcohol with aromatics (menthol, camphor, phenol, and eucalyptol)

Pilocarpine Ocular Therapeutic System (Ocusert)
Polymeric membrane: providing pilocarpine outflow of 20 μg/8hr (Ocusert Pilo-20) or 40 μg/hr (Ocusert Pilo-40), plus or minus 20%

Carbachol (Carbacel, Isopto Carbachol)

Carbachol is a useful alternative to pilocarpine, especially when the client is not sufficiently responsive to pilocarpine or experiences irritation or hypersensitivity. Carbachol is potent but penetrates the intact cornea only poorly. If the corneal epithelium is abraded, the effect of carbachol is greatly increased, so corneal abrasion is a contraindication for its use.

Benzalkonium chloride is included in carbachol preparations as a wetting agent to improve penetration of the active drug. Absorption is also enhanced by gentle massage of the cornea through the eyelid. Carbachol is a little more resistant to destruction by acetylcholinesterase than is pilocarpine, producing its miotic action for up to 8 hours. Adverse effects of carbachol are the same as those for pilocarpine.

Preparations and Administration

Carbachol (Carbacel, Isopto Carbachol)
Drops, ophthalmic solutions
Recommended Doses: 1–2 drops, 2–3 times daily.

Cholinesterase Inhibitors

Mechanisms and Effects Cholinesterase inhibitors are indirect-acting cholinomimetics, resembling the choline esters in their pharmacology but differing in mechanism and pharmacokinetics. These agents inhibit the enzyme acetylcholinesterase (true cholinesterase), thereby intensifying the actions of endogenous actylcholine. Physostigmine (Eserine) and demecarium (Humorsol) act only on true cholinesterase whereas isoflurophate (Floropryl) and echothiophate (Echodide, Phospholine Iodide) inhibit cholinesterase of plasma and erythrocytes (pseudocholinesterase) as well. As with choline esters, the pupil is constricted, the ciliary muscle is contracted (causing lens accommodation), and outflow of aqueous humor is augmented. These effects result in decreased intraocular pressure, but they also cause diminished night vision and myopia and nurses should so advise clients. Some physicians prescribe instillation of sympathomimetics along with cholinesterase inhibitors for open-angle glaucoma. Sympathomimetics counteract the pupillary constriction and redness produced by cholinesterase inhibitors while at the same time enhancing the therapeutic benefit of reduced intraocular pressure.

Pharmacokinetics Of the four cholinesterase inhibitors used in glaucoma, three are long-acting. Only physostigmine (Eserine) is a reversible, short-acting type of inhibitor. Physostigmine must be instilled three times daily and offers no advantage over choline esters.

The long-acting, irreversible cholinesterase inhibitors are demecarium, echothiophate, and isoflurophate. The effect of these drugs extends for 1 week or longer. Because of the extended half-lives of these drugs, there is a risk of accumulation and resultant toxicity. *Clients should be warned that the full effect may not be seen until after several weeks.*

Clinical Indications Because of its short duration of action, physostigmine is not widely used and is indicated only for reducing intraocular pressure during acute episodes of congestive glaucoma. The long-acting inhibitors are indicated for therapy of chronic, open-angle glaucoma that does not respond adequately to primary drug choices (pilocarpine, timolol, epinephrine, carbachol). Long-acting cholinesterase inhibitors are also useful after iridectomy, accommodative esotropia, and other conditions amenable to miotic therapy. Cholinesterase inhibitors are seldom useful in closed-angle glaucoma and should not be used in clients with active uveal inflammation or hypersensitivity to cholinesterase inhibitors.

Adverse Effects and Contraindications Systemic adverse effects of the long-acting cholinesterase inhibitors occur with overdosage and to a lesser extent even with normal doses. *When instilling eyedrops, compressing the lacrimal sac for 1 or 2 minutes after instillation prevents drainage into the nasal passages and subsequent systemic absorption. The client should avoid squeezing the eyelids together.*

Signs of systemic cholinesterase inhibition include increased salivation, diarrhea, nausea, muscle weakness, urinary incontinence, respiratory difficulty, or cardiac irregularities, especially bradycardia. Any of these symptoms are indications that use of these drugs should be discontinued. Atropine and even pralidoxime may be required to alleviate systemic toxicity. *Nurses should especially observe clients who are using cholinesterase inhibitors if these individuals have other conditions such as bronchial asthma, gastrointestinal spasms, peptic ulcer, parkinsonism, or epilepsy. In addition, special attention should be given clients who have had a myocardial infarct, or who have congestive heart failure, bradycardia, or hypotension.*

Latent infections may be activated causing iritis or uveitis; cysts may form or enlarge on the iris. Client complaints of "fuzzy vision" or "a curtain coming down over my eye" may be indicative of retinal detachment. Vitreous hemorrhage may also occur occasionally. *With initial instillation of cholinesterase inhibitors, tonometric readings should be taken every hour for the first 3–4 hours to detect a rise in intraocular pressure (that can result from unexpected angle closure) or a sudden drop in intraocular pressure (indicating possible retinal detachment).*

Tolerance may develop to these drugs and long-term use can lead to obstruction of the nasolacrimal canals, lens opacities, conjunctival thickening, and posterior synechiae to the lens; this last effect can be avoided by maximal dilation of the pupils with a mydriatic every 6 months to 1 year. Paradoxical increases in intraocular pressure occur occasionally due to pupillary block of flow from the ciliary processes into the main anterior chamber. Use of long-acting cholinesterase inhibitors should be discontinued at least 3 weeks prior to ocular surgery.

Drug Interactions Cholinesterase inhibitors interact with a variety of other drugs to the extent that they are systemically absorbed. Effects of succinylcholine on ganglia and neuromuscular synapses are greatly potentiated. Effects of systemic anticholinesterase drugs (employed in myasthenia gravis) will be additive with systemic effects of topically administered ocular anticholinesterases. Clients who work with pesticides and insecticides that contain organophosphate or carbamate cholinesterase inhibitors may experience additive toxicity, depending on the amount of spray or dust inhaled during use. They should wear respiratory masks and gloves, and wash gloves and clothing frequently. Alcohol can increase the severity of systemic toxicity produced by cholinesterase inhibitors. *Nurses should advise clients receiving any of these drugs to avoid use of alcohol.*

Preparations and Administration Careful dosage adjustment should be made to minimize adverse effects and maximize the therapeutic benefit. *Clients should have tonometric readings during therapy to determine the optimum concentration of drug to be used and the frequency. Clients may be advised to instill drops at bedtime so that daytime visual disturbances will be minimized.* The first instillation is often done by the physician.

When echothiophate is employed, miosis occurs within 30 minutes and may last from several days up to 4 weeks after drug elimination. Echothiophate iodide solutions are stable only up to 1 month at room temperature. However, since cold solution can be uncomfortable when applied to the eye, the client should keep a small amount that is in active use at room temperature, and any additional supply under refrigeration. Demecarium should be stored in tight, light-resistant containers. *Nurses should advise clients who use soft contact lenses to remove the lens before instilling echothiophate eye drops because the soft lenses may be damaged either by the drug or by the preservatives in the medication.*

After administration of isoflurophate, miosis occurs within 20 minutes and a decrease in intraocular pressure within a few hours. The ointment should be applied to the conjunctival sac with the client supine, avoiding contact between the tip of the tube and the cornea. The hands should be washed immediately after administration since isoflurophate can cause contact dermatitis. Isoflurophate hydrolyzes in the presence of water and therefore the tube should be kept tightly closed between applications of drug. The tip of the tube should not be washed or allowed to touch moisture in the conjunctival sac.

Demecarium Bromide (Humorsol)
Ophthalmic solutions
Recommended Doses: Frequency of administration ranges from 1 drop twice a week to 1 or 2 drops twice a day. When initially administered, intraocular pressure should be monitored at least hourly for 3–4 hours to determine if an initial rise in intraocular pressure occurs. Twice a day provides the best control in severe cases or when diurnal fluctuations in intraocular pressure are noted.

Echothiophate Iodide (Echodide, Phospholine Iodide)
Powder for ophthalmic solutions with diluent
Recommended Doses: One drop in each eye twice a day is an ideal schedule but less frequent administration can be effective.

Isoflurophate (Floropryl)
Ointment in polyethylene mineral oil gel
Recommended Doses: For initial treatment of glaucoma, a quarter-inch strip of ointment is applied to the eye every 8–72 hours as required.

Physostigmine (Eserine)
Ophthalmic solutions and ointment

Sympathomimetics

The relationship between sympathetic receptors and glaucoma is not a clear one. Mydriasis caused by sympathetic stimulation is known to be mediated by α-receptors. Nonselective sympathomimetics such as epinephrine cause mydriasis but nevertheless have a beneficial effect in open-angle glaucoma. The main efficacious effect of epinephrine is to decrease the rate of formation of aqueous humor, and experimental evidence indicates that this effect is achieved by an action on beta-receptors. Yet timolol, an antagonist at β_1- and β_2-receptors, also decreases production of aqueous humor. Thus we are presented with the pharmacologic conundrum that both a beta-agonist and a beta-antagonist decrease the rate of formation of aqueous humor. The role of alpha-receptors is no less puzzling. When given for prolonged periods, epinephrine begins to exhibit a second beneficial effect in open-angle glaucoma: a modest increase in drainage of aqueous humor, which appears to be mediated by α-receptors. Yet α-blockers have also been observed to lower intraocular pressure. These seemingly incongruous observations are unresolved at present. The empirical fact is that both sympathomimetics and certain beta-blockers reduce intraocular pressure in open-angle glaucoma.

Sympathomimetic agents dilate the pupil of the eye, constrict ocular blood vessels, and increase drainage of aqueous humor by their alpha-effects; they inhibit formation of aqueous humor and relax the ciliary muscle by beta-mediated activity. The sympathomimetics are indicated alone or in combination with cholinomimetics for open-angle glaucoma, but are contraindicated in angle-closure glaucoma or in eyes capable of angle-closure in response to mydriatics.

Although systemic absorption is not great after topical application, caution must be exercised when using sympathomimetics in clients with hypertension, diabetes, heart disease, cerebral arteriosclerosis, bronchial asthma, hyperthyroidism, or those receiving monoamine oxidase inhibitors or tricyclic antidepressants. Systemic adverse effects may include palpitation, tachycardia, extrasystoles, cardiac dysrhythmias, hypertension, faintness, anxiety, trembling, sweating, and pallor. *Systemic toxicity can be minimized by applying pressure to the lacrimal duct for 1 minute after instillation and not squeezing the eyes.*

Adverse responses resulting from ocular effects include headache, browache, and a slight stinging when the drug is initially instilled. *Nurses should inform clients that these symptoms may occur but usually subside as the client continues use of the medication. If the symptoms persist, the client should consult with the physician. Clients should be advised to report immediately any occurrence of edema, itching, discharge, or crusting of the eyelids.*

If a sympathomimetic is applied to an eye from which the lens has been removed, there is a risk of hemorrhages about the macula and gradual loss of visual acuity. *Often the first indication that a client is los-*

ing vision comes when he or she suggests a need for a change in glasses. The two sympathomimetics employed for glaucoma are epinephrine and dipivefrin.

Epinephrine

Epinephrine is available as the hydrochloride, bitartrate, or borate salts. A 2% solution of the bitartrate form is equivalent to 1.1% of either the hydrochloride or borate salts. Administration frequency and concentration is adjusted by tonometry. Clients with heavily pigmented eyes tend to be more resistant to the effects of epinephrine than those with light pigmentation and therefore generally require stronger concentrations. *When epinephrine is used with a cholinomimetic, the latter drug should be applied first. Because of the limited capacity of the conjunctival sac, the client should be instructed to wait 2–5 minutes before instilling the epinephrine. Clients using soft lenses should be advised to remove them prior to instilling eye drops since soft lenses may be damaged either by the drug or the preservative. Epinephrine solutions are light sensitive and should be stored in a cool, dark location; those that have turned brown or formed precipitates should be discarded.*

Preparations and Administration

Epinephrine Bitartrate (Mytrate, Epitrate, E)
Ophthalmic solutions
Recommended Doses: One drop in each eye once or twice daily as an initial regimen.

Epinephrine Borate (Epinal, Eppy/N)
Ophthalmic solutions
Recommended Doses: One drop in each eye once or twice daily as an initial regimen.

Epinephrine Hydrochloride (Epifrin, Glaucon)
Ophthalmic solutions
Recommended Doses: One drop in each eye once or twice daily as an initial regimen.

Dipivefrin (Propine)

Dipivefrin is an epinephrine prodrug converted in the eye by hydrolysis to epinephrine and pivalic acid. It has the advantage of better absorption and is substantially more lipophilic than epinephrine, penetrating the cornea 17 times more effectively. Substantially lower concentrations of drug are required because of the improved penetration, and successful therapy can be achieved with fewer adverse effects. The response to 0.1% dipivefrin twice daily is comparable to that of 2% pilocarpine, 4 times daily and only slightly less than 2% epinephrine twice daily.

Adverse effects of dipivefrin are substantially less frequent than with either 2% epinephrine or 2% pilocarpine. Dipivefrin does not cause miosis, ciliary spasm, blurred vision, or night blindness. Burning and stinging may occur upon instillation in some clients (about 6%) as well as conjunctival injection. Systemic toxicity resembles that of epinephrine but occurs less frequently. Dipivefrin can be used effectively with cholinomimetics.

Preparations and Administration

Dipivefrin (Propine)
Ophthalmic solution
Recommended Doses: One drop in each eye under treatment, initially every 12 hours.

Beta-Adrenergic Blockers

Three beta-adrenergic blockers are available in ophthalmic solutions for use in glaucoma: timolol, levobunolol, and betaxolol.

Mechanisms and Effects Timolol and levobunolol are antagonists at both β_1- and β_2-receptors, while betaxolol is selective for β_1-receptors. None of these drugs possess intrinsic sympathomimetic activity nor local anesthetic activity like some of the other beta-blockers. Beta-blockers decrease the rate of formation of aqueous humor, thereby lowering intraocular pressure. They have little or no effect on pupil size, accommodation, night vision, or visual acuity. Timolol, administered twice a day in concentrations of 0.25% or 0.5%, produces a reduction in intraocular pressure greater than that achieved with pilocarpine solutions as high as 4%, 4 times per day, or epinephrine solutions up to 2%, twice a day. After a single dose, the effects of timolol or betaxolol are observed in approximately 30 minutes, while that of levobunolol occurs within 1 hour. The peak effect occurs in 1–2 hours for timolol or betaxolol and between 2 and 6 hours for levobunolol. Significant reduction of intraocular pressure persists for up to 12 hours for betaxolol and up to 24 hours for timolol and levobunolol. Tolerance has not been observed in as much as 1 year of use.

Clinical Indications Beta-blockers are used alone or in combination with cholinomimetics or carbonic anhydrase inhibitors for chronic open-angle glaucoma, secondary glaucoma, aphakia with glaucoma, and ocular hypertension. Addition of a beta-blocker to an existing regimen when the response is inadequate frequently results in further reduction of intraocular pressure.

Adverse Effects and Contraindications Adverse reactions to ophthalmic beta-blockers are minimal. Mild ocular irritation may occur and rarely lo-

Nursing Observations for Antiglaucoma Drugs

THERAPEUTIC GOAL	Reduction of intraocular pressure by decreasing formation of aqueous humor, increasing its drainage, or both.
PREADMINISTRATION ASSESSMENT	
Baseline Data	Assess for ocular pain, frequent headaches, reduced visual acuity, loss of peripheral vision and, later, central vision, widely dilated pupils, steamy cornea, or ciliary injection. Evaluate intraocular pressure.
EVALUATION OF DRUG RESPONSE	
For Therapeutic Benefit	Monitor changes in intraocular pressure and alleviation of symptoms associated with elevated intraocular pressure, such as pain, headache, or visual impairments.
For Adverse Effects	When cholinomimetics are employed, monitor for visual disturbances, including myopia, loss of visual acuity, impairment of distance vision, impairment of vision in dim light, conjunctival vascular injection, temporal or superorbital headaches, contact dermatitis, or folliculitis. Watch for systemic toxicity in predisposed individuals, including symptoms of bradycardia, bronchospasms, congestive heart failure, peptic ulcer, gastrointestinal spasm, thyroid storm, or parkinsonism. When sympathomimetics are employed, monitor for diminished visual acuity, hypertension, and aggravation of diabetes. Monitor pulse pressure when timolol is given.
For Compliance	Evaluate the client's compliance with all facets of the therapeutic regimen by careful observation, interviewing, and review of progress. Report compliance problems to the physician and act as client-advocate when changes in the therapeutic regimen seem indicated.

cal hypersensitivity. Systemic side effects have included bradycardia and acute bronchospasms in clients with asthma. Betaxolol poses less risk than timolol or levobunolol for clients with restricted pulmonary function because of its selectivity for β_1-receptors. The only contraindication for use of these agents is hypersensitivity to the drug itself. Beta-blockers have additive systemic and ocular effects with oral beta-blocking medications. Concomitant use of beta-blockers and epinephrine has been observed to cause mydriasis.

Preparations and Administration *Prior to administering a beta-blocker, the nurse should record the client's pulse. The nurse should teach the client how to record pulse rate and to report any change in rate or rhythm. Blood pressure should also be monitored, particularly in clients with heart disease, and any occurrence of hypotension or palpitation should be reported immediately. Clients should also be advised to report any difficulty with respiration.* When beta-blockers are substituted for other agents, the previous regimen should be continued on the first day of treatment with the beta-blocker and then discontinued. As with other antiglaucoma medications, a finger should be lightly pressed against the lacrimal sac for 1–2 minutes after drug administration.

Betaxolol (Betoptic)
Ophthalmic solution
Recommended Doses: One drop in each affected eye initially, twice daily.

Levobunolol (Betagan)
Ophthalmic solution
Recommended Doses: One drop initially in the affected eye(s), once or twice daily.

Timolol (Timoptic)
Ophthalmic solution
Recommended Doses: One drop of the 0.25% solution initially, twice a day, in each eye requiring treatment.

Carbonic Anhydrase Inhibitors

Mechanisms and Effects Carbonic anhydrase (CA) inhibitors, once widely used as diuretics, are now mainly used to lower intraocular pressure in acute attacks of closed-angle glaucoma. They are used less frequently as adjunctive treatment for

Nursing Diagnoses and Interventions for Antiglaucoma Drugs

Nursing Diagnoses	*Related Interventions*
TO ENHANCE DRUG BENEFITS OR REDUCE DRUG REQUIREMENTS	
Alteration in comfort related to increased intraocular pressure	Pain and headache associated with increased intraocular pressure should resolve with adequate treatment; analgesics may be useful but should not be used as a substitute for treating the glaucoma.
Anxiety or fear related to possible loss of vision	Provide emotional support and reassurance. Provide information related to the effectiveness of current drug therapy.
Increased risk of injury related to impaired vision	Provide safety measures as required; encourage client to adjust activities appropriately.
Self-care deficit or impaired home maintenance management related to visual impairment	Advise the client regarding community services that may be available.
TO MINIMIZE DRUG SIDE EFFECTS OR INTERACTIONS	
Sensory-perceptual alterations related to glaucoma or anti-glaucoma drugs	Advocate adjustments in the drug regimen as required.
TO ENSURE SAFE AND EFFICACIOUS DRUG USE	
Knowledge deficit related to drug regimen	Teach clients about the nature of glaucoma and the rationale for the therapeutic regimen. They should understand that glaucoma can be controlled but not cured by drug therapy.
	Teach clients how to instill drugs in the eye properly. After instillation of most ocular preparations, a finger should be pressed lightly against the lacrimal sac for about 1 minute to prevent drainage of the drug into the nasal chamber. Excess solution should be wiped away.
	Warn clients that ophthalmic preparations may sting for a few seconds upon initial instillation. This response should diminish with continued use.
	Show clients how to install the pilocarpine ocular therapeutic system if this is prescribed.
	Advise clients with darkly pigmented eyes that they will probably require higher doses of a sympathomimetic if one is prescribed.
	Provide client with a list of adverse effects and drug interactions for each drug in the regimen and explain what to do if any of these occur.
	Warn clients that they should not drive immediately after instilling glaucoma medications.
	Instruct clients not to discontinue drugs for glaucoma simply because overt symptoms have disappeared. Advise them to consult with the physician before changing or discontinuing their regimen.

chronic open-angle glaucoma. Aqueous humor is rich in bicarbonate ions. Formation of bicarbonate ions by the ciliary processes involves hydration of carbon dioxide by the enzyme carbonic anhydrase. The decrease in bicarbonate and hydrogen ions in the aqueous humor produced by CA inhibitors results in a movement of water by osmosis from the anterior chamber into the posterior chamber. The result is a decrease in intraocular pressure.

Clinical Indications Use of carbonic anhydrase inhibitors is generally confined to short-term relief of acute congestive glaucoma attacks because of the difficulties they present when used for extended periods of time.

Adverse Effects and Contraindications Carbonic anhydrase inhibitors are nonbacteriostatic sulfonamides. All of the adverse effects commonly associated with sulfonamides occur with these drugs: fever, skin eruptions, crystalluria, renal calculi, and aplastic anemias of all types (pancytopenia, leukopenia, agranulocytosis, hemolytic anemia, or thrombocytopenic purpura). Diuresis induced by CA inhibitions may result in hyperchloremic acidosis, hypokalemia, and dehydration. These drugs should not be used in clients with depressed serum electrolyte levels, marked kidney or liver disease, adrenocortical insufficiency, chronic angle-closure glaucoma, or in the first trimester of pregnancy. Nor should they be used in clients with pulmonary distress, since acidosis ordinarily stimulates increased ventilation to achieve compensation. CA inhibitors may produce additive diuresis when given with diuretics in other classes, and will aggravate digitalis toxicity by depleting potassium.

Other side effects include tingling sensations, pruritus, urticaria, skin eruptions, photosensitivity reactions, loss of appetite, polyuria, dry mouth, weight loss, nausea, vomiting, constipation, urinary frequency, drowsiness, weakness, sedation, lassitude, depression, dizziness, confusion, headache, and loss of taste and smell sensations. Aplastic anemias have also been reported. *Nurses should advise clients against driving or involvement in other dangerous tasks requiring alertness while taking CA inhibitors. Gastrointestinal disturbances can be minimized by taking these medications with food.*

Preparations and Administration The available carbonic anhydrase inhibitors are acetazolamide, dichlorphenamide, and methazolamide. Acetazolamide tablets (Diamox, Ak-Zol) have an onset of action in 60–90 minutes, a peak effect in 2–4 hours, and a duration of 8–12 hours, for lowering intraocular pressure. Dichlorphenamide (Daranide, Oratrol) reduces intraocular pressure within 1 hour after administration, reaches peak effect in 2–4 hours, and lasts from 6–12 hours. Methazolamide (Neptazane) acts in 2–4 hours, pressure reduction peaks in 6 to 8 hours, and subsides in 10–18 hours.

Acetazolamide (Diamox, Ak-Zol)
Tablets, sustained release capsules, powder for injection solutions
Recommended Doses: 250 mg PO, once a day, up to 1,000 mg per day in divided doses.

Dichlorphenamide (Daranide, Oratrol)
Tablets
Recommended Doses: 100–200 mg PO initially as a priming dose, followed by 100 mg every 12 hours until an adequate reduction of intraocular pressure is achieved. After that, 25–50 mg is given 1–3 times daily if maintenance therapy is required.

Methazolamide (Neptazane)
Tablets
Recommended Doses: 50–100 mg PO, 2 or 3 times daily.

Hyperosmotic Agents

The hyperosmotic agents, mannitol, urea, glycerin, and isosorbide, increase the osmolarity of serum and cause a shift of fluid from the anterior chamber of the eye into the plasma. **Mannitol** is a nearly inert sugar alcohol that is rapidly excreted by the kidneys. It is always administered by intravenous infusion through an in-line filter since mannitol can crystallize. Cardiovascular status must be evaluated before administration of mannitol because the sudden expansion of the extracellular compartment produced by rapid infusion of mannitol can precipitate congestive heart failure. Adverse effects of mannitol infusion have included pulmonary congestion, fluid and electrolyte imbalances, acidosis, osmotic nephrosis, dizziness, headache, nausea, vomiting, rhinitis, fever, chills, thrombophlebitis, urticaria, skin necrosis, anginal pain, hypo- or hypertension, and tachycardia.

Urea is used in a similar fashion by intravenous infusion of a 30% solution at a rate not to exceed 4 ml/minute. Adverse effects include headaches, nausea and vomiting, syncope, disorientation, confusional states, and occasional chemical phlebitis at the site of injection. As with mannitol, electrolyte and fluid imbalances may occur.

Glycerin is employed as an oral hyperosmotic agent to reduce intraocular pressure, most often 60–90 minutes before surgery for glaucoma or cataracts. Intraocular pressure begins to respond in about 10 minutes, reaches a maximum reduction in 30–120 minutes, and returns to the predrug level in 4–6 hours. Side effects include nausea, vomiting, diarrhea, headache, confusion, and disorientation. Severe dehydration, cardiac dysrhythmias, and hyperosmolar, nonketotic coma have occurred in rare cases. Caution should be exercised in clients who are hypervolemic, dehydrated, diabetic, confused or senile, or who have congestive heart failure. Glycerin can be used successfully in conjunction with intravenous hyperosmotic agents or cholinomimetics.

Isosorbide, like glycerin, is an oral hyperosmotic drug. It is indicated for short-term reduction of intraocular pressure before and after intraocular surgery and in some cases of glaucoma. Nausea, vomiting, diarrhea, anorexia, gastric discomfort, lethargy, lightheadedness, vertigo, thirst, hypernatremia, hyperosmolality, hiccoughs, and skin rashes are the reported adverse reactions. Isosorbide should not be employed in clients with kidney disease, severe pulmonary edema, severe dehydration, or ocular hemorrhage. Repetitive doses may result in fluid and electrolyte imbalance. Onset of action occurs in 30 minutes, peak effect in 1–1.5 hours, with a duration of 5–6 hours.

Preparations and Administration

Glycerin (Osmoglyn, Glyrol)
Oral solutions
Recommended Doses: 1.0–1.5 g/kg PO.

Isosorbide (Ismotic)
Oral solution
Recommended Doses: 1.5 g/kg PO initially.

Mannitol (Osmitrol, generics)
Injection solutions
Recommended Doses: For reduction of intraocular pressure, 1.5 to 2 g/kg IV as a 15–25% solution administered over 30 minutes for a prompt and maximal effect.

Urea
Recommended Doses: For reduction of intraocular pressure in adults, 1.0–1.5 g/kg IV.

Marihuana

Marihuana and its main active-constitutent, delta-9 tetrahydrocannabinol (Δ_9-THC), lower intraocular pressure by an unknown mechanism. Some clients refractory to pilocarpine respond well to Δ_9-THC. Other ocular functions are affected very little by Δ_9-THC, but the prominent CNS effect represents a side effect when Δ_9-THC is employed for glaucoma either orally or by smoking marihuana. Preliminary evaluation of a congener, Δ_{10}-THC, suggests that it can decrease intraocular pressure with less tendency to produce euphoria than Δ_9-THC. Interactions with other antiglaucoma drugs have not been determined. It remains to be seen whether an effective topical preparation can be developed. Although use of THCs or marihuana has been permitted by legal agencies for a small number of individuals, it is not yet known whether this drug will become a significant addition to the treatment arsenal for glaucoma.

Important Nursing Implications for Drugs for Glaucoma

- ☐ Obtain baseline data about the client's cardiovascular function before initiating therapy with cholinomimetics or sympathomimetics for glaucoma.
- ☐ Warn clients that topical cholinomimetic drugs for glaucoma may cause blurring of vision and impairment of night vision. Advise them to avoid night driving or other hazardous activities.
- ☐ Advise clients that they may experience browaches or headaches shortly after administration of cholinomimetics to the eye. An analgesic may be used to relieve the head pain.
- ☐ Advise clients of possible adverse ocular effects, such as stinging or burning. Teach clients how to distinguish between normal irritation from instillation of drops and signs of more severe irritation that may necessitate discontinuation of the medication.
- ☐ Examine clients for evidence of activation of latent infections of the eye structures when drops are employed. Advise clients to report any fuzzy vision or itching.
- ☐ Note that clients who are allergic to carbonic anhydrase inhibitors are also likely to be cross-allergic to drugs of related structure including thiazide diuretics, sulfonylureas, and sulfonamide antibiotics. Such allergies should be carefully recorded in the medical chart and clients should be warned about these likely cross-sensitivities.
- ☐ Teach clients the proper techniques for inserting and checking the pilocarpine ocular system.
- ☐ Teach clients to press the lacrimal sac for 1 minute after inserting drops into the eye to prevent leakage into the nasal passages.
- ☐ When sympathomimetics and cholinomimetics are used together for treatment of glaucoma, teach the client to apply the cholinomimetic

first, followed by the sympathomimetic after 2–5 minutes.

- ☐ Check the client's pulse prior to administering a beta-blocker, even a topical one for glaucoma. If the pulse is less than 60, contact the prescriber.

Mydriatics

Mydriatics are drugs that dilate the pupil of the eye. Mydriasis can be achieved either by reducing parasympathetic influence on the pupil or by augmenting sympathetic influence. Although the parasympatholytic and sympathomimetic drugs share in common the ability to dilate the pupil, they differ with respect to other ocular effects (Table 54–3) and, consequently, in clinical utility.

Parasympatholytic Mydriatics

Mechanisms and Effects Parasympatholytic agents are anticholinergic drugs that act in particular as antagonists at muscarinic receptors. Muscarinic receptors of the eye regulate the sphincter muscle of the iris and the ciliary muscles of the ciliary bodies. The action of antimuscarinic drugs at these sites is to produce mydriasis and paralysis of accommodation, also called *cycloplegia.* The anticholinergic mydriatics are sometimes designated as *cycloplegic mydriatics.* It is useful to induce both mydriasis and cyclopegia in certain diagnostic procedures involving the eye. For example, induction of mydriasis and cycloplegia permits accurate measurement of refractive errors, a necessary step for proper determination of lens requirements for eyeglasses. Pupillary dilation is also useful in inflammatory conditions of the iris and uveal tract.

Adverse Effects and Contraindications Adverse reactions to topically applied cycloplegic mydriatics are largely referable to the eye itself. Anticholinergic drugs may increase intraocular pressure. The drops may sting transiently upon instillation and if used for extended periods may cause local irritation, characterized by follicular conjunctivitis, vascular congestion, edema, and exudation. Photophobia and corneal staining can also occur. *Clients should be advised to discontinue drops if eye pain occurs. They should also be warned that they may experience blurring of vision and increased light sensitivity and should be advised to avoid driving if visual acuity is affected.*

Systemic adverse effects rarely accompany short-term use but are more common with prolonged use. Systemic toxicity encompasses all features of the classic anticholinergic syndrome such as

Table 54–3
Effects of Mydriatics

Drugs	Mydriasis	Cycloplegia	Ocular vasoconstriction
Parasympatholytics			
Atropine	Yes	Yes	No
Cyclopentolate	Yes	Yes	No
Homatropine	Yes	Yes	No
Scopolamine	Yes	Yes	No
Tropicamide	Yes	Yes	No
Sympathomimetics			
Direct-acting			
Ephedrine	Yes	No	Yes
Epinephrine	Yes	No	Yes
Naphazoline	Yes	No	Yes
Phenylephrine	Yes	No	Yes
Tetrahydrozoline	Yes	No	Yes
Indirect-acting			
Cocaine	Yes	Yes	Yes
Hydroxyamphetamine	Yes	No	Yes

dry mouth, inhibited sweating, dry skin, flushing, tachycardia, fever, abdominal distention, constipation, urinary retention, headache, somnolence, confusion, hallucinations, ataxia, restlessness, incoherent speech, disorientation, and psychosis. *Systemic absorption is reduced by compression of the lacrimal sac for 1 minute after instillation of drops.* Anticholinergic medications are contraindicated in clients with glaucoma or a known sensitivity to anticholinergic medications. Infants, children with spastic paralysis, and persons with brain damage or Down's syndrome are also likely to be highly sensitive to anticholinergic drugs.

Preparations and Administration Care should be taken not to touch the eye or eyelids with the dropper tip to avoid contamination. Intraocular tension should be determined before and during therapy. Atropine produces weaker mydriatic effects in people with dark eyes whereas those with blue eyes tend to be highly sensitive to the drug. Nurses need to be particularly cognizant of the potential side effects among this group.

Atropine Sulfate
Ophthalmic solutions, ophthalmic ointment
Recommended Doses: For diagnostic procedures, 1 or 2 drops in each eye, 1 hour before examination. For uveitis, 1 or 2 drops instilled up to 3 times daily.

Cyclopentolate Hydrochloride (Cyclogyl, Ak-Pentolate)
Ophthalmic solutions
Recommended Doses: For diagnostic procedures: if the 0.5% solution is employed, one drop is applied followed by a second drop 5 minutes later; one drop of the 1.0% or 2.0% solution is sufficient. Individuals with darkly pigmented eyes usually require one drop of the 2.0% solution. Complete recovery occurs in 24 hours but can be shortened to 3–6 hours by instillation of 1–2 drops of 1–2% pilocarpine. Maximal mydriasis and cycloplegia occurs in 15–45 minutes.

Homatropine Hydrobromide (Homatrocel, generic)
Recommended Doses: For long-lasting mydriasis and cycloplegia (up to 2 days), 1 or 2 drops, repeated in 5–10 minutes if necessary. For treatment of uveal tract inflammations, 1 or 2 drops every 3–4 hours. Peak mydriasis occurs within 10–30 minutes and peak cycloplegia in 30–90 minutes.

Scopolamine Hydrobromide (Hyoscine, Murocoll-2, generic)
Ophthalmic solutions, ophthalmic ointment
Recommended Doses: For refraction, 1 or 2 drops 1 hour before testing. For uveitis, 1 or 2 drops up to 3 times daily. Scopolamine effects last several days.

Tropicamide (Mydriacyl)
Ophthalmic solution
Recommended Doses: For induction of cycloplegia and mydriasis for measurement of refraction, 1 or 2 drops of 1% solution, repeated in 5 minutes. Tropicamide produces maximal effects in about 25 minutes; recovery occurs in 4–6 hours.

Sympathomimetic Mydriatics

Mechanisms and Effects Sympathomimetic mydriatics do not induce cycloplegia, but they constrict ocular blood vessels, decrease formation of aqueous humor, increase outflow of aqueous humor, and relax the ciliary muscle to some extent. The use of epinephrine and dipivefrin in glaucoma was discussed earlier. Here, we consider the topical sympathomimetics used for (1) constricting blood vessels and reducing infiltration in conjunctivitis and uveitis, (2) inducing mydriasis for diagnostic purposes, (3) controlling bleeding or inducing mydriasis during ocular surgery, and (4) relieving ocular congestion and irritation caused by hay fever, colds, swimming, use of contact lenses, eye strain, smoke, smog, dust, wind, or glare.

Adverse Effects and Contraindications Adverse effects related to the eye include transitory stinging upon initial instillation, headache, brow ache, conjunctival allergic reactions, pigmentation of the lids, conjunctiva, or cornea, and rebound miosis. *Nurses should advise clients that after instillation, the pupils of the eye will be very large and highly sensitive to light. Therefore use of sun glasses will be necessary. If the sensitivity persists beyond 12 hours, the drug should be discontinued and the physician notified.* Systemic adverse effects are rare but include hypertension, palpitation, tachycardia, extrasystoles, other dysrhythmias, anxiety, fear, trembling, sweating, and pallor. *Nurses should warn clients not to swallow the material since this will result in profound systemic effects.*

Preparations and Administration **Epinephrine** hydrochloride, in addition to its previously discussed use in glaucoma, finds use as a 0.1% solution for control of bleeding or induction of mydriasis during ocular surgery and for alleviating infiltration of conjunctivitis.

Phenylephrine hydrochloride is a widely used decongestant mydriatic. Phenylephrine is light-sensitive and oxidizes when exposed to air. Solutions that are brown or which contain a precipitant should be discarded. Phenylephrine is incompatible with butacaine.

Hydroxyamphetamine Hydrobromine (Paredrine)
Ophthalmic solution
Recommended Doses: 1 to 2 drops instilled to induce pupillary dilation that lasts up to 6 hours.

Naphazoline Hydrochloride
Ophthalmic solutions (AK-Con, Albalon, Naphcon, Vasocon, VasoClear, Allerest Eye Drops, Clear eyes, Degest); ophthalmic decongestant combinations with antihistamines, including pheniramine (Naphcon-A) and antazoline phosphate (Albalon-A, Vasocon-A)
Recommended Doses: For topical ocular vasoconstriction, 1 or 2 drops in each affected eye every 3–4 hours.

Phenylephrine Hydrochloride
Ophthalmic solutions: 0.08%, 0.12%, 0.15%, 2.5%, and 10%.
Combinations for minor eye irritations: 12% phenylephrine with the antiseptic zinc sulfate (Neozin, Phenylzin, Zincfrin, Prefrin-Z), zinc sulfate and the local anesthetic piperocaine (M-Z Ophthalmic), or the antihistamine, pheniramine maleate, and the weak local anesthetic, antipyrine.
Recommended Doses: For decongestant applications (relief of minor eye irritations due to allergies, colds, or environmental irritants), the weaker solutions (0.08–0.15%) are employed. The 2.5% solution is indicated for inducing mydriasis for surgery or diagnostic procedures. The 10% solution is employed in uveitis, in wide-angle glaucoma, and for inducing profound mydriasis during surgery. One drop of a suitable solution is applied in each eye.

Tetrahydrozoline Hydrochloride
Ophthalmic solutions (Clear and Brite, Murine Plus, Opt-Ease, Tetracon, Tetrasine, Visine)
Recommended Doses: For use as an ocular decongestant, 1 or 2 drops are applied in each eye up to 2–3 times per day.

Antimicrobial and Anti-Inflammatory Ophthalmics

Topical ophthalmic preparations of antimicrobial and anti-inflammatory drugs are used in the ocular inflammatory diseases, which more often than not are caused by infection. Inflammatory diseases of the eye include conjunctivitis, keratitis, inflammations of eyelid structures, and uveitis.

Conjunctivitis is the most common inflammation involving structures of the eye. Acute conjunctivitis is undoubtedly the most benign ocular inflammation as well. This disorder, commonly known as "pink eye," is characterized by superficial corneal and scleral injection (reddening of the eye) and a mucopurulent discharge of sparse or copious volume. The features that distinguish acute conjunctivitis from the other two most common acute eye disorders are summarized in Table 54–4. Acute conjunctivitis is usually caused by bacterial, viral, or fungal organisms. Less frequently, mechanical or chemical irritants, allergies, or systemic diseases are

Table 54–4
Characteristic Features of Acute Eye Disorders

Feature	Acute glaucoma	Acute conjunctivitis	Acute iritis
Pupil	Dilated	Normal	Constricted, irregular
Iris	Congested, bulging	Normal	Swollen, muddy
Cornea	Steamy	Normal	Transparent, hazy with precipitates
Anterior chamber	Shallow	Normal	Normal
Injection	Circumcorneal and episcleral	Superficial corneal	Ciliary (deep), circumcorneal
Lacrimation	Yes	No	Yes
Discharge	None	Mucopurulent	None
Eyeball tension	Elevated	Normal	Normal or low
Vision	Severely impaired	Normal	Slightly impaired
Pain	Very severe	Mild burning or itching	Moderately severe

implicated. Identification of the cause is important because topical steroids are contraindicated if the conjunctivitis is caused by herpes virus but are helpful if the condition is caused by allergies. The characteristic features of bacterial, viral, and allergic conjunctivitis appear in Table 54–5. Irritant causes include excessive lacrimation, eye drops, and eye makeup. Acute conjunctivitis is usually self-limited, resolving in 7–10 days without treatment or 3–5 days with treatment. Chronic conjunctivitis is similar in appearance but is characterized by periodic exacerbations and remissions.

Keratitis, an inflammation of the corneal surface, may be caused by bacterial or viral infections, especially herpes viruses. Topical antibiotics should be given promptly, ideally after identification of the causative organisms. Photophobia often accompanies keratitis and can be controlled with dark glasses. Topical anesthetics should not be used to control pain since these may delay recovery. Systemic analgesics may be required.

Eyelid inflammations include **blepharitis, hordeolum,** and **chalazion.** Blepharitis is usually caused by staphylococcal infections and involves the lid margins; erythema, thickening, scaling, crusting, and shallow ulcerations occur. Hordeolum, or sty, is a localized inflammation of the glands of the eyelid, usually due to staphylococcal infections. Chalazion is an inflammation of the eyelid caused by occlusion of the ducts of the meibomian glands. All three conditions are responsive to topical antimicrobials.

Uveitis is an inflammation of any part of the uveal tract, which encompasses the iris, ciliary body, and choroid. **Anterior uveitis** includes **iritis** (see Table 54–4), **cyclitis,** or the combined inflammation of the iris and ciliary body called **iridocyclitis. Posterior uveitis** may be limited to the choroid (**choroiditis**) or may involve the retina as well (**chorioretinitis**). Viral or bacterial infections or hypersensitivity reactions are potential causes. Anterior uveitis responds well to topical steroids. A potential complication of anterior uveitis is the formation of adhesions between the iris and lens, called **posterior synechiae.** These are prevented by maintaining pupillary dilation with mydriatics until the inflammation resolves. Posterior uveitis requires systemic steroids.

Antibacterial Agents

Antibacterial agents are available either as drops or ointments for topical application to the eye. Drug selection should normally be based on determination of the causative organisms by laboratory isolation. The relatively benign character of most conjunctivitis infections, however, renders laboratory determination unnecessary.

The main problem associated with topical use of ophthalmic antibiotics is hypersensitivity. Reactions include stinging, burning, itching, urticaria, edema, and maculopapular dermatitis. Prolonged or frequent use should be avoided. Selection of antibiotics not normally used systemically will minimize the risk of sensitization to antibiotics that may later be employed systemically. Secondary infections may occur due to superinfection when ophthalmic antibiotics are employed.

When applying antibiotics topically to the eye, the eyelid is first cleaned of any discharge by gently wiping the closed lid from inside to outside with a clean cloth or sterile gauze pad. The head is tilted back and the drops or ointment placed in the conjunctival sac. The eyes should then be closed and a finger applied lightly against the lacrimal sac for 1 minute following instillation. Care should be taken

Table 54–5
Characteristic Features of Various Types of Conjunctivitis

Feature	Bacterial	Viral	Allergic
Appearance of discharge	Purulent	Clear	Clear
Principal cell type involved in inflammatory response	Neutrophils	Monocytes	Eosinophils
Degree of lid swelling	Moderate	Minimal	Moderate or severe
Preauricular node involvement	No	Yes	No
Pruritus	No	No	Severe

not to contaminate the tip of the tube or dropper. Drops are instilled 2–4 times daily and ointments approximately every 3–6 hours.

Chloramphenicol (Chloroptic, Econochlor, Antiopto, Ophthochlor) is broadly effective against gram-positive and gram-negative bacteria but is seldom used systemically because of risk of aplastic anemia. Since systemic absorption may occur to a small extent after topical application to the eye, its use should be limited to a short period. **Polymyxin B** (Aerosporin) is a broad-spectrum antibiotic also seldom used systemically. It is especially effective against *Pseudomonas aeruginosa,* and hypersensitivity reactions are very rare. **Bacitracin** (Baciguent and generic) is effective against gram-positive bacteria and produces minimal toxicity. **Neomycin** (Myciguent) is a broad-spectrum antibiotic but produces fairly frequent hypersensitivity reactions, including contact dermatitis. **Erythromycin** (Ilotycin) is active against a broad-spectrum of bacteria. **Gentamicin** (Garamycin, Genoptic) is effective against gram-negative and gram-positive bacteria, especially *Pseudomonas, Proteus, Klebsiella,* and *Escherichia coli* organisms. **Tobramycin** (Tobrex), another aminoglycoside, is a broad-spectrum agent but produces hypersensitivity reactions frequently.

Tetracyclines are used for superficial ocular infections and exert bacteriostatic action against a broad microbial spectrum. **Sulfonamides** have a broad-spectrum bacteriostatic effect when applied to the eye. They are indicated for superficial ocular infections caused by sensitive bacteria. Hypersensitivity is rare, but a careful history taking may reveal a history of allergic reactions to drugs of this family. Purulent exudates will interfere with the action of sulfonamides. Sulfacetamide is available only for topical use and is therefore to be preferred unless irritation occurs.

Preparations and Administration

Bacitracin
Ointments (Bacitracin, Baciguent), combinations with polymyxin B listed.

Chloramphenicol (Chloroptic, Econochlor, Antibiopto, Ophthochlor)
Ophthalmic solution, powder for reconstitution in diluent (Chloromycetin), ointment (Chloromycetin, Chloroptic, Econochlor), combination with polymyxin B (Chloromyxin)

Chlortetracycline (Aureomycin)
Ointment

Erythromycin (Ilotycin)
Ophthalmic ointment

Gentamicin (Garamycin, Genoptic)
Ophthalmic ointment, ophthalmic solution

Neomycin (Myciguent)
Ophthalmic ointment, and combination ointments listed under polymyxin.

Oxytetracycline
Combination with polymyxin B

Polymyxin B (Aerosporin and generic)
Powder, combination drops or ointment with chloramphenicol (Chloromyxin), with neomycin (Statrol), with neomycin and gramicidin (Neosporin), with bacitracin (Polysporin), with neomycin and bacitracin (Neosporin, Neotal, Mycitracin), or with oxytetracycline (Terramycin with Polymyxin B).

Sulfacetamide
Ophthalmic solution (AK-Sulf, Bleph-10, Opthacet, Sodium Sulamyd, Sulf-10, Isopto Cetamide, Sulfacel-15, generic), ointment (Cetamide, Sodium Sulamyd, generic); antibiotic/decongestant combination ophthalmic solution with phenylephrine (Vasosulf)

Sulfisoxazole (Gantrisin)
Ophthalmic drops or ointment

Tetracycline (Achromycin)
Ophthalmic drops, ophthalmic ointment

Tobramycin (Tobrex)
Ophthalmic solution

Antiviral Agents

Three antiviral ophthalmic agents control the eye lesions of herpes simplex virus: idoxuridine, vidarabine, and trifluridine. These agents are also used for dermatologic lesions caused by herpes simplex type I virus. Keratoconjunctivitis, the ocular lesion caused by herpes viruses, is effectively treated with antiviral agents in most cases. The complete pharmacology of these drugs is presented in Chapter 53.

Preparations and Administration

Idoxuridine (Dendrid, Stoxil)
Ophthalmic drops
Recommended Doses: One drop every hour during the day and every 2 hours at night, or as ointment 5 instillations per day (every 4 hours while awake with the last instillation at bedtime). Therapy should be continued 3–5 days after healing is complete. Improvement should occur in 7–8 days, healing in no more than 21 days.

Trifluridine (Viroptic)
Ophthalmic drops
Recommended Doses: One drop every 2 hours while awake, up to 9 drops daily. If no improvement is

seen in 7 days, or if complete reepithelialization has not occurred within 14 days, alternative therapy should be considered. Trifluridine should be continued at one drop every 4 hours for 1 week after complete reepithelialization.

Vidarabine (Vira-A)
Ointment
Recommended Doses: Half-inch ointment strips applied to the eye at 3-hour intervals, 5 times daily. If improvement is not seen in 7 days or complete reepithelialization in 21 days, another form of treatment should be considered.

Antifungal Agents

Fungal conjunctivitis is most often caused by *Candida albicans, Aspergillus, Fusarium,* and *Cryptococcus.* Frequently, it is a facet of systemic fungal infection, in which case treatment may be effected by systemic antifungal medications. Antifungal drugs are applied topically to the eye to augment systemic antifungal therapy or as the primary mode for local ocular infections. The antifungal drugs used topically include amphotericin B (Fungizone), flucytosine (Ancobon), nystatin (Mycostatin, Nilstat) and natamycin (Natacyn).

Amphotericin B is fungistatic and sometimes fungicidal for *Blastomyces, Coccidioides, Histoplasma,* and *Candida.* It is usually administered to the eye as a 2.5–5.0 mg/ml ophthalmic solution. Adverse reactions are minimal, including rare hypersensitivity reactions or slight local irritation.

Although **flucytosine** is usually employed orally, a 1% solution applied topically is well tolerated and effective against *Candida* and *Cryptococcus.* **Nystatin** is effective only as a topical administration applied as a solution or an ointment. Nystatin is useful for infections caused by *Aspergillus* or *Candida.*

Natamycin acts against a number of yeasts and fungi including *Aspergillus, Candida,* and *Fusarium.* It is the drug of choice for keratitis caused by *Fusarium solanae.* Topical administration to the eye provides adequate antifungal concentrations within the cornea but not in the intraocular fluid. It is therefore indicated for fungal blepharitis, conjunctivitis, and keratitis caused by susceptible organisms. Susceptibility should be established by laboratory evaluation. Adverse effects are uncommon, but conjunctival chemosis (edema) and hyperemia of probable allergic origin have been reported.

Preparations and Administration

Natamycin (Natacyn)
Ophthalmic suspension
Recommended Doses: For fungal keratitis, 1 drop in the conjunctival sac every 1–2 hours. After 3–4 days, frequency of application can be reduced to one drop 6–8 times daily. If improvement does not occur in 7–10 days, infection is probably not due to a susceptible organism. Treatment should be continued for 2–3 weeks or until there is resolution of active fungal keratitis, and then gradually discontinued to assure complete elimination of the organism. For fungal conjunctivitis or blepharitis, initial treatment can be less frequent, perhaps 4–6 instillations per day.

Antiseptics

The use of antiseptics in the eye has declined with the advent of specific antimicrobial agents. Antiseptic irrigating solutions may be used following tonometry or gonioscopy, for removal of secretions, mucus, or foreign bodies; or to soothe and cleanse the eye in conjunction with use of hard contact lenses. Many of the irrigating solutions consist of salt solutions with **benzalkonium chloride.** Benzalkonium chloride is a surface-active antiseptic. Products that consist of salts with benzalkonium chloride include Dacriose, Eye-Stream, Lavoptik, and aqua-FLOW.

Another antiseptic commonly encountered in irrigating solutions is **borate,** in the form of boric acid, sodium borate, or both. Borate is the principal antiseptic in Lauro, Zoptic, Collyrium, Blinx, and Triosol. Borate is found with benzalkonium chloride in Neo-Flo and Irigate and with thimerosal in AK/Rinse and M/Rinse. Ophthalmic irrigants are available in the form of lotions or solutions.

Thimerosal is a mercurial antiseptic with bacteriostatic and fungistatic activity. Thimerosal is seldom employed because it does not completely eliminate the infecting organisms, it does not act on spores, and it can cause irritation and hypersensitivity reactions. Thimerosal is available as an ophthalmic ointment (Merthiolate) and in the irrigant solution mentioned above (AK/Rinse, M/Rinse).

Silver salts are sometimes used in newborn infants as prophylaxis against gonococcal ophthalmia neonatorum. Application of silver nitrate to the eyes of newborns is a legal requirement in some states. Two drops of a 10% solution are applied to each eye after birth. The solution must remain in contact with the conjunctival sac for at least 30 seconds and should not be rinsed out by irrigation. Use of silver nitrate is not without controversy: the agent is irritating and produces a chemical conjunctivitis; rarely, sensitivity reactions develop. Some physicians prefer to employ antimicrobials, but these may cause sensitization. A second silver preparation is mild silver protein, which is indicated for ophthalmia neonatorum, eye infections, or preoperatively with eye surgery. It is useful for removing mucus, which it coagulates. With prolonged use, discoloration of the skin or sclera may occur.

Preparations and Administration

Mild silver protein (Argyrol)
Ophthalmic solution
Recommended Doses: For preoperative asepsis, 2 or 3 drops followed by a rinse with an irrigating solution. For eye infections, 1–3 drops every 3 or 4 hours for 2 days.

Steroidal Anti-Inflammatory Drugs

Topical steroids exert a local anti-inflammatory effect including suppression of hyperemia, vascularization, cellular infiltration, fibroblastic proliferation, photophobia, and pain of inflammation. Topical application of steroids to the eye is indicated in acute inflammatory conditions, involving the sclera, eyelid, conjunctiva, cornea, and anterior uveal tract (iris and ciliary body). However, the following principles should be observed in determining the advisability of steroid therapy:

1. Steroids are indicated *only* for inflammations caused by allergies or irritation and are contraindicated for purulent inflammations (since purulence is an indication of infection) because they inhibit defense mechanisms and increase susceptibility to pathogenic organisms, especially fungi and viruses.
2. Steroids should not be used for minor abrasions, since these drugs increase the opportunity for penetration and colonization by microorganisms.
3. Steroids should not be used for extended periods, since prolonged ocular steroid therapy can cause glaucoma, cataracts, optic nerve damage, or systemic toxicity such as adrenal suppression.
4. Steroids should not be used in clients who have exhibited ocular hypersensitivity reactions to the drug.

Although systemic adverse effects occur only with extensive use, ocular reactions are not uncommon. Adverse ocular effects of glucocorticoids include reduced visual acuity and field defects, cataract formation, optic nerve damage, glaucoma, secondary infections, and occasional stinging or burning.

Glucocorticoids are applied as drops or ointment into the conjunctival sac with the head tilted back. The eyes are then closed and a finger pressed lightly against the lacrimal sac for a minute following instillation. Brief stinging, burning, or itching is to be expected. Care should be taken not to contaminate the tip of the application tube by touching the eye or lid. Some ophthalmologists believe that corticosteroid drops provide better drug contact with the eye than do ointments.

Preparations and Administration

Cortisone
Ophthalmic ointment with neomycin (Neosone)

Dexamethasone
Ophthalmic drops with benzalkonium chloride (Decadron, Maxidex); ophthalmic ointment (Decadron, Maxidex); combination drops or ointment with neomycin (NeoDecadron), or with neomycin and polymyxin B (Maxitrol).
Recommended Doses: Same as hydrocortisone.

Fluorometholone
Ophthalmic suspension with benzalkonium chloride (FML)

Hydrocortisone
Ophthalmic solution (Optef), ophthalmic ointment (generics); eye drop combinations with chloramphenicol (Chloromycetin Hydrocortisone), oxytetracycline (Terra-Cortril), neomycin (Ak-Neo-Cort, Cort-Oticin, Neo-Cortef, Ophthel), and neomycin and polymyxin B (Cortisporin); ointment combinations with neomycin (Neo-Cortef), neomycin, bacitracin, and polymyxin B (Cortisporin, Coracin), and chloramphenicol and polymyxin B (Ophthocort).
Recommended Doses: Drops are initially instilled one or two at a time every hour during the day and every 2 hours at night. This can be reduced to a frequency of every 4 hours and then to every 6 hours if a favorable response is obtained. Ointments are applied 3 or 4 times daily at first, then 2 times daily after a response is obtained.

Medrysone
Ophthalmic suspension with benzalkonium chloride (HMS)

Methylprednisolone
Ophthalmic ointment with neomycin (Neo-Medrol)

Prednisolone
Ophthalmic suspension (Predulose); suspension with benzalkonium chloride (Pred Mild, Econopred Plus, Pred Forte); ophthalmic solutions with benzalkonium chloride (Inflamase, Ak-Pred, Hydeltrasol, Metreton); solution with benzalkonium chloride (Ak-Tate, Inflamase Forte, Ak-Pred); ophthalmic ointment (Hydeltrasol); combinations with antimicrobials, including drops with neomycin (Neo-Delta-Cortef, Neo-Hydeltrasol), neomycin and polymyxin B (Poly-Pred), or sodium sulfacetamide (Metimyd, Ophtha P/S, Opti-

myd, Isopto Cetapred, Sulfapred, Blephamide, and Vasocidin); and ointments with neomycin (Neo-Delta-Cortef, Neo-Hydeltrasol), chloramphenicol (Chloroptic-PS.O.P.), or sodium sulfacetamide (Metimyd, Vasocidin, Cetapred, or Blepharmide).

Recommended Doses: Same as for hydrocortisone.

Nonsteroidal Anti-Inflammatory Drugs

A nonsteroidal anti-inflammatory agent, flurbiprofen (Ocufen), was marketed in 1986 in an ophthalmic solution. Its mechanism of action is the same as other aspirin-like drugs, namely inhibition of the enzyme prostaglandin synthetase that catalyzes production of prostaglandins. In the eye, prostaglandins contribute to many of the symptoms of ocular inflammations including dilation and permeability of the ocular microvasculature, leukocytosis, increased intraocular pressure, and miosis. The approved clinical indication for flurbiprofen is for inhibition of the miosis that typically accompanies cataract surgery.

The principal adverse effect of flubiprofen is a transient stinging sensation upon installation in the eye. After topical application to the eye, a portion of the dose is absorbed systemically, but there is no evidence of significant systemic side effects. Flurbiprofen is contraindicated for clients with active herpes simplex keratitis and should be used cautiously in clients with a prior history of this condition because it inhibits the inflammatory response that helps to suppress the infection. Flurbiprofen is contraindicated for clients with a history of allergy to the drug. There is also a likelihood of cross-sensitivity in clients with known allergies to aspirin or other nonsteroidal antiinflammatory drugs.

Preparations and Administration

Flurbiprofen (Ocufen)
Ophthalmic solution
Recommended Doses: One drop every 0.5 hours beginning 2 hours before surgery for a total of four administrations.

Other Ophthalmic Agents

Topical Anesthetics

Local anesthetics are indicated for induction of corneal anesthesia of short duration to facilitate tonometry, gonioscopy, removal of foreign objects or sutures from the cornea, or for short corneal or conjunctival procedures. Local anesthetics should not be applied repeatedly to painful irritations because these drugs delay wound healing. They may also cause stinging, burning, photophobia, conjunctival injection, corneal opacity, and (rarely) softening, erosion, or perforation of the cornea. Systemic toxicity is not a problem when local anesthetics are applied topically to the eye. Cocaine was once widely used but has given way to other agents because of toxicity to the central nervous system and the need to regulate its distribution carefully.

Tetracaine acts in 2–3 minutes. Epithelial damage occurs with prolonged use. Tetracaine is incompatible with mercury or silver salts found in some ophthalmic preparations. **Proparacaine** is employed in a manner similar to tetracaine. It causes less stinging or burning of the eyeball but otherwise shares the adverse effects of tetracaine.

Preparations and Administration

Proparacaine (AK-Taine, Alcaine, Ophthaine, Ophthetic)
Ophthalmic solution

Tetracaine (Pontocaine)
Ophthalmic solutions
Recommended Doses: For removal of sutures or foreign bodies, 1 or 2 drops of a 0.5% solution. For deep anesthesia, one drop is instilled every 5–10 minutes to a maximum of 5–7 doses.

Enzyme: Chymotrypsin

Chymotrypsin is a proteolytic enzyme used occasionally as an aid in removal of cataracts. It is injected behind the iris into the front of the posterior chamber where it dissolves the zonules that hold the lens, which permits removal of the lens. Following dilation of the pupil with a mydriatic and incision under anesthesia, 1–2 ml of chymotrypsin solution is injected. The enzyme acts in 2–4 minutes and is washed out by irrigation. After removal of the lens, the pupil is contracted with a miotic. Chymotrypsin is provided with a diluent for reconstitution immediately prior to use. Chymotrypsin is available as 750 units with 10 ml of diluent (Alpha Chymar), 750 units with 9 ml of diluent (Zolyse), 300 units with 2 ml of diluent (Catarase 1:5000), or 150 units with 2 ml of diluent (Catarase 1:10,000).

Lubricants

Ocular lubricants provide temporary relief of minor eye irritation. The ocular lubricants include zinc sulfate, rose petal aqueous infusion, petrolatum, and artificial tears. Lubricants are useful for use with contact lenses and artificial eyes. Artificial tears are especially useful for relief of dry eyes due to deficient lacrimation. Artificial tear formulations generally consist of methylcellulose or other polymers with an antiseptic, usually benzalkonium chloride. Available preparations include Isopto Tears, Tears Plus, Visculose, Tears Naturale, and many others.

Zinc sulfate is provided in 0.217% drops with boric acid (Eye-Sed) or 0.25% drops with benzalkonium chloride (BufOpto, Op-Thal-Zin). Two drops may be administered, twice daily. Rose Petal Aqueous Infusion (Estivin) is a 0.01% aqueous solution with thimerosal. One drop is recommended 3–4 times daily for minor irritations. Petrolatum, lanolin, and mineral oil ointment combinations are indicated for lubrication of the eye and protection in exposure keratitis or recurrent corneal erosions. Available products are Lacri-Lube and Duratears Lubricant Ointment.

Hyperosmolar Preparations

Hypertonic solutions may be used to reduce corneal edema by osmotic attraction of water. One or two drops of solution or a small amount of hyperosmolar ointment is applied every 3–4 hours. Available hyperosmolar preparations are 2% or 5% hypertonic sodium chloride drops (Adsorbonac, Hypersal, Muro 128) or ointment (Muro 128), glycerin drops (Ophthalgan), or 40% glucose ointment (generic).

Diagnostic Aids

Mydriatics and local anesthetics are diagnostic aids in some of their applications. In addition, fluorescein dye is an aid to visualization of corneal abrasions, foreign bodies, and conjunctival ulcerations. After instillation of fluorescein into the eye, areas of corneal abrasion are stained a bright green. Foreign bodies are surrounded by a green ring; conjunctival lesions are stained yellow-orange. Fluorescein can also be used as an aid to fitting hard lenses. Areas of contact between the lens and cornea will appear black under ultraviolet light while other areas of the cornea exhibit the green fluorescein color. Fluorescein should not be used with soft lenses because it will stain the lens. Fluorescein can also be used by injection to facilitate examination of the iris vasculature, fundus, and aqueous flow and to differentiate between viable and nonviable tissue or malignant and nonmalignant tumors.

After topical instillation, adverse effects are limited to occasional hypersensitivity reactions. Also, fluorescein solutions may become contaminated by *Pseudomonas aeruginosa.* After injection, side effects are more common. Nausea, headache, gastrointestinal disturbances, hypotension, cardiac arrest, convulsions, and syncope have occurred. Clients may complain of allergic reactions such as transient dyspnea, urticaria, pruritus, or fever. Nurses should advise clients that the dye may cause skin discoloration for 6–12 hours after injection and invariably imparts a bright yellow color to the urine. Fluorescein strips contain impregnated dye and are moistened just before use. This obviates concern about *Pseudomonas* contamination. Fluress also contains a local anesthetic, benoxinate, and is a useful preparation for removal of foreign objects. Fluorexon is a large molecular form of fluorescein that can be used for fitting soft contact lenses without staining the hydrogel lens.

Preparations and Administration

Fluorescein Dye

Topical solutions (Fluoreseptic, Fluress), topical strips (Ful-Glo, Fluor-I-Strip), solution of large molecular weight fluroescein (Fluoresoft), injection solution (Fluorescite, Funduscein, AK-Fluor)

Recommended Doses: One drop of 2% solution followed by irrigation to promote distribution or touching a moistened strip to the conjunctiva by closing the eyelid. For ophthalmologic procedures, inject into the antecubital vein. A small test dose should be given first to test for possible allergic manifestations. Epinephrine, an antihistamine, and oxygen should be available in the event of severe allergic reactions.

Ocular Toxicity of Drugs

Drugs and chemicals can impair vision in numerous ways. For example, chemicals or drugs may be the principal cause of conjunctivitis or keratitis, or a disorder may be further aggravated by the drug. Since many of the prescription and nonprescription eye remedies have potential for ocular toxicity, a careful history of drugs used in the eye is an important part of nursing assessment. Other irritants may be encountered in the workplace, at home, or as environmental allergens. When questioning the client about drugs or exposure to chemicals, it is useful for the nurse to have a list of drugs or chemicals that affect the eye (Table 54–6).

Some ocular side effects (usually from ophthalmic medications) are predictable and reversible, such as the myopia, blurring of vision, and light-sensitivity that occur with mydriatics. On the other hand, certain visual side effects require the immediate attention of the physician, such as opacities, inflammations, ocular pain, or any disturbance of the visual field. The client should always be given clear information about the symptoms that are normal responses to a prescribed medication and those that need to be brought to the attention of the treatment team.

Table 54–6
Ocular Toxicities of Drugs and Chemicals

Type of toxicity	Drugs or chemicals
Corneal and conjunctival toxicities	
Chemical burns/tissue necrosis	Alkylating agents, cardiac glycosides, caustics, detergents, poison ivy, rare-earth salts, solvents, sulfur dioxide, surfactants, tissue fixatives
Conjunctivitis and/or keratitis	Alkylating agents, aminosalicylic acid, antimitotic drugs, arsenicals, barbiturates, bromides, carbimazole, chloral hydrate, chlorpropamide, cocaine, copper, corticosteroids, epinephrine, fluorescein solutions, gold, hydantoins, methotrexate, methoxsalen, novobiocin, oral contraceptives, penicillamine, penicillin, phenolphthalein, phenothiazines, phensuximide, phenylbutazone, silver salts, sulfonamides, and topical anesthetics
Follicular conjunctivitis	Atropine, bacitracin, idoxuridine, miotics, neomycin, penicillin, and scopolamine
Conjunctival hyperemia (injection)	Cholinesterase inhibitors, dibenzyline, ethylene glycol, local anesthetics, marihuana, reserpine, sulfonamides
Corneal and/or conjunctival discoloration	Aniline, benzoquinone, hydroquinone, iron minerals, mepacrine, nitrobenzene, silver salts, sympathomimetics
Corneal edema	Anticholinergics, dichloroethane, diethyl diglycolate, ethylenediamines, N-ethylmorpholine
Corneal deposits	
Epithelial deposits	Bismuth, chloroquine, chlorpromazine, hydroxychloroquine, indomethacin, mepacrine, triparanol
Calcification	Beryllium, vitamin D hypervitaminosis
Stromal Deposits	Cholesterol, gold, mercury, silver
Corneal opacities	Chloroquine, chlorpropamide, indomethacin, local anesthetics, sympathomimetics, tolbutamide
Eyelid toxicities	
Ptosis	Barbiturates, botulism, bretylium, chloral hydrate, corticosteroids, guanethidine, marihuana, mephenesin, phenoxybenzamine, primidone, reserpine, tetraethylammonium, thallium, venoms, vincristine
Lid retraction	Amphetamines, cocaine, methoxamine, phenylephrine
Lid edema	Chloral hydrate, hydralazine, spider venoms
Lid twitches	Cholinesterase inhibitors
Lid discoloration	Chloroquine, hydroxychloroquine, mercuric oxide, nitrofurazone, physostigmine, sympathomimetics, thiotepa, triparanol
Alopecia of lids	Actinomycin D, thallium, triparanol, vitamin A
Lacrimal toxicities	
Lacrimation	Arsenicals, bethanechol, cholinesterase inhibitors, diazoxide, dimercaprol, heroin, hydralazine, mercury, narcotic withdrawal, reserpine, sulfathiazole, zoxazolamine
Lens, iris, and anterior chamber toxicities	
Cataracts and lens opacities	Allopurinol, carbamazepine, chlorpropamide, corticosteroids, dinitrophenol, hydroxychloroquine, miotics, mitotane, radiation, sugars, triparanol
Reversible white clouding of lens	Imipramine, levorphanol, methoxsalen, narcotics, phenothiazines, sympathomimetics
Lens discoloration	Copper, iron, mercury, phenothiazine, phenylmercuric salts, silver salts
Weakness of accommodation	Anticholinergics, hydroxychloroquine, isoxsuprine, narcotics, sympathomimetics, vasoconstrictors
Myopia	Acetazolamide, alpha-blockers, arsenicals, methylene blue, miotics (cholinomimetics, cholinesterase inhibitors), phenothiazines, sulfonamides
Idiosyncratic myopia	Acetazolamide, clofenamides, phenformin, phenothiazines, spironolactone, sulfonamides, tetracyclines, thiazides
Anterior chamber shallowing	Acetazolamide, sulfanilamide, urea
Increased intraocular pressure	Anticholinergics, caffeine, caustics, chymotrypsin, cocaine, copper, corticosteroids, cyclopentolate, decamethonium, flavoxate, iron, isoxsuprine, ketamine, oxybutynin, phenol, suxamethonium, sympathomimetics, tolazoline, tropicamide, wasp stings

Table 54–6
Ocular Toxicities of Drugs and Chemicals (*continued*)

Type of toxicity	Drugs or chemicals
Lens, iris, and anterior chamber toxicities (*continued*)	
Decreased intraocular pressure	Acetazolamide, ascorbic acid, diclofenamide, digitalis, dihydroergotamine, ethanol, glycerol, isosorbide, mannitol, pargyline, phentolamine, propranolol, propylene glycol, quinine, sugars, thiopental, urea
Uveitis	Colchicine, naphthalene, wasp stings
Iris atrophy	Quinine
Posterior synechia	Miotics
Posterior chamber and optic nerve toxicities	
Impaired light adaptation/photophobia	Digitalis, heroin, hydroxychloroquine, local anesthetics, mecury, mydriatics, nalidixic acid, penicillamine, sulfathiazole, trimethadione
Impaired dark adaptation	Carbon dioxide, carbon disulfide, carbon monoxide, digitalis, miotics, narcotics
Pigmented retinopathy	Chloroquine, copper, hydroxychloroquine, indomethacin, iron, oxygen, phenothiazines (especially thioridazine), quinine
Retinal edema	Chloramphenicol, cyanide, diiodohydroxyquin, glue sniffing, methanol, quinine, radiopaque contrast media
Retinal hemorrhages	Arsphenamine, benzene, chloramphenicol, dicumarol, ethambutol, lead, licorice, methyl bromide, phenylbutazone, radiopaque contrast media, snake venoms, sulfonamides, vitamin A, warfarin
Retinal angiopathy	Alloxan, licorice, oxygen
Retinal detachment	Cobalt, deferoxamine, epinephrine, mercuric chloride, naphthalene, oxygen, pyrazolones, pyrithione
Papilledema	Arsphenamine, aspirin, bee stings, chenopodium oil, chloramphenicol, ethylene glycol, isoniazid, lead, methylene blue, nalidixic acid, oral contraceptives, penicillamine, penicillin, phenylenediamines, phosphorus, sulfonamides, tetracyclines, triamcinolone, vitamin A
Optic neuritis	Arsenicals, bee stings, botulism, chloramphenicol, digitalis, dinitrobenzene, ethambutol, ethchlorvynol, ethionamide, isoniazid, lead, methanol, penicillamine, phenothiazines, phosphorus, pyrazolones, quinine, rabies vaccine, streptomycin, sulfonamides, thallium
Retrobulbar neuritis	Chloramphenicol, chlorpropamide, digitalis, diiodohydroxyquin, dinitrobenzene, dinitrotoluene, disulfiram, ethambutol, isoniazid, lead, thallium
Optic atrophy	Arsenicals, carbon dioxide, carbon disulfide, chloramphenicol, dinitrobenzene, diiodohydroxyquin, ethambutol, ethylene glycol, hexamethonium, isoniazid, lead, methanol, methylene blue, quinine, streptomycin, thallium
Scotoma	Caffeine, camphor, carbon dioxide, carbon disulfide, chloramphenicol, chloroquine, clomiphene, digitalis, dinitrobenzene, dinitrotoluene, disulfiram, emetine, ethambutol, ethchlorvynol, ethanol, Gila monster venum, hydroxychloroquine, isoniazid, lead, methanol, pyrazolones, quinacrine, quinidine, quinine, streptomycin, sulfonamides, thallium, tobacco, wasp stings
Visual field constriction	Arsenicals, bee stings, botulism, carbon dioxide, carbon monoxide, chloramphenicol, emetine, ethambutol, hydroxychloroquine, methanol, methylmercury compounds, naphthalene, oxygen, quinine
Eye movement toxicities	
Weakness/palsy of extraocular muscles	Barbiturates, curare, digitalis, ethanol, gold salts, hydroxychloroquine, lead, pentaquine, phenothiazines, pyrazolones, rabies vaccine, streptomycin, sulfonamides, thallium, venoms, vincristine, vitamin A
Nystagmus	Barbiturates, bufotenin, carbamazepine, carbon disulfide, diazepam, dieldrin, ethanol, ethylene glycol, ergot, fenfluramine, glutethimide, hydantoins, methyl halides, primidone, streptomycin, tripelennamine
Oculogyric crisis	Butyrophenones, phenothiazines, other antipsychotic agents
Convergence defects	Barbiturates, carbon dioxide, carbon monoxide, chloral hydrate

(*continued*)

Table 54–6
Ocular Toxicities of Drugs and Chemicals (*continued*)

Type of toxicity	Drugs or chemicals
Eye movement toxicities (*continued*)	
Diplopia	Botulism, carbamazepine, carbon disulfide, carbon monoxide, diazepam, ethanol, ethylene glycol, hydantoins, imipramine, lead, lidocaine, mephenesin, nitrofurantoin, primidone, vitamin A
Orbital toxicities	
Orbital edema	Phenylenediamine, sulfonamides
Exophthalmos	Corticosteroids, thyroid hormones, vitamin A
Orbital necrosis	Thalidomide
Referred pain	
Headache/browache	Cholinesterase inhibitors, sympathomimetics
CNS visual toxicities	
Cortical blindness	Barbiturates, carbon monoxide, lead, methadone
Visual hallucinations	Anticholinergics, cannabis, carbamazepine, carbon monoxide, digitalis, diphenhydramine, disulfiram reactions, ephedrine, ethanol, harmaline, LSD, mescaline, pentazocine, psychedelics, thiocyanate, tricyclic antidepressants, trihexyphenidyl
Color vision alterations	Cannabis, carbon dioxide, chlorothiazide, digitalis, dihydrostreptomycin, ethambutol, furosemide, pentylenetetrazol, thiocyanate, trimethadione
Ocular teratogenicity	
Teratisms	Thalidomide; in animals — caffeine, colchicine, quinine, salicylates, vinblastine, vincristine

Case Study: Glaucoma

W. F., a 64-year-old, white woman was brought to the ophthalmology unit from the emergency room, where she had been brought by her husband. W. F. was experiencing severe pain on the right side of her head and in the right eye. She complained of nausea and had vomited three times in the last 6 hours. She reported that her vision was blurred and that she saw halos around the lights.

The nurse examined W. F. and noted that her eyes were red and the pupil in the right eye was dilated and watery. The cornea appeared cloudy. The nurse conducted a finger-pressure test and found the eyeball noticeably firm. The nurse observed that W. F. was distraught about her condition. Vital signs were recorded as follows: blood pressure 145/90, pulse 95, temperature 98.6°F, and respiration 22. The nurse learned from Mr. F. that his wife had been taking aspirin several times daily for the last week for head pain in a similar location though less severe than at present. W. F. admitted that she suspected that she might have glaucoma since her father had gone blind late in life from this condition. She had avoided going for a visual examination, fearing what she might be told. The nurse reassured her that glaucoma would not usually culminate in blindness if properly managed but that lifelong drug therapy or possibly surgery would probably be required. W. F. had no history of chronic ailments.

After examining the eyes, conducting a tonometric evaluation, and reviewing the nurse's findings, the ophthalmologist concluded that W. F. was experiencing an acute attack of closed-angle glaucoma. Medication orders were for 4% pilocarpine by instillation in the right eye every hour, 1.5 g/kg of 20% mannitol by intravenous infusion over 30 minutes, bedrest, a low-sodium diet, and 20 mEq of oral potassium chloride. Routine blood tests and urinalysis were conducted. The nursing diagnoses in this case were (1) alteration in comfort: pain related to elevated intraocular pressure, (2) sensory-perceptual alterations related to elevated intraocular pressure, (3) anxiety related to worry about possible future blindness, and (4) potential alteration in cardiac output in response to mannitol infusion.

The nurse administered the pilocarpine, mixed the potassium chloride in orange juice and gave it to W. F. Before infusing the mannitol, the nurse reviewed the lab measurements of serum electrolytes (all normal) and made sure that a filter was in place in the intravenous line. During the infusion, blood pressure, pulse, heart sounds, and respiratory sounds at 5-minute intervals were monitored, and W. F. was instructed to report any shortness of breath, chills, or chest pain. Intake-output monitoring was also initiated. The nurse checked the right eye for its response to pilocarpine and noted pupillary constriction but no sign of inflammation or irritation. The nurse made certain to maintain an attitude of efficient confidence, talked reassuringly with W. F., and kept her room quiet but well-lighted.

After 1 hour, the nurse noted that the redness and teariness of the right eye had been relieved. W. F. reported she was feeling better and had no pain. Blood pressure was not 125/85 (usual for W. F.) and pulse rate at 80. Heart and lung sounds were normal.

1. Which of the initial symptoms were likely attributable to the acute attack of closed-angle glaucoma?
2. Which of the nurse's observations during physical assessment and history taking support the diagnosis?
3. What is the likely reason for the elevation in blood pressure and pulse at initial evaluation?
4. Why did the ophthalmologist order pilocarpine instead of carbechol or epinephrine?
5. What is the rationale for the use of mannitol in this situation?
6. Why did the nurse check serum electrolytes and presence of an in-line filter before beginning the mannitol?
7. Why did the nurse monitor blood pressure, heart rate, heart sounds, and pulmonary sounds during mannitol infusion?
8. What interventions did the nurse employ to address each of the nursing diagnoses?

Answers appear at the end of the book.

Recommended Readings

Boyd-Monk H: Conjunctivitis. *Nursing* 1982;12(11):67.

Chiou GC, Watanabe K: Drug delivery to the eye. *Pharmacol Ther* 1982;17(2):269–278.

Condl ED: Ophthalmic nursing. *Nurs Clin North Am* 1970;5:467–476.

Ellis PP: *Ocular Therapeutics and Pharmacology,* ed 6. St Louis, CV Mosby Co, 1981.

Gittinger JW: *Ophthalmology, a Clinical Introduction.* Boston, Little Brown & Co, 1984.

Katz I: Beta blockers and the eye: An overview. *Ann Ophthalmol* 1978;10:847–850.

Quail C, Waddleton C: Treating the glaucomas. *Nurs Drug Alert* 1980;4(12):93–96.

Schwartz B: The glaucomas. *N Engl J Med* 1978;299:182–184.

Smith JF: *Ophthalmologic Nursing.* Boston, Little Brown & Co, 1980.

Zimmerman TL et al: Advances in ocular pharmacology. *Annu Rev Pharmacol Toxicol* 1980;20:415–428.

CHAPTER 55

Drugs Used for Disorders of the Ear and Sinuses

Drugs Used for Disorders of the Ear

External Otitis

The external ear canal is protected from infection by a layer of epithelial cells and the wax, or cerumen, produced by apocrine and sebaceous glands in the outer third of the external ear canal. External otitis, an infection of the outer ear canal, occurs when these defense mechanisms have been compromised.

Wetness contributes to external otitis by creating a moist environment conducive to microorganisms. Frequent flushing of the ear during summer swimming washes away protective cerumen, increasing susceptibility to infection. The frequent incidence of external otitis among swimmers is called **swimmer's ear.** Other predisposing factors include chemical irritants, such as cosmetics (hair spray or dye) and industrial irritants; trauma, most often self-inflicted by insertion of a cotton swab, a fingernail, or other objects into the ear canal; and allergies and dermatoses of the scalp, such as psoriasis and seborrhea. External otitis can also develop from middle-ear infections if the eardrum is perforated.

A relatively small number of pathogens account for most cases of external otitis. The organism *Pseudomonas* is the single most common cause. When *P. aeruginosa* is the causative agent of external otitis in elderly or diabetic clients, the condition may be malignant, spreading to blood vessels and temporal bone. Therefore, when external otitis occurs in these clients, it must be treated vigorously with systemic (usually intravenous) antibiotics.

Other gram-negative microbes frequently implicated are *Escherichia coli* and *Proteus vulgaris*. *Staphylococcus aureus* is the main gram-positive bacterium that is found in ear infections, producing a localized infection called *furuncles*. Fungal infections are less common and are recognized by clinical appearance in which the skin has a characteristic soft cotton-like texture and is multicolored. Most cases of external otitis caused by fungi are due to *Aspergillus* or *Candida*. Fungal colonizations are often secondary infections that develop after using antimicrobials or steroids. Antimicrobials typically found in otic preparations for external otitis are summarized in Table 55–1.

Clients with external otitis have tenderness and pain of the ear canal, erythema, pruritus, and edema. A discharge with a foul odor may be present as well as congestion of the ear canal and an associated reversible impairment of hearing. Furuncles in the ear canal, which are especially painful, are not responsive to topical treatment but drain spontaneously. Dry heat applied to the ear and systemic analgesics provide interim relief. Generalized external otitis usually responds well to topical antibiotics and steroids.

Antibacterial Agents

The antibacterial agents found in topical otic preparations are chloramphenicol, neomycin, and the polymyxins. **Chloramphenicol** has broad activity against the principal bacterial causes of external otitis, including *Pseudomonas, Escherichia coli, Proteus,* and *Staphylococcus aureus*. Hypersensitivity to chloramphenicol results in a variety of local irritant effects, such as itching, burning, urticaria, or maculopapular eruptions. Hypersensitivity is the only contraindication for use of chloramphenicol. Prolonged or too frequent use of chloramphenicol can cause serious systemic toxicity, such as bone marrow suppression that leads to aplastic anemia or hypoplastic leukopenia. Superinfection may result from the colonizing of nonsusceptible fungal or bacterial organisms. Chloramphenicol is available as a 0.5% solution (Chloromycetin Otic) for application to the external auditory canal. Two or three drops are instilled 3 times daily.

Neomycin is effective against *Escherichia coli, Proteus,* and *Staphylococcus aureus*, and has modest activity against *Pseudomonas*. Neomycin is an aminoglycoside, and like all members of this class can produce ototoxicity when used systemically; ototoxicity has also been reported after topical application. Clients with a perforated eardrum should be considered at special risk of ototoxicity. Cutaneous hypersensitivity reactions and superinfections may also occur. Neomycin is the sole antibiotic in Otobiotic Otic, a formulation designated as "possibly effective." More often, neomycin is found in combination with polymyxin B and hydrocortisone (My Cort Otic, Otocort, Otoreid, Cortisporin, Pyocidin-Otic, Otobione), with

Table 55–1

Spectra of Activity of Antimicrobial Drugs Commonly Employed in External Otitis Against Pathogens Commonly Responsible

Microorganism	Acetic acid	Chloramphenicol	Neomycin	Polymyxins	Amphotericin B
Gram-negative bacteria					
Pseudomonas aeruginosa	++	++	+	++	No
Escherichia coli	?	++	++	++	No
Proteus vulgaris	?	++	++	No	No
Gram-positive bacilli					
Staphylococcus aureus	?	++	++	No	No
Streptococci	?	No	++	No	No
Fungi					
Aspergillus	++	No	No	No	No
Candida	++	No	No	No	++

acetic acid and hydrocortisone (Neo-Cort-Dome), with hydrocortisone (Ortho), or with colistin and hydrocortisone (Coly-Mycin S). These preparations consist of solutions and suspensions.

Two **polymyxins** are utilized in otic formulations: polymyxin B and colistin (polymyxin E) and are effective against *Pseudomonas aeruginosa* and *Escherichia coli* but are not effective against *Proteus* or gram-positive bacteria. Hypersensitivity irritation and superinfection are the main adverse effects. Polymyxin B is not always effective when used alone (Lidosporin Otic) because of its limited spectrum but is usually combined with other antibiotics. It is found in combination with oxytetracycline as an ointment (Terramycin with Polymyxin B), with hydrocortisone and neomycin in the preparations listed above, and with hydrocortisone as a solution (Pyocidin-otic).

Antibacterial agents should be applied after thorough but gentle cleansing of the ear canal. The ideal vehicle for otic antibacterial preparations is a solution or suspension in propylene glycol that will mix with the film of wax and fatty acids that compose the cerumen and also provide aqueous penetration if there is a watery exudate.

Antifungals and Antiseptics

Amphotericin B, which is especially effective against *Candida,* is available in a lotion (Fungizone) that can be applied to the ear canal. Otherwise, treatment of the uncommon fungal infections is conducted with antiseptics found in otic preparations that have antifungal activity. These include mainly acetic acid and parachlorometaxylenol.

Acetic acid solutions at 2% have both antifungal and antibacterial activity and are especially active against *Pseudomonas aeruginosa, Candida,* and *Aspergillus.* Acetic acid does not cause hypersensitivity reactions, does not promote formation of resistant organisms, and is well tolerated. Acetic acid is available in combination with parachlorometaxylenol and benzalkonium chloride as drops (Otic-Plain or Benxodyne). It is applied by use of a saturated wick (cotton plug), 3–4 times daily. Acetic acid is also available alone (Domeboro) and with parachlorometaxylenol (Orlex Otic).

Parachlorometaxylenol is another antiseptic with antifungal activity. This drug is marketed with acetic acid (mentioned above), benzocaine and epinephrine (Myringacaine), and with benzocaine and benzethonium chloride (Hesathricin). However, use of local anesthetics in the ear is ill advised because they cause irritation and may mask sensitivity to symptoms of infection or irritation. Local anesthetics also provide unpredictable activity.

Corticosteroids

Corticosteroids are marketed in combination with the various antimicrobials mentioned above. They suppress the inflammatory component of external otitis caused by bacteria. Steroids are contraindicated for infections caused by fungi because they suppress bodily defenses against these organisms. Corticosteroids are also contraindicated in clients who exhibit hypersensitivity to steroids or have viral infections such as herpes simplex.

Otitis Media

The middle ear is separated from the external ear canal by the tympanic membrane. Otitis media is an infection of the middle ear that usually develops secondarily to upper respiratory tract infections. Microorganisms may migrate from the nasopharynx to the middle ear via the eustachian tube. Nasopharyngitis or rhinitis can occlude the eustachian tube and cause congestion and stasis within the tube and the inner ear that creates an environment favorable for growth of organisms. Usually, bacteria are the organisms involved in otitis media even though upper respiratory tract infections are most often viral. Nasopharyngeal cultures do not correlate reliably with the etiological agent in otitis media; thus otitis media is more often due to a secondary infection than to spread of infection.

Otitis media is most common in young children, from 3 months to 3 years of age, because the small channels of the inner ear are more easily occluded. Gram-negative bacilli are usually implicated, notably *Escherichia coli* and *Staphylococcus aureus.* Between ages 3 and 8, inner ear infections are most often caused by *Streptococcus pneumoniae, Hemophilus influenzae, Staphylococcus aureus,* and group A beta-hemolytic streptococci. After age 8, Streptococci and *Staphylococcus aureus* are the most frequent causative agents.

The characteristic symptom of otitis media is a severe and persistent earache. In young children, the earache is often accompanied by fever and sometimes by nausea, vomiting, or diarrhea. With an otoscope, the bulging tympanic membrane can be observed. It can rupture if the infection is severe. If the tympanic membrane is perforated, a discharge that is clear, bloody, or purulent may flow into the outer ear canal. Untreated otitis media can lead to serious complications, including hearing loss, meningitis, facial paralysis, brain abscess, otitic hydroencephalus, or lateral sinus thrombosis, which are indicated by such symptoms as headache, vertigo, chills, fever, and hearing loss.

Oral antibiotics are used to treat otitis media and serve the dual purpose of hastening resolution of the disorder and reducing risks of complications. Ampicillin is widely employed in children under age 8 because of its effectiveness against likely pathogens, including *H. influenzae.* The agents usually responsible for otitis media after age 8 are responsive to penicillin. Decongestants instilled topically in the nasal passages have an effect on the eustachian tubes similar to that on the nasal mucosa and may improve function of the eustachian tubes, promoting drainage.

Cerumen-Softening Agents

Cerumen is the waxy secretion of the apocrine and sebaceous glands of the external ear canal that provides a protective coat that is hydrophobic, bacteriostatic, and fungistatic. Under normal circumstances, it is removed from the ear at a rate commensurate with its rate of production. Cerumen can accumulate, however, if the ear canal is unusually dry, narrow, tortuous, or hairy, so that the normal process of wax removal may require facilitation.

When wax is hard but not impacted, **light mineral oil** provides the best means of softening cerumen to promote its removal. The ear canal can be filled with mineral oil and plugged with cotton overnight for 1–3 nights. Mineral oil has the advantage of being nonallergic and is also inexpensive.

The wax is then removed by irrigating the external canal with water or saline warmed to body temperature or a solution of carbamide peroxide in glycerin (Benadyne Improved, Debrox, Murine). Glycerin softens wax while carbamide peroxide provides an effervescence that promotes loosening of wax and tissue debris. Following the irrigation, the ear should be thoroughly dried with a blow dryer or by rinsing with a 70% isopropyl alcohol solution. The glycerin procedure may have to be repeated twice a day for 3 or 4 days to remove large deposits of hardened wax.

If wax is impacted, the most effective technique for removal is use of a ring curette under visual observation. If this is not feasible, wax softeners are employed as described above. The extreme tactic is the use of the ceruminolytic agent, triethanolamine polypeptide oleate-condensate in propylene glycol (Cerumenex). The effectiveness of this agent has not been clearly established and it may cause contact dermatitis. It is instilled in the ear with a dropper, allowed to sit for 15–30 minutes, and flushed out. When external otitis is accompanied by impacted wax, antimicrobial preparations may have the double value of softening the cerumen while combating the infection.

Ototoxicity

Ototoxicity is the impairment of auditory or vestibular function due to the effect of a drug on the inner ear. Ototoxic drugs are invariably agents excreted by the kidneys; therefore, renal impairment is a predisposing factor in ototoxicity. It is more likely to occur in elderly individuals because of preexisting hearing deficits and diminished renal function.

An obscure relationship exists between the cochlea and the renal tubule. The two structures have antigenic similarity. Autoimmune disorders involving the one frequently involve the other as well, so that hearing loss is often associated with renal pathology. Both structures are intimately engaged in active transport of electrolytes. In the cochlea, the scala media (a fluid compartment) maintains an electrolyte composition similar to intracellular fluid (rich in potassium, low in sodium) while the scala vestibuli and scala tympani (the remaining fluid compartments) maintain a fluid composition resembling extracellular fluid. The concentration gradient between these compartments is responsible for the endocochlear potential that is required for initiation of generator potentials in primary auditory afferents. The cochlear potential is maintained by active exchange of K^+ for Na^+ across a specialized membrane. For this reason, the potent loop diuretics can disrupt auditory function just as they alter renal transport of electrolytes.

Ototoxic Drugs

Among the **loop diuretics,** ethacrynic acid has the greatest ototoxicity, producing permanent deafness in some cases. Furosemide has only recently been observed to produce permanent deafness; most cases of ototoxicity from this drug have been transient. Bumetanide is less ototoxic than the other loop diuretics. Hearing of high-frequency sound is affected first by loop diuretics.

Nonsteroidal anti-inflammatory agents, including aspirin, indomethacin, naproxen, fenoprofen, phenylbutazone, and ibuprofen have long been known to cause tinnitus, vertigo, and rarely reversible hearing loss. **Cinchona alkaloids,** including quinine and quinidine, produce a similar temporary ototoxicity. Permanent deafness has occurred in only a few cases. The best evidence currently available suggests that these drugs cause ototoxicity by producing vasoconstriction and transient ischemia within the inner ear. In the infrequent cases of permanent deafness, evidence suggests that the ischemia progresses to anoxic necrosis.

Perhaps the most important of the ototoxic agents are the **aminoglycoside antibiotics.** Strepto-

Nursing Observations for Drug Therapy for Otitis

THERAPEUTIC GOAL	To prevent and alleviate inflammation of the ear canal.
PREADMINISTRATION ASSESSMENT	
Baseline Data	Assess extent of earache, tenderness, pain, erythema, pruritus, congestion, nausea, vomiting, vertigo, diarrhea, or unusual discharge or edema in the ear canal. Observe for adjustments in bodily position as compensations for hearing loss (such as leaning forward or cocking the head). Evaluate appearance of ear canal and determine presence of fever. Assess hearing and functions.
EVALUATION OF DRUG RESPONSE	
For Therapeutic Benefit	Monitor for reduction of inflammation, itching, congestion, and impairments of hearing or balance.
For Adverse Effects	Monitor for allergic reactions (itching, burning, urticaria, or rash) to topical otic antimicrobials. Observe for ototoxicity if neomycin is employed topically. Watch for aggravation of otic fungal infections if steroids are administered.
For Compliance	Evaluate the client's compliance with all facets of the therapeutic regimen by careful observation, interviewing, and review of progress. Report compliance problems to the physician and act as client-advocate when changes in the therapeutic regimen seem indicated.

mycin exerts toxicity primarily on the vestibular portion of the inner ear structure. Vertigo and inability to maintain balance are the clinical manifestations. Hearing loss occurs in up to 15% of clients and becomes permanent if treatment is prolonged. Neomycin on the other hand is toxic mainly to the cochlea. It is not used systemically but is found in some of the antibacterial preparations used topically for external otitis. Ototoxicity has been reported when neomycin has been employed in this way and is especially likely if there is rupture of the tympanic membrane. Among the newer aminoglycosides that are used systemically, the incidence of cochlear toxicity varies. Toxicity is greater with kanamycin than with amikacin, which is much more likely to produce toxicity than gentamicin or tobramycin. Vancomycin has caused hearing loss, and viomycin has caused both cochlear and vestibular toxicity. The ototoxicity of aminoglycosides is additive to that produced by loop diuretics. Clinical evidence indicates that more careful adjustment of dosage by the monitoring of plasma levels significantly reduces aminoglycoside-induced ototoxicity. A new aminoglycoside netilmicin, appears to have very little ototoxicity.

An interesting footnote about the functional parallels between the cochlea and the nephron is that ototoxicity and nephrotoxicity are the two major problems associated with use of aminoglycosides. High-frequency hearing is affected first by aminoglycosides, gradually extending into lower frequencies. Morphologically, the basal region of the cochlea is affected first with gradual spread to the upper turns. Although ototoxicity is not normally associated with use of erythromycin, it has occurred in a few instances after administration of high doses.

Tinnitus and deafness have been observed in clients receiving **anticancer drugs** such as nitrogen mustard, 6-aminonicotinamide, and cis-diamminedichloroplatinum. High-frequency hearing loss occurs first and is reversible if the drug is discontinued; otherwise, deafness may ensue. Cis-diamminedichloroplatinum is also nephrotoxic. Industrial chemicals have been implicated in ototoxicity as well. Occupational exposure to **alkylmercurials** can produce Hunter Russell disease, which includes ataxia and hearing loss among its characteristic symptoms. **Organic solvents,** including benzene, ethanol, gasoline, methanol, and propanol, have produced deafness and cochlear lesions (both benzene and methanol are known to cause tinnitus).

A loose connection may exist between **female sex steroids** and ototoxicity. Some females experience a sensation of congestion in the inner ear channels during pregnancy or when using oral contraceptives. Elevation of steroids in these circumstances appears to alter the characteristic of the epithelium of the eustachian tubes. Also, during and after menopause, some females experience vertigo; in addition, an association has been noted between hereditary anovulation and deafness.

Application of drugs to the external ear canal presents a serious risk of ototoxicity if the tympanic membrane is perforated. Ototoxicity by this means has been reported with polymyxin B, chloramphenicol, erythromycin, tetracycline, antiseptics, and local anesthetics. Ear drops should therefore be avoided in clients with perforation of the tympanic membrane or a history of ear surgery.

Hearing loss is common in hypothyroidism. Replacement therapy with thyroid hormones often brings about improvement.

Administration of Otic Medications

Physicians often prescribe ear drops or ointments to treat disorders involving the ear, and nurses are the health care professionals most likely to be called upon to instruct the client in proper methods for instillation.

When drops are prescribed, the nurse should in-

Nursing Diagnoses and Interventions for Drug Therapy for Otitis

Nursing Diagnoses	*Related Interventions*
TO ENHANCE DRUG BENEFITS OR REDUCE DRUG REQUIREMENTS	
Alteration in comfort: pain related to otic infection and otitis	Encourage the client to rest and provide a nonnarcotic analgesic if required.
Impaired social interactions related to difficulty in participating in conversations; Impaired verbal communication related to difficulty understanding others because of impaired hearing; Sensory-perceptual alterations related to hearing impairment; Social isolation related to embarrassment about hearing loss	Consider referral to an audiologist for evaluation and possible hearing aid. Encourage client to explain the hearing limitation to others and to request that they speak louder to accommodate the deficit. Avoid use of ototoxic drugs that can aggravate hearing impairment. Take time to speak slowly and clearly with the client as required by the hearing deficit.
Increased risk of injury related to disturbances of balance and hearing	Provide safety measures as required. Encourage the client to adjust activities appropriately.
TO ENSURE SAFE AND EFFICACIOUS DRUG USE	
Knowledge deficit related to drug regimen	Teach clients about the nature of otitis and the rationale for the treatment regimen. Educate clients about preventive measures such as keeping water from getting in the ears while swimming or showering. Teach clients to avoid irritants that may contribute to otitis such as certain hair sprays, dyes, or industrial chemicals. Teach clients proper use of cotton swabs so as to avoid traumatizing the ear canal. Advise clients not to insert a fingernail or implements into the ear. Warn clients about possible pain during air travel due to reduced ability to adjust air pressure in the auditory canals and sinuses. Teach clients how to properly administer medications to the ear when required. Provide the client with a list of adverse effects and drug interactions for each drug in the regimen and explain what to do if any of these occur.

struct the client to position him or herself with the head tilted to one side so that the affected ear is upward. The auricle should then be drawn back and upward to straighten the acoustic canal. The medication to be administered should be warmed to room or even body temperature but not overheated and dropped into the external acoustic meatus without touching the dropper to the ear. The nurse should then place mild pressure on the tragus to force the fluid forward.

If an ointment is used, the nurse should teach the client to employ a cotton tip, applying the ointment with a twirling motion deep into the external acoustic meatus. The procedure should be carried out with care, and clients cautioned against using the applicator to scratch the external acoustic meatus. To be effective, ear medications should be placed in clean, dry ears.

Drugs Used for Disorders of the Paranasal Sinuses

The paranasal sinuses consist of four pairs of cavities surrounding the nasal passages. The frontal sinuses lie above the eyes, the ethmoid sinuses behind the nasal bridge, the sphenoid sinuses beneath the inner ear canthus, and the large maxillary sinuses adjacent to the nose. Acute sinusitis develops most often in a manner similar to otitis media, as a secondary infection precipitated by acute viral upper respiratory infections. Less commonly, sinusitis is caused by an allergic reaction. The usual microbes implicated in acute sinusitis are streptococci, pneumococci, and staphylococci. Maxillary sinusitis is sometimes caused by spread of dental infections. Most commonly, sinusitis follows occlusion of the ostium of the paranasal sinuses by swelling of the nasal mucosa. With colonization of bacteria and the influx of leukocytes to combat the bacteria, a positive pressure develops, which leads to referred pain that is usually experienced in or around the eye sockets. A frontal headache frequently develops, and rhinorrhea is a common accompanying symptom.

The object of treatment for sinusitis is improved drainage of the infected sinus. A nondrug approach is steam inhalation, which promotes constriction of nasal blood vessels and shrinkage of swollen membranes. Most drug preparations for sinusitis consist of nasal decongestants or combinations of decongestants and antihistamines. The most widely used decongestants are pseudoephedrine (Sudafed, Afrin), phenylpropanolamine, and phenyltoloxamine. Pseudoephedrine is marketed in combination with antihistamines such as dexbrompheniramine (Drixoral), triprolidine (Actifed), and chlorpheniramine (Chlor-Trimeton D). Phenylpropanolamine is found in combination with acetaminophen (Sinaid); acetaminophen and phenyltoloxamine (Sinutab); and calcium carbaspirin, pheniramine, and pyrilamine (Ursinus). The addition of an antihistamine would have value in sinusitis of allergic origin but would have no obvious value in the more common instances of infectious origin. Topical decongestants should not be continued beyond 7 days because of the risk of rebound nasal constriction. Oral decongestants can be used for longer periods of time without the problem of rebound, but lack consistent efficacy.

Systemic antibiotics such as penicillin G and erythromycin are occasionally indicated in acute sinusitis and should be taken for at least 10–12 days. Chronic sinusitis occasionally responds to prolonged courses of antibiotic therapy lasting 4–6 weeks. If it does not, treatment is limited to acute exacerbations, with short courses of broad-spectrum antibiotics such as ampicillin or tetracyclines.

Case Study: Sinusitis

P. B., a 42-year-old female, had a history of recurrent sinusitis. Episodes usually occurred shortly after onset of acute respiratory infections. During an episode, P. B. experienced headache in the region of the forehead, a runny nose, and a feeling of pressure and congestion in the head. She found that these attacks interfered with the mental activities required in her job and decided to discuss the problem with a friend who was a nurse.

The nurse told P. B. that steam inhalation was often helpful in promoting shrinkage of swollen membranes and that nonprescription preparations for sinusitis were available that she could obtain from a pharmacist.

The pharmacist told P. B. that the available preparations generally contain two drugs: one an antihistamine and the other a decongestant. The decongestant would help to drain the sinuses, while the antihistamine might be helpful if the sinusitis was due to an allergic mechanism. The pharmacist recommended a commonly used oral preparation and advised P. B. to seek medical help if the condition persisted.

1. What is sinusitis? What are the usual causes?
2. How rational are the products marketed for sinusitis?
3. If P. B. had selected a decongestant in the form of a nasal spray, what warning should the pharmacist have given her?

Answers appear at the end of the book.

Recommended Readings

Brummett RE: Drug-induced ototoxicity. *Drugs* 1980;19:412–428.

Moran E et al: The use of antihistamine decongestant in conjunction with an anti-infective drug in the treatment of acute otitis media. *J Pediatr* 1982;101(1):132–136.

Parkin JL: Antimicrobial treatment of otitis media: penicillins, cephalosporins, sulfonamides. *Otolaryngology and Head and Neck Surgery* 1981;89:376–380.

Rybak LP: Drug ototoxicity. *Annu Rev Pharmacol Toxicol* 1986;26:79–100.

UNIT XII

Cancer Chemotherapy

CHAPTER 56

Drugs and Malignancies

The Nature of Cancer

The term *cancer* encompasses more than a hundred distinct disease conditions. Cancer is a malignant hyperproliferation of cells, leading to growth of one or more solid cellular masses (called *tumors* or *neoplasms*) or accumulation of one or more types of blood cells. These new and abnormal growths can develop in the lungs, nasopharynx, larynx, mouth, gastrointestinal tract, genitourinary system, liver, breast, bone, brain, spinal cord, epithelium, adrenal gland, thyroid gland, bone marrow, or lymphatic tissue.

A number of terms are used to designate particular types of cancers. *Carcinomas* are cancers of the epithelial cells of mucocutaneous tissue, including tumors of the alimentary tract, genitourinary system, and skin. Specific examples of carcinomas include **choriocarcinomas** arising from the embryonic cells of the testes or ovaries, **basal cell carcinomas** and **squamous cell carcinomas** of the skin, and tumors arising from the melanocytes, called **melanomas. Carcinoid syndrome** results from tumors of the mucosal epithelium, usually in the ileum, which secrete serotonin, prostaglandins, bradykinin, and other autacoids.

Cancers of the bone, muscles, or connective tissue are designated **sarcomas. Leukemias** are malignant diseases of the blood-forming tissues, principally the bone marrow. **Lymphomas** are tumors of the lymphoid tissue, including the lymph nodes and lymphocytes. Hodgkin's disease is an example of a chronic, progressive lymphoma.

Neoplasms can be benign or malignant (cancerous). **Benign tumors** are tissue growths composed of cells that resemble the cells of the tissue from which they derive. Benign neoplasms grow evenly from their center to form a cohesive mass, and they do not spread to other tissues. After surgical removal, benign tumors seldom recur. **Malignant tumors,** by contrast, are composed of atypical cells, with aberrant chromosomes and rapid rates of cell division. They grow irregularly and invade surrounding tissue. They are highly vascularized and may rupture causing hemorrhage. The malignant tumor is characterized by its ability to spread to distant sites; the process referred to as *metastasis*. Malignant cells are disseminated through the body by the lymph and blood. Millions of cells may be shed by a malignant tumor each day. Some will colonize at new sites, adhering initially to endothelial cells of capillaries and ultimately breaking through the blood vessel walls into the interstitial spaces where new tumors can be established.

The incidence and mortality rates for cancers in various tissue locations differ between men and women (Figure 56–1). In men, lung cancer occurs most commonly (22% of all cancers in men), followed by cancer of the prostate (19%), cancer of the colon and rectum (14%), other gastrointestinal cancers (12%), cancers of the urinary tract (9%), leukemias and lymphomas (8%), and oral cancers (4%). In women, breast cancer is most common (26%), followed by cancer of the colon and rectum (16%), lung cancer and cancer of the uterus (11% each), leukemias and lymphomas (7%), ovarian cancer and cancers of the urinary tract (4% each). All told, some 930,000 persons were expected to be newly diagnosed as having cancer in 1986 in the United States. In the 50 years during which cancer statistics have been kept, the death rate of lung cancer has increased tenfold (4–42 deaths per 100,000 population) while the death rates for other forms of cancer have remained level (breast, colon and rectum, prostate cancers) or have dropped dramatically (uterine, stomach, and liver cancers).

The cure rate (5-year survival rate) for cancer is approximately 40–45%, a figure higher than for most chronic diseases. About two-thirds of clients with cancer have tumors that are localized at the time of diagnosis, and for these the cure rate is better than 60%. About one-third of individuals with cancer have tumors that have **metastasized** (spread from the original site) before diagnosis. For these people, the cure rate is only about 12%. Early diagnosis is thus an important factor in survival.

The Etiology of Cancer

The abnormal proliferation of cancer cells appears to be caused by presence of abnormal chromosomes, called **oncogenes.** Many factors contribute to formation of oncogenes: environmental agents, diet, oncogenic viruses, parasitic infections, chronic mechanical or thermal trauma, genetic predisposition, and aging. Environmental agents that promote cancer are termed **carcinogens.** Carcinogens are **mutagens,** or substances that cause mutations (or changes) in DNA, promoting formation of oncogenes. Carcinogenic agents include radiation, ultraviolet light, drugs, industrial chemicals, industrial pollutants, and substances in cigarette smoke. Workers likely to be exposed regularly to **radiation** include miners exposed to radon and radiologists exposed to x-rays. Leukemia, in particular, can be caused by irradiation. Survivors of Hiroshima and Nagasaki, exposed to radiation from the atomic bombs detonated there during World War II, have a high incidence of leukemia. Ultraviolet light from the sun is a major factor in occurrence of skin cancer.

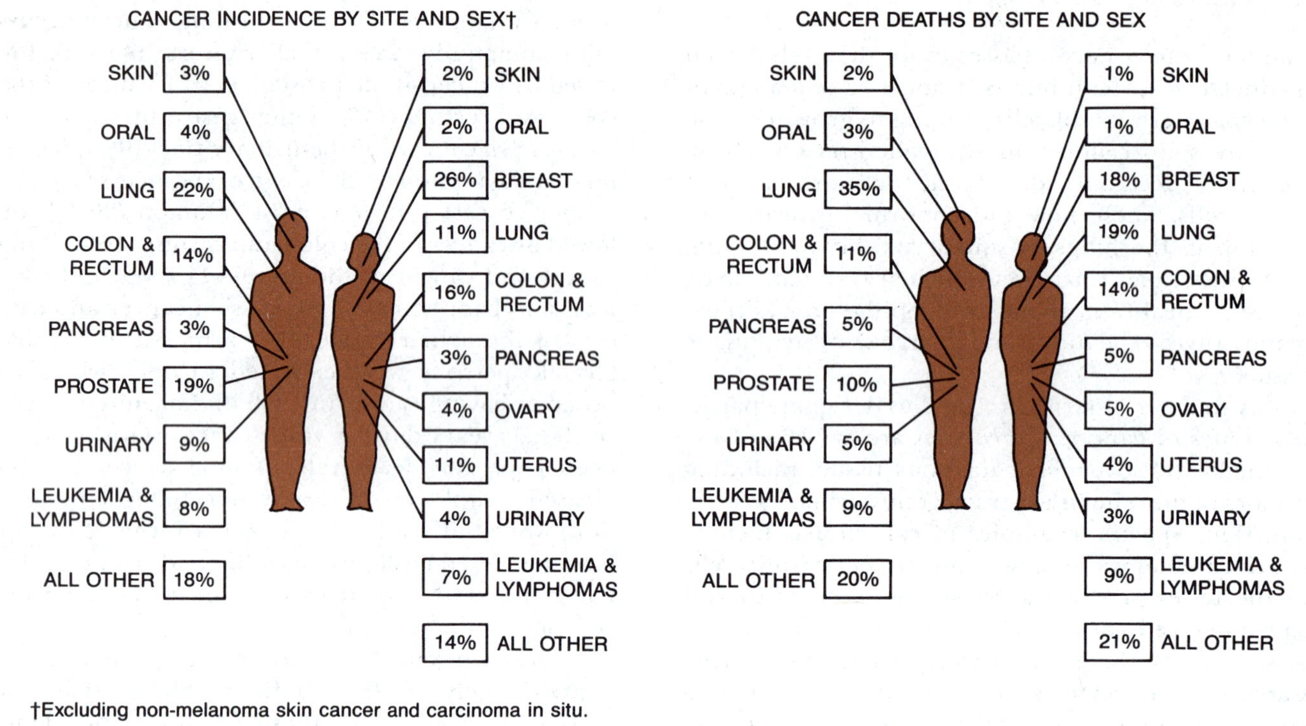

Figure 56–1
Incidence of the various kinds of cancer in males and females. Courtesy of the American Cancer Institute, New York, 1986.

Most drugs with carcinogenic potential are removed from clinical use once the risk is identified. However, griseofulvin, metronidazole, and diethylstilbestrol are important therapeutic agents with limited carcinogenic potential which continue to be used. Many of the drugs used to treat cancer are themselves potentially mutagenic because of their interactions with DNA molecules of tissue cells.

Among the industrial chemicals with identified carcinogenic potential are the polycyclic hydrocarbons, aromatic amines, arsenic, alkylating agents, nitrosamines, nitrosocompounds, benzene, and polyvinyl chloride. Individuals who live in areas of high industrial pollution have a twofold to tenfold increased risk of cancer. Polycyclic hydrocarbons are especially potent carcinogens and are found in cigarette smoke and automobile exhaust. Cigarette smoke contains fifteen identified carcinogens. Some of the environmental chemicals identified as contributing to carcinogenicity are, strictly speaking, precarcinogens rather than carcinogens, being converted in the body to the ultimate carcinogen.

The links between diet and cancer are not well established except as related to alcohol and nitrites. Alcohol ingestion increases risks of cancers of the mouth, pharynx, larynx, and esophagus, probably as a result of chemical irritation of the mucosal membranes of these tissues. Nitrites, commonly found as food additives, are converted in the body to nitrosocompounds that are carcinogenic. Aflatoxin B, a mold found on corn, peas, rice, barley, soybeans, fruits, nuts, milk, and cheddar cheese, has been linked with liver cancer in humans. Betel nuts have been linked to cancers of the mouth. Diets low in fiber tend to increase risk of cancer of the colon while diets rich in foods that are salted or smoked increase risk of stomach cancer. Other connections between diet and cancer are at best tenuous.

There is a strong relationship between viral infections and a few forms of cancer, including the link between Epstein-Barr virus and occurrence of Burkitt's lymphoma and carcinoma of the nasopharynx. Some viruses, called **retroviruses,** have been shown to promote formation of oncogenes. Often there is a long latency period between initial viral infection and the neoplastic transformation that results in hyperplasia.

Habits relating to sexuality can influence occurrence of cancer of the cervix. Women who begin sexual activity at a young age and who have multiple partners are at greater risk of cervical cancer. Breast cancer is more common in women who have early menarche, late menopause, and those who do not have children. The **genetic influence** on susceptibility to cancer is not great and there is no significant population of people that is free of risk, but some kinds of tumors (such as breast and colon tumors) tend to run in families.

Clinical Manifestations

In the early stage of development of a tumor, clinical symptoms may be absent. The tumor may simply not be large enough to interfere with bodily functions. This is especially likely if the tumor is in a region of the body where there is space and distensibility. A small tumor in the abdomen is likely to be asymptomatic whereas a tumor of similar size within the cranium might produce severe dysfunction.

As a tumor continues to grow, local symptoms develop as a result of (1) interference with blood flow, (2) interference with tissue function, and (3) activation of immunologic and inflammatory responses. Pressure exerted by the tumor against blood vessels tends to reduce tissue perfusion, depriving the tissue of oxygen and nutrients and allowing accumulation of metabolic wastes. Blood vessels may become eroded by local accumulation of lactic acid, leading to bleeding. Tissue ischemia and necrosis may occur.

Soft tissue such as the lungs or colon are especially prone to disturbances of function caused by tissue compression as a tumor expands. Bronchial compression may cause atelectasis. Bowel tumors may cause obstruction of the bowel. Bowel compression results in constipation and compensatory hyperperistalsis, leading to painful cramps. Pressure against nerves or nerve terminals may cause continuous pain. Sensations of pain that are continuous or gradually intensifying are hallmarks of neoplasms. Immunologic and inflammatory activity against the tumor may result in inflammatory irritation of the tissue to which the tumor is fixed.

Systemic manifestations of cancer are varied. In clients with leukemias and lymphomas, the demands placed on the metabolic resources of the body by the proliferative activity may result in fatigue and lethargy. Symptoms not caused directly by the tumor or metastatic neoplasms are called **paraneoplastic symptoms.** Among the first systemic symptoms are nausea, anorexia, weight loss, and general malaise. Later symptoms can be neurologic (ataxia, dementia, muscle weakness, spasticity, hyperreflexia or areflexia, sensory loss, altered taste sensitivity, paralysis), hematologic (anemia, coagulation defects), gastrointestinal (malabsorption, liver dysfunction, obstruction), or metabolic (lactic acidosis, hyperlipidemia). Endocrine tumors, whether attached to an endocrine gland or metastatic, produce distinctive systemic symptoms. Thus, lung tumors may be ACTH-secreting and resulting in Cushing's syndrome; calcitonin-secreting thyroid tumors may cause hypocalcemia, and parathyroid-secreting parathyroid tumors may produce hypercalcemia; intestinal carcinomas may secrete serotonin and histamine to cause carcinoid syndrome; and adrenal-like tumors may secrete adrenal medullary hormones to cause pheochromocytoma.

Treatment of Malignant Neoplasms

The three types of treatment for cancer are surgery, radiation therapy, and chemotherapy. Surgery is the usual treatment for cancers that have not metastasized at the time of diagnosis. For example, of the half-million cases of localized cancer diagnosed in 1980, 212,000 were cured by surgery alone, 90,000 with a combination of surgery and radiation, and 12,000 with surgery and chemotherapy. Surgery is of little use in the one-third of new cases of cancer in which metastasis has already occurred by the time of diagnosis.

Radiation can be administered either as x-rays or in radioactive drugs. The usefulness of x-ray therapy, like that of surgery, is limited to localized cancer. Drugs are important in radiation therapy either as the source of radiation (radioisotopes) or as adjuncts to x-ray therapy (radiosensitizers or radioprotectors).

Chemotherapy is the most important form of therapy when metastasis of a cancer has already begun. Since these are also the clients with the poorest prognosis, chemotherapy is generally associated with lower success rates than surgery or radiation. The antineoplastic agents currently available can be grouped into six broad categories: (1) alkylating agents, (2) antimetabolites, (3) vinca alkaloids, (4) cytotoxic antibiotics, (5) hormones and hormone antagonists, and (6) a miscellaneous group that includes L-asparaginase, platinum complexes, hydroxyurea, mitotane, and procarbazine. A spin-off of cancer research has been the development of useful immunosuppressives that are drugs of the alkylating or antimetabolite categories. The most widely used immunosuppressive, azathioprine, is discussed in Chapter 50. It is an antimetabolite agent related to methotrexate. Although not yet available for clinical use, immunomodulators such as interferons and interleukins are likely to play an important role in cancer chemotherapy in the future.

Interleukin-2 and Lymphokine-activated killer cells

A novel approach to the treatment of cancer currently undergoing clinical investigation is the administration of interleukin-2 and lymphokine-activated killer (LAK) cells. Interleukin-2, one of the lymphokines released by sensitized T lymphocytes during immunological reactions, promotes formation of LAK cells and stimulates their activity. LAK cells can attack and destroy malignant cells (but not normal cells) and in healthy individuals help to prevent malignant cells from developing into established tumors.

Recombinant DNA technology has recently made possible the production of interleukin-2 in large quantities. This has opened the way for clinical trials using interleukin-2 for renal cell carcinomas, melanomas, and, colon cancer. However, only certain patients are eligible for such trials. They must have normal white blood cell counts, hemoglobin and hematocrit values, an absence of infections, no other cancers (except skin cancer), and uncompromised renal, cardiac, or respiratory function. The primary neoplastic disorder for which the interleukin is given must be progressive, clinically measurable, and nonresponsive to standard treatments.

Interleukin-2 is usually coadministered with LAK cells by the following procedure. Interleukin-2 is initially given to patients intravenously every eight hours for three days. Twenty-four to thirty-six hours after the last dose, LAK cells that have been produced in the person as a result of interleukin-2 stimulation are removed from the blood by a filtering process called leukopheresis. The LAK cells removed from the patient are then incubated for three days with interleukin-2 to increase their number. The newly generated LAK cells are then infused into the patient through a central venous catheter along with interleukin-2. The concurrent administration of LAK cells with interleukin-2 greatly increases its antineoplastic efficacy. Tumor regression has already been demonstrated with this therapy, but the full extent of benefits or problems is yet to be established.

Side effects of interleukin-2 are quite diverse. Fever and chills, headache, and nausea are most common. Meperidine (Demerol) may be required to manage chills, prochlorperazine (Compazine) for nausea, and acetominophen for headache and fever. Pancytopenia, anemia, or thrombocytopenia may occur. Another potential problem is capillary-permeability-leak syndrome, which can result in hypovolemia, vasodilation, hypotension, and potentially dangerous pulmonary edema.

The optimum route for administration of interleukin-2 is not yet known. It has been given by IV infusion, IV bolus, subcutaneous injection, peritoneal infusion, and intrahepatic infusion.

Principles of Cancer Chemotherapy

In the last two decades, cancer chemotherapy has come into its own as an alternative or adjunct to surgery and radiation. No drugs yet available are truly selective for malignant cells. All antineoplastic agents exert substantial toxicity on normal tissue cells. In comparison with antimicrobial chemotherapy, cancer chemotherapy less frequently provides true cures, is less selective for pathogenic versus normal cells, has a narrow margin of safety, requires prolonged treatment, and more often induces drug resistance. Neoplastic cells are more similar to normal host cells than are microbial cells, so that finding agents that are selectively toxic against malignant cells is difficult. In spite of these shortcomings, chemotherapy can sometimes cure some forms of cancer, including choriocarcinoma, acute lymphocytic leukemia in children, Hodgkin's disease, diffuse histiocytic lymphoma, nodular mixed lymphoma, testicular carcinoma, ovarian carcinoma, acute myelogenous leukemia, Wilm's tumor, Burkitt's lymphoma, embryonal rhabdomyosarcoma, and Ewing's sarcoma.

Cell Proliferation and Cytotoxicity of Antineoplastic Drugs

Antineoplastic drugs work by inhibiting cell proliferation. These drugs are selective only to the extent that they are more toxic to cell groups that are proliferating rapidly. Tumors with a large **growth fraction** (a large proportion of cells engaged in cell division) are most susceptible to antineoplastic agents. Young tumors have a high growth fraction and are therefore susceptible to chemotherapy, another reason to try to achieve early diagnosis. Cures can often be effected when therapy begins while a tumor is young. Older tumors, with a relatively low growth fraction, seldom respond adequately to chemotherapy. Lymphomas and lymphocytic leukemias have very high growth fractions, melanomas and carcinomas of the colon have moderate growth fractions, and breast cancers have a low growth fraction.

Adverse effects of antineoplastic agents are determined by the same principle. Tissues with high rates of cell proliferation are the most susceptible to toxic effects of anticancer drugs. Normal tissues with a high rate of proliferation include the bone marrow, the hair follicles, and the mucosal membranes of the alimentary tract, from the mouth to the rectum. The resulting adverse effects are leukopenia, alopecia, and ulcerative lesions with nausea and vomiting. These are adverse effects shared by all antineoplastic agents.

The cycle of cell division provides the basis for categorizing the mechanisms of anticancer drugs. Cell growth occurs in five phases (Figure 56–2): (1) the resting state (G0), (2) the postmitotic gap, during which the building blocks of DNA are synthesized (G1), (3) the synthetic phase, the synthesis of DNA itself (S), (4) the premitotic gap, the preparation of the mitotic spindle (G2), and (5) mitosis, or cell division (M). Cells are most vulnerable to the action of antineoplastic drugs during the two active phases, the synthetic phase and mitosis. Most antineoplastic agents can act only on cells that are in a specific stage in their cycle. Such drugs are termed **cell-cycle specific.** Antimetabolites and cytotoxic antibiotics act only on cells in the synthetic phase, whereas vinca alkaloids act only on cells in the mitotic phase. Alkylating agents and cisplatin, by contrast, are **cell-cycle nonspecific;** they can act on the cell during any phase. Their toxic effects do not become apparent, however, until the cell enters into the active phases of the cell cycle.

Acquired Tumor Resistance

The objective of cancer chemotherapy is the eradication of all malignant cells, **total cell-kill.** Anything short of total cell-kill cannot be considered a clinical cure because a single surviving malignant cell can ultimately multiply sufficiently to kill the host. The immune system cannot be depended upon to complete the task of total eradication as it can in the case of antimicrobial chemotherapy. For one thing, tumor cells are more likely to escape the notice of the host defense mechanisms because of their derivation from normal host cells. For another, the integrity of the immune system may itself be compromised by the use of antineoplastic agents.

Tumor cells have a greater capacity to develop drug resistance than microbial cells. Anything less than total cell-kill promotes development of resistance as the hardy survivors proliferate selectively. Tumor resistance can develop to any of the available antineoplastic agents, and there is no way at present to ensure the success of cancer chemotherapy in a given instance.

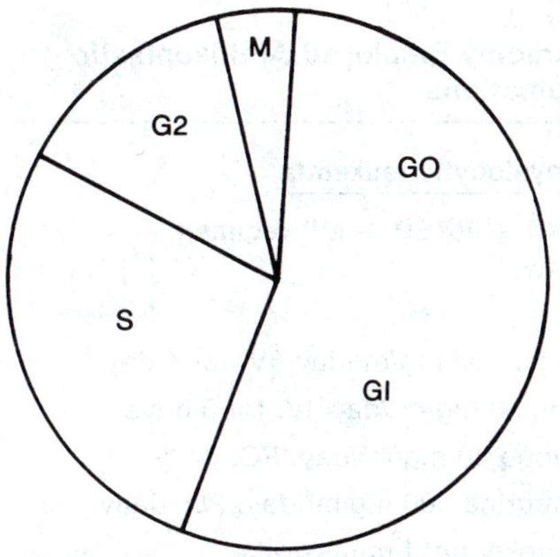

Figure 56–2
The cell cycle resting state (GO); postmitotic gap (GI); synthetic phase (S); premitotic gap (G2); mitosis (M).

Tumor resistance can be due to any of several mechanisms. Some tumor cells exhibit **cytokinetic resistance** because they are proliferating slowly. Tumors develop **schedule resistance** to some antineoplastic drugs when they are used too infrequently. Efficacy of hydroxyurea, cytarabine, and bleomycin is seriously compromised if the drugs are given intermittently instead of frequently or by continuous infusion. A brain tumor may exhibit drug resistance because it is located in a kind of **pharmacokinetic sanctuary** within the blood-brain barrier.

All of these examples of resistance are inherent characteristics of certain tumors in relation to certain drugs. Tumor cells may also develop **acquired resistance,** biochemical changes that improve the cells' ability to withstand the action of a drug. Sometimes tumor cells enhance cellular activities involved in repair of damaged DNA. Other times, tumor cells will reduce their uptake of an antineoplastic agent. Some tumor cells synthesize substances that provide alternate binding sites for the drug or develop alternate metabolic pathways when antimetabolite drugs are employed. A successful drug regimen must preclude the development of tumor resistance.

Use of Combination Regimens for Cancer

One tactic for minimizing resistance development is the use of multidrug regimens. Combinations are advantageous only if the drugs chosen act by different mechanisms on different phases of the cell cycle. Drugs used in combinations are occasionally given in alternating short courses rather than concurrently, which appears to further retard acquisition of resistance. Examples of widely used combination regimens are described in Table 56–1.

Table 56–1
Some Commonly Employed Antineoplastic Drug Combinations

For acute myelocytic leukemia

Ara-C + DNR + PRED + MP regimen (Children only)

Induction

- Daunorubicin 25 mg/m^2/day, IV, for 1 day
- Cytarabine 80 mg/m^2/day, IV, for 3 days
- Prednisolone 40 mg/m^2/day, PO, daily
- Mercaptopurine 100 mg/m^2/day, PO, daily
- Repeat weekly until remission

Maintenance

- Daunorubicin 25 mg/m^2/day, IV, for 1 day
- Cytarabine 80 mg/m^2/day, IV, for 3 days
- Prednisolone 40 mg/m^2/day, PO, daily
- Mercaptopurine 100 mg/m^2/day, PO, daily
- Repeat every month or 28 days

Ara-C + 6-TG regimen

Induction

- Cytarabine 100 mg/m^2/every 12 hours, IV, for 10 days
- Thioguanine 100 mg/m^2/every 12 hours, PO, for 10 days
- Repeat every 30 days until remission

Maintenance

- Cytarabine 100 mg/m^2/every 12 hours, IV, for 5 days
- Thioguanine 100 mg/m^2/every 12 hours, PO, for 5 days
- Repeat every month

For acute lymphocytic leukemia, induction therapy

VP regimen

Vincristine 2.0 mg/m^2, IV, once weekly for 4–6 weeks

Prednisone 60 mg/m^2/day, PO, in divided doses for 4 weeks; taper weeks 5–7; or 2.2 mg/kg, PO, days 1–28

For breast cancer

CAF regimen

Cyclophosphamide 100 mg/m^2/day, PO, days 1–14

Doxorubicin 30 mg/m^2/day, IV, days 1 and 8

Fluorouracil 400 mg/m^2/day, IV, days 1 and 8

Repeat every 4 weeks to maximum of 450 mg/m^2 of doxorubicin, then substitute methotrexate, 40 mg/m^2, IV, for doxorubicin and increase fluorouracil to 600 mg/m^2/day, IV

cAMP regimen

Cyclophosphamide 300 mg/m^2/day, IV, days 1 and 8

Doxorubicin 20 mg/m^2/day, IV, days 1 and 8

Methotrexate 15 mg/m^2/day, IV, days 1 and 8

Procarbazine 100 mg/m^2/day, PO, days 1–10

Repeat every 28 days

CMFP regimen

Cyclophosphamide 100 mg/m^2/day, PO, days 1–14

Methotrexate 60 mg/m^2/day, IV, days 1 and 8

CMFP regimen (*continued*)

Fluorouracil 700 mg/m^2/day, IV, days 1 and 8

Prednisone 40 mg/m^2/day, PO, days 1–14

Repeat every 28 days

For disseminated testicular cancer

VBP regimen

Vinblastine 0.2 mg/kg/day, IV, days 1 and 2 (every 3 weeks, 5 times)

Cisplatin 20 mg/m^2/day, IV infusion over 15 minutes beginning 6 hours after vinblastine, day 1–5 (every 3 weeks, 3 times)

Bleomycin 30 units/wk, IV, 6 hours after vinblastine on day 2 of each week for 12 weeks up to a total dose of 360 units

For chronic lymphocytic leukemia

CHL + PRED regimen

Chlorambucil 0.4 mg/kg/day, PO, for 1 day every other week

Prednisone 100 mg/day, PO, for 2 days every other week

For Hodgkin's disease, induction

MOPP regimen

Mechlorethamine 6 mg/m^2/day, IV, days 1 and 8

Vincristine 1.4 or 2 mg/m^2/day, IV, days 1 and 8 (max. 2.0 mg)

Procarbazine 100 mg/m^2/day, PO, days 1–14

Prednisone 40 mg/m^2/day, PO, days 1–14

Repeat every 4 weeks for 6 cycles

For lung cancer

cAMP regimen

Cyclophosphamide 200 mg/m^2/day, IV, days 1 and 8

Doxorubicin 20 mg/m^2/day, IV, days 1 and 8

Methotrexate 15 mg/m^2/day, IV, days 1 and 8

Procarbazine 100 mg/m^2/day, PO, days 1–10

Repeat every 4 weeks

MACC regimen

Methotrexate 40 mg/m^2/day, IV, day 1

Doxorubicin 40 mg/m^2/day, IV, day 1

Cyclophosphamide 400 mg/m^2/day, IV, day 1

Lomustine 30 mg/m^2/day, PO, day 1

Repeat every 3 weeks

POCC regimen

Procarbazine 100 mg/m^2/day, PO, days 1–14

Vincristine 2.0 mg/m^2/day, IV, days 1 and 8 (max. 2.0 mg)

Cyclophosphamide 600 mg/m^2/day, IV, days 1 and 8

Lomustine 60 mg/m^2, PO, day 1

Repeat every 4 weeks

Table 56–1
Some Commonly Employed Antineoplastic Drug Combinations (*continued*)

For multiple myeloma

M-2 protocol

Vincristine 0.03 mg/kg/day, IV, day 1 (max. 2.0 mg)

Carmustine 0.5 mg/kg/day, IV, day 1

Cyclophosphamide 10 mg/kg/day, IV, day 1

Melphalan 0.25 mg/kg/day, PO, days 1–4

Prednisone 1.0 mg/kg/day, PO, days 1–7; then taper to day 21

Repeat every 5 weeks until progression of the disease

For non-Hodgkin's lymphomas

CVP regimen

Cyclophosphamide 400 mg/m²/day, PO, days 2–6

CVP regimen (*continued*)

Vincristine 1.4 mg/m², IV, day 1 (max 2.0 mg)

Prednisone 100 mg/m²/day, PO, days 2–6

Repeat every 3 weeks for 6 cycles

For urinary tract carcinomas

CISCA regimen

Cyclophosphamide 650 mg/m²/day, IV, day 1

Doxorubicin 50 mg/m²/day, IV, day 1

Cisplatin 100 mg/m²/day, IV infusion over 2 hours, day 2

Repeat every 3 weeks. Discontinue doxorubicin when total dose reaches 450 mg/m² and increase cyclophosphamide to 1,000 mg/m², IV

Shared Adverse Effects of Antineoplastic Drugs

As we indicated earlier, antineoplastic drugs produce toxic effects most readily in tissues that are dividing rapidly. Thus the bone marrow, the epithelial cells of the alimentary tract, and the hair follicles are among the tissues most frequently damaged by anticancer drugs.

Bone Marrow Suppression

Most of the antineoplastic agents produce bone marrow suppression, but they vary in the extent of this effect and in their relative influence on the production of granulocytes, thrombocytes, red blood cells, and lymphocytes. For example, both mechlorethamine and cyclophosphamide sharply suppress granulocytes, but cyclophosphamide has much less effect than mechlorethamine on platelets. The drugs also vary in how rapidly the bone marrow suppression develops and how long it persists (Table 56–2). *The nurse needs to be aware of the likely time course of bone marrow suppression in order to provide accurate information to the client. Also, before treatment, the nurse should obtain complete blood cell information on the client to provide a basis for later evaluation of treatment response.*

When short courses of antineoplastic agents are employed, increased susceptibility to infection generally persists only for as long as the drug is being given. Even though the white blood cell (WBC) count may be depressed for a period after the last drug treatment, the antigen-stimulated rise in WBCs occurs normally during the posttreatment period of leukopenia. During short treatment courses and for extended periods of chronic treatment, susceptibility to infection presents a major difficulty. *The nurse should advise clients who are receiving antineoplastic agents to avoid contact with infected individuals and should educate family members concerning this need for relative isolation. It is also important to protect the client from stress and trauma, situations that place added demands on the impaired defense mechanisms. Sore throat, fever, chills, or respiratory infection should be reported to the physician immediately. The skin and mucous membranes should be examined for signs of overgrowth by infectious organisms because drug-induced leukopenia can activate latent infections such as herpes zoster or candidiasis.*

If the drug is one that can cause thrombocytopenia, the nurse should monitor the client regularly for signs of occult bleeding and enlist the aid of the client and significant family members in the effort. Common signs of bleeding include petechiae, ecchymoses, tarry stools, blood in the vomitus, easy bruising, or bleeding of the gums or nose. Fatigue and pallor may indicate anemia resulting from myelosuppression.

Epithelial Ulcerations

The cells of the mucosal epithelium are particularly vulnerable to the cytotoxic effects of antineoplastic agents because of their rapid rate of turnover. Nausea and vomiting are commonplace responses to anticancer drugs and stomatitis, gastrointestinal bleeding, ulcerations, and desquamation are not uncommon.

Nausea may be so severe that clients may refuse further treatment, especially when cisplatin is employed. Even when nausea is bearable, it may undermine nutritional status by causing distaste for food, anorexia, and loss of nutrients from frequent vomiting. *When possible, drug administration should be scheduled so that mealtimes and peak periods of nausea do not coincide. Meals can be rescheduled if necessary. Frequent small meals may be better tolerated than three normal meals. Cold foods may be better tolerated than hot foods. Breakfast*

Table 56–2
Severity and Time Course of Leukopenia Caused by Antineoplastics

Drug	Severity	Onset (days)	Maximum (days)	Recovery (days)
Alkylating agents				
Nitrogen mustards				
Mechlorethamine	+++	4-8	10	14-28
Cyclophosphamide	+++	7-10	10-14	21
Chlorambucil	+++	7-14	10-28	42
Melphalan	+++	7-14	10-21	28-42
Uracil mustard	+++	7	14-28	28-42
Nitrosureas				
Lomustine	++++	14-35	21-49	42-56
Carmustine	++++	14-35	21-49	35-56
Streptozocin	+	7	14	21
Triazenes				
Dacarbazine	++	7-10	10-14	21-24
Alkyl sulfonates				
Busulfan	++++	7-10	14-28	28-56
Ethylenimines				
Thiotepa	+++	10-14	14-21	28-49
Antimetabolites				
Folate antagonists				
Methotrexate	+++	4-7	10-14	14-21
Pyrimidine analogues				
Fluorouracil	+++	7-10	9-14	16-30
Cytarabine	++++	4-7	7-18	21
Purine analogues				
Mercaptopurine	++	7-10	10-14	21-28
Cytotoxic antibiotics				
Dactinomycin	++++	7-10	14	21-28
Doxorubicin	++++	10	14	21-24
Bleomycin	+	4-7	10	14-18
Mithramycin	+++	7-10	14	21-28
Mitomycin	++++	10-21	21-36	42-56
Vinca alkaloids				
Vinblastine	+++	4-7	10	17-21
Vincristine	+	4-7	10	17-21
Miscellaneous				
Cisplastin	++	7-10	14-21	21-35
Hydroxyurea	+++	4	7	10-14
Procarbazine	+++	10-14	14-21	21-28
Etoposide	++	4-10	8-16	21

Key: +, least severe, ++++, most severe.

may be the best tolerated meal of the day. The nurse should consult with a dietician if necessary and advise the client's family as to how to help the client maintain nutrition. Dietary preferences of the client should be catered to in order to improve appetite. Presentation of food in an appealing, attractive layout can have a positive effect on appetite. Dietary supplements may be required if adequate nutrition cannot be achieved through food sources alone.

Prolonged vomiting, especially if accompanied by diarrhea, may cause fluid and electrolyte problems as well as poor nutrition. *The nurse should look for indications of dehydration such as poor skin turgor, a dry or shrunken tongue, weakness, postural hypotension, decreased urine output, or confusion. Indications of dehydration should be reported to the physician.*

Antinausea drugs may be helpful in controlling nausea and vomiting. Chlorpromazine or prochlorperazine can be employed for this purpose. Tetrahydrocannabinol (the active chemical in marihuana) was available from the National Cancer Institute for a number of years for treatment of nausea and vomiting associated with cancer chemotherapy that is refractory to other drugs. In 1985 it became commercially available under the name of dronabinol (Marinol) in 2.5 mg, 5 mg, and 10 mg liquid capsules. The recommended initial dose is 5 mg/m^2, 1–3 hours prior to chemotherapy, repeated every 2–4 hours up to 4–6 doses/day. The maximum recommended dose is 15 mg/m^2/dose.

Oral hygiene should be meticulous during cancer chemotherapy to minimize risk of oral lesions, superinfection, and demineralization of teeth caused by deficient salivation. *Oral membranes should be kept hydrated by frequent rinsing. A saliva substitute such as Xero-Lube or Moi-stir can be employed to relieve dry mouth. Teeth should be flossed and brushed with a soft-bristled brush after every meal as long as platelet count is above 15,000. Flossing should be discontinued if platelet counts fall below 15,000 and brushing as well if platelet count drops below 10,000. When platelet counts are too low to permit brushing and flossing, oral hygiene can be maintained with a cotton swab and a gentle stream of warm water. If ulceration does occur in the oral membranes, foods that are hot, cold, sour, spicy, or gritty should be avoided. Use of tobacco and alcohol beverages should be discouraged. A lip balm or petrolatum should be used to relieve cracked lips. An anesthetic solution can be swished in the mouth just prior to meals to reduce sensitivity to irritation.*

Other Shared Adverse Effects

Three other adverse effects that occur with many of the antineoplastic agents are **alopecia** (loss of hair), **vesication** (blistering), and **inhibition of spermatogenesis**. Some of the anticancer drugs also cause **amenorrhea** in female clients. *Clients should be warned that antifertility effects of antineoplastic agents may be long-lasting and frequently irreversible.* Most antineoplastic agents are teratogenic. *Nurses should encourage female clients to use an effective contraceptive measure during treatment with antineoplastic agents, and for several months thereafter.*

Alopecia is almost always reversible. The nurse should keep in mind that for many individuals, hair is an important element in self-image and feelings of sexual attractiveness. In addition, some clients may develop changes in skin color. *Clients should be encouraged to seek cosmetic remedies if alopecia or skin changes are an important personal concern.*

Many of the antineoplastic agents have vesicant (blister-producing) properties (Table 56–3). To avoid serious local reactions, nurses must exercise utmost care not to contact the drug or its vapors and to avoid extravasation of the drug during injection. Contact with the skin or other tissue before the drug has been diluted by dispersion through the body fluids can result in blistering, pain, and tissue necrosis. Guidelines relating to the vesicant properties of antineoplastic drugs are provided in Table 56–3.

Antineoplastic agents that cause rapid cytolysis of malignant cells or white blood cells can produce **hyperuricemia** from breakdown of cell constituents. Joint and flank pain may result. It may be necessary to institute therapy with allopurinol or a uricosuric agent, such as probenecid (Benemid). Some antineoplastic agents require dosage adjustment if probenecid is given concurrently.

Although hepatic, renal, and pulmonary side effects are not as widely shared by antineoplastic drugs as bone marrow suppression, gastrointestinal irritation, and alopecia, each can occur in response to several of the available antineoplastic agents. **Hepatic toxicity** is especially likely with methotrexate, mercaptopurine, and azathioprine. Dacarbazine, doxorubicin, carmustine, and lomustine are also significantly hepatotoxic. **Renal toxicity** is most often caused by cyclophosphamide, cisplatin, streptozocin, and methotrexate. **Pulmonary toxicity** occurs most readily in response to cyclophosphamide, busulfan, methotrexate, and bleomycin. **Cardiotoxicity** occurs mainly when doxorubicin or daunorubicin are used. **Neurotoxic effects** are most likely when the regimen includes vincristine, vinblastine, procarbazine, L-asparaginase, fluorouracil, methotrexate, or cytarabine.

Special Hazards of Anticancer Drugs to Health Care Professionals

While most nurses recognize that anticancer drugs are toxic to healthy cells, they rarely consider these dangers as they relate to themselves. The toxicity of antineoplastic agents includes carcinogenicity and

Table 56-3
Guidelines Related to the Vesicant Properties of Antineoplastic Agents

Antineoplastic agents with vesicant properties	Recommended antidotes if extravasation occurs
Carmustine	Sodium bicarbonate 8.4%
Dactinomycin	Sodium thiosulfate 10% or ascorbic acid 50 mg/ml
Daunorubicin	Sodium bicarbonate 8.4% and dexamethazone
Doxorubicin	Sodium bicarbonate 8.4% and dexamethazone
Mechlorethamine	Sodium thiosulfate 10%
Mithramycin	EDTA 150 mg/ml
Mitomycin C	Sodium thiosulfate 10% or ascorbic acid 50 mg/ml
Vinblastine	Sodium bicarbonate 8.4% or heat and hyaluronidase
Vincristine	Heat and hyaluronidase

Guidelines

1. Exercise utmost care not to contact the drug or its vapors. Wear rubber gloves during preparation and administration of the drug. Any areas of skin accidentally exposed to a vesicant drug should be immediately washed with an appropriate antidote (listed above). If the drug or its vapors come into contact with the eyes, flush them immediately with ample quantities of normal saline.

2. Dilute the drug with the proper amount of diluent. Do not use vesicant drugs at higher than recommended concentrations. If more than one antineoplastic drug is being given, inject nonvesicant agents first.

3. Select an appropriate infusion site. The forearm is best, followed in order of preference by the dorsum of the hand, the wrist, and the antecubital fossa.

4. Employ a double syringe technique to minimize vesicant effects at the site of injection. Discard the needle used to withdraw the drug from the container. Insert a 20–23 gauge butterfly needle into the selected vein. Tape the tubing distal to the needle so that the injection site is not obscured.

5. Before giving the drug, inject 5 ml of saline and then withdraw a small amount of blood to test the integrity of the site. Observe for any signs of extravasation. If extravasation occurs, select a new site (but not a distal point on the same vein).

6. When a patent site has been established, inject the vesicant drug slowly over at least 3 minutes at about 5 ml/min. Pause by drawing back on the plunger after each milliliter of drug solution and ask the patient if pain or burning is present along the vein. When the injection is completed, flush out the drug remaining in the tubing with 5–10 ml of saline.

7. Alternatively, vesicant drugs may be injected into a free-running saline infusion to minimize risks of extravasation.

8. If extravasation occurs during injection of a vesicant drug, stop the injection immediately, leaving the needle in place. Withdraw 3-5 ml of blood and solution if possible, administer 25 mg of cortisone, and remove the needle.

9. With a 27-gauge tuberculin syringe, remove as much extravasated fluid as possible from around the injection site. Administer the appropriate antidote (listed above) into the area of extravasation in 4–5 injections.

10. Apply 1 hour of cold compresses (to allow the antidote to act), followed by 1 hour of warm compresses.

11. Reexamine the site several times at appropriate time intervals (weekly for most vesicants but sooner with mechlorethamine), observing for inflammation or necrosis.

mutagenicity. Research shows that repeated handling of parenteral neoplastic agents is a health threat. Chromosomal damage has been noted in cells in the urine of nurses who have been preparing and administering drugs for only a few days. Nurses who have not used adequate protection when handling antineoplastic drugs have reported incidence of lightheadedness, dizziness, hair loss, nausea, and nasal and mucosal sores.

How hazardous the drug is depends on several factors. The chemical properties of the drug may make it more or less toxic. Alkylating agents are generally more toxic than antimetabolites: thiotepa is more toxic than methotrexate. The individual's susceptibility is a factor. Dietary habits and smoking may increase susceptibility. The amount and duration of exposure are also important factors, as well as the type of exposure.

Exposure can occur in any number of ways. Breaking a vial or ampul may produce droplets of spray which are then inhaled, absorbed through the skin or mucous membranes, or splattered onto glasses or cups used for drinking. One line of defense is to assure that eating and drinking utensils are not nearby when preparing these medications. Leaky syringes, stopcocks, or tubing connections are another potential source of contamination. Vomitus, urine, or fecal material from a patient receiving antineoplastic drugs may be contaminated.

There are additional methods nurses should take to minimize exposure. Avoid preparing antineoplastic drugs if possible. The hospital pharmacy, with a vertical laminar airflow hood, is the appropriate place for drug preparation. If the nurse must prepare these drugs, he or she should make certain to receive proper training. A nurse who is pregnant, breast-feeding, or attempting to become pregnant should not prepare or administer parenteral antineoplastic drugs.

Preparation of these medications should be done under a vertical laminar flow hood or, if this is not available, in a work area away from heating and cooling vents and other people. The work area should be covered with a disposable plastic liner. The nurse should wear gloves made of latex. (Gloves made of polyvinyl chloride are permeable to some cytotoxic drugs.) The nurse should wash his or her hands both before and after removing the gloves. The nurse should also wear a disposable, nonpermeable surgical gown with a closed front and knit cuffs that completely cover the wrists.

Syringes and intravenous equipment should have Luer-Lok fittings and be disposable. Priming of IV sets requires special care. Before withdrawing the reconstituted drug from a vial, the vial should be vented to lower internal pressure and thus to reduce the risk of spilling or spraying when the needle is removed from the diaphragm of the vial. When the nurse withdraws the drug from the vial, a sterile alcohol wipe should be used around the needle and vial top. When expelling air bubbles from the syringe, a sterile alcohol wipe should be placed around the needle. When the top of a glass ampul is to be broken, the neck of the ampul should be wrapped with a sterile alcohol wipe to prevent spraying and to protect fingers from cuts and lacerations.

Once drugs have been prepared, the external surfaces of the syringes and IV bottles should also be wiped with an alcohol sponge. Disposable equipment should be placed in separate disposable plastic bags for incineration and labeled "chemotherapy."

Nurses should also wear latex gloves when disposing of urine, vomitus, or feces from patients receiving cytotoxic drugs. For outpatients, it is just as important for those providing care in the home to be taught protective measures before undertaking disposal of vomitus or feces. In cleaning a client following episodes of vomiting or diarrhea, the nurse or other attendant should wear gloves.

If any solution gets on the hands or skin, the nurse (or care provider in the home) should wash the hands thoroughly with soap and water. If the drug gets into the eyes, the nurse should flush with copious amounts of isotonic saline eyewash (or water, if saline is not immediately available). The incident should be recorded and reported to the health department and medical attention sought immediately. The identity of the drug and type and duration of exposure should be documented.

Clients' Anxieties about Cancer and Chemotherapy

Clients about to begin chemotherapy must deal with anxiety concerning the therapy itself as well as the disease to be treated. Nurses who are responsible for teaching clients about the particular malignancy and the chemotherapy need to remember that anxiety tends to interfere with the clients' ability to absorb information. Nurses will often need to explain repeatedly the rationale for therapy and encourage the client by pointing out that the drug is efficacious. The nurse needs to explore the clients' preconceptions about chemotherapy and clarify issues that

Nursing Observations for Cancer Chemotherapy

THERAPEUTIC GOAL	Remission or, failing that, delayed progression of the neoplasm.
PREADMINISTRATION ASSESSMENT	
Baseline Data	Observe for abnormal growths; constipation and compensatory hyperperistalsis, malabsorption, or intestinal obstructions; continuous, gradually intensifying pain; atelectasis; inflammation of affected tissue; lethargy and fatigue; anorexia and weight loss; elevated blood cell counts; neurological symptoms (ataxia, dementia, weakness, sensory loss, altered reflexes); symptoms of endocrine disorders. Conduct a complete baseline physical examination. Obtain laboratory tests including complete blood cell counts, renal and liver function, and clotting tests.
Contraindications/ Precautions	Pregnancy, lactation, bone marrow depression, allergies, renal or hepatic failure.
EVALUATION OF DRUG RESPONSE	
For Therapeutic Benefit	Monitor tumor regression.
For Adverse Effects	Monitor blood cell counts, gastrointestinal irritation, nutritional status, occurrence of infections, and renal function.
For Drug and Dietary Interactions	Monitor for interactions specific for each antineoplastic agent (see individual drug discussions).
For Compliance	Evaluate the client's compliance with all facets of the therapeutic regimen by careful observation, interviewing, and review of progress. Report compliance problems to the physician and act as client-advocate when changes in the therapeutic regimen seem indicated.

arise. Clients need to be assured that each instance of cancer chemotherapy presents unique factors and that the experiences of others do not indicate the kind of response the individual client will have. Some clients will respond well to participation in groups with others who are undergoing similar therapy or who have experienced remissions as a result of chemotherapy.

In providing information, it is important to ascertain whether the client is emotionally capable of hearing only the bare essentials required for safe treatment or will want to know all the information available. Some clients are not content until they read and understand their laboratory reports and know every detail about the drugs to be used. In addition, clients' families must have current information to enable them to be supportive and help monitor clients during therapy.

Alkylating Agents

The alkylating agents represent the largest group of antineoplastic drugs, encompassing thirteen individual drugs in five chemical groups (Table 56–4). The five chemical groups of alkylating agents are (1) nitrogen mustards, (2) nitrosureas, (3) ethylenimines and methylmelamines, (4) alkyl sulfonates, and (5) triazenes. Differences in the pattern of adverse effects of the various alkylating agents are summarized in Table 56–5.

Table 56–4
Routes of Administration and Clinical Indications for Antineoplastic Agents

Drug	Routes	Indications
Alkylating agents		
Nitrogen mustards		
Mechlorethamine	IV	Lymphomas (especially Hodgkin's disease), bronchogenic carcinoma, lymphocytic leukemia, polycythemia vera, mycosis fungoides
Cyclophosphamide	PO, IV	Hodgkin's disease, other lymphomas, multiple myeloma, lymphocytic leukemia, solid tumors
Chlorambucil	PO	Chronic lymphocytic leukemia, lymphomas, ovarian and breast carcinomas
Melphalan	PO	Multiple myeloma, malignant melanoma, ovarian carcinoma
Uracil mustard	PO	Lymphocytic leukemia, non-Hodgkin's lymphomas, myelogenous leukemia, polycythemia vera, mycosis fungoides
Nitrosureas		
Lomustine	PO	Brain tumors, advanced Hodgkin's disease, lung cancer
Carmustine	IV	Brain tumors, multiple myeloma, MOPP-refractory Hodgkin's disease, other lymphomas, metastatic or progressive carcinoma of the prostate
Semustine	PO	Lymphomas, brain tumors, malignant melanomas, tumors of stomach, colon, or kidney
Streptozocin	IV	Metastatic islet cell carcinoma
Triazenes		
Dacarbazine	IV	Metastatic malignant melanoma, some sarcomas, refractory Hodgkin's disease
Alkyl sulfonates		
Busulfan	PO	Lung cancer, chronic myelogenous leukemia

Table 56–4
Routes of Administration and Clinical Indications for Antineoplastic Agents (*continued*)

Drug	Routes	Indications
Alkylating agents (*continued*)		
Ethylenimines and methylmelamines		
Thiotepa	IV	Adenocarcinoma of breast or ovary, superficial papillary tumors (topical irrigation), serous effusions of body cavities
Hexamethylmelamine	PO	Ovarian and small-cell lung carcinomas
Antimetabolites		
Folate antagonists		
Methotrexate	PO, IM, IV, IA, IT	Acute lymphocytic leukemia; choriocarcinoma; carcinomas of cervix, breast, testes, neck, lung, or head; osteogenic sarcoma
Pyrimidine analogues		
Fluorouracil or floxuridine	IV	Cancer of breast, colon, stomach, pancreas, ovaries, head, neck, bladder, and skin (topically)
Cytarabine	IV, SC, IT	Acute lymphocytic or granulocytic leukemias
Azaribine	PO	Mycosis fungoides, polycythemia vera
Purine analogues		
Mercaptopurine	PO	Acute lymphocytic or granulocytic leukemias, chronic granulocytic leukemia
Thioguanine	PO	Acute lymphocytic or granulocytic leukemias, chronic granulocytic leukemia
Cytotoxic antibiotics		
Anthracyclines		
Doxorubicin	IV	Sarcomas, lymphomas, acute leukemias, cancer of breast, genitourinary tract, thyroid, lung, stomach, neuroblastoma
Daunorubicin	IV	Acute granulocytic and lymphocytic leukemias
Other		
Dactinomycin	IV	Testicular carcinoma, Wilm's tumor, sarcoma, choriocarcinoma
Bleomycin	IV, IM, SC	Squamous cell carcinomas (head, neck, skin, esophagus, cervix, vulvovaginal area, rectum, pelvis), lymphomas
Plicamycin	IV	Squamous cell carcinomas of testes, malignant hypercalcemia
Mitomycin	IV	Squamous cell carcinomas (stomach, cervix, colon, breasts, pancreas, bladder, rectum), adenocarcinoma of breast
Vinca alkaloids		
Vinblastine	IV	Hodgkin's and non-Hodgkin's lymphomas, cancers of breast, testes, or renal cells
Vincristine	IV	Acute lymphocytic leukemia, neuroblastoma, breast carcinoma, sarcomas, Wilm's tumor, lymphomas

(*continued*)

Table 56–4
Routes of Administration and Clinical Indications for Antineoplastic Agents (*continued*)

Drug	Routes	Indications
Hormone and hormone antagonists		
Glucocorticoids Prednisone, hydrocortisone	PO, IV	Acute and chronic lymphocytic leukemias, breast cancer, lymphomas, multiple myeloma
Progestins Medroxyprogesterone	PO, IV	Endometrial, breast, prostate, or renal cell tumors
Androgens Fluoxymesterone	PO	Advanced breast cancer
Estrogens Diethylstilbestrol	PO	Breast cancer, cancer of prostate
Antiestrogens Tamoxifen	PO	Breast cancer
Miscellaneous		
L-Asparaginase	IV, IM	Acute lymphocytic leukemia
Cisplatin	IV	Germinal cell neoplasias of testes, lymphomas, ovarian carcinomas, squamous cell carcinomas of head or neck, neuroblastoma, osteogenic sarcoma
Etoposide	IV	Testicular carcinoma
Hydroxyurea	PO	Chronic granulocytic leukemia, malignant melanoma, advanced ovarian carcinoma
Interferon Alfa-2	IM, SC	Hairy-cell leukemia
Mitotane	PO	Adrenal cortical carcinoma
Procarbazine	PO	Lymphomas, bronchogenic carcinoma, malignant melanoma, brain tumors

Key: IA, intraarterially; IM, intramuscularly; IT, intratumor; IV, intravenously; PO, orally; SC, subcutaneously.

Mechanisms and Effects Alkylating agents act by forming highly reactive carbonium ions which react with cellular molecules to form covalent linkages. The formation of these bonds is referred to as alkylation. Alkylating agents form bonds with the guanine bases of DNA and either split the molecule or form cross links between the parallel DNA chains (Figure 56–3).

Alkylating agents, unlike many other antineoplastic agents, are not cell-cycle specific. They can react with cellular DNA at any stage in the cycle. However, the cytotoxic effect is not manifested until a cell enters into the active phase of synthesis that leads up to mitosis. The progression of the alkylated cell through the stages of the proliferation cycle is arrested at the premitotic phase and cell death occurs.

Resistance develops fairly commonly in tumor cells to the action of alkylating agents. When it occurs, there is cross-resistance to other drugs in the group of alkylating agents. Although alkylating agents share the same fundamental mechanism, differences exist with respect to reactivity at different pH's, stability in solution, and extent of absorption after oral administration.

Adverse Effects The hematopoietic system is especially sensitive to cytotoxic effects of alkylating agents. Marked leukopenia is the most serious side effect. White blood cell counts typically reach their nadir about 2 days after the first dosage, but leukopenia may be delayed as long as 4–5 weeks after a series of daily doses of an alkylating agent. Production of new blood cells in the bone marrow and lymphoid tissue begins within 6–8 hours after administration of an alkylating agent. Lymphocytopenia becomes apparent within 24 hours, grows progressively more severe for the next 5–7 days, and recovers only after about 4–6 weeks. *Immunosuppression*

Table 56–5
Comparison of Adverse Effects of Alkylating Agents

Drug	Leukopenia	Thrombo-penia	Nausea & vomiting	Other
Nitrogen mustards				
Mechlorethamine	+++	+++	+++	Vesicant
Cyclophosphamide	+++	+	++	Alopecia, cystitis
Chlorambucil	+++	+++	+	Bronchopulmonary fibrosis, antifertility effect
Melphalan	+++	+++	+	
Nitrosureas				
Lomustine	++++	+++	+++	Alopecia, stomatitis, liver impairment, pulmonary fibrosis
Carmustine	++++	+++	+++	Alopecia, stomatitis, liver impairment, pulmonary fibrosis
Streptozocin	+	+	+++	Renal impairment
Ethylenimines				
Thiotepa	+++	++++	+	
Alkyl sulfonates				
Busulfan	++++	++	+	Pulmonary fibrosis, gynecomastia
Triazenes				
Dacarbazine	++	+++	+++	Flu-like symptoms

Key: +, least severe; ++++, most severe.

produced by alkylating agents can result in activation of latent infections such as herpes zoster. Nurses need to instruct clients to look for other signs of candida overgrowth such as furry patches on the tongue or oral membranes, diarrhea, foul-smelling stools, or vaginal itch. Nurses should also make certain that clients have been advised not to receive vaccination during treatment with antineoplastic drugs. Granulocytopenia develops more slowly than leukopenia and is less long-lasting. It becomes evident within a few days and lasts 10–21 days. Platelet and red blood cell counts decline less dramatically if at all, with maximum reductions occurring in the second or third week. Myelosuppression is often used as the basis for dosage adjustment in order to maintain the leukocyte count between 3,000 and 4,000/mm^3.

Alkylating agents produce toxic effects on other rapidly proliferating tissues as well. Epithelial cells exhibit arrest of mitosis, frequently resulting in desquamation and lesions. Hair follicles may be affected to the extent that alopecia occurs, but hair loss is usually reversible. In males, spermatogenesis is inhibited resulting in a depletion of spermatozoa. In females, anovulation and amenorrhea may occur and persist for up to several months after treatment with an alkylating agent. Infertility is likely to become permanent if chemotherapy with an alkylating

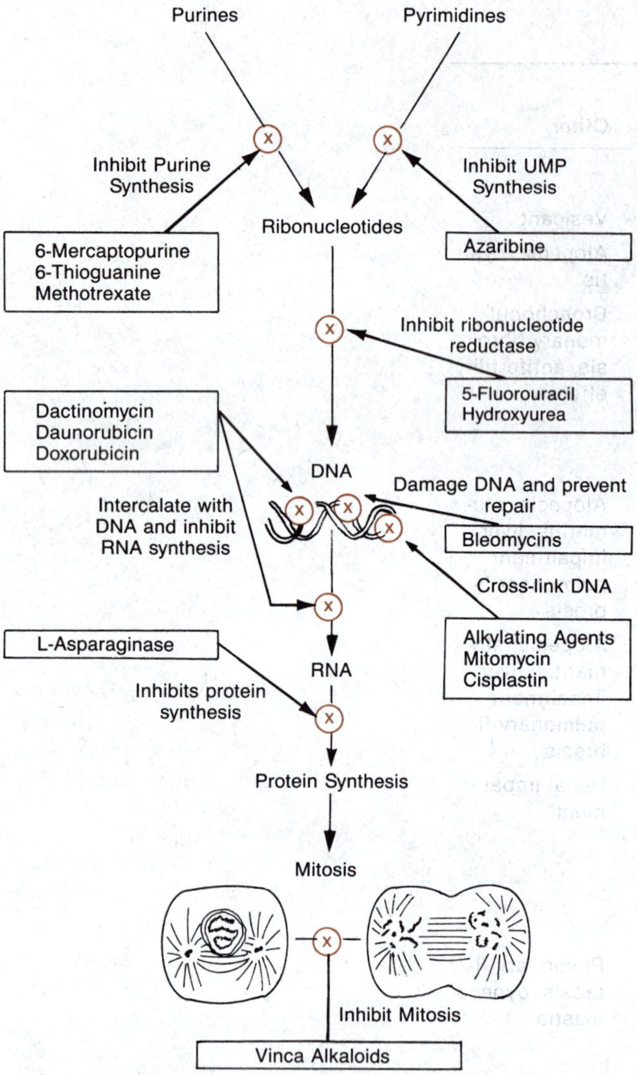

Figure 56–3
Mechanisms of antineoplastic drugs.

agent continues for 6 months or more. *Clients need to be informed of these possibilities prior to instituting therapy.* Hepatoxicity sometimes occurs, most commonly in clients with prior liver impairment. *Nurses should instruct clients to report signs of possible hepatoxicity such as presence of frothy dark urine, light colored stools, jaundice, or pruritus.* Alkylating agents are potential teratogens. *Female clients should be advised to employ a contraceptive method during treatment and for at least 4 months thereafter. Nurses should be alert to the neurologic toxicities that alkylating agents can cause, including nausea, convulsions, and muscular paralysis. Rapid cytolysis of tumor and blood cells caused by alkylating agents may result in uric acid accumulation causing clients to complain of joint and flank pain.*

Nitrogen Mustards

The nitrogen mustard group of alkylating agents were developed in the mid-nineteenth century, but the anticancer potential of these drugs did not become apparent until 1942. Highly secretive research on nitrogen mustards was conducted during World War II, when these drugs were viewed as potential agents of chemical warfare. Mechlorethamine (nitrogen mustard) was the first of the anticancer drugs.

Mechlorethamine (Mustargen)

A disadvantage of mechlorethamine is that it is highly unstable in solution. Solutions of the drug must be prepared within a few minutes of injection. After injection mechlorethamine has a half-life of less than 10 minutes.

Mechanisms and Effects Mechlorethamine and other nitrogen mustards have a *vesicant* (blister-producing) effect on the skin, eyes, and respiratory tract. Procedures relating to avoidance of vesicant effects are itemized in Table 56–3.

Clinical Indications The foremost indication for mechlorethamine is for clients with Hodgkin's lymphoma, who may be given the drug in conjunction with vincristine (*O*ncovin), *p*rocarbazine, and *p*rednisone (the MOPP regimen). Other less reactive nitrogen mustards are now preferred for other lymphomas, leukemias, and solid tumors.

Preparations and Administration *Mechlorethamine must be reconstituted immediately prior to injection. The solution should be discarded if discolored.* It may be injected directly or into tubing of a rapidly flowing IV infusate consisting of normal or half-normal saline. Mechlorethamine is sometimes administered intracavity. Before intracavity administration, most of the fluid in the cavity is removed. Injection of mechlorethamine into the intrapleural or intrapericardial spaces is conducted through a thoracentesis needle. Intraperitoneal injections are given through a rubber catheter fitted into a paracentesis trocar or an 18 gauge needle. Intraperitoneal injection often results in pain, nausea, and vomiting. Cardiac irregularities may accompany intrapleural injection, so cardiac function should be monitored.

Mechlorethamine Hydrochloride (Mustargen)
Powder for injection
Typical Regimens: When given alone, mechlorethamine is administered at a dose of 0.4 mg/kg once every 4–6 weeks. More frequently, mechlorethamine is employed in the MOPP regimen for Hodgkin's disease, in conjunction with vincris-

tine, procarbazine, and prednisone. In this regimen, mechlorethamine is given at a dose of 6 mg/m^2/day, IV, on days 1 and 8 along with vincristine, 2 mg/m^2/day (maximum 2.0 mg), IV, on days 1 and 8; procarbazine, 100 mg/m^2/day, PO, on days 1–14; and prednisone, 40 mg/m^2/day, PO, on days 1–14. The MOPP regimen is repeated every 28 days for 6 cycles.

Cyclophosphamide (Cytoxan, Neosar)

Mechanisms and Effects Cyclophosphamide is a prodrug, requiring metabolic activation by liver enzymes to produce the active metabolites, phosphoramide mustard and acrolein, that promote alkylation.

Pharmacokinetics Cyclophosphamide can be given orally or by IM or IV injection. The half-life of the parent compound is about 6.5 hours. It is only 10–15% bound by plasma proteins, but the active metabolites are about 50% bound. Peak levels of the active metabolites usually occur about 2–3 hours after administration of cyclophosphamide. Inducers of liver enzymes, such as phenobarbital, can hasten formation of the active derivatives.

Clinical Indications Cyclophosphamide is the most useful of the alkylating agents. It is indicated for Hodgkin's disease and other lymphomas, multiple myeloma, lymphocytic leukemia, and certain solid tumors.

Adverse Effects and Contraindications Cyclophosphamide has the advantage of not causing the neurotoxic effects associated with some of the nitrogen mustards. Also, cyclophosphamide produces less thrombocytopenia and is not a vesicant. However, nurses should warn clients that cyclophosphamide is especially likely to cause alopecia. It can also produce cystitis in up to 20% of treated individuals. *Thus it is important to advise clients to report immediately any occurrence of dysuria or blood-tinged urine. Clients should be encouraged to drink at least 3 quarts of fluid per day to decrease risk of cystitis. Oral cyclophosphamide should be taken in the morning so that the drug will be cleared from the system by night and not remain in the bladder overnight. When cyclophosphamide is given intravenously in large doses, prehydration and sometimes posthydration with intravenous fluids is required.*

Large doses of cyclophosphamide have been reported to cause renal impairment as well. Hemorrhagic subendocardial necrosis, dysrhythmias, congestive heart failure, and interstitial pulmonary fibrosis have also occurred at high doses.

Preparations and Administration Solutions are stable for 6 days under refrigeration and for 1 day at room temperature. *Cyclophosphamide is usually taken on an empty stomach. If nausea and vomiting are severe, cyclophosphamide may be taken with a meal.*

Cyclophosphamide (Cytoxan, Neosar)
Tablets, powder for preparing parenteral solutions (in sterile water) or oral solutions (in Aromatic Elixir, USP)
Typical Regimens: Cyclophosphamide is employed in the CVP regimen with *v*incristine and *p*rednisone; in place of mechlorethamine in the MOPP regimen described above; and in the CMF regimen with *m*ethotrexate and 5-*f*luorouracil. Cyclophosphamide is an alternative to azathioprine for immunosuppression (see Chapter 50). The usual oral dose for cyclophosphamide is 2–3 mg/kg/day or 50–100 mg/m^2/day.

Chlorambucil (Leukeran)

Chlorambucil is a nitrogen mustard with somewhat less reactivity than mechlorethamine. It is used primarily for chronic lymphocytic leukemia, lymphomas, and carcinomas of the breast and ovaries. Bone marrow suppression is the most important toxic effect of chlorambucil. Other adverse effects are those common to the class of drugs, including nausea, vomiting, sterility, and bronchopulmonary fibrosis.

Preparations and Administration

Chlorambucil (Leukeran)
Tablets
Recommended Doses: 0.1–0.2 mg/kg/day. It is usually employed in short courses of therapy lasting for 3–6 weeks.

Melphalan (Alkeran)

Melphalan is the least reactive of the nitrogen mustards. It is used orally for treatment of clients with multiple myeloma or carcinomas of the breast and ovary. Melphalan is less likely than cyclophosphamide to produce alopecia. The major adverse effects are bone marrow suppression, gastrointestinal irritation, dermatitis, pulmonary fibrosis, and hypersensitivity reactions. When melphalan is employed in clients with multiple myeloma, there is a special risk of severe leukopenia because the effect of the drug adds to the reduced capacity of clients with this disease to produce normal quantities of antibodies. Myelosuppression with melphalan is usually maximal within a few weeks. *The tablets should be stored in a light-resistant airtight container. Nurses may need to encourage such clients to persist in therapy. Introducing clients with multiple myeloma to one another and plan-*

ning joint instructional sessions or conferences may prove effective in helping those who become discouraged to continue therapy.

Preparations and Administration

Melphalan (Alkeran)
Tablets
Typical Regimen: The usual dose is 0.1–0.2 mg/kg/day PO for 5 days. *Melphalan should be taken with meals to minimize nausea and vomiting.* The course of treatment is repeated every 4–6 weeks as required. Clients with multiple myeloma who take oral melphalan improve very gradually over a period of many months.

Uracil Mustard

Uracil mustard is readily absorbed after oral administration. It is indicated for use in lymphocytic leukemias, non-Hodgkin's lymphomas, myelogenous leukemia, polycythemia vera, and mycosis fungoides. Like other alkylating agents, it produces hematopoietic toxicity and is carcinogenic. Uracil mustard increases levels of uric acid in the blood and in the urine. *Patients should be advised to drink plenty of fluids and to urinate frequently during treatment with uracil mustard to prevent formation of urate crystals.*

Preparations and Administration

Uracil Mustard
Capsules
Typical Regimen: 0.15 mg/kg PO in adults or 0.3 mg/kg in children, once weekly, for 4 weeks.

Nitrosoureas

The nitrosoureas include four agents: lomustine, carmustine, semustine, and streptozocin. The family of drugs is an important series of antitumor agents with a wide spectrum of effective applications

Lomustine (CeeNu), Carmustine (BiCNU), and Semustine

Mechanisms and Effects Lomustine, carmustine, and semustine share a high level of lipid solubility. They are thus able to penetrate into the brain and are useful in treatment of brain tumors. Lomustine is also indicated for clients with advanced Hodgkin's disease. Carmustine is employed in clients who have multiple myelomas, Hodgkin's disease that is refractory to the MOPP regimen, or other non-Hodgkin's lymphomas. Semustine has been used for clients with lymphomas, malignant melanomas, and tumors of the stomach, colon, or renal cells.

Pharmacokinetics The half-life of nitrosoureas is very brief, 5–15 minutes. However, isocyanate metabolites produced are somewhat more persistent and contribute to the antitumor effect. The parent compounds produce active chlorethyl moieties and the isocyanate metabolites produce carbamyl moieties, both of which promote alkylation and cross-linking of DNA. Nitrosoureas penetrate into the cerebral spinal fluid (CSF) reaching levels about 15–30% of plasma concentrations.

Adverse Effects Nurses need to warn clients that nitrosoureas will produce nausea and vomiting with considerable frequency and intensity. Usually it begins 3–4 hours after drug administration and lasts less than 24 hours. *Nausea can be controlled by having the client fast or take an antiemetic drug prior to administration of the nitrosourea. It may also help if the nitrosourea is taken at bedtime because clients sleep through mild nausea.* Anorexia generally persists for 2–3 days after a dosage.

Bone marrow depression is also severe; however, the effect is often a delayed one, with leukopenia and thrombocytopenia occurring only after 4 or 5 weeks. *Blood cell counts should be monitored at least weekly for the first 6 weeks.* Nitrosoureas should not be repeated in less than 6 weeks because hematologic responses may be delayed and cumulative. A new course of therapy should not be undertaken until leukocytes exceed 4,000/mm^3 and platelet count is over 100,000/mm^3. Other adverse reactions include alopecia, stomatitis, mildly impaired liver function, and pulmonary fibrosis.

Preparations and Administration Carmustine has vesicant properties and can cause phlebitis when given intravenously. *In administering carmustine, nurses should take care to avoid extravasation and to utilize the other precautions related to vesicants (Table 56–3).*

Pharmacists may sometimes need to prepare the prescribed dose of semustine or lomustine by combining capsules of various strengths. A given dose may therefore include capsules of different colors and this will have to be explained to the client.

Carmustine (BiCNU)
Powder for injection with sterile diluent
Typical Regimen: Once every 6 weeks, IV. When utilized with vincristine, melphalan, cyclophosphamide, and prednisone in the M-2 regimen for multiple myeloma, carmustine is given in a dose of 0.5 mg/kg, IV, on day 1 of the 35-day cycle. When employed in the BCVPP regimen with *c*yclophosphamide, *v*inblastine, *p*rocarbazine, and *p*rednisone for Hodgkin's disease, the recommended dose of carmustine is 100 mg/m^2, IV, on day 1 of the 28-day cycle.

Lomustine (CeeNu)
Capsules, dose packs containing two 100 mg capsules, two 40 mg capsules, and two 10 mg capsules
Typical Regimen: 130 mg/m^2 PO as a single dose, every 6 weeks. Subsequent doses are adjusted according to blood cell counts.

Semustine
Capsules
Typical Regimen: 200 mg/m^2 once every 6 weeks by the oral route.

Streptozocin (Zanosar)

Streptozocin differs from the other nitrosoureas in being highly water soluble. It is indicated for use, alone or preferably in combination with fluorouracil, for treatment of metastatic islet cell carcinoma. Streptozocin produces remission in 50–60% of islet cell carcinomas.

Nurses should advise clients to expect severe nausea and vomiting reactions to streptozocin. It usually begins about 4 hours after drug administration and lasts for 24 hours. Most clients experience some renal toxicity, such as proteinuria, hypophosphatemia, or renal tubular necrosis. The renal toxicity is cumulative and dose dependent. Therefore other nephrotoxic drugs should not be used concurrently. Hematologic reactions are less common than with most other antineoplastic agents. Mild anemia is the most common blood cell effect. Streptozocin may cause hypoglycemia. Like other alkylating agents, streptozocin should be considered teratogenic and clients should be advised to practice contraception when using this medication.

Streptozocin is not absorbed after oral administration. It is therefore given intravenously. *The drug should be stored under refrigeration.*

Preparations and Administration

Streptozocin (Zanosar)
Powder for injection
Typical Regimen: 500 mg/m^2/day for 5 days, repeated every 2–4 weeks; or 1.0–1.5 g/m^2 once weekly.

Ethylenimines and Methylmelamines

Triethylenethiophosphoramide (Thiotepa)

Triethylenethiophosphoramide is an ethylenimine. The original agents of this class were developed as industrial chemicals to aid in the finishing of rayon fabrics. Since ethylenimines, like nitrogen mustards, generate ethylenimonium ions, an effort was made in the 1950s to develop alkylating agents from this chemical group. Thiotepa is the sole drug in this group that remains clinically available. It is less reactive than nitrogen mustards; thiotepa has been supplanted by cyclophosphamide and other nitrogen mustards. It is most effective in cancers of the ovaries, breasts, and bladder. Thiotepa is given by intravenous, intratumor, intracavitary, or intravesical injection because oral absorption is too erratic. The principal adverse effects are bone marrow suppression, gastrointestinal reactions, and inhibition of spermatogenesis. Thiotepa powder should be refrigerated at 2–8° C. *After reconstitution, solutions are stable under refrigeration for 5 days. The solution should be clear or slightly opaque but without a precipitate.*

Preparations and Administration

Triethylenethiophosphoramide (Thiotepa)
Powder for injection
Typical Regimen: 0.3–0.4 mg/kg at 1- to 4-week intervals.

Hexamethylmelamine

Although it was developed and set aside in the early 1960s, there has recently been renewed interest in use of the melamine derivative hexamethylmelamine (HMM). HMM, like thiotepa and nitrogen mustards, generates ethylenimonium ions. It has useful activity against ovarian, breast, pulmonary, cervical, and renal carcinomas. HMM is not water soluble and thus is marketed only as an oral formulation. It is readily absorbed after oral administration, reaching peak levels in about 1 hour. The drug is metabolized and the metabolites are eliminated by urinary excretion. Adverse effects of hexamethylmelamine include nausea, vomiting, diarrhea, bone marrow suppression, and peripheral neuropathies.

Preparations and Administration

Hexymethylmelamine
Capsules
Typical Regimen: HMM is most often used in combination therapy for ovarian cancer, along with cyclophosphamide, cisplastin, and doxorubicin. A typical dose is 4–12 mg/kg/day for several months. When employed in combination regimens for ovarian or small-cell lung carcinomas, the usual dose is 100–200 mg/m^2/day for 7–14 days, repeated every 3–4 weeks.

Alkyl Sulfonates

Busulfan (Myleran)

Busulfan is the most active of a group of alkanesulfonic acid esters studied as possible alkylating agents. Busulfan has the special property of being relatively selective in its cytotoxic action for the bone marrow. Busulfan is indicated for treatment of chronic myelogenous leukemia and for lung cancers. Daily oral administration produces cell lysis and relieves symptoms in the chronic phase of leukemia. When used alone, busulfan tends to cause uric acid accumulation due to excessively rapid cell lysis, but coadministration of allopurinol prevents this adverse effect. Busulfan causes the usual antineoplastic drug side effects of anemia, thrombocytopenia, nausea, alopecia, and sterility. Unique side effects of busulfan include gynecomastia, increased skin pigmentation, and interstitial pulmonary fibrosis with possible cough or dyspnea.

Preparations and Administration

Busulfan (Myleran)
Tablets
Typical Regimen: The recommended initial daily dose is 4–8 mg, which is often reduced to 1–3 mg for maintenance purposes.

Nursing Diagnoses and Interventions for Cancer Chemotherapy

Nursing Diagnoses	*Related Interventions*
TO ENHANCE DRUG BENEFITS OR REDUCE DRUG REQUIREMENTS	
Physiologic Diagnoses	
Activity intolerance related to fatigue secondary to cancer	Provide adequate rest. Assist client in maintaining bedtime routines.
Alteration in bowel elimination: constipation related to disease treatments, immobility, or changes in food intake	Provide bulk foods and maintain a high level of fluid intake. Encourage establishing a regular time for bowel elimination.
Alteration in urinary elimination related to incontinence caused by the disease	Provide access to bedpan. Provide hygienic measures. Instruct clients to report any change in urinary output. Instruct clients to practice stop and start of urinary stream several times during voiding.
Impairment of skin integrity related to poor nutrition, immobility and poor circulation secondary to cancer	Provide skin care. Apply oils or linaments. Encourage adequate nutrition.
Psychosocial Diagnoses	
Alteration in family processes related to role disturbances, uncertain future, stress, and schedule of treatments; Disturbance in self-concept related to role disturbances, uncertain future, and drug side effects; Grieving related to anticipated loss of life or restriction in quality of life; Impaired social interactions related to rejection or fear of rejection; Powerlessness related to uncertain prognosis and helplessness; Sexual dysfunction related to the disease, pain or fatigue produced by treatments, grieving, changes in body image or role responsibilities, or antifertility effects of anticancer drugs	Assist clients and families in coping with the disease; provide emotional support and appropriate reassurance. Help the client remain at home and to continue working as long as possible. Assist clients in maintaining an appropriate balance between time alone and time with friends and relatives; encourage continuing support from friends and relatives. Keep hospital room cheerful and pleasant; provide comfortable places for clients to congregate. Advise clients about cosmetic compensations for hair loss. Encourage clients to associate with others with similar problems as well as healthy people.
Self-care deficits related to pain, fatigue, or depression	Assess the client's self-care capabilities (wholly compensatory, partly compensatory, or supportive-educative).
TO MINIMIZE DRUG SIDE EFFECTS OR INTERACTIONS	
Alteration in bowel elimination: diarrhea related to cancer chemotherapy	Assist client to maintain fluid intake in spite of diarrhea; provide low-residue foods; advise client about

	perineal hygiene and application of vasoline or vitamin A and D ointment.
Alteration in comfort related to disease or treatments	For hospitalized clients, provide comfort measures such as extra pillows, skin care, frequent changes of position, and exercise within the limits imposed by the condition. Teach clients and families similar measures for use at home.
Alteration in nutrition: intake less than requirements related to nausea, vomiting, anorexia, and fatigue because of the disease process and treatments	Assess the state of nutrition of the client and determine relevant factors; modify nutritional status; provide nutritional support. Encourage clients to take small frequent meals and to take antiemetic drugs immediately before meals. Suggest light, bland foods and alkaline-ash foods such as citrus fruits to minimize hyperuricemia caused by anticancer drugs. Tell client to avoid greasy foods. Encourage client to eat favorite foods when possible.
Alteration in oral mucous membranes related to the cancer or treatment with radiation or antineoplastic drugs	Intensify oral hygienic measures; instruct clients to use a soft toothbrush. Urge clients to discontinue use of tobacco or alcohol. Relieve pain due to mouth sores with a local anesthetic or systemic analgesic.
Fluid volume deficits related to vomiting, diarrhea, and adipsia secondary to disease or treatments	Assess the state of hydration of the client. Provide adequate fluid replacement. Encourage client to drink the fluids that are best tolerated.
Increased risk of infection related to immunosuppression caused by antineoplastic drugs	Protect hospitalized clients from exposure to infection and teach those at home the importance of avoiding exposure during the period of maximum immunosuppression. Monitor white blood cell counts. Provide a clean environment. Administer antimicrobial agents as required.
Increased risk of injury related to weakness, disorientation, muscle deterioration, and bleeding tendencies caused by disease or drugs	Provide safety measures as required; monitor clients for evidences of bleeding; monitor platelet counts; instruct clients to inform their dentists that they are receiving cancer chemotherapy.
TO ENSURE SAFE AND EFFICACIOUS DRUG USE	
Knowledge deficit related to drug regimen	Teach clients to avoid contact with carcinogens such as industrial pollutants, unnecessary drugs, automobile exhaust, cigarettes, and radiation. Explain to clients the importance of early detection and teach clients techniques such as self-examination of the breasts to facilitate early detection. Explain the nature of the type of cancer that a client has to the client and family and clear up any misconceptions or generalizations based on previous experiences with other forms of cancers in other individuals. Explain the rationale for the particular mode of therapy selected. Teach clients with cancer and who are at home how to assess their physical condition for changes. Provide the client with a list of adverse effects and drug interactions for each drug in the regimen and explain what to do if any of these occur. Reinforce the importance of adhering precisely with the therapeutic regimen.

Triazenes

Dacarbazine (DTIC-Dome)

Dacarbazine is a prodrug that is activated by N-demethylation or photoactivation. After IV administration, the parent compound disappears rapidly from the blood with a half-life of 19–20 minutes as the drug is taken up and metabolized by the liver. The elimination half-life is about 5 hours. Dacarbazine is not significantly protein bound in plasma and enters the CSF only to the extent of about 14% of plasma concentrations. Dacarbazine is effective in treating clients with metastatic malignant melanoma, selected sarcomas, or Hodgkin's disease that is refractory to standard regimens. Dacarbazine is a primary choice for metastatic melanoma, producing a 20% remission rate. For sarcomas or Hodgkin's disease, it is typically given in combination with doxorubicin. Adverse effects of dacarbazine include severe nausea and vomiting, leukopenia and thrombocytopenia (usually about 2 weeks after initiation of therapy), and flu-like symptoms (fever, malaise, and myalgias). Alopecia and renal or hepatic dysfunction can also occur. After reconstitution, solutions are stable for up to 72 hours at 4° C or for 8 hours at room temperature. Dacarbazine is a vesicant. *When administering decarbazine, nurses should avoid extravasation and employ other precautions for vesicant drugs (Table 56–3).*

Preparations and Administration

Dacarbazine (DTIC-Dome)
Powder for injection
Typical Regimen: The usual dose is 250 mg/m^2/day, by IV injection, for 5 days, repeated every 3–4 weeks.

Antimetabolites

The antimetabolites used in cancer chemotherapy include a folic acid antagonist, purine analogues, and pyrimidine analogues. Drugs of this type interfere with production of purine or pyrimidine bases or their incorporation into ribonucleotides, RNA, and DNA. Purine and pyrimidine analogues may in the process be incorporated into nucleic acid to produce aberrant DNA or RNA. As a result, antimetabolites interfere with cell proliferation. Most antimetabolites are cell-cycle specific, acting only on cells during the synthetic phase that precedes division. Fluorouracil and floxuridine may be cell-cycle nonspecific.

Folate Antagonists

Methotrexate (Folex, Mexate, and generic)

Mechanisms and Effects Methotrexate has been recognized as an inhibitor of the vitamin folic acid (or folate) since 1948. Methotrexate inhibits the enzyme dihydrofolate reductase that converts dietary folate to the active coenzyme form, tetrahydrofolic acid (THF). Deficiency of the coenzyme inhibits production of nucleic acids and proteins. Cells actively engaged in synthesis of these macronucleotides in preparation for mitosis are most severely compromised by lack of THF, and cell death typically occurs in the S-phase.

Pharmacokinetics Methotrexate is well absorbed after oral administration of doses up to 30 mg/m^2 but is only incompletely absorbed at higher doses. Peak plasma concentrations occur in 1–2 hours. The drug is approximately 50% bound by plasma proteins, and it can be displaced by concurrent use of salicylates, sulfonamides, phenytoin, or other highly bound drugs. Methotrexate distributes to some extent into body fluids of the pleural and peritoneal cavities. If the fluids in these compartments are expanded, as in ascites, such fluids may act as a depot for the drug resulting in a prolonged elimination half-life and toxicity. Normally, disappearance from the blood is triphasic, with the first phase representing rapid distribution into tissue (half-life 45 minutes), the second phase renal elimination of the remaining plasma fraction (half-life 2–3.5 hours), and the third phase gradual secondary redistribution and elimination of tissue stores (half-life about 10 hours). Toxicity appears to correlate especially with prolongation of the third phase.

Clinical Indications Methotrexate first came to attention for its ability to achieve long-lasting remissions, including virtual cures, in women with choriocarcinoma, an uncommon malignancy. Methotrexate is currently used in an effective combination regimen for acute lymphocytic leukemia, Burkitt's lymphoma, or trophoblastic choriocarcinoma. The combination is frequently curative. However, methotrexate is more often employed for maintenance of induced remissions, in combination with mercaptopurine and sometimes cyclophosphamide as well. Methotrexate is particularly effective in acute lymphoblastic leukemias in children. It is used in combination with other antineoplastic agents for women with breast cancer (the CMFP regimen, for example, combines *c*yclophosphamide, *m*ethotrexate, *f*luorouracil, and *p*rednisone) and people having lung cancer (the CAMP regimen combines *c*yclophosphamide, doxorubicin (*A*driamycin), *m*ethotrexate, and *p*rocarbazine). Methotrexate is also used for the nonmalignant, hyperproliferative skin condition psoriasis when it is severe and recalcitrant to other drug regimens (see Chapter 53).

Drug resistance occurs commonly to methotrexate. Three distinct mechanisms of resistance have been observed: (1) cells may exhibit reduced transport of methotrexate into the cell interior, (2) cells may produce modified dihydrofolate reductase that is more resistant to the drug, (3) cells may produce an excess of dihydrofolate reductase.

Adverse Effects and Contraindications The common adverse reactions to methotrexate are those common to antineoplastic agents: alimentary distress (including nausea, vomiting, stomatitis, and ulceration), bone marrow suppression, and alopecia. *Clients should be taught the hygienic measures indicated for minimization of stomatitis.* In addition, allergic skin eruptions may occur (rash, pruritus, urticaria, photosensitivity), renal failure, hepatic necrosis, interstitial pneumonitis (possibly fatal), or neurologic difficulties (arachnoiditis, transient paresis, or leukoencephalopathy). *Hepatic and renal function tests should be performed before initiating therapy.*

Nurses should be certain to advise clients receiving methotrexate to avoid use of alcohol or salicylates since these can aggravate gastrointestinal irritation. Alcohol can also add to the hepatoxicity of methotrexate. *Nurses should also be certain to advise clients to avoid use of sun lamps or excessive exposure to sunlight because of the risk of photosensitivity. Clients should be told of possible drug eruptions and gastrointestinal reactions and to report these if they occur.* For example, the onset of bloody diarrhea necessitates interrupting drug therapy to prevent perforation and hemorrhagic enteritis.

Methotrexate can precipitate diabetes. *Nurses should encourage clients to obtain periodic blood glucose tests when blood cell counts are being conducted. They should also have clients report increased thirst or increased voiding.*

Because of potential teratogenicity, clients should be urged to avoid pregnancy by contraception for at least 8 weeks following termination of methotrexate therapy.

Clients and their families should be provided with a list of symptoms that should be reported to the physician if they occur: diarrhea; tarry stools; abdominal pain; fever; chills; persistent sore throat; bleeding; bruising; sores in the mouth; discoloration of the eyes, skin, or urine; bloody urine; swelling of the feet or legs; joint or flank pain; or difficult respiration.

Drug Interactions A new development in the use of methotrexate is so-called "rescue" therapy. This technique allows administration of higher doses of methotrexate than could otherwise be tolerated and is effective in promoting remissions (in about 30% of clients) with metastatic osteogenic sarcomas that otherwise cannot be treated. In this method, a high dose (50–250 mg/kg, IV) of methotrexate is given followed 6–24 hours later by administration of leucovorin (folinic acid) and/or thymidine. Leucovorin is a derivative of folic acid that is already reduced and ready to function as a coenzyme. Thymidine is a precursor of thymidylate that can be utilized without requirement for THF. Leucovorin and thymidine thus antagonize the effects of methotrexate to rescue normal tissue cells from the cytotoxic actions of the antimetabolite. Rapidly proliferating tumor cells are damaged by 24 hours of THF deficiency, but slowly proliferating tissue cells can tolerate THF deficiency for this time period.

Organic acids such as salicylates, probenecid (Benemid), and sulfonamides compete with methotrexate for renal secretion as well as displacing it from plasma proteins. This can result in increased methotrexate toxicity.

Vitamin preparations containing folic acid, on the other hand, may inhibit the efficacy of methotrexate. Since clients receiving methotrexate for treatment of a tumor may feel tired and weak both because of the disease and the drug therapy, they often want to take vitamin preparations. *Nurses should advise them to avoid using multivitamin formulations containing folic acid and show them how to read the label to determine if this substance is present before purchasing a product.* Concurrent use of folate antagonists employed as antimicrobials (pyrimethamine, sulfonamides, trimethoprim) will result in additive toxicity. Methotrexate can increase the effect of oral anticoagulants due to its ability to cause hypoprothrombinemia.

Preparations and Administration

Methotrexate (Mexate, Folex, and generic)
Tablets, injection solution, powder for injection
Typical Regimens: Methotrexate is normally employed by IV or IM injection, but intrathecal administration is also feasible. The usual doses when methotrexate is used as a single drug regimen are 75 mg/m^2/day for treatment of solid tumors. For intrathecal administration, the recommended dose is 6–12 mg/m^2/week. When rescue therapy is undertaken, doses of 50–250 mg/kg, IV, are employed. The drug is infused in a large volume of IV fluid containing bicarbonate to maintain renal fluid at a pH greater than or equal to 7.0 to ensure solubility of methotrexate in the renal filtrate and urine. Leucovorin rescue is undertaken after 24 hours.

Pyrimidine Analogues

The pyrimidine analogues include drugs used systemically as antineoplastics (fluorouracil, floxuridine, cytarabine, azaribine), systemically for immunosuppression (cytarabine), systemically for psoriasis (azaribine), topically for eye infections caused by herpes zoster (cytarabine), and topically for skin and eye infections caused by herpes simplex (idoxuridine). Only the systemic applications for suppression of neoplasms will be discussed here.

Fluorouracil (Adrucil) and Floxuridine (FUDR)

Mechanisms and Effects Fluorouracil is a halogenated analogue of the pyrimidine bases that are constituents of nucleic acids. Fluorouracil does not itself compete with pyrimidine bases, but must first be metabolically activated to the nucleotide level. Fluorouracil is converted in a series of steps to 5-fluoro-2′-deoxyuridine-5′ phosphate (F-dUMP). F-dUMP is the active antimetabolite, competing with the natural substrate, deoxyuridine-5′ phosphate (dUMP), for incorporation into nucleic acids.

Floxuridine was prepared for use as a drug with the idea of circumventing the series of steps needed to activate fluorouracil. This compound can be converted directly to F-dUMP in a single step. However, a large part of an administered dose of floxuridine is converted rapidly to fluorouracil and must be activated in the same manner as administered fluorouracil.

Pharmacokinetics Fluorouracil and floxuridine are erratically absorbed after oral administration, necessitating administration by intravenous injection. These drugs are cleared rapidly from the plasma (within 20 minutes) being taken up by tissue cells. Metabolic degradation occurs primarily in the liver and is significantly compromised in persons with liver impairment. Less than 20% of the parent compounds are excreted unchanged.

Clinical Indications Fluorouracil and floxuridine are used in palliative therapies for people with carcinomas of the breast, gastrointestinal tract (colon, stomach), pancreas, ovaries, head, neck, or bladder. There is little reason to believe that use of these drugs results in any significant prolongation of life expectancy however. Fluorouracil is also used in topical application to the skin for multiple superficial basal-cell carcinomas and premalignant keratoses, but only when conventional surgical techniques are impractical.

Adverse Effects and Contraindications The principal adverse effects of fluorouracil and floxuridine are those common to all antineoplastic drugs. Cytotoxic effects on the gastrointestinal tract may be manifested as anorexia, nausea, stomatitis, and diarrhea. Some clients will experience dysphagia, retrosternal burning, or proctitis. Bone marrow suppression results in leukopenia, anemia, and thrombocytopenia. Leukopenia is most often somewhat delayed, reaching its maximum extent 9–14 days after the first injection. Blood cell values usually return to normal by the thirtieth day after administration. Adverse epidermal effects include dermatitis, alopecia, nail changes, increased pigmentation, and atrophy of the skin. Photophobia and lacrimation may occur. *Dark glasses can be suggested to the client to protect against photophobia.*

Topical use of fluorouracil is associated with both local and systemic adverse effects. Local adverse effects include pain, pruritus, hyperpigmentation, dermatitis, scarring, scaling, swelling, and photosensitivity. *Clients should be warned about unsightly effects that may occur, such as hyperpigmentation and scarring and should be instructed to avoid prolonged exposure to ultraviolet rays when the drug is being used.* Use of an occlusive dressing increases the risk of irritant effects on adjacent normal skin.

Preparations and Administration

Fluorouracil (generic, Adrucil)
Injection solution, topical solution, cream
Typical Regimens: For internal carcinomas, fluorouracil is given intravenously. The recommended initial dose of fluorouracil is 12 mg/kg (maximum 800 mg), IV, once daily for 4 successive days. If toxicity is not observed, additional doses are given on alternate days, on days 6, 8, 10, and 12. The dose of fluorouracil is reduced by 50% in individuals at risk because of poor nutritional status or impaired liver function. Elderly individuals may also exhibit increased toxicity. The first course of therapy should be conducted in a hospital setting or under rigid supervision.

Maintenance therapy can be instituted in clients if significant toxicity has not been manifested to the initial course of therapy. Maintenance therapy can be conducted by repeating the initial course of therapy once every 4 weeks or by giving 10–15 mg/kg or 600 mg/m^2 once weekly by rapid IV injection.

For treatment of actinic keratoses, apply topically to the lesions twice daily in an amount sufficient to cover the lesion. Use is discontinued when the skin reaches the ulcerative stage, usually in about 2–4 weeks, and healing then ensues in 1–2 months. For basal cell carcinoma, fully cover the lesion with the 5% preparation, twice per day. Treatment is continued for at least 3–6 weeks but can last up to 12 weeks.

Floxuridine (FUDR)
Powder for injection
Typical Regimens: Floxuridine is usually employed by intraarterial infusion. Floxuridine is employed in schedules similar to fluorouracil at twice the doses or by continuous intraarterial infusion at 0.1–0.6 mg/kg/day.

Cytarabine (Cytosar-U)

Mechanisms and Effects Cytarabine is an analogue of the pyrimidine nucleoside, cytidine, and is incorporated into nucleic acids to produce dysfunctional molecules. Cytarabine is activated by the enzyme deoxycytidine kinase and inactivated by the enzyme cytidine deaminase. The responsivity of various tissue or tumor cells to cytarabine depends in large part on the ratio of activity of these two enzymes in the cells. Some tumor cells acquire resistance to cytarabine by reducing their complement of deoxycytidine kinase or by generating modified forms of the enzyme that are less active for the cytarabine substrate.

Pharmacokinetics Cytarabine is not reliably or well absorbed from the alimentary tract and is therefore employed intravenously. After IV injection, cytarabine is cleared from the plasma within 20 minutes. Less than 10% of a dose of cytarabine is excreted unchanged by the kidney. Most is metabolized by cytidine deaminase to arabinoxyl uracil. Cytarabine enters the cerebrospinal fluid. If administered intrathecally, cytarabine is cleared from the CSF with a half-life of 2 hours.

Clinical Indications Cytarabine is indicated for clients who have acute lymphocytic or granulocytic leukemias, in adults or children. It is employed primarily for initial induction of remission, alone or with other drugs such as thioguanine and daunorubicin. The cytotoxic effect of cytarabine is particularly exerted against the bone marrow, giving it a degree of selectivity for use in leukemias. Cytarabine has useful immunosuppressive properties but has been largely replaced by azathioprine and other newer agents for immunosuppression in conjunction with organ transplants (see Chapter 50).

Adverse Effects and Contraindications Because the effect of cytarabine is relatively selective for the bone marrow, toxicity of cytarabine is mainly due to excessive bone marrow suppression. Leukopenia, anemia, and thrombocytopenia are likely to develop. *Blood cell counts should be conducted daily during initial therapy.* Lymphocytes are less affected than other white blood cells. Other side effects of cytarabine include gastrointestinal disturbances, stomatitis, and rarely thrombophlebitis at the site of injection, hepatic dysfunction, fever, or dermatitis. Cytarabine may cause severe nausea, requiring pretreatment with an antiemetic.

Preparations and Administration *Cytarabine powder should be refrigerated until use. Solutions are stable at room temperature for 48 hours. Hazy solutions should be discarded.* Nurses should anticipate that alterations of drug dosage will frequently be necessary when cytarabine is employed because of toxicity. This should be explained to clients so that changes in the drug protocol are fully understood. Noncontinuous drug schedules are sometimes established to allow clients to tolerate larger amounts of drug.

Cytarabine (Cytosar)
Powder for injection
Typical Regimens: There are two alternative dosage schedules. One schedule calls for rapid IV injection of 100–200 mg/m^2/day for 5–7 days. The alternative schedule is 5–100 mg/m^2/day by continuous IV infusion for 5–7 days. For maintenance therapy, 1 mg/kg is given weekly or biweekly, but cytarabine is less effective in maintenance applications than for induction of remissions.

Azaribine (Triazure)

Mechanisms and Effects Azaribine is a prodrug that is converted to the active form, azauridine (AzUR), after administration. Azaribine provides two advantages over administration of azauridine. It is better absorbed from the intestines and it is less susceptible to metabolism by intestinal microorganisms to azauracil, a metabolite that contributes to CNS toxicity.

Pharmacokinetics Azaribine is well absorbed after oral administration. It is rapidly deacetylated to AzUR, which reaches peak plasma levels in 2–4 hours. AzUR disappears from the blood with a half-life of 6–8 hours by renal extraction and tissue uptake. AzUR undergoes intracellular conversion to 6-azauridylic acid (AzUMP), which inhibits formation of the uridylic acid required for DNA and RNA production by rapidly proliferating cells.

Clinical Indications Azaribine has therapeutic benefit in people afflicted with psoriasis, mycosis fungoides, or polycythemia vera. However, a possible link between use of the drug and occurrence of thromboembolic disorders has caused concern. Azaribine (Triazure) is currently available for investigational use only.

Adverse Effects and Contraindications The chief toxicity of azaribine is anemia, reticulocytopenia, and elevations in serum iron concentrations.

Preparations and Administration

Azaribine (Triazure)
Tablets
Typical Regimen: Doses of 270 mg/kg daily are employed in polycythemia vera in order to reversibly suppress erythropoiesis.

Purine Analogues

The purine analogues include drugs used systemically for treatment of leukemias (mercaptopurine and thioguanine); the leading immunosuppressive agent (azathioprine); a drug used parenterally for treating skin infections due to herpes simplex virus, type 1, or herpes zoster (vidarabine); and a drug used topically or parenterally for skin infections due to herpes simplex viruses, types 1 or 2, or herpes zoster (acyclovir). Vidarabine is discussed in Chapter 48 and acyclovir in Chapters 48 and 53; azathioprine is taken up in Chapter 50. Here we consider only the purine analogues employed in treatment of leukemias.

Mercaptopurine (Purinethol)

Mechanisms and Effects Mercaptopurine is an analogue of hypoxanthine. Mercaptopurine was the first effective immunosuppressive and antileukemia agent, and its introduction was an important advance in pharmacology. Like most other antimetabolites, mercaptopurine must be activated *in vivo* by conversion to its nucleotide form. This nucleotide inhibits the synthesis of the natural purines, with the result that these purines are not available for nucleic acid synthesis. Mercaptopurine is activated by the enzyme hypoxanthine-guanine-phosphoribosyltransferase (HGPRTase) and is inactivated by alkaline phosphatase or by xanthine oxidase. Resistance can develop to mercaptopurine due to either a decrease in HGPRTase or an increase in alkaline phosphatase.

Pharmacokinetics Mercaptopurine is readily absorbed after oral administration, reaching peak plasma levels in less than 2 hours. In the plasma, mercaptopurine is about 20% bound by plasma proteins. Allopurinol, an inhibitor of xanthine oxidase, will greatly potentiate the effect of mercaptopurine by blocking one avenue by which it is normally metabolized. The elimination half-life of mercaptopurine is about 90 minutes.

Clinical Indications Mercaptopurine is used primarily in maintenance therapy for acute leukemia, both lymphocytic and granulocytic varieties. It has been more effective in children than in adults, producing remissions in 40% of treated children. Mercaptopurine also has usefulness in maintenance therapy for chronic granulocytic leukemia but is less effective than busulfan. Mercaptopurine, like its congener, azathioprine, is an effective immunosuppressive agent.

Adverse Effects The principal adverse effect of mercaptopurine is excessive bone marrow suppression. Liver toxicity and gastrointestinal disturbances occur occasionally.

Preparations and Administration

Mercaptopurine (Purinethol)
Tablets
Typical Regimen: The usual dose is 2.5 mg/kg/day for induction and consolidation therapy for acute leukemia. For maintenance therapy, 1.5–2.5 mg/kg/day is employed. The total daily dose is given at one time.

Thioguanine

Mechanisms and Effects Thioguanine is an analogue of the purine base guanine. Thioguanine is activated by conversion into the nucleotide form, which may then be incorporated into DNA and RNA to produce dysfunctional nucleic acids. It may also produce a feedback suppression on synthesis of the natural purine bases. Malignant white blood cells occasionally develop resistance to thioguanine by decreasing activation of thioguanine.

Pharmacokinetics Thioguanine is employed orally. After oral administration, thioguanine is absorbed slowly, reaching peak levels only after 6–8 hours. Since xanthine oxidase does not play a major role in metabolism of thioguanine, concurrent administration of allopurinol does not significantly alter its activity or toxicity.

Clinical Indications Thioguanine is used principally for induction of remissions in acute lymphocytic or granulocytic leukemias, often in conjunction with cytarabine. It has been used in chronic granulocytic leukemias, but is less valuable than busulfan for this application. It is not useful for treatment of solid tumors.

Adverse Effects and Contraindications Thioguanine toxicity includes excessive bone marrow suppression.

Preparations and Administration

Thioguanine
Tablets
Typical Regimens: The initial starting dose of 2 mg/kg/day PO can be increased after 4 weeks to 3 mg/kg/day if there is no reduction in leukocytes or platelets at the lower dose. The daily dose is usually rounded off to the nearest multiple of 20 mg for simplicity of dosing. The daily dose is taken at one time.

Vinca Alkaloids

Mechanisms and Effects Two alkaloids derived from the periwinkle plant have been used in cancer chemotherapy: vincristine (Oncovin) and vinblastine (Velban). Vinca alkaloids bind to a type of cellular protein called *tubulin,* which is a constituent of the microfilaments that form in preparation for mitosis. Administration of vinca alkaloids has the effect of arresting the cell cycle as the cells begin cell division. Other cell functions that depend on the microtubules are likewise impaired, including phagocytosis, degranulation, intracellular transport, and motility. Vinca alkaloids are cell-cycle specific, exerting their cytotoxic effect exclusively on cells in the M-phase or, less commonly, in the S-phase.

Pharmacokinetics Vincristine and vinblastine are given by intravenous injection. Removal of vincristine and vinblastine from the blood is triphasic, involving primary tissue distribution (half-life of 4 minutes), liver extraction and biliary excretion (half-life of 52 minutes), and secondary redistribution (half-life of 18 hours). Toxicity of vinca alkaloids is exaggerated in individuals with obstructive jaundice.

Clinical Indications Clinical uses of the two vinca alkaloids are not identical (Table 56–6), despite their similar mechanism of action. Both agents are employed in combination regimens for Hodgkin's and non-Hodgkin's lymphomas. The MOPP regimen, for example, combines vincristine with mechlorethamine, procarbazine, and prednisone. Other applications are distinctive. Vincristine is used in treating people with cancers of the breast, lung, or cervix; in clients having sarcomas; and in children with a variety of solid tumors, including Wilm's tumor, Ewing's sarcoma, neuroblastoma, and rhabdomyosarcoma. Vinblastine, by contrast, is used in individuals with cancers of the testes, breast, or renal cells.

Adverse Effects The vinca alkaloids produce all the toxic manifestations characteristic of antineoplastic drugs — bone marrow suppression, alopecia, and gastrointestinal disturbances. In addition, neurologic toxicity is a limiting feature of the vinca alka-

Table 56–6
Comparison of Clinical Uses and Adverse Effects of the Two Vinca Alkaloids

Characteristic	Vincristine	Vinblastine
Clinical indications		
Lymphomas	Yes	Yes
Solid tumors of breast, lung, cervix	Yes	No
Pediatric tumors: Wilm's tumor, Ewing's sarcoma, neuroblastoma, rhabdomyosarcoma	Yes	No
Cancers of testes, breasts, and renal cells	No	Yes
Adverse effects		
Bone marrow suppression	+	++++
Neurotoxicity	++++	+
Alopecia	++	++
GI disturbances	+	+

Key: +, least severe; ++++, most severe.

loids. Common manifestations of neurotoxicity from vinca alkaloids include sensorimotor peripheral neuropathies, paresthesias, generalized weakness, hyporeflexia, and autonomic neuropathies resulting in pain, constipation, or urinary retention, diplopia, ptosis, facial weakness, jaw pain, depression, insomnia, and rarely, convulsions. *The nurse can monitor neurologic toxicity by checking reflexes and grip strength, looking for signs of ptosis, hoarseness, or motor difficulties, and chatting with the client in order to assess mental acuity.*

Neurologic toxicity is more severe with vincristine than vinblastine (Table 56–6) and is not always reversible when the drug is discontinued. On the other hand, vincristine produces relatively little suppression of the bone marrow, in comparison with vinblastine or the antineoplastic agents. Vincristine is thus an attractive drug for use in combinations with other antineoplastic agents that suppress the bone marrow to a significant extent. With vinblastine, leukopenia is often severe and is the most common adverse effect of this drug. Leukopenia caused by vinblastine reaches its peak intensity between 4 and 7 days after treatment and subsides in 14–18 days. Thrombocytopenia may also occur.

Preparations and Administration The reconstituted solution of vincristine is stable for up to 14 days under refrigeration. Vinblastine solutions are stable for up to 30 days if refrigerated. *The nurse should take care to avoid extravasation of the drug when injecting vinca alkaloids because both drugs are potent vesicants.*

Vinblastine (Velban)
Powder for injection
Typical Regimens: The usual dose is 0.1 to 0.2 mg/kg, IV, once weekly. Doses of both vincristine and vinblastine must be adjusted if hepatic disease or biliary obstruction is present.

Vincristine (Oncovin)
Powder for intravenous injection with diluent
Typical Regimen: The usual adult dose is 1.4 mg/m^2 in a single weekly dose; the maximum adult dose is 2.0 mg/m^2. In the MOPP regimen, the dose of vincristine is 2.0 mg/m^2, IV, on days 1 and 8.

Cytotoxic Antibiotics

Cytotoxic antibiotics are agents derived from fungi of the *Streptomyces* group. The first drugs in this group were the actinomycins of which dactinomycin (actinomycin D) is the only example in clinical practice.

Dactinomycin (Cosmegen)

Mechanisms and Effects Dactinomycin is a chromopeptide produced by a species of *Streptomyces.* Dactinomycin binds noncovalently to strands of DNA and thus inhibits DNA-directed RNA synthesis. Like the alkylating agents, dactinomycin is not cell-cycle specific, but its cytotoxic effect is exerted more on rapidly proliferating than on resting cells. Resistance sometimes occurs to the action of dactinomycin as a result of diminished uptake of the drug by tumor cells.

Pharmacokinetics Dactinomycin is given by intravenous injection. It is not significantly bound to plasma proteins and is rapidly cleared from the plasma. Dactinomycin does not enter the brain. It is excreted in both the bile and the urine, mostly (96%) as the unchanged drug. The elimination half-life is 36 hours.

Clinical Indications Dactinomycin is indicated for use in clients with testicular tumors and is employed in effective combinations for those with Wilm's tumor, Ewing's sarcoma, rhabdomyosarcoma, or gestational choriocarcinoma. The VAC Standard regimen for soft tissue sarcomas and rhabdomyosarcoma employs dactinomycin (*a*ctinomycin D) with *v*incristine and *c*yclophosphamide. Dactinomycin is active against other solid tumors but has been largely replaced for such applications by other agents.

Adverse Effects The major adverse effects of dactinomycin are the ones common to all neoplastic agents: bone marrow suppression, gonadal suppression, nausea and vomiting, and alopecia. Stomatitis, diarrhea, and mucositis also occur. Dactinomycin can cause severe erythema and even desquamation of skin areas previously exposed to radiation, a phenomenon referred to as "radiation recall."

Drug Interactions The nurse should anticipate drug interactions between dactinomycin and antigout drugs, since dactinomycin elevates uric acid levels. Dosage adjustments of antigout agents may be needed to control hyperuricemia and gout. Dactinomycin also decreases the effects of vitamin K, leading to prolonged clotting time and potential hemorrhage.

Preparations and Administration *Water containing preservatives such as benzyl alcohol or parabens should not be used to reconstitute dactinomycin, since these substances can cause precipitation of dactinomycin.* The reconstituted solution can be added to a 5% dextrose or saline infusate. *Cellulose ester membrane filters should not be employed during infusion of dactinomycin, since these can result in partial removal of the drug. Dactinomycin solutions are light-sensitive. Any unused portion of reconstituted solution should be discarded. When dactinomycin is injected directly, a double needle technique should be used because dactinomycin is a powerful vesicant.*

Dactinomycin (Cosmegen)
Powder for injection
Typical Regimen: 15 mcg/kg or 0.5 mg/m^2, IV, for 5 days, repeated every 3 or 4 weeks.

Doxorubicin (Adriamycin) and Daunorubicin (Cerubidine)

Mechanisms and Effects Doxorubicin and daunorubicin are closely related anthracycline antibiotics obtained from *Streptomyces peucetius.* Like dactinomycin, these cytotoxic antibiotics bind to DNA strands and inhibit DNA-directed RNA synthesis. The action of these agents is not cell-cycle dependent, but cells are most affected as they enter the S-phase of the cell cycle. Resistance occurs by an alteration in active transport of these substances into tumor cells.

Pharmacokinetics Both doxorubicin and daunorubicin are employed by intravenous injection, being very poorly absorbed after oral administration. After IV injection, uptake into all tissues except the brain occurs rapidly (half-life 12 minutes). The elimination half-life is rather long, about 30 hours for doxorubicin. A substantial fraction of doxorubicin is excreted in the bile unchanged, but daunorubicin is first metabolized in the liver before biliary excretion. Metabolites of both drugs appear mainly in the bile. Since hepatic clearance is the major factor in elimination of these drugs, toxicity is increased in individuals with hepatic dysfunction.

Clinical Indications Doxorubicin is among the most useful agents for treatment of people with carcinomas of the breast, ovaries, endometrium, bladder, genitourinary tract, thyroid, lungs, or stomach. It is also used in combination regimens for lymphomas and sarcomas. It is employed in the CAMP regimen with cyclophosphamide, methotrexate, and procarbazine or the MACC regimen with methotrexate, cyclophosphamide, and lomustine for lung cancer. It is also used in the CAF regimen with cyclophosphamide and fluorouracil for breast cancer. The CISCA regimen, in which doxorubicin is used with cyclophosphamide and cisplastin, is effective in treatment of clients with urinary tract cancers. Daunorubicin is used principally for treating people with acute granulocytic and lymphocytic leukemias. It is used in a combination regimen with cytarabine, prednisolone, and mercaptopurine for acute myelocytic leukemia in children.

Adverse Effects The most important toxic effects of doxorubicin and daunorubicin are cardiac toxicity and bone marrow suppression. These agents can cause transient cardiac arrhythmias and myocardial depression or chronic cardiotoxicity in up to 30% of individuals receiving more than 550 mg/m^2 of doxorubicin. *A baseline ECG should be conducted before therapy. The nurse should assess clients for early signs of cardiotoxicity: dyspnea, rapid pulse, hypotension, dysrhythmias, or steady weight gain.* Therapy with these drugs should be discontinued at the first sign of congestive heart failure. Bone marrow depression is manifested as leukopenia and a lesser degree of thrombocytopenia. Leukopenia reaches its peak intensity 10–14 days after initiation of therapy and subsides after 3 weeks. Gastrointestinal effects of daunorubicin and doxorubicin include nausea, vomiting, stomatitis, and esophagitis. Like dactinomycin, these drugs can cause dermatitis and radiation recall. Phlebitis and sclerosis can occur at the site of injection. Doxorubicin can impart a deep red coloration to the urine.

Preparations and Administration *The nurse should avoid contact of the drug with the skin during preparation of doxorubicin solutions. Reconstituted solutions are stable for 24 hours at room temperature or 48 hours under refrigeration (4–10° C). The solution is light-sensitive. Any remaining solution should be discarded after use.* Intravenous injections should be given slowly, over no less than 3–5 minutes. Doxorubicin is a vesicant and extravasation can lead to local reactions. Local erythematous streaking along the vein and/or facial flushing may be indicative of too rapid an infusion rate.

Nurses should wear gloves while preparing solutions of daunorubicin. After reconstitution, the solution is stable for 24 hours at room temperature or 48 hours under refrigeration. The solution is light-sensitive. Daunorubicin is a vesicant. *Nurses administering daunorubicin should observe the precautions for vesicants (Table 56–3).*

Doxorubicin (Adriamycin)
Powder for injection
Typical Regimen: 60–75 mg/m^2 for 3 weeks when the drug is used alone or 30–50 mg/m^2 when used in combination regimens.

Daunorubicin (Cerubidine)
Powder for injection
Typical Regiman: The recommended IV dose is 30–60 mg/m^2 daily for 3 days. When used in combination with cytosine arabinoside, daunorubicin is given at 45 mg/mm^2/day IV on days 1, 2, and 3 with 100 mg/m^2/day of cytosine arabinoside by IV infusion daily for 7 days for the initial course. For subsequent courses, daunorubicin is given only on days 1 and 2, and cytosine arabinoside for 5 instead of 7 days.

Bleomycin (Blenoxane)

Mechanisms and Effects The bleomycins were isolated from a Japanese actinomycete called *Streptomyces verticillus.* Bleomycins are copper-chelating glycopeptides that interact with molecular oxygen to produce superoxides that cut DNA chains. Bleomycins also bind to DNA strands to inhibit RNA synthesis.

Pharmacokinetics Bleomycin is poorly absorbed and thus is employed parenterally, by IM, IV, or SC routes. After parenteral administration, bleomycin distributes widely. Its disappearance is biphasic: the initial phase half-life is about 1.3 hours and the terminal phase half-life is about 9 hours. Renal excretion accounts for about two-thirds of elimination, but in some tissues, bleomycin is metabolized by bleomycin hydrolase. This enzyme is lacking from the skin and lungs, so these tissues develop higher concentrations of bleomycin and are major sites of toxicity. The toxicity of bleomycin is increased in clients experiencing pronounced renal impairment.

Clinical Indications Bleomycin has a wide range of antitumor activity against squamous-cell carcinomas. It is employed in the VBP regimen in combination with *v*inblastine and cisplatin (*P*latinol) for testicular tumors, a combination that provides a high cure rate in this form of cancer. Bleomycin is also useful in treatment of clients with squamous-cell carcinomas of the head, neck, esophagus, genitourinary tract, cervix, vulva, scrotum, penis, rectum, and vulvovaginal area.

Adverse Effects A positive feature of bleomycin is the low incidence of bone marrow suppression. However, mucocutaneous reactions occur with a high frequency, including stomatitis, ulceration, alopecia, hyperpigmentation, hyperkeratosis, erythema, pruritus, and vesiculation. *Early signs of mucocutaneous irritation include complaints of swelling and hyperesthesia of the hands and redness or swelling over pressure points of the body. The nurse should monitor the client's skin condition and provide for skin care and periods of mobility. Oral membranes should be inspected regularly. If bucal membranes become ulcerated, nurses should advise clients to rinse the mouth frequently with warm water, and to use a soft toothbrush for the teeth and an unwaxed dental floss for flossing at least once a day. Clients should be advised to avoid highly acidic food and drinks or coarse foods.* Mucocutaneous symptoms may recur when other antineoplastic agents are employed within 6 weeks after bleomycin.

Bleomycin can also cause anaphylactoid reactions. Therefore, chills, sweating, dehydration, or anuria should be immediately recorded and reported. A test dose of 2 units of bleomycin may be given prior to the first full dose to determine if the client is hypersensitive, especially in clients with lymphomas since they have increased risk of anaphylactoid reactions. Diphenhydramine may be given prophylactically as a precaution; epinephrine is given if an anaphylactoid reaction develops.

Pulmonary fibrosis occurs in up to 20% of those treated with bleomycin and can be fatal. Monitoring of diffusion capacity for carbon monoxide can help reveal early subclinical pulmonary toxicity. *The nurse should question the client about occurrence of dyspnea, chest pain, or cough, and check for rales by auscultation.* Individuals over 70 and those who have received prior radiation therapy directed to the chest area are at increased risk of severe pulmonary fibrosis. Pulmonary toxicity is also increased when cumulative doses exceed 400 units; therefore total doses greater than 400 units should be given with extreme caution.

Although adverse reactions involving hematopoietic tissue are rare in response to bleomycin, the nurse should instruct clients to report any unexplained bleeding or bruising promptly.

Preparations and Administration The potency of bleomycin is standardized by bioassay. *After reconstitution in sterile water (for IM or SC injection) or in normal saline or glucose (for IV solutions), bleomycin is stable for 24 hours at room temperature.*

Bleomycin Sulfate (Blenoxane)
Powder for injections
Typical Regimens: The recommended dose is 10–20 units/m^2/week by IV or IM injection; or 10–15 units/m^2 for 3–7 days by continuous IV or intraarterial infusion. The latter method provides better response.

Plicamycin (Mithramycin)

Mechanisms and Effects Plicamycin is another chromomycin antibiotic. It is produced by *Streptomyces tanashiensis.* Plicamycin binds to DNA to inhibit

DNA-regulated transcription. It also appears to have a direct effect on bone, blocking the effect of administered parathyroid hormone. The effect on bone appears to be exerted directly on osteoclasts. A single injection of plicamycin (25 μg/kg) can lower serum calcium significantly in 24–48 hours.

Clinical Indications Plicamycin is limited by severe toxicity to use in advanced embryonal tumors of the testes and life-threatening hypercalcemia associated with tumors or Paget's disease.

Adverse Effects and Contraindications The relatively low doses (12.5–25 μg/kg, every 4–7 days) of plicamycin employed in hypercalcemia produce few side effects — mainly nausea and mild thrombocytopenia. The higher doses (25–50 μg/kg for 5 days or on alternate days for 2 weeks) used for clients with testicular cancer produce severe toxicity, including a high degree of thrombocytopenia, hemorrhage, and azotemia. Mortality rates from plicamycin-induced hemorrhage, may be as high as 25% when high doses are employed. Hemorrhage is caused by a combination of suppression of clotting factor synthesis, thrombocytopenia, and vascular effects. *The nurse should watch closely for indications of bleeding; purpura, hemoptysis, oral bleeding, or tarry stools.* Antineoplastic doses of plicamycin can also cause liver and kidney damage, hypocalcemia, and hypophosphatemia. Rebound hypercalcemia may occur following plicamycin-induced hypocalcemia.

Preparations and Administration Plicamycin is a vesicant; extravasation may result in local tissue necrosis.

Plicamycin (Mithracin)
Powder for injection
Typical Regimen: 25–30 μg/kg/day for 8–10 days, not to exceed 30 μg per dose or 10 days duration.

Mitomycin (Mutacycin)

Mechanisms and Effects Mitomycin is derived from *Streptomyces caespitosus.* Mitomycin is an alkylating agent, producing cross-links in DNA between guanine and cytosine base pairs. It exerts its cytotoxic effect when cells enter the early S-phase of the cell cycle.

Pharmacokinetics After IV injection, mitomycin rapidly leaves the plasma, entering most tissues but not the brain.

Clinical Indications Mitomycin has limited value, exerting a palliative effect in squamous-cell carcinomas of the head, neck, lungs, breasts, and cervix, and adenocarcinomas of the stomach, pancreas, colon, and breasts.

Adverse Effects and Contraindications The major toxic effect of mitomycin is severe, long-lasting bone marrow suppression (reaching peak intensity in 4–6 weeks). It also produces nausea and vomiting, neurotoxicity, renal toxicity (glomerular damage), flu-like symptoms (malaise, fever), dermatologic reactions, and interstitial pneumonia. *Complete blood cell counts should be conducted frequently for at least 7 weeks after administration of mitomycin. The client should be closely monitored for signs of infection. The nurse should monitor the client's fluid intake and output and ensure hydration because of the risk of nephrotoxicity.*

Preparations and Administration The drug solution is light-sensitive. Extravasation will cause local irritation.

Mitomycin (Mutacycin)
Powder for injection
Typical Regimen: The recommended dose is 10–20 mg/m^2, IV, once every 6–8 weeks.

Hormone and Hormone Antagonists in Cancer Chemotherapy

Hormones and hormone antagonists have limited value in cancers related to tissues that are targets of endocrine regulation. Hormones sometimes employed for treatment of specific cancers include glucocorticoids, progestins, androgens, estrogens, and gonadotropin-releasing hormone analogs. Antiestrogens are the only hormone antagonists currently employed in cancer chemotherapy.

Glucocorticoids

Glucocorticoids suppress proliferation of lymphocytes and leukocytes and are thus useful in acute and chronic lymphocytic leukemia, lymphomas, and multiple myelomas. In addition, glucocorticoids are useful in certain nonhematologic tumors such as breast and prostatic carcinomas. Glucocorticoids are especially useful in providing symptomatic relief of the hemolytic anemia, thrombocytopenia, and hemorrhage that often accompany lymphomas and lymphocytic leukemias. Glucocorticoids also help to improve the psychological status of clients with malignancies because of their mood-elevating influence.

Prednisone is the most widely used glucocorticoid for neoplasms, but dexamethasone or parenteral hydrocortisone are suitable alternatives. Prednisone is widely used in combination regimens (Table 56–7). Adverse effects of glucocorticoids are discussed in Chapter 32. In general, adverse effects with short courses of therapy are minimal but with long courses, serious toxicity can develop, including adrenal suppression.

Progestins

Progestins are used in treating clients who have endometrial carcinomas, renal cell carcinomas, or breast carcinomas. Progestins produce an involution (shrinkage) of tissues that are target tissues for this hormone. Progestins are relatively free of adverse effects even at the high doses used for neoplastic disorders. Progestins may increase the incidence of thromboembolic disorders such as thrombophlebitis, myocardial infarcts, and pulmonary embolisms. The progestational agents most frequently used in cancer chemotherapy are medroxyprogesterone acetate (Depo-Provera), hydroxyprogesterone caproate (Delalutin), and megestrol acetate (Megace). Medroxyprogesterone and hydroxyprogesterone are given intramuscularly; megestrol is given orally.

Table 56–7
Some Antineoplastic Combination Regimens Utilizing Prednisone

Indication	Regimen	Other drugs	Dose of prednisone
Acute lymphocytic leukemia, induction	VP	Vincristine	60 mg/m²/day, PO, for 4 weeks, taper during weeks 5–7
Acute myelocytic leukemia in children	ADPM	Cytarabine	40 mg/m²/day, PO, daily until remission
Breast cancer	CMFVP	Cyclophosphamide Methotrexate Fluorouracil Vincristine	0.75 mg/kg/day, PO, days 1–21, then taper
Chronic lymphocytic leukemia	CP	Chlorambucil	100 mg/day, PO, 2 days every other week
Hodgkin's disease, induction	BCVPP	Carmustine Cyclophosphamide Vinblastine Procarbazine	60 mg/m²/day, PO, days 1–10 of 28-day cycle
	MOPP	Mechlorethamine Vincristine Procarbazine	40 mg/m²/day, PO, days 1–14 of 28-day cycle
Multiple myeloma	MP	Melphalan	75 mg/m²/day, PO, days 1–7 of 28-day cycle
	M-2	Vincristine Carmustine Cyclophosphamide Melphalan	1.0 mg/kg/day, PO, days 1–7, then taper 8–21 of 35-day cycle
Non-Hodgkin's lymphoma	CVP	Cyclophosphamide Vincristine	100 mg/m²/day, PO, days 2–6 of 21-day cycle
	CHOP	Cyclophosphamide Doxorubicin Vincristine	60 mg/day, PO, days 1–5 of 21- or 28-day cycle

Androgens

Androgens have been used in treating women who have advanced breast cancer because they produce a regression of metastatic breast tumors. Hormonal therapy with androgens or estrogens for breast cancer is reserved for clients who cannot be treated effectively with surgery or radiotherapy. Androgens are employed only in premenopausal women. Tumor regression occurs in approximately 25–30% of women treated with androgens. Fluoxymesterone (Halotestin) has been the agent most widely employed. Calusterone (Methosarb) and testolactone (Teslac) are also employed. These drugs are less virilizing than testosterone itself or its esters. Nevertheless, masculinization is a potential adverse effect. Other adverse effects of androgens include nausea and vomiting (which can be minimized by starting with low doses), salt and water retention, hypercalcemia, hepatotoxicity, and increased libido.

Preparations and Administration

Calusterone
Tablets
Typical Regimen: The recommended dose is 200 mg/day orally in 4 divided doses.

Fluoxymesterone (Halotestin, Ora-Testryl, and generic)
Tablets
Typical Regimen: The recommended dose for breast cancer is 20–30 mg/day PO in 3 divided doses for at least 2 months.

Estrogens

Estrogens are used to promote involution of carcinomas of the breast and prostate. Estrogen-induced remissions average 6 months to a year, but average survival time is not increased by therapy with estrogens. Responsiveness of women with breast cancer to estrogen therapy is dependent on hormonal status and presence or absence of estrogen receptors (ER). Postmenopausal clients who are ER-positive based on biopsy evaluation are most likely to respond to estrogen therapy. ER-negative clients seldom respond. In premenopausal women, estrogens may accelerate the neoplastic process. Premenopausal women are most likely to benefit from oophorectomy (removal of the ovaries).

The use of estrogens in cancer of the prostate is based on their ability to antagonize the influence of androgens on this gland. It has long been recognized that androgens produced by the testes maintain the prostate gland and contribute to neoplastic proliferative activity of malignant prostate cells. Treatment of prostatic carcinoma is based on the concept of androgen-control therapy. If prostatic cancer is identified prior to metastasis, combined use of estrogens and bilateral orchiectomy provide the greatest chance of remission. If metastasis has already occurred, estrogen and orchiectomy offers no advantage over orchiectomy alone.

Diethylstilbestrol and ethinyl estradiol are the estrogens most often employed. Diethylstilbestrol is used in doses of 15 mg/day in 3 divided doses for breast cancer and 1 mg/day for prostatic cancer. Male clients may experience gynecomastia, women may experience changes in libido, and both sexes may experience nausea, vomiting, fluid retention, and hypercalcemia.

Estramustine (Emcyt)

Estramustine is a molecule that combines estradiol and nornitrogen mustard. It is indicated for use in metastatic or progressive carcinomas of the prostate. It is marginally more effective in this application than diethylstilbestrol and is effective in about 20% of males with advanced prostatic cancer that is refractory to estrogens.

Estramustine produces adverse effects typical of the estrogens, such as increased risk of thrombosis and myocardial infarction and electrolyte imbalances involving calcium and phosphorus. Estramustine has mutagenic potential.

Preparations and Administration

Estramustine (Emcyt)
Capsules
Typical Regimen: The recommended dose is 14 mg/kg/day PO in 3 or 4 divided doses for 30–90 days. Therapy may be further extended if a favorable response is obtained.

Antiestrogens

Antiestrogens, tamoxifen (Nolvadex) and nafoxidine, have proven useful in breast cancer. Antiestrogens are most useful if biopsy is ER-positive. Approximately 15% of breast tumors in premenopausal women are ER-positive, while two-thirds are ER-positive in postmenopausal women. Antiestrogens bind to the estrogen receptors and suppress growth of estrogen-dependent tumors. Antiestrogens are useful in combination with oophorectomy since estrogen continues to be produced by the adrenal glands. Approximately 40% of clients respond to tamoxifen to some degree and 10–15% experience complete remissions.

Tamoxifen is slowly but well absorbed after oral administration, reaching peak blood levels (about 0.1 mEq/ml) in 4–7 hours. The drug accumulates selectively in estrogen sensitive tissues. The terminal half-life for elimination is 7 days. Adverse effects of tamoxifen include leukopenia, hot flashes, nausea and vomiting, skin rashes, pruritus vulvae, headache, lassitude, dizziness, dysgeusia, and leg cramps. *Blood cell counts should be monitored periodically. Neurologic symptoms such as confusion or somnolence should be reported immediately to the physician. Clients may experience a marked increase in bone pain due to metastatic disease during the first few days of tamoxifen therapy and may require increased doses of pain medication during that time.* The increase in pain is sometimes correlated with a positive response to the treatment. *Tamoxifen tablets should be stored between 59 and 86° F and protected from light.*

Preparations and Administration

Tamoxifen (Nolvadex)
Tablets
Typical Regimen: The recommended dose is 20–40 mg PO daily in 2 divided doses. Tumor regression typically occurs after 4–10 weeks. Therapy should be continued at least 6 weeks to determine responsiveness.

Gonadotropin-Releasing Hormone Analogue

Leuprolide (Lopron) is an analogue of gonadotropin-releasing hormone (GRH) that desensitizes the receptors for GRH in the pituitary gland when given chronically in therapeutic doses. The result is a suppression of gonadotropin secretion by the pituitary and a consequent reduction in gonadal steroids—testosterone in males and estrogens in females. The reduction in gonadal hormones occurs after 2–4 weeks of daily treatment and is preceded by a transient increase in these hormones. In males, the ultimate extent of suppression of androgens is comparable to that achieved by castration. In females, estrogen secretion in premenopausal women is reduced to postmenopausal levels.

Leuprolide is currently approved as a palliative treatment for patients with advanced prostatic cancer, as an alternative to orchiectomy or estrogens when these are either not indicated or unacceptable to the individual. The most frequent adverse effect of leuprolide, hot flashes, occurs in half of treated individuals. Other side effects are uncommon and generally comparable to those produced by the estrogenic agent diethylstilbestrol: edema (in 8% of clients), gynecomastia or breast tenderness (3% of clients), impotence (2%), neurologic symptoms (paresthesias, pain, headache, dizziness), and gastrointestinal symptoms (nausea, vomiting, anorexia, and constipation). Rare but serious adverse reactions have included cardiac dysrhythmias, hematuria and reduced hematocrit, dyspnea, and gastrointestinal bleeding. Because of the transient rise in gonadal hormones, leuprolide may briefly increase symptoms of prostatic cancer. *Nurses should advise clients not to discontinue medication without consultation with the physician. Clients should be warned about possible pain at the site of injection and should be instructed to notify the physician if this becomes severe. Leuprolide should be refrigerated until use.*

Preparations and Administration

Leuprolide acetate (Lopron)
Injection solution
Typical Regimen: The usual regimen is 1 mg SC once daily.

Miscellaneous Antineoplastic Drugs

L-Asparaginase (Elspar)

Mechanisms and Effects Some tumor cells are unable to manufacture the amino acid L-asparagine and must take it up from the blood in order to continue proliferation. Such cells can be inhibited by depleting the blood of L-asparagine. This can be accomplished by administration of the enzyme L-asparaginase. L-asparaginase catalyzes conversion of asparagine to aspartic acid and ammonia. The L-asparaginase used in cancer chemotherapy is derived from two bacterial species: *Escherichia coli* and *Erwinia carotovora.* The commercially available product comes from *Escherichia coli.* Erwinia L-asparaginase is available from the National Cancer Institute.

Pharmacokinetics L-Asparaginase is given by IV or IM injection. After absorption, the drug is largely retained within the vasculature compartment, where it is gradually metabolized. Some inactivation also occurs due to binding to antibodies. L-asparaginase does not distribute significantly into the cerebrospinal fluid and is not filtered by the kidneys. Its elimination half-life ranges from 6 to 30 hours.

Clinical Indications L-Asparaginase is employed principally for treatment of acute lymphocytic leukemia, less frequently for lymphomas. Complete remissions are achievable with this drug in up to 60% of clients. L-asparaginase is useful in combination regimens because it produces little of the bone marrow suppression that is typical of other antineoplastic agents and because it does not produce cross-resistance with other drugs. For example, L-asparaginase is a useful addition to the VP regimen for acute lymphocytic leukemia which employs vincristine and prednisone.

Adverse Effects The principal adverse effects of L-asparaginase are hypersensitivity reactions. This is not surprising since this drug is a foreign protein. Urticarial skin rashes occur in up to 20% of clients treated with L-asparaginase and severe anaphylactic reactions in 5–10%. Individuals given L-asparaginase should be hospitalized and pretreated with antihistamines. *The nurse should observe closely for signs of an allergic reaction such as angioderma, urticaria, skin eruptions, dyspnea, bronchospasm, or hypotension. In addition, the nurse should make certain that epinephrine and a glucocorticoid are at hand during treatment.*

Gastrointestinal symptoms occur commonly with L-asparaginase, including nausea, anorexia, and weight loss. Gastrointestinal ulcerations do not occur, but pancreatitis, often leading to hyperglycemia, is a frequent problem. *Therefore, nurses should teach clients the signs of pancreatitis and advise diabetic clients that L-asparaginase can elevate blood sugar levels.* Mild fever is frequently reported. L-Asparaginase also causes varying degrees of hepatic dysfunction, including diminished levels of clotting factors and albumin proteins, and elevations in serum transaminases. Severe hepatoxicity may occur, but in less than 5% of cases. *The nurse should encourage clients to report immediately symptoms such as itching, yellowed skin, discoloration of the sclera, or joint pain that may indicate hepatic toxicity.* CNS toxicity occurs in varying degrees in about 30% of clients. CNS symptoms include drowsiness, cognitive impairment, confusion, and coma. *Clients should be warned that neurologic symptoms may continue for several weeks after discontinuation of the drug.*

Preparations and Administration L-Asparaginase (Elspar) is derived from *E. coli*. *Before initiating therapy, an intradermal skin test is performed.* Desensitization must be conducted in individuals who exhibit a positive reaction to the skin test. A negative skin test does not preclude an allergic reaction to the treatment dose.

L-Asparaginase (Elspar)
Powder for injection
For individuals allergic to L-asparaginase derived from *E. coli*, Erwinia asparaginase is available from the National Cancer Institute.

Typical regimens: 1,000 IU/kg/day, IV, for 10–14 days or 6,000 IU/m^2, IM, 3 times daily for 3–4 weeks. When employed with the VP regimen, the recommended dose of L-asparaginase is 10,000 units/m^2/day, IV, for 14 days.

Cisplatin (Platinol)

Mechanisms and Effects Cisplatin is a novel antineoplastic agent. It is an inorganic complex of the metallic ion platinum. It is a potent antineoplastic agent with broad antitumor activity but severe toxicity. Cisplatin binds to DNA in a manner similar to alkylating agents, and like the alkylating agents, its action is not cell-cycle specific.

Pharmacokinetics After IV administration, cisplatin is highly bound (79%) in the plasma by proteins but is taken up by tissues with a distribution half-life of 25–50 minutes. Cisplatin does not enter the brain to a significant degree. Cisplatin is eliminated only very slowly by renal excretion with a half-life of 2–4 days.

Clinical Indications Cisplatin is indicated especially for metastatic tumors of the testes and ovaries. It is widely used in the VBP regimen with bleomycin and vinblastine for testicular cancer; with doxorubicin for ovarian tumors; and in the CISCA regimen with cyclophosphamide and doxorubicin for carcinomas of the urinary tract. Cisplatin exhibits activity against tumors of the head, neck, cervix, prostate, and lungs as well. It has been employed successfully in treating clients with osteogenic sarcoma. The VBP regimen for testicular cancer produces complete remissions in 50–70% of clients.

Adverse Effects Like other heavy metal compounds, cisplatin can produce renal toxicity. Clients with compromised renal function should not be given this drug. Renal function tests, including creatinine clearance and blood urea nitrogen (BUN) should be conducted before initiation of therapy. During the first few days of treatment, increases in BUN and creatinine can be expected. Proteinuria and excretion of renal enzymes is also likely to occur. However, because of excess magnesium loss, nurses may expect clients to experience hypomagnesia, weakness, and tetany. *Creatinine clearance should be reevaluated before each dose of cisplatin and the drug should be withheld if the measured value is less than 50 ml/minute. Vigorous hydration and the use of an osmotic diuretic can reduce the incidence of renal toxicity from 30% to 5% of clients. Nurses should monitor the intake and output of clients receiving cisplatin.*

Nausea and vomiting caused by cisplatin are particularly severe. Even with vigorous antiemetic therapy, nausea and vomiting may be severe enough to require hospitalization. Some clients refuse further cisplatin therapy because of the severity and persistence of the nausea produced.

Cisplatin produces less bone marrow toxicity than most other antineoplastics. Leukopenia reaches peak intensity 2–3 weeks after drug administration and subsides after 3–5 weeks. Thrombocytopenia and anemia also occur. RBC transfusions may be required. *Blood cell counts should be monitored for 3 weeks after each treatment.*

Cisplatin is ototoxic, frequently causing high-frequency hearing loss and less frequently midrange hearing loss. *Clients should be instructed to report occurrence of tinnitus or loss of auditory acuity.* Anaphylactic reactions to cisplatin have been reported. Peripheral neuropathies, such as paresthesias, weakness, and tremors may occur.

Preparations and Administration The dry powder is stable up to 2 years if refrigerated at 2–8° C. After reconstitution (in sterile water), the solution is stable for 20 hours at room temperature.

Cisplatin (Platinol)
Powder for injection
Typical Regimens: Cisplatin is given by IV infusion. In the VBP regimen for testicular tumors, cisplatin is given in a dose of 20 mg/m^2/day, IV, for 5 days every 3 weeks for 3 courses. When used with doxorubicin for ovarian tumors, the recommended dose is 50 mg/m^2, IV, once every 3 weeks (along with doxorubicin, 50 mg/m^2, IV, once every 3 weeks). When used alone, cisplatin is administered at 100 mg/m^2, IV, once every 4 weeks.

Hydroxyurea (Hydrea)

Mechanisms and Effects Hydroxyurea is a derivative of urea that has antitumor potency in granulocytic leukemia. Its benefit is its ability to sharply and rapidly reduce levels of circulating granulocytes. It is used for this purpose for clients who have acute and chronic myelocytic leukemia. It is also used to a limited extent in those with renal cell carcinomas, malignant melanomas, and advanced ovarian cancer. The mechanism of action of hydroxyurea is not established, but the drug appears to exert an inhibitory effect on DNA synthesis without altering RNA production.

Pharmacokinetics Hydroxyurea is readily absorbed after oral administration, reaching peak serum levels in under 2 hours. It is eliminated mainly by renal excretion with a half-life of 2–3 hours. About one-third of the administered dose is excreted unchanged. The drug should be used with extreme caution if renal function is significantly impaired.

Adverse Effects Bone marrow suppression is a prominent adverse effect. White blood cells are especially depressed. Leukopenia occurs typically 4–7 days after a 2-week treatment protocol and subsides 10–14 days after the termination of drug therapy. Thrombocytopenia occurs only occasionally. Hydroxyurea can also adversely affect production of red blood cells, but only transiently, causing a self-limited megaloblastic erythropoiesis. *Blood cell counts should be determined frequently, prior to and during therapy. Hydroxyurea should be discontinued if WBC count falls below 2,500/mm^3 or if platelets fall below 100,000/mm^3.*

Alimentary symptoms are not frequent with hydroxyurea but can include nausea, vomiting, anorexia, diarrhea, constipation, or stomatitis. Dermatologic reactions such as rash, facial erythema, and alopecia are likewise infrequent. Neurologic reactions are very rare and mild, consisting of headache, dizziness, disorientation, hallucinations, and convulsions. Hydroxyurea has been reported to cause transient impairment of renal tubular function. Periodic measurements of blood urea nitrogen and creatinine should be conducted.

Preparations and Administration

Hydroxyurea (Hydrea)
Capsules
Typical Regimen: For resistant chronic myelocytic leukemia, the recommended schedule is 20–30 mg/kg/day in a single oral dose. For solid tumors of the head and neck (excluding the lip) hydroxyurea is used either in the 20–30 mg/kg/day continuous regimen or in an intermittent regimen of 80 mg/kg, in a single oral dose, every third day. Hydroxyurea can be combined with radiation therapy in the treatment of solid tumors of the head and neck, in which case the intermittent regimen is employed. The recommended trial period is 6 weeks after which therapy can be continued indefinitely if response is satisfactory.

Mitotane (Lysodren)

Mechanisms and Effects Mitotane is a derivative of the insecticide DDT. Its exclusive clinical application is for carcinomas of the adrenal cortex. Mitotane is toxic to adrenocortical cells and thereby produces a reduction in tumor size and secretory activity. The action of mitotane is exerted equally on malignant and normal cells of the adrenal cortex. It therefore has the capacity for inducing adrenocortical insufficiency. Production of corticosteroids should be monitored during therapy. Corticosteroid supplementation is frequently required and mineralocorticoids are sometimes administered as well.

Pharmacokinetics Mitotane is employed orally, but its absorption is incomplete. Like its insecticide relative, mitotane tends to accumulate in adipose tissue.

Clinical Indications Mitotane is indicated only in the treatment of clients with inoperable adrenocortical carcinoma and Cushing's syndrome. Mitotane treatment is purely palliative; it does not provide a cure in any treated individuals. Brain damage and functional impairment may result from administration of high doses of mitotane. Intermittent courses of therapy generally result in failure to respond after three or four courses.

Adverse Effects and Contraindications Mitotane causes nausea and vomiting, diarrhea, and dermatitis. With long-term use, neurologic effects may occur, including lethargy, depression, brain damage, dizziness, and somnolence. Ocular toxicities occur rarely, including blurred vision, diplopia, lens opacities, and retinopathy.

Preparations and Administration

Mitotane (Lysodren)
Tablets
Typical Regimen: Therapy is usually initiated at 2–10 g/day in 3 or 4 divided doses. The maximum tolerated dose ranges from 2–6 g/day but is usually in the 8–10 g range.

Procarbazine (Matulane)

Mechanisms and Effects Procarbazine is a synthetic hydrazine derivative first recognized as having antitumor activity in the 1960s. During its metabolism, procarbazine initially forms azo-procarbazine, hydrogen peroxide, and hydroxyl free radicals. The latter two products react with DNA to inhibit DNA synthesis and DNA-directed transcription and translation. There is no cross-resistance between procarbazine and other antineoplastic drugs.

Pharmacokinetics After oral administration, procarbazine is rapidly and completely absorbed. Procarbazine readily crosses the blood-brain barrier, equilibrating between plasma and the cerebrospinal fluid. Procarbazine is rapidly eliminated from plasma by uptake into tissues but is excreted slowly, mainly in the urine as metabolites.

Clinical Indications Procarbazine is employed most frequently in treatment of Hodgkin's and non-Hodgkin's lymphomas. Originally it was employed in single-drug regimens and was observed to produce tumor regression in over half of treated individuals. Unfortunately, the remissions were short-lasting, typically 1–3 months. It is now used mainly in combination regimens such as the MOPP regimen for Hodgkin's disease with mechlorethamine, vincristine, and prednisone; and in the POCC regimen for lung cancer with vincristine, cyclophosphamide, and lomustine. The MOPP regimen produces complete remissions in approximately 80% of clients with Hodgkin's disease.

Adverse Effects and Contraindications Procarbazine frequently produces leukopenia, anemia, and thrombocytopenia due to bone marrow suppression. *The nurse should assess the client for bleeding, noting such indications as petechiae, purpura, epistaxis, hemoptysis, hematemesis, or melena. Clients should be advised to report unusual bleeding or bruising tendencies.* Infections may occur during treatment due to leukopenia, with symptoms such as cough, pneumonitis, sore throat, and hoarseness. *Clients should be advised to report immediately to the physician symptoms of cough, shortness of breath, thickening of bronchial secretions, fever or chills, or sore throat.*

Procarbazine commonly causes nausea and vomiting, and less frequently stomatitis, dysphagia, diarrhea, and constipation. *Nurses should advise clients to expect loss of appetite. In addition, nurses should instruct them to report tarry stools or bloody vomitus.* Nausea and vomiting is minimized by utilizing reduced doses (2–4 mg/kg/day) for the first week of procarbazine therapy. Tolerance to the nausea-inducing effect of procarbazine often occurs after the first week.

Flu-like symptoms may occur with initial therapy, including myalgia and arthralgia, chills and fever, sweating, lethargy, weakness, and fatigue. *These should be recorded and reported.* Dermatologic reactions to procarbazine include rash, pruritus, hyperpigmentation, alopecia, and herpes infections. Procarbazine can cause photosensitivity and photophobia. *Clients should be advised to avoid prolonged exposure to sunlight.* Mild hypotension may occur and is additive with that produced by potent diuretics.

Neurologic effects are a particular problem with procarbazine. *Nurses should instruct clients to report headache, dizziness, tremors, or paresthesia.* Convulsions, coma, or evidence of ataxia should be reported as well as any behavioral changes such as confusion. Psychiatric symptoms may include depression, apprehensiveness, insomnia, hallucinations, and nightmares. *Clients should be warned that driving or other potentially hazardous tasks may be especially dangerous while receiving procarbazine because of drowsiness, blurred vision, confusion, or dizziness caused by the drug.* CNS toxicity is increased by concurrent use of sedative-hypnotics, alcohol, antihistamines, narcotics, neuroleptics, or other CNS depressants. Procarbazine should be discontinued if significant neurotoxicity occurs, such as paresthesias, confusion, or neuropathies. Procarbazine is a potential teratogen. *Clients should be urged to employ contraceptive measures during treatment with procarbazine.*

Drug and Nutrient Interactions Procarbazine inhibits monoamine oxidase (MAO) and has a disulfiram-like action. Tricyclic antidepressants, MAO inhibitors, sympathetic amines, phenothiazines, and tyramine-containing foods should not be employed during procarbazine administration. *Clients should be instructed to refrain from use of alcohol (especially sherry, chianti wines, and beer), aged and natural cheeses, yogurt, yeast extract, sour cream, chocolate, coffee, colas, pickled herring, meat tenderizers, chicken liver, avocados, broad beans, pineapple, raisins, figs, or ripe bananas — all sources of tyramine.* The pressor effect of tyramine is greatly exaggerated when this amine is ingested by a person receiving a drug with MAO-inhibiting properties. Procarbazine may increase the hypoglycemic effect of insulin and oral hypoglycemic agents.

Preparations and Administration

Procarbazine (Matulane)
Capsules
Typical Regimens: The recommended regimen is 4–6 mg/kg/day until WBC count falls below 4,000/mm^3, platelets drop below 100,000/mm^3, or a maximum response is achieved. During the first week of therapy, use of smaller doses (2–4 mg/kg/day) helps to reduce the incidence of nausea and vomiting. If a favorable response is achieved with procarbazine, the dose can be reduced for maintenance to 1–2 mg/kg/day. When employed in the MOPP regimen for Hodgkin's disease or the POCC regimen for lung cancer, the recommended dose of procarbazine is 100 mg/m^2/day, orally, on days 1–14 of the 28-day cycle.

Etoposide (VePesid)

Mechanisms and Effects Etoposide was approved in 1983 for use in combinations with other antineoplastic agents for refractory testicular tumors. This drug is a derivative of podophyllotoxin, a naturally occurring alkaloid found in American mandrake. Etoposide prevents the progression of cells into mitosis and is most lethal to cells in the S-phase or G_2-phase of the cell cycle.

Clinical Indications The combination of etoposide with bleomycin and cisplatin is highly effective in achieving remissions in testicular carcinomas.

Adverse Effects and Contraindications Adverse effects of etoposide include significant bone marrow suppression (leukopenia and thrombocytopenia), nausea and vomiting (in 30% of clients), allergic reactions (in 1% of clients), reversible alopecia (in 100% of clients), and hypotension when the drug is given by rapid intravenous injection. Leukopenia reaches peak severity in 8–10 days and subsides after 3 weeks.

Preparations and Administration

Etoposide (VePesid)
Powder with a vehicle composed of polyethylene glycol, ethyl alcohol, and polysorbate.
Typical Regimen: After dilution in 5% dextrose or normal saline to a concentration of 0.2–0.4 mg/ml, a dose of 50–100 mg/m^2/day is given in a 30–60 minute IV infusion for 5 days every 3–4 weeks. Alternatively, 100 mg/m^2/day can be given on days 1, 3, and 5.

Interferon Alfa-2

Mechanisms and Effects Interferons are a family of endogenous proteins released by macrophages, T lymphocytes, and tissue cells. The natural interferons have antiviral activity (see Chapter 48) and modulate immune responses (see Chapter 46). The natural interferons are classified into three types: alpha, beta, and gamma. The alpha type, which has at least sixteen subtypes, is released by macrophages and tissue cells. It is very potent in inhibiting viral penetration into uninfected cells and in stimulating natural killer cells to suppress proliferation of tumor cells. Beta interferon is less potent in inhibiting viral penetration but has similar antitumor activity. Gamma interferon differs from the other two types. It is a lymphokine released by sensitized T lymphocytes that serves mainly to stimulate activity of macrophages. In a limited number of clinical trials, gamma interferon has not exhibited significant antitumor activity.

Recently, techniques have been developed for producing alpha interferon by recombinant DNA technology. This is accomplished by isolating the gene from human T cells responsible for directing synthesis of alpha interferon, removing the relevant segment of the DNA chain, and splicing it into the DNA of an *Escherichia coli* cell. As the *E. coli* cells reproduce, they also make interferon. After a period of incubation, the cells are killed and the interferon is extracted and purified. Two subtypes of alpha interferon, called interferon alfa-2a and interferon alfa-2b, have now been marked as anticancer agents. Thus far, there is no evidence of differences between the two in any of their effects.

Pharmacokinetics After IM or SC injection, peak concentration occurs in about 4 hours for interferon alfa-2a and in 6–8 hours for interferon alfa-2b. Interferons are cleared from the blood primarily by renal excretion. Doses must therefore be adjusted quickly at the first indication of renal impairment. In healthy people, the elimination half-life averages 5 hours for interferon alfa-2a and 6–7 hours for interferon alfa-2b.

Clinical Indications Currently, the two interferon preparations are approved only for the treatment of hairy-cell leukemia in patients 18 years or older. This relatively rare type of cancer gets its name from the presence of hairlike projections on the lymphoid cells that line peripheral blood vessels and the bone marrow and which proliferate excessively to cause this chronic form of leukemia. The symptoms of hairy-cell leukemia are fatigue, anemia, frequent infections, and easy bruising, all of which are attributable to pancytopenia. Prior to the advent of interferon, clients with hairy-cell leukemia required splenectomy and later, in most cases, frequent transfusions of red blood cells and platelets. Hairy-cell leukemia responds to doses of interferon that are smaller than those required to achieve regression of most other kinds of tumors. Some complete remissions of hairy-cell leukemia have occurred after interferon therapy, but most responses are partial and relapse usually occurs after interferon injections are discontinued. After additional clinical studies, other indications will probably be approved for interferon.

Adverse Effects and Contraindications A flu-like syndrome occurs initially in nearly every client treated with interferon, including symptoms of fever, chills, headache, muscle aches, and fatigue. *Nurses will need to forewarn clients and their families about this reaction, because it comes on abruptly (about 3 to 6 hours after interferon administration) and would otherwise be quite alarming.* The flu-like symptoms can be minimized by giving acetaminophen immediately before the interferon dose and every 3 to 4 hours thereafter as required. Aspirin and other antipyretics are not recommended since these can interfere with the effect of interferon. *Since the initial chills are followed by a rise in temperature (usually reaching a peak of 102° to 104° F), nurses should refrain from overdoing the provision of warm beverages or additional blankets when the patient experiences chills, since these measures can aggravate the subsequent rise in temperature. Provision of oral fluids to replace fluid lost from sweating is important during the period of fever.* Low-grade fever may persist up to 20 hours after interferon. Cardiovascular symptoms accompanying the flu-like syndrome can be significant if the client has a prior history of cardiovascular difficulties. Hypotension, hypertension, tachycardia, chest pain, and, rarely, myocardial infarction and sudden cardiac death have all been reported following interferon administration.

Other common neurological side effects include confusion, nervousness, impatience, and depression. *Clients should be cautioned against engaging in hazardous activities following administration of interferon.* At high doses, more severe neurological toxicities include paranoia, feelings of impending doom, and cognitive deficits (which can be evaluated by assessing the client's performance of simple calculations).

Gastrointestinal symptoms include alterations in taste, anorexia, nausea, and diarrhea. Anorexia caused by interferon may result in significant weight loss, but the weight is recovered after the drug is discontinued. *Nurses should ensure that clients receiving interferon are provided with nutritional counseling to avoid potential nutritional deficits.* Potential dermatological responses to interferon therapy include rash, pruritus, dry skin, diaphoresis, and reactivation of herpes infections.

Brief reductions in all classes of blood cells have been observed after interferon administration. However, these hematological reactions are much less severe with interferon than with other antineoplastic drugs. Other side effects reported in response to interferon have included impotence, peripheral neuropathy, and transient elevations of serum transaminases (indicative of mild liver toxicity). Most adverse effects of interferon are dose dependent and therefore occur less often when the drug is being used for hairy-cell leukemia, since this condition responds to relatively low doses of the drug. Administration of interferon preparations is contraindicated for clients who are allergic to any component of the particular product. Safety of interferon preparations has not been established for children under 18 or for women who are pregnant or are breast-feeding infants.

Preparations and Administration Clients who are receiving long-term maintenance therapy with interferon may be expected to inject themselves. *Nurses will need to teach these clients injection techniques similar to those employed for subcutaneous injection of insulin (see Chapter 33), including site selection, rotation of sites, accurate measurement of doses, and handling of syringes.*

Interferon Alfa-2a (Roferon-A)
Injection powder or solution
Recommended Doses: For hairy-cell leukemia, 3 million International Units (IU), IM or SC, for 16 to 24 weeks. For maintenance in hairy-cell leukemia, 3 million IU three times per week.

Interferon Alfa-2b (Intron A)
Injection powder
Recommended Doses: For hairy-cell leukemia, 2 million International Units (IU)/sq meter, IM or SC, three times per week.

Important Nursing Implications for Antineoplastic Agents

- ☐ Obtain complete baseline data before initiating cancer chemotherapy, including blood tests, weight, and intake/output ratio.
- ☐ Determine the likely course of bone marrow suppression for each drug being employed. Instruct clients accordingly to avoid risk of infection, stress, and trauma during periods of bone marrow suppression. Monitor blood cell counts and examine the skin for signs of candida overgrowth.
- ☐ If the drug causes thrombocytopenia, monitor the client for indications of occult bleeding such as petechiae, ecchymoses, tarry stools, easy bruising, or bleeding of the gum or nose.
- ☐ During periods of nausea, serve solids and liquids separately and avoid greasy or heavy foods.
- ☐ Advise clients to maintain meticulous oral hygiene during cancer chemotherapy with frequent rinsing. A soft-bristled brush should be employed. Advise clients to discontinue flossing if the platelet count falls below 15,000 and brushing as well if the platelet count falls below 10,000.
- ☐ Since antineoplastic drugs can activate latent infections, teach clients to monitor for and recognize indications of candida overgrowth, such as furry patches on the tongue or oral membranes, foul-smelling stools, vaginal or rectal itchiness, or diarrhea.
- ☐ Teach clients to report signs of hepatotoxicity such as frothy, dark urine, light-colored stools, yellowing of the skin or sclera, and pruritus.
- ☐ Advise women receiving antineoplastic agents to utilize an effective means of birth control throughout the period of treatment and for several months thereafter. Nurses who are pregnant or breast-feeding should not be involved in preparing solutions of antineoplastic agents.
- ☐ Warn younger clients that antifertility effects of antineoplastic drugs are sometimes irreversible.
- ☐ Avoid extravasation when administering antineoplastic drugs by infusion. Avoid contact of drug solutions with the skin. Wear latex gloves while preparing solutions. If contact does occur with the skin or mucous membranes, immediately irrigate the tissue with large amounts of water.
- ☐ Carefully follow instructions for storage and reconstitution for each antineoplastic agent.

Radiopharmaceutics

Radioisotopes in Cancer Therapy

Radioisotopes should be used only by physicians and associated health professionals specifically trained in their use and handling under licensure by appropriate government agencies.

Phosphorus ^{32}P

Phosphate is required by all cells for metabolism, especially during cell proliferation. Administered phosphate tends to accumulate in those tissues where cells have a rapid rate of proliferation, including neoplastic cells and normal cells of the bone marrow and lymphatic tissue. Ultimately, the largest proportion of administered phosphate is accumulated by bone, but initially the drug appears in the soft tissues. Sodium phosphate-^{32}P emits a beta particle that irradiates and kills the cells in which the drug has accumulated. Unfortunately, the effect is not adequately selective and radioactive bombardment of the bone marrow and bone tissue after a dose of sodium phosphate-^{32}P can lead to bone marrow suppression, leukopenia, anemia, and thrombocytopenia.

Nurses need to assess clients who have received phosphate-^{32}P therapy for signs of infection as well as bleeding tendencies. If infection is likely, clients need to be placed in well-ventilated, reverse isolation units. Air is not recircu-

lated and nurses and other care providers must wear gowns and gloves. Visitors must either wear mask and gown or visit through windows. Food must be sterilized prior to eating as must all utensils that come into client contact. The loneliness accompanying this isolation often leads to depression and a feeling of powerlessness. The nurse will need to provide emotional support.

Sodium phosphate-^{32}P has been used primarily for treatment of clients with polycythemia vera, chronic myelocytic leukemia, and chronic lymphocytic leukemia. Chemotherapy is preferred. Use of sodium phosphate-^{32}P can itself result in neoplasm of the bone marrow. The potential hazards of ^{32}P with respect to pregnancy, fertility, and lactation are not established. When employed in clients with severe polycythemia vera, the recommended intravenous dose of sodium phosphate-^{32}P is 2.5–5 millicuries (mCi). In chronic leukemia, doses from 6–15 mCi are employed. *Nurses should administer oral doses of this drug when the client has had no food for several hours in order to increase the amount absorbed.*

Radioactive phosphate-^{32}P can also be delivered to target tissues in the form of chromic phosphate-^{32}P. This compound is used in treatment of peritoneal or pleural effusions caused by metastatic disease. It is administered by intraperitoneal or intrapleural instillation. It should not be used in the presence of ulcerative tumors. The dose for intraperitoneal instillation is 10–20 mCi; for intrapleural instillation the dose is 6–12 mCi.

Iodine ^{131}I

In addition to its uses in diagnosing thyroid conditions and in treating hyperthyroidism, ^{131}I is indicated in treatment of selected cases of carcinoma of the thyroid. After administration of sodium iodide-^{131}I, the radioactive iodide is rapidly accumulated by the thyroid. The stomach and salivary glands concentrate iodide to a lesser extent. Radioactive iodide produces irradiation that is 90% due to beta radiation and 10% due to gamma radiation.

When using ^{131}I, patients, visitors, and medical personnel must be protected from exposure to radiation. Use of ^{131}I should be avoided in women during pregnancy, and, when possible, in any women under 30 of childbearing potential. Radioiodide is excreted in breast milk; therefore, breast-feeding should be discontinued for the duration of ^{131}I therapy.

Adverse effects of ^{131}I include depression of the hematopoietic system (with large doses), nausea and vomiting, chromosomal abnormalities, and acute thyroid crisis. *The nurse should assess the patient for signs of tenderness or swelling of the neck, pain upon swallowing, sore throat, or cough. These symptoms usually occur about 3 days after treatment. Analgesics can be given to alleviate such symptoms.* Some patients experience delayed thinning of the hair, 2 or 3 months following therapy. The nurse should reassure clients that this is a transient side effect. Doses of ^{131}I for carcinoma must be determined individually, but the typical dose is 50–150 mCi.

Gold ^{198}Au

Gold-198 is an isotope with a brief half-life of 2.7 days, emitting both beta and gamma radiation. It has been employed infrequently in treatment of brain tumors because of its lack of diffusibility. The ^{198}Au is injected directly into the tumor. The procedure is dangerous and offers no advantages over chemotherapy.

Radiosensitizers and Radioprotectors

Radiosensitizers and radioprotectors are currently experimental. The ionizing effects of radiation are most pronounced on cells that are well oxygenated. Cancer cells that are located deep within tumors are often poorly vascularized and somewhat hypoxic and thus are poorly responsive to radiation therapy. **Radiosensitizers** are chemicals that are free radicals. They selectively attach to hypoxic cells, substituting for oxygen in sensitizing the cells to the effects of radiation. One such agent being tested experimentally for use as a radiosensitizer is misonidazole.

Radioprotectors operate in the opposite way. They are free radical scavengers. Radioprotectors selectively enter the well-oxygenated cells that are more characteristic of normal tissue. Radioprotectors have the effect of protecting normal tissue cells from radiation.

Case Study: Cancer

J. A., a 57-year-old married woman, discovered a lump in her left breast during a self-examination and made an appointment with her physician to have it evaluated. The physician scheduled her for a biopsy, which revealed a carcinoma 3 cm in diameter with involvement of two lymph nodes. J. A. agreed to a radical mastectomy and postsurgical chemotherapy. J. A. was 6 years postmenopausal but the tumor tissue was estrogen receptor negative. The physician elected to employ the CAF regimen for eight cycles (see Table 56–1). This meant that J. A. would be in the hospital for an 8-day period during each 4 weeks over the next 6 months. The nurse worked out a calendar with J. A.

Before the first cycle of chemotherapy, the nurse obtained complete blood cell counts and an ECG. She recorded J. A.'s height and weight and from these calculated her body surface area. The nurse discussed with J. A. the potential adverse effects of the drugs that were to be employed. She told her that she might experience loss of hair, but that her hair would grow back, although it might be different in color or texture. She told her to be careful not to brush her hair vigorously during the period of cancer chemotherapy as this would increase hair loss. She explained to J. A. that her skin and fingernails might become darker and her skin more sensitive to light. She advised J. A. to avoid exposure to sunlight during this period of therapy.

She explained to J. A. that she would have an increased risk of infection during the period that she was receiving the antineoplastic drugs and should avoid contact with crowds and people with colds. She told J. A. to report any occurrence of sore throat, cold symptoms, or fever. J. A. was also advised that the drugs being employed could increase bleeding tendencies and that she should report any bruising or evidence of bleeding.

The nurse told J. A. that one of the drugs being given might cause her urine to turn red but that this was harmless. However, in order to minimize the possibility of bladder irritation, J. A. should drink at least 1.5 quarts of water daily while receiving drug therapy and should report any painful urination.

During the periods of hospitalization, J. A. received doxorubicin and fluorouracil by intravenous infusion. The nurse took care to prevent extravasation and told J. A. to report any pain or inflammation at the site of infusion. The nurse gave J. A. prochlorperazine an hour before initiating the infusions. During the infusions, a scalp tourniquet was applied to minimize subsequent alopecia.

The nurse also told J. A. that she should observe for swelling of the ankles, shortness of breath, congestion in the lungs, or productive cough and report these to the physician or nurse immediately. J. A. was also told to note and report any abdominal pain, nausea during the period that the drugs were not being taken, and sores in the mouth.

To reinforce these points of client education, the nurse provided J. A. with a card itemizing the instructions relating to her regimen. The nurse talked with J. A. each time she came to the hospital about the mastectomy, the reaction of her husband, family, and friends, and the chemotherapy. During these conversations the nurse had the opportunity to assess J. A.'s adjustment to her medical difficulties, which was very positive under the circumstances. The nurse took care to promote a cheerful atmosphere in J. A.'s hospital room during the therapy and J. A. received frequent visits and excellent support from her family.

After the completion of the eighth cycle of CAF therapy, J. A. was examined regularly at 6-month intervals. She remained in remission with no recurrence of breast cancer after 5 years.

1. What is the CAF regimen?
2. Why did the nurse obtain baseline blood cell counts and ECG?
3. Why do antineoplastic drugs cause hair loss? Gastrointestinal disturbances? Increased risk of infection?
4. What did the nurse have in mind when she instructed J. A. to report any swelling of the ankles, shortness of breath, congestion in the lungs, or productive cough?
5. Why did the nurse administer prochlorperazine an hour before the infusion of doxorubicin and fluorouracil?

Answers appear at the end of the book.

Recommended Readings

American Cancer Society: *Cancer Facts & Figures.* New York, American Cancer Society, 1986.

Anderson RW et al: Risks of handling injectable antineoplastic agents. *Am J Hosp Pharm* 1982;39:1881–1887.

Ballentine R: Nursing implications of cancer chemotherapy. *Nursing* 1983;13(7):56A–56B.

Barlock AL, Howser DM, Hubbard SM: Nursing management of adriamycin extravasation. *Am J Nurs* 1979; 79(1):94–96.

Bergemann D: Handling antineoplastic agents. *Amer J I.V. Therapy Clin Nutrition* 1983;10:13.

Bubela H: Is your client at risk for respiratory complications? *Can Nurse* 1983;79(3):46–48.

Burns N: *Nursing and Cancer.* Philadelphia, WB Saunders, 1982.

Carter SK: Cancer chemotherapy: New developments and changing concepts. *Drugs* 1980;20:375–397.

Chabner B: *Pharmacologic Principles of Cancer Treatment.* Philadelphia, WB Saunders, 1982.

Daeffler R: Oral hygiene measures for patients with cancer (parts 1 & 2). *Cancer Nurs* 1980;3(5):347–356, 3(6):427–432.

D'Arcy PF: Reactions and interactions in handling anticancer drugs. *Drug Intell Clin Pharm* 1983;17:532–538.

Elbaum N: With cancer patients, be alert for hypercalcemia. *Nursing* 1984;14(8):58–59.

Fredette SL, Gloriant FS: Nursing diagnoses in cancer chemotherapy in theory. *Am J Nurs* 1981;81(11):2013–2019.

Gever LN: Cisplastin. A breakthrough for the cancer patient. A nursing challenge for you. *Nursing* 1980; 10(12):53.

Gever LN: Metoclopramide — relief for cancer chemotherapy patients. *Nursing* 1984;14(4):87.

Horton J, Hill E (eds): *Clinical Oncology.* Philadelphia, WB Saunders, 1977.

Hughes CB: Giving cancer drugs: Some guidelines. *Am J Nurs* 1986;86(1):34–38.

Koch PM: Thrombocytopenia. *Nursing* 1984;14(10):54–57.

Larson D: Treatment of tissue extravasation by antitumor agents. *Cancer* 1982;49(5):1796–1799.

Lurn JLJ et al: Nursing care of oncology patients receiving chemotherapy. *Nurs Res* 1978;27:340–346.

McHugh MK: Deciphering diagnostic studies: White blood cell tests. *Nursing* 1982;12(1):10–15.

Miller SA: Nursing actions in cancer chemotherapy administration. *Oncology Nursing Forum* 1980;7:8–16.

Schaffner A: Safety precautions in home chemotherapy. *Amer J Nurs* 1984;84(3):374.

Smith FP, McCabe MS: Preventing chemotherapy-induced alopecia. *Am Fam Physician* 1983;28(1):182–184.

Thomas NP et al: Preparing cancer patients to administer medication. *Patient Counsel Health Educ* 1982;3(4): 137–143.

Tobin BK: Hazards hidden on the job: parenteral antineoplastic drugs. *Nursing Life* 1985;5(5):45–49.

Valentine AS, Stewart JA: Oncologic emergencies. *Am J Nurs* 1983;83(9):1282–1285.

Wroblewski SS, Wroblewski SH: Caring for the patient with chemotherapy-induced thrombocytopenia. *Am J Nurs* 1981;81:746–749.

UNIT XIII

Toxicology

CHAPTER 57

Toxicology: Principles and Applications

Toxicology and pharmacology are allied disciplines. Toxicology differs from pharmacology in two respects. First, toxicology is concerned with adverse effects of substances on the body, while pharmacology addresses all actions, beneficial, harmful, or neutral. In this regard, the focus of toxicology is narrower than that of pharmacology. Second, toxicology concerns itself with all classes of chemicals, while pharmacology is concerned only with drugs. In this respect, toxicology has a broader range of concern than pharmcology. All drugs are potentially toxic, but certain drugs, because of widespread availability or low therapeutic index, are more frequently encountered in poisonings than others. These are the drugs most likely to be studied by the toxicologist. One type of toxic reaction to chemicals, the adverse drug reactions, were discussed in Chapter 3. This chapter addresses principles of toxicology and treatment of poisonings, which are reactions to excessive amounts of drugs or other chemicals, usually from inadvertent contact or ingestion.

Principles of Toxicology

Risk Assessment

The concept of risk assessment is as fundamental to toxicology as the dose-response principle is to pharmacology. In fact, the two concepts are interrelated. The reader should review the portions of Chapter 3 pertaining to the dose-response relationship, graded and quantal dose-response curves, and determination of the LD_{50}, ED_{50}, and therapeutic index of a drug (pp. 23–45). The LD_{50} of a drug (the dose that is lethal to 50% of a population of laboratory animals) provides a preliminary indication of the potential of a substance for toxicity, but there is a vast range of possible adverse effects that do not necessarily bear a predictable relationship to the LD_{50}. In addition, the LD_{50} of a drug may vary substantially from species to species even after differences in mass or surface area are taken into account. For example, the LD_{50} when expressed in milligrams per kilogram of body weight, is typically about 10 times smaller in humans than in common laboratory animals such as rats, mice, rabbits, cats, or dogs.

Most adverse effects are dose dependent, occurring with increasing frequency and severity as doses of a drug or extent of contact with environmental chemicals is increased. However, allergic and idiosyncratic reactions are exceptions to the concept of dose dependency. Allergic reactions are responses of the immune system to drugs and generally occur with a severity that is largely independent of the amount of substance taken into the body or contacting the skin. Idiosyncratic reactions are genetically determined adverse responses of unusual severity that occur in a group of individuals who possess the particular genes. Responses in this group of individuals are statistically distinct from the distribution of responses for the remaining population. Examples include sensitivity of individuals with glucose-6-phosphate dehydrogenase deficiency to oxidant drugs and exaggerated reaction of individuals with a deficiency of pseudocholinesterase to succinylcholine.

Toxicity that either is delayed after acute exposure to a drug or that occurs only with chronic exposure presents special difficulties with respect to assessment. Carcinogenic effects of chemicals may not be manifested until 20–30 years after exposure. Moreover, occurrence of cancer may, in some instances, reflect the accumulated toxic influences on nucleic acids that have been exerted by many different mutagenic compounds encountered over several decades. The most popular of the social drugs, alcohol, nicotine, and caffeine, are notable for their severe toxic effects on various bodily tissues when employed chronically in spite of the relative absence of acute adverse effects associated with these drugs.

The toxicity of a drug can only be evaluated in the context of the doses required for its beneficial effects. Similarly, the toxicity of nondrug substances must be appraised in light of estimates as to the extent of exposure of individuals to the substance when it is employed for its useful applications. Toxicity is thus an expression of expected incidence and severity of adverse reactions to a substance at the levels of exposure typically encountered clinically or environmentally. The concept of toxicity is closely related to **margin of safety** or **therapeutic index** of drugs as described in Chapter 3. No chemical substance is entirely free of the potential for toxicity. All drugs and nondrug substances produce adverse effects that could ultimately cause death at some level of exposure.

If the chemical substance in question is one that is employed or proposed for employment for commercial, cosmetic, nutritional, or medical applications, the likely level of exposure is that which is required to achieve the intended beneficial application. Risk assessment, under these circumstances, is a two-step process. The first step is the evaluation of likely adverse consequences to individuals, society, and the environment. The second step is the assessment of the extent to which the estimated risk is acceptable in light of the anticipated benefits to be derived from use of the compound. The assessment of risk can be a complex sociopolitical phenomenon, involving questions of need for substances, alternatives, extent of use, economic impacts, and environmental impacts. With respect to drugs, a higher level of risk is acceptable when the drug is one that is used for a potentially fatal disease for which there may not be adequate alternative treatments than when the drug is proposed for palliative treatment of a self-limited condition. We routinely employ drugs in cancer chemotherapy that have a potential for toxicity that would be totally unacceptable in a preparation for the common cold.

Preclinical Evaluation of Drug Toxicity

Every new drug under development is required by law to proceed through several kinds of preclinical studies (Table 57–1). Acute studies proceed first because of their relative simplicity and low cost. The drug is tested acutely in at least four species of laboratory animals — usually mice, rats, rabbits, and dogs — to determine its LD_{50} in each species. At least two routes of administration are employed including the one most likely for ultimate clinical use. A substantial percentage of compounds being screened for possible clinical use can be ruled out on the basis of the acute studies alone, if the LD_{50} is low in relation to the dose required for the proposed beneficial effect.

Subchronic studies are conducted next. In this kind of study, the drug is usually administered for 90 days in two species, usually rats and dogs. Three dosage levels are studied, the proposed therapeutic dose, a somewhat higher dose, and one frankly toxic but nonlethal dose. Such studies help to determine

Table 57–1
Preclinical Evaluation of Drug Toxicity

1. Acute studies	Determination of the LD_{50} in four animal species (typically mice, rats, rabbits, and dogs).
	At least two routes of administration (typically IP and PO), including the one(s) expected to be employed clinically.
2. Subchronic studies (typically 90 days)	Determination of hematology, organ toxicity, and other parameters of toxicity.
	Three dosage levels (therapeutic level, intermediate level, and a frankly toxic but not fatal level).
	Two species (usually rats and dogs).
3. Chronic studies (6 months to 2 years)	Same parameters as in subchronic study.
	At least two dosage levels (therapeutic and somewhat toxic levels).
	Length of study determined by intended length of exposure in proposed clinical applications, but at least 6 months.
	Usually in rats and mice.
	Can be concurrent with clinical trials.
4. Special tests	Teratogenicity
	Perinatal and postnatal toxicity
	Effects on fertility
	Mutagenicity
	Carcinogenicity
	Corrosiveness

if there is cumulative toxicity from repeated administration of the drug. At the end of the study, each experimental animal is examined by a pathologist. Measurements include hematologic evaluation, clinical chemistry, gross and histopathologic evaluation of various organs, and measurement of body weight.

Chronic studies are often undertaken concurrent with clinical trials and may last up to 2 years. At least two dosage levels are studied. The parameters measured are the same as those for the subacute studies.

In addition, special tests of toxicity may be required for certain drugs depending on the proposed applications. Special tests may evaluate potential influences on reproductive function including fertility effects, teratogenicity, or prenatal and postnatal development. The need to evaluate teratogenicity of drugs was made painfully apparent by the thalidomide tragedy of the late 1950s and early 1960s in which administration of the drug thalidomide to women during their first trimester of pregnancy resulted in birth defects, mainly phocomelia (see Figure 57–1), in hundreds of babies. Drugs proposed for topical use will be studied for local toxicity on the eyes, skin, or other tissue to which the drug might be applied.

The mutagenic and carcinogenic (cancer-causing) potential of drugs requires special attention because such effects are frequently irreversible and could occur with a single exposure. Since carcinogenic influences of drugs may occur after an extended latency period, standard acute, subacute, or even chronic studies may not reveal carcinogenic po-

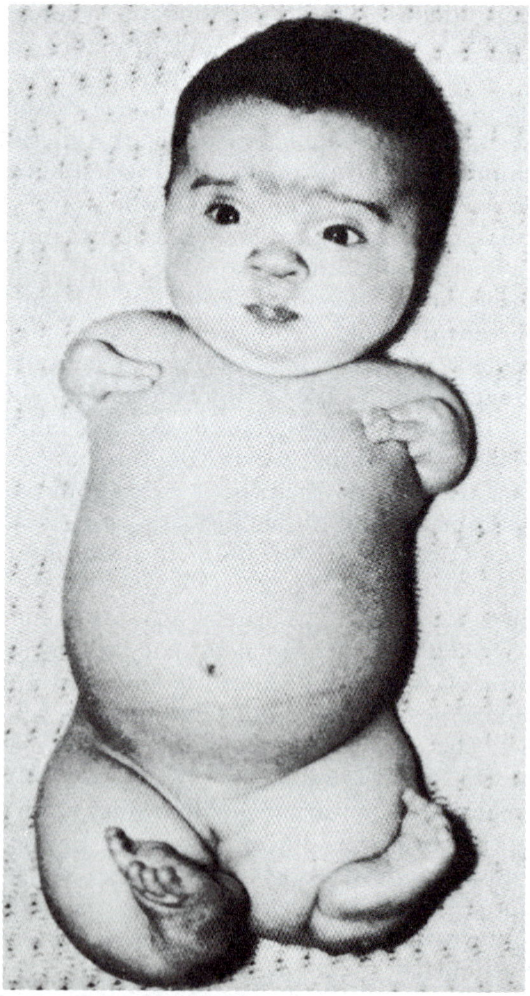

Figure 57–1
Phocomelia in a 6-month-old female as a result of thalidomide teratogenicity. From Department of Medical Illustrations, Welsh National School of Medicine, Cardiff.

tential of drugs. Some drugs (primary carcinogens) are carcinogenic in their own right, but more frequently drugs act as procarcinogens, yielding carcinogenic metabolites after activation by liver enzymes. Thus, it is important that both new drugs and their metabolites be tested. The likelihood that a drug will cause cancer is often judged by testing its mutagenicity (that is, its ability to cause changes in DNA) since this is often closely correlated with its carcinogenicity.

Incidence of Poisonings

Although there are no firm data on the overall incidence of poisonings in the United States, estimates indicate that there are 2–5 million poisonings a year. Only a small fraction of poisonings and overdoses culminate in death. The mortality statistics published by the U. S. Department of Health and Human Services, Public Health Service for 1981 (Table 57–2), the latest data available, indicates that 6,499 drug overdoses occurred, 882 fatal poisonings by other solid or liquid substances, and 3,970 poisonings by gases, mainly carbon monoxide. This resulted in a total of over 11,000 fatal poisonings of which 5,400 were suicides, about 5,000 accidental deaths, and 48 homicides. Narcotic overdoses show unusual yearly fluctuations based on the relative success of law enforcement efforts in relation to drug trafficking of illegal opiates. Barbiturate overdoses have been declining gradually with the ascendancy of benzodiazepine hypnotics, which are less likely to produce toxicity.

Mortality associated with chronic drug toxicity is far more widespread than acute poisonings (Table 57–3). Alcohol is responsible for an estimated 80% of the more than 30,000 deaths each year due to liver cirrhosis, as well as more than 5,000 deaths attributed to alcohol dependence, 300 to delirium tremens, and 30 associated with alcohol psychosis. Tobacco is thought to be responsible for 90% of the current epidemic of lung cancer fatalities. In addition, alcohol, caffeine, and nicotine contribute to heart disease; alcohol contributes to arteriosclerosis; nicotine and caffeine to peripheral vascular disorders; and nicotine and alcohol to cerebrovascular accidents, all important factors in mortality. Alcohol use is estimated to be involved in more than 50% of automobile fatalities, 18% of fatal home accidents, and 13% of fatal occupational accidents. Cigarettes are responsible for one-third of fatalities associated with household fires.

A positive note in the toxicity statistics is a 60% reduction in poisoning in children over the last 8 years. Accidental poisonings occur most commonly in children in the 2- to 3-year-old age group. The agents most often involved are aspirin, insecticides, plants, soaps, solvent cleaners, detergents, bleaches, and cold pills. In about half of cases, the substance responsible for the poisoning was not in its original container. Most of the reduced incidence of poisoning in infants and toddlers is thought to be due to improved packaging of drugs, household cleansers, and other household chemicals. Better education of parents has also contributed. *Advising parents to keep drugs and other toxic chemicals out of the reach of children is an important nursing responsibility. Nurses should also advise parents to record the telephone number of the nearest poison control center in a handy location.*

Principles of Treatment for Poisonings

Telephone Assessment

Often the first contact with a victim of poisoning (or the parent if the victim is a child) is by telephone. In many cases, exposure to a chemical does not result in poisoning and it would be inappropriate to send every individual to an emergency room. Telephone assessment is therefore an important initial screening that requires thoughtful evaluation of the potential severity of poisoning. The following information should be obtained:

1. the name and telephone number of the caller
2. the age of the victim of possible poisoning
3. the identity of the substance or product (by trade or brand name and category) ingested or otherwise contacted
4. the ingredients of the substance if specified on the label; if not, the name and address of the manufacturer
5. the estimated quantity ingested
6. the estimated time of exposure
7. symptoms being exhibited by the victim
8. any medical conditions the victim has
9. medications being used by the victim
10. treatment steps taken thus far

If telephone assessment indicates that emergency treatment is warranted, the person acting on behalf of the victim should be instructed to take along the container of the substance suspected to be involved in the poisoning. When poisoning results from a suicide attempt, it should be borne in mind that such victims frequently provide inaccurate information concerning the ingested substance.

Table 57–2
Incidence of Fatal Poisonings by Substances in 1981

Substance or Class	Self-administered	During medical intervention	Suicides	Homicides	Undetermined accidental or intentional	Total	Percentage males
Sedative-hypnotics	155		500		83	738	46.7
Barbiturates	81		387		59	527	46.1
Alcohol	6					6	83.3
Other	68		113		24	205	47.3
Analgesics and antipyretics	768	8	295		214	1285	46.5
Narcotics	405						
Salicylates	74						
Other	289						
Psychotherapeutic agents	243		806		138	1193	39.9
Antidepressants	130						
Phenothiazines	27	4					
Benzodiazepines	50						
Other tranquilizers	13	2					
Hallucinogens	3						
Stimulants	20						
Anesthetics						170	72.4
General		8					
Local	156	6					
Other CNS drugs	42	4				46	71.7
Autonomic drugs	11	2				13	84.6
Endocrine drugs	22	12				34	58.8
Cardiovascular drugs	202	7				209	41.6
Hematologics and antigout	44	9				53	37.7
Anti-infectives	57	23				80	46.3
All other drugs	956	116	1,129		363	2,564	42.7
Total all drugs	2,656	201	2,730	31	881	6,499	50.2
Other solids and liquids	569		248	3	62	882	66.6
Gases	1,280		2,453	14	223	3,970	72.2
Carbon monoxide	(985)			(1,676)	(206)	(2,867)	
Venoms	54					54	85.2
ALL FATAL POISONINGS	4,559	201	5,431	48	1,116	11,405	59.6

Table 57–3
Relationship of Drugs to Principal Causes of Mortality

Cause of mortality	Percentage of total	Contribution of drugs to incidence
Heart disease and failure	38	Liability is increased by alcohol, caffeine, or nicotine.
Tumors	21	Tobacco smoke contains 15 identified carcinogens. Caffeine use has been linked to cancer of the pancreas.
Cerebrovascular disease	9	Nicotine and alcohol each increase liability.
Trauma	8	
Motor vehicle accidents	(33)	More than half are alcohol related.
Accidents (falls, suffocations, drownings, blows, wounds, etc.)	(30)	Alcohol is involved in about 18% of home accidents and 13% of occupational accidents.
Burns	(4)	One-third of all household fires are started by cigarettes.
Poisonings	(3)	50% involve drugs; 50% other substances and gases.
Suicides	(17)	Drugs are used for more than 3,000/year (>10%) in the United States; drugs contribute to >50% of cases of depression, the usual prelude to suicide
Homicides	(13)	Many are related to drug trafficking.
Vascular	4	Alcohol contributes to arteriosclerosis; nicotine and caffeine can cause peripheral vascular disorders; all three of these drugs contribute to hypertension.
Infections	4	Chronic drug abuse increases susceptibility to infections; IV drug users are at risk of AIDS.
Congenital diseases and diseases of infancy	3	Congenital defects are often related to use of drugs by the mother during pregnancy.
Chronic obstructive pulmonary disease	3	Many cases are due to use of tobacco.
Cirrhosis	2	More than 80% of cases are alcohol related.
Neurologic/psychiatric:	2	
Organic brain disorders	(30)	Alcohol can cause or aggravate organic brain syndromes
Drug dependence	(20)	Alcohol accounts for 90% of cases.
Spinal and peripheral neuropathies	(12)	

(continued)

Table 57–3
Relationship of Drugs to Principal Causes of Mortality (*continued*)

Cause of mortality	Percentage of total	Contribution of drugs to incidence
Neurologic/psychiatric (*continued*)		
Paralysis agitans	(11)	
Meningitis and other inflammations	(7)	
Epilepsy	(7)	Risk of seizures increases during drug withdrawal
Multiple sclerosis	(5)	
Other	(8)	
Diabetes	1	Alcohol use complicates control of diabetes.
Peptic ulcers	1	Caffeine, nicotine, alcohol, and aspirin are all ulcergenic.
Other	4	

First Aid

The central theme underlying first aid in poisoning is removal of the toxic substance. When the poison has been swallowed, inhaled, or injected (as in snakebite) the objective is to minimize absorption of the substance. For poisons acting on external surfaces, such as in skin contamination, chemical burns, or contact with the eye, removal of the substance and thorough rinsing of the contact site is usually the first concern.

When the poison has been swallowed, vomiting should usually be induced using an emetic, such as ipecac. Vomiting should *not* be induced if the client is comatose or convulsing, or if the poisonous substance is a corrosive poison (potent acids and bases). Dilution of acids or bases is safer than neutralization since the exothermic neutralization reaction can add a temperature burn to whatever chemical burn has already occurred to mucosal membranes. Milk or water are appropriate diluents. Dilution should not be attempted for poisons ingested in solid form since this will only hasten absorption. A sample of vomitus should be saved as an aid to identifying the toxin. Poison containers or uningested poison should also be saved.

When the poison has been inhaled, the patient should immediately be carried out into the fresh air. Clothing should be loosened and, if necessary, artificial respiration applied. The victim should be wrapped in a warm blanket if chilling occurs, and he or she should remain quiet. If convulsions occur, the person should be protected from injury and occlusion of the airway and, if possible, placed in bed in a darkened, quiet room.

For snakebite, absorption should be minimized by having the person remain as inactive as possible and applying a tourniquet. The tourniquet should not be so tight as to obliterate the pulse below the tourniquet, and it should be loosened for 1 minute in each 15 minutes. An ice pack is applied periodically to the bite, but not left for any length of time to avoid local injury.

For poisoning of a topical nature, the skin or eye is washed with large quantities of water. Speed is of the essence. Applications of creams or ointments should be avoided. Chemical burns are covered loosely with a clean cloth.

When a hospital is located nearby, the client should be taken to the emergency room as quickly as possible after first aid has been administered.

Medical Treatment of Poisonings

Medical treatment of poisonings encompasses five aspects: (1) physical assessment and history with special emphasis on identifying the poison, (2) removal of any residual poison, (3) symptomatic and supportive therapy, (4) systemic elimination of the poison by promoting excretion or by renal dialysis, and (5) administration of an antidote when appropriate. The order and extent of implementation of these five components of treatment depends on the circumstances of each individual case. Usually if a poisoning victim is asymptomatic or mildly symptomatic but alert, treatment centers on assessment and removal of any residual poison. If, however, the person is semicomatose or comatose, the full gamut of measures may be required. Symptomatic and supportive treatment, with special emphasis on maintaining respiratory and cardiovascular function, is the first priority.

Physical Assessment and History

In the best of circumstances, the identity of a poisoning substance may be known with certainty by the victim or a person bringing the victim for treatment. At other times, extensive questioning may be required to determine the substance or narrow the possibilities. Under these circumstances physical assessment provides important clues to the substance involved and supportive measures required. Physical assessment of the victim of poisoning includes observation of signs and symptoms and measurement of concentrations of common intoxicants in serum or urine samples. Observable signs and symptoms help to narrow the range of possible poisons (Table 57–4).

Table 57–4
Signs and Symptoms of Drug Overdose and Likely Causative Agents

Signs and symptoms	Likely agents
Ocular	
Dilated pupils	Amphetamine-like stimulants, anticholinergics (including antihistamines with anticholinergic properties, tricyclic antidepressants, neuroleptics, atropine-like drugs), cocaine, opiate withdrawal, psychedelics, respiratory depressants if anoxia has developed (e.g., sedative-hypnotics, narcotics).
Constricted pupils	Narcotics, cholinesterase inhibitors, mushrooms containing cholinomimetic alkaloids, pilocarpine
Nystagmus	Phencyclidine, phenytoin, sedative-hypnotics
Blurred vision	Alcohol, anticholinergics, botulin, methanol, organophosphates
Neurologic/psychiatric	
Ataxia	Alcohol, carbon monoxide, heavy metals, neuroleptics, organic solvents, phenytoin, psychedelics, sedative-hypnotics, tricyclic antidepressants
Muscle twitches/ convulsions	Amphetamine, antihistamines, chlorinated hydrocarbon insecticides, cocaine, cyanide, hemlock, isoniazid; lead, organophosphate insecticides, phencyclidine, phenothiazines, salicylates, sedative-hypnotic/ alcohol withdrawal, strychnine, theophilline
Somnolence/coma	Alcohol, anticholinergics, antihistamines, narcotics, neuroleptics, sedative-hypnotics, tricyclic antidepressants
Neurologic/psychiatric (*continued*)	
Muscle paralysis	Botulin, heavy metals
Psychosis	Alcohol, amphetamine-like stimulants, cannabis, cocaine, phencyclidine, psychedelics
Hallucinations	Alcohol, amphetamine-like stimulants, anticholinergics, cocaine, psychedelics
Pulse rate	
Rapid	Alcohol, amphetamines, anticholinergics, phencyclidine, salicylates
Slow	Beta-blockers, digitalis, narcotics, sedative-hypnotics
Respiration	
Rapid	Amphetamines, barbiturates (initially), carbon monoxide, methanol, petroleum distillates, salicylates
Slow	Alcohol, narcotics, sedative-hypnotics
Wheezing/pulmonary edema	Narcotics, organophosphate insecticides, organic solvents
Breath odor	
Acetone/fruity	Isopropyl alcohol, ketoacidosis, methanol, phenol
Alcohol	Ethanol
Ammonial	Ammonia
Bitter almond	Cyanide
Garlicky	Arsenic, dimethyl sulfoxide (DMSO), organophosphate insecticides, phosphorus

(*continued*)

Table 57–4
Signs and Symptoms of Drug Overdose and Likely Causative Agents (*continued*)

Signs and symptoms	Likely agents
Breath odor (*continued*)	
Gasoline	Gasoline, kerosene, petroleum distillates
Pear-like	Chloral hydrate
Pungent	Ethchlorvynol
Violets	Turpentine
Wintergreen	Methyl salicylate
Mouth	
Dry	Anticholinergics, antihistamines, narcotics
Salivation	Arsenic, corrosives, mercury, mushrooms containing cholinomimetic alkaloids, organophosphates, strychnine
Gum discoloration	Arsenic, lead, mercury
Gastrointestinal	
Constipation	Lead, narcotics
Cramps	Arsenic, heavy metals, lead, mushrooms containing cholinomimetic alkaloids, narcotic withdrawal, organophosphate insecticides
Diarrhea	Arsenic, boric acid, iron, mushrooms containing cholinomimetic alkaloids, organophosphates
Gastrointestinal (*continued*)	
Emesis	Boric acid, caffeine, corrosives, heavy metals, iron, isopropyl alcohol, phenol, salicylates, theophylline
Skin	
Blue-gray, dry, warm	Silver salts
Bullae	Barbiturates, carbon monoxide
Cherry red	Carbon monoxide (severe)
Cyanosis	Amyl nitrate, carbon monoxide, cyanide, nitrites, strychnine
Diaphoresis	Alcohol, amphetamine, atropine, barbiturates, cholinomimetics, cocaine, organophospate insecticides, salicylates
Flushed	Alcohol, antihistamines, atropine, boric acid, carbon monoxide
Jaundice	Acetaminophen, arsenic, carbon tetrachloride
Needle marks	Amphetamines, cocaine, narcotics, phencyclidine
Purpura	Salicylates, snake or spider bites

Measurement of drug concentrations in the serum confirms the presence of potentially toxic levels of the poison (Table 57–5). Poisoning, especially when associated with suicide attempts, may involve multiple substances which can result in complicated physical findings. Some toxic substances produce a series of physical responses in sequence rather than concurrently. This often occurs with toxicity associated with cocaine and related drugs, where initial cardiac and central nervous system excitation may give way to profound depression in both systems. Some symptoms, such as hepatotoxicity, are often delayed. Moreover, all symptoms of toxicity may be delayed if gastric emptying time is prolonged if the poison is absorbed mainly from the intestines. Liquids are usually absorbed more rapidly than substances ingested as solids.

Removal of Residual Poison

If the poison has not been completely removed by first aid, completing the removal is the top priority if the client is asymptomatic or mildly symptomatic and alert. When the contact has occurred on the skin surface or in the eye, the process of rinsing the poison from the contact surface with water or another suitable fluid is completed. If the toxin is an insecticide, green soap is recommended for decontamination of the skin. It contains alkaline substances that hydrolyze organophosphates and alcohol that dissolves hydrocarbons. If green soap is not available, plain soap can be used with alcohol rinses. Personnel conducting decontamination of skin exposed to pesticides should wear disposable gloves, aprons, and shoe covers.

If the substance has been ingested, there are four kinds of measures that can be employed to facilitate removal of unabsorbed poison: (1) emesis, (2) gastric lavage, (3) chemical absorption, neutralization, or inactivation, and (4) catharsis. Emesis and lavage are the most important clinical tools for removal of unabsorbed drug.

Emesis (vomiting) is the method of choice for removing ingested substances from the stomach in most circumstances. It is more effective than lavage because a portion of the stomach contents is held in pouches that are inaccessible to a lavage tube. How-

Table 57–5
Therapeutic, Toxic, and Lethal Blood Levels of Common Intoxicants

Drug	Therapeutic level	Toxic level	Lethal level
Alcohols and glycols			
Ethanol	100 mg/dl	100–200 mg/dl	350 mg/dl
Ethylene glycol	—	150 mg/dl	200–400 mg/dl
Isopropanol	—	340 mg/dl	—
Methanol	—	20–80 mg/dl	75–125 mg/dl
Analgesics			
Acetaminophen	10–20 μg/ml	150 μg/ml	1,500 μg/ml
Pentazocine	0.14–0.6 μg/ml	2–5 μg/ml	10–20 μg/ml
Propoxyphene	50–200 ng/ml	5–20 μg/ml	50–80 μg/ml
Salicylates	10–30 mg/dl	30–50 mg/dl	50–80 mg/dl
Antiepileptics			
Phenytoin	5–22 μg/ml	20–50 μg/ml	100 μg/ml
Primidone	5–12 μg/ml	50–80 μg/ml	100 μg/ml
Antihistamines			
Diphenhydramine	5 μg/ml	10 μg/ml	—
Cardiovascular			
Digoxin	0.6–1.3 ng/ml	2.9 ng/ml	—
Procainamide	3–8 μg/ml	12 μg/ml	—
Quinidine	2–6 μg/ml	10 μg/ml	30–50 μg/ml
Heavy metals			
Arsenic	—	1.0 μg/ml	15 μg/ml
Iron	50–150 μg/ml	500–600 μg/ml	—
Lead	—	0.7 μg/ml	2.0 μg/ml
Psychedelic			
Phencyclidine	—	0.5 μg/ml	1.0 μg/ml
Psychotherapeutic agents			
Benzodiazepines	0.5–6 μg/ml	5–30 μg/ml	50 μg/ml
Chlorpromazine	0.1–0.5 μg/ml	1–2 μg/ml	3–12 μg/ml
Lithium	0.5–1.5 mEq/L	2 mEq/L	2–5 mEq/L
Meprobamate	5–30 μg/ml	50–100 μg/ml	200 μg/ml
Thioridazine	1–1.5 μg/ml	10 μg/ml	20–80 μg/ml
Tricyclic antidepressants	50–300 ng/ml	300–1,000 ng/ml	2,000 ng/ml
Sedative-hypnotics			
Barbiturates (long-acting)	10–25 μg/ml	40–60 μg/ml	80–150 μg/ml
Barbiturates (short-acting)	0.1–1 μg/ml	7–20 μg/ml	20–30 μg/ml
Ethchlorvynol	5 μg/ml	20 μg/ml	150 μg/ml
Methyprylon	10 μg/ml	30–60 μg/ml	100 μg/ml
Methaqualone	5 μg/ml	10–30 μg/ml	30 μg/ml
Stimulants			
Amphetamines	20–30 ng/ml	—	2.0 μg/ml
Caffeine	—	—	100 μg/ml
Theophylline	10–20 μg/ml	>50 μg/ml	—

ever, emesis is specifically contraindicated if (1) the client is stuporous, delirious, or comatose, (2) if the agent ingested is corrosive or caustic, or (3) if the poison is a CNS stimulant likely to cause convulsions. When the ingested poison is a corrosive or caustic, emesis may result in gastric perforation or further burning of the esophagus. Treatment should be based on dilution with moderate amounts of water, milk, or both. If the substance is a petroleum distillate, emesis may result in aspiration of the substance, which can cause pneumonitis. Treatment varies depending on which of the many petroleum distillates is involved but is usually based primarily on symptomatic support. If the agent ingested has the potential for producing convulsions, emesis could precipitate convulsions as a result of the added stimulation.

Ipecac is the most useful of the emetic sustances. Syrup of ipecac is preferable to the fluid extract, which is 14 times more concentrated. The recommended dose for emergency room use is 10 ml orally for children under 1 year old, 15 ml for children 1–5 years old, 15–30 ml for children over 5, and 30 ml for adults. Ipecac syrup should be followed immediately by 1–2 glasses of water. Emesis should follow in 15–30 minutes. A second dose should be given after 20–30 minutes if emesis has not occurred. The pharmacology of ipecac and other emetics is presented in Chapter 51. Apomorphine is another emetic but is generally less desirable than ipecac because of its central nervous system effects.

Gastric lavage is often indicated when emesis is not, such as in clients who are comatose, lethargic, or in seizures or postictal depression. Under most circumstances, a cuffed endotracheal tube is first put in place to protect the airways. Then a gastric tube of maximum diameter is inserted. Warm tap water is typically employed as the lavage fluid, but other solutions may be used for specific intoxicants (Table 57–6). The total volume of lavage fluid should usually not exceed 200–250 ml in adults or 10 ml/kg in children so as not to unduly hasten gastric emptying. Gastric lavage should only be performed if vital functions are adequate or adequately supported. Lavage can be useful as long as 3–12 hours after ingestion of the poison, depending on how rapidly the substance is absorbed.

After emesis or lavage, administration of **activated charcoal** will help to prevent absorption of any toxin remaining in the stomach or intestines. Most drugs are well absorbed by activated charcoal (Table 57–7). Activated charcoal is especially useful for drugs ingested in sustained-release formulation or those subject to enterohepatic recycling. Activated charcoal is more effective than commercially available alternatives such as **universal antidote.** A few substances are not well absorbed by activated charcoal (Table 57–7). The recommended dose of activated charcoal is 30–60 g in children and 50–100 g in adults. The charcoal may be mixed in water to produce a slurry that the client drinks; in some facili-

Table 57–6
Special Lavage Solutions for Specific Poisons

Poison	Lavage solution
Ferrous sulfate	1.5% sodium bicarbonate to form complex
Fluorides or oxalic acid	15-30 mg/ml calcium gluconate to form precipitate
Iodine	75-80 mg/ml solution of cornstarch

Table 57–7
Absorption of Substances By Activated Charcoal

Well absorbed	
Acetaminophen	Methyl salicylate
Amphetamine	Morphine
Antihistamines	Nicotine
Arsenic	Opium
Aspirin	Oxalic acid
Atropine	Parathion
Barbiturates	Penicillin
Camphor	Phenol
Chloroquine	Phenolphthalein
Chlorpheniramine	Phenothiazines
Cocaine	Phenylpropanolamine
Colchicine	Phenytoin
Digitalis	Phosphorus
Ethchlorvynol	Primaquine
Glutethimide	Propantheline
Iodine	Propoxyphene
Ipecac	Quinidine
Isoniazid	Quinine
Malathion	Strychnine
Mefenamic acid	Sulfonamides
Meprobamate	Theophylline
Mercuric chloride	Tricyclic antidepressants
Not well absorbed	
Alcohols	
Caustic alkalis	
Corrosives	
Cyanide	
Ferrous sulfate	
Iron	
Lead	
Lithium	
Mineral acids	
Petroleum distillates	

ties, a commercially available suspension in water and sorbital is employed. Charcoal can be administered through a lavage tube if the client is comatose. Activated charcoal should not be administered concomitantly with ipecac. Although activated charcoal tastes bad, it should not be mixed with milk, ice cream, or sherbets, since these reduce its absorptive capacity. Activated charcoal must be stored in sealed containers to prevent absorption of gases from the atmosphere.

Catharsis is generally of little value as a primary mode of preventing absorption of drugs from the gastrointestinal tract. However, catharsis may be useful when a drug is ingested in the form of an enteric coated tablet and an hour or more has elapsed since ingestion. A cathartic is often given after activated charcoal administration to reduce the transit time for the charcoal and absorbed toxin. Sodium sulfate, magnesium sulfate, magnesium citrate, or sorbitol can be employed for this purpose.

Symptomatic and Supportive Therapy

The old adage "Treat the client, not the poison" sums up the significance of this phase of treatment of toxicity victims. If the victim is semicomatose or comatose, symptomatic and supportive therapy takes first precedence. Among the measures that nurses may be required to use are artificial respiration and maintenance of blood pressure. In the emergency room, nurses may be involved in replacement of fluids intravenously, treatment of acid-base disturbances, or administration of anticonvulsants and vitamin, nutrient, or electrolyte supplements. Emotional support is often of utmost importance. In many cases the nurse will be responsible for providing supportive treatment. Nurses should note that the most common physiologic disturbances associated with poisonings are CNS depression, convulsions, hypotension, hypoxia, cardiac dysrhythmias, fluid or electrolyte imbalances, and edema (especially cerebral or pulmonary).

When the victim is comatose or semicomatose, emergency treatment attends first to respiratory and cardiovascular functions. The nurse should examine the mouth and clear it of any material such as food, vomit, or dentures. The nurse should position the victim on the left side with head down to reduce risk of aspiration. Mechanical ventilation is initiated if necessary. The nurse takes pluse, blood pressure, and temperature measurements. If the individual is in shock, therapy is initiated first with intravenous fluids or plasma expanders, followed by vasopressors or vasodilators as indicated.

Promoting Systemic Elimination

Elimination of absorbed poison can be promoted by stimulating diuresis, altering urinary pH, or by dialysis. Excretion of drugs that are freely filtered by the renal glomeruli can be enhanced, though not much, by administration of an osmotic diuretic such as mannitol. Mannitol is given intravenously at 1.5 g/kg in a 20% solution up to a total of 100 g/day. It is important that good hydration be maintained during mannitol therapy. Forced diuresis is contraindicated when the victim suffers from renal insufficiency, pulmonary edema, heart failure, or shock. The nurse should monitor fluid intake and output if forced diuresis is employed.

Forced diuresis is most efficacious when used in conjunction with urinary acidification or alkalinization for appropriate drugs (weak acids or bases). Drugs that exhibit increased rates of excretion as a result of urinary acidification or alkalinization are listed in Table 57–8. Urinary acidification has been employed mainly in overdoses involving amphetamines, urinary alkalinization in barbiturate and salicylate overdoses. Acidification of the urine is best accomplished with ascorbic acid or ammonium chloride. Alkalinization of the urine is achieved most efficiently with 1–2 mEq/kg of sodium bicarbonate or sodium lactate.

Dialysis can be accomplished by peritoneal lavage or by use of an artificial kidney. Dialysis is used to hasten elimination or, in the case of nephrotoxic substances, as a temporary substitute for a dysfunctional kidney. Nephrotoxins that may require use of an artificial kidney include carbon tetrachloride, ethylene glycol, mercury, and sulfonamides. Other dialyzable substances include alcohol, ammonia, amphetamines, anilines, antibiotics, barbiturates, bromides, calcium, chlorates, cinchona alkaloids, phenytoin, ethchlorvynol, ethylene glycol, ethinamate, halogens, meprobamate, narcotics, paraldehyde, piperidinediones, potassium, salicylates, and thio-

Table 57–8
Drug Elimination in Relation to Urinary pH

Drugs eliminated more rapidly after urinary alkalinization	Drugs eliminated more rapidly after urinary acidification
Arsenic	Amphetamines
Aspirin	Phencyclidine
Isoniazid	Phosphorus
Lithium	Quinine
Meprobamate	Quinidine
Naphthalene	Strychnine
Phenobarbital	
Salicylates	

Table 57–9
Dialyzability of Common Drugs

Drug class	Negligible	Slight	Substantial
Anti-infectives	Amphotericin B	Aminoglycosides	Ampicillin
	Chloroquine	Isoniazid	Carbenicillin
	Clindamycin		Cephalosporins
	Colistimethate		Chloramphenicol
	Erythromycin		Ethambutol
	Lincomycin		5-Fluorocytosine
	Methicillin		PAS
	Quinine		Penicillin G
	Rifampin		Sulfonamides
	Vancomycin		Trimethoprim
CNS drugs	Chloral hydrate	Diazepam	Acetaminophen
	Chlordiazepoxide	Ethchlorvynol	Aspirin
	Meprobamate	Short-to-intermediate acting barbiturates	Lithium
	Phenothiazines		Long-acting barbiturates
	Phenytoin		
	Propoxyphene		
	Tricyclic antidepressants		
Cardiovascular drugs	Digitoxin	Diazoxide	Methyldopa
	Digoxin		Procainamide
	Guanethidine		
	Lidocaine		
	Propranolol		
	Quinidine		
	Reserpine		
Antineoplastics			Cyclophosphamide
			5-Fluorouracil
Anti-inflammatory drugs	Gold	Colchicine	Aspirin
	Indomethacin	Glucocorticoids	
	Phenylbutazone		
	Probenecid		

cyanates. The dialyzability of a number of drugs is listed in Table 57–9.

Antidotes

Antidotes can act either within the alimentary tract or systemically, although most act systemically. The use of acids to neutralize bases, and vice versa, in the gastrointestinal tract, is out of favor because neutralization produces heat.

The major examples of systemic antidotes are listed in Table 57–10. Many of these have been discussed in appropriate chapters throughout the book. Those that pertain to heavy metals are presented in the following section.

Teaching Clients About Poisoning

Nurses, by virtue of their training and experience and their accessibility to clients in a variety of settings can play an important role in preventing accidental poisoning and in providing immediate assis-

Table 57–10
Antidotes for Specific Toxins

Toxin	Antidote
Acetaminophen	Acetylcysteine
Anaphylactoids	Epinephrine, antihistamines
Arsenic	Dimercaprol, penicillamine
Black widow spider venom	Antivenin (Lactrodectus mactans)
Calcium	Disodium edetate
Carbon monoxide	Oxygen
Cholinomimetics	Atropine
Convulsant drugs	Diazepam
Copper	Penicillamine
Coumarin-type anticoagulants	Vitamin K
Curariform agents	Edrophonium
Cyanide	Amyl nitrite pearls, sodium nitrite, sodium thiosulfate
Digitalis	Potassium chloride, phenytoin, disodium edetate, digoxin immune FAB
Disulfiram	Ascorbic acid
Ethylene glycol (antifreeze)	Ethanol
Folic acid antagonists	Leucovorin
Gold	Dimercaprol
Heparin	Protamine
Insulin	Glucagon
Iron	Deferoxamine
Isoniazid	Pyridoxine
Lead	Calcium disodium edetate, dimercaprol
Lithium	Sodium
Mercury	Dimercaprol, penicillamine
Methanol	Ethanol
Narcotics	Naloxone
Nitrites	Methylene blue
Organophosphate insecticides	Atropine, pralidoxime
Pit viper venom	Antivenin (Crotalidae) polyvalent
Strychnine	Mephenesin
Sympathetic amines	Alpha-blockers, beta-blockers

tance to clients and family members until an expert can arrive on the scene.

An obvious role in prevention involves teaching parents about the toxic effects chemicals may have upon their children and warning them to keep household chemicals out of children's reach. Household cleansers, disinfectants, detergents, and other substances should be kept out of the reach of children. This means not only putting things high up on shelves but, given the normal childhood urge to climb, locking up the substances as well. Other materials such as medications should also be placed in locked cabinets and the key put where the child cannot obtain it. Vitamins, cold remedies, minerals obtained from the local health food store, antihistamines, and herbs can all be hazardous to children. In fact, evidence suggests that the accidental ingestions and fatalities that occur among children are most likely to involve substances that parents would not generally classify as poisons.

The nurse should also teach clients to read carefully the labels on containers, noting what to do in case of ingestion. It is also a good idea to print on cards directions concerning what to do and make certain that family members and babysitters know where to find such cards in case of emergency.

Nurses should also advise parents concerning drug dosages for children. Parents should be warned not to use adult standards of drug dosage for children. Furthermore, adults should not assume that a bad taste will deter children from eating a substance. Adults should not refer to medication as candy. The child should know it is medicine and is necessary for health or recovery.

School nurses and community health nurses are in a unique position to establish education programs to inform the public about measures to prevent accidental poisoning and treatment of those who have been poisoned. Nurses should include instructions concerning the location of poison centers. Regional networks of poison control centers can be contacted at any hour of the day or night for information about poisons. Nurses should advise people to post the telephone number of the local poison control center in an immediately accessible location. Pediatricians and pharmacists often have stickers with the nearest poison control hotline telephone number, which parents may affix directly to the telephone.

Nurses should include in their course the admonition that drugs never be taken in the dark. Labels should always be read, and old or unused drugs should be discarded in the toilet rather than trash cans where children might find them. If the drug being taken requires using syringes and needles, these implements should be mutilated prior to being discarded. Also included in the teaching sessions should be the names of plants that are poisonous (such as the leaves of philodendren and rhubarb) and which therefore should not be grown where there are young children.

Nursing Observations for Poisonings

THERAPEUTIC GOAL	Removal of residual poison, support of vital functions and relief of symptoms, and elimination and/or antidoting of absorbed poison.
PREADMINISTRATION ASSESSMENT	
Baseline Data	Observe for dilated or constricted pupils, nystagmus, blurred vision, ataxia, muscle twitches, convulsion, somnolence, coma, muscle paralysis, psychosis, hallucinations, rapid or slow pulse, rapid or slow respiration, wheezing, breath odor, increased or decreased salivation, constipation or diarrhea, intestinal cramps, emesis, cyanosis, altered skin color, diaphoresis, flushing, jaundice, purpura, or needle marks. Evaluate vital signs, pupils, muscle tone, neurologic status, psychological status, breath odor, salivation rate, bowel function, skin color, and skin texture. Obtain laboratory tests including analysis of vomitus, urine, and serum for identification of poison and measurement of its concentration.
EVALUATION OF DRUG RESPONSE	
For Therapeutic Benefit	Monitor alleviation of the symptoms of poisoning and reductions in serum levels of the poison.
For Adverse Effects and Interactions	Monitor for adverse effects or interactions of any antidotes administered (see individual drug discussions).

Heavy Metals and Antagonists

Heavy metals are a group of chemical elements that form divalent, trivalent, or pentavalent cations and many of them are highly toxic. They may be encountered as components of drugs but are more likely to be ingested as environmental pollutants or constituents of nondrug chemicals. Two of the heavy metals have been discussed in other chapters because of special relationships to particular body systems—copper in Chapter 22 in relation to Wilson's disease and the extrapyramidal system and iron in Chapter 41 in relation to anemia. Other toxic heavy metals include lead, mercury, arsenic, antimony, gold, silver, beryllium, thallium, bismuth, and cadmium.

Heavy Metals

Lead is the most common cause of poisoning among the heavy metals. **Lead** poisoning occurs indirectly in certain occupations and in children who ingest lead-containing substances. Children frequently eat chipped paint containing lead. Many paints applied before World War II contain high concentrations of lead, but standards adopted in 1955 limit concentrations of lead in paint to 1%, so the incidence of poisoning from paint is declining. Lead contamination of the environment has occurred because of combustion of gasoline containing tetraethyllead. Contamination of food and beverages by lead occurs occasionally when containers are improperly glazed. Children are especially susceptible to lead toxicity. The syndrome includes encephalopathy, abdominal pain, muscle weakness, a persistent metallic taste, headache, and neurologic impairments. Complaints of abdominal colic, pallor, anemia, and blue-black pigmentation should cause nurses to suspect lead poisoning, especially in areas where cases of lead poisoning have been previously reported. A combination of dimercaprol and calcium disodium edetate is a useful antidote in acute poisonings involving lead. Lead has no therapeutic uses.

Mercury poisonings were sometimes associated with the use of mercurials as diuretics (for example, mersalyl) or antiseptics (for example, merbromin), but neither drug is in use in modern medicine. However, methylmercury derived from mercurial waste products of industry has become incorporated into the environment and the food chain to an alarming extent. The toxic effects of mercury poisoning include kidney damage, ulcerations, and inflammations of the gastrointestinal tract, and hypersensitivity reactions. Clients become lethargic, agitated, and develop hypovolemia. Chronic mercury intoxication is a major concern, since mercury in the form of methylmercury accumulates in tissues. Dimercaprol is an effective antidote for acute mercury poisoning.

Nursing Diagnoses and Interventions for Poisonings

Nursing Diagnoses	*Related Interventions*
TO ENHANCE BENEFITS OF ANTIDOTAL THERAPY	
Alteration in comfort related to chemical burns, gastrointestinal irritation, hyperpyrexia, or other toxic effects	Remove poison. Provide comfort measures. Administer analgesics if prescribed.
Alterations in respiratory function or cardiac output	Maintain respiration with mouth-to-mouth resuscitation or mechanical assistance if required. Clear the mouth of obstructions. Maintain blood pressure with pressor drugs if required. Monitor the ECG and vital signs.
Anxiety or fear related to treatments such as lavage, emesis, or dialysis	Provide client with emotional support and reassurance.
Increased risk of injury related to convulsions, bleeding, or diminished judgment and orientation	Administer anticonvulsants if required; control bleeding and replace fluid if required. Provide safety measures to protect from trauma injury.
Parental anxiety related to guilt and uncertain outcome	Provide parents with emotional support and reassurance.
TO ENSURE SAFE AND EFFICACIOUS DRUG USE	
Knowledge deficit related to poisonings	Teach clients proper storage of household chemicals and drugs, recognition of local poisonous plants, and risks of drug abuse.
	Teach clients how to administer first aid in the event of household poisonings.
	Advise clients of the location and telephone numbers of local poison control and information centers.
	Explain to clients who have ingested a poisonous substance the nature of the medical problem and the reason for treatments.

Arsenic and **arsenicals,** although once widely used as antimicrobials, are now encountered mainly in environment and industrial sources. The toxic effects of arsenic include liver damage, bone marrow suppression, neuritis, skin eruptions, gastrointestinal disturbances and inflammations, and injury to capillaries. The most useful antidote for arsenic is dimercaprol. **Antimony** compounds are used occasionally in parasitic diseases, such as schistosomiasis (see Chapter 48). Toxic symptoms resemble those of arsenic; indeed, the two metals are chemically similar. Dimercaprol is useful in treatment of poisoning caused by the trivalent form of antimony.

Gold is used in treatment of rheumatoid arthritis (Chapter 45). Toxic effects commonly include pruritus and mucous membrane ulcerations. Blood dyscrasias and thrombocytopenia occur less frequently. Other effects include encephalitis, neuritis, and hepatitis. Dimercaprol and penicillamine are effective antidotes for gold toxicity but may impair the therapeutic effectiveness as well. **Silver** salts are used as topical antiseptics. These include silver nitrate, silver sulfadiazine, and silver allantoinate. The latter two are insoluble and are not absorbed systemically. Ingested silver nitrate can be chemically inactivated with sodium chloride solution, since silver chloride is an insoluble precipitate. However, the treatment of choice is an activated charcoal slurry. Silver nitrate ingestion can cause hypochloremia. The principal toxic effect of silver nurses can expect to observe is development of a bluish tint to the skin and conjunctiva, called argyria. It also occurs in internal organs. This condition can occur with topical or systemic use of silver colloids or salts. Treatment is difficult at best.

Beryllium can produce a disease called berylliosis, characterized by granulomata in the lungs (Chapter 52). Beryllium dust inhalation or accidental ingestion of beryllium compounds can occur in certain industrial situations. Berylliosis can be acute or chronic. In acute cases, corticosteroids have been used effectively to produce both clinical and physiologic improvement. **Thallium** poisoning may result from ingestion of ant or rat poison containing the metal. Alopecia and erythema occur with chronic sublethal doses. Acute toxicity is characterized by gastrointestinal irritation, motor paralysis, and respiratory failure.

Heavy Metal Antagonists

Dimercaprol

Mechanisms and Effects Dimercaprol, also called British anti-Lewisite (BAL), is a simple organic substance having adjacent sulfhydryl groups. It forms a stable ring structure with various heavy metals.

Clinical Indications Dimercaprol is useful for treatment of poisonings with arsenic, gold, mercury, and antimony. It is also indicated in conjunction with calcium disodium edetate for acute lead poisoning.

Adverse Effects and Contraindications Dimercaprol is contraindicated in poisonings involving cadmium or selenium and has no value in iron poisoning. Dimercaprol is toxic in its own right. At high doses it inhibits most enzymes requiring metal cofactors. Side effects at therapeutic doses include nausea, headache, muscle aches, and hypertension. Such symptoms typically occur within a few minutes after injection and may last up to two hours. *Nurses should inform clients that the drug can impart an unpleasant garlicky odor to the breath.* At higher doses, coma, convulsions, and capillary damage may occur. Contact of the drug with the skin may produce erythema, edema, and dermatitis. *Nurses should therefore handle the drug with care.*

Nurses should monitor client intake and output since dimercaprol is potentially nephrotoxic. If renal insufficiency develops, the drug should be discontinued or used with extreme caution. Nurses should work to keep the client's urine alkaline to reduce potential renal damage that may occur during elimination of dimercaprol chelate. In addition, nurses should have the client's urine examined daily for albumin, blood, casts and pH.

Preparations and Administration Dimercaprol (BAL in oil) is given only by deep intramuscular injection. *The site of injection must be rotated to avoid local pain, gluteal abscesses, and skin sensitivity. If calcium disodium edetate is to be given concurrently, the two antidotes must be injected at different sites. Urine and blood levels of the heavy metal involved in the poisoning should be measured and employed as a guide for dosage adjustments.* Since irreversible tissue damage can occur quickly when heavy metal poisoning occurs, dimercaprol therapy needs to be initiated as quickly as possible after the metal is ingested — generally within 1–2 hours for optimal value.

Dimercaprol (BAL in Oil)
Injection solution
Recommended Doses: For arsenic or gold poisoning, 2.5 to 3 mg/kg every 4 hours for 2 days, then twice on the third day, and once per day for 10 additional days. For acute mercury poisoning, 5 mg/kg initially, followed by 2.5 mg/kg once or twice daily for 10 days.

Calcium Disodium Edetate

Mechanisms and Effects Calcium disodium edetate (CaEDTA) chelates (forms a complex) with lead, zinc, copper, chromium, cadmium, manganese, and nickel, rendering these metals harmless. The complex formed by lead and the drug is excreted slowly by the kidneys.

Adverse Effects and Contraindications Adverse reactions to calcium disodium edetate include gastrointestinal irritation, renal damage, bone marrow suppression, and hypersensitivity reactions.

Nurses must carefully monitor clients' intake and output. Inadequate urinary output could cause nephrotoxicity since the drug is excreted almost exclusively from the kidneys. Any marked decrease in urinary output or absence of urine is an indication the therapy should be stopped immediately and the physician notified. Nurses must teach clients at home (and their families) how to keep accurate records of fluid intake and urinary output, how to recognize signs and symptoms of renal dysfunction, and whom to contact.

Before onset of therapy, a routine urinalysis and tests for coproporphyrine should be conducted; these should be repeated daily during the course of treatment. If epithelial cells, blood, or protein appear in the urine, the drug should be terminated immediately. Also BUN, serum creatinine, calcium, and phosphorus determinations should be done prior to and during the course of therapy.

Since calcium disodium edetate chelates copper, zinc, and magnesium as well as other metals, nurses should assure that clients on prolonged therapy with this chelator are periodically checked for deficiencies of these trace elements.

Preparations and Administrations When clients are to be given calcium disodium edetate, the nurse should prepare them by assuring adequacy of urinary output by administering intravenous fluids. While fluid intake is generally increased to enhance urinary excretion of chelates, excess fluid intake must be avoided, especially in those clients who have had encephalopathy, because it may further increase intracranial pressure. Thus, infusion rates must be closely monitored assuring they run as prescribed by the physician. An excessively rapid infusion could cause cerebral edema and death.

Calcium Disodium Edetate
Tablets
Recommended Doses: For treatment of lead poisoning in adults, 4 g/day PO in divided doses administered by slow intravenous infusion over 2–3 days. For children, 1 g/35 lb/day in divided doses. Allow at least 2 days between courses.

Pencillamine

Mechanisms and Effects Penicillamine (Cuprimine, Depen) is a chelating agent used in copper poisoning and in Wilson's disease, a condition in which copper accumulates in the body, causing damage to the liver and lenticular nucleus of the brain. Wilson's disease is associated with hepatic degeneration and extrapyramidal symptoms (see Chapter 22). Although penicillamine also chelates certain other metals, it is the drug of choice only for copper toxicity.

Adverse Effects and Contraindications Penicillamine can produce hypersensitivity reactions and renal dysfunction. *Prior to instituting therapy with penicillamine, nurses should assure that the following laboratory tests are completed: white and differentiated blood counts, direct platelet counts, hemoglobin, urinalysis, and liver function tests. These should be repeated every 3 days during the first month of therapy and every 2 weeks thereafter. Nurses should monitor clients for thrombocytopenia, leukopenia, and agranulocytosis and report any indications of these immediately. They should also instruct clients to report any unusual bruising or bleeding, as well as sore mouth or throat, fever, or skin rash.*

If the client expects to undergo surgery, the nurse should make certain the physician is aware that the client is taking penicillamine since the drug tends to retard healing by inhibiting the formation of collagen and elastin. Penicillamine also interferes with the metabolism of vitamin B_6. Therefore physicians may wish to order B_6 prophylactically.

Preparations and Administration The dose of penicillamine for Wilson's disease is determined by monitoring urinary excretion of copper. Since the low copper diet utilized in Wilson's disease will usually limit copper intake to less than 1.0 mg daily, the objective of penicillamine therapy is to achieve excretion of a similar quantity: 0.5–1.0 mg of copper daily. The usual maximum dosage required to achieve this objective is 2 g/day for adults or 1 g/day for children, taken orally. It may be necessary to initiate therapy at doses as low as 250 mg/day to minimize adverse effects that occur at the beginning of therapy. Doses over 500 mg/day are given in divided doses. The optimum dosage of penicillamine for clients with Wilson's disease is determined by quantitative analysis of urinary copper. *Nurses need to take care that neither they nor clients confuse penicillamine with penicillin. Clients should be advised to collect urine in a copper-free container.*

Penicillamine (Cuprimine, Depen Titratabs)
Capsules, tablets
Recommended Doses: see discussion above.

Trientine (Cuprid)

Trientine is an effective copper chelator indicated for treatment of Wilson's disease when clients are intolerant to penicillamine. The effectiveness of trientine is comparable to that of penicillamine. The principal adverse effect that has been reported when trientine is employed in clients with Wilson's disease is iron deficiency.

Preparations and Administration

Trientine (Cuprid)
Capsules
Recommended Doses: For adults, 750–1,250 mg/day PO initially, in 2 to 4 divided doses daily. The total daily dose may be increased as required up to 1,500 mg/day. Trientine must be taken on an empty stomach, at least 1 hour before or 2 hours after meals.

Deferoxamine (Desferal)

Deferoxamine is a chelating agent that binds iron in the ferric form. It is injected intramuscularly or infused intravenously in iron toxicity or hemochromatosis. The iron bound by deferoxamine is excreted in the urine. *Nurses should warn clients that the drug imparts a reddish color to urine.* Adverse effects include skin rashes and hypotension. With extended therapy, cataracts, blurred vision, fever, and allergic reactions have occurred.

Preparations and Administration

Deferoxamine (Desferal)
Powder for injection
Recommended Doses: 1 g IM intially, followed by 0.5 g 4 and 8 hours later. If necessary, additional 0.5 g doses can be given at 4-hour intervals up to 6 g daily.

Pesticides

Pesticides are chemicals employed to destroy one or another life form deemed to be a nuisance to humans. This includes insecticides, rodenticides, fumigants, herbicides, and fungicides. Mortality associated with poisoning by pesticides declined sharply from annual rates of about 150 in the mid-fifties to about 30 per year by the late seventies, probably due to greater awareness on the part of treatment centers and improved treament measures rather than reduced exposure to these toxins.

Insecticides

The principal classes of insecticides are the organophosphates and the chlorinated hydrocarbons. The **organophosphates** have the advantage of low carcinogenicity and do not persist in the environment as do the chlorinated hydrocarbons, but they produce much greater acute toxicity in humans. The acute dermal toxicity of organophosphates is 100 fold greater than for the chlorinated hydrocarbons. In October 1984 leakage of a derivative of malathion from an American Cyanamid tank in Linden, New Jersey led to hospitalization of 100 exposed individuals. The pharmacology of organophosphates and treatment measures for toxic exposure are discussed in Chapter 28.

The **chlorinated hydrocarbons** were widely employed in the two decades following World War II. Some of the most commonly used agents were chlorophenothane (DDT), hexachlorocyclohexane (lindane), chlordane, and dieldrin. Chlorinated hydrocarbons have very low water solubility, being highly lipophilic. They are readily absorbed from the gastrointestinal tract and through the skin. Once absorbed, they accumulate in fat tissue, possibly resulting in cumulation toxicity. With acute exposure, accumulation of chlorinated hydrocarbons in lipid tissue has a protective effect, reducing the concentration of toxic substance to which the brain (the major target of toxicity) is exposed. But the high level of lipid solubility also contributes to **biomagnification** of toxicity within a food chain. Chlorinated hydrocarbons tend to increase in concentration in tissue of organisms at successive levels in a food chain, affecting those at the top of a chain (such as humans) to the greatest extent. This mechanism is thought to be responsible for the decline in populations of fish-eating birds. Excretion of chlorinated hydrocarbons occurs only slowly. For example, it is estimated that only 1% of the body stores of DDT are excreted daily.

Acute toxic manifestations caused by chlorinated hydrocarbons are attributable to their action on the central nervous system. DDT stimulates the CNS by prolonging excitatory potentials. Symptoms include hypersensitivity to stimuli, irritability, apprehensiveness, tremor, and convulsions. However, acute fatalities are virtually nonexistent with these compounds. Treatment of acute poisoning with chlorinated hydrocarbon insecticides is limited to removal of the drug (by emesis unless the patient is convulsing, by catharsis, and by washing the skin) and supportive treatment.

Rodenticides

Rodenticides include warfarin, brodifacoam, red squill, sodium fluoroacetate, and thallium. Warfarin is minimally toxic to humans because its effects depend upon chronic intake. However, brodifacoam and other long-acting and potent anticoagulants can produce their effects acutely. Red squill contains scillaren glycosides, which have a cardiotonic action. Fortunately, these glycosides trigger emesis in humans, thus minimizing risk of toxicity. Rodents such as rats lack an emetic mechanism. Sodium fluoroacetate and thallium are highly toxic in humans as well as rodents but are strictly regulated.

Fumigants

Fumigants are used mainly to control insects and rodents. **Cyanide** and methyl bromide are often employed and present considerable risks to humans. Cyanide toxicity is also encountered in use of laetrile. Household sources of cyanide include fruit pits (in large quantities) and silver polish, as well as insecticides and rodenticides. Cyanide has been used for executions in gas chambers because of its rapid action. It was employed in the suicide/murders in Jonestown, Guyana which resulted in 900 deaths on November 18, 1978. In 1982 capsules of Tylenol brand acetaminophen sold in the Chicago area were found laced with cyanide, causing the deaths of seven individuals. Other instances of drug tampering involving cyanide contamination occurred in 1985 and 1986. Cyanide is also encountered as hydrocyanide gas. Another gaseous cyanide derivative, methylisocyanate, was responsible for 2,500 deaths and 100,000 injuries in December 1984 in Bhopal, India when the gas escaped from storage tanks.

Cyanide inhibits cellular respiration by inactivating cytochrome oxidase. Treatment must be rapid, since death occurs quickly after lethal doses. Gastric lavage is used to remove unabsorbed cyanide. In addition, three steps are taken to tie up cyanide that has already been absorbed systemically. Amyl nitrite is administered immediately by inhalation while a solution of sodium nitrite is being prepared. Sodium nitrite is injected as soon as it is ready. Both of these drugs generate methemoglobin, an alternate binding site for cyanide. Methemoglobin has a higher affinity for cyanide than does cytochrome oxidase. Finally, sodium thiosulfate is injected intravenously to promote conversion of cyanide to thiocyanate, a much less toxic substance that is rapidly excreted by the kidneys. Artificial respiration and 100% oxygen are often utilized as well.

Methyl bromide is another toxic fumigant. Because of the severe potential of toxicity with methyl bromide, chloropicrin, a drug that causes tearing, is added to methyl bromide as a warning device against exposure. Toxic symptoms include headache, nausea, vomiting, malaise, and visual disturbances.

Herbicides and Fungicides

The herbicide most widely encountered is 2,4-dichlorophenoxyacetic acid (**2,4-D**). Animals or humans ingesting plants sprayed with this compound can experience stiffness, paralysis, ataxia, coma, or ventricular fibrillation. The herbicide is well absorbed by activated charcoal. Contact dermatitis can occur with topical exposure.

Another herbicide, **paraquat,** received considerable notoriety when it was used to spray marihuana and opium crops in Mexico to discourage illicit production. Marihuana containing paraquat appeared on the black market in the late 1970s. Paraquat can cause respiratory distress and death when ingested and lung damage when smoked.

The principal fungicides include dithiocarbamates, hexachlorobenzene, and pentachlorophenol. Dithiocarbamates are minimally toxic to humans. Hexachlorobenzene can cause an increase in hepatic weight. At least two deaths have occurred by this agent.

Organic Solvents

Organic solvents are widely used and exhibit varying degrees of toxicity. **Gasoline** and kerosene frequently cause poisonings because they often are stored in containers previously used for beverages, which leads children to ingest the substances. Toxic symptoms produced by these substances resemble those caused by alcohol: confusion, disorientation, incoordination, ataxia, or coma. Liver and kidney damage may be severe. The most serious toxic symptoms occur from inhalation of vapors in high concentrations, which can result in chemical pneumonitis, pulmonary edema, and even immediate death. Gastric lavage and emesis are usually contraindicated after petroleum ingestion. Treatment is symptomatic.

Carbon tetrachloride is less often encountered than formerly when it was widely used in carpet cleaners and spot removers. Moderate exposure leads to irritation of mucosal membranes of the eyes, nose, and throat, nausea and vomiting, dizziness, and headache. Higher concentrations can cause convulsions, stupor, or coma.

Benzene and **toluene** are widely employed industrial solvents. Acute exposure to benzene causes dizziness, euphoria, headache, nausea, vomiting, weakness, ataxia, tremors, dyspnea, paralysis, or unconsciousness. Chronic exposure to benzene has been linked to occurrence of leukemia and aplastic anemia. Toluene does not cause these chronic actions but can cause CNS depression and euphoria acutely.

Toxicity can occur from ingestion of alcohols such as **methanol** and **isopropanol,** or glycols such as **ethylene glycol** (encountered in antifreeze). Ethyl alcohol is a useful antagonist when poisoning is due to any of these substances. Isopropanol produces severe gastritis and intestinal bleeding and prolonged CNS depression. Ethylene glycol causes narcosis and renal injury. Methanol and ethylene glycol yield metabolites that are more toxic than the parent compounds: formic acid in the case of methanol and glyoxylic acid, oxalic acid, and finally formic acid in the case of ethylene glycol. Alcohol is used to slow the formation of these toxic metabolites by competitive inhibition of alcohol dehydrogenase. Metabolic acidosis caused by the metabolites is treated with sodium bicarbonate. Dialysis can be used for these agents.

Air Pollution and Poisonous Gases

Air Pollution

Air pollution has become a major problem of modern, industrialized and motorized society. Five pollutants account for 98% of air pollution: carbon monoxide (52%) sulfur oxides (18%), hydrocarbons (12%), particulate matter (10%), and nitrogen oxides (6%). Five sources account for most of pollution: automobiles (60%), industry (18%), electric power plants (13%), home heating (6%), and refuse disposal (3%). However, the sources differ in the type of pollutant produced. Automobiles account for over 90% of annual carbon monoxide emissions (excluding natural sources), 63% of hydrocarbons, and 46% of nitrogen oxides, but less than 10% of particulate pollution and less than 5% of sulfur oxides. Carbon monoxide, hydrocarbons, and nitrogen oxides produce an **oxidizing type of pollution.** Particulate pollution and sulfur oxides produce a **reducing type of pollution** and is more than 75% attributable to industry and electric power plants.

The reducing kind of pollution can become acutely dangerous when atmospheric temperature inversions occur in a heavily polluted area for more than a couple of days. Three famous instances resulted in 65 deaths in Belgium in 1930, 20 deaths in Donora, Pennsylvania in 1948, and 4,000 deaths in London in 1952. Sulfur oxides are also major contributors to acid rain that is threatening the survival of ponds, lakes, and forests as natural habitats. Rain passing through air containing sulfur oxides becomes acidified. The resulting acid rain can be deadly to fish and plant life alike. Ultimately, it is heavy metals, such as aluminum, leached from the drainage basin soil by acid rain and carried into pond and lake water, that kill fish. Many former freshwater fish habitats in the United States, Canada, Scandinavia, and Europe no longer sustain fish because of the effects of acid rain. Some bodies of fresh water are more resistant than others to the effects of acid rain because of presence of limestone, which neutralizes acid rain, in the drainage basin soil. The toxic sulfur oxides include sulfur dioxide, sulfuric acid, and paticulate sulfates. Sulfur dioxide and sulfuric acid cause bronchial constriction and thickening of the mucosal layer of the bronchi.

Particulate matter in the atmosphere is derived principally from incomplete combustion of fossil fuels. Particles larger than 5 μ are filtered by the nares or deposited in the upper airways. Particles 2–5 μm are deposited in the tracheobronchial trees and are removed by the mucociliary escalator mechanism and by coughing and sneezing. Particles less than 2 μm become lodged in the alveoli. Removal of these particles by phagocytic cells and the lymphatic ducts is slow and sometimes incomplete. Excessive rates of particulate sedimentation or inadequate rates of removal lead to pulmonary impaction. Some particulate matter poses special risks of toxicity, such as dusts composed of silica, asbestos, beryllium, and coal. The disorder associated with pulmonary toxicity of these substances is discussed in Chapter 52.

Pollution produced by automobiles is mainly the oxidizing type of pollution, also called photochemical pollution. The smog that occurs in Los Angeles is of this type. Oxidizing pollutants include **nitrogen dioxide,** a lung irritant. Individuals exposed to elevated concentrations of NO_2 are at risk of pulmonary damage. For example, farmers who maintain silos may develop silo-filler's disease from NO_2 produced from ensilage. NO_2 also provides a source of **ozone.** Ozone is the most abundant oxidant in polluted air and is a potent lung irritant. At concentrations about 2 parts per million (ppm), it causes desquamation of epithelial cells throughout the respiratory tract.

Another group of oxidizing pollutants are the hydrocarbons, which yield aldehydes as a result of photooxidation. Two of these aldehydes, formaldehyde and acrolein, are potent airway irritants that increase resistance to airflow. These substances contribute to the noxious odor of polluted highway and city air. Concentrations of 0.5–1 ppm are detectable by odor, concentrations of 2–3 ppm are irritating, and concentrations of 4–5 ppm are extremely noxious and hazardous.

Carbon Monoxide

Carbon monoxide (CO) is the single most common cause of fatal poisonings by a wide margin, accounting for 1,191 accidental deaths and 1,676 suicides in 1981, 25% of all deaths due to substance intoxications. The average atmospheric concentration is 0.1 ppm. Most of the CO in the atmosphere comes from natural sources including atmospheric oxidation of methane, carbon monoxide-producing microorganisms of the ocean, and forest fires. About 10% comes from human activities, especially automobiles. However, the requirement for installation of catalytic converters should have a positive impact since these devices reduce CO emissions from 90 g/mile to 3.4 g/mile.

Carbon monoxide is toxic because it reacts with hemoglobin. Carbon monoxide affixes more tightly to hemoglobin than does oxygen, dissociating at only 1/2,200th the rate of oxygen from the carrier substance. The effect of CO exposure is to reduce the oxygen carrying capacity of the blood. A CO concentration of 0.1% (1,000 ppm, close to 1/2,200th the concentration of oxygen) will result in a 50% reduction in oxygen carrying capacity, a potentially fatal deficit. Exposure to a CO concentration of 0.01% (100 ppm) would reduce oxygen carrying capacity by 5%. Concentrations of 100–200 ppm are typical in heavy traffic, and concentrations of 75 ppm are likely to occur on expressways. Even in residential areas, concentrations average about 25 ppm.

When 0–10% of hemoglobin is in the form of carboxyhemoglobin (COHb), clinical symptoms are absent, but even at levels of 5–10%, deficits can be demonstrated on tests of vigilance and cardiac cells may shift from aerobic to anaerobic metabolism. When COHb levels reach 10–20% of total hemoglobin, cutaneous dilation and vascular headaches occur. At levels of 20–30%, headache intensifies. At 30–40% COHb, weakness, dizziness, visual impairments, nausea, and vomiting ensue. Loss of consciousness is likely at levels of 40–50% COHb. Pulse and respiration increase at 50–60% COHb; convulsions, cardiac depression, and respiratory depression occur at 60–70% COHb; and death at 60–80% saturation. When individuals are rapidly exposed to high concentrations of CO, loss of consciousness may occur without warning symptoms. Patients who are unconscious for more than 21 hours after CO exposure are unlikely to regain full neurologic function. In older individuals, coma in excess of 11 hours after CO poisoning is seldom followed by full recovery of function.

It is usually evident from the circumstances surrounding an episode of carbon monoxide poisoning that CO is the causative substance. If not, signs such as pallor and cyanosis (due to hypoxia) are revealing indications. If exposure is severe and especially at lethal levels of exposure, the skin may be bright red because of the cherry color of COHb. Blood levels of COHb provide definitive diagnosis or postmortem determination of cause of death.

Treatment of CO poisoning is based on promoting respiratory excretion of the gas. In normal room air, the elimination half-life of CO is 320 minutes. This can be reduced to 80 minutes by administering 100% oxygen or to 23 minutes by administering hyperbaric 100% oxygen. The latter technique is preferred for unconscious patients. If a pregnant woman is exposed to excessive CO, the fetus is vulnerable to toxicity with possible brain damage.

Case Study: Poisoning

C. B., a 4-year-old boy, was brought to the emergency room of a hospital by his mother after he had gotten into medication left on the counter while visiting at his aunt's house. The admitting nurse quickly learned that his mother had found him near the open bottle and had observed that some of the capsules were spilled out over the counter but had assumed that none had been ingested. Forty-five minutes later, C. B. began to act intermittently lethargic and restless. He began complaining of fuzzy vision and kept asking for water. The mother gave him a glass of water, which caused him to vomit after a few seconds. At this point the mother had rushed him into her car to go to the hospital. On the drive to the hospital, the mother observed the child appear to "pass out" twice for periods of about one-half minute each time.

The physician was called and, in the meantime, the nurse had the child lie down on the examining table. She noted that his pupils were dilated. His pulse was 95, blood pressure 75/50, temperature 97.5° F, and respirations 16/minute. The child was covered with a blanket to prevent hypothermia. The nurse asked the mother if she knew what kind of capsules had been in the bottle. The mother had not looked but went to telephone her sister to find out. The nurse observed that the child's reflexes were hyperactive and muscles were rigid. The nurse auscultated the abdomen for bowel sounds, which were absent. As the nurse began to remove the child's shirt to attach ECG electrodes, she noted that the child appeared to faint for a few seconds and then regained consciousness when the head was lowered again. As the physician arrived, the child began to convulse. The nurse quickly reviewed her observations and the physician ordered immediate administration of diazepam, 5 mg IV. The seizure subsided in 5 minutes. The physician asked how long it had been since the child ingested the capsules and if he had vomited. It had been 2 hours since the time of poisoning. The nurse attached electrodes for cardiac monitoring while another nurse placed an intravenous line. The ECG showed a prolongation of the QRS complex. The physician ordered preparation of a syringe with 0.5 mg of physostigmine salicylate, a blood sample for determination of pH and serum potassium concentrations, and a syringe with 2 mg sodium bicarbonate. At this point the mother returned with the information that the bottle contained Elavil.

The sodium bicarbonate was administered as a bolus. The physostigmine was not given but was kept on hand in the event that the condition did not respond adequately to initial therapy. After a few minutes the QRS wave shortened to normal, pulse rate declined, and respiratory rate increased. The pretreatment blood assessment was received at this point, indicating a pH of 7.28 (normal: 7.33–7.41) and potassium level of 4.8 mEq/L (normal: 3.8–5.6 mEq/L). A second blood sample taken 10 minutes after completion of the sodium bicarbonate injection gave a pH of 7.46. After 30 minutes, the child was exhibiting improved neurologic status and blood pressure. Vital signs and ECG continued to be monitored for the next 12 hours with no additional problems.

1. Explain each of the following symptoms with reference to the properties of the drug contained in Elavil: lethargy and restlessness, fuzzy vision, severe thirst, vomiting immediately after a glass of water, fainting, dilated pupils, pulse of 95, blood pressure 75/50, temperature 97.5° F, respirations 16/minute, hyperactive reflexes, muscle rigidity, absence of bowel sounds, convulsions and prolonged QRS.
2. Why didn't the physician order gastric lavage? If he had elected to do so, what would have been the appropriate time?
3. Explain the pretreatment serum pH of 7.28. Is it alarming that the posttreatment pH was 7.46?
4. Why wasn't physostigmine given immediately?

Answers appear at the end of the book.

Recommended Readings

Dreisbach RH: *Handbook of Poisonings, Diagnosis, and Treatment,* ed 8. Los Altos, Calif, Lange Medical Publications, 1980.

Frank-Stromborg M et al: Carcinogens: Are some risks acceptable? *Am J Nurs* 1986;86(7):814–817.

Gosselin RE et al: *Clinical toxicology of Commercial Products,* ed 5. Baltimore, Williams & Wilkins Co, 1984.

Goulding R, Volans GN: Emergency treatment of common poisonings: Emptying the stomach. *Proc Roy Soc Med* 1977;70:766–770.

Haddad LM, Winchester JF (eds): *Clinical Management of Poisoning and Drug Overdose.* Philadelphia, W B Saunders, 1983.

Horoshak I: What to do in a poison emergency. *RN* 1977;40:44–50.

Mennear JH: The poisoning emergency. *Am J Nurs.* 1977;7:842.

Newton M, Bartek JK, Fitzgerald A, Cawthorn-Sippel M, Schnell C: General treatments of household poisonings. *J Emerg Nurs* 1987;13(1):12–15.

Newton M, Bartek JK, Fitzgerald A, Cawthorn-Sippel M, Schnell C: Specific treatments of poisoning by household products and medications. *J Emerg Nurs* 1987;13(1):16–26.

Answers to Case Study Questions

Chapter 5 Case Study: Importance of Accurate Charting of Medication

1. Ms. P.'s legal responsibilities were: to ensure that the right drug had been administered to the right patient; to learn the normal dosage of the drug, the anticipated patient responses, the potential adverse reactions, and the symptoms a patient would be most likely to complain about; to accurately record the drug once it was administered.

2. She had cross-checked all orders with the Kardex and medication card against the doctor's order. Before administering the drug, Ms. P. reviewed literature pertaining to it, and so she knew the patient responses she might expect. Before giving the drug, Ms. P. called the patient by name and checked the patient's arm band. Following the actual administration she charted the drug in the correct place on the patient's chart. Further, she refused to follow a physician's order to readminister the drug, knowing that doing so would constitute administering an overdose of the drug. Not only did Ms. P. follow proper legal procedure, she adhered to the ethical principle of doing no harm.

3. Legal grounds supporting Ms. P's action are based on the fact that she is responsible for all drugs she administers. Acceding to the physician's demands would have resulted in the patient's receiving an overdose of the drug and in potential harm to the patient.

Chapter 6 Case Study: Altered Pharmacokinetics in a Child

1. The chapter appendix indicates that the recommended dosage range for phenytoin in infants or children is 3 to 8 mg/kg/day PO. The prescribed dose of 6 mg/kg/day PO is within this range.

2. One factor that may have contributed to subtherapeutic serum levels of phenytoin (Dilantin) was uncovered by the nurse's assessment: the mother had failed to shake the suspension before pouring the dose. Another possible factor was the rapid rate of metabolism in children, which has the effect of shortening the half-life of drugs that are inactivated largely by metabolism. The physician reduced the interval between drug administrations to compensate for the more rapid rate of drug metabolism.

3. Increasing the total dose of drug administered is a less satisfactory compensation for the rapid rate of drug metabolism in children because it elevates the peak as well as the trough plasma concentrations, the likely result being excessive adverse effects during the time of peak plasma concentrations.

Chapter 7 Case Study: Increased Drug Sensitivity in a Geriatric Client

1. The normal adult IM dosage for meperidine (Demerol) is 50–150 mg IM, every 3–4 hours, as necessary.

2. Meperidine frequently causes exaggerated responses in the elderly. For one thing, the capacity of the liver to metabolize many drugs, and meperidine in particular, is often reduced in elderly clients. For another, the fraction of meperidine in the plasma that is bound to inactive binding sites on plasma proteins or red blood cells is less than in younger adults. In H. B.'s case, measurement of the serum concentration of meperidine revealed a higher than therapeutic level. Since measurements of this kind measure both bound and unbound drug, the principal factor in this case must have been a diminished rate of metabolism of the drug by the liver.

Chapter 8 Case Study: Assessment of a Client's Preparedness for Client Education

1. The immediate focus of concern of the case as presented is client education. Presumably, then, the nurse has made a nursing diagnosis of "Knowledge deficit." The

case study describes elements of her assessment of M. R.'s preparedness for learning that she will utilize in tailoring a nursing plan to address the knowledge deficit. In addition, the case implies that additional nursing diagnoses have been made related to nutrition, such as "Alterations in Nutrition, glucose intake in excess of body requirements." Although not directly addressed in the case presented, a variety of additional nursing diagnoses are likely to apply when clients are diagnosed as having diabetes mellitus (see Chapter 33).

2. Clients are more likely to comply with the prescribed regimen if they have a thorough understanding of the nature of the disorder and the rationale for the treatment. In this case, the nurse will need to avoid underestimating M. R.'s capacity for understanding while at the same time not overestimating his ability to comprehend the necessary information from a single oral presentation. The nurse may need to repeat information and use simple terms to communicate effectively with M. R. Providing M. R. with written material about his condition and treatment that he can reread several times could be helpful. Ultimately, whatever methods are used, the nurse should test M. R.'s actual comprehension by asking him to explain back to her the essential points.

Chapter 10 Case Study: Irrational Drug Utilization

1. Drug abuse is a subcategory of drug misuse. Instances of drug misuse must meet three criteria to also qualify as abuse: (1) the drug is self-administered; (2) the motivation for using the drug is to produce an altered mental state; and (3) the use of the drug impairs or is likely to impair the user's physical or mental health or ability to function in a social context. The examples of drug misuse cited in the case do not meet the second criterion. The example involving the grandson also does not meet the first criterion. So the case illustrates examples of drug misuse that do not qualify under the stricter definition of drug abuse.

2. An appropriate nursing diagnosis relating to E. P.'s misguided use of drugs would be "Knowledge deficit relating to use of nonprescription drugs." A nursing plan needs to be developed that will provide E. P. with the education she requires concerning appropriate use of medications.

Chapter 12 Case Study: Barbiturate Intoxication

1. Body temperature was low, respirations were slow, and pulse was rapid. The hypothermia is due to heat loss from peripheral vasodilation; slow respirations is due to the effect of the barbiturate on the respiratory center of the medulla oblongata; the rapid pulse is a reflex compensation on the part of the heart to mild hypoxia.

2. Both the pH and the Po_2 was below normal. The low pH is indicative of respiratory acidosis due to depressed respirations. The low Po_2 and high Pco_2 indicate hypoxia and hypercapnia respectively, also due to depressed respirations.

3. The loss of reflexes and pain response and the slow respiration are indicative of grade IV barbiturate intoxication.

4. Naloxone (Narcan) reverses respiratory depression only when it is caused by a narcotic (see Chapter 25). Analeptics were once widely used to treat barbiturate overdoses, but they may produce convulsions even before they reverse respiratory depression. Dialysis is not usually necessary in a barbiturate overdose, unless hepatic dysfunction is evident. In the absence of hepatic impairment, treatment is based on support of vital functions and letting the liver take care of inactivating the drug.

5. Nursing diagnoses in this case might include:

alteration in family processes: marital discord and inability to perform role functions related to drug abuse.

impaired social interaction related to intoxication.

increased risk of injury related to impaired judgment and coordination during intoxication.

ineffective individual coping: mood changes, irritability, and argumentativeness during intoxication.

social isolation related to loss of family contacts.

Chapter 13 Case Study: Alcohol Troubled Person

1. The first priority in treating C. S. is alleviation of delirium tremens, since this is a potentially life-threatening condition. Chlordiazepoxide (Librium), 50 mg PO, should be administered. Fluids will need to be given to correct dehydration. Thiamine and a multivitamin preparation should be given orally to alleviate any nutritional deficiencies that may be present. If epigastric distress is evident, an antacid might be employed. Diazepam (Valium) should be at hand in case seizures develop.

2. The conditions described in the case meet several of the criteria typically used for determining admissions of emergency room patients with alcohol withdrawal (see Table 13–1): two significant metabolic problems (acidosis and hypoglycemia), anemia (reduced hematocrit), and significant dehydration. In addition, the prolonged prothrombin time could be due to impaired hepatic synthesis of clotting factors, suggesting possible liver dysfunction from alcohol consumption. Further nursing assessment might also reveal, in this case, a lack of satisfactory opportunity for care for C. S. as an outpatient, since his wife is institutionalized with Alzheimer's disease.

3. Acidosis in this case is probably due to inhibition of lactic acid conversion to pyruvate by alcohol. Low blood sugar levels are likely due to additive hypoglycemic effects of alcohol and insulin. Dehydration is commonplace in alcohol withdrawal since most alcoholic beverages are hyperosmotic and because alcohol promotes diuresis. The low hematocrit is indicative of anemia, which could be due to functional deficiencies in vitamin B_{12} and folic acid (a frequent problem in chronic alcoholics) or

might indicate occult blood loss. Prolonged prothrombin time may indicate liver dysfunction resulting in decreased production of clotting factors.

4. Alcohol inhibits conversion of lactic acid to pyruvate, an early step in gluconeogenesis. Thus, alcohol tends to cause hypoglycemia that can be additive to that caused by other hypoglycemic drugs, including insulin. Symptoms of hypoglycemia include tremulousness, flushing, faintness, palpitations, hunger, nervousness, headache, confusion, visual disturbances, ataxia, weakness, aphasia, and ultimately coma or convulsions (see Chapter 33).

5. After the immediate medical emergency is dealt with, C. S. should be encouraged to enter an alcohol treatment program. The son might benefit from participation in a program for family members of alcohol troubled persons.

Chapter 14 Case Study: Attention Deficit Disorder

1. For M. T., "Attention deficit disorder, with hyperactivity." For B. T., "Attention deficit disorder, residual type."

2. M. T. exhibits several of the characteristics that have been found to correlate with successful response to stimulant therapy: observable hyperkinetic behaviors, a low threshold for seizure discharge activity, and the deficit in visual memory.

3. B. T.'s heavy use of coffee and her "paradoxical" response to it (it helps her slow down) suggest that she has residual attention deficit disorder and has accidentally discovered a crude means of self-medicating for the problem with coffee.

4. Since prolonged therapy with methylphenidate (Ritalin) can cause blood cell abnormalities (especially a decrease in platelets), the nurse obtained this initial blood analysis to provide a baseline for later evaluation of adverse reactions.

Chapter 15 Case Study: Bad Trip

1. STP is a street name for 2, 5 dimethyl-4-ethylamphetamine. It is a substituted phenylalkylamine, similar in structure to mescaline, amphetamine, and norepinephrine.

2. Pupillary dilation occurs with psychedelics. By contrast, narcotics constrict the pupil. PCP and barbiturates have no effect on pupillary diameter. PCP would typically elevate blood pressure and cause nystagmus. Barbiturates and narcotics could be expected to slow respiration. Marihuana would typically cause ptosis.

3. Chlorpromazine (Thorazine) is an antipsychotic drug and is useful in controlling delirium or hallucinosis caused by psychedelic drugs related to mescaline or LSD. It is usually contraindicated for toxic psychoses caused by depressant drugs (because of additive depressant effects) or by PCP (because it can intensify feelings of isolation). It should not be used for toxic psychoses caused by anticholinergic drugs because of potential additive anticholinergic effects.

4. The answer to this question is a matter of personal judgment, depending on your views of the relative value of different kinds of treatment approaches: individual psychotherapy, group therapy with others having drug abuse problems, a residential program for drug abusers, and so forth. Family therapy is not a viable option in this case, since E. P. is lacking a stable family commitment.

Chapter 16 Case Study: Surgical Procedure

1. Meprobamate was used to alleviate preoperative apprehensiveness. Atropine was used for its hyporeflexic properties to suppress respiratory secretions. The combination of halothane-oxygen and nitrous oxide provided the anesthetic coma during the surgical procedure. Nitrous oxide provides better analgesia than halothane but does not provide sufficiently deep anesthesia by itself. Meperidine, a narcotic, provided analgesia. Curare provided skeletal muscle relaxation. During recovery, ampicillin was used as a precaution against infection. Meperidine and acetaminophen were used for pain control.

2. Postoperative hypothermia can occur following anesthesia because of peripheral vasodilation and inhibition of shivering from the depressant influence of general anesthetics.

3. A common adverse effect of meperidine is orthostatic hypotension, which could add dangerously to the hypotension already present.

Chapter 17 Case Study: History of Allergic Reaction to a Local Anesthetic

1. Novocaine is a trade name for procaine, which is a generic name.

2. Procaine belongs to the ester group of local anesthetics. The client is very likely to be allergic to any drug in the ester group but has only a 10% chance of being allergic to an amide type local anesthetic. Drugs in the amide group of local anesthetics include lidocaine, dibucaine, bupivacaine, etidocaine, mepivacaine, and prilocaine.

Chapter 18 Case Study: Acute Schizophrenic Episode

1. H. L. exhibits several of the overt symptoms of schizophrenia: auditory hallucinations, incoherence, inappropriate affect, and grossly disorganized behavior. There is a deterioration of previous level of functioning, H. L. is less than 45 years of age, and there is no evidence presented indicating preceding depression, mania, organic brain syndrome, or mental retardation. From the case description, it appears that this psychotic state does not meet the duration criterion for schizophrenia of at least 6

months and is therefore more accurately characterized as schizophreniform disorder.

2. The fact that his mother had a nervous breakdown and one of his sisters had nervous problems suggests a familial influence; but without further evidence, it is not possible to determine whether the familial trend is generated by genetic factors, interpersonal factors, or both.

3. The nurses are protecting H. L. from possible effects of orthostatic hypotension, such as dizziness and faintness, in advising him not to change position rapidly and helping him to the bathroom. Intake and output monitoring as well as monitoring of frequency of urination is advisable when therapy is begun with chlorpromazine, because phenothiazines can cause urinary retention (as an anticholinergic side effect). Bowel elimination should also be monitored to check for constipation (another anticholinergic effect). Since neuroleptics also have the potential of producing extrapyramidal side effects, the nurses observed H. L. for changes in motor patterns.

4. The symptoms exhibited by H. L. beginning on the sixth day are akathisias. Benzodiazepines, such as diazepam (Valium), are effective in reducing akathisias. Anticholinergic drugs are also effective but add to the anticholinergic properties of the neuroleptic and sometimes aggravate the psychotic condition. Levodopa would not be an appropriate choice for akathisias. It would provide no benefit and would aggravate the psychosis.

5. Less sedating antipsychotic drugs include the piperazine phenothiazines and butyrophenones.

6. Akathisias are self-limited, disappearing after a few weeks of therapy with an antipsychotic drug. Since diazepam was begun to control akathisias, there is no reason to continue it indefinitely. It could be begun again if akathisias recur.

7. There is a high risk of recurrence of psychosis during the first 6 months after an acute psychotic episode. Antipsychotic drugs are usually continued for 6 months after recovery to guard against recidivism.

8. For outpatients, once-a-day regimens result in better compliance than do regimens requiring several administrations each day. The small advantage that divided doses provide with respect to more stable blood levels is more than matched by the benefit of improved compliance.

Chapter 19 Case Study: Post-traumatic Stress Disorder

1. Delayed.

2. Likely contributing factors include T. P.'s being laid off from his job, the television shows about the Vietnam War, and the traumatic events he experienced during the war.

3. Diazepam (Valium) is an effective antianxiety drug for up to 3 months of daily use. Since T. P.'s anxiety symptoms were acutely severe at the time of initial treatment, a prescription for an antianxiety drug was appropriate.

4. Benzodiazepine anxiolytics should not be continued indefinitely or for periods longer than 2–3 months because they lose effectiveness and because the risk of dependence increases with prolonged use.

Chapter 19 Case Study: Generalized Anxiety Disorder

1. Factors likely to be contributing to anxiety for R. S. include raising three teenage children, a nonsupportive spouse, menopause, and excessive use of caffeine.

2. High blood pressure, or hypertension, is usually a result of multiple factors. One of the factors that contributes to hypertension is elevated tone in the sympathetic nervous system, which in turn is often related to chronic stress and anxiety.

3. There is no substantial evidence in this case to indicate that the stresses in R. S.'s life are more severe at this time than they are likely to be in 2 or 3 months. Since diazepam (Valium), taken on a regular daily schedule (such as the 2 mg tid regimen prescribed for R. S.), is effective at most for 2–3 months, little is gained by its prescription. A regimen calling for minimal use of the drug on an as-needed basis would have been more appropriate. In the long run, improvement in R. S.'s condition will depend on her responses to the suggestions from the nurse for adjustments in life-style. The prescription of the drug could have the undesirable effect of encouraging R. S. to depend too much on the easy chemical solution in lieu of the more difficult adjustments in daily living. The nurse in this case, to her credit, provided a degree of counseling that was a good deal more complete than is usually provided in treatment of anxiety clients.

4. Excessive use of caffeine is the most frequent drug factor contributing to anxiety states and its role is often unappreciated by clients and clinicians alike.

5. Alcohol and certain nonprescription drugs (such as antihistamines) have additive depressant effects with benzodiazepines. Antacids delay the absorption of diazepam.

Chapter 20 Case Study: Depression

1. C. R.'s condition is best characterized as major depression. The case description provides indications of dysphoric mood extending beyond 2 weeks, lethargy ("feeling tired"), decreased appetite and weight loss, apathy ("bored with his job"), and low self-esteem ("felt rather useless").

2. The lack of any obvious precipitating event suggests an endogenous origin.

3. Use of alcohol is one of the most frequent contributing factors in depression. Even moderate use should be discontinued when depression is evident.

4. The various laboratory tests were to assess for possible causes of secondary depression. Complete blood cell counts might reveal anemia, urinalysis might indicate an electrolyte imbalance or uremia, serum glucose determination could uncover evidence of hypoglycemia or dia-

betes mellitus, and thyroid function tests might indicate hypothyroidism or hyperthyroidism.

5. Imipramine is more sedative than protriptyline and is preferred in clients who exhibit agitation or anxiety along with depression. C. R. did not exhibit these symptoms.

6. The nurse can be expected to discuss the potential anticholinergic side effects that occur with tricyclic antidepressants, such as blurred vision, dilated pupils, dryness of mouth, sweating, constipation, urinary retention, and mental confusion. The nurse should also discuss potential changes in sexual function (possible impotence or loss of libido). The nurse should discuss the potential for orthostatic hypotension and the measures that should be used to combat this side effect. The nurse should discuss the potential for gastrointestinal irritation and instruct C. R. to take his medication with meals.

7. Measurement of protriptyline (Vivactil) levels has the double value of evaluating compliance and determining if therapeutic plasma concentrations are being achieved by the prescribed regimen. Tricyclic antidepressants exhibit variable pharmacokinetics but produce clinical benefits predictably when doses are adjusted to achieve plasma concentrations within the drug's therapeutic window.

Chapter 21 Case Study: Bipolar Affective Disorder

1. Very low. Once bipolar disorder is evident in a given individual, spontaneous remission is unlikely.

2. Yes. Chlorpromazine (Thorazine) alters the distribution of lithium between the inside and outside of cells. Molindone (Moban) does not.

3. When lithium therapy is begun, a loading dose is used initially to saturate body tissues; then smaller maintenance doses are employed.

4. Antipsychotic drugs such as chlorpromazine are used in treatment of mania only as a short-term, interim regimen until lithium begins to take effect.

5. Not necessarily. Thirst and tremor are side effects of lithium that occur commonly at normal therapeutic doses. If more severe side effects occur, the dose of lithium could be divided into more frequent, smaller administrations over the course of the day. In addition, certain side effects can be treated by other means: for example, propranolol for tremor or thyroid hormone for lithium-induced hypothyroidism.

6. Noncompliance is a frequent problem in lithium therapy for mania. For one thing, with effective therapy, symptoms of mania are controlled to an extent that it is no longer apparent to the client that he or she needs to continue the medication. For another, mania is often experienced by clients as pleasurable or useful during periods when there are extensive demands on them. They may purposefully discontinue lithium to reclaim the elevated mood and high energy level that are hallmarks of mania.

7. Lithium produces beneficial effects in mania only after 1 week or so of administration. The rapid response when R. R. was treated with chlorpromazine and lithium was attributable to the chlorpromazine.

Chapter 22 Case Study: Parkinson's Disease

1. Benztropine (Cogentin) is most effective in alleviating the action tremor and the muscle rigidity that accompany Parkinson's disease, while levodopa is more effective in alleviating the resting tremor and akinesia. The two drugs together, therefore, provide more improvement in motor function than either alone. Carbidopa has no beneficial effect in its own right in treating clients with Parkinson's disease, but it increases the fraction of the dose of levodopa that gets into the brain. This results in more response to levodopa and less severe peripheral side effects.

2. Unfortunately, clients treated with antiparkinsonian drugs frequently develop resistance to the beneficial effects of the medications as the condition progresses.

3. Vitamin B_6, pyridoxine, interferes with the efficacy of levodopa in parkinsonism.

4. Amantadine (Symmetrel) is a dopamine agonist. It is often used as an add-on to an existing regimen for Parkinson's disease when the client has developed resistance to the regimen. Amantadine often provides additional benefit for a period of time, but frequently resistance develops as well to the effect of amantadine.

Chapter 22 Case Study: Acute Dystonic Reaction

1. Trifluoperazine (Stelazine) is a piperazine phenothiazine. This subgroup of antipsychotic drugs is especially likely to produce extrapyramidal reactions. Moreover, the dose of trifluoperazine being employed at the opening of the case study (15 mg IM, tid) is excessive (the normal IM dose in hospitalized patients is 1–2 mg every 4–6 hours). The symptoms exhibited by R. K. are best characterized as an acute dystonic reaction. Although some of the features also resemble tardive dyskinesias, the time course makes it clear that the symptoms are an acute dystonic reaction.

2. Benztropine (Cogentin) is an anticholinergic drug used in treating clients with Parkinson's disease and for alleviating extrapyramidal reactions to antipsychotic drugs, such as the acute dystonic reaction evident here.

3. Extrapyramidal reactions are less common with aminoalkyl phenothiazines such as chlorpromazine (Thorazine), with dihydroindolones such as molindone (Moban), and especially with piperadine phenothiazines such as thioridazine (Mellaril).

Chapter 23 Case Study: Grand Mal Epilepsy

1. It is not especially surprising that there was no abnormality apparent in the EEG. This is frequently the case in diagnosing epilepsy, because the seizure focus may lie

deep in the cortical tissue, where its influence will not be evident in the EEG. The EEG is helpful but not definitive in diagnosing epilepsy.

2. Other factors that can contribute to precipitation of seizures include changes in blood gases, changes in serum electrolytes, changes in serum pH, changes in blood sugar levels, hormone imbalances, fatigue, and nutritional deficiencies.

3. Protection from injury is the first priority in managing a client during a major seizure. The client should not be restrained, but a pillow or blanket should be placed under the head to protect it from concussion. If available, a padded tongue depressor or other firm, soft object should be used to protect the tongue. After the convulsion subsides, the individual should be turned onto his or her side to facilitate drainage of fluids from the respiratory tract.

4. Diazepam (Valium) is the drug of choice for stopping most kinds of seizures that are in progress. Intramuscular injection is not the preferred route of administration for diazepam under most circumstances, because absorption after IM injection is irregular. However, during a seizure, oral administration is contraindicated and intravenous administration is seldom practical, so the IM route is used by default. Deep injection maximizes the likelihood that an IM dose will be absorbed rapidly.

5. Phenytoin (Dilantin) has an antivitamin effect with respect to vitamin D. Although supplementation of the other vitamins contained in a multivitamin preparation is not a clear necessity, it is a reasonable and harmless precaution to provide vitamins at the recommended daily allowances for clients who suffer from a chronic disease such as epilepsy.

6. From the analysis of serum concentration of phenytoin, it is apparent that the serum level achieved by the prescribed regimen is within the range that is reliably effective (10–20 μg/ml). Were it lower than 10 μg/ml, it would be sensible to increase the dose of phenytoin before adding a second drug. But given that the plasma concentration is within the effective range, addition of phenobarbital to the regimen is more likely to provide additional therapeutic benefit without risking toxic concentrations of either drug.

7. Additive CNS depression should be expected from the interaction of phenytoin and phenobarbital.

Chapter 23 Case Study: Petit Mal Epilepsy

1. Petit mal often first comes to clinical attention as an apparent learning disability because the frequent seizures characteristic of petit mal tend to interrupt the continuity of learning activities for the child.

2. Heavy use of alcohol (or other sedative-hypnotics) can be a factor in triggering seizures, because the seizure threshold is lowered after CNS depression during the subsequent withdrawal phase. Marihuana can have variable effects on seizure threshold as well.

3. Adolescents are especially sensitive about how they appear in the eyes of their peers. The requirement to take medication may itself cause the child to feel self-conscious and different. Any side effects that alter appearance, such as skin eruptions, skin discolorations, or changes in hair distribution, will be especially unacceptable to adolescents.

Chapter 24 Case Study: Acute Exacerbation of Chronic Organic Brain Syndrome

1. M. S.'s husband indicated that M. S. had been drinking heavily of late but not during the day immediately preceding the onset of psychotic symptoms. If this report is accurate, the timing is consistent with occurrence of alcohol withdrawal symptoms and inconsistent with acute toxic psychosis, which occurs while alcohol blood levels are very high after a drinking bout.

2. Hypokalemia is always a potential consequence of therapy with diuretic drugs such as hydrochlorthiazide. There is no indication from the case study that M. S. is making use of potassium-rich foods or using potassium supplements to prevent hypokalemia. Hypokalemia is a potential cause of acute organic brain syndrome or, as in this case, acute aggravation of existing chronic organic brain syndrome.

3. Thiamine is vitamin B_1. Chronic alcoholism often results in a thiamine deficiency; its prescription is a precaution against this possibility. Dihydroergotoxine (Hydergine) is a stimulator of cerebral metabolism. It is used to enhance cognitive function in clients with chronic organic brain syndrome.

4. We have already noted that hydrochlorthiazide can aggravate chronic organic brain syndrome to the extent that hypokalemia occurs. Alcohol and flurazepam, both CNS depressants, can increase the cognitive impairments of chronic organic brain syndrome.

5. The physician was checking for other factors that might contribute acutely to organic brain syndrome: hypoxia, anemia, acidosis, or hypoglycemia.

6. Chlordiazepoxide (Librium) is often used for treatment of alcohol withdrawal. It substitutes for alcohol, preventing development of the withdrawal syndrome. Although the client must later undergo withdrawal from chlordiazepoxide, this syndrome is less severe and is far less life-threatening than withdrawal from alcohol. Potassium chloride was given to alleviate hypokalemia.

7. Alcohol and flurazepam (Dalmane) would produce additive depressant effects with chlordiazepoxide.

Chapter 25 Case Study: Pain and Analgesia

1. Morphine has only limited oral effectiveness. Meperidine (Demerol) provides a comparable analgesic benefit and is orally effective. Oral administration, when feasible, is safer, easier, and generally more acceptable to clients.

2. Codeine is a narcotic analgesic of intermediate potency, while meperidine is a high-potency drug. Since

abuse liability is determined by potency, it is best to use the narcotic of least potency, at the lowest possible dose, that provides an adequate level of analgesia.

3. The analgesia produced by codeine can be augmented by addition of a nonnarcotic analgesic, such as acetaminophen, as soon as oral administration is feasible.

Chapter 26 Case Study: Migraine Headache

1. The periodic occurrence of the headaches and the occurrence of prodromal symptoms (nausea, lightheadedness, and blindspots).

2. Hypertension, vasospastic peripheral vascular disorders, sepsis, hepatic or renal disease, severe pruritus, or known hypersensitivity to ergot alkaloids.

3. Effectiveness of ergotamine in migraine is directly related to how quickly it is taken after onset of symptoms.

4. Propranolol (Inderal) is the drug most often used for this purpose in the United States. Methysergide (Sansert) is another option. A variety of other drugs have been used experimentally and in Europe (see text).

Chapter 28 Case Study: Shock

1. Low blood pressure, rapid pulse, rapid respirations, recent history of urinary tract infection, fever, abdominal pain, painful urination, and flu-like symptoms.

2. Administration of fluids is the first priority in overcoming shock.

3. Pressor drugs raise blood pressure by constricting peripheral blood vessels. In shock, tissue perfusion is already impaired and constriction of peripheral vessels could further aggravate tissue anoxia.

4. Alpha blockers dilate peripheral vessels to improve tissue perfusion.

5. Since an alpha-blocker will lower blood pressure, it cannot be given until blood pressure has been increased sufficiently by fluid therapy.

6. When the alpha-blocker is administered, it must be given slowly to prevent an untoward reduction in blood pressure.

Chapter 29 Case Study: Myasthenia Gravis

1. Myasthenia gravis was indicated by muscular weakness, drooping eyelids, and easy fatigability, but there are many other medical conditions that can lead to similar symptoms of muscle weakness and fatigue.

2. Neostigmine is a reversible cholinesterase inhibitor. It has the effect of elevating endogenous levels of acetylcholine by blocking its breakdown. In the event of an overdose, an anticholinergic drug, such as atropine, could be given.

3. Intravenous titration is more rapid.

4. Excess salivation, gastrointestinal hyperactivity (resulting in nausea, vomiting, diarrhea, or cramps), and increased respiratory secretion are indications of excess muscarinic activity. Since swallowing difficulties often occur in myasthenia gravis, an excess of fluids in the trachea can pose special problems for F. B.

5. Diuretics increase elimination of potassium, possibly resulting in hypokalemia. Hypokalemia aggravates myasthenia gravis and complicates its drug management.

Chapter 30 Case Study: Isolated Growth Hormone Deficiency

1. Isolated growth hormone deficiency is a type of pituitary insufficiency and is not an inherited condition. Hereditary factors are involved in only about 40% of all cases of short stature in children.

2. Growth hormone is a protein and will denature when exposed to temperature extremes.

3. Although growth hormone is potently anabolic, its growth-promoting influence is supported by lipid metabolism rather than glucose metabolism. Growth hormone actually reduces glucose metabolism, which tends to raise blood sugar levels and produce glucose intolerance.

4. Although the current evaluation of R. G. has indicated an isolated deficiency of growth hormone, the condition could later generalize to other anterior pituitary hormones such as thyroid-stimulating hormone, the hormone that regulates thyroid function.

Chapter 31 Case Study: Thyroid Disorders

1. Emotional instability, rapid pulse, fine tremor of the hand, increased reflexes, warm moist skin, exophthalmos, and low weight.

2. Serum total T_4 may also be raised when levels of thyroid-binding globulin have been increased by estrogen even though the client is euthyroid. T_3 resin uptake may be elevated when thyroid-binding globulin has been lowered by certain drugs (such as anabolic steroids or phenytoin), even though the client is euthyroid. See Table 31–1.

3. Antithyroid drugs can cross the placental barrier and cause hypothyroidism in the fetus.

4. Some of the symptoms of hyperthyroidism are attributable to supersensitivity of beta-adrenergic receptors induced by thyroid hormones (see Table 31–4). Propranolol (Inderal) blocks beta-adrenergic receptors, alleviating these symptoms.

5. Propylthiouracil often takes 3 days to 6 weeks to produce beneficial effects because it may take that long to deplete the existing stores of thyroid hormone. However, those symptoms related to adrenergic supersensitivity can be alleviated immediately by administration of propranolol.

6. Overly vigorous therapy for hyperthyroidism with propylthiouracil can result in symptoms of hypothyroidism, including fatigue and weight gain.

7. Six months of propylthiouracil therapy results in extended remission of hyperthyroidism in a fraction of clients (variably estimated at between 16% and 50%).

8. Iodine is used prior to thyroid surgery as a means of inducing involution (shrinkage) of the gland to facilitate surgery.

9. T_3 has a shorter half-life than T_4 and therefore allows for more rapid dosage adjustment. After dosage adjustment, substitution of T_4 allows for less frequent drug administration because of its longer half-life. T_3 must be continued for 3 days during the switchover period to avoid a period of hypothyroidism during initial accumulation of T_4.

10. The removal of part of the parathyroids could result in hypocalcemia because of the important role of parathyroid hormone in calcium homeostasis. Ergocalciferol is a form of vitamin D, which plays an important role in calcium absorption.

11. Cramps and paresthesias are classic indications of hypocalcemia.

12. Anxiety, warmth, and weight loss are symptoms of hyperthyroidism, indicating a need for downward adjustment of the dosage of T_3.

Chapter 32 Case Study: Cushing's Syndrome

1. Redistribution of fat is a hallmark of Cushing's syndrome. This feature was indicated by the puffy eyelids, rounded cheeks, and obesity on the torso but not on the extremities. Easy bruisability, presence of red striae, and psychotic symptoms are additional indications of Cushing's syndrome in this case.

2. The elevation of plasma and free cortisol levels, the absence of the normal diurnal rhythm, and the low-dose dexamethasone test are all indicative of Cushing's syndrome but do not distinguish between the various possible etiologies. The lack of response to the high-dose dexamethasone test and the metapirone test rule out a pituitary adenoma. The low serum level of ACTH rules out both a pituitary adenoma and ectopic ACTH syndrome. The ACTH challenge test made the final differentiation between an adenoma and an adenocarcinoma. See Table 32–3 for a summary of test results that occur for each type of test.

3. The only alternative to surgical intervention for Cushing's syndrome is administration of inhibitors of steroid synthesis.

4. Insufficient glucocorticoid activity results in hypoglycemia, decreased cold tolerance, and weakness. Glucocorticoid excess results in the full range of symptoms of Cushing's syndrome: hyperglycemia, suppression of lymphocytes, monocytes, and eosinophils, cataracts and increased intraocular pressure, psychotic symptoms, susceptibility to infection, easy bruisability, acne, redistribution of fat, muscle wasting, and osteoporosis. Mineralocorticoid deficiency results in hypotension, hyponatremia, hyperkalemia, hypovolemia, and ultimately circulatory collapse. Mineralocorticoid excess produces opposite effects, including hypernatremia, hypokalemia, alkalosis, hypervolemia, hypercalcemia, hypertension, and congestive heart failure.

Chapter 32 Case Study: Addison's Disease

1. Low blood pressure, syncope upon standing, weakness and fatigue, nausea and vomiting, and increased skin pigmentation are indications of Addison's disease.

2. Overly vigorous therapy with a diuretic could have accounted for some of the symptoms and electrolyte changes.

3. The low serum level of sodium (hyponatremia) and elevated level of potassium (hyperkalemia) are direct consequences of insufficient aldosterone activity, since aldosterone's normal role is to stimulate reabsorption of sodium and secretion of potassium. The low fasting blood sugar level and elevated blood urea nitrogen are caused by deficiency of glucocorticoid activity, which results in reduced carbohydrate metabolism and elevated protein catabolism. The low white blood cell count is another typical finding in Addison's disease.

4. The physician is anticipating replacement therapy that will include a glucocorticoid. These drugs increase susceptibility to infection and can convert latent tuberculosis into fulminating or disseminated tuberculosis.

5. The lack of a rise in plasma 17-hydroxysteroids in response to metyrapone is indicative of primary Addison's disease. The levels would rise sharply if the condition were secondary.

6. A regular plan of exercise minimizes the need for the fine tuning of glucose levels in which glucocorticoids play a role. A. B. should maintain a high-protein diet to offset the catabolic influence of the glucocorticoids in his regimen. The fundamental physiological role of glucocorticoids is in preparing the body to respond to stressful circumstances, so higher doses of glucocorticoids are required for physiological replacement during times of stress.

7. Hydrocortisone ester, given by injection, provided a rapid response during initial therapy, but an oral preparation is more practical for maintenance therapy after discharge.

8. The replacement regimen provided for a larger dose in the morning than in the afternoon in order to more closely simulate the normal diurnal rhythm of the glucocorticoids.

9. Prednisone provides little mineralocorticoid activity. Flurocortisone has mainly mineralocorticoid activity and provides replacement for aldosterone that is lacking in Addison's disease.

Chapter 33 Case Study: Diabetes Mellitus

1. Typically in treating clients who have diabetes mellitus with insulin, an intermediate- or long-acting insulin is used daily to provide a baseline replacement, and a short-acting preparation is used for fine tuning glucose control to compensate for variations in daily activities or food intake.

2. Allergic reactions are more common to insulins obtained from animal sources because of presence of small amounts of animal proteins in the preparations.

3. The midday symptoms are indicative of hypoglycemia. Since E. S. takes an intermediate-acting and a short-acting insulin preparation in the morning, hypoglycemia is most likely to develop at midday when the short-acting drug is producing its peak action. The evening symptoms are ones associated with hyperglycemia. E. S. would be

most apt to experience such symptoms in the evening, because the effects of the morning dose of the short-acting preparation have substantially worn off by that time. It is not surprising that E. S. experiences symptoms of both hypo- and hyperglycemia at different times of the day, because insulin injections do not adequately mimic the fine control normally exerted by the pancreas over insulin release and blood glucose levels.

4. For the person with diabetes, exercise is equivalent to a dose of insulin in its effect on blood glucose levels. Thus, exercise plus a normal dose of insulin is equivalent to an excessive dose of insulin, which leads to hypoglycemia.

5. Use of alcohol or tobacco complicates management of diabetes with insulin.

6. Increasing the dose of the long-acting drug will provide for more effect in the evening to combat hyperglycemia. Reducing the dose of the short-acting drug will decrease the overall effect at midday to alleviate the hypoglycemia.

7. Most types of learning have to be reinforced from time to time. Moreover, client education provided at the time when a medical condition is initially diagnosed is often poorly retained by the client, because the stress of learning that one has a significant medical problem interferes with acquisition of information.

8. Oral hypoglycemics are not effective in the insulin-dependent type of diabetes mellitus and would thus not provide adequate control of blood sugar levels for E. S.

9. Ketoacidosis is treated with a rapid-acting form of insulin (such as Humulin R) to provide the quickest possible benefit. Sodium bicarbonate is given to alleviate acidosis. Fluid therapy and potassium chloride were provided to alleviate cellular dehydration and electrolyte imbalances that frequently accompany ketoacidosis.

10. State-of-the-art treatment of severe diabetes mellitus can delay but does not indefinitely prevent the complications associated with the disorder. The more carefully blood sugar levels are regulated, the slower the complications develop. There is no indication from the information presented that E. S. received anything less than very good medical care by current standards of treatment for this disorder.

Chapter 34 Case Study: Contraception with a Combination Oral Contraceptive

1. The presenting symptoms are ones related to estrogen deficiency (see Table 34–5).

2. Ortho-Novum 2 mg provides high estrogenic activity and medium progestin activity, and should thus alleviate the symptoms of estrogen deficiency that occurred with Norlestrin 2.5/50.

3. The nurse should not have advised S. S. to double up on the next few doses after missing 3 days. Doubling up is employed only when the client misses the first two pills. A single missed pill is taken as soon as remembered without doubling up. The cycle should not be extended beyond its normal end point when any number of pills are skipped.

4. When three or more pills are missed at the beginning of a cycle, contraception is unreliable. If there is any likelihood of pregnancy, birth control pills should be discontinued immediately, because their use presents a risk of teratogenic effects to the fetus.

Chapter 34 Case Study: Pregnancy and Postpartum

1. The added metabolic demands placed on a woman by pregnancy justify supplementation of vitamins even if the diet is one that would be normally adequate.

2. Alcohol and tobacco have teratogenic potential. Alcohol use during pregnancy can cause the fetal alcohol syndrome, characterized by elevated incidence of birth defects such as ptosis, hirsutism, craniofacial anomalies, skeletal defects, and congenital heart disease. Tobacco use during pregnancy is associated with decreased birthweight and increased frequency of spontaneous abortion.

3. Tetracyclines form complexes with calcium and can impair the development of the fetal skeleton.

4. Thiazide diuretics cross the placental barrier and, although their effects on the fetus are unknown, they are no longer favored for routine use in pregnancy. Increased bedrest helps to alleviate edema by reducing pooling of fluid in the extremities. Lying on the left side increases venous return to the heart, improving cardiac output.

5. Swelling that does not respond to bedrest, blood pressure in excess of 140/90, and albuminuria are indications of preeclampsia.

6. When preeclampsia develops after 34 or 35 weeks of pregnancy, labor may be induced to protect the health of the mother. Oxytocin stimulates the smooth muscle of the uterus to produce contractions similar to natural labor.

7. Meperidine (Demerol), a narcotic, was given to F. W. during labor for pain relief. Naloxone (Narcan) was given to the neonate to antagonize the depressant effect of meperidine on respiration.

8. Symptoms of preeclampsia do not resolve immediately with delivery of the child.

9. In addition to the psychological benefits to mother and child alike when mothers breastfeed, breast milk provides the optimum nutritional support for early development and provides transfer of immunological competence from mother to child. See Chapter 44 for comparisons of breast milk and formulas.

Chapter 35 Case Study: Abuse of Anabolic Steroids

1. The NCAA forbids the use of performance enhancing drugs in intercollegiate sports and has initiated a program of drug testing at championship events.

2. Women using androgens have the special liability of masculinization, including such symptoms as growth of facial hair, deepening of the voice, increased musculature,

male-pattern baldness, and hypertrophy of the clitoris. Hypogonadal males treated with androgenic drugs may initially experience priapism—persistent, painful erections.

Chapter 37 Case Study: Congestive Heart Failure

1. Weak pulse is a direct indication of diminished cardiac output. Breathlessness, painful respiration, wheezes, and rales are classic backward manifestations of left heart failure indicating congestion of fluid in the lungs. Cyanosis is a forward manifestation of left heart failure and is caused by insufficient perfusion of peripheral tissues. Cardiomegaly and rapid pulse are compensatory responses.

2. Furosemide (Lasix) is used to reduce edema and pulmonary congestion, which helps to reduce cardiac workload. Rotating tourniquets has the effect of reducing venous return to further reduce the work requirements of the heart. Digoxin is a cardiac glycoside used to increase cardiac output in congestive heart failure.

3. Digoxin increases contractility of the myocardium. This is its positive, inotropic effect. Its immediate action is inhibition of the sodium-potassium pump, which increases intracellular sodium. Since sodium can be exchanged for calcium, intracellular calcium levels also increase. Calcium has an important role in initiating contraction of cardiac smooth muscle.

4. Normal hemoglobin ruled out the possibility that anemia was the cause of the dyspnea and breathlessness. Elevated blood urea nitrogen and slight hypokalemia are signs of impaired renal output, probably secondary to reduced renal blood flow.

5. Loading doses of digoxin are used initially to saturate body tissues; maintenance doses are lower.

6. Without potassium supplementation, hydrochlorthiazide causes hypokalemia. Hypokalemia increases the effect and toxicity of cardiac glycosides. Lidocaine (Xylocaine) and phenytoin (Dilantin) are antidysrhythmic drugs used to control dysrhythmias related to toxicity of cardiac glycosides.

7. The electrolyte imbalance that was aggravating the toxicity of digitoxin was corrected by intravenous fluid therapy.

8. J. D. altered his administration pattern from taking the drug on an empty stomach to taking it after lunch with a glass of cold milk. Absorption of digoxin is reduced when it is taken with foods. Cold foods in particular prolong gastric emptying time, delaying absorption of digoxin. Different brands of digoxin may vary significantly in pharmacokinetic characteristics.

Chapter 38 Case Study: Ventricular Fibrillation

1. Contributing factors in development of ventricular fibrillation in this case most likely included the physical exertion of several sets of tennis, the history of tobacco smoking, the history of alcohol consumption, the stress of changing jobs, and P. L.'s age.

2. Ventricular fibrillation is fatal unless terminated quickly. During ventricular fibrillation, circulation of blood may be impaired to the extent that delivery of drug to the heart after injection or even intravenous infusion can not be assumed. In any case, cardioversion by direct current is the treatment of choice for ventricular fibrillation and provides the best hope of recovery.

3. Sympathetic activity accompanying stress and anxiety could precipitate recurrence of cardiac dysrhythmia. Diazepam (Valium) is employed as required to provide sedation.

4. Yes. Frequent PVBs are frequently harbingers of ventricular tachycardia or fibrillation. Lidocaine (Xylocaine) is used to depress myocardial excitability when frequent PVBs occur to forestall more serious tachydysrhythmias.

5. Tocainide (Tonocard) is orally effective. Lidocaine is effective only by injection and is therefore limited to in-hospital use.

6. Administration of tocainide with food slows its absorption but does not alter the ultimate extent of absorption.

Chapter 38 Case Study: Cinchonism

1. The nurse recognized that the disturbance in vision, nausea, photophobia, and elevated temperature were possible indications of cinchonism. Even though D. S. did not volunteer the information, the nurse was astute enough to question him about the presence of such symptoms. The complaints were recorded and reported immediately to the physician.

2. In her assessment, the nurse observed the change in the client's reading habits and that the reason given suggested an alteration in visual function. Further assessment revealed that D. S. was experiencing photophobia, nausea, and hyperthermia. The analysis phase included a review of blood studies already conducted, the medication chart, and literature in the ward library. In establishing a plan to address the drug side effects that D. S. was experiencing, the nurse recognized that the prescribing physician and other members of the health care team would need to be involved. She implemented her plan by meeting with the health care team to report her findings. After quinidine therapy was discontinued, the nurse evaluated D. S. for improvement in the symptoms noted earlier during assessment and observed that the symptoms ultimately resolved.

Chapter 39 Case Study: Essential Hypertension

1. Risk factors for hypertension in R. H.'s case included his age, gender, and race. Contributing factors may have included his use of alcohol and caffeinated beverages and an uncontrolled diet high in sodium, saturated fats, and cholesterol.

2. Hypertension is one of several potential causes of vascular headaches (see Chapter 26).

3. High blood pressure initially produces no substantial health deficits, but over a period of years contributes to arteriosclerosis, congestive heart failure, myocardial infarction, and mortality in general. Effective therapy for high blood pressure by dietary adjustments, exercise, and drugs not only lowers pressure, but also protects the individual from the associated long-term complications.

4. The usual second step in treatment of hypertension is addition of a beta-blocker. Other drugs that might be added to the regimen ultimately include centrally and peripherally acting sympatholytics, vasodilators, and inhibitors of angiotensin-converting enzyme.

5. Counting pills is one straightforward means of assessing compliance.

6. Regular monitoring of blood pressure should be conducted in order to evaluate whether the client continues to comply with the regimen and if the regimen continues to provide sufficient control of blood pressure.

Chapter 40 Case Study: Ischemic Heart Disease

1. R. B.'s angina is best characterized as typical (it is exercise induced) and unstable (it is gradually getting worse).

2. Dipyridamole (Persantine) is a long-acting nitrite used for prophylaxis of angina pectoris. Nitroglycerin is used to alleviate acute attacks.

3. Angina tends to be aggravated by heavy meals ("on way from restaurant") and cold weather ("blustery February night"). Myocardial infarction often develops from an acute aggravation of preexisting angina.

4. Warfarin (Coumadin) is an oral anticoagulant that may be employed electively in an effort to prevent further clot formation that could result in secondary complications such as pulmonary embolism, extension of the infarct, or thrombophlebitis. There is no irrefutable evidence that oral anticoagulants succeed in diminishing these complications (see Chapter 41).

5. Lidocaine (Xylocaine) and procainamide (Pronestyl) are antidysrhythmic drugs employed in this instance to eliminate ventricular premature beats that might progress to dangerous ventricular tachydysrhythmias.

6. Procainamide causes gastrointestinal reactions (such as anorexia, nausea, vomiting, and diarrhea), neurological symptoms (such as confusion, hallucinations, nightmares, and depression), and allergic reactions (including skin rashes, febrile reactions, bone marrow suppression, and a dangerous lupus erythematosus-like syndrome). See Chapter 38 for a complete discussion of procainamide.

7. Propranolol (Inderal) has been shown to reduce 6-month mortality rates when given during the recovery period following a myocardial infarct.

Chapter 41 Case Study: Iron-Deficiency Anemia

1. Iron-rich foods include liver, egg yolks, oysters, brewer's yeast, wheat germ, dried beans, fruits, and spinach.

2. Ferrous sulfate is the iron salt most often used to provide iron supplementation. Oral preparations include tablets, timed release capsules, liquids, syrups, and elixirs. Other salts of iron sometimes used include ferrous gluconate and ferrous fumarate.

3. Daily intake of iron is barely adequate to replace losses under the best of circumstances because of its relative scarcity in foods and its poor absorption. Any factor adversely affecting the balance between iron intake and requirements can result in a frank deficiency. Such factors include pregnancy, menstruation, bleeding, use of nonsteroidal anti-inflammatory drugs, malabsorption syndrome, elevated dietary starch, or disorders of iron reutilization.

Chapter 41 Case Study: Pulmonary Embolism Secondary to Deep Vein Thrombosis

1. The most common cause of pulmonary embolism is dislodgement of a clot from a deep vein in the thigh or calf. After dislodgement, the clot typically passes freely to and through the heart and is passed to the lungs where it becomes lodged in a small pulmonary blood vessel.

2. Rapid pulse, rapid respirations, and slight hyperthermia.

3. When pulmonary perfusion is reduced by embolism, exchange of gases is impaired. The result is hypoxia and respiratory alkalosis due to accumulation of CO_2 in the blood. The immediate objective of treatment with an oral anticoagulant is to increase prothrombin time by a factor of 2, from the normal value of 11–12 seconds to 20–25 seconds. The initial measurement provides a baseline value for later assessment of the drug effect.

4. Heparin is rapidly effective but can be given only by injection. The effect of Warfarin (Coumadin) begins only after 8–12 hours, but it is more useful for extended therapy because of its oral effectiveness.

5. Heparin therapy can be monitored by use of Lee-White whole blood clotting time or an activated partial thromboplastin time. The prothrombin test is not affected by heparin.

6. Use of estrogen-containing oral contraceptives has been linked to an increased risk of thromboembolism. This risk is especially great for women who have had a previous embolism.

7. Use of anticoagulants increases the risk of bleeding and the risk that bleeding will be severe if it occurs. Hemorrhage is the foremost concern when anticoagulants are employed.

8. Elevated intake of vitamin K will antagonize the action of oral anticoagulants. Therefore, the nurse probably instructed B. E. to avoid vitamin preparations con-

taining vitamin K and excessive consumption of spinach, kale, cabbage, or collard greens.

9. Heparin cannot be administered practically outside of a hospital setting, because it lacks oral effectiveness.

Chapter 42 Case Study: Dehydration

1. Symptoms indicative of dehydration in this case include flushed and warm skin, inelasticity of the skin, rapid weight loss, low blood pressure, diminished urinary output, dark coloration of urine, feeling weak, and elevated temperature.

2. The nurse helped the client develop a plan that would enable him to care for himself at home. The plan made use of fluids that L. T. enjoyed drinking.

Chapter 42 Case Study: Hypokalemia

1. Hypokalemia can result in paralytic ileus, a condition in which the motor activity of the intestines is suppressed, resulting in constipation and adominal distention. Hyperkalemia can also result in motor paralysis. In G. A.'s case, ascites caused by chronic alcohol ingestion may be another factor contributing to abdominal distention.

2. Potassium solutions provide the least risk of intestinal lesions. Time release tablets are next safest, then regular tablets, and enteric coated products most likely to cause ulcerations.

3. Foods rich in potassium include bananas, citrus fruits, tomatoes, potatoes, and lima beans (also see Table 42–7). Cola beverages also contain large amounts of potassium. In addition to potassium salts used to provide potassium supplementation, the most important potassium-containing drug is potassium penicillin G.

4. Laxatives promote loss of potassium-rich gastrointestinal secretions, contributing to or aggravating hypokalemia.

5. Potassium levels are important for cardiovascular, neurological, and motor function. Potassium levels also influence the activity and toxicity or other drugs, including diuretics and cardiac glycosides.

Chapter 43 Case Study: Diabetes Insipidus

1. M. T. has neurogenic diabetes insipidus, which is deficient production of antidiuretic hormone (vasopressin) by the pituitary gland.

2. Antidiuretic hormone (ADH) is also known as vasopressin, and this alternative name emphasizes the activity of ADH on vascular smooth muscle. ADH is a potent vasoconstrictor. ADH also bears a structural resemblance to oxytocin, its companion hormone in the posterior pituitary, and has weak oxytocic activity. It is this oxytocic activity that results in uterine contractions. Bradycardia in response to ADH is a reflex compensatory response to rising blood pressure.

3. Antidiuretic hormone decreased output of water in the urine, thereby promoting fluid retention. An excessive ADH action can result in water intoxication.

Chapter 43 Case Study: Diuretic Therapy

1. Swelling and pain in the right big toe joint is a classic indication or uric acid retention.

2. Calcium is normal; chloride is low (hypochloremia); bicarbonate is elevated (metabolic alkalosis); potassium is depleted (hypokalemia); magnesium is low (hypomagnesia); sodium is on the low side of the normal range; phosphate is normal; pH is elevated (alkalosis); the BUN is elevated; creatinine is normal; and glucose is normal. The imbalances that are present are typical consequences of vigorous thiazide therapy without adequate potassium supplementation. The elevated BUN indicates uric acid retention.

3. An appropriate diagnosis would be hypochloremic, hypokalemic alkalosis caused by diuretic therapy without adequate potassium supplementation. The neurological symptoms are most likely a reflection of hypokalemia.

4. The normal sodium and creatinine values indicate an appropriate, therapeutic degree of diuresis.

5. Since the type IV pumps secrete either potassium or hydrogen in exchange for sodium, elevating the availability of potassium also reduces the necessity for secreting hydrogen ions.

6. Aspirin tends to stimulate respiration and can cause respiratory alkalosis as a result. This influence could tend to aggravate the existing metabolic alkalosis.

7. Colchicine is useful for acute relief of hyperuricemia because it blocks uric acid receptors.

8. Dyazide contains a potassium-sparing diuretic as well as hydrochlorthiazide. The potassium-sparing diuretic reduces the potassium-depleting effect of the thiazide but provides additive diuretic efficacy.

9. When a potassium-sparing diuretic is included in the regimen, there is a risk that hyperkalemia will develop if potassium intake is excessive.

Chapter 44 Case Study: Low-Cholesterol Diet

1. Serum cholesterol levels correlate positively with the likelihood of heart attacks. Regimens that succeed in lowering serum cholesterol reduce the incidence of heart attacks.

2. It is often difficult for clients to adhere to dietary restrictions to achieve a therapeutic goal such as reducing serum cholesterol when there is no observable benefit. The nurse working with G. T. attempted to make the dietary adjustments as palatable as possible by including his favorite food, Polish sausage.

3. This question invites your personal observations based on your own philosophy of nursing.

Chapter 44 Case Study: Hypervitaminosis A

1. Symptoms in this case that are consistent with a diagnosis of hypervitaminosis A include abdominal discomfort, lack of energy, poor appetite, dry skin, pruritus, brittle nails, hair loss, and irritability.

2. Excess intake of vitamin D also leads to a clinical syndrome. Disorders of vitamin excess are most often seen with fat-soluble vitamins, since these vitamins tend to accumulate in fat depots of the body. Water-soluble vitamins seldom produce symptoms of excess, because amounts ingested in excess of requirements are rapidly excreted in the urine.

Chapter 45 Case Study: Rheumatoid Arthritis

1. Yes. Pain, tenderness, and immobility are the hallmark symptoms of rheumatoid arthritis.

2. Mild anemia (normochromic, normocytic) is typical in many chronic diseases, including rheumatoid arthritis. Use of aspirin can also contribute by increasing occult blood loss.

3. The demonstration of presence of RF factor is the most direct evidence. X-ray evaluation revealing changes typical of rheumatoid arthritis is also valuable.

4. Excess weight places undue strain on joints already damaged by rheumatoid arthritis. Provision of adequate rest periods reduces wear and tear on the affected joints.

5. Gastrointestinal distress, tinnitus, and increased bleeding tendencies are likely adverse responses to nonsteroidal anti-inflammatory drugs such as aspirin.

6. P. C. appears to be complying with the therapeutic regimen based on the evaluation of serum salicylate concentration and on the general improvement in her physical mobility.

7. Nonsteroidal anti-inflammatory drugs are effective in alleviating pain and immobility associated with rheumatoid arthritis but do not correct existing deformity. Thus, the lack of change in the extent of deformity is to be expected and does not adversely reflect on therapeutic progress.

Chapter 47 Case Study: Pneumonitis—Bacterial vs. Viral

1. The symptoms that are probably related to pneumonia include chills, shakes, fever, nonproductive cough, rapid pulse, rapid respirations, and nasopharyngeal inflammation. The x-ray finding of opacity in the lower left lung, the presence of leukocytosis, and the sputum culture revealing presence of *Staphylococcus aureus* supported a diagnosis of pneumonia.

2. Cloxacillin is a penicillinase-resistant drug that is effective against most strains of *Staphylococcus aureus*. Methacillin has a similar antibacterial spectrum but lacks oral effectiveness.

3. Allergic reactions are common with use of anti-infective drugs. A 30-minute period of observation after administration of the first dose is a reasonable precaution against occurrence of potentially serious hypersensitivity reactions.

4. Completing the full course of antibacterial therapy is of crucial importance to the ultimate success of the regimen. Symptoms may resolve after most of the bacteria have been eliminated, but premature discontinuation of the drug regimen may allow the remaining hardy survivors to proliferate and produce a reinfection that will be harder to treat than the original one.

5. Round-the-clock administration of antibacterial agents maximizes their effectiveness in eradicating the pathogenic bacteria.

6. Each antimicrobial drug is effective only against certain organisms. For most kinds of viral infections, including influenza, type A, there are no effective drug remedies.

Chapter 48 Case Study: Candidiasis

1. Perlèche is inflammation in the corner of the lips, with exudation, maceration, and fissuring. Thrush is candidiasis of the oral mucous membranes, with possible ulceration.

2. No, because *Candida albicans* is part of the commensal flora—always present to some extent—but causes opportunistic infections.

3. The opportunity for proliferation of *Candida* was most likely provided by L. R's poor nutritional habits and elevated stress.

4. Other drugs active in candidiasis include amphotericin B (Fungizone), nystatin (Mycostatin), miconazole (Monistat), and flucytosine (Ancobon). Amphotericin B and miconazole must be given by injection. Nystatin can be given orally, but only for intestinal infections. Flucytosine is useful orally, but not sufficiently effective to be used alone.

5. Ketoconazole (Nizoral) is a mildly basic drug and requires adequate stomach acid for dissolution and absorption. Antacids therefore impair absorption of ketoconazole. Taking ketoconazole with food minimizes nausea and vomiting.

6. An antiemetic drug can be administered with ketoconazole to alleviate nausea and vomiting.

7. Ketoconazole, being mildly basic, could irritate the oral mucosa.

8. Yellow skin or sclera, pale stools, dark urine, or pruritus are indications of possible allergic jaundice.

Chapter 49 Case Study: Immunizations

1. DPT is a triple vaccine consisting of diphtheria and tetanus toxoids and pertussis vaccine. MMR is another triple vaccine, for measles, mumps, and rubella.

2. Current evidence suggests that when measles epidemics occur among late adolescents or young adults, those who have had the disease in childhood are as likely to get the disease as are those who did not. Christine might

gain protection from an immunization at age 17 even if she had measles (or if she had been immunized) as a child.

3. The protection afforded by immunization has begun to dissipate by late adolescence, leaving these individuals susceptible to outbreaks. Symptoms of measles are more intense and more often life-threatening in older children and young adults than in prepubescent children. This is especially the case for individuals immunized during childhood with the original killed measles vaccine, since these people are susceptible to a severe atypical measles syndrome that involves elevated fever, headache, abdominal pain, and cough.

4. Most vaccines are grown in a medium of duck or chick embryos and contain small amounts of animal proteins that could cause allergic reactions in sensitive individuals. Sensitivity to eggs is an almost certain indication that a reaction will occur to vaccination. Individuals who are receiving steroid therapy (specifically, glucocorticoids) should not be given measles vaccine because these drugs suppress the immune system and could result in an exaggerated reaction to vaccination.

5. Measles vaccination is contraindicated during pregnancy because natural measles is known to increase fetal risk of pneumonia, otitis media, encephalitis, or death.

6. Immediate allergic reactions.

Chapter 50 Case History: Systemic Lupus Erythematosis (SLE)–Like Reaction to Medication

1. B. B. exhibited facial erythema, photosensitivity, oral ulceration, arthritis without deformity, lupus erythematosus (LE) cells, pleuritic pain, and hemolytic anemia.

2. Hydralazine is known to produce an SLE-like syndrome in some individuals.

3. The clinical course of SLE is highly variable and unpredictable although the prognosis for drug-induced SLE is a good deal more positive than for idiopathic SLE. Discontinuation of the causative agent, in this case hydralazine, often results in alleviation of symptoms within a few weeks and complete remission. But even in drug-induced SLE, the condition can recur spontaneously after many months or even years.

4. Other drugs associated with occurrence of SLE-like reactions are procainamide (Pronestyl), methyldopa (Aldomet), and chlorpromazine (Thorazine). Nurses should monitor clients receiving one of these drugs for arthralgia, myalgia, calf tenderness, pleuritic pain, pulmonary infiltration, fever, renal changes, anemia, leukopenia, psychosis, convulsions, or pericarditis. Nurses should also watch for occurrence of a characteristic facial skin rash, "butterfly rash"—a rash on both cheeks connected across the bridge of the nose. Serological tests should be ordered periodically (measuring antinuclear antibodies and LE cell factor) since the onset of drug-induced SLE may be insidious and may be mistaken for complications of the underlying disorder at which drug therapy is directed.

Chapter 50 Case Study: Pollen Allergy

1. Pseudoephedrine is a sympathomimetic agent. Sympathomimetics produce physiological changes that oppose those occurring in type I allergic reactions. Chlorpheniramine is an antihistamine. It blocks the effects of histamine, one of the mediators of type I allergic reactions.

2. Pseudoephedrine acts on the brain to produce a moderate amphetamine-like stimulation. When L. C. switched to a product that contains only an antihistamine, without a sympathomimetic, the "buzz" did not occur.

3. Yes. Diphenhydramine belongs to the ethanolamine group of antihistamines, the group that produces the greatest degree of sedation (see Table 50–4).

4. The nurse might suggest use of an antihistamine with less tendency to produce sedation, such as chlorpheniramine. L. C. had previously used this drug, but in combination with a sympathomimetic. Chlorpheniramine is also marketed as an individual agent.

Chapter 51 Case Study: Peptic Ulcer

1. Peptic ulcer is indicated by occurrence of gnawing epigastric pain, epigastric tenderness, and presence of blood in the stools. Pyloric obstruction is suggested by vomiting shortly after food ingestion. Anemia is indicated by the subnormal hematocrit, hemoglobin, and serum iron levels.

2. Use of digoxin, aspirin, tobacco, alcohol, and coffee can each contribute to gastric irritation. In addition T. C. is currently experiencing stressful circumstances in his life.

3. Iron absorption from the diet is barely sufficient to meet requirements under the best of circumstances. An impairment of the gastrointestinal system, such as ulcers, may significantly reduce availability of iron from absorption.

4. Cimetidine is an H_2-blocker. It blocks the receptors through which histamine produces its stimulation of gastric acid production, thereby reducing secretion of this ulcergic substance. Antacids act to increase pH in the stomach by neutralizing a portion of the hydrochloric acid that is secreted.

5. Anticholinergic drugs also suppress secretion of hydrochloric acid in the stomach but are specifically contraindicated when pyloric obstruction is present, because they inhibit opening of the pyloric valve, thus aggravating pyloric obstruction.

6. Acetaminophen produces less irritation of the gastrointestinal mucosa than does aspirin.

7. When the ulcer is in the duodenum, it is helpful to delay gastric emptying time by measures such as lying down after meals, as suggested by the nurse. In gastric ulcer, there is nothing to be gained by delaying gastric emptying time except when an antacid is administered, in order to maximize its opportunity to work in the stomach.

8. Symptoms decline in peptic ulcer before the ulcers are completely healed. Premature discontinuation of medication increases the likelihood that ulcers will recur.

Chapter 52 Case Study: Asthma

1. R. D.'s asthma is best characterized as mixed, because it involves both intrinsic, or nonallergic, factors (stress, respiratory infection) and extrinsic, or allergic, factors (pollen, dander, and upper respiratory infections).

2. More of the drug is delivered to the site of therapeutic action, and less is available for adverse systemic effects.

3. Yes. Theophylline is known to irritate the gastrointestinal mucosa.

4. The stress of having to give a seminar, an upper respiratory tract infection, and congestion from the infection preventing effective aerosol therapy.

5. The nurse was making sure that the administered dose would not produce a dangerous additive effect with residual drug from a previous administration.

6. The laboratory values at the height of the attack are indicative of impaired respiration: hypercapnia and hypoxia. After treatment, the values have been normalized except that P_{CO_2} remains slightly elevated.

Chapter 53 Case Study: Burn Injury

1. Yes, Alice's burn is minor because it is superficial and covers less than 10% of the surface area of the body.

2. For treatment of minor burns, the protectant applied should have moisturizing and lubricating properties. Petrolatum is useful, having both of these properties. Powders, such as talcum powder, are neither lubricating nor moisturizing, producing instead a drying effect.

3. If a local anesthetic is applied, it should be a preparation containing a local anesthetic within its safe and effective concentration range. Only small amounts can be safely applied to injured skin, but the anesthetic will be effective because of easy penetration. Higher concentrations will be required if the preparation is applied to intact skin.

4. The nurse's recommendation regarding use of a topical antibacterial drug was reasonable because these preparations have questionable value and may cause development of resistant organisms or allergic reactions. It is usually better to leave a minor wound open rather than to apply a closed dressing unless it is impossible to protect the wound from contamination while it is open.

Chapter 54 Case Study: Glaucoma

1. Presenting symptoms that could be attributed to glaucoma include severe eye pain, nausea, vomiting, blurred vision, and seeing halos.

2. Dilated pupils, red and watery eyeballs, cloudy cornea, and firmness of the eyeball to touch were physical findings that supported the diagnosis of glaucoma. Confirmation was provided by tonometric evaluation.

3. Blood pressure elevation and rapid pulse were most likely responses to pain and stress of glaucoma.

4. Pilocarpine is the usual first drug in treatment of persons with glaucoma. Carbechol is more potent and is reserved for clients who do not respond adequately to pilocarpine or who experience unusually severe adverse reactions. Epinephrine is specifically contraindicated in angle-closure glaucoma.

5. Mannitol is an osmotic diuretic that produces fluid contraction by drawing water into the renal tubule for ultimate excretion in the urine. The resultant hypotension draws fluid from the anterior chamber of the eye into the circulation, producing rapid correction of acutely elevated intraocular pressure.

6. Mannitol can cause electrolyte imbalance or aggravate existing imbalances. The nurse reviewed the serum electrolyte measurements prior to beginning mannitol therapy to ensure that no preexisting imbalances were present. Mannitol is always administered through an in-line filter since it can crystallize.

7. To guard against potential adverse responses to mannitol-induced hypotension.

8. The nursing measures employed for each of the nursing diagnoses were as follows:

Nursing Diagnoses: Related Measures

Alteration in comfort; pain related to intraocular pressure: Administered pilocarpine; monitored response to pilocarpine.

Sensory-perceptual alterations related to elevated intraocular pressure: Administered pilocarpine; monitored response to pilocarpine.

Anxiety related to worry about possible future blindness: Maintained confident, efficient manner; talked reassuringly with W. F.

Potential alteration in cardiac output in response to mannitol infusion: Administered potassium chloride (to prevent hypokalemia); reviewed serum electrolyte measurements; monitored blood pressure, heart sounds, and respiratory sounds during the infusion; instructed W. F. to report any shortness of breath, chills, or chest pain; monitored intake and output.

Chapter 55 Case Study: Sinusitis

1. Sinusitis is inflammation of the paranasal sinuses. It can be caused by allergy or infection. Typical organisms involved in infectious sinusitis are streptococci, pneumococci, and staphylococci.

2. Most drug preparations for sinusitis contain a decongestant and an antihistamine. The decongestant may help to promote drainage of congested sinuses. The antihistamine could be expected to have value only if sinusitis is of allergic origin.

3. Topical nasal decongestants should not be used for more than a few days at a time to guard against occurrence of rebound nasal stuffiness.

Chapter 56 Case Study: Cancer

1. The CAF regimen utilizes cyclophosphamide (100 mg/m^2/day, PO, days 1–14), doxorubicin (30 mg/m^2/day, IV, days 1 and 8), and fluorouracil (500 mg/m^2/day, IV, days 1 and 8).

2. Baseline blood cells counts and an ECG provide means of comparison should adverse effects develop after the regimen is instituted. All three of these antineoplastic agents are likely to cause leukopenia. Doxorubicin may cause transient cardiac dysrhythmias and myocardial depression.

3. Antineoplastic drugs produce adverse effects most often involving normal tissues with rapid rates of proliferation, including the hair follicles, the gastrointestinal mocosa, and the bone marrow, resulting in hair loss, gastrointestinal irritation, and leukopenia, respectively.

4. Pulmonary congestion (productive cough, shortness of breath) and edema (swelling of the ankles) are early signs of cardiotoxicity that can occur with doxorubicin.

5. Prochlorperazine (Compazine) is an effective antinausea drug that helps to minimize nausea associated with cancer chemotherapy.

Chapter 57 Case Study: Poisoning

1. Elavil contains imipramine, a tricyclic antidepressant in the tertiary amine subgroup, with anticholinergic and depressant properties. The anticholinergic properties of imipramine account for many of the toxic symptoms, including blurred ("fuzzy") vision, dry mouth (severe thirst), paralytic ileus (lack of bowel sounds and rapid vomiting after oral fluids), dilated pupils, tachycardia, and the prolonged QRS. Imipramine in toxic doses also acts as a CNS depressant, causing depression of respiration, lethargy, and coma. Orthostatic hypotension caused by imipramine was responsible for the fainting and low blood pressure. Imipramine produces extrapyramidal side effects, accounting for the muscle rigidity. It also lowers the seizure threshold, producing hyperreflexia or even outright convulsions.

2. The physician presumably felt that there would be little of the drug remaining in the stomach since 2 hours had elapsed and the child had already vomited. In addition, lavage could not have been performed while the child was in seizures or before vital signs were adequately stabilized or supported. Since the child responded well to the treatment protocol, lavage was not felt necessary.

3. The low serum pH was indicative of respiratory acidosis attributable to depressed respirations. It was corrected with sodium bicarbonate. Maintaining serum pH at a slightly elevated level (> 7.45) during the treatment phase after tricyclic poisoning guards against development of cardiac dysrhythmias.

4. Physostigmine is an anticholinesterase drug that permits a buildup of levels of acetylcholine in cholinergic synapses to combat the anticholinergic effects of imipramine. In children, a dose of 0.5 mg can be repeated as required at 5-minute intervals up to a total dose of 2.0 mg. Apparently, the number of capsules swallowed by C. B. was not great, since physostigmine needed to be repeated only once and sodium bicarbonate not at all.

Index

Boldface page numbers indicate the main entry for a topic. Trade names are followed by their generic name in parentheses. Page numbers for trade names refer to preparations sections only; see the generic name for full coverage.